AF527158

Surgery
Core Principles and Practice

Surgery

Core Principles and Practice

Second Edition

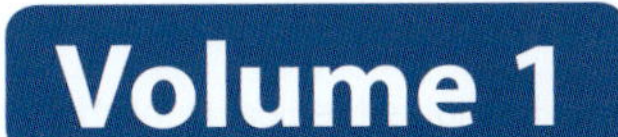

Editors

John D Corson MBChB FRCS (Eng) FRCS (Edin) FACS
Clinical Professor
Department of Surgery
The University of New Mexico
School of Medicine
Albuquerque, New Mexico, USA
Former Professor of Surgery and Director of Vascular Surgery
The University of Iowa Hospitals and Clinics
Iowa City, Iowa, USA

Robin CN Williamson MA MB MD MChir (Cantab) FRCS (Eng)
FRCS (Ed) Hon FRCS (Thailand) Hon DMedSci (Mahidol)
Professor of Surgery, Imperial College
Chairman
The London Clinic
Former Professor and Director of Surgery
Royal Postgraduate Medical School and
Hammersmith Hospital
London, England, UK

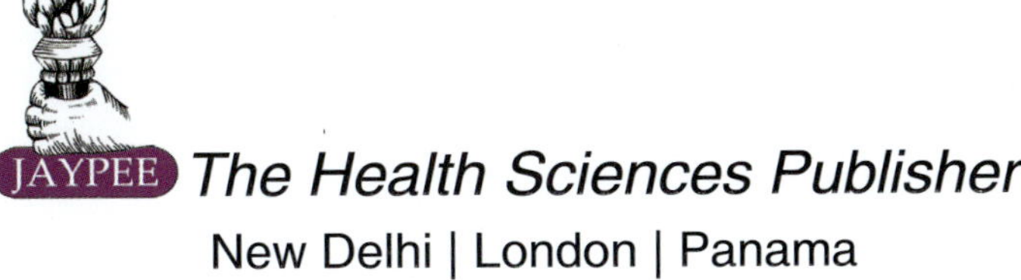

The Health Sciences Publisher
New Delhi | London | Panama

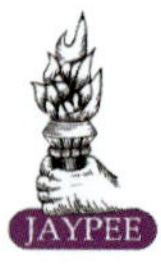

Jaypee Brothers Medical Publishers (P) Ltd

Headquarters

Jaypee Brothers Medical Publishers (P) Ltd
4838/24, Ansari Road, Daryaganj
New Delhi 110 002, India
Phone: +91-11-43574357
Fax: +91-11-43574314
Email: jaypee@jaypeebrothers.com

Overseas Offices

J.P. Medical Ltd
83, Victoria Street, London
SW1H 0HW (UK)
Phone: +44 20 3170 8910
Fax: +44 (0)20 3008 6180
Email: info@jpmedpub.com

Jaypee-Highlights Medical Publishers Inc
City of Knowledge, Bld. 235, 2nd Floor, Clayton
Panama City, Panama
Phone: +1 507-301-0496
Fax: +1 507-301-0499
Email: cservice@jphmedical.com

Jaypee Brothers Medical Publishers (P) Ltd
17/1-B, Babar Road, Block-B, Shaymali
Mohammadpur, Dhaka-1207
Bangladesh
Mobile: +08801912003485
Email: jaypeedhaka@gmail.com

Jaypee Brothers Medical Publishers (P) Ltd
Bhotahity, Kathmandu, Nepal
Phone +977-9741283608
Email: kathmandu@jaypeebrothers.com

Website: www.jaypeebrothers.com
Website: www.jaypeedigital.com

Inquiries for bulk sales may be solicited at: jaypee@jaypeebrothers.com

Surgery: Core Principles and Practice (Vol. 1)

First Edition: 2000 (Published by Mosby)
Second Edition: **2017**

ISBN 978-93-86261-11-3

Printed at Replika Press Pvt. Ltd.

Dedication

This work is dedicated to our gallant patients.

Section Editors

Göran Åkerström MD PhD
Professor Emeritus Endocrine Surgery
Institution of Surgical Sciences
Uppsala University Hospital
Uppsala, Sweden

J Andrew Bradley PhD FRCS FMedSci Fellow
Professor of Surgery
and Head of Department
Department of Surgery
University of Cambridge
Honorary Consultant Surgeon
Addenbrooke's Hospital
Cambridge, England, UK

Andrew de Beaux MD FRCS
Consultant General and Upper
Gastrointestinal Surgeon
and Honorary Clinical Senior Lecturer
Department of General Surgery
Royal Infirmary of Edinburgh
Edinburgh, Scotland, UK

John D Corson MBChB FRCS (Eng) FRCS (Edin) FACS
Clinical Professor
Department of Surgery
The University of New Mexico
School of Medicine
Albuquerque, New Mexico, USA
Former Professor of Surgery and Director
of Vascular Surgery
The University of Iowa Hospitals and Clinics
Iowa City, Iowa, USA

Mahesh Desai MBBS MS FRCS
Medical Director
Department of Urology
Muljibhai Patel Urological Hospital
Nadiad, Gujarat, India

J Michael Dixon OBE BSc (Hons) MBChB MD FRCS FRCSEd FRCPEd (Hon)
Professor of Surgery
and Consultant Surgeon
Edinburgh Breast Unit
Western General Hospital
Edinburgh, Scotland, UK

Donald E Fry MD FACS
Adjunct Professor of Surgery
Department of Surgery
Northwestern University
Feinberg School of Medicine
Chicago, Illinois
Emeritus Professor
Department of Surgery
University of New Mexico School of
Medicine
Albuquerque, New Mexico, USA

Andrew Hart BSc MD PhD MRCS FRCS
Stephen Forrest Professor of Plastic
Surgery Research
College of Medical, Veterinary and Life
Sciences
The University of Glasgow
Consultant Hand and Plastic Surgeon
Canniesburn Plastic Surgery Unit and
The Scottish National Brachial
Plexus Service
Glasgow Royal Infirmary
Glasgow, Scotland, UK

MRB Keighley MS FRCS
Emeritus Professor of Surgery
University of Birmingham
Consultant Surgeon
BMI The Priory Hospital
Birmingham, England, UK

Timothy F Kresowik MD FACS
Professor of Surgery
University of Iowa College of Medicine
Iowa City, Iowa, USA

James W Maher MD
Professor of Surgery
Department of Surgery
Virginia Commonwealth University
School of Medicine
Richmond, Virginia, USA

Michael J Reardon MD FACS
Allison Family Distinguished Chair of
Cardiovascular Research
Professor of Cardiothoracic Surgery
Houston Methodist Research Institute
DeBakey Heart and Vascular Center
Houston, Texas, USA

Anthony D Sandler MD FACS
Senior Vice President and
Surgeon-in-Chief
Joseph E Robert, Jr, Center for
Surgical Care
Children's National Health System
Diane and Norman Bernstein Professor in
Pediatric Surgery
Principal Investigator, Immunology
Initiative
Sheikh Zayed Institute for Pediatric
Surgical Innovation
Washington, DC, USA

William I Wei FRCS FRCSE FRACS (Hon) FACS (Hon)
Emeritus Professor
Department of Surgery
The University of Hong Kong
Head, Department of Surgery
Director
Li Shu Pui ENT Head & Neck Surgery
Centre
Hong Kong Sanatorium & Hospital
Hong Kong SAR, China

Robin CN Williamson MD MChir FRCS
Chairman
The London Clinic
Former Professor and Director of
Surgery
Royal Postgraduate Medical School and
Hammersmith Hospital
London, England, UK

Section Editors

Contributors

Brian C Adams MD
Vascular Surgery Fellow
Department of Vascular Surgery
University of Iowa
Iowa City, Iowa, USA

Sumeet Ahuja MD
Resident
Department of Neurosurgery
Rush University Medical Center
Chicago, Illinois, USA

Catherine Akay MD
Assistant Professor
Surgical Oncology
MD Anderson Cancer Center
Houston, Texas, USA

Roxie M Albrecht MD FACS FCCM
Professor
Department of Surgery
University of Oklahoma Health Science Center
Oklahoma City, Oklahoma, USA

John C Alverdy MD
Professor of Surgery
Department of Surgery
University of Chicago
Chicago, Illinois, USA

Al Aly MD FACS
Professor of Plastic Surgery
Surgical Subspecialties Institute
Cleveland Clinic Abu Dhabi
Abu Dhabi, United Arab Emirates

Irum Amin MB BChir MA MRCS MChir
Transplant Surgery Registrar
Department of Surgery
University of Cambridge
Cambridge, England, UK

Parth B Amin MD
Assistant Professor
Department of Cardiovascular Surgery
Western Michigan University
Kalamazoo, Michigan, USA

Christopher P Armstrong FRCS
Consultant Surgeon
Department of General Surgery
Southmead Hospital
North Bristol NHS Trust
Bristol, England, UK

Kenneth S Azarow MD FACS
Helen B Tracy Professor of Pediatric Surgery
Division of Pediatric Surgery
Oregon Health and Science University
Portland, Oregon, USA

Adrian Barbul MD FACS
Professor
Department of Surgery
Vanderbilt University School of Medicine
Nashville, Tennessee, USA

Philip S Barie MD FACS
Professor of Surgery
Weill Cornell Medical College
Attending Surgeon
New York-Presbyterian/Weill Cornell Medical Center
New York City, New York, USA

Philip Barker MB BS MS FRCS (Eng)
Emeritus Defence Professor of Surgery
Defence Medical Services and Royal College of Surgeons
England, UK
Surgeon to the International Committee of the Red Cross
Geneva, Switzerland

David CC Bartolo MS (London) FRCS FRACS
Professor of Surgery
University of Western Australia
Department of Colorectal Surgery
Fiona Stanley Hospital
Murdoch, Western Australia, Australia

Alfred E Baylor MD
Assistant Professor
Department of Surgery
Wayne State University School of Medicine
Detroit, Michigan, USA

David E Beck MD FACS FASCRC
Professor and Chairman Emeritus
Department of Colon and Rectal Surgery and Ochsner Clinical School
Ochsner Clinic and University of Queensland
New Orleans, Louisiana, USA
Brisbane, Queensland, Australia

Amit Bhattu MS DNB Urology
Fellow in Endourology and Lapararobotic Urology
Consultant Urologist
Muljibhai Patel Urological Hospital
Nadiad, Gujarat, India

James G Bittner IV MD
Assistant Professor of Surgery
Director
VCU Minimally Invasive Surgery Center
Program Director
Advanced Gastrointestinal
Minimally Invasive Surgery Fellowship
Department of Surgery
Virginia Commonwealth University
Medical College of Virginia
Richmond, Virginia, USA

Kirby I Bland MD FACS
Professor
Department of Surgery
The University of Alabama at Birmingham
Birmingham, Alabama, USA

John MA Bohnen MD FRCSC FACS
Professor
Department of Surgery
University of Toronto
Toronto, Ontario, Canada

Eleanor M Bolton PhD
Assistant Director of Research
Department of Surgery
University of Cambridge
Cambridge, England, UK

Neil Borley FRCS FRCS (Ed) MS
Consultant Colorectal Surgeon
Department of Colorectal Surgery
Cheltenham Hospital
Gloucestershire Hospitals NHS Foundation Trust
Gloucestershire, England, UK

Mark W Bowyer MD FACS DMCC
Ben Eiseman Professor of Surgery
Chief Division of Trauma and Combat Surgery
The Norman M Rich Department of Surgery
Uniformed Services University of the Health Sciences
Bethesda, Maryland, USA

J Andrew Bradley PhD FRCS FMedSci Fellow
Professor of Surgery and Head of Department
Department of Surgery
University of Cambridge
Honorary Consultant Surgeon
Addenbrooke's Hospital
Cambridge, England, UK

Marco Braga MD
Professor of Surgery
San Raffaele University
Milan, Italy

Ian Brown MD
Assistant Professor
Department of Surgery
University of California
Sacramento, California, USA

Robin A Brown DCH (SA) FCS (SA) FRCS (Edn) MPhil (Ancient Cultures)
Adjunct Professor
Department of Pediatric Surgery
University of Cape Town
Cape Town, South Africa

Joseph A Buckwalter MD FACS
Professor
Orthopedics and Rehabilitation Department
The University of Iowa Health Care
Iowa City, Iowa, USA

Dudley J Bush MBBS FRCA
Anesthesiology Consultant
Department of Pain Management
Leeds Teaching Hospitals
Leeds, West Yorkshire, England, UK

AJ Butler MBBS FRCS
Consultant Transplant Surgeon
Addenbrooke's Hospital
Cambridge, England, UK

Michael D Cadogan BA MA MB
ER Attending
Department of Emergency Medicine
Sir Charles Gairdner Hospital
Perth, Western Australia, Australia

Chris Callaghan PhD FRCS
Consultant Transplant Surgeon
Department of Nephrology and Transplantation
Guy's Hospital
London, England, UK

David Cameron MD FRCS
Professor
Edinburgh Cancer Research Centre
The University of Edinburgh
Edinburgh, Scotland, UK

Michael J Campbell MD
Assistant Professor
Department of Surgery
University of California
Sacramento, California, USA

Guilherme M Campos MD FACS
Professor and Chair
Division of Bariatric and Gastrointestinal Surgery
Department of Surgery
School of Medicine
Virginia Commonwealth University
Richmond, Virginia, USA

Sally E Carty MD FACS
Professor of Surgery
Department of Surgery
Division of Endocrine Surgery
University of Pittsburgh
Pittsburgh, Pennsylvania, USA

Anees B Chagpar MD MSc MPH MBA FACS FRCS (S)
Associate Professor
Department of Surgery
Director
The Breast Center-Smilow Cancer Hospital at Yale-New Haven
Assistant Director
Global Oncology
Yale Comprehensive Cancer Center
Program Director
Yale Interdisciplinary Breast Fellowship
Yale University School of Medicine
New Haven, Connecticut, USA

Francis KL Chan MD
Professor of Medicine and Therapeutics
Department of Medicine and Therapeutics
The Chinese University of Hong Kong
Sha Tin, Hong Kong SAR, China

Jimmy Yu Wai Chan MD
Associate Professor
Division of Head and Neck Surgery
Department of Surgery
University of Hong Kong
Hong Kong SAR, China

Richard M Charnley DM FRCS
Consultant Hepatobiliary and Pancreatic Surgeon
The Freeman Hospital
The Newcastle upon Tyne Hospitals NHS Foundation Trust
Newcastle upon Tyne, England, UK

John Chen MBBS PhD FRACS
Attending Surgeon
Hepato-Pancreato-Biliary Unit
Department of Surgery
Flinders Medical Centre
Flinders University
Adelaide, South Australia, Australia

Ming-Huei Cheng MD MBA
Professor
Division of Plastic and Reconstructive Microsurgery
Department of Plastic and Reconstructive Surgery
Chang Gung Memorial Hospital
Taoyuan, Taiwan

Ian C Chetter MD FRCS
Professor
Department of Vascular Surgery
University of Hull
East Yorkshire, England, UK

Ben K Chew MBChB MRCS MPhil FRCS (Plast)
Consultant Plastic Surgeon
Canniesburn Plastic Surgery Unit
Glasgow Royal Infirmary
Glasgow, Scotland, UK

Adrian Chung MBBS (Hons) FRACP
Attending Physician
Department of Gastroenterology
Flinders Medical Centre
Adelaide, South Australia, Australia

Jordan M Cloyd MD
Surgical Resident
Department of Surgery
Stanford University
Stanford, California, USA

Christine Cocanour MD FACS FCCM
Professor
Department of Surgery
University of California
Sacramento, California, USA

Dawn M Coleman MD
Assistant Professor of Surgery
Section of Vascular Surgery
University of Michigan
Ann Arbor, Michigan, USA

David Cooper MA MB BChir FRCS
Consultant Vascular and Endovascular Surgeon
Department of Vascular Surgery
Gloucestershire and Swindon Vascular Network
Cheltenham, England, UK

Eleanor Cornford MRCP FRCR
Consultant Radiologist
Nottingham Breast Institute
Nottingham University Hospitals
Nottingham, England, UK

John D Corson MBChB FRCS (Eng) FRCS (Edin) FACS
Clinical Professor
Department of Surgery
The University of New Mexico School of Medicine
Albuquerque, New Mexico, USA

Graeme W Couper MD MBChB FRCS
Consultant Upper Gastrointestinal Surgeon
Department of Surgery
University of Edinburgh
Edinburgh, Scotland, UK

Albert E Cram MD FACS
Former Professor of Surgery and Director
Section of Plastic and Reconstructive Surgery
University of Iowa College of Medicine
Iowa City, Iowa, USA

H Gill Cryer MD FACS
Professor of Surgery, Department of Surgerys
Chief of Trauma and Acute Care Surgery
University of California
Los Angeles
Ronald Reagan-UCLA Medical Center
Los Angeles, California, USA

Brad M Cushing MD FACS
Professor
Tufts University School of Medicine
Department of Surgery
Maine Medical Center
Portland, Maine, USA

Andrew M Davidoff MD FACS
Professor
Department of Surgery
St. Jude Children's Research Hospital
Memphis, Tennessee, USA

Andrew de Beaux MD FRCS
Consultant General and Upper Gastrointestinal Surgeon and Honorary Clinical Senior Lecturer
Department of General Surgery
Royal Infirmary of Edinburgh
Edinburgh, Scotland, UK

Jan De Waele MD PhD
Professor
Department of Critical Care Medicine
Ghent University Hospital
Ghent, Belgium

Chris Deans MD FRCS
Consultant General and Upper Gastrointestinal Surgeon
University Department of Surgery
Edinburgh Royal Infirmary
Edinburgh, Scotland, UK

Jennifer R DeFazio MD
Resident
Department of Surgery
University of Chicago
Chicago, Illinois, USA

Elias Degiannis MD PhD FRCS (Glasg) FCS (SA) FACS
Professor of Surgery
Trauma Directorate
Chris Hani Baragwanath Academic Hospital
University of the Witwatersrand
Johannesburg, South Africa

Mahesh Desai MBBS MS FRCS
Medical Director
Department of Urology
Muljibhai Patel Urological Hospital
Nadiad, Gujarat, India

J Michael Dixon OBE BSc (Hons) MBChB MD FRCS FRCS (Ed) FRCP (Ed) (Hon)
Professor of Surgery and Consultant Surgeon
Edinburgh Breast Unit
Western General Hospital
Edinburgh, Scotland, UK

Gerard Doherty MD FACS
Utley Professor and Chair
Department of Surgery
Boston University
Boston, Massachusetts, USA

Heather S Dolman MD
Assistant Professor
Department of Surgery
Wayne State University School of Medicine
Detroit, Michigan, USA

Quan-Yang Duh MD FACS
Professor
Department of Surgery
University of California, San Francisco
San Francisco, California, USA

Jonothan J Earnshaw FRCS
Consultant in Vascular Surgery
Department of Vascular Surgery
Gloucestershire Hospitals NHS Foundation Trust
Gloucestershire, England, UK

Charles E Edmiston PhD CIC FIDSA FSHEA
Emeritus Professor of Surgery
Director
Surgical Microbiology and Hospital Epidemiology Research Laboratory
Division of Vascular Surgery
Department of Surgery
Medical College of Wisconsin
Milwaukee, Wisconsin, USA

Jonathan L Eliason MD FACS
Associate Professor of Surgery
Lindenauer Professor of Vascular Surgery
University of Michigan
Ann Arbor, Michigan, USA

Michael J Englesbe MD FACS
Associate Professor of Surgery
University of Michigan Health Systems
Ann Arbor, Michigan, USA

D Gareth Evans MD FRCP
Professor
Department of Genetic Medicine
University of Manchester
Manchester, England, UK

Jordan Fishman MPH
Chief Administrative Resident
Department of Surgery
Rutgers New Jersey Medical School
Newark, New Jersey, USA

Irma Fleming MD
Resident
Department of General Surgery
The University of Chicago Medicine
Chicago, Illinois, USA

Lewis Flint MD FACS
Editor-in-Chief
Selected Readings in General Surgery
Division of Education
American College of Surgeons
Chicago, Illinois, USA

Sascha Flohé MD
Professor of Surgery
Heinrich-Heine-Universität Düsseldorf
Düsseldorf, NRW, Germany

Thomas Frohlich MD
Cardiovascular Surgeon
Sutter Health
Oakland, California, USA

Donald E Fry MD FACS
Adjunct Professor of Surgery
Department of Surgery
Northwestern University
Feinberg School of Medicine
Chicago, Illinois, USA
Emeritus Professor
Department of Surgery
University of New Mexico School of Medicine
Albuquerque, New Mexico, USA

Raguram Ganesamoni MS MRCS MCH
Fellow
Endourologist and Laparorobotic Surgeon
Ganesamoni Hospital
Nagercoil, Tamil Nadu, India

Arvind P Ganpule MBBS MS DNB
Vice Chairman
Department of Urology
Chief
Division of Laparoscopic and Robotic Surgery
Muljibhai Patel Urological Hospital
Nadiad, Gujarat, India

Nitin Garg MBBS MPH
Assistant Professor
Department of Vascular and Endovascular Surgery
Wake Forest University
Winston-Salem, North Carolina, USA

Lindsay Gates MD
Vascular Surgery Attending
Department of Vascular Surgery
Yale New Haven Hospital
New Haven, Connecticut, USA

Puja Gaur MD FACS
Assistant Professor
Department of Thoracic Surgery
Weill Cornell Medical College
Houston Methodist Hospital
Houston, Texas, USA

Glenn W Geelhoed MD FACS
Professor of Surgery, International Medical Education, Microbiology, Immunology, and Tropical Medicine
Office of the Dean
George Washington University
Washington, DC, USA

Bruce L Gewertz MD FACS
Surgeon-in-Chief and Chairman
Department of Surgery
Cedars-Sinai Medical Center
Los Angeles, California, USA

Joshua Gierman MD
Assistant Professor of Surgery
Department of Surgery
University of Oklahoma
Oklahoma City, Oklahoma, USA

Thomas G Gleason MD FACS
Ronald V Pellegrini Professor of Cardiothoracic Surgery
Department of Cardiothoracic Surgery
University of Pittsburgh
Pittsburgh, Pennsylvania, USA

Peter Gloviczki MD FACS
Joe M and Ruth Roberts Professor of Surgery
Division of Vascular and Endovascular Surgery
Mayo Clinic
Rochester, Minnesota, USA

James M Goff Jr MD FACS
Professor of Surgery
Chief
Surgical Service
New Mexico VA Health Care System
Albuquerque, New Mexico, USA

Sarah Goodbrand MBBS
Specialist Registrar
Department of Surgery
Royal Infirmary
Edinburgh, Scotland, UK

Dirk J Gouma MD
Professor of Surgery
Department of Surgery
Academic Medical Center
University of Amsterdam
Amsterdam, The Netherlands

Jacob A Greenberg MD EdM
Assistant Professor of Surgery
Department of Surgery
University of Wisconsin School of Medicine and Public Health
Madison, Wisconsin, USA

Jose G Guillem MD MPH FACS
Associate Professor of Surgery/Attending Colorectal Surgeon
Department of Surgery
Colorectal Service
Memorial Sloan-Kettering Cancer Center
New York City, New York, USA

Sheng-Po Hao MD FACS FICS
Professor and Chairman
Department of Otolaryngology Head and Neck Surgery
Shin-Kong Wu Ho-Su Memorial Hospital
School of Medicine
Fu Jen University
Taipei, Taiwan

Alden H Harken MD FACS
Professor and Chair
Department of Surgery
University of California, San Francisco-East Bay
Oakland, California, USA

SJF Harper MBChB MD FRCS
Clinical Lecturer and Specialist Registrar
University of Cambridge
Addenbrooke's Hospital
Cambridge, England, UK

Andrew Hart BSc MD PhD MRCS FRCS
Stephen Forrest Professor of Plastic Surgery Research
College of Medical Veterinary and Life Sciences
The University of Glasgow
Consultant Hand and Plastic Surgeon
Canniesburn Plastic Surgery Unit and The Scottish National Brachial Plexus Service
Glasgow Royal Infirmary
Glasgow, Scotland, UK

George E Havelka MD
Vascular Surgery Fellow
Department of Vascular Surgery
Northwestern University
Chicago, Illinois, USA

William S Havron III MD FACS
Assistant Professor
Department of Surgery
University of Oklahoma
Oklahoma City, Oklahoma, USA

Per Hellman MD PhD
Professor
Department of Surgical Sciences
Uppsala University
Uppsala, Sweden

J Michael Henderson MD FACS
Chief Medical Officer
University of Mississippi Medical Center
Jackson, Mississippi, USA

James C Hewes FRCS
Consultant Surgeon
Department of General Surgery
Southmead Hospital
North Bristol NHS Trust
Bristol, England, UK

Charles R Hickam MD FACR
Consultant Radiologist (retired)
Albuquerque, New Mexico, USA

Paul Hollington MBBS PhD FRACS
Consultant Colorectal Surgeon
Department of Surgery
Flinders University of South Australia
Adelaide, South Australia, Australia

Philip M Hopkins MBBS MD FRCA
Professor of Anesthesia
Director
Leeds Institute of Biomedical and Clinical Sciences
University of Leeds
Leeds, England, UK

Eric Hoste MD PhD
Professor
Department of Intensive Care Medicine
Ghent University
Ghent, Belgium
The Research Foundation-Flanders (FWO)
Brussels, Belgium

Anthony Howell MD
Professor
Institute of Cancer Sciences
University of Manchester
Manchester, England, UK

Vanessa W Hui MD
Clinical Research Fellow
Department of Surgery
Colorectal Service
Memorial Sloan-Kettering Cancer Center
New York City, New York, USA

John G Hunter MD FACS
Professor and Chair
Department of Surgery
Oregon Health and Science University
Portland, Oregon, USA

Jared Huston MD FACS
Assistant Professor of Surgery
Department of Surgery
Hofstra North Shore-LIJ School of Medicine
Manhasset, New York, USA

Jitendra V Jagtap MD DNB (Urology)
Endourology Fellow
Department of Urology
Muljibhai Patel Urological Hospital
Nadiad, Gujarat, India

Glyn Jamieson MD FRACS FACS FRCS
Emeritus Professor
Division of Surgery
University of Adelaide
Adelaide, South Australia, Australia

Ramin Jamshidi MD FACS
Assistant Professor
Department of Surgery and Department of Child Health
University of Arizona
Pediatric Trauma Medical Director
Maricopa Integrated Health System
Phoenix, Arizona, USA

Mike Jane FRCS
Consultant Orthopedic Surgeon
NHS Greater Glasgow and Clyde
Glasgow, Scotland, UK

Long R Jiao MD FRCS
Professor
Surgery and Cancer
Hammersmith Hospital
Imperial College London
London, England, UK

Gregory J Jurkovich MD FACS
Chief of Surgery
Denver Health and Hospital Authority
Department of Surgery
University of Colorado
Denver, Colorado, USA

Jeanwan Kang MD FACS
Associate Staff
Department of Vascular Surgery
Cleveland Clinic
Cleveland, Ohio, USA

Manish K Kasliwal MD
Chief Resident
Department of Neurosurgery
Rush University Medical Center
Chicago, Illinois, USA

Gerald P Kealey MD FACS
Professor
Department of Surgery
University of Iowa
Iowa City, Iowa, USA

MRB Keighley MS FRCS
Emeritus Professor of Surgery
University of Birmingham
Consultant Surgeon
BMI The Priory Hospital
Birmingham, England, UK

John M Kellum MD FACS
Chair
Division of General Surgery
Professor
Department of Surgery
Virginia Commonwealth University
Richmond, Virginia, USA

Erika R Ketteler MD MA RPVI FACS
Associate Professor
Department of Surgery
University of New Mexico
Chief
Vascular Surgery
Raymond G Murphy VAMC
Albuquerque, New Mexico, USA

Makarand V Khochikar MS FRCS (Urol) DNB (Urol) Dip Urol (London)
Fellow European Board of Urology
Chief Uro-oncologist
Shri Siddhivinayak Ganapati Cancer Hospital
Miraj, Maharashtra, India

Brigid K Killelea MD MPH FACS
Assistant Professor of Surgery (Oncology)
Yale School of Medicine
New Haven, Connecticut, USA

Vasilis Kosmoliaptsis MD PhD FRCS
Clinical Lecturer
Department of Surgery
University of Cambridge
Addenbrooke's Hospital
Cambridge, England, UK

Marcus R Kret MD
Clinical Fellow
Division of Vascular Surgery
Stanford University School of Medicine
Stanford, California, USA

Anna Kundel MD
Assistant Professor
Department of Endocrine Surgery
New York University
New York City, New York, USA

Peter Lamb MBBS MD FRCS
Consultant General and Upper Gastrointestinal Surgeon and Honorary Clinical Senior Lecturer
Department of Surgery
Royal Infirmary Edinburgh and University of Edinburgh
Edinburgh, Scotland, UK

Jacob C Langer MD FACS
Professor
Department of Surgery
University of Toronto
Toronto, Ontario, Canada

Mark Langsfeld MD FACS
Chief
Division of Vascular Surgery
Clinician Ed-Professor
Department of Surgery
Assistant Professor
Department of Radiology
University of New Mexico School of Medicine
Albuquerque, New Mexico, USA

Oliver B Lao MD MPH
General and Pediatric Attending Surgeon
Mary Bridge Children's Hospital
Tacoma, Washington, USA

Konstantinos G Lasithiotakis MD
General Surgeon
Department of General Surgery
York Teaching Hospital
NHS Foundation Trust
York, North Yorkshire, England, UK

Joseph WY Lau MD FRCS FACS FRACS (Hon)
Choh-Ming Li Research Professor of Surgery
Emeritus Professor
Faculty of Medicine
The Chinese University of Hong Kong
Hong Kong SAR, China

David J Leaper MD ChM FRCS FACS FLS
Emeritus Professor of Surgery
University of Newcastle upon Tyne
Professor of Clinical Sciences
Institute of Skin Integrity and Infection Prevention
University of Huddersfield
Queensgate, Huddersfield, England, UK

Jason T Lee MD FACS
Associate Professor of Surgery
Division of Vascular Surgery
Stanford University Medical Center
Stanford, California, USA

Amos Loh MD
Deputy Chairman
Division of Surgery
Senior Consultant Pediatric (Hepatobiliary Surgery)
Department of Pediatric Surgery
KK Women's and Children's Hospital
Singapore

Daniel Lollar MD
Trauma/Acute Care Surgery Fellow
Department of Surgery
Denver Health Medical Center
University of Colorado Hospital
Denver, Colorado, USA

E Jane Macaskill MBChB MD FRCSEd
Consultant Breast Surgeon and Honorary Clinical Senior Lecturer
Department of Breast Surgery
Ninewells Hospital and Medical School
Dundee, Scotland, UK

R Douglas Macmillan MBChB MD FRCS
Consultant Breast and Oncoplastic Surgeon
Nottingham Breast Institute
Nottingham, England, UK

Marc Maegele MD
Professor
Department of Traumatology and Orthopedic Surgery
Cologne-Merheim Medical Center
Institute for Research in Operative Medicine
Universitat Witten/Herdecke
Campus Cologne-Merheim
Cologne, Germany

James W Maher MD
Professor of Surgery
Department of Surgery
Virginia Commonwealth University School of Medicine
Richmond, Virginia, USA

Andrew J Malouf MD
Colorectal Attending Surgeon
Shelharbour Private Hospital
Barrack Heights, New South Wales
Australia

John Marek MD FACS
Professor of Surgery
Division of Vascular Surgery
University of New Mexico
Albuquerque, New Mexico, USA

Nick Matharu FRCS PhD
Consultant Vascular and Endovascular Surgeon
Department of Vascular Surgery
University Hospital Coventry and Warwickshire
Warwickshire, England, UK

Peter T McCollum MB MCh FRCSI
Chair
Vascular Surgery
The Hull York Medical School
University of York, Heslington,
York, North Yorkshire, England, UK

Kelly L McCoy MD
Assistant Professor
Department of Surgery
Division of Endocrine Surgery
University of Pittsburgh
Pittsburgh, Pennsylvania, USA

Funda Meric-Bernstam MD FACS
Professor
Division of Cancer Medicine and Surgery
Chair
Department of Investigational Cancer Therapeutics
The University of Texas MD Anderson Cancer Center
Houston, Texas, USA

Fred A Mettler Jr MD FACR
Professor Emeritus
Department of Radiology
University of New Mexico
Albuquerque, New Mexico, USA

Sara Mijal MD FACS
Vascular Surgery Attending
Affiliated Surgeons of Rockford
Rockford, Illinois, USA

Alastair JW Millar FRCS FRACS (Paed Surg) FCS (SA)
Emeritus Professor of Pediatric Surgery
Department of Pediatric Surgery
Red Cross War Memorial Children's Hospital and University of Cape Town
Cape Town, South Africa

Shashikant Mishra MBBS MS DNB
Consultant Urologist
Muljibhai Patel Urological Hospital
Nadiad, Gujarat, India

Rohin Mittal MS
Associate Professor
Surgery Unit II (Colorectal Surgery)
Christian Medical College
Vellore, Tamil Nadu, India

John Moawad MD FACS
Vascular Surgery Attending
Akron Vascular Associates
Northeast Ohio Medical University
Akron, Ohio, USA

Ashley Morgan MD
Surgical Resident
University of California, San Francisco-East Bay
San Francisco, California, USA

Neil Mortensen MD FRCS
Professor
Department of Colorectal Surgery
University of Oxford Hospitals
Oxford, England, UK

Vinodh Murali MBBS
Resident
Department of Urology
Muljibhai Patel Urological Hospital
Nadiad, Gujarat, India

Rachael Nicholson MD FACS
Clinical Associate Professor
Department of Surgery
Division of Vascular Surgery
University of Iowa
Iowa City, Iowa, USA

Jamison S Nielsen DO MBA FACS
Surgical Critical Care Fellow
Oregon Health and Science University
Portland, Oregon, USA

James V O'Connor MD FACS
Professor
Department of Surgery
University of Maryland School of Medicine
Baltimore, Maryland, USA

Patrick J O'Hara MD FACS
Professor of Surgery
Cleveland Clinic Lerner College of Medicine
Staff Vascular Surgeon
Emeritus Department of Vascular Surgery
Cleveland Clinic Foundation
Cleveland, Ohio, USA

Olga Oikonomidou PhD MD BSc
Clinician Scientist in Medical Oncology
Department of Oncology
The University of Edinburgh
Edinburgh, Scotland, UK

Katja Ott MD
Professor and Attending Upper Gastrointestinal Surgeon
General, Vascular and Thoracic Surgery Clinic
RoMed Klinikum Rosenheim
Rosenheim, Germany

Nancy Parks MD
Assistant Professor
Department of Surgery
The University of California
California, USA

Luigi Pascarella MD
Clinical Assistant Professor of Surgery
The University of Iowa
Carver College of Medicine
Iowa City, Iowa, USA

Janice L Pasieka MD
Clinical Professor
Department of Surgery and Oncology
University of Calgary
Calgary, Alberta, Canada

Rajesh Patel MBChB FRACS
Endocrine Surgery Fellow
Foothills Medical Centre
University of Calgary
Calgary, Alberta, Canada

Hugh M Paterson MD FRCSEd
Clinical Senior Lecturer in Colorectal Surgery
Colorectal Surgery Unit
University of Edinburgh
Edinburgh, Scotland, UK

William H Pearce MD FACS
Professor of Surgery
Department of Surgery
Northwestern University
Chicago, Illinois, USA

Benjamin Perakath MS FRCS (G)
Professor
Department of Surgery
Christian Medical College
Vellore, Tamil Nadu, India

Ioannis E Petrakis MD PhD
Consultant, General Surgeon
Department of General Surgery
University Hospital of Heraklion
Crete, Greece

Graeme J Pitcher MBBCh FCS (SA) FACS
Associate Professor
Division of Pediatric Surgery
University of Iowa
Iowa City, Iowa, USA

Ian M Pope BA BM BcH MD FRCS
Surgical Attending
Department of HPB Surgery
University Hospitals Bristol
Bristol, England, UK

RK Praseedom MBBS MA FRCS
Consultant HPB-Transplant Surgeon
Department of Surgery
Addenbrooke's Hospital
University of Cambridge
Cambridge, England, UK

Emad A Rakha MD PhD FRCP
Clinical Associate Professor and Honorary Consultant Pathologist
University of Nottingham and Nottingham University Hospitals NHS Trust
Nottingham, England, UK

Basel Ramlawi MD FACS
Associate Professor of Surgery
Cardiovascular Surgery
Houston Methodist Hospital
Houston, Texas, USA

Michael J Reardon MD FACS
Allison Family Distinguished Chair of Cardiovascular Research
Professor of Cardiovascular Surgery
Houston Methodist Research Institute
DeBakey Heart and Vascular Center
Houston, Texas, USA

Thomas A Reekie MBChB MRCS
Senior Clinical Research Fellow
Canniesburn Plastic Surgery Unit
Glasgow Royal Infirmary
Glasgow, Scotland, UK

David Rice MBBCh BAO FRCSI
Professor
Department of Thoracic and Cardiovascular Surgery
Division of Surgery
The University of Texas MD Anderson Cancer Center
Houston, Texas, USA

John J Ricotta MD FACS
Professor of Surgery
Georgetown University
Chair
Surgery
Washington Hospital Center
Washington, DC, USA

Layton F Rikkers MD FACS
Emeritus Professor
Department of Surgery
University of Wisconsin
Madison, Wisconsin, USA

Thomas S Riles MD FACS
Frank C Spencer Professor of Surgery
Department of Vascular Surgery
New York University Langone Medical Center
New York City, New York, USA

John H Robertson MD FRCS
Attending Surgeon
Department of Colorectal Surgery
Victoria Hospital
Kirkcaldy, Fife, Scotland, UK

Ravindra B Sabnis MBBS MS MCh
Professor and Chairman
Department of Urology
Muljibhai Patel Urological Hospital
Nadiad, Gujarat, India

Mikel Sadek MD
Assistant Professor
Division of Vascular Surgery
Department of Surgery
New York University Langone Medical Center
New York City, New York, USA

Kourosh Saeb-Parsy MA MB BChir PhD FRCS
University Lecturer and Consultant Transplant Surgeon
Department of Surgery
University of Cambridge
Cambridge, England, UK

Edgardo S Salcedo MD FACS
Assistant Professor of Surgery
Division of Trauma and Acute Care Surgery
University of California
Sacramento, California, USA

Anthony D Sandler MD
Senior Vice President and Surgeon-in-Chief
Joseph E Robert, Jr., Center for Surgical Care
Children's National Health System
Diane and Norman Bernstein Professor in Pediatric Surgery
Principal Investigator
Immunology Initiative
Sheikh Zayed Institute for Pediatric Surgical Innovation
Washington, DC, USA

Abeezar I Sarela MSc MS MD FRCS
Consultant Surgeon and Honorary Senior Lecturer in Surgery
Department of Upper Gastrointestinal Surgery
St James' University Hospital
Leeds, England, UK

Thomas M Scalea MD FACS
Professor
Department of Surgery
University of Maryland School of Medicine
Baltimore, Maryland, USA

Mark Schaverien MBChB MD MSc Med FRCS (Plast)
Specialist Registrar in Plastic Surgery
Department of Plastic Surgery
Ninewells Hospital
Dundee, Scotland, UK

Paul J Schenarts MD FACS
Professor and Vice Chair for Academic Affairs
Chief Trauma Surgery
Department of Surgery
University of Nebraska Medical Center
College of Medicine
Omaha, Nebraska, USA

Carol R Schermer MD MPH FACS
Professor *(Former)*
Department of Surgery
University of California
Sacramento, California, USA

Lewis B Schwartz MD FACS
Attending Vascular Surgeon
Department of Surgery
Lutheran General Hospital
Park Ridge, Illinois, USA

John Scott MB ChB FRCS
Consultant Plastic and Reconstructive Surgeon
Department of Plastic Surgery
Glasgow Royal Infirmary
Glasgow, Scotland, UK

Aamir S Shah MD
Associate Professor of Surgery
Cardiothoracic and Vascular Surgery
Cedars-Sinai Medical Center
Los Angeles, California, USA

Jon Shenfine MBBS FRCS FRACS PhD
Consultant Surgeon
Royal Adelaide Hospital
Honorary Senior Lecturer
Department of Surgery
University of Adelaide
Adelaide, South Australia, Australia

Susanna H Shin MD FACS
Assistant Professor
Department of Surgery
Georgetown University
Washington, DC, USA

JR Siewert MD
Senior Medical Director and Chairman of the Board
University Medical Center Freiburg
Freiburg, Germany

Kristen C Sihler MD MS
Assistant Professor
Department of Surgery
Maine Medical Center
Tufts University School of Medicine
Portland, Maine, USA

Erik D Skarsgard MD FRCSC FACS FAAP
Professor
Department of Surgery (Pediatric Surgery)
University of British Columbia
Vancouver, British Columbia, Canada

Martin D Smith MBBCh FCS
Professor
Department of Surgery
University of the Witwatersrand
Johannesburg, South Africa

Stig Sømme MD
Assistant Professor
Division of Pediatric Surgery
Department of Surgery
University of Colorado
Aurora, Colorado, USA

Panos Souroullas MBChB MRCS (Eng) PGCert (ResMet)
Clinical Research Fellow in Vascular Surgery
Department of Vascular Surgery
Hull Royal Infirmary
Hull-York Medical School
Hull, East Riding of Yorkshire, England, UK

Peter Stålberg MD PhD
Professor
Department of Surgery
Endocrine Surgical Unit
Uppsala University
Uppsala, Sweden

James C Stanley MD FACS
Handleman Professor
Section of Vascular Surgery
University of Michigan
Ann Arbor, Michigan, USA

Bauer Sumpio MD PhD FACS
Emeritus Chief of Vascular Surgery
Yale New Haven Hospital
Professor of Surgery and Radiology
Yale University School of Medicine
New Haven, Connecticut, USA

Mia Talmor MD FACS
Associate Professor of Clinical Surgery
Department of Surgery
Weill Cornell Medical College
New York City, New York, USA

Raymond SY Tang MD
Clinical Professional Consultant
Institute of Digestive Diseases
The Chinese University of Hong Kong
Hong Kong SAR, China

Jeremy JT Tate FRCS FRACS FACS
Lead Clinician
General Surgery Unit
Royal United Hospitals Bath
Bath, England, UK

Geoffrey B Thompson MD FACS
Professor of Surgery
Department of Surgery
Mayo Clinic
Rochester, Minnesota, USA

Sérgio A Toledo-Valdovinos MD
Resident
Department of General Surgery
Oregon Health and Science University
Portland, Oregon, USA

Vincent C Traynelis MD FACS
Professor
Department of Neurosurgery
Rush University Medical Center
Chicago, Illinois, USA

Dhaval Trivedi MD
Assistant Professor of Surgery
Department of Cardiothoracic Surgery
University of Pittsburgh
Pittsburgh, Pennsylvania, USA

Bruce R Tulloh MD FRACS FRCS (Ed)
Consultant Surgeon
Department of Surgery
Royal Infirmary of Edinburgh
Edinburgh, Scotland, UK

Gilbert R Upchurch, Jr MD FACS
William H Muller Jr Professor of Surgery
Department of Surgery
University of Virginia
Charlottesville, Virginia, USA

Selman Uranüs MD
Professor and Head
Section for Surgical Research
Department of Surgery
Medical University of Graz
Graz, Austria

Alex B Valadka MD FACS
Chairman and Chief Executive Officer
Seton Brain and Spine Institute
Austin, Texas, USA

Thomas M van Gulik MD
Professor
Department of Surgery
Academic Medical Center
University of Amsterdam
Amsterdam, The Netherlands

Martin Veller MD
Dean
School of Medicine
Professor
Department of Surgery
University of the Witwatersrand
Johannesburg, South Africa

Jean-Louis Vincent MD PhD
Professor
Department of Intensive Care
Erasme Hospital
Université Libre de Bruxelles
Brussels, Belgium

Daniel S Vryhof MD
Resident
Grand Rapids Medical Education Partners
Grand Rapids, Michigan, USA

Seth Waits MD
Resident
Department of Surgery
University of Michigan Health System
Ann Arbor, Michigan, USA

Matthew Waltham MA PhD FRCS
Senior Lecturer
Academic Department of Surgery
St Thomas' Hospital
London, England, UK

Thomas N Wang MD PhD
Associate Professor, Department of Surgery
Division of Surgical Oncology
University of Alabama at Birmingham
Birmingham, Alabama, USA

David I Watson MBBS MD FRACS FAHMS
Professor, Department of Surgery
Flinders University of South Australia
Adelaide, South Australia, Australia

Laurence A Webber MBBS FRACS
General Surgeon, Department of Surgery
Albany Regional Hospital
Albany, Western Australia, Australia

Kristin L Weber MD
Attending Surgeon, Division of Oncology
Children's Hospital of Philadelphia
Philadelphia, Pennsylvania, USA

William I Wei FRCS FRCSE FRACS (Hon) FACS (Hon)
Emeritus Professor, Department of Surgery
The University of Hong Kong
Head, Department of Surgery,
Director
Li Shu Pui ENT Head & Neck Surgery Center
Hong Kong Sanatorium and Hospital
Hong Kong SAR, China

James ML Williamson MRCS MSc
Specialty Training Registrar
Department of General Surgery
Bristol Royal Infirmary
Bristol, England, UK

Robin CN Williamson MD MChir FRCS
Professor of Surgery, Imperial College
Chairman
The London Clinic
Former Professor and Director of Surgery
Royal Postgraduate Medical School and
Hammersmith Hospital
London, England, UK

Robert F Wilson MD FACS
Professor
Department of Surgery
Wayne State University School of
Medicine
Detroit, Michigan, USA

Sherry M Wren MD FACS FCS (ECSA)
Professor of Surgery
Director of Global Surgery
Department of Surgery
Center for Innovation and Global Health
Stanford University
Stanford, California, USA

Kyle L Wu MD MBA
Resident
Department of Surgery
Georgetown University Hospital
Washington, DC, USA

Tugba H Yilmaz MD
Attending Surgeon
Department of General Surgery
Baskent University
Izmir, Turkey

Elias Zigiriadis MD FC Cardio (SA)
Cardiothoracic Surgeon
Division of Cardiothoracic Surgery
Charlotte Maxeke Johannesburg
Senior Specialist
University of the
Witwatersrand
Johannesburg, South Africa

David H Zonies MD MPH FACS
Associate Professor of Surgery
Trauma, Critical Care, and Acute Care
Surgery
Oregon Health and Science University
Portland, Oregon, USA

Preface to the Second Edition

Seventeen years have passed since the first edition of our award-winning surgical textbook was published by Mosby. That first edition was novel in many respects and, accordingly, was met with much enthusiasm from surgical colleagues and educators due to the textbook's distinguishing features, notably the format consisting of sections coded by different colors; the clear, consistent and well-rendered illustration program; the illustrious editorial and author pool; global content; and the integration of clinical cases with basic science and surgical knowledge.

The long gap between that inaugural edition and this second edition did afford us the opportunity to analyze objectively what worked best in the first edition and what could be changed. Practitioners and surgeons in training from North America, Europe, and India evaluated copies of the first edition thoroughly, from stem to stern. As you can imagine, surgical reviewers were quite candid in their comments, and we thank all of these international colleagues for their input.

We used the results of this analysis to develop the new edition, keeping many of the original features, such as the Key Points and Case Studies (titled Practical Problems in the first edition), which were appreciated by readers, while discarding the oversize and unwieldy trim size and idiosyncratic system used for numbering pages and chapters. A new cohort of section editors and contributors has infused the new edition with their expertise, especially in terms of global content, and *we are proud that this work features more contributions from international experts than from any other surgical textbook available.*

The overall thrust and goal of the book remain the same: to provide a comprehensive textbook on surgery, recognizing that for many surgeons, the range of conditions encountered in an emergency context is broader than the scope of their elective practice. It is a well-known axiom that the pace of medical advances remains astonishing for surgical practice as well as other medical specialties. Barely 150 years have passed since modern anesthesia and antisepsis permitted most of the operations now regarded as commonplace. Since the publication of the first edition of this textbook, surgical practice has evolved considerably, not least in the progressive adoption of minimally invasive techniques in many different fields of surgery to supplement (and often to challenge) the tried and tested role of "open" operations. The core principles of surgery may have changed rather less than the technical aspects of the profession, but there have still been many discoveries in the scientific knowledge that underpin our practice. The introductory section devoted to Principles of Surgery and Critical Care was an integral part of the first edition and has been retained and indeed expanded in this new edition of the book. In this regard, we are especially grateful to Dr Donald E Fry, who has again acted as the relevant section editor.

How to do justice to the growth of knowledge without producing a book that bends the shelf is a challenge to all editors of modern medical textbooks. One method involves the ruthless excision of older facts that seem to have been supplanted; yet this exercise can be overdone. Many doctors stumble across what they believe to be a new discovery only to find that it has previously been described somewhere in the literature. Coleridge's saying – "The dwarf sees farther than the giant when he has the giant's shoulder to mount on" – reminded us not to ignore the established body of knowledge when updating the chapters. In the present book, we have chosen to help limit the book's overall size by separating many of the lengthier entries in reference lists from the text and making these references available online. This maneuver has provided space to retain several popular features of the first edition: the Key Points at the start of each chapter, the wealth of illustrative material, and the Case Studies that serve to amplify the text. Additionally, we have moved to a two-volume format.

This edition features several new clinical photographs, radiographs, and other images while the explanatory diagrams have been redrawn. For the first time, the print work will also be available as an ebook, as well as available online at www.emedicine360.com. As before, there is a liberal use of color. It is our plan to produce a companion volume the next year that will incorporate the past, present, and some additional Case Studies since many readers have told us that they enjoy these illustrative examples of the real patient cases.

The extent of subjects covered is faithful to the first edition of the book. Based on the recommendations of our surgical colleagues, we consolidated much of the content in the sections on Transplantation, Breast Surgery, and Vascular Surgery, while expanding content in the Trauma section and in the Principles of Surgery and Critical Care sections. The book is designed to appeal to surgical trainees as well as those in independent practice. The initial chapters on core principles, critical care and trauma are followed by the major components of general surgery: gastrointestinal, vascular, breast, endocrine and transplantation. The book ends with a more limited coverage of those allied surgical specialties – pediatric, head and neck, genitourinary, skin and soft tissue, cardiothoracic – that from time to time will be relevant to those caring for patients in a "general" surgical ward or clinic.

We have been helped by an outstanding team of surgeons from around the world, led by a cadre of 15 section editors who have overseen about 100 full chapters and nearly 50 Case Studies. Of all surgical textbooks available, *Surgery: Core Principles and Practice* is the most international in terms of content and contributors, featuring contributions from surgical colleagues within Europe (Austria, Belgium, Germany, Greece, The Netherlands, Sweden and Switzerland) and Asia (China, India, Turkey and Taiwan) as well as Australia, Canada, South Africa and, of course, our own nations: the United States and Great Britain.

John D Corson MBChB FRCS (Eng) FRCS (Edin) FACS
Albuquerque, New Mexico, USA

Robin CN Williamson MD MChir FRCS
London, UK, 2017

Preface to the First Edition

Some may question the wisdom of developing a new textbook of surgery. Is the market not already saturated with adequate treatises that contain the appropriate body of surgical knowledge? What is different about this new surgical text that justifies its birth? Does the enormous expansion in technological communications not spell the end of the traditional surgical textbook? Will anyone actually read the book? These and many similar questions were discussed at length before the initiation of this project over four years ago.

It seems fitting that the first publication of *Surgery* would be at the start of the new millennium, an event that coincides with rapid evolution if not revolution in our surgical practice. The resetting of the calendar seems to offer a chance to close a previous chapter in the history of surgery and provide for a new beginning. We must continue to progress in our surgical learning and understanding and adapt the current knowledge base of surgery for the next century so as to make it available to a new generation of surgeons.

Indeed we do live in exciting times as we struggle with many issues in our daily surgical lives that are novel and challenging. Modern surgery is relatively young and is continuing to undergo rapid transformations. Current methods of imaging offer us preoperative information that our predecessors would have given their eye teeth to possess. New techniques and discoveries abound and force us to question earlier beliefs and treatments. Evidence-based medicine is here to stay. These facts all make for a unique educational experience, yet it is frustratingly hard to keep up with the pace of all the new information. We must have good teaching aids and resources to stay in touch with the explosion of knowledge.

The integration of clinical skills with a sound grasp of basic science is essential for the modern surgeon and is an important aspect of our text. The challenge to the editors of this book has not only been to provide space for all this new knowledge but also to define those components of a traditional surgical text that could be safely jettisoned to make room for the new material and still publish a single-volume, comprehensive textbook. The development of surgical specialties and the fragmentation of general surgery have impacted on the organization of our text, which we believe retains a core of knowledge required of all surgeons. Excellent subspecialty texts abound for those whose careers progress down a subspecialty path. Our overall theme has been to present principles of knowledge in subspecialty areas that provide a sound foundation for future learning.

The fact that the book is aimed at the general surgeon may seem out of touch with the theme of modernity since the future of this species is under threat. Yet all surgical trainees are exposed to a common stem of training that includes the diverging subspecialties of general surgery, namely gastroenterology and its component parts, vascular surgery, breast, endocrine and transplantation surgery. Moreover, there are several important branches of surgery that are so closely allied to 'general' surgery that both trainees and those in independent practice will encounter relevant patients on a regular basis. These allied surgical disciplines are pediatric, head and neck, plastic, cardiothoracic and urologic surgery, and they are covered in extensive, yet not exhaustive, detail in the final section of the book. However subspecialist our elective surgery, most of us will bear responsibility for a wider range of emergency conditions and can scarcely afford to let slip our knowledge of these related areas. This fact explains the large section on trauma in the book.

Another major issue throughout the project has been an attempt to make the book very user-friendly. The ratio of text to illustrative material is carefully balanced to break up the tedium of textual absorption by reinforcement of visual images. The use of color throughout the textbook is another major departure from existing surgical texts and one that should allow for more enjoyable studying. Color-coding of the various sections will facilitate the use of the book. Practical problems at the end of the various sections are intended to rehearse important clinical lessons. The book is liberally referenced so that the reader can have an entrée into the relevant literature on almost any topic.

Since worldwide travel and communication enable knowledge to be rapidly shared, we felt obliged to offer an international rather than an insular (or continental) perspective and have utilized surgical writing talent from many parts of the world. For authors, we have attempted to focus on potential future surgical leaders, who have a certain familiarity and understanding of modern science that might be lacking in their senior colleagues, who grew up in a vastly different surgical era. Our team of section editors represents an outstanding group of well-recognized academic surgeons and educators. Prominent among them has been Dr Joel Roslyn, who died before the completion of the book. Without their collaboration, this type of comprehensive text would not be possible. We are indebted to them for dedicating their time and expertise to this project.

John D Corson
Robin CN Williamson
Iowa City and London, 2000

Acknowledgments

A special thanks must be extended to our respective families, who provided support (and patience!) during the many long hours spent planning this work as well as editing the content. *Warm thanks to our wives, Christina and Judy.*

It is a pleasure to acknowledge the constant help and encouragement that we have received from the publishers, notably Marco Ulloa, Barton Dudlick, and Tom Gibbons, along with their leader, Joe Rusko, all based in Jaypee's Philadelphia office. To all of these individuals, we owe a considerable debt of gratitude. We hope that the resulting book will entertain as well as educate.

Finally, this second edition would not have been possible without the excellent contributions of the initial group of section editors and contributors, who paved the way for the current work. We both appreciate the substantial efforts of those involved in the groundbreaking first edition team.

We would like to thank Mr Jitendar P Vij (Group Chairman), Mr Ankit Vij (Group President), Ms Chetna Malhotra Vohra (Associate Director-Content Strategy), and the Production team of Jaypee Brothers Medical Publishers (P) Ltd., New Delhi, India for the successful completion of this project.

Contents

Volume 1

Volume 2

Section 4: Vascular Surgery

Section Editors: *John D Corson, Timothy F Kresowik*

Part 4A: Principles of Vascular Surgery

Part 4B: Arterial Disease

Part 4C: Miscellaneous Circulatory Disorders

Part 4D: Common Vascular Emergencies

Section 1

Principles of Surgery

Section Editor: *Donald E Fry*

Parts

1

The Acquisition of Surgical Knowledge

Lewis Flint

Key Points

- Acquisition of surgical knowledge from patients requires "effective listening" including attentiveness, concentration, and directed questioning.
- Learning from colleagues and healthcare professionals requires dedicated attention to the message being sent. Interruptions should be minimized.
- Learning from the surgical literature requires cautious application of the principles of evidence-based medicine.
- When evaluating evidence from the surgical literature, remember the hazards inherent in the term "statistically significant."
- Surgical simulation offers the opportunity for "deliberate practice" that will improve certain skills. Data are not yet available to support improved patient outcomes after simulation training.

INTRODUCTION

Surgeons use knowledge, technical skill, compassion, and judgment to achieve the best outcomes for each patient. Ideally, compassion is an inborn characteristic that may evolve over time as surgeons learn to integrate knowledge, compassion, empathy, and communication into what is currently termed "patient-centered practice." The most critical challenge facing surgeons in the application of the principles of "patient-centered practice" is to use knowledge and judgment to inform the patient and guide his or her choices toward the treatment that will achieve the best result for them. Achieving the best result may, at times, require advising against a surgical procedure. Effective communication to the patient and family members is a key element in the process of teaching them about therapeutic choices and obtaining the "buy-in" from both patient and family into the plan of treatment. Communication is a dynamic, not a static process since patient perceptions and preferences change as the disease state changes and the treatment and its complications progress.

This chapter will review the sources of surgical knowledge, the techniques of evaluating information, methods for quantifying the reliability of available information, and ways of communicating the certainties and uncertainties inherent in applying knowledge to the individual patient.

Table 1.1 Four sources of surgical knowledge.
Patients
Other healthcare professionals
The medical literature
Experience and simulation

Similar to the techniques of the concert violinist, technical skill in surgery improves with deliberate practice. New skills may be acquired and existing skills honed using simulation. The strengths and limitations of technical skill acquisition through simulation will also be reviewed.

Four main sources of surgical knowledge are easily available and are identified in Table 1.1. As we progress through this chapter, we will consider each of these sources in sequence.

LEARNING FROM PATIENTS

Patients and their families are rich sources of medical knowledge. They are the ones who experience the illness and the surgical treatment used to produce an improved state of health. Facilitating the transfer of knowledge from patient to surgeon can be challenging. Surgeons are well aware of the fact that pain and suffering must be inflicted on the patient and will be necessary to achieve the improved state of health. An editorial by Alpert[1] in 2011 provides advice for the surgeon that will make the transfer of the patient's experience easier so that knowledge acquisition can occur. Most important for the surgeon is to practice effective listening, embracing attentiveness, concentration, and directed questions. During the transfer of knowledge from patient to surgeon, the surgeon will be a teacher as well as a learner. A time-honored axiom states that the best way to learn something is to teach it. When teaching patients about their illness and its treatment, surgeons have a unique opportunity to learn the patient's perspectives, values, cultural context, and needs. From these experiences, knowledge can be gained that will be useful in the care of future patients.

Many professional organizations have begun to emphasize the importance of effective communication between patients and healthcare professionals. The Committee on Healthcare for Underserved Women and the Committee on Patient Safety and Quality improvement of the American College of Obstetrics and Gynecology produced an opinion statement on the elements of effective communication between patients and healthcare professionals.[2] The committees recommend using the "partnership" model of communication wherein the healthcare professional seeks to equalize the time spent speaking by both parties participating in the knowledge exchange. The committee statement goes on to emphasize the importance of several personal characteristics that help ensure high-quality information exchange and knowledge acquisition. These characteristics are comfort, acceptance, responsiveness, and empathy. Comfort and acceptance relate to the healthcare professional's ability to deal with difficult topics without becoming uneasy or disorganized. Responsiveness and empathy relate to the ability to detect and interpret subtle and indirect messages from the patient that may be transmitted by body language or indirect verbal messaging. An example contained in the committee opinion is helpful: a patient may be tearful but minimize the problem saying, "I'm just having a bad day." An effective approach would be for the healthcare professional to offer an opportunity to discuss issues leading to the "bad day." The committee recommendations close with suggestions that healthcare professionals adopt patient-centered interviewing techniques, that patients be encouraged to write questions in advance of the information exchange, and that training in cultural sensitivity may be beneficial. A final recommendation is that electronic communication with patients be adopted in compliance with national guidelines from organizations such as the American Medical Association.

The adoption and practice of effective communication skills has to be coupled with persistence. It is obvious to most practitioners that patient attitudes are dynamic and vary with changes in the illness status, the development of complications of treatment, and numerous other factors. Being alert to changes will help optimize information exchange and knowledge acquisition.

LEARNING FROM COLLEAGUES

Interactions between healthcare professionals can provide a meaningful opportunity for knowledge transfer and learning if specific measures are taken to ensure timely, accurate, and understandable information. This information can be in the form of conversation or narrative contained in the medical record. Other opportunities for professional interaction occur in the forms of educational presentations and seminars.

The characteristics of high-quality verbal exchanges between healthcare professionals are reviewed in the editorial by Alpert.[1] Central to achieving accuracy of information transfer and maximum understanding of the meaning and importance of the conversation is a mutual attitude of respect between the participants. Alpert stresses that each participant must be willing to be attentive to the process of information transfer. Actions such as the checking of emails on a smartphone should be avoided. If possible, interruptions for receiving telephone calls and answering pages should be minimized. The healthcare professional who wishes to provide information to a physician or surgeon should be the central focus of attention. Important parts of the information being transferred will be omitted if the person delivering the information perceives that the listener is not paying attention. It is also important for the listener to understand the level of importance that is placed on the information to be transferred by the person bringing the information. The listener needs to transmit to that person, through direct or indirect means, that the listener believes the information to be important. One effective way to send this message is to look attentively at the person delivering the information.

Alpert stresses that effective listening is critical to understanding questions that are being posed and the exact content needed by the requestor. The response to a question posed by a colleague or other healthcare professional should be framed to answer the question specifically without additional supplementary information. Inquiring of the questioner as to whether the response provided effectively answered the question is also an important component of the conversation.

Important medical information is presented and received by use of the medical record. For this mode of knowledge transfer to be used effectively, certain writing skills need to be used. Reviewing these skills, Simon[3] emphasizes the importance of clarity when entries are made into the medical record. Good narrative writing will be useful to the surgeon when she/he returns to the medical record after a time interval. Simon notes that effective entries in the medical record can "bring the patient to life" when the record is opened for a future patient encounter. Effective and clear narrative is increasingly important because of the fact that patients now have full access to their medical records. Patient access to medical records has benefits and hazards. The benefits are that patients can add perspective to their medical histories and correct errors. Hazards include the risk for causing fear and anxiety if the medical record contains frightening material that is presented without clarification or written without a balanced perspective. Several pieces of advice offered in the article include an admonition to "write with pride," with narrative designed to present information clearly and with compassion. Writers are encouraged to "be personal," using the patient's name frequently. It is useful to include direct quotes from the patient. As use of electronic medical records increases, it is important to resist the urge to "cut and paste" when constructing a narrative. One critical point to remember is to proofread notes. An approach that I find valuable is to read narrative aloud. If it then sounds correct and good, the narrative will probably be meaningful when read by the patient or another healthcare professional.

Surgical knowledge can be acquired during formal education presentations and seminars. During presentations by expert surgeons it is important that surgeons receiving the information maximize their opportunity to receive it accurately by using efficient listening. Direct questions to the presenter can be helpful to integrate the information into "real-world" practice situations. Alpert[1] includes useful advice for presenters in his editorial. He emphasizes that slide presentations should not include too much detailed information on each slide. Four or five clearly stated points presented on slides that are easy to read without too much color and/or extraneous material will ensure that the message is transmitted with the maximum clarity.

LEARNING FROM THE MEDICAL LITERATURE

There is current consensus that surgeons should use an "evidence-based" approach to clinical practice. Central to the successful implementation of evidence-based practice by surgeons and surgical teams is the ability to use information from the medical literature to improve patient outcomes. The principles of evidence-based practice include a hierarchy of research quality. The highest quality research is the prospective, randomized, double-blinded clinical trial. Randomized trials that evaluate surgical interventions are difficult to perform and are expensive to conduct. As a consequence, the evidence supporting most aspects of surgical practice cannot be considered strong. Conducting randomized trials in any area of medicine is challenging because of the difficulty in obtaining sufficient patient enrollment. Because results of medical treatments have improved over time, the selected endpoints of a research trial occur infrequently and treatment effects are often small in magnitude. This fact means that enrollment will need to be large, and many studies are concluded and published with suboptimal enrollment. This problem has been countered, to some extent, by the use of meta-analytic research techniques. Meta-analysis combines available research studies and uses specific statistical and categorization techniques to analyze combinations of studies. The result is the production of a group of research subjects that is large enough to have the necessary statistical power to evaluate the impact of an intervention and to facilitate the introduction of the intervention into practice. In an exchange of views on the utility of small trials that are later combined into meta-analytic studies by Guyatt et al.[4] the authors emphasize the hazard of interpreting small trials that are underpowered. They also stress the importance of high-quality meta-analyses.

For a meta-analysis to be valuable it has to meet certain requirements. Ideally, the plan to conduct the meta-analysis should be published as a research protocol ahead of the analysis itself or registered on a Web site such as PROSPERO (www.crd.ac.york.uk/NIHR/PROSPERO/). Also, meta-analyses should examine publications in languages other than English and evaluate unpublished data. Recommendations for the items to be included in a meta-analysis are found in the *Preferred Reporting Items for Systematic Reviews and Meta-analyses* (www.prisma-statement.org). Unfortunately, most publications that purport to be systematic reviews or meta-analyses fail to meet these requirements. In the era of "comparative effectiveness" research, the challenge is to prevent "metabias," which is the biased interpretation that can result from the evaluation of a group of flawed meta-analyses.[5] Despite the flaws in many published reports, the meta-analyses and systematic reviews pertaining to surgical topics can, if published in a peer-reviewed surgical journal and reviewed carefully and critically by the reader, contribute meaningfully to the improvement of surgical practice. One particularly strong source of meta-analyses and systematic reviews that meet all of the proposed evidence quality requirements are those published by the Cochrane Collaboration (www.cochrane.org). In future, it is likely that carefully performed meta-analysis will greatly ameliorate the problem of small randomized trials. Thus, there is no reason to discourage the conduct of carefully structured small randomized trials.

Another source of data to assist in the acquisition and application of surgical knowledge is observational research. High-quality observational, nonrandomized research studies can provide outcomes that are similar to high-quality randomized trials.[6,7] The most valuable observational studies are cross-sectional analyses, cohort analyses, and case–control studies. Cross-sectional studies evaluate characteristics of a sample of research subjects from a population of interest at a single point in time. Cohort studies select a sample of subjects from a population of interest and follow these subjects over time to record changes in health status. Case–control studies select a sample of research subjects from a population of interest and record baseline data. An intervention is used in each subject, and the change in health status for each subject over time is recorded. In case-control studies each subject serves as her/his own control.

Unfortunately, high-quality observational research studies pertaining to surgical topics are small in number. In fact, most reports of surgical topics consist of retrospective case series, multicenter prospective nonrandomized trials, and literature reviews. Surgical textbooks and periodic literature reviews (such as the publication I edit) fall into the lowest category of medical literature evidence, namely expert opinion. Practicing surgeons need to evaluate retrospective case series and prospective single or multicenter trials carefully. If several retrospective case series from differing locations reach the same conclusion, and the conclusion reached harmonizes with the experience of a surgeon or group of surgeons, the evidence has a good chance of being dependable and valuable. Focused literature reviews can be valuable if all viewpoints are acknowledged and estimates of the quality of the evidence reviewed are included. To have accurate data from the practice of an individual surgeon so that a "reality check" of published data can be conducted, it is important that individual surgeons record clinical data from their patient care experiences. The Surgeon-Specific Registry sponsored by the American College of Surgeons is a convenient and confidential way to record these data and easily retrieve them for analysis. At the hospital level, accurate risk-adjusted data that can be used to document outcomes can be acquired by participation in the National Surgical Quality Improvement Project sponsored by the American College of Surgeons.

Successful use of the medical literature requires an understanding of the strengths and weaknesses of published research. One successful method for evaluating and applying information from the medical literature is found in the reference work by Guyatt.[8] Several important pitfalls in interpretation of medical literature publications are presented in this book, and readers are encouraged to review them.

Caution is indicated when interpreting information published in the medical literature because of shortcomings in the design of published research studies, including misleading use of the term "statistical significance," inadequate sample size, and bias. It is common for authors to suggest that a hypothesis is supported because of a "*p* value" of $<.05$ obtained from use of statistical analysis software; the implication of this interpretation of "statistical significance" is that there is at least a 95% chance that the null hypothesis (there was no benefit from the tested intervention) is false. In fact, a p value of <0.05 means that the null hypothesis will be true, on average, in 5% of the population represented by the reported sample. Statistical significance is easily demonstrated in large samples, but the observed results may not be clinically significant. For example, the use of a particular intervention may lead to a shortened recovery time as indicated by return to work in 5 days compared to 6 days in patients who did not have the intervention. In a sample of $>1,000$ patients this outcome will be statistically significant, but the clinical relevance of a 1-day difference given the varying practices of employers in permitting return to work is questionable. Guyatt et al. emphasize that authors should make efforts to ensure that data are expressed in more detailed ways that make interpretation of the reported observations easier. Some of these practices include reports of risk reduction, number needed to treat, and 95% confidence intervals. Risk reduction is determined by analyzing the difference in the risk of an event (death, for example) in patients who did not have an intervention compared with patients who had the intervention. This approach is best applied to data from a prospective randomized controlled trial. The frequency of the event in question in the control group is considered the baseline risk. Assuming that the frequency of the event in the treatment group is reduced compared with the control group, one can express the potential benefit in the treated patients in various ways. Risk reduction is frequently reported as absolute risk reduction, relative risk reduction, or odds ratios. Each reporting method is acceptable, but differences between them can be important. For example, the absolute risk reduction is basically the difference in the frequency of the event in the control and treated groups. The relative risk reduction refers to the proportion of the baseline frequency of the unwanted event that is removed when the treatment is applied. Odds ratios express the odds of an event occurring or not. Groups can be compared to determine the differences in odds of an event when the two groups are compared. Odds ratios should be used with caution; however, Guyatt et al. present an example of a treatment that reduces the odds of an event by 30% in each of three groups of patients. If the baseline risk of the event is 30% the treatment reduces the odds of the event to 20%. If the baseline risk is 1%, however, the risk is reduced to 0.67%. In the group with the lowest baseline risk (1%), a treatment with a 10% or more risk of a disabling complication would probably not be offered to the group with the lowest baseline risk.

Another way of interpreting data about a potentially beneficial treatment is to use an estimate of the number of patients who would receive the treatment to prevent one occurrence of the event in question (death, for example). If the difference in the risk of death with treatment compared with the risk without treatment is, for example, 20%, then 20 events would be avoided in every 100 patients treated. The number that would need to be treated to avoid one event is 100 divided by 20 or 5 patients. A final way of expressing data about treatment effectiveness is the use of 95% confidence intervals. These intervals are calculated to provide an estimate of the range of values where the true benefit of treatment may be located. Trials with larger samples will, in general, have smaller 95% confidence intervals. If confidence intervals are wide and especially if the lower boundary is a negative number and the higher boundary is a positive number, the observed effect of treatment is at risk for inaccuracy. Confidence intervals can facilitate application of research data to clinical situations. If the lower bound of the confidence interval indicates a treatment benefit that exceeds the minimum acceptable benefit from the patient's perspective, then a treatment would be chosen. An example of a surgical prospective randomized trial where confidence intervals were helpful in confirming benefit was the North American Symptomatic Carotid Endarterectomy Trial reported in 1998.[9] This trial showed a stroke risk reduction benefit of 22% ($p < .05$) with a confidence interval of 7%–52%. This finding indicates that the lowest stroke reduction risk that could be expected from a successful carotid endarterectomy in a symptomatic patient is 7%, with a possible maximum risk reduction of 52%. The risk of perioperative stroke in this study was 2.1% at 90 days after operation and 6.7% at 8 years. Calculation of the number needed to treat indicated that 15 patients would have to undergo carotid endarterectomy to prevent one stroke. This study had >99% long-term follow-up that strengthened the evidence of benefit considerably. Another randomized prospective trial comparing three methods for control of methicillin-resistant *Staphylococcus aureus* colonization in critically ill patients reported confidence intervals for risk reduction for bloodstream infection using universal decolonization measures; the intervention reduced risk of bloodstream infection by 44%.[10] The confidence interval calculation indicated that the lowest estimated risk reduction was 35%, with the highest being 51%. Even if the actual risk reduction was 35%, this finding would represent significant improvement in control of this prevalent infection in critically ill patients. Confidence intervals are useful also to provide support of a decision not to use a treatment. Guyatt et al.[4] emphasize that evaluation of the lower bound of the confidence interval may assist decisions about whether or not to use a treatment. If the lower bound of benefit approaches a minimal reduction in risk, then use of a toxic or expensive treatment would be rejected.

It is tempting to believe that large samples provide "better" data than small samples. Interpretation of data from large sample studies such as multicenter trials and use of data from administrative databases should take into consideration several important factors. In large sample patient studies, especially retrospective studies, data concerning time of enrollment in the study and follow-up intervals should be reported. Patients enrolled in a trial over a prolonged interval may differ depending on time of enrollment because of changes in baseline risk of the event that have occurred over time with changing health status of the population being analyzed or the use of more recent adjunctive treatments. Data reported from large administrative databases can be unreliable because of missing values or because the data were gathered for a reason that does not relate to the research question being examined. For example, data from hospital billing records are influenced by the behavior of billing personnel. If the billing data are expressed with a view toward maximizing reimbursement, then disease descriptor data points may not reflect actual patient characteristics. Administrative data that are rigorously controlled for accuracy of patient characteristics and complete data entry (for example, the National Surgical Quality Improvement database) can provide meaningful clinical information. A review of some of the hazards of using administrative datasets is provided in an article by Ioannidis.[11] This editorial reviews in detail the sources of error that can be encountered when using data from administrative datasets. Ioannidis notes that all analyses from large administrative datasets are overpowered to detect clinically meaningful differences. Tiny, clinically insignificant differences can be "statistically significant" with the large numbers of subjects in administrative databases. Ioannidis suggests inclusion of "falsification endpoints" or analyses of associations that are known to be null. The use of this technique is reviewed in detail by Prasad and Jena[12] who give an example of the use of falsification endpoints. In an analysis of the use of proton pump inhibitors in a large patient database, a falsification endpoint might be to analyze associations of the use of these drugs with associations known not to exist such as increased risk of soft tissue infection. If these associations are statistically significant, then other significant associations may be undependable. Other sources of error include misclassification of variables, erroneous modeling of variables, and unmeasured variables. Finally, identifying modifiable characteristics from administrative data is extremely challenging.

A major challenge to the use of administrative datasets in surgical research is the problem of unknown confounding variables. The impact of variables such as socioeconomic status, nonprescription drug use, or direction of a certain type of patient to one or another healthcare institution on the basis of diagnosis cannot be adjusted for in the administrative dataset. Two methods of adjusting for unknown confounding variables are the use of statistical techniques such as instrumental variables and propensity scores.[13,14] An example of this practice is research studies that evaluate the effectiveness of trauma systems.[15] In trauma systems, severely injured patients are preferentially directed to designated centers. This factor produces a mortality bias in favor of nontrauma center hospitals, making comparisons of outcomes in trauma centers and nontrauma center hospitals difficult. Adjusting for such confounder characteristics is possible using one of these approaches. Each of these techniques is an acceptable way to adjust for unknown confounding variables. A detailed discussion of these is beyond the scope of this chapter. Interested readers are referred to the other articles cited.

Guyatt[8] notes that bias can influence the results of medical research at several points during the conduct of a study. Biased results will be obtained if there are differences in the control and experimental groups at the beginning of a study. Actions to reduce the impact of this form of bias include randomizing patients or conducting preintervention matching of pairs of patients based on clearly defined characteristics. Surgical research studies are frequently reported using "before and after" research models. In this type of study, the intervention group is compared with an historical control group. Bias is a major hazard with this type of study design. Although the two groups may be similar in terms of demographic data, important differences will often go undetected.

During the conduct of a study, bias can emerge because of placebo effects (a problem particularly in studies where the results are reported by the patient) because some patients may have differing compliance characteristics or receive cointerventions that others do not. These factors produce bias in assessment of outcomes. Ideally, such bias can be countered by "blinding" of patients, clinicians, data collectors, and other participants to the treatment applied. Blinding is a challenge in surgical research studies because of the difficulty in concealing the fact that the patient had an operation.

At the end of the research study bias can be introduced if significant numbers of patients are lost to follow-up, if the study is ended prematurely because of perceived increased frequency of adverse effects or because of an unexpectedly large treatment effect emerging in a small number of patients, and if patients "cross over" from the control group to the treatment group. This is a particular problem in trials evaluating surgical procedures because patients' and caregivers' desires to have the surgical procedure may increase during the conduct of the study. This problem is remedied by the use of "intent to treat" analysis, which requires that each patient be counted in the group to which that patient was originally assigned. Bias can affect the results of surgical research in several ways. One of the most common is bias introduced because of reporting of retrospective data from the experience of a single surgeon or single institution. Another common form of bias is selection bias. Excellent results of using surgical procedures or medical treatments can be obtained if patients with minimal risk for adverse outcomes are reported in a clinical research article and moderate to high-risk patients are excluded. This type of bias would obviously tend to overestimate the benefit of a procedure or treatment.

Bias can also be introduced by the use of composite endpoints. Because most research on medical treatments produces small benefits of one treatment versus another, there is interest in attempting to obtain results that show statistical strength. Composite endpoints that are each interpreted as "beneficial" can, when combined, increase the number of patients in whom benefit is observed. Precautions that need to be taken when trying to interpret composite endpoints are reviewed by Guyatt.[8] They note that the composite endpoint should consist of outcomes that are important to patients and that the frequency with which each endpoint occurred should be reported in the results section of the research article. Uncertainty as to the quality of a treatment benefit can occur when there is imbalance in the frequency of each of the composite endpoints. Consider a research study of a surgical intervention that uses a composite endpoint of death within 90 days of operation, readmission to the hospital, and quality of life at 6 months after the operative procedure. If mortality risk and quality of life scores are equivalent in the two comparison groups, but the surgical intervention is associated with fewer readmissions to the hospital, it would be difficult to conclude that benefit in terms of outcomes important to the patient were achieved.

Obviously, the most insidious and dishonest form of bias is the deliberate withholding or alteration of data. This has been a serious problem in the production of pharmaceutical research data. A review of the extent and depth of this form of biased research is found in an article by Washington.[16] The wrongdoing cited in this article stimulated the increased use of research study registries where names of investigators, study protocols, and the data from the research are stored and are available for review. The obvious limitation of the registries is the fact that many, if not the majority, of ongoing studies are not registered.

A final way of acquiring surgical knowledge from the medical literature is through the use of practice guidelines. Practice guidelines are produced by national professional organizations and are intended to provide practical guidance to physicians and surgeons who are striving to practice on the basis of the highest quality of available evidence. Practice guidelines usually include detailed explanations of the evidentiary basis for the guidelines and the degree of consensus achieved by the group producing the guidelines. The strength of the evidence supporting the guidelines is assessed and presented in the guidelines document. Entities such as the United States Preventive Services Task Force, the American College of Chest Physicians, and the Oxford Center for Evidence Based Medicine have produced manuals that provide rules and practices for grading the strength of evidence and producing practice guidelines. The production of practice guidelines documents is labor intensive and expensive. Because of the fact that additional scientific evidence is being generated continuously as medical science evolves, there needs to be a commitment by the sponsoring organization periodically to update and revise the guidelines. Some of the problems encountered when trying to ascertain the quality and consistency of practice guidelines are reviewed in an article by Kavanagh.[17] The author notes that one set of practice guidelines, the International Guidelines for the Management of Severe Sepsis and Septic Shock,[18] has been broadly adopted and graded as high-quality guidelines. Close examination of the guidelines documents produced in 2004 and 2008 show that at least one recommendation presented with a low evidence grade in the early document was repeated with the same supporting data in the 2008 version with a high grade of evidence. The author concludes that current approaches to assigning quality grades to practice guidelines need to be improved.

An additional concern with the application of practice guidelines is a possible conflict of the guidelines with the standards of patient-centered practice. These issues are reviewed in an article by Goldberger and Buxton.[19] The authors note that a pitfall in the interpretation of data supporting the practice guideline can occur if subgroup analyses in a clinical trial detect a group of patients in whom an intervention is not effective, but this group is included as eligible for treatment according to the practice guideline. The authors cite data from one randomized clinical trial that identified nonbenefit in 19% of patients enrolled in the trial, and these patients could be identified using clinical characteristics. Despite the fact that no benefit occurred, using the intervention in such patients was supported by the guideline. The authors emphasize that, ideally, inclusion of this patient subgroup in the guidelines should only be done after additional prospective research focusing on patients with the characteristics of the subgroup. In the instance cited, further trial research was not done. Practitioners seeking to practice personalized, patient-centered medicine would, on the basis of the evidence, withhold the intervention from the patients in whom no benefit was identified, but these practitioners would then be guilty of noncompliance with guideline-based practice. A potential conflict exists, therefore. They recommend that practitioners remember that guidelines (and trial data) refer to groups of patients and not individual patients. Guidelines are intended to provide suggestions for clinical practice and should not be viewed as rules for practice.

The question that remains for practitioners is: how do I apply data and guidelines in my practice if I don't have time to review all of the data that were used to support the guidelines? There is no single answer. Surgeons will need to assimilate guidelines and data from the literature into their personal body of knowledge and apply this information carefully to their patients. Maintenance of a personal practice database containing information on patient outcomes will help provide a real-world view of the effects of interventions in an individual surgeons practice. Amalgamating surgeon-specific and institutional data on risk-adjusted patient outcomes will serve to guide the use of knowledge gleaned from the literature.

LEARNING FROM EXPERIENCE AND FROM USING SIMULATION

A time-honored axiom of surgical practice is that "good judgment comes from experience and experience comes from bad judgment." Research into the topic of learning from experience has shown that expertise does not increase linearly with the time spent in medical practice. Current thought regarding the acquisition and maintenance of expertise over time are reviewed by Ericsson.[20] He notes that the fundamental tenets of the roles of genetics and deliberate practice in the acquisition of expertise were established by the work of Galton in the 19th century. Subsequent research cited by Ericsson has shown that expertise does not increase over time but actually decays in the absence of deliberate, repetitive practice. Ericsson notes that early learners tend to concentrate on achieving a level of expertise that will permit performance of the desired task without errors. For activities such as typing, playing golf, and driving an automobile, approximately 50 hours of practice are necessary to achieve this level of expertise. The task performance then becomes automated. During the automation period, the subject is generally unable to make conscious changes in the way the tasks are performed, and expertise then reaches a plateau and does not increase with time. Ericsson notes that the main difference in acquisition of medical expertise is the time course of the acquisition. Once a level of medical expertise is attained (at the end of residency training, for example), further improvement in expertise is not recognized without deliberate practice. The author cites research that documents the increase in expertise in a specialist who sees many patients with the same or similar diagnosis or a surgeon who does a small number of operations repeatedly, compared with a practitioner in a general community practice who encounters a variety of patients or who performs a variety of procedures. Ericsson notes that introduction of a new set of surgical techniques such as with the introduction of laparoscopic surgery produced a "field experiment" that documented the value of deliberate practice in the acquisition of expertise.

The use of surgical simulators has produced an environment in which the use of deliberate practice can facilitate the acquisition of expertise. This topic is the focus of a report by Crochet et al.,[21] who conducted an analysis of skill acquisition after a training course on a virtual reality laparoscopic simulator followed by an interval of deliberate practice. Acquisition of expertise was measured by determining the time required to complete a set of tasks and the number of movements needed to complete each subtask sequentially over the course of several practice sessions. Twenty-two candidates were evaluated. One group was assigned to deliberate practice activities between virtual reality simulator sessions, whereas the control group did not practice. The analysis showed that the deliberate practice group began to improve in terms of time required and movements required after the 10th virtual reality session, and improvements continued from that point onwards. These results confirmed the value of deliberate practice. Deliberate practice has been associated with improved performance in clinical situations. A study of this topic is by Stefanidis et al.[22] The authors randomly assigned subjects to a deliberate practice group or a traditional training group. The task was to perform the suturing maneuvers necessary to complete a laparoscopic Nissen fundoplication. The deliberate practice group used the suturing simulation exercise contained within the Fundamentals of Laparoscopic Surgery course sponsored by the American College of Surgeons. This experience was supplemented by training using a porcine model of a laparoscopic Nissen fundoplication. The intervention group practiced until "automaticity" had been achieved as judged by suturing accuracy and time required to complete a secondary task. When compared to the conventional training group, suture task completion scores during the performance of a laparoscopic Nissen fundoplication in a second porcine model were significantly improved. The data in these two articles support the conclusion that deliberate practice using simulation can improve performance of defined skills tasks.

One distinct advantage of the use of simulation in aviation has been the ability to train pilots in the management of emergency situations. Ericsson[20] cites data from military experience that confirm improved outcomes in actual emergencies when pilots had undergone simulator training for that emergency. Whether skills acquisition for the management of surgical emergencies can be acquired with simulator training has been a source of ongoing discussions. One effort to use simulated emergency surgical situations to train surgeons for care of life-threatening emergencies encountered in the operating room is the Advanced Trauma Operative Management Course sponsored by the Committee on Trauma of the American College of Surgeons. In this course problems of bleeding and operative exposure that are actually encountered during the care of injured patients are simulated in a porcine animal model. Participants are coached by experienced instructors through several encounters of various operative problems such as retrohepatic bleeding, inferior vena cava laceration, and penetrating cardiac injury. Assessments of candidate perceptions of improvement have been conducted.[23] Participant perceptions of improved understanding of the management of operative emergency situations have been consistently shown. An article describing the implementation of the Advanced Trauma Operative Management course in a surgical residency program is by Ali et al.[24] The analysis of questionnaire responses and instructor evaluations showed that participants improved significantly in their knowledge of important technical maneuvers for the care of life-threatening emergencies in injured patients. Instructors documented improved performance by participants with repeated simulations and participants expressed satisfaction with the improved levels of knowledge acquired during the course.

A final study of simulation to improved responses to emergency events in the operating room is described in an article by Acero et al.[25] The authors conducted simulator training for an exsanguination emergency in the operating room. A mannequin simulator was used to produce signs and symptoms that would be encountered in a pregnant patient with a carotid artery laceration. Specific instruction was given in the conduct of care of the patient to 171 operating room staff members who were divided into teams. The team members then practiced resuscitation and advanced cardiac life support interventions on the mannequin. At baseline, 50% of participants believed they knew the appropriate roles and interventions for successful management of the simulated patient. At the close of the instructional period and the practice sessions, this perception had risen to 98%.

The available data indicate that simulation training is an effective means of providing deliberate practice that leads to improvements in performance of structured tasks. What remains is to conduct research to confirm that the acquired expertise results in improved clinical outcomes. Simulation provides a viable means for surgeons to perform deliberate practice that should result in improved levels of expertise.

CONCLUSION

Teachers of surgery often say: "the more you know, the easier the practice of surgery is." While this is true, digesting the knowledge gained from the sources discussed in this chapter will continue to be challenging for surgeons, but the effort will supply the intellectual stimulation that will make the practice of surgery rewarding for the entirety of the surgeon's professional life.

REFERENCES

1. Alpert JS. Some simple rules for effective communication in clinical teaching and practice environments. Am J Med. 2011;124(5):381-2.
2. American College of Obstetricians and Gynecologists Committee on Health Care for Underserved Women: Committee on Patient Safety and Quality Improvement. ACOG Committee Opinion No. 492: Effective patient-physician communication. Obstet Gynecol. 2011;117(5):1254-7.
3. Simon HB. The write stuff: how good writing can enhance patient care and professional growth. Am J Med. 2013;126(6): 467-71.

4. Guyatt GH, Mills EJ, Elbourne D. In the era of systematic reviews, does the size of an individual trial still matter. PLoS Med. 2008;5(1):e4.
5. Goodman S, Dickersin K. Metabias: a challenge for comparative effectiveness research. Ann Intern Med. 2011; 155(1):61-2.
6. Concato J, Horwitz RI. Beyond randomised versus observational studies. Lancet. 2004;363(9422):1660-1.
7. Concato J, Lawler EV, Lew RA, et al. Observational methods in comparative effectiveness research. Am J Med. 2010; 123(12 Suppl 1):e16-23.
8. Guyatt GH. Users' Guides to the Medical Literature. Chicago, Illinois: McGraw-Hill Medical; 2008.
9. Barnett HJ, Taylor DW, Eliasziw M, et al. Benefit of carotid endarterectomy in patients with symptomatic moderate or severe stenosis. North American Symptomatic Carotid Endarterectomy Trial Collaborators. N Engl J Med. 1998; 339(20):1415-25.
10. Huang SS, Septimus E, Kleinman K, et al. Targeted versus Universal Decolonization to Prevent ICU Infection. N Engl J Med. 2013;368(24):2255-65.
11. Ioannidis JP. Are mortality differences detected by administrative data reliable and actionable? JAMA. 2013;309(13): 1410-1.
12. Prasad V, Jena AB. Prespecified falsification end points: can they validate true observational associations? JAMA. 2013; 309(3):241-2.
13. Durham R, Pracht E, Orban B, et al. Evaluation of a mature trauma system. Ann Surg. 2006;243(6):775-83; discussion 83-5.
14. Martens EP, Pestman WR, de Boer A, et al. Instrumental variables: application and limitations. Epidemiology. 2006; 17(3):260-7.
15. Joffe MM, Rosenbaum PR. Invited commentary: propensity scores. Am J Epidemiol. 1999;150(4):327-33.
16. Washington H. Flacking for big Pharma. Am Sch. 2011. Available at: http://theamericanscholar.org. [Accessed May 19, 2013].
17. Kavanagh BP. The GRADE system for rating clinical guidelines. PLoS Med. 2009;6(9):e1000094.
18. Dellinger RP, Levy MM, Rhodes A, et al. Surviving Sepsis Campaign: international guidelines for management of severe sepsis and septic shock, 2012. Intensive Care Med. 2013;39(2):165-228.
19. Goldberger JJ, Buxton AE. Personalized medicine vs guideline-based medicine. JAMA. 2013:1-2.
20. Ericsson KA. Deliberate practice and the acquisition and maintenance of expert performance in medicine and related domains. Acad Med. 2004;79(10 Suppl):S70-81.
21. Crochet P, Aggarwal R, Dubb SS, et al. Deliberate practice on a virtual reality laparoscopic simulator enhances the quality of surgical technical skills. Ann. Surg. 2011;253(6):1216-22.
22. Stefanidis D, Scerbo MW, Montero PN, et al. Simulator training to automaticity leads to improved skill transfer compared with traditional proficiency-based training: a randomized controlled trial. Ann Surg. 2012;255(1):30-7.
23. Jacobs LM, Burns KJ, Kaban JM, et al. Development and evaluation of the advanced trauma operative management course. J Trauma. 2003;55(3):471-9; discussion 9.
24. Ali J, Ahmed N, Jacobs LM, et al. The advanced trauma operative management course in a Canadian residency program. Can J Surg. 2008;51(3):185-9.
25. Acero NM, Motuk G, Luba J, et al. Managing a surgical exsanguination emergency in the operating room through simulation: an interdisciplinary approach. J Surg Educ. 2012; 69(6):759-65.

2

Perioperative Risk Assessment and Care of the Surgical Patient

Robert F Wilson, Alfred E Baylor, Heather S Dolman

Key Points

- Assessment of operative risk is important in the determination of risk–benefit decisions in operative care. The recognition of specific clinical variables that are associated with adverse outcomes is essential when making surgical judgments.
- Objective evaluation of the cardiovascular, pulmonary, renal, and hepatic systems and of nutritional status is an essential basis to determine risk variables and to optimize the patient's condition for operation.
- Management of blood volume, judgments about the need for transfusion and evaluation, and management of coagulation disorders are fundamental to sound perioperative care.
- Preventive strategies for thromboembolic and infectious complications are necessary for patients undergoing major thoracic and abdominal operations.
- Perioperative patients require a variety of tubes and intravascular devices for management and monitoring. Each has benefits but carries potential risks.

INTRODUCTION

Thorough preoperative risk assessment and appropriate perioperative management of patients are essential for optimal surgical outcomes. After an accurate diagnosis has been made and a surgical treatment strategy developed, appropriate perioperative care includes a complete evaluation of risk factors, preoperative optimization of the patient, and intraoperative and postoperative monitoring of the patient. Postoperative care involves the recognition and management of intercurrent complications. This chapter will address physiologically based strategies for meeting these perioperative needs. By necessity, the content of this chapter will overlap with many other chapters of this volume that have more descriptions of the problems and management of specific perioperative issues in the surgical patient. The reader will be referred to these appropriate chapters for a more detailed discussion.

ASSESSMENT OF OPERATIVE RISK

Perioperative and postoperative complications can be divided into two risk periods following the operation. There is the period of initial 48 hours postoperatively with specific complications that include myocardial infarction, arrhythmias, congestive heart failure, stroke, respiratory failure, metabolic derangements, and technical problems from the operation. The period from 3–30 days after the operation is associated with complications of pulmonary embolism, surgical site infection, peritonitis, sepsis, hypermetabolism, and multiorgan dysfunction.

The risk of specific morbid events depends upon the type of procedure and patient-specific variables. The functional status of the patient's cardiovascular, pulmonary, hepatic, renal, and other systems can be classified preoperatively into risk categories using the American Society of Anesthesiologists (ASA) Physical Status Scale (Table 2.1).[1] Although subjective, the ASA categories have been proven to be accurate for predicting death or complications in large groups of patients.

The goal of the preoperative evaluation is to identify and optimize conditions that might otherwise increase perioperative morbidity and mortality. For elective operations, past medical and surgical history is obtained, current medications are defined, and functional status is assessed. For an unstable, critically ill patient, this history will need to be gathered in parallel with immediate clinical management and will commonly need to be obtained from family or others.[2]

A thorough physical examination is very important and must be done before any laboratory or imaging studies are undertaken. Recent practice guidelines recommend that

Table 2.1 American Society of Anesthesiologists (ASA) classification.

ASA class	*Description of disease state*	*Examples*
1	No systemic or organic disease that poses an anesthetic risk	Elective inguinal hernia repair in a healthy 20-year-old patient
2	Mild or moderate systemic or organic disease that may or may not be related to reasons for operation	Elective abdominal operation in patient who has mild heart disease, essential hypertension, or morbid obesity
3	Severe systemic or organic disease that is related or not to indications for operation that restrict activity	Elective operation in poorly controlled diabetic patient with severe hypertension and pulmonary disease
4	Life-threatening systemic or organic disease that is life-threatening, independent of need for operation and is incapacitating	Operation in a patient who has heart, lung, liver, or renal failure
5	Moribund patient with little chance of survival with or without an operation	Operation for uncontrolled hemorrhage (e.g. from ruptured aneurysm, gunshot wound)
6	A declared brain dead patient whose organs are being removed for donor	Fatal head injury undergoing organ donation
Emergency operation (E)	The designation "E" indicates that the procedure is undertaken as an emergency	Emergency laparotomy for perforated diverticulum in an elderly diabetic patient

Commonly used classification recommended by the ASA to determine the risk in patients undergoing operations requiring general anesthesia.

testing in patients should be guided by a pertinent clinical history and physical examination to avoid needless and unnecessary studies.[3] The clinical information from the history and physical examination will also direct necessary preoperative consultation including anesthesiology assessment to optimize the results of surgical care.[4]

Preoperative laboratory testing will usually include a basic battery of studies for major operations. The extent of these studies is governed by the expectation that results will alter preparation to minimize risk, complexity of the operation to be undertaken, assess effects from drugs that the patient is taking (e.g. diuretics or nonsteroidal anti-inflammatory drugs), and to evaluate specific markers of organ function when clinical information suggests that a problem may be present. By convention, complete blood counts with coagulation evaluation, electrolytes, creatinine, and fasting blood sugar are customarily performed for major inpatient operations, but may not be done for favorable risk patients undergoing ambulatory procedures. A urinalysis is performed if there is a history of prostatic disease or prior urinary tract infection, but is not generally of use as a routine study without clinical indications.

Special Problems of the Elderly

The elderly represent the fastest-growing segment of the population. Individuals over the age of 65 years constitute a high proportion of healthcare expenditures and account for > 40% of all surgical procedures. Evidence indicates that this group is heterogeneous with respect to perioperative risk.[5] Age and a simple list of comorbidities (hypertension, diabetes, etc.) often fail to capture the nuances of loss of function and strength in this population, and cannot adequately predict morbidity and mortality.[6] Indeed, in patients > 80 years old, functional dependence was associated with a threefold increased risk of death.[7]

Accurate preoperative risk stratification is an essential element in the choice of the surgical procedure and determination of the appropriate location of postoperative care (intensive care or general ward).[8] Recent cohort studies have reported 3–4% mortality rates associated with surgery in the elderly in both European[9] and North American[10] patient populations. In the prospective European Surgical Outcomes Study, wide international variability in mortality was observed, suggesting that it may be possible to implement measures to improve surgical outcome. In particular, 73% of the elderly patients who died were not admitted to critical care, and unplanned critical care admissions were associated with higher mortality than when planned. Identifying the subgroup of patients at high risk of mortality preoperatively may allow more focused attention with management, critical care resources, and evidence-based interventions. Retrospective studies from the United Kingdom suggest that approximately 12% of patients are in a high-risk group, and these patients account for 80% of perioperative deaths.[11]

Postoperative morbidity is more common than mortality (16–18% in recent case series) and presents important healthcare and social burdens.[12] Postoperative complications not only increase short-term costs by prolonging length of stay (LOS) in hospital but also have long-term implications for mortality. Furthermore, they may lead to repeated hospital admissions and chronic ill health. The avoidance of postoperative complications is consequently of great importance. Postoperative complications arise more commonly from medical issues rather than direct technical or surgical site complications, and their

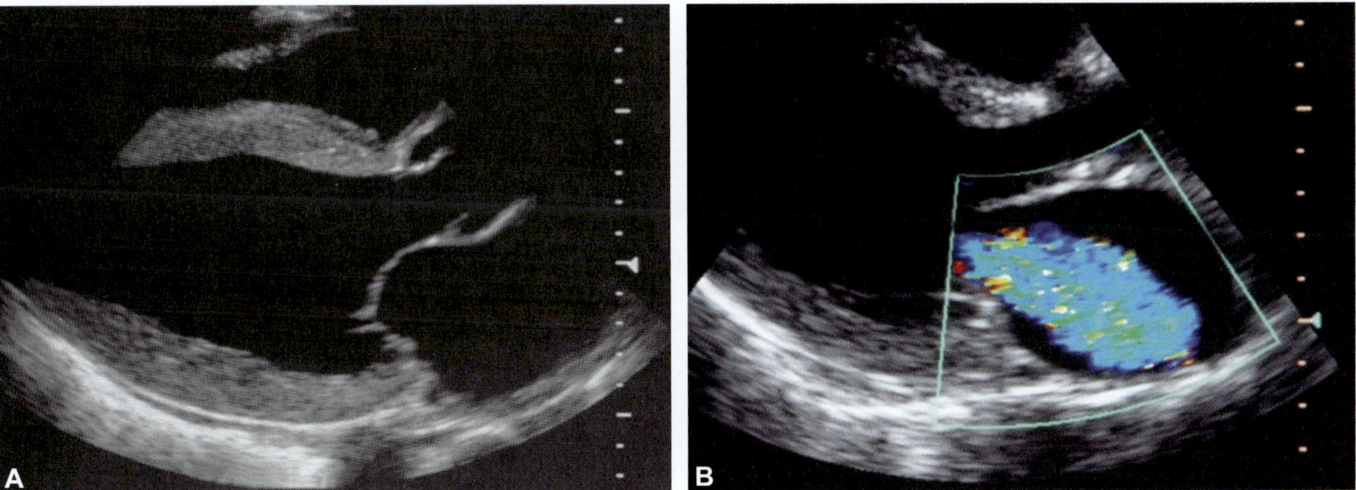

Figs. 2.1A and B: Normal and abnormal two-dimensional echocardiograms. (A) Systolic frame showing a normal study. (B) Color Doppler enhanced systolic frame showing mitral regurgitation.

increased rate is associated with advanced physiological age, multiple morbidities, and geriatric syndromes, including frailty, sarcopenia, and delirium.

Specific organ system risks are of particular importance in the elderly. General cardiovascular assessment should be consistent with principles that are detailed in Chapters 18, ("Surgical Management in the Elderly") and 27 ("Cardiac Assessment and Support of the Surgical Patient"). Because the elderly are at increased risk for cardiac valvular disease, the presence of a murmur on physical examination should prompt an echocardiographic evaluation to assess valvular pathology and cardiac function (Figs. 2.1A and B). Since peripheral vascular disease and limited exercise capacity are more prevalent in the elderly, dipyridamole thallium scanning and dobutamine stress echocardiography can be useful tools in evaluating the high-risk elderly patient. The importance of correct risk stratification and appropriate preoperative evaluation is further emphasized by >50% mortality rate associated with a perioperative myocardial infarction.[12]

Important pulmonary changes occur with aging. The inability to carry out activities of daily living (ADL) independently is a predictor of postoperative pneumonia, as there is a >10% weight loss within the last 6 months. These two factors may assume greater relevance than smoking and chronic obstructive pulmonary disease (COPD). Smoking within 12 months of operation is also a risk factor for complications.

There can be an almost 40% decrease in the size of the liver in 80-year-old patients. In proportion to the decrease in liver size, there is a corresponding decrease in splanchnic blood flow. The reduction in mass is not associated with hepatic insufficiency in the absence of intrinsic liver disease (e.g. cirrhosis).

There is a high rate of pre-existing renal dysfunction in elderly patients. There is loss of both renal mass and glomeruli, with almost half the glomeruli present in a young patient gone or nonfunctional by the time the patient reaches his ninth decade. There is also a significant decrease of renal blood flow caused by loss in renal mass and changes in the renal vasculature. Although there is a significant decrease in creatinine clearance with aging, there is usually not a corresponding increase in serum creatinine because of skeletal muscle atrophy. As the patient ages, there is decreased urine concentrating ability, impaired absorption of glucose, and decreased responsiveness to antidiuretic hormone.

Frailty is the multidimensional state of weakness and decreased physiologic reserve. Frailty is especially important in the perioperative period because of high levels of physiologic stress and inflammation. Recently, two types of frailty have been described: the "frailty phenotype" of Fried and colleagues[13] and the "frailty index" of Mitnitski and coworkers.[14] The frailty phenotype views frailty as a complex biological syndrome, characterized by decreased levels of physical ability, endurance, strength, and speed, accompanied by sarcopenia and/or weight loss. The Survey of Health Aging and Retirement in Europe (SHARE) has adapted the frailty phenotype for clinical use. The SHARE frailty instrument employs a patient survey and one performance-based measure (handgrip strength) to assess the domains outlined by Fried et al.

In contrast, the frailty index represents a multidimensional risk state measured by the quantity of "deficits" an individual has accumulated. It incorporates 30–70 dichotomized deficits including comorbidities, ADL, and physical and neurological deficits. Since the frailty index is a continuous measure, it is capable of reflecting dynamic changes. Although this scale can be cumbersome, it is readily converted for clinical use to be part of an electronic medical record.

Walking speeds significantly predict postoperative morbidity and mortality.[15] Moreover, a history of one or more falls in the 6 months prior to operation is strongly associated with operative complications. Of note, these approaches to detect frailty require minimal training and can often be performed and recorded in < 1 minute.

Robinson and associates[16] assessed frailty using six clinical markers: Mini-Cog score of three or less, an albumin level of ≤ 3.3 g/dL, more than one fall in the last 6 months, a hematocrit level of < 35%, dependence for at least one ADL, and the presence of at least three comorbidities. The presence of at least four of these markers predicts 6-month mortality with a sensitivity of 81% and specificity of 86%.

"Prehabilitation" is the process of enhancing functional capacity preoperatively to improve a patient's ability to withstand physiologic stress. Indeed, prehabilitation was effective in improving functional recovery in older orthopedic patients. Many of these studies used a single intervention such as strength training to improve or correct frailty. In a recent study of patients having colorectal surgery, 80% of the older patients who were enrolled in a trimodal prehabilitation program, including protein supplementation, anxiety reduction, and an exercise program, returned to baseline function at 8 weeks compared to only 40% in the preintervention control group. Details of prehabilitation, depression, and delirium in the elderly are addressed in Chapter 18. Dementia increases in prevalence with age, and its clinical significance ranges from subtle cognitive deficits to complete functional dependence. However, cognitive impairment is not "normal" and does not occur universally. Many older patients are cognitively intact, whereas others may present normally but have subclinical dementia that nevertheless requires vigilance for postoperative complications and increased support with the postoperative transition.[1]

Obesity

Obesity has been defined as a body mass index (BMI) >30 kg/m^2, and morbid obesity has been referred to as a BMI > 40 kg/m^2, or a BMI > 35 kg/m^2 with an obesity-related comorbidity. With these definitions, about 34% of adults in the United States are obese. Anatomically, obesity is defined by the presence of excess stored fat. Physiologically, adipocytes are metabolically very dynamic cells and obesity is a multisystem proinflammatory disorder.[17]

The pathophysiological issues that must be considered in the obese surgical patient are many. The metabolic syndrome typically includes obesity, hyper- or dyslipidemia, an insulin-resistant state, and hypertension. Clinical problems of glucose control can be anticipated in these patients even if clinical diabetes has not been diagnosed in the preoperative period. The metabolic syndrome translates into increased risks of atherosclerotic cardiovascular disease, congestive heart failure, and potential complications from peripheral vascular occlusive disease. Obesity has an impact upon diaphragmatic and chest wall mechanics and leads to the obstructive sleep apnea syndrome.

Despite a large lipid store, major operations will unmask underlying nutritional deficiencies in the obese patient. Iron deficiency occurs in 6–29% of these patients, with 3–18% also having vitamin B12 deficiency.[18] There is also a significant risk of deficiencies of folate, zinc, selenium, magnesium, and thiamine. Deficits of vitamins A, D, and K are also possible, but vitamin K deficiency is not usually severe enough to cause abnormalities in coagulation testing.

Cognitive Assessment

Baseline alteration in cognitive function, both acute and chronic, places the patient at increased risk for postoperative delirium and resulting complications. Baseline cognitive impairment has been associated with a 2 to 17-fold increased risk of postoperative delirium.[18] Screening tools for dementia and delirium may be utilized to identify patients at risk and allow the surgery team to optimize the timing of surgery as well as provide adequate support during the perioperative period.[1]

Cardiac Risk

In the United States, as many as 15.4 million Americans aged ≥20 years suffer from coronary artery disease. In 2009, about one in every six deaths in the United States was caused by coronary artery disease.[19] Major clinical factors associated with perioperative cardiac events are unstable coronary syndromes, decompensated heart failure (Fig. 2.2), important dysrhythmias, and severe valvular heart disease. Obviously high-risk aortic or peripheral

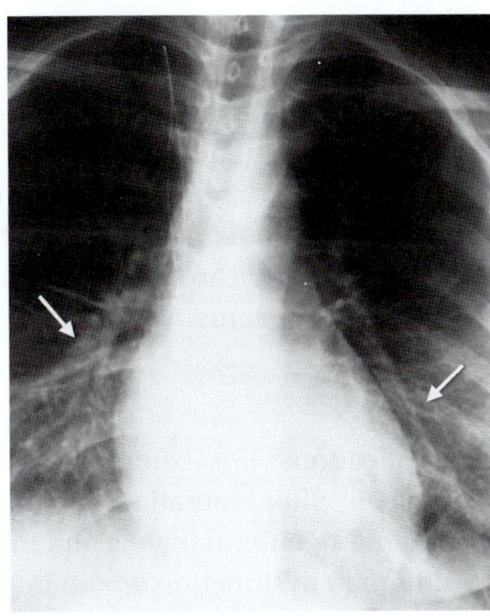

Fig. 2.2: Congestive heart failure in a preoperative patient. There are increased bronchovascular markings bilaterally running down from both the hila (seen better on the right) (arrows). One can sometimes also find thin white peripheral horizontal densities called Kerley's B lines on the chest X-ray. These are usually seen best in the costophrenic sulci and are thought to represent edematous interlobular septa.

vascular procedures are associated with high risk for these complications. Perioperative use of antiplatelet agents in patients with coronary stents involves a multidisciplinary approach that depends on the type of stent, how long it has been present, and the type of surgical procedure. Preoperative initiation of β-blocker therapy in high- and intermediate-risk patients reduces the incidence of perioperative cardiac events, but it should be started weeks before the operation.

It is estimated that cardiovascular complications cause at least half of all the morbidity and mortality experienced in the perioperative period for patients undergoing noncardiac surgery, with even higher rates among vascular patients having major vascular surgery. Every year, approximately 27 million patients undergo a noncardiac operation in the United States; of these, about 8 million (30%) have major underlying coronary artery disease or other cardiac problems. Of people undergoing noncardiac surgery, 1 million, or 3%, will experience perioperative cardiac complications. The mortality rate after perioperative myocardial infarction is as high as 40–50%.

The goal of the preoperative evaluation is to screen broadly for undiagnosed disease and to find evidence of known conditions that are poorly controlled. The preoperative evaluation also helps determine if additional work up is necessary. The risk of cardiac events has been divided into low-, intermediate-, or high-risk groups, with cardiac event rates being <1%, 1–5%, or >5%, respectively.[20] The recently published guidelines by the American College of Cardiology and American Heart Association should be followed in the evaluation of these patients.[21] Chapter 27 provides a detailed presentation for the evaluation of patients for cardiac risk. The importance of the evaluation is to fully utilize noninvasive and clinically practical methods, and reserve invasive testing and imaging only for those patients with unstable cardiac disease where clinical interventions may be necessary to enhance the patient's risk. Common symptoms encountered in patients requiring further evaluation of ischemic heart disease are angina, dyspnea, cough, edema, palpitations, and syncopal episodes. Patients with advanced, chronic ischemic heart disease often present with unstable coronary syndromes, prior myocardial infarction, arrhythmias, history of decompensated heart failure, or presence of pacemaker or implantable defibrillators. The ECG remains a common method of the evaluation of ischemic heart disease (Table 2.2).

Table 2.2 Relative risk of a surgical procedure for patients who have cirrhosis.

	Class A	*Class B*	*Class C*
Serum albumin g/dL (g/L)	>3.5	3.0–3.5	<3.0
	>35	30–35	<30
Bilirubin mg/dL (μmol/L)	<2.0	2.0–3.0	>3.0
	<34.2	34.2–51.3	>51.3
Ascites	None	Easily controlled	Poorly controlled
Encephalopathy	None	Mild	Advanced
Nutritional status	Excellent	Good	Poor
Prothrombin time (seconds above control)	<3.0	3.0–5.0	>5.0
Operative mortality for porto-systemic shunt operation (%)	2	10	50

This shows classification of cirrhosis patients into three classes (A, B, and C) and the relative risk of portosystemic shunt for each class.

Current medications must be completely and accurately recorded. Medications that are particularly important include: β-blockers, antiplatelet agents, renin–angiotensin–aldosterone antagonists, lipid-lowering agents, nitrates, and α2-agonists. Their interaction with other medications (including anesthetic agents) and side effects must be taken into consideration in formulating plans for perioperative management.

Some items of perioperative care that are particularly important in these patients undergoing noncardiac surgery include (1) continuation of β-blockers in patients with titration of medication as needed to achieve a resting heart rate of 60–65 bpm, (2) continuation of statins in patients already taking a statin, and (3) management of postoperative arrhythmia, including rate control (β-blocker, calcium channel blocker, or digoxin) and treatment of any underlying causes.

Hypertension Risks

In the United States, it is estimated that about 30% of the US population over 25 years of age have hypertension. Although guidelines exist for the treatment of hypertension, there are few accepted guidelines for the perioperative evaluation and care of these patients. Of particular importance is defining the patients most vulnerable to complications and the indications for immediate and rapid antihypertensive treatment. Scheduled elective operations may need to be deferred until the hypertension is brought under control.[22]

The association between hypertension and adverse surgical outcomes remains unclear. Recent studies have failed to establish a link between perioperative complications with either pre-existing hypertension or an elevated arterial pressure of <180/110 mm Hg during surgery. In fact, even at these higher pressures, there is not good evidence to support a causal relationship between the hypertension and surgical risk. As a result, the level of evidence to support delaying surgery to allow treatment of a poorly controlled arterial pressure is poor.[23] Furthermore, attempts at blood pressure control perioperatively may cause an increased risk of hypotension, ischemic organ damage, and adverse drug reactions.[24] Guidelines have identified that mild-to-moderate hypertension <180 mm Hg systolic or <110 mm Hg diastolic is not an independent risk factor for perioperative cardiovascular complications.[25]

Cerebrovascular Risk

Any history of a cerebrovascular problem is generally an indicator for study prior to moderate major surgery, especially if there is any reasonable chance of developing hypotension. The significance of any otherwise incidentally found carotid bruit is unclear. The presence of a carotid bruit is a poor predictor of carotid stenosis, although it can indicate the presence of generalized cerebrovascular and atherosclerotic disease. The Framingham Heart Study showed that carotid bruits are associated with a double risk of stroke, but that most of these strokes occurred in vascular territories other than the bruit.[26]

Patients with symptomatic carotid stenosis or a prior stroke or transient ischemic attack are at elevated risk of a perioperative cerebrovascular event. Ultrasonography of the cervical vessels should be performed preoperatively if a bruit is present, and in patients about to undergo major arterial surgery. There is no evidence of a correlation between asymptomatic carotid murmurs and perioperative cerebrovascular events.

Pulmonary Risk

Pulmonary complications are common after surgical operations, especially after operations on the chest or upper abdomen, among older patients, and in those with pre-existing pulmonary dysfunction. Preoperative evaluation of the lungs includes chest X-rays and arterial blood gas analysis. Pulmonary function tests before and after a bronchodilator can be important in patients who will have lung resections. In patients who may require a pulmonary resection, split-lung function studies may also be required. Factors that can contribute to postoperative pulmonary insufficiency include pain from thoracic or abdominal incisions and the depressive effects of anesthetic gases and pain medications. General anesthesia may predispose the patient to aspiration of oropharyngeal and/or gastric contents. The anesthetic agents may also decrease the efficacy of mucociliary clearance mechanisms.

Routine preoperative chest radiography in asymptomatic, otherwise healthy patients is not indicated. If the patient has new or unstable cardiopulmonary signs or symptoms, chest radiography is clearly needed. Although abnormal findings on preoperative screening radiography are fairly common, these findings are usually chronic and predictable from the history and physical examination; furthermore, they only rarely alter perioperative management.

The sensitivity of anteroposterior chest X-rays for cardiopulmonary disease is low. They should only be obtained if there is clinical suspicion of a condition that could affect decision-making in the perioperative period, e.g. pneumonia, pleural effusion, or a relevant anatomical abnormality. The most frequent pre-existing lung diseases seen in patients having operations are COPD (e.g. emphysema and chronic bronchitis), asthma, acute bronchitis, and pneumonia.

Patients who have chronic emphysema ("blue bloaters") have an increased residual volume and inefficient pulmonary gas exchange. They tend to retain carbon dioxide and develop hypoxia because of inefficient ventilation and increased dead space. Patients who have chronic bronchitis ("pink puffers") tend to have copious bronchial secretions, but often have relatively normal blood gases. Postoperatively, these patients have an increased tendency to atelectasis and pneumonia.

Patients who smoke over ten cigarettes per day preoperatively have an increased incidence of cardiovascular and pulmonary perioperative complications. Cessation of smoking 12–18 hours preoperatively lowers carboxyhemoglobin concentrations and may decrease heart rate, arterial blood pressure, and catecholamine concentrations. However, stopping smoking may not markedly reduce perioperative pulmonary complications unless the smoking is discontinued at least 2–4 weeks before operation.

Impaired consciousness also increases the risk of postoperative pulmonary complications. No matter how good the ventilatory support, it is seldom as good as spontaneous deep breaths and coughs. In addition, although comatose patients can be turned from side-to-side, this is not nearly as effective for improving pulmonary toilet and function as spontaneous sitting, standing, and walking.

Current evidence does not support routine preoperative evaluation of pulmonary function; however, strategies to prevent pulmonary complications include identifying patients at risk and optimizing perioperative care directed at specific risk factors. These include smoking cessation, preoperative inspiratory muscle training, and evaluation for undiagnosed and/or untreated obstructive sleep apnea.

Some physicians encourage patients to practice perioperative lung expansion techniques, such as incentive spirometry, intermittent positive-pressure breathing, continuous positive-pressure airway pressure, and chest physiotherapy. Other considerations include efforts to optimize anesthetic and postoperative pain management. Avoidance of long-acting neuromuscular blockade and use of regional anesthetic techniques can be helpful. Surgical options, such as the use of minimally invasive techniques and surgical incision size and placement should also be considered that minimize their negative influences on pulmonary mechanics.

Abnormal findings on pulmonary function tests can help predict an increased incidence of pulmonary complications after surgical procedures that do not involve the lungs. Patients scheduled for extrathoracic surgery should undergo pulmonary function testing only if they have a known or suspected pulmonary disease that has not been studied adequately.

Hepatic Risk

A thorough history and physical examination is usually sufficient to detect an underlying hepatic problem. If there are no symptoms or signs of hepatic dysfunction, no special testing is required preoperatively in most elective operations. Risk factors that may be detected by history include previous transfusions, excessive alcohol intake, multiple sexual partners, a family or personal history of jaundice, anemia, or hereditary liver disease. Additionally, any physical signs of muscle wasting, jaundice, spider nevi, palmar erythema, ascites, or hepatosplenomegaly should make one suspect underlying hepatic disease (Table 2.2).

Scoring systems that correlate with operative morbidity and mortality include the modified Child-Turcotte-Pugh and the model for end-stage liver disease.[27] Other risk factors include male gender, age >70 years, upper gastrointestinal bleeding ascites, intraoperative hypotension, COPD, elevated creatinine, preoperative infection, and cirrhosis. High-risk surgeries for patients with hepatic disease include abdominal surgery, open cholecystectomy, cardiothoracic surgery, trauma laparotomy, esophageal surgery, and emergency surgery.[28]

A newer liver test that can be performed noninvasively for hepatic fibrosis (Fibroscan) can show early disease.[29] If the scans are indeterminate, a liver biopsy should be done. The highest-risk group with liver dysfunction will show an increased international normalized ratio, low platelets, splenomegaly, and an irregular liver. This high-risk group should also have a Fibroscan. If cirrhosis is seen, these patients should be screened for esophageal varices and hepatocellular carcinoma.

Renal Risk

The perioperative evaluation of acute or chronic kidney disease is difficult due to multiple indices used to address it. There is an age-related susceptibility to dehydration and electrolyte disturbances due to restricted access to fluid and polypharmacy (diuretics and other drugs). There are several preoperative acute kidney injury (AKI) risk factors for noncardiovascular operations, including age (>59 years), BMI >32, emergency surgery, high-risk surgery, peripheral vascular disease, COPD, and liver disease. These were categorized from class I–IV that correspond to 0–≥3 risk factors, respectively, and confer an AKI frequency of 0.3–4.3%.[30] Preoperative function of the kidneys and other factors mentioned are critical in assessing the risk of developing postoperative AKI. In noncardiac patients with normal renal function, AKI is generally <1%. During surgery, one must protect the kidney by sufficient renal perfusion via adequate intravascular volume and arterial pressure. The ability to maintain and optimizing intravascular volume and cardiac output is by preventing hypotension and lactic acidosis. Optimization of cardiac output and oxygen delivery in high-risk surgery decreased perioperative AKI.

Postoperatively, it is extremely important to maintain adequate renal perfusion. If administration of fluid and blood is not adequate to maintain a mean blood pressure of at least 65 mm Hg, inotropes and/or vasopressors can be used. Urinary obstruction and/or sepsis should be treated promptly.

Although several biomarkers for early detection of AKI show promise, serum creatinine is the gold standard. Neutrophil gelatinase-associated lipocalin is a urine and plasma protein found to be elevated as much as 48 hours prior to a rise in creatinine.[31] This marker was the most specific (81%) and sensitive (68%) for AKI and all had an excellent negative predictive value (>95%).

Coagulation Risk

Details of the medical history that are especially important for detecting bleeding or clotting problems include previous problems with operations or trauma, family history of bleeding disorders, and a drug history, including antiplatelet agents and anticoagulants. In patients with a negative history, it is not necessary to perform a routine coagulation screen.

In general, coagulation tests [prothrombin time (PT), activated partial thromboplastin time (aPTT), and platelet count] are performed preoperatively in patients with medical conditions associated with impaired hemostasis (e.g. liver disease, diseases of hematopoiesis), patients taking anticoagulants, and those whose history and examination suggest an underlying coagulation disorder (e.g. history of spontaneous bruising or excessive surgical bleeding, family history of a known heritable coagulopathy). Besides clot formation, clot stability is important, and is governed by factor XIII and the activity of the fibrinolytic system. Point of care tests, such as viscoelastic tests of coagulation with thromboelastography and rotational thromboelastometry, can analyze whole blood to give a complete assessment of hemostasis from clot formation to fibrinolysis.[32]

Platelet count is part of the routine full blood count, with a normal range of 150–400 × 10^9 per liter; however, patients with a normal platelet count can have functional disorders of adhesion, activation, or action, either as a result of disease or antiplatelet drugs. Increasingly, patients with drug-eluting coronary stents are presenting for operation and are required to continue their antiplatelet drugs to avoid the risk of stent thrombosis. There is also marked individual variability in response to antiplatelet drugs, with 30% of patients having little or no platelet inhibition from clopidogrel, and the time for offset of effects is not always predictable. Platelet function can be assessed by a variety of tests, including light transmission aggregometry, flow cytometry, and impedance aggregometry.

It is recommended that patients at high risk for thromboembolic events receive bridging anticoagulation while warfarin is held. For patients with coronary stents, guidelines recommend the following: bare-metal coronary stents, one should delay elective operations for 30–45 days, and continue aspirin perioperatively. For drug-eluting stent, one should delay elective surgery for a year and continue aspirin perioperatively.[2] For patients with known hemostatic derangements, including anticoagulant drug therapies, consultation with a hematologist is generally recommended.

PERIOPERATIVE CARE

The overall principles in the management of the surgical patient in the perioperative period should include maintenance of adequate intravascular volume, medication adjustment in anticipation of hypotension or other untoward consequences, judicious continuation of β-blockers and other cardiac drugs, optimum pain control, and prevention of polypharmacy and excessive testing. Specific issues of perioperative care are highlighted below. Specific chapter references are supplied elsewhere in this volume to provide the reader with more details.

Because the issues of perioperative management have become so extensive, a variety of management strategies and protocolized care pathways have been developed during the last several decades in an effort to reduce the time required to recover from surgery. The "enhanced recovery" concept is based on the belief that traditional perioperative management practices, such as fasting in the preoperative period, liberal fluid administration in the intraoperative period, and the use of nasogastric tubes and opioid pain-management strategies in the postoperative period, deserve re-evaluation and modification in light of the best available evidence-based medicine. More than 10 case-control studies including >3000 subjects have demonstrated that an average 2–3 days reduction in LOS can be achieved with the use of an enhanced recovery program in a variety of surgical patient populations.[33] The enhanced recovery protocol has also been able to reduce the amount of opioids administered perioperatively by nearly 80%; LOS was also reduced by 2–3 days from 6.8 ± 4.7 to 4.6 ± 3.6 days ($p = 0.0002$). Despite leaving 2.2 days earlier, 30-day readmissions of patients on enhanced recovery protocols have not increased. While these protocols have been useful in providing direction and structure to perioperative management, individualization of management for the specific issues in a patient's care still requires in-depth knowledge in the management of patients after operation.

Blood Volume

Anesthetic agents are associated with vasodilation that may lead to reductions in cardiac output and clinical hypotension. The consequences of these hypotensive events may be severe if not attended to promptly, and may have grave consequences of infarction or organ failure if the patient has major coronary, cerebral, or renal artery disease.

A history of fluid loss (e.g. vomiting or diarrhea) before operation, symptoms of gastrointestinal ileus, or prolonged status without oral intake before elective procedures may create hypovolemia. Prolonged vasoconstriction (e.g. hypertensive patients) or patients on preoperative diuretics often have a contracted blood volume. A normal hemoglobin value does not necessarily indicate a normal blood volume, especially in elderly patients or those with recent blood loss when laboratory values are obtained prior to adequate equilibration time.

Volume replacement should be continued until vital signs are normal and urine output is at least 0.5 mL/kg/h. Balanced salt solutions (Ringer's lactate) should be used for the replacement of extracellular water deficits. In many patients, it will be desirable to monitor the central venous pressure to assist in volume replacement (*see* Chapter 14).

Anemia

Anemia [hemoglobin >10 g/dL (100 g/L)] has generally been viewed as increasing operative risk. It is now generally accepted that patients who are otherwise healthy and with minimal expectation of additional blood loss can tolerate a hemoglobin concentration to a level of 7 g/dL (70 g/L; hematocrit 20–22%).[34] For patients who have cardiac or pulmonary problems, a hemoglobin of 10 g/dL (100 g/L) is probably adequate. Because of rheological changes, patients who have platelet dysfunction due to uremia tend to have less bleeding if the hematocrit is ≥30%.[35]

For an elective operation in an anemic patient, it is prudent to delay the operation for evaluation and management of any underlying problem so as to avoid transfusion. Because correction of "correctable" anemias (due to iron, folate, or vitamin B_{12} deficiency or transient bone marrow depression) can take several days or weeks, blood transfusion may be the only option for urgent procedures.

"Uncorrectable" anemias (e.g. due to myelodysplasia, chronic disease, uremia, and thalassemia) often require blood transfusions. In such situations, any additional interventions that may be indicated for renal failure, gastrointestinal bleeding, or alcoholism must be planned. All perioperative blood management should comply with the ASA guidelines.[36]

Leukocyte Abnormalities

The clinical importance of leukopenia depends upon the cell type, the severity of the cell count, and understanding the underlying disorder. The major consequence in surgical patients is the impairment of the cellular response of the innate immune response and the attendant susceptibility to bacterial infection.

If severe leukopenia is due to bone marrow suppression by antineoplastic agents or radiation, recovery usually begins about 14–21 days after exposure. If it is due to idiosyncratic reactions or other diseases, recovery may take weeks or months, or there may be no improvement. Elective procedures should be deferred until the granulocyte count has increased to above 1000/mm^3.

If recovery from leukopenia is not expected or an operation is urgently needed, there is an increased risk of infection. Antibiotic therapy is not indicated for leukopenia alone, but broad-spectrum coverage should be instituted at the first sign of infection. Granulocyte–monocyte stimulating factor has become available for stimulating the production of white blood cells and may be used for severe leukopenia.[37]

Leukocytosis is often an indicator of an underlying inflammatory, infectious, or a neoplastic process, but neutrophilia may be due to corticosteroid use.[38] Only in rare circumstances, when the leukocyte count is >100,000/mm^3 in leukemia, will symptoms occur directly due to leukostasis in cerebral or pulmonary vessels. If an operation is urgently needed, the best results are obtained by using immediate chemotherapy along with leukocytopheresis to reduce the white blood cell count to <50,000/mm^3.[39]

Hemostasis Abnormalities

Hemostasis and management of coagulation disorders are discussed in detail in Chapter 6, "Hemorrhage, Hemostasis, and Transfusion". The hemostatic system should be evaluated by an appropriate clinical examination and laboratory tests before any operation in which marked blood loss is anticipated or if a bleeding diathesis is suspected. The history should include questions about easy bruising, bleeding, or petechiae that occur spontaneously or have followed previous operations, trauma, pregnancy, or menstrual cycles. On physical examination, check carefully for ecchymosis or petechiae.

If there is any suspicion of a bleeding diathesis, the standard preoperative screening tests include the platelet count, aPTT, and PT. Suspected problems of platelet function (e.g. uremia or use of antiplatelet drugs) require documentation of the bleeding time. If the bleeding time is prolonged, a platelet count is necessary. Renal function should be assessed. More sophisticated studies of platelet function may be necessary for prolonged bleeding times that cannot be explained.

If the PT is prolonged, check for use of vitamin K antagonists (e.g. warfarin) or any other substances interfering with the production or function of coagulation factors. Malnutrition or diseases involving the liver, biliary tract, or small bowel may interfere with absorption and use of vitamin K. If none of these problems is present and if the aPTT is also normal, more sophisticated clotting studies, including a factor VII assay, are indicated.

If the aPTT is prolonged, ensure that the patient is not on heparin or that blood was drawn from an indwelling vascular catheter. Because only 25–30% of most coagulant factors are needed for a normal aPTT, addition of an equal amount of normal plasma should result in a normal aPTT if the problem is a deficiency of coagulation factors. If poor clotting persists, then an inhibitor is probably present. If the aPTT is greatly prolonged but the PT is normal, there may be a factor XII deficiency, which does not usually increase the risk of bleeding intraoperatively. In vitamin K deficiencies or mild liver disorders, the PT is usually prolonged but aPTT may be normal. In severe liver disease, the PT and aPTT both usually are prolonged and are commonly unresponsive to vitamin K therapy, but the thrombin time, platelet count, and bleeding time may be normal. In disseminated intravascular coagulation, all coagulation studies are abnormal, and fibrin split products and D-dimer concentrations are also increased.

Coagulopathy

Fresh frozen plasma (FFP) contains all of the clotting factors. If a patient has severe factor deficiencies, at least 4–6 units of FFP (250 mL each) given rapidly will be needed to begin restoration of aPTT and PT. With continuing consumption of clotting factors, at least 8–12 units of FFP may be needed to restore clotting factor concentrations to normal; however, if there is concomitant coagulation factor consumption, even greater amounts of FFP are required. Specific coagulation factors should be given to manage those coagulation disorders that are refractory to FFP (*see* Chapter 6, "Hemorrhage, Hemostasis, and Transfusion").

If reversal of heparin (half-life of 90 minutes) is not urgent, discontinuation of heparin 3 hours before an operation results in the presence of only about 25% of the original anticoagulant effect. If complete reversal is necessary (e.g. neurologic or ophthalmic operations), it should be discontinued 6 hours preoperatively.

The specific antidote to heparin is protamine sulfate, which must be infused slowly intravenously to prevent cardiac depression and hypotension. In a heparinized patient who needs an immediate operation, 10 mg of protamine sulfate dissolved in 50 mL of normal saline is infused intravenously over 10 minutes, followed by 20 mg of protamine dissolved in 50 mL of normal saline infused intravenously over 30 minutes.

The specific antidote for warfarin anticoagulation is phytomenadione (vitamin K_1): 5–10 mg of phytomenadione in 50–100 mL of 5% dextrose in water or 0.9% saline is infused over 30–60 minutes, or 2.5–5 mg is injected subcutaneously. If phytomenadione is infused too rapidly, it may cause allergic reactions or even anaphylaxis. If hepatic function is normal, the PT is usually corrected within 18–24 hours. With life-threatening bleeding from warfarin, the recommended treatment is at least 4–6 units of FFP. If an elective operation is to be undertaken for a patient taking warfarin, the management of the anticoagulation depends upon the relative risks of bleeding versus the risks of thrombosis or thromboembolism.

Thromboprophylaxis

Primary risk factors for the development of deep venous thrombosis (DVT) and pulmonary embolus (PE) include advanced age, prolonged operation, operation involving the abdomen, pelvis, or lower extremities; and previous DVT or PE. Secondary risk factors include prolonged

Table 2.3 Classification of the risk of postoperative deep vein thrombosis (DVT) and pulmonary embolism (PE) in patients undergoing operations.

Risk category	*Calf DVT (%)*	*Proximal DVT (%)*	*PE (%)*
High risk	**40–80**	**10–20**	**1–5**
Age >40 years			
Duration of operation >30 minutes			
Orthopedic operation			
Pelvic or abdominal cancer operation			
Previous DVT or PE			
Secondary risk factors (obesity, immobilization, malignancy, varicose veins, estrogen use paralysis)			
Hereditary or acquired coagulopathies (protein C and protein S deficiencies, antithrombin III deficiency, anticardiolipin antibodies)			
Moderate risk	**10–40**	**2–10**	**0.1–0.7**
Age >40 years			
Duration of operation >30 minutes			
Secondary risk factors (obesity, immobilization, malignancy, varicose veins, estrogen use, paralysis)			
Low risk	**<10**	**<1**	**<0.01**
Age <40 years			
Surgery minor, <30 minutes duration			
No secondary risk factors			

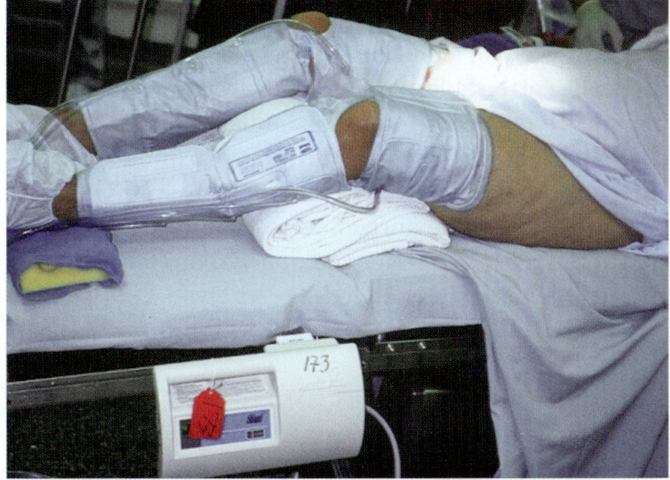

Fig. 2.3: Sequential compression stockings. Operating room photograph showing the use of sequential compression stockings in a patient. They are best applied before the procedure and then kept on until the patient is fully ambulatory postoperatively.

immobilization, paralysis, malignancy, obesity, varicose veins, and estrogen use. Using these and other factors, patients can be classified as having a low, moderate, or high risk for developing DVT. Risk factors for DVT are identified in Table 2.3. Methods for the prevention of DVT and PE include perioperative heparin, sequential compression stockings (Fig. 2.3), and in selected cases full anticoagulation with warfarin. These methods are discussed in detail in Chapter 6, "Hemorrhage, Hemostasis, and Transfusion".

Prevention of Infection

Prevention and management of infection in the surgical patient is discussed in Chapter 7, "Infection, Inflammation, and Antibiotics". Factors increasing the risk of postoperative infections include preoperative infections, severe malnutrition, uncontrolled diabetes mellitus, obesity, poor circulation, marked intraoperative contamination, prolonged operation, periods of hypotension, multiple blood transfusions, and many others.

Antimicrobial prophylaxis is generally recommended for operations that have high infection rates (e.g. colon surgery), that employ prosthetic material (e.g. total joint replacement), and have severe consequences of infection (e.g. median sternotomy). Antimicrobial prophylaxis protects the patient against infection at the surgical site, but is not of benefit in the prevention of hospital-acquired infections at other sites in the body.

An effective prophylactic regimen should be directed against the most-likely infecting organisms. For clean cultures where gram-positive organisms are likely pathogens, cefazolin has a long record of effectiveness. In institutions where methicillin-resistant *Staphylococci* are important postoperative pathogens, vancomycin can be used. For colorectal operations and appendectomy, any agent or combination that is effective against both *Escherichia coli* (and other gram-negative aerobes) and enteric anaerobes (especially *Bacteroides fragilis)* can be used. A single dose of an appropriate antibiotic given 30 minutes before the skin incision provides adequate tissue concentrations throughout the operation. If the operation lasts for >3–4 hours, if there is major blood loss or if the antimicrobial has a short half-life (such as cefoxitin), one or more additional doses are advisable during the procedure. One or two doses can also be given postoperatively.

Optimization of Organ Reserve

Cardiac Function

The overall goals of the perioperative assessment and care of the cardiovascular system in high-risk patients include optimizing cardiac output and oxygen delivery, decreasing myocardial oxygen requirements by normalization of the systolic blood pressure and heart rate, maintaining coronary blood flow by keeping the aortic diastolic pressure at normal or slightly higher levels and keeping the heart rate as slow as possible, and reducing the risk of arrhythmias.

Evidence of coronary artery disease requires a preoperative ECG (Fig. 2.4). A stress test or cardiac catheterization may be required, but only in patients with cardiac symptomatology (*see* Chapter 27, "Cardiac Assessment and Support of the Surgical Patient"). Cardiac catheterization with coronary arteriography is indicated to delineate accurately the extent of any heart disease and the site and severity of any coronary artery lesions. In the postoperative patient, clinical indicators of unstable ischemic heart disease, elevated cardiac enzymes, or ECG changes require further evaluation.

Patients who have evidence of heart failure must be carefully evaluated to determine the optimal preload, need for afterload reduction, and need for inotropic agents. Volume overload is a constant hazard in patients who have chronic heart failure (Fig. 2.5). In addition, patients who have chronic cardiac failure have usually been treated with a low-salt diet and diuretics and may have decreased blood volume and serum sodium, potassium, and magnesium levels. These electrolyte abnormalities may be manifested clinically by weakness, lethargy, hypotension, and arrhythmias.

Hypertension is the leading cause of congestive heart failure. Because patients who have chronic severe hypertension may need higher blood pressures than normal, the blood pressure should be reduced gradually in the preoperative period to ensure perfusion of the heart, brain, kidneys, and other organs. Diuretic-associated reductions in extracellular water volume may be necessary in the preoperative hypertensive patient but care must be exercised to avoid over-diuresis and potential hypotension with the induction of anesthesia.

Nearly 5% of clinical hypertension is secondary to surgically correctable causes. Surgically correctable causes include renal artery stenosis, unilateral renal parenchymal disease, pheochromocytoma, Cushing's disease, aldosteronoma, hyperthyroidism, hyperparathyroidism, or coarctation of the aorta. Severe, new-onset hypertension is the reason to suspect that a workup for surgically correctable disease is needed.

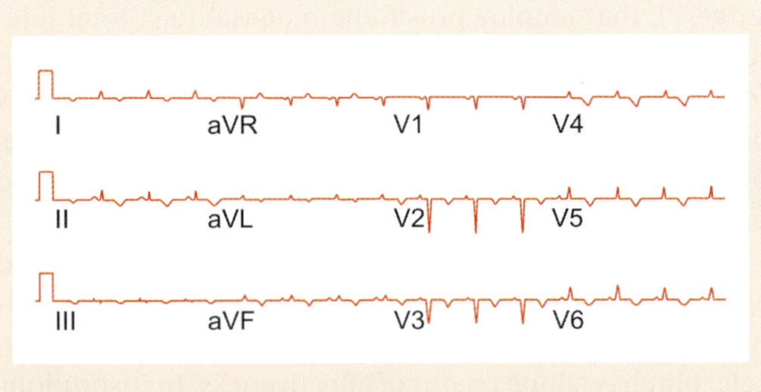

Fig. 2.4: Preoperative cardiac ischemia. This 12-lead preoperative ECG demonstrates anterior and inferolateral ischemic findings and a possible recent anterior infarction. Abnormal ECGs, such as this, help to determine the extent of cardiac evaluation that should be pursued in the preoperative patient. (The inverted T-waves in the V1–V6 are consistent with anterior ischemia, and inverted T-waves in II, III, and aVF are consistent with inferior ischemia. The lack of any R waves in V1–V3 is consistent with a possible recent anterior infarction).

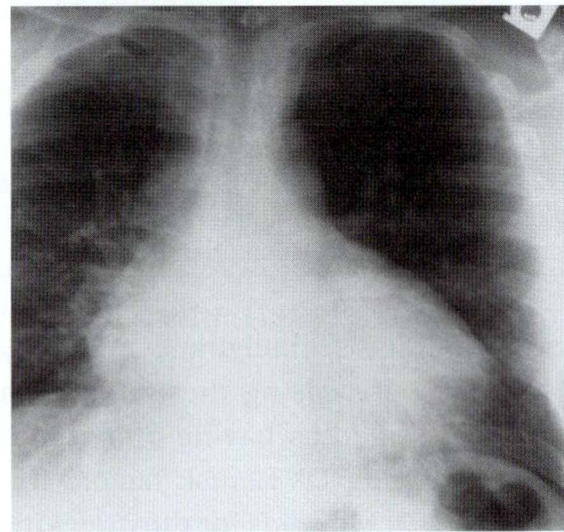

Fig. 2.5: Cardiomyopathy. This patient had a known cardiomyopathy from chemotherapy preoperatively. The cardiac shadow is considerably wider than normal, which is less than half the width of the chest at its widest point. Patients with cardiomyopathy with an enlarged heart on preoperative chest radiography have a major risk of developing congestive failure perioperatively.

Premature ventricular contractions and premature atrial contractions should be corrected preoperatively because they are associated with an increased risk of a perioperative cardiac death. Many anesthetic agents increase the tendency to arrhythmias by a direct effect on the conduction tissue or by enhancing the arrhythmogenic activity of epinephrine (adrenaline).

Atrial fibrillation can reduce ventricular filling by 20–50%, particularly if a rapid ventricular rate is observed.[22] Consequently, sinus rhythm should be restored as rapidly as possible. If this is not possible, the ventricular rate should at least be controlled preoperatively.

Heart block may be aggravated by vagal stimulation, digitalis, α-adrenoceptor antagonists, calcium antagonists, and anesthetic agents. Indeed, anesthesia may precipitate the development of complete heart block in patients who have underlying atrioventricular or intraventricular conduction disorders by altering intracellular and serum potassium concentrations. Even spinal anesthetics may not be safe in patients who have conduction disorders because absorption of local anesthetics can cause sinus bradycardia and induce heart blocks, especially in patients who have an underlying bundle branch disorder.

Temporary pacing should be considered if the patient has a block with a bradycardia that is unresponsive to atropine or if first-degree heart block is accompanied by a bundle branch block.[22] Temporary pacing is necessary for Mobitz type I (Wenckebach) block only if the patient is symptomatic. However, temporary (or permanent) pacing is necessary in Mobitz type II second-degree heart block and third-degree heart block.

Most permanent pacemakers are implanted prophylactically for complete atrioventricular blocks or sick sinus syndrome, but they are increasingly being implanted to control recurrent tachyarrhythmias. The risk of interference by electrocautery during operation is minimized by placing the diathermy plate away from the pacemaker and limiting the duration of electrocautery use.

Beta-blockers are useful for patients who have ischemic heart disease, hypertension, hypertrophic cardiomyopathies, and some types of arrhythmias. They are particularly helpful for protecting the heart from the ischemic effects of tachycardia and enhanced contractility. For many years, β-blockers were discontinued before elective operation. However, detailed intraoperative hemodynamic studies have shown that arterial pressure and cardiac output are well-maintained during anesthesia in patients receiving these drugs. The β-blockers also tend to blunt hypertensive responses to intubation and reduce the incidence of arrhythmias and myocardial ischemia. Withdrawal of the β-blockers before and following the operation for these patients is associated with increased cardiac mortality rates.[40] If patients have been on β-blockers before the operation, they should be continued on the drug through the perioperative period of time.[41] While β-blockade that is started within 24 hours of noncardiac surgery is associated with the prevention of nonfatal myocardial infarction, this immediate preoperative initiation of the drug is associated with increased deaths, stroke, and hypotensive events and cannot be recommended.[42]

Calcium channel blockers are used extensively in the management of supraventricular arrhythmias, angina, and arterial hypertension; however, these agents also potentially impair compensatory tachycardic, inotropic, and vasoconstrictor responses. For these reasons, there has been concern about the need to discontinue these drugs prior to major operations. Also, halogenated anesthetics tend to reduce calcium fluxes in cardiac cells and may potentiate the negative inotropic and chronotropic effects of calcium antagonists. A meta-analysis concludes that calcium channel blockers are beneficial and should be continued for elective operation, but careful monitoring is necessary to avoid potential complications such as postoperative bleeding.[43]

Angiotensin-converting enzyme inhibitors are used extensively to treat hypertension. The risk–benefit of continuing or withholding these drugs immediately before major operation continues to be debated. These drugs have been consistently associated with an increased incidence of intraoperative hypotension.[44] Recent studies have identified no risk of intraoperative or immediate postoperative hypertension when these medications were withheld preoperatively.[45]

Pulmonary Function

Chronic pulmonary problems are common comorbidities for major surgical patients. Pulmonary evaluation is important so that patients may have their pulmonary condition optimized before operation[46] and operations should be deferred if possible for those patients with any respiratory acidosis ($P\text{CO}_2 > 46$ mm Hg with a pH < 7.37), $P_a\text{O}_2 < 60$ mm Hg (8.4 kPa) or $P_{A\text{-}a}\text{O}_2 > 55$ mm Hg (7 kPa) on room air, purulent bronchial secretions, or spirometry values $< 50\%$ of expected. Determinations of pulmonary vascular resistance or the maximum oxygen consumption with exercise (which should be at least 10 ml/kg/min and preferably > 20 mL/kg/min) may help determine the extent of the postoperative pulmonary risk.

Aggressive preoperative intervention (including stopping smoking, bronchodilators and pulmonary toilet and antibiotics as needed for purulent bronchial secretions) reduces the incidence of postoperative complications. In patients with asthma, a short course of corticosteroids may be helpful. All patients should be encouraged to stop smoking. Although the cardiovascular effects of smoking may disappear within 24–48 hours, the associated airway inflammation may take several weeks to resolve.

Postoperatively, most studies have shown that analgesia provided by thoracic epidural analgesia is much preferable to that provided by parenteral narcotics.[47] A postoperative regimen that uses patient-controlled or local or regional analgesic techniques is preferable to physician-scheduled analgesic medication. Deep breathing and coughing help to decrease the incidence and severity of postoperative pneumonia, atelectasis, and respiratory failure, which contribute to greatly prolonged hospitalization and increased mortality rates. Incentive spirometry remains of uncertain value despite decades of use in postoperative patients.[48]

Stress Gastritis Prophylaxis

Stress gastritis has traditionally been one of the most important causes of postoperative gastrointestinal hemorrhage. Stress ulceration is commonly identified among critically ill patients, but the actual incidence of clinical bleeding has declined in recent years. Stress ulcerations are characteristically asymptomatic, multiple, superficial, and located in acid-producing areas of the stomach (fundus and body).

Stress gastric bleeding typically occurs 3–7 days after an operation in untreated patients. Traditional mortality rates of up to 80% have been reported when surgical intervention is required for managing the bleeding episode, which is why prevention strategies are so important. Risk factors for bleeding from stress ulceration include central nervous system (CNS) injury (Cushing's ulcers), extensive burns (Curling's ulcers), hypotension, uremia, sepsis, coagulopathy, and respiratory failure.

The cornerstone of prophylaxis is neutralization of the gastric luminal pH that may be achieved with intragastric infusion antacids, sucralfate, histamine H_2-receptor antagonists, or proton pump inhibitors. The use of antacids has generally fallen into disfavor because of the logistics of frequent administrations and side effects of diarrhea, alkalosis, and other electrolyte problems. The H_2-receptor antagonists maintain a suitably high gastric pH and may be more effective when given as a continuous infusion. Choices of H_2-receptor antagonists include famotidine, nizatidine, cimetidine, and ranitidine. Proton-pump inhibitors are considered the most effective agent in the inhibition of acid production and include omeprazole, esomeprazole, and pantoprazole. Recent data would favor proton-pump inhibitors as the most effective systemic medication for prevention of stress ulceration.[49]

Sucralfate administered as a 1 g slurry q6h by nasogastric tube appears to be as effective in preventing bleeding from stress ulcers as antacids and H_2-receptor antagonists. There was initially an expected lower risk of pneumonia with sucralfate because it does not raise the gastric pH.[50] However, it is now generally felt that there is no significant difference in pneumonia rates related to the method of stress ulceration prophylaxis that is employed.

Renal Function

Renal failure in the perioperative surgical patient may be secondary to pre-existent chronic disease or the acute renal injury may be present either because of the patient's fundamental disease process or because of complications of care. Patients who have chronic renal disease are unable to concentrate their urine appropriately even when hypovolemic. Therefore, a good urine output in a patient who has chronic renal disease does not necessarily indicate an adequate volume status. When there are high insensible losses or so-called "third-spacing" of fluids or bleeding, the patient who has chronic renal failure may continue to make relatively high urine volumes, which can contribute to an increasing hypovolemia. Acute kidney injury is covered in detail in Chapter 28, "Acute Kidney Injury".

Aminoglycosides have been a common nephrotoxic agents used by surgeons, but their use has declined in favor of alternative agents in recent years.[51] Aminoglycoside nephrotoxicity can be avoided or limited by reduction in the total amount of the drug that is used. Commonly accepted risk factors for aminoglycoside-related acute renal failure include pre-existing renal insufficiency, advanced age, use of other nephrotoxic drugs, dehydration, and hypokalemia. Peak and trough drug concentrations following the third dose should be obtained. Careful attention to peak and trough drug concentrations may also lessen the risk of ototoxicity, which is primarily vestibular and not often appreciated. It can, however, be severe and may be irreversible. Toxicity of aminoglycosides can be reduced by limiting use to ≤5 days. Aminoglycosides may also be less toxic when given only once a day.

The increased incidence of methicillin-resistant *Staphylococci* has increased the use of vancomycin. Although vancomycin may potentiate the nephrotoxicity and ototoxicity of aminoglycosides, its own nephrotoxic potential is relatively small. Nevertheless, dosage adjustments in patients who have renal failure are imperative. When sustained and high-dose therapy with vancomycin is necessary, pharmacokinetic dosing may also be necessary. The uncertain pharmacokinetics and clearance of vancomycin has led to recommendations for continuous infusion for inpatients to optimize drug concentrations and therapeutic efficacy.[52]

Contrast-induced nephropathy continues to be a complication among patients who are elderly, those with degree of reduced glomerular filtration, and those that have hypovolemia.[53] Contrast agents are hypertonic and can induce an osmotic diuresis, which aggravates dehydration and a further decline in renal function. The nephrotoxicity of these agents may be minimized by hydration and maintaining a brisk diuresis during the procedure by using loop diuretics and mannitol. In clinically well-hydrated azotemic patients, 1000–1500 mL of 0.9% saline is given over 8–12 hours before and again for 8–12 hours following the procedure. Mannitol (12.5–25 g) and furosemide (10–20 mg) can also be administered at completion of the study.

Nutritional Support

A complete discussion of the vast area of nutritional support of the perioperative patient is presented in Chapter 25, "Nutritional Support". Patients who are severely malnourished should be given nutritional support before operation.[54] Enteral nutrition is preferred, but with poor gut function or lack of gut continuity due to disease, then total parenteral nutrition is used. The objective of preoperative nutritional support is transition of the malnourished patient into positive nitrogen balance, enhance wound healing, and enhance immunologic responsiveness for the anticipated operation. The amount of nutritional support that is necessary to optimize outcomes remains largely a clinical decision.

Postoperative nutritional support for patients with preoperative protein-calories malnutrition and those with complex surgical problems that will likely require prolonged inpatient care is usually begun as soon as possible following operation with the expectation that complications of care will be reduced and that overall recovery will be enhanced.[55] For abdominal surgery, enterostomy is a prudent consideration for the patient where postoperative feeding is anticipated. Nasojejunal access is a preferred route for enteral feeding to avoid risks for aspiration from intragastric delivery and the increased rates of pneumonia that are observed with intragastric delivery.[56] Intragastric feeding can be enhanced by use of percutaneous endoscopic gastrostomy. If intragastric feeding results in evidence of potential reflux, reduce the amount or frequency of gastric feedings, attempt to improve gastric emptying with propulsive agents, and/or attempt to pass the feeding tube into the duodenum.

While most clinical evidence supports enteral feeding when feasible, there are clinical circumstances where parenteral feeding is the preferred option.[57] Parenteral nutrition is usually initiated in the patient as soon as hemodynamic stability is achieved. Details of this feeding strategy are presented in Chapter 25, "Nutritional Support".

Endocrine Function

Perioperative hyperglycemia is a persistent problem in surgical patients. While hyperglycemia has traditionally been associated with diabetes, many other clinical conditions are associated with perioperative hyperglycemia. The systemic inflammatory response syndrome, increased hepatic gluconeogenesis, insulin resistance, and excessive exogenous glucose administration are all variables in addition to the patient's diabetic stasis that make glucose control problematic.[58] The consequences of perioperative hyperglycemia are increased rates of infection and associated fluid-electrolyte abnormalities. Glucose management in the postoperative period is largely performed by frequent measurements of the blood glucose and titration with insulin. The problem in the glucose management issue is not that hyperglycemia has adverse consequences, but what is the safe target for the goal of treatment. Some have advocated targets as low as 80–110 mg/100 mL (4.4–6.1 mmol/L),[59] while others have identified increased complications of efforts to reduce the blood glucose to this level.[60] At present, a reasonable target of 150–200 mg/100 mL (8.3–11.1 mmol/L) appears to have benefit but minimizes the risks of hyperglycemia. For diabetic patients, it is desirable to resume their preoperative management as quickly as possible following the operation.

Perioperative hyperthyroidism can be extremely subtle, especially in the elderly. Some elderly patients present with "apathetic hyperthyroidism" with nonspecific failure to thrive, muscle weakness, arrhythmias, unexplained congestive heart failure, psychiatric dysfunction, or apathy. Intraoperative hyperthermia, tachycardia, or hypertension makes thyroid storm part of the differential diagnosis.

Treatment includes α-adrenergic blockers for hypertension and β-adrenergic blockers for tachycardia and tremor. Corticosteroids, oxygen, glucose, and potassium iodide may also be helpful.

Hypothyroidism may be missed clinically, but should be suspected in anyone who has a thyroid problem. Drugs with CNS effects should be administered with great care to such individuals. In severely myxedematous patients, thyroid hormone replacement should be given as soon as possible before emergency operation. Thyroxine in doses of 0.3–0.5 mg given intravenously or through a nasogastric tube can quickly saturate tissue and carrier protein binding sites, and standard replacement doses can then be given daily.[61]

Hydrocortisone in stress doses of 100 mg intravenously every 8 hours should be considered if the patient becomes hypotensive because of a suspected decreased adrenal reserve. A more common scenario is the patient who has received daily steroid doses in excess of the basal state of 30 mg hydrocortisone or 7.5 mg prednisone for more than a few weeks prior to operation. These levels of steroid administration suppress hypothalamic corticotropin-releasing hormone and pituitary adrenocorticotropic hormone secretion. Current preoperative recommendations for perioperative steroid administration are only a single 25 mg dose of hydrocortisone for procedures of <1 hour that are conducted under local anesthesia and then continue the patient's usual steroid dosing. Moderate stress procedures of joint replacement or elective laparotomy should receive 50–75 mg of hydrocortisone preoperatively and then continuation of the usual steroid dose following the procedure. For major thoracotomy or median sternotomy procedures, 50 mg hydrocortisone is given preoperatively and every 8 hours following the procedure for 48–72 hours with resumption of the usual daily steroid dosing at that point.[62]

PERIOPERATIVE TUBES AND MONITORING

Routine use of nasogastric decompression in the postoperative period for patients having abdominal operations is a matter of debate. Even in patients who have small intestinal or colonic anastomoses, use of the nasogastric tube postoperatively does not affect patient outcome. Nevertheless, nasogastric decompression is appropriate for patients who develop nausea, vomiting, or severe ileus.

Foley catheters are routine during and after major abdominal operations. Bladder catheterization allows precise monitoring of urine output, which can be an important guide to the adequacy of tissue perfusion. A Foley catheter left in place for more than a few days can cause a number of complications, including urinary tract infection or strictures, especially in young men.

Perioperative peripheral intravenous lines are necessary to administer drugs and various fluids. These intravenous catheters should be inserted with aseptic technique. The catheters should also be secured to reduce the risks of infiltration. In general, veins in the center of the forearm are used. Catheters at the wrist or elbow can be easily dislodged, and those on the back of the hand are often painful. These catheters should be rotated to another site after 48 hours. If there is any question of extravasation or infection, they should be removed earlier.

Central Venous Catheters

A detailed description of central catheter placement and management is given in Chapter 14, "Vascular Access". When peripheral access is not available, long-term vascular access is needed, or if the hemodynamic condition of the patient suggests a need for central venous pressure measurements, then central venous catheterization is necessary (Fig. 2.6). Such catheters are associated with a number of complications, particularly pneumothorax at the time of placement, thrombosis, and infection. Complication rates are similar with subclavian versus internal jugular placement, although both are considered preferable to femoral access.[63] Ultrasound-assisted central catheter placement is identified with fewer acute complications.[64] Peripherally inserted central catheters have fewer acute placement complications, but may not have any advantages over long-term

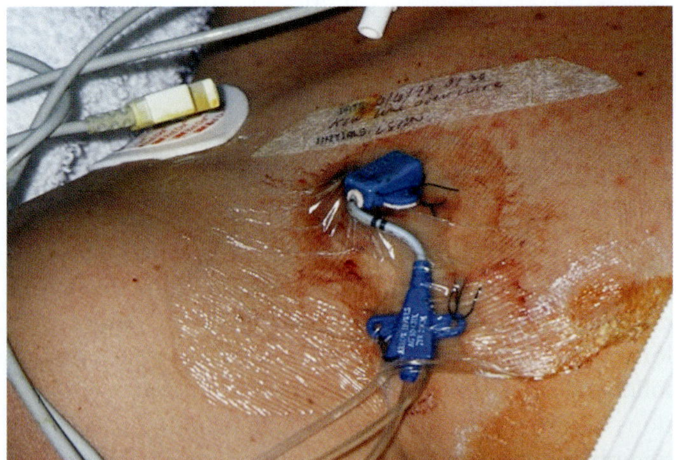

Fig. 2.6: Newly placed central venous catheter via the subclavian access route.

complication rates.[65] As is discussed in Chapter 14, "Vascular Access", infectious complications of central venous catheters can be dramatically reduced by adherence to strict infection control practices in the placement and in the management of these lines.

Pulmonary Artery Catheters

The pulmonary artery catheter achieved a broad level of usage in the management of the critically ill surgical patient. Benefits from the hemodynamic data that was derived from this invasive method gave clinicians assurances about hemodynamic profiles of the patient and of clinical responses to therapeutic interventions. However, actual clinical improvement in outcomes has been challenged, complications of the pulmonary artery catheter have been critically appraised, and alternative but less invasive methods for monitoring cardiac output have been gaining favor.[66] This invasive monitoring technique is only used in very specific circumstances for the management of critically ill surgical patients at present.

Arterial Lines

The indications and methods for placement of arterial lines are detailed in Chapter 23, "Assessment and Monitoring in Critical Illness". Arterial lines are used for continuous measurement of arterial blood pressure in intensive care unit patients and for frequent arterial access for blood gas determinations. The use of the arterial line has become a standard for care in the intensive care unit even though benefits in improved outcomes of care have really not been rigorously evaluated. A recent propensity-matched study has challenged whether arterial lines improve outcomes in critically ill patients.[67] Arterial lines certainly have acute placement complications and infections associated with management after placement. While considered a standard of care by most in the management of intensive care unit patients, objective evaluations of the arterial line are necessary.

REFERENCES

1. American Society of Anesthesiologists. ASA physical status classification system. http://www.asahq.org/resources/clinical-information/asa-physical-status-classification-system.[Online] Accessed May 31, 2015.
2. Scandrett KG, Zuckerbraun BS, Peitzman AB. Operative risk stratification in the older adult. Surg Clin North Am. 2015;95:149-72.
3. Feely MA, Collins CS, Daniels PR, et al. Preoperative testing before noncardiac surgery: guidelines and recommendations. Am Fam Physician. 2013;87:414-8.
4. Fitz-Henry J. The ASA classification and peri-operative risk. Ann R Coll Surg Engl. 2011;93:185-7.
5. Bettelli G. Anaesthesia for the elderly outpatient: preoperative assessment and evaluation, anaesthetic technique and postoperative pain management. Curr Opin Anaesthesiol. 2010;23:726-31.
6. Amrock LG, Deiner S. The implication of frailty on preoperative risk assessment. Curr Opin Anaesthesiol. 2014;27:330-35.
7. Turrentine FE, Wang H, Simpson VB, et al. Surgical risk factors, morbidity, and mortality in elderly patients. J Am Coll Surg. 2006;203:865-77.
8. Levett DZ, Grocott MP. Cardiopulmonary exercise testing for risk prediction in major abdominal surgery. Anesthesiol Clin. 2015;33:1-16.
9. Pearse RM, Moreno RP, Bauer P, et al. Mortality after surgery in Europe: a 7 day cohort study. Lancet. 2012;380:1059-65.
10. Khuri SF, Henderson WG, DePalma RG, et al. Determinants of long-term survival after major surgery and the adverse effect of postoperative complications. Ann Surg. 2005;242:326-41.
11. ATS/ACCP Statement on cardiopulmonary exercise testing. Am J Respir Crit Care Med. 2003;167:211-77.
12. John AD, Sieber FE. Age associated issues: geriatrics. Anesthesiol Clin North Am. 2004;22:45-58.
13. Fried LP, Tangen CM, Walson J, et al. Frailty in old adults: evidence for a phenotype. J Gerontol Med Sci. 2001;56:M146-M156.
14. Mitnitski A, Song X, Skoog I, et al. Relative fitness and frailty of elderly men and women in developed countries and their relationship with mortality. J Am Geriatr Soc. 2005;53:2184-9.
15. Robinson TN, Wu DS, Sauaia A, et al. Slower walking speed forecasts increased postoperative morbidity and 1-year mortality across surgical specialties. Ann Surg. 2013;258:582-8.
16. Robinson TN, Eiseman B, Wallace JI, et al. Redefining geriatric preoperative assessment using frailty, disability and co-morbidity. Ann Surg. 2009;250:449-55.
17. Cullen A, Ferguson A. Perioperative management of the severely obese patient: a selective pathophysiological review. Can J Anaesth. 2012;59:974-96.
18. Schweiger C, Weiss R, Berry E, et al. Nutritional deficiencies in bariatric surgery candidates. Obes Surg. 2010;20:193-7.
19. Odonkor PN, Grigore AM. Patients with ischemic heart disease. Med Clin North Am. 2013;97:1033-50.
20. Halub ME, Sidwell RA. Cardiac Risk stratification and protection. Surg Clin North Am. 2015;95:217-35.
21. Fleisher LA, Fleischmann KE, Auerbach AD, et al. 2014 ACC/AHA guideline on perioperative cardiovascular evaluation and management of patients undergoing noncardiac surgery: a report of the American College of Cardiology/American Heart Association Task Force on practice guidelines. J Am Coll Cardiol. 2014;64:e77-137.
22. Lien SF, Bisognano JD. Perioperative hypertension: defining at-risk patients and their management. Curr Hypertens Rep. 2012;14:432-41.
23. Howell SJ, Sear JW, Foex P. Hypertension, hypertensive heart disease and perioperative cardiac risk. Br J Anaesth. 2004;92:570-83.

24. Marik PE, Varon J. Perioperative hypertension: a review of current and emerging therapeutic agents. J Clin Anesth. 2009;21:220-9.
25. Fleisher LA, Beckman JA, Brown KA, et al. ACC/AHA 2007 guidelines on perioperative cardiovascular evaluation and care for noncardiac surgery: a report of the American College of Cardiology/American Heart Association Task Force on Practice Guidelines. Circulation. 2007;116:e418-499.
26. Lanzino G, Rabinstein AA, Brown RD, Jr. Treatment of carotid artery stenosis: medical therapy, surgery, or stenting? Mayo Clin Proc. 2009;84:362-87.
27. Befeler AS, Palmer DE, Hoffman M, et al. The safety of intra-abdominal surgery in patients with cirrhosis: model for end-stage liver disease score is superior to Child-Turcotte-Pugh classification in predicting outcome. Arch Surg. 2005;140:650-4.
28. Kiamanesh D, Rumley J, Moitra VK. Monitoring and managing hepatic disease in anaesthesia. Br J Anaesth. 2013;111(Suppl 1):i50-61.
29. Afdhal NH. Fibroscan (transient elastography) for the measurement of liver fibrosis. Gastroenterol Hepatol (NY). 2012;8:605-7.
30. Kheterpal S, Tremper KK, Englesbe MJ, et al. Predictors of postoperative acute renal failure after noncardiac surgery in patients with previously normal renal function. Anesthesiology. 2007;107:892-902.
31. Bagshaw SM, Bennett M, Haase M, et al. Plasma and urine neutrophil gelatinase-associated lipocalin in septic versus non-septic acute kidney injury in critical illness. Intensive Care Med. 2010;36:452-61.
32. Clevenger B, Mallett SV. Preoperative assessment of coagulation and bleeding risk. Br J Hosp Med (Lond). 2014;75: C71-74.
33. Thiele RH, Rea KM, Turrentine FE, et al. Standardization of care: impact of an enhanced recovery protocol on length of stay, complications, and direct costs after colorectal surgery. J Am Coll Surg. 2015;220:430-43.
34. Carson JL, Grossmann BJ, Kleinman S, et al. Red blood cell transfusion: A clinical practice guideline from the AABB. Ann Intern Med. 2012;157:49-58.
35. Remuzzi G, Livio M, Marchiaro G, et al. Bleeding in renal failure: altered platelet function in chronic uraemia only partially corrected by haemodialysis. Nephron. 1978;22:347-53.
36. American Society of Anesthesiologists Task Force on Perioperative Blood Management: Practice guidelines for perioperative blood management. Anesthesiology. 2015;122:1-35.
37. Shi Y, Liu CH, Roberts AI, et al. Granulocyte-macrophage, colony stimulating factor (GM-CSF) and T-cell responses: what we do and don't know. Cell Res. 2006;16:126-33.
38. Hoagland HC. Hematologic complications of cancer chemotherapy. Semin Oncol. 1982;9:95-102.
39. Schwartz J, Winters JL, Padmanabhan A, et al. Guidelines on the use of therapeutic apheresis in clinical practice-evidence-based approach from the Writing Committee of the American Society for Apheresis: the sixth special issue. J Clin Apher. 2013;28:145-284.
40. Shammash JB, Trost JC, Gold JM, et al. Perioperative beta-blocker withdrawal and mortality in vascular surgical patients. Am Heart J. 2001;141:148-53.
41. Fleisher LA, Fleischmann KE, Auerbach AD, et al. 2014 ACC/AHA guideline on perioperative cardiovascular evaluation and management of patients undergoing noncardiac surgery: a report of the American College of Cardiology/American Heart Association Task Force on practice guidelines. J Am Coll Cardiol. 2014;64:e77-137. doi: 10.1016/j.jacc.2014.07.944. Epub 2014 Aug 1.
42. Wijeysundera DN, Duncan D, Nkonde-Price C, et al. Perioperative beta blockade in noncardiac surgery: a systematic review for the 2014 ACC/AHA guideline on perioperative cardiovascular evaluation and management of patients undergoing noncardiac surgery: a report of the American College of Cardiology/American Heart Association Task Force on practice guidelines. J Am Coll Cardiol. 2014;64:2406-25. doi: 10.1016/j.jacc.2014.07.939. Epub 2014 Aug 1.
43. Wijeysundera DN, Beattie WS. Calcium channel blockers for reducing cardiac morbidity after noncardiac surgery: a metaanalysis. Anesth Analg. 2003;97:634-41.
44. Rosenman DJ, McDonald FS, Ebbert JO, et al. Clinical consequences of withholding versus administering renin-angiotensin-aldosterone system antagonists in the preoperative period. J Hosp Med. 2008;3:319-25.
45. Twersky RS, Goel V, Narayan P,et al. The risk of hypertension after preoperative discontinuation of angiotensin-converting enzyme inhibitors or angiotensin receptor antagonists in ambulatory and same-day admission patients. Anesth Analg. 2014;118:938-44.
46. American Thoracic Society: Surgery in and for COPD. Available from http://www.thoracic.org/copd-guidelines/for-health-professionals/management-of-stable-copd/surgery-in-and-for-copd/surgery-in-the-copd-patient.php [Online] [Accessed May 20, 2015].
47. Popping DM, Elia N, Marret E, et al. Protective effects of epidural analgesia on pulmonary complications after abdominal and thoracic surgery: a meta-analysis. JAMA Surg. 2008;143:990-9.
48. do Nascimento Junior P, Módolo NS, Andrade S, et al. Incentive spirometry for prevention of postoperative pulmonary complications in upper abdominal surgery. Cochrane Database Syst Rev. 2014;2:CD006058. doi: 10.1002/14651858.CD006058.pub3.
49. Alhazzani W, Alenezi F, Jaeschke RZ, et al. Proton pump inhibitors versus histamine 2 receptor antagonists for stress ulcer prophylaxis in critically ill patients: a systematic review and meta-analysis. Crit Care Med. 2013;41:693-705.
50. Driks MR, Craven DE, Celli BR, et al. Nosocomial pneumonia in intubated patients given sucralfate as compared with antacids or histamine type 2 blockers. The role of gastric colonization. N Engl J Med. 1987;317:1376-82.

Additional references appear in the online version of this book.

3

The Operating Room Environment

Charles E Edmiston, David J Leaper

Key Points

- The layout of a general operating room (OR) is based upon an optimal area of 400 ft^2 (37 m^2), which is provided with electrical and plumbing connections and adjacent facilities for scrub-up, anesthesia, and specialist surgical equipment.
- Integrated hybrid ORs are larger (900–1200 ft^2) and incorporate state-of-the-art imaging, communication and ergonomic technology.
- Positive-pressure air flow should allow a minimum of 20 total changes of air per hour without recirculation; temperature and humidity must be controlled.
- Drapes and gowns should be designed to provide an adequate barrier to microorganisms and fluids; alternatives to the standard latex gloves are needed for personnel or patients who are allergic.
- Decontamination of the patient's skin involves a detergent scrub followed by an antiseptic solution such as chlorhexidine or an iodophore with or without 70% isopropyl alcohol. Alternatively, an antiseptic alcoholic solution alone is acceptable.
- Absorbable sutures (for gastroenterological or urological procedures) are prepared from animal tissue or synthetic polymers; silk, nylon, and polypropylene are examples of nonabsorbable sutures (although the unacceptable host reaction to all "natural" materials has made them less suitable); modern needles are swaged onto the suture.
- Safety precautions entail the avoidance of (1) OR fires and burns to personnel and patients by the proper use of electrocautery and lasers; (2) exposure to ionizing radiation; (3) injury from surgical instruments; and (4) transmission of healthcare-associated infections.
- The OR environment should embrace a culture of safe surgery as advocated by the World Health Organization (WHO) checklist.

INTRODUCTION

The modern operating room (OR) is a dynamic, technology-driven environment in which multidisciplinary teams can perform complex surgical procedures with delivery of safe and effective surgical care. ORs have been characterized as the "financial engine" of the hospital with the average OR income of approximately $1,500 per hour,[1] but this is dependent upon the efficiency of design and control of operational overheads. A major issue associated with construction of the modern OR must also be patient and staff safety, especially in an era of value-based purchasing, where failure to mitigate risk has an adverse impact on procedural reimbursement.[2]

A primary goal of the modern OR is to provide a controlled space, which can offer flexibility and utility across a breadth of operative procedures. The complexity of this process is influenced by several factors, including:

- The total projected number of eligible surgical cases per surgical service
- Will the room be used for unscheduled cases such as trauma emergency or limited to day and/or evening hours?
- Average case time as measured by "wheels-in and wheels-out"
- Estimated compared with actual turn-around time between cases
- Will the room have permanent instrumentation or equipment dedicated to that specific room limiting service utility?
- Does the design enhance the quality of care by allowing future adaptability without compromising the intrinsic infection prevention characteristics?
- Finally, and most importantly, does the facility provide a safe and effective environment for the patient?

This chapter reviews the OR environment in detail, in addition to the ancillary components required for a "safe, surgical patient-care experience".

OPERATING ROOM CHARACTERISTICS (PATIENT TRANSFER: ARRIVAL TO RECOVERY)

The number of ORs needed in an operating suite needs to match the projected elective and emergency workload, and the types of surgery undertaken, for its foreseeable future. The use of OR time differs between countries; if it has to be compensated for by time/case then planning OR periods has to be more accurate and to recognize extra time needed for training purposes. The OR suite should also include a reception area, changing rooms, anesthetic rooms, preparation and storage rooms, cleaning and sterilization facilities, and a recovery area with space for parents or other relatives. A "common room", which can be used for writing notes or having case conferences, as well as a rest area, is also required. Ideally, the OR suite should be centrally placed in the hospital with easy, rapid access to transport, the emergency and radiology departments and intensive care unit (ICU) facilities.

Typically, the OR area is 400 ft^2 (approximately 37 m^2), which allows major and minor invasive procedures to be performed (Figs. 3.1 and 3.2). However, this dimension has increased substantially with the development of the integrated hybrid OR. Space requirements must also be made to include ceiling lighting, cabinets, shelving, white boards, and adequately sized X-ray boxes or other IT systems. ORs intended for cardiovascular, orthopedic, neurosurgery, trauma, and other special procedures often require at least 600 ft^2 (55 m^2) for the associated additional personnel and large equipment storage in or adjacent to the OR. This space includes extracorporeal pumps for open heart procedures; built-in radiology equipment and lead lining for endovascular surgical procedures; and, in orthopedic ORs, enclosed storage space for exhaust suit equipment, splints, and traction equipment. In some ORs (mandated for most orthopedic procedures) laminar air flow is often built into the heating-ventilation-air

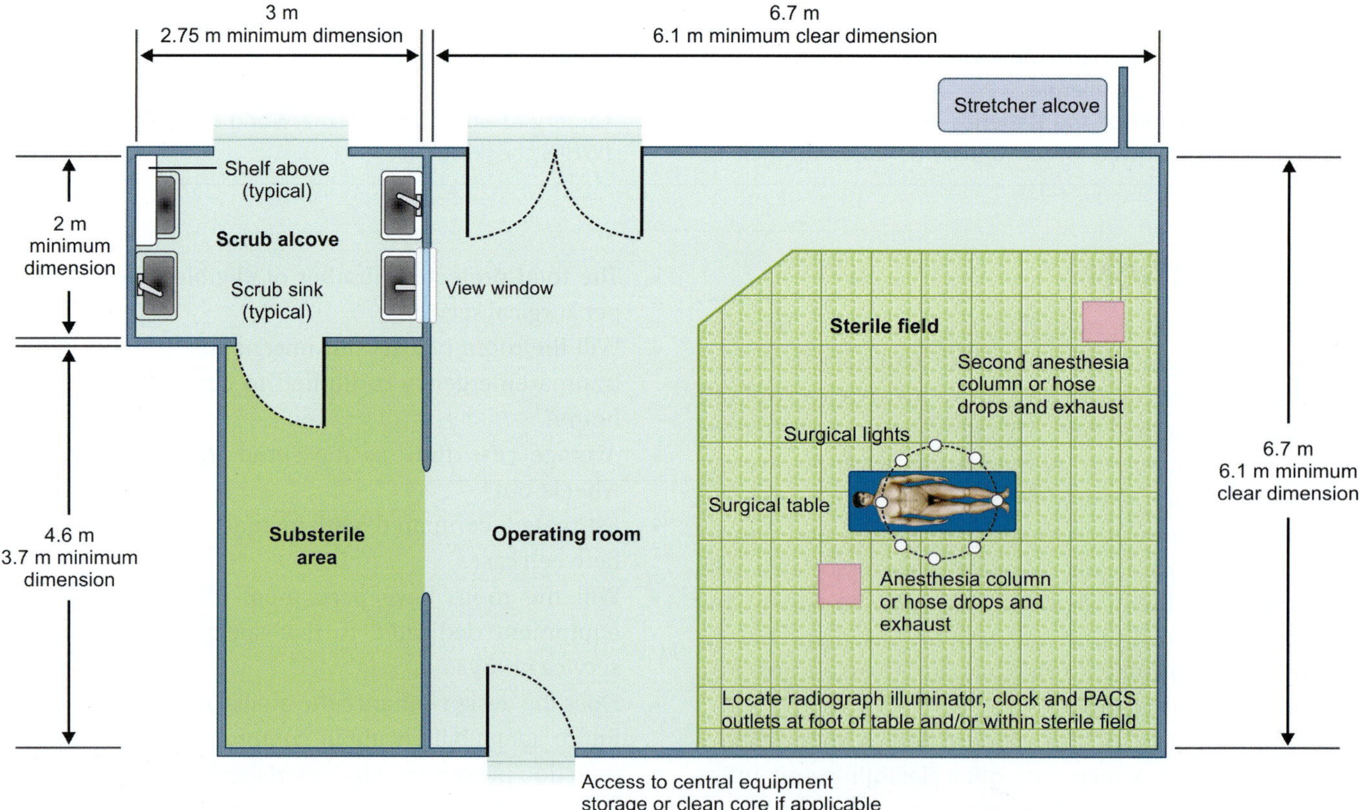

Fig. 3.1: General operating room format.

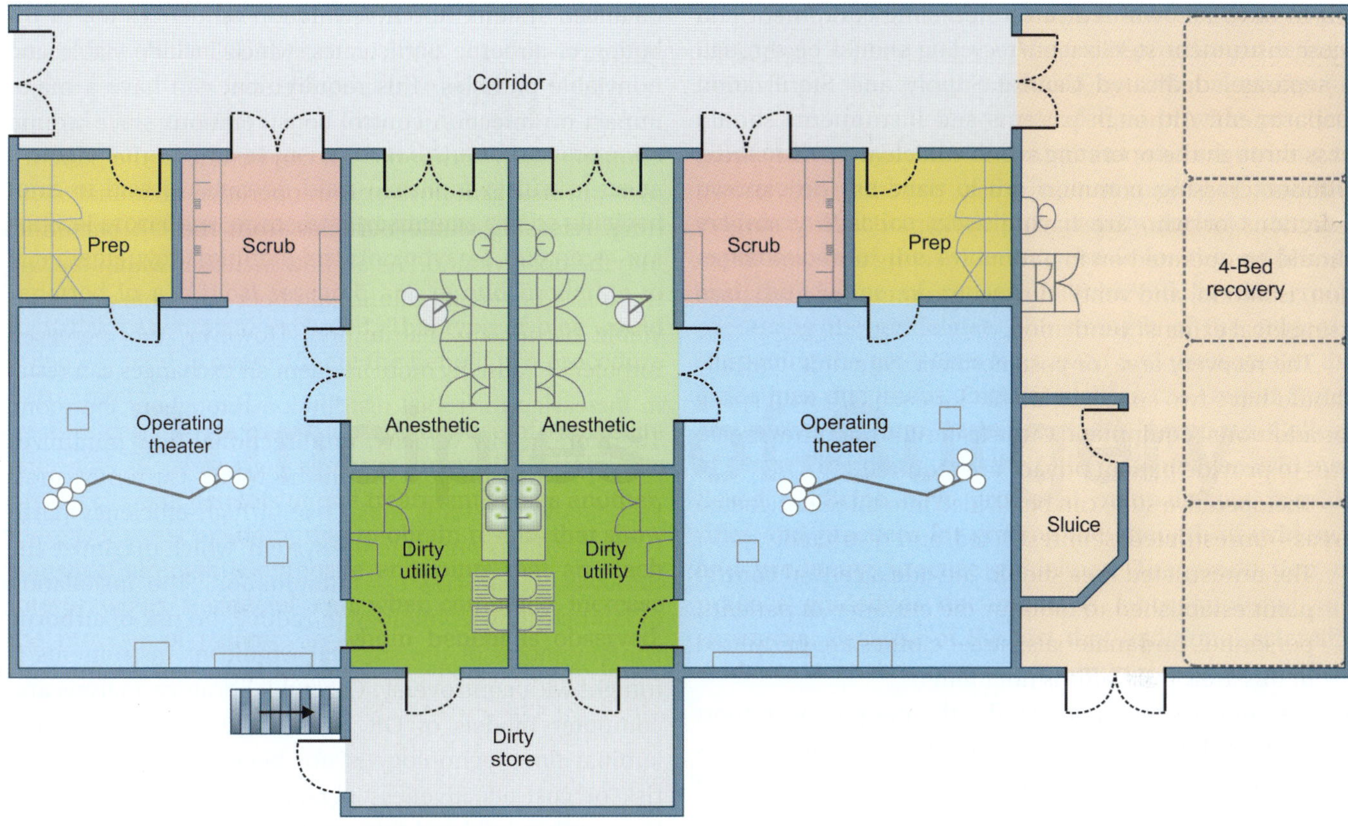

Fig. 3.2: Operating room layout suitable for day case surgery.

conditioning (HVAC) system, and these ORs may need to be ring fenced for this purpose, as trauma and emergency lists are, often on 24 hour availability.

When outpatient, day case, surgical care is provided in an acute care hospital or other medical facility, the facility ought to be specifically designed for this use and adjacent but separate from the main OR suite. Day case ORs may be smaller in size but need equal attention to design that accommodates workload, which may include provision of endoscopy, as well as specialized reception and recovery areas.

In an OR suite designed with a sterile core, there must be no cross traffic of staff and supplies from soiled areas to the sterile clean areas: a "clean-to-dirty" pathway. A nursing control station should be located to monitor all traffic into the OR suite visually. There should be appropriate space for the OR supervisor and other essential personnel who may require office or work areas, space to store and distribute medications, and access to hand washing facilities.

Two or three scrub positions should be provided near the entrance to each OR. These positions may serve adjacent ORs if they are close to the entrance of each room. However, additional sinks are usually needed, and these facilities should be arranged to minimize incidental splatter. Scrub sinks should be recessed out of the way of main traffic areas, preferably in an OR anteroom, and should be located outside the sterile core of the OR. A clean work room is required whenever clean materials are assembled in the OR before use or following decontamination. This room should contain a work counter, storage facility for clean supplies, space to package reusable items, and a hand washing fixture. It should be separate from the area in which sterile supplies are stored.

Facilities outside the OR for soiled and decontaminated processing, assembly, and preliminary cleaning before sterile recycling should be designed to separate the flow of goods and personnel from clean and sterile to dirty areas without compromising aseptic technique. An enclosed, soiled work room for the exclusive use of the OR suite should be located in the restricted area and should contain a flushing-rim clinical sink, a hand washing fixture, a work counter, and space for soiled linen receptacles. This room should not have a direct connection with the ORs or other sterile activity rooms. It is not necessary for each

OR to have its own dedicated sterilizing equipment and most instrument sterilization/recycling should be through a separate, dedicated Central Supply and Sterilization Department. Although patients and instruments should pass through the operating suite from clean to dirty areas without crossing common areas, patients with known infections or who are having anticipated dirty surgery should be operated on in a room meeting airborne infection, isolation, and ventilation requirements or in a space using local exhaust ventilation.

The recovery area, or postanesthetic care unit, typically should have two spaces available for each OR, with space for additional equipment. Cubicle curtains or other measures to provide patient privacy are required.

The operative suite can be divided into three designated areas—unrestricted, semirestricted, and restricted:

- The unrestricted area should include a central control point established to monitor the entrance of patients, personnel, and materials; street clothes are permitted in this area and traffic is not limited.
- A semirestricted area includes the peripheral support areas of the operative suite and includes storage areas for clean and sterile supplies, areas for processing of instruments and corridors leading to the restricted areas of the operative suite; traffic is limited, and personnel are required to wear surgical attire and cover head and facial hair.
- The restricted area includes the ORs, procedure rooms, the clean core between ORs and scrub sink areas; surgical attire and hair coverings are required, and masks are required where sterile supplies have been opened or scrubbed persons are located.

OPERATING ROOM DESIGN

State and federal codes in the USA govern the minimum total and outdoor air exchange rates for ORs, requiring a minimum of 20 air exchanges and 4 air exchanges of outdoor air when the room is in use.[3] However, 20–25 total air exchanges are usually required to maintain room temperature, to ensure efficient particulate removal, and to manage the dissipation of room heat associated with the lights and other equipment load within a typical OR. Mechanical and ventilation codes require that the ORs maintain a positive air pressure relative to surrounding spaces, whether or not the room is occupied. One air handling unit, most often, services multiple ORs; therefore, precise pressure monitoring is required to maintain a balanced system. Room ventilation influences the distribution of airborne particulates, which include viable and nonviable particles. This requirement can have a major impact on infection control considerations since wound contamination within the OR can be due to the patient's own intrinsic skin flora or intraoperative microbial shedding, releasing viable particles from the OR personnel into the open wound.[4] As air flow increases within the OR, there is a beneficial dilutional effect on viable and nonviable particulate distribution. However, the increased turbulence cause by more frequent air exchanges can result in increasing microbial distribution throughout the room. Therefore, a low velocity, unidirectional flow minimizes microbial distribution within the room. Currently, most recirculation systems make use of high-efficiency particulate air filters built into the system, which maximize the removal of particulate contamination. The installation of laminar flow technology to reduce the risk of airborne contamination of the surgical wound or instruments is fraught with controversy. Careful laboratory analysis and computer models of OR air recirculation suggest that laminar-flow technology is not beneficial from either a risk or cost-effectiveness perspective.[5,6] Clinical studies have further validated this perspective.[7,8] In addition, consideration should be given to disruption of laminar air flow systems by the use of forced-air intraoperative devices, used for maintaining core temperature.

Many studies have validated the benefits of keeping patients warm during the perioperative interval. However, the recommended temperature within the OR during an operation is between 68°F and 73°F (20°C and 23°C), and maintaining the appropriate temperature within the OR can be challenging. Because of the use of heavy, multilayer surgical gowns and length of some operative procedures, many surgeons request that the temperature within the OR be maintained somewhere between 60°F and 65°F (15°C and 18°C) or lower. This often leads to condensation issues (increased humidity) since many of the ORs are maintained at temperatures that are much cooler than the HVAC system was originally designed to sustain. The presence of excess condensation can have an impact on personnel comfort and potentiate infection control issues, associated with the buildup of moisture on lights, instrumentation, and surgical instruments, thereby compromising sterility. The recommended relative humidity for the OR environment based upon American Institute of Architects recommendations is 30–60%.

THE INTEGRATED (HYBRID) OPERATING ROOMS OF THE FUTURE

The ORs of the future will encompass ergonomics, real-time imaging and navigation, medical informatics, and training through simulation.[9] The development of an integrated hybrid OR started over 20 years ago with the transition from open to minimally invasive surgery in several surgical procedures. For the first time the concept of ergonomic alignment has become relevant within the surgical suite. The advancements associated with more complex, minimally invasive procedures and allowing real-time imaging have introduced another element to OR pressure. The placement of monitors, ceiling booms (C-arms), and communication technology to facilitate telesurgery all necessitate ergonomic decisions that improve the surgical work flow while minimizing risk and improving patient outcomes. The design of new integrated ORs minimizes the clutter that accrues when standard ORs are reconfigured, and they are typically two to three times the square footage (900–1200 ft^2) of standard ORs to accommodate the extra technology (Figs. 3.3 and 3.4). With the introduction of sophisticated imaging or computer-assisted surgical platforms (robotic surgery) into the OR, additional infection control considerations are warranted, because they must not be a source of contamination within the sterile field. Therefore, the ORs of the future also need new processes for cleaning between cases or following contaminated procedures, and terminal cleaning at the end of the day.

OPERATING ROOM CLEANING

Although new OR designs require a change in methods of cleaning and decontamination, fundamental principles must remain to reduce the microbial burden within the

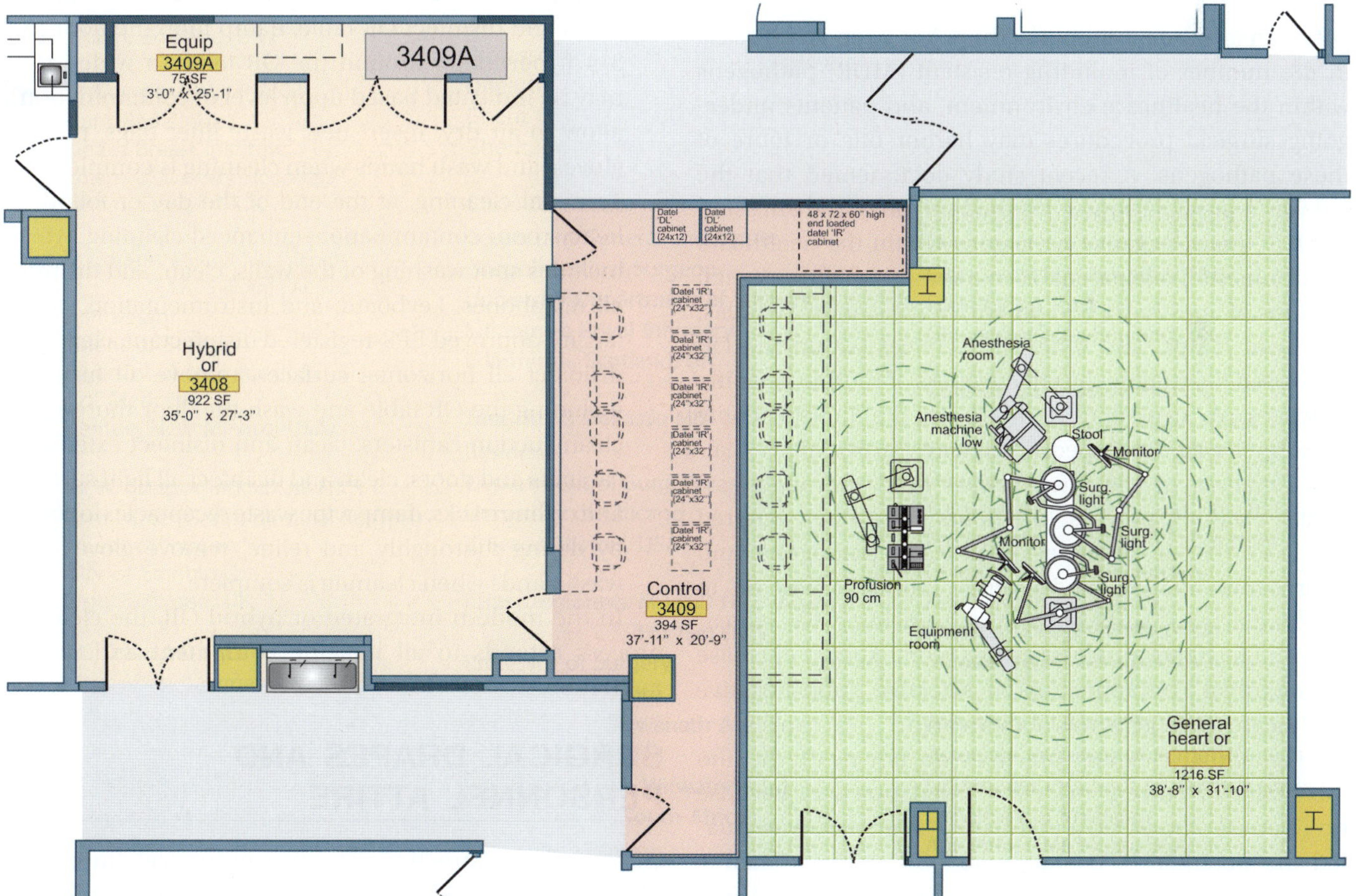

Fig. 3.3: Schematic drawing of back-to-back integrated (hybrid) operating rooms. The room on the left is hybrid vascular-intervention radiology suite (922 ft^2), note communication/computer console on the right in separate cubicle. The room on the right is Heart/CT operating room (1216 ft^2), note communication/computer consoles on the left of room in separate cubicle.

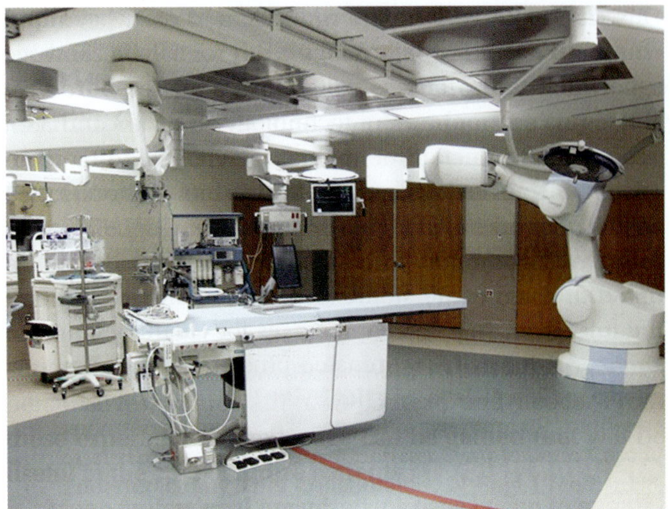

Fig. 3.4: Hybrid vascular–endovascular operating room; note large expansive area (900 ft^2) accommodating multiple ceiling booms and CV-arms.
(By courtesy of Froedtert Hospital, Milwaukee, Wisconsin USA).

OR to an absolute minimum. There has been an increase in the number of multidrug-resistant (MDR) pathogens within the healthcare environment, and patients undergoing surgical procedures may harbor one or more of these pathogens. A recent study documented that the OR was a possible source for the horizontal transmission of MDR, gram-negative pathogens within the healthcare environment. Transparent UV markers and environmental cultures of anesthesia equipment, Mayo stands, IV poles, overhead lamps, and other flat services within the OR were used to evaluate the effectiveness of routine cleaning practices. A structural feedback to the housekeeping personnel was developed; in essence providing a real-time analysis of the effectiveness (and thoroughness) of the cleaning process. OR floors were often ignored as a source of potential healthcare pathogens and floor contamination inadvertently found its way on to horizontal work surfaces. Through an intensive education and feedback process (using UV markers) a decrease in microbial contamination of selective gram-negative healthcare pathogens was documented.[10]

Traditional cleaning practices do not neatly fit into the realm of current evidence-based practice, because no rigorous studies exist that have systematically evaluated the potential of contaminated OR surfaces leading to higher rates of hospital-acquired infection. However, studies conducted within the critical care patient population (ICU) have demonstrated that interventional housekeeping practices can reduce the transmission of methicillin-resistant *Staphylococcus aureas*, other MDR pathogens and *Clostridium difficile*. The current Association of Operating Room Nurses (AORN) recommendations represent a "best practice" approach to environment cleaning in the OR and, until a more thorough correlation between process and outcome is established, these recommendations continue to guide current housekeeping practices.[11] Briefly, the process of environmental cleaning of the OR can be broken down into three phases [personal protective equipment (PPE) must be worn when disposing of waste that may be contaminated with blood or body fluids]:

- At the beginning of each day, prior to first procedure—clean all horizontal surfaces with a cloth dampened with a facility-approved Environmental Protection Agency (EPA)-registered disinfectant
- Cleaning of OR between cases—clean all horizontal surfaces with a cloth dampened with a facility-approved EPA-registered disinfectant, clean suction canisters, clean and disinfect OR table, damp mop the floor in a 3–4 ft perimeter around the OR table (a wider zone may be indicated based upon level of contamination), allow to air dry, insert new waste liner bags, remove gloves, and wash hands when cleaning is complete.
- Terminal cleaning, at the end of the day or following heavy room contamination-enhanced cleaning, which includes spot washing of the walls, clean, and disinfect all telephones, keyboard, and instrumentation with a facility-approved EPS-registered disinfectant, clean and disinfect all horizontal surfaces, remove all furniture including the OR table and wash the floor thoroughly, clean suction canisters, clean and disinfect exterior of cabinets and doors, clean and disinfect all light surfaces and ceiling tracks, damp wipe waste receptacles followed by drying thoroughly and reline, remove gloves, and wash hands when cleaning is complete.

In the modern integrated or hybrid OR, the cleaning process extends to all imaging equipment and instrumentation.

SURGICAL DRAPES AND PERSONNEL ATTIRE

Historically, the functional purpose of surgical drapes and gowns was to provide barrier protection of the sterile field from extrinsic bacterial contamination. With promulgation of the Occupational Safety and Health Administration Final Standard on Occupational Exposure to Bloodborne

Table 3.1 Suggested use of gowns for the surgeon and first assistant.

Site	*Estimated blood loss* *Minimal (<100 mL)*	*Moderate (100–500 mL)*	*High (>500 mL)*
Skin and subcutaneous	Standard	Reinforced	Plastic-reinforced
Head and neck	Standard	Reinforced	Plastic-reinforced
Chest	Standard	Plastic-reinforced	Plastic-reinforced
Abdomen	Reinforced	Plastic-reinforced	Plastic-reinforced
Extremities	Reinforced	Reinforced	Plastic-reinforced
Trauma	Reinforced	Plastic-reinforced	Plastic-reinforced

Pathogens and the Use of Personal Protective Equipment, the surgical gown became a frontline device to protect the healthcare professional from exposure to blood and body fluids.[12] Sterile surgical drapes should have the following characteristics:

- Provide an appropriate barrier to microorganisms, particulate matter and fluids
- Be able to maintain adequate integrity and durability and withstand the physical conditions presented during a given operation
- Be resistant to tears, punctures, and other usual wear
- Be free of toxic ingredients and
- Be of low-lint production.

Tightly woven fabrics lose their protective qualities after repeated processing. Laundering and steam sterilization cause fibers to change in size and eventually loosen, thereby allowing microorganisms to pass through the barriers, both by wicking or pressure differentials. It is important to follow the manufacturers' instructions for the handling, processing, and suggested limitations of these materials, which should also be resistant to combustion. In general, most institutions have accepted disposable drapes as the preferred type of barrier. Some operative procedures are undertaken using "incise" drapes, which adhere to the patient's skin, the rationale being that drapes, which are clipped to the skin, are subject to "drape-lift" from the edges of the surgical wound. Drapes that fit tenaciously to the skin may theoretically prevent horizontal migration of skin contaminants into the surgical wound. This supposition has never been proven by evidence-based research, and incise drapes are accepted as being convenient and less traumatic to the skin. However, if they are not impregnated with an antiseptic they may increase surgical site infection (SSI) risk through a "greenhouse" effect. Several manufacturers have suggested that their drapes and gowns offer superior barrier protection to others, and while certain laminates or polypropylene-treated gowns do possess enhanced barrier protection over single-layer nonwoven fabrics, assessing barrier effectiveness in an objective, comparative manner is difficult. Gowns and drapes composed of 100% woven cotton, while reusable, provide the least barrier protection. Furthermore, repetitive laundering of reusable, single layer fabrics increases microbial transmission through the fabric, whereas reinforced fabrics are more resistant.[13,14]

Nearly all gowns become contaminated externally during the course of an operation. The most frequently contaminated areas are the forearms (36%), chest (25%), and abdomen (18%).[15] Gowns are often reinforced in these areas to prevent penetration of blood to the inside of the gown. Blood penetration as a result of heavy contamination is less for plastic, reinforced gowns than for single-layer, unreinforced gowns.

To determine the type of gown to wear during an operation, the following factors need to be considered:

- Duration of the operation
- Anticipated blood loss and
- Operative site.[16]

In addition, factors such as personal comfort and cost may influence the type of gown worn. Importantly, the surgeon and first assistant are the most likely to be accidentally exposed to blood during an operation. Cardiothoracic, trauma, and cesarean section operations are most likely to subject the surgeon to blood exposure.[17] Penetration occurs most often when there is heavy contamination on the outside of the gown. Table 3.1 serves as a guide when deciding upon the type of gown needed by the surgeon and first assistant for a particular procedure. Other assistants and the scrub nurse and technician should wear at least one level of protection less. Disposable gowns come in three basic types:

- Standard disposable gowns consist of a single layer of material
- Reinforced gowns have a second layer of material on the front panel and from the sleeve cuffs to the elbow and
- Plastic-reinforced gowns have a layer of plastic laminated onto the gown material in the same areas as the reinforced gowns.

When a reusable gown is chosen, it should be of high or very high thread count and reinforced over the risk areas. Reusable gowns are made of fabric that either incorporates expanded polytetrafluoroethylene (PTFE) laminated between two layers of polyester fabric or consists of a high thread count woven polyester fabric that has been treated with a fluid repellent. These gowns can also be reinforced over the front panel and arms. The PTFE gowns provide protection and comfort equal to those of a disposable gown.

Sleeve covers should be worn when it is anticipated that the forearms of the gown may become saturated during an operative procedure. Saturation happens most frequently during long-duration abdominal operations and operations in which there is excessive bleeding (e.g. operations for major abdominal trauma and ruptured abdominal aortic aneurysms). The sleeve cover should be made of an impermeable material rather than cloth fabric.

Whenever possible, surgical team members should be involved in the evaluation of gowns that are being considered for use in the OR. While the type of gown used by members of the surgical team is a matter of personal preference, the choice of gown should be governed by its selective barrier properties, especially when the risk is high of exposure to blood and body fluids.

Gloves and Masks

Latex is the most common material used for surgical gloves. Latex-free gloves should be provided for personnel who are allergic to latex and should also be used when treating patients who have latex allergies. Additional types of gloves that are available usually have had one or more irritant chemicals eliminated during processing and can help avoid certain types of contact dermatitis among OR personnel.

Glove failure or leakage can occur even with short periods of use because of strains and stress. A substantial risk of injury and blood exposure among surgical personnel in approximately 50% of elective surgical procedures has been reported.[18] Another survey found that in 63% of glove failures the surgical practitioners observed visible blood on their skin upon glove removal,[19] and a further study found that glove failure rates during surgery vary from 9.2% to 37.7%.[20] The practice of wearing two gloves is an acceptable approach to reducing the risk of blood exposure during high-risk surgical cases, in which the rubber-like elasticity of the glove facilitates a "wiping-like" effect by creating a mechanical constriction around any object penetrating the glove. For suture needle puncture the volume of residual blood left on a suture or needle has been estimated to be reduced by as much as 95% after passage through two glove layers.[21,22] Despite the data supportive of double gloving as an effective risk reduction strategy, many surgeons feel that double gloving reduces tactile sensitivity and manual dexterity, which has led to limited application in practice. The benefits of double gloving are twofold; first, it provides protection against disease transmission from healthcare professional to the patient (mostly skin organisms, which may contribute to SSIs); and second, it protects against disease transmission (HIV and HBV) from patient to healthcare professional.

Wearing surgical masks during surgery is traditional, the main rationale being the reduction of droplet contamination by members of the operative team into the wound. This rationale has been the subject of much controversy since several published studies have suggested that the wearing of surgical masks does not prevent SSIs[23,24] but nasopharyngeal shedding or "venting" does occur through the sides of the mask, leading to contamination of the surgical wound.[25,26] The dynamics of this have been investigated, using molecular epidemiology during prolonged vascular procedures, and clearly documented dispersion of nasopharyngeal flora throughout the OR, which originated from vascular team members.[26] Despite the inconclusive evidence, the wearing of a surgical mask is now viewed as an element of one's PPE, providing protection to the lower face against splashes from blood or body fluids. This perspective is clearly embraced by the Centers for Medicare & Medicaid Services, and institutions have been criticized for not enforcing the wearing of a protective surgical mask when there is a perceived risk of exposure to blood and body fluids during surgical operations. Many surgical masks now also come with an attached face shield that provides additional protection for the eyes against exposure to blood or body fluids.

PREPARATION OF THE PATIENT'S SKIN AND ANTISEPSIS

Decontamination of the patient's skin before operation is one of the most effective practices to prevent postoperative incisional infection. The patient's skin microflora presents an important reservoir for bacterial contamination of incisions. A preoperative shower or cleansing with an antiseptic agent using a standardized regimen prior to admission has been documented to reduce the incidence of SSIs after clean operative procedures.[27-29] If hair is to be removed from the operative site, it is now mandated by the Surgical Care Improvement Project that it be removed by clipping with a disposable head, using an electric razor rather than a traditional blade since nicks or scratches can lead to increased bacterial colonization of the skin, which may increase the risk of SSI.[30]

The surgical site and surrounding area should always be prepared with a Food and Drug Administration (United States FDA)-approved antiseptic agent. The area of skin preparation should:

- Be large enough to accommodate any extension of the incision, the need for additional incisions and all potential drain sites and
- Extend far enough to avoid wound contamination through inadvertent movement of drapes during the operative procedure.

The antiseptic agents used for surgical skin preparation should be applied in a sterile fashion from single-use containers using sterile gloves and a no-touch technique.[11] The microbial burden on the skin varies depending upon the body region. Bacterial concentrations range from $1 \times 10^2/cm^2$ on the forearms to $1.5 \times 10^6/cm^2$ on the skin around the perineum or groin. Factors such as skin moisture, pH, desquamation, and skin disease can affect the concentration of the skin microflora.[31] The most common bacteria cultured from the skin of healthy individuals are *Staphylococcus epidermidis*, corynebacteria, *Propionibacterium acnes*, and lactobacilli, which are commensal organisms and rarely responsible for infection in humans. The skin may also become contaminated with transient bacteria from a variety of sources including the hospital environment. Transient bacteria often include more virulent MDR pathogens. It is these transient bacteria that are most effectively removed by skin preparation.

Initially, a detergent-based scrub may be required to remove excessive soil from the surface of the skin. Following this, all detergent must be removed from the operative site and an antiseptic solution applied in concentric circles starting at the proposed incision site outward. Currently, some skin antiseptic agents come in a sterile foam-tipped applicator in which case the agent is applied to the skin in an outward motion, originating from the incisional site. The current recommendation suggest using either an iodophor such as 7.5% povidone iodine (PI), 2–3% chlorhexidine gluconate (CHG) or preferably an alcoholic formulation of CHG or PI.[32] While the iodophore skin antiseptic agents have been used traditionally to prepare the skin surface prior to surgery, CHG with or without 70% alcohol has emerged as an evidence-based alternative to PI.[33,34] CHG is a cationic bisbiguanide that exhibits excellent antimicrobial activity on contact against gram-positive, gram-negative, and selected fungal pathogens. In addition to its broad spectrum activity, CHG binds to the cells of skin, accumulating over time to provide a residual activity not observed with PI. Finally, CHG is not inactivated by the presence of blood or tissue protein, which may confer a selective advantage over other skin-prepping agents. One cautionary comment is warranted: when using any skin antiseptic agent containing alcohol, sufficient time must be allowed for the antiseptic agent to dry (2–3 minutes) prior to draping to reduce the likelihood of a fire occurring during electrocautery.

PATIENT SAFETY IN THE OPERATING ROOM

The OR exposes both the surgeon and patient to a substantial risk of injury. These hazards include:

- OR fires
- Exposure to infectious body fluids
- Injury from both manual and power tools
- Burns from electrocautery or laser units

Fires in the OR pose the most risk of serious injury to the patient and surgical staff.[35] The incidence of fires in the OR has decreased as noninflammable anesthetic agents have been introduced; however, 20–30 OR fires still occur each year in ORs in the United States. Lasers or an electrocautery unit can ignite excess antiseptic skin agent that contains an alcohol base that has soaked the immediate operative field. The resultant fire can spread to surrounding drapes and plastic equipment, which serve as further fuel for the fire. Although usually treated with fire retardant materials, disposable drapes burn readily once ignited. The OR personnel may also be injured when disposables are ignited. Endotracheal tubes are particularly prone to ignition because of the high flow of oxygen used during surgical procedures. Incision or coagulation of the trachea with an electrocautery unit is the cause of most endotracheal tube fires. The resultant fire may spread rapidly to surgical drapes. It is essential that the patient is immediately extubated when such a fire is recognized and promptly reintubated with another endotracheal or tracheostomy tube.

The risk of an OR fire can be minimized by observing the following guidelines:[36]

- Electrocautery units should be kept in their holster when not in use
- Alcohol-based antiseptic preparations must be thoroughly dry before initiation of the surgical procedure
- Care should be taken to avoid spilling excess alcohol-based preparations on the operative drapes
- Electrocautery should not be used to incise the trachea or coagulate bleeding from the tracheal edges
- The potential risk of the laser must be recognized
- Safety protocols must be established and followed
- All OR personnel should be instructed about the proper response to a fire.

Exposure to radiation is another obvious hazard in the OR environment. Sources include portable radiograph machines, fluoroscopy, and intraoperative radiation therapy. A dosimeter should be worn by anyone who frequently works in the vicinity of X-ray exposure. Precautions to minimize X-ray exposure include minimizing the number of personnel near the patient during the exposure, maximizing the distance from the X-ray machine, and wearing lead aprons when feasible. The patient must also be adequately shielded when appropriate.

Suture needles, scalpel blades, and syringes are most often associated with intraoperative injuries and, compared with other areas of the hospital, ORs are less compliant in adopting safer surgical practices to reduce the risk of sharps injury. Percutaneous sharp injury rates vary from 1.7% to 15.4% depending upon the surgical procedure.[37,38] Transmission of hepatitis B, hepatitis C, and HIV have been of greatest concern. Historically, hepatitis B infection has been the greatest cause of morbidity and death.[39] It has been estimated that after needle-stick exposure hepatitis B occurs in 30% of individuals, hepatitis C in 2.5–10%, and HIV infection 0.3%.[40] All OR personnel should be familiar with the protocols within their institution for reporting sharp-related injury and should follow appropriate recommendations for evaluation of risk, which may include immunoprophylaxis.

The OR personnel are exposed to a measurable amount of surgical smoke or laser plumes. The US National Institute of Occupational Safety and Health (NIOSH) has demonstrated an appreciable mutagenic potential of electrocautery smoke from samples taken during surgical procedures.[41,42] It has been estimated that the mutagenic potential of smoke produced from 1 g of electrocauterized tissue is equivalent to that of 3–6 cigarettes. The AORN has long been an advocate for the development of smoke control policies, which promote respiratory protection.[43] Exposure to surgically generated smoke can be significantly decreased by using local exhaust ventilation technology or NIOSH-approved respirator masks.

Prevention of Hypothermia

As the OR temperature (typically 22°C) and relative humidity (typically 55%) are low, patients lose heat rapidly unless steps are taken to maintain normothermia. In addition, if body cavities are open with exposure of viscera, this heat loss can be even more substantial. Perioperative hypothermia is common and occurs in about half of all surgical patients.[44] Research into perioperative temperature homeostasis has unraveled a wide range of pathophysiological adverse effects that hypothermia has on surgical patients, which extends beyond the immediate postoperative period. Avoidance of hypothermia has also been shown to be an effective way of avoiding or treating many of these complications and improving outcomes. The complications of hypothermia include hematologic and immune effects, particularly coagulopathy, acidosis, cardiac dysrhythmias and infarction, and an increased risk of infection and poor healing. There is level I evidence that perioperative warming significantly reduces SSI, the need for blood transfusion, cardiac events and is cost-effective in reducing morbidity, mortality, and hospital stay.[45] A National Institute for Clinical Excellence guideline (in the United Kingdom) has been issued to address hypothermia as a predictor of poor postoperative outcome.[46]

The use of conventional blankets, even if warmed or reflective, is insufficient and it could be argued now that it is a critical incident to have perioperative hypothermia (<36°C) and anesthesia; surgery should not proceed without its correction. Many strategies can be used to maintain patient temperature and have included:

- Intravenous fluid warmers and warmed inhaled anesthetic gases
- Warm irrigation fluids, particularly warmed thoracic and abdominal lavage
- Warmed ORs (which are uncomfortable for the operating team)
- Forced warm-air devices placed on the patient in areas outside the sterile field, although they may disrupt laminar air flow[47,48]
- Local and systemic warming using resistive polymer mattresses and overblankets

The latter two methods have been shown to be the most effective.[49,50]

Prevention of Decubitus Ulcers

The in-patient incidence of pressure sores in secondary care is approximately 10–15%; half of these are nosocomially acquired and mostly of an early stage, where there is nonblanchable erythema (stage I), which may progress to partial thickness skin loss involving epidermis and dermis (stage II). Pressure ulcers are defined by the National Pressure Ulcer Advisory Panel as being a localized injury to skin and/or underlying tissue, usually over a bony prominence, as a result of pressure in combination with shear.[51,52] Elderly patients undergoing operation are at particular risk, more so when they are hypothermic or have other risk factors such as obesity or severe cachexia or neurological impairment. During operation and in the recovery period, all patients need protection of their bony prominences: ischium, trochanters, sacrum, heels, and malleoli. Protection includes pressure dispersion mattresses and cushions, regular turning when possible and skin care to avoid moisture and soiling. Stage III and IV pressure ulcers, respectively, involve tissue loss into the subcutaneous tissues or deeper to muscle and bone. They are a cause of considerable morbidity and mortality and present a large microbial reservoir needing extensive debridement, wound dressing, and nurse care.

Prevention of Peripheral Nerve and Arterial Injuries

During the operation all superficial nerve points at risk, such as the ulnar and peroneal nerves at the elbow and knee, must be protected against injury. There is a higher risk during prolonged limb surgery, and pressure-dispersing boards used to position limbs during surgery must be checked regularly for risk of traction injury. Vascular injuries and compartment syndromes can be avoided by supervised tourniquet times and the avoidance of tight bandaging or antiembolic stockings, particularly in patients with known arterial compromise. Failure to prevent these injuries is associated with considerable litigation.

SURGICAL INSTRUMENTS

Appropriate surgical instruments must be readily available during the operative procedure and may be tailored for specific surgeon preference. Difficulties can be minimized by attention to the WHO "safe surgery saves lives" checklists. Instrumentation may be made available by equipping ORs for certain procedures, thereby avoiding redundancy between prepared instrument trays, and be stocked with specialty equipment, such as for eye operations or laparoscopy. Experienced personnel and equipment for specific services need to match the increases in surgical technology, such as robotic surgery. However, this dedication decreases any desired flexibility in OR assistants and is only feasible if the number of surgical procedures and case mix are large.

Laparoscopic surgery is associated with an increase in the use of disposable instrumentation, with attendant concerns of waste disposal and cost-effectiveness.[53,54] Single-use instruments have the advantage of availability, increased sharpness, and decreased reprocessing costs; disadvantages include increased cost, wastage when instruments are opened but not used, and space requirements for the increased inventory.

Sutures and Needles (Including Blunt Needle Technology)

There is evidence of surgical closure of wounds using sutures in an Egyptian scroll from 3,500 BCE. The Egyptians used thorns and needles, with various threads, and adhesive linen strips to close wounds. By 1,000 BCE, the surgeons of India were using sutures of horsehair, cotton, and leather. In Roman times, linen and silk together with metal clips called fibulae were commonly used on gladiators. By the turn of the late 19th century, the developments in the textile industry led to major advances in suture material and silk and catgut became popular as suture materials. The sterilization of suture material, introduced by Lord Lister, made it possible to bury permanent sutures in clean wounds without resultant infection. Although individual preferences play a major role in suture selection, certain guidelines must be followed to achieve optimal wound healing; interestingly, silk and catgut are no longer widely used because of the inflammatory reaction they promote with uncertain loss of integrity. These natural materials have been replaced by synthetic absorbable and non-absorbable polymers, which can be tailored for their individual use as monofilaments or braids; coated to allow smooth passage through tissues and to knot securely; with the smallest diameter to minimize the amount of suture material placed in tissue (which can be a nidus for biofilm and infection); and have an ability to retain tensile strength as long as required.[55] Suture diameters vary from 0.02–0.8 mm, corresponding to 0.2–8 on the metric system (millimeters times ten) and 10/0–5 on the British Pharmacopoeia (BP) system.

The incorporation of the antiseptic triclosan into sutures either as a coating (such as polyglactin) or impregnation (as in polydioxanone) has shown promise as an effective risk reduction strategy for prevention of SSIs. A meta-analysis has documented that the use of triclosan-coated (impregnated) braided or monofilament sutures represents Cochrane 1a evidence as an effective strategy for reducing the risk of SSI in clean and clean-contaminated surgical procedures.[56]

Metal Sutures, Clips, and Staples

Stainless steel wire is the strongest and least reactive permanent suture. Despite its strength, however, wire is not particularly durable and fracture of wire with time is not uncommon. Its handling characteristics are also poor and great care must be taken to prevent cutting through the tissue, and its current usage is primarily restricted to operations involving ligaments, tendons, or bone. Metal clips for skin also allow quick, accurate closure. Disposable units are more expensive than Michel clips, although the saving in operative time more than makes up for their expense. All clips are easy to remove and give cosmetically acceptable scars.

A linear mechanical stapling device was first used successfully by Humer Hültl in Hungary for gastric surgery, but now there is now a wide choice of linear, side-by-side, and end-to-end stapling devices that give strong, predictable suture lines. The staplers also allow access to difficult areas, such as transthoracic or esophagogastric anastomoses, or after anterior resection to allow a very low anastomosis without the need for a colostomy. Their use in surgery is described in the appropriate sections of this book. Most staple units are entirely disposable, but this makes them expensive to use. There are three basic types of gastrointestinal stapling device:

1. *Linear staplers*, which give a linear, terminal, everting staple line: used for end closure of a viscus (e.g. duodenal stump closure in polya gastrectomy).
2. *Side-to-side staplers*, with or without a knife blade, for transection of a viscus between staple rows: a linear inverting anastomosis with transection (used for side-to-side intestinal anastomoses such as gastroenterostomy); a linear staple line without transection: used for fashioning enteric reservoirs (e.g. ileal pouch), or a linear staple line with transection used for closure of a viscus (e.g. small bowel resection).
3. *End-to-end staplers* are used for circular, inverting, end-to-end gastrointestinal anastomosis (e.g. closure of colostomy following Hartmann's procedure). These also incorporate a circular knife blade.

Ligating and dividing surgical staplers are used for simultaneously ligating and dividing blood vessels with metal staples (particularly useful for dividing mesenteric or omental vessels). Advances in laparoscopic surgery in recent years also owe much to the refinement of clip and stapling devices designed to be used with laparoscopic instruments and are addressed in the appropriate parts of this book.

Needles

The choice of surgical needle is as important as the choice of suture. Cutting needles have at least two sharp cutting edges and are used for suturing skin and bone. Tapered or round needles pierce and spread tissue without cutting and are used for approximating soft tissue, hollow organs and vascular structures. The needle holder also needs to be appropriate to the needle to prevent breakage or bending. A large needle holder can damage a small needle, and a large needle is unmanageable in a small needle holder. Virtually all needles used today are swaged onto the accompanying suture, thus minimizing the size discrepancy between needle and suture. Swaged needles can be easily detached from the suture, which can be avoided by careful placement of the needle holder. The passage of a needle through tissue should follow the curvature of a needle. This minimizes tissue damage. The appropriate size and shape of cutting, or round-bodied atraumatic needle, needs to be chosen for the least traumatic passage through tissue. Shaped needles allow easier access for suturing. Examples are the J-shaped needle in low-approach femoral hernia repair, or the compound curve in ophthalmic surgery. Hand needles should be avoided because of the risk of needlestick injury. The tips of laparotomy closure needles are deliberately blunted by some of their manufacturers to reduce the risk of needlestick injury. Needles may come with a loop suture (to avoid a knot at the end of a laparotomy) or as double-ended sutures.

Electrocautery

Electrocautery (diathermy) became widely used in after the development of inflammable inhalational anesthetics in the 1950s. There are two types of electrocautery:

- Monopolar
- Bipolar

Both types draw high-voltage, high-frequency current from an electric generator, the major difference being the

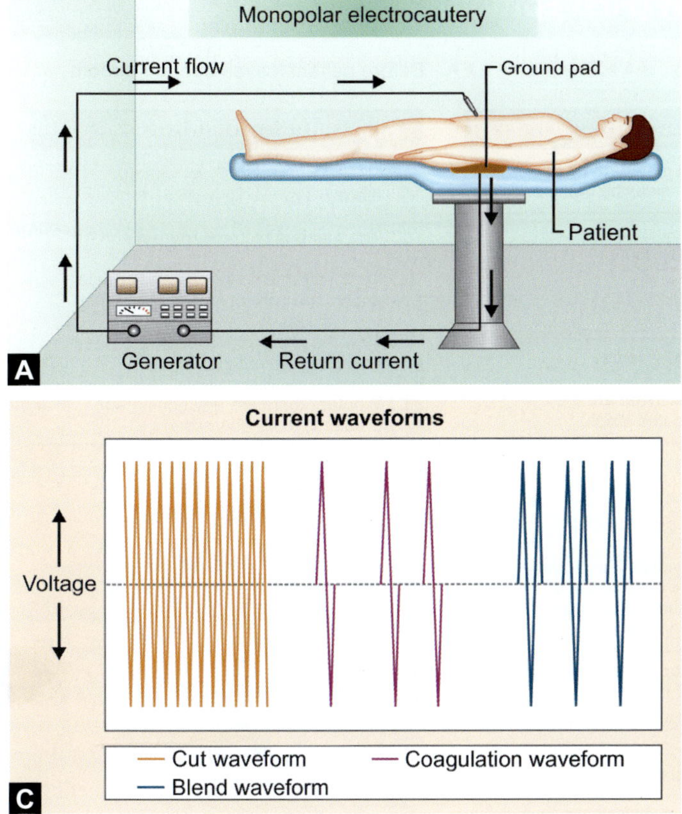

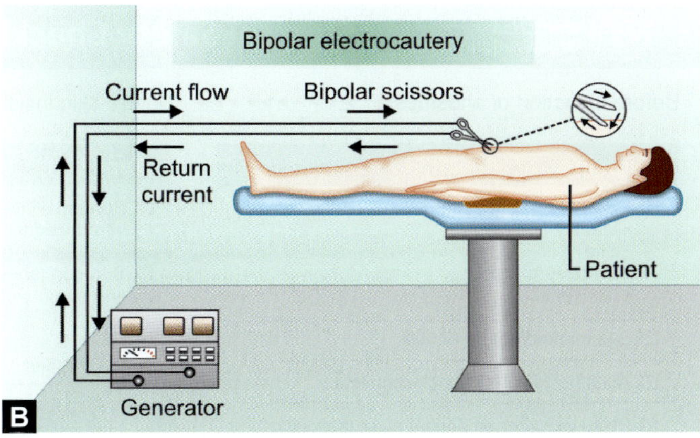

Figs. 3.5A to C: (A) *Monopolar electrocautery*, in which the current passes from the instrument, through the patient, and back to the generator through the grounding pad. (B) *Bipolar electrocautery* in which the current passes from one electrode to the other and back to the generator. The patient is part of the circuit. (C) *Current waveforms*, the constant current in the cutting diathermy wave form maintains the temperature needed for dissection. The pulsed coagulation wave form produces a lower current density and less heat allowing coagulation rather than vaporization of tissue. The blended waveform combines both cutting and coagulation characteristics, which can be adjusted by the surgeon.

method of grounding the current. A monopolar instrument consists of a single active electrode, which distributes the high-voltage current from the generator. The grounding pad is attached distally to the patient and returns current to the generator (Fig. 3.5A). Therefore, in monopolar electrocautery the patient is part of the circuit. In bipolar diathermy the handheld instrument has both an active and return electrode. Current travels from one electrode back to the other and passes only through the small section of tissue that lies between the two electrodes (Fig. 3.5B). Therefore, in bipolar electrocautery the patient is not part of the circuit.

The advantages of monopolar electrocautery are ease and versatility as it can provide effective and rapid hemostasis. However, monopolar circuits can create the potential for patient injury, for example, as a result of incomplete grounding, which exposes the patient to a burn injury. As the patient is part of the circuit, monopolar electrocautery can also deprogram implanted pacemakers.

By contrast, bipolar electrocautery is highly focused to the surgical wound, which reduces the risk of burn injury. Lower voltage and power settings can be used, because the electrodes are close, with less tissue destruction. The disadvantage is that, with these lower energy outputs, longer time is needed to coagulate larger vessels effectively and it is ineffective in tissue dissection.

Changes in current frequency give waveforms, which are useful for cutting tissue or coagulating tissue (Fig. 3.5C). The cutting constant waveform produces heat very rapidly to achieve tissue vaporization. There is very little thermal effect beyond the immediate area receiving the current, and therefore there is almost no coagulation or hemostasis. A coagulating waveform varies in voltage and current size. In contrast to cutting diathermy the temperature produced by a coagulating current, about 70°C, is too low to vaporize cells. Heat penetration is deep, with thermal damage to surrounding tissue with the burnt tissue forming a coagulum. By varying the waveform, it is possible to blend the cutting and coagulation characteristics to meet specific needs.

The use of electrocautery can markedly impair cardiac pacemaker function. When it cannot be avoided in a patient who has an implantable pacemaker, several intraoperative precautions should be observed: bipolar

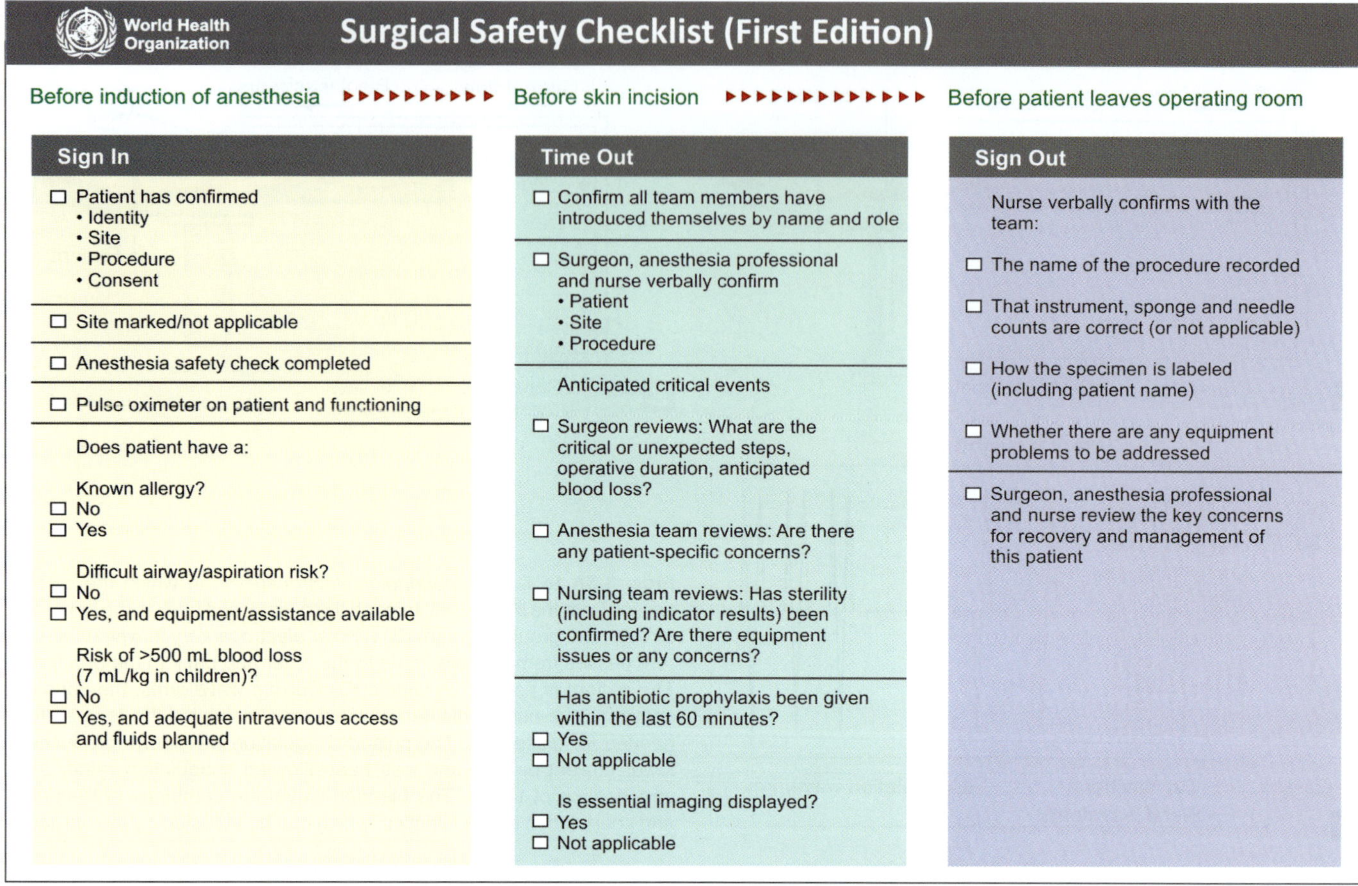

World Health Organization

Surgical Safety Checklist (First Edition)

Before induction of anesthesia ▶▶▶▶▶▶▶▶▶▶ Before skin incision ▶▶▶▶▶▶▶▶▶▶▶▶▶ Before patient leaves operating room

Sign In

- ☐ Patient has confirmed
  - Identity
  - Site
  - Procedure
  - Consent
- ☐ Site marked/not applicable
- ☐ Anesthesia safety check completed
- ☐ Pulse oximeter on patient and functioning

Does patient have a:

Known allergy?
- ☐ No
- ☐ Yes

Difficult airway/aspiration risk?
- ☐ No
- ☐ Yes, and equipment/assistance available

Risk of >500 mL blood loss (7 mL/kg in children)?
- ☐ No
- ☐ Yes, and adequate intravenous access and fluids planned

Time Out

- ☐ Confirm all team members have introduced themselves by name and role
- ☐ Surgeon, anesthesia professional and nurse verbally confirm
  - Patient
  - Site
  - Procedure

Anticipated critical events
- ☐ Surgeon reviews: What are the critical or unexpected steps, operative duration, anticipated blood loss?
- ☐ Anesthesia team reviews: Are there any patient-specific concerns?
- ☐ Nursing team reviews: Has sterility (including indicator results) been confirmed? Are there equipment issues or any concerns?

Has antibiotic prophylaxis been given within the last 60 minutes?
- ☐ Yes
- ☐ Not applicable

Is essential imaging displayed?
- ☐ Yes
- ☐ Not applicable

Sign Out

Nurse verbally confirms with the team:
- ☐ The name of the procedure recorded
- ☐ That instrument, sponge and needle counts are correct (or not applicable)
- ☐ How the specimen is labeled (including patient name)
- ☐ Whether there are any equipment problems to be addressed
- ☐ Surgeon, anesthesia professional and nurse review the key concerns for recovery and management of this patient

This checklist is not intended to be comprehensive. Additions and modifications to fit local practice are encouraged.

Fig. 3.6: The World Health Organization checklist.

diathermy instruments minimize the electrical field around the cautery unit, and if monopolar cautery is used, the grounding pad should be placed as far from the pacemaker as possible.

CONCLUSION

The range of operative procedures is wide and increasingly complex and continues to widen to a level inconceivable a generation ago. As surgery progresses, so must the development of the OR environment for the safety of operating staff and, more importantly, our patients. Cultural change may be needed, just as it has in the aviation industry, to ensure best and safest performance. The use of checklists has been advocated by the WHO (Fig. 3.6) and their adoption, together with the use of care bundles and audited compliance, will help ensure this.[57-59]

REFERENCES

1. Cima RR, Brown MJ, Hebl JR, et al. Use of lean six sigma methodology to improve operating room efficiency in a high-volume tertiary care academic medical center. J Am Coll Surg. 2011;213:83-92.
2. Weston A, Caldera K, Doron S. Surgical care improvement project in the value-based purchasing era: more harm than good? Clin Infect Dis. 2013;56:424-7.
3. ANSI/ASHRAE/ASHE Standard. Ventilation of Healthcare Facilities Standard 170-2008. ASHRAE Standards Committee, January 29, 2011, Atlanta, GA.
4. Edmiston CE, Seabrook GR, Cambria RA, et al. Molecular epidemiology of microbial contamination in the operating room environment: is there a risk for infection? Surgery. 2005;138:573-82.
5. Diab-Elschahawi M, Berger J, Blacky A, et al. Impact of different-sized laminar air flow versus no laminar air flow on bacterial counts in the operating room during orthopedic surgery. Am J Infect Control. 2011;39:e25-9.
6. Memarzadeh F, Manning AP. Comparison of the operating ventilation systems in the protection of the surgical site. ASHRAE Trans. 2002;108(pt. 2):1-13.
7. Brandt C, Hott U, Sohr D, et al. Operating room ventilation with laminar airflow shows no protective effect on the surgical site infection rate in orthopedic and abdominal surgery. Ann Surg. 2008;248:695-700.

8. Lipsett PA. Do we really need laminar flow ventilation in the operating room to prevent surgical site infections? Ann Surg. 2008;248:701-3.
9. Bharathan R, Aggarwal R, Darzi A. Operating room of the future. Best Pract Res Obstet Gynecol. 2013;27:311-22.
10. Munoz-Price LS, Bimbach DJ, Lubarsky DA, et al. Decreasing operating room environmental pathogens contamination through improved cleaning practice. Infect Control Hosp Epidemiol. 2012;33:897-904.
11. Association of Operating Room Nurses. Standards, recommended practices, guidelines: 2012. Denver: AORN Publications; 2012.
12. Occupational Safety & Health Administration. Occupational Exposure to Blood-borne Pathogens (Final Rule, 29CFR, Part 1910.1030). Fed Regist. 1991;56(sec 6):64040-182.
13. Leonas KK. Effect of laundering on barrier properties of reusable surgical gown fabric. Am J Infect Control. 1008; 26:495-501.
14. Belkin NL. Evaluating the protective value of hospital gowns. Am J Infect Control. 1999;27:178-9.
15. Quebbeman EJ, Telford GL, Hubbard S, et al. In-use evaluation of surgical gowns. Surg Gynecol Obstet. 1992;174: 369-75.
16. Telford GL, Quebbeman EJ. Barriers protecting the operating room personnel. In: Malangoni MA (Ed). Critical Issues in Operating Room Management. Philadelphia: Lippincott-Raven Publishers; 1997. pp. 191-202.
17. Popejoy SL, Fry DE. Blood contact and exposure in the operating room. Surg Gynecol Obstet. 1991;172:480-3.
18. Quebbeman EJ, Telford GL, Hubbard S, et al. Risk of blood contamination and injury to operating room personnel. Ann Surg. 1991;214:614-20.
19. Wright JG, McGeer AJ, Chyatte D, et al. Mechanisms of glove tears and sharps injuries among surgical personnel. JAMA. 1991;266:1668-71.
20. Driever R, Beie M, Schmitz E, et al. Surgical glove perforation in cardiac surgery. Thorac Cardiovasc Surg. 2001;49:328-30.
21. Hartley JE, Ahmed S, Milkins R, et al. Randomized trial of blunt-tipped versus cutting edge needles to reduce glove puncture during mass closure of the abdomen. Br J Surg. 1996;83:1156-7.
22. Thomas S, Agarwal M, Mehta G. Intraoperative glove perforation: single gloves versus double-gloving in protection against skin contamination. Postgrad Med J. 2001;77:458-60.
23. Hendricksen D, Miller RF, Quigg DL, et al. Effect of cap and mask on infection rates. Ir Med J. 1984;165:397-9.
24. Mitchell J, Hunt S. Surgical face mask in the modern operating room. A costly and unnecessary ritual? J Hosp Infect. 1991;18:239-42.
25. Lypp A, Edwards P. Disposable surgical face mask: a systematic review. Can Oper Room Nurs J. 2005;23:20-38.
26. Edmiston CE, Seabrook GR, Cambria RA, et al. Molecular epidemiology of microbial contamination in the operating room environment: is there a risk for infections? Surgery. 2005;138:572-88.
27. Edmiston CE, Krepel CJ, Seabrook GR, et al. The preoperative shower revisited: can high topical antiseptic levels be achieved on the skin surface prior to surgical admission? J Am Coll Surg. 2008;207;233-9.
28. Eiselt D. Presurgical skin preparation with a novel 2% chlorhexidine gluconate cloth reduces rates of surgical site infection in orthopaedic surgical patients. Orthop Nurs. 2009;28;141-5.
29. Lipke VL, Hyott AS. Reducing surgical site infections by bundling multiple risk reduction strategies and active surveillance. AORN J. 2010;92:288-96.
30. Jones RS, Brown C, Opelka F. Surgeon compensation: "Pay for Performance": the American College of Surgeons National Surgical Quality Improvement Program, the Surgical Care Improvement Program and other programs. Surgery. 2005;138:829-36.
31. Fry DE, Telford GL, Fectceau DL, et al. Prevention of blood exposure: body and facial protection. Surg Clin North Am. 1995;75:1141-57.
32. Mangram AJ, Horan TC, Pearson ML, et al. The Hospital Infection Control Practice Advisory Committee, Guidelines for the prevention of surgical site infections. Am J Infect Control. 1999;27:97-132.
33. Darouiche RO, Wall MJ, Itani KM, et al. Chlorhexidine-alcohol versus povidone-iodine for surgical-site antisepsis. N Eng J Med. 2010;362:18-26.
34. Lee I, Agarwal RK, Lee BY, et al. Systematic review and cost analysis comparing use of chlorhexidine with use of iodine for preoperative skin antisepsis to prevent surgical site infection. Infect Control Hosp Epidemiol. 2010;31: 1219-29.
35. Padnos YD, Williams RA. Fires in the operating room. Bull Am Coll Surg. 1997;82:14-7.
36. Duensing RA, Mueller GP, Williams RA. Hazards in the operating room. In: Malangoni MA (Ed). Critical Issues in Operating Room Management. Philadelphia: Lippincott-Raven; 1997. pp. 231-51.
37. Hussair SA, Latif ABA, Choudhary A. Risk to surgeons: a survey of accidental injuries during operations. Br J Surg. 1988;75:314-6.
38. Quebbeman EJ, Telford GL, Wadsworth K, et al. Double gloving: protecting surgeons from blood contamination in the operating room. Arch Surg. 1992;127:213-6.
39. Fry DE, Flint LM. Hepatitis: an overview of important issues. Bull Am Coll Surg. 1997;82:8-13.
40. Howard RJ, Fry DE, Davis JM, et al. Hepatitis C virus infection in healthcare worker. J Am Coll Surg. 1997;184: 540-52.
41. Gatti JE, Bryant CJ, Noone RB, et al. The mutagenicity of electrocautery smoke. Plast Reconstr Surg. 1992;89:781-4.
42. Tomita Y, Mihashi S, Nagata K, et al. Mutagenicity of smoke condensation induced by CO_2 laser irradiation and electrocauterization. Mutat Res. 1981;39:145-9.
43. Edward BE, Reiman RE. Comparison of current and past surgical smoke control practices. AORN J. 2012;95:337-50.
44. Kumar S, Wong PF, Melling AC, et al. Effects of perioperative hypothermia and warming in surgical practice. Int Wound J. 2005;2:193-204.

45. Mahoney CB, Odom J. Maintaining intraoperative normothermia: a meta-analysis of outcomes with costs. Am Assoc Nurse Anesth J. 1999;67:155-63.
46. Inadvertent perioperative hypothermia: the management of inadvertent perioperative hypothermia in adults. [online] NICE Guideline CG65. 2008. (www.nice.org.uk/CG065fullguideline). Accessed April 5, 2013.
47. Kurz A, Sessler DI, Lenhardt R. Perioperative normothermia to reduce the incidence of surgical wound infection and shorten hospitalization. N Engl J Med. 1996;334:1209-15.
48. McGovern PD, Albrecht M, Belani KG, et al. Forced-air warming and ultra-clean ventilation do not mix. An investigation of theatre ventilation, patient warming and joint replacement infection in orthopaedics. J Bone Joint Surg. 2011;93-B:1537-44.
49. Melling AC, Ali B, Scott EM, et al. Effects of preoperative warming on the incidence of wound infection after clean surgery: a randomised controlled trial. Lancet. 2001;358:876-80.
50. Wong PF, Kumar S, Bohra A, et al. Randomised clinical trial of perioperative systemic warming in major elective abdominal surgery. Br J Surg. 2007;94:421-6.

Additional references appear in the online version of this book.

4

Wound Healing

Adrian Barbul, Jordan Fishman

Key Points

- There are four separate but overlapping phases of wound healing.
- Both deficiencies and excess in wound healing are major clinical problems that surgeons encounter frequently in their practice.
- Appropriate antibiotic prophylaxis significantly reduces the incidence of postoperative wound infections.
- Clinicians should be alert to patients who are susceptible to the development of chronic wounds as preventive prophylactic therapy may avoid the development of these lesions, which are difficult to heal once they have developed.

INTRODUCTION

Successful wound healing is fundamental and essential to all surgical disciplines. The resection of diseased tissue and restoration of function to an organ involve the creation of a wound. The process of wound healing is similar, whether the procedure is removal of a portion of the brain or an anastomosis between two segments of the gastrointestinal tract. Surgeons are often called upon to manage accidental wounds resulting from trauma and burns, and to care for wounds that arise from chronic disease and debilitation. As mammals are generally incapable of tissue regeneration, repair of an injured organ depends upon a complex process that involves inflammatory cell migration and cytokine actions, collagen and extracellular matrix deposition, and scar remodeling. All wound healing results in the formation of scar and, therefore, by definition it remains an imperfect, albeit effective, process. The process of wound repair differs little from one tissue to another and is generally independent of the nature of injury. The body has a number of elaborate and redundant mechanisms that complement one another to facilitate healing and multiple factors influence the wound-healing process. Poor wound healing leading to an adverse outcome can result from:

- Surgical technique
- Host factors and
- Factors in the external environment

Understanding the process of healing and the factors that favor or impede healing has direct application to the care of surgical patients. The surgeon can have a positive impact on healing by:

- Selecting and creating an appropriate incision
- Choosing appropriate suture materials, and
- Attending to host and local factors that influence wound outcome.

HISTORICAL PERSPECTIVE AND OVERVIEW

Long before the practice of medicine necessitated the creation of therapeutic (surgical) wounds, ancient healers were tasked with the care of mostly traumatic wounds. Despite popular misconception, "primitive" wound care was often superior to that practiced until at least the late 16th century. The earliest extant medical text, a Sumerian tablet from 2,100 BCE, describes "the three healing gestures": cleaning the wound, the application of protective topical agents, and dressing the wound. These basic tenets of wound healing were practiced by the Egyptians (as described in the Ebers Papyrus, ca 1,400 BCE), the Greeks (as codified in the Hippocratic Collection) and in the ancient Levant (Luke, 10:34). By the first century CE, Roman wound care, as described by Cornelius Celsus and Galen, had advanced to include the successful treatment of large, traumatic wounds with hemostasis by ligation.

Many of the components of historic wound salves (wine, honey, myrrh, and frankincense, to name a few) have been shown to possess antiseptic and bactericidal properties, and some are still in use today.[1]

Knowledge of effective wound care was lost following the fall of the Roman Empire. Throughout the Middle Ages, standard treatment was to allow the wound to "rot a bit" in the hopes that it would be colonized by less virulent bacteria, instead of one that would cause rapid wound sepsis and death. Wound care practices further deteriorated with the introduction of gunpowder and bullet wounds. The contemporary explanation for the rapidity with which bullet wounds became gangrenous, and therefore lethal, was that poison was introduced from the gunpowder into the wound. Treatment paradigms consisted of efforts to remove this poison, often by pouring burning oil onto the wound. In 1545 Ambroise Paré exhausted his supply oil and treated a wound with egg yolk and turpentine. Expecting his patient to die, he returned the next morning to find him faring better than his companions.[2] Three hundred years later, Joseph Lister introduced wound dressings soaked in carbolic acid, and for the first time in recorded history, complex wounds that were previously uniformly fatal healed by primary intention without mortality.[3]

Further advances in medical science with understanding of the pathophysiologic response to injury and cellular repair mechanisms have led to an increase in survivability of major catastrophic wounds such as burns and destructive ballistic injuries. While much has been accomplished since the Ebers Papyrus, wound care still presents many unsolved clinical and research challenges.

Although most mammalian tissues do not regenerate, some organs compensate for lost mass by hypertrophy or hyperplasia. This phenomenon is most notable in the liver. It is a complex process governed by both cellular and humoral factors. The major healing pathway in mammals is scar formation, which has the advantage that it is quick, predictable and functionally acceptable. Scar formation can overwhelm and overtake the process of hypertrophy, as occurs in patients with liver cirrhosis in which the injured liver tissue is replaced by scar.

The observation that exuberant cellular and biochemical responses triggered by injury are remarkably similar to tissue responses in neoplastic growth has paved the way for new and potentially significant insights into the factors that control cellular growth and may have an impact on the understanding of carcinogenesis. Many of the participating cells, their surface receptors and responses to ligands and cytokines are similar in both these processes. Characteristically, in wounds there is an orderly "phasing down" of this cellular response with the onset of the remodeling phase, which leads to a strong, supple, and cellular scar. In this respect, tumors are "wounds that do not heal"[1] because their early cellular, vascular, and inflammatory responses are not replaced by a remodeling phase but instead continue unabated. Many investigators of wound healing believe that to decipher the "on" and "off" signals for wound repair will provide significant advances in the understanding and treatment of neoplastic disorders.

Chronic disease states, such as diabetes, vascular insufficiency, and paralysis, often result in the generation of acute and chronic wounds recalcitrant to current wound care strategies. As more is understood of the complex biology underlying the wound-healing process, wound care treatments will likely progress past the three healing gestures.

PHASES OF WOUND HEALING

Injury triggers an organized and complex cascade of cellular and biochemical events resulting in a healed wound. The wound-healing response can be divided into four separate, but overlapping, phases:

- Hemostasis and inflammation
- Proliferation
- Maturation and remodeling and
- Wound contraction[4]

Failure or prolongation in any one phase may result in delay of healing or nonclosure of the wound.

Hemostasis and Inflammation

The obligatory rupture of vessels that accompanies injury exposes the subendothelial collagen to platelets, which results in aggregation of platelets and activation of the intrinsic part of the coagulation cascade. The contact between collagen and platelets as well as the presence of thrombin, fibronectin, and their fragments results in the release of cytokines and growth factors from platelet a-granules, such as platelet-derived growth factor (PDGF), transforming growth factor-beta (TGF-β), platelet-activating factor, fibronectin, and serotonin (Table. 4.1). The locally formed fibrin clot serves as a scaffolding for invading cells such as neutrophils, monocytes, fibroblasts, and endothelial cells. Inadequate clot formation, such as

Table 4.1 Hemostatic and platelet-derived factors associated with wound healing.

Hemostatic factors	*Function*
Fibrin, plasma fibronectin	Coagulation, chemoattractant, adhesive, serves as scaffolding for cell migration
Factor XIII (fibrin stabilizing factor)	Induces chemoattraction, induces adhesion
Circulatory growth factors	Regulation of chemoattraction, mitogenesis, fibroplasia
Complement	Antimicrobial activity, chemoattractant
Platelet-derived factors	Function
Cytokines, growth factors (TGF-β, PDGF)	Regulation of chemoattraction, mitogenesis, fibroplasia
Fibronectin	Early matrix, ligand for platelet aggregation
Platelet-activating factor	Platelet aggregation
Thromboxane A_2	Vasoconstriction, platelet aggregation, chemotactic factor
Platelet factor IV	Chemotactic for fibroblasts and monocytes, neutralizes activity of heparin, inhibits collagenase
Serotonin	Induces vascular permeability, chemoattractant for neutrophils
Adenosine dinucleotide	Stimulates cell proliferation, migration, induces platelet aggregation
PDGF, platelet-derived growth factor; TGF-β, transforming growth factor-β	Orchestrate collagen deposition and maturation

observed in factor XIII (fibrin stabilizing factor) deficiency, is associated with impaired wound healing secondary to either decreased adhesion of cells into the inflammatory area or decreased chemotaxis.

The inflammatory phase is an essential event of healing, characterized by increased vascular permeability, chemotaxis of cells from the circulation into the wound milieu, local release of cytokines and growth factors, and activation of migrating cells. Within 6 hours of injury circulating immune cells migrate into the wound. Polymorphonuclear leukocytes (PMNs) are the first blood leukocytes to enter the wound site and their numbers increase steadily, peaking at 24–48 hours. Increased vascular permeability caused by inflammation and release of prostaglandin, together with a concentration gradient of chemotactic substances such as complement factors, interleukin-1 (IL-1), tumor necrosis factor-alpha (TNF-α), TGF-β, platelet factor 4, and bacterial products stimulate neutrophil migration. The main function of the PMNs is phagocytosis of bacteria and tissue debris. The presence of PMNs is not essential for healing to take place provided bacterial contamination has not occurred.[5]

The next cellular immune elements to enter the wound are the macrophages. These cells, derived from circulating monocytes, migrate within the wound 48–96 hours after injury, and their number reaches a peak around the third day after injury. Wound macrophages have a much longer life span than the PMNs and persist in the wound until healing is complete. Their appearance is followed by that of lymphocytes, which occur in significant numbers around the 5th day after injury, with peak numbers on about the 7th day after injury. In contrast to PMNs, the presence and activation of both macrophages and lymphocytes in the wound is critical to progression of the normal healing process.[6,7]

Chemotaxis of cells into the wound milieu is followed by cellular activation, which signifies the phenotypic alteration of cellular, biochemical, and functional properties induced by local mediators. Although neutrophils, macrophages, and lymphocytes predominate during inflammation, the contribution of each cell population to successful wound healing is variable.

Activation of macrophages has fundamental implications in several aspects of wound healing, such as debridement, matrix synthesis, and angiogenesis. The initial and brief release of factors from platelets is a first and strong stimulus of macrophage activation. Activated macrophages release cytokines, which mediate angiogenesis and fibroplasia[8] and synthesize nitric oxide (NO), which has antimicrobial properties and stimulates collagen synthesis.[9,10] Many other cells, including endothelial cells, fibroblasts, monocytes, and lymphocytes, can be activated to produce NO. Synthesis of NO is reduced during impaired wound healing,[11] and this inhibition results in diminished healing responses.[12] Macrophages evolve phenotypically as healing progresses, for example, switching from NO synthesis and inflammatory function to arginase expression and more synthetic functions.[13] Activation of cells during wound healing also means profound phenotypic changes in certain cell populations such as the fibroblasts[14,15] and epidermal cells. Fibroblasts derived from the wound environment—wound fibroblasts—demonstrate increased collagen synthesis, increased matrix contraction, and decreased proliferation when compared with normal dermal fibroblasts.[16] These phenotypic alterations occur within the wound environment secondary to the action of macrophage-derived cytokines or surrounding matrix molecules such as fibronectin.[17,18]

The inflammatory phase of healing is vital to the proper evolution of the subsequent phases of healing. Reduced inflammatory responses profoundly affect subsequent healing, as observed clinically in patients who have diabetes mellitus or secondary to corticosteroid treatment.[19]

Proliferation

The proliferative phase involves a number of events and important cellular elements.

Angiogenesis

Revascularization of the wound proceeds in parallel with fibroplasia. Capillary buds sprout from blood vessels adjacent to the wound and extend into the wound space. On the second day after injury endothelial cells from the side of the venule closest to the wound begin to migrate in response to angiogenic stimuli. These capillary sprouts eventually branch at their tips and join to form capillary loops, through which blood begins to flow. New sprouts then extend from these loops to form a capillary plexus.[20,21]

The soluble factors responsible for angiogenesis remain incompletely defined. It appears that angiogenesis occurs by a combination of proliferation and migration. Putative mediators for endothelial cell growth and chemotaxis include cytokines produced by platelets, macrophages and lymphocytes in the wound,[22,23] low oxygen tension,[24] lactic acid,[25] and biogenic amines.[26] Of the potential cytokine mediators of neovascularization, vascular endothelial growth factor (VEGF) is one of the most potent; basic fibroblast growth factor (bFGF), acidic fibroblast growth factor, TGF-β, epidermal growth factor (EGF), and TGF-β have all been shown to play a role in stimulating new blood vessel formation.[27-30] Mesenchymal cells themselves can be induced to release growth factors and cytokines in an autocrine manner, so continuing the angiogenic process.

Fibroplasia

Fibroplasia is the process of fibroblast proliferation and matrix synthetic activity. Significant numbers of fibroblasts first appear in the wound on the 3rd day after injury and achieve peak numbers around the 7th day.[31] Fibroblasts in the surrounding tissue need to become activated from their quiescent state in which they are nonreplicative (Table 4.2). Growth factors such as PDGF or EGF induce chemotaxis and proliferation of fibroblasts. The rapid expansion in the fibroblast population at the wound site results from a combination of proliferation and migration.[32] Fibroblasts are derived from local mesenchymal cells, particularly those associated with blood vessel adventitia.[33] They are attracted to the wound and induced to proliferate by cytokines released initially from platelets and subsequently from macrophages and lymphocytes. Fibroblasts are the primary synthetic element in the repair process and are responsible for producing the majority of structural proteins necessary for tissue reconstruction. The main protein product of fibroblasts is collagen, a family of triple-chain glycoproteins that form the main constituent of the extracellular wound matrix; these are ultimately responsible for imparting tensile strength to the scar. Collagen is first detected in the wound around the 3rd day after injury.[34,35] The levels then increase rapidly for approximately 3 weeks. It continues to accumulate at a more gradual pace for up to 3 months after wounding. Recently, a circulating population of fibrocytes (<0.5% of nonerythrocytic circulating cells) has been defined as contributing to the healing fibroblastic population and contributing to collagen synthesis.[36]

Collagen is initially deposited in a seemingly haphazard fashion. Subsequently, the individual collagen fibrils are reorganized by cross-linking into regularly aligned bundles oriented along the lines of stress in the healing wound. Fibroblasts are also responsible for the production of other matrix constituents, including fibronectin, hyaluronic acid, and the glycosaminoglycans.[37]

Table 4.2 Functional characteristics of wound-activated fibroblasts when compared with those of resident tissue fibroblasts.

Function	*Change in wound-activated fibroblasts*
Proliferation	↓
Collagen synthesis	↓
Protein synthesis	↔
Matrix ground substance synthesis	↑
Matrix contraction	↑
Nitric oxide synthesis	↑

Epithelialization

While granulation tissue and collagen synthesis are proceeding deep in the wound, epithelial integrity is being restored at the wound surface. Reepithelialization of the wound begins within a few hours of injury. Epithelial cells arising from either the wound margins or residual dermal epithelial appendages within the wound bed begin to migrate under the scab and over the underlying viable connective tissue. The epidermis immediately adjacent to the wound edge begins thickening within 24 hours after injury. Marginal basal cells at the edge of the wound lose their firm attachment to the underlying dermis, enlarge, and begin to migrate across the surface of the provisional matrix filling the wound. Fixed basal cells in a zone near the cut edge undergo a series of rapid mitotic divisions and migrate by moving over one another in a leapfrog fashion until the defect is covered.[38,39] Once the defect has been bridged, the migrating epithelial cells loose their flattened appearance, become more columnar in shape, and increase their mitotic activity. Layering of the epithelium is reestablished and the surface layer eventually keratinized.[40] Reepithelialization is complete in < 48 hours in approximated incised wounds but may take substantially longer in larger wounds in which there is a major tissue defect.

If only the epithelium is damaged, such as occurs in split-thickness skin graft donor sites and superficial second-degree burns, repair consists primarily of reepithelialization with minimal or absent fibroplasia and granulation tissue formation. The stimuli for reepithelialization remain incompletely defined, but it appears that the process is mediated by a combination of loss of contact inhibition, exposure of constituents of the extracellular matrix, particularly fibronectin,[41] and cytokines produced by immune mononuclear cells such as macrophages and lymphocytes.[42] In particular EGF, TGF-β, bFGF, PDGF, and insulin-like growth factor-1 have been shown to promote epithelialization. Macrophages and keratinocytes themselves are sources of cytokines and growth factors that act in autocrine and paracrine fashions. Although the mechanisms by which these factors enhance epithelialization are not clear, they all stimulate in vitro epithelial cell mitogenesis and/or chemotaxis.

Although much interest has been focused on the signals that "turn on" the proliferative phase, little is known about the signals that bring this phase to a controlled end. Stimuli for the activation of cells do not have to be long-lasting,[43] but the induced phenotypic alterations are often not maintained in vitro over time.[16,44] It is probable that negative feedback mechanisms play a role.

The destiny of some cells remains unclear after completion of their function in the wound-healing cascade. Neutrophils undergo apoptosis and are ingested by macrophages. Macrophages also undergo apoptosis and in the process release arginase, which influences wound metabolism.[45] Macrophages also play a role in decreasing the cellularity of healed wounds by ingesting apoptotic fibroblasts.[13]

Maturation and Remodeling

Matrix Deposition in the Wound

Changes in wound matrix composition follow a certain pattern over time: initially, the wound matrix is composed mainly of fibrin and fibronectin that originate from the hemostatic cascade and macrophages;[37] another protein expressed early is thrombospondin-1, which also supports cellular recruitment in the wound milieu.[46] Glycosaminoglycans, proteoglycans, and other proteins such as secreted protein acidic rich in cysteine are synthesized next and support future matrix deposition and remodeling.[46,47] Subsequently, collagens become the predominant scar protein.

The intact dermis is predominantly composed of collagen I (80–90%) and III (10–20%). In granulation tissue the proportion of type III collagen is increased (30%), whereas in the mature scar the proportion of type III collagen is low (10%).[48-50] The early appearance of type III collagen coincides with the presence of fibronectin—it has been proposed that the coating of denatured collagen with fibronectin facilitates its phagocytosis.[37,51] However, the role of the early deposition of type III collagen, which does not significantly contribute to the strength of the wound, remains unclear.[52,53]

Net collagen synthesis is increased for at least 4–5 weeks after wounding.[34,35] The increased rate of collagen synthesis during healing arises not only from the increased number of fibroblasts in the wound, but also from a net increase in collagen production by each cell.

The structure of the matrix changes with time as well. Normal dermis shows a basket-weave pattern, whereas in a healing wound thinner collagen fibers are arranged parallel to the scar. These thinner collagen fibers gradually thicken after wounding and organize along the stress line of the wound. This process is accompanied by increased scar strength, which indicates a positive correlation between fiber thickness and orientation with tensile strength.[54]

Biochemically, collagen derived from granulation tissue differs from collagen derived from nonwounded skin, with more hydroxylation and glycosylation of lysine residues, which correlates with a thinner fiber diameter.[55]

Despite a prolonged ongoing remodeling phase (up to 1 year), the orientation of collagen fibers in the healed scar tissue does not become as organized as in the intact dermis. As a functional corollary, scar breaking strength is always less than the strength of unwounded skin. A time course of the breaking strength shows that after 1 week the wound has only 3% and after 3 weeks 20% of its final strength.[49] After 3 months the scar has approximately 80% of the strength of unwounded skin and no further increase occurs.[56]

Collagen Metabolism

Collagen, the most abundant protein in the body, plays a critical role in the successful completion of wound healing. Its deposition, maturation, and subsequent remodeling are critical to the functional integrity of the wound.

Biochemically, each chain of collagen is composed of a glycine residue in every third position. The second position in the triplet is made up of proline or lysine during the translation process. The polypeptide chain that is translated from mRNA contains approximately 1,000 amino acid residues and is called protocollagen. Release of protocollagen into the endoplasmic reticulum results in the hydroxylation of proline into hydroxyproline and of lysine into hydroxylysine by specific hydroxylases. Prolyl hydroxylase requires oxygen and iron as cofactors, α-ketoglutarate as cosubstrate and ascorbic acid (vitamin C) as an electron donor. In the endoplasmic reticulum, the protocollagen chain is glycosylated by the linking of galactose and glucose at specific hydroxylysine residues. These steps of hydroxylation and glycosylation alter the hydrogen bonding forces within the chain, which imposes steric changes so that the protocollagen chain assumes an α-helical configuration. Three α-helical chains then entwine to form a right-handed superhelical structure called procollagen. This structure contains nonhelical peptide domains, named "registration peptides" at both ends. Although initially joined by weak ionic bonds, the procollagen molecule becomes much stronger through the covalent cross-linking of lysine residues. Collagen biosynthesis and its posttranslational modification are highly complex biochemical events (Table 4.3). Each step in this process requires its own set of enzymes, cofactors, and substrate for successful completion.

Table 4.3 Major steps in the synthesis of collagen and their cellular localization.

Step	*Location*
Transcription	Nucleus
Translation	Cytoplasm/RER
Hydroxylation of proline and lysine	RER lumen
Glycosylation	RER lumen
α-chain association	RER lumen
Helix formation	RER lumen
Secretion	—
Registration peptide cleavage	Extracellular
Polymerization	Extracellular
Cross-linking	Extracellular

(RER: Rough endoplasmic reticulum).

Before the procollagen molecule is extruded extracellularly, the nonhelical registration peptides are cleaved by a procollagen peptidase. After completion of the posttranslational modifications, the triple helix is secreted as procollagen into the extracellular environment in which the propeptide ends are specifically cleaved by procollagen-C proteinases and procollagen-N proteinases. This cleaving process is directly responsible for decreasing the solubility of the molecule. Now the process of fibril formation starts. The cross-linking of fibrils occurs after the free amino acid groups of several lysine and hydroxylysine residues have been transformed into aldehyde residues by the enzyme lysyl oxidase. Cross-linking occurs between the aldehyde groups and amino acid groups of the nontransformed lysine or hydroxylysine residues. The resultant collagen monomer is further polymerized and cross-linked by the formation of intra- and intermolecular covalent bonds.

Collagen breakdown during healing begins early and is very active during inflammation. Sources of collagenase in the wound are inflammatory cells,[57] endothelial cells,[58] as well as fibroblasts[59] and keratinocytes.[60] Collagens are almost exclusively digested extracellularly by specific collagenases. These specific enzymes are able to degrade the normally very stable triple helical structure of the collagen at specific sites, rendering the molecule more susceptible for degradation by other proteases.[55,61]

The activity of collagenases is tightly controlled by cytokines. Many cytokines actually exert their effect on matrix metabolism in the wound not only by inducing new gene transcription, but also by decreasing collagenase activity (e.g. TGF-β1). Based on in vitro work it has been suggested that collagenase is also regulated by the organization of the cytoskeleton of the cell and by the extracellular matrix.[62,63]

Proteoglycans

Glycosaminoglycans comprise a large portion of the "ground substance" within the granulation tissue. Rarely found free, they are coupled with proteins and therefore form proteoglycans. The polysaccharide chain is made up of repeating disaccharide units composed of glucuronic or iduronic acid and a hexosamine that is usually sulfated. The disaccharide composition of proteoglycans varies from about 10 units (heparin sulfate) to as many as 2,000 units (hyaluronic acid).

In wounds, the major glycosaminoglycans are dermatan and chondroitin sulfate. Fibroblasts synthesize these compounds and their concentration in wounds greatly increases during the first 3 weeks of healing. The interaction between collagen and proteoglycans is currently being studied. It is thought that the assembly of collagen subunits into fibrils and fibers is dependent on the lattice provided by the sulfated proteoglycans. Furthermore, it appears that the extent of sulfation is critical in determining the configuration of the collagen fibrils. As the scar collagen is deposited, the proteoglycans are incorporated into the collagen scaffolding. However, with scar maturation and collagen remodeling, the content of proteoglycan gradually diminishes.

The main feature of the maturation phase is the deposition of collagen in the wound. From a clinical point of view this is the most important phase of healing because the rate, quality, and total amount of matrix deposition determine the strength of the scar. Many healing deficiencies become clinically manifest secondary to poor collagen deposition, although the underlying cause may vary. The poor matrix deposition in diabetes mellitus, for instance, in part arises from altered and ineffective inflammation. On the other hand, excessive collagen synthesis, such as in a hypertrophic scar or a keloid, remains a clinical problem with few therapeutic options because the pathophysiology is not well enough understood.[64-66]

Wound Contraction

Wound contraction is the approximation of the wound edges together, whereas wound contracture is the shortening of the scar itself. Healing by primary or secondary intention determines the role of wound contraction in the healing process. Several theories have been proposed for the mechanisms of wound contraction.[67] It has been postulated that a special cell, the myofibroblast, is responsible for contraction, whereas another theory suggests that the locomotion of all fibroblasts leads to reorganization of the matrix and contraction.

The cytoskeletal structure of the myofibroblast differs from that of the normal fibroblast. Typically, the myofibroblast expresses a-smooth muscle actin in thick bundles called stress fibers, which allow it to contract.[68] The α-smooth muscle actin is nondetectable until day 6 and is then progressively expressed for the next 15 days of wound healing.[69] After 4 weeks this expression fades and the cell is believed to undergo apoptosis.[70] The appearance of the myofibroblast does not correspond perfectly with the time course of wound contraction, which starts almost immediately after wounding and continues for the next 2–3 weeks.[69] Fibroblasts placed in a collagen lattice actively move in the lattice and can contract it without expressing stress fibers. This finding led Ehrlich to hypothesize that the movement of the cells and the concomitant reorganization of the cytoskeleton are responsible for contraction.[71] More recently, the contraction function has been shown to be preserved in the absence of the myofibroblasts.[72]

GROWTH FACTORS AND WOUND HEALING

The transition from the immediate postinjury chaos through the structured initial stages of hemostasis, early repair, and finally an organized stable scar is orchestrated by an ever more complex network of growth factors, cytokines, and chemokines. The immediate release of cell signaling molecules following injury appears to trigger the inflammatory cascade with subsequent recruitment of inflammatory cells. Cell-mediated phagocytosis, reepithelialization, granulation tissue formation, and angiogenesis are all heralded and signaled by changes in the local growth factor and cytokine milieu. With the increasing sophistication of molecular assays, an evergrowing list of growth factors, and their downstream cellular targets, has been described.

Eight growth factors/growth factor families deserve special attention for their role in the wound-healing process: EGF, TGF-β, FGF, VEGF, granulocyte macrophage colony stimulating factor (GM-CSF), PDGF, connective tissue growth factor, and wound associated proinflammatory cytokines [interleukin family (IL) and TNF-α]. Only one growth factor family member, PDGF-BB, has been Food and Drug Administration (FDA)-approved

Table 4.4 Growth factors with possible or approved clinical use.

Growth factor (Family name)	*Secreted by*	*Actions*	*Clinical use*
PDGF-B (Platelet derived growth factor family)	Platelets, macrophages, keratinocytes, fibroblasts, endothelial cells	Enhances cellular migration and wound healing at wound site, causes secretion of VEGF which increases angiogenesis, improves extracellular matrix production.	Becaplermin (Regranex) is a PDGF-BB recombinant human protein. FDA approved for the treatment of lower extremity diabetic ulcers. Increased incidence of complete wound closure and decreased healing time.[73]
FGF-7 (Fibroblast growth factor family)	Fibroblasts and keratinocytes	Promote keratinocyte recruitment and activation. Upregulate matrix metalloproteinases production. Stimulate TGF-α secretion. May have cytoprotective effect by inducing antioxidant defense proteins.	Palifermin (Kepivance) is a human recombinant protein FDA approved for treatment of oral mucositis. While early phase II trails were promising for patients with venous stasis ulcers, ultimately did not change incidence of wound healing.[79]
FGF-2 (Fibroblast growth factor family)	Inflammatory cells, vascular endothelial cells, fibroblasts, keratinocytes.	Promote reepithelializaiton, angiogenesis. Contribute to extracellular matrix remodeling and synthesis.	Evaluated in diabetic foot ulcers and found ineffective. Early, promising data from clinical trials with pressure ulcers.[74]
FGF-1 (Fibroblast growth factor family)	Inflammatory cells, vascular endothelial cells, fibroblasts, keratinocytes.	Promote reepithelializaiton, angiogenesis.	May decrease wound healing times seen in burns.[74]
KGF-2/FGF-10 (Fibroblast growth factor family)	Fibroblasts and keratinocytes	Promotes reepithelialization	May accelerate chronic venous ulcer healing.[79]
EGF (Epidermal growth factor family)	Platelets, macrophages, fibroblasts, mesenchymal cells	Promotes epithelialization, angiogenesis, and fibroblast growth and survival.	Early stages, has shown some benefit in animal burn models.[74]
TGF-β3 (Transforming growth factor super family)	Macrophages, keratinocytes, fibroblasts, platelets	Recruit inflammatory cells, fibroblasts, and keratinocytes. May decrease scar formation.	In clinical trials for pressure ulcers as well as excessive scaring.[74]
Granulocyte macrophage-colony stimulating factor (cytokine)	Macrophages, T-cells, mast cells, NK cells, endothelial cells, fibroblasts	Activate and recruit neutrophils. Activate keratinocytes, promotes epithelialization. May augment angiogenesis.	May be effective in diabetic foot ulcers and in burn wounds.[74]

(in the USA) for the treatment of diabetic ulcers. Unfortunately, there is a noted dose-dependent increase in neoplasm risk that has hindered widespread adaptation.[73] Several studies of chronic, nonhealing wounds have demonstrated correlations with insufficient levels of FGF, VEGF modulators, EGF, and TGF-β.[74] While animal and some early phase-I trials have shown promising results, these were not confirmed in phase II trials. A summary of the various growth factors, their mechanisms of action, and potential clinical use can be found in Table 4.4.

Three members of the EGF family have roles in wound healing: EGF, heparin-binding EGF, and TGF-α.[75] These growth factors are released by a variety of cells found in the wound during the early repair process such as macrophages, lymphocytes, keratinocytes, platelets, fibroblasts, and vascular smooth muscle cells. Downstream effects include stimulation of migration of keratinocytes, epithelialization, angiogenesis, fibroblast proliferation, and survival. The EGF family is implicated also in the induction of the early inflammatory response as well as its regulation through the generation of anti-inflammatory mediators.

The TGF-β is part of a large superfamily of growth factors that have been implicated in regulatory and modulatory roles during the healing process, specifically TGF-β1, TGF-β2, TGF-β3, the bone morphogenic proteins (BMPs), and the activins.[74] TGF-β1 and 2, produced by macrophages, platelets, keratinocytes, and fibroblasts, serve to recruit inflammatory cells and fibroblasts and help transform fibroblasts into myofibroblasts. Interestingly, TGF-β3 inhibits scar formation and likely has a role in the counterregulatory system that ensures appropriate, but not excessive scar formation. BMPs are found throughout normal skin and influence keratinocyte differentiation. Activins, expressed by fibroblasts, endothelial cells, and keratinocytes, induce keratinocyte differentiation, and stimulate fibroblasts to deposit matrix substances.[76]

Fibroblast growth factors 1, 2, 7, 10, and 22, all members of the fibroblast growth factor family, have multiple roles in the wound healing. Produced by inflammatory cells, vascular endothelial cells, fibroblasts, and keratinocytes, these factors are involved with reepithelialization, angiogenesis, granulation tissue formation, as well as production and remodeling of the extracellular matrix.[77]

The VEGF family, composed of six known members, is primarily responsible for the angiogenesis seen during the early phases of wound healing. Not surprisingly, concentrations in normal skin are negligible and expression is dramatically upregulated in response to hypoxia and other growth factors. VEGF is actively expressed by keratinocytes, macrophages, fibroblasts, and platelets with primarily paracrine mediated action on endothelial cells. VEGF stimulation increases vascular permeability, basement membrane breakdown, migration of endothelial cells, and ultimately, early vascular progenitor cell proliferation. Monocyte migration and activation, as well as smooth muscle migration and proliferation have also been associated with VEGF.[78]

The GM-CSF, a specific cytokine shown to increase granulocytes, is increased in epidermal cells following injury. It is believed to increase the number and activity of neutrophils in the early inflammatory phase. In addition, this cytokine is thought to upregulate keratinocyte proliferation, and via endothelial cell migration and proliferation, promote angiogenesis.[74]

A four member family, PDGF is one of the first factors expressed during wounding and remains constitutively expressed throughout the entire wound-healing process. Consequently, PDGF is released by all cells involved in the wound-healing process, from platelet to vascular endothelium. PDGF is chemotactic for early inflammatory cells (neutrophils and macrophages) as well as fibroblasts and smooth muscle cells. Furthermore, PDGF triggers the release of TGF-β from macrophages and increased secretion of VEGF. PDGF has also been described as independently contributing to angiogenesis, reepithelialization, and the synthesis of the extracellular matrix.[75]

Connective tissue growth factor, an integrin-specific protein that is synthesized by fibroblasts, is increased following acute injury. Interestingly, the major target of this cytokine is the fibroblast itself. It has been associated with increased granulation tissue formation, extracellular matrix formation and remodeling, and reepithelialization. Knockout studies have demonstrated that this growth factor is required for wound healing.[74]

Inflammatory cytokines, responsible for the growth and differentiation of early inflammatory cells, are essential for successful wound healing. IL-1, IL-6, and TNF-α are actively secreted throughout the inflammatory phase. Produced by neutrophils, monocytes, macrophages, keratinocytes, these factors serve to promote early chemotaxis of neutrophils, proliferation of keratinocytes, as well as activation of fibroblasts.[74]

Given the multiple effects of growth factors and our ability to characterize, sequence, and produce them it is not surprising that much hope has been placed in their possible role in enhancing wound healing, particularly for impaired healing or chronic wounds. Only five defined growth factors have been found to have a positive effect on wound healing in humans (*see* Table 4.4).

The failure of the clinical application of individual growth factors is most likely due to the following:

- Multiple factors coexist within the wound environment
- They probably modulate the response of other growth factors and
- Their presence or absence at a particular course in time has a definite effect on the overall cellular reaction at the healing site.

However, it is not known how and when such interactions occur during the wound-healing cascade. In terms of chronic wounds, although the concept of an exogenously applied growth factor to reverse the nonhealing process is highly attractive, it seems more likely that such an approach alone would not often be successful. More likely of success would be a combination of interventions:

- Correct the local and systemic imbalance in factors that have led to impaired wound healing
- Aggressive surgical debridement of all the devitalized tissue and
- Exogenous application of growth factors.

FETAL WOUND HEALING

Rowlatt's initial observation, first published in 1979, was that fetal skin is able to heal without scarring. Subsequent confirmation in animal and human models raised the hope that scarless healing could be accomplished in adult patients.

Table 4.5 Major differences between fetal and adult wound healing.

Fetal wounds	Adult wounds
No scar, maintains original strength	Scar formation, 70% of original tensile strength
Replaces dermal components (hair follicles, sweat glands, etc).	Dermal components absent
Faster	Slower
Type III/IV collagen predominates	Type I collagen predominates
Increased hyaluronic acid content	Decreased hyaluronic acid content
Increased MMPs found in ECM	Decreased ECM adhesion molecules
Relative absence of inflammatory cells	Inflammation required for successful wound healing
More abundant and more active fibroblasts	Increased fibroblast to myofibroblast conversion

In truth, scarless fetal healing is observed for a limited timeframe during human gestation, and only if the wound is sufficiently small. Scarless fetal healing is characterized by a nondisrupted collagen matrix as well as the ability to generate normal dermal structures (hair follicles, sweat, and sebaceous glands). Fetal scarring begins to occur at approximately 24 weeks of gestation; however, large wounds may produce scar even earlier. The 24 gestational week mark roughly corresponds to the point at which fetal skin undergoes rapid growth.[80]

The major differences between fetal and adult wound healing are summarized in Table 4.5. A major difference between the adult wound and the fetal wound is the extracellular matrix. The fetal extracellular matrix encourages cellular migration and proliferation. Adult wounds have a preponderance of type I collagen throughout early scar formation. While type I collagen provides more strength and rigidity, it is believed to restrict cellular migration. This is in direct contrast to the fetal wound, which is composed primarily of type III collagen. There are important differences also in the level of hyaluronic acid, a glycosaminoglycan, and a major component of the extracellular matrix. Fetal skin, and therefore, fetal wounds contain increased amounts of hyaluronic acid compared with adult skin and wounds. Fetal fibroblasts have increased hyaluronic acid receptors and there are fewer cytokines known to reduce hyaluronic acid levels. Scarless fetal healing was initially attributed to the sterile, hyaluronic acid rich intrauterine environment. This hypothesis, however, was disproven in a number of elegant experiments.[81] Nevertheless, hyaluronic acid and/or its derivatives are being used clinically to prevent the excessive scarring that characterizes adhesion formation or corneal injury.

Other differences in fetal extracellular matrix include differing levels of modulators of collagen fibrillogenesis and an increase in matrix metalloproteinases, the latter believed to help organize the extracellular matrix. Fetal wounds demonstrate an increased ability to express adhesion proteins that may function to better stabilize the nascent extracellular matrix.[82,83]

Another major difference is the relative paucity of inflammatory cells and mediators in fetal wounds. Unlike adult wounds, which are dependent on inflammatory cells for healing, fetal wounds that heal without scar do so without an associated inflammatory phase. Conversely, if inflammation is induced into a fetal wound, scar is generated. Early cellular mediators of inflammation, such as platelets, are scarce in fetal wounds. There is decreased platelet aggregation and degradation, and consequently, less platelet-released growth factors (PDGF, TGF, etc.). As fetal wounds approach 24 weeks of gestation, an increase in platelet response is observed. Neutrophils are decreased in numbers in fetal wounds as well.[84]

There are differences in fibroblast function between fetus and adult. Fetal fibroblasts synthesize more type III and IV collagen, as opposed to adult fibroblasts, which are secrete more type I collagen. Unlike adult fibroblasts, which can either secrete collagen or undergo rapid mitosis, fetal fibroblasts are able to accomplish both simultaneously. Furthermore, wounds made early during the fetal period, and therefore, less likely to form scar, have few myofibroblasts present. An increased number of myofibroblasts is observed in wounds created closer to the 24 week gestation mark.[85]

WOUND MANAGEMENT

By definition, all wounds created by a surgical operation are classified as acute wounds. Accidental wounds arise from a variety of mechanical insults including abrasions, avulsions, crush injuries, lacerations, projectile penetrations, and combinations of these. Burn wounds result from exposure to extremes in temperatures, corrosive or denaturing chemicals, electrical current, and ionizing radiation. Finally, ulcers and similar wounds caused by infection, neoplasm, and circulatory insufficiency present first as acute wounds, which progress to chronicity (*see* Chronic Wounds).

All wounds when left unattended attempt to heal by inflammation, deposition of collagen and extracellular matrix by fibroblast proliferation, contraction, epithelialization and subsequent remodeling of the resultant scar. Reestablishment of an intact epithelial barrier reestablishes water vapor barrier, whereas collagen remodeling improves the wound's tensile strength. These processes occur in a linear overlapping sequence and are accompanied by changes in the cellular and cytokine constituents of the wound milieu, as described in the section Phases of Wound Healing. The result of this process is formation of scar with the attendant morbidity of adhesion and contracture, as well as keloid and stricture formation.

HOST FACTORS

Wound healing may be complicated by a variety of comorbid systemic and local conditions. A careful history and physical examination are therefore essential before undertaking the care of patients who have acute wounds. Table 4.6 summarizes patient comorbid factors that affect wound healing.

Wound healing is critically dependent upon an intact inflammatory response for the initial formation of wound matrix and subsequent maintenance of a sterile environment. Consequently, patients who have impaired immune function secondary to diabetes mellitus, uremia, jaundice, malnutrition, sepsis, and immunosuppression have an increased risk for wound dehiscence, poor healing, and wound infection.

Collagen forms more slowly in patients receiving corticosteroids, chemotherapy, or radiation therapy. Although these wounds eventually heal, wound strength increases more slowly and wound repairs must be reinforced and protected. These factors should be carefully considered in all surgical decision making.

ACUTE WOUNDS

Broadly speaking, acute wounds can be classified into one of two main categories: surgical wounds and acute accidental wounds. Acute accidental wounds can be further divided on the basis of the mechanism of injury and/or the extent and type of tissue injury. While general principles of wound care apply equally to both acute accidental wounds and operative wounds, for the purposes of this discussion, operative wounds are addressed separately.

Operative Wounds

Operative wounds are classified through a schema developed by the US National Academy of Sciences and the National Research Council that is predictive of postoperative surgical site infections (SSIs) and based on levels of bacterial contamination. The likelihood of subsequent SSI can be helpful in selecting the most appropriate wound care strategy. This information is summarized in Table 4.7.

Clean wounds are defined by an incision into noninfected, noninflamed tissue without entry into a visceral organ. Examples of clean wounds are inguinal hernia repairs and mastectomies. Prospective studies evaluating

Table 4.6 Comorbid factors that impair wound healing.

Tissue ischemia
Inadequate arterial inflow (atherosclerosis, radiation-induced arteriolar fibrosis, obesity, vasoconstriction caused by nicotine)
Decreased blood oxygen content (impaired pulmonary diffusion, anemia, acid-base disturbances)
Impaired venous outflow (venous stasis disease, tissue edema, chronic pressure, tissue fibrosis)
Impaired inflammatory response
Diabetes mellitus
Uremia
Jaundice
Malnutrition
Immunosuppression (AIDS, transplant recipients)
Impaired collagen formation
Corticosteroid therapy
Chemotherapy
Radiation therapy
Elderly

Table 4.7 National Academy of Sciences and the National Research Council operative wound classification scheme.[90]

Operative wound classification[90]		
Description	*Wound infection rate*	*Surgical examples*
Clean (type I)	1-2%	Inguinal hernia repair, lumpectomy
Clean-contaminated (type II)	>30% (organ system dependent)	Laparoscopic cholecystectomy, uncomplicated appendicectomy
Contaminated (type III)	Up to 60%	Reversal of loop ileostomy, right hemicolectomy
Infected	>60%	Hartmann's procedure for perforated diverticulitis, above knee amputation for an wet gangrene

clean wounds have documented the risk of SSI at 1–2%. Given the low likelihood of future infection, clean wounds can be safely closed with primary intent.[86]

Clean contaminated wounds are those carried out through a noninfected, noninflamed tissue plane with a controlled entry into a visceral organ without spillage or contamination of contents. Examples of clean contaminated wounds include the laparoscopic entry sites used in a laparoscopic cholecystectomy or a thoracotomy incision used for a wedge resection. Depending on the organ system entered, clean-contaminated wounds have a potential wound infection risk of up to 30%. Given the low incidence of SSI, primary closure remains the recommended wound care strategy.[86]

Contaminated wounds are defined as those in which unintentional hollow viscus penetration has occurred, a large break in sterile technique, incision into an area of purulence or inflammation, and operations in which gross spillage of enteric contents occurs. Examples of contaminated wounds include the cutaneous wound following colostomy or ileostomy reversal and surgical incisions in which there is an inadvertent enterotomy. Contaminated wounds are associated with an up to 60% incidence of SSI, and frequently, decisions on wound management are made on a case-by-case basis. Many surgeons will choose to close these wounds primarily with the express understanding that >50% will require subsequent reopening and healing by secondary intention. Other surgeons are unwilling to risk SSI and allow all contaminated wounds to heal by secondary intention. One additional strategy is to allow the wound to heal by tertiary intention (delayed primary closure). In this technique, the sutures for closure are placed but not tied and the wound remains open for the first 3–5 postoperative days. In the absence of visible infection, the sutures are tied, usually at the bedside, and the wound is allowed to heal.[86]

The final category of operative wounds, dirty (infected), include those wounds in which an incision is made through devitalized or grossly infected tissue, wounds whereby the abdomen is entered with a perforated viscus or gross fecal contamination, or wounds that contain a foreign body. Given the variability of the contamination and bacterial burden, these wounds have a large (>60%) incidence of subsequent SSI and are best closed by either secondary intention or delayed primary closure.[86]

Most surgical wounds that will become infected do so within 72 hours. The physician should observe for signs of localized wound infection, specifically erythema, induration, and increased pain; these will frequently herald wound infection well before suppuration, which typically occurs between 7 and 10 days. Once an SSI is suspected, the wound should be opened by removal of sutures or staples and inspected for drainage. Gram stain and culture of the wound bed should be taken at this time to guide future antimicrobial therapy, if required. Local wound care, consisting of saline-soaked sterile gauze applied in a wet-to-dry fashion, will provide a moist wound-healing environment, a mechanical barrier to premature closure, and effective superficial debridement. In lieu of wet-to-dry dressings, other dressing options (hydrocolloids, hydrocellular or polyurethane foam, alginate, hydrogels, hydrofiber, dextranomer, paraffin gauze, nonadherent, hyaluronic acid-impregnated, silver-coated, activated charcoal, and protease-modulating matrix) may be used that are equally or more effective in creating a moist, covered wound-healing environment. No study to date has documented superiority of these dressing options over wet-to-dry dressings in time to wound closure; however, they may be more comfortable and less unsightly to the patient.[87]

If the extent of the infection or devitalized tissue is large and sufficient debridement cannot be accomplished at the bedside, operative debridement may be necessary. Once clean, viable granulation tissue is observed and a quantitative wound culture with a bacterial count $<10^5/mm^3$ is achieved, there is highly likelihood of successful closure with wound reapproximation. For those patients with wounds that remain colonized or those who are deemed poor candidates for delayed primary closure, the wound can be allowed to close via secondary intention.[88,89]

One of the most feared SSI is the necrotizing soft tissue infection. While infrequent, these infections can be rapidly fatal if not recognized and treated appropriately. Unlike nonnecrotizing SSI, these infections evolve rapidly, typically within the first 24–48 hours and are associated with wound pain, crepitance, and either a clear dishwater or foul-smelling brownish discharge. Common organisms for these infections include the clostridial species, group A Streptococcus, *Staphylococcus aureus*, and Bacteroides species. Associated laboratory findings include leukocytosis and hyponatremia. These conditions require urgent and wide surgical debridement and rapid broad spectrum antibiotic therapy.[89]

Acute Accidental Wounds

Acute accidental wounds can be effectively categorized on the basis of the mechanisms of occurrence and presentation. Major categories include abrasions, lacerations,

Table 4.8 Wound features associated with tetanus risk.[92]

Feature	*Low tetanus risk*	*High tetanus risk*
Depth	≤1 cm	>1 cm
Shape	Linear	Stellate, jagged edges, avulsed, or abraded
Time since injury	≤ 6 hours	>6 hours
Mechanism	Laceration	Tissue trauma (crush, projectile), thermal injury (burn, frostbite)
Visible infection	Absence of	Presence of
Nonviable tissue	Absence of	Presence of
Foreign body	Absence of	Presence of

Table 4.9 Recommendation for tetanus immunization for acute wounds.[92]

Immunization History	Wound is not tetanus prone	Wound is tetanus prone
Uncertain	Toxoid only	Toxoid and immunoglobulin
0–2 previous doses	Toxoid only	Toxoid and immunoglobulin
≥3 previous doses	If last toxoid was ≥10 years, additional toxoid dose. Otherwise, no prophylaxis	If last toxoid was ≥5 years, additional toxoid dose. Otherwise, no prophylaxis.

and thermal injury. Despite different wound management techniques, the overall approach to wound care is similar. The fundamental goal is to foster rapid healing with optimal cosmetic result and minimal functional impairment. To accomplish this goal, secondary complications (such as infection and hypertrophic scarring) should be minimized and the healing environment should be optimized.[89]

Prior to treatment, a thorough understanding of the mechanism, extent of, and timeframe surrounding the injury should be obtained. Wounds that are associated with specific infection (rabies and tetanus for example) should undergo additional screening and treatment. In addition, any factors that might impair wound healing should be ascertained (diabetes, medications known to delay wound healing). Guidelines for tetanus prophylaxis and treatment are outlined in Tables 4.8 and 4.9. A detailed examination of the wound then follows with particular attention to the depth of injury, the extent of contamination and the amount of nonviable tissue.[91]

All wounds should be thoroughly irrigated, ideally with water or saline. Wounds with a high degree of contamination should undergo additional irrigation, with either a commercially available high pressure system or through a syringe and a splatter shield. Wounds should not be irrigated with liquids other than water or saline (such as hydrogen peroxide or Betadine), as such substances have not been shown to decrease the incidence of subsequent infection and may actually retard the healing process. If irrigation is painful or uncomfortable, the wounds can be effectively anesthetized with either lidocaine (1% solution) or bupivacaine (0.25%) injected in the area around the wound. Epinephrine (adrenaline) may be added to either of the above solutions with the advantage of providing local hemostasis and decreasing the total volume of local anesthetic needed by decreasing systemic absorption. Epinephrine should not be used in parts of the body supplied by end arterioles (fingers, toes, ear lobes, nose, or penis) as there is theoretical risk of necrosis. Following this, grossly infected or devitalized tissue should be removed to facilitate healing.[91]

All hematomas present within wounds should be carefully evacuated and any remaining bleeding sources controlled by ligature or cautery. If the viability of remaining tissues is suspect or if the wound has resulted in the formation of a marginal flap of skin or tissue, capillary perfusion should be assessed using intravenous fluorescein and ultraviolet light, or tissue oxygen tension should be measured before closure. If marginally perfused tissues remain, these should be resected or revascularized before further wound repair and closure.

Patients who sustain crush or electrocution injuries are at high risk of having an occult deep-tissue injury and of developing a compartment syndrome. Surgeons who care for these patients must maintain a high index of suspicion for compartment syndrome and be prepared to perform appropriate fasciotomies to minimize additional tissue loss. Patients who develop a compartment syndrome also have a risk of developing myonecrosis and subsequent myoglobinuria. Urine output should be carefully monitored and the presence of urine myoglobin aggressively treated with alkalinization using hydration and acetazolamide.

Finally, patients who are injured by air, grease, or paint guns generally present with small circumscribed wounds. The extent of the subcutaneous and deep tissue penetration in these wounds is seldom evident at the surface. These patients require extensive exploration of their wounds and careful debridement of all injected foreign material.

Wounds heal best in a moist environment: It serves to prevent further tissue loss through desiccation, as well as to promote collagen synthesis and angiogenesis. Many wound dressings can provide an optimal moist environment; these include semiocclusive dressings, topical wound agents, or various commercial wound dressings. There is no clinical evidence to support one type of dressing over another; the clinician can therefore choose the dressing to best fit the individual patient and the wound location.[91]

Once wounds have been sufficiently inspected, appropriate prophylaxis has been administered, the wound has been cleaned and anesthetized, and devitalized/infected tissue has been removed, consideration can turn to closure. Although there is an association between the time a wound remains open and the incidence of wound infection, the optimal timeframe within which primary closure should not occur has not been fully elucidated. Wounds open for 12–24 hours can be safely closed assuming there is low risk for infection. Wounds in which there is a high likelihood of infection should be closed within 6 hours.[91]

In general, acute closure can be attempted on lacerations, skin tears, and some bite wounds. Complicated wounds, such as those caused by thermal injury (either burn or frostbite), deep dermal abrasions, or chemical injury present challenging management problems and can frequently be associated with systemic illness. A comprehensive review of the care for these specific injuries is beyond the scope of this chapter, and frequently, care involves a multidisciplinary approach for optimal results.

Wound edges should be approximated with as little tension as possible. This technique will serve to decrease the likelihood of hypertrophic scars, the incidence of wound breakdown, and the incidence of poor wound healing. If the skin edges cannot be approximated in a tension free fashion, subcuticular sutures can be used to maintain wound strength and integrity. If the wound edges cannot be approximated with appropriate tension despite placement of subcuticular sutures, advanced wound closure strategies, such as local advancement flaps or tissue transfer, may be needed. Synthetic absorbable sutures, which are frequently less reactive and have the ability to retain their tensile strength, are ideal for placement in subcuticular tissue. The optimal suture for skin is nonabsorbable, and one should use the smallest suture possible that can still approximate the edge. Skin should be closed so that the wound edges are everted and tension free. This maneuver will result in a normal scar appearance once remodeling has flattened the wound.

Table 4.10 Advantages and disadvantages of skin closure methods.

Device	*Advantages*	*Disadvantages*
Suture	Maximum applicable tension Customizable strength	Painful application Hard to evert edges Time consuming
Skin staples	Easy to evert edges Quick	Unattractive scarring if left too long Unsightly appearance during healing—“Frankenstein look”
Dermal glue	Easy to apply Waterproof No removal needed No dressing needed	Hard to evert edges Difficult to use with wounds under tension
Wound tape	Rapid application Easier to evert edges	Difficult to align wound edges Needs additional dressing Requires removal

Other options for skin closure include staples, dermal glue (cyanoacrylate), and wound tape. Wound closure methods should be selected on the basis of the need of the patient and the physician closing the wound. Benefits and detriments of the skin closing options are outlined in Table 4.10.

Antimicrobial Prophylaxis and Therapy for Acute Wounds

Exhaustive studies have been undertaken to examine the appropriateness of antibiotic prophylaxis in the treatment of operative wounds. Normal bacterial contaminants of skin are prevented from entry into deep tissues by an intact epithelium. A surgical incision breaches the intact epithelium, allowing bacteria access to these tissues and the bloodstream. Antibiotic prophylaxis is most effective when an adequate concentration of antibiotic is present in the tissues at the time of the incision. Addition of antibiotics after operative contamination has been encountered has been clearly shown to be ineffective in the prevention of postoperative wound infection.

In studies that compared operations performed with and without antibiotic prophylaxis, class II, III, and IV procedures treated with appropriate prophylactic antibiotics were shown to have only one third the wound infection rate than that in previously reported series without antibiotic coverage. More recently, studies have demonstrated that repeat dosing of antibiotics is essential to decrease the incidence of postoperative wound infections for operations that take longer than the biochemical half-life of the antibiotic or in which there is large-volume blood loss and fluid replacement. In such cases, for those in which prosthetic implants are used or when unexpected contamination is encountered, additional doses of antibiotic may be administered for 24 hours postoperatively.[93]

Patients who have prosthetic heart valves or any implanted vascular or orthopedic prostheses should receive antibiotic prophylaxis before any procedure in which significant bacteremia is anticipated. Dental procedures require prophylaxis with broad-spectrum penicillins or amoxicillin, whereas patients who undergo urologic instrumentation should be pretreated with a secondgeneration cephalosporin. Patients with prostheses who undergo gastrointestinal operations should receive broad-spectrum penicillins, whereas those with penicillin allergies should receive vancomycin.[94]

Selection of antibiotic for use in prophylaxis should be tailored to:

- Type of operation to be performed
- Expectation for encountering operative contamination and
- Profile of resistant organisms present at the institution in which the operation is performed

The continuing widespread appearance of methicillin-resistant *Staphylococcus aureus* and vancomycin-resistant enterococci has significantly restricted the selection of these agents for routine use.

Choice of antibiotic treatment for other acute wounds must be based upon the expected organisms within the infected wound and the patient's overall immune status. When a single-specific organism is suspected, treatment may be commenced using a single antibiotic. Conversely, when multiple organisms are suspected, as with enteric contamination or when a patient's immune function is impaired by diabetes mellitus, chronic disease or medication, treatment should commence with multiagent broad-spectrum antibiotics. Lastly, the location of the wound and the quality of tissue perfusion have an important effect on wound healing.

As with surgical wounds, fresh wound drainage material should be obtained and submitted for Gram stain, culture, and assessment of bacterial antibiotic sensitivity. Debridement of any remaining necrotic tissue can aid in converting an infected wound into a contaminated wound. As discussed above, a careful history is essential to predict accurately the likely bacterial contaminants of acute wounds (see the section Acute Accidental Wounds). Patients who are injured in farm accidents or who receive penetrating injuries through shoes should be treated for mixed gram-positive and -negative infections.

Bite wounds, particularly human bites, carry an extremely heavy bacterial load and patients who receive penetrating human bites should be treated for mouth flora and *Eikenella corrodens*. Patients who have injuries from dogs and cats are subject to lower bacterial loads at the time of injury, but remain susceptible to a variety of organisms, most notably *Pasteurella multocida*.

All patients who sustain animal bites, particularly from high-risk wild animals, such as bats, coyotes, raccoons, and skunks, should be considered for antirabies immunization. Frequently, the offending animal escapes, but when available, it should be observed for 7–10 days or, if behaving erratically, killed and examined for rabies by immunostaining brain tissue.

Once organisms have been identified and assayed for sensitivity, broad-spectrum antibiotic therapy should become more specific according to the results. Patients who are infected by an organism that has a known resistance pattern, such as *Pseudomonas aeruginosa*, should ideally be treated with two agents, selected for their different mechanisms of action.

As medical practice and reimbursement have led to shortened inpatient stays, surgeons have been under pressure to discharge patients who have surgical and acute wound infections home quickly. To this end, when there is an adequate antibiotic response, it is advantageous to select an agent that can easily be administered on an outpatient basis.

CHRONIC WOUNDS

Chronic wounds are generally defined as those that fail to heal following 3 months of conservative wound therapy. Upon examination, these wounds demonstrate a failure of central migration of epithelial tissue, leaving a central eschar or moist fluid losing center. The etiology of the development and maintenance of the chronic wound is multifactorial; it involves bacterial contamination, ongoing tissue ischemia, inadequate inflammatory response, and failure of wound protein synthesis. Advanced age, immobility, and malnutrition are further contributors to this process.

Chronic wounds cause major morbidity and add tremendously to the costs of medical care. Many chronic wounds may be avoidable, and clinicians should be attentive to prophylactic issues and exiting risk factors in patients who are susceptible to developing chronic wounds. Treatment requires a multisystem approach and can frequently bring relief to the patient and ultimate healing of the wound.

Pressure Sores

Pressure ulcers have commonly been referred to as "bed sores," although this designation is inaccurate in describing the etiology of their development or the susceptible patients. The overall surgical, nursing, and medical costs for the care of pressure sores are estimated to be up to $5 billion annually in the USA.

Pressure sores arise from ischemia created by continuous perpendicular pressure and parallel shear forces upon tissues that overlie bony prominences. The bony prominences most frequently involved are the ischium, sacrum, greater trochanters, heels, elbows, knees, and posterior scalp; however, any location subject to continuous pressure can be affected. Continuous pressure impairs flow through the tissue microvasculature and tissue loss can begin when the pressure exceeds 25 mm Hg.

Patients who are immobilized because of neurologic disease or debilitation are at particular risk for developing pressure sores. Furthermore, these patients frequently manifest tissue loss secondary to malnutrition or disuse atrophy, which further increases the risk for developing pressure sores as the bony prominences have less overlying padding. Patients who have neurologic injuries have the added difficulty of sensory deficits, which prevent them from recognizing chronic pressure.

As with all chronic wounds, prevention is an essential component of caring for these patients. In acute care facilities, current financial policy penalizes institutions when pressure ulcers occur de novo. Debilitated and quadriplegic patients in long-term care settings should be treated with meticulous attention to frequent turning schedules, and more recently automatic rotation low-airloss beds have shown some benefits in caring for such patients. Nevertheless, even with the best preventive care, these patients frequently develop sores. Paraplegic patients must be advised to shift their positions frequently, and their chairs and beds should be equipped with pressure-dispersing cushions to supplement their care.

Pressure sore wounds frequently demonstrate a pattern of small, well-circumscribed skin loss, with more extensive necrosis of the underlying fat and muscle. Immobilized patients who have isolated pressure sores should be offered surgical excision as the treatment of choice. However, extensive tissue loss may require radical debridement and creation of musculocutaneous flaps, typically taken from the patient's thigh, or coverage with split-thickness skin grafts. Although successful in closing the wounds, durability is very limited.

Pressure sores following an acute illness in an otherwise mobile patient can be treated with local debridement and dressing changes. These wounds proceed to heal by secondary intention, with subsequent epithelial migration from the wound edges. As scar is less resilient to pressure necrosis than repaired normal or transposed skin, this approach is seldom as effective in patients who have ongoing debilitation and immobilization.

Arterial and Venous Leg Ulcers

The vast majority of leg ulcers result from valvular incompetence and venous insufficiency. Venous insufficiency leads to increased venous pressure in the capillary beds and generalized edema of the extremity. This pressure increase combined with edema results in decreased transcapillary flow and inadequate tissue perfusion, especially in the gaiter region of the leg. Arterial insufficiency and various vasculitides impair the inflow of oxygenated arterial blood to the tissues, but this is not typically associated with extensive tissue edema.

In patients with venous insufficiency, surgical treatment may alleviate venous back pressure. Patients who have venous stasis ulcers are well managed by frequent and regular Unna's boot dressing changes combined with an overlying elastic bandage. The Unna boot bandage (or zinc paste dressing) maintains a moist environment, whereas the elastic bandage ensures venous return and provides compression. The surgeon may follow the wound's progress on a weekly basis; however, many patients cannot tolerate the continuous presence of the bandage and the difficulty with bathing. Fitted compression stockings are essential to use after healing has been achieved.

Treatment of ischemic ulcers begins with assessment and treatment of the underlying vascular problem. This therapy is followed by careful debridement of the ulcer to remove eschar and fibrin, and to provide a clean epithelial edge for healing. Treatment of any underlying vasculitis should also occur. After revascularization chronic ischemic ulcers, refractory to conservative therapy, may require surgical excision and primary closure or, more typically, coverage with split-thickness skin grafts.

Diabetic Foot Ulcers

In the USA diabetic foot ulcers are thought to occur in 15–20% of all diabetics, resulting in 50,000–75,000 amputations each year and accounting for nearly $20 billion in medical costs, rehabilitation expense and loss of productivity.

Contrary to notions popular in the medical community, no studies have convincingly demonstrated that diabetic foot ulcers result from obliteration of the microvasculature. Instead, tissue loss arises from decreased oxygenation caused by glycosylation of hemoglobin and erythrocyte membranes and obstructed infrapopliteal arteries. Glycosylation results in increased hemoglobin oxygen affinity. Similarly, glycosylation of cell membranes decreases erythrocyte deformation, increases blood viscosity, and decreases flow. Simultaneously, diabetics develop peripheral neuropathies that render their feet insensate. The combination of undetected prolonged pressure and inadequate tissue oxygenation leads to tissue loss, most typically over the clawed metatarsal heads.

Recent studies show that meticulous regulation of blood glucose levels can decrease some of the end-organ complications of diabetes. Diabetics must be taught meticulous foot care, including daily inspection, avoidance of tight shoes, and frequent removal of callus. Patients who have severe peripheral neuropathy can be treated with shoe orthotics that transfers pressure away from the metatarsal heads.

Revascularization can be helpful in some cases. Magnetic resonance angiography has become increasingly useful in identifying appropriate vessels for distal bypass. Local debridement and dressing changes can lead to healing of these wounds; however, many patients proceed to loss of digits, feet, and limbs if these local measures are unsuccessful.

THERAPEUTIC ADJUNCTS

Dressings

Dressings are used to:

- Cover wounds and protect them from contamination while epithelial integrity is reestablished
- Absorb any blood or tissue transudate, thereby proving a dry and sanitary covering
- Protect against desiccation and mechanical injury by providing a padded covering and
- Act as psychological supports, shielding patients from viewing their wounds and identifying where the injury or operation has taken place.

Ideal dressings should fulfill each of the above requirements and should additionally be inexpensive, require infrequent changes, and be easy to change when required. At present, over 150 different dressings are commercially available. To date, none has been conclusively shown to be more effective in the promotion and completion of healing than standard dressing materials, despite active and aggressive promotion by the pharmaceutical and biotechnology companies. The seven major types of wound dressings and their appropriate use are summarized in Table 4.11.

Table 4.11 The seven choices of wound dressings.

Wound dressings

Type	*Description*	*Uses*
Film	Semipermeable plastic	Primarily a closed wound with no drainage. Impermeable to fluid and bacteria. Prevents desiccation
Foam	Hydrophilic or hydrophobic; nonocclusive	Wound that is secreting a large non occlusive quantity of tissue fluid and requires frequent debridement
Gel	>80% water in a cross-linked synthetic polymer	Wound in which there is minimal tissue fluid. Maintains moist wound environment, but requires additional dressing cover
Hydrocolloid	Hydrophilic particles (synthetic and natural)	Wound in which there is some tissue fluid requiring debridement of soft nonviable tissue
Impregnated	Impregnated gauze (various antibacterial or moisturizing compounds)	Wound in which there is minimal exudate. Provides antibacterial or moisture properties. Does not adhere to wound. Additional dressing cover may be needed
Powder or paste	Hydrophilic particles (synthetic and natural)	Wound in which there is a large amount of exudate. Debrides nonviable tissue

Hyperbaric Oxygen

The use of hyperbaric oxygen in the treatment of a variety of wound types has been debated through the past decades. Hyperbaric oxygen therapy is based upon the principle of supranormal oxygen delivery to wounded tissues. The increase in oxygen delivery is presumed to act through improved oxygenation at the cellular level, whereas increased oxygen concentration promotes the formation of toxic oxygen-derived radicals. Although some studies have shown some promise for hyperbaric oxygen therapy, it is not appropriate for routine use.

EXCESSIVE SCARRING

Excessive scarring can be considered as an overaggressive wound-healing response and can be as problematic clinically as insufficient healing. While excessive scarring affects all tissue types and organs (consider cirrhosis of the liver), two broad categories of excessive scarring are managed by the general surgeon: dermal scars and intra-abdominal scars.

The Dermis: Keloids and Hypertrophic Scars

Hypertrophic scarring is best characterized as an inappropriately robust response to a traumatic dermal event. The characteristic hypertrophic scar is elevated, erythematous, and contained within the original site of injury. This scar type often occurs following major dermal trauma such as burn injury, as well as in areas closed under high tension, such as the neck, knees, ankles, and in incisions through skin creases. Most appear within 4 to 8 weeks after initial injury, and a large percentage of these scars gradually regress to a flat scar over a period of years. Histology, hypertrophic scars are composed of an abundance of collagen, specifically type III, that are oriented parallel to the surface of the epithelium in wavy bundles. Hypertrophic scars also contain small nodular structures composed of myofibroblasts, small vessels, and fine collagen fibers.[95]

In contrast to the excessive, but organized, picture seen in hypertrophic scars, keloids are described as excessive and disorganized. Keloid scars also present as elevated and erythematous, with a shiny surface, but pathognomonically extend beyond the margins of the original wounds. There seems to be no defined relationship between the extent of the initial injury and the appearance of keloids, and interestingly, keloids have been described in areas that have not been wounded. Unlike hypertrophic scars, keloids have a predilection for the anterior chest, earlobes, and upper arms. There is a strong familial association with the disease, as well as a higher incidence in dark-skinned patients. Histologically, keloids are devoid of organized collagen bundles, and instead, are composed of disorganized sheets of type I and type III collagen haphazardly arranged with respect to the epithelial surface.[95,96]

There is substantial evidence to suggest that both hypertrophic scarring and keloids are associated with a prolonged inflammatory response, with a greater number of inflammatory cells present. Consistent with theories of ongoing inflammation, the immune cell infiltration decreases over time in hypertrophic scars; this, however, does not occur in keloid scars. In addition to an increased inflammatory response, both keloid and hypertrophic scarring are associated with an increased and aberrant fibroblast response. Keloid fibroblasts have upregulated growth factor receptors, respond more intensely to growth factors, and reduced expression of downregulatory gene proteins.[95,96]

Current treatment paradigms for excessive scarring reflect our current understanding of the disease. The most effective treatment paradigm remains prevention: surgeons should pay meticulous attention to avoid excessive tissue trauma, incisions should not be placed over skin creases or in areas of high tension, and wounds should not be closed under tension. Two well-studied additional prophylactic treatments include continuous pressure and silicone gel sheeting. These techniques are especially well suited to patients with a history of excessive scar formation or an injury that predisposes itself to excessive scarring (burns, for example). If excessive scar formation has already occurred, one must first differentiate hypertrophic scars from keloids as they are treated differently. Hypertrophic scars should be allowed to regress, and if they remain symptomatic after sufficient time, they are usually amenable to simple scar excision and closure without tension. This technique is not appropriate for keloids as there is a >50% recurrence rate and often, further growth of keloid beyond the original keloid. First-line therapy for keloids involves intralesional injection of corticosteroids (typically triamcinolone acetonide). Additional treatment modalities are extensive, but include cryotherapy, radiotherapy, laser therapy, and chemotherapeutics, each with varying degrees of success.[96]

Intra-Abdominal Adhesions

An intra-abdominal adhesion is the result of injury to the peritoneal lining that results in a localized inflammatory process and ultimately, intra-abdominal scar formation. In most cases, the early adhesive band is reabsorbed within 10 days. Often, however, these scars can become organized, thicker, and fibrotic. Once organized, they are unlikely to resolve. Intra-abdominal adhesions are frequently responsible for disease states, notably small bowel obstruction, and they pose technical challenges at any subsequent operation.

Like scarring in any other part of the body, intra-abdominal scarring is principally mediated by inflammation, infection, ischemia, and foreign bodies. As there are no effective treatment modalities for adhesions, prevention is paramount. Careful attention must be paid while operating with the peritoneal cavity to avoid excessive tissue tension, tissue devitalization, and ischemia. Furthermore, foreign bodies prone to inflammation, like silk suture, should be used sparingly and judiciously. Gloves with talcum powder should be avoided: talcum powder is an effective agent for pleurodesis because of its inflammatory response. In addition, Seprafilm, a sodium hyaluronate-based bioresorbable membrane, has been FDA approved for the prevention of intra-abdominal adhesions. Widespread adoption of this product is limited as there is an increased incidence of anastomotic breakdown with its use.[97] Laparoscopic procedures result in lesser adhesion formation, and their wider and wider use should ultimately result in decreased numbers of operation for adhesion-related pathology.[98]

REFERENCES

1. Broughon G, Janis JE, Attinger CE. A brief history of wound care. PRS. 2006;117:6S-11S.
2. Hamby WB. Ambroise Paré, Surgeon of the Renaissance. St. Louis: W. H. Green; 1967. p. 251.
3. Illingworth C. The lister lecture, 1964: wound sepsis—from carbolic acid to hyperbaric oxygen. Can Med Assoc J. 1964;91:1041-5.
4. Schilling JA. Wound healing. Surg Clin N Am. 1976;56: 859-74.
5. Simpson DM, Ross R. The neutrophilic leucocyte in wound repair. A study with antineutrophil serum. J Clin Invest. 1972;51:2009-23.
6. Leibovich SJ, Ross R. The role of the macrophage in wound repair. A study with hydrocortisone and antimacrophage serum. Am J Pathol. 1975;78:71-100.
7. Barbul A, Breslin JR, Woodyard JP, et al. The effect of in vivo T helper and T suppressor lymphocyte depletion on wound healing. Ann Surg. 1989;209:479-83.
8. Polverini PJ, Cotran PS, Gimbrone MA Jr, et al. Activated macrophages induce vascular proliferation. Nature. 1977;269:804-6.
9. Malawista SE, Montgomery RR, van Blaricom G. Evidence for reactive nitrogen intermediates in killing of staphylococci by human neutrophil cytoplasts. A new microbicidal pathway for polymorphonuclear leukocytes. J Clin Invest. 1992;90:631-6.
10. Schaffer MR, Efron PA, Thornton FJ, et al. Nitric oxide, an autocrine regulator of wound fibroblast synthetic function. J Immunol. 1997;158:2375-81.
11. Bulgrin JP, Shabani M, Chakravarthy D, et al. Nitric oxide synthesis is suppressed in steroid-impaired and diabetic wound healing. Wounds. 1995;7:48-57.
12. Schaeffer MR, Tandry U, Gross SS, et al. Nitric oxide regulates wound healing. J Surg Res. 1996;63:237-40.
13. Brancato SK, Albina JE. Wound macrophages as key regulators of repair. Am J Pathol. 2011;178:19-25.
14. Fries KM, Blieden T, Looney RJ, et al. Evidence of fibroblast heterogeneity and the role of fibroblast subpopulations in fibrosis. Clin Immunol Immunopathol. 1994;72:283-92.
15. Sempowski GD, Borrello MA, Blieden TM, et al. Fibroblast heterogenity in the healing wound. Wound Rep Reg. 1995;3:120-31.
16. Regan MC, Kirk SJ, Wasserkrug HL, et al. The wound environment as a regulator of fibroblast phenotype. J Surg Res. 1991;50:442-8.
17. Colige AC, Lambert CA, Nusgens BV, et al. Effect of cell–cell and cell–matrix interactions on the response of fibroblasts to epidermal growth factor in vitro. Expression of collagen type 1, collagenase, stromelysin and tissue inhibitor of metalloproteinases. Biochem J. 1992;285:215-21.
18. Serini G, Gabbiani G. Modulation of α–smooth muscle actin expression in fibroblasts by transforming growth factor–β isoforms: an in vivo and in vitro study. Wound Rep Reg. 1996;4:278-87.
19. Fahey TJ 3rd, Sadaty A, Jones WG 2nd, et al. Diabetes impairs the late inflammatory response to wound healing. J Surg Res. 1991;50:308-13.
20. Ausprunk DH, Folkman J. Migration and proliferation of endothelial cells in preformed and newly formed blood vessels during tumor angiogenesis. Microvasc Res. 1977; 14:53-65.
21. Burger PC, Chandler DB, Klintworth OK. Corneal neovascularization as studied by scanning electron microscopy of vascular casts. Lab Invest. 1983;48:169-80.
22. Knighton DR, Silver IA, Hunt TK. Regulation of wound healing angiogenesis: effect of oxygen gradient and inspired oxygen concentration. Surgery. 1981;90:262-70.
23. Harlan JA. Consequences of leucocyte vessel wall interactions in inflammatory and immune reactions. Semin Thromb Hemost. 1987;13:434-44.
24. Remensnyder JP, Majno G. Oxygen gradients in healing wounds. Am J Pathol. 1969;52:301-19.

25. Imre G. Role of lactic acid. Br J Ophthalmol. 1964;48:75-82.
26. Zauberman H, Michaelson IC, Bergmann F, et al. Stimulation of neovascularization in the cornea by biogenic amines. Exp Eye Res. 1969;8:77-83.
27. Schreiber AB, Winkler ME, Derynck R. Transforming growth factor alpha: a more potent angiogenic mediator than epidermal growth factor. Science. 1986;232:1250-3.
28. Lynch SE, Colvin RB, Antoniades HN. Growth factors in wound healing. Single and synergistic effects on partial thickness porcine skin wounds. J Clin Invest. 1989;84:640-6.
29. Gospodarowicz D, Cheng J, Lui GM, et al. Angiogenic factor is related to fibroblast growth factor. Endocrinology. 1985;117:2383-91.
30. Gospodarowicz D, Ferrara N, Schweigerer L, et al. Structural characterization and biological function of fibroblast growth factor. Endocrinol Rev. 1987;8:95-114.
31. Ross R, Benditt EP. Wound healing and collagen formation. I. Sequential changes in components of guinea pig skin wounds observed in the electron microscope. J Biophysiol Biochem Cytol. 1961;11:677-700.
32. Clarke RAF. Overview and general considerations of wound repair. In: Clarke RAF, Henson PM (Eds). The Molecular and Cellular Biology of Wound Repair. New York: Plenum Press; 1988. pp. 3-23.
33. Ross R, Everett NB, Tyler R. Wound healing and collagen formation. VI. The origin of the wound fibroblast studied in parabiosis. J Cell Biol. 1970;44:645-50.
34. Diegelmann RF, Rothkopf LC, Cohen IK. Measurement of collagen biosynthesis during wound healing. J Surg Res. 1975;19:239-42.
35. Madden JW, Peacock EE. Studies on the biology of collagen during wound healing I. Rate of collagen synthesis and deposition in cutaneous wounds of the rat. Surgery. 1969;64:288-94.
36. Blakaj A, Bucala R. Fibrocytes in health and disease. Fibrogenesis Tissue Repair. 2012;5(suppl 1):S6.
37. Kurkinen M, Vaheri A, Roberts PJ, et al. Sequential appearance of fibronectin and collagen in experimental granulation tissue. Lab Invest. 1980;43:47-51.
38. Winter GD. Formation of the scab and role of epithelization in the skin of young domestic pigs. Nature. 1962;193:293-4.
39. Stenn KS, Depalma L. Re-epithelialization. In: Clarke RAF, Henson PM (Eds). The Molecular and Cellular Biology of Wound Repair. New York: Plenum Press; 1988. pp. 321-35.
40. Johnson FR, McMinn RMH. The cytology of wound healing of the body surface in mammals. Biol Rev. 1960;35:364-412.
41. Woodley DT, Bachman PM, O'Keefe EJ. The role of matrix components in human keratinocyte reepithelialization. In: Barbul A, Caldwell MD, Eaglstein WH, et al. (Eds). Clinical and Experimental Approaches to Dermal and Epidermal Repair. Normal and Chronic Wounds. New York: Wiley-Liss; 1991. pp. 129-40.
42. Lynch SE. Interaction of growth factors in tissue repair. In: Barbul A, Caldwell MD, Eaglstein WH, et al. (Eds). Clinical and Experimental Approaches to Dermal and Epidermal Repair. Normal and Chronic Wounds. New York: Wiley-Liss; 1991. pp. 341-57.
43. Korn JH. Fibroblast prostaglandin E_2 synthesis. Persistence of an abnormal phenotype after short-term exposure to mononuclear cell products. J Clin Invest. 1983;71:1240-6.
44. Vande Berg JS, Rudolph R, Woodward M. Comparative growth dynamics and morphology between cultured myofibroblasts from granulating wounds and dermal fibroblasts. Am J Pathol. 1984;114:187-200.
45. Albina JE, Mills CD, Henry WL Jr, et al. Temporal, expression of different pathways of l-arginine metabolism in healing wounds. J Immunol. 1990;144:3877-80.
46. Reed MJ, Puolakkainen P, Lane TF, et al. Differential expression of SPARC and thrombospondin 1 in wound repair: immunolocalization and in situ hybridization. J Histochem Cytochem. 1993;41:1467-77.
47. Bentley JP. Rate of chondroitin sulfate formation in wound healing. Ann Surg. 1967;165:186-91.
48. Bailey AJ, Sims TJ, Le Lous M, et al. Collagen polymorphism in experimental granulation tissue. Biochem Biophys Res Commun. 1975;66:1160-5.
49. Ehrlich HP, Krummel TM. Regulation of wound healing from a connective tissue perspective. Wound Rep Reg. 1996;4:203.
50. Miller EJ. Biochemical characteristics and biological significance of the genetically distinct collagens. Mol Cell Biochem. 1976;13:165-92.

Additional references appear in the online version of this book.

5

Fluids and Electrolytes

Edgardo S Salcedo, Carol R Schermer

Key Points

- A solid understanding of the normal and abnormal physiology of water and electrolyte homeostasis is critical to recognizing and managing abnormalities.
- Water and electrolyte homeostasis are disrupted with surgical operations and illness, so it is important to understand derangements to provide appropriate therapy.
- Although crystalloids are often considered interchangeable, fluids really are drugs: some are alkalinizing some acidifying and they do not all behave equally.
- How much is too much? Avoiding fluid overload: new data support that the concept "swell to get well" may be harmful.
- Balanced fluids: physiologic fluids that have electrolyte composition similar to plasma are associated with better outcomes. sodium chloride 0.9% is not physiologic for most surgical disease states.

INTRODUCTION

Knowledge of fluids and electrolytes is critical to caring for the surgical patient. The patient's requirements vary throughout the perioperative period and under different clinical circumstances such as sepsis, trauma, or in the setting of comorbid conditions. Appropriate management requires a fastidious practitioner, as some of the derangements in fluid and electrolyte balance and their complications are iatrogenic in nature. The chapter begins with a discussion of normal water and electrolyte balance, and the changes associated with dynamic nature of the surgical patient will be covered. Disturbances of specific electrolytes, seen in the surgical patient and how to manage them will also be reviewed. The chapter concludes with a discussion of more recent issues in fluid and electrolyte therapy regarding fluid overload and balanced fluid therapy, and concludes with a brief summary of acid-base balance that commonly accompanies the management of fluid and electrolyte abnormalities.

Total Body Water and Compartments

Total body water (TBW) comprises intracellular fluid (ICF) and extracellular fluid (ECF). ICF accounts for approximately two thirds of TBW, with the remaining one third in ECF. ECF is divided further into plasma and interstitial fluid. Interstitial fluid accounts for a 75% of the water found in ECF with the remaining in plasma.[1,2]

Fifty percent to 60% of an adult's body weight approximates TBW. Compartmentalizing the body weight estimate into ICF and ECF shows that ICF is 40% of body weight, plasma is 5% of body weight, and interstitial fluid is 15% of body weight.[1,2] The breakdown of TBW is presented graphically in Figure 5.1.

Electrolyte Composition and Compartments

Water, freely diffusible across cell membranes, will flow between fluid compartments based on osmolality. The osmotic force driving the movement of water depends only on the number of particles in the ICF and ECF independent of their electrical charge or size. Because the ICF compartment has a greater number of particles than the ECF compartment, the ICF compartment has a greater volume of water to equalize the osmolality of ECF and ICF.[2]

In the case of the human body, the solutes are the different electrolytes, proteins, and molecules, and the solvent is water. Electrochemical gradients govern the concentrations of the electrolytes distributed throughout the body's compartments. The number of electrical charges

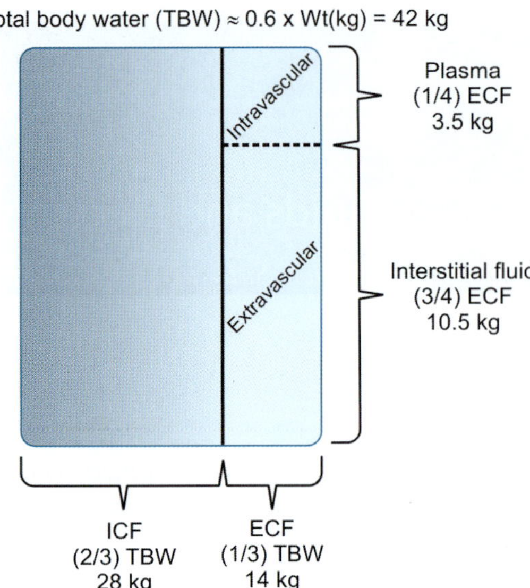

Fig. 5.1: Total body water distribution across all compartments. Estimated weights are calculated assuming 70 kg adult.
(TBW: Total body water; ICF: Intracellular fluid; ECF: Extracellular fluid).

per unit of volume is expressed in milliequivalents per liter (mEq/L). The number of solutes per kilogram of solvent is osmolality (mOsm/kg). Osmolarity, a term used much more frequently than osmolality, is the number of solutes per liter of solvent. In vivo clinically, osmolality and osmolarity (and their measurement units) are interchangeable because 1 L of water weighs 1 kg. The calculation for plasma osmolality (P_{osm}) arises from taking the sum of the major components of plasma per liter of serum water:

$$P_{osm} = 2 \times [Na^+](mEq/L) + (BUN\ (mg/dL)/2.8) + (Glucose(mg/dL)/18)$$

Blood urea nitrogen and glucose require correction factors to convert their measurements in serum to the appropriate units for osmolality. Sodium is doubled because each mOsm contribution of Na^+ has a corresponding negatively charge mOsm, most commonly chloride, which contributes to osmolality. Osmolality is also a measure of osmotic pressure, which can be measured directly in the laboratory with an osmometer. The normal range for plasma osmolality is 285 to 295 mOsm/kg.[3] The difference between the calculated plasma osmolality and the measured osmolality is referred to as the osmolal gap. A normal osmolal gap is <10 mOsm/kg. Abnormal elevations in the osmolal gap reflect elevated plasma levels of alcohols, sugars, lipids and proteins found in situations of toxicity, medication administration, or in a variety of disease conditions.

The normal distribution of electrolytes is specific to each compartment and obeys the principle of electroneutrality wherein there is a balance of cations and anions. In the ECF compartment, composed of plasma and interstitial fluid, the principal cation is sodium balanced by the principal anions, chloride, and bicarbonate. The ICF compartment's principal cations are potassium and magnesium, balanced by anionic phosphate, sulfate, and proteins.

The balance of these two major electrochemical forces results in the electrolyte compositions for each fluid compartment summarized in Figure 5.2.[4]

Perturbations of the balance due to disease states or interventions result in a movement of water and electrolytes between fluid compartments of the body. Because water is freely diffusible but electrolytes have restricted movement through the semipermeable cell membrane, changes in plasma osmolality will trigger an adjustment of water distribution to equalize osmolality in the compartments.[5] For example, when plasma osmolality decreases after an infusion of hypotonic solution, water will diffuse from the ECF compartment to the ICF compartment to lower intracellular osmolality and cause cellular swelling. The opposite occurs when plasma osmolality increases, drawing water out of the ICF compartment. The semipermeable nature of the cell membrane maintains sodium as the primary extracellular cation and potassium as the primary intracellular cation. Changes in electrolyte concentrations will trigger ion transport across the cell membrane mostly via energy-requiring processes that occur subsequent to the relatively rapid initial adjustments made through water diffusion.

WATER

Water homeostasis is a balance of intake, primarily ingested, and loss. Normal daily water intake is approximately 2 L/day. Water is lost through the urine, stool, and insensible losses. Insensible water loss occurs through the skin and lungs. As such, these losses are a function of total body surface area and will fluctuate in a variety of conditions including exercise or variations in environmental temperature. Typical, daily losses for a 70 kg adult include 1 L through urine, 300 mL through stool, and 600 mL in insensible losses.

Circulating levels of antidiuretic hormone (ADH) (arginine vasopressin)[2] are the primary mechanism controlling renal free water elimination. The posterior pituitary gland or neurohypophysis secretes ADH in response

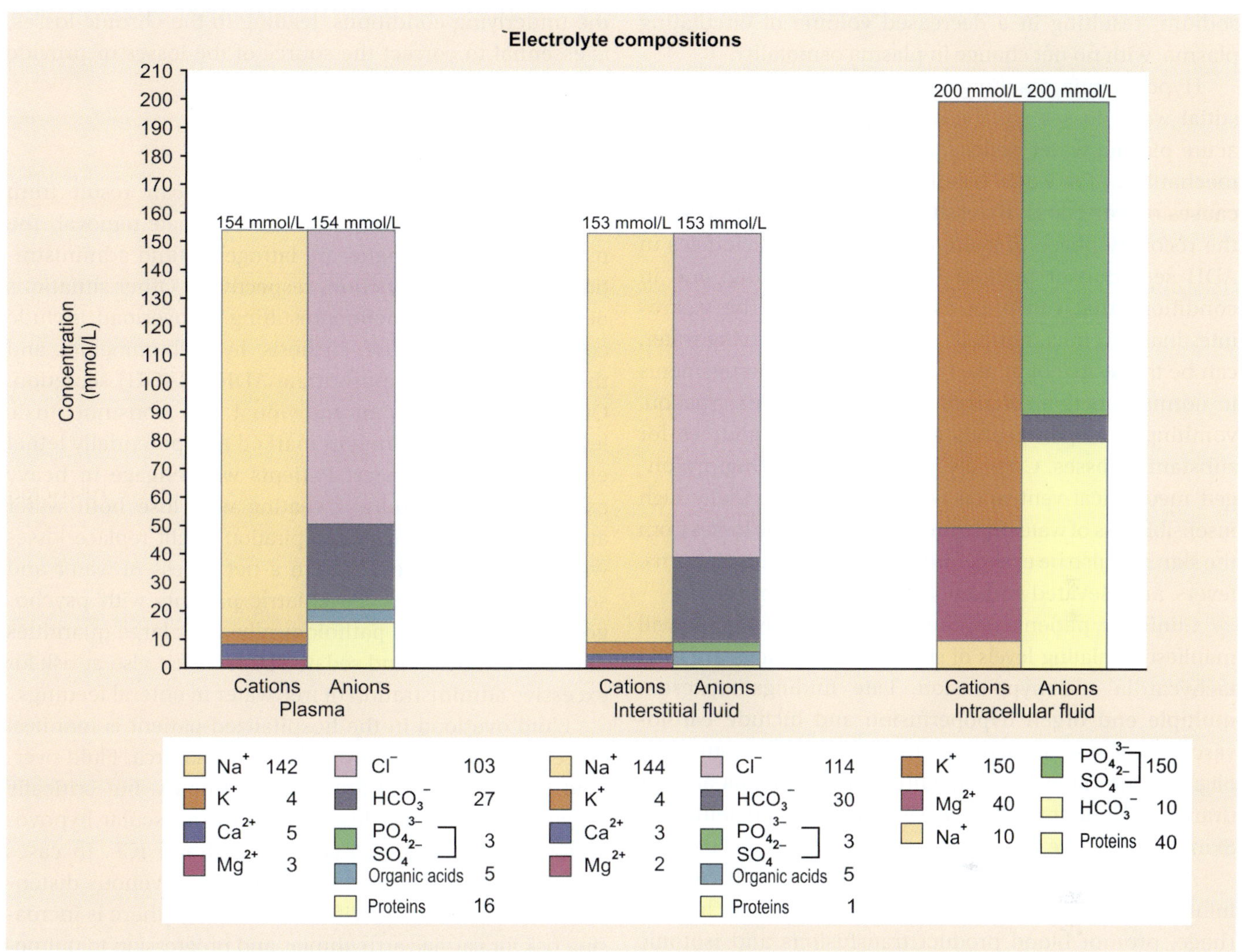

Fig. 5.2: Electrolyte composition of plasma, interstitial fluid, and intracellular fluid. All values are expressed in mmol/L.
Source: Data from Gamble JL. Chemical anatomy, physiology and pathology of extracellular fluid. Cambridge: Harvard University Press; 1947.

to dehydration or volume depletion, triggering the kidneys to conserve water, resulting in an increase in urine osmolality and the sensation of thirst to promote increased intake of water. In the setting of dehydration, plasma osmolality will increase because of the higher plasma concentration of sodium in a smaller amount of water. ADH secretion is highly sensitive to changes in plasma osmolality through receptors located in the anterior hypothalamus. Conversely, if plasma osmolality decreases ADH secretion will be suppressed resulting in increased water diuresis and a lower urine osmolality. However, the range of normal urine osmolality is quite broad (300 to 900 mOsm/kg).[3]

Stretch receptors, or baroreceptors, located in the aortic arch, carotid sinus, and atria of the heart sense changes in hemodynamics. Reductions in blood pressure will result in an increase in ADH secretion and renal water conservation to restore intravascular volume and to normalize hemodynamics. The sensitivity of the baroreceptor contribution to the feedback system is not as fine as the one for the osmoreceptor, hence changes are more likely to be driven by alterations in osmolarity than blood pressure. Moreover, changes in blood pressure will not prompt ADH secretion until relatively major reductions occur.

Water and Volume Deficit

When describing water deficits it is important to describe the degree of water loss and relative sodium loss. Dehydration is primarily loss of water in excess of sodium resulting, in an increased serum sodium concentration. Isotonic water loss refers to equal losses of water and sodium, resulting in a decreased volume of circulating plasma, with no net change in plasma osmolality.

Hypovolemia resulting from hemorrhage and interstitial water losses are the most common etiologies for acute plasma water deficits. Disturbances in the normal mechanisms for water balance account for the chronic causes of water loss. Excessive water losses can occur in the recovery phase of acute renal failure, deficiencies in ADH secretion or malfunctions in its signaling, and in conditions that cause an osmotic diuresis. The gastrointestinal (GI) tract, normally excellent at conserving water, can be the source of marked water loss with derangements in normal function. Diarrhea, enteric fistulas, obstruction, vomiting, and pancreatitis are all potential sources for substantial losses. Critically ill patients requiring prolonged mechanical ventilation will have an abnormally high insensible loss of water from the lungs. Insensible losses from the skin can also be exaggerated with open wounds, burns, fevers, and elevated ambient temperature or humidity.

Clinically, patients developing acute hypovolemia will manifest escalating levels of shock. Early findings are mild tachycardia and hypotension. Late findings represent multiple end organ hypoperfusion and include cardiovascular collapse, tachypnea, obtunded mental status, and oliguria. The clinical signs of chronic hypovolemia are less dramatic. Patients will be easily fatigued and lethargic. Skin turgor will be poor and mucosal surfaces will be dry.

Acutely hypovolemic patients require intravenous infusions to replace the acute losses. In those with hemorrhage, prompt blood product transfusions and isotonic fluid replacement can be life saving. Therapy is aimed at restoring normal hemodynamic parameters and preserving organ function. Addressing any surgical causes for the acute hemorrhage is critical to successful therapy. In cases of acute hypovolemia in other conditions, isotonic losses should be replaced with isotonic fluids with a similar electrolyte composition to the lost fluid. Hence, highly acidic losses resulting in alkalosis (nasogastric suction, vomiting) should be replaced with a high-chloride fluid (acidifying due to its chloride content), for example, isotonic saline with potassium, alkaline losses such as the bicarbonate losses seen with diarrhea result in acidosis and should be replaced with alkalinizing fluids such as Ringer's lactate or Plasma-Lyte.

Chronically hypovolemic patients will require similar replacement of losses. These patients will usually not require the replacement as rapidly, but they may require larger volumes for adequate replacement. Addressing the underlying conditions, leading to the chronic losses, is essential to correct the source of the losses or provide adequate ongoing replacement.

Water and Volume Excess

Water intoxication or fluid overload can result from excessive intake of fluids or from inadequate removal. The most common etiologies are iatrogenic fluid administration and renal dysfunction, respectively. Other situations of end-organ dysfunction resulting in overload include congestive heart failure, cirrhosis, hypoalbuminemia, and the syndrome of inappropriate ADH (SIADH) secretion. On rare occasions, an individual can consume toxic levels of water, resulting in marked and potentially lethal electrolyte disturbances. Patients who engage in heavy exertion with profound sweating who lose both water and electrolytes through perspiration might replace losses with water alone, resulting in a net excess of water and severe hyponatremia. Psychiatric patients with psychogenic polydipsia will pathologically drink large quantities of water. Intubated and sedated patients are also at risk for excessive administration of free water in enteral feedings.

Fluid overload in the hospitalized patient is manifest by generalized edema progressing to anasarca. Fluid overload can occur in all fluid compartments, but critically ill patients often manifest signs of intravascular hypovolemia while having excess interstitial and ICF. In cases where the fluid overload is intravascular, venous distension will be observed. With fluid overload there is increasing risk for cardiac arrhythmias and progression to pulmonary edema and congestion. Patients suffering from water toxicity from excessive ingestion will typically present with the acute mental status changes associated with the profound hyponatremia that accompanies marked intake of free water. Water restriction is the only therapy required for mild, asymptomatic cases. Diuretics may be required for more severe cases.

Initial management for fluid overload is fluid restriction, aiming for net negative volume status until normal fluid balance is restored. Diuretic therapy can be used to achieve the necessary excretion of fluid. When renal dysfunction is severely impaired, hemofiltration may be required. Appropriate fluid and water administration requires daily assessment and adjustment as the patient's clinical status dictates. This principle is particularly important given the dynamic, and sometimes unpredictable, nature of the surgical patient. Particular issues of fluid overload of the surgical patient are discussed further in the fluid overload section.

SODIUM

Sodium is the principal extracellular cation; sodium balance refers to the difference between sodium intake and output. Intake sources are daily ingestion and fluid administration. Output mechanisms include primarily renal elimination and to some degree GI losses and insensible losses through the skin and lungs. Excess losses can result from disturbances in renal and GI function. Inflammation and injury will also modulate insensible losses of sodium and water and will alter the sodium distribution between compartments.

The normal range for plasma sodium is 136 to 145 mEq/L.[3] Nearly all the body's stores of sodium are located in the ECF compartment. Significant deviations from normal levels of sodium are typically manifest in neurological disturbances and changes in mental status. Sodium balance is closely tied to water and volume balance due to the semipermeable cell membrane separating the intracellular and extracellular spaces. Sodium is the primary plasma solute responsible for triggering the osmoreceptors to signal the kidneys to conserve or diurese water, functioning as the driving force in maintaining extracellular and thereby intravascular fluid volume.

Hypernatremia

Elevations in plasma sodium levels are sometimes caused by excessive ingestion, but most cases are due to a net loss of free water from the ECF compartment.[6] Hypernatremia may also result from iatrogenic causes such as excessive administration of hypertonic solutions (increased intake) or osmotic diuretics (increased water loss). Patients with traumatic brain injury will often have induced hypernatremia as part of their therapy in an effort to draw fluid out of the ICF compartment to control brain edema.[7] Inadequate free water replacement in critically ill patients with underappreciated insensible losses due to the ventilator is another iatrogenic etiology.

Diabetes insipidus, sometimes resulting from brain trauma, involves dysfunction of the ADH pathway in which ADH is not appropriately secreted resulting in hypernatremia due to excessive water losses.

Hypernatremia is defined as a plasma level >145 mEq/L. The main clinical findings associated with hypernatremia are related to the central nervous system, a reflection of the altered brain fluid content as a result of elevated sodium levels, and they are typically observed at levels >160 mEq/L. The main clinical findings include restlessness and irritability, with progression to convulsions and coma at marked levels of hypernatremia. Symptoms may also become apparent at lower levels when there are rapid changes in sodium levels.

Treatment for hypernatremia is aimed at correcting the underlying cause and reducing plasma hypertonicity by replacing the free water deficit. Careful reviews of the patient's medications and nutritional supplementation regimen are essential. Free water deficit is calculated using the following equation:

$$\text{Free water deficit} = 0.6 \times \text{weight (kg)} \times [(\text{measured Na}^+/140)-1]$$

Total body water is estimated from the patient's weight. Some argue that the equation above underestimates free water deficit. An alternate equation for the calculation is:[8]

$$\text{Free water deficit} = 0.6 \times \text{weight (kg)} \times [1 - (290/P_{osm})]$$

No estimate is perfect, and close monitoring to titrate water replacement is required. The free water deficit represents the amount of water required, in liters, to restore plasma sodium levels to 140 mEq/L. Enteral replacement is the preferred administration route with asymptomatic hypernatremia. When patients exhibit clinical symptoms of hypernatremia, more rapid correction of plasma sodium is necessary with intravenous infusions of hypotonic solutions. However, lowering sodium levels too rapidly can result in diffusion of water back into brain cells resulting in cerebral edema, which can be lethal.[6] Dextrose or hypotonic saline solutions should be used to replace the calculated free water deficit over a 48-hour period. To determine the rate at which the water should be administered, some use the equations:

$$\text{Hours to correct} = (\text{serum Na}^+ - 140)/05$$

$$\text{Infusion rate} = \frac{\text{Free water deficit}}{\text{Hours to correct}}$$

The lower the sodium content of infused solutions, the less volume it will take to reduce the plasma sodium level. Serum sodium levels should not be lowered at a rate faster than 0.5–1 mEq/L/h to prevent this complication. A safe goal is to aim for reducing serum plasma levels by 10 mEq/L/day. While starting a hypotonic infusion, serum sodium levels should be monitored closely every 1 to 2 hours to assure adequate but not overly rapid correction and can then be reduced d to every 4–6 hours until below 150 mEq/L.

Hyponatremia

Hyponatremia is the most common electrolyte disturbance observed in hospitalized patients.[9] Hypotonic or dilutional hyponatremia is the result of increased relative levels of water. In outpatients, the most common etiology for this condition is impaired renal water elimination. SIADH will cause excessive renal resorption of water.[10] In the inpatient setting hyponatremia is most commonly due to excessive fluid administration. Children are at particularly high risk of hyponatremia due to the infusion of hypotonic fluids. A number of deaths due to cerebral edema occur annually due to iatrogenic water intoxication of children. The problem is so great that in 2007 the UK National Health Service issued a safety alert cautioning the use of hypotonic fluids in children due to deaths caused by IV infusion of hypotonic fluids in children.

Hyponatremia can also be due to excessive sodium losses in the urine, which can result from diuretic use, adrenal insufficiency or cerebral salt wasting seen in brain-injured or neurosurgical patients. Pseudohyponatremia occurs when nonsodium plasma solutes increase plasma osmolality sufficiently to draw water from the intracellular space into the extracellular space, as seen with marked hyperglycemia (most common) or hyperlipidemia.

Hyponatremia is defined as a plasma level < 136 mEq/dL. Just as with hypernatremia, the main clinical findings are related to central nervous system dysfunction. Clinical findings are related to both the severity of the hyponatremia, typically apparent at levels < 120 mEq/L, and also the rapidity of the sodium decrease. Symptoms start with fatigability and nausea and progress to confusion, lethargy, seizures, and coma.

The underlying cause must be identified and corrected. Similar to hypernatremia, plasma sodium should not be corrected too rapidly or it can result in central pontine myelinolysis.[11] Most cases of dilutional hyponatremia can be treated with free water restriction. Patients with fluid excess and hyponatremia will respond to a combination of free water restriction and diuresis. For patients with SIADH, when free water restriction is insufficient, some patients may require demeclocycline, which blocks the secretion of vasopressin in the kidney. For patients with euvolemic or hypervolemic hypernatremia, such as those with severe congestive heart failure or cirrhosis who fail to respond to diuresis and fluid restriction, a vasopressin receptor antagonist may be required for water elimination. This class of drugs is commonly referred to as Vaptans. Patients with markedly reduced sodium levels associated with marked hypovolemia will also respond to isotonic saline and hypertonic saline. Hypertonic saline solutions are reserved for patients with the most severe clinical symptoms such as seizures and coma. Sodium requirement and correction infusion rate are calculated using the following equations:

$$\text{Na}^+ \text{ requirement (mmol)} = \text{TBW} \times (\text{desired Na}^+ - \text{serum Na}^+)$$

$$\text{Infusion rate} = [\text{Na}^+ \text{ requirement (mmol)} \times 1000]/[\text{infusate Na}^+ \text{ (mmol/L)} \times \text{time (hours)}]$$

Sodium levels should not be corrected faster than 0.5–1 mEq/L/h or approximately 12 mEq/L/day.

POTASSIUM

Potassium is primarily an intracellular electrolyte, with 98% of total body potassium found within the cells. The remaining extracellular potassium is found in the extracellular space and plays a critical role in cardiac and neuromuscular activity. It follows that disturbances in potassium balance manifest clinically as derangements of cardiac and neuromuscular function.[2]

Normal plasma concentrations of potassium are in the range of 3.5–5.0 mEq/L.[3] Movement of potassium to and from the intracellular space is critical to maintain this narrow range of plasma levels. Although K is primarily intracellular, its extracellular (plasma) concentration is maintained in a very narrow range. Small changes in extracellular potassium can have profound physiologic effects despite normal intracellular potassium levels.

Hyperkalemia

Elevated levels of potassium, defined as > 5.0 mEq/L,[3] are potentially lethal if left untreated. Broadly, hyperkalemia can result from sudden increases in extracellular potassium concentrations. Acute elevations in serum potassium can arise from excesses in exogenous intake and/or inadequate renal clearance from circulation. Also, because potassium is primarily intracellular, biochemical changes may result in rapid shifts of these large stores to the extracellular space, which can cause acute hyperkalemia.

Acute increases in extracellular potassium may result from multiple etiologies. Increased oral or intravenous intake and cell destruction can increase potassium levels beyond the normal range. Hemolysis, rhabdomyolysis, extensive soft tissue injury after trauma (typically crush injury), or burns are all conditions that result in cell lysis and the release of potassium from the intracellular space. Medications such as angiotensin-converting enzyme-inhibitors, potassium-sparing diuretics, and depolarizing neuromuscular blockade agents (succinylcholine) can also cause hyperkalemia, especially in the presence of impaired renal function. Acute changes in pH, as in diabetic ketoacidosis (DKA) and hyperchloremic acidosis due to excessive saline infusion, will also cause a shift from intracellular to extracellular space and contribute to hyperkalemia, though transiently.[12]

Clinical symptoms may not be present even at significant levels of hyperkalemia. When present, they manifest as GI complaints, neuromuscular changes, and cardiac abnormalities. Electrocardiogram (ECG) findings are most helpful with diagnosis.[13] Peaked T waves are noted with early hyperkalemia, progressing to widened QRS complexes and depressed or inverted ST segments. At higher levels of hyperkalemia the ECG will appear sinusoidal and eventually progress to ventricular fibrillation. ECG changes do not generally become apparent until potassium levels reach or exceed 7.0 mEq/L.

Prompt therapy is essential to avoid the catastrophic consequences of unrecognized or untreated hyperkalemia. There are three goals for treatment: stabilizing the myocardium, rapidly reducing plasma levels of potassium, and removing excess potassium from the body.[12]

Preventing heart conduction abnormalities is the first priority because these effects are the most immediately life threatening. Infusion of calcium will antagonize the effects of potassium on the myocardium. It is administered in 10 mL doses of 10% calcium gluconate, with the first 1 to 2 g given over 10 to 20 minutes. Faster administration may result in cardiac dysfunction and even arrest. If needed, calcium gluconate can also be administered intramuscularly. Calcium, also available as calcium chloride, has three times the amount of calcium per dose. Although calcium chloride is an acceptable option for cardiac stabilization, extravasation of calcium chloride can cause tissue necrosis precluding intramuscular administration and requiring close monitoring when given peripherally. For the same reason, infusion through a central line is preferred.

Insulin infusion achieves rapid reduction of plasma potassium levels by moving potassium back into the intracellular space. Glucose is administered simultaneously to mitigate the hypoglycemic consequences of an insulin bolus. The recommended dose is 10 units of regular insulin administered intravenously with 50 mL of D50 (50% dextrose) immediately after the insulin. Albuterol, a B2 agonist, can also be used to lower plasma potassium levels and can be administered intravenously or through an inhaler or nebulizer. Treatment with B2 agonists however may result in an increase in glucose levels and heart rate. Though these measures reliably decrease plasma potassium levels, they are not definitive or permanent: they do not result in removal of potassium from the body, but only change the compartmentalization of potassium within the body.

Loop diuretic administration will achieve potassium removal from the body through renal elimination. Furosemide 20–40 mg intravenously is the recommended drug and dose and should be given along with fluid administration depending on volume status. Sodium polystyrene sulfonate (Kayexalate) is a cation exchange resin that binds potassium in the GI tract. It is often mixed into solution with 20% sorbitol, and it induces an osmotic diarrhea when administered orally as a 15–30 g dose. When given rectally the dose is 30–60 g, but this should not be mixed with sorbitol. It takes 4 to 24 hours to observe the effect of the resin, which should therefore be used for longer term elimination and not for transient hyperkalemia. For patients with renal failure, or in situations in which hyperkalemia is persistent and refractory to medical management, hemodialysis is indicated.

Patients with DKA or those in a hyperglycemic hyperosmolar state experience rapid shifts in potassium during resuscitation, potentially triggering life-threatening arrhythmias. Death during initial resuscitation of patients with DKA is often caused by hyperkalemia, whereas hypokalemia is a common cause of death after treatment initiation. Serum potassium should be checked every 2 hours until it is stable in all patients with a hyperglycemic crisis. Initial insulin therapy and volume replacement will rapidly drive potassium back into the intracellular space, thereby correcting the acute hyperkalemia. However, because DKA patients are often potassium deficient, as intracellular levels are restored while the hyperglycemic crisis is controlled, plasma levels will normalize and eventually decrease; the process requires close monitoring and repletion.

Hypokalemia

Low levels of potassium, defined as <3.5 mEq/L, are most commonly caused by GI losses and diuretic administration. Vomiting, prolonged gastric suctioning, diarrhea, and enterocutaneous fistulae are all routes for potassium loss. Inadequate monitoring and insufficient potassium supplementation can lead to marked hypokalemia. Diuretic administration increases renal losses of potassium. As mentioned in the therapy for hyperkalemia, administration of insulin and albuterol can also cause a transient hypokalemia.[12]

Patients with hypokalemia may present with muscle weakness, fatigability or cramping, and GI disturbances including ileus or constipation. Importantly, cardiac electrical abnormalities may be noted on ECG. These changes include flattened or inverted T waves, U waves, wide QRS complexes, and prolonged PR intervals.[14]

Treatment for hypokalemia is aimed at correcting the underlying cause and replacing potassium losses.[12] All medications potentially contributing to do hypokalemia should be held. Enteral replacement therapy is rapid and effective but not always possible in the surgical patient. Potassium chloride can safely be administered intravenously at a rate of 10 mEq/h, but faster rates up to 1/3 mEq/kg/h can be used for severe cases as long as the patient is being monitored. Magnesium replacement is often necessary during refractory hypokalemia and will minimize urinary K losses.

CALCIUM

Most of the calcium in the body is stored in the bone and teeth. Less than 1% of calcium in the body is found in the soft tissues and ECF. Circulating levels of parathyroid hormone (PTH) primarily control plasma levels of calcium. PTH promotes calcium absorption from the intestines, calcium reabsorption in the kidney, and calcium release from bones. PTH levels increase in response to decreasing calcium levels, thereby protecting the body from hypocalcemia. Calcitonin, a hormone produced in the parafollicular cells of the thyroid, opposes the effects of PTH and inhibits bone resorption by inhibiting osteoclast activity.

The normal range for total calcium is 9 to 10.5 mg/dL.[3] Approximately half of measurable calcium is protein bound, primarily to albumin. Total calcium measurements will fluctuate directly with albumin levels, requiring correction when albumin is abnormally elevated or decreased. The corrected total calcium level will increase or decrease by 0.8 mg/dL (0.2 mmol/L) for every 1 g/dL (1 U/L or 150 umol/L) above or below normal levels of albumin. The calculation for calcium correction is less accurate for surgical critical care patients.[15]

Forty percent to 45% of calcium is free or ionized calcium, which is the physiologically active form. The normal range for ionized calcium is 4.5 to 5.6 mg/dL (1.1–1.4 mmol/L).[3] Ionized calcium levels can also be measured directly and are more accurate than total calcium levels. Ionized calcium levels do not change with albumin levels, but they are inversely related to pH. The remaining small percentage of calcium is bound to other plasma proteins.

Hypercalcemia

An increased level of circulating PTH, as a result of primary hyperparathyroidism, is the most common cause of hypercalcemia. Primary hyperparathyroidism can arise from parathyroid adenomas or hyperplasia. Metastatic lesions to bone will also cause hypercalcemia. Certain types of malignancies can produce PTH-related protein (PTHrP), which shares most of the same activity with PTH. Other causes of hypercalcemia include sarcoidosis, vitamin D toxicity, milk-alkali syndrome, and thiazide diuretic use. As introduced in the previous section, total calcium levels may be falsely elevated in the setting of hyperalbuminemia (e.g. severe dehydration). More calcium is bound to albumin, but ionized and active calcium levels may remain normal. Patients with hypercalcemia present with a variety of complaints ranging from abdominal pain, nausea and vomiting, bone and muscle aches, polyuria, renal stone development, and psychiatric conditions (mostly depression). ECG will reveal a short QT interval and widened T wave.[14] Symptoms usually do not arise until calcium levels reach 12 mg/dL. Severely elevated calcium levels to 15 mg/dL may present with markedly depressed mental status and carry a high risk of cardiac arrest.

Treatment is reserved for symptomatic patients or when serum levels exceed 12 mg/dL. Therapy is aimed at volume expansion followed by diuresis with loop diuretics to promote calcium elimination in the urine. Normal saline is infused rapidly and is titrated to a urine output of 150 to 200 mL/h. The recommended dose for furosemide, only after adequate volume resuscitation is achieved, is 40 to 80 mg, intravenously every 6 hours. Bisphosphonates can also be used in conjunction with volume and diuresis to inhibit osteoclast activity and therefore bone resorption. Calcitonin administration will also inhibit osteoclast activity, but its effect is transient when compared with the sustained effect of bisphosphonates.

Hypocalcemia

Hypocalcemia is defined as calcium levels below 9 mg/dL or an ionized calcium <4.5 mg/dL (1.1 mmol/L). It is important to remember that only ionized or free calcium in the plasma is subject to the hormonal regulation systems described above, whereas albumin-bound calcium is not. In the setting of malnutrition or hypoalbuminemia, total calcium levels may be low although ionized calcium levels are normal. True cases of hypocalcemia result from low levels of PTH from hereditary hypoparathyroidism or, more commonly, acquired hypoparathyroidism from surgical excision of the parathyroid glands. Other causes of hypocalcemia include severe acute pancreatitis, severe necrotizing soft tissue infections, hypomagnesemia, and vitamin D deficiency. Even in the absence of any of these conditions, hypocalcemia is common in surgical and critically ill patients.[16] It is one of the most common electrolyte disturbances seen in the intensive care unit (ICU), affecting 80% to 90% of patients, and has been linked to increased mortality in this population. Proposed etiologies for these cases include precipitation within tissues, citrate interactions after blood transfusions and disruptions of the humoral regulation system secondary to inflammatory mediators. Trauma patients may develop hypocalcemia from resuscitation-induced hemodilution[17] and large amounts of citrate in preserved blood.

Acutely hypocalcemic patients may present with severe clinical manifestations including muscle spasm, tetany, and neuromuscular irritability manifest by positive Chvostek's and Trousseau's sign and altered mental status or seizures. ECG will demonstrate a prolonged QT interval.[14] Dysrhythmias and hemodynamic instability may ensue with severe hypocalcemia.

Treatment for hypocalcemia is aimed at replacing deficits commensurate with their severity and speed of onset. Mild hypocalcemia can be treated with oral calcium supplementation and vitamin D supplementation when necessary, whereas severe acute onset hypocalcemia after total parathyroidectomy requires more aggressive management. In the latter case, treatment with 1 to 2 g of intravenous calcium gluconate should be started promptly. Ongoing calcium administration is titrated to symptom resolution and measured total serum calcium levels between 7 and 9 mg/dL. Magnesium levels should also be checked and corrected as needed.

MAGNESIUM

Nearly 99% the total body content of magnesium is intracellular, with over half found in the skeleton. It is the fourth most common cation in the body and essential for important cellular processes including energy metabolism and protein synthesis. Magnesium homeostasis and activity is closely tied to the calcium homeostasis and function.

Normal serum levels of magnesium are between 1.7 and 2.2 mg/dL.[3] Approximately, 50% to 60% of the body's magnesium is found in bone, which serves as its main storage site. Only 1% of total body magnesium is in the extracellular space, rendering serum levels poorly suited to assess overall magnesium body stores. However, similar to potassium, extracellular levels are important. Approximately, 30% of magnesium in the plasma is bound to albumin and inactive. Magnesium is absorbed through the intestines and excreted through the kidneys. A small amount of ingested, but unabsorbed magnesium, is eliminated in feces.[18]

Hypermagnesemia

The kidneys are highly efficient at excreting magnesium in times of excess. Upon reaching a threshold level of serum magnesium, the kidneys readily excrete additional filtered magnesium. It follows that hypermagnesemia, a relatively rare condition, results from excessive magnesium intake and impaired renal function. Patients with chronic renal failure are most at risk, but renal function must be severely compromised to make a major contribution to hypermagnesemia. Medications such as antacids, cathartics, or enemas taken in excess or intravenous magnesium administered to pregnant women with preeclampsia can also cause elevated magnesium levels. Excessive magnesium administration is also possible through total parenteral nutrition (TPN). Conditions with extensive tissue damage can release the normally intracellular magnesium, giving rise to symptomatic hypermagnesemia.

Magnesium toxicity, if unrecognized or untreated, is potentially lethal. Signs and symptoms will typically become evident when magnesium levels reach 4 to 6 mg/dL, increasing in severity with rising levels. Findings include facial flushing, nausea, vomiting, lethargy, and eventually coma. Patients will also develop hypotension, hyporeflexia, and paralysis of increasing severity. On ECG, PR and QT intervals will be prolonged with widened QRS complexes and bradycardia. Cardiac arrest may result.[14]

Treating hypermagnesemia in a patient with normal renal function usually only requires removing any sources of excess magnesium intake and supportive care. For markedly elevated levels, intravenous fluid administration and diuresis with furosemide is the mainstay of therapy. Intravenous administration of 1 g of calcium is also helpful to counteract the effects of magnesium on neuromuscular and cardiac tissue. For the most severe cases or for patients with renal failure, hemodialysis may be required.[2]

Hypomagnesemia

Hypomagnesemia results from inadequate intake or excessive extrarenal or renal losses.[18] Decreased intake of magnesium can result from poor diet (often noted in chronic alcoholics), intestinal malabsorption, or inadequate dosing in TPN. GI fistulas, diarrhea, or prolonged nasogastric suction are extrarenal etiologies for hypomagnesemia. Cutaneous losses of magnesium can also be noted after periods of prolonged and intense exertion. Renal losses of magnesium are observed with diuretic use, fluid overload, hyperaldosteronism and hypercalcemia. Hypomagnesemia can also be seen in patients with DKA, major burns, acute pancreatitis, and hungry bone syndrome. It is common among the critically ill and postoperative populations and has been associated with a two-to-threefold increase in mortality.

Clinical manifestations of hypomagnesemia are similar to those seen in hypocalcemia. Patients develop tremors and muscle twitches progressing to tetany. Similar to hypocalcemia, Trousseau's and Chvostek's signs are positive. ECG findings include prolonged QT and PR intervals, ST segment depression and deterioration to torsades de pointes.[14]

Intravenous administration of magnesium for replacement is preferred when the diagnosis is certain.[16] The recommended dose is 1 to 2 g of magnesium sulfate administered rapidly over 2 to 4 minutes. Slower rates of infusion minimize the threshold effect of magnesium excretion, improving the efficiency of replacement therapy. Cessation of any medications contributing to renal magnesium wasting should be held. Concomitant calcium and potassium electrolyte repletion is usually required as hypomagnesemia is often noted with both hypokalemia and hypocalcemia. Careful examination of nutritional support is required to maintain adequate supplementation after the acute deficit is addressed. Oral magnesium salts are available, with a recommended daily dose of 300 mg/day. Adjustments are made depending on the presence and severity of extrarenal loss pathways discussed above.[2]

PHOSPHORUS

Phosphate is the major intracellular anion. It is integral to a range of cellular functions, chiefly involving energy metabolism, and is found in the energy transport molecule, adenosine triphosphate. The kidneys and PTH are the main regulators of serum phosphate levels.[19]

Normal serum levels of phosphate are between 3 and 4.5 mg/dL.[3] Approximately, 85% of an adult's phosphate is found in the bones. Only 1% is found in the plasma, of which approximately one-third exists as inorganic phosphates in the form of $H_2PO_4^-$ or HPO_4^{2-}. Less than 20% of inorganic phosphate found in serum is bound to protein. Phosphorus is absorbed in the intestines and eliminated through the kidney. To a lesser degree, it is exchanged from the plasma into both the intracellular space and bone as part of phosphate homeostasis.[2]

Hyperphosphatemia

Elevated levels of serum phosphate can result from excessive intake, impaired renal excretion, or acute shifts from the intracellular space into the extracellular space. Though diets high in phosphorus rarely cause clinically significant hyperphosphatemia medications such as phosphate-containing laxatives or unmonitored TPN can provide enough ingested phosphate to result in toxicity. Acute and chronic renal disease will limit phosphate excretion resulting in elevated serum levels. Hypoparathyroidism (hereditary or acquired) or pseudohypoparathyroidism can cause hyperphosphatemia because of the deficit or ineffectiveness of PTH to inhibit phosphate reabsorption. Hypocalcemia is also seen in these patients. Conditions such as tumor lysis syndrome, rhabdomyolysis, or severe trauma where massive cell destruction occurs can result in marked phosphate toxicity. Conditions that produce an acidosis, such as DKA, lactate production, or respiratory acidosis can trigger an efflux of intracellular phosphate into the extracellular space.

Most of the clinical manifestations of hyperphosphatemia—neuromuscular irritability, spasms, and tetany—are related to hypocalcemia. The calcium-phosphate product is calculated by multiplying the serum total calcium level by the serum level of phosphate. An elevated calcium-phosphate product may be associated with increased risk of death in patients with end-stage renal disease on dialysis. A calcium-phosphate product level >70 increases the risk of metastatic calcifications. This type of extraosseous calcification results from the precipitation of calcium and phosphate in small arteries and soft tissue leading to necrosis.

Treatment of acute hyperphosphatemia with associated hypocalcemia begins with volume expansion to promote renal phosphate excretion. All exogenous phosphate sources should be held. Treatment aimed at correcting any underlying causes of acidosis will help resolve the hyperphosphatemia. Severe cases of phosphate toxicity, particularly with impaired renal function, may require hemodialysis. Treatment for chronic hyperphosphatemia involves diet modification and the use of phosphate-binding compounds such as aluminum hydroxide gels. Aluminum-containing phosphate binders should be avoided in patients with renal failure because of toxicity.

Table 5.1 Common solution compositions.[20]

Solution	Na^+	Cl^-	K^+	Ca^{2+}	pH	Osm	Other
0.9% normal saline	154	154	0	0	5.6	308	
Hartmann's or Lactated Ringer's	130	110	4	3	6.5	273	Lactate 28 mEq
D5½ normal saline	77	77	0	0	4	406	Dextrose 50 g
D5¼ normal saline	34	34	0	0	4	321	Dextrose 50 g
3% hypertonic saline	513	513	0	0	5.8	1,030	
Plasma-Lyte A	140	98	5	0	7.4	294	Acetate 27 mEq Gluconate 23 mEq Magnesium 3 mEq

(All electrolytes are measured in mEq/L. Osm = osmolarity (mOsm/L)).

Hypophosphatemia

Hypophosphatemia is common in ICU patients, affecting approximately one-third of patients, and is even more common in septic patients, affecting approximately two thirds. The condition can result from poor intake, as seen in chronic alcoholics and inadequate TPN, or impaired absorption with excessive use of phosphate-binding antacids. Losses from the GI tract in diarrhea or through the kidneys will also contribute to low serum levels of phosphate. Rapid shift of extracellular phosphate to the intracellular space triggered by respiratory alkalosis, by hungry bone and refeeding syndromes, and by insulin administration can also cause hypophosphatemia.[16]

Clinical manifestations of hypophosphatemia are related to the importance of phosphate for cellular energy processes. Symptoms such as malaise and fatigue start to appear at severely low levels of serum phosphate. Left untreated, muscle weakness can progress to paralysis, hypoventilation, or impaired cardiac contractility leading to death. Hemolysis will occur secondary to diminished red cell flexibility, exacerbating decreased oxygen delivery associated with increased hemoglobin-oxygen affinity.

Treatment for hypophosphatemia is aimed first at reversing the underlying cause followed by replenishing any deficits. Replacement therapy is available in oral and intravenous formulations, constituted with sodium or potassium, with dosing in mmol of phosphate. The typical dose for moderate to severe hypophosphatemia is 30 mmol once to twice per day to replenish deficits over the course of a week.[2]

FLUID AND ELECTROLYTE THERAPY

Appropriate administration of intravenous fluids is critical to patient care and should be evaluated and reevaluated on a daily basis given the dynamic nature of surgical patients. The two main goals of fluid and electrolyte therapy are to restore any existing deficits and to replace ongoing losses for maintenance therapy. A variety of solutions are available, with advantages and disadvantages specific to each, and with ongoing controversy surrounding the ideal approach to optimize surgical outcomes. The remainder of the chapter will review the most commonly used solutions for therapy as well as management strategies. The compositions of several commonly used intravenous fluids are summarized in Table 5.1.[20]

Resuscitation Fluid Therapy

Acute intravenous fluid resuscitation in the setting of sepsis, trauma, and other forms of shock will be discussed in detail elsewhere in this book. Briefly, in clinical circumstances requiring the rapid restoration of intravascular volume, isotonic crystalloid solutions are the mainstay of therapy. In cases highly suspicious for, or with known, hemorrhagic shock prompt transfusion of blood products should not be delayed.[21] In general, end points of resuscitation include restoration of normal blood pressure and resolution of significant tachycardia with good hourly urine output to assure adequate organ perfusion.[22] Invasive monitoring to assess central venous pressure and cardiac function will also aid with resuscitation efforts. Echocardiography is an acceptable alternative to assess cardiac parameters in lieu of a pulmonary artery catheter. These adjuncts are particularly useful in patients with impaired renal function or when fluid resuscitation is not restoring acceptable hemodynamic parameters as expected. Fastidious monitoring of electrolyte and acid-base balance is of particular importance when large volumes of 0.9% normal saline are infused. Aggressive fluid resuscitation or prolonged infusions with this solution can cause hyperchloremic acidosis in patients.[23]

Although beyond the scope of this chapter, the use of colloid solutions as an alternative resuscitation fluid for critically ill patients has been studied extensively. A large meta-analysis does not support the use of colloid over crystalloid for resuscitation in critically ill patients.[24] One recent large multicenter randomized trial showed no clinical benefit to the albumin group over the saline group.[25] Subgroup analyses in studies to follow have shown there could be increased mortality associated with its administration to trauma patients, especially those with severe traumatic brain injury.[26]

Maintenance Fluid Therapy

Healthy patients who are nil by mouth and awaiting an operation or recovering uneventfully after an operation should receive maintenance intravenous fluid therapy. For the preoperative patient, assuring adequate intravascular volume is critical to avoiding complications of anesthesia, specifically induction. For the postoperative patient, maintenance therapy is employed until the patient can safely meet intake needs by mouth.[27] For patients with normal renal function, supplemental potassium can be added. Despite much surgical dogma, there is no standard fluid composition or rate for maintenance intravenous fluid therapy. However, a good starting point for most patients is one that meets basic sodium and potassium and water needs: D5 0.45% normal saline with 20 mEq/L of potassium chloride. In children, the rate for the fluid therapy can be calculated using the following weight-based approach:

For 0 to 10 kg : 4 mL/kg/h

For 11 to 20 kg: 2 mL/kg/h + 40 mL/kg/h (from the 1st 10 kg)

For 21 kg and up:

1 mL/kg/h + 60 mL/kg/h (from the 1st 20 kg)

Those values can then be applied to an adult. For example, for an adult weighing 60 kg, the fluid rate would be:

4 mL/h (for the first 10 kg) + 20 mL/h (for the second 10 kg) + 40 mL/h (for the remaining 40 kg) = 100 mL/h

As most adults weigh >20 kg, it follows that maintenance fluids should run at a rate of 1 mL/kg/h + 60 mL/kg/h. This is also known as the 4/2/1 rule for maintenance intravenous fluids. Daily electrolytes should be monitored to assess the adequacy of the fluid and supplemental electrolyte composition, with strict recording of intake and urine output to titrate the fluid rate. Contrary to older teachings, children should be maintained on an isotonic formulation as they are at risk of hyponatremia.[28,29]

Table 5.2 Gastrointestinal secretions.

Fluid	*Na^+*	*K^+*	*Cl^+*	*HCO_3^-*	*H^+*	*Output*
Saliva	50	20	40	30	–	1,000
Gastric	100	10	140	–	30–100	1,500
Bile	140	5	100	60	–	1,000
Pancreatic	140	5	75	100	–	1,500
Small bowel	140	5	70	50	–	2,000
Colon	60	70	15	30	–	200

All electrolytes are measured in mEq/L. Output is given in mL.

Patients in the immediate postoperative period will have more third-space fluid, i.e. fluid that is extravascular but still within the body in the interstitial space. Patients who have sustained major injuries or burns or who have large open wounds or soft tissue defects will exhibit similar disruptions in fluid physiology. These patients should be treated with an isotonic solution such as 0.9% normal saline, lactated Ringer's (LR), or Plasma-Lyte for the first 24 to 48 hours postoperatively. After this time period, anticipated third-space fluid will return to the intravascular space, typically triggering a brisk autodiuresis, signaling when it is acceptable to decrease infusion rates and switch to maintenance fluid solutions. Once the patient is able to tolerate adequate oral intake, the maintenance fluid rate can be further decreased and ultimately discontinued.

Surgical patients will often present with pathology that contributes to ongoing losses, which require adjustment of maintenance fluid therapy. The GI tract, normally highly efficient at absorbing fluids and water, when deranged can be a source of appreciable daily losses. Diarrhea, persistent vomiting or gastric suctioning, the presence of fistula, or marked ileus all require an assessment of output to adequately keep pace with fluid and electrolyte losses.

Normal daily fluid production for GI secretions and their electrolyte content is summarized in Table 5.2. Any pathology resulting in marked ongoing losses from a particular part of the GI tract should be monitored and replaced with a solution tailored to restore these losses.

RECENT EVIDENCE-BASED CONTROVERSIES

Surgeons have often worked under two assumptions: (1) too much fluid is better than too little and (2) 0.9% saline is harmless and that all crystalloids behave similarly in vivo. There was a period of time in which fluid volumes for resuscitation became high enough to cause compartment syndrome within the abdomen or within noninjured extremities. Large volumes of fluids were sometimes given in the ICU to avert renal failure and other end-organ perfusion problems, but good data were not available to guide when to reduce infusion rates or even to diurese the patient. Newer data in the ICU show that fluid overload is quite harmful and affects outcomes. In addition, data over the last decade shows that not all crystalloids are created equal. The differences in the solutions are the basis of more than esoteric questions or personal preference. The section below addresses these two topics.

Perioperative Fluid Therapy and Fluid Overload

The goal of perioperative fluid therapy is to maintain intravascular volume to preserve tissue perfusion and thereby prevent end-organ failure and complications. Historically, in surgical practice large volume infusions have been used to assure that adequate fluid volumes are maintained in the belief thatthere are few, if any, risks when compared with the benefits of preserving renal function. Surgical trainees were historically taught the concepts of "you need to swell to get well" and "it is easier to treat pulmonary failure than renal failure."

Recent literature suggests that fluid overload is unnecessary and may put perioperative patients at increased risk of complications.[30] Randomized controlled trials have shown that fluid therapy plans aimed at limiting perioperative fluid therapy may confer better patient outcomes.[31,32] Specifically, one study examined the effect of limiting salt and water infusions immediately postoperatively in elective hemicolectomy patients.[33] The restricted perioperative fluid regimen group showed faster return of bowel function as measured by tolerating liquid then solid food and passage of flatus then stool. Overall hospital stays were shorter, with no renal or other complications noted in the restricted fluid regimen group. An additional multicenter, randomized trial[31] demonstrated a reduction in major complications and suggested a mortality benefit when a restricted fluid regimen was employed intraoperatively and postoperatively in elective colorectal surgical patients. Notably, cardiopulmonary and tissue-healing complications were significantly reduced with the restricted fluid regimen. Rates of postoperative hypotension were similar in both groups. While postoperative low urine output was more frequent with the restricted fluid regimen, there was no difference in clinically significant renal complications.

The ARDSnet group conducted a randomized controlled trial in a large series of patients diagnosed with acute lung injury.[34] Though no difference in mortality rate was noted for conservative (restricted) versus liberal (standard) fluid therapy, there were statistically significant improvements in respiratory function and decreases in ventilator-free days and ICU lengths of stay among patients in the restricted group. Again, no differences in clinically important renal complications were noted. A post hoc subgroup analysis limited to surgical patients demonstrated similar findings.[35]

Allowing patients to remain volume depleted has known risks of serious postoperative complications. However, mounting evidence suggests that fluid overload may be similarly dangerous.[32,36] Indeed, the optimal fluid management plan in the perioperative period may lie somewhere in the middle, aiming for a more even level of fluid balance. Historically, such an approach might appear to be focused on inadequately restoring intravascular volume, as evidenced by recent trials naming these strategies "restricted" or "conservative" versus "standard" or "liberal." In reality, the goal is not to withhold any necessary restoration of volume, but rather to avoid fluid overload.[30]

Differences among Crystalloids: Balanced Solutions

Different solutions are available for fluid therapy, including crystalloids and natural and artificial colloids. Although historically most clinicians have believed that the varied crystalloid solutions behave similarly in vivo, the pharmacological properties of these solutions are markedly different. The ideal crystalloid, whether given on its own or functioning as a diluent for colloids, should not exert any negative effects on acid–base homeostasis or organ function.

Balanced versus Unbalanced Fluids

Crystalloids with an electrolyte composition similar to plasma are often referred to as "balanced" or "physiological" fluids. Balanced crystalloid solutions have been available for many years (e.g. Hartmann's solution/Ringer's lactate, Plasma-Lyte, Normosol, Isolyte S.) but are often not used due to relative hypotonicity (LR) or because of a perceived harm due to their potassium content along with lack of benefit or cost differences.

Although the acidifying effect of 0.9% sodium chloride has been known for nearly a century,[37] "normal saline" is still the most commonly used isotonic crystalloid in the world. Both preclinical and clinical studies have shown that when 0.9% saline is given in large volumes, the result is a predictable hyperchloremic metabolic acidosis.[38-40] Moreover, the acidosis associated with 0.9% saline infusion may also give rise to adverse effects including immune dysfunction[41] GI dysfunction,[40] and decreased renal blood flow.[42,43]

Balanced fluids that contain inorganic ions (calcium, potassium, or magnesium), and buffer components, such as bicarbonate, lactate, acetate, or gluconate along with a physiologic chloride concentration, are not associated with similar acidosis. Human and animal data suggest that the acidosis associated with saline infusion may be clinically important. Patients randomized to balanced solutions as opposed to saline-based fluids have less impairment of acid–base disorders, less impairment of hemostasis,[44,45] and improved gastric perfusion,[40] with better preservation of electrolyte levels.[45,46] Renal function may also be better preserved with balanced fluids (Figs. 5.3A to C).[42,47]

The overwhelming majority of studies performed comparing balanced fluids to saline are in favor of balanced fluids. There are a few cogent arguments against LR due to its hypotonicity and calcium content. Because isotonic saline has a higher osmolarity than LR solution, there is a potential disadvantage of using LR in patients with traumatic brain injury. Moreover, LR is not approved by the Association of American Blood Banks[48] for infusion with citrate-preserved packed red blood cells because of the presence of calcium in the fluid. Chelation of the calcium by citrate can result in the clotting of blood filters and small bore IV catheters. In addition, when LR is administered to patients with hemorrhagic shock, sepsis, or during renal transplant[49] or hepatic surgery[46] LR causes a small increase in serum lactate levels, although the clinical importance of this increased lactate is unknown. Plasma-Lyte, Normosol, and Isolyte all contain acetate, which in the high doses tested for dialysis may cause hypotension. However, human studies of these solutions that contain a much lower dose of acetate do not show adverse effects.

Effect of Other Electrolytes in Balanced Solutions

All of the balanced fluids contain potassium in a physiologic range, so clinicians are concerned that infusion will exacerbate or cause hyperkalemia. Many clinicians are trained under the concept of "no Pee, no K" and hence avoid potassium containing solutions in dehydrated patients. However, because the acidifying chloride is replaced with alkalinizing bases (lactate or acetate), no studies have shown that humans with normal renal function or those undergoing renal transplantation will increase their potassium levels. Normal saline has been compared with LR or Plasma-Lyte in healthy volunteers,[50] patients undergoing major abdominal[51] and pelvic surgery, and patients undergoing transplant surgery,[49,52] and none have developed hyperkalemia in the balanced group. In fact, two studies in kidney transplant recipients[52,53] showed that hyperkalemia occurred in patients receiving saline because the saline-induced acidosis caused a shift of potassium into the extracellular space.

Three randomized trials of patients undergoing renal transplantation[49,52,53] compared saline to balanced fluids. In all three studies, patients who received saline had a lower pH and serum bicarbonate level during and at the end of operation. Two trials showed no differences in potassium between the groups. The Khajavi trial showed elevated potassium in the saline group. In the O'Malley trial, although there was no difference in the mean potassium at the end of operation, the study was terminated because there were more elevated serum potassium levels in the saline group.

In a small randomized trial of patients undergoing elective abdominal aortic aneurysm surgery,[51] patients were randomized to receive LR or saline to maintain the cardiac filling pressures within 10% of baseline. Blood, colloid, and bicarbonate use were all standardized. Patients in the saline group had significantly higher chloride levels and osmolarity and required more blood products and bicarbonate than LR patients. Patients in the saline group had significantly lower pH on arrival to the ICU. In a propensity-matched cohort analysis, Shaw et al. compared the use of saline to Plasma-Lyte in patients undergoing major open abdominal surgery. They showed that saline recipients received more buffers and had more electrolyte abnormalities than Plasma-Lyte recipients.

Effect on the Kidney

Reid et al. randomized healthy volunteers to receive 2 L of LR or saline. They found that infusion of LR resulted in higher urine output and less fluid retention than saline infusion. Subjects who received saline had significantly higher chloride levels and lower bicarbonate levels at the end of the study without any difference in serum

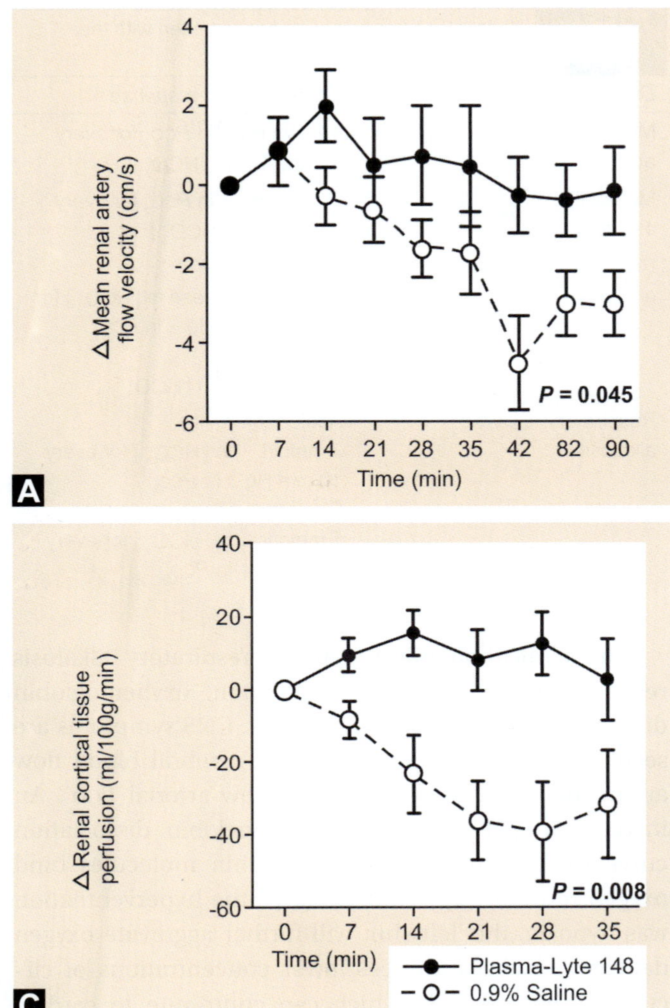

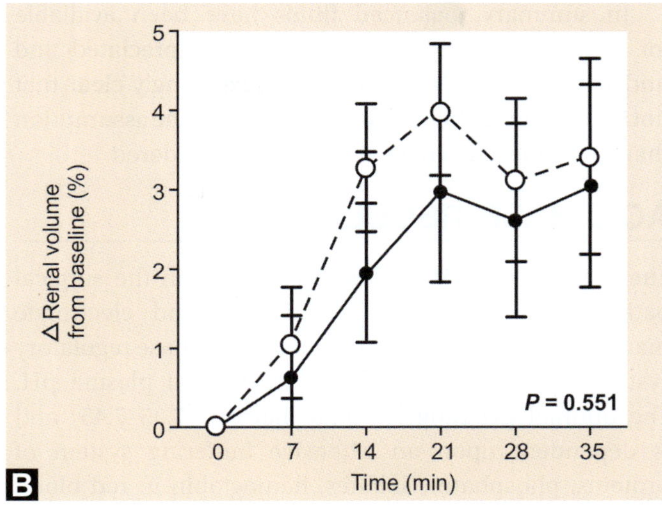

Figs. 5.3A to C: Changes in renal artery blood flow velocity, renal volume, and renal cortical tissue perfusion after infusion of 2 L of 0.9% saline and Plasma-Lyte 148 over 1 hour. All vales are mean (SEM). *P* values are for the test of 0.9% saline versus Plasma-Lyte 148 using the analysis of variances and repeated measures model.
Source: Figure and data from Chowdhury AH, Cox EF, Francis ST, et al. A randomized, controlled, double-blind crossover study on the effects of 2-L infusions of 0.9% saline and Plasma-Lyte(R) 148 on renal blood flow velocity and renal cortical tissue perfusion in healthy volunteers. Ann Surg. 2012;256(1):18-24.

osmolarity. The same research group later conducted a similar trial of Plasma-Lyte 148 against saline with similar findingsregarding acidosis and hyperchloremia.[42] In addition, the second trial also showed that saline infusion decreased renal artery blood flow velocity and renal cortical perfusion (Figs. 5.3A to C). A propensity-matched cohort analysis comparing the use of Plasma-Lyte versus saline in major abdominal surgery showed that patients receiving saline were more likely to require renal dialysis.

In addition to direct effects on the kidney, the Chowdhury et al. study comparing Plasma-Lyte to saline showed that although blood volume changes were identical between groups, there was greater expansion of the extravascular fluid volume after saline. Both the randomized trials in human volunteers showed a shorter time to first micturition in the balanced fluid group along with a greater postinfusion urinary volume.

Effect on Fluid Balance and Complications and Costs

The large propensity-matched cohort analysis of saline versus Plasma-Lyte by Shaw et al. showed that treatment with balanced fluid was associated with fewer complications (odds ratio 0.79). Postoperative infection, renal failure requiring dialysis, blood transfusion, acidosis investigation, and intervention were all more frequent in patients receiving 0.9% saline.

In both the Shin et al. study comparing Plasma-Lyte to LR in hepatic surgery and in the Young et al. study that compared Plasma-Lyte to saline in trauma patients, magnesium levels were maintained within the normal range in the Plasma-Lyte groups. The trauma study showed that the cost of magnesium replacement alone offset the cost difference in fluid acquisition.[54]

In summary, balanced fluids have been available for a long time and are highly underappreciated and underutilized. Data are becoming increasingly clear that not all crystalloids behave similarly in vivo. The assumption that 0.9% saline is benign should be reconsidered.

ACID-BASE REGULATION

The management of acid-base problems in the surgical patient is closely aligned with fluid and electrolyte management. The primary role of the acid-base regulatory system is the maintenance of an optimal plasma pH. The optimal pH range is quite narrow (7.35–7.45) and is dependent upon an extensive buffering system of proteins, phosphates, sulfates, hemoglobin in red blood cells and a tight relationship between dissolved carbon dioxide (CO_2) and HCO_3^-. This interaction is described by the Henderson Hasselbalch equation:

$$pH = pK_a(6.1) + \log_{10}([HCO_3^-]/[H_2CO_3]).$$

Clinical abnormalities of acid-base equilibrium result in a compensatory response. The two most common mechanisms for compensation involve changes in ventilation or renal function. Respiratory compensation occurs quickly and results in a rapid change in arterial $P\text{CO}_2$ and renal compensation occurs by altering the excretion of H^+ and resorption of HCO_3^-. The renal compensatory mechanism is a much slower but a more effective response and reflects a chronic change from the normal acid-base equilibrium. The different compensatory changes are indicated in Table 5.3.

Table 5.3 Various compensatory responses seen with the primary acid-base disturbances.

Disorder	*Primary change*	*Compensatory response*
Metabolic acidosis	$\downarrow[HCO_3^-]$	1.2 mm Hg ↓ in $P\text{CO}_2$ for every 1 mmol/L ↓ in $[HCO_3^-]$
Metabolic alkalosis	$\uparrow[HCO_3^-]$	0.7 mm Hg ↑ in $P\text{CO}_2$ for every 1 mmol/L ↑ in $[HCO_3^-]$
Respiratory acidosis	↑$P\text{CO}_2$	Acute: 1 mmol/L increase in $[HCO_3^-]$ for every 10 mm Hg ↑ in $P\text{CO}_2$ Chronic: 3.5 mmol/L ↑ in $[HCO_3^-]$
Respiratory alkalosis	↓ $P\text{CO}_2$	Acute: 2 mmol/L ↓ in $[HCO_3^-]$ for every 10 mm Hg ↓ in $P\text{CO}_2$ Chronic: 5 mmol/L ↓ in $[HCO_3^-]$ for every 1 mm Hg ↓ in $P\text{CO}_2$

Respiratory Alkalosis

Respiratory alkalosis is the most common acid-base disorder and is due to hyperventilation with a resultant decrease in arterial $P\text{CO}_2$.[55] The most common cause is hypoxemia resulting in an increased respiratory drive. Other causes include pregnancy, pain, sepsis, iatrogenic over-breathing of an intubated patient who is on a ventilator, and central nervous system (CNS) injury due to trauma or a "cerebrovascular accident". When a CNS injury is the cause, alkalosis is due to the loss of regulatory control of respiration and not a decrease in local pH. The pathogenesis of the alkalosis is the generation of increased minute ventilation due to an increased respiratory rate and/or increased ventilator tidal volume out of proportion to the stimulus to breathe secondary to the arterial $P\text{CO}_2$. The resultant fall in $P\text{CO}_2$ causes a reduction in HCO_3^- concentration.

The clinical manifestations of respiratory alkalosis result in alterations of CNS function, oxyhemoglobin dissociation and cardiac conduction. CNS symptoms are secondary to a decline in effective cerebral blood flow autoregulation that occurs with a low arterial $P\text{CO}_2$. An increase in pH shifts the oxyhemoglobin dissociation curve to the left, making hemoglobin molecules bind oxygen more firmly. If the cause of the hyperventilation was hypoxia, this left shift will further aggravate oxygen delivery. Alkalosis induces lower concentrations of circulating K^+ and Ca^{2+}, which can contribute to cardiac conduction disturbances. These abnormalities are exaggerated with body K^+ losses and therapeutic digoxin. Clinically, respiratory alkalosis presents with skeletal muscle cramps, dizziness, paresthesias, and syncope.

Management

The management of respiratory alkalosis requires specific clinical interventions. If inappropriate mechanical ventilation is the cause, ventilator adjustments are required to reduce the excess minute volume. If hypoxemia is the cause, then normalizing both pH and arterial oxygen saturation will be required. Administration of intravenous KCl and $CaCl_2$ will help to minimize the risk of arrhythmia. Manipulation of the arterial $P\text{CO}_2$ can be achieved by increasing ventilatory dead space.

Respiratory Acidosis

Respiratory acidosis is an increased arterial $P\text{CO}_2$ and is due to an imbalance between total body production of CO_2 and elimination of CO_2 by the lungs, usually due to hypoventilation.[56] The most common causes can be separated into acute and chronic problems. Acute respiratory acidosis results from a hypoventilatory mechanical event (such as airway obstruction due to trauma, tumor or foreign body aspiration), hypoventilation secondary to inappropriate ventilator settings with low minute ventilation, over sedation (e.g. narcotics), or an acute exacerbation of pulmonary disease (e.g., asthma or acute respiratory distress syndrome). Chronic respiratory acidosis is usually related to severe chronic obstructive pulmonary disease, severe muscle weakness, or the patient's body habitus (e.g. morbid obesity or severe skeletal abnormalities). Patients who have chronic respiratory acidosis ordinarily will have evidence of renal compensation that results in an elevation in HCO_3^- concentration.

Management

Treatment of respiratory acidosis is directed at correcting hypoventilation. For acute onset respiratory acidosis correction requires ensuring a patent airway and normalizing minute ventilation. For patients who have chronic respiratory acidosis, it may not be necessary to correct the increased Pco_2 until it exceeds 55–60 mm Hg, particularly if the HCO_3^- concentration exceeds 30 mEq/L (30 mmol/L). When changes are made, the elevated Pco_2 should be corrected more slowly to avoid CNS problems caused by sudden alterations in pH. Patients with respiratory acidosis from hypoventilation may also be hypoxemic and this will require supplemental oxygen. Supplemental oxygen therapy must be approached with caution in the patient with chronic respiratory acidosis since hypoxemia may be the driver for CNS ventilation and increasing the PO_2 acutely may lead to apnea.

In patients receiving parenteral nutrition with hypertonic glucose solutions, a high respiratory quotient may present with hypercapnia if there is hypoventilation. It may be necessary to reduce the glucose quantity that is employed and use lipids as an alternative calorie source.

Metabolic Alkalosis

Metabolic alkalosis is the result of a loss of H^+ and Cl^- with a relative increase in HCO_3^-.[57] The most common site of H^+ and Cl^- losses is the upper gastrointestinal tract. Vomiting from gastric outlet obstruction or long-term nasogastric tube use with inadequate Cl^- replacement accounts for the majority of cases. Metabolic acidosis may also result from excess renal excretion of Cl^- secondary to chronic diuretic (particularly chlorothiazide) use or excess hormonal stimulation of the kidney by aldosterone- or cortisol-producing tumors.

Metabolic alkalosis is further compounded by a low serum K^+ concentration. K^+ is the primary exchange ion for the resorption of Na^+ by the kidney under the normal stimulation of aldosterone. Inadequate K^+ as an exchange ion results in H^+ becoming the alternative exchange ion for Na^+ reabsorption. When the cause is related to diuretic use, patients are frequently volume contracted. Common causes of metabolic alkalosis are shown in Table 5.4.

Table 5.4 Causes of metabolic alkalosis.

Causes
Loss of H^+
Gastrointestinal loss
Removal of gastric secretions—vomiting or nasogastric suction*
Antacid therapy, particularly with cation-exchange resins
Chloride-losing diarrhea
Renal loss
Loop or thiazide-type diuretics
Mineralocorticoid excess*
Postchronic hypercapnia*
Low chloride intake
High-dose carbenicillin or other penicillin derivative
Hypercalcemia, including the milk-alkali syndrome
H^+ movement into cells
Hypokalemia*
Refeeding carbohydrates after fast
Retention of HCO_3^-
Massive blood transfusion
Administration of $NaHCO_3$
Sweat losses in cystic fibrosis

*Most common causes

Clinical manifestations of metabolic alkalosis include muscle weakness and fatigue, mild CNS abnormalities, cardiac arrhythmias secondary to hypokalemia and significant loss of gastrointestinal motility (paralytic ileus). The compensatory response for metabolic alkalosis may be problematic because hypoventilation may not be well tolerated.

Management

The effective treatment for metabolic alkalosis is the prevention of additional losses of H^+ and the restoration of lost Cl^- by aggressive fluid administration with NaCl and KCl solutions. The likelihood of success with this therapy can be assessed by measuring Cl^- excretion in the urine. Those patients who have values equal to or less than 10–15 m Eq/L (10–15 mmol/L) will respond to Cl^- replacement therapy, but those who have levels greater than 20 m Eq/L (20 mmol/L) will probably not respond to intravenous therapy alone.

Aggressive KCl replacement is an essential part of restoring normal pH. For patients who have hypokalemic hypochloremic alkalosis, correction of alkalosis is dependent upon correction of the hypokalemia. Failure to replace K^+ will be associated with a continued paradoxical aciduria and the patient will continue to have a systemic metabolic acidosis. If the alkalosis is more chronic, additional therapy using acetazolamide, a carbonic anhydrase inhibitor may be necessary.

If carbonic anhydrase therapy is ineffective, the only remaining choice is replacement of H^+ using an NH_4Cl or 0.31% HCl (100 mmol/L) solution. The HCl solution must be administered through central venous access usually at a rate of up to 100 mL/h. This will restore H^+ at a rate of approximately 10 mEq/h (10 mmol/h). Calculations similar to those used to calculate Na^+ or water replacement can be used to provide an estimate of the Cl^- deficit. When using HCl, it is essential to monitor the arterial pH frequently and discontinue therapy as soon as it approaches normal.

If excess mineralocorticoid concentrations are the cause of metabolic acidosis (Cl^- > 20 mmol/L in urine), it is unlikely that replacement with NaCl or KCl will be sufficient. Cessation of cortisol therapy or surgical extirpation of the adrenal lesion after preoperative preparation with spironolactone will be necessary to resolve the alkalosis.

Metabolic Acidosis

Metabolic acidosis is a common abnormality of acid-base balance.[58,59] Metabolic acidosis is due to the production of excess organic or inorganic acids and/or excessive losses of HCO_3^-. Acute excess acid production is most frequently related to systemic hypoxia secondary to a low-flow state with impaired tissue perfusion (e.g. lactic acidosis). Other acute causes of excess acid load include renal failure, diabetic ketoacidosis and poison ingestion (e.g. salicylates, methanol, ethylene glycol). Other causes of excessive HCO_3^- may occur from pancreatic or enterocutaneous fistulas, diarrhea, and renal losses of HCO_3^- due to drugs, renal tubular acidosis and hypoaldosteronism.

The clinical manifestations of acute metabolic acidosis due to a low flow state involve deterioration in the function of all systems and include decreased cardiac output, reduced arterial pressure, and hemodynamic collapse. The compensatory response of the patient is the elimination of CO_2 through hyperventilation. Those patients with metabolic acidosis secondary to ketoacidosis or exogenous poisoning may have a significantly impaired mental status but without the hemodynamic changes associated with shock.

Management

The management of shock requires aggressive volume and blood resuscitation for the patient who has lactic acidosis. It is not necessary to use bicarbonate therapy in these patients until the pH drops to less than 7.2 and there are obvious physiologic derangements. There are serious consequences of excessive $NaHCO_3$ therapy, including hypernatremia, a hyperosmolar state, and a "rebound" alkalosis. Rebound alkalosis occurs when large amounts of HCO_3^- are given during the acute phases of metabolic acidosis such as occurs in acute hemorrhagic shock. When oxygenation and tissue perfusion have been restored, oxidation of lactate will lead to internal correction of the acid load and net alkaline effects. Metabolic alkalosis from excessive exogenous HCO_3^- can be the result. Therefore, the use of alkalizing agents should be limited to those patients who have failed to respond to all routine measures.

Alternatives to HCO_3^- therapy include Carbicarb, which is a mixture of $NaHCO_3$ and sodium carbonate. The buffering capability of this agent is potentially better, but it carries the same risk for hypernatremia and hyperosmolar state mentioned above. Another agent is tris (hydroxymethyl) aminomethane (THAM), which is a non-Na^+ containing buffer. Finally, dichloroacetate, which blocks lactate production by inhibiting protein kinase, is also available.

The treatment of non-anion gap metabolic acidosis should be directed at the cause, specifically correction of losses from the gastrointestinal tract, reversal of Addison's disease with mineralocorticoids or alteration of treatment for drug-induced renal tubular acidosis. Treatment of anion gap acidosis includes intravenous insulin for diabetic ketoacidosis, and dialysis for those patients who have severe acidosis secondary to poisoning. It may not be necessary to dialyze patients who have renal failure unless their acidosis becomes refractory to other treatments.

REFERENCES

1. Edelman IS, Leibman J. Anatomy of body water and electrolytes. Am J Med. 1959;27:256-77.
2. Taal MW, Chertow GM, Marsden PA, et al. Brenner and Rector's The Kidney. Philadelphia, PA: Elsevier Saunders; 2011.
3. Kratz A, Ferraro M, Sluss PM, et al. Case records of the Massachusetts General Hospital. Weekly clinicopathological exercises. Laboratory reference values. N Engl J Med. 2004;351(15):1548-63.
4. Gamble JL. Chemical anatomy, physiology and pathology of extracellular fluid. Cambridge: Harvard University Press; 1947.
5. Leaf A, Chatillon JY, Wrong O, et al. The mechanism of the osmotic adjustment of body cells as determined in vivo by the volume of distribution of a large water load. J Clin Invest. 1954;33(9):1261-8.
6. Adrogue HJ, Madias NE. Hypernatremia. N Engl J Med. 2000;342(20):1493-9.
7. Wright WL. Sodium and fluid management in acute brain injury. Curr Neurol Neurosci Rep. 2012;12(4):466-73.
8. Cheuvront SN, Kenefick RW, Sollanek KJ, et al. Water-deficit equation: systematic analysis and improvement. Am J Clin Nutr. 2013;97(1):79-85.
9. Bagshaw SM, Townsend DR, McDermid RC. Disorders of sodium and water balance in hospitalized patients. Can J Anaesth. 2009;56(2):151-67.
10. Bartter FC, Schwartz WB. The syndrome of inappropriate secretion of antidiuretic hormone. Am J Med. 1967;42 (5): 790-806.
11. Ball SG. Hyponatraemia. J R Coll Physicians Edinb. 2010;40 (3):240-5.
12. Schaefer TJ, Wolford RW. Disorders of potassium. Emer Med Clin N Am. 2005;23(3):723-47, viii-ix.
13. Pepin J, Shields C. Advances in diagnosis and management of hypokalemic and hyperkalemic emergencies. Emer Med Prac. 2012;14(2):1-17; quiz -8.
14. Diercks DB, Shumaik GM, Harrigan RA, et al. Electrocardiographic manifestations: electrolyte abnormalities. J Emer Med. 2004;27(2):153-60.
15. Byrnes MC, Huynh K, Helmer SD, et al. A comparison of corrected serum calcium levels to ionized calcium levels among critically ill surgical patients. Am J Surg. 2005;189(3):310-4.
16. Sedlacek M, Schoolwerth AC, Remillard BD. Electrolyte disturbances in the intensive care unit. Semin Dial. 2006;19(6):496-501.
17. Vivien B, Langeron O, Morell E, et al. Early hypocalcemia in severe trauma. Crit Care Med. 2005;33(9):1946-52.
18. Musso CG. Magnesium metabolism in health and disease. Int Urol Nephrol. 2009;41(2):357-62.
19. Amanzadeh J, Reilly RF Jr. Hypophosphatemia: an evidence-based approach to its clinical consequences and management. Nat Clin Pract Nephrol. 2006;2(3):136-48.
20. Medicine USNLo. (1993). DailyMed Current Medication Information. [online] Available from http://dailymed.nlm.nih.gov/dailymed/about.cfm [last accessed November 26, 2012].
21. Dutton RP. Haemostatic resuscitation. Br J Anaesth. 2012; 109(Suppl 1):i39-i46.
22. Holley A, Lukin W, Paratz J, et al. Review article: part one: goal-directed resuscitation--which goals? Haemodynamic targets. Emerg Med Australas. 2012;24(1):14-22.
23. Blanloeil Y, Roze B, Rigal JC, et al. [Hyperchloremic acidosis during plasma volume replacement]. Ann Fr Anesth Reanim. 2002;21(3):211-20.
24. Roberts I, Blackhall K, Alderson P, et al. Human albumin solution for resuscitation and volume expansion in critically ill patients. Cochrane Database Syst Rev. 2011;(11): CD001208.
25. Finfer S, Bellomo R, Boyce N, et al. A comparison of albumin and saline for fluid resuscitation in the intensive care unit. N Engl J Med. 2004;350(22):2247-56.
26. Myburgh J, Cooper DJ, Finfer S, et al. Saline or albumin for fluid resuscitation in patients with traumatic brain injury. N Engl J Med. 2007;357(9):874-84.
27. Pearse RM, Ackland GL. Perioperative fluid therapy. BMJ. 2012;344:e2865.
28. Alves JT, Troster EJ, Oliveira CA. Isotonic saline solution as maintenance intravenous fluid therapy to prevent acquired hyponatremia in hospitalized children. J Pediatr. 2011; 87(6): 478-86.
29. Choong K, Arora S, Cheng J, et al. Hypotonic versus isotonic maintenance fluids after surgery for children: a randomized controlled trial. Pediatrics. 2011;128(5):857-66.
30. Lobo DN. Fluid overload and surgical outcome: another piece in the jigsaw. Ann Surg. 2009;249(2):186-8.
31. Lobo SM, Ronchi LS, Oliveira NE, et al. Restrictive strategy of intraoperative fluid maintenance during optimization of oxygen delivery decreases major complications after high-risk surgery. Crit Care. 2011;15(5):R226.
32. Varadhan KK, Lobo DN. A meta-analysis of randomised controlled trials of intravenous fluid therapy in major elective open abdominal surgery: getting the balance right. Proc Nutr Soc. 2010;69(4):488-98.
33. Brandstrup B, Tonnesen H, Beier-Holgersen R, et al. Effects of intravenous fluid restriction on postoperative complications: comparison of two perioperative fluid regimens: a randomized assessor-blinded multicenter trial. Ann Surg. 2003;238(5):641-8.
34. Wiedemann HP, Wheeler AP, Bernard GR, et al. Comparison of two fluid-management strategies in acute lung injury. N Engl J Med. 2006;354(24):2564-75.
35. Stewart RM, Park PK, Hunt JP, et al. Less is more: improved outcomes in surgical patients with conservative fluid administration and central venous catheter monitoring. J Am Coll Surg. 2009;208(5):725-35; discussion 35-7.
36. Bagshaw SM, Brophy PD, Cruz D, et al. Fluid balance as a biomarker: impact of fluid overload on outcome in critically ill patients with acute kidney injury. Crit Care. 2008;12(4):169. PubMed PMID: 18671831.

37. Hartmann AF. Chemical changes occurring in the body as a result of certain diseases in infants and children: I. The effects of diarrhea, vomiting, dehydration and oliguria on the acid-base balance of the plasma of infants with mastoiditis. Am J Dis Child. 1928;35(1):557-75.
38. McFarlane C, Lee A. A comparison of Plasmalyte 148 and 0.9% saline for intra-operative fluid replacement. Anaesthesia. 1994;49(9):779-81.
39. Scheingraber S, Rehm M, Sehmisch C, et al. Rapid saline infusion produces hyperchloremic acidosis in patients undergoing gynecologic surgery. Anesthesiology. 1999;90 (5):1265-70.
40. Wilkes NJ, Woolf R, Mutch M, et al. The effects of balanced versus saline-based hetastarch and crystalloid solutions on acid-base and electrolyte status and gastric mucosal perfusion in elderly surgical patients. Anesth Analg. 2001;93(4):811-6.
41. Kellum JA, Song M, Li J. Science review: extracellular acidosis and the immune response: clinical and physiologic implications. Crit Care. 2004;8(5):331-6.
42. Chowdhury AH, Cox EF, Francis ST, et al. A randomized, controlled, double-blind crossover study on the effects of 2-L infusions of 0.9% saline and Plasma-Lyte(R) 148 on renal blood flow velocity and renal cortical tissue perfusion in healthy volunteers. Ann Surg. 2012;256(1):18-24.
43. Hansen PB, Jensen BL, Skott O. Chloride regulates afferent arteriolar contraction in response to depolarization. Hypertension. 1998;32(6):1066-70.
44. Todd SR, Malinoski D, Muller PJ, et al. Lactated Ringer's is superior to normal saline in the resuscitation of uncontrolled hemorrhagic shock. J Trauma. 2007;62(3): 636-9.
45. Young JB, Utter GH, Schermer CR, et al. Saline vs. Plasma-Lyte A in initial resuscitation of trauma patients: a randomized trial. Ann Surg. 2014;259(2):255-62.
46. Shin WJ, Kim YK, Bang JY, et al Lactate and liver function tests after living donor right hepatectomy: a comparison of solutions with and without lactate. Acta Anaesthesiol Scand. 2011;55(5):558-64.
47. Shaw AD, Bagshaw SM, Goldstein SL, et al. Major complications, mortality, and resource utilization after open abdominal surgery: 0.9% saline compared to Plasma-Lyte. Ann Surg. 2012;255(5):821-9.
48. AABB. (2009). Circular of information for the use of human blood and blood components. [online] Available from http://www.aabb.org/resources/bct/pages/aabb_coi.aspx#_blood [Accessed January 16, 2009].
49. Hadimioglu N, Saadawy I, Saglam T, et al. The effect of different crystalloid solutions on acid-base balance and early kidney function after kidney transplantation. Anesth Analg. 2008;107(1):264-9.
50. Reid F, Lobo DN, Williams RN, et al. (Ab)normal saline and physiological Hartmann's solution: a randomized double-blind crossover study. Clin Sci. 2003;104(1):17-24.

Additional references appear in the online version of this book.

6

Hemorrhage, Hemostasis, and Transfusion

Marc Maegele

Key Points

- Hemostasis is achieved by a complex interaction of coagulation proteins, platelets, and the vascular endothelial cells. These hemostatic mechanisms are counterbalanced by a sophisticated fibrinolytic system, which prevents potentially detrimental excessive thrombosis.
- The recently introduced "cell-based model of coagulation" has led to a major improvement in our understanding of hemostasis.
- Disordered hemostasis may be the consequence of blood loss or disease processes such as disseminated intravascular coagulation (DIC). Furthermore, patients may present with an array of intrinsic abnormalities of the hemostatic mechanisms, which must be identified and corrected.
- Specific diagnostic tools are available to evaluate the various components of the hemostatic mechanism, and each must be thoroughly understood.
- The benefits of transfusion must be weighed against its risks. Current guidelines recommend adhering to a restrictive transfusion strategy (hemoglobin <7 to 8 g/dL) in hospitalized, nonbleeding, and stable patients.
- Blood transfusion has complications that must be fully understood to minimize any associated morbidity. Unnecessary blood transfusions should be avoided.

MECHANISMS OF BLOOD COAGULATION

Blood coagulation refers to the process of clot formation to limit and/or stop bleeding. It is part of an important host defense mechanism termed hemostasis, which promotes the cessation of blood loss from a damaged vessel. There are three interacting factors involved in clot formation:

1. Vessel wall (vasoconstriction)
2. Humoral clotting ("The cascade model of coagulation")
3. Platelets (platelet plug formation).

The recently introduced "cell-based model of coagulation" has led to improvement in our understanding of hemostasis. This novel concept incorporates the role of cells for an integrated understanding of the complex mechanisms behind coagulation.

Vessel Wall (Vasoconstriction)

The blood vessel wall is involved in hemostasis in two ways. The first and simpler are mechanical changes, which result from the vascular trauma itself; the second involves the active participation of the vascular endothelium.

Vasoconstriction

Vasocontriction is the body´s first response to injury to the vascular wall. When injury occurs, vessel walls constrict, causing reduced blood flow at the site of the injury. This response reduces local blood loss, whereas the other hemostatic mechanisms become active. Vessel constriction results in intimal buckling and retraction of the vessel wall within the adventitial lining. This process is most prominent in muscular arteries and can often lead to complete hemostasis, even with large vessel transection. The normal intact small arteriole has an endothelial lining (muscularis) and external serosal coat. If there is complete transection of the arteriole, contraction of the muscularis withdraws the endothelial-lined intima within the serosal "sleeve." The covering serosa over the end of the transected vessel combined with the formation of a mature clot provides for hemostasis. The importance of mechanical factors decreases with decreasing muscularity of the vessel, although even relatively small veins exhibit this behavior. These mechanical changes in the vessel wall are really only effective for injuries that fully transect the vessel. Partial transection of the arteriole results in contraction of the

Table 6.1 Thrombophobic and thrombophilic properties of the endothelium.

Thrombophobic properties	*Thrombophilic properties*
Prostacyclin—prevents platelet aggregation	von Willebrand's factor—promotes platelet adhesion
Thrombomodulin—membrane bound glycoprotein interacting with thrombin. The resulting complex is responsible for activation of protein C	Plasminogen activator inhibitor I—regulates fibrinolytic activity; increased production when endothelial cells are injured
Heparan sulfate—anticoagulant activity. Binding of ATIII to heparan sulfate of endothelial surface results in effective inhibition of thrombin	Adenosine diphosphate—promotes platelet aggregation
Tissue plasminogen activator—lysis of fibrin through fibrinolytic system	Fibronectin—adhesive protein for platelets
Glycocalyx—mucopolysaccharide preventing the interaction of platelet and coagulation proteins	Collagen—exposure of or injury to collagen promotes platelet aggregation and activation of plasma coagulation factors
Urokinase—activates plasminogen	

muscularis at the site of vessel disruption, but the intact segment prevents full contraction, leaving a wide open defect with continued bleeding. This contraction of the muscularis in the incomplete injury therefore proves to be a liability for hemostasis.

Vascular Endothelium

The endothelium is the thin layer of cells lining the interior surface of blood vessels. It represents a cellular system containing 10^{11} cells with approximately 720 g of weight. The endothelium normally provides a nonthrombogenic surface because it contains, for example, heparan sulphate, which acts as a cofactor for activating antithrombin (AT), a protease that inactivates several coagulation factors. Apart from its thrombophobic and anticoagulatory properties, the endothelium also owns thromophilic and thus procoagulatory properties that may become relevant in cases of vascular injury. Table 6.1 summarizes the most important thrombophobic and thrombophilic properties of the vascular endothelium. Similar charging between endothelial and platelet membranes during inactive states as well as a thin layer of plasma on the surface of the endothelium prevents binding of nonactive platelets to the intact endothelium. If platelets are activated, they are capable of binding onto the intact endothelium via glycoprotein IIb/IIIa, fibrinogen, and vitronectin. The basement membrane and intracellular matrix also have component parts that play important and specific roles in balancing procoagulant and anticoagulant states, initiating and regulating fibrinolytic activity, and mediating platelet adherence.[1]

Humoral Clotting ("The Cascade Model of Coagulation")

Although mechanical factors can be quite effective at achieving hemostasis under optimal circumstances, most of the leak-sealing function is achieved by the formation of fibrin clot. Fibrin clot is formed through complex interaction between more than a dozen individual factors and cells. If a critical mass of fibrin is generated, these soluble fibrin molecules will polymerize into fibrin strands, thus resulting in an insoluble matrix.

In the 1960s, the "cascade model of coagulation" was introduced consisting of a sequence of steps in which enzymes would cleave zymogen substrates (proenzymes) to generate the next enzyme in a cascade manner.[2] This model was helpful in understanding how enzymatic steps occur in plasma-based coagulation in vitro. The vast majority of cleaving steps within this model occur on phospholipid membrane surfaces in the presence of calcium. This calcium dependency resulted in the use of calcium chelators to prevent clotting during blood sampling.

Basically, the "cascade model of coagulation" consists of two independent activation arms converging on a common final pathway. Figure 6.1 shows the major factors involved in this cascade and their position in the initiating sequence. The enzyme components of the clotting cascade are soluble proteins, most of which are produced by the liver. The concentration and half-life vary from factor to factor (Table 6.2). Most are proteases that exist in an inert proenzyme form. Upon activation a given factor serves as theenzyme (which acts in concert with other mediators) toconvert the next factor in the chain from its inactive to its active form. Over the years the original "cascade model of coagulation" was modified to recognize observations that some procoagulants were in fact cofactors and did not possess their own enzymatic activity. The interactions of the activated factors were intricate and interrelated, leading to many levels of feedback control, some autocatalytic, and some inhibitory.

Table 6.2 Characteristics of the protein factors that are components of the "cascade model of coagulation".

Factor	*Common name*	*Cell of origin*	*Half-life*	*Normal concentration*	*SI units*
I	Fibrinogen	Liver	3–6 days	200–400 mg/dL	6–12 mmol/L
II	Prothrombin	Liver	3–5 days	100 mg/dL	1.4 mmol/L
V	Labile factor	Liver	12–36 hours	5–12 mg/dL	15–36 nmol/L
VII	Stable factor	Liver	4–6 hours	0.5 mg/dL	10 nmol/L
VIII-C	Antihemophilic factor	Liver	10–20 hours	0.1 mg/dL	0.3 nmol/L
VIII-vWF	von Willebrand's factor	Endothelium, platelets	10 hours	10 mg/dL	40 nmol/L
IX	Christmas factor	Liver	18–36 hours	2–7 mg/dL	36–125 nmol/L
X	Stuart--Prower factor	Liver	1–3 days	6–10 mg/dL	100–170 nmol/L
XI	Plasma thromboplastin antecedent	Liver	2–4 days	2–7 mg/dL	12–44 nmol/L
XII	Hageman factor	Liver	2–3 days	30–40 mg/dL	375–500 nmol/L
XIII	Fibrin stabilizing factor	Liver, platelets	6–7 days	15–25 mg/dL	47–78 nmol/L

Within this model, the clotting cascade is activated by either the extrinsic or intrinsic pathway (Fig. 6.1). The extrinsic system is localized "outside" of the blood and consists of tissue factor (TF) and coagulation factor FVIIa. The extrinsic pathway may be thought of as the prothrombin time (PT) pathway, as activation of factor VII (FVII) is the initiation step for this assay. Therefore, the PT is affected by pathology that alters either the extrinsic pathway or the common pathway. In contrast, the intrinsic system is localized "inside" within the blood and is initiated via contact activation of coagulation factor FXII on negatively charged surfaces with exposed collagen at the site of endothelial damage. Other factors capable of activating factor FXII include complement fragments and kallikrein. The activation of factor FXII by complement cleavage products and by kallikrein, and, in turn, the reciprocal activation of complement, prekallikrein to kallikrein, and mast cell degranulation by activated factor FXII demonstrates that activation of the coagulation cascade via the intrinsic pathway is also important in the initiation of human inflammation. The partial thromboplastin time (PTT) is an assay that primarily measures intrinsic pathway function, but is also affected by dysfunction of the common pathway.

The two pathways join at the level of factor FX to form a common final pathway.[3] In the common pathway, activated factor FX combined with activated factor FV forms the enzyme complex that converts factor FII (prothrombin) into its active form (thrombin), which then cleaves fibrinogen to form fibrin. Thrombin is often called the central element in the clotting cascade. Thrombin is primarily responsible for converting fibrinogen into fibrin, which then polymerizes to form the stable clot. However, thrombin is also a critical element in feedback control of the clotting cascade as well as a major factor in controlling the fibrinolytic system.[4]

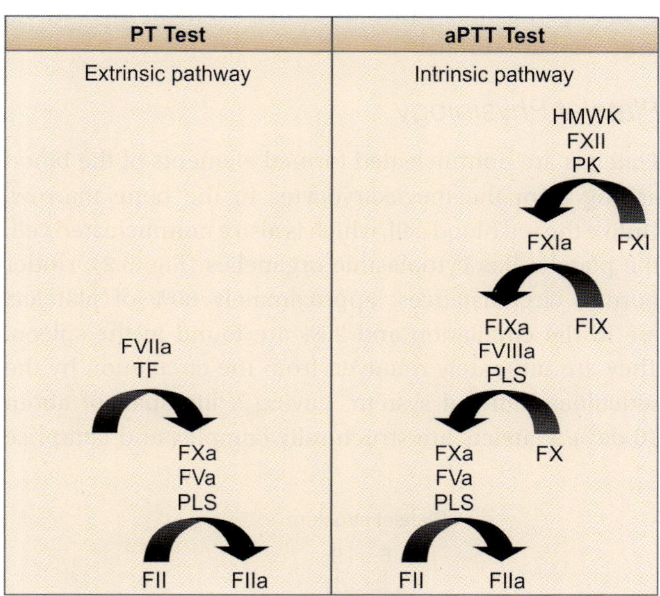

Fig. 6.1: The "cascade model of coagulation" and fibrin formation dividing the coagulation system into separate and redundant extrinsic and intrinsic pathways. Both pathways convert to one common final pathway leading to the formation of the factor FXa–FVa complex, which signs responsible for thrombin generation and subsequent cleavage of fibrinogen to fibrin. Many of the enzymes and enzyme complexes require calcium and binding to phospholipid surfaces (PLS) to generate full activity. The pathways are clinically assessed via the prothrombin time (PT) or the activated partial thromboplastin time (aPTT). (HMWK: High molecular weight kininogen; PK: Prekallikrein).

Platelets (Platelet Plug Formation)

Platelets are the critical elements in the initial steps of hemostasis. The humoral clotting mechanism can work

independently of platelets, but is far less efficient in controlling hemorrhage. Platelets have three primary functions:
1. Adherence and aggregation
2. Release of procoagulant factors
3. Provision of phospholipid surface for the assembly of enzyme complexes.

The expression of phosphatidylserine (PS) and phosphatidylethanolamine (PE) on the cell surface has been shown to exert profound impact on the procoagulant properties of the cell membrane surface. It is known that the presence of PS on the membrane dramatically increases the speed of some coagulation reactions, whereas less PS is required for the maximum speed if PE is present.[5] Both PS and PE are shuffled from the cell membrane´s inner to the outer leaflet, which turns the cell membrane into a procoagulant surface.[6]

Platelet Physiology

Platelets are nonnucleated formed elements of the blood arising from the megakaryocytes in the bone marrow. Unlike the red blood cell, which is also a nonnucleated cell, the platelet has cytoplasmic organelles (Fig. 6.2). Under normal circumstances, approximately 80% of platelets are in the circulation and 20% are found in the spleen. They are ultimately removed from the circulation by the reticuloendothelial system, having a life span of about 10 days. Platelets are structurally complex and comprise three separate layers, each having a specific role in overall platelet function:[7]
1. Outermost peripheral or adhesion zone contains the receptors needed for interaction with the vessel wall or other platelets.
2. Cytoplasmic or gelsol zone contains the cytoskeletal elements necessary for the changes in platelet shape that occur with activation.
3. Organelle zone contains the secretory apparatus for the various platelet factors.

Platelets have three different types of secretory granules,containing a number of agents including general procoagulant substances such as adenosine diphosphate (ADP), adenosine triphosphate (ATP), fibrinogen, and von Willebrand's factor (vWF), as well as a number of platelet-specific actors (Table 6.3).[8]

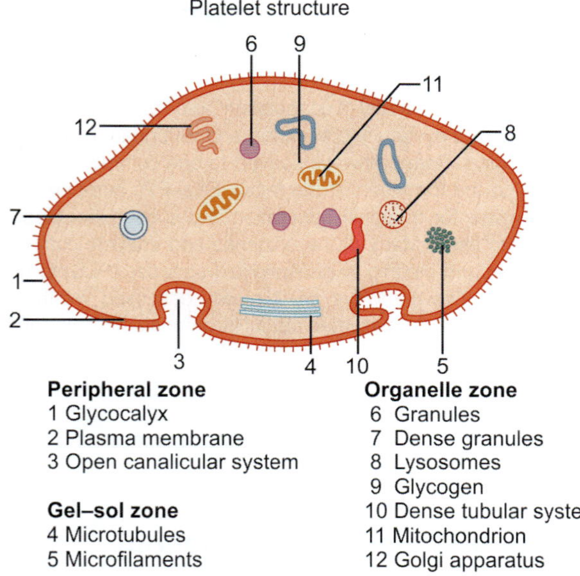

Fig. 6.2: Platelets are 2–3 mm in diameter, nonnucleated cells containing organelles within each of their three separate zones.

Clot Formation

Under normal conditions, platelets circulate and do not adhere to each other or to the undamaged vascular endothelium. However, they rapidly adhere to sites of endothelial damage and lead to the formation of stable hemostatic structures composed of aggregates of activated platelets bound by fibrin. Platelets identify areas of vessel damage through the loss of the normal endothelial lining.

Adhesion of platelets to areas of damage is accomplished through specific receptors, mediated by vWF. The mechanism is complex and dependent upon the flow characteristics in the particular blood vessel. It is likely that different mechanisms of platelet adherence may be active at different points within the circulatory system, depending upon vessel size and flow velocity.[9] Once adherent to the vessel wall, the platelets become activated by exposure to collagen and other TFs. Platelet activation results in:
1. Synthesis of thromboxane A_2
2. Release of the contents of platelet secretory granules.

Table 6.3 Types of platelet granule and their contents.

Type of granule	*Contents*
Alpha granules	Platelet-derived growth factor (PDGF) Platelet factors 1–7 β-Thromboglobulin Other plasma hemostatic proteins
Dense body granules	Adenosine diphosphate/adenosine triphosphate Calcium/magnesium Serotonin Epinephrine/norepinephrine (adrenaline/noradrenaline)
Lysosomal bodies	Acid hydrolases

The release of both thromboxane A_2 and granule contents cause platelets to aggregate in large numbers, forming a platelet plug. This plug is stabilized by platelet interaction with fibrinogen through cell surface receptors. In addition, the process of activation leads to a rearrangement of the platelet membrane so that a procoagulant phospholipid layer is exposed. This surface provides a platform for assembling the enzyme complexes necessary for the humoral clotting cascade. Stable cross-linked fibrin clot is rapidly formed under these circumstances.[10] According to the novel concept of "cell-based coagulation" (*see* below), the platelet has been recognized as probably the only cell type on which specific phases of coagulation, for example the so-called "propagation" phase can occur effectively. The surface of platelets once activated is able to host and coordinate the assembly of the most relevant steps for coagulation including the "tenase" (FIXa/FVIIIa) and the "prothrombinase" (FXa/FVa) complexes.

Deficiencies of the "Cascade Model of Coagulation"

The description of the Y-shaped "cascade model of coagulation" has advanced the understanding on how enzymatic coagulation processes occur in plasma-based in-vitro coagulation where fluid is static, not interacting with vascular walls or cell surfaces, and for the interpretation of laboratory tests for plasma coagulation abnormalities, for example the PT for deficiencies in the extrinsic or common pathways, and the activated PTT (aPTT) for deficiencies in the intrinsic or common pathways.[11] However, this model suggesting independent and redundant extrinsic andintrinsic pathways fails adequately to explain the hemostatic process as it occurs in vivo.[12] Clinical manifestations of selected isolated coagulation factor deficiencies in both the intrinsic and extrinsic pathways seem to contradict the concept that these enzymatic systems function as independent FXa generators. For example, initial deficiencies in components of the intrinsic pathway (FXII, high molecular weight kininogen or prekallikrien) were associated with markedly prolonged aPTTs but not with increased bleeding tendencies.[13] In contrast, deficiencies in further downstream intrinsic components may result in severe bleeding tendencies as observed for coagulation factors FVIII and FIX in clinical hemophilia A and B despite anintact extrinsic pathway.[13] Vice versa, deficiencies in extrinsic factor FVII may be associated with severe bleeding despite an intact intrinsic pathway.[14]

The "Cell-Based Model of Coagulation" (and Fibrin Formation)

A major development over the past one-and-half decades toward a better understanding of the mechanisms by which coagulation may occur within the dynamic vascular system was the integration of the role of cells, including the specific platelet binding sites for coagulation proteins.[15-17] The model suggests that the extrinsic and intrinsic systems are in fact parallel FXa generators but occurring on different cell surfaces rather than in redundant independent pathways.[15] For effective coagulation, thrombin has to be generated directly on the surface of activated platelets rather than just on the surface of the TF-bearing cells. This concept further considers that some coagulation proteases that contribute to the enzymatic cascade of coagulation may also function outside of hemostasis, for example, in inflammation, vessel wall function, and proliferation. The evaluation of the "cell-based model of coagulation" currently suggests that coagulation in vivo occurs in distinct overlapping phases as shown in Figures 6.3A to C. Three phases are distinguished:

1. Initiation
2. Amplification
3. Propagation

These require the joint participation of two cell types:

1. TF-bearing cells
2. Platelets.

Initiation (of Coagulation on TF-Bearing Cells)

There is strong evidence to date that the single relevant initiator of coagulation in vivo is TF. Cell expressing TF are usually localized outside the vasculature, which prevents coagulation under normal circumstances with an intact endothelium. There is always some amount of circulating blood-borne TF, but under normal conditions this TF is considered to be inactive or encrypted. Its exact role is still debated. In case of injury, the flowing blood is exposed to a TF-bearing cell and coagulation factor FVIIa rapidly binds to TF. FVIIa is the only coagulation protein that routinely circulates with the bloodstream in both its active (1% of total FVII) and inactive form. The TF–FVIIa complex then recruits additional FVIIa from FVII for even more TF–FVIIa complex activity, which then actives FIX and FX. Activated coagulation factor FXa binds to its cofactor FVa on the surface of the TF-bearing cell to form the so-called "prothrombinase" complex, which subsequently cleaves prothrombin thus generating small amounts of thrombin.

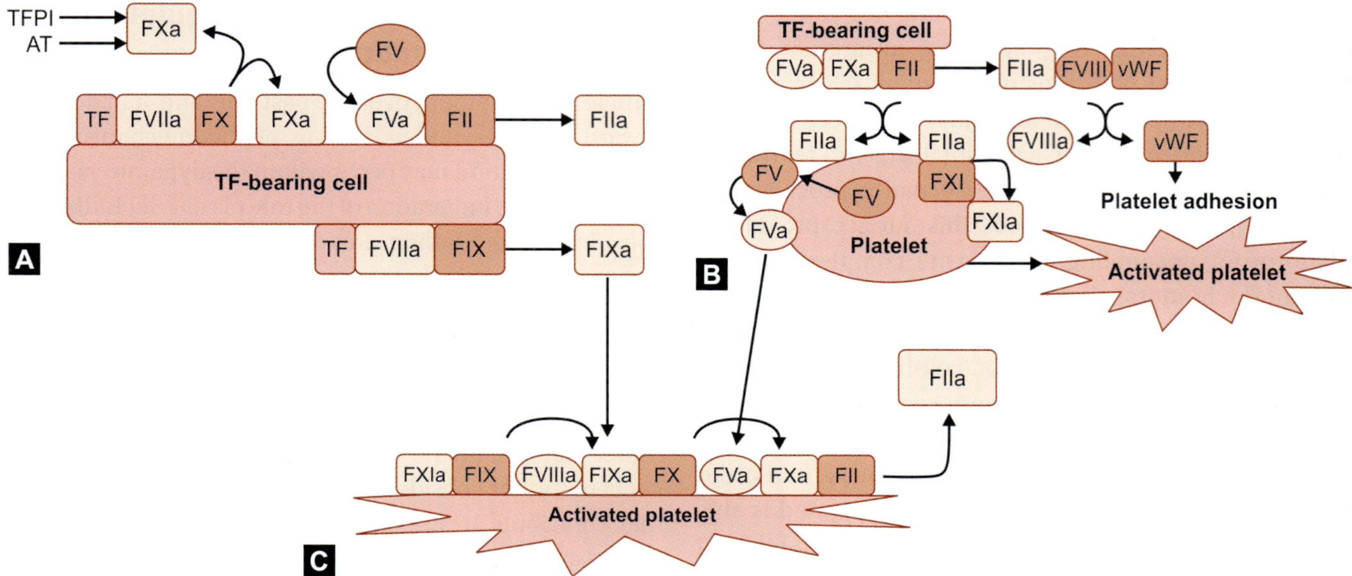

Figs. 6.3A to C: The "cell-based model of coagulation," which incorporates various cell surfaces as well as tissue factor (TF)-bearing cells and platelets to fibrin formation. In this model thrombin generation occurs in distinct overlapping phases: (A) initiation, (B) amplification, and (C) propagation. The initiation (A) is localized to the TF-bearing cell when injury to the vessel exposes the TF-bearing cell to the blood flow. During this phase small amounts of factor FIXa and thrombin are generated that diffuse to the platelet. During the second phase referred to as amplification (B) the small amount of thrombin generated during (A) activates platelets, releases von Willebrand's factor (vWF) and triggers the generation of activated factors FVa, FVIIIa, and FXIa. During the last phase, also referred to as propagation (C) the different enzymes generated during (A) and (B) assemble on the procoagulant surface membrane of activated platelets to form the so-called intrinsic "tenase" complex (FIXa–FVIIIa) resulting in factor FXa generation. In the last step "prothrombinase" complex (FXa–FVa) is formed promoting burst thrombin generation directly on the activated platelet.

Since any of the factor FXa that dissociates from the membrane surface of the TF-bearing cell is immediately inactivated by either TF pathway inhibitor (TFPI) or AT, the generated factor FXa activity is effectively restricted to the surface of the TF-bearing cell on which the factor was generated. In contrast, factor FIXa is able to dissociate and may interact with nearby platelets or other cells, since it is not inhibited by TFPI and only very slowly by AT.

Since TF is always in the perivascular space, any FVIIa within the bloodstream leaving the vasculature through minor endothelial breaks will bind to TF, thus potentially triggering the coagulation process. Low levels of the activation peptides of the coagulation factors are detectable in the blood of healthy individuals. This phenomenon has been referred to as "basal coagulation" or "idling." Under normal conditions, this ongoing process does not lead to clot formation since the larger components of the coagulation process (e.g. platelets, FV, fibrinogen) are kept sequestered in the vascular space. Under normal conditions, endothelial barrier gaps are very small (e.g. FVII 50,000 Da). Thus, coagulation beyond the small amounts of thrombin progresses only if injury allows platelets and other larger proteins to leave the vascular space into the extravascular area to adhere to the TF-bearingcells.[15]

Amplification

After the initiation phase, thrombin diffuses away from the TF-bearing cell and is available for the activation of platelets that have leaked from the vasculature at the site of the vessel damage. Platelets stick to the site of injury, forming a plug at the injured vessel wall and become activated via binding of thrombin. This binding of thrombin via specific platelet surface receptors induces profound changes to the surface of the platelets, resulting in shape change, flopping of membrane phospholipids from the inner to the outer membrane leaflet to provide a procoagulant membrane surface and the release of granule contents, thus further promoting the coagulation process and platelet activation. The presence of calcium may promote clustering of platelets and the binding of coagulation factors on the membrane surface. Another function of thrombin produced during the initiation phase is the activation of cofactors FV and FVIII on the activated platelet surface. In this process, thrombin cleaves vWF off factor FVIII to mediate additional platelet adhesion and aggregation at the site of the injury. vWF and factor FVIII usually circulate bound together, and the released factor FVIII is subsequently activated to factor FVIIIa.[2] Small amounts of thrombin also activate factor XI to XIa on the platelet surface during this phase. This mechanism may explain why factor FXII and other contact factors are not always necessary for coagulation as postulated for the "cascade model of coagulation."

Propagation

The propagation phase occurs on the surface of activated platelets. Once activated, platelets release granule contents and express ligands on their surface, thus recruiting additional platelets to the injured vessel site and promoting cell-to-cell interaction and aggregation. During this phase, factor FIXa generated during initiation by TF-FVIIa can bind to cofactor FVIIIa produced during amplification on the platelet surface to form the so-called "tenase" complex (FIXa–FVIIIa). Additional factor FIXa can be generated by platelet-bound factor XIa. Once this intrinsic complex is formed, it rapidly generates FXa on the platelet. Since factor Xa cannot shift effectively from the TF-bearing cell to the activated platelet as it is rapidly inhibited if it moves away from the TF-bearing cell surface, factor FXa must be provided directly on the platelet surface via cleavage by the intrinsic "tenase" complex. The factor FXa generated on platelets then rapidly associates with its cofactor FVa (which is produced by thrombin during the amplification phase) to cleave prothrombin to thrombin. The completion of this so-called "prothrombinase" complex (FXa–FVa) results in thrombin burst, leading to cleavage of fibrinopeptide A from fibrinogen. If a sufficient amount of thrombin is produced at sufficient speed to result in a critical mass of fibrin, soluble fibrin will spontaneously polymerize into fibrin strands thus to form an insoluble fibrin matrix.[2]

Additional Aspects of Hemostasis

The generation of sufficient amounts of thrombin resulting in effective clot formation does not determine the end of the coagulation process. A number of steps relevant to hemostasis occur after the formation of the fibrin gel. Almost 95% of thrombin is generated even after fibrin polymerization to play an important role for the structure and stability of the clot that is formed. Thrombin additionally cleaves factor FXIII to FXIIIa, which modifies the polymerized fibrin to generate cross-links between the fibrin strands. These cross-links substantially modify the stability of the clot that is formed.[18] Hemostatic abnormalities due to deficiencies in hemostatic function that occur following initial fibrin polymerization are not accessible via the standard coagulation assays such as PT and aPTT. Small amounts of thrombin may bind to endothelial thrombomodulin (TM) thus activating thrombin activatable fibrinolysis inhibitor.

BALANCE OF CLOTTING AND FLUIDITY

Although it is essential that injuries to the vascular system are sealed as rapidly as possible, it is equally essential that the clotting mechanism is controlled to keep the circulating blood in a fluid state. Without such a balance, a single nidus of clot formation would progress to clotting of the entire blood volume. Once the stable fibrin-platelet clot has been generated at the site of the vessel injury, the process of further coagulation must be limited to prevent widespread systemic fibrin formation. There is always some diffusion of proteins from activated platelets downstream, but the lack of procoagulant surfaces on resting endothelial membranes prevents thrombin generation at distant sites by any factor FXa diffusing into the vasculature. Both, factor FXa and thrombin are also inhibited by endothelial surface-bound anticoagulant systems such as TFPI and AT. The principle mechanisms that work to keep blood fluid are described in the following.

Fibrinolytic System

Fibrin clot is rapidly degraded by the enzyme plasmin. Plasmin is a serine protease generated from the precursor plasminogen by an enzyme called plasminogen activator. This enzyme is released by the vascular endothelium as well as other tissues. In general, many of the same elements of the clotting cascade that amplify the clotting stimulus also activate the fibrinolytic system. The tendency toward clot formation and the lysis of the formed clot are therefore kept in balance. Thrombin is central to this interaction. The pathways of activation of the fibrinolytic system are shown in Figure 6.4. Specific activators of plasminogen, including streptokinase and urokinase, have been isolated and commercially produced for the therapeutic lysis of fibrin clot. Breakdown of fibrin results in specific identifiable compounds that can be assayed in the blood. These assays allow for quantification of fibrinolysis. Plasmin has a much less selective spectrum than thrombin, which is its parallel in the procoagulant cascade. Although the chief function of plasmin is to breakdown fibrin, plasmin also hydrolyzes fibrinogen and several of the enzyme factors on the procoagulant side. Therefore, activation of the fibrinolytic system leads to a broad-based pattern of enzyme

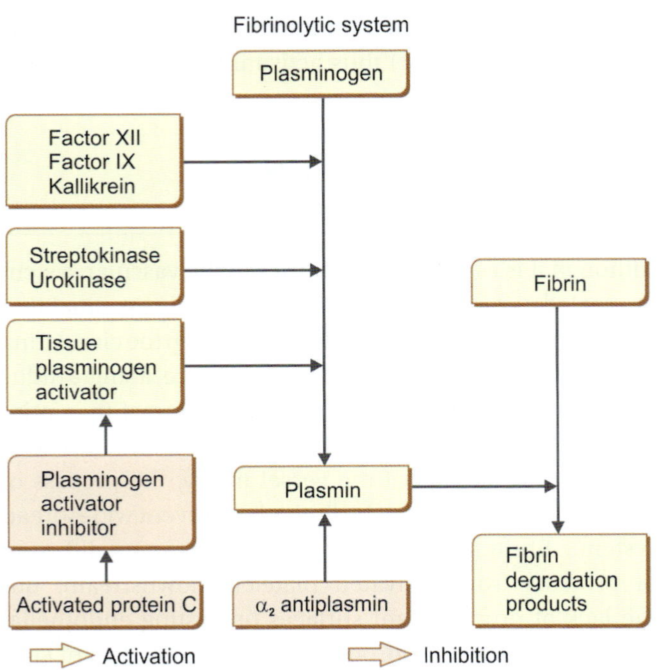

Fig. 6.4: Fibrinolytic system showing the pathways of plasmin activation.

degradation in addition to the primary function of fibrin degradation. This fact is of particular importance in certain pathologic conditions in which there is a generalized activation of plasmin.

The fibrinolytic system provides one method for regulating the clotting system, but it is effective only once the coagulation process has been initiated. The balance between fluidity and clot formation is also aided by the presence of anticoagulant properties of endothelial cells and circulating factors that inhibit the coagulation cascade, and so prevent the initiation of clot formation.

Anticoagulant Properties of Endothelial Cells

Apart from observations that resting endothelial membranes, in general, do not support coagulation reactions, nonactivated endothelial cells express quite a number of anticoagulant proteins on their surface.

Heparan Sulfated Proteogylcans (HSPGs)

Heparan sulfated proteoglycans (HSPGs) are localized in small amounts on the luminal surface of the endothelial cell in direct contact with the bloodstream. Via binding HSPGs fully activate AT to inactivate thrombin in the vicinity of HSPGs. The mechanism is similar to that induced by heparin-AT when clinically administering soluble forms of heparin.

Tissue Factor Pathway Inhibitor

Tissue factor pathway inhibitor is localized on the endothelial surface and prevents additional thrombin generation by inhibiting both factor FXa and FVIIa. TFPI binds irreversibly to factor FXa, generating a complex together with FVIIa and TF and thus inactivating these proteines from participation in further thrombin generation.[14]

Thrombomodulin

Nonactivated resting endothelial cells also express TM on their surface. Thrombin converts TM into an anticoagulant by binding to it and generating the so-called "thrombin–TM" complex, which converts protein C (PC) to activated PC (aPC) together with its cofactor protein S (ProS). aPC then irreversibly cleaves factors FVa and FVIIIa to inhibit their role in further thrombin generation. It has been observed that aPC–ProS is much more effective at inactivating factor FVa on the endothelial surface as compared with the platelet surface. This finding indicates that aPC–ProS is very efficient in limiting thrombin generation on uninjured resting endothelial cells but not on activated platelets.[19] aPC–ProS also inactivates plasminogen activator inhibitor-1 (PAI-1), which ultimately leads to increased fibrinolysis. It has been reported that TM expression in the capillary endothelium is 100-fold higher than TM expression in major vessels.[20]

Circulating Anticoagulants

Antithrombin

Antithrombin is a large glycoprotein and one of the central factors of the natural anticoagulant system. It binds to thrombin, directly inhibiting the cleavage of fibrinogen and decreasing the ability of thrombin to activate other elements of the clotting cascade, including platelets. To a lesser extent, AT directly inhibits other components of the coagulation cascade as well. Heparin exerts its anticoagulant effects via interaction with AT.

Protein C–Protein S

Protein C is synthesized in the liver through a vitamin K-dependent pathway. It has a shorter half-life than the vitamin K-dependent elements of the procoagulant pathway. In its active form, it inhibits the action of the enzyme complexes responsible for the formation of activated factor FX and thrombin. In addition, PC decreases inhibition of tissue plasminogen activator and increases the tendency toward thrombolysis. ProS is a cofactor promoting the activation of PC.

CLINICAL MONITORING OF HEMOSTASIS

Specific patient needs in the management of clinical bleeding disorders require practical means for monitoring the coagulation cascade and platelet function:

1. Hemostatic mechanisms may be evaluated preoperatively to avoid unnecessary intraoperative blood loss.
2. Coagulation efficiency may need to be monitored intraoperatively or, in the case of acute trauma/injury, if there is or has been major blood loss.
3. Special types of procedures are associated with deliberate (e.g. cardiac bypass procedures) or anticipated (e.g. liver transplantation) coagulation abnormalities.

Standard Laboratory Tests

The standard laboratory screening tests to assess coagulation are the PT and the activated aPTT. Levels of fibrinogen and times for thrombin clotting are also reported. Poor sampling technique such as underfilling of the sampling tube may dramatically impair the test results and may prolong clotting times artefactually due to over-anticoagulation. To prevent clotting of the sample, whole blood is usually mixed with calcium-chelating agents such as EDTA or citrate in a 9:1 ratio. The standard coagulation tests are usually performed on centrifuged platelet-poor plasma samples. The time to fibrin strand formation is usually detected via photo-optical or electromechanical devices.

Prothrombin Time (PT)

Prothrombin time (PT) is the time to fibrin strand formation when platelet-poor plasma is recalcified in the presence of thromboplastin (TF and phospholipid). Different thromboplastins provide different reference ranges for PT. The international normalized ratio (INR) standardizes the thromboplastin reagent. It is the ratio of the patient´s PT to a control plasma PT raised to the power of a correction factor (ISI = international sensitivity index), which is specific for each thromoplastin reagent. The PT measures the vitamin K-dependent elements of coagulation, which includes the extrinsic pathway (factors FI, FII, FV, FVII), but it is also affected by the common pathway. The INR is most sensitive to a decrease in factor FVII. It is used preoperatively or postoperatively for:

1. Patients who have intrinsic liver disease (e.g. cirrhosis) or preexistent nutritional problems (vitamin K deficiency)
2. Patients on warfarin anticoagulation and
3. DIC and high doses of heparin.

Traditional reporting of PT is in seconds (usually about 12 seconds), with the patient specimen being compared with a control to account for variation resulting from the use of local reagents. An INR of 1.0 is normal, and ratios larger than this indicate impaired coagulation.

Activated Partial Thromboplastin Time (aPTT)

"Partial thromboplastin" indicates that the reagent contains phospholipids to substitute the platelet membrane but no TF. In addition, the reagent contains a contact activator of negatively charged particles (kaolin, or ellagic acid). In principle, all procoagulant factors are measured by this test except factors FVII and FXIII. This test is used:

1. To monitor unfractionated heparin (UFH) therapy
2. As a screening tool for hemophilia A, B, and coagulation inhibitors

The aPTT is prolonged when procoagulant activity is reduced to < 30–40% of normal by a specific clotting factor inhibitor, heparin or lupus anticoagulant acting as a nonspecific intrinsic pathway inhibitor. The results are measured in seconds, with the 95% confidence interval being 26–40 seconds in duration. The aPTT is more sensitive to heparin than the PT.

Thrombin Time (TT)

This is a simple test to assess fibrin polymerization. Citrated, platelet-poor plasma is mixed with a standard concentration of human thrombin and the time to clotting is measured. Clot formation requires only fibrinogen and the absence of thrombin inhibitors. This test is independent of all other factor deficiencies. The most common thrombin inhibitor is heparin. TT is prolonged in hypo-(dys) fibrinogenemia and by fibrin degradation products. It is also used to monitor fibrinolytic therapies and toassess resistance to heparin.

Plasma Fibrinogen Concentration

Dilutional effects upon coagulation secondary to massive bleeding and hemodilution are best measured by the plasma fibrinogen concentration. Fibrinogen concentrations > 1.5 g/L are required for effective coagulation. There are a number of tests available to assess fibrinogen levels in plasma, but the two commonest are the Clauss assay and the PT-derived fibrinogen level (PT-Fg). The Clauss method adds high concentrations of thrombin to diluted test plasma, and the clotting time is compared to a calibration curve generated by serial dilution and reference plasma of known fibrinogen concentration. The result is expressed in gram per liter (g/L). PT-Fg is an indirect measurement of fibrinogen, comparing the PT of a test sample with a reference curve generated as mentioned above.

Platelet Count

The adequacy of platelets in surgical patients is usually only estimated by the platelet count. Platelet counts are easily performed, unlike other platelet tests, which attempt to assess platelet function. The normal platelet count is 150,000–450,000/μL. Clinical bleeding is seldom secondary to an inadequate platelet unless the count is < 50,000/μL.

Near-Patient Tests of Coagulation (POC = Point-of-Care-Testing)

Near-patient tests of coagulation usually have shorter turnaround times, require less preparation, personnel and transport, and also use only minimal quantities of whole blood.[21] Clinical decision making and therapeutic interventions can be made more rapidly, improving convenience for staff and patients.[22] Over the years, a variety of tests have been introduced. For example, the hemochrom-activated clotting time (HACT) for situations in which assessment of systemic heparinization is required almost instantaneously. The Hemochron Jr. signature is a handheld device for ACT, aPTT, and PT. The results are displayed as the INR. The Roche CoaguCheck S uses 10 μL of capillary blood or venous whole blood to derive an INR with reference to that obtained from a control solution using reflectance photometry.

Platelet Function Analyzing Monitor

The platelet function analyzing monitor (PFA-100) may be considered a near-patient test, although the analysis has to be performed 30–120 minutes after blood sampling. The PFA-100 is a system to analyze platelet function in which citrated whole blood is aspirated at high shear rates through disposable cartridges containing an aperture within a membrane coated with either collagen and epinephrine (CEPI) or collagen and ADP (CADP). This biochemical and shear stress leads to platelet adhesion, activation, and aggregation, resulting in a rapid occlusion of the aperture and cessation of blood flow termed as the closure time (CT). Sealing of the aperture is sensed by a pressure transducer and occurs in 81–166 seconds with CEPI and 54–109 seconds with CADP. The test is used to distinguish the effect of aspirin from other abnormalities of platelet function. If the PFA-100 result is normal with CEPI, normal platelet function can be assumed. A prolonged result with CEPI, which normalizes with CADP, is indicative of an aspirin effect. If both assays are prolonged, more complex assessment for thrombocytopathy is indicated.

Multiplate Analyzer (Impedance Aggregometry)

The Multiplate analyzer is a platelet function analyzer utilizing whole blood via impedance aggregometry. The adhesion and aggregation of platelets on the sensor surface enhances the electrical resistance (impedance) between two sensor electrodes. At the end of incubation of diluted whole blood, the agonist is added. The increase of impedance due to the attachment of platelets to the electrodes is detected for each sensor and is transformed to aggregation units (AUs) plotted against time. Approximately 8 AU corresponds to 1 ohm. The aggregation measured with this device is quantified as area under the curve (AUC). Multiplate is highly sensitive for the detection of aspirin, clopidogrel, prasugrel, IIb/IIIa receptor antagonists, and other platelet inhibitors. The test is further sensitive and clinically predictive for perioperative platelet function disorders as well as screening for platelet defects (e.g. Glanzmann´s thrombasthenia, GT) and functional detection of heparin-induced thrombocytopenia (HIT).

Viscoelastic Point-of-Care Hemostatic Assays (VHA)

The necessity to analyze whole blood accurately to identify relevant coagulopathies has led to a revival of VHA such as Thromboelastography (TEG) and Rotation Thromboelastometry (ROTEM). Thromboelastography was first described in 1948 by Hartert[23] as a method to assess the viscoelastic properties of coagulation in whole blood under low shear conditions.[24] The VHA produces a trace, which quantifies the kinetics of clot formation and dissolution from the point of initial fibrin formation through to clot retraction and lysis. This approach is different from most other coagulation tests, which use time to fibrin formation as endpoint disregarding what happens thereafter. VHA assess the interplay between fibrinogen, platelets, and clotting factors within one single test.[25]

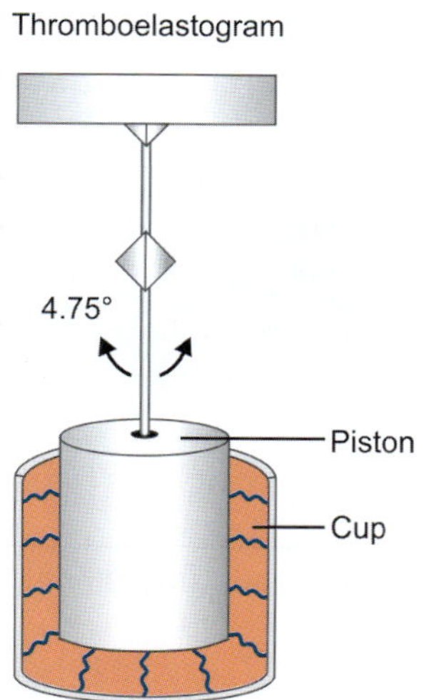

Fig. 6.5: Basic mechanics of the thromboelastogram. A fine stainless steel piston is suspended into a stainless steel cup with a small space between the two. A specimen of 0.36 mL of blood is placed into the space between the cup and the piston, and the piston is then rotated back and forth through 4.75°. The torque that develops on the suspended piston is then quantitated on an attached recorder. Characteristic patterns are identified for specific hemostatic function abnormalities.

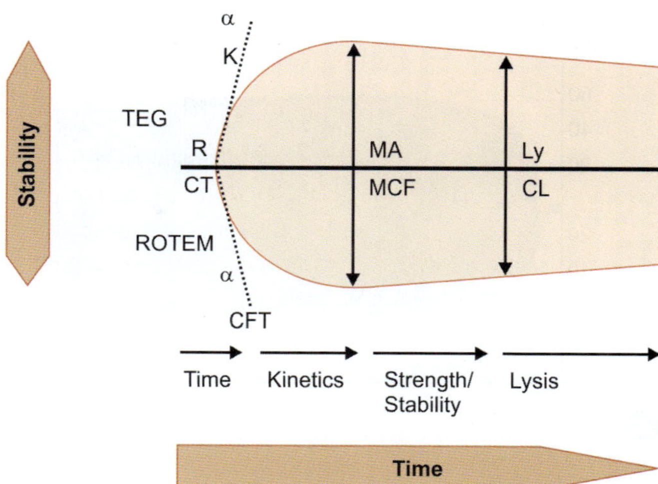

Fig. 6.6: Schematic trace for TEG (upper panel) and ROTEM (lower panel). Note that the nomenclature for both is slightly different. Commonly reported variables include: (A) clotting time indicating time to 2-mm amplitude [TEG: R (reaction time)/ROTEM: CT (clotting time)]; (B) clot formation time indicating time from 2- to 20-mm amplitude [TEG: K (kinetics)/ ROTEM: CFT (clot formation time)]; (C) alpha angle [TEG: a (slope between R and K)/ ROTEM: α (slope of tangent at 2-mm amplitude)]; (D) maximum clot strength [TEG: MA (maximum amplitude)/ ROTEM: MCF (maximum clot firmness)]; and (E) clot lysis indicating lysis at fixed time points [TEG: Ly30/Ly60 (reduction in amplitude at 30 and 60 minutes after MA)/ ROTEM: CL30/CL60 (reduction in amplitude at 30 and 60 minutes after MCF)]. TEG: Thromboelastography; ROTEM: Rotation Thromboelastometry.

Modified from Johansson PI, Stissing T, Bochsen L, et al. Thromboelastography and tromboelastometry in assessing coagulopathy in trauma. Scand J Trauma Resusc Emerg Med. 2009;17:45.

Whole blood is incubated at 37°C in a prewarmed cup. Within the cup is suspended a pin connected to a detector system (a torsion wire in TEG and an optical detector in ROTEM). The cup and pin are oscillated relative to each other through an angle of 4.75° (Fig. 6.5). The movement is initiated from either the cup (TEG) or the pin (ROTEM). As fibrin forms between the cup and pin, the transmitted rotation from the cup to pin (TEG) or the impedance of the rotation of the pin (ROTEM) are detected at the pin and a trace is generated (Fig. 6.6). The trace is divided into different parts reflecting different stages of the hemostatic process (clotting time, kinetics, strength, and lysis) with slightly different nomenclature for TEG and ROTEM. Examples of traces generated from normal as well as selected pathological states are shown in Figures 6.7A to D. VHA can either be performed at the bedside using native nonanticoagulated blood if the sample is analyzed within 5 minutes or it can be performed in a laboratory setting, where citrated blood samples are employed. The results are quickly available making them relevant for clinical decision making. Although this test is primarily used in liver transplantation, it has potential applications in monitoring anticoagulation in open heart surgery and in other settings involving massive blood loss and coagulopathy, such as trauma-induced coagulopathy.[26]

VHA and the Cell-Based Model of Coagulation

The VHA may reflect the three different phases of cell-based hemostasis. Recent work using scanning electron microscopy demonstrated that the clotting time [R (reaction time) in TEG/CT (clotting time) in ROTEM] corresponds to the initiation phase, whereas clot formation time [K (kinetics) in TEG/clot formation time (CFT) in ROTEM] reflects the amplification phase.[27] Other work has shown that the thrombin burst is reflected by the α-angle (TEG/ROTEM) and determines the clot strength and stability.[28] The capacity of VHA to reflect thrombin generation has clinical utility because coagulation factor deficiencies secondary to massive bleeding, dilution, consumption, and thrombocytopenia, and cytopathy may result in impaired thrombin generation and impaired clot strength (maximum amplitude in TEG/maximum clot firmness in ROTEM).

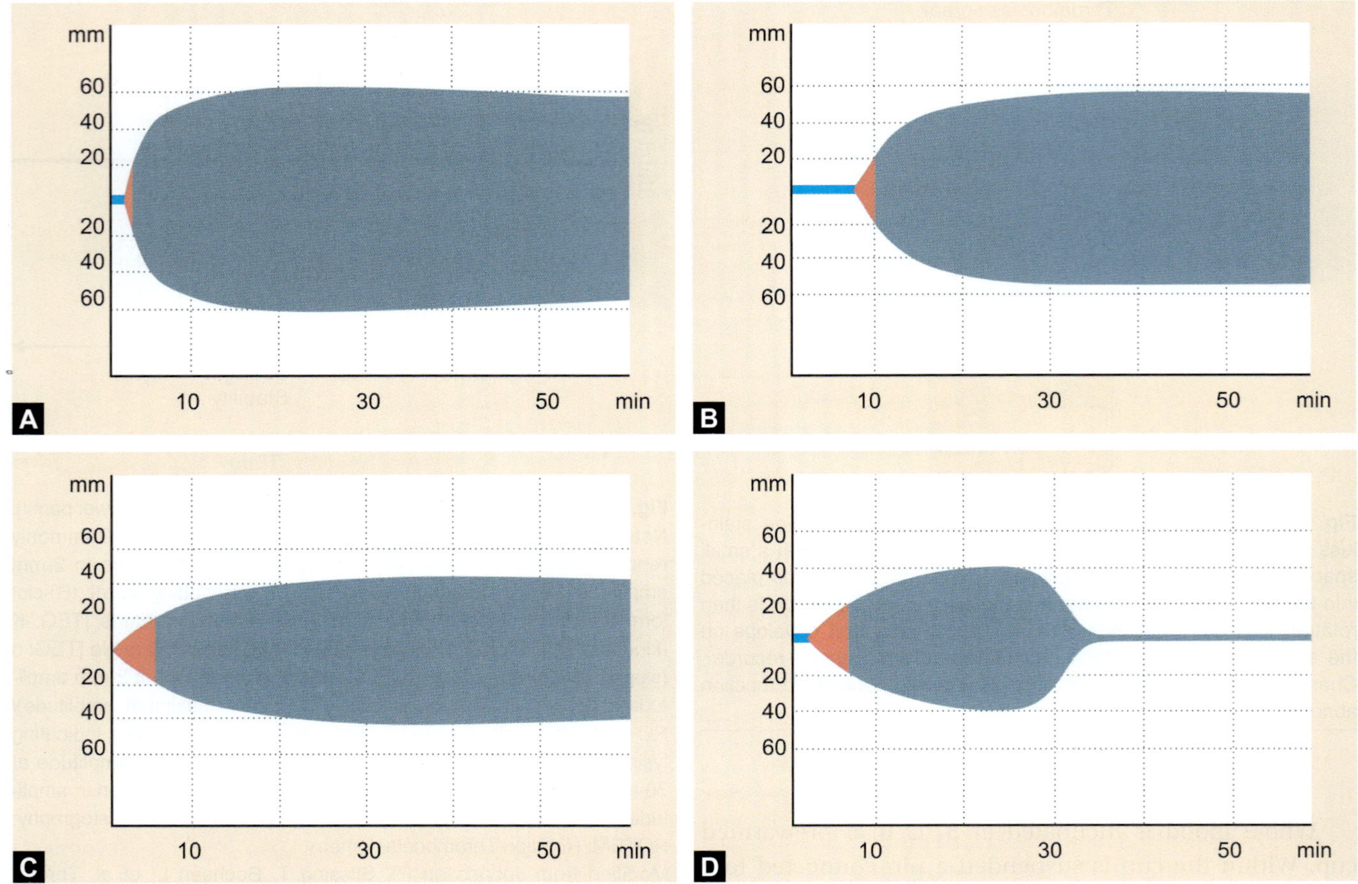

Figs. 6.7A to D: Exemplar ROTEM traces in the EXTEM test: (A) normal test result; (B) delayed coagulation (CT↑); (C) reduced clot strength (MCF↓), and (D) hyperfibrinolysis. (ROTEM: Rotation thromboelastometry; CT: Clotting time; MCF: Maximum clot firmness).
Modified from Schöchl H, Maegele M, Solomon C, et al. Early and individualized goal-directed therapy for trauma-induced coagulopathy. Scand J Trauma Resusc Emerg Med. 2012;20:15.

VHA in the Surgical Setting

To date, < 20 clinical studies have reported on the potential benefit of VHAs versus standard coagulation testing to identify coagulopathy and guide transfusion therapy. The studies include three randomized clinical trials involving > 4,500 patients undergoing major surgery. The majority of studies have been performed in patients undergoing liver or cardiac surgery, all reporting the benefit of VHA over standard tests as shown by reductions in transfusion requirements and need for reexploration. No study to date has reported a benefit of using plasma-based standard tests to predict bleeding or guide transfusion therapy when compared to VHA, thereby supporting the rationale of whole blood viscoelastic assays in this setting. Ten studies including more than 700 patients have evaluated the benefits of VHA in trauma patients.[24]

DISSEMINATED INTRAVASCULAR COAGULATION (DIC)

Failure of hemostasis after massive transfusion or after a systemic inflammatory insult has been recognized for many years. Prior to the era of laboratory assays for clotting function, severely decreased levels of fibrinogen and severe thrombocytopenia were associated with this condition. The syndrome has been called consumptive coagulopathy because the cause of hemostatic failure was thought to be consumption of the active factors required for clot formation.[29]

Factors and platelets may be consumed by:

1. Ongoing extravascular clotting
2. Situations of persistent bleeding
3. DIC, which involves the diffuse formation and rapid degradation of clot within the microcirculation.

The analysis of DIC has largely focused on the tendency to bleed, but most of the associated mortality and morbidity are probably related to microvascular thrombosis leading to end-organ failure.

Pathophysiology

Disseminated intravascular coagulation is an acquired coagulation disorder resulting from excessive activation of the coagulation system. The consumption of coagulation factors is due to an ongoing stimulus for intravascular clot formation including the generation of fibrin strands, which lead to thrombosis within the microcirculation with subsequent organ failure. In some circumstances, the ongoing stimulus is the presence of persistent bleeding from macroscopic injuries and large amounts of clotted and clotting blood. This circumstance provides a reservoir of activated factors promoting ongoing clot formation. In addition to this physiologic stimulus triggered by ongoing bleeding, the coagulation process can be initiated and maintained by other circumstances involving various proinflammatory stimuli. Bacterial endotoxin is a strong initiator of the coagulation process, as are cellular fragments created by trauma or hemolysis. Whatever the cause, the process of ongoing clot formation and clot lysis leads to a depletion of critical factors and subsequent hemostatic failure. Rapid decreases in platelet counts occur in sepsis and after hemolytic transfusion reactions or major ongoing bleeding. Parallel decreases in protein factors, especially fibrinogen, are also seen and can be marked. Table 6.4 provides an overview of clinical conditions that may be associated with DIC according to the International Society for Thrombosis and Haemostasis (ISTH).[30] According to severity, two forms of DIC are distinguished: (1) fulminant DIC (overt DIC) and (2) compensated nonovert DIC.

Table 6.4 Frequent causes of DIC according to the International Society for Thrombosis and Haemostasis.
Sepsis and severe infection (the most common cause of DIC; >50% of cases)
Trauma (polytrauma, CNS-trauma, burns)
Organ destruction (e.g. pancreatitis)
Malignancy (acute promyelocytic leukemia, acute myelomonocytic or monocytic leukemia, disseminated prostatic carcinoma, solid tumors)
Obstetric complications (placental separation and amnotic fluid embolism may result in release of placental TF, with excess thrombin generation)
Vascular abnormalities (e.g. hemangiomas, aortic aneurysm, empyema)
Liver disease/failure (acute hepatic necrosis, fatty liver of pregnancy, insertion of a LeVeen shunt in a patient with chronic liver disease and ascites)
Toxic (e.g. heatstroke, lightning strike, snakebite, recreational drugs, e.g. cocaine)
Severe immunological reactions (e.g. transfusion with ABO incompatible blood cells, transplant rejection)

(DIC: Disseminated intravascular coagulation; CNS: Central nervous system; TF: Tissue factor).
Adapted from Taylor FB, Toh CH, Hoots WK, et al. Towards a definition, clinical and laboratory criteria, and a scoring system for disseminated intravascular coagulation. J Thromb Haemost. 2001;86:1327-30.

Diagnosis

There is no single laboratory test that can confirm or rule out DIC. The diagnosis of DIC should, therefore, encompass both clinical and laboratory information. A diagnosis of DIC must be considered in any patient who shows evidence of a new onset of hemostatic failure. It is most common in the clinical settings of ongoing poorly controlled bleeding, multisystem trauma, and systemic sepsis. The most common clinical finding is renewed bleeding at sites that had previously stopped bleeding. This bleeding is usually noted at percutaneous needle puncture sites and skin wounds and in the gastrointestinal tract. Intraoperatively, areas within the surgical field that were previously dry may begin to ooze diffusely. Pooled blood will generally not clot. The ISTH has developed standards toward clinical and laboratory criteria including a scoring system for DIC, which is shown in Table 6.5.[30] The ISTH DIC scoring system provides objective measurement of DIC. Where DIC is present, the score correlates with key clinical observations and outcomes.

Treatment

The type and likely efficacy of treatment for DIC depends upon its etiology.[31] The prime aim is treatment of the underlying condition and to remove the ongoing stimulus to clot formation.[32] If the initiating stimulus cannot be controlled, successful treatment is highly unlikely. Examples are the administration of antibiotics and/or surgical drainage in patients where DIC is due to severe infection or sepsis. When diffuse activation of the clotting system results from an inflammatory insult, it may be impossible to identify and remove the stimulus. Basic principles include an active search for and aggressive treatment of sources of ongoing sepsis, as well as other efforts to moderate the systemic inflammatory response to injury or

Table 6.5 ISTH diagnostic scoring system for DIC.

Scoring system for overt DIC
Risk assessment: Does the patient have an underlying disorder known to be associated with DIC?
If yes: proceed
If no: do not use this algorithm
Order global coagulation tests [prothrombin time (PT), platelet count, fibrinogen, fibrin-related marker]
Score the test results
• Platelet count (>100 = 0; < 100 = 1; < 50 = 2) • Elevated fibrin-related marker (e.g. soluble fibrin monomers/ fibrin degradation products) (no increase = 0; moderate increase = 2; strong increase = 3) • Prolonged PT (<3 s = 0; >3 s. But < 6 s = 1; > 6 s = 2) • Fibrinogen level (> 1.0 g/L = 0; < 1.0 g/L = 1)
Calculate score
Sum score ≥ 5 = compatible with overt DIC; repeat scoring daily
Sum score < 5 = suggestive (not affirmative) for nonovert DIC; repeat next 1–2 days

(ISTH: International Society for Thrombosis and Haemostasis; DIC: Disseminated intravascular coagulation).
Adapted from Taylor FB, Toh CH, Hoots WK, et al. Towards a definition, clinical and laboratory criteria, and a scoring system for disseminated intravascular coagulation. J Thromb Haemost. 2001;86:1327-30.

illness. These efforts are followed by replacing the coagulation factors. If the factors are replaced without removing the stimulus to clot formation, the process will be perpetuated rather than halted. In the surgical arena, the usual stimulus is ongoing bleeding. The vital first step is therefore to control hemorrhage and evacuate large collections of clotted blood. Once macroscopic hemostasis has been achieved, the depleted factors can be replaced.

The transfusion of platelets or plasma in DIC patients should not primarily be based upon laboratory findings and should, in general, be reserved for bleeding patients. In case of platelet counts < 50,000/μL, the transfusion of platelets should be considered. In bleeding patients with DIC and prolonged PT and aPTT, the administration of fresh-frozen plasma (FFP) concentrates may be beneficial. In nonbleeding patients, prophylactic administration of platelets is not indicated unless the patient is at high risk of bleeding. There is no evidence that infusion of plasma stimulates the ongoing activation of coagulation. In cases in which FFP administration is not possible, for example, in patients with bleeding due to fluid overload, factor concentrates such as prothrombin complex concentrate (PCC) may be considered, however, recognizing that these concentrates contain selected factors only. In DIC, there is global deficiency of coagulation factors. Hypofibrinogenemia (<1 g/L) despite FFP administration may be additionally treated with fibrinogen concentrate or cryoprecipitate. In selected DIC cases, thrombosis may be predominant. In these cases, therapeutic doses of heparin may be considered. Monitoring aPTT in these cases may be difficult, and clinical observation of bleeding is important. For critically ill patients with absent bleeding, prophylaxis of venous thromboembolism using heparin is recommended. The use of AT cannot be recommended, and patients with DIC should generally not be treated with antifibrinolytics. If DIC is characterized by a primary hyperfibrinolytic state combined with severe bleeding, lysin analogs such as tranexamic acid may be considered.

SURGICALLY RELEVANT PLATELET DISORDERS

Pathophysiology

Dilution

Advances in blood banking and the wide availability of large volumes of blood components mean that massive transfusion, in which the circulating blood volume is replaced many times over, is not uncommon. This replacement consists almost exclusively of packed red blood cells (pRBCs) and crystalloid solutions, both of which are essentially devoid of platelets and soluble clotting factors. As a result, massive transfusion leads to a profound decrease in the platelet count. This dilutional thrombocytopenia is the most common clotting disorder seen in patients receiving large-volume resuscitation. To optimize hemostasis, the platelets must be replaced. To make optimal use of the transfused units of platelet concentrate, the replacement therapy should begin only after major surgical bleeding has been controlled.

Consumption

The process of ongoing bleeding and attempts at clot formation also decreases the platelet count through consumption. Large numbers of platelets become adherent to damaged tissues or are incorporated in fibrin clot. A low circulating platelet count may also arise from peripheral sequestration or accelerated peripheral destruction of platelets through antibody-mediated mechanisms unrelated to acute trauma or bleeding. Hypersplenism,autoimmune disorders, or immunization to homologous platelets from a previous transfusion can result in a highly accelerated rate of platelet destruction. In these circumstances, the platelet count can be very low despite normal marrow function. Thrombocytopenia of this type is often profound and can be refractory to transfusions of random donor platelets.

Abnormal Function (Thrombocytopathy)

Thrombocytopathy is an abnormality of platelets and can be congenital or acquired. Abnormalities in platelet function may cause thrombotic or bleeding tendencies or may be part of wider and more complex disorders such as myelodysplasia. Defects within the platelet system manifest themselves rather as primary hemostatic phenomena in the form of increased bleeding times, petechiae or purpura, rather than secondary hemostatic phenomena, for example hemarthrosis, and muscle hematomas.[33] Table 6.6 summarizes frequent causes for inherited and acquired platelet function disorders.

Congenital

The most common congenital cause of platelet dysfunction results from deficiencies in the function of vWF, which is abnormal function of receptors on the platelet surface. This protein mediates platelet adhesion to the endothelium and protects factor FVIII from degradation. The platelets themselves are normal, but they are unable to interact with vWF, so the critical initial adherence and aggregation necessary for clot initiation cannot occur. von Willebrand's disease is inherited as an autosomal dominant condition. Bernard-Soulier syndrome (BSS) is characterized by a deficiency of platelet glycoprotein Ib, which mediates the early action of platelets on the subendothelial surface through the von Willebrand's protein. It is a rare but severe bleeding disorder. GT is a deficiency of the glycoprotein IIb–IIIa complex, which inhibits platelets to aggregate. Type I is characterized by complete absence of the glycoprotein IIb–IIIa complex, while in type II, some of the glycoprotein IIb–IIIa complex is still present. Both BSS and GT respond to platelet transfusion, but this should be restricted to severe problems as alloantibodies may form.

Acquired

Acquired abnormalities of platelet function are most commonly due to the administration of aspirin or nonsteroidal anti-inflammatory drugs (NSAIDs). These agents interfere with the prostaglandin metabolism, inhibiting the formation of thromboxane A_2 through various mechanisms. The result is decreased platelet aggregation and inefficient platelet plug formation. Aspirin causes acetylation of a serine residue in the active site of cyclooxygenase. As platelets are incapable of regenerating cyclooxygenase, the effect of aspirin is permanent; it lasts for the life of the platelet (approximately 10 days). The effect of other NSAIDs may be transient. Chronic renal insufficiency also interferes with platelet function, apparently through abnormal interaction with vWF. This form of platelet dysfunction usually improves with dialysis, although its underlying cause is not completely understood. Clopidogrel is a thienopyridine class antiplatelet agent that works by irreversibly inhibiting P2Y12, an ADP chemoreceptor on platelet cell membranes. This mechanism is important for platelet activation and cross-linking for fibrin.

Diagnosis

A thorough history/examination is recommended to detect potential underlying conditions. The simplest laboratory test to perform is the peripheral platelet count. This test alone is sufficient to identify most coagulopathies due to dilution, consumption, or destruction of platelets. Hemostasis is generally considered to be adequate if the platelet count is >50,000/μL. Spontaneous bleeding becomes a high risk with counts of <15,000/μL. The initial laboratory screening should further include full blood count with a differential and a blood film, PT, aPTT, renal function, and thyroid function tests.

Bleeding Time

If there is an adequate number of platelets, a functional assay is required to determine the adequacy of platelet function objectively. The bleeding time measures the time required for bleeding to stop from a fresh superficial cut (1-mm deep and 1-cm long) made on the volar surface of the forearm, using a template under standard conditions. A normal platelet count with a prolonged bleeding time suggests a problem of platelet function. However, the bleeding time is very operator dependent and has poor reproducibility, sensitivity, and specificity.

Platelet Function Analyzers

The PFA-100 and the Multiplate analyzer are described above. The PFA-100 may be used for screening, but results

Table 6.6 Frequent causes for inherited and acquired platelet function disorders.

Inherited disorders	*Acquired disorders*
Severe disorders of platelet function • Wiskott–Aldrich syndrome • Glanzmann's thrombasthenia • Bernard–Soulier syndrome	Medications and chemicals • Aspirin and other nonsteroidal anti-inflammatory drugs • Clopidogrel • Dipyridamole • Beta-lactam antibiotics • Some herbal supplements
Disorders of receptors/signal transduction • Platelet cyclooxygenase deficiency • Thromboxane synthase deficiency • Thromboxane A2 receptor defect • ADP receptor defect	Organ diseases • Chronic kidney disease • Heart valve disease • Cardiopulmonary bypass • ECMO(extracorporeal membrane oxygenation)
Disorders of platelet adhesion • von Willebrand's disease	Myeloproliferative/dysplastic disorders • Essential thrombocythemia • Polycythemia vera
Disorders of the platelet granules • Idiopathic dense-granule disorder • (d-storage pool disease) • Hermansky–Pudlak syndrome • Chediak–Higashi syndrome • Gray platelet syndrome • Paris–Trousseau/Jacobsen syndrome	Paraproteins • Multiple myeloma • Waldenström's macroglobulinemia
Disorders of phospholipid exposure • Scott syndrome	Antibody-induced platelet dysfunction • Idiopathic thrombocytopenic purpura

have to be considered with caution and in the context of the clinical circumstances as the test is not diagnostic or sensitive for mild platelet disorders. The Multiplate analyzer is highly sensitive for the detection of aspirin, clopidogrel, prasugrel, IIb/IIIa receptor antagonists, and other platelet inhibitors. The test is further sensitive and clinically predictive for perioperative platelet function disorders as well as screening for platelet defects (e.g. GT) and functional detection of HIT.

Specific assays of inherited platelet dysfunction may include light transmission aggregometry, flow cytometry, measurement of total and released nucleotides, enzyme-linked immunosorbent assay (ELISA), electron microscopy, and molecular genetic diagnosis.

Treatment

Management depends on the underlying cause of the platelet dysfunction. Treatment of coagulopathy due to low platelet count consists primarily of replacement therapy. In addition, every effort must be made to ensure adequate surgical hemostasis and control of external hemorrhage. Platelet transfusion will also be effective when there is a defect in innate platelet function due to, for example, chronic aspirin use or uremia. In contrast, they are usually unnecessary for mild-to-moderate bleeding entities. Platelet transfusions should be used selectively and sparingly due to the potential risk of alloimmunization against human leucocyte antigen (HLA) and/or platelet glycoproteins. HLA-matched single donors of platelets may reduce the risk. Alternatively, leukocyte-depleted blood components may be used. The vasopressin analog desmopressin can be used to cause a transient increase in platelet function through interaction with vWF. Desmopressin increases plasma levels of vWF and coagulation factor FVIII, thus increasing platelet adhesiveness and aggregation associated with reductions in bleeding time. It is effective in controlling bleeding in uremic patients and in neurosurgical patients.

HYPERCOAGULABLE STATES

The greatest emphasis is often placed on the procoagulant aspect of the hemostatic system and its ability to stop bleeding. The existence of the innate balancing system of circulating anticoagulants has been known for a much shorter time, and these systems are much less well understood. Hypercoagulable states commonly manifest as lower extremity deep venous thrombosis (DVT), with its high morbidity in the involved extremity and associated risk of embolic phenomena. More than 60% of patients with an unprovoked venous thromboembolism have an underlying inherited hypercoagulable abnormality. Arterial thrombosis is less common, but usually more acutely damaging. Thrombosis at the level of the microcirculation has been implicated as a major cause of organ system failure in critical illness. The concept of a state of hypercoagulability dates back to 1854 when Virchow suggested that thrombosis resulted from, and in turn precipitated, three interrelated factors (Virchow's triad):

1. Decreased blood flow (venous stasis)
2. Inflammation of or near the blood vessels (vascular endothelial injury)
3. Intrinsic alterations in the nature of the blood itself.[34]

Hypercoagulable states can be either inherited or acquired and are associated with: (1) a predisposition to venous thrombosis, including upper/lower extremity DVT with or without pulmonary embolism; (2) cerebral venous thrombosis; (3) intra-abdominal venous thrombosis; (4) arterial thrombosis, including myocardial infarction (MI), stroke, acute limb ischemia, and splanchnic ischemia; or (5) combinations of both. Thrombocytosis, enhanced platelet aggregation and activity levels of coagulation factors as well as excess plasma levels of fibrinolytic inhibitors may lead to pathologic thrombosis. Both quantitative and qualitative deficiencies of a natural anticoagulant coagulation factor, resistance to inactivation by natural anticoagulants, and deficiencies of fibrinolytic protein may all be associated with hypercoagulability. Many diverse clinical scenarios lead to an increased tendency toward thrombosis. Known risk factors include trauma, malignancy, advanced age, a variety of drugs (especially oral contraceptives), and conditions predisposing to venous stasis. Table 6.7 provides an overview of potential hypercoagulable states.

The prevalence of hypercoagulable states follows the following order: factor V Leiden mutation > prothrombin G20210A mutation > AT deficiency = PC deficiency = ProS deficiency. aPC resistance secondary to factor V Leiden, prothrombin G20210A mutation, and deficiencies of natural anticoagulants are examples of inherited conditions, whereas antiphospholipid antibodies (APAs) represent an acquired set of disorders. Hyperhomocysteinemia can be precipitated by both genetic defects and acquired medical conditions, including vitamin deficiency states. The risk of a first venous thromboembolic event (VTE) varies according to the hypercoagulable state being present.

Table 6.7 Overview of established or potential hypercoagulable states.
Activated protein C resistance
Alpha-macroglobulin deficiency
Anticardiolipin antibodies
Antithrombin deficiency
Dysfibrinogenemia
Factor V Leiden
Factor V deficiency and excess
Factor VII excess
Factor VIII excess
Factor XI excess
Heparin cofactor II deficiency
Hyperhomocysteinemia
Hyperfibrinogenemia
Lupus anticoagulants
PAI-1 excess
Plasminogen deficiency
Protein C deficiency
Protein S deficiency
Prothrombin G20210A
tPA deficiency
TFPI deficiency
Thrombomodulin deficiency

(PAI-1: Plasminogen activator inhibitor-1; TFPI: Tissue factor pathway inhibitor; tPA: Tissue plasminogen activator).

The most common clinical entities associated with hypercoagulable states are described below.

Factor V Leiden Mutation

Factor V Leiden, or factor V G1691A, is a single-point mutation in the gene coding for coagulation factor FV transmitted through autosomal dominant inheritance. The mutation renders coagulation factors FV and FVa resistant to inactivation by aPC and accounts for 92% of cases of aPC resistance (APC-R). The remaining 8% result from oral contraceptive use, pregnancy, malignancies, selected APAs, and other factor FV point mutations.[35] Thus, APC-R represents an independent risk factor for VTE, even in the absence of factor V Leiden. Because factor FVa functions as a cofactor for prothrombin conversion to thrombin, the mutation results in greater amounts of factor Va, thus shifting the hemostatic balance toward more thrombin generation. The relative risk of a first VTE in patients with Factor FV Leiden is 2-10; if combined with prothrombin G20210A ("double heterozygous") 20,0.

Prothrombin G20210A Mutation

Prothrombin G20210A is an autosomal dominant single-point mutation resulting in elevated concentrations of plasma prothrombin. The prothrombin G20210A mutation is the second most common inherited predisposition to hypercoagulability and results in elevated concentrations of plasma prothrombin, which is the immediate precursor of thrombin. The underlying mechanisms are unknown. Hypercoagulability seems to be derived from greater availability of prothrombin for conversion to thrombin.[35] The relative risk of a first VTE in patients with prothrombin G20210A mutation is 2-6.

Antithrombin (AT) Deficiency

An increased propensity to thrombosis as a result of AT deficiency was first described in 1981. Deficiency can be either congenital or acquired. AT is the primary inhibitor of thrombin and of other serine proteases, such as coagulation factors FXIIa, FXIa, FXa, and FIXa. Therefore, AT deficiencies are associated with enhanced thrombin formation. Complete AT deficiency most likely leads to unfettered thrombin formation and hypercoagulability to degrees that are fatal in utero. In congenital cases, the homozygous genotype is usually fatal in infancy. The heterozygous genotype is associated with markedly decreased levels of AT and usually presents with an episode of spontaneous thrombosis by 45 years of age. Acquired deficits are related to inadequate hepatic synthesis due to disease or malnutrition, or increased consumption due to DIC, catabolism, or nephrosis. A diagnosis of AT deficiency should be considered in patients who develop recurrent spontaneous venous or arterial thrombosis, especially in the absence of other known risk factors. As heparin exerts its anticoagulant effect by interacting with AT, these episodes are characterized by an inability to achieve therapeutic anticoagulation on heparin and often occur in the course of a heparin infusion. The diagnosis can be made by direct assay of serum AT. Both absolute levels and function should be assessed. Serum assays should be carried out with the patient off all anticoagulants and may be impossible to assess in the acute setting due to AT consumption by ongoing thrombosis. The relative risk of a first VTE in patients with AT deficiency is 5-40.

Protein S and Protein C Deficiency

Deficiencies in PC and ProS are commonly implicated in hypercoagulable states.[36] PC, in its activated form (aPC), controls the formation of thrombin in the presence of its cofactor, ProS. Thus, in the setting of PC or ProS deficiency, thrombin formation is also enhanced and leads to hypercoagulability.[37] PC deficiency can be either congenital or acquired. In the congenital case, homozygous inheritance usually results in death during infancy due to widespread clotting of the microcirculation. Heterozygous inheritance leads to levels that are about half those of normal, but upper levels of heterozygous deficiency may overlap lower limits of normal. Acquired deficiency is usually due to altered hepatic synthesis, which can be secondary to warfarin administration. The diagnosis should be considered in repetitive episodes of thrombosis, especially when the episodes occur before 45 years of age. Measurement of levels during an acute thrombotic episode is likely to be inaccurate. The relative risk of a first VTE in patients with PC deficiency is 6.5-31; for patients with ProS deficiency 2-26, respectively.

Antiphospholipid Antibodies (APA)

There are two major APA subgroups: (1) the lupus anticoagulants and (2) the anticardiolipin antibodies. Lupus anticoagulants are assessed by their ability to prolong phospholipid-dependent coagulation assays in vitro (e.g. aPTT and dilute Russell viper venom time) via a competitive blocking mechanism. Anticardiolipin antibodies are assessed via ELISA.[38] APAs that are associated with autoimmune disorders (e.g. systemic lupus erythematosus, Sjögren's syndrome, rheumatoid arthritis, and mixed connective tissue disease) or malignancies are considered secondary. The lupus anticoagulant is found in <5% of patients with systemic lupus erythematosus. APAs detected in the absence of any underlying condition are considered primary. APAs have also been observed in the context of idiopathic autoimmune hemolytic anemia, malaria, syphilis, Q fever, mycobacteria, pneumocystis, cytomegalovirus (CMV), and drugs such as neuroleptics, quinidine, and procainamide. The mechanisms by which APAs promote thrombosis are unknown. To date, the suggested mechanisms include acquired aPC resistance, stimulation of platelet adhesion, activation, aggregation, upregulation of TF, enhanced expression of cell adhesion molecules and reduction of ProS levels. The relative risk of a first VTE in patients with lupus anticoagulants is 11; for patients with anticardiolipin antibodies 3,2, respectively.

Hyperhomocysteinemia

Inherited severe hyperhomocysteinemia (>100 μmol/L), as seen in classic homocystinuria, may result from homozygous methylenetetrahydrofolate reductase (MTHFR) or cystathionine β-synthase (CBS) deficiencies and, more rarely, from inherited failures of cobalamin (vitamin B12) metabolism.[39] Mild-to-moderate forms (15–100 μmol/L) may result from heterozygous deficiencies, but most commonly from an autosomal recessive single-point mutation for the MTHFR binding site leading to the substitution of valine for alanine and resulting in a thermolabile variant of the MTHFR (tlMTHFR). Acquired hyperhomocysteinemia may be related to folate deficiency, vitamin B6 and B12 deficiencies, renal failure, diabetes mellitus, hypothyroidism, carcinoma, pernicious anemia, inflammatory bowel disease, and methotrexate, theophylline, or phenytoin therapy. The mechanisms by which hyperhomocysteinemia causes thrombosis are also unclear. The suggested mechanisms include vascular injury, increased TF activity, inhibition of PC activation, increased platelet activation and aggregation, suppression of TM, and impaired fibrinolysis via inhibition of tPA binding to its endothelial cell receptor.[40] The relative risk of a first VTE in patients with hyperhomocysteinemia is 2,4.

Diagnosis

There are no specific signs or symptoms associated with hypercoagulable states, but laboratory tests for hypercoagulability may detect an inherited abnormality in > 60% of patients presenting with a first VTE. However, testing is expensive and rarely affects treatment. Therefore, and in the absence of evidence-based guidelines, testing should be restricted to selected patients in whom results are most likely to influence treatment. These are patients with:

1. Idiopathic VTE
2. VTE at age < 45 years
3. Recurrent VTE
4. VTE at unsusual sites
5. VTE combined with strong family history of VTE
6. Recurrent pregnancy loss.

The assessment for hypercoagulability is recommended in stages, beginning with highest yield assays (e.g. aPC-R, PCR for prothrombin G20210A mutation, and activity assays for AT, PC, and ProS).

Treatment

There are no specific therapies to reverse most hypercoagulable states. Recombinant factor concentrates of AT and aPC exist and may be useful in selected cases. Plasmapheresis or immunosuppressive therapies for APAs have not been successful. Increased plasma homocysteine levels in hyperhomocysteinemia can be lowered by folic acid or other vitamin B-complex supplementation. However, it is not known if normalization of homocysteine plasma levels may reverse hypercoagulability completely. Aggressive prophylaxis against VTE is mandatory in patients with a predisposition to hypercoagulability during high-risk situations such as major abdominal or orthopedic surgery as up to 70% of all VTEs occur following a situational risk factor.[41] In contrast, oral anticoagulation for primary VTE prophylaxis in asymptomatic carriers of any hypercoagulable state has not been advised, mainly because the annual absolute risk of idiopathic VTE is low or not high enough to be favorably balanced against the annual risk of major and fatal hemorrhage related to oral anticoagulation. The presence of a hypercoagulable state should not affect acute VTE treatment, i.e. initial anticoagulation with intravenous UFH or subcutaneous low molecular weight heparin followed by oral anticoagulation with warfarin—in most patients, except for those with a lupus anticoagulant as these antibodies may prolong aPTT. The monitoring of UFH therapy in this scenario should be performed by heparin assay (protamine titration or anti-factor Xa activity assay).

Currently, there are no data for the optimal duration of anticoagulation therapy in patients with specific hypercoagulable states. Any decision regarding the duration of therapy must therefore consider the estimates of VTE recurrence for a given disorder, the nature of the index VTE, and the risk of bleeding associated with prolonged oral anticoagulation. At the moment, The Sixth American College of Chest Physicians Guidelines to Antithrombotic Therapy do not recommend continuation of anticoagulation therapy beyond 3 to 6 months after a situational VTE in patients with heterozygous factor V Leiden or prothrombin G20210A mutation, and suggest that such therapy should last "1 year to lifetime" only in individuals with active cancer, persistently elevated anticardiolipin antibodies, and AT deficiency.[42] It may also be reasonable to consider long-term anticoagulation therapy in conditions known to be associated with increased VTE rates of recurrence, such as persistent lupus anticoagulants, homozygous factor V Leiden, and perhaps patients with a deficiency of PC or ProS, or with double heterozygosity for factor V Leiden and prothrombin G20210A mutation. In general, the outcomes of patients with hypercoagulable states are dependent on VTE recurrence associated with the different disorders. To date, no data suggest reduced survival in patients who carry an inherited predisposition to hypercoagulability.

HEPARIN-INDUCED THROMBOCYTOPENIA (HIT)

Heparin-induced thrombocytopenia is an antibody-mediated adverse drug reaction to heparin that can be associated with devastating thromboembolic complications involving the arterial system, the venous system, or both, including pulmonary embolism, ischemic limb necrosis necessitating limb amputation, acute MI, DVT, skin necrosis, end organ damage, and cerebrovascular accidents. Studies quote HIT frequencies as high as 1–5%. Most studies that have reported HIT frequencies to be as high as 5% were performed in postoperative orthopedic patients who had received UFH thromboprophylaxis for 10–14 days.[43] HIT appears to occur more frequently with UFH compared to low molecular weight heparin. Affected individuals are likely to have a 20–50% risk of developing new thromboembolic events and mortality rates of approximately 20% have been reported, with an additional approximate 10% of patients requiring amputations or suffering from other major morbidity.[44]

Two different mechanisms of HIT have been described, differing in their timing, degree of thrombocytopenia, and clinical course.[45] The first type is caused by a direct interaction between heparin and platelets, leading to platelet aggregation. The platelet count drops early in the course of heparin administration, almost always within the first 2–5 days. Platelet counts rarely drop < 100,000/μL, and often recover spontaneously even if heparin treatment is continued. There seems to be little clinical risk of thrombosis, and no need for clinical intervention. This phenomenon is sometimes called type 1 HIT. It is well known that type 1 HIT is a nonimmune disorder, and it occurs with the direct effect of heparin on platelet activation. Type 2 HIT is triggered by an antibody-mediated immune response, which typically occurs 4–10 days after exposure to heparin, and it is the serious type with its life- and limb-threatening prothrombotic complications. In general medical practice, HIT refers to type 2 HIT. The platelet count usually drops to 50–70,000/μL. It may take several weeks for the platelet count to recover after heparin is stopped. The target of the antibody response is probably a complex of heparin bound to tetrameric platelet factor 4 (PF4).[46] Plasma from more than 90% of patients with HIT contains anti-PF4-heparin antibodies. A few studies have identified immunoglobulin G (IgG) antibodies, but more recent studies demonstrate IgM and IgA antibodies as well. Immune complexes of HIT antibodies and PF4/heparin bind to the surface of platelets and induce their activation by cross-linking Fc IIA receptors and bind to the surface of the endothelium, triggering procoagulant activity. Platelets activated with HIT IgG increase their release and surface expression of PF4, and a positive feedback loop is installed as further PF4 release occurs with platelet activation. Low molecular weight heparins are much less likely to stimulate antibody formation compared to UFH, but once the antibody is formed, both unfractionated and low molecular weight heparins will react and trigger platelet aggregation.

Diagnosis

Bleeding complications of HIT are rare; the immune-mediated type HIT actually produces a hypercoagulable state. Three characteristic features of HIT can distinguish it from other causes of thrombocytopenia:

1. Timing of the onset of thrombocytopenia, with a platelet count that decreases between days 5 and 14 after initiation of heparin treatment
2. Severity of the thrombocytopenia (usually mild-to-moderate) and
3. Large-vessel venous or arterial thrombosis in association with thrombocytopenia.

The possibility of HIT should be considered if venous thromboembolism (VTE) develops during or soon after UFH use; if thrombocytopenia is present, alternative anticoagulation is recommended until HIT is excluded. Delayed-onset HIT develops several days after heparin cessation. In patients with previous heparin exposure, HIT may have a rapid onset within a few hours of reexposure. HIT should be presumed in any patient who develops new or progressive thrombosis after the initiation of heparin therapy.

To date, there are four diagnostic tests available for HIT:

1. Serotonin release assay (SRA)
2. Heparin-induced platelet aggregation assay (HIPA)
3. Solid-phase immunoassay (H-PF4 ELISA)
4. Particle gel immunoassay.

Most laboratories use HIPA, which is considered highly specific but less sensitive than the SRA. The SRA is considered the "gold standard" for the detection of heparin-dependent antibodies, with sensitivity as high as 90% and specificity as high as 100%.[47] SRA is based on HIT antibodies causing platelet aggregation and the release of serotonin. The HIPA is a platelet-activation test in which the patient's serum is combined with donor platelets in the presence of heparin. Aggregation of the donor platelets indicates the presence of antibodies to the heparin-PF4 complex. Both the SRA and the HIPA are functional assays. The ELISA measures PF4-antibodies bound to heparin, whereas the particle gel immunoassay measures agglutinated microbeads after patient serum and heparin–PF4-coated microbeads are incubated.[48] In addition to these tests, both clinical vigilance and judgment are highly important. Suspicion should be triggered by a drop in platelet count of 30–50% from baseline that is associated with heparin administration. The antibody to heparin–PF4 complex can be detected and quantified, but the presence of antibody, even in high concentration, does not predict thrombosis. Various assays of platelet function are also used, but these methods lack sensitivity and specificity.

Treatment

The treatment of HIT is evolving, and the approach depends on two factors:

1. The need for ongoing anticoagulation
2. The likelihood of thrombotic complications.

The immediate cessation of all forms of heparin therapy is essential in patients with clinically suspected HIT. Simply discontinuation of heparin may not necessarily prevent heparin exposure because UFH is commonly used to flush catheters. If the patient does not require ongoing anticoagulation and there is no evidence of thrombosis, the need for treatment beyond cessation of heparin administration has not been established. There is a theoretical risk of thrombosis, which has led some to suggest addition of alternative anticoagulant therapy. If the patient requires ongoing anticoagulation (and most do), or if there is evidence of new thrombosis, it is mandatory to begin administration of a nonheparin anticoagulant in addition to cessation of heparin administration.

Warfarin has been associated with increased thrombotic complications and venous gangrene when used in the acute phase of HIT. This fact is likely to reflect warfarin-induced decreases in PC concentration, which can precede the drop in thrombin levels. Therefore, warfarin should not be used as the initial treatment for HIT-induced thrombosis and should be postponed until sufficient platelet recovery.[48] Preferably, warfarin should not be started before the thrombocyte count is > 150,000/μL. If warfarin has already been started, vitamin K should be given. An investigation for lower limb DVT should be undertaken. Warfarin can be safely used for chronic anticoagulation, if its administration is overlapped with another anticoagulant. Once the patient has been fully anticoagulated by other means, there is no additional risk associated with warfarin. Low molecular weight heparins are of no value in this situation, as they will cross react with the existing antibodies. Platelet transfusions should be avoided in HIT, as they may increase the thrombogenic effect.

Fortunately, there are several agents that can inhibit the action of thrombin. The agent with the largest clinical experience is danaparoid sodium, which is an extract of pig intestine containing a number of low molecular weight glycosaminoglycans. It acts primarily to inhibit activated factor FX and to a lesser degree interacts with AT to inhibit thrombin. In vitro, there is an approximately 10–20% rate of cross-reactivity with the heparin–PF4 antibody, but sequelae of this cross-reactivity are uncommon in the clinical application. Danaparoid sodium has two major drawbacks in clinical use. It does not cause abnormalities in the PT or PTT, and so clinical monitoring of the degree of anticoagulation is difficult. An assay for activity against activated factor FX can be used, but the assay is comparatively complex. In addition, danaparoid sodium has a long duration of action, leading to slow response to decreases in dosage. Danaparoid does not cross the placenta.

Lepirudin (Refludan) is recombinant hirudin derived from yeast cells. It forms irreversible 1:1 complexes with thrombin and thereby blocks the thrombogenic activity of thrombin. It is a highly specific direct inhibitor of thrombin. The mode of action is independent of AT, and PF4 does not inhibit lepirudin. The half-life, which is 80 minutes with normal renal function, increases substantially with renal failure. The activity of lepirudin is measured in a chromogenic assay. One AT unit is the amount of lepirudin neutralizing one unit of WHO preparation 89/588 of thrombin. As a result, all thrombin-dependent coagulation assays are affected for a target aPTT of 1.5–2.5 times of baseline.[48]

Another potential agent is argatroban, a synthetic dipeptide agent that acts by direct competitive inhibition of thrombin. It inhibits fibrin formation, platelet aggregation, and activation of coagulation factors FV, FVIII, FXIII, and PC. Argatroban is used to treat both HIT with thrombosis and isolated HIT. The dose is adjusted by aPTT, with a target of 1.5–3 times the baseline. The initial dose should be reduced in liver dysfunction. The INR is prolonged more prominently with argatroban compared with lepirudin. The agent is the alternative to heparin for patients receiving dialysis, because it does not require dose adjustment. This agent may represent an improvement over hirudin due to superior pharmacokinetics and decreased immunogenicity.

For the duration of treatment, therapeutic doses of alternative anticoagulants should be continued until the platelet count recovers to a stable plateau in cases of only isolated thrombocytopenia. Due to the remaining high risk of thrombosis for 2–4 weeks after initiation of treatment, anticoagulant therapy with an alternative agent or warfarin should be continued for up to 4 weeks. In cases of HIT with thrombosis, therapy with an alternative anticoagulant should be followed by a transition to warfarin, but only after platelet counts have recovered to >150,000/μL. Oral anticoagulants should be started at low doses, and an overlap with a direct thrombin inhibitor for at least 5 days should be kept until therapeutic INR is established for at least 48 hours. Surgical care could be considered individually on the basis of the complications of HIT.[49]

THROMBOCYTOSIS

Thrombocytosis is a condition of an abnormally high platelet count, generally defined as >500,000/μl (500 $\times 10^9$/L). Platelet counts <1,000,000/μL are thought to pose a minimal risk of spontaneous thrombosis. Platelet counts >1,000,000/μL (1,000 $\times$ 10^9/L) are an indication for either specific therapy or extreme vigilance. Two types of thrombocytosis can be distinguished: primary and secondary. Primary thrombocytosis, also known as essential thrombocythemia, is a disease in which abnormal cells in the bone marrow cause an increase in platelets. The cause is yet unclear. The most common cause of a high platelet count is general bone marrow upregulation, usually as a response to inflammation, infection, sepsis, or systemic stress. In otherwise healthy individuals, platelet counts in the range of 500,000–750,000/μL are commonly seen. This is termed secondary thrombocytosis. There does not seem to be an appreciable risk of thrombosis. Thrombocytosis is quite common after splenectomy, with platelet counts often rising >1,000,000/μl. Other causes for secondary thrombosis include anemia due to iron deficiency, malignancies, and recent surgical operation. Usually, increased platelet counts do not cause clinical symptoms. When symptoms do appear, they may include skin bruising or bleeding from various sites such as the nose, mouth, and gums, or the stomach and intestinal tract. Abnormal blood clotting may also occur, leading to stroke, heart attack, and unusual clotting in abdominal vessels.

Treatment

The assessment of potential underlying conditions (e.g. iron deficiency anemia, malignancy, or infection) may support the diagnosis and treatment of thrombocytosis. Bone marrow aspiration and other blood tests can confirm the diagnosis. Secondary thrombocytosis subsides when the underlying process causing the elevated platelet count resolves. In the absence of any secondary cause, the patient is presumed to have essential thrombocythemia. Patients who have no symptoms may remain stable and only require routine checkups. The risk of thrombosis is unknown, and platelet counts <1,000,000/μL are rarely treated. If the platelet count is >1,000,000/μL some form of antiplatelet therapy should be considered. Aspirin is most commonly used in this setting, although there is no clear evidence of clinical efficacy. The low dose used for this purpose does not usually cause stomach upset or bleeding. Various myeloproliferative disorders are associated with thrombocytosis. Treatment is aimed at controlling the underlying disorder. Antineoplastic agents are given to suppress platelet synthesis. As in other forms of thrombocytosis, the risk of thrombosis and indications for antiplatelet therapy are poorly defined. In cases of essential thrombocythemia, medications such as hydroxyurea or anagrelide are used to suppress platelet production by the bone marrow. Usually, these medications have to be taken indefinitely. In cases of severe life-threatening thrombocytosis, plateletpheresis may be performed immediately to lower platelet numbers to safer levels.

BLOOD TRANSFUSION

Red Blood Cells

The red cell is a highly specialized cell, which originates from the bone marrow by a sophisticated maturation process. The mature red cell is a biconcave disc that measures 7–8 μm in diameter and 1.5–2.5 μm in thickness. In the final step of maturation, it exudes its nucleus and all intracellular organelles, leaving only a flexible membrane sac of hemoglobin. There is no further synthesis of hemoglobin because the nucleus and ribosomes have all been expelled. Similarly, all energy production is by anaerobic glycolysis because all mitochondria have also been exuded. However, the red cell does retain all of its surface carbohydrate and protein antigens, which are fundamental to compatible transfusion. The red cell has a life span of 120 days and is eliminated by the fixed reticuloendothelial system with senescence.

Blood Types

The life-saving potential of blood transfusion was obvious in the earliest days of medicine and a variety of human

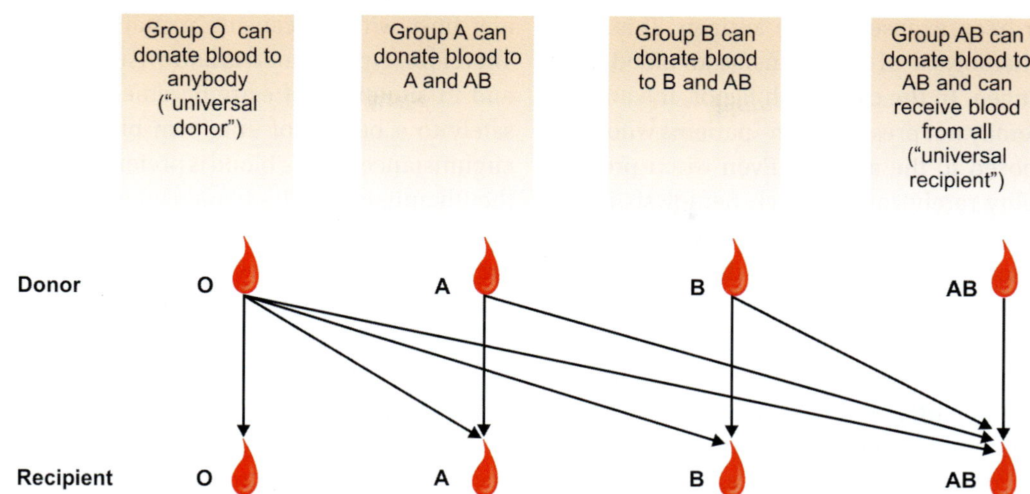

Fig. 6.8: Matched blood types for safe transfusion.

and nonhuman donors were used. Although all blood is made of the same basic elements, not all blood is alike and the immune consequences of transfusing the "wrong" type of blood are catastrophic.[50] Blood transfusions were successfully accomplished between individuals who had compatible blood types as a result of being related to each other or "good luck" long before a scientific basis for success or failure was known. The major ABO blood types were first described by Landsteiner around 1901.

Blood cells, both red cells and leukocytes, express antigens on their cell surfaces that are important in self-recognition and immunologic surveillance. Since some antigens can trigger a patient's immune system to attack the transfused blood, safe blood transfusions ultimately depend on careful blood typing and cross-matching. There are a large number of these surface antigen systems, but the dominant system involved in blood transfusion is the ABO system. In this system, the two major antigens on the surface of red blood cells have been designated A and B. Depending upon genotype, blood cells independently express or do not express either of these antigens. This produces four distinct combinations, which yields the four basic ABO blood types:

1. Group A—has only A antigen on red blood cells (and B antibody in plasma).
2. Group B—has only B antigen on red blood cells (and A antibody in plasma).
3. Group AB—has both A and B antigens on red blood cells (and neither A nor B antibody in plasma).
4. Group O - has neither A nor B antigens on red blood cells (but both A and B antibodies in plasma).

The specific ways in which blood types must be matched for safe transfusion are shown in Figure 6.8. Not all ethical groups have the same mix of blood types. For example, Hispanic people have a relatively high number of type O, whereas Asian people have more frequently type B. Another antigen system, the Rh factor, is also routinely used in standard blood typing. Independent of the basic ABO blood type, the Rh factor may either be expressed or not expressed. The Rh status is commonly expressed as a "+" or "–" (alternatively, "Rh+" or "Rh–") after the basic ABO type. In general, Rh- blood is given to Rh- patients, and either Rh+ blood or Rh- blood is given to Rh+ patients. These two antigen systems yield eight combinations of blood types, as shown in Table 6.8. The universal red blood cell donor has Group O negative blood type; the universal plasma donor has Group AB positive blood type.

Table 6.8 The eight different combinations of ABO and Rh antigen.

Blood type		*A antigen*	*B antigen*	*Rh antigen*
Type O	Rh+	–	–	+
	Rh–	–	–	–
Type A	Rh+	+	–	+
	Rh–	+	–	–
Type B	Rh+	–	+	+
	Rh–	–	+	–
Type AB	Rh+	+	+	+
	Rh–	+	+	–

If a given antigen is expressed on the cell surface, the body recognizes this as self and therefore does not produce antibodies against that antigen. On the other hand, if the particular antigen is not expressed on the cell surface, the body will form antibodies against that antigen. For the antigens of the ABO complex, these antibodies are present in the serum in high concentration even if the body has never been exposed to the antigen. This leads to immediate hemolysis of any transfused blood cells carrying the antigen. In the case of Rh factor, the anti-Rh antibody is generally not present in Rh– patients who have never been exposed to the antigen. Even when present, Rh incompatibility rarely causes much hemolysis in the adult transfusion recipient. The primary danger associated with immunization against Rh factor is the risk of severe hemolysis in the Rh+ fetus of an immunized Rh- mother. In addition to the major ABO antigens and the Rh factor, many other minor antigens are expressed on blood cells that present the potential for rare naturally occurring antibodies or acquired alloantibodies from a previous transfusion. The Lewis, Ii, and P antigens are carbohydrate antigens for which there may be naturally occurring IgM antibody in the transfused host. Kidd, Duffy, and Kell antigens are proteins that require previous exposure and immunization. These alloantibodies are IgG.[51] Usually, patients who have never received a homologous blood transfusion will not have preformed antibody in their serum. Patients with a previous history of transfusion and the rare patient with no such history will have preformed antibodies against minor antigens. Clinical problems can then develop during transfusion, depending upon the existence and concentration of these antibodies.

Blood Typing and Crossmatching

When a patient's blood sample is analyzed for a future transfusion, the ABO and Rh type is determined by standard means. This step is known as blood typing. The sample can then be checked for the presence of several common preformed antibodies, called the screen or antibody screen. For maximum safety, a small aliquot of the patient's blood is tested directly with each potential donor unit, in a step called the crossmatch. Crossmatching is the final step in pretransfusion testing. It is commonly referred to as compatibility testing, or "Type and Cross." If there is no reaction, the unit is deemed safe for transfusion. The initial ABO typing and antibody screen can usually be performed within about 15 minutes and do not require testing of donor units to determine compatibility. The crossmatch step is significantly slower and more laborious. It must be carried out for each donor unit and usually requires 45–60 minutes to complete.

Blood Type O—"Universal Donor"

Blood type O cells do not express any of the major ABO antigens on their cell surface and can be transfused into any host without causing a major hemolytic reaction. Therefore, type O blood is known as the "universal donor" and in situations of extreme emergency it can be given safely to a patient of unknown blood type. Under these circumstances O Rh– blood is preferred as the cells also lack the Rh antigen; O Rh+ blood can also be used without an appreciable danger of hemolysis, but if possible should be limited to males and postmenopausal or sterilized women to prevent Rh immunization and subsequent danger to a potential Rh+ fetus. Because it can be safely transfused without previous testing, O Rh– blood is an extremely valuable resource that is inherently limited in quantity. In addition, problems with subsequent blood typing can occur with large-volume administration of O Rh– blood to patients with blood types other than O because the patient's blood will contain significant populations of red cells of both type O and the native type. For these reasons, the use of unmatched O Rh– blood should be restricted to immediately life-threatening situations where type-matched blood is not available.

Classes of Blood Transfusion

Units of blood for transfusion can be considered to belong to one of three classes based on the time required for preparation, availability, and potential risks of transfusion reaction. The first is O—universal donor. This donor type can be administered immediately, without testing the recipient. The major drawback is the limited supply, so other options should be used as soon as available. The second class is type-specific blood. In this circumstance, the major ABO and Rh type are determined and the patient's blood is screened for major antibodies. The donor units are matched by type, but are not individually tested. In general, type-specific blood can be available in 10–15 minutes. Experience has shown that the administration of uncrossmatched type-specific blood is quite safe in the general population. The final option is cross-matched blood. Individual donor units are tested for compatibility with the recipient (*see* above).

Rapid Massive Transfusion

Rapid massive transfusion is usually defined as the rapid administration of large volumes of blood in a 24-hours period. In adults, this may be >5 L, ≥10 units of pRBCs, or > 1 blood volume. Rapid massive transfusion may result in several adverse effects, which must be monitored and corrected to minimize morbidity and mortality. It has been shown that both morbidity and mortality increase with

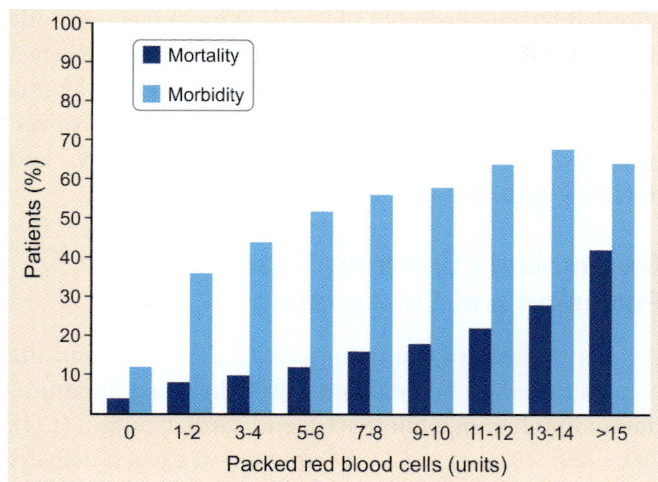

Fig. 6.9: Unadjusted morbidity and mortality by numbers of packed red blood cells (pRBCs) received in intraoperative blood transfusion. Modified from Ferraris VA, Davenport DL, Saha SP, et al. Surgical outcomes and transfusion of minimal amounts of blood in the operating room. Arch Surg. 2012;147(1):49-55.

every unit of pRBCs administered and that even minimal amounts of blood products may increase mortality, wound problems, pulmonary complications, postoperative renal dysfunction, systemic sepsis, composite morbidity, and postoperative length of stay (Fig. 6.9).[52] Once the patient's blood volume has been replaced, the importance of potential minor antibodies is greatly reduced. Because there is little or none of the patient's own serum left, there is no value in the crossmatch process until the patient has recovered sufficiently to manufacture antibody in significant quantity. Therefore, further acute transfusion should be carried out with type-specific units and crossmatching is resumed once the massive transfusion has ended. The possible complications associated with massive transfusion are related to the number of units transfused, the rate of transfusion, and factors intrinsic to the patient. They can be divided into three categories:

1. Hypothermia (massive transfusion may result in clinically relevant hypothermia body temperature < 35°C)
2. Metabolic (may include hypocalcemia, hypomagnesemia, metabolic alkalosis, hyperkalemia, or hypokalemia) and
3. Hemostatic (due to dilution and depletion of coagulation proteins/platelets).

INDICATIONS FOR TRANSFUSION

The advantages of a component approach to transfusion therapy are compelling. Currently, the transfusion of whole blood is rare and there are only very few indications for this, e.g. situations in which blood transfusion is required immediately for rapid, life-threatening hemorrhage when red blood cell component therapy is not available. In this case, irradiated blood and the use of a leukocyte filter should be used. Upon donation, a unit of blood is usually separated into:

1. pRBCs, consisting primarily of red and white cells
2. Platelet fraction
3. Serum fraction.

When used directly, the serum fraction is known as "fresh frozen plasma". Further processing of the cellular components can yield leukocyte-rich preparations and further processing of the serum fraction can yield specific factor concentrates. Each individual blood component is available for separate administration, depending upon factor-specific indications.

Packed Red Blood Cells (pRBCs)

After donated blood is collected, the components are separated in a centrifuge, then a small amount of an anticoagulant is added to prevent the pRBCs from clotting. The blood is kept in a refrigerator and is good for approximately 42 days from the date of donation. pRBCs must be compatible and matched to the recipient. The transfusion of pRBCs is indicated to provide adequate oxygen-carrying capacity in patients who have a low red blood cell mass due to acute hemorrhage, hemolysis, or chronic anemia. In patients with active ongoing bleeding, pRBCs must be administered at a rate sufficient to keep up with the losses until hemostasis can be achieved. Patients in advanced hemorrhagic shock should receive an initial transfusion of O Rh– blood if available, and this is typically limited to 4–8 units. At the same time, the patient's own blood should be analyzed for ABO type and rapid antibody screen. Ongoing emergency transfusion should be converted to type-specific donor units as soon as available, usually within 10–15 minutes. Type-specific units should be used for the remainder of the transfusion(s) until initial stability has been achieved. It has been shown that transfusion of old blood (> 12 days) may be associated with worsening oxygen delivery because stored red blood cells lose their deformability and hence their ability to pass through the microvasculature and unload oxygen.

Nonemergency Transfusion

The decision to transfuse a patient has to balance the known risks of transfusion with the need to provide adequate tissue oxygenation and the appropriate utilization of blood as a resource of limited availablity.[53] The minimum tolerated hemoglobin level is not well established, and considerable variation exists in transfusion practices. The traditional transfusion trigger of 10 g/dL has been challenged over the recent years by reports indicating that aerobic metabolism is supported by hemoglobin levels of 5 g/dL or even less. There is also evidence from randomized trials demonstrating that withholding transfusions may result in improved outcomes. Anecdotal reports documenting the course of Jehovah's Witness patients who have experienced major bleeding episodes confirm the ability to tolerate hemoglobin levels well below those conventionally accepted by physicians. To date, many centers have lowered their trigger for blood transfusion from 8 to 7 g/dL in normovolemic, symptomatic chronic anemia patients. The current AABB (formerly, the American Association of Blood Banks) Guideline recommends adhering to a restrictive transfusion strategy (7 to 8 g/dL) in hospitalized, stable patients.[54]

Multiple variables must be evaluated by the clinician, and the final decision to give a transfusion depends upon individual physiologic need and clinical circumstances rather than on arbitrary numeric hemoglobin triggers. These physiologic triggers can be based on signs and symptoms of impaired global oxygenation (lactate, venous O_2 saturation [SvO_2]) or, even better, of regional tissue oxygenation (electrocardiographic ST-segment, electroencephalographic P300 latency).[55] Clinical aspects to consider before transfusion may also include the duration of anemia and the probability of additional blood loss. Patients with chronic renal failure will usually tolerate hemoglobin concentrations of 5–6 g/dL without adverse sequelae. Adaptation of oxyhemoglobin–oxygen dissociation mechanisms affords efficient oxygen delivery to tissues despite the profound hemodilution. However, a 7 g/dL threshold is commonly used as an indicator for transfusion for acute hemodilution secondary to acute blood loss, although in young patients with ability for cardiac compensation, acute blood loss to a hemoglobin as low as 5 g/dL may be well tolerated. The toleration of 7 g/dL requires careful consideration of the additional clinical variables defined below. If a patient has had an acute blood loss from gastrointestinal bleeding or acute injury and there is the prospect for continued or recurrent blood loss (e.g. due to acute bleeding peptic ulcer, pelvic fracture), then higher hemoglobin concentrations may be more desirable. Patients at risk of additional major loss of red cell mass need a larger physiologic reserve than is afforded by a hemoglobin of 7 g/dL. Vice versa, it is hotly debated in the literature how many transfusions are in fact "unnecessary." Older studies report a low rate, ranging from 1.4% to 4% of transfusions. These rates are, however, probably "inappropriate" rather than "unnecessary," and thus they underestimate the overuse of blood.[56]

Mechanisms Ensuring Tissue Perfusion and Oxygenation

Oxygen delivery to the tissues (DO_2) depends upon the concentration of hemoglobin (Hb), the percent saturation of that hemoglobin (SaO_2), and cardiac output (CO): $DO_2 = Hb \times \% \ SaO_2 \times CO$. A reduction in oxygen delivery below a critical level deprives tissues of the oxygen necessary for oxidative metabolism and results in a shift to anaerobic metabolism. If there is hemodilution from acute blood loss, the intravascular volume must be normalized. This process is usually achieved by the administration of adequate crystalloid volume, but the hemoglobin concentration can then decline to dangerously low levels (e.g. <5 g/dL). Nevertheless, despite the risk of further hemodilution, restoration of intravascular volume is essential to ensure adequate tissue perfusion.

The primary mechanism for preserving oxygen delivery with acute hemodilution (i.e. anemia) is the compensatory increase in cardiac output (Fig. 6.10).[57] Isovolemic hemodilution, although reducing the oxygen-carrying

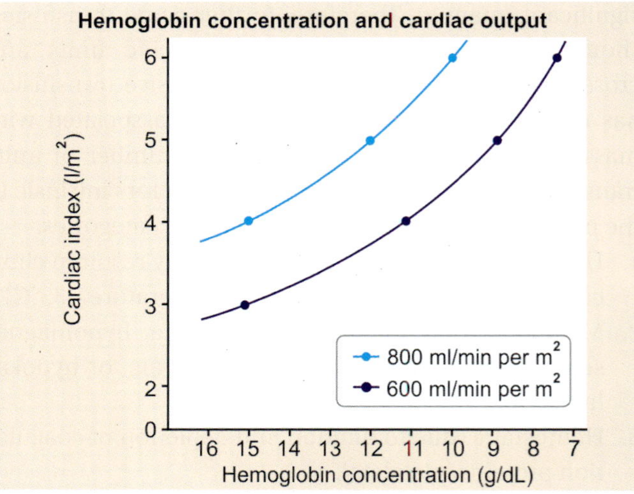

Fig. 6.10: Relationship between hemoglobin concentration in isovolemic hemodilution and cardiac output necessary to deliver a specific amount of oxygen per unit of time. The delivery of 600 mL/min/m² is an approximation of normal oxygen delivery in adults. The delivery of 800 mL/min/m² is the desired delivery in circumstances of stress and sepsis.

capacity of the blood, actually improves the rheologic properties of the blood. Systemic vascular resistance to flow is diminished and, given an appropriate cardiac preload, results in an increase in cardiac output. Although oxygen-carrying capacity/unit volume of blood is diminished, oxygen delivery can be preserved by increased rates of flow. Increased flow rates with isovolemic hemodilution are achieved without appreciable tachycardia. Cardiac work is principally driven by cardiac rate, so isovolemic hemodilution compensated by an increased cardiac output can be safely achieved in most patients. Greater tachycardia with rates > 100/minute either reflect hypovolemia or a reduced cardiac reserve that does not allow the increase in cardiac output needed to preserve peripheral oxygen delivery.

Toleration to Hemodilution

Cardiac output is the principal compensatory mechanism for acute hemodilution, but the degree of hemodilution that can be tolerated also depends upon:

1. Patient's intrinsic cardiac function
2. Presence of myocardial or cerebrovascular disease and
3. Presence of pulmonary disease.

Patients who have heart disease and in whom cardiac output cannot be increased become tachycardic and develop lactic acidosis or become hypotensive from congestive failure. These patients require higher hemoglobin concentrations and cannot tolerate lower concentrations. The current AABB Guideline recommends adhering to a restrictive strategy in hospitalized patients with preexisting cardiovascular disease and considering transfusion for patients with symptoms or a hemoglobin level of 8 g/dL.[54] The guideline does not recommend for or against a liberal or restrictive transfusion threshold for hospitalized, hemodynamically stable patients with acute coronary syndrome. Likewise, patients with lung disease may not be able to maintain an adequate hemoglobin saturation and will require higher hemoglobin concentrations. The AABB Guideline suggests that transfusion decisions be influenced by symptoms as well as hemoglobin concentration.

Intraoperative Transfusion

Indications for intraoperative administration of blood are similarly based upon:

1. Maintenance of normovolemia
2. Estimates of blood loss
3. Expectations of further losses during the procedure
4. Cardiopulmonary reserve of the patient.

Crystalloid volume resuscitation to maintain volume and intraoperative monitoring of hemoglobin concentration to corroborate estimates of blood loss are important. Hemoglobin concentrations between 7 and 10 g/dL warrant transfusion if further blood loss is anticipated during the remainder of the procedure. Hemoglobin concentrations between 8.5 and 10 g/dL at the time of completion of a procedure would ordinarily not warrant transfusion, but must be closely monitored for further immediate postoperative equilibration. A hemoglobin concentration of 7 to 8 g/dL at completion of the procedure will usually result in transfusion of older patients and patients with vascular or cardiac disease. In younger patients without anticipated additional losses, an expectant strategy can be pursued with close monitoring of the hemoglobin concentration.

ALTERNATIVES TO TRANSFUSION

Autotransfusion

Autotransfusion is commonest alternative strategy used during surgical procedures.[58] The shed blood is captured during and after operation using an intraoperative blood salvage device (such as a "cell saver"); it is then anticoagulated to allow readministration to the patient. This approach is used in operations in which there is expected to be a large volume blood loss (e.g. aneurysm, total joint replacement, and spinal surgeries). Citrate phosphate dextrose is the common anticoagulant used. Excessive anticoagulation and hypocalcemia can be problems with this strategy. Blood must be filtered during collection and reinfusion. Bacterial contamination from bowel injury in trauma patients results in a risk of microbial dissemination. Concern about the potential dissemination of malignant cells has limited the use of antotransfusion during major abdominal or thoracic cancer operations.

Direct Donation

Self-donation of blood in the preoperative period has been used to reduce the need for transfusion from blood donors.[59] During the month prior to a major elective procedure, patients may autodonate one or two units and have them available for transfusion during the subsequent procedure (e.g. total hip replacement). This method has proved useful for selected procedures. Designation of a specific friend or relative as the blood donor has also been used as a means to reduce the need for transfusion from blood donors. However, designated donations have not been shown to be any safer than transfusion from carefully screened blood bank units.

Preoperative Hemodilution

Preoperative acute normovolemic hemodilution (ANH) involves withdrawal of whole blood with concurrent infusion of fluids to maintain normovolemia. This strategy has been used in cardiac and other vascular procedures.[60] Two to four units of blood are removed in the immediate preoperative period, and each removed unit is simultaneously replaced with a volume expander. Ringer's lactate, dextran or certain polystarch plasma expanders have been used for this method. The patient's preoperative hemoglobin is reduced to the 10 g/dL range and autotransfusion of the patient's blood is begun on a unit for unit basis during the operation. Such a strategy should allow a four-unit blood loss without any need for additional transfusion. A recent meta-analysis indicated only modest benefits from preoperative ANH, with the safety of this approach left unproven.[61] ANH is contraindicated in cardiac disease, impaired renal function, baseline hemoglobin <11 g/dL, low levels of coagulants, and the absence of appropriate monitoring capability.

Blood Substitutes

The attempt to develop and introduce viable blood substitutes spans back over the last seven decades. Most activity in this field has been focused on the capacity of red blood cells to transport and deliver oxygen. Therefore, most of the products tested so far in advanced clinical trials are hemoglobin derivates known as HBOCs (hemoglobin-based oxygen carriers).[62] Tested substances so far included perfluorocarbon emulsions, stroma-free hemoglobin, and polyethylene glycol hemoglobin. To date, there is no approved oxygen-carrying blood substitute. Most of the initial attempts failed due to adverse effects including hypertension, abdominal pain, skin rash, diarrhea, jaundice, hemoglobinuria, oliguria, fever, stroke, and laboratory anomalies.

Recombinant Erythropoietin

Recombinant erythropoetin is a glycoprotein hormone that controls erythropoiesis. It has been used as an alternative to transfusion, particularly in those who have chronic renal failure.[63] However, its use has not yet shown benefits in avoiding transfusion in postoperative surgical or acute trauma patients.

FRESH-FROZEN PLASMA (FFP)

Fresh-frozen plasma relates to the liquid portion of human blood, which has been frozen and preserved after blood donation. FFP contains components of the coagulation, fibrinolytic, and complement systems. It also contains proteins that maintain and modulate oncotic pressure and immunity as well as fats, carbohydrates, and minerals. The indications for transfusing FFP are limited. When transfused it can have unpredictable adverse effects. The risks of transmitting infection are similar to those of other blood components unless a pathogen-reduced plasma is used.[64] Of particular concern are allergic reactions and anaphylaxis, transfusion-related acute lung injury (TRALI), and hemolysis from transfused antibodies to blood group antigens, especially A and B.

FFP should be used to replace single inherited clotting factor deficiencies, notably factor FV, for which no virus-safe fractionated product is available. FFP and platelets are indicated when there are demonstrable multifactor deficiencies associated with severe bleeding and/or DIC. It is not indicated in DIC with no evidence of bleeding. There is no evidence that prophylactic replacement regimens prevent DIC or reduce transfusion requirements. FFP has only a partial effect, is not the optimal treatment, and should never be used for the reversal of warfarin anticoagulation in the absence of severe bleeding. FFP should not be used to correct prolonged clotting times in ICU patients; vitamin K is superior. Its use is advocated by some for the prevention of bleeding in patients with liver disease and a prolonged PT, although the response may be unpredictable and complete normalization of the hemostatic defect does not always occur. Whether and how much FFP should be used for treating a patient with massive blood loss should be guided by timely tests of coagulation, including near-patient tests (see above). Volume replacement alone in the absence of coagulation abnormalities is generally not considered to be an appropriate indication. When FFP is administered, it should be with an end point of improved coagulation function. Coagulation studies should be obtained before and after FFP transfusion to assess the efficacy and adequacy of replacement.[64]

PLATELET CONCENTRATE

Platelets are collected from units of whole blood and pooled to make a therapeutic dose, or by apheresis. Up to eight units of platelets, each from a separate donor, can be pooled into a single bag for transfusion. All units are from the same ABO type. If ABO compatible platelets are unavailable, ABO incompatible platelets can be substituted with very little risk. Apheresis platelets are prepared from a single donor and are equivalent to 4–6 pooled units. An apheresis platelet concentrate contains 200–400 mL of plasma. Platelets are stored under constant agitation at 20–24°C. Platelets collected by either method have a very short shelf-life, typically 5 days.

The primary indication for platelet transfusion is thrombocytopenia with active bleeding or risk of bleeding. The threshold of thrombocytopenia at which bleeding may occur will vary depending on the patient's clinical condition. Platelet counts >50,000/μL are generally sufficient for hemostasis in circumstances of ongoing bleeding, although higher levels may be targeted to help ensure hemostasis. Platelet counts <20,000/μL are associated with a definite risk of spontaneous bleeding and platelet transfusion is generally indicated to keep the platelet count > 20,000/μL. In a surgical patient, the necessary platelet count varies according to the procedure. In some circumstances, such as chronic uremia, a deficit in platelet function results in a bleeding tendency despite a normal platelet count. Platelet transfusion may be necessary to control acute bleeding in these circumstances as well. The platelet count is of no value in directing therapy, and functional assessments or clinical observations of adequate hemostasis are used instead. Abnormal platelet function may be congenital, or due to medications, sepsis, malignancy, tissue trauma, obstetric complications, extracorporeal circulation, or organ failure such as liver or kidney disease. Spontaneous bleeding may then occur at higher platelet counts.

SPECIFIC FACTOR CONCENTRATES

In certain circumstances, specific factor concentrates such as factor FVIII concentrate or cryoprecipitate (which is extremely rich in fibrin) may allow more precise replacement than that obtained using FFP alone. Sophisticated fractionation methods have been developed to allow specific isolation of protein components of the plasma (Fig. 6.11).[65] Fractionation allows specific replacement for specific medical indications. Specific granulocyte-rich fractions are used in patients with profound granulocytopenia. Use of such special concentrates should be targeted to the precise replacement of the specific deficit, and careful assessment is needed using appropriate laboratory assays.

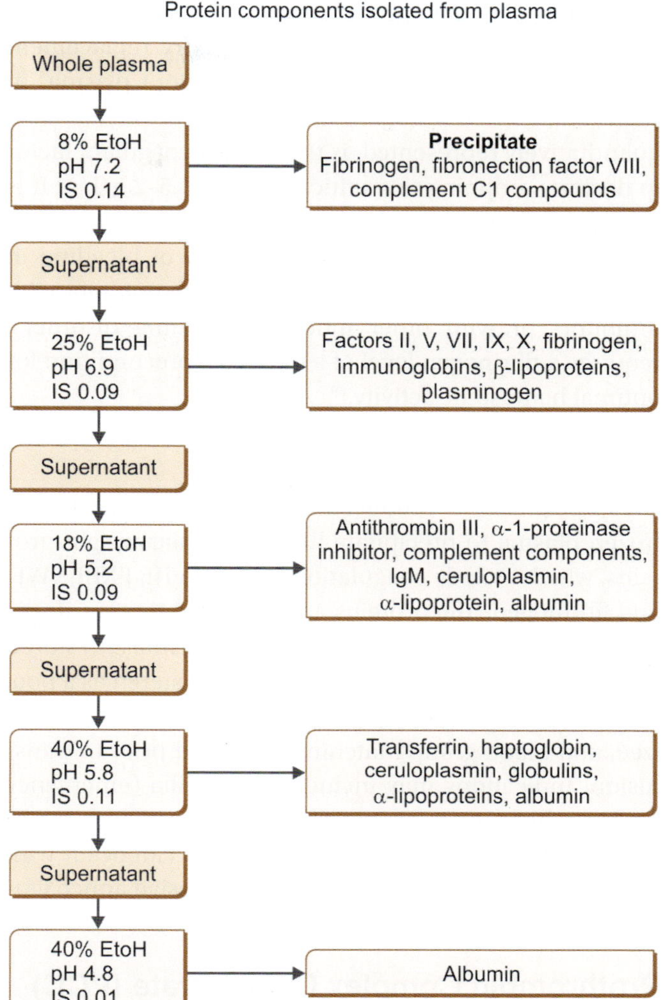

Fig. 6.11: Methods used to separate the specific protein components of plasma. The technique uses various concentrations of ethanol (EtOH), pH, and the ionic strength (IS). The fractionation method has allowed specific protein components to be given for specific indications.

Fibrinogen Concentrate

Fibrinogen concentrate is prepared from pooled human plasma using the Cohn/Oncley cryoprecipitation procedure.[66] The concentration of fibrinogen is standardized; the product is stored as a lyophilized powder at room temperature and can be reconstituted quickly, allowing for rapid administration without delays for thawing or crossmatching. In contrast to FFP and cryoprecipitate, viral inactivation steps by solvent/detergent exposure or pasteurization are routinely included in the manufacturing process for fibrinogen concentrate, thus minimizing the risk of viral transmission.[67] Fibrinogen replacement is indicated as prophylaxis and therapy of hemorrhage in congenital and acquired fibrinogen deficiency, being associated with liver failure, DIC, massive transfusions, and cardiac surgery. Hypofibrinogenemia is defined by a decreased level of normal fibrinogen between 0.5 g/L and the lower limit of the normal range for the local laboratory (usually 1.5 g/L). Fibrinogen deficiency can develop in the event of massive transfusion in the context of loss and dilution coagulopathy due to primary replacement by crystalloids, colloids, and pRBCs without plasma. In such situations fibrinogen, the coagulation factor most quantitatively represented, is the first procoagulant factor to decline, dropping to a critical level of 1.5–2 g/L .[68] It is noteworthy that recombinant activated factor FVII, which is used for the treatment or prevention of bleeding in patients with acquired and congenital hemophilia with inhibitors or with other inherited bleeding disorders, requires a fibrinogen level of ≥1 g/L as a precondition for optimal hemostatic activity.[69]

Cryoprecipitate

Cryoprecipitate is produced by controlled thawing of frozen plasma to precipitate high molecular weight proteins, which include coagulation factors FVIII, FXIII, vWF, and fibrinogen. The proteins are separated by centrifugation, resuspended in a small volume of plasma and stored frozen.[70] Cryoprecipitate is usually administered as a pool of 4–6 units. Its fibrinogen concentration is not standardized, and blood group matching is needed prior to transfusion. Indications may include hemophilia (emergency backup when factor concentrates are not available), hypofibrinogenemia (low fibrinogen levels), as can occur with massive transfusions, bleeding from excessive anticoagulation, massive hemorrhage, and DIC.

Prothrombin Complex Concentrate (PCC)

Prothrombin complex concentrate is a plasma protein fraction containing a combination of vitamin K-dependent coagulation factors FII, FVII, FIX, and FX, as well as PC and ProS. PCC is produced by ion-exchange chromatography from the cryoprecipitate supernatant of large plasma pools after removal of AT and factor XI.[71] Different processing techniques enable the production of either three-factor (i.e. factors FII, FIX, and FX) or four-factor (i.e. factors FII, FVII, FIX, and FX) concentrates with a final overall clotting factor concentration approximately 25 times higher than in normal plasma.[72] Four-factor PCCs are most frequently used for replacement of vitamin K-dependent clotting factors and inhibitors proteins C and S in patients bleeding after phenprocoumon or warfarin overdose, in vitamin K-deficient patients presenting with life-threatening bleeding (gastrointestinal or intracranial hemorrhage), and liver disease. PCC is an important option when urgent reversal of anticoagulation is required. PCC appears to correct clotting factor deficiencies more rapidly and completely than plasma and seems to be associated with a lower incidence of volume overload carrying minimal risk of viral transmission.[73]

COMPLICATIONS

The benefits of transfusion must be weighed against its risks. Transfusion is in essence a transplant of allogeneic cells, and its risks, although modest, are not negligible. Although hard data are not available, it is likely that leukodepletion has reduced the frequency of symptomatic adverse events associated with transfusion.[74] Complications of blood transfusion range from simple febrile reactions to fatal hemolytic reactions. Most unavoidable reactions are minor, whereas catastrophic hemolytic transfusion reactions are most commonly the result of preventable errors in patient identification.[75] Complications can be organized by consequences, mechanisms, symptoms, time of onset, and other variables. Table 6.9 arbitrarily distinguishes immediate and delayed types of transfusion complications.

Hemolytic Transfusion Reactions

Immediate hemolytic transfusion reactions, either as a result of ABO incompatibility or reaction with other antigens, cause a rapid onset of systemic symptoms. Extensive immune destruction of red cells leads to:

1. Activation of complement
2. Initiation of the clotting cascade
3. Platelet activation
4. Production of bradykinin.

Table 6.9 Types of transfusion complications.

Immediate (≤ 24 hours after transfusion)	*Delayed (days to months after transfusion)*
Acute hemolytic (immune)	Alloimmunization
Acute hemolytic (nonimmune)	Delayed hemolytic
Air embolism	Iron overload
Allergic	Post-transfusion purpura
Anaphylactic	Transfusion-associated graft-versus-host disease
Bacterial sepsis	Transfusion-transmitted diseases
Circulatory overload	
Febrile nonhemolytic	
Isolated hypotension	
Medication/solution interactions	
Massive transfusion	
– Hemostatic complications	
- Metabolic complications	
- Hypothermia complications	
Transfusion-related acute lung injury	

The activation of the complement cascade may lead to intravascular hemolysis with hemoglobinemia and hemoglobinuria, release of vasoactive complement components resulting in hypotension and shock, thrombin and platelet activation culminating in DIC and renal failure. Chills and fever are the most common symptoms, and other features are back and chest pain, tachycardia, and hypotension. Diffuse bleeding may ensue as a result of DIC triggered by the hemolysis. Acute hemolytic reactions are rarely fatal if the transfused volume is <100 mL.[76] With large volumes of incompatible blood, uncontrollable bleeding, renal, and liver failure may ensue.

The primary treatment for a major hemolytic transfusion reaction is to stop the infusion. After the transfusion has been stopped, the treatment is largely supportive and aimed at blunting the effects of widespread activation of the inflammatory system. Adequate intravascular volume should be maintained, along with an osmotic diuresis to assist in pigment clearance by the kidneys. Care should be taken to avoid fluid overload in patients with impaired cardiac or renal function. Patients may also develop hemolytic reactions several days after a transfusion as a result of an anamnestic response to antigens encountered in previous transfusions. Such reactions are usually mild. The patient is often asymptomatic and presents with evidence of low-grade hemolysis, which is self-limited. Further transfusions should not be given until completed serologic investigation and determination of the cause of the reaction.

Minor Transfusion Reactions

Nonhemolytic transfusion reactions consist primarily of fever and chills beginning within the first few hours of transfusion. Such reactions may affect as many as 1–2% of all transfusions.[77] These nonhemolytic reactions are thought to be due to antigens on transfused leukocytes and are more common in patients who are multiparous or have received previous transfusions. Minor transfusion reactions are treated symptomatically once the possibility of a major hemolytic reaction has been excluded. Febrile reactions can be partially prevented by pretreatment with acetaminophen (paracetamol) or corticosteroids, and by filtering of donor units to remove leukocytes before transfusion.

Allergic-Type Reactions

Allergic-type reactions with itching and urticaria occur infrequently. Such symptoms alone are not due to reaction with the cellular components of transfused blood. Urticarial transfusion reactions are thought to be caused by preexisting recipient IgE antibody to proteins in the plasma of the transfused blood component. Anaphylactic reactions to blood transfusion have been reported, but the incidence is very low. Allergic transfusion reactions occur on a continuum of severity. When bronchospasm and laryngeal edema occur, the allergic reactions are often called anaphylactoid. When severe hypotension and shock occur, the reaction is designated as anaphylactic. If symptoms are light, the transfusion may be temporarily interrupted and the patient be given an antihistamine. When the reaction subsides, the transfusion may be continued but at a slower infusion rate. In patients known for this type of reaction, antihistamines may be prescribed before transfusion. In case of an anaphylactic transfusion reaction, the transfusion must be immediately stopped and the reaction is treated as a severe allergic reaction with fluids, epinephrine, antihistamines, bronchodilators, and vasopressors as appropriate.

Transfusion-Related Acute Lung Injury (TRALI)

TRALI is characterized by acute respiratory distress following transfusion and has a frequency ranging between 1/1,120 and 1/57,810 units transfused according to definition. All plasma-containing blood products have been implicated. TRALI is associated with high rates of morbidity and mortality (5–10%). Clinical symptoms develop quickly during or within 6 hours of a transfusion, with the rapid onset of dyspnea and tachypnea. Chest X-rays typically show bilateral pulmonary edema in the absence of heart failure (noncardiogenic pulmonary edema), which may progress to complete "white out." TRALI is to be distinguished from TACO and cardiogenic pulmonary edema by the absence of circulatory overload (normal central venous pressure and normal pulmonary capillary wedge pressure). The treatment is usually supportive including supplemental oxygen therapy or, in severe cases, mechanical ventilation, and ICU support. There is no role for diuretics or corticosteroids. Although several pathways may lead to TRALI, passive transfusion of leukocyte antibodies is currently the most important association.[78] Since donor-derived antibodies may be one of its causes, the frequency of TRALI may be reduced by the judicious use of blood components only for indications that are justified.

Infectious Complications

Infectious disease transmission, especially viral diseases, is the most common clinical complication of transfusion in spite of careful selection of donors and testing of blood. Donor selection criteria usually screen out individuals who are at risk for human immunodeficiency virus (HIV), human T-cell lymphotropic virus (HTLV), and hepatitis infection. Donor samples are usually tested for antibodies to HIV-1 and HIV-2, HTLV-I/II, hepatitis C virus (HCV), HB core antigen, the presence of hepatitis B surface antigen (HBsAg), syphilis, and the presence of viral RNA (HIV-1, HCV and WNV).

Hepatitis

Among the possible infections, hepatitis B and C remain the most common. Over the recent years, antibody screening of donor blood has dramatically reduced transmission of this infection. The risk of having a donation that carries hepatitis B is about 1 in 205,000; the risk for hepatitis C is 1 in 2 million. The major complication associated with both hepatitis B and C infections is the risk of developing chronic infection. About 10% of acute infections for hepatitis B follow transfusion, and 90% of hepatitis C infections become chronic.

HIV Infection

Since the beginning of HIV testing of donor blood in the 1980s, the transmission of HIV during transfusion has dropped sharply. The development of a nucleic acid test for the HIV-1 RNA has lowered the rate of donor blood seropositivity to about 1 in 3 million units. As transmission of HIV does not necessarily mean HIV infection, the latter could still occur, at an even lower rate.

Cytomegalovirus Infection (CMV)

Cytomegalovirus is a common agent found in banked blood, but rarely causes problems in immunocompetent recipients. CMV-related disease is usually confined to immunosuppressed patients. The most common clinical settings are in neonates and posttransplant patients. Although routine screening of blood for CMV is considered impractical, it should be considered for those who are profoundly immunosuppressed, such as bone marrow transplant recipients and infants who have a birth weight of <1,500 g. To reduce the frequency of CMV transmission, leukoreduced cellular components may be used. For some patients at particularly high risk of severe CMV disease, transfusion of components from CMV-seronegative donors may be considered in addition to the use of leukoreduced components.

Other Infectious Diseases

In the United States and Western Europe, transfusion is rarely associated with other infectious diseases, and it is therefore extremely difficult to assess these risks with accuracy. Estimates are further complicated because symptoms may not appear for many years and are difficult to link to prior transfusion. Other infectious diseases that can be transmitted by blood transfusions include malaria, syphilis, Epstein–Barr virus infection, and *Trypanosoma cruzi* or Chagas' disease. There have been documented cases of transfusion-transmitted Chagas' disease in North America. Recent studies indicate that variant Creutzfeldt–Jakob disease may be transmitted by blood transfusion. The potential for transmission of unidentified viruses is unknown.

Bacterial Contamination

Blood products may rarely be contaminated with bacteria resulting in life-threatening infection, also referred to as transfusion-transmitted bacterial infection. The risk of severe bacterial infection is estimated at about 1 in 50,000 platelet transfusions and 1 in 500,000 red blood cell transfusions.[79] Potential sources of contamination may include the donor´s blood and skin, the phlebotomist's skin, and from containers. The contaminating organisms vary greatly and usually comprise skin flora, gut flora, or environmental organisms.

Paratransfusion Complications

Dilutional Effects

Transfusion of large volumes of blood and fluid at rapid rates can lead to a number of complications. Dilutional thrombocytopenia is probably the most common, and a transfusion of platelet concentrate may be required to achieve adequate hemostasis. Dilution of soluble factors is thought to be unusual. Similarly, although hypocalcemia is a potential complication of transfusion with citrated blood, it is rarely seen, and empiric administration of calcium is no longer recommended. In each case, replacement therapy should be guided by the measured deficiency. Hyperkalemia is another potential complication that is rarely seen in clinical practice.

Hypothermia

The most prevalent and perhaps the most dangerous complication of massive transfusion is hypothermia. Although not specific to the use of blood products, hypothermia can be a serious problem during complex surgical operations and in major trauma. A blood temperature of <33°C markedly affects coagulation by reducing the pace of plasma coagulation factor biochemical reactions[80] as well as decreasing cardiac contractility and increasing frequency of ventricular arrhythmia. The reaction pace of coagulation factors is slowed down by approximately 5% with each 1°C drop in temperature. The vWF-glycoprotein Ib interaction that activates platelets is absent in 75% of individuals at 30°C.[81] It has also been shown that hypothermia may cause a potential deficit in fibrinogen availability and a delay in thrombin generation, consequently inhibiting coagulation function.[82] Hypothermia is best prevented by careful attention to both passive and active warming of the patient, including warming of fluids administered during the course of massive transfusion. In some circumstances, an extracorporeal circulation may be required to provide core heating.

Immunosuppression/Modulation

Over the recent years there has been increasing interest in the idea that transfusions may cause immunosuppression.[83] This syndrome has been referred to as transfusion-related immunomodulation (TRIM). TRIM was first demonstrated in renal transplantation when improved allograft survival was observed in patients who had received transfusions before transplantation. In contrast, several authors have reported reduced survival of cancer patients associated with blood transfusion,[84] whereas others have reported transfusion to be an independent risk factor for nosocomial infections, recurrence of malignancy, and short-term mortality.[85] To date, there remains much controversy regarding the possible mechanisms of TRIM and its clinical significance. Potential mechanisms may be specifically human leucocyte antigen dependent or related to nonspecific bioactive soluble factors. It is likely that transfused allogeneic white blood cells (WBCs) are responsible for the majority of TRIM effects. After transfusion there is impaired natural killer cell function, decreased macrophage phagocytic function, suppression of lymphocyte production, and effective antigen presentation. Studies in cardiac surgery have demonstrated an increase in short-term mortality, of unspecified cause, in patients receiving non-WBC-reduced allogeneic blood transfusions. Recent studies on the risk of bacterial infection and transfusions have been conflicting, but most tended to report negative findings. Universal WBC reduction is increasingly common, although its role in mitigating TRIM remains controversial.[85]

PATIENT BLOOD MANAGEMENT (PBM)

Preoperative anemia is a common phenomenon in patients scheduled to undergo orthopedic and other major operations , and it is frequently associated with a higher risk of perioperative and postoperativemorbidity (including complications of transfusion) and mortality. Almost half of all patients who undergo major orthopedic operations receive perioperative pRBC transfusions,[86] making this the primary surgical indication for transfusion.[87] Both clinical and economical disadvantages of transfusions have triggered the search for altervatives based on "own blood" rather than blood derived from donors. Patient Blood Management (PBM) is a clinical, multidisciplinary, multimodal and patient-centered concept aiming to reduce and prevent peri/postoperative anemia and blood loss and to adopt more rational use of blood products to prevent unneccessary transfusions.[88] Several programs have been implemented around the world, for example in Australia, Austria and Germany.

There are three pillars to PBM:

1. Optimize/stimulate hemopoesis
2. Minimize blood loss and bleeding
3. Harness and optimize tolerance of anemia.

Before operation, PBM involves the assessment of anemia and potential bleeding risk to allow for detection and correction in a timely manner (Fig. 6.12). Blood tests and the use of antiplatelet and anticoagulant drugs should be restricted to a minimum, and indications should be carefully verified. Hemoglobin levels prior to elective orthopedic operations should be targeted to reference ranges defined by the World Health Organization (WHO): females ≥12 g/L and males ≥13 g/L. Iron deficiencies should be treated with iron supplementation. Underlying disorders causing anemia should be identified and treated. Intraoperative measures to prevent or minimize blood loss include blood-sparing surgical techniques, anesthetic blood-conserving strategies and the application of both topical and systemic hemostatic agents. After a recent resolution of the WHO, PBM implementation has been encouraged in all member states.

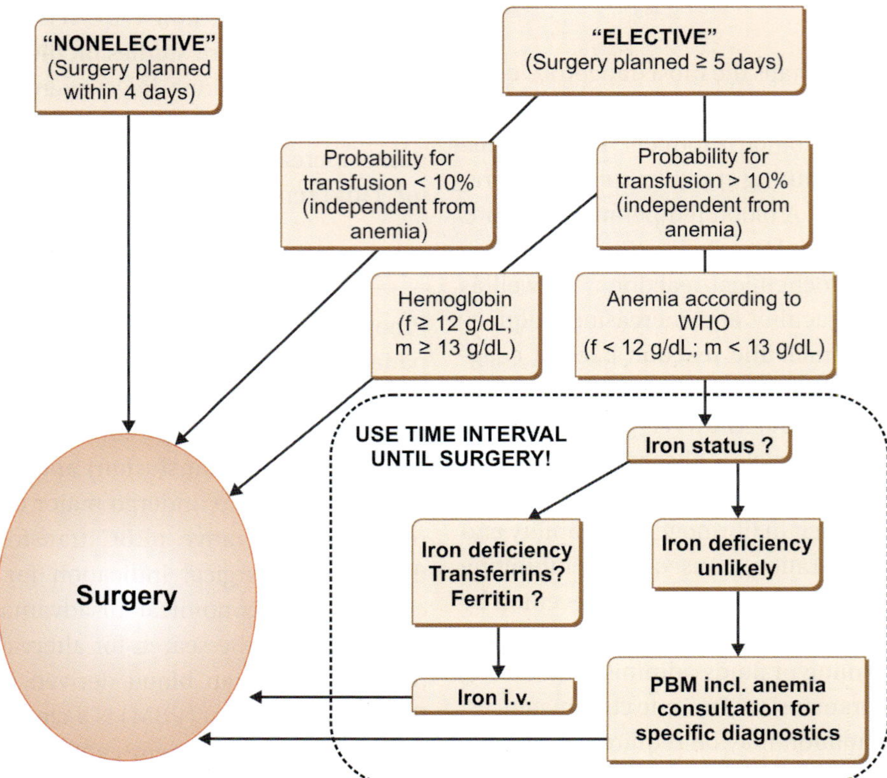

Fig. 6.12: Preoperative anemia algorithm according to Patient Blood Management (PBM). Modified from www. patientbloodmanagement.de/.

MANAGEMENT OF PREOPERATIVE/ PREINJURY INTAKE OF ANTICOAGULANTS AND ANTIPLATELET DRUGS

For the past decades, warfarin (phenprocoumon; coumadin) has been the main oral anticoagulant in atrial fibrillation and the prevention of stroke. The effects of warfarin can easily be reversed by vitamin K and prothrombin complex concentrates (PCC). To date, new oral anticoagulants (NOACs), such as rivaroxaban apixaban and dabigatran, offer an alternative to warfarin and are likely to replace warfarin and other vitamin K anatgonists for most of their indications in the future. Rivaroxaban and apixaban are inhibitors of activated factor Xa, whereas dabigatran directly inhibits thrombin.[89] However, NOACs are associated with risks as there are yet no specific antidotes available and the coagulation status cannot be monitored by INR, making reversal during emergency surgery and bleeding difficult and challenging.[90] Moreover, the number of surgical patients on these drugs in constantly increasing. The anticoagulant effect of NOACs reaches maximum concentrations approximately 3 hours after intake and decreases rapidly 12 to 24 hours after intake, but it is substantially prolonged in renal insufficiency. Therefore, all NOACs require dose reductions according to renal function, and knowledge about the time point of the last NOAC intake, dose and renal function is of utmost clinical importance. The pharmacological characteristics of the three drugs are summarized in Table 6.10. Bridging is recommended in high-risk patients with atrial fibrillation and is treated with vitamin K antagonists, but not in patients on NOACs as the diminuation of anticoagulant effect is predictable, enabling a rather short-term interruption prior and restart after operation. For elective surgery with no imminent risk of bleeding, NOACs may be discontinued for 18–24 hours prior to operation and restarted 6 hours after operation. In elective surgery with a risk of minor bleeding and no renal insufficiency, NOACs are stopped at least 24 hours prior to operation. For elective surgery with a high risk of bleeding, NOACs should be discontinued 48 hours prior to operation.[89] For unplanned emergency or trauma procedures, supportive care and withholding further doses are most likely to be sufficient in most cases but, if possible, operation should be postponed for at least 12, or better, 24 hours. Once sufficient hemostasis has been regained, NOACs may

Table 6.10 Pharmacological characteristics of NOACs.

	Rivaroxaban	*Apixaban*	*Dabigatran*
Mechanism of action	Factor Xa inhibitor	Factor Xa inhibitor	Direct thrombin inhibitor
Prodrug	no	no	yes
Dosing	1 × day	2 × day	2 × day
Half-life (hours)	5–9	8–15	12–14
Bioavailability (%)	80	66	6,5
Concentration (max; hours)	2–4	3–3.5	1.25–3
Clearance	30% renal, hepatic	25% renal, hepatic, 50% intestinal	80% renal
Plasma protein binding (%)	95	87	35
Interactions	CYP3A4	CYP3A4	p-glycoprotein

Modified from Lai et al.[89]

be restarted 24 hours after low-risk operations and after 48–72 hours after high-risk operations. In immobilized patients, low molecular heparins (LMWHs) may be given 6–8 hours popstoperatively, with NOACs being restarted at 48-72 hours.[89] Hemodialysis may be considered for quicker elimination of dabigatran in cases of bleeding.

When taken as a lifelong therapy for secondary prevention after stroke, acute coronary syndrome, myocardial infarction, or coronary revascularization, aspirin should not be interrupted for operation as it does not increase the perioperative risk, except for patients with diabetes.[91] If patients are under dual antiplatelet therapy, e.g. aspirin plus clopidogrel, all elective operations should be postponed and only vital procedures should be perfomed. For operations with only minor or moderate risk of bleeding, dual antiplatelet therapy should not be interrupted. If clopidogrel intake is interrupted for high-risk operatiopns, aspirin must be continued without interruption. Antiplatelet therapy should be restarted within 12–24 hours postoperatively by using a clopidogrel loading dose. Current data suggest that the risk for cardiovascular events when stopping these agents preoperatively is higher than the risk of surgical bleeding when continuing these drugs, except for operative procedures in closed spaces (e.g. intracranial, posterior eye chamber) or those associated with massive bleeding and difficult hemostasis.[91]

REFERENCES

1. Ware JA, Heistad DD. Platelet-endothelium interactions. N Engl J Med. 1993;328:628-35.
2. Hoffmann M. Remodelling the blood coagulation cascade. J Thromb Thrombolysis. 2003;16(1-2):17-20.
3. Colman RW, Clowes AW, George JN, et al. Overview of hemostasis. In: Hemostais and Thrombosis, 5th edition. Philadelphia: Lippincott Williams & Wilkins; 2006. pp. 3-16.
4. Fenton JW, Ofosu FA, Brezniak DV, et al. Understanding thrombin and hemostasis. Hematol Oncol Clin North Am. 1993;7:1107-19.
5. Neuenschwandert PF, Bianco-Fisher E, Rezaie AR, et al. Phosphatidylethanolamine augments factor VII-tissue factor activity: enhancement of sensitivity to phosphatidylserine. Biochemistry. 1995;34(43):13988-93.
6. Yamaji-Hasegawa A, Tsujimoto M. Asymmetric distribution of phospholipids in biomembranes. Biol Pharm Bull. 2006;29(8):1547-53.
7. Henry RL. Platelet function in hemostasis. In: Murano G, Bick RL (Eds). Basic Concepts of Hemostasis and Thrombosis. Boca Raton: CRC Press; 1980. pp. 17-41.
8. Niewiarowski S, Holt JC. Biochemistry and physiology of secreted platelet proteins. In: Colman RW, Hirsh J, Marder VJ, Salzman JB, (Eds). Hemostasis and Thrombosis. Basic Principles and Clinical Practice, 2nd edition. Philadelphia: JB Lippincott; 1987. pp. 618-30.
9. Ruggeri ZM. Mechanisms initiating platelet thrombus formation. Thromb Hemost. 1997;78:611-6.
10. Hassouna HI. Laboratory evaluation of hemostatic disorders. Hematol Oncol Clin North Am. 1993;7:1161-249.
11. Mann KG, Brummel K, Butenas S. What is all that thrombin for? J Thromb Haemost. 2003;1(7):1504-14.
12. Furie B, Furie BC. In vivo thrombus formation. J Thromb Haemist. 2007;5(Suppl 1):12-7.
13. Gailani D, Renne T. The intrinsic pathway of coagulation: a target for treating thromboembolic disease? J Thromb Haemost. 2007;5(6):1106-12.
14. Morrissey JH, Mutch NJ. Tissue factor structure and function. In: Hemostasis and Thrombosis, 5th edition. Philadelphia: Lippincott Williams & Wilkins; 2006. pp. 91-106.
15. Roberts HR, Hoffman M, Monroe DM. A cell-based model of thrombin generation. Semin Thromb Hemost. 2006;32 (Suppl 1):32-8.
16. Becker RC. Cell-based models of coagulation: a paradigm in evolution. J Thromb Thrombolysis. 2005;20(1):65-68.
17. Smith S. The cell-based model of coagulation. J Vet Emerg Med Crit Care. 2009;19(1):3-10.
18. Nugent DJ. Prophylaxis in rare coagulation disorders-factor XIII deficiency. Thromb Res. 2006;118(Suppl 1):S23-8.

19. Oliver JA, Monroe DM, Church FC, et al. Activated protein C cleaves factor Va more efficiently on endothelium than on platelet surfaces. Blood. 2012;100(2):539-46.
20. Sagripanti A, Carpi A. Antithrombotic and prothrombotic activities of the vascular endothelium. Biomed Pharmacother. 2000;54(2):107-11.
21. Curry ANG, Pierce JMT. Conventional and near-patient tests of coagulation. Cont Educ Anaesth Crit Care Pain. 2007;7:45-50.
22. Jahn UR, Van Aken H. Near-patient testing-point-of-care or point of costs and convenience? Br J Anaesth. 2003;90 (4):425-7.
23. Hartert H. Blutgerinnungsstudien mit der Thrombelastographie, einem neuen Untersuchungsverfahren. Klin Wochenschr. 1948;26:577-83.
24. Johansson PI, Stissing T, Bochsen L, et al. Thrombelastography and tromboelastometry in assessing coagulopathy in trauma. Scand J Trauma Resusc Emerg Med. 2009;17:45.
25. Mallett V, Cox DJA. Thrombelastography. Br J Anaesth. 1992;69:307-13.
26. Schöchl H, Maegele M, Solomon C, et al. Early and individualized goal-directed therapy for trauma-induced coagulopathy. Scand J Trauma Resusc Emerg Med. 2012;20:15.
27. Kawasaki J, Katori N, Kodaka M, et al. Electron microscopic evaluations of clot morphology during thromboelastography. Anesth Analg. 2004;99:1440-4.
28. Johansson PI, Svendsen MS, Salado J, et al. Investigation of the thrombin-generating capacity, evaluated by thrombogram, and clot formation evaluated by thrombeolastography of platelets stored in the blood bank for up to 7 days. Vox Sang. 2008;94:113-8.
29. Rodriquez-Erdman F. Bleeding due to increased intravascular blood coagulation: hemorrhagic syndromes caused by consumption of blood-clotting factors (consumption coagulopathies). N Engl J Med. 1965;273:1370-8.
30. Taylor FB, Toh CH, Hoots WK, et al. Towards a definition, clinical and laboratory criteria, and a scoring system for disseminated intravascular coagulation. J Thromb Haemost. 2001;86:1327-30.
31. Bick RL. Disseminated intravascular coagulation: objective clinical and laboratory diagnosis, treatment, and assessment of therapeutic response. Semin Thromb Hemost. 1996; 22:69-88.
32. Levi M, Toh GH, Thachil J, et al. Guidelines for the diagnosis and management of disseminated intravascular coagulation. Br J Haematol. 2009;145:24-33.
33. Thiagarajan P. Overview of Platelet Disorders. Medscape, May 2011.
34. Kitchens CS. Concept of hypercoagulability: a review of its development, clinical application, and recent progress. Semin Thromb Hemost. 1985;11:293-315.
35. Deitcher SR, Caiola E, Jaffer A. Demystifying two common genetic predispositions to venous thrombosis. Cleve Clin J Med. 2000;67:825-6.
36. Eldrup-Jorgensen J, Flanigan DP, Brace L, et al. Hypercoagulable states and lower limb ischemia in young adults. J Vasc Surg. 1989;9:334-41.
37. Seligsohn U, Lubetsky A. Genetic susceptibility to venous thrombosis. N Engl J Med. 2001;344:1222-31.
38. Levine JS, Branch DW, Rauch J. The antiphospholipid syndrome. N Engl J Med. 2002;346:752-63.
39. De Stefano V, Casorelli I, Rossi E, et al., Interaction between hyperhomocysteinemia and inherited thrombophilic factors in venous thromboembolism. Semin Thromb Hemost. 2000;26:305-11.
40. Guba SC, Fonseca V, Fink LM. Hyperhomocysteinemia and thrombosis. Semin Thromb Hemost. 1999;25:291-309.
41. Kearon C, Crowther M, Hirsh J. Management of patients with hereditary hypercoagulable disorders. Annu Rev Med. 2000;51:169-85.
42. Hyers TM, Agnelli G, Hull RD, et al. Antithrombotic therapy for venous thromboembolic disease. Chest. 2001;119:176S-93S.
43. Warkentin TE, Eikelboom JW. Who is (still) getting HIT? Chest. 2007;131(6):1620-2.
44. Nand S, Wong W, Yuen B, et al. Heparin-induced thrombocytopenia with thrombosis: incidence, analysis of risk factors, and clinical outcomes in 108 consecutive patients treated at a single institution. Am J Hematol. 1997;56(1):12-6.
45. Warkentin TE, Greinacher A. Heparin-induced thrombocytopenia: recognition, treatment, and prevention. The Seventh ACCP Conference on Antithrombotic and Thrombolytic Therapy. Chest. 2004;126(Suppl 3):311S-37S.
46. Visentin GP, Ford SE, Scott JP, et al. Antibodies from patients with heparin-induced thrombocytopenia/thrombosis are specific for platelet factor 4 complexed with heparin or bound to endothelial cells. J Clin Invest. 1994;93(1):81-8.
47. Sheridan D, Carter C, Kelton JG. A diagnostic test for heparin-induced thrombocytopenia. Blood. 1986;67(1):27-30.
48. Meyer O, Salama A, Pittet N, et al. Rapid detection of heparin-induced platelet antibodies with particle gel immunoassay (ID-HPF4). Lancet. 1999;354(9189):1525-6.
49. Warkentin TE. Heparin-induced thrombocytopenia: diagnosis and management. Circulation. 2004;110(18):e454-8.
50. Oberman HA. The history of blood transfusion. In: Petz LD, Swisher SN (Eds). Clinical Practice of Blood Transfusion. New York: Churchill Livingstone; 1981. pp. 9-28.

Additional references appear in the online version of this book.

7

Infection, Inflammation, and Antibiotics

Donald E Fry

Key Points

- Surgical site infection (SSI) is the prototype infection in surgical patients. Determinants of infection are the extent of bacterial contamination, the virulence of these organisms, the microenvironment of the wound, and the integrity of host defenses.
- Preoperative prophylactic antibiotics will reduce SSI rates and are selected according to their antimicrobial activity, toxicity, and elimination half-life within the body. Prolonged administration after the completion of the procedure is counterproductive.
- Infections of the skin and skin structures are very diverse in severity and require surgical debridement of devitalized tissue, drainage of pus, and systemic antibiotics.
- Intra-abdominal infection requires surgical control of the source of microbial contamination, vigorous supportive care to ensure tissue perfusion and oxygenation, and antibiotic therapy to cover the polymicrobial microflora associated with these infections.
- Postoperative pneumonia, urinary tract infection (UTI), intravascular device infection, and *Clostridium difficile* infection (CDI) are hospital-acquired events that are major problems in the surgical patient and require specific prevention and management strategies.
- Fungal and viral infections are an increasing issue in the surgical patient.
- The main groups of antibiotics are discussed together with their spectrum of activity and disadvantages.

INTRODUCTION

Infection is a major challenge in surgery. It is commonly a community-acquired disease that requires surgical management, it may be a complication at the surgical site, and it is also a common complication in the surgical patient at anatomic sites remote from the operative site. Despite the development of broad spectrum and highly effective antibiotics, and refined techniques for prevention, infection remains one of the most problematic areas of surgical care. The expanded vistas of surgical care now include multiorgan transplantation, reconstructive vascular surgery of the heart, and total joint replacement. These expansions of surgical care into an older or a less healthy population of patients mean that infectious complications remain common but also have severe morbidity for these vulnerable populations. Infection in the surgical patient is the consequence of a complex interaction between microbial contaminants and the critical elements of host defense.

Infection is the local activation of the human inflammatory response secondary to the proliferation of microorganisms. The clinical event that separates colonization from infection is not microbial proliferation alone because microbes are constantly proliferating on the skin, in the mouth, and in the intestinal tract. The defining event of clinical infection is the local activation of the inflammatory cascade rather than either the presence or the proliferation of the microbe. Therefore, the study of infection and its sequelae is necessarily a study of inflammation. The clinical findings associated with infection at each anatomic site are evidence of inflammation. When the domain of proliferating organisms becomes systemic, then inflammation becomes generalized and is clinical sepsis. This chapter explores this host-pathogen interrelationship to define the diagnostic, preventive, and treatment strategies necessary to manage the protean manifestations of clinical infection.

SURGICAL SITE INFECTION

Determinants of Infection

Surgical site infections occur at the site of conduct of the operative procedure. This includes those infections of

Table 7.1 The generally accepted definitions of surgical site infection by the Centers for Disease Control and Prevention, Atlanta, Georgia, USA.

Superficial incisional SSI: Infection occurs within 30 days after the operation and infection involves only skin or subcutaneous tissue of the incision and at least one of the following:
1. Purulent drainage, with or without laboratory confirmation, from the superficial incision.
2. Organisms isolated from an aseptically obtained culture of fluid or tissue from the superficial incision.
3. At least one of the following signs or symptoms of infection: pain or tenderness, localized swelling, redness, or heat and superficial incision is deliberately opened by surgeon, unless incision is culture negative.
4. Diagnosis of superficial incisional SSI by the surgeon or attending physician.
Do not report the following conditions as SSI:
1. Stitch abscess (minimal inflammation and discharge confined to the points of suture penetration).
2. Infection of an episiotomy or newborn circumcision site.
3. Infected burn wound.
4. Incisional SSI that extends into the fascial and muscle layers (see deep incisional SSI).
Deep incisional SSI: Infection occurs within 30 days after the operation if no implant* is left in place or within 1 year if implant is in place and the infection appears to be related to the operation and infection involves deep soft tissues (e.g. fascial and muscle layers) of the incision and at least one of the following:
1. Purulent drainage from the deep incision but not from the organ/space component of the surgical site.
2. A deep incision spontaneously dehisces or is deliberately opened by a surgeon when the patient has at least one of the following signs or symptoms: fever (>38°C), localized pain, or tenderness, unless site is culture negative.
3. An abscess or other evidence of infection involving the deep incision is found on direct examination, during reoperation, or by histopathologic or radiologic examination.
4. Diagnosis of a deep incisional SSI by a surgeon or attending physician.
Notes:
1. Report infection that involves both superficial and deep incision sites as deep incisional SSI.
2. Report an organ/space SSI that drains through the incision as a deep incisional SSI.
Organ/space SSI: Infection occurs within 30 days after the operation if no implant* is left in place or within 1 year if implant is in place and the infection appears to be related to the operation and infection involves any part of the anatomy (e.g. organs or spaces), other than the incision, which was opened or manipulated during an operation and at least one of the following:
1. Purulent drainage from a drain that is placed through a stab wound† into the organ/space.
2. Organisms isolated from an aseptically obtained culture of fluid or tissue in the organ/space.
3. An abscess or other evidence of infection involving the organ/space that is found on direct examination, during reoperation, or by histopathologic or radiologic examination.
4. Diagnosis of an organ/space SSI by a surgeon or attending physician.

*National Nosocomial Infection Surveillance definition: a nonhuman-derived implantable foreign body (e.g. prosthetic heart valve, nonhuman vascular graft, mechanical heart, or hip prosthesis) that is permanently placed in a patient during surgery.
†If the area around a stab wound becomes infected, it is not an SSI. It is considered a skin or soft tissue infection, depending on its depth.
(SSI: Surgical site infection).
Adapted from Horan TC, Gaynes RP, Martone WJ, et al. CDC definition of nosocomial surgical site infections, 1992; a modification of CDC definitions of surgical wound infections. Infect Control Hosp Epidemiol. 1992;13:606-8.

the surgical incision, of the body cavities entered by the operation, and of prosthetic devices surgically placed into the patient. The severity of SSI may be superficial incisional, deep incisional, or an organ-space infection (Table 7.1).

The surgical incision violates the skin, which is the primary host defense against infection. External microbes contaminate the open wound by the incisional process, from contaminants carried into the wound by the surgeon or surgical instrumentation, and from the environment of the operating room. The procedure may then enter into colonized areas of the body (e.g. the colon), which become a major source for microbial contamination of the surgical site. Regardless of the mechanism, all surgical sites are contaminated. However, all do not become infected. The determinants of SSI are:

- Quantity of bacterial contamination
- Virulence of the bacterial contaminants
- Microenvironment of the wound
- Integrity of host defenses.

The probability of infection in an incision increases as the number of bacterial contaminants increases. Quantitative cultures of even clean wounds will identify bacteria. Infection commonly develops when the quantity of bacterial contaminants exceeds a specific critical threshold. The quantity of bacteria necessary to cause infection has commonly been recognized to be 10^5 organisms per gram of tissue, but the exact number is likely to vary for each bacterial species.

Different bacterial species have different virulence factors. Virulence factors include both production of exotoxins by the bacteria and structural components of the bacterial cell (e.g. endotoxins). The numerous exotoxins include hemolysins, leucocidins, coagulase, and collagenase. Specific strains of organisms that elaborate these exotoxins are more virulent and require fewer contaminants to cause clinical infection. Fewer coagulase-positive *Staphylococcus aureus* are required to cause wound infection than coagulase-negative *Staphylococcus epidermidis.* The production of the Panton-Valentine leukocidin is a particularly important exotoxin of community-acquired methicillin-resistant *S. aureus*[1] (CA-MRSA). Among cell structural components that are virulence factors, endotoxin of the outer membrane of gram-negative bacteria is most notable. Endotoxin with the lipid A moiety (e.g. *Escherichia coli)* is more likely to cause infection than endotoxin without the lipid A component (e.g. *Bacteroides fragilis*).

A third determinant of SSI is the microenvironment at the operative site. For example, hemoglobin within the surgical incision produces a rich pabulum of essential nutrients for bacterial proliferation, of which ferric iron may be the most important. Ferric iron may be a rate-limiting factor in bacterial growth and wound hematoma is a rich source of this iron. Dead tissue and foreign bodies are potent promoters of infection. Braided suture material and surgically placed prosthetic devices become examples of foreign bodies that enhance the probability of infection.

A fourth determinant of infection is the systemic host response, which may be impaired by either intrinsic or acquired defects. Genetically programmed differences are likely to exist between different patients, but they are not easily measured.[2] Acquired host impairment has been associated with shock, hypoxemia, hypothermia, acute and chronic alcoholism, recent blood transfusion, and current corticosteroid therapy. The clinical associations with SSI are numerous and reflect the important role of optimization of the patient's physiological condition at the time of operation.[3]

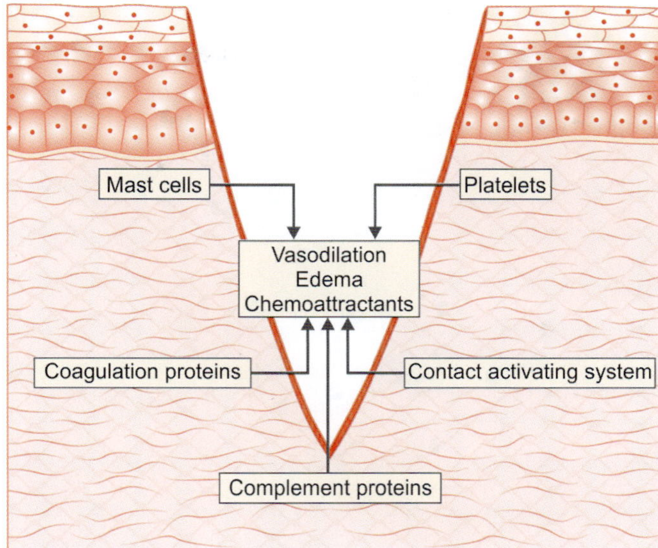

Fig. 7.1: Initiator events of the inflammatory response activated by the creation of a surgical wound.

Pathogenesis

The pathogenesis of SSI begins with the incision. Tissue disruption activates the coagulation cascade, platelets, mast cells, complement proteins, and the contact activating system (Fig. 7.1). Activation of the five initiators of the inflammatory response results in local tissue vasodilation and increased vascular permeability. Vasodilation increases the total perfusion to the area of injury but slows flow velocity to allow neutrophil delivery and efficient margination of neutrophils. Increased vascular permeability allows suffusion of plasma proteins and plasma volume into the injured area and results in tissue edema. Tissue edema delivers opsonic proteins into the area and provides aqueous channels for phagocytic cell migration.

Activation of the initiators of inflammation and the attendant increased local perfusion delivers chemoattractant factors, which serve as chemical "beacons" to attract phagocytic cells to the area of injury and contamination (Fig. 7.2). These chemoattractant factors include activated Factor XII from the coagulation cascade, inflammatory proteins from mast cells and platelets, complement cleavage products and bradykinin from the contact activating system. Chemokines are specific chemoattractant cytokines that are also produced by several cell populations.[4] Diffusion of the chemoattractant factors from the epicenter of injury upregulates adhesion molecules on endothelial cells, which initially slow neutrophils by causing "rolling" across the epithelial surface. The rolling then

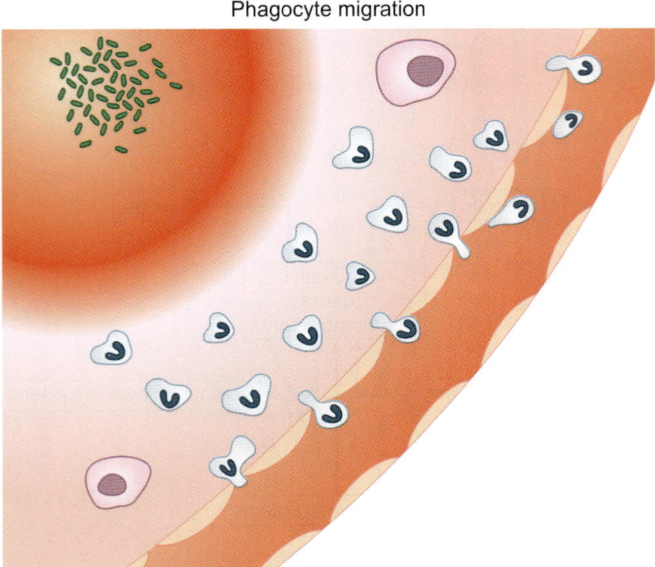

Fig. 7.2: Process of phagocytic cell migration into an area of infection.

allows complete margination of the neutrophil to the endothelial cell by the interaction of neutrophil integrins with intercellular adhesion molecule on the epithelial cell surface. Neutrophil diapedesis toward the chemotactic gradient of the area of injury and contamination then initiates phagocytosis.

Neutrophil mobilization occurs within 12–24 hours of tissue injury and contamination. At 24–48 hours, the monocyte cell is similarly mobilized into the area of injury. If injury and contamination is minimal, as sensed by the intensity of the chemoattractant signals, the monocyte may be a minimal participant in the process as normal phagocytic function of the neutrophil eradicates pathogens from the wound. In the absence of strong chemotactic signals, the monocyte becomes instrumental in the elaboration of important cytokine signals, which initiate the process of wound healing. If large concentrations of chemoattractant signals are present as a reflection of severe injury and microbial proliferation, the monocyte elaborates proinflammatory cytokines, which include tumor necrosis factor (TNF), interleukin-(IL)-l, IL-6, and IL-8 -TNF, and other proinflammatory signals that mediate an intense upregulation of neutrophil phagocytic activity. Extracellular release of acid hydrolases and reactive oxygen intermediates from the neutrophil considerably enhance local inflammation. The end result of digested tissues, dead neutrophils, microbial cells, and thick proteinaceous exudate is generally known as pus. Clinical signs in the incision of advancing cellulitis, erythema, induration, wound tenderness, and pus define the state of active clinical infection.

Prevention

Prevention of SSI begins by reducing the number of potential contaminants that gain access to the open incision. Preoperative showering or bathing of the proposed surgical site with an antiseptic soap is advocated by many but has not had conclusive evidence to support generalized use.[5] The surgical site is scrubbed and painted with an antiseptic as part of the preoperative preparation in the operating room, with recent evidence favoring the use of chlorhexidine as the topical agent.[6] Hair removal should only be done with electric clippers and may be avoided completely in patients with limited hair at the site. Shaving with a straight razor has been associated with increased SSI rates and should be avoided. Cuts and abrasions of the skin from straight razor shaving serve as sites for local microbial proliferation and increased rates of infection.

The duration of preoperative hospitalization increases the rate of wound infection.[7] Several preoperative days are likely to result in colonization of the patient with hospital-based bacteria that prove more pathogenic and less sensitive to preventive strategies. Elective procedures on hospitalized patients are best postponed until a period of "recolonization" with normal microflora has occurred outside the hospital.

Intraoperative strategies to prevent SSI include both attention to infection control practices and refined surgical techniques to avoid creating local conditions that favor infection. Scrubbing the hands, surgical gloves, gowns, caps, masks, and all barriers in the operating room are designed to reduce microbial access to the open wound. Tissues should be handled gently to avoid the trauma that creates necrosis. Excessive and indiscriminate use of the electrocautery increases the quantity of necrotic tissue and the probability of infection. Parsimony in the use of suture material in the wound avoids the adjuvant effects provided by these foreign bodies. The adjuvant effects of the electrocautery and sutures for hemostasis must be weighed against the hematoma risks of poor hemostasis. Finally, excessive dead space allows serum collections within the wound and increases infection rates. Closed suction drains that enter the wound space through a separate stab wound can reduce infection rates. Passive (Penrose) drains and those exiting through the incision should be avoided.

Systemic variables are likely to affect infection rates, but they may not be easily manipulated. Malnourished patients may need nutritional support before the procedure but the duration and composition of feeding necessary to impact outcomes continues to be a source of investigation.[8] It may not be practical to discontinue preexistent corticosteroid therapy. However, adequate intraoperative oxygenation, appropriate intravascular volume, and appropriate arterial pressure help prevent wound infection. Although still having some controversy, maintenance of core body temperature and reasonable glycemic control may also reduce SSI rates.[9,10]

Wound irrigation with saline is a common practice that is of limited value. Irrigation eliminates tissue debris, shreds of fibrin, and small clots within the wound, and by eliminating these adjuvants potentially reduces some risk of SSI. However, low velocity irrigation does not reduce bacterial colony counts. Pulsed lavage may be useful for wounds during lengthy procedures or those associated with overt contaminating events because the higher velocity irrigation may remove the fibrin peel from the surface of the wound. This fibrin peel contains most of the bacteria likely to cause infection.

Preventive Antibiotics

Preventive systemic antibiotics have an important role in the prevention of SSI. Systemic antibiotics given before surgical incision create a "safety net" of active drugs in the wound. As contaminants strike the wound and the fibrin matrix is precipitated around the microbes, antibiotic also becomes imbedded within the fibrin. Active antibiotic in the wound at the time of contamination reduces the viable contaminants and infection rates. Systemic preventive antibiotics for the surgical wound are indicated when:

- The risk of infection is great because a colonized or infected area of the body is being entered by the procedure
- Infection rates are low, but the consequences of infection are catastrophic (e.g. open heart operations, total joint replacements, major prosthetic vascular reconstruction, and virtually any procedure that uses synthetic materials).

The use of preventive systemic antibiotics for routine clean elective procedures, such as inguinal hernia repair or breast operations, is unclear. As is illustrated in Figure 7.3, preventive antibiotics have least benefit when the magnitude of contamination is either small or very excessive. In the clean surgical incision, it is likely that adherence to

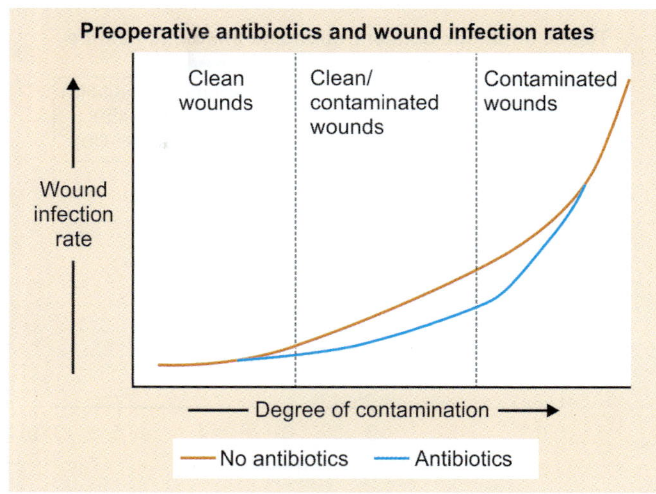

Fig. 7.3: Preoperative preventive antibiotics and rates of surgical site infections for operative procedures of different risk.

rigorous infection control to avoid contamination is the most important consideration. One large study reports benefit for the use of preoperative systemic antibiotics in clean operations.[11]

Critical considerations in the selection of a preventive systemic antibiotic include antimicrobial activity, toxicity, and biologic elimination half-life. First, the antibiotic must have activity against the pathogens likely to beencountered. Preventive antibiotics for colonic procedures should cover the common aerobic and anaerobic colonic microflora, whereas those for biliary tract procedures should cover *E. coli* and *Klebsiella* spp. and those for cardiac procedures and major vascular cases should provide antistaphylococcal coverage. Second, the drugs should have limited toxicity. As penicillins have the greatest risk of causing hypersensitivity or anaphylaxis events after a single dose, they should be used sparingly for preventive indications. Finally, the systemic preventive antibiotics must produce tissue concentrations within the wound for the period of risk. Short half-life antibiotics are rapidly eliminated and require frequent intraoperative redosing. Longer half-life antibiotics should be selected (Fig. 7.4).

The emergence of CA-MRSA has created the dilemma for covering this pathogen in hospitals with high prevalence rates. This debate for and against using MRSA coverage is further compounded by the increasing pattern of resistance trends of this pathogen to vancomyin and the absence of an alternative antibiotic choice. A randomized prospective clinical trial in cardiac surgery demonstrated that vancomycin versus cefazolin resulted in comparable

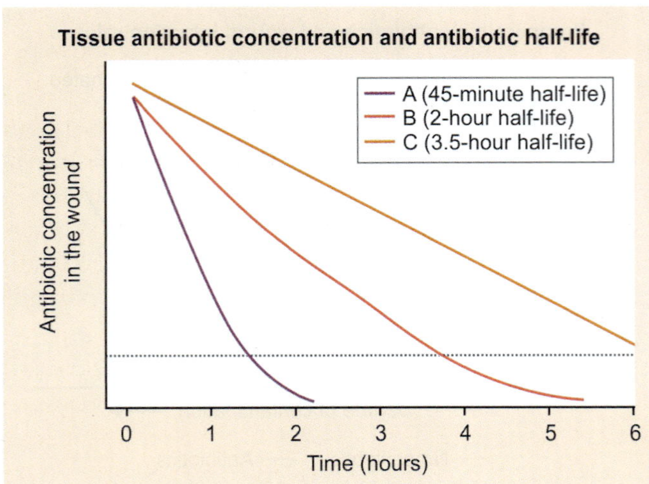

Fig. 7.4: Antibiotics with longer half-lives will have more sustained tissue concentrations and longer periods of effectiveness for longer procedures.

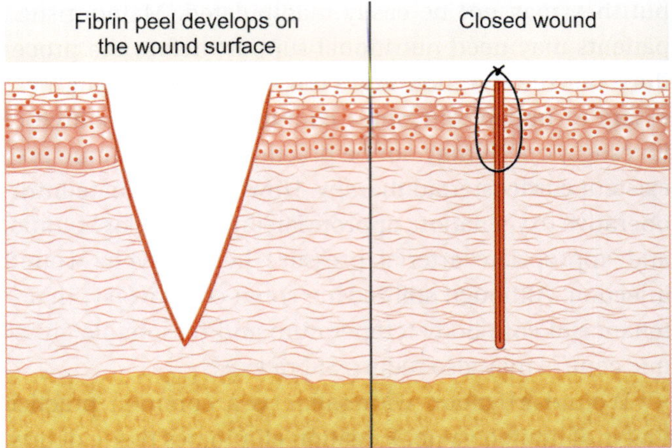

Fig. 7.5: The dense fibrin matrix and the "halo" of tissue edema and increased hydrostatic pressure, which prevent postoperatively administered antibiotics from making contact with pathogens within the closed surgical wound.

overall SSI rates.[12] The interesting part of this clinical trial is that patients receiving cefazolin had higher MRSA infection rates while patients receiving vancomycin had higher methicillin-sensitive *S. aureus* (MSSA) infection rates. The story remains unresolved but it certainly appears that systemic preventive coverage for MRSA will require a continuing reassessment and that vancomycin even when used for susceptible MRSA contamination may be inadequate for MSSA.

Preventive systemic antibiotics are not of value when given postoperatively. Once the wound is closed and intraoperative contamination is over, the period of systemic antibiotic penetration into the wound has also passed (Fig. 7.5). The mature fibrin matrix of the closed surgical wound is impervious to systemic antibiotics. The progression of tissue edema in the freshly closed surgical wound creates a "halo" of increased hydrostatic pressure around the wound, which makes the wound interface relatively ischemic. Probably, the most common error in the clinical use of preventive antibiotics is to continue the drugs for several days postoperatively.

Another important consideration in the use of preventive systemic antibiotics is that they are only of value when the period of bacterial contamination is short. An operation begins and ends within a few hours. Antibiotics can reduce the viable bacterial contamination during this period of time. However, when the period of bacterial contamination spans multiple generation times of the microbes, then prolonged systemic antibiotic use favors the emergence of resistant pathogens. Use of systemic antibiotics cannot prevent infection in open wounds, burns, endotracheal tubes, Foley catheters, intravenous catheters, and all other indwelling treatment and monitoring devices.

The use of poorly absorbed, orally administered antibiotics for patients who undergo elective colorectal surgery deserves special consideration. Elective colon procedures have the highest wound infection rates of any elective procedure because the colon has the highest microbial concentration of any body cavity. The concept of bowel preparation is to give the patient a thorough mechanical bowel preparation 24–48 hours before operation followed by three preoperative doses of a poorly absorbed antibiotic with activity against the colonic organisms. The current practice is to use neomycin (1 g) and erythromycin base (1 g) at three time intervals, on the afternoon and evening preceding the operation for the following day. The oral antibiotic bowel preparation has been demonstrated to reduce SSI rates of elective colorectal procedures and should be used with an appropriate preoperative systemic antibiotic.[13]

Much has been written over the last decade about the ineffectiveness of mechanical bowel preparation alone in the prevention of SSI in colon surgery.[14] Mechanical bowel preparation alone without the use of oral antibiotics is not effective, but it is a necessary requirement for the effective use of oral antibiotics!

Preventive systemic antibiotics may have some value in the management of contaminated traumatic wounds. The contamination of the traumatic wound has already occurred before the antibiotic can be started, but the immediate use of a systemic antibiotic that targets the likely contaminants at the time of wound debridement, irrigation, and closure should provide a beneficial wound concentration of the drug. This similarly applies for the management of open fractures as well.[15] Continued administration of preventive systemic antibiotics after wound closure is not beneficial.

Interest continues to focus upon the use of topical antiseptics and topical antibiotics in the incision at the time of operation. Evidence to support the use of topical agents in the incision is lacking at this time.

Diagnosis

A diagnosis of SSI is primarily made from the physical examination. The prototype incisional infection shows the classic signs of inflammation, which include induration, erythema, warmth, and tenderness. Systemic findings of fever and leukocytosis may or may not be present depending upon the severity of the SSI.

The defining evidence of infection is the discharge of pus from the wound, although the definition has been expanded (Table 7.1). Commonly, the area of wound induration may need to be probed with a surgical instrument or cotton-tipped probe to identify pus. Serous drainage from the wound may be cloudy or blood tinged and leaves uncertainty about the diagnosis. In general, it is best to treat all incisional discharge as though infection is present.

Routine cultures of the infected incision have traditionally been suspect. As will be discussed, most incisional SSIs do not require systemic antibiotic treatment. Gram's stains of the wound pus commonly identify gram-positive cocci and confirm that staphylococcal infection is present. However, the emergence of CA-MRSA has increased the frequency of resistant SSI pathogens and has made cultures a necessity for most cases.

Management

The treatment of SSI is to open and drain the infection. Cutaneous sutures or staples are removed and the skin edges are separated to permit evacuation of pus. A common error is to be too limited in opening the full extent of the wound to achieve complete drainage. Fibrinous debris and sutures should be removed. Necrotic tissue needs to be debrided. Extensive necrosis or pain from local debridement may necessitate a return to the operating room for adequate debridement.

When infected abdominal incisions are opened they must be carefully inspected to determine fascial involvement. An incisional SSI may be the seminal event that heralds a fascial dehiscence. Fascial dehiscence with incisional SSI usually means a return to the operating room for debridement.

Systemic antibiotics are not necessary for most superficial SSIs. Antibiotics are required for extensive cellulitis around the wound, although the cellulitis commonly resolves quickly once the infection has been drained. Systemic antibiotics are also required if there is necrosis of the subcutaneous tissues or evidence of fascial necrosis. Gram-positive infections can be determined by Gram's stain and require antistaphylococcal antibiotic therapy, but sensitivity data are necessary to define the presence of CA-MRSA. Infections of surgical wounds after colonic surgery usually result from polymicrobial enteric flora and should be treated with appropriate antibiotics.

The Burst Abdomen

A major complicating event in patients with deep SSI in abdominal surgery is necrosis of fascia and muscle. The result is dehiscence of the fascial closure, which is commonly called the "burst abdomen" when there is actual evisceration of abdominal contents. Evisceraton has the real risk of injury to intra-abdominal structures. While the burst abdomen may be the consequences of technical failure (e.g. broken suture) or closure with excessive tension especially in obese patients, the reality is that invasive infection is responsible in the majority of cases.

Prevention of the burst abdomen can be achieved by the liberal use of delayed primary closure or secondary closure when massive contamination is encountered in the index procedure. Some have recommended the use of retention sutures but this method remains controversial in terms of true efficacy for prevention. When contamination is accompanied by marked intestinal edema, then the completely open abdomen may be chosen to avoid abdominal compartment syndrome and the consequences of invasive infection in the fascia that is closed under tension.

The diagnosis of fascial dehiscence is commonly heralded by acute "soaking" of the abdominal wound dressing. Careful inspection identifies the extravasation of peritoneal fluid and potentially pus from between the skin closure sutures or staples. Direct inspection identifies the separated fascia. Sutures will usually be noted to have pulled through the fascia. Deep infection in the surgical wound is usually accompanied by suppuration but also the presence of necrotic fascia and associated muscle. While a local area of fascial separation can be managed conservatively with local care if the closure was performed with an interrupted technique, most separations of the fascia are the true burst abdomen and require a return to the operating room for management.

There are multiple components to the management of the burst abdomen.[16] Management of the burst abdomen requires debridement of the necrotic muscle and fascia until only bleeding and clearly viable tissue remains. Debridement cannot be minimized in the interest of trying to primarily close the remaining fascial wound. Debrided tissue should be sent for cultures and not simply the superficial exudate of the wound. Initial antibiotic therapy will likely require a broad spectrum of coverage to included MRSA and gram-negative pathogens. If the infection is following a colonic operation, then anaerobic coverage is also advised. Antibiotic therapy is then deescalated once culture results are available.

Management of the fascial defect in the burst abdomen has a temporary and a long-term component. With invasive infection in the fascia, reoperation may be required. Thus, temporary absorbable meshes or other temporary wound closure strategies are chosen. When the infection has been resolved, consideration is then given to a permanent fascial replacement. Granulation tissue over the temporary absorbable mesh may lead to split-thickness skin grafting and the acceptance that a ventral hernia will have to be managed months later. Separation of parts, polypropylene mesh, biological meshes, and other materials have been chosen for fascial replacement with skin flap coverage for subsequent repair of the ventral hernia once the patient has completely recovered from the multiple operations and the complications of care.

SOFT-TISSUE INFECTIONS

Skin and Skin Structure Infections

Infections of the skin and related skin structures [skin, skin structure, and related soft-tissue infections (SSSTIs)] are the most common of all infections. These have a broad continuum of severity with some being self-limited and requiring no treatment. Others may be severe and need hospitalization with extended surgical and medical treatment.

Cellulitis is an invasive infection that is confined to the skin and subcutaneous tissues. It is characterized by an advancing, blanching erythema. The infection is usually streptococcal. The epicenter of the infection may be following a minor cut, abrasion, or burn. It may arise from glandular elements within the skin. When these infections are staphylococcal in origin, they may have a central pyogenic focus about the primary injury site or skin structure of origin. The infection is a clinical diagnosis. If a black eschar is identified about the epicenter, then CA-MRSA is suspected and cultures are necessary. Penicillin remains the antibiotic treatment for streptococcal cellulitis. MSSA infections are treated with an oral penicillin (dicloxacillin) or a cephalosporin. CA-acquired MRSA is often effectively treated with oral trimethoprim–sulfamethoxazole or clindamycin. Severe MRSA infections require hospitalization, potentially local debridement, and parenteral vancomycin therapy.

Erysipelas is a streptococcal infection confined to the skin only. It has an advancing deep red rash with a clear line of demarcation about the perimeter of the infection. It is exquisitely painful. *Peau d'orange* reflecting skin edema, lymphadenitis, and lymphangitis may be seen. It is a clinical diagnosis and may be treated with penicillin, clindamycin, or a fluoroquinolone. Hospitalization and parenteral therapy may be required for severe cases, which are usually seen in the elderly or immunocompromised hosts.

Pyogenic SSSTIs include impetigo, furuncles, and carbuncles. They are most commonly *S. aureus* infections and usually arise from infections of the follicle or glandular elements of the skin. Impetigo is seen in children as small skin abscesses of nonfollicular origin that suppurate, drain, and crust over. Evacuation of pustules and cleansing of crusts is treatment and is commonly followed by topical bacitracin or other local antibiotic treatment. Systemic antibiotics are reserved for severe cases. CA-MRSA is seen with impetigo.

A *furuncle* is an abscessed hair follicle and a *carbuncle* is multiple, confluent pyogenic infections of adjacent hair follicles. They are treated by local incision and drainage. Antistaphylococcal therapy is needed in severe cases. Local tissue necrosis with eschar suggests CA-MRSA.

There are an extensive array of cellulitic and pyogenic infections that follow any cutaneous injury. Among these are human and animal bites that are associated with an array of anaerobic pathogens. These infections after bites commonly require antibiotic therapy with amoxicillin–clavulanate.

Necrotizing Fasciitis

A particularly virulent form of soft tissue infection is necrotizing fasciitis, which should more appropriately be called *necrotizing soft tissue infection (NSTI)* to more accurately reflect the character of the disease.[17] These infections may be monomicrobial infections caused by *Clostridium perfringens*, group A streptococci, or *S. aureus*. NSTIs may be polymicrobial infections, which are commonly a combination of gram positive, gram negative, and obligate anaerobes. These infections may complicate a variety of cutaneous injuries and may be complications of surgical wound infection or diabetic cutaneous infections.

Despite the variety of causative organisms, these infections share a common pathogenesis. The perifascial space is a potential space between the posterior surface of the subcutaneous fat and the investing fascia overlying the muscle underneath (Fig. 7.6). This potential space contains a loose areolar tissue. When a surgical or traumatic wound produces infection at the fascial level or when more superficial infection invades vertically to gain access to this potential space, infection can spread very rapidly. The result is the loss of penetrating nutrient vessels to the skin and subcutaneous tissue leading to necrosis. The necrosis may involve the investing fascia itself or the underlying muscle itself, depending upon whether the initial wound penetrated the fascia.

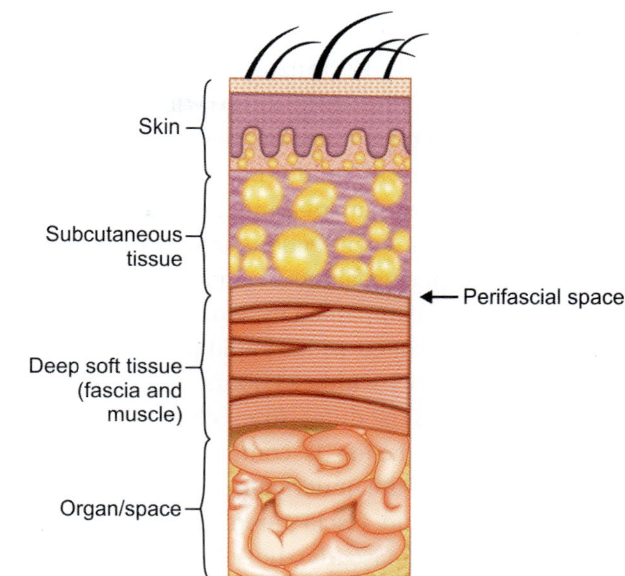

Fig. 7.6: The location of the perifascial space, which lies immediately beneath the subcutaneous fat but superficial to the investing fascia of the underlying skeletal muscle.

Clostridial NSTIs

Clostidium perfringens is the pathogen associated with gas gangrene as the most aggressive of the NSTIs. *C. perfringens* exists as a spore in the environment and transforms into the vegetative infectious state when introduced into injured tissues with optimum conditions for growth. The organism is an obligate anaerobe and requires an oxygen-free environment to cause invasive infection. Thus, dead tissue and hematoma become environmental requirements for infection to occur. Given appropriate environmental conditions, the organisms rapidly proliferate and produce an array of exotoxins that kill adjacent soft tissues. Proliferating organisms then invade the adjacent dead tissue, more toxin is produce, and more dead tissue follows in this rapidly progressing disease.

Clostridial NSTI progression has the characteristic feature of pain and tenderness that extends beyond the anticipated symptoms of the inciting injury. Infection may involve extensive muscle necrosis but have only mild external evidence that infection exists. Overlying skin and subcutaneous edema may be modest. Some skin sloughing or cutaneous necrosis may be present at the site of injury. A "dishwater" drainage can be identified from the inciting wound and will commonly have gram-positive rods on Gram stain. Blood and tissue cultures are inevitably positive but not in time to make a clinical difference in these rapidly progressing and lethal (>50% mortality) infections. Fundamentally, clostridial NSTI requires a high index of suspicion in a patient with a penetrating injury and rapidly evolving pain and tenderness with systemic signs of infection. The treatment is extensive surgical debridement of dead tissue; aggressive supportive care with volume, ventilator, and inotropic support; and antibiotics. Antibiotic management includes high-dose aqueous penicillin (24 million units per day) in combination with clindamycin (1,200–1,500 mg every 6–8 hours). Clindamycin is added to inhibit toxin production from the pathogen.[18] Many recommend hyperbaric oxygen but evidence for improved outcomes is inconclusive.

Rarely, one will see clostridial NSTI that is not associated with a penetrating injury but is rather a blood-borne disease when *Clostridium* spp. will lodge in skeletal muscle from a remote site. *Clostridium septicum* is associated with colonic pathology (e.g. colon cancer) as the portal of entry into the blood for distant seeding, whereas *Clostridium sordellii* from infection within the uterus (e.g. septic abortion) is seen rarely in younger women with distant myonecrosis from clostridial NSTI. Patients who survive these unusual clostridial infections require evaluation for the source of the organisms.

Streptococcal NSTIs

Group A streptococcal necrotizing fasciitis can follow injuries as trivial as minor abrasions or needle puncture wounds.[19] It can complicate any cutaneous injury, including varicella infections in children. It is most commonly seen in diabetics, obese patients, and in ischemic extremities, but about one third of infections arise in patients who do not have predisposing factors. As many as 50% of these infections may be accompanied by a toxic shock-like syndrome and are associated with a rapid progression from injury to systemic shock within 24 hours.

Streptococcal NSTIs differ from clostridial myonecrosis in that the infection is commonly superficial to the investing fascia of the underlying skeletal muscle. The underlying muscle and fascia remain alive (hence the misnomer necrotizing fasciitis), but the overlying subcutaneous tissue has extended necrosis with the tan, frothy exudate within the perifascial space. Surface necrosis of skin with bullae, blisters, and rapidly advancing cellulitis is present in infection that is superficial to the investing muscle fascia. Myonecrosis may be present if the inciting injury penetrated the fascia, in which case the disease behaves very similar to clostridial myonecrosis.

The diagnosis of streptococcal NSTI is a clinical diagnosis of expanding pain and tenderness out of proportion to the associated injury in a patient with rapidly evolving clinical infection. External advancing infection is very helpful in establishing the diagnosis if present, and touch plates of weeping surfaces or exudates from wounds will commonly have gram-positive cocci in chains. Cultures are positive but too late for clinical value. Treatment requires extensive debridement with the same supportive care and the same antibiotic regimen that is used with clostridial NSTIs.

Streptococcal gas gangrene will occur from blood borne seeding of muscle or other peripheral injury sites without an attendant local cutaneous injury. These uncommon infections are likely from a hypopharyngeal entry site with distant lodgment. Rapidly expanding pain and tenderness in a patient with evolving systemic symptoms of infection and no surface injury requires an acute index of suspicion if effective treatment is to be delivered.

Staphylococcal NSTIs

Staphylococci have emerged as a relatively new monomicrobial pathogen for NSTIs.[20] While the presence of coagulase in *S. aureus* has given a phenotype of localized pyogenic infection, CA-MRSA has exotoxin characteristics that have made these pathogens part of the constellation of NSTIs. Signs and symptoms are similar to streptococcal NSTIs except that the presentation can be more heterogenous with some infections less aggressive than others. A pyogenic character is commonly identified at the site of injury. Nevertheless, the characteristic pain out of proportion to the primary site of injury or cutaneous infection is present. The diagnosis is largely a clinical one with the Gram stain of wound drainage demonstrating gram-positive cocci in clusters. Cultures are important to define the presence of MRSA. Blood cultures may be positive but are less frequently so compared to streptococcal NSTI. Treatment requires debridement of all necrotic tissue and appropriate antibiotics (Table 7.2). Empiric selections before culture data are available should cover MRSA, with antibiotic therapy subsequently contoured to the results of sensitivities.

Polymicrobial NSTIs

Polymicrobial NSTIs are a heterogenous group of infections that are characterized by multiple pathogens on culture of the infected tissues.[21] These are most commonly seen after surgical or traumatic wounds with extensive environmental or intestinal tract contamination. Myonecrosis and complete fascial necrosis from infection in traumatic and surgical wounds result in full-thickness loss of the extremity or truncal tissues. Other variants of polymicrobial NSTIs include Melaney's synergistic gangrene with anaerobic streptococcal and staphylococcal pathogens, the diabetic fetid foot, the burrowing necrotic infection of pressure ulcers, and Fournier's gangrene of the perineum.

These polymicrobial NSTIs tend to be less aggressive in invading adjacent tissues when compared with streptococcal or clostridial infections, but again the pattern is very heterogeneous with selected infections having very aggressive behavior. The diagnosis is clinical recognition. Cultures are of real value since prediction of the array of pathogens in the infection cannot be ascertained by the clinical evidence. Deep tissue cultures of infected tissue are necessary, since the sampling of superficial exudate and debris of the wound will yield an inadequate sample and may isolate surface contaminants that are not participants in the infection.

The treatment is surgical debridement of necrotic tissue and broad-spectrum antibiotic therapy. Debridement of the infected site will usually have to be repeated every 24 hours to ensure complete removal of all dead tissue.

Table 7.2 Adult dosing of antibiotic choices for the treatment of MRSA infections.

Antibiotic choice: all MRSA	*Adult dosage*	*Commentary*
Vancomycin	2 g daily in divided doses of 500 mg q 6 h, or 1 g q 12 h.	Only available IV for treatment of MRSA; Requires 60 min for infusion; used for surgical prophylaxis and therapy
Linezolid	600 mg q 12 h either IV or oral	Oral preparation has bioavailability similar to IV preparation; has a broad base of gram-positive activity. No prophylaxis indication
Daptomycin	4 mg/kg q 24 h	Only available as IV preparation; only for treatment of skin/soft tissue infections; poor lung penetration; long half-life permits once daily treatment. No prophylaxis indication
Tigecycline	100 mg loading dose followed by 50 mg q 12 h	Only available as IV preparation; has very broad gram-positive and gram-negative activity; no prophylaxis indication
Telavancin	10 mg/kg q 24 h	Only available as IV preparation; only for skin and soft tissue infections; requires 60 min for dose administration; no prophylaxis indication.
Ceftaroline	600 mg IV q 12 h	Only available as IV preparation; indicated for skin and soft tissue infection but not MRSA pneumonia. Covers enterobacteriaceae and gram positives. No prophylaxis indication
Antibiotic choice: only CA-MRSA		
Trimethoprim–sulfamethoxazole	Tablets of 80 mg trimethoprim and 400 mg sulfamethoxazole: 1–2 tablets q 12 h	Only an oral preparation
Clindamycin	300–600 mg q 6 h	IV and oral preparation
Doxycycline	100 mg q 12 h for day 1, then 50 mg q 12 h	IV and oral preparation
Minocycline	200 mg initial dose, then 100 mg q 12 h	IV preparation only

(MRSA: Methicillin-resistant *Staphylococcus aureus*; CA-MRSA: Community-acquired methicillin-resistant *Staphylococcus aureus*; IV: Intravenous).

It is customary to have broad gram positive, gram negative, and anaerobic coverage with the initial antibiotic regimen. Both sensitive and resistant gram negatives will be encountered depending upon the patient's prior exposure to antibiotics and to the healthcare environment. Staphylococci including CA-MRSA may be participants in these infections especially if the patient has had prior antibiotic exposure (e.g. diabetic fetid foot). Poor responsiveness of the infection reflects inadequate debridement and usually requires reculturing of the wound since secondary pathogens can be an issue especially for intensive care unit patients.

While the classification of the four common bacteriological patterns of NSTIs account for the majority of these cases, it should be emphasized that virtually every bacterial and even fungal pathogens have been associated with these infections. Any pathogen that can cause infection in the soft tissue and can access the perifascial space in an immunocompromised patient can result in an NSTI. Unusual patterns of infection will be observed. Pain and tenderness that is in excess of findings anticipated by any soft tissue injury requires the consideration for NSTI and also means that the culture identification of the pathogen is essential.

Toxic Shock Syndrome

Toxic shock syndrome (TSS) occurs from infections by specific strains of *S. aureus* or *Streptococcus pyogenes* that produce potent superantigens. These superantigens bind to T-lymphocyte targets, which lead to a massive release of proinflammatory cytokines and the resultant fulminate systemic inflammatory response syndrome (SIRS).[22] TSS is associated with marked tachycardia, tachypnea, hypotension, and multiple organ dysfunction syndrome (MODS). These infections with staphylococci are associated with a diffuse maculopapular rash with subsequent desquamation.

Early reports of staphylococcal TSS were associated with foreign body exotoxin production. The prototypical cases occurred in vaginal tampons during the menses but also occur in foreign bodies (e.g. nasal packing) and surgical wounds (Table 7.3). Local evidence of inflammation is minimal and bacteremia with staphylococci is uncommon in TSS.

Table 7.3 Anatomic sites and operative procedures reported to be complicated by toxic shock syndrome secondary to infection with *Staphylococcus aureus*.

Abdominal surgery wounds	Inguinal hernia repair
Abdominoplasty	Mastitis (postpartum)
Arthroplasty	Nasal packing/nasosinus surgery/ sinusitis
Breast biopsy	Ovarian cyst drainage
Breast reconstruction (muscle flaps and prostheses)	Peritoneal dialysis Pharyngitis
Burns	Pilonidal cystectomy
Dermabrasion/skin abrasions	Poison oak dermatitis
Diagnostic peritoneal lavage	Salivary gland surgery
Ear piercing	Septic hip
Enterocolitis	Stab wounds
Fractures: external fixators	Tooth abscess
Hand surgery	Varicella
Human bites	

Treatment of staphylococcal TSS requires removal of the foreign body, drainage of exudates, antibiotic therapy, and systemic supportive care. Nafcillin or a first-generation cephalosporin is used for MSSA and vancomycin is used for MRSA. The systemic consequences of the toxin may persist well after the primary site has been appropriately managed and requires continued supportive care.

A similar TSS is seen with invasive streptococcal infection. The associated toxins have protein homology to the staphylococcal toxins. The clinical presentation is similar, although the streptococcal TSS is associated with invasive infection without the presence of a foreign body. With streptococcal NSTI, the clinical picture of rapidly evolved systemic inflammation, shock, and MODS is dramatic. Positive blood cultures are commonly seen with streptococcal TSS. Treatment of streptococcal TSS requires debridement of the site of infection, antibiotics, and supportive care. Streptococcal TSS blood stream infection is seen within a clinical site of origin in nearly 15% of bacteremic cases.[23]

For both staphylococcal and streptococcal TSS, there is considerable interest in the development of immunoglobulin therapy to neutralize the toxin. Although some of these efforts have shown promise, the biology of the superantigen binding to lymphocytes to stimulate the massive release of proinflammatory cytokines means that immunotherapy will need to be administered very early in the process to improve outcomes.

INTRA-ABDOMINAL INFECTION

Acute Peritonitis

The peritoneal space has a surface area that approaches 40% of the external surface area of the patient. The large surface area provides ample opportunity for microbial invasion into soft tissues. Inflammation and invasive infection in this compartment cause large fluid shifts of plasma and extracellular water and can rapidly lead to a life-threatening event. A diagnosis of acute peritonitis and its sequelae must be understood to allow effective treatment.[24]

Infection within the peritoneal cavity begins when bacteria gain access to the cavity, adhere to the mesothelial lining cells, proliferate, and elicit a host inflammatory response. Uncommonly, *primary peritonitis* may occur from hematogenous or lymphatic spread from a remote site. Free fluid within the peritoneal cavity appears to enhance the vulnerability to bacteremic or lymphatic seeding from a remote site. The most common scenario for primary peritonitis is the cirrhotic patient with ascites. Postpartum women have increased free peritoneal fluid in the 4–6 weeks after delivery and will occasionally develop streptococcal primary peritonitis. Primary peritonitis is usually a monomicrobial infection with either a gram-positive or gram-negative pathogen or even fungi but not anaerobes. Treatment is with specific antibiotics.

Secondary peritonitis is the most common intra-abdominal infection in the surgical patient. In this setting peritonitis develops secondary to another disease process within the abdomen. A perforated appendix, a perforated peptic ulcer, a colonic perforation from diverticulitis or cancer, and perforation of the biliary tract are the processes leading to peritonitis. Following perforation in secondary peritonitis, dynamic forces within the peritoneal cavity result in dissemination of the contamination throughout the entire space. Gravity and body position tend to move the contaminant toward dependent spaces. Movement of the diaphragm with ventilation results in a relatively negative pressure with expiration that disseminates peritoneal fluid.

Dissemination reduces the microbial density at the site of perforation and increases the interface between the bacterial pathogens and host defense mechanisms. It also mobilizes the microbial contaminants toward the diaphragmatic surface, where vast numbers of diaphragmatic fenestrations evacuate peritoneal fluid and bacterial contaminants into the thoracic duct lymph. Clearance of bacteria into the lymphatic system is an important mechanism for microbial elimination from the peritoneal space.

After perforation and dissemination, inflammation is activated. The magnitude of the inflammatory response is governed by the chemical reaction to the foreign body effect of bile, peptic enzymes and acid, and fecal material. The severity of peritonitis is governed by the inoculum of bacterial pathogens released with a perforation. The inoculum depends upon the site of perforation and the duration during which the perforation has free communication into the peritoneal space. For example, the bacterial density within the colon approaches 10^{10}–10^{12} bacteria per gram of human stool, whereas a perforated peptic ulcer in younger patients is virtually free of bacterial colonization because of acid production.

Prevention of peritonitis is best achieved by recognition and treatment of the disease process before perforation. Prompt diagnosis of acute appendicitis before perforation is achievable for most patients. The appropriate medical management of peptic ulcer disease is associated with fewer perforations. Appropriate medical and elective surgical management of diverticulitis may prevent peritonitis.

A diagnosis of acute peritonitis is a clinical one. These patients usually have a history of a seminal event that denotes the perforation. All perforations are characterized by acute abdominal pain. A perforated appendix may be identified by the acute relief of distension and pressure within the acutely obstructed appendix before diffuse pain begins. The diagnosis of peritonitis is defined by physical examination. Rebound tenderness indicates peritoneal inflammation and constitutes justification to proceed with abdominal exploration. Fever and leukocytosis are usual, but these are sometimes minimal or absent in elderly patients. Abdominal and upright chest radiographs may or may not identify free air. Computed tomography (CT) imaging with contrast is a useful method to validate clinical findings and can be most beneficial with equivocal presentations.

The underlying treatment of acute peritonitis is:

- Containment of the bacterial source
- Debridement of nonviable tissue
- Drainage of pus and exudates
- Antibiotic therapy addressed to the likely pathogens participating in the infection
- Supportive care to maintain systemic oxygenation and perfusion.

First, the site of perforation must be managed. This may include resection, plication, primary repair, or exteriorization of the perforated segment of the intestinal tract. Without source control of the contamination, all other treatments will fail. Second, all necrotic and purulent

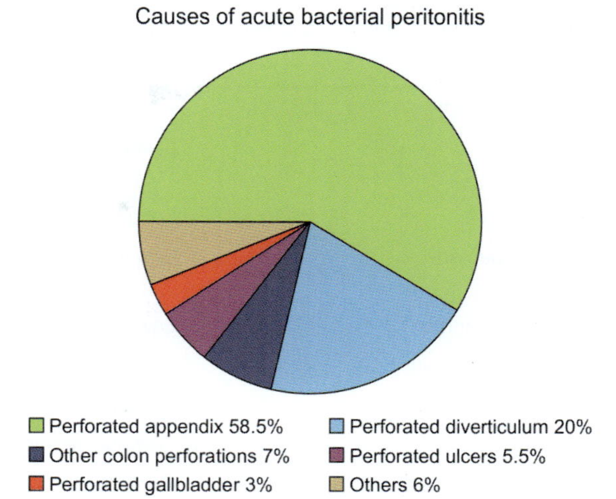

Fig. 7.7: The location of perforations within the abdomen that are responsible for secondary peritonitis.

materials must be evacuated. Foreign material and debris should similarly be removed.

Antibiotic therapy should be based upon expected pathogens. Aerobic gram-positive and enteric gram-negative bacterial coverage is potentially useful for perforated peptic ulcers. Coverage of *E. coli* and *Klebsiella* spp. is adequate for biliary tract and proximal gastrointestinal perforations. Distal small bowel and colonic perforations require antibiotic therapy for aerobic gram-negative bacteria (e.g. *E. coli)* and obligate enteric anaerobes *(B. fragilis)*. Because the specific diagnosis responsible for acute peritonitis is commonly not discernible until the abdomen has been opened, and because the colon and appendix are responsible for most cases of acute bacterial peritonitis (Fig. 7.7), empiric antibiotic management should assume the need for both gram negative and obligate anaerobic coverage (Table 7.4). Antibiotic coverage of enterococci is not supported by current trials for acute bacterial peritonitis.

A traditional practice has been to culture the peritoneal cavity of patients who have acute bacterial peritonitis. This practice continues despite the facts that:

- Surgeons still cover the anticipated pathogens that are likely to be present.
- Surgeons ignore or have no confidence in the results of intraoperative cultures.
- Changing the antibiotic after the critical first 3 days of antibiotic therapy does not appear to change patient outcome.

Cultures of acute peritonitis are not of value in patients with community-acquired perforations in patients without healthcare exposure immediately prior to the perforating event. Patients with recent antibiotic exposure, recently

Table 7.4 Advantages and disadvantages of antibiotics to treat acute bacterial peritonitis.

Antibiotic	*Advantages*	*Disadvantages*
Single-agent therapy		
Cefoxitin	Low toxicity; extensive record of use	Short half-life (40–45 min); some aerobic and anaerobic resistance
Cefotetan	Long half-life allows q12 h dosing	Resistance among nonfragilis *Bacteroides* spp.
Ampicillin–sulbactam	Low toxicity	Short half-life (1 h); emerging gram-negative resistance
Ticarcillin–clavulanate	Low toxicity	Short half-life (1 hr)
Piperacillin–tazobactam	Low toxicity; *Pseudomonas* spp. activity	Short half-life (1 h)
Imipenem	Comprehensive spectrum	CNS toxicity; short half-life (1 h)
Meropenem	Comprehensive spectrum	Short half-life (1 h)
Ertapenem	Comprehensive spectrum but no *Pseudomonas* spp. activity	Long half-life permits once daily dosing
Double-agent therapy		
Aminoglycoside (gentamicin, tobramycin or amikacin) + clindamycin or metronidazole	Excellent gram-negative coverage	Nephro- and ototoxicity; unpredictable pharmacokinetics
Aztreonam + clindamycin or metronidazole	Low toxicity	Limited clinical data in peritonitis
Ciprofloxacin + clindamycin or metronidazole	Low toxicity	Limited clinical data in peritonitis
Triple-agent therapy		
Aminoglycoside or quinolone + clindamycin or metronidazole + ampicillin	Presumes that there is value to adding enterococcal coverage	Expensive cost of administration; toxicity of aminoglycosides

hospitalized patients, nursing home residents, and chronic dialysis patients will be colonized with more resistant microbes and should have peritoneal cultures performed.

One of the most difficult issues in the treatment of peritonitis is the duration of antibiotic therapy. Some investigators advocate continuation of antibiotics until the patient is afebrile and the white blood cell count is normal. For many patients this therapeutic plan leads to an excessive duration of treatment because complete normalization of body temperature and leukocyte counts are protracted processes as a result of resolution of residual inflammation and open wounds. An overall clinical assessment of the patient, including a return to ambulation, resumption of feeding, and normal bowel habits all reflect recovery from the infection and justify discontinuation of antibiotics.

Continued leukocytosis and spiking fevers during the postoperative period while the patient is receiving appropriate antibiotic therapy represent potential failure of the initial management. The natural tendency is to change the antibiotic strategy. Sustained evidence of clinical infection in the postoperative peritonitis patient usually means that an abscess or an undrained purulent collection is present and that mechanical drainage is necessary.

Intra-abdominal Abscess

An intra-abdominal abscess occurs when the contamination within the abdominal cavity has been successfully contained by the inflammatory process, but the numbers of bacteria present at the focus exceed the phagocytic capacity of the host. An abscess is likely when contamination from the primary perforation event is massive or surgical intervention is delayed. Abscesses tend to form in the dependent areas of the peritoneal cavity, including the subphrenic, subhepatic, paracolic, and pelvic spaces.

The prevention of abdominal abscess formation is best achieved by early and effective management of acute peritonitis, as detailed above. Prompt surgical intervention and aggressive systemic antibiotic therapy are important. Omission of antibiotic coverage during the management of acute peritonitis has been shown to result in an increased probability of abscess formation in both clinical and experimental studies. *Bacteroides fragilis* in particular has a capsular polysaccharide that retards phagocytosis and promotes abscess formation.

Vigorous irrigation with or without topical antibiotics at the time of management of acute peritonitis is commonly thought to reduce abscess rates, but little evidence validates this contention. Irrigation of the peritoneal cavity may remove clot and fibrinous debris but does little to reduce bacteria that are adherent to tissue surfaces. Pulsed irrigation may be more effective than conventional irrigation, but again the evidence is largely testimonial. Continuous peritoneal irrigation in the postoperative period with antibiotics through operatively placed irrigation catheters has been advocated but remains of unproven value.

Various drains have been used in patients who have acute peritonitis to prevent abscess formation, including Penrose drains, sump drains, and closed suction drains. Diffuse peritonitis in the peritoneal cavity cannot be effectively drained with any of these systems. Drains become conduits for external contamination to gain access to the peritoneal cavity and may actually increase abscess rates. Closed suction drains are often employed in dependent areas about precarious suture lines of the intestinal tract in the hopes of creating controlled fistula rather than abscess if leakage occurs.

A diagnosis of abdominal abscess is associated with the clinical syndrome of persistent leukocytosis, spiking fever, sustained gastrointestinal ileus, glucose intolerance, and hemodynamic patterns consistent with the septic response. Patients may have early evidence of organ dysfunction. The constellation of symptoms is variable for different patients, so that the clinician must have an index of suspicion about abscess formation in any postoperative patient who is being treated for acute peritonitis. The physical examination is of limited value when patients have abdominal incisions that create tenderness with abdominal palpation. The dependent nature of abscess formation in the supine patient means that palpation seldom helps identify an abdominal mass. Rectal examination still has value in the recognition of pelvic abscesses.

CT scans with contrast of the abdomen are the standard imaging study to diagnose an abdominal abscess. Abscesses in the abdomen tend to occur in the dependent drainage basins of the abdominal cavity: the subphrenic, subhepatic, pericolic, and pelvic spaces. CT scans provide excellent anatomic resolution of abscesses and their relationship to other anatomic structures. Abscesses within the pelvis (Fig. 7.8), retroperitoneum (Fig. 7.9), and solid visceral organs (Fig. 7.10) are all readily identified.

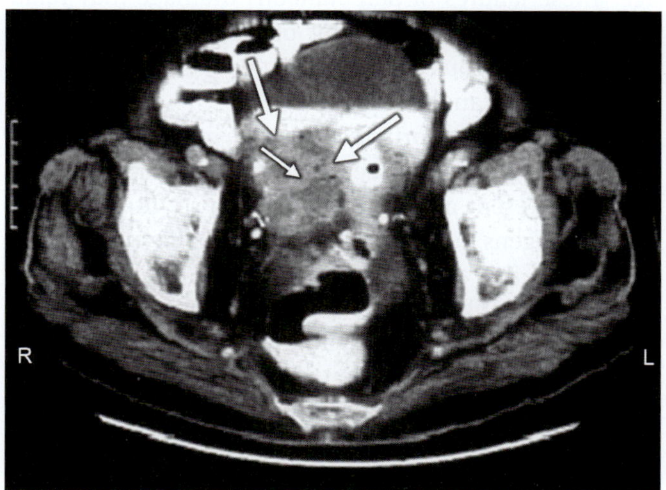

Fig. 7.8: Computed tomography scan illustrating a pelvic abscess (arrows).

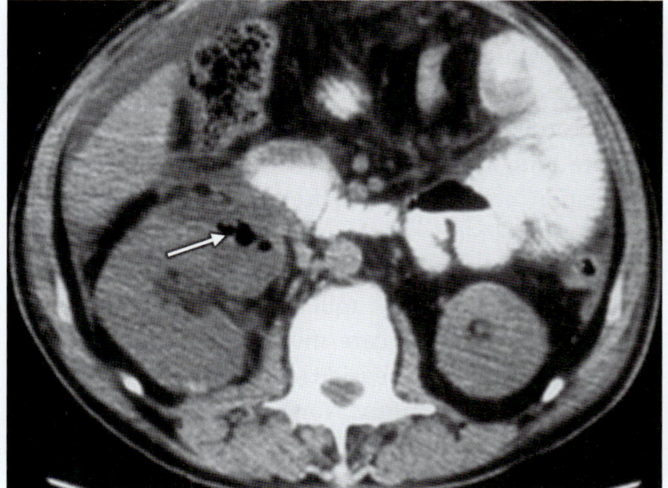

Fig. 7.9: Computed tomography scan illustrating a retroperitoneal abscess (arrow) that is anterior and superior to the right kidney.

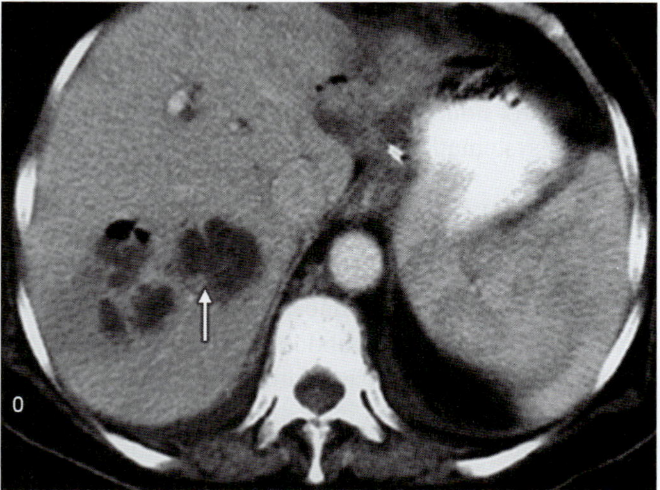

Fig. 7.10: Computed tomography scan illustrating an intrahepatic abscess (arrow).

Treatment of an abdominal abscess is mechanical evacuation of the pus. Percutaneous drainage under CT guidance has become a preferred treatment method that can be employed in many patients at the time of diagnosis. Open exploration and drainage may still be required if percutaneous drainage requires penetration of another visceral structure, there are multiple intra-abdominal collections, there is poor loculation of the fluid collection, or there are other indications (e.g. leaking suture line) that requires reoperation. Empiric reoperation of the postoperative patient may be necessary if the CT scans are equivocal or nondiagnostic. Finally, reexploration may be necessary if the patient continues to have a septic course following apparent successful percutaneous drainage. These failures of percutaneous drainage may relate to nondependent positioning of the catheter drainage system, or a viscous collection that does not readily drain from the percutaneous drain.

Cultures are important at the time of percutaneous or open drainage of an abscess. When large inocula of bacteria are present at the initial peritonitis episode, recovered pathogens may be sensitive to the antibiotics already employed. The abscess pathogens may be affected by antecedent antibiotic therapy and other variables (e.g. use of drains). Very broad antibiotic therapy needs to be employed initially and then should be tailored to the cultured organisms once the information is available. The duration of antibiotic therapy is based upon the clinical response.

Continued clinical infection after either percutaneous or open drainage of an abscess means that drainage may have been incomplete. The abscess may have been inadequately drained, the density of microbes may have resulted in recurrence, or a second abscess may have been missed. Repeat abdominal CT scanning is warranted. Furthermore, nonabdominal causes of infection should always be systematically evaluated as possibilities.

Tertiary Peritonitis

A limited number of patients develop a severe fibrinopurulent infection of the peritoneal cavity after massive contamination and repeated abdominal explorations.[25] The diffuse inflammatory process within the abdomen results in a thick exudative peel over the serosa of the gut, the intestinal mesentery, and the parietal peritoneum. This condition is termed "tertiary" peritonitis. The severity of the intra-abdominal infection in these cases combined with associated soft tissue infection and necrosis of the abdominal wall necessitates that the surgical wound and fascia are commonly left completely open on completion of the abdominal exploration. The severity of the morbidity in such cases is associated with intestinal fistulas and abdominal wall stomas, which contribute further contamination.

Tertiary peritonitis evolves from severe secondary peritonitis. Thoughtful judgment in the use of resection, diversion, and exteriorization in the management of the source lesion is of value to prevent tertiary peritonitis. The avoidance of leaking suture lines and wound dehiscence becomes an important preventative strategy.

A diagnosis of tertiary peritonitis is an arbitrary one. Tertiary peritonitis is generally considered to be present when primary closure of the abdominal wall is no longer feasible or desirable because of severe fibrinopurulent infection of the abdominal wall and the peritoneal cavity. Densely adherent exudate is present over all anatomic components of the peritoneal cavity. Efforts to sharply debride this fibrinopurulent peel result in considerable bleeding and risks entering into the lumen of intestinal structures with the attendant subsequent risk of fistula. These abdominal cavities become large inflammatory wounds with fibrin, pus, and granulation tissue.

Tertiary peritonitis is caused by hospital-acquired microbes. The microbiology bears no resemblance to those pathogens responsible for the original secondary peritonitis. Exposure to broad-spectrum antibiotics and the resident microflora of the critical care environment means that resistant gram-negative bacteria, *Enterococcus* spp. and *Candida* spp., MRSA, and *Staphylococcus epidermidis* are commonly cultured microbes. Anaerobic bacteria are common in secondary peritonitis, but not in tertiary peritonitis.

Treatment of tertiary peritonitis is primarily mechanical. Vigorous local wound care is required to remove exudate and fibrin. Wet dressings that prevent wound desiccation combined with frequent dressing changes are essential. Frequent returns to the operating room for wound cleansing and debridement under general anesthesia may be necessary until bedside dressing changes are practical. Extreme care must be taken in both the operating room and in bedside management of the wound to prevent intestinal injury. Nonadherent gauze may provide an interface between moist gauze dressings and the bowel surface to prevent intestinal injury. A variety of dressings and bioabsorbable meshes are used to avoid bowel injury but still permit drainage of the peritoneal infection. Synthetic meshes are associated with increased fistulization in the experience of some investigators. Permanent reconstruction is not considered until the intra-abdominal infection has resolved.

The role of antibiotics in the treatment of tertiary peritonitis is unclear. If the patient has evidence of invasive infection, antibiotics are clearly important. Bacteremia, abdominal wall erythema, progressive tissue necrosis, and active exudate production between dressing changes reflect clinical evidence of ongoing acute infection. However, interpretation of fever, leukocytosis, and septic hemodynamic parameters can be very deceptive because of the large open wound and other nosocomial infections. The recovery of culturable bacteria alone from the surface of the large wound must not be interpreted as a need for systemic antibiotics. The open granulating surface is never free of bacteria. Progressive granulation of the wound and the elimination of new exudate mean that invasive infection has been controlled.

HOSPITAL-ACQUIRED INFECTIONS

Postoperative Pneumonia

Postoperative pneumonia has the highest associated mortality rate of any nosocomial infection. It occurs in a variety of different clinical scenarios in the surgical patient after operation. Postoperative pneumonia occurs in elderly patients after major procedures, following traumatic injury, and is associated with critical illness. It occurs by different mechanisms in surgical patients.

Nonventilator-associated pneumonia (N-VAP) occurs as a consequence of inadequate tidal volumes in the postoperative patient. The combination of prolonged general anesthesia, narcotic analgesia for pain, splinting of breathing patterns secondary to painful laparotomy or thoracotomy incisions and preexistent lung disease from tobacco use results in inadequate ventilation and subsequent atelectasis. In addition to atelectasis, many of these patients with altered sensorium will have microaspiration of saliva or refluxed gastric contents to be a source of bacteria that are introduced into the lung. The collapse of alveoli and small airways entraps the normal bacterial flora or those from microaspiration, resulting in local microbial proliferation and inflammation. Invasion of these proliferating microbes into the adjacent pulmonary tissues defines pneumonia.

Prevention of N-VAP is by prevention of atelectasis. Coughing, deep breathing, and early ambulation of the postoperative patient expand collapsed segments of atelectatic lung. Postural changes (moving patients from side to side and getting them out of bed and sitting) are also useful. Nasotracheal suctioning can be useful, because the process induces a paroxysm of coughing, which reexpands the lung. Fever on the first night after an operation is most commonly the host response to atelectasis. Vigorous reexpansion of the lung quickly resolves the febrile illness and avoids invasive infection (Figs. 7.11A and B).

A diagnosis of N-VAP is made by correlating clinical, radiographic, and microbiologic data. The N-VAP patient usually has an early postoperative fever, followed by tachypnea, tachycardia, fever, and leukocytosis. Coughing

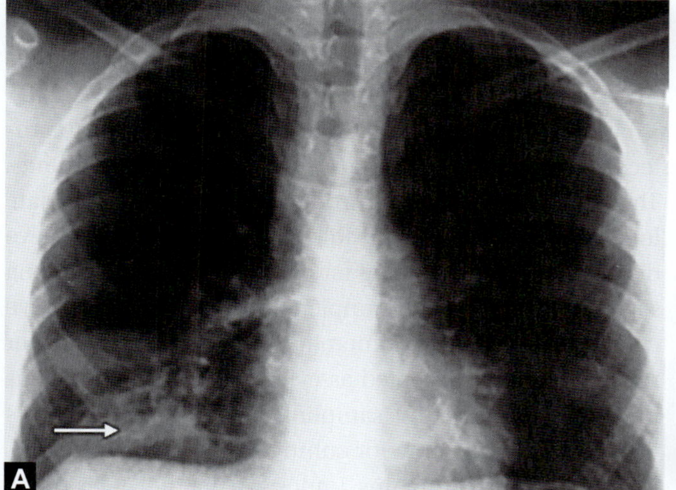

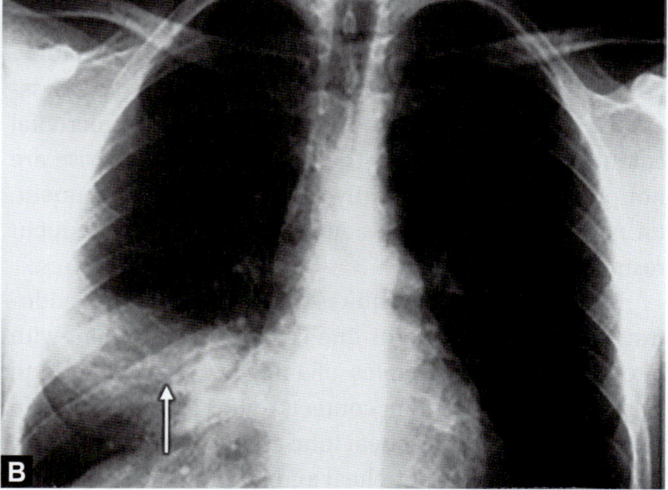

Figs. 7.11A and B: (A) Atelectasis seen in the right lung of a postoperative patient (arrow). (B) Without effective treatment, the atelectasis proceeds in 24 hours to invasive pneumonia of the right middle lobe (arrow).

usually results in purulent sputum. Identification of a new lung infiltrate then completes the diagnosis.

The microbiology of N-VAP can be variable and depends upon two key issues. As N-VAP arises from entrapped bacteria, the duration of preoperative hospitalization and preoperative antibiotic therapy affects the patient's lung colonization. Patients who have short or no preoperative hospital days and no preoperative antibiotics have pneumonia caused by *Streptococcus pneumoniae* or *Haemophilus influenzae.* Those who have had previous antibiotic therapy, or hospitalization for several days before the procedure, or those with other healthcare-associated environmental exposure (e.g. nursing homes) have more resistant gram-negative infections. Documentation of the pathogen by culture is necessary.

N-VAP requires treatment with antibiotics specific for the responsible pathogen. Penicillin is the traditional treatment for pneumonia secondary to pneumococcus, but the emergence of resistance has led to increased use of cephalosporins and quinolones. *H. influenzae* is treated with a penicillin plus β-lactamase inhibitor or an advanced generation cephalosporin. Gram-negative pneumonia requires sensitivity documentation for treatment.

Ventilator-associated pneumonia (VAP) is a common complication of the intensive care unit surgical patient. Ventilator support is required following prolonged anesthesia, excessive lung water from resuscitation or contusion from trauma, or secondary to intrinsic lung disease from tobacco use. Ventilator support means that an endotracheal or tracheostomy tube breaches the lungs' first line of defense (i.e. the glottis). Direct communication of the internal lung air spaces to the environment of the critical care unit results in bacterial contamination of the impaired lung. Furthermore, the use of H-2 histamine antagonists and proton-pump inhibitors to avoid stress-associated gastritis is associated with resistant microbial colonization of the orogastric mucosa that otherwise are not present in the ordinarily acidic gastric environment. From all of these variables, infection is an all-to-frequent result.

Prevention of VAP requires management of the endotracheal appliance and in-line ventilator equipment with attention to the principles of infection control.[26] Hand washing between patient contacts and the use of gloves in the care of the endotracheal tube are essential. Aggressive suctioning to remove tracheal and large airway secretions is important to remove their contribution to microbial proliferation. However, the most important preventive strategy for VAP is early weaning of the patient from ventilator support. The likelihood of pneumonia increases as the number of ventilator days increase, regardless of the effectiveness of infection control practice. Early removal of the endotracheal tube to prevent bacterial contamination and barotrauma from ventilation is paramount.

Innovative methods have been used in ventilator patients to prevent infection. Oral mouth washes with antiseptic (e.g. chlorhexidine) solutions have been employed to reduce mouth colonization with pathogens that access the lower airway. Antibiotic pastes containing neomycin and other antibiotics have similarly been used. Aerosolization of antibiotics that are delivered to the lung via the ventilator have been studied and have been identified with short-term benefits in prevention of pneumonia. However, resistant bacteria commonly emerge and the consequences of aerosolization of antibiotics into the environment of the intensive care unit have the prospects for the enhancement of resistant bacteria. There is no role for systemic antibiotics for the prevention of VAP.

A diagnosis of VAP can be elusive (Figs. 7.12A and B).[27] Many patients in the critical care unit have abnormal chest radiographs that may not reflect pneumonia. Underlying lung disease, fluid resuscitation, lung contusion, and ventilator barotrauma can all create pulmonary infiltrates. Expansion of lung infiltrates is presumptive evidence of pneumonia. Fever and leukocytosis are usual, but they are nonspecific findings in the critical care unit patient. After 48 hours of ventilator support, virtually all suction samples from the lung contain culturable bacteria and colonization versus pneumonia cannot be differentiated by culture of tracheal aspirates alone. Efforts have been made to use quantitative lung cultures of tracheal aspirates to differentiate colonization from invasive infection, but their predictability remains poorly defined.

Culturing techniques have been advocated using protected brushings or bronchoalveolar lavage (BAL) methods. The protected brush is introduced into the appropriate lung segment using a flexible bronchoscope to achieve distal sampling of the lung for culture. With BAL, the lung segment is lavaged and sampled for cultures. Quantitative cultures of the BAL specimen that are $\geq 10^4$ organisms per mL are generally accepted as evidence that pneumonia is present.[28] Because the sampling and culturing process with BAL requires time for culture results to be available, clinical evidence remains important in the decision to initiate antibiotic therapy. Fever, leukocytosis and changing or new pulmonary infiltrates in a patient who has purulent

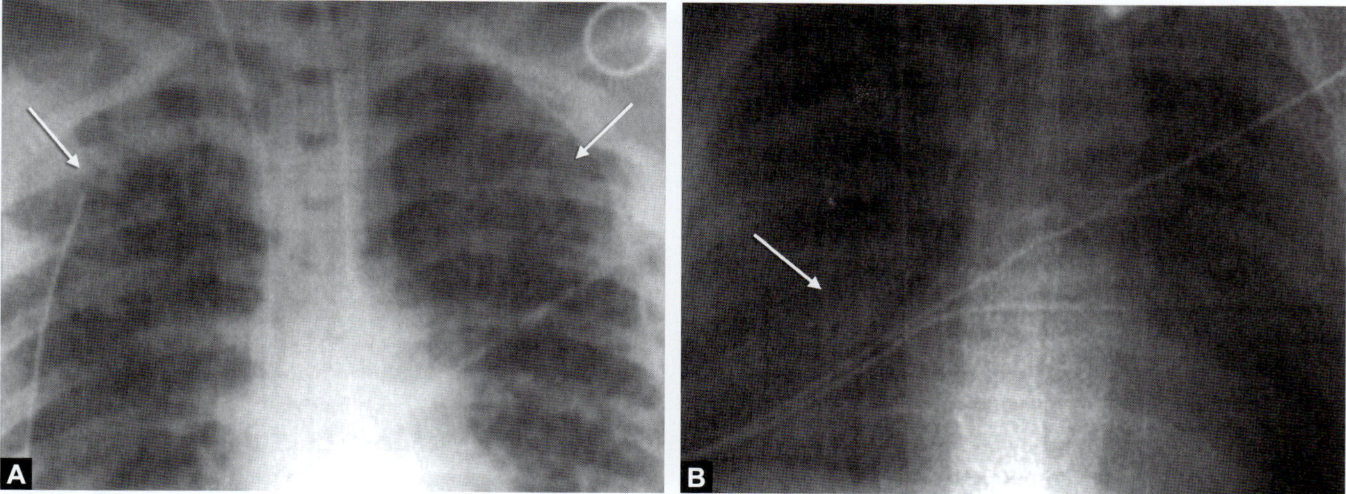

Figs. 7.12A and B: Ventilator-associated pneumonia. (A) Chest radiograph of a patient who has a culture-proven ventilator-associated pneumonia (arrows). The radiographic findings seen can also be seen with chest trauma or from ventilator barotrauma and are not specific for pneumonia. (B) Chest radiograph of a ventilated patient who has adult respiratory distress syndrome. The symmetrical findings bilaterally of the fine infiltration (arrow) are characteristic of adult respiratory distress rather than pneumonia.

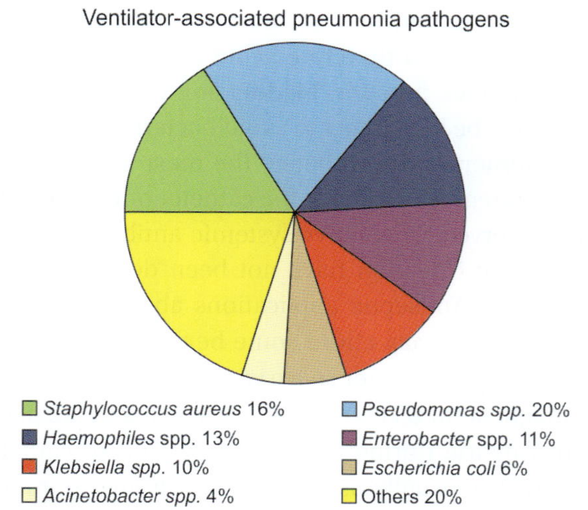

Fig. 7.13: The estimated frequency of pathogens identified in ventilator-associated pneumonia.

pulmonary secretions would generally be recognized as sufficiently diagnostic to permit the initiation of treatment.

Management of VAP requires aggressive antibiotic therapy for the demonstrated pathogen. Gram-negative pathogens with a pattern of antibiotic resistance usually predominate, but staphylococcal isolates have increased in recent years with the prevalence of MRSA (Fig. 7.13). Antibiotic therapy commonly requires combination of drugs that have appropriate synergistic actions against the bacterial pathogens. An aminoglycoside and an expanded-spectrum penicillin (e.g. piperacillin) would be one such strategy. Quinolones, ceftazidime, cefepime, and aztreonam may similarly be used. The use of carbapenem antibiotics such as imipenem–cilastatin, meropenem, or doripenem are commonly used for resistant bacteria. When gram-positive organisms are identified, vancomycin is usually required for coverage of MRSA until all culture results are available. Multiple antibiotics are commonly employed at the beginning of treatment and therapy is typically deescalated once sensitivity data are available.

The duration of antibiotic management in these patients is problematic. Cultures rarely revert to being completely negative. Radiographic changes occur more slowly than clinical improvement. An important measure in the progress of VAP is the ability to wean the patient from the ventilator. Improving arterial oxygenation is evidence that VAP is improving. Successful weaning means that antibiotic therapy can soon be discontinued. Current evidence indicates that systemic antibiotics can be discontinued after 7–10 days of therapy.

Aspiration pneumonia has traditionally been the consequence of inhalation of vomited components from the stomach. This gross aspiration occurs in the clinical setting of the patient who has an altered sensorium who regurgitates gastric contents into the mouth. The aspirated contents establish a chemical pneumonitis that then makes the lung vulnerable to secondary invasive pneumonia (Figs. 7.14A and B). The chemical pneumonitis immediately after aspiration is usually so severe that intubation and ventilator support is necessary. Infection becomes a secondary event.

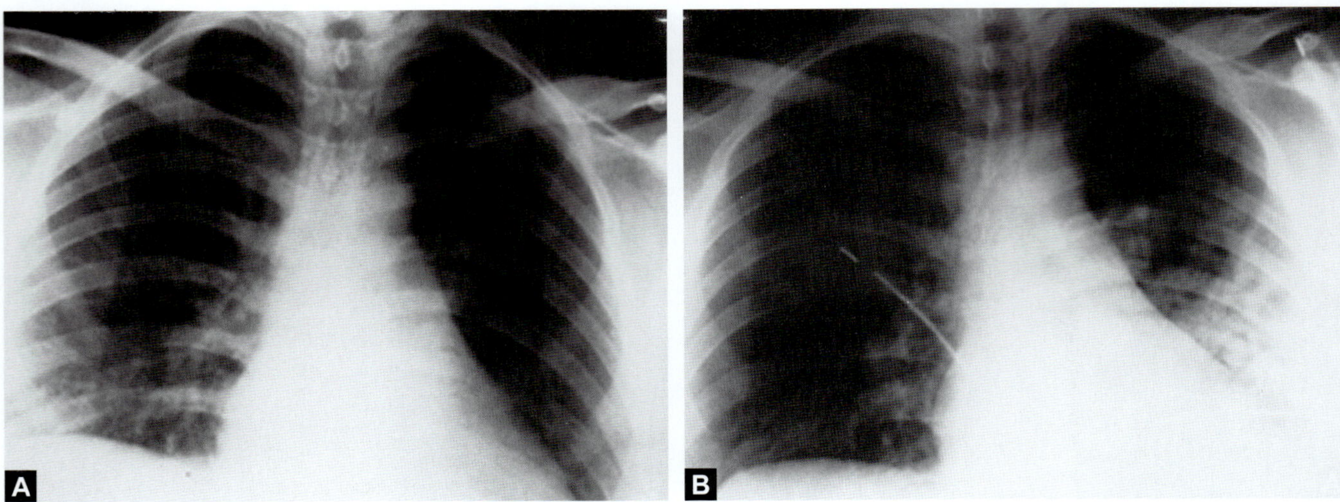

Figs. 7.14A and B: Acute aspiration. (A) Chest radiograph of a patient immediately after an acute aspiration event. (B) A second chest radiograph 12 hours later demonstrates the evolving infiltration.

Prevention of gross aspiration pneumonia begins with gastric decompression during the early postoperative period or after admission for major trauma patients to reduce vomiting and aspiration. Elevation of the head of the bed is potentially helpful. Once the gross aspiration event has occurred and ventilatory assistance has been initiated, preventive strategies follow the guidelines for VAP as noted above.

A diagnosis of gross aspiration is suspected by observation of a vomiting event. Chest radiographs demonstrate a diffuse pattern suggestive of aspiration. Bronchoscopy confirms that aspiration has occurred and also provides the opportunity to remove particulate matter. The use of corticosteroids is not beneficial. Preventive systemic antibiotics are not indicated at the time of the acute aspiration event. Once bacteria are recovered from the lung with quantitative cultures following BAL, a diagnosis of pneumonia is established. Since severe aspiration requires ventilator support, treatment of aspiration pneumonia follows the pattern of VAP.

Urinary Tract Infection

Urinary tract infection in postoperative patients is usually associated with the use of a Foley catheter. A Foley catheter establishes a direct conduit between the bladder lumen and the external environment. Retrograde microbial migration around the catheter results in bacterial access. The balloon of the Foley catheter erodes the protective transitional cell epithelium of the bladder and facilitates bacterial adherence and invasive infection.

Prevention of UTI begins with effective infection control practices at the time of placement of the catheter.[29] The catheter should be anchored to prevent movement of the catheter and therefore avoid the sump effect that draws microbes into the bladder lumen. The drainage system must be kept intact to avoid bacterial access to the internal lumen of the catheter. The most important preventive strategy is to remove the catheter once its purpose has been served. Preventive systemic antibiotics or topical antibiotic irrigation have not been demonstrated to prevent UTI. Antiseptic applications about the external urethral meatus may afford some benefit from microbes entering the pericatheter space within the urethra.

A diagnosis of UTI is clinically suspected in the patient who has pyuria during or after the period of catheterization. UTI is usually associated with fever, suprapubic tenderness, or costovertebral pain or tenderness. Microorganisms may be seen on Gram stain, but cultures are easily obtained and the diagnosis is generally accepted if over 10^5 bacteria/mL of urine with a single pathogen are identified in patients with clinical symptoms. It should be emphasized that the threshold of 10^5 bacteria/mL is based upon criteria developed from community-acquired UTI and may not be completely applicable to the catheterized patient.

The microbiology of postoperative UTI follows a different pattern than that of community-acquired UTI (Fig. 7.15). Infections trend to a variety of gram negatives, enterococci, and Candida spp.[30] Resistant hospital-acquired bacterial pathogens are seen. The presence of these resistant pathogens is directly related to the duration

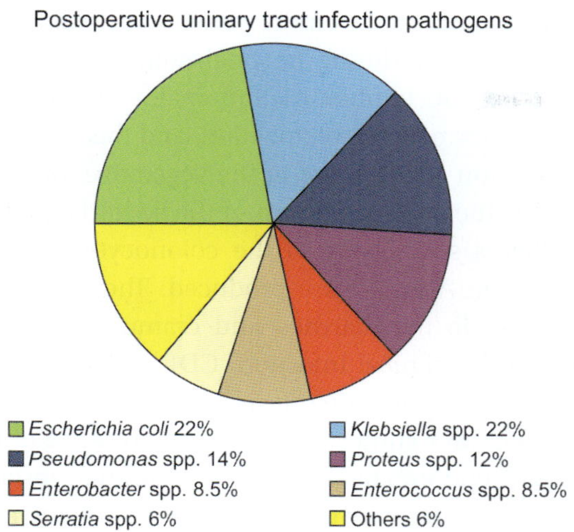

Fig. 7.15: The frequency of likely pathogens to be seen in postoperative urinary tract infections.

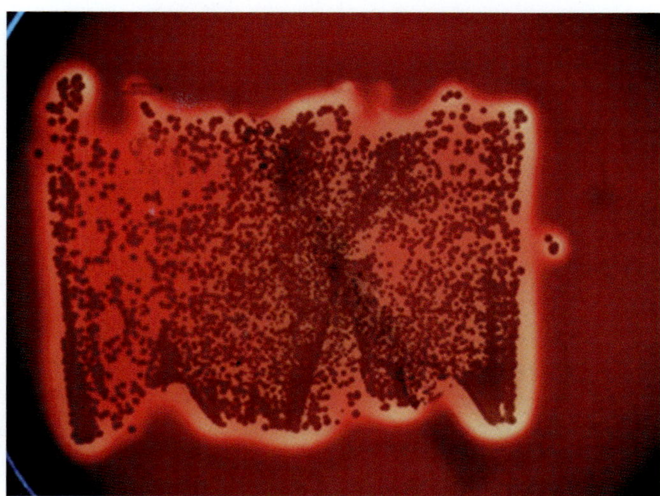

Fig. 7.16: A positive semiquantitative culture from an infected peripheral intravenous catheter. The removed catheter is rolled *over* the surface of a blood agar culture plate. A positive culture is defined as >15 colony forming units.

of hospitalization and the microbiologic pressure created by antecedent antibiotic therapy.

Treatment of UTI requires systemic antibiotic therapy. Fluoroquinolones have become very popular in the treatment of these infections, but sensitivity data are always necessary because of the unanticipated resistant pathogen. Removal of the foreign body from the bladder is desirable. Prerenal volume administration to increase urine flow after removal of the catheter has been associated with the clearance of bacteriuria in younger patients.

Intravascular Device Infections

The numerous intravascular devices in the surgical patient are all portals of direct access for bacteria or fungi into the intravascular compartment. The catheter or device that penetrates the skin and passes into the vein (or artery) results in colonization of the subcutaneous tunnel, either from microbes introduced during placement or from microbial migration around the barrel of the device. Catheter penetration of the vessel wall results in an intravascular thrombus that supports microbial proliferation. Bacterial growth in the thrombus or organisms on the device itself can then be responsible for a bacteremic event.

Prevention of infections from intravascular devices begins with standardized infection control practices in placement.[31] Standard barrier protections with caps, masks, gowns, and gloves are necessary for central line placement. The femoral access site is avoided for central line placement. Various antibiotic or antiseptic ointments have been used over the site of catheter penetration at the time of placement. Chlorhexidine preparations appear to provide the best topical antiseptic agent. Tunneling the catheter has been used to reduce infections. Silver or antibiotic impregnated catheters continue to be evaluated. An occlusive dressing is employed over the placed device. Systemic antibiotics are not appropriate for the prevention of infection in intravascular devices. For peripheral intravenous catheters, removing the device and changing the site of venous access every 72 hours is the best method for prevention.

A diagnosis of intravascular device infection requires a high index of suspicion. All intravascular device sites of patients who have fever and leukocytosis without identified sites of infection must be suspected. New fever on the third or subsequent day following placement suggests that an intravascular device is the source. A positive blood culture for *S. aureus* is a device-related infection until proven otherwise in the postoperative patient.

Infection from a central line catheter is presumed when patients have clinical signs of infection, which resolve with catheter removal. The definitive diagnosis is made with the semiquantitative culture of the offending device (Fig. 7.16).[32] Obviously, the blood culture pathogen and the catheter tip culture should be positive for the same organism. *S. aureus* and *S. epidermidis* are the most common pathogens (Fig. 7.17).[33] Over 50% of *S. aureus* infections are MRSA. Central catheters can be removed over a guidewire and the tip cultured if clinical evidence implicating the catheter is marginal and replacement of the catheter will be a formidable undertaking. If the culture

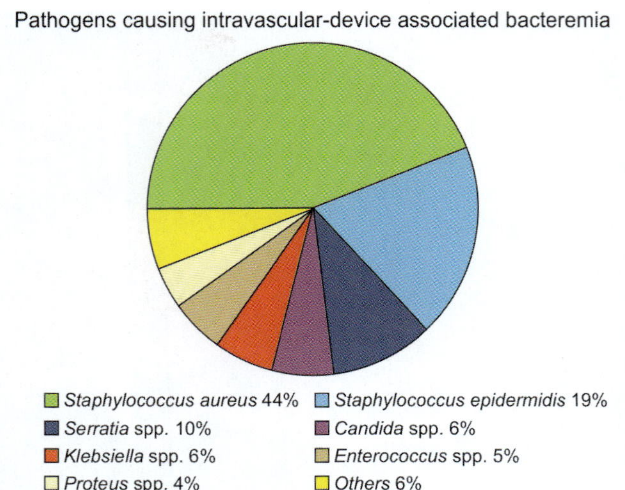

Fig. 7.17: Pathogens identified in semiquantitative cultures from patients who had documented intravascular device-associated blood stream infection.

is positive, the new catheter should be removed and a new access site should be established.

Treatment of intravascular device infections begins with removal of the device. It is inappropriate to suspect a catheter infection, keep the device in place, and administer antibiotics. Only limited antibiotic therapy of a few days is required for gram-negative infections becauseremoval of the catheter generally proves to be definitive. For *S. aureus* bacteremia, 14 days of antibiotic therapy is generally recommended to reduce the risks of metastatic infection (e.g. endocarditis). Candidal fungemia from a device requires continued antimicrobial therapy until resolution of clinical infection.

Persistent bacteremia after removal of the device usually indicates the presence of septic thrombophlebitis. This is suspected when pus is expressed from the catheter site. Continued bacteremia requires excision of the infected vein for peripheral septic thrombophlebitis. Long-segment resections of the infected vessel may be necessary. Central catheter septic thrombophlebitis is a much more difficult situation and surgical removal may not be an option. Continued bacteremia may reflect endocarditis and echocardiography should be carried out. Echocardiography may be desirable before the cessation of antibiotic therapy, even for relatively uncomplicated cases of septic thrombophlebitis.

Clostridium difficile Infection

Clostridium difficile infection is always a consideration when diarrhea in the postoperative surgical patient occurs. This infection occurs when the patient has been exposed either prior to, or during hospitalization, to *C. difficile* spores. Systemic antibiotics and major surgical stress change the normal gut colonization, and this may lead to transformation of the spore to the vegetative form of the bacterium. The vegetative form of the bacterial pathogen then adheres specifically to the colonocyte and enteropathic Toxin A and B are produced. The enteropathic toxins result in the diarrhea and cramping abdominal as signs of the clinical infection. CDI is associated with recent or concurrent antibiotic use, patient age > 70, and in the postoperative surgical patient. The presence of nasogastric and endotracheal tubes are potential portals for access of the spores from the hospital environment into the patient's alimentary tract. Drug therapy with H-2 histamine antagonists, proton-pump inhibitors, and nonsteroidal anti-inflammatory drugs have been associated with CDI.

Prevention of *C. difficile* infection is best achieved by shorter courses of antibiotics. Prevention requires maintenance of relatively normal gut colonization with prudent antibiotic use and enteral feeding. Probiotics and prebiotics have been proposed for prevention, but these strategies have yet to be proven effective. The preemptive use of *C. difficile*-directed antibiotic therapy in postoperative patients for prevention of the infection is not recommended. Infection control practices of adherence to hand washing practices between patient contacts will also reduce the dissemination of spores from patient-to-patient and reduce the risk of this infection.

A diagnosis of CDI is suspected from diarrhea in patients who are receiving antibiotics or have received antibiotics previously during hospitalization. Cramping abdominal pain and varying degrees of abdominal distention are usually present. The diagnosis is confirmed by detection of the toxin for *C. difficile* in fresh stool specimen by enzyme immunoassay methods. Polymerase chain reaction detection of toxin B gene is rapidly becoming the preferred method for diagnosis because of better accuracy.[34] Cultures are generally not used for the diagnosis.

Treatment of CDI is oral antibiotic therapy with metronidazole for mild to moderately severe cases, and with vancomycin for severe cases. Fidaxomycin is a new drug that is used in the treatment of CDI.[35] It has not resulted in better outcomes in acute infections but may result in fewer cases of relapsing infection. Relapsing and recurring CDI is a problem in 20–30% of cases and many of these will require repeated treatment. The difficulty in eradication of recurring CDI in selected patients has even required fecal transplantation as a treatment option.[36]

In very severe cases, a toxic megacolon syndrome can occur and surgical resection of the colon may be necessary. A new mutant strain of *C. difficile* has resulted in a dramatic increase in toxin production that has led to a rapid evolution of severe disease and the need for surgical intervention.[37] Patients with SIRS in association with the rapid evolution of CDI must be considered for laparotomy. CDI is an increasing problem in the United States with more postoperative cases identified each year. CDI has now become a community-acquired infection and requires that surgeons entertain this diagnosis in elderly patient presenting with diarrhea, cramping abdominal pain, and abdominal distention even when no recent antibiotic or hospital exposure has been present.

OTHER BACTERIAL INFECTIONS

Perirectal Abscess

Perirectal abscess is the consequence of infection and inflammation within the cryptoglandular structures at the junction of the rectal mucosa and the anal verge. Inflammation and invasive infection penetrates the full thickness of the rectal wall and invades the perirectal space. Infection usually spreads between the tissue planes, and the abscess "points" externally in the perianal area. However, the process is unpredictable and the infection may track proximally into the pelvis. Perirectal abscess can be extensive and, in diabetic or other immunocompromised patients, can be fatal. Recognized configurations of abscesses include "horseshoe" and intersphincteric collections.

A diagnosis of perirectal abscess is made from the physical examination. A fluctuant mass at the margin of the anal opening is the usual presentation. The sphincter mechanism is palpable between the anal opening and the abscess cavity. Rectal examination may give an indication of the proximal extent of the abscess. Anoscopic examination may identify the internal opening of the fistula tract. Occasionally, induration or depth of the abscess within the perineal tissue may obscure fluctuance, with only a hard palpable mass being present. Needle aspiration confirms the presence of pus in these cases.

Treatment of perirectal abscess is drainage of the pus. A radial incision is made laterally from the medial aspect of the fluctuant mass. An ellipse of skin is taken to ensure patency of the opening. The abscess cavity is digitalized to break up any loculations. The fistula tract may not be seen at drainage and no attempt is made at fistulotomy or fistulectomy at the time of abscess drainage. The cavity is loosely packed with a gauze wick. The wick is removed the next day and sitz baths are initiated three times per day.

Antibiotic therapy is usually not essential for most cases, but it is commonly used. The abscess yields gram-negative rods and obligate anaerobes of colonic origin, but cultures are only necessary for infections among high-risk groups of patients. Proximal extension of the abscess may occur into the pelvic musculature and even to the floor of the pelvis. Complete drainage is necessary and closed suction drains may need to be advanced into large proximal cavities of the pelvic musculature. Patients with diabetes may require extensive debridement of nonviable tissue and repeated operations to achieve complete debridement.

Breast Abscess

Breast abscess most commonly occurs in the immediate postpartum period. Stasis of lactation flow combined with bacteria in the duct system sets the stage for bacterial proliferation and abscess. *S. aureus* is the most common pathogen.

A diagnosis of breast abscess is clinical. The patient complains of severe pain and tenderness in the breast and is usually febrile. Cutaneous erythema and marked induration is commonly present.

Treatment of breast abscess is drainage. Severe pain may require general anesthesia. Loculations within the abscess cavity need to be disrupted. An ellipse of skin is commonly taken at the time of drainage to ensure continued. Cultures are necessary to assess the presence of CA-MRSA. Antibiotics for staphylococci (cefazolin or nafcillin) are used for MSSA and trimethoprim–sulfamethoxazole is commonly used for CA-MRSA. Severe MRSA infections may require hospitalization and vancomycin therapy.

Empyema of the Chest

Empyema of the pleural space most commonly follows placement of a chest tube in trauma patients with hemothorax, or as a postoperative complication after thoracotomy. Bacteria gain access to the pleural space after thoracotomy or tube thoracostomy in the presence of undrained blood or tissue fluids. It may uncommonly be a complication of pulmonary tuberculosis or bacterial pneumonia.

Prevention of empyema requires adherence to infection control practices in the placement of chest tubes. Complete evacuation of blood from the pleural space after blunt or penetrating hemothorax is essential. Retained pleural clot from failed tube drainage may need to be surgically, or thoracoscopically, evacuated to avoid empyema. The probability of empyema increases with the duration of chest tube presence. Early tube removal is important. The use of preventive antibiotics at the time of tube placement may be of value in prevention. Continuing systemic antibiotics following tube placement is not of value.

The diagnosis of empyema is suspected by fever and leukocytosis after thoracotomy or following chest tube placement. Purulent drainage from the chest tube may or may not be present. Chest radiographs show evidence of inflammation or pleural effusion. CT generally proves quite accurate in establishing the diagnosis, and percutaneous drainage may accompany the CT imaging procedure.

Treatment of empyema is drainage of the infection. Replacement of a chest tube into the infected collection or CT placement of catheters has been very successful. Rib resection and placement of an empyema tube may be required for complex collections that are incompletely drained by tube or CT-directed methods. The large-bore empyema tube is then left to drain into a large bulky dressing or into a stomal bag. Entrapment of the lung may require decortication to restore full lung compliance. Antibiotic therapy is tailored to the culture results from drainage but may not add a great deal when drainage of the infection has been effectively done.

Mediastinitis

Mediastinitis is a complication of severe SSI of the sternum following cardiac surgery. It may also occur from esophageal perforations either from trauma or iatrogenic injury. Infection commonly extends into one or both pleural spaces. Mortality rates may approach 50% and require prompt recognition and intervention. Prevention of infection following median sternotomy is achieved by infection control practices during the operation and effective perioperative systemic antibiotics.

The diagnosis is made by purulent discharge from the sternal wound and by instability in the sternal closure. Mediastinitis after esophageal injury or anastomotic leaks after esophageal surgery is made by contrast studies usually at the time of CT examination of the chest. Infections from esophageal leaks commonly are identified with pleural space collections.

Treatment of mediastinitis is complete drainage of the area plus systemic antibiotics. Tube drainage of the mediastinum and the pleural space are necessary to avoid purulent collections. Antibiotic therapy is tailored to the cultured pathogens. SSIs of the sternum are commonly staphylococci but may be gram negatives. Once open drainage of the infected site has occurred, it is not uncommon to have gram-negative pathogens from the hospital environment be secondarily present. Antibiotic therapy is commonly sustained for multiple weeks and is discontinued based upon clinical response of the infection.

Vascular Graft Infections

Prosthetic grafts are extensively used for arterial reconstruction. Although synthetic grafts have greatly expanded the opportunities for vascular reconstruction, infection is more common than with autogenous grafts. Infections of the synthetic graft material can occur early or remote from the time of placement. Graft infections may result in loss of life or limb.

Infection of vascular grafts occurs primarily from intraoperative contamination. Although there is always concern about the potential for remote secondary hematogenous seeding of the graft, prevention of these infections is primarily focused upon the reduction of bacterial contamination during the procedure as discussed earlier.

Prevention of graft infection begins with meticulous surgical technique at the time of graft placement. The prosthetic graft should not make direct contact with the skin during the procedure. Precise hemostasis is required to avoid hematoma. Ligation of lymphatic channels in the groin dissection is also important to avoid lymphoceles.

Preventive systemic antibiotics have been shown to reduce wound infection and, by inference, graft infections. The antibiotics are initiated immediately before the procedure and should be discontinued within 24 hours of the procedure. There is no value for giving multiple days of antibiotics after the procedure. The fibrin matrix, which encases the graft after placement, means that systemic antibiotics given after wound closure are unlikely to reach the graft–fibrin interface at which operative contamination resides.

A diagnosis of graft infection can be obvious or obscure. Purulent discharge from the surgical wound indicates that a wound infection is present and the diagnosis is confirmed if the pus communicates with the graft. Sinography, ultrasonography, and CT scans are used to identify fluid around the graft but only provide indirect evidence of infection. The presence of perigraft fluid is strong evidence favoring graft infection. Radionuclide isotope scans have also been used but remain of uncertain value.

Graft thrombosis and pseudoaneurysm are commonly the consequence of graft infection.

The microbiology of early graft infection is *S. aureus*. The wound drainage appears from cloudy to frank pus. Gram's stains confirm the presence of gram-positive cocci. Infections with *S. epidermidis* are declared later, are more subtle, but are nevertheless from intraoperative contamination. Wound drainage is commonly clear, Gram's stains may reveal no visible bacteria, and cultures are negative. *S. epidermidis* strains produce a biofilm that encases the organisms on the surface of the graft and as a result organisms may not be found in the inflammatory exudate. Sonication of removed graft material may be required to recover these organisms. Gram-negative pathogens are also seen in graft infection, particularly if there has been appreciable preoperative hospitalization or antecedent antibiotic therapy. Diabetic or ischemic ulcers that exist distally on the extremity being revascularized increase the likelihood of gram-negative infection.

Treatment of graft infection requires removal of the prosthetic material. Occasional infections have been successfully treated without graft removal and extended antibiotics, but these are the exception. The consequences of removal of the graft pose special problems because of the critical importance of the disrupted vasculature. Reconstruction is a very complex process requiring consideration for autogenous tissue, extraanatomic bypass, and many other considerations.

Systemic antibiotics for the cultured or anticipated pathogen are used for treatment. When *S. aureus* is the pathogen, MRSA is always a consideration in antibiotic coverage. Since many of these patients will have had extensive interaction with the healthcare system and with prior antibiotic therapy, gram negatives with resistant antibiotic sensitivities will make the choice of antibiotics driven by culture results.

Postsplenectomy Sepsis

A function of the spleen is to clear encapsulated bacteria from the circulation. In the absence of the spleen clearance of transient bacteremic events, likely to be from the respiratory or upper aerodigestive tracts, it is required to have opsonization for hepatic clearance. Therefore, younger patients who do not have specific immunity for the various encapsulated microbes have a risk of developing fulminant postsplenectomy sepsis syndrome following splenectomy. Similarly, older splenectomy patients who have an immunocompromised state are at risk.

Prevention of postsplenectomy sepsis has occurred by the use of greater efforts to avoid splenectomy. Indications for splenectomy in trauma have become quite restrictive for patients < 30 years of age. When splenectomy is necessary, specific vaccination is carried out for the common serotypes of encapsulated bacteria (e.g. pneumococcus, meningococcus, and *H. influenzae*). The risk remains for these patients because the vaccines contain only the antigens for the most common serotypes of bacteria.

Postsplenectomy sepsis is characterized by a fulminant infection that rapidly progresses to septic shock. Patients, the family, and the physician must be keenly aware of this risk in the splenectomized patient. A prompt response is necessary for any febrile illness, especially those of respiratory origin. Antibiotics to cover the likely pathogen need to be initiated promptly. Blood cultures usually document the infection, but they are not available until too late in the process.

Treatment of postsplenectomy sepsis is aggressive antibiotic therapy. General supportive care, including intravascular volume support and oxygenation, are very important during the early phases of this rapidly evolving infection.

FUNGAL INFECTIONS OF SURGICAL IMPORTANCE

The advent of antibiotics with greater spectra of activity and the increasing number of immunocompromised patients means that fungal infections are now more common in surgical patients. These infections have principally been complications of inpatient management. Although surgeons may be involved in the care of patients who have community-acquired fungal infections (e.g. blastomycosis, histoplasmosis, cryptococcal infections), the nosocomial fungal infections with *Candida* spp. are most common.

Candida albicans Infections

Candida infections occur by several different mechanisms. First, *Candida albicans* may directly infect an anatomic site in much the same way that bacterial infections do. Sites of candida infection include oropharyngitis (thrush), esophagitis, meningitis, osteoarthritis, endocarditis, and endophthalmitis. *C. albicans* is seen among infections in the peritoneal cavity and the urinary tract. The key factors for these infections are long-term broad-spectrum antibiotic therapy and an immunocompromised host. Second, candidemia occurs as a blood-borne infection from central vein intravascular devices. Finally, candidemia occurs from translocation of the fungus from the proximal gastrointestinal reservoir. Protein–calorie malnutrition, antineoplastic chemotherapy, corticosteroid therapy, and broad-spectrum systemic antibiotic therapy are the predisposing factors. Prevention of *C. albicans* infection is best achieved by reductions in the number and duration of broad-spectrum antibiotics, by enteral feeding to enhance normal gut colonization, and avoidance of the central vein catheter. Chemotherapeutic prophylaxis is considered for high-risk patients (e.g. transplantation recipients) with fluconazole.

A diagnosis of candida infection generally requires isolation of the fungus from two separate anatomic sites. Cultures of the pharynx, peritoneal cavity, or urinary tract readily grow *C. albicans* if present. Blood cultures are considered necessary to establish a diagnosis of candidemia. For visceral candidiasis, biopsy (e.g. liver) may be necessary for histologic confirmation. Positive blood cultures should immediately trigger concern that a central catheter is responsible. Removal of central catheters and catheter-tip cultures are necessary.

The treatment of choice is the echinocandins: caspofungin (50 mg daily), anidulafungin (50–100 mg daily), or micafungin (50–150 mg daily).[38] If *C. albicans* is the pathogen then fluconazole is commonly added. Fluconazole does not add benefit to the echinocandins for non-*albicans* candidal infections.

Aspergillus Infections

Aspergillus fumigatus is an airborne opportunistic pathogen as a pulmonary, sinus, or ear infection in immunosuppressed or debilitated patients. A recognized form of this pulmonary infection is a matted ball of vegetations known as an "aspergilloma." This pathogen can disseminate and be associated with endocarditis, endophthalmitis, and even solid organ infections. The organism is easily cultured and isolation from the suspected lung or sinus establishes the diagnosis. Tissue biopsy is occasionally necessary for diagnosis.

Treatment of these infections is with voriconazole (4 mg/kg every 12 hours).[39] Severe hemoptysis may require lung resection. Drainage and debridement may be necessary for invasive sinus infections.

Mucormycosis

Mucormycosis is an uncommon fungal infection of the sinuses, lung, and even soft tissue or burn wounds. There are over 100 different fungal species that cause these infections, but they are collectively referred to as mucormycosis. These ubiquitous fungi are airborne or from the soil. The severely immunocompromised or the severe diabetic is the typical host. The diagnosis is usually suggested by a black discharge or eschar at the infected site. Tissue biopsy and histologic recognition of invasive fungal infection is most reliable, since cultures are inconsistently positive. The infections are managed by local surgical debridement and systemic lipid formulations of amphotericin B (3–6 mg/kg daily).

VIRAL INFECTIONS OF SURGICAL SIGNIFICANCE

Viruses are assuming a greater role in infections of significance to surgeons. They can be infectious complications in immunosuppressed patients (e.g. transplantation). They are recognized as having an increasing role in oncogenesis. Viruses continue to be an occupational risk to surgeons from blood exposure.

Hepatitis

Multiple distinct hepatitis viruses have been characterized, and there is reason to believe that additional strains remain to be defined. Hepatitis A and E are transmitted by the fecal–oral route, are self-limited acute infections that can be quite severe, but are not associated with a chronic persistent state. They are not associated with postnecrotic cirrhosis. Hepatitis D is an incomplete RNA virus that must have acute or chronic hepatitis B (HBV) infection present for it to have clinical relevance as a synergistic pathogen. Hepatitis G appears to be a variant of hepatitis C (HCV) and is not clearly associated as having an independent role in human hepatitis infection, although the virus may be carried by 2% of the US population. The TT (Transfusion Transmitted) and SEN viruses have been reported, but their role in human hepatitis remains to be clarified. It is HBV and HCV as blood-borne viruses that have the greatest clinical relevance to surgeons.

Hepatitis B

HBV is a DNA virus that is transmitted by the blood-borne route. It is most commonly associated with intravenous drug abuse or sexual transmission. The virus binds to the liver cell as the target site for the infection. Infection of the host only results in clinical disease in about 25 % of documented infections. In 5% of infections, the patient develops chronic HBV and is infectious to others for life.

Table 7.5 Details characteristics of the eight human herpesviruses.

HHV-type	Common name(s)	Site of latency	Surgical significance
1	Herpes simplex virus-1	Sensory nerves	Reactivation disease in immunosuppressed patients
2	Herpes simplex virus 2, or genital herpes	Sensory nerves	Reactivation disease in immunosuppressed patients
3	Varicella (chickenpox), herpes zoster (shingles)	Sensory nerves	Varicella associated with necrotizing soft tissue infections; zoster is reactivation disease in immunosuppressed, cancer, and transplant patients
4	Epstein–Barr virus	B-cells and endothelial cells	Burkitt's lymphoma, nasopharyngeal cancers, posttransplantation lymphoproliferative syndrome
5	Cytomegalovirus	Lymphocytes and endothelial cells	Reactivation disease in transplant patients
6	Roseola infantum	Lymphocytes	Reactivation disease in immunosuppressed patients
7	Pityriasis rosea	Lymphocytes	Reactivation disease in transplant recipients
8	Kaposi's sarcoma virus	Endothelial cells	Kaposi's sarcoma in HIV and other immunosuppressed populations; associated with Castleman's disease.

The natural history of the disease in selected cases is for the chronically infected host to proceed to cirrhosis, portal hypertension, hepatocellular carcinoma, or end-stage liver disease. A number of infected cases have chronic persistent infection and do not have progressive liver disease but nevertheless remain infectious to others. It is currently estimated that over 350 million people in the world have chronic HBV.

Prevention of HBV infection is by vaccination of populations at-risk for the infection. A safe and effective vaccine against HBV is readily available. The three-dose vaccination process over 6 months confers an antibody response and protection for 95% of individuals who receive it. Antibody titers should be confirmed after completion of the vaccination process to document seroconversion. Those not seroconverting on the initial vaccination should have the entire three-dose process repeated. Expanding the population of people to receive the vaccine will hopefully yield a progressive reduction of acute and chronic infections. For unvaccinated people or those not seroconverting to repeated vaccination attempts, avoidance of high-risk personal conduct is the means to avoid infection.

The diagnosis of HBV infection is made by detection of antibody to the core antigen of the virus. A positive serology confirms that infection has occurred and detection of the antigen for HBV indicates whether the individual has current infection. The presence of the antigen that is temporally remote from the acute infection becomes the measure for defining chronic HBV.

There are currently seven different drugs that are employed for the treatment of chronic HBV infection (Table 7.5).[40] Combinations of these treatments have been documented to reduce the burden of the virus with the hope that this will result in an arrested progression of the chronic disease. The treatments at this point are not considered curative.

HBV has been a recognized occupational risk to surgeons and other healthcare workers since 1950.[41] Prospective studies have noted that as many as 30% of unvaccinated and previously uninfected healthcare workers will acquire acute HBV as a result of a single needlestick exposure from an antigen-positive patient. The best method for protection from occupational HBV infection is for all surgeons and all healthcare personnel to be vaccinated against HBV. Because chronic HBV infection in surgeons has been demonstrated to result in transmission of infection to patients, vaccination avoids the problem of whether the chronically infected surgeon should continue in surgical care.

Hepatitis C

Hepatitis C (HCV) is a blood-borne RNA virus that was characterized in 1989. HCV is the major constituent of what was formerly known as non-A, non-B hepatitis. It too is a virus that targets the hepatocyte in the exposed host. Like HBC, HCV infection is clinically occult with acute infection is 70–75% of cases. Unlike HBV, chronic disease persists in 60–80% of patients. HCV infection is primarily identified with percutaneous exposure to infected blood or blood products. It has been associated with multiple sexual partners. The natural history of the disease is unpredictable with some patients spontaneously clearing the virus, and as many as 20% progressing to end-stage liver disease or hepatocarcinoma. Chronically infected patients are infectious to others. There is no vaccine for HCV, so avoidance of blood exposure is the only preventive strategy.

The diagnosis of HCV infection is presumed when persistent antibody is found for HCV. Chronic infection is confirmed by reverse-transcriptase polymerase chain reaction for detection of viral RNA. Patients with persistence of liver enzyme elevations should undergo liver biopsy to evaluate hepatic fibrosis.

Like chronic HBV infection, dramatic improvements have been made in the treatment of chronic HCV infection.[42] Overall viral eradication has been achieved in 80% of all treated patients and in 60% of type-1 chronic HCV with the use of the protease inhibitor treatments. The expense of treatment continues to be an issue for wider deployment of these new anti-HCV treatments.

Chronic HCV infection exists in 150 million people worldwide and accounts for over 350,000 deaths annually.[43] It remains an occupational risk for surgeons. Transmission from infected patients to surgeons and from infected surgeons to patients has been documented. Since there is no vaccine, surgeons, and all healthcare workers need to adopt behaviors that avoid blood exposure in patient care. Because of effective treatment for HCV infection, all exposed individuals in the operating room should be screen for evidence of transmission so that early therapy can be initiated.

Human Immunodeficiency Virus (HIV) Infection

Human immunodeficiency virus (HIV) is the RNA blood-borne retrovirus of the acquired immunodeficiency syndrome (AIDS). The infection preferentially attacks the CD4 T-cells of the host and causes a deficiency in cell-mediated immunity. The untreated natural history of the disease results in unusual infections and neoplasia. Without treatment the disease is considered to be uniformly fatal after the latent period of infection that may last for a decade. There are estimated to be about 35 million people in the world who are living with HIV infection.

Transmission of HIV infection is from exposure to infected blood or body fluids. Sexual contact and intravenous drug abuse are the most common causes. Vertical transmission to the child from an infected mother has dramatically reduced in frequency with peripartum, antiretroviral treatments. Effective blood screening has virtually eliminated transfusion as a means of transmission.

The diagnosis of HIV infection is initiated by detection of anti-HIV specific antibodies. A western blot is then performed to confirm the diagnosis. Indeterminate diagnoses requiring direct viral detection have become infrequent with refinements in diagnostic procedures.

Dramatic improvements in treatment for HIV infection have led to the development of the highly-effective anti-retroviral therapy (HEART). The potential treatments are from six different categories of drugs. Three or more drugs will be chosen from different categories based upon mechanism of action for initial treatment of the naïve patient. New guidelines have been recommended for earlier treatment to avoid disease progression.[44] Progress is monitored with CD4 cell counts and by direct measurement of viral RNA units in blood. Additional drugs are added and others are replaced based upon monitoring of the patients progress with treatment. Extensive expertise is required in the management of these multiple treatment options.

Recognition of HIV infection as a blood-borne disease resulted in enormous concern about the occupational risks to surgeons and other healthcare workers. A total of 57 healthcare workers have been documented to have acquired occupational HIV infection, but none have been surgeons.[45] There are a small number of cases (>10) that have been evaluated as probable transmissions for this entire period of time. The advent of HEART has further reduced the risk by having HIV patients coming to operation with very low viral counts. The fears of the past appear unwarranted with respect to occupational risks of HIV for healthcare workers. Nevertheless, there remains a risk for HIV transmission with percutaneous exposure. Blood exposure must be viewed as a potential risk for HCV and other potential pathogens within the blood supply.

Human Herpesviruses (HHVs)

The eight human herpesviruses (HHVs) are summarized in Table 7.5. These are very common viral infections. Acute infection is self-limited, but the virus is retained within nerve cells for life. Thus, reactivation of clinical infection is a characteristic of the HHVs. For most patients they do not have any long-term sequelae. HHV-3 is the responsible virus for herpes zoster, which is commonly seen in adult surgical patients. HHV-4 (EB virus) has been associated with mononucleosis and Burkitt's lymphoma. HHV-8 is the virus responsible for Kaposi's sarcoma, which has become a recognized entity in immunosuppression in patients with advanced HIV infection. It is cytomegalovirus (CMV) (HHV-5) infection that will be primarily discussed here.

Cytomegalovirus is a ubiquitous virus that can cause a mild mononucleosis-like syndrome with acute infection, but it has greatest clinical consequences as an infection in immunosuppressed transplant, cancer, and AIDS patients. The virus appears to be chronically carried among

60–70% of individuals, but it is not associated with any clinical infection. Transmission of infection occurs by blood exposure, sexual contact, transfusion, and organ transplantation. Clinical infection emerges in the surgical patient from either activation of preexistent latent virus in the host after the development of immunosuppression, or acute new viral infection derived from transfusion or organ transplantation.

Prevention of CMV infection has been actively pursued, especially for transplant patients. It is important to know if an organ recipient is seronegative for CMV so that preventive antiviral therapy can be used for 3–6 months after exposure. Ganciclovir, valacyclovir, and valganciclovir are used for prevention.

Acute CMV infection or reactivation in the immunosuppressed host has the clinical appearance of any severe infection. Fever and the clinical septic picture are not unlike those of bacterial or fungal infections. The patients develop a febrile mononucleosis-like disease associated with an interstitial pneumonitis and hepatitis-like syndrome. CMV ulceration of the gastrointestinal tract may lead to perforation of the gut. Retinitis and encephalitis may also develop. The clinical diagnosis is confirmed by antigen detection, DNA detection, or even viral isolation. In general, serologic methods of diagnosis have had limited usefulness because a 4-week period may be required for acute antibody responses. Also, antibody titers remain high for a sustained period after reactivation and current detection may reflect a prior event.

Treatment of CMV infection involves efforts to improve the patient's immunosuppressed status and antiviral drug therapy. For transplant patients, it may be necessary to reduce immunosuppression drug therapy. Appropriate nutritional support measures to improve host responsiveness are also necessary. Ganciclovir or valganciclovir is the treatment of choice for confirmed active CMV infection.

Human Papillomavirus (HPV)

Human papillomavirus (HPV) infects human epithelium. These viruses are transmitted by direct contact with another infected patient and to some degree by environment contact. Infection of the basal layer keratinocyte occurs when a break in the overlying epidermal layers permit access of the viral contaminant to the basal layer where infection occurs. The virus then is propagated as the keratinocytes divide. There is no acute inflammatory response and no acute clinical infection. In the vast majority of the cases, the infection either completely resolves or may become latent. In selected cases, benign or malignant epithelial lesions evolve.

There are over 100 unique types of HPV. They are numbered individually and are identified by detection of unique DNA sequences. Types 16 and 18 are most commonly associated with invasive squamous cancer, whereas types 6 and 11 are most commonly associated with benign anogenital warts. Cutaneous warts are very common in the population and are due to an array of other HPV types. Sexual contact is the major route for transmission for HPV-associated cancers and anogenital warts.

HPV infection is the cause of virtually all human cervical carcinoma and a large percentage of vaginal, labial, and anal carcinomas. In recent years, HPV has become an increasingly associated cause of head and neck squamous cancers. It appears that HPV as a cause of head and neck cancer may be exceeding traditional causes of tobacco and alcohol, and HPV head and neck cancers are likely to eclipse cervical cancer in frequency if current trends continue. In 50% of cases, penile carcinoma is associated with HPV infection.

The diagnosis of HPV infection has traditionally been made with the identification of epidermal pathology. Warts and genital lesions have been identified and treatments have been implemented. Pap smears have been used to identify abnormal cytology that is characteristic of premalignant dysplastic lesions of the cervix. Biopsy of suspicious areas based upon high-risk behavior or clinical concern about abnormalities has identified intraepithelial neoplasia that is precursor of invasive cancer. Direct detection of HPV-types 16 and 18 are being used to identify the presence of the cancer-associated viral types and permits biopsies and clinical assessments to be intensively pursed for those patients with known infection.

Prevention of HPV infection by vaccination is being used. A bivalent vaccine, which covers HPV-types 16 and 18, and a quadrivalent vaccine that also includes types 6 and 11, are presently being used. The vaccines must be administered prior to sexual activity and already established HPV infection. They have been shown to reduce rates of detected infections with the targeted HPV-types and to reduce the development of cervical intraepithelial neoplasia. These vaccines continue to be studied to identify whether actual invasive cancer rates will be less and to evaluate the longevity of protection. The extension of the vaccination program to males is being recommended since they become the source of transmission for female HPV infection. Because males appear to have a threefold

Table 7.6 Therapies for the management of anogenital warts. None of medical therapies are proven safe for pregnant patients.

Treatment	*Preparation*	*Commentary*
Imiquimod	5% cream	Self-administered three times per week for up to 16 weeks. Treated area should be washed 6–10 h after application. Treatment is immune enhancer and will have local inflammatory reactions.
Podofilox	0.5% solution or gel	Self-administered application twice per day for 3 days with 4 days off. Repeated for four cycles if necessary. Mild pain and discomfort. Only for wart burden < 10 cm^2.
Podophyllin resin	10–25% in tincture of benzoin	Applied weekly by healthcare provider. Applied to only 10 cm^2 per treatment episode. Air drying is necessary at application to avoid contact with normal skin from clothing. Area of treatment should be washed 1–4 h after application.
Sinecatechins	15% ointment	Self-administered green tea extract. Applied three times daily for up to 16 weeks. Local burning and pain. Not recommended for immunosuppressed (e.g. HIV) patients.
Trichloroacetic or bichloroacetic acid	80–90% solution	Chemical coagulation of proteins. Applied by healthcare provider once per week. Must dry to avoid injury to adjacent tissues. Pain and irritation.
Cryotherapy	Liquid nitrogen	Liquid nitrogen application by healthcare provider. Care must be taken to avoided injury to adjacent tissues. Effective therapy will have pain. Repeat applications are commonly necessary.
Surgical removal	Electrocautery, laser, tangential excision, curettage.	Surgical removal by excision or electrocautery is reserved for large burden of warts. Topical therapy may be required for small residual lesions.

higher rate of HPV-associated head and neck cancer, vaccination may have a longer-term benefit for men.

The treatment of the several HPV-associated cancers is covered elsewhere in this book. The treatment of benign anogenital lesions are managed by podophyllin preparations, imiquimod cream, freezing, electrocautery, and by surgical excision (for large bulk lesions)[46] (Table 7.6). The treatment of cutaneous warts has been best with topical salicylic acid, although a host of other treatments have been used in the management of these lesions.[47]

PROTOZOAN INFECTIONS OF SURGICAL SIGNIFICANCE

Protozoan infections are relatively infrequent in surgical patients. Most are community-acquired infections from the ingestion of contaminated food or water.

Entamoeba histolytica Infection

Amebic colitis is a worldwide problem. Fecal-oral transmission occurs when infective cysts are ingested from contaminated water or food and the cysts mature to trophozoites (Fig. 7.18), which then penetrate and damage the colonocyte lining. The infection may then spread to other organs, most notably the liver, in which amebic abscess is the result. Prevention is only achieved by avoiding cyst ingestion.

A diagnosis of amebic colitis is suggested by an acute onset of diarrhea and abdominal pain. Localized or generalized tenderness is present. Fever is not a predictable finding. The diagnosis is most dependably made by identification of the *Entamoeba histolytica* trophozoites in a fresh stool specimen. Detection of amebic proteins or DNA is an evolving diagnostic strategy. Coloscopy commonly demonstrates characteristic flask-shaped mucosal ulcerations. These amebomas of the colon may resemble colon neoplasms. Endoscopic scrapings of ulcerative lesions are excellent specimens to identify trophozoites. Right upper quadrant pain and hepatomegaly suggest

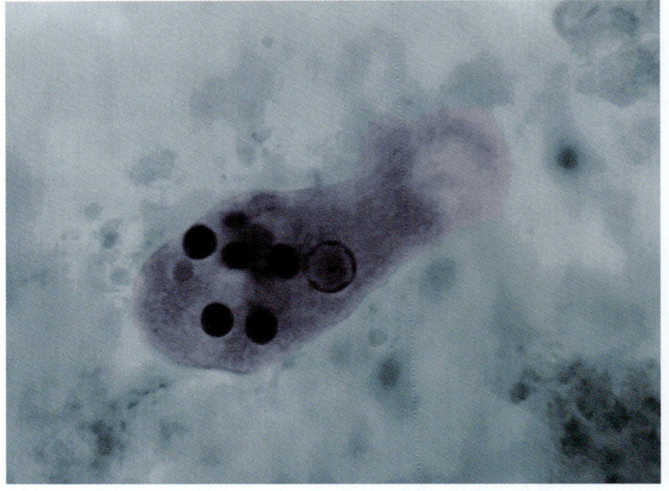

Fig. 7.18: This photomicrograph (trichrome stain) illustrates *an Entamoeba histolytica* trophozoite with internalized red blood cells. From the Public Health Image Library, Centers for Disease Control, Atlanta, Georgia. Contributed by Dr. Mae Melvin. http://phil.cdc.gov/phil/quicksearch.asp.

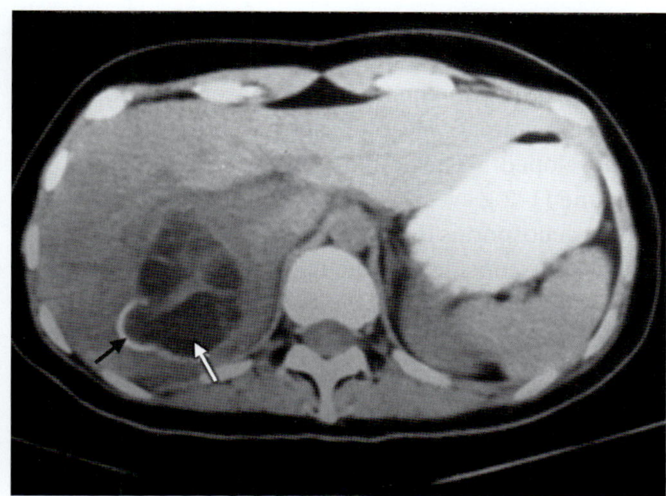

Fig. 7.19: Abdominal computed tomography scan showing a hydatid cyst (white arrow) of the liver. Cyst wall is indicated by black arrow.

amebic abscess of the liver. CT scans identify the round or oval abscess, which tends to be near the periphery of the liver.

Treatment of amebic colitis and abscess is systemic metronidazole. Liver abscesses generally respond promptly to metronidazole treatment and do not requiremechanical drainage. Some evidence supports that tinidazole may have better results has been presented,[48]metronidazole is still the recommended treatment. Some recommend percutaneous drainage of large abscesses (>10 cm in diameter) or those that are unusually symptomatic and generate concern about possible rupture. The occasional case may not respond to amebicidal therapy and require drainage. Fulminate colitis or colonic rupture can occur and require surgical interventions.

Echinococcal Infection

Echinococcal infection most commonly results from *Echinococcus granulosus* infection. Ingestion of contaminated food or water containing the ova of the echinococcus results in the development of the mature oncosphere. The oncosphere penetrates the intestinal mucosa and enters the portal circulation. It lodges in the liver to form a hydatid cyst. Hydatid cysts can also occur in the lung, brain, and other tissues.

The diagnosis is suspected in people who have a culture or occupation that involves simultaneous exposure to dogs and sheep together. Symptoms tend to be nonspecific and relate to the hydatid cyst. Cysts are commonly found by ultrasound evaluation for cholelithiasis. CT scans identify the characteristic cystic lesion in the

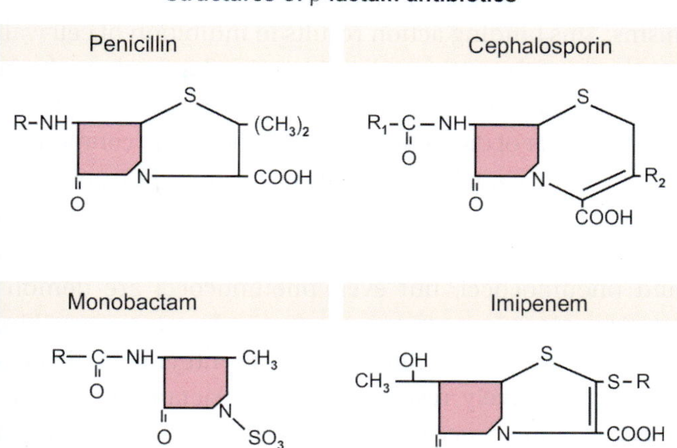

Fig. 7.20: Similar structures of the different β-lactam antibiotics. The shaded area identifies the common β-lactam ring. Enzymatic disruption of this ring neutralizes the activity of the antibiotic.

liver. Calcification of a portion of the cyst wall is not uncommon (Fig. 7.19). Various serologic studies are employed for confirming the diagnosis when it is suspected by imaging studies.

Treatment of hydatid liver cysts is evacuation of the lesion and removal of the cyst membrane. At operation the cyst is injected with hypertonic saline or formalin. The cyst is carefully evacuated with a trocar. The endocyst lining is removed. Liver resection may be required for particularly difficult or large cysts. Systemic albendazole therapy is used before and in the period after cyst evacuation. Albendazole therapy (400 mg twice daily by mouth) is used without surgical intervention in selected patients with small hepatic cysts and in patients with extrahepatic disease. Albendazole therapy is extended for ≥ 3 months.

ANTIBIOTICS

Since the introduction of penicillin and sulfa in the early 1940s, a vast array of different types of antibiotics have been introduced into surgical practice. Each of these antibiotics has a different mechanism of action, a different spectrum of antimicrobial coverage and a different scope of potential toxicity. Doses indicated for each drug are adult recommendations that are intravenously administered unless indicated otherwise.

Penicillins

Penicillin antibiotics are in the broad class of β-lactam antibiotics (Fig. 7.20). The biologic action of penicillin antibiotics results from binding to specific penicillin-binding proteins on the plasma membrane of target microorganisms. This binding action results in inhibition of cell wall synthesis of the actively dividing microbes and results in lysis of the actively dividing microorganisms.

A number of different intravenous penicillin compounds are currently available. Penicillin G (12–24 million units/day in divided doses) has primary activity against common gram-positive organisms, such as pyogenic streptococci and pneumococci, but even pneumococci are demonstrating some increasing resistance of recent. Oxacillin, nafcillin, and methicillin are semisynthetic penicillins that are relatively resistant to the β-lactamase production by staphylococcal organisms, although only nafcillin (500 mg–1 g every 4 hours) is commonly used at present. Ampicillin (1–2 g every 4–6 hours) was the first penicillin antibiotic to have gram-negative coverage. Advanced-generation penicillins, such as ticarcillin and piperacillin, have extensive gram-negative coverage to include *Enterobacter* spp. and even some strains of *Pseudomonas* spp. The addition of β-lactamase inhibitors, such as clavulanic acid with ticarcillin (3.1 g every 4–6 hours), sulbactam with ampicillin (1.5–3.0 g every 6 hours), and tazobactam with piperacillin (3.375 g every 6 hours) have resulted in expanded spectrums of activity.

The toxicity of the penicillins is principally hypersensitivity reactions, which can vary from mild allergic rashes to anaphylaxis. Every patient should be asked about a history of penicillin allergy when considering antibiotic therapy.

Cephalosporins

The cephalosporins are β-lactam drugs that have been used extensively in surgical practice. Cephalothin was the first of the cephalosporins and had activity against most aerobic gram-positive organisms including *S. aureus,* and *E. coli* and *Klebsiella* spp. among the gram-negatives, but is no longer used. Cefazolin (1 g every 6–8 hrs) is a longer half-life first-generation cephalosporin that has similar activity to cephalothin and continues to be extensively used for surgical prophylaxis when gram-positive organisms are sources of concern.

The second-generation cephalosporins have a broader scope of activity than cefazolin. These include cefamandole (500 mg–1 g every 4–8 hours), cefuroxime (750 mg–1.5 g every 8 hours), cefoxitin (1–2 g every 6–8 hours), and cefotetan (1–2 g every 12 hours). Cefoxitin and cefotetan have anaerobic activity.

Advanced-generation cephalosporins include cefotaxime (1–2 g every 6–8 hours) and ceftriaxone (1–2 g daily), which have excellent activity against common gram-negative aerobes but reduced gram-positive activity. Activity against *Pseudomonas* spp. was observed among these advanced-generation cephalosporins, but resistance rapidly developed. Ceftazidime (1 g every 8–12 hours) and cefepime (1–2 g every 8–12 hours) are advanced-generation cephalosporins that have essentially no gram-positive activity but considerable activity against gram-negative pathogens including *Pseudomonas aeruginosa.* Ceftaroline (600 mg every 12 hours) and ceftobiprole (500 mg every 8 hours) are new advanced-generation cephalosporins with activity against MRSA but are not available in all countries. As a general rule, the advanced-generation cephalosporins have limited activity against anaerobic bacteria.

Like the penicillins, the cephalosporins bind to penicillin-binding proteins on the plasma membrane of the target organism. Inhibition of cell wall synthesis is the result. Hypersensitivity to the cephalosporins is less common than with the penicillins.

Carbapenems

The carbapenem antibiotics include imipenem/cilastatin (500 mg–1 g every 6–8 hours), meropenem (500 mg–1 g every 8 hours), doripenem (500 mg every 8 hours), and ertapenem (1 g daily). These antibiotics have activity against gram-positive, gram-negative, and obligate anaerobic organisms. Ertapenem does not have activity against *Pseudomonas* sp. The carbapenems are commonly used when empiric therapy is required for broad-spectrum coverage or if resistant organisms are anticipated. The toxicity of carbapenems has been principally CNS toxicity with high dosing schedules.

Monobactams

Aztreonam (1–2 g every 6–8 hours) is the prototype monobactam antibiotic. It binds to penicillin proteins and inhibits cell wall synthesis. Aztreonam has use against gram-negative aerobic microorganisms but has no activity against obligate anaerobes. It has no unique toxicity.

Aminoglycosides

The aminoglycosides have been used extensively to treat gram-negative infections in surgical patients. They have been particularly active against *Serratia, Enterobacter,* and *Pseudomonas* spp. and other nosocomial gram-negative infections in the intensive care unit. Gentamicin (1 mg/kg every 8 hours), tobramycin (1 mg/kg every 8 hours), and amikacin (5 mg/kg every 8 hours, or 7.5 mg/kg every 12 hours) are the principal aminoglycoside antibiotics. The aminoglycosides bind irreversibly to the ribosomes in the cytoplasm of the target microorganism. The irreversible binding to ribosomes and the inhibition of protein synthesis by the aminoglycosides translates into bactericidal activity. A postantibiotic effect is seen secondary to this irreversible binding in that continued drug effect is seen even after a given dose has been completely eliminated.

The aminoglycoside antibiotics have both nephrotoxicity and ototoxicity. The toxicity combined with the precarious and unpredictable pharmacokinetics of the aminoglycosides necessitates pharmacokinetic dosing to minimize toxicity. The toxicity of the aminoglycosides resulted in reduced utilization over recent years. This reduced usage has led to improved activity of these drugs against many gram-negative isolates and may lead to a resurgence of use.

Tetracyclines

The tetracyclines bind in a reversible fashion to cytoplasmic ribosomes of target organisms and inhibit protein synthesis. The reversible binding of the tetracyclines makes them bacteriostatic antibiotics. The principal activity of the tetracyclines has been against the common gram-negative bacteria, but they have some activity against obligate enteric anaerobic bacteria. The tetracyclines have been relatively safe with rare hypersensitivity reactions. Tetracycline is seldom used intravenously at present and is dosed at 1 g daily in 2–4 divided doses. Doxycycline (50–100 gm every 12–24 hours) is a tetracycline derivative that continues to be used for selected gram-positive and gram-negative infections and does have some use for CA-MRSA.

Tigecycline is a glycylcycline antibiotic that shares structural features of the tetracycline group. It has a broad spectrum of activity that includes gram-positive, gram-negative, and anaerobic pathogens. It also has MRSA activity. It has a wide range of clinical uses because of its very broad spectrum of activity. It is dosed at 100 mg initially with 50 mg every 12 hours to follow.

Erythromycin

Erythromycin binds in a reversible fashion to ribosomes and inhibits protein synthesis. It has activity against common gram-negative aerobic organisms and extensive anaerobic activity. It is locally toxic when administered via the intravenous (500 mg every 6 hours) or intramuscular route and this has limited its use. The most common use is the erythromycin base preparation for the oral antibiotic bowel preparation with neomycin for patients who undergo elective colonic surgery. Hypersensitivity and other systemic toxicity are uncommon.

Clindamycin

Clindamycin (600–900 mg every 8 hours) reversibly binds to cytoplasm ribosomes and inhibits protein synthesis. It has activity against streptococci and also has some staphylococcal coverage. It has activity against 70% of community-associated MRSA, but it is not active against healthcare-associated MRSA. Because of its activity against anaerobic bacteria (e.g. *Bacteroides fragilis*) it has been extensively used with the aminoglycosides for patients who have peritonitis and other polymicrobial infections. It is also recommended in NSTIs due to *Streptococcus pyogenes* or *C. perfringens* to inhibit toxin production. Clindamycin has few hypersensitivity problems, but its use is associated with the development of *C. difficile* enterocolitis.

Sulfonamides

The sulfonamides are inhibitors of folic acid metabolism. A related compound that works at a separate step in folic acid metabolism is trimethoprim. The trimethoprim–sulfamethoxazole preparation is commonly used for treating gram-negative urinary infections and has 90% coverage of community-associated MRSA. It is administered as an oral drug in doses of 160-mg trimethoprim and 800-mg sulfamethoxazole in a single or divide dose daily. The principal toxicity of sulfonamides is hypersensitivity.

Glycopeptides

Vancomycin (500 mg–1 g every 6–12 hours up to 2 g daily) is the most commonly used glycopeptide; it binds to the plasma membrane (not penicillin-binding proteins) of susceptible organisms and inhibits cell wall synthesis. It is used for the treatment of all strains of MRSA. It is also active against enterococci, although vancomycin-resistant enterococci and a few strains of vancomycin-resistant *S. aureus* have now emerged.[49] The concentration of vancomycin necessary to inhibit the growth of MRSA has gradually demonstrated a measureable increase over time which may translate into outcome problems if this trend continues. Vancomycin has nephrotoxicity and may require pharmacokinetic dosing. Rapid infusion of intravenous vancomycin is associated with a systemic hyperemia known as the "red man" syndrome from histamine release. Telavancin (10 mg/kg/daily), oritavancin (1,200 mg for 7 days of treatment), and dalbavancin (1,000 and 500 mg at day 7 if necessary) are new and long half-life glycopeptides that are being evaluated for the treatment of MRSA infections but have not displaced vancomycin.Optimum dosing of these new long half-life drugs are still being investigated.

Metronidazole

Metronidazole penetrates the bacterial cell and mediates damage to the DNA and other macromolecular structures within the cell. It was originally used to treat amebic colitis. It was subsequently found to have excellent activity against obligate intestinal anaerobes (e.g. *B. fragilis)*. Metronidazole (7.5 mg/kg every 6 hours not to exceed 4 g daily) is commonly used with quinolones, aztreonam, or aminoglycosides to treat polymicrobial infections. Metronidazole has been used extensively for several decades and has had limited development of resistance. It has limited toxicity but can produce seizures if given in excessively high doses.

Fluoroquinolones

Fluoroquinolones inactivate the gyrase enzyme systems involved in microbial replication. Ciprofloxacin, levofloxaxin, gatifloxacin, moxifloxacin, ofloxacin, norfloxacin, and many others have been used or are currently being used in patient care around the world. Ciprofloxacin (500 mg every 12 hours) and levofloxacin (500—750 mg daily) are the most commonly used. They commonly used for the treatment of community- and hospital-acquired pneumonia and UTIs. Fluoroquinolones generally lack enteric anaerobic activity (except moxifloxacin) but have been used with metronidazole or clindamycin for the treatment of moderately severe intra-abdominal infections. Oral quinolones are absorbed very efficiently. Neurotoxicity, rupture of tendons (e.g. Achilles), and association with *C. difficile* infections have been identified.

Oxazolidinones

Linezolid (600 mg every 12 hours) is the oxazolidinone used in clinical practice. It is broadly active against gram-positive pathogens, and its clinical use has largely focused on MRSA infections. It inhibits protein synthesis. It is generally viewed as a safe drug but is quite expensive. Other antibiotics in this class that are under evaluation are tedizolid, eperezolid, posizolid, and radezolid.

Lipopeptides

Daptomycin (4–6 mg/kg daily) is the prototype of the lipopeptides. The molecule inserts into the cell membrane of the bacterial cell and results in holes and depolarization of the plasma membrane. It is active against gram-positive bacteria and is primarily used for MRSA infection. It is administered only intravenously. It has poor penetration of the lung and is not used for pneumonia, but it is used for severe soft tissue and blood stream infections. It is relatively safe but associated with an increase in creatine kinase, which is of uncertain significance in standard courses of treatment. A number of additional lipopeptides have been discovered and are being entertained for clinical development.

INFECTION AND THE SYSTEMIC INFLAMMATORY RESPONSE

Infection is the local activation of the inflammatory response by the proliferation and invasion of microbes into host tissues. The evolutionary role of inflammation in tissue injury, contamination, and local infection is containment and eradication of potential pathogens to prevent systemic dissemination. However, failure of containment by the local inflammatory response results in dissemination of bacteria, bacteria cell products and toxins, and proinflammatory cytokines. The inflammatory processes are beneficial for the host at the local tissue level but become deleterious at the systemic level, and set into motion the SIRS.[50]

Flowchart 7.1 schematically illustrates the theoretical construct of systemic inflammation secondary to invasive infection.[51] Invasive infection, intense local inflammation, and necrosis of tissue result in upregulation of the systemic inflammatory cascade through damage-associated molecular pathways (DAMPs). DAMPs are further subdivided into those that are alarmins, which are cellular products from injured or necrotic cells, and pathogen-associated molecular pathways (PAMPs), which are from the pathogens themselves. Alarmins activate systemic inflammation through RAGE receptors and PAMPs through toll-like receptors. All DAMPs activate the nonspecific initiators of the inflammatory response in the coagulation cascade, platelets, mast cells, bradykinin, and complement proteins. The activation of the nonspecific initiators results in the systemic vasodilation, increased vascular permeability, and systemic edema that is seen in SIRS. The activation of RAGE and toll-like receptors on macrophage/monocyte populations of cells is the proinflammatory

Flowchart 7.1: Schematic representation of the systemic inflammatory response where activation of the various steps of inflammation results in septic shock, peripheral tissue necrosis, and the multiple organ dysfunction syndrome.

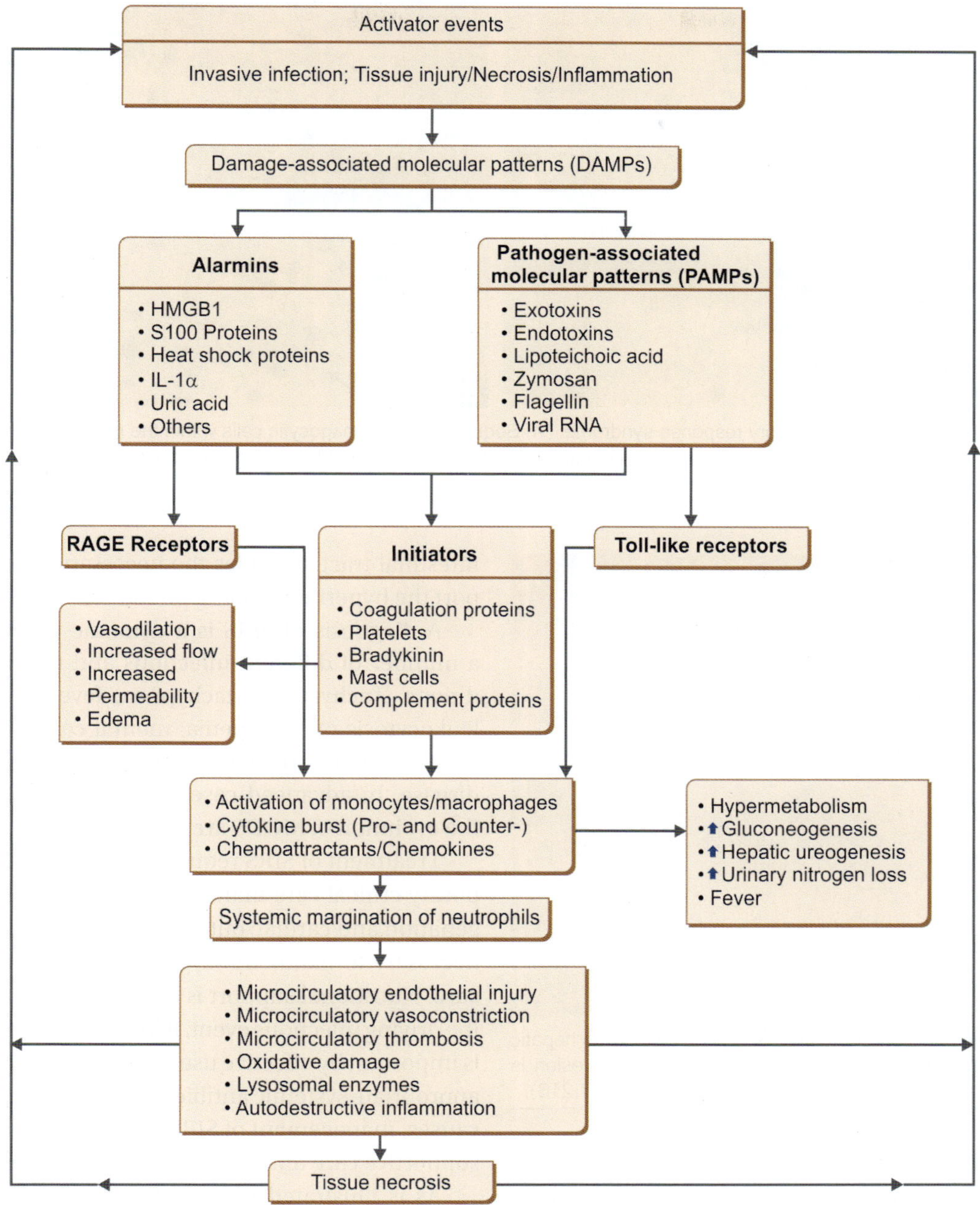

burst of cytokines. An abundance of chemoattractant and chemokine proteins are released and margination of leukocytes through the microcirculation of visceral tissues (Figs. 7.21A and B). The hypermetabolic sequelae are activated and the local tissue destructive events of unleashed inflammation results in local tissue necrosis. These foci of local tissue necrosis refuel the DAMPs that originally activated the process and set into motion a viscous cycle of systemic inflammation, which yields tissue necrosis, which in turn reactivates the entire systemic inflammatory process (Fig. 7.22). The exaggerated vascular changes of inflammation yield septic shock and progressive tissue injury yields the multiple organ dysfunction seen in these patients.

Prevention of septic shock and MODS is the prevention of SIRS. Local infection, regardless of anatomic site, must be recognized and promptly treated. The drainage of pus, debridement of dead infected tissue and systemic use

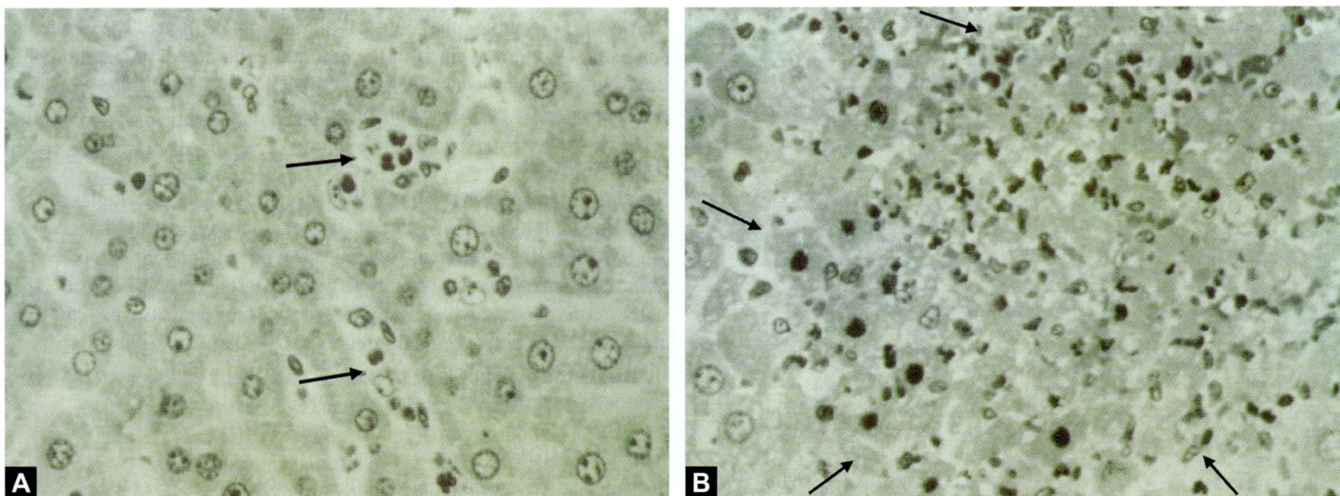

Figs. 7.21A and B: Systemic inflammatory response syndrome. (A) Sequestration of phagocytic cells within the microcirculation of the hepatic sinusoids 5 hours after a bacteremic event (arrows). (B) Focal necrosis of hepatocytes (arrows), presumably as a result of the tissue-based consequences of systemic inflammation.

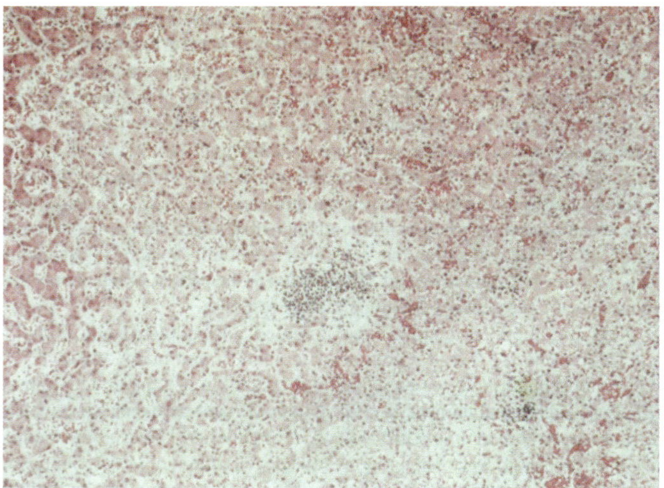

Fig. 7.22: Histologic section of the liver of a patient who has hepatic failure and intra-abdominal sepsis. The focal inflammatory lesion is analogous to that seen in experimental bacteremia (*see* Fig. 7.21B).

of antibiotics are required to contain and eradicate local infection before systemic dissemination. In many cases, SIRS has been activated when the patient is first seen. Prevention of SIRS progression to septic shock and MODS requires the same efforts at containment and eradication. In addition, systemic support of cardiac output through preload administration with crystalloid solutions and red cell mass (as needed) maintain tissue perfusion. Adequate oxygenation must be maintained. Hypovolemia and hypoxemia have additive effects to the microcirculatory injury of progressive SIRS to create both tissue and cellular injury. Aggressive nutritional support, if possible via the intestinal tract, provides the necessary substrates to support the hypermetabolic septic state.

A diagnosis of SIRS is a dynamic process that spans a number of different infectious and noninfectious conditions. Tachycardia, tachypnea, fever or hypothermia, leukocytosis or leukopenia, mental confusion, diaphoresis, hypoxemia, and oliguria are common symptoms of the disease. In advanced cases, systemic lactic acidosis and the evolution of MODS are seen.

Treatment of SIRS requires the application of contemporary critical care management methods. Systemic oxygenation and cardiac output must be maintained at levels necessary to maintain oxygen delivery and arterial pressure. Nutritional support is likewise important. Control of the driving infectious event, if infection is the driving event, is important by effective use of drainage, debridement and appropriate systemic antibiotic therapy. For noninfectious causes, management of SIRS requires aggressive systemic supportive care until the process has resolved.

As is illustrated in Flowchart 7.1, there is a biologic threshold beyond which the inflammatory process becomes a self-cycling and self-energizing process. The realization that control of infection may not "turn off" fully activated SIRS has led to the pursuit of treatments that attack specific elements of the inflammatory response. There have been a host of biological treatment strategies that have included antiendotoxin antibodies, anticytokine antibodies, receptor antagonists, and others that have failed to change the clinical outcome in these patients. Recombinant activated protein C appeared to have promise as treatment, but that too has not sustained the test of prolonged evaluation and usage in clinical practice.

A new paradigm is needed in the treatment of SIRS. As more is being learned about the counterinflammatory signaling in critically ill patients, many believe that future treatments require reestablishment of a clinical balance between the pro- and counterinflammatory responses may be the best approach to achieving physiologic homeostasis. Recent investigation into the neuroinflammatory reflex indicates that modulation of the inflammatory response is important and that loss of balance between pro- and counterinflammatory mechanisms can result in run-away systemic inflammation, or excessive counterinflammatory signaling in profound immunosuppression of the host. Until a new treatment model can be established, control of infection and systemic supportive care of the SIRS patient remain the foundation of management.

REFERENCES

1. Shallcross LJ, Fragaszy E, Johnson AM, et al. The role of the Panton-Valentine leucocidin toxin in staphylococcal disease: a systematic review and meta-analysis. Lancet Infect Dis. 2013;13:43-54.
2. Sørensen TI, Nielsen GG, Andersen PK, et al. Genetic and environmental influences on premature death in adult adoptees. N Engl J Med. 1988;318:727-32.
3. Fry DE. Fifty ways to cause surgical site infections. Surg Infect. 2011;12:497-500.
4. Cardona SM, Garcia JA, Cardona AE. The fine balance of chemokines during disease: trafficking, inflammation, and homeostasis. Methods Mol Biol. 2013;1013:1-16.
5. Webster J, Osborne S. Preoperative bathing or showering with skin antiseptics to prevent surgical site infection. Cochrane Database Syst Rev. 2012;9:CD004985.
6. Darouiche RO, Wall MJ Jr, Itani KM, et al. Chlorhexidine-Alcohol versus povidone-iodine for surgical-site antisepsis. N Engl J Med. 2010;362:18-26.
7. Vogel TR, Dombrovskiy VY, Lowry SF. In-hospital delay of elective surgery for high volume procedures: the impact on infectious complications. J Am Coll Surg. 2010;211:784-90.
8. Braga M. Perioperative immunonutrition and gut function. Curr Opin Clin Nutr Metab Care. 2012;15:485-8.
9. Beltramini AM, Salata RA, Ray AJ. Thermoregulation and risk of surgical site infection. Infect Control Hosp Epidemiol. 2011;32:603-10.
10. May AK, Kauffmann RM, Collier BR. The place for glycemic control in the surgical patient. Surg Infect. 2011;12:405-18.
11. Platt R, Zaleznik DF, Hopkins CC, et al. Perioperative antibiotic prophylaxis for herniorrhaphy and breast surgery. N Engl J Med. 1990;322:153-60.
12. Finkelstein R, Rabino G, Mashiah T, et al. Vancomycin versus cefazolin prophylaxis for cardiac surgery in the setting of a high prevalence of methicillin-resistant staphylococcal infections. J Thorac Cardiovasc Surg. 2002;23:326-32.
13. Fry DE. Colon preparation and surgical site infection. Am J Surg. 2011;202:225-32.
14. Güenaga KF, Matos D, Wille-Jørgensen P. Mechanical bowel preparation for elective colorectal surgery. Cochrane Database Syst Rev.2011;(9):CD001544.
15. Dellinger EP. Antibiotic prophylaxis in trauma: penetrating abdominal injuries and open fractures. Rev Infect Dis. 1991;13(Suppl 10):S847-57.
16. van Ramshorst GH, Eker HH, Harlaar JJ, et al. Therapeutic alternatives for burst abdomen. Surg Technol Int. 2010;19: 111-9.
17. Fry DE. Skin, skin structure, and soft tissue infections. In: Fry DE, (Ed). Surgical Infections. London: JP Medical Publishers; 2013., Chapter 5, pp. 63-74.
18. Stevens DL, Aldape MJ, Bryant AE. Life-threatening clostridial infections. Anaerobe. 2012;18:254-9.
19. Steer AC, Lamagni T, Curtis N, et al. Invasive group a streptococcal disease: epidemiology, pathogenesis and management. Drugs. 2012;72:1213-27.
20. Miller LG, Perdreau-Remington F, Rieg G, et al. Necrotizing fasciitis caused by community-associated methicillin-resistant Staphylococcus aureus in Los Angeles. N Engl J Med. 2005;352:1445-53.
21. Kao LS, Lew DF, Arab SN, et al. Local variations in the epidemiology, microbiology, and outcome of necrotizing soft-tissue infections: a multicenter study. Am J Surg. 2011; 202:139-45.
22. Brosnahan AJ, Schlievert PM. Gram-positive bacterial superantigen outside-in signaling causes toxic shock syndrome. FEBS J. 2011;278:4649-67.
23. Davies HD, McGeer A, Schwartz B, et al. Invasive group a streptococcal infection in Ontario, Canada. N Engl J Med. 1996;335:547-54.
24. Mazuski JE, Solomkin JS. Intra-abdominal infections. Surg Clin North Am. 2009;89:421-37.
25. Herzog T, Chromik AM, Uhl W. Treatment of complicated intra-abdominal infections in the era of multi-drug resistant bacteria. Eur J Med Res. 2010;15:525-32.
26. Kollef MH. Ventilator-associated complications, including infection-related complications: the way forward. Crit Care Clin. 2013;29:33-50.
27. Ashraf M, Ostrosky-Zeichner L. Ventilator-associated pneumonia: a review. Hosp Pract. 2012;40:93-105.
28. DiCocco JM, Croce MA. Ventilator-associated pneumonia: an overview. Expert Opin Pharmacother. 2009;10:1461-7.
29. Hooton TM, Bradley SF, Cardenas DD, et al. Diagnosis, prevention, and treatment of catheter-associated urinary tract infection in adults: 2009 International Clinical Practice Guidelines from the Infectious Diseases Society of America. Clin Infect Dis. 2010;50:625-63.
30. Burton DC, Edwards JR, Srinivasan A, et al. Trends in catheter-associated urinary tract infections in adult intensive care units-United States 1990–2007. Infect Control Hosp Epidemiol. 2011;32:748-56.
31. O'Grady NP, Alexander M, Burns LA, et al. Guidelines for the prevention of intravascular catheter-related infections. Am J Infect Control. 2011;39(4 Suppl 1):S1-34.

32. Crnich CJ, Maki DG. Intravascular device infection. In: APIC Text of Infection Control and Epidemiology, 3rd edition. Washington, DC: Association for Professionals in Infection Control and Epidemiology, Inc.; 2009. Chapter 24, pp. 1-22.
33. O'Grady NP, Alexander M, Burns LA, et al. Guidelines for the prevention of intravascular catheter-related infections. Am J Infect Control. 2011;39:S1-S34.
34. Gerding DN, Johnson S. Clostridium difficile infection in 2010: advances in pathogenesis, diagnosis and management of CDI. Nat Rev Gastroenterol Hepatol. 2011;8: 67-8.
35. Crook DW, Walker AS, Kean Y, et al. Fidaxomicin versus vancomycin for Clostridium difficile infection: meta-analysis of pivotal randomized controlled trials. Clin Infect Dis. 2012;55(Suppl 2):S93-103.
36. Kassam Z, Lee CH, Yuan Y, et al. Fecal microbiota transplantation for Clostridium difficile infection: systematic review and meta-analysis. Am J Gastroenterol. 2013;108: 500-8.
37. Cartman ST, Heap JT, Kuehne SA, et al. The emergence of 'hypervirulence' in Clostridium difficile. Int J Med Microbiol. 2010;300:387-95.
38. Pappas PG, Kauffman CA, Andes D, et al. Clinical practice guidelines for the management of candidiasis: 2009 update by the Infectious Diseases Society of America. Clin Infect Dis. 2009;48:503-35.
39. Walsh TJ, Anaissie EJ, Denning DW, et al. Treatment of aspergillosis: guidelines of the Infectious Diseases Society of America. Clin Infect Dis. 2008;46:327-60.
40. Tujios SR, Lee WM. New advances in chronic hepatitis B. Curr Opin Gastroenterol. 2012;28(3):193-7.
41. Fry DE. Occupational risks of blood exposure in the operating room. Am Surg. 2007;73:637-46.
42. Liang TJ, Ghany MG. Current and future therapies for hepatitis C virus infection. N Engl J Med. 2013;368(20):1907-17.
43. World Health Organization. Hepatitis C. [online] Available from http://www.who.int/mediacentre/factsheets/fs164/en/[Accessed July 1, 2013].
44. World Health Organization. WHO issues new HIV recommendations calling for earlier treatment. [online] Available from http://www.who.int/mediacentre/factsheets/fs164/en/ [Accessed July 1, 2013].
45. Centers for Disease Control. Occupational HIV transmission and prevention among healthcare workers. [online] Available from http://www.cdc.gov/hiv/resources/factsheets/hcwprev.htm [Accessed July 1, 2013].
46. Centers for Disease Control and Prevention. (2010). Sexually transmitted diseases: treatment guidelines 2010, genital warts. [online] Available from http://www.cdc.gov/std/treatment/2010/genital-warts.htm [Accessed July 10, 2013].
47. Kwok CS, Gibbs S, Bennett C, et al. Topical treatments for cutaneous warts. Cochrane Database Syst Rev. 2012;9: CD001781.
48. Gonzales ML, Dans LF, Martinez EG. Antiamoebic drugs for treating amoebic colitis. Cochrane Database Syst Rev. 2009;(2):CD006085.
49. Fry DE, Barie PS. The changing face of *Staphylococcus aureus*: a continuing surgical challenge. Surg Infect. 2011; 12:191-203.
50. American College of Chest Physicians/Society of Critical Care Medicine Consensus Conference. Definition for sepsis and organ failure and guidelines for the use of innovative therapies in sepsis. Crit Care Med. 1992;20:864-70.

Additional references appear in the online version of this book.

8

Minimal Invasive Surgery

Sérgio A Toledo-Valdovinos, John G Hunter

Key Points

- Minimal invasive surgery (MIS) is the current surgical approach in which the surgical outcome is equal or superior to the open procedures with a reduced trauma to the access tissue.
- The mechanical and humoral effects of a pneumoperitoneum affect homeostatic mechanisms, and the operating team must be aware of these potential physiologic changes.
- An immediate conversion to an open operative procedure may be required to treat a complication of minimal access surgery. Delays in converting to an open procedure may be associated with an increased procedural morbidity and mortality.

INTRODUCTION

Over the last two decades, a new trend in the mindset about surgical approaches has been established, in which the former aphorism "Big surgeons, big incisions" is no longer accurate.

Minimal invasive surgery (MIS) is a concept in which major operations can be performed, usually using high-tech instruments and technology, through small incisions without compromising the outcome. This way of thinking has been fostered by the rapidly growing technological developments (e.g. novel imaging techniques, digitalization, and computerized information systems) and the patient demands for a less troublesome recovery and a more aesthetic result. Although the open and MIS procedures can be essentially the same, the surgeons need to acquire and master a new set of skills to be proficient in the MIS approach.

This chapter aims to introduce the principles of MIS, especially as they apply to laparoscopy. MIS is not a specialty in itself, but a new approach to traditional surgery that has been embraced by a number of distinct disciplines. Radiologists who use computed tomography or ultrasound guidance to gain access to particular anatomic spaces for drainage and gastroenterologists who use endoscopic retrograde cholangiography to stent obstructed biliary trees are as much "minimal invasive surgeons" as general surgeons who use laparoscopy to perform antireflux procedures. All minimal access surgeons aim for the common goal of optimal therapy with the least morbidity, discomfort, and inconvenience to the patient with an earlier return to normal activities after operation.

HISTORY

Laparoscopic surgery has common origins with endoscopy, and these date back to their first description in the School of Hippocrates (460-375 BC) where a rectal speculum was created. A similar vaginal speculum is described in the Babylonian Talmud (500 BC). But it was not until 1805 when a German obstetrician, Philipp Bozzini, designed the "Der Lichtleiter" (light conductor), a device to look into the rectal and vaginal cavities using the light of a candle and mirrors to reflect it. Antonio Desormeaux performed the first "true" endoscopy while presenting his "modern" cystoscope to the Academy of Medicine in Paris in 1865. Five years later (1870), after attending a sword show, Adolph Kussmaul performed an esophagoscopy using a rigid tube with mirrors. While in Vienna, Maximilian Nitze, an urologist from Berlin, worked closely with a medical instrument maker, Joseph Leiter, to create a cystoscope, which was lit with rheostat-controlled electrically heated platinum filaments, a water-cooling system and telescopic lenses for visualization.[1] Using Nitze's device, combined with Thomas Alva Edison's 1880 invention, the light bulb, the German surgeon Georg Kelling performed on September 23, 1901, the first laparoscopic peritoneal cavity examination in a dog, using cotton-wool filtered oxygen to inflate the abdomen and named the procedure "Kölioscopie."[2] Various gases were used for insufflation until the mid-1930s, when carbon dioxide (CO_2) became popular. Soon after, Hans Christian Jacobeus executed the first celioscopy in humans and accumulated a series of 115 patients who had ascites during 1 year. He also coined the term "laparoscopy."[3]

A major practical obstacle to laparoscopy was the transmission of sufficient light into the abdomen to illuminate the abdominal organs without creating excessive heat. In 1952, the British physicist Harold H. Hopkins developed a method of illumination by cold light through a series of short-sculpted quartz rods. The development of fiberoptics at about the same time allowed transmission of light around corners and curves, so opening up the field of flexible endoscopy. Over the following 20 years the technology of flexible endoscopy for both diagnosis and therapy evolved rapidly. Meanwhile during the 1960s and 1980s, the laparoscopic armamentarium was enormously increased under the leadership of the German gynecologist Kurt Semm, who also performed the first laparoscopic appendectomy. Developments included automatic insufflators with abdominal pressure monitoring and several laparoscopic instruments (e.g. hook scissors, irrigation/aspiration apparatus, thermocoagulation instruments, endoloop applicators, etc).[1]

In the 1980s, a major advance in MIS (a term coined by the British urologist John E. A. Wickham in 1983) occurred with the development of small high-resolution charge-couple device (CCD) video cameras, which could be fixed to the end of flexible or rigid scopes. Combining these technologies with high-resolution video monitors resulted in the development of the videoendoscope, which has dramatically changed the current practice of surgery.

TRAINING

Technical skills are essential to the practice of surgery. Historically, procedures were learned by apprenticeship using the Halstedian model: "see one, do one, and teach one." With the advent of MIS training issues arise, and this philosophy is no longer applicable. Many minimal invasive procedures like laparoscopic cholecystectomy replaced existing procedures rather than expanded the indications for operative intervention. Patient demand forced the practicing general surgeons to acquire new MIS skills rapidly or be faced with a dwindling practice.

The challenge is not simply to learn a new operation but to master a new technique, a technique that eliminates the tactile sense that surgeons had traditionally relied on and removes the three-dimensional (3D) perspective. Initially, trainees have acquired their MIS skills on patients through several surgical exposures with a variable grade of complexity until they dominate the procedures. This type of teaching has faced several hurdles that are shifting the surgical residents' learning experiences, including patient safety concerns, ethical concerns of "practicing on patients," operation room costs, pressure to increase productivity, and limited resident work hours.[4,5]

The MIS education is now more established. The Society of American Gastrointestinal Endoscopic Surgeons developed the Fundamentals of Laparoscopic Surgery (FLS) program, a comprehensive web-based education module that develops the fundamental knowledge and technical skills required in basic laparoscopic surgery. These goals are achieved through hands-on skills training and assessment tool components using "box trainers," which are simulated abdominal cavities with a video camera, monitor, and working ports to execute several tasks with targeted models. These box trainers can be very primitive or sophisticated (e.g. virtual simulators) as preferred. The use of live animals and human cadavers provides other options that can add more realism to the training.

It has been shown that performance in the simulators improves progressively with practice and correlates with performance in the operating room.[5] Therefore, the American Board of Surgery requires FLS certification for general surgeons to qualify for the board examination.

With the new technology revolution the surgical approaches were not the only ones that changed; the teaching field was in a desperate need of improvement and evolution. The traditional training paradigms were time-based curricula, in which a specific training time was set, or a repetition-based curriculum, in which a minimum number of repetitions were set to consider the task complete. With different baseline skills among trainees and different types of motivation, which directly impact on acquisition of skills, the above mentioned curricula may end in either inadequate training or overtraining. Currently, the proficiency-based training is considered the best model. In this model, a specific set of training goals is given, which allows learners to achieve a performance objective along with performance feedback. The apprentice can compare their performance, and this promotes motivation and self-practice and enhances the overall results.[4]

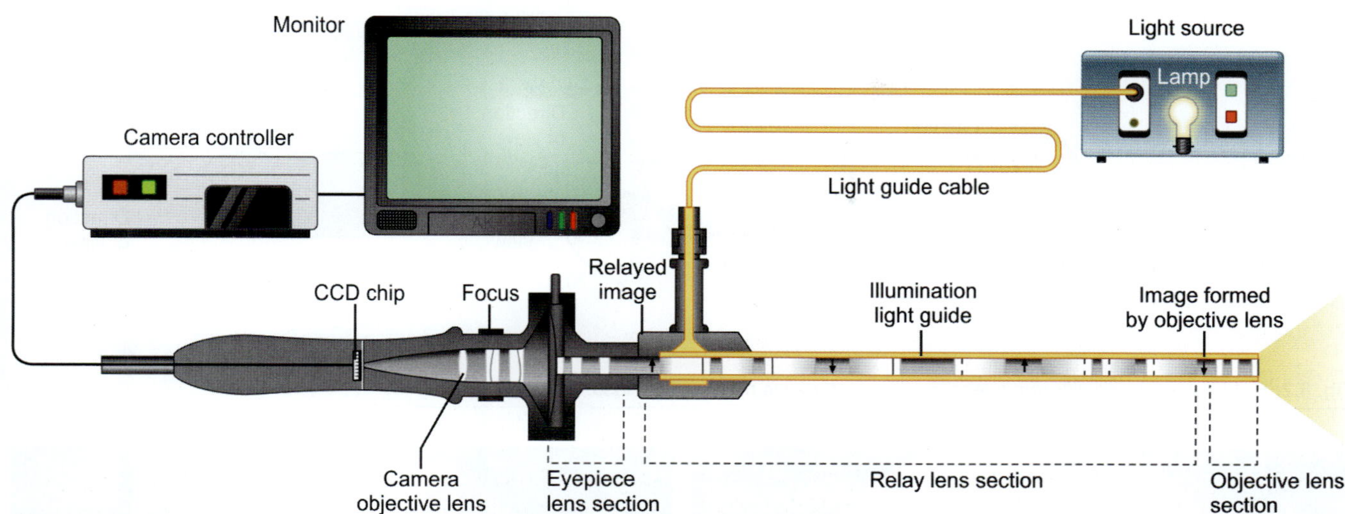

Fig. 8.1: Typical laparoscopic imaging system—Illumination increases with the square of the telescope diameter. CCD: Charge-couple device.

The conquest of complicated manual skills has three sequential stages:

1. *Cognitive stage*: Understanding the manual task through reading and watching demonstrations
2. *Associative stage*: Putting into practice the acquired knowledge with actual practice of the task. The initial outcome will be poor and erratic, but with practice movements become smoother and more efficient
3. *Autonomous stage*: Psychomotor movements are achieved in an automated manner with minimal demands on attention, which can then be utilized in a higher cognitive aspect of the operation, like elucidating the anatomy or forecasting.[5]

INSTRUMENTATION

Successful MIS requires sophisticated instrumentation. The wide array of instruments that is now common in most operating rooms demonstrates the rapid response of industry to the introduction of laparoscopy. Minimal instrumentation for MIS includes quality video imaging systems, energy sources, and hand instruments to carry out the desired procedure in a minimal and safe environment.

Imaging Systems

The major development in the imaging system devices is the use of a CCD, which is a formation of photosensitive sensors (pixels) that transform the incoming light into an electric charge. This charge will be later converted to an image. In earlier flexible endoscope versions, the CCD was mounted at the proximal (external) end of a bundle of fiberoptic cables. Nowadays, most standard endoscopes contain a CCD at the distal end of the flexible scope. The situation is different with rigid laparoscopes, in which the light and images are delivered through quartz rods coupled to a CCD on the external end. Telescopes vary in diameter from 2 to 12 mm. The larger the scope diameter, the larger the cross-sectional area for light transmission (Fig. 8.1).

Telescopes are usually 30 cm in length, but longer ones are available especially for bariatric patients. They may have a flat end that provides a straight view (0°) or an angled end that provides an oblique view (30° or 45°). Angled ends result in a small loss of light intensity, but greater flexibility in the viewing area (Fig. 8.2). Rotation of the angled scope alters and the field of view, which is very useful in certain laparoscopic procedures (Figs. 8.3A to C).[6]

Light delivery to the scope is achieved through fiberoptic cables, which carry light from an external light source. Extremely bright xenon, mercury, or halogen light sources of ≥ 300 W are required because of the high degree of light lost in the delivery system (≥ 90%).[7]

There are some rules with the video imaging systems that are needed during MIS to ensure a safe surgical procedure: first illumination, second resolution (capacity to distinguish between two line pairs), and third color. Without the first two elements the safety of the operation is compromised. Almost all laparoscopic cameras have red, green, and blue inputs or three-chip cameras, which provide the best color resolution (Fig. 8.4). Old one-chip cameras convert gray scale inputs to approximate colors, which were adequate for most operative procedures but

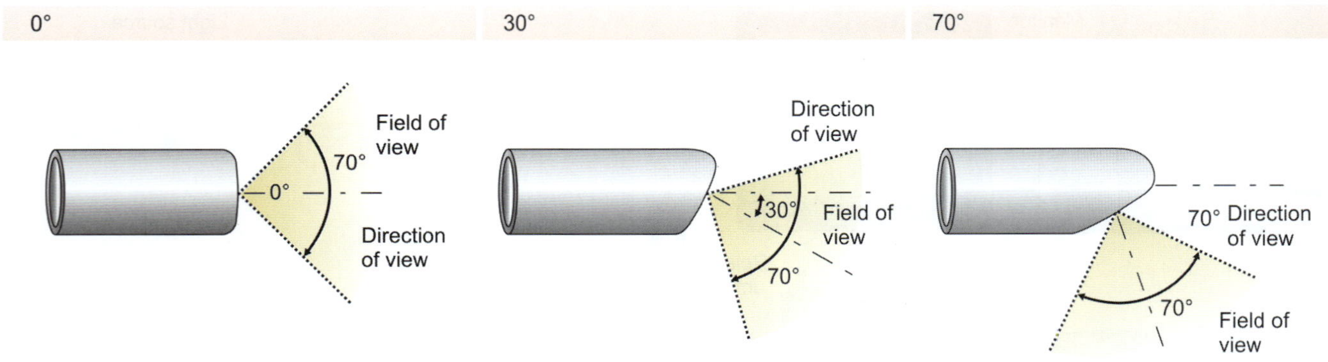

Fig. 8.2: Fields of view with different telescopes. Larger angles result in light loss.

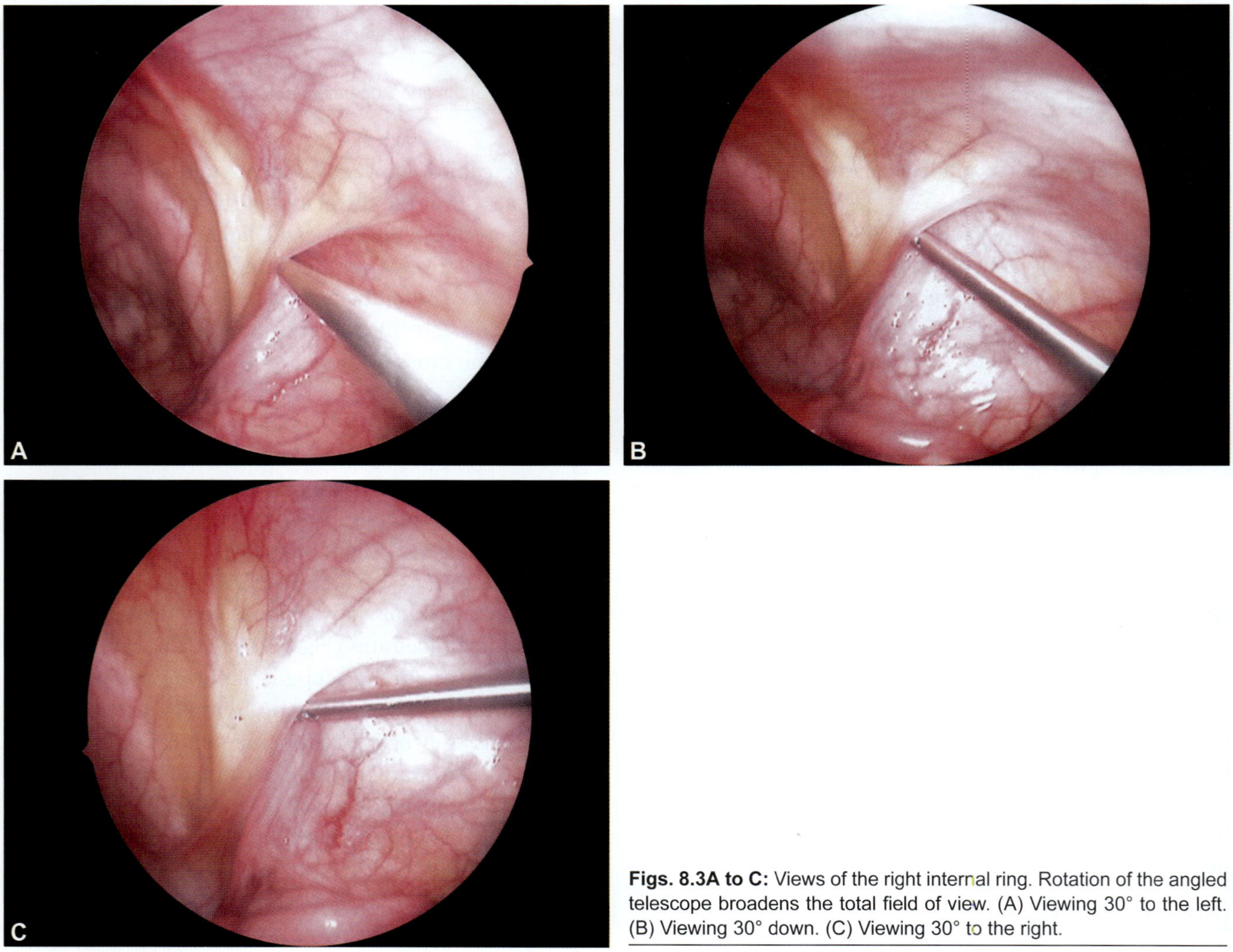

A
B
C

Figs. 8.3A to C: Views of the right internal ring. Rotation of the angled telescope broadens the total field of view. (A) Viewing 30° to the left. (B) Viewing 30° down. (C) Viewing 30° to the right.

create a video image that is less color accurate. Analog images can now be digitally enhanced, an additional feature of many video cameras, by adding contrast at color interfaces between two adjacent pixels, making images appear more "crisp." New laparoscopic cameras have a high-definition (HD) chip, which increases the resolution up to seven times, but to have the clarity of HD imaging, HD monitors are necessary. Combined with digital enhancement, HD monitors can confer up to eight times more resolution than standard monitors.

Three-dimensional technology is also available to add depth to a standard two-dimensional (2D) image. Its interest has come and gone. The image quality is not as sharp as 2D imaging; in fact, the image edges become blurry with resolution loss due to the oscillation between the two similar images. To overcome this issue optical accommodation is necessary and might be tiring and even induce cephalea if one uses the system for a long period of time. 3D images may facilitate tasks for inexperienced laparoscopists but are of little advantage to experienced laparoscopists.

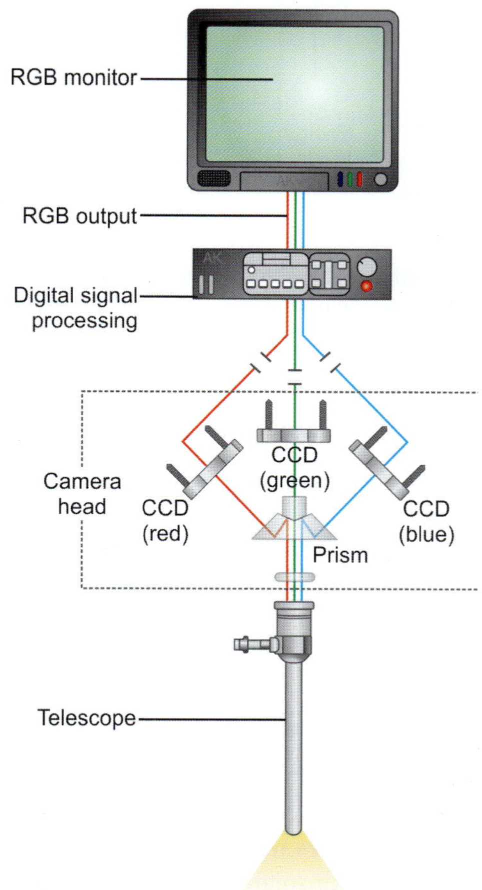

Fig. 8.4: Prisms direct red (R), green (G), and blue (B) light to separate charge-couple devices in a three-chip camera system. The RGB video signals are subsequently sent to a video monitor.

Energy Sources

Video surgery requires a relatively bloodless field to allow good visualization of critical anatomy. This fact boosted new ways of applying energy. The phases through which the tissues progress after the application of heat are coagulation (60°C), vaporization and desiccation (100°C), and carbonization (>200°C).[8]

Electrosurgery

Radio frequency (RF) electrosurgery is the most commonly used energy delivery system for both open operations and MIS and one that has been shown to be safe and less expensive than other sources.[9] RF electrosurgery is essentially an alternating current at a high-frequency 500,000 cycles/s (Hz). The high frequency causes electron reverberation that creates heat without extensive membrane depolarization. RF energy is delivered through either monopolar or bipolar electrodes.

Monopolar electrosurgery delivers electrons from the energy source through a single fine-tipped electrode to a large ground plate [commonly a gel pad placed on the patient's thigh (Figs. 8.5A and B)]. High-frequency current with a sinusoidal waveform has a cutting effect and

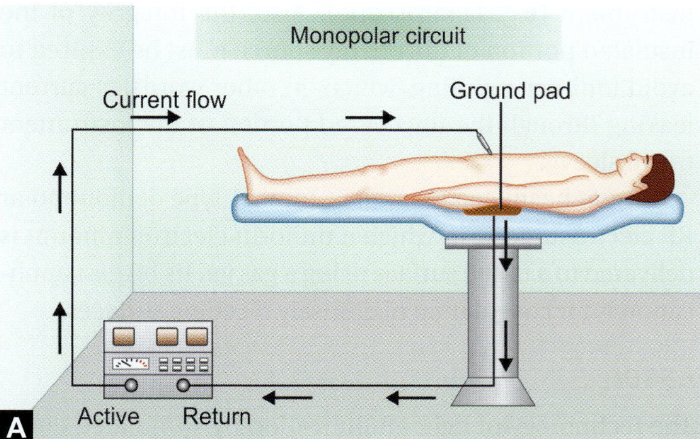

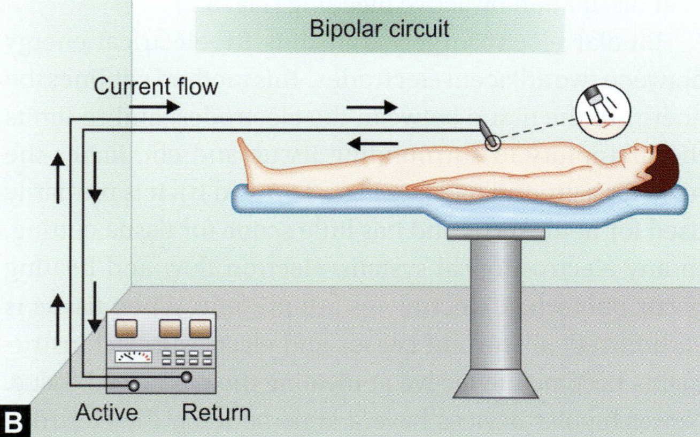

Figs. 8.5A and B: Cautery—In monopolar cautery current flows from a small active electrode and dissipates to a broad surface grounding pad. In bipolar cautery a grounding pad is not needed because current flows between two active electrodes, cauterizing only the tissue between the two electrodes.

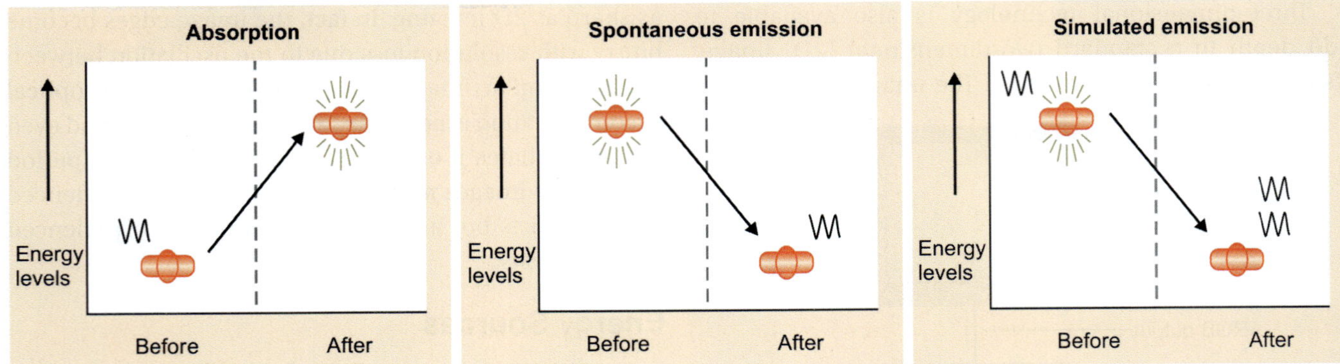

Fig. 8.6: Energy transfer—This results in elevation of an electron (represented by a colored oval shape) to an unstable energy state. A photon of light (represented as wavy lines) is emitted as the electron returns to a stable ground state. The photon then strikes another excited electron to cause a stimulated decay, which results in two photons in phase across time and space.

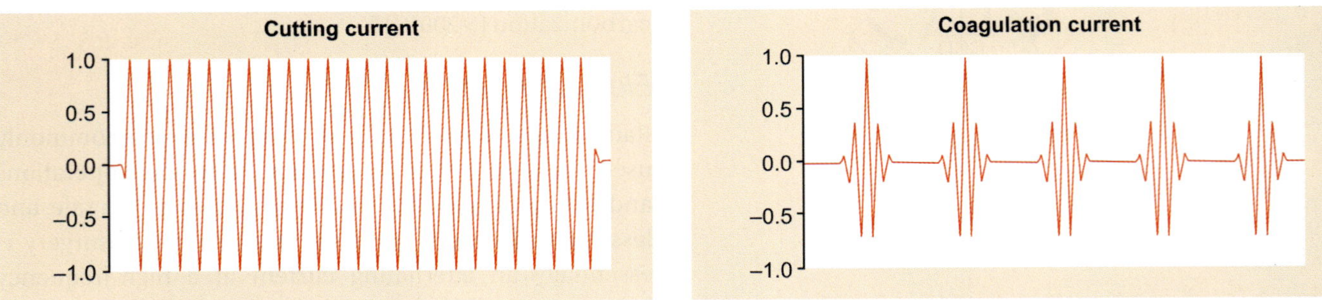

Fig. 8.7: Cutting and coagulation current waveforms—Cutting current results in tissue vaporization. Coagulation current results in tissue desiccation and formation of a coagulum of cellular debris.

produces very little coagulation. High-energy transfer (Fig. 8.6) over a very small surface causes tissue vaporization and desiccation with little coagulation. Surface coagulation is best achieved by intermittent pulses of high-voltage current. The high-voltage discharge drives deeper tissue penetration of heat, with less opportunity for heat dissipation by active bleeding (Fig. 8.7).[8]

Bipolar electrosurgery transmits RF electrical energy between two adjacent electrodes. This method confines the energy to the tissue between the electrodes, and so limits thermal injury to surrounding tissue and eliminates the need for a ground pad (*see* Figs. 8.5A and B). It is primarily used for hemostasis and has little scope for tissue cutting. In any electrosurgical system, electron flow and heating occur only when electrolytes are present. When tissue is carbonized, all current ceases and electrosurgical instruments become ineffective at dividing the desiccated tissue. Newer bipolar devices have a knife between the electrode forceps jaws of the instrument and are able to coagulate and cut larger vessels (up to 7 mm in diameter). The downside of these devices is the slowness with which they work.

It is essential to have within the surgical field of view a full display of the uninsulated portion of the instrument. One should also keep away from another tool when energy sources are applied, to avoid direct thermal injuries to adjacent structures or direct coupling, which is the transmission of current to the viscera through another instrument (e.g. laparoscope). Also, the integrity of the insulated portion of the energy source must be assured to avoid indirect coupling, which, in other words, is current leaking through the uncovered portion of the instrument metal sleeve.[8]

Argon beam coagulation is another type of monopolar RF electrosurgery, in which a uniform electron amount is delivered to a tissue surface using a gas jet. Its biggest application is for coagulation of diffusely bleeding surfaces.

Laser

The technology of light amplification by stimulated emission radiation (known by its acronym *laser*) has evolved rapidly since the early 1960s. Despite this evolution, the level of interest in its application has been variable.

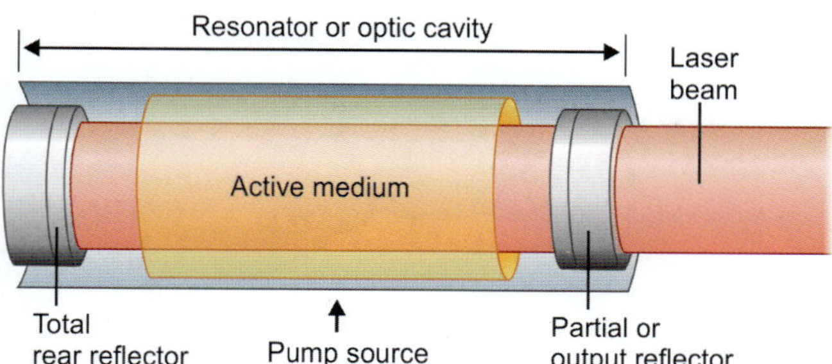

Fig. 8.8: Laser activation—The laser medium is activated by an external energy source. Coherent light is formed within the optical cavity and released through an output reflector at one end of the cavity.

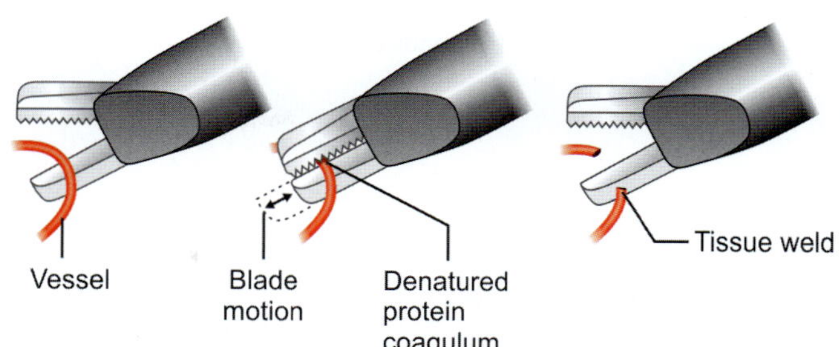

Fig. 8.9: Harmonic scalpel shears—Vibration of the active blade results in the formation of a "sticky" coagulum. Pressure from the non-active blade causes the vessel to "weld" closed.

The characteristics of a laser beam depend upon the active medium used to generate the beam and the amount of energy applied (Fig. 8.8).[9] The active medium can be:

- Gas (CO_2)
- Metal vapor (copper or gold)
- Liquid dye [coumarin (green) or rhodamine (red)] or
- Solid-doped crystalline medium [most commonly yttrium-aluminum-garnet (YAG) mixed with neodymium (Nd:YAG)]

Laser applications for endoscopy and laparoscopy have undergone dramatic changes. Currently, lasers have limited use in MIS because equally effective and less expensive alternatives are available.[10] New technology looks promising for the development of "tunable" lasers that will allow the surgeon to pick the laser wavelengths most effective at destroying or heating the target tissue.[11] Currently, it is necessary to compromise, using the laser that has the closest wavelength to that desired. At present hospitals have to buy several fixed wavelength lasers to meet all their needs.

Ultrasonic Energy

A major breakthrough in the energy technology is the use of ultrasonic energy. This energy modality uses fast oscillation instruments (55,500 Hz) that, through friction, produce tissue heating and protein denaturation. Protein denaturation results in the formation of a sticky coagulum, which, if subjected to direct pressure, results in tissue welding (Fig. 8.9). The harmonic scalpel is an example of this technology. It allows the surgeon to occlude, weld, and divide vessels without the use of hemostatic clips or sutures and without the need to first skeletonize the vessel. This high-tech machinery has greatly facilitated many laparoscopic procedures by combining vessel occlusion and division (especially for medium-size vessels) into one step with a minimal collateral damage.[12]

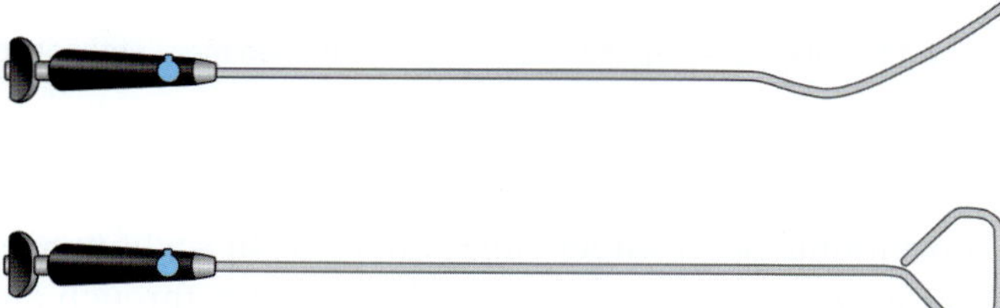

Fig. 8.10: Flexible retractor—The straight floppy position (top) allows introduction through a cannula, whereas the closed position (bottom) allows tissue retraction.

Hand Instruments

Many commonly used instruments in open surgery have had to be reconfigured for laparoscopic surgery. Retractors, for example, had to be developed to provide a broad atraumatic retracting surface yet still pass through a 5- or 10-mm port. A number of retractor designs ensued. Early designs featured a fan of blades, which when closed could be passed through a port and then expanded in the abdominal cavity to provide a broad retracting surface. Other designs included inflatable retracting surfaces, which were less traumatic but slightly less rigid.

Other innovative design comprises a series of cylindric segments linked by internal cables. The snake-like instruments can be passed through a 5-mm port. Once in the abdominal cavity, the cables are tightened with a screw mechanism at the end of the handle. As the cables tighten, the segments take on a triangular or circular configuration, which are reasonably stiff yet relatively atraumatic (Fig. 8.10).

Laparoscopic retraction can be hazardous because the retractor is outside the endoscopic view for most (>75%) of the operation. Inadvertent movement can result in appreciable tissue injury, bleeding, or loss of exposure. If possible, external fixation of the retractor is recommended to avoid accidental movement. It also frees the assistant's hand for other tasks.

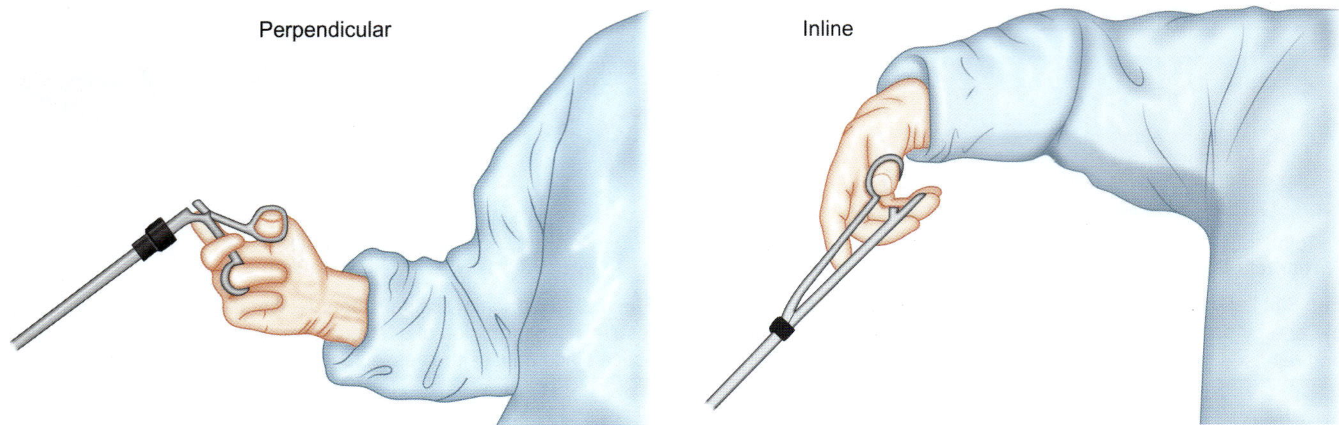

Fig. 8.11: Handles—Perpendicular handles are often more ergonomically friendly for the surgeon than inline handles.

Many hand instruments for MIS are duplicates of conventional open surgery instruments with slight modifications in the shaft and tip to allow passage through an access port. Standard-length instruments have a 30-cm long and 5-mm wide shaft, but longer instruments (45 cm) were developed for bariatric surgery. More specialized instruments are wider, like dissectors (10 mm) or staplers (up to 12 mm), but instruments can also be shorter and thinner for pediatric and arthroscopic procedures. Forceps and clamps have been replaced by a variety of different graspers, their function being determined by configuration of the jaw. Care must be taken when using graspers because the pressure applied to the tissues is greater and in a smaller area, with an increased risk of damaging them. On the other hand, these long thin instruments are more difficult to clean and maintain (e.g. scissors sharpening). Disposable instruments eliminate the problems of cleaning as well as the costs of maintenance and repair. Reusable instruments may be more difficult to clean but are much less expensive for hospitals in which a moderate-to-high volume of MIS is carried out. A number of manufacturers produce "reposable" instruments, which consist of a reusable shaft and disposable tip and appear to be an affordable compromise for high-maintenance items such as laparoscopic scissors.

Laparoscopic handles have undergone many innovations. The two configurations are: handle in a perpendicular position to the instrument shaft (pistol grip) and the "inLine," as well as a locking or nonlocking mechanism. Most instrument handles are pistol grips, which are often more ergonomically friendly when the instrument must be held with an elevated arm, away from the body (Fig. 8.11). However, this configuration is very different from the "inline" handle design of most conventional instruments. Many situations, such as knot tying, require more precise movements, which are easier to perform with the handle in the "inline" position. Therefore, needle drivers and suturing devices are now primarily designed with "inline" configurations. Other instruments such as scissors and graspers, are also available with these handles. Several instrument manufacturers now produce handles that can be flipped from an "inline" to a perpendicular position, depending upon the surgeon's need.

Room Setup

Laparoscopic surgery requires a great deal of equipment. Even the simplest procedure requires:

- At least one video monitor
- Insufflation (or mechanical lift device)
- Light source
- Camera system
- Energy source and
- Specialized instruments

Add to this a second energy source (lithotriptor or ultrasonic generator), a second monitor, a video recorder, and it becomes clear that a large organized room is necessary.[13] Most basic laparoscopy equipment can be organized on a single cart that carries a monitor, insufflator, camera, video recorder, and electrosurgery energy source. It is not essential to have one, but the development of MIS suites made a great contribution to the field because they simplify the performance of complex procedures. The core equipment (imaging, monitors, and insufflators) is set in ceiling mobile consoles maximizing cable organization, facilitating the personnel movement around the room, and allowing and expedite and continuous adjustments during the operation.

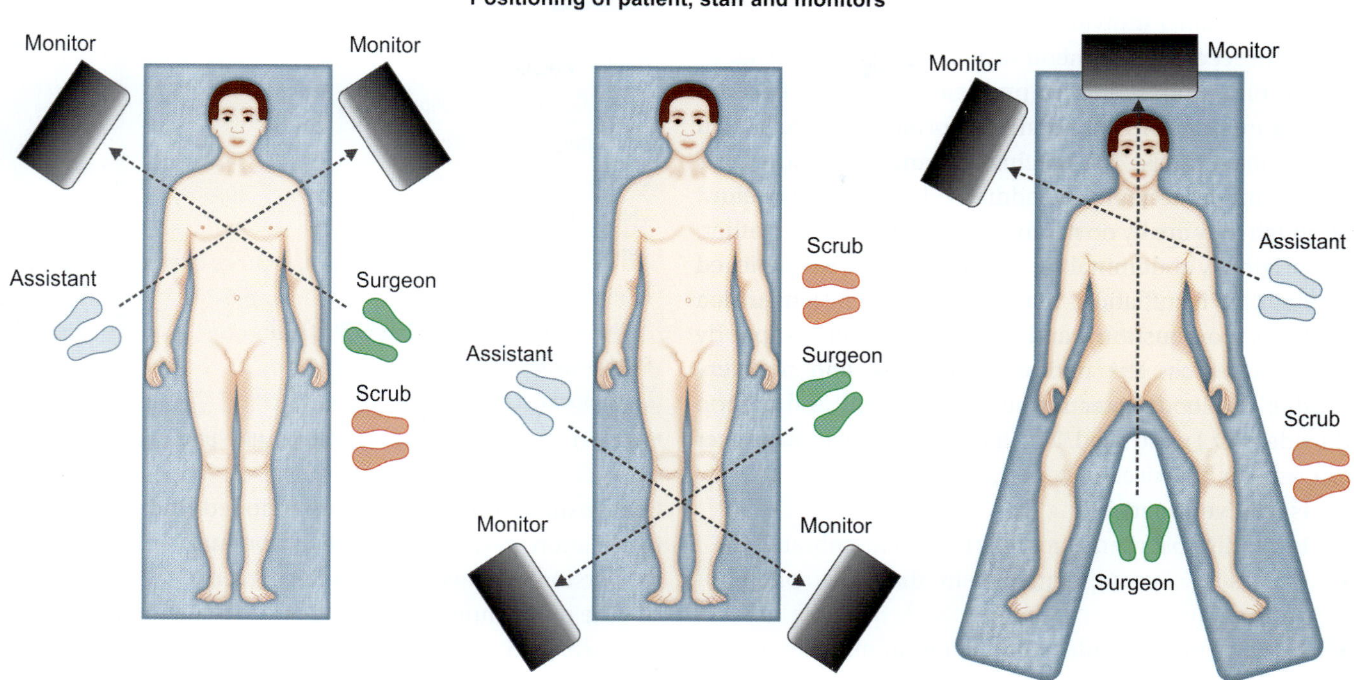

Fig. 8.12: Patient positions that allow the monitor to be placed across the table from the surgeon and assistant.

The patient should be placed between the surgeon and the video monitor. A second or "slave" monitor is helpful for the surgical assistant across the operating table from the surgeon. The insufflation and monitoring equipment should also be placed within the surgeon's view if possible. This setup allows the surgeon to work in a direct line between his hands and the video image, so minimizing fatigue (Fig. 8.12). Eyestrain is directly related to the monitors' distance and height between the surgeons. The preferable viewing distance ranges between 80 cm (for standard 19 in CRT monitors) to 120 cm (for 21 in HD monitors) so that the extensive accommodation and conversion by the extraocular musculature will be avoided. The monitors should be desirably placed <15° of the horizontal plane to avoid excessive spine axial rotation and in the vertical plane to the eye level or up to 15° downward, which is the most comfortable eye position.[14]

Some procedures require more than one videoscopic image (e.g. laparoscopic common bile duct exploration or endoscopic retrograde cholangiopancreatography). In these situations, the two monitors should be as close together as possible or the images merged into a "picture in picture" using a video mixer.

The table height should be positioned so that the surgeon works with his or her arms relaxed at the shoulders; the elbows are kept close to the side and bend in a 90° angle. This position will minimize both fatigue and frustration. The "wing out" position with the shoulder abducted at 60–90° cannot be maintained for more than half an hour without producing extreme fatigue and tremor.

PHYSIOLOGY OF MINIMAL INVASIVE SURGERY AND ANESTHETIC CONSIDERATIONS

Laparoscopy

Although there are numerous benefits to abdominal MIS, these procedures are often particularly challenging for the anesthesiologist. The insufflation of gas into the peritoneal cavity during laparoscopic procedures has a profound effect on homeostatic mechanisms.[15,16] The increased intra-abdominal pressure exerted by the gas as well as the nature of the insufflation gas alter hemodynamics through mechanical and humoral mechanisms. Coupled with these alterations is the change in patient position to extreme Trendelenburg and/or reverse Trendelenburg positions, which may cause further cardiovascular flux. The physiology of pneumoperitoneum, therefore, dictates the anesthetic requirements.

The effects of pneumoperitoneum are well tolerated in young healthy individuals. The introduction of laparoscopic procedures to general surgery has led to a reexamination of the physiology of pneumoperitoneum because procedures are longer and are performed on older, often sicker, individuals. The mechanical and humoral effects of pneumoperitoneum are addressed individually below, although they are by no means independent of each other.

Originally abdominal cavity visualization was achieved through air insufflation, but air contains oxygen (which supports combustion) and nitrogen, which is poorly absorbed across the peritoneal surfaces and not very soluble in blood. Later nitrous oxide (N_2O) and carbon dioxide (CO_2) were used. N_2O has several advantages over CO_2 and air because it:

- Is relatively inert
- Is rapidly absorbed across peritoneal membranes
- Causes less postoperative pain than CO_2 pneumoperitoneum and
- Reduces the end-tidal volume and minute ventilation required to maintain homeostasis compared with CO_2[17]

Carbon dioxide is still the preferred gas used for insufflation because it:

- Is rapidly absorbed across the peritoneal membranes
- Does not support combustion and
- Is safer to use than N_2O[18]

The largest body buffer lies in the bones, with a CO_2 absorption capacity of up to 120 L, which minimizes the hypercarbia and respiratory acidosis (generation of carbonic acid from CO_2) during short laparoscopic procedures.[19] In more prolonged surgeries absorption of CO_2 overwhelms the body's buffer system, and the respiratory system assumes the duty of carbon dioxide absorption. Increased ventilation then becomes the only elimination route for CO_2.[20] This process is rarely a problem for patients who have normal ventilatory function and is managed by increasing the ventilatory rate and vital capacity. Decreasing the pressure of the pneumoperitoneum to 8–10 mm Hg (1.1–1.3 kPa) also helps. Progressively higher respiratory rates (>20) may result in increased "dead space" ventilation and hypercapnia. Although mild respiratory acidosis is rarely a problem, increasingly severe acidosis may cause:

- Tachycardia
- Increased systemic vascular resistance
- Cardiac ischemia and
- Life-threatening arrhythmias

In these situations, evacuation of the pneumoperitoneum to allow CO_2 "wash out" is imperative. Occasionally, CO_2 insufflation must be abandoned for a different insufflation gas, mechanical abdominal wall "lifts," or conversion to conventional open surgery.

Table 8.1 Physiologic effects of carbon dioxide pneumoperitoneum.

Physiologic parameter	*Effect*
Cardiac output	↑↓*
Systemic vascular resistance	↑
Pulmonary vascular resistance	↑
Central venous pressure	↑
Venous resistance	↑
Venous return	↑↓*
Heart rate	↑↓*
Partial pressure of carbon dioxide (Pco_2)	↑
Peak inspiratory pressure	↑
Urine output	↓

* Depends upon volume status and insufflation pressure

The most important management issue for anesthesia is a clear and thorough understanding of the physiology of CO_2 pneumoperitoneum, as summarized in Table 8.1. Although the physiologic consequences of CO_2 insufflation are well tolerated by healthy individuals, problems may arise with those who have compromised cardiovascular function. Good communication between the surgeon and anesthesiologist is imperative because the surgeon can greatly influence cardiovascular performance by dropping insufflation or retracting abdominal organs.

Preload may be affected in a number of ways depending upon:

- Hydration
- Cardiac function
- Vascular resistance

Studies in dogs have found that small (i.e. low-pressure) increases in intra-abdominal pressure increase venous return by "squeezing" blood from abdominal organs into the central venous system. This effect, coupled with a relatively small increase in mean arterial pressure, may actually increase venous return. As intra-abdominal pressure is further increased (generally >20 mm Hg), venous return decreases because of increments in both venous and systemic vascular resistance.[21] Increased external pressure on the vena cava results in sluggish blood flow in the lower extremity venous system, especially in procedures where the patient is in reverse Trendelenburg, creating an ideal situation for deep venous thrombosis (DVT). Therefore, DVT prophylaxis is recommended, especially in procedures above 90 minutes in duration.

Insufflation may also induce cardiac arrhythmias as a result of positive pressure, hypercapnia, or both. Bradycardia is the most common cardiac arrhythmia associated with laparoscopy. Peritoneal stretch results in an increase in vagal tone, which may induce bradycardia. Bradycardia that results in hypotension should be treated with:

- Rapid desufflation of the abdominal cavity
- Intravascular volume resuscitation and
- Atropine

Pneumoperitoneum raises not only intra-abdominal pressure but also intrathoracic pressure if there is a surgically paralyzed diaphragm, resulting in increased peak inspiratory pressure. Although this fact theoretically increases the likelihood of barotrauma, this has not proved to be a major problem at moderate insufflation pressures [< 20 mm Hg (2.7 kPa)].

Fluid Balance

Other anesthetic considerations during laparoscopy are fluid loss and assessment of volume status. Much of the evaporative fluid loss that occurs in open surgery is virtually eliminated during laparoscopic procedures. Insufflated air is humidified by some insufflators, which further decreases fluid loss, so supplemental intraoperative intravenous fluid administration is very rarely needed.

Urine production cannot be usefully monitored as an indicator of volume status during laparoscopic procedures. Increased intra-abdominal pressure from the insufflated gas decreases renal blood flow, which results in decreased glomerular filtration and urine output.[22] This drop in renal blood flow elicits a secondary release of renin and antidiuretic hormone, resulting in sodium and free water reabsorption with the end result of oliguria. Postoperatively, the urine output often remains low for over 1 hour until the hormonal mediators restore homeostasis. A lack of understanding of the effects of pneumoperitoneum on urine output can result in fluid overload and congestive cardiac failure in patients with cardiac function.

Thoracoscopy

Video-assisted thoracoscopic surgery (VATS) is minimally invasive thoracic surgery and has some differences compared with the abdominal MIS. The use of positive pressure in the thorax will result in a decreased venous return and mediastinal shift. Since the thorax has a rigid bony structure, the use of positive pressure can be spared.[23] To create a working space it is necessary to use a double-lumen endotracheal tube to collapse the lung from the ipsilateral hemithorax. The trocars used for VATS differ from laparoscopic ones in their valve absence because there is no positive pressure to contain, and also the use of standard open thoracotomy instruments is possible.

Extracavitary Minimal Invasive Surgery

The MIS concept has been taken to other parts of the body besides the thorax and the abdominal cavity. In these places there is a lack of a true anatomical space, and a working area needs to be created. This working space is generally achieved using a balloon inflation technique followed by a low-pressure gas inflation device (usually < 10 mm Hg) to maintain the created space. This approach has a lower physiologic impact compared with pneumoperitoneum, but the carbon dioxide can cause subcutaneous emphysema with consequent metabolic acidosis due to the wide spreading of the gas through the tissues.[24]

Some of the areas and organs that are approached with extracavitary MIS are the laparoscopic inguinal hernia repairs, laparoscopic or robotic prostatectomy, laparoscopic nephrectomy, and lower extremities vascular procedures (e.g. saphenous vein harvesting).

The MIS extracavitary approach has a smaller working space than laparoscopy; on the other hand, it eliminates the intestinal injury risk and the postoperative adhesion formation.[25]

ABDOMINAL ACCESS, TROCAR INSERTION, PLACEMENT, AND CLOSURE

Laparoscopy is not free from risks. One of the most dangerous parts of a laparoscopic procedure is gaining access to the peritoneal cavity and trocar placement. Trocars are the working ports (tubes) through which the instruments are inserted into the patient's body. They insure against loss of the working space containing the insufflated gas through its one-way valves (sealing mechanism), and they also avoid damage to the skin and muscle.

The least safe technique of access the abdominal cavity is direct trocar puncture without insufflation. Although still practiced by some surgeons, it should be abandoned because the risk of visceral or vascular injury is greater than with other methods. The two accepted methods for peritoneal insufflation are the closed and open techniques. The most common access site is the umbilicus, where the abdominal wall is thinnest. Another relatively safe area for access is Palmer's point, 3 cm below the left costal margin, lateral to the rectus muscle in the midclavicular line. A right-sided approach can be used as well.[26] However, it is important to judge the safest site for the primary puncture in a previously operated abdominal cavity as well as the best placement site for the camera to facilitate completion of the procedure.

Closed Access Technique

The closed access technique involves a small stab wound through the skin, which is followed by insertion of a spring-loaded needle cannula (Veress needle).[27] The needle surrounds a blunt protective inner stylet, which retracts under pressure to expose the sharp needle tip and then springs back beyond the needle tip when the resistance of the abdominal wall is lost upon entering the peritoneal cavity (Fig. 8.13). This method is relatively safe in patients who have not had previous surgery. Upward traction is placed on the abdominal wall to lift it away from the underlying viscera, and the Veress needle is inserted with steady pressure. Two characteristic "pops" are felt as the needle passes through the fascia and peritoneum. Aspiration helps check the position of the needle:

- If blood is aspirated, the needle is repositioned
- If the blood return is pulsatile, a great vessel may be injured and laparotomy should be performed immediately
- If bile or bowel contents are aspirated, the needle should be repositioned and the damage assessed laparoscopically
- If nothing is aspirated the needle is flushed with saline, which should flow freely into the peritoneal cavity

If saline is reaspirated, the needle is probably preperitoneal in location and a saline drop test is carried out. A drop of saline is placed at the top of the needle and the abdominal wall is lifted further–the drop should descend, confirming intraperitoneal placement. In the Palmer test the full barrel of a syringe is attached to the Veress needle after the plunger has been removed. Observation of the flow rate from a 10-mL syringe provides quantifiable information on intraperitoneal needle placement and is our preferred method for confirming position.

Carbon dioxide insufflation is then begun at a low flow rate (1.5 L/min). An initial high-pressure reading (>6 mm Hg) or sudden jump to a high pressure suggests that the needle tip is either inappropriately placed outside the peritoneal cavity, abutting omentum or viscera, or that the patient is not relaxed. High flow can be instituted if none of these problems arise at low-flow insufflation. After an adequate pneumoperitoneum has been achieved [approximately 15 mm Hg (2.0 kPa)], the needle is removed, the skin incision is enlarged, and a 5- or 10-mm trocar is carefully advanced until the abdominal cavity is entered, directing the tip away from the great vessels and the sacral promontory. The trocar is removed, a laparoscope is inserted, and the abdominal contents are inspected. Further trocar site insertions are selected, the abdominal wall is transilluminated to avoid large abdominal wall vessels and its entrance to the abdominal cavity is followed under direct visualization.

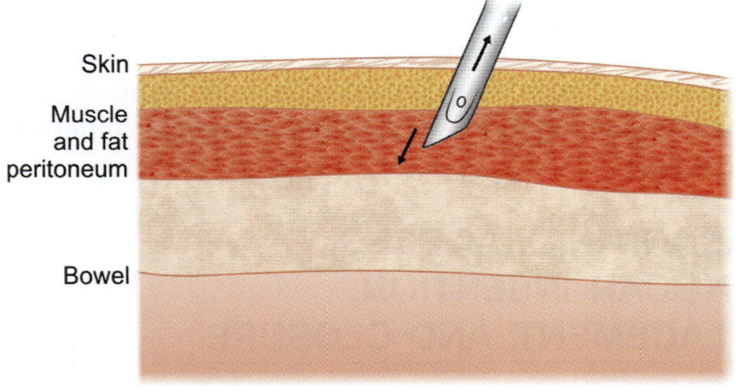

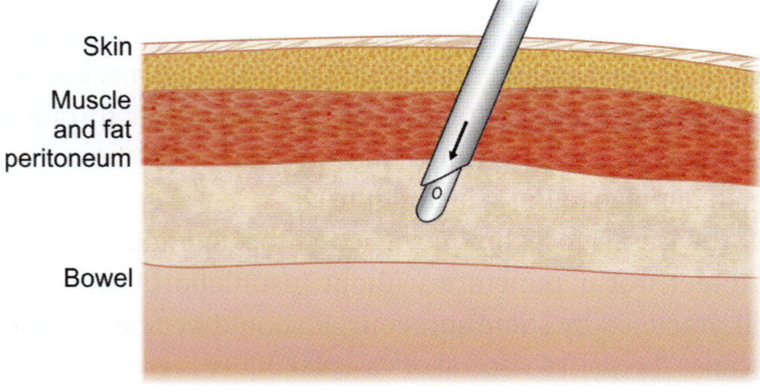

Fig. 8.13: Veress needle—The spring-loaded inner stylet of the Veress needle retracts under the pressure of the abdominal wall, exposing the sharp needle tip, but rebounds into its protective position once the abdominal wall resistance is lost upon entering the peritoneal space.

Open Access Technique

A blunt-tipped (Hasson) cannula is required for the open technique.[28] This technique is particularly useful in patients who have a history of previous surgery and suspected intra-abdominal adhesions. In many centers, this access method is preferred, as it is felt to be safer.

The umbilicus is the preferred site of primary entry, as the abdominal wall is thinnest at this point. Infiltration of the skin and underlying tissue helps separate the layers and aids postoperative analgesia. A skin incision is made either in the inferior periumbilical region or through the umbilicus itself. The lateral skin edges can be elevated slightly to aid subsequent closure if desired. The skin edges are then elevated and retracted laterally. A Kocher clamp is placed on each side of the midline, and the fascia and peritoneum are opened under direct vision. A finger may be inserted into the peritoneal cavity and used to sweep away any adhesions from the port site before inserting the Hasson cannula. Large absorbable sutures (usually 0-0) are placed on either side of the fascial opening. The cannula is placed in position by fixing the "plug" to the fascial slitches, which maintains an air seal and thus minimizes pneumoperitoneum leakage around the cannula. The laparoscope can then be inserted to ensure intraperitoneal placement, and insufflation can be initiated at a high flow.

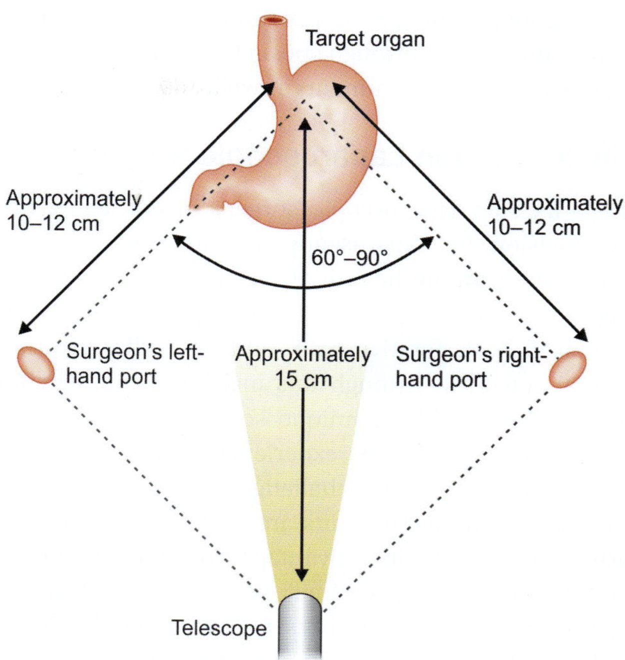

Fig. 8.14: Positioning of the operating and camera ports—These should be placed to form a diamond with the area of operation at one apex and the telescope at the other. The operating instruments are placed through the lateral ports. This configuration facilitates two-handed dissection with minimal fatigue and contortion.

Abdominal Wall Lift Technique

A third option for abdominal access is the abdominal wall lift technique.[29] In this technique, retractors are inserted into the peritoneal cavity through a small open incision. The retractors are then fixed to a mechanical lift device, which elevates the anterior abdominal wall like a tent to create a working space below. This technique has the advantage of not requiring intraperitoneal gas insufflation, avoiding the physiologic changes from pneumoperitoneum, alleviating the problems of gas leaks, and port-instrument incompatibilities.

Trocar Placement

In general, trocars should be placed to form an equilateral triangle with the surgeon's operating hands approximately 10 cm apart and the camera port between and behind them. The operative field should occupy a mirror position to the camera port. The two adjacent triangles form a diamond, which gives the surgeon the greatest degree of freedom for instrument manipulation, with few if any awkward contortions (Fig. 8.14).

There are many trocar types available. They may be disposable or nondisposable with unique characteristics, but the main difference is the introductory mechanism they possess. They can be tipbladed and nonbladed. Bladed trocars have a retractable shield and cut the muscular fascia while entering. The blade is exposed while under pressure during penetration of the abdominal wall layers, and it will be covered with the shield once the peritoneal cavity is reached and the pressure is gone. Nonbladed trocars make smaller fascia defects and come in a wide variety. Some have rough plastic edges in the tip that divide the tissues while entering the abdomen wall, other have a Veress needle system (dilating system) with an expandable sheath attached. Once the peritoneal cavity is entered, the Veress needle is removed and a blunt-tipped trocar is introduced through the expandable sheath to guide it to the cavity. Nonbladed trocars tend to make smaller cuts in the muscular fascia, minimizing the bleeding risk, creating a tighter seal for the pneumoperitoneum and decreasing the risk of an incisional hernia.[30]

Hand-Assisted Laparoscopy

The combination of strengths of the open surgery (the tactile advantage) and the MIS makes the hand-assisted laparoscopy an interesting option, especially as a step before conversion to an open procedure in difficult cases or as an adjuvant tool for the steep learning curve a surgeon faces in advanced laparoscopic procedures.[31]

To contain the pneumoperitoneum, the surgeon's hand is introduced through specialized hand ports allowing the use of MIS instruments as well.

Single-Incision Laparoscopic Surgery

Single-incision laparoscopic surgery means using only one incision for laparoscopy; the incision is usually 2–3-cm long and in the umbilicus. This approach has the theoretical advantage of an almost scarless procedure, decreased postoperative pain, and an earlier return to normal activities. Through this incision a multichannel port is placed. This technique seems to be adoptable, feasible, and safe for the experienced MIS surgeon, but it carries more technical challenges. The positions of the camera and the instruments are parallel to each other, losing the triangulation advantage from the laparoscopy and diminishing the optimal field of view. Also, this instrument position produces a "sword fight" because of the working space reduction and coaxial entry of the surgical instruments. Many measures have been taken trying to address these issues. Some of them involve the manufacture of roticulating instruments, utilizing instruments of different seizes and crossing the hands while operating.[32,33]

Port Closure

At the conclusion of the procedure, all trocars must be withdrawn under direct visualization and bleeding should be assessed.

To avoid the risk of port-site hernia, it is recommended to close the muscular fascia in incisions ≥10 mm made with bladed trocars. This statement does not necessarily hold true with nonbladed trocars in which the created defect is smaller or if the port placement is off the midline and above the transverse mesocolon. As a general consensus, 5-mm size trocar sites do not require to be sutured.

COMPLICATIONS

Complications Associated with Abdominal Access and Trocar Placement

Between one third and one half of all MIS major complications occur at the time of the surgical entry, regardless of the method (open vs closed access technique) used, with an overall incidence of 1.1 per 1,000 cases.[34]

Wound infections are less common in MIS than open surgery. Both open and closed laparoscopic access have similar wound infection rates of 0.1–3%.[35] Wound infections are determined by the procedure rather than the method of access. When they occur they are generally minor and easily treated with hygienic wound care, antibiotics, and drainage if necessary.

Port-site hernias are uncommon (0.5%) and occur regardless of the access method. The possibility for a hernia development is higher when the size of the port is bigger (≥ 12 mm), when bladed trocars are used or with a higher body mass index and older age.[36] Herniation is more common in the midline where the abdominal wall is the thinnest. Oblique port angulations through the abdominal muscles may reduce the likelihood of subsequent hernia formation.

Bladder Injury

This type of lesion is especially feared when performing a pelvic procedure. The risk increases with suprapubic trocar insertions. When a port placement below the umbilicus is anticipated, a Foley catheter should be placed to decompress the bladder and minimize the injury potential.

The minor serosal tears or small cystotomies can either be managed expectantly with continuous bladder drainage for 7 to 10 days, or they can be sutured with a 2-0 or 3-0 absorbable braided suture. Diathermy lesions or those >1 cm should be repaired with running or interrupted stitches in two layers to ensure a watertight closure, which has to be tested by backfilling the bladder and assessing any leakage. The indwelling Foley catheter is kept in place up to 7 days and, before removing it, the bladder integrity is confirmed with a cystogram.

Suspected bladder lesions can be evaluated with the intravenous administration of 5-mL indigo carmine. After 10 minutes the blue dye will be excreted through the urine, and the bladder can be assessed for dye spillage.[34]

Vascular Injury

The reported rate of vascular complication ranges from 0.1 to 6.4 per 1,000 laparoscopic cases. The lesion can may not be immediately appreciated due to the bleeding either into the mesentery of the retroperitoneum. Laceration of the mesenteric vessels is the most common vascular complication during the introduction of the Veress needle or with the placement of the first trocar, especially if there are several adhesions. During the placement of lateral trocars the most common vascular lesion is laceration of the inferior epigastric artery.[37,38]

The most devastating complication of trocar placement is injury to major retroperitoneal vessels, with a reported rate of 0.3% to 1% of MIS procedures; almost 80% of these occur during primary needle insertion or trocar placement. The aorta is more likely to be injured in upper abdominal procedures, whereas for gynecologic or colorectal procedures the iliac vessels are more prone to injury, especially on the right side, which may be related to a right-handed surgeon introducing the Veress needle or to a trocar inserted from the patient's left side. Early diagnosis and treatment are crucial because the reported mortality rate is as high as 23%, either from exsanguination or massive air embolism.[34,39,40] An obvious gush of blood through the Veress needle or trocar requires immediate exploration in most cases. A constant welling of blood in the abdominal cavity also suggests major vessel injury and is usually an indication for laparotomy. The offending trocar or needle should be left in place to provide some form of compression and aid rapid localization of the injury. Veress needle injuries can be subtle and present as hemodynamic instability secondary to an expanding retroperitoneal hematoma. Venous injury is slightly more difficult to appreciate because the pneumoperitoneum may tamponade the injury. Lowering the insufflation pressure in suspected cases may make bleeding more apparent and allow prompt treatment.

Abdominal wall vessels are also at risk of lesion. Epigastric vessel injury may occur from secondary ports. These injuries may present as a slow steady dripping of blood down the trocar shaft or may not be apparent until the trocar is removed. It is therefore imperative to inspect all port sites after ports have been removed to ensure hemostasis. Most of the bleeding points can be detected and treated with monopolar electrosurgery. If bleeding continues a Foley catheter can be inserted through the trocar site, inflated to produce compression to the bleeding vessel and then held in place for 5 minutes. If all these maneuvers fail, full-thickness abdominal wall stitches (U-stitches) with a braided absorbable suture can be placed under direct laparoscopic visualization using endoscopic closure devices; sometimes the skin incision needs to be extended to control the bleeding. If missed, these injuries can form massive abdominal wall hematomas or may continue to bleed into the peritoneal cavity. The latter may prove fatal if unrecognized or not properly treated.

Visceral Injury

Visceral injury from needle or trocar insertion is slightly more common than vascular injury, with an incidence of 1%. The small bowel is the most common gastrointestinal structure to be damaged. Visceral injury is often missed at the initial operation in 15%–77% of cases) and presents late in the postoperative period with sepsis; it carries a mortality rate as high as 28%.[34,41]

Signs of obvious bowel injury include aspiration of bowel contents from the Veress needle, feculent odor from trocar sites, and the overt spillage of bowel contents. A bowel injury should also be suspected if the opening "intra-abdominal" pressure is between 8 and 10 mm Hg. Veress needle punctures can be managed expectantly, but the area of injury must be carefully inspected to ensure that a laceration has not occurred. Trocar injuries, on the other hand, usually require primary repair because the injuries are more commonly full-thickness lacerations, which need to be repaired in a two-layer fashion. However, if the injury is a partial thickness laceration, interrupted sutures with a 3-0 delayed-absorbable suture can be placed. Antibiotics should be given if a laceration is confirmed.

Gastric decompression, avoidance of N_2O anesthetic, and bladder decompression before needle or trocar insertion help minimize the risk of visceral injury. Although the open technique of access is associated with fewer complications in the hands of the novice laparoscopist, it is not risk free. Strict adherence to proper principles and techniques minimizes the risk of complications for both open and closed access techniques.

Complications of Pneumoperitoneum

The complications of pneumoperitoneum are usually a consequence of:

- Physiologic effects of the insufflated gas (CO_2)
- Mechanical effects of the pressure exerted by the gas.

The physiology of pneumoperitoneum is addressed in relation to the anesthetic requirements (see above). Patients who have poor cardiac or respiratory reserve are more prone to complications. Arrhythmias are quite common during laparoscopy:

- Bradyarrhythmias secondary to vagal stimulation from peritoneal stretching may lead to sinus arrest[42]
- Other arrhythmias, which include tachycardia and premature ventricular contractions caused by hypercapnia;[43] these are generally well tolerated unless the arterial partial pressure of CO_2 is allowed to increase above 60 mm Hg (8.0 kPa).

Subcutaneous emphysema is the presence of CO_2 gas outside the peritoneum and muscular fascia. It can extend from as high as the submandibular area to as low as the inguinal area, including the scrotum. This extraperitoneal insufflation may occur when the trocars are under a great deal of torque, particularly when they are inserted at a wrong angle or in obese patients (thus stretching the incision and allowing the gas to escape from the peritoneal cavity), or when trocars or gas inflow slips into the thickness of the abdominal wall. Subcutaneous emphysema is identified as a crepitus under the skin or when a slowly rising CO_2 level is detected during the operation. Usually, it causes no harm to a patient and will spontaneously regress within 1 to 2 days, but severe swelling around the neck can cause airway compression.

Pneumothorax and/or pneumomediastinum are rare (< 1%), but may make hypercarbia difficult to control with hyperventilation.[44]

Death has been reported from excessive pneumoperitoneum pressure [> 40 mm Hg (5.3 kPa)] caused by an extreme reduction in venous return, cardiac output, and blood pressure.[44] This cardiac depression is analogous to that seen in tension pneumothorax.

As mentioned above, lower limb venous flow decreases during laparoscopy. It is therefore recommended to use DVT prophylaxis, such as sequential compression devices alone or in conjunction with subcutaneous heparin or low molecular weight heparin for procedures over 90 minutes in duration. With this approach, the incidence of DVT after laparoscopy is <0.05%.[45]

Hypothermia may also occur in prolonged procedures that require large volumes of gas exchange.[46]

A rare (0.002–0.02%) but often fatal complication of pneumoperitoneum is venous gas embolism.[47,48] Small amounts of gas can be absorbed and never identified, but clinically important gas embolism can occur with venous injury. It usually occurs during abdominal wall access, when the gas is insufflated into the venous system, thus placing a vapor lock in the cardiac pump. This accident results in:

- Acute hypotension
- Premature ventricular contractions
- Cyanosis
- Hypoxia
- A classic "mill wheel" murmur.

Treatment is immediate release of the pneumoperitoneum and placement of the patient in a steep Trendelenburg and left lateral decubitus position, so the gas gets trapped in the apex of the right ventricle. This gas is then aspirated through a central venous catheter.

Postoperative abdominal or shoulder pain is a consequence of pneumoperitoneum. Its frequency ranges from 35% to 80%. It can vary from mild to severe and usually lasts 1 to 3 days, but gas has been observed in the peritoneal cavity up to 1 week postoperatively without evidence of gastrointestinal perforation. The exact mechanism of pain after laparoscopy is unclear; the leading hypothesis is that CO_2 combines with water to form carbonic acid, which irritates the peritoneum and induces phrenic nerve irritation, causing referred pain projected to the shoulder via the C4 nerve root. The irritation might be caused by local acidosis, distension and stretching of the peritoneum and diaphragm, or irritation secondary to CO_2 remaining in the abdomen. Operations using standard pneumoperitoneum pressures (14 mm Hg) and incomplete evacuation may exacerbate this pain by eliminating the "vacuum" of the hepatodiaphragmatic space. These complications can be minimized by using low pressure pneumoperitoneum (<10 mm Hg), adequate irrigation, and evacuation of CO_2 from the peritoneal cavity.[49-51]

LAPAROSCOPY IN CHILDREN

The use of laparoscopy in the pediatric population is rapidly increasing to the point at which the MIS approach is becoming the standard for a variety of procedures (e.g. appendix, gallbladder, ovaries). With the development of instruments appropriate to this age that are shorter in length (15 to 20 cm) and diameter (3 mm), the benefit of MIS in the pediatric population may be more marked than in the adult population.

Although smaller diameter telescopes (3–5 mm) provide less illumination than larger telescopes, sufficient illumination is provided because the abdominal cavity in a child is smaller. Angled scopes (from 30° to 70°) are frequently used in children because the angle allows the telescope to keep out of the way of instruments in these small spaces.

Children over 6 months of age can usually tolerate pneumoperitoneum pressures of 15 mm Hg (2.0 kPa). Those under 6 months of age usually tolerate pressures of 10–12 mm Hg (1.3–1.6 kPa) for several hours. Fortunately, because the abdominal wall is much thinner and pliable in these patients, adequate visualization can typically be achieved with a lower intra-abdominal pressure [5–10 mm Hg (0.6–1.3 kPa)]. However, most children can tolerate transient pneumoperitoneum pressure increases up to 25 mm Hg (3.3 kPa), which is especially useful for trocar placement. The hypercapnia associated with CO_2 insufflation is generally well controlled with hyperventilation in children and does not cause major respiratory problems.[52,53]

Trocar positions for common adult procedures may not be the same for children because of their small size. Also, the distance between organs and the abdominal wall is much less in a child, so extra care must be taken with trocar insertion. Certain preoperative steps should be taken to remove as much intestinal gas as possible. Preoperative nasogastric suction is helpful for stomach and small bowel decompression in children who weigh < 10–15 kg. Cathartics are helpful for colonic decompression, and paregoric results in colonic contraction. Urinary catheters are not usually necessary if a Crede's maneuver is performed at the end of anesthesia.

Smaller patients should be taped onto the operating table to allow table positioning to optimize visualization. The same principles of patient positioning as for adults apply to pediatric patients.

Deep vein thrombosis is a rare clinical situation in children, and prophylaxis is only recommended only on those patients with multiple risk factors undergoing prolonged surgical procedures.[54]

LAPAROSCOPY IN PREGNANCY

Laparoscopy in the pregnant woman was absolutely contraindicated until 1990. Then, gradually and with much reluctance, the MIS approach gained currency. In the last decade there has been a paradigm shift, to the point that MIS is becoming the preferred method to treat most surgical situations in the gravid patient; data show the safety and efficacy of laparoscopy during all trimesters for many surgical situations, with similar outcomes compared with open operations. However, some of the constant controversies include timing, safest abdominal access and appropriate fetal, and maternal monitoring.[52,55]

Between 1 in 500 and 1 in 635 pregnant patients will require a nonobstetrical abdominal operation. The most common situation is acute appendicitis, with a similar incidence to that the nonpregnant female population (1 in 1,500). Performing the appendectomy with MIS carries the same preterm delivery and 1-month preterm birth rate (i.e. delivery 1 month after operation) as open appendectomy. Symptomatic cholelithiasis or biliary disease is the second most common nonobstetric condition present during pregnancy. Again, with the MIS approach, the outcomes (risk of spontaneous abortion and preterm labor) are equivalent to those of the open procedure.[52]

The benefits of MIS compared with open surgical techniques in pregnancy are:

- Magnified and improved view of the surgical field
- Decreased postoperative pain with lower narcotic use, faster ambulation, and lower thromboembolic events
- Decreased fetal depression with reduced maternal narcotic use
- Decreased postoperative maternal pulmonary complications
- Decreased uterine manipulation
- Decreased bowel manipulation with faster bowel function return and a possible decrease in adhesion formation, ileus, and bowel obstruction
- Decreased uterine irritability with lower rates of spontaneous abortion and preterm delivery
- Fewer wound complications (e.g. wound infection, incisional hernias, wound dehiscence with uterine growth)
- Faster postoperative recovery and return to regular activities[52]

The physiologic changes observed during pneumoperitoneum are accentuated in the pregnant population, especially in the cardiovascular and respiratory systems. The displacement of the diaphragm due to the enlarging uterus, coupled with pneumoperitoneum, promotes a decreased compliance, reduces the functional reserve capacity, and increases the peak airway pressure along with ventilation-perfusion mismatching, alveolar-arterial oxygen gradient, and pleural pressure. All these changes are more pronounced with the Trendelenburg position. On the other hand, the reverse Trendelenburg position reduces the cardiac index up to 50% and produces hypotension secondary to aortocaval compression from the gravid uterus and the pneumoperitoneum. To minimize the vena cava compression it is advisable to place the patient in the left lateral decubitus position during the surgical procedure, thus improving the venous return and cardiac output.[52,55]

An additional concern is decreased uterine blood flow during pneumoperitoneum. This is unlikely given the far greater pressure changes that safely occur during maternal coughing, straining, and midpregnancy uterine contractions. In fact, the pressure of pneumoperitoneum may be far safer than manual uterine retraction during open surgery.

MIS procedures can be performed at any time during pregnancy. The first trimester poses the least technical challenge, because the uterus is well below the point of initial trocar entry and visualization is optimal. However, the risk of teratogenesis is the greatest. Also, it is wise to wait until the most frequent period for spontaneous abortions has passed. Operation performed in the second trimester of pregnancy poses less risk to the fetus, but it is technically more difficult. The third trimester requires more surgical skills since the gravid uterus hinders optimal visualization and the potential for preterm labor is latent. Because of the higher risks to the fetus, either in the first or third trimester of pregnancy, it seems obvious that the second trimester is the safest interval for operative intervention for elective cases.

The decision on the abdominal access technique for MIS and placement of the trocars will be determined by the uterine size (fundal height) and previous incisions (Fig. 8.15). The open technique (Hasson) is the most popular in this setting, but when using the closed technique (with the Veress needle) Palmer's point is often used as the introduction area beyond the first trimester. To improve Veress needle safety and trocar insertion, either ultrasound guidance or a subxiphoid entry point can be employed. Alternatively, the gasless technique, lifting the abdominal wall with mechanical devices, has some followers, but more data are necessary to support this method.[52,55]

In the pregnant patient the use of vaginal instrumentation, cervical clamps, and uterine manipulator is prohibited.

The optimal pneumoperitoneum pressure is controversial, with some authors recommending a pressure < 12 mm Hg to decrease the cardiovascular impact on the pregnant patient, but CO_2 insufflation between 10 and 15 mm Hg can be safely used during MIS.[55]

Even though there is no proof of detrimental effects from pneumoperitoneum on human fetuses, the potential harm due to acidosis led to the recommendation of perioperative CO_2 monitoring by capnography, since the fetal pH follows maternal pH in a linear fashion. With this method maternal blood gas monitoring is unnecessary. The end-tidal CO_2 should be maintained between 32 and 34 mm Hg when carbon dioxide is used as the insufflation gas. This goal can be achieved by increasing the respiratory rate and tidal volume. The blood pressure should be maintained within 20% of baseline. Fetal heart monitoring in the pre- and postoperative periods is considered sufficient.[52,55]

To decrease the risk of DVT in the hypercoagulable state of pregnancy compounded by the pneumoperitoneum exacerbating venous stasis, the use of prophylactic pneumatic compression devices is recommended during the surgical event plus early ambulation in the postoperative period. The routine use of unfractioned heparin or low molecular heparin lacks literature support and should be used on a case-by-case basis.[55]

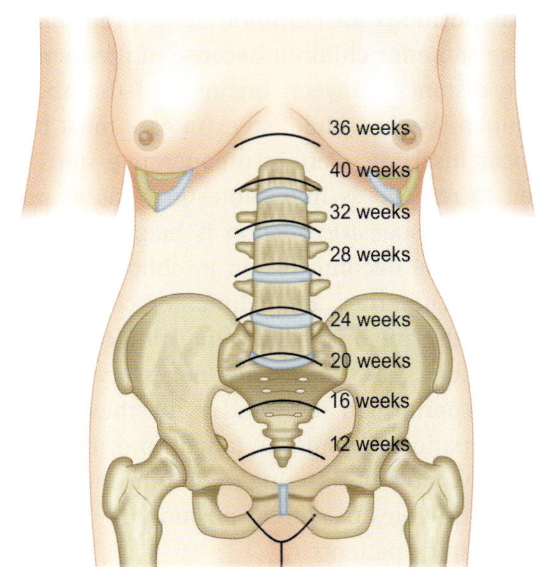

Fig. 8.15: Height of the uterus at various months of pregnancy.

LAPAROSCOPY IN THE ELDERLY

Although the operative risk should be judged on the basis of physiologic rather than chronologic age, many elderly patients are denied symptomatic relief from troublesome ailments because they are considered too fragile to undergo laparotomy.[56] MIS has allowed these individuals to undergo necessary interventions with minimal morbidity and mortality rates. This population requires more extensive anesthetic and postoperative management than younger patients.[57]

The anesthetic management and monitoring of the elderly may be more challenging when the procedure is performed laparoscopically as opposed to by an open technique because of the effects of the CO_2 pneumoperitoneum. In addition, many elderly patients have impaired cardiac and respiratory function that requires more invasive monitoring techniques such as Swan-Ganz catheters and arterial lines.

Much of the operative morbidity in the elderly is associated with postoperative impairments in mobility and hypoventilation. Pulmonary, urinary tract, wound, and thrombotic complications are often attributed to a lack of mobilization. MIS surgery allows a far more rapid return to normal activity, and often circumvents these complications.

Not all elderly infirm patients are suitable for an MIS approach, and these patients are more likely to require a conversion to an open procedure due to their disease chronicity.[58] Other patients with severe cardiac or respiratory disease may be better served by nonoperative interventions such as therapeutic endoscopy or radiographically guided stenting or drainage.

LAPAROSCOPY IN CIRRHOSIS AND PORTAL HYPERTENSION

Assessing which patient with cirrhosis is well enough to undergo an operation continues to be a quandary, and the outcomes are directly related to the underlying hepatic function. Most of these patients have a very low physiologic reserve, so that putting them under the stress of a surgical procedure can lead to hepatic failure. Therefore, it is of utmost importance to know the exact severity of liver damage. The Child-Turcotte-Pugh (Child) classification, which predicts the postoperative mortality risk, was commonly used in the prelaparoscopic era to address this issue. The mortality rate for Child A patients was 10%, as opposed to a 30% mortality rate for Child B cirrhosis and a 75% mortality rate for Child C cirrhosis.[59] Later, the Model of End-stage Liver Disease (MELD), which predicts 90-day mortality after operation in patients with liver disease, was adopted because of its reliability and superiority compared to Child's classification. In one study, preoperative Meld scores >14 were a better predictor of postoperative death than Child C status,[60] but in another study, the association between preoperative MELD score and 30-day postoperative mortality rate was broken down in a more stratified way, and the rates are as follows[61]:

- MELD score of ≤ 7—5.7% mortality
- MELD score of 8-11—10.3% mortality
- MELD score of 12-15—25.4% mortality
- MELD score of 16-20—44% mortality
- MELD score of 21-25—53.8% mortality
- MELD score of > 26—90% mortality

Regardless of these classifications, a low hemoglobin level (< 10 mg/dL) is an independent factor for poor surgical outcome in cirrhotic patients, who should therefore receive a corrective transfusion prior to operation.[60]

One of the biggest concerns in a cirrhotic patient undergoing operation is the bleeding risk at any stage (e.g. trocar insertion, dissection field) because of the subjacent coagulopathy. Also, the risk of bacterial infections is higher, especially with ascites leakage: reason enough to close the trocar sites in a watertight manner.

Portal hypertension is a relative contraindication to MIS, which must be delayed until the pressure in the portal system has been reduced. Most of these individuals are intravascularly depleted, and insufflation pressures should be reduced to avoid a decrease in the cardiac output.

ROBOT-ASSISTED LAPAROSCOPY

The term robot comes from the Czech word "*robota*" that means forced labor. A surgical robot is a computer-controlled instrument that can be programmed to accomplish specific tasks and aid in the disposition or handling of the instruments.

Since the 1980s surgical robots have been developed to help surgeons and try to overcome some of the limitations of laparoscopy such as ergonomics, visualization enhancement, and using instruments with a higher degree of freedom without losing all the advantages of MIS.[62] The first robot use in the surgical field was in 1985. It was the PUMA 560 developed to orient a needle for a brain biopsy under computerized tomography. Later in 1988 Imperial College, London, launched another robotic system that had been created to aid in transurethral prostate resections. It was called the PROBOT. The orthopedic field wanted to be part of this emerging technology, and in 1992 International Business Machines created the ROBODOC, a prototype for precise hole drilling during hip replacement operations. Two years later, the first "intelligent" camera holder was developed, the Automated Endoscopic System for Optimal Positioning (AESOP), which was designed to maneuver the telescope on voice commands. The goal was to give a steadier and better image, obviating the need for a surgical assistant to hold the camera.

The biggest achievement in robotic-assisted devices was definitively the master-slave platform creation. It was initially designed by the Stanford Research Institute, the National Aeronautics and Space Administration, and the Department of Defense to satisfy military needs in the battlefield. Soon after, the technology was acquired by Intuitive Surgical, who commercialized and spread the device, initially in Europe in 1999 and later in the United States after Food and Drug Administration approval in 2001, under the name of da Vinci Surgical System. Meanwhile Computer Motion, the creators of AESOP, launched ZEUS as a competing system for the da Vinci. ZEUS was discontinued in 2003 following the merger of Computer Motion and the rival company Intuitive Surgical.[63]

The major advantages of robotic-assisted laparoscopy over standard laparoscopy are:

- Improved image quality and conversion from a 2D to a 3D view
- Mechanical improvements with increased degrees of freedom (7) similar to the human hand, as opposed to the standard laparoscopic instruments with 4 degrees
- Stabilization of instruments in the surgical field, thus minimizing the tremor that develops during conventional laparoscopy
- Improved ergonomics for the surgeon sitting in a comfortable position during the operation, while an assistant stands at the surgical table and changes the instruments as needed. In the conventional MIS approach poor ergonomics can lead to fatigue and joint strains for the surgeon, especially when operating on an obese patient.[63-65]

The limitations faced by robotic-assisted laparoscopy are:

- Additional training
- Lack of haptics
- Limited instrumentation (e.g. irrigation and suction device, less energy sources)
- Limited to two abdominal quadrants at a time, with increased difficulty in changing the patient's position
- Increased cost and operating times
- Bulkiness of the devices
- Risk of mechanical or information transmission failure.[66]

Currently, robotic-assisted laparoscopy is widely used in urologic and gynecologic surgery but has had a lesser impact on cardiac and general surgery.[67,68]

The final application of this type of approach is yet to be determined, but it surely opens the way for telesurgery under hostile circumstances (battlefield, polar expeditions) or in complicated environments (space missions, deep sea explorations).[69]

NATURAL ORIFICE TRANSLUMINAL ENDOSCOPIC SURGERY (NOTES)

Natural Orifice Transluminal Endoscopic Surgery has been one of the hottest emerging approaches in MIS since Kalloo et al. described the procedure in 2000.[70] The concept is to access the peritoneal cavity, chest, or mediastinum via a hollow viscus using a flexible endoscope to perform diagnostic and therapeutic procedures.

The initial NOTES approaches were transgastric, but transvaginal, transurethral/transcystic, transcolonic, and transesophageal have been done.[71,72]

Defenders of the NOTES claim the following advantages:

- A hole in a hollow viscera is better tolerated by the body than one made in the abdominal wall, with potentially fewer complications (e.g. pain, ileus, adhesions, hernias) than standard laparoscopy
- Better cosmetic outcome with a scarless procedure (to some patients the most important outcome)
- Easier access in certain patients such as those who are obese
- Potentially faster recovery with a shorter hospital stay.

The procedures continue to be challenging mainly because the endoscopes and instruments are not the most appropriate, and this also makes them lengthier than standard laparoscopic operations. Efficient and affordable processes of disinfection and sterilization are still a challenge, so that a continuous potential threat in NOTES is bacterial contamination of the cavity due to the viscerotomy and prolonged manipulation even in the absence of a leak.[73]

During standard MIS laparoscopy the amount of pressure applied to the peritoneal cavity is controlled with pressure sensors, but with NOTES those sensors are absent and the risk of overinsufflation is latent, with the potential for decreased venous return to the heart.[74]

Major complications occur in any surgical procedure, such as bleeding or damage to adjacent organs and structures (e.g. bowel perforation or bile leak), but the ability to manage these situations with NOTES seems unlikely. Thus it might be necessary to convert to a standard laparoscopic or open procedure.

Today, most of the NOTES procedures are still hybrid, using the aid of standard MIS to ensure adequate exposure, retraction, and closure of the viscera. Although NOTES is still considered primarily experimental and it is too early to predict its ultimate role and value, it has dramatically changed our perception of how to approach gastrointestinal surgery.

ECONOMICS OF MINIMAL ACCESS SURGERY

The issue of procedure cost is a continuously moving target in the current era of changing healthcare reimbursements. Managed care contracts, private insurance contracts, hospital contracts with instrument suppliers, and federally funded healthcare all impact on costs and patient charges. Nevertheless, MIS must continue to be cost-effective in the current healthcare environment to survive.

Most MIS procedures offset the higher equipment costs by reducing the duration of hospitalization. The duration of hospital stay of complex and advanced laparoscopic procedures (e.g. fundoplication, adrenalectomy, or esophagectomy) compared with their open equivalents is so much shorter that this outweighs the additional instrument costs, making these procedures cost-effective.[75-78]

Benefits are less clear cut when the procedure results in the same duration of hospital stay regardless of access. For example, both laparoscopic and open hernia repair are outpatient procedures, but equipment costs are far greater with a laparoscopic repair.[79] Therefore, there appear to be no cost savings. Some have argued that the cost to society as a whole is lower with a laparoscopic repair because of the more rapid return to work and rejoining the pool of productive members of society. This philosophic argument is, however, beyond the scope of the present chapter.

If the use of disposable instrumentation is minimized and hospital resources and inpatient stays are used effectively, most MIS procedures are more cost-effective than their open counterparts.[80]

REFERENCES

1. Nano M. A brief history of laparoscopy. G Chir. 2012; 33(3):53-7.
2. Kelling G. Zur Kölioscopie. Arch Klin Chir. 1923;126:226-9.
3. Jacobeus HC. Kurze Übersicht über meine Erfahrungen mit der laparoskopie. Munch Med Wochenschr. 1911;58: 2017-9.
4. Stefanidis D. Optimal acquisition and assessment of proficiency on simulators in surgery. Surg Clin North Am. 2010;90(3):475-89.
5. Sroka G, Feldman LS, Vassiliou MC, et al. Fundamentals of laparoscopic surgery simulator training to proficiency improves laparoscopic performance in the operating room-a randomized controlled trial. Am J Surg. 2010;199(1): 115-20.
6. Prescher T. Video imaging. In: Toouli J, Gossot D, Hunter JG (Eds). Endosurgery. New York: Churchill Livingstone; 1996. pp. 41-54.
7. Margulies DR, Shabot MM. Fiberoptic imaging and measurement. In: Hunter JG, Sackier J (Eds). Minimally Invasive Surgery. New York: McGraw-Hill; 1993. pp. 7-14.
8. Odell RC. Laparoscopic electrosurgery. In: Hunter JG, Sackier J (Eds). Minimally Invasive Surgery. New York: McGraW-Hill; 1993. pp. 33-4l.
9. Enderby CEO Laser Instrumentation. In Dixon JA (Ed). Surgical Applications of Lasers, 2nd edition. Chicago: Year Book Medical Publishers; 1987. pp. 52-78.
10. Hunter JG. Controversies in laparoscopic cholecystectomy exposure, dissection, and laser versus electrosurgery. Am J Surg. 1993;165:492-6.
11. Hunter JG, Bruhn E, Godman G, et al. Reflectance spectroscopy predicts safer wavelengths for pulsed laser lithotripsy of gallstones [Abstract]. Gastrointest Endosc. 1991;37:273.
12. Laycock WS, Trus TL, Hunter JG. New technology for the division of short gastric vessels during laparoscopic Nissen fundoplication. A prospective randomized trial. Surg Endosc. 1996;10:71-3.
13. Buess G. The endoscopic operating room. In: Toouli J, Gossot D, Hunter JG (Eds). Endosurgery. New York: Churchill Livingstone; 1996. pp. 3-8.
14. van Det MJ, Meijerink WJ, Hoff C, et al. Optimal ergonomics for laparoscopic surgery in minimally invasive surgery suites: a review and guidelines. Surg Endosc. 2009; 23(6):1279-85.
15. Safran O. Physiologic effects of pneumoperitoneum. Am J Surg. 1994;167:281-6.
16. Ho HS, Wolfe BM. The physiology and immunology of endosurgery. In: Toouli J, Gossot D, Hunter JG (Eds). Endosurgery. New York: Churchill Livingstone; 1996. pp. 163-7l.
17. Tsereteli Z, Terry ML, et al. Prospective randomized clinical trial comparing nitrous oxide and carbon dioxide pneumoperitoneum for laparoscopic surgery. J Am Coll Surg. 2002;195:173.
18. Cheng Y, Lu J, Xiong X, et al. Gases for establishing pneumoperitoneum during laparoscopic abdominal surgery. Cochrane Database Syst Rev. 2013;1:CD009569.
19. Callery MP, Soper NJ. Physiology of the pneumoperitoneum. Baillieres Clin Gastroenterol. 1993;7(4):757-77.
20. Tan PL, Lee TL, Tweed WA, et al. Carbon dioxide absorption and gas exchange during pelvic laparoscopy. Can J Anaesth. 1992;39:677-8l.
21. Kashtan J, Green JF, Parsons EQ, et al. Hemodynamic effects of increased abdominal pressure. J Surg Res. 1981;30: 249-55.
22. Harman PK, Kron IL, McLachlan HD, et al. Elevated intra-abdominal pressure and renal function. Ann Surg. 1982;196:594-7.
23. Gossot D. Access modalities for thoracoscopic surgery. In: Toouli JG, Gossot D, Hunter JG (Eds). Endosurgery. New York/London: Churchill-Livingstone; 1996. p. 743.
24. Horvath KD, Kao LS, Wherry KL, et al. A technique for laparoscopic-assisted percutaneous drainage of infected pancreatic necrosis and pancreatic abscess. Surg Endosc. 2001;15:1221.
25. Himpens J. Laparoscopic preperitoneal approach to the inguinal hernia. In: Toouli JG, Gossot D, Hunter JG (Eds). Endosurgery. New York/London: Churchill-Livingstone; 1996. p. 949.
26. Palmer R. Safety in laparoscopy. J Reprod Med. 1974;13(1): 1-5.
27. Veress J. Neues Instrument Zur Ausführung Von Brust Über Bauch Punktionen. Dtsch Med Wochenschr. 1938;41: 1480-3.
28. Hasson HM. A modified instrument and method for laparoscopy. Am Obstet Gynecol. 1971;110:886-7.
29. Araki K, Namikawa K, Yamamoto H, et al. Abdominal wall retraction during laparoscopic cholecystectomy. World J Surg. 1993;7:105-7.

30. Yim SF, Yuen PM. Randomized, double-masked comparison of radially expanding access device and conventional cutting tip trocar in laparoscopy. Obstet Gynecol. 2001;97:435-8.
31. Targarona EM, Gracia E, Rodriguez M, et al. Hand-assisted laparoscopic surgery. Arch Surg. 2003;138:138.
32. Romanelli JR, Earle DB. Single-port laparoscopic surgery: an overview. Surg Endosc. 2009;23:1419.
33. Canes D, Desai MM, Aron M, et al. Transumbilical single-port surgery: evolution and current status. Eur Urol. 2008;54:1020.
34. Makai G, Isaacson K. Complications of gynecologic laparoscopy. Clin Obstet Gynecol. 2009;52(3):401-11.
35. Crist DW, Gadacz TR. Complications of laparoscopic surgery. Surg Clin North Am. 1993;3:265-89.
36. Swank HA, Mulder IM, la Chapelle CF, et al. Systematic review of trocar-site hernia. Br J Surg. 2012;99:315.
37. Shirk GJ, Johns A, Redwine DB. Complications of laparoscopic surgery: how to avoid them and how to repair them. J Minim Invasive Gynecol. 2006;13(4):352-9.
38. Magrina JF. Complications of laparoscopic surgery. Clin Obstet Gynecol. 2002;45:469.
39. Yuzpe AA. Pneumoperitoneum needle and trochar injuries in laparoscopy: a survey on possible contributing factors and prevention. J Reprod Med. 1990;35:485-90.
40. Sandadi S, Johannigman JA, Wong VL, et al. Recognition and management of major vessel injury during laparoscopy. J Minim Invasive Gynecol. 2010;17:692.
41. Ahmad G, Duffy JM, Phillips K, et al. Laparoscopic entry techniques. Cochrane Database Syst Rev. 2008;CD006583.
42. Doyle DJ, Mark PW. Laparoscopy and vagal arrest (letter). Anaesthesia. 1989;44:448.
43. Cimino L, Petitto M, Nardon G, et al. Holter dynamic electrocardiography during laparoscopy (letter). Gastrointest Endosc. 1988;34:72.
44. Arthure H. Laparoscopy hazard. Br Med J. 1970;04:492-3.
45. Jorgenson JO, Hanel K, Lalak NJ, et al. Thromboembolic complications of laparoscopic cholecystectomy [Letter]. Br Med J. 1993;306:518.
46. Ott DE. Correction of laparoscopic hypothermia. J Laparoendosc Surg. 1991;1:183-6.
47. Loffer FD, Pent D. Indications, contraindications and complications of laparoscopy. Obstet Gynecol Surv. 1975; 30:407-27.
48. Mintz M. Risk and prophylaxis in laparoscopy: a survey of 100,000 cases. J Reprod Med. 1977;18:269-72.
49. Sandhu T, Yamada S, Ariyakachon V, et al. Low-pressure pneumoperitoneum versus standard pneumoperitoneum in laparoscopic cholecystectomy, a prospective randomized clinical trial. Surg Endosc. 2009;23(5):1044-7.
50. Phelps P, Cakmakkaya OS, Apfel CC, et al. A simple clinical maneuver to reduce laparoscopy-induced shoulder pain: a randomized controlled trial. Obstet Gynecol. 2008; 111(5):1155-60.

Additional references can be found in the online version of this book.

9

Informatics, Outcomes, and Economics of Surgical Care

Donald E Fry

Key Points

- Informatics, outcomes, and economics of surgical care are interrelated and interactive areas that will be increasing areas of major change for the delivery and evaluation of healthcare for the future.
- Informatics includes all of the hardware, software, and organization networks that are necessary for the transformation of the huge amounts of data within healthcare into useful information.
- Objective measures of outcomes of care must be used to assess the results of those clinical methods that are currently employed and to assess new technology that is introduced into surgical care. The development of objective measures of complications of care and of postdischarge events is essential in an environment where the duration of inpatient care is becoming progressively shorter.
- Healthcare costs are continuing to increase at rates that are faster than general economic inflation. Surgeons will need to adopt practices that will not only give the best outcomes, but they will also need to exercise economic stewardship in the expenditure of healthcare resources.
- It is likely that payment models of the future will link outcomes and economics of surgical care together via intricate informatics structures. Episode-based payment models may well replace conventional fee-for-services reimbursement with the goal of realignment of hospital and surgeon incentives in the provision of surgical care.

The last 50 years have witnessed an enormous growth in the size and complexity of healthcare. The amount of healthcare-related data, science, and technology that exists has had an exponential growth during this time. To paraphrase Leape et al.,[1] this highly technical system of physicians, nurses, other healthcare professionals, health product manufacturers, administrators, and government policy makers has resulted in a complex structure that almost defies a clear understanding.

The complexity of this healthcare structure has made the organization of data, the interpretation of outcomes of care, and the overall assessment of necessary costs for the delivery of care exceedingly difficult. The consequence has been a large number of technologies, operations, and medical treatments that have accelerated costs, but with an associated uncertainty regarding clinical benefit. Similarly, the dramatic growth in medical literature and publications has created an unsustainable circumstance for maintaining currency in medical knowledge for the individual clinician. The net effect of the explosion of healthcare information has been the further subspecialization of physicians and now the subspecialization of hospitals. The complexity of care and the subspecialization of all providers have led to a fragmentation of care that is necessarily driven by the vast information and data of healthcare but makes coordinated management of patients a formidable and expensive task.

This chapter will attempt to summarize the areas of informatics, outcome, and economics of surgical care. It is understood that each of these areas are in themselves very large subdisciplines of healthcare and that any effort can only be an overview and a perspective. These three areas are very interrelated and interactive and cannot be addressed independent of one another.

TOOLS OF INFORMATICS

Healthcare informatics is the processes by which the vast amounts of data are distilled into information (Flowchart 9.1). It is about processes for the development of information that can be used to guide and direct patient care, processes that can measure the various outputs and results of healthcare delivery, and processes that provide information about the economics of healthcare

Flowchart 9.1: The multiple components of healthcare informatics.

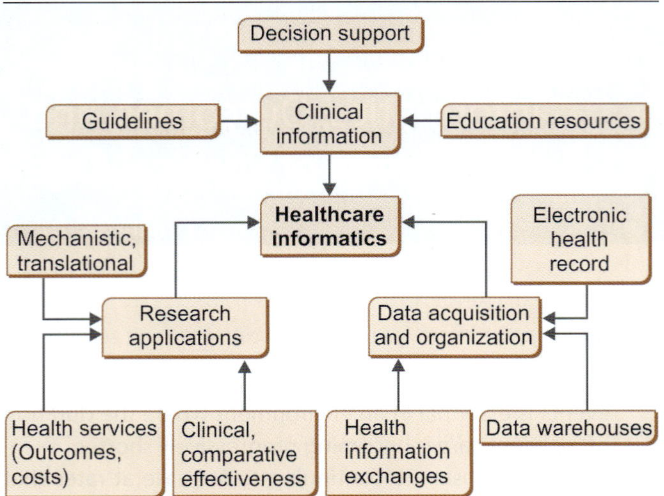

performance. Information output from informatics is fashioned into scientific and educational materials to direct a new generation of ideas and clinical direction.

Data are not information. Raw data extracted from a single episode of inpatient care consume by historical standards a large amount of computer memory, and when printed into hard copy become a confusing morass of endless observations and documentation. The itemized cost reports of that single episode of care become equally daunting in size and complexity. Similarly, the surgeon compelled to research a clinical issue in laparoscopic cholecystectomy, total joint replacement, or coronary artery bypass grafting will be confronted by large numbers of published works and opinions that address appropriate but very narrowly focused treatises that lack an overall context in patient management. Healthcare informatics is about the systems and methods to organize the meaningful elements within the vast amounts of data into a meaningful format for interpretation. Informatics is currently not making decisions and interpretations but rather providing the necessary structure to allow information to emerge that will direct decision making. With the development of neural networks[2] and artificial intelligence,[3] there are many who believe that informatics may soon be a major participant in clinical decisions as the vast amount of medical information continues to expand.

The anatomy of informatics is founded in hardware. Hardware is the structure that permits the processing of data into information. Hardware is an array of electronic circuitry that executes transferring, processing, and storing data. Hardware spans a vast continuum of complexity. Computer systems are the prototypes of hardware. Initially, large mainframes of computing power could be accessed by multiple users, but the real age of hardware proliferation in healthcare and in society in general had its genesis with the personal computer. The desktop computer became the opportunity to disseminate independent computing capability to individuals. Word processing, clinical and research data repositories, rapid computational capacity, and the efficient production of audiovisual materials for educational objectives became the day-to-day products of the personal computer.

The movement in hardware over 30 years has been progressive miniaturization. Desktop units have become progressively smaller at the same time that speed of computing has increased and the sophistication of applications has expanded. Storage capacity with an everincreasing size of hard drives has now resulted in terabytes of size that would have been unthinkable a couple of decades ago. The continued miniaturization has yielded very portable notebooks and tablet devices. The applications of the cell phone have resulted in devices that are likely to become full service microcomputers in due time. The evolution of Universal Serial Bus (USB) has generated a remarkable capacity for the storage and transportation of large quantities of data and information.

The physiology of informatics is software. Software programs provide the instructional base that informs the hardware to perform specific tasks. The operating system within the computer provides the flexibility for use of multiple specific functions of different software units. Operating systems such as Windows and Macintosh provide a structure to the hardware circuitry to perform the numerous tasks requested by the operator. Software programs cover a very large number of applications. Common software programs in personal computing include word processing, database management, and slide preparation programs for educational and presentation purposes. Large numbers of analytic programs are available for complex computations and analyses of very large databases. Mobile telephones now have a vast array of installed applications ("apps") that permit an untold number of functions that can be performed in our mobile society. Information access is achievable by Google, Yahoo, Bing, and other search engines.[4] Accessing medical literature through Pubmed[5] and other literature reference services has revolutionized the search for healthcare information.

Computer networking permits the exchange of data, information, and correspondences among individual computer units. Traditionally, these networks have been defined as local area networks that are within an office or building, or wide area networks that have a broader geographical sweep of connectivity among computer units across cities or regions. These traditional networks use cable media within an office environment, or dedicated phone or cable lines for wide area networks. Local area networks continue to exist within office units for common resource server units, FAX machines, and printers.

The evolution of wireless connectivity has introduced portability for computer systems that allows even handheld portable computer units as well as accessibility to the central server unit in a fashion that has only been a dream in the past. Accessing data, information, software, and all saved documents can be done from remote sites and independently of land-based cable or telephone lines. In an increasingly mobile society the efficient acquisition, storage, retrieval, and utilization of information have become essential components of healthcare informatics.

HEALTH INFORMATICS

The foundation component of health informatics is the clinical record of each patient care event. The clinical record of patient care becomes the source of data that are then fashioned into the several outcomes by the processes of health informatics. Traditionally, the comprehensive records of a patient's aggregate care events have been disconnected from each other. Office records of physicians, hospital records for inpatient events, pharmacy records of dispensed drugs, and utilization of laboratory or imaging studies are not in a central repository, let alone being integrated into a meaningful structure for interpretation. The recorded information is often too brief, without a common structure, and all too often is not legible when handwritten. Audits of both inpatient and outpatient clinical events are consistently identified as having inaccuracies and omitting critical information. Treatment orders for inpatients are frequently not documented, and tracking of documented orders to actual administration of drugs continues to be problematic. Health information technology will integrate the fragmented pieces of the healthcare record and is likely to have its greatest impact upon measurements of outcomes and upon payment—cost considerations in care delivery.[6]

ELECTRONIC HEALTH RECORD (EHR)

The centerpiece for health informatics is to have medical encounters electronically recorded so that an electronic health record (EHR) can be a legible, accurate, and current chronicle of the patient's healthcare history. The EHR is the aggregated health information for a single individual and is inclusive of all clinical, demographic, and administrative information for that patient. An ideal model would be to have an electronic record that was generated for each patient encounter so that the aggregate records from all physician, therapist, hospital, pharmacy, radiology, and clinical laboratory are integrated together with a standard organizational design. The EHR could then be accessed by care providers and by patients to optimize patient safety, improve outcomes of care, and enhance efficiency in the use of health expenditures.

Flowchart 9.2: Illustrates the multiple proposed functions of the electronic health record.

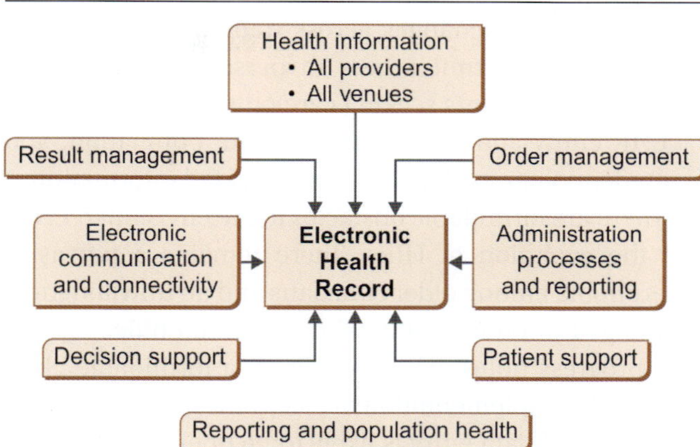

The Institute of Medicine has outlined eight basic capabilities for an EHR (Flowchart 9.2).[7] The envisioned benefits to be derived from EHRs include improved documentation of clinical data and care that is actually provided by facilitating the recording processes of patient encounters. Additional benefits would include:

- Decision support for providers could be achieved by a standardized organizational structure for the entered clinical information, which would enhance tracking and recovery as need for patient care.
- Alerts and reminders could be programmed into the electronic system to identify drug allergies and drug interactions and provide prompts for necessary preventive and recurrent services that are need.
- Practice guidelines could similarly be available in the electronic network to direct the details of care.
- Patients could organize personal health records (PHRs) around information within the EHR.
- Quality assessments and clinical research would be greatly enhanced.

- EHR information could be integrated into health information exchanges (HIEs), which would permit information exchanges across traditional boundaries that would permit access to personal health information of patients seeking care outside of the primary EHR entity and allow public health, population, and epidemiology evaluations of aggregated information.

There are formidable obstacles to the envisioned EHRs and the evolution of HIEs. There remains a pervasive cyberphobia among older clinicians and an unwillingness to change from the traditional handwritten office or hospital progress notes, which will pose a formidable challenge in the implementation of electronic documentation. The quality of data entry is likely to be uneven in terms of detail and accuracy, and data usability will be compromised in the rollout phase of EHR implementation. Getting accepted standards and interoperability of data structure has been an issue in early efforts at EHR implementation. Accessible EHRs and HIEs will have privacy and confidentiality issues. A substantial capital investment is required for physicians to have the necessary hardware and support staff to be an integral part of the EHR and its integration with other sources of patient data. Finally, ensuring that the entire EHR structure meets Meaningful Use to achieve all of the potential benefits will be necessary.

The structure of data storage within the EHR will be important for accessibility and utility of necessary information. Inpatient episodes of care are likely to continue to follow the traditional construct of the individual elements in Figure 9.1. A critical part of each hospitalization will be the appropriate discharge summary that provides a reasonably concise overview of the high points of the inpatient episode. The quality and accuracy of the discharge summary has been inconsistent over the years, and inaccuracies or oversights in the discharge summary commonly become false information that is perpetuated into the future of the patients care.

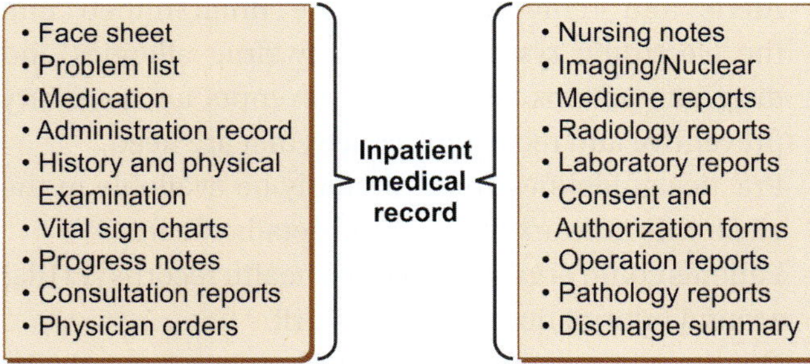

Fig. 9.1: Multiple components of the inpatient medical record.

The administrative summary of the patient's hospitalization becomes a useful document in the EHR. The UB-O4 is a universal standard for all US hospitalization, which gives a summary of the demographic details of the patient and coded details of the patient's diagnoses and procedures performed during the inpatient event (Fig. 9.2). These coded details have traditionally been in the International Classification of Disease, 9th Revision, Clinical Modification (ICD-9-CM) in the United States, but they are being transitioned to the ICD-10-CM version to provide greater detail to the diagnoses, procedural events, and complications of the hospitalization and to be consistent with coding practices in Western Europe and Canada. The inclusion of present-on-admission flags for each of the inpatient diagnosis codes will facilitate the compartmentalization of those diagnoses that already existed at the time of hospitalization from those clinical conditions that were hospital acquired.[8] A similar administrative document is employed for noninstitutional episodes of care (CMS-1500), which also uses ICD-10-CM coding for detailing the medical reasons and treatments provided (Fig. 9.3). The combination of these administrative records with the documentation from the actual clinical encounter will greatly enhance the interpretation of care for research and quality evaluation.

Computerized Provider Order Entry (CPOE)

An important component of EHR is the computerized provider order entry (CPOE). The timely and accurate execution of physician orders for inpatient care remains a major source of errors. Hand-written orders are commonly not legible, excessive, or inadequate services may be requested, and drug orders may contain dosing errors that jeopardize patient safety. Orders are commonly not recorded for services that may have been verbally ordered by the clinician. Written orders may be missed by transcribers or simply not completed due to a host of different reasons. CPOE allows point of care entry of orders and in mature systems can lead to direct communication with hospital services centers that provide the specific services. Efficiency in order delivery, menus of services that allow physicians to customize their commonly used services or drugs, safeguards against ordering medications with existing allergies or ordering incorrect dosing, and decision support features to guide drugs and services not commonly employed by the clinician are all positive features. CPOE will greatly facilitate billing and tracking of service utilization for all inpatients. Computerized

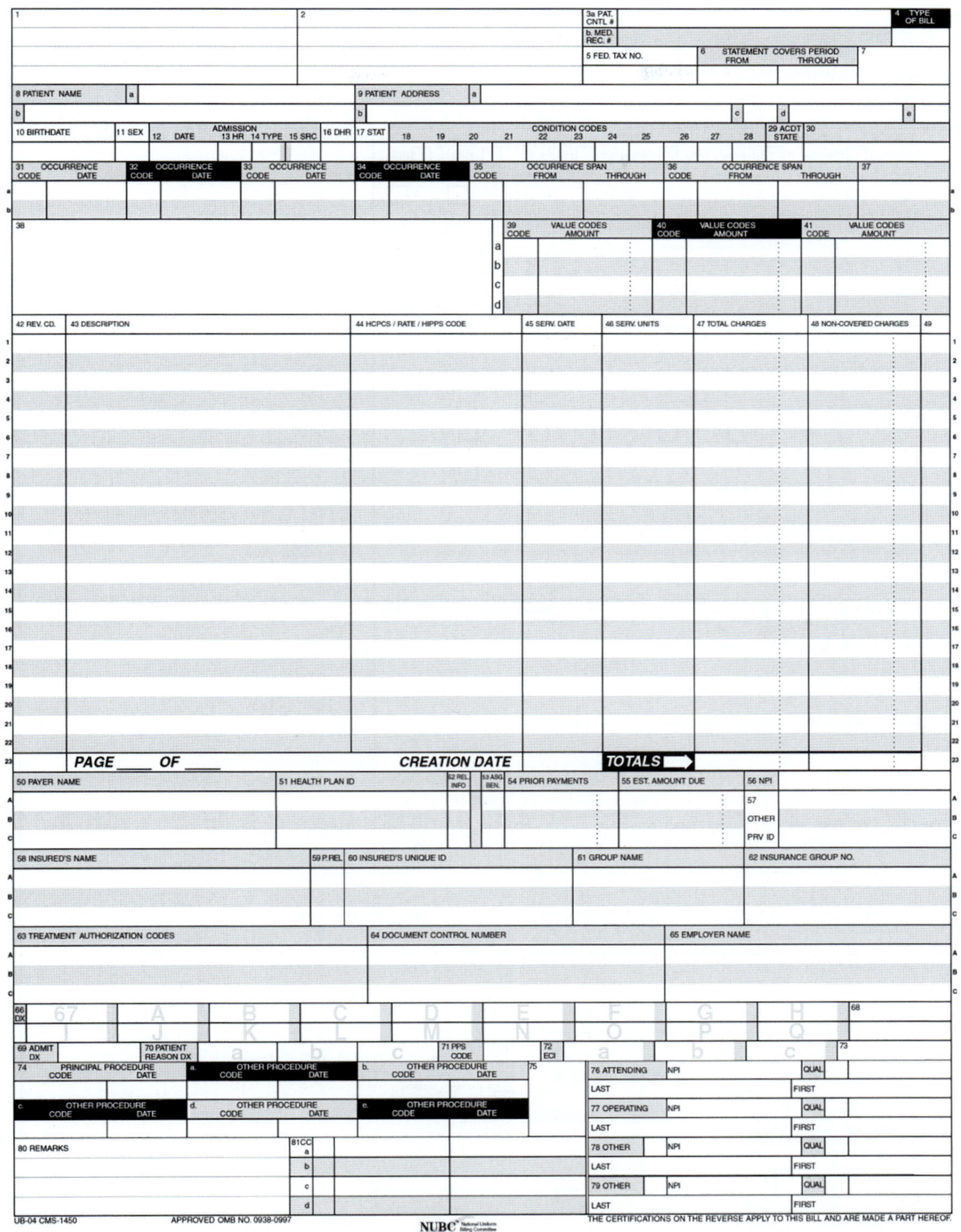

1 | 2 | 3a PAT. CNTL # | 4 TYPE OF BILL
b. MED. REC. #
5 FED. TAX NO. | 6 STATEMENT COVERS PERIOD FROM THROUGH | 7
8 PATIENT NAME a | 9 PATIENT ADDRESS a
b | b | c | d | e
10 BIRTHDATE | 11 SEX | ADMISSION 12 DATE 13 HR 14 TYPE 15 SRC | 16 DHR | 17 STAT | CONDITION CODES 18 19 20 21 22 23 24 25 26 27 28 | 29 ACDT STATE | 30
31 OCCURRENCE CODE DATE | 32 OCCURRENCE CODE DATE | 33 OCCURRENCE CODE DATE | 34 OCCURRENCE CODE DATE | 35 OCCURRENCE SPAN CODE FROM THROUGH | 36 OCCURRENCE SPAN CODE FROM THROUGH | 37
38 | 39 VALUE CODES CODE AMOUNT | 40 VALUE CODES CODE AMOUNT | 41 VALUE CODES CODE AMOUNT
a b c d
42 REV. CD. | 43 DESCRIPTION | 44 HCPCS / RATE / HIPPS CODE | 45 SERV. DATE | 46 SERV. UNITS | 47 TOTAL CHARGES | 48 NON-COVERED CHARGES | 49
1 2 3 4 5 6 7 8 9 10 11 12 13 14 15 16 17 18 19 20 21 22 23
PAGE ___ OF ___ CREATION DATE TOTALS
50 PAYER NAME | 51 HEALTH PLAN ID | 52 REL. INFO | 53 ASG. BEN. | 54 PRIOR PAYMENTS | 55 EST. AMOUNT DUE | 56 NPI
A B C | 57 OTHER PRV ID
58 INSURED'S NAME | 59 P. REL | 60 INSURED'S UNIQUE ID | 61 GROUP NAME | 62 INSURANCE GROUP NO.
A B C
63 TREATMENT AUTHORIZATION CODES | 64 DOCUMENT CONTROL NUMBER | 65 EMPLOYER NAME
A B C
66 DX | 67 A B C D E F G H | I J K L M N O P Q | 68
69 ADMIT DX | 70 PATIENT REASON DX a b c | 71 PPS CODE | 72 ECI a b c | 73
74 PRINCIPAL PROCEDURE CODE DATE | a. OTHER PROCEDURE CODE DATE | b. OTHER PROCEDURE CODE DATE | 75 | 76 ATTENDING NPI QUAL LAST FIRST
c. OTHER PROCEDURE CODE DATE | d. OTHER PROCEDURE CODE DATE | e. OTHER PROCEDURE CODE DATE | 77 OPERATING NPI QUAL LAST FIRST
80 REMARKS | 81CC a b c d | 78 OTHER NPI QUAL LAST FIRST | 79 OTHER NPI QUAL LAST FIRST
UB-04 CMS-1450 APPROVED OMB NO. 0938-0997 NUBC National Uniform Billing Committee THE CERTIFICATIONS ON THE REVERSE APPLY TO THIS BILL AND ARE MADE A PART HEREOF.

Fig. 9.2: The UB-04 form that is completed for the administrative abstraction of all hospital discharges in the United States.

linkages to the responsible ordering provider will enhance comparative utilization patterns and provide feedback to clinicians relative to their personal practices. An impediment to the implementation of CPOE has been the reluctance of clinicians to adopt the computerized ordering systems, establishing standardized orders to minimize having extended selection menus, and the time and expense of training all to use the system, and other

1500

HEALTH INSURANCE CLAIM FORM

APPROVED BY NATIONAL UNIFORM CLAIM COMMITTEE 08/05

PICA — PICA — CARRIER

1. MEDICARE (Medicare #) MEDICAID (Medicaid #) TRICARE CHAMPUS (Sponsor's SSN) CHAMPVA (Member ID#) GROUP HEALTH PLAN (SSN or ID) FECA BLK LUNG (SSN) OTHER (ID)

1a. INSURED'S I.D. NUMBER (For Program in Item 1)

2. PATIENT'S NAME (Last Name, First Name, Middle Initial)

3. PATIENT'S BIRTH DATE MM DD YY SEX M F

4. INSURED'S NAME (Last Name, First Name, Middle Initial)

5. PATIENT'S ADDRESS (No., Street)

6. PATIENT RELATIONSHIP TO INSURED Self Spouse Child Other

7. INSURED'S ADDRESS (No., Street)

CITY STATE

8. PATIENT STATUS Single Married Other

CITY STATE

ZIP CODE TELEPHONE (Include Area Code) ( )

Employed Full-Time Student Part-Time Student

ZIP CODE TELEPHONE (Include Area Code) ( )

9. OTHER INSURED'S NAME (Last Name, First Name, Middle Initial)

10. IS PATIENT'S CONDITION RELATED TO:

11. INSURED'S POLICY GROUP OR FECA NUMBER

a. OTHER INSURED'S POLICY OR GROUP NUMBER

a. EMPLOYMENT? (Current or Previous) YES NO

a. INSURED'S DATE OF BIRTH MM DD YY SEX M F

b. OTHER INSURED'S DATE OF BIRTH MM DD YY SEX M F

b. AUTO ACCIDENT? YES NO PLACE (State)

b. EMPLOYER'S NAME OR SCHOOL NAME

c. EMPLOYER'S NAME OR SCHOOL NAME

c. OTHER ACCIDENT? YES NO

c. INSURANCE PLAN NAME OR PROGRAM NAME

d. INSURANCE PLAN NAME OR PROGRAM NAME

10d. RESERVED FOR LOCAL USE

d. IS THERE ANOTHER HEALTH BENEFIT PLAN? YES NO ***If yes**, return to and complete item 9 a-d.*

READ BACK OF FORM BEFORE COMPLETING & SIGNING THIS FORM.

12. PATIENT'S OR AUTHORIZED PERSON'S SIGNATURE I authorize the release of any medical or other information necessary to process this claim. I also request payment of government benefits either to myself or to the party who accepts assignment below.

SIGNED DATE

13. INSURED'S OR AUTHORIZED PERSON'S SIGNATURE I authorize payment of medical benefits to the undersigned physician or supplier for services described below.

SIGNED

PATIENT AND INSURED INFORMATION

14. DATE OF CURRENT: MM DD YY ILLNESS (First symptom) OR INJURY (Accident) OR PREGNANCY(LMP)

15. IF PATIENT HAS HAD SAME OR SIMILAR ILLNESS. GIVE FIRST DATE MM DD YY

16. DATES PATIENT UNABLE TO WORK IN CURRENT OCCUPATION MM DD YY FROM TO

17. NAME OF REFERRING PROVIDER OR OTHER SOURCE

17a.

17b. NPI

18. HOSPITALIZATION DATES RELATED TO CURRENT SERVICES MM DD YY FROM TO

19. RESERVED FOR LOCAL USE

20. OUTSIDE LAB? YES NO $ CHARGES

21. DIAGNOSIS OR NATURE OF ILLNESS OR INJURY (Relate Items 1, 2, 3 or 4 to Item 24E by Line)

1. ___ . ___ 3. ___ . ___

2. ___ . ___ 4. ___ . ___

22. MEDICAID RESUBMISSION CODE ORIGINAL REF. NO.

23. PRIOR AUTHORIZATION NUMBER

24. A. DATE(S) OF SERVICE From MM DD YY To MM DD YY	B. PLACE OF SERVICE	C. EMG	D. PROCEDURES, SERVICES, OR SUPPLIES (Explain Unusual Circumstances) CPT/HCPCS MODIFIER	E. DIAGNOSIS POINTER	F. $ CHARGES	G. DAYS OR UNITS	H. EPSDT Family Plan	I. ID. QUAL.	J. RENDERING PROVIDER ID. #
1								NPI	
2								NPI	
3								NPI	
4								NPI	
5								NPI	
6								NPI	

25. FEDERAL TAX I.D. NUMBER SSN EIN

26. PATIENT'S ACCOUNT NO.

27. ACCEPT ASSIGNMENT? (For govt. claims, see back) YES NO

28. TOTAL CHARGE $

29. AMOUNT PAID $

30. BALANCE DUE $

31. SIGNATURE OF PHYSICIAN OR SUPPLIER INCLUDING DEGREES OR CREDENTIALS (I certify that the statements on the reverse apply to this bill and are made a part thereof.)

SIGNED DATE

32. SERVICE FACILITY LOCATION INFORMATION

a. NPI b.

33. BILLING PROVIDER INFO & PH # ( )

a. NPI b.

PHYSICIAN OR SUPPLIER INFORMATION

NUCC Instruction Manual available at: www.nucc.org APPROVED OMB-0938-0999 FORM CMS-1500 (08-05)

Fig. 9.3: The CMS 1500 form that is completed for noninstitutional ambulatory care provided in the United States.

unanticipated consequences.[9] A fully mature CPOE has taken considerable time to complete, but the promise of greater efficiency and better surgical care has been identified in those hospitals that have completed the process.[10]

In a fully integrated system, point of service CPOE from the physician office or clinic creates a similar level of efficiency in the delivery of services. A common computer system employed for both outpatient and inpatient ordering and testing results avoids the repetitive waste that accompanied the traditional ordering processes. The use of e-Prescribing ensures the accuracy of dosing and patient instructions for utilization. Direct communications to hospital or private pharmacies minimizes delays in dispensing of medications for patients. The electronic format also provides clinical support in the identification of drug costs, dosing errors, and incompatibility with other drugs that the patient is using. Finally, the e-prescribing strategy eliminates the problems of nonlegible prescriptions and provides a permanent record of both the prescribed and the dispensed drugs.

Radio Frequency Identification (RFID)

The era of wireless communication and sensing has led to the proposed use of radio frequency identification (RFID) in healthcare.[11] This sophisticated system automates the specific identification of objects, persons, or information by a tag. The tag is commonly a small transponder with a memory chip, which a receiver can detect as the tag passes through an electromagnetic zone. The RFID tag is so small that it has been used to track the behavior of insects. Tracking people, products, and information can be easily done when the unique tag is within the area of the receiver. The medical application of RFID tags is in its infancy, but the potential applications are vast. Many feel that the RFID tag may replace the commonly used bar code in the identification of commercial products when the cost of these tags drops to an acceptable level (>$0.01 US/tag). Unlike bar codes, RFID tags can be identified at a distance without contact or direct line of site. Obviously, the RFID technology risks an uncomfortable interface with privacy of the individual and individual personal information. It can be anticipated that government regulations will infiltrate the world of RFID tags and their utilization.

Meaningful Use of EHRs

The rate of integration of EHR into clinical practice has been highly variable by country. In the United States, adoption of EHR has been slow because of the capital investment in the hardware and software necessary to operate a system and because of the decentralized nature of private practice. Educational requirements and reluctance to abandon the traditional paper system of medical records has also been an issue. To achieve this transition to EHR, the US Government has enacted "Meaningful Use" legislation to provide an incentive for physicians and hospitals to adopt certified EHR in a three-stage process.[12] Stage 1 requires that physician practices and hospitals meet performance criteria (e.g. e-prescribing). Stage 2 requires that the EHRs have a structure to permit electronic exchange of healthcare information. Stage 3 of the EHR rollout must demonstrate evidence that quality of care has been improved. Beginning in 2011, financial incentives have been instituted to reward physicians who met targets for implementation of EHRs in a meaningful way. All Core Objectives and five of the Menu Objectives are to be met for Stage 1 of the program and are presented in Table 9.1. Participation in the Meaningful Use program is voluntary, but by 2015 physicians not adopting and using a certified EHR will be subject to financial penalties for payments by Medicare. While the acceptance and adoption has been slow, financial rewards and penalties are likely to enhance the pace of EHR implementation and use. The impact of Meaningful Use legislation upon clinical practice has been less in surgery than in medical specialties, but the administrative and compliance costs are still considerable.

Personal Health Records

By the sixth decade of life, most patients have accumulated a substantial history of prior illnesses, prior operations, previous diagnostic studies, and current/past medications. Most patients who are queried at the time of a new clinical condition are usually poor historians in recounting their prior medical issues. Information gaps can be critical omissions in going forward in the patient's care.

The PHR is a proposed method to solve the problem of a patient's health history.[13] As opposed to the EHR, which is controlled by a medical institution (e.g. hospital) or by a clinical practice, the PHR is controlled by the patient. The organizational categories of a proposed PHR are identified in Table 9.2. The data could be kept in a paper file, but electronic storage seems a more practical consideration with the proliferation of electronic media. Some have suggested that such information could be kept on a personal storage device (e.g. USB) or that web portals could be established and maintained by the patient. The portal could be accessed with a password by the patient, a family member, or an authorized provider at the appropriate time. Networking between the patient's EHR and their PHR is envisioned as a method for keeping information current. A likely problem with this concept will be patient compliance with keeping information current, but the concept of the PHR is gaining traction in many areas and will likely expand in use in upcoming years.

Table 9.1 The 13 core objectives and 10 menu objectives (of which 5 are chosen by the eligible professional) of stage 1 of the Meaningful Use of electronic health record (EHR) established by law in the United States. The minimal measure of compliance for each objective is also detailed.

Core objectives	*Measures of compliance*
Computerized provider order entry (CPOE)	≥30% if patients ≥ 1 medication ordered by CPOE
Drug–drug and drug allergy interactive checks	Enabled for entire report period
Maintain current problem list of diagnoses	≥80% of unique patients
Generate and transmit electronic prescriptions	≥40% of all prescriptions
Active medication list	≥80% of unique patients
Active medication allergy list	≥80% of unique patients
Demographics (preferred language, gender, race, ethnicity, date of birth)	≥50% of unique patients
Vital Signs (height, weight, blood pressure, body mass index, growth charts for children)	≥50% of unique patients
Smoking status of adolescents and adults	≥50% of unique patients
Report ambulatory clinical quality measures to CMS	Successfully report quality measures
Implement clinical decision support rule	Successful implementation
Provide patients with electronic copy of health information	≥50% of all patients requesting health information within 3 business days
Provide clinical summaries for patients for each office visit	≥50% of summaries provided
Protect electronic health information by EHR certified technology	Conduct security analysis
Menu objectives	
Implement drug formulary checks	Enabled to access ≥ 1 internal or external formulary for entire period
Incorporate clinical lab-test results into EHR	≥40% of all clinical lab results incorporated into EHR as structured data
Lists of patients by condition for quality measurements, reduction of disparities, research, outreach	Generate ≥ 1 report of patients with a specific condition
Send patient reminders for prevention/follow-up care	≥20% of patients ≥ 65 years of age, or ≤ 5 years of age sent an appropriate reminder
Provide patients with timely electronic access	≥10% of patients with electronic access to health information
Identify patient-specific education resources	≥10% of unique patients sent specific educational resources
Medication reconciliation in patients from another provider	≥50% reconciliation of medications among all patients transitioned into the eligible professional's care
Summary care record for patients transitioned to another provider	≥50% compliance with summary care records for transitioned patients
Submit electronic data to immunization registry	≥1 test of EHR capacity to send electronic data to immunization registry and follow-up submission if successful
Capability to submit electronic syndromic surveillance data to public agencies	≥1 test of EHR capacity to send syndromic surveillance data and follow-up submission if successful

Other Healthcare Information Systems

The discussion about EHRs has largely focused upon the generation of information around a healthcare entity of hospitals and physicians. Traditionally, the medical information of a patient has been retained by the hospital or by the physician and has only been shared with other healthcare providers within that environment unless an outside physician, hospital, or even the patient goes through a formal process to request the information. In recent years, electronic transfer of information upon request between providers or between a provider and the patient has been facilitated with email, although this method of transferring medical information has attendant problems with security. Other forms of information transfer between providers is expanding at a rapid rate with telemedicine and telehealth initiatives that permit real-time transfers of patient images and medical information in the interest of solving current medical management issues.

The HIEs have emerged in recent years as an effort to allow health information to be shared across the traditional boundaries. At the community level, HIEs permit interactions between hospitals, hospitals and clinicians,

Table 9.2 Categories of information that should be included in a comprehensive personal health record (PHR). The PHR is the patient's responsibility to organize and maintain.

PHR organizational categories	*Content*
Personal identification data	Gender, height, weight, ethnicity, blood type, occupation, and others
Emergency contacts	Primary and secondary contacts for emergent conditions
Healthcare providers	Physicians, dentists, and others providing current care
Insurance providers	Current insurance information
Legal documents/medical directives	Advanced directives, living will, power of attorney
Personal medical history	These are identified from a comprehensive checklist; this should include infectious diseases of the past (e.g. hepatitis) and immunizations
Allergies/drug sensitivities	History of proven or suspected drug reactions
Family history	This should be checklist driven by family member
Lifestyle/habits	Tobacco, alcohol, and other recreational drugs; should include exercise profile
Personal health log	Recent major illnesses; this should include pregnancies and childbirth information. Recent diagnostic studies (e.g. computerized tomography scan)
Medications	All prescription, over-the-counter medicines and vitamins, and alternative/herbal medications
Physician visits	All visits here should be linked to a healthcare provider identified above
Hospitalizations	This should provide a succinct identification of the diagnosis, hospital, physician, and complications of care
Operations	This should include the operation, hospital, surgeon, and complications of care
Laboratory/imaging results	Ideally, laboratory results would be in a structured format for easy searching
Medical devices	Pacemakers, implants, prosthetic devices, inhalers
Physical/occupational therapy	Provider and indications should be identified
Vision	Glasses, contacts, LASIK procedures; provider identified above
Dental health	Major dental issues; dentist should be identified under healthcare providers above

imaging centers, and laboratories with the care providers. Similar sharing of information can occur between providers of care with pharmacies to permit the free-flow of information to enhance the efficiency and quality of services. HIEs have been created at the state or regional level to create a central repository of patient information, which can be accessed for a patient seeking care outside their ordinary venue. For example, a patient with an acute medical problem in an emergency department remote from a customary site of care could give authorization for providers to access health information through the exchange. Similarly, a Nationwide Health Information Network (NHIN) is being created as an Internet information highway that connects HIEs from different communities or regions into a national network for the management of patients, but also to provide the foundation for a large-scale data repository for clinical information to be used for epidemiological, population, and health services research.[14] The maturation and growth of the NHIN is anticipated from the efforts of the Meaningful Use initiate in the United States. The challenges in the evolution of HIEs are considerable because of the technology, standards, legalities, confidentiality, and governance issues that have to be addressed as the network expansion covers a broader geographic area and larger populations of patients. Funding remains a major impediment to the evolution of the several HIEs that have been launched.[15] Nevertheless, while in their infancy at present, the growth and evolution of HIEs should parallel the expansion and sophistication of EHRs.

Healthcare Databases

The enormous volume of clinical data that is being organized into standard structure and formats from EHRs, HIEs, and other healthcare information systems means that accessible databases will be a requirement to transform the data into meaningful information. Databases become the medium for the organization of clinical data from multiple patients into a structure that permits population, epidemiologic, and health services research. Clinical databases permit evaluation of outcomes and costs of care. Databases permit efforts at comparative effectiveness research of different treatments.

There are multiple structures for database organization. Flat files identify record lines with a large number of fields for each line. This structure works well for identification of single binary or single continuous variable observations in a specific episode of care across a large number of patients. The flat file does not work well for complex queries of data where multiple different diagnoses are present or multiple continuous variables are observed over time intervals. Hierarchical data are structured like a filing system on the computer. A folder for diagnostics would have subfiles of clinical examination, laboratory studies, and imaging. Under the subfile of laboratory studies would be each of the respective hematology and clinical chemistry values over time. Relational databases are commonly used for healthcare where the data are aggregated into multiple tables. Each table is composed of rows and fields, with each table being analogous to a flat field of data nested within a larger database. Many other complex database structures are designed and may have data stored in different locations and within different computer systems. Available data bases such as the various components (e.g. National Inpatient Sample) of the Healthcare Cost and Utilization Project[16] and the Research Identifiable Files of CMS[17] illustrate the large data sets that can be constructed and are available for analytic evaluation. As EHRs and HIEs expand in use, the opportunities for innovation and new structure of healthcare data are just beginning.

Public Media

The accessibility of clinical information to inform healthcare professionals is extensive. The volume of published treatises covering all aspects of care is greater than even a specialist in surgery in a narrowly defined area can know. Tools for the retrieval of information in a timely fashion are essential to permit effective decision making but also to build a foundation of knowledge. Traditional textbooks have become less effective in serving this role because the rapid growth of information makes this medium incomplete or out of date at the time of publication. Utilization of the Internet with any of a number of search engines permits access to general information on a broad array of medical themes, but it has the hazard of inadequate safeguards governing the integrity of all posted materials. However, the Internet does provide access to Medline, PubMed, and other healthcare literature indexing so that focused inquiries of recent and past medical literature can be reviewed. Guidelines for care can be accessed through warehouses, or through surgical societies with special interests in specific areas of care. The Internet even permits direct contact via email with those who have authored specific publications and opinions to have questions addressed. While the explosion in published literature on most subjects of surgical interest has made current knowledge on a specific theme very difficult, the electronic media have made access to reliable sources of information quite efficient.

An exciting and emerging tool in maintaining current knowledge has been the interactive webinar. Programs of 1 hour or an entire day can be presented with a very structured educational format and can be viewed from the office or from home. These webinars are commonly interactive with either written or telephoned questions and answers between the participants and the presenters. The efficiency of these presentations means that virtual societies are likely to emerge in the future in which the entire program will be decentralized for presentations from different locations and webcast to the multiple participants for learning and discussion without leaving home. While the networking that has traditionally been associated with regional and national surgical meetings is likely to continue, highly specialized content will probably find a place in the webinar conference.

OUTCOMES

Improvement in the quality of surgical care has been the goal since the inception of the profession. Quality in surgical care means that services provided are superior to alternative care. Quality of care at the present time is usually examined in the context of value. Value is the product of quality and price. Value places an economic parameter on quality.

In healthcare, the metric by which quality should be measured is the outcome; the results of the clinical enterprise that improve the longevity or the functionality of the patient. The outcome must be an objective determination and have minimal influence or bias that gives the impression that the end result appears to be better or worse because of prejudices that the observer may have.

For purposes of analysis and value judgment, outcomes of care need to be viewed as binary events: the outcome was either good or suboptimal. The analytic process needs to use objective, reproducible, and transparent tools for the measurement of good or suboptimal outcomes. Despite the fact that senior clinicians know a good result when they see it, good outcomes have been difficult to quantitate within a population of patients receiving a common operation or management of a similar disease entity.

Because the measurement of outcomes has been difficult, many government and other oversight agencies have resorted to using process measures as surrogates for measuring outcomes. The supposition is that if you complied with selected processes that have been associated with improved outcomes, then you have met the test of quality performance. The use of process measures is rife with shortcomings, not the least of which is the assumption that compliance with one or two processes within a complex matrix of interactive variables in clinical care will make a difference. In no other area has the use of process measures been more prevalent than in the prevention of surgical site infection (SSI). The objective measurement of SSI has proven difficult for reasons that will be subsequently discussed. In lieu of objective measurements, the Surgical Care Improvement Project (SCIP) has identified a series of process measures that have strong scientific foundations in the prevention of SSI (Table 9.3). Hospitals and surgeons are given good evaluations if they have high degrees of compliance with these SCIP measures and are given poor evaluations for lesser degrees of compliance. Multiple clinical studies have demonstrated that there is little or no correlation between hospital compliance with SCIP measures and actual improvements in SSI rates.[18] Similar process measures for the prevention of SSI have been promulgated by the National Institute for Health and Care Excellence in the United Kingdom.[19] The reality of SSI is that a multitude of different clinical variables and prevention methods influence the observed rate of infection and that manipulation of one or two variables in a complex system may not influence outcomes. Improvement in outcomes requires a systems approach to manage the entire array of events that influence the end product. Process measures are not outcomes and should not be used as a surrogate for clinical quality.

Risk Adjustment

A critical consideration in the assessment of outcomes is risk adjustment. All would agree that there are complications of surgical care that are preventable if only the correct clinical methods had been used in the management of the

Table 9.3 The current process measures used by the Surgical Care Improvement Project in the United States. The process measures for hair removal and intraoperative hypothermia have been suspended.

Process measures	*Comments*
Prevention of surgical site infection (SSI)	
Systemic prophylactic antibiotics administered within 1 hour of incision	Antibiotics must be administered prior to the incision. Short half-life antibiotics can be administered too soon and be eliminated while contamination still occurs in the operation
Appropriate antibiotic selected for the procedure being performed	The antibiotic must have activity against the anticipated bacterial contaminants
Prophylactic antibiotics discontinued within 24 hours after surgery end time	Antibiotics given after wound closure have been repeatedly documented to not prevent SSI
Cardiac surgery patients with controlled 6 AM postoperative serum glucose	Glycemic control in cardiac surgery has been documented to be of value during the operation and early in the postoperative period
Postoperative urinary catheter removal on postoperative Day 1 or 2	Removal of the urinary catheter is desirable but may not be achievable in elderly males with prostatic hypertrophy
Prevention of cardiac events	
Surgery patients on a beta-blocker prior to arrival that received a beta-blocker during the perioperative period	It is not recommended that patients not already on a beta-blocker should receive perioperative beta blockade
Prevention of venous thromboembolism	
Surgery patients with recommended venous thromboembolism prophylaxis ordered	Numerous methods are acceptable including heparin derivatives, anticoagulants, Factor Xa inhibitors, pneumatic compression devices, and aspirin
Surgery patients who received appropriate venous thromboembolism prophylaxis within 24 hours prior to surgery to 24 hours after surgery	The complete perioperative interval of time should be covered by the chosen preventive strategy

patient. However, all surgeons have had the experience of major complications and even deaths following operations where all techniques and clinical treatments appeared to be appropriate. Thus, adverse outcomes of surgical care may be preventable, or they may relate to high-risk patient variables that yield a suboptimal outcome in a definable percentage of cases, or they may be a probable result of the disease process being managed. Furthermore, as the processes of care have become more complex and the degree of patient illness has become more severe, it is likely that in selected circumstances the clinician may be confronted with clinical circumstances in which we have reached the current limits of our management technology.

Effort to quantitate the intrinsic risk to the patient is the process of risk adjustment. An analogy can be made that individual patients with specific diseases are like a card game. The patient is dealt their cards for the disease episode. Some hands of cards are always winners, and some more likely than not to be losers. Between the two extremes is a vast array of hands that will win or lose depending upon how the cards are played. Thus, an assessment of an outcome depends upon the probabilities of winning or losing given the composition of the cards and the skills of the contestants in playing out the hand. In fact, the analytic process may require the evaluation of a large sample of card games and evaluation of a large number of players to identify the probabilities of outcomes.

The process of risk adjustment may be a univariate or a multivariate approach. In both cases, independent variables or risk factors are assembled. The term "variable" is used in many contexts, and numerous different types of variables can be employed in risk adjustment (Table 9.4). Risk factors for surgical care are those clinical conditions that exist at the beginning of the episode of care with the potential to affect the outcome independent of the quality of care that is provided. Risk factors may be chronic diseases or they may be acute clinical conditions present at the time of surgical intervention. Table 9.5 identifies chronic conditions that this author has commonly used in risk adjustment for elective surgical care. The univariate approach examines the statistical significance of any one independent variable with the dependent outcome of interest. Thus, if postoperative death or SSI or postoperative pulmonary embolism was the dependent variable of interest, then its association with any risk factor (e.g. diabetes) can be assessed by examining the study population of patients undergoing a single operation.

For example, in a study of 1,000 patients undergoing an elective operation, 50 (5%) cases had an SSI. There were 200 patients with diabetes in the study population, and

Table 9.4 The definition for the different types of variable descriptions used in the development of prediction models.

Description of variable	*Definition*
Binary/dichotomous	A variable that can only exist in two possible states usually identified as "0" or "1" (e.g. a disease exists or it does not exist).
Categorical/nominal	A variable that can exist in a defined number of possible groups (male or female).
Polychotomous	Categorical variables with more than two possible groups (e.g. married, single, divorced, widowed).
Ordinal	Categorization of data by rank, such as cancer staging. Each category is greater or lesser than others but differences are not necessarily equal between categories
Continuous/interval	A variable that ranges across a low and a high value with large numbers of points depending upon the sophistication of the measurement.
Discrete	A continuous variable that is expressed only as integers, not fractions or decimals.
Dependent/criterion/outcome/responding	The effect or consequence of another variable or variables. It is the outcome of interest in an experimental study.
Independent/manipulated/treatment/predictor	The cause(s) or influence on the dependent outcome of interest in an experimental study.
Latent	A variable assumed to exist but cannot be measured. Personal income can be assumed (not reported) in an administrative data set by the mail zip code, which is reported.
Dummy	A dependent variable created by converting multiple categorical variables into a binary relationship. A surgeon or a hospital is labeled as "1" while all others are aggregated together "0."
Confounding	A variable that has positive or negative effects upon both the dependent variable but also upon one or more independent variables.
Intervening/mediating	A variable that has a causal link between two other variables.

Table 9.5 Candidate variables that might be used as risk factors for elective surgical care in addition to age and gender.

Alcohol abuse	Congestive heart failure*	Neurohypoadrenal dysfunction
Aplastic anemia*	Dementia/Alzheimer's	Other neurological disease
Blood loss anemia*	Depression*	Obesity
Deficiency anemia	Diabetes mellitus	Paralysis*
Hemolytic anemia*	Diabetic complications	Parathyroid disease
Other anemia*/hypersplenism	Drug abuse (nonalcohol)	Chronic peptic ulcer
Aortic aneurysm	Esophageal reflux/esophagitis	Chronic peripheral vascular disease
Lymph/hematopoietic cancer	Esophageal varices	Polycythemia/hypercoagulability
Metastatic cancer	Gout	Psychosis
Primary cancer	Hepatic cirrhosis	Chronic pulmonary disease
Ischemic cardiac disease	Chronic hepatic disease	Inflammatory bowel disease
Cardiomyopathy	HIV/AIDS	Chronic renal disease
Cardiac arrhythmias	Hyperlipidemia	Chronic skin ulcer
Chronic cerebrovascular disease	Hypertension	Chronic steroid use
Transient ischemic attacks*	Hypothyroidism	Urinary tract obstruction*
Clotting abnormality	Malabsorption	Valvular heart disease
Collagen vascular disease/rheumatoid arthritis	Malnutrition/weight loss*	Varicose veins

The "*" identifies those conditions that could potentially be complications of care in an administrative database and should be identified as diagnoses that are present on admission.

they had 24 (12%) SSIs. Both the independent variable (diabetes) and the dependent variable (SSI) are binary variables, so the significance of diabetes being associated with SSI would be determined by a chi-square calculation. In this clinical scenario, the chi-square is 25.8 ($p < .001$ with 1 degree of freedom) for diabetes being a risk factor in the prediction of SSI in this operation.

In any analysis using the univariate assessment of independent variables with a dependent outcome, multiple variables may achieve statistical significance and it becomes desirable to use quantitative *measures of association* to which variables have the greater influence on the outcome of interest. In the example above, the measures of association may be ratios or absolute differences.

The relative risk ratio (RRR) is easily understood. In our example, it is the ratio of the observed rate of SSI among patients with diabetes (24/200 = 12%) compared with the observed rate of SSI among patients without diabetes (26/800 = 3.25%). For this study population, diabetes has an RRR of 12%/3.25%, or 3.7. Patients with diabetes are 3.7 times more likely to have an SSI than patients without diabetes.

The odds ratio (OR) is less easily understood. It is a ratio of a ratio. It is the ratio of diabetics with SSIs to diabetics without SSIs, compared with the ratio of nondiabetics with SSIs to nondiabetics without SSIs. In the example, the OR is 24/176 compared with 26/774, or 4.1. The OR is higher than the RRR, but asymptotically approaches the RRR as the rate of the dependent variable (e.g. SSIs) gets smaller. The OR is most commonly used in case-control trials in which 800 patients with diabetes undergoing the operation with a 12% SSI rate are compared with 800 matched patients without diabetes with a 3.25% SSI rate. This case-control example yields 96 diabetic SSIs: 704 diabetics without SSIs, compared with 26 nondiabetics SSIs: 774 nondiabetics without SSIs. The OR again computes to 4.1. The RRR cannot be used in the case-control study because the number of patients with diabetes to patients without diabetes has been set equal and does not reflect the actual incidence of the independent variable in the study group.

Another measure of association is attributable risk. The attributable risk is the degree to which the risk factor increases the dependent outcome of interest. In the illustration above the absolute increased risk of SSI because of diabetes is 12%–3.25%, or 8.75%. Stated another way, the percentage of attributable risk for diabetes in this operation is 8.75%/12%, or 73%. In large population studies, absolute attributable risk and percentage attributable risk are used to identify the epidemiologic impact of a given clinical variable upon outcomes of patient management.

The problem with univariate analysis is that it assumes that the single independent variable is acting solely in its association with the dependent outcome of interest. In the diabetes example that was just used, it is likely that the patient's current renal function, overall vascular disease, and glycemic control at the time of operation would be clinical variables that are linked to diabetes. Their presence or absence would be significant modifiers of the influence of diabetes as an underlying condition with SSI rates. In addition, if the patient smoked cigarettes it is easy to envision synergistic relationships among variables. It is easy to understand that with the complex number of comorbidities and other risk factors that are present, it is likely that there are interactions among the numerous variables that could potentially influence the outcome of a major operation.

Multivariate analysis has become the most common method for the assessment of risk adjustment in inpatient surgical populations. Because the number of candidate variables in the assessment of risk of a given patient is large (Table 9.5), regression analysis is ordinarily used. Logistic regression is used if the dependent variable is a dichotomous or binary event (e.g. dead or alive), and linear regression is used when the dependent outcome of interest is a continuous or discrete variable (e.g. length of hospital stay).

With logistic regression, the dependent variable is expressed as the probability of the index event occurring on a scale from 0 to 1. With continuous independent variables, these are expressed as OR and the relationship with the probability of the outcome is not a linear relationship but assumes a linear configuration when the slope of the regression is expressed as a natural logarithm (Fig. 9.4). The coefficient of independent variables in a logistic regression is expressed as a natural logarithm. The natural logarithm coefficient of statistically significant variables can then be expressed as the OR of that variables association with the outcome of interest by the formula: OR = exp(coefficient). Thus, a natural logarithm coefficient of 1.0 for an independent variable has an OR = 2.71828..., or the base number for natural logarithms.

Linear regression is much more easily understood since both the dependent variable and the independent variables are expressed as conventional numbers. The dependent variable is a continuous variable, and the independent variables in the regression may be binary or continuous. When using linear regression, it is usually an appropriate practice to perform a scatter plot of the data to ensure that a linear relationship exits. With selected cases, the relationship between the dependent and independent variables deviates from linear at extremely high or low values and can skew the slope and the intercept in the analysis. Some investigators will convert the dependent variables to a logistic value to address the extremes, whereas others may winsorize the data and remove the extreme values and use only the linear component of the relationship for completion of the analysis.

Regardless of the methods, risk adjustment is only as good as the database from which the frequency of risk factors and complications of care are derived. Administrative data employing the information from the UB-04 or other similar abstractions are commonly used for risk adjustment. These documents are commonly lacking in the full scope of comorbid conditions and other pertinent clinical information. Furthermore, if selected diagnoses are not differentiated as being present-on-admission, it is difficult in emergency admissions to the hospital to segregate risk factors from complications of care. Full chart clinical abstraction will usually provide the best data, but the process can be costly and time intensive. Selected clinical elements of care (e.g. admission laboratory tests) have been shown to improve the discrimination of prediction models for surgical care, especially when combined with accurate present-on-admission coding and may prove to be an effective alternative to full chart abstraction.[20,21]

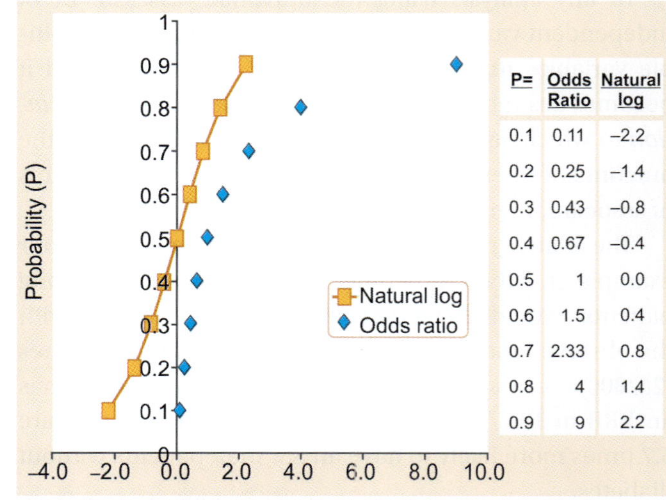

P=	Odds Ratio	Natural log
0.1	0.11	–2.2
0.2	0.25	–1.4
0.3	0.43	–0.8
0.4	0.67	–0.4
0.5	1	0.0
0.6	1.5	0.4
0.7	2.33	0.8
0.8	4	1.4
0.9	9	2.2

Fig. 9.4: The linear transformation of the odds ratio by conversion to natural logarithms.

Objective Measures of Outcomes

Objective measures of outcomes are essential to permit judgments about the quality of care provided, but effective metrics with methods for monitoring outcomes have proven to be elusive.[22] Outcome measurement segregates patients into good or suboptimal categories and should be approached as a nonprejudicial determination. At a preliminary level of consideration, complications of care should be viewed with a "no-fault" mentality so that all are identified and all can be evaluated. Prevailing attitudes that complete identification and full reporting can yield the appearance of substandard care may lead to events being incompletely identified. It is essential that objective measures of outcomes be well defined, consistently identified by different observers, and be appropriately risk adjusted to avoid attempts at comparison of fundamentally different cohorts of patients.

Surgical Mortality Rates

Deaths following elective or emergency surgical care would be recognized by all as representing an adverse outcome of care. Among all measures of outcomes, death is most easily identified and consistently reported during the inpatient episode of care. Rates of risk-adjusted deaths following elective and emergency operations have been clearly documented to differ among countries,[23] hospitals,[24] and surgeons.[25] When large volumes of cases for study are available and when sophisticated risk adjusted is employed, differences in rates indicate that preventable deaths do occur and that there are performance differences between hospitals and between surgeons.

These observed differences have raised the issue of death rates being used as a major quality metric to gauge provider performance. Selected government and other quality review organizations have proposed public disclosure of mortality rates as methods to inform patients in making choices about which hospital and which surgeon to choose for a specific operation. These mortality rates are commonly expressed as ratios of Observed (O) Deaths/Predicted (P) Deaths. Most public disclosures of mortality rates have attempted to represent risk adjustment in public disclosure efforts, although the quality of those efforts has been highly variable. There is no evidence that public disclosure of outcomes by hospital or by clinician affects patient decisions.[26]

Risk-adjusted mortality rates are measureable outcomes, but pose many problems when being interpreted in the context of being a quality measure in surgical care. For elective surgery, overall mortality rates are quite low (Table 9.6). Sample sizes of patient populations between hospitals or between surgeons have to be large to assess statistically significant differences. For example, in Table 9.6 the inpatient mortality rate of elective colon resection in Medicare patients in the United States was identified as 2.7%. The 95% confidence interval for a surgeon with 50 cases in a year will have an upper limit of 7.2%; for a surgeon with 20 cases, the 95% confidence interval is 9.8%. Defining the upper limit for suboptimal care can hinge on events in one or two cases and may be the consequence of random chance rather than suboptimal care.[27] Furthermore, public reporting of low volume outcome will pose real problems for the public to interpret an operative mortality rate of 9% in a small volume surgeon as not being a statistically significant outcome.

The problem of small numbers has led some to recommend pooling the entire experience of a hospital or an individual surgeon. With predicted values that can be tailored to each operation, an overall expected value for a given group of different cases can be determined. It is likely

Table 9.6 Upper and lower limits of the 95% confidence interval for mortality rates identified among Medicare patients (2009–2010) when evaluating patients from a hospital or a surgeon.

			95% confidence interval for N = 100 cases	
Elective operation	*Cases*	*Deaths (%)*	*Lower limit, %*	*Upper limit, %*
Craniotomy	6,634	116 (1.75)	0	4.37
Lung and thorax	30,208	755 (2.50)	0	5.62
Coronary artery bypass	127,675	3,085 (2.42)	0	5.49
Aortic surgery	6,499	234(3.60)	0	7.33
Colonic surgery	57,272	1,555 (2.72)	0	5.97
Liver/biliary Tract/pancreas	10,815	224 (2.07)	0	4.92
Total Joint Replacement	681,141	725 (0.11)	0	0.77

that performance in different operations by a surgeon may be different and that the assessment of a heterogeneous group of operations would regress to the mean and not be of value in estimates of quality performance.

Deaths occurring during the hospitalization for the index operation are always considered postoperative deaths, but the appropriate postdischarge interval of time for inclusion in the total mortality rate of an operation remains uncertain. Many death rates are reported for only those that occurred during the hospitalization itself. More recently, several organizations including the National Surgical Quality Improvement Project of the American College of Surgeons have been employing a 30-day death rate from the date of the operation. Recently, 90-day postdischarge death rates among discharged US Medicare patients after elective surgery was found to be larger than that of deaths that occurred during the index hospital stay.[28] A correct interval for inclusion of postdischarge deaths requires more study but must be standardized to permit comparisons among provider groups.

Finally, there are system issues within a hospital unit that make outcomes indexed to the surgeon very difficult. The quality of anesthesiology services, the availability of critical care beds, the quality of critical care services, the presence of surgical trainees, and nursing mishaps are all variables that can influence the outcomes of a given surgeon. The surgeon's performance in the operating room is not the only variable to influence suboptimal outcomes. Mortality rates as a metric of quality outcomes are best applied at the hospital level. Hospitals have the responsibility to apply rigorous clinical review to assign accountability for postoperative deaths. That accountability should extend into a reasonable period of time after discharge from the hospital (e.g. 90 days).

Complications of Surgical Care

Observations of the frequency of complications following surgical episodes have the face value of being a logical means to assess the outcomes of surgical care. A reference standard for the frequency of these complications can be derived from quality performing hospitals, and each hospital can compute whether their rates are more or less frequent. The profile of complications can be aggregated together and an overall complication rate can be determined.

However, what is a complication of surgical care?[29] Table 9.7 identifies those postoperative events that would generally be viewed as complications after operations. Those that are listed are generic complications in that they would have a definable frequency in virtually any major operation. Each specific operation obviously has events that are unique such as mechanical dysfunction of a prosthesis following total joint replacement or mediastinitis after open heart surgery. While a definition can be provided for each of the coded complications in Table 9.7, there would be considerable debate about whether definitions should be very narrow in spectrum and only encompass those events directly related to the operation, or whether they should include decompensation of other chronic medical conditions that coincide with the postoperative period of time. For purposes of this discussion, this author would define a complication as an unexpected event associated with a surgical operation and its attendant postoperative care that would likely not have occurred had the operation not occurred. It is temporally related to the operation and the aftermath of the pathophysiologic sequelae of the operation and its management. Complications are not restricted to the inpatient episode but should be inclusive of a defined period of postoperative care until the patient resumes the normal activities of living. This is obviously an all-inclusive definition that would not be accepted by every surgeon.

The reality in differences of opinion about the definition underscores one of the problems of using complication frequencies as a measure of outcomes in surgical care, but there are several others. First, there is the problem of effective surveillance. Like mortality rates, SSI rates and other infectious complications following operations are being publicly reported by government and other oversight organizations. Hospitals that are thorough in assessing SSIs and other specific complications will likely have higher rates than those with less rigorous surveillance methods. The coded rates for all complications of surgery have highly variables rates of being reported in the literature, and published rates are frequently at great variance from those that are identified in administrative data of abstracted hospital discharges. Accordingly, underreported complication events makes the reference rates from epidemiologic studies lower than reality and makes hospitals with valid reported rates appear to be of lesser quality. High rates may not reflect inferior performance but be the unintended consequences of effective capture of all unintended events.

A second problem in tallying complication rates is the inclusion period of time after operation. Many rates are only available for the hospitalization time, but significant

Table 9.7 The most common generic complications that are reported in the coded complication events following elective surgical procedures.

Infectious complications	*Cardiopulmonary/coagulation*	*Other complications*
Clostridium difficile infection	Acute myocardial infarction	Noninfectious surgical site complications
Streptococcal infection	Acute congestive heart failure	Fluid/electrolyte/acid–base complications
Staphylococcal infection	Acute cerebrovascular accident	Acute renal failure
Methicillin-resistant *Staphylococcus aureus* infection	Cardiac arrest	Anemia
Gram-positive infection	Ventricular fibrillation	Hypotension/shock
Gram-negative infection	Unspecific cardiac complications	Alcohol/drug withdrawal
Unspecified bacteremia	Pulmonary embolism	Encephalopathy
Systemic inflammatory response syndrome/septic shock	Deep venous thrombophlebitis	Peripheral vascular complications
Classified postoperative infection	Pulmonary failure	Gastrointestinal complications
Soft tissue/musculoskeletal infection	Pulmonary effusion	Acute hepatic decompensation
Pneumonia	Pneumothorax	Mechanical urinary tract complications
Bacterial endocarditis	Pulmonary collapse (atelectasis)	Paralytic ileus
Candida infection	Coagulation/platelet complications	Decubitus ulcer
Urinary tract infection		Rhabdomyolysis
Central line-associated blood stream infection		Transfusion reaction

complications of care follow discharge. SSIs, *Clostridium difficile* infection, acute myocardial infarction, deep venous thrombophletitis/pulmonary embolism, and others may not become clinically evidence until the postdischarge period of time. Increased recognition of complication events in the United States and other countries has occurred after discharge because of the increased emphasis on earlier hospital discharges. As was identified in Chapter 7, SSIs may need 30 days or even 90 days of postoperative surveillance. For other complications (e.g. myocardial infarction), this duration of follow up is not standardized, nor is it clear when events like myocardial infarction are consequences of the patient's underlying coronary artery disease and may be independent of any association with the operation.

Finally, postoperative complication events span a wide continuum of severity. SSIs may be only a mild stitch abscess or a superficial area of wound drainage that quickly resolves with minimal or no specific treatment. SSI may also be necrotizing infection of the fascia with dehiscence of the abdominal incision. *C. difficile* infection may be a transient episode of diarrhea that is quickly recognized and treated with no morbidity for the patient, but it may also be associated with transmural necrosis of the colon. Most complicating events are considered binary events, but the consequences of the events are very heterogeneous.

The monitoring of complications of care is very useful within a given hospital. The definitions and duration of monitoring can be standardized. The occurrence of these events can be compared to historical controls within the hospital for months and years in the past to identify whether progress in control of postoperative complications is being achieved. Comparison of rates between or among different hospitals really runs the risk of misrepresenting the outcomes of surgical care.

Risk-Adjusted Postoperative Length of Stay (RApoLOS)

Excessive length of postoperative hospitalization has been proposed as a potential objective measure of complications of surgical care. Specifically, hospitalization that exceeds an upper limit of duration that is adjusted for the patient's overall comorbid conditions and overall risks could potentially be a surrogate marker for significant morbidity after the operation. An argument against this concept would be that events other than complications may result in excessive lengths of stay. While this argument is valid in the context of emergency admissions and emergency operations because of problems of disposition for recovering patients, in the setting of elective surgery the postoperative disposition of the patient should have been amply considered preoperatively and this is an unlikely reason to explain excessive RApoLOS.

The determination of RApoLOS requires the use of statistical process control (SPC) methods as developed by Shewhart for application in manufacturing quality control.[30] SPC is the foundation upon which the concept of "Six-Sigma" has been developed.[31] SPC is founded on the premise that with any product or service that is provided, there will be *common cause variation*. Even with precise manufacturing techniques, there will be minor variation, which does not affect the functional character of the final output. However, *special cause variation* represents an undesired outcome that may be caused by failed processes or systematic issues. In elective surgical care, the measurement of RApoLOS can be used as a measure of special cause variation by using the Moving Range (XmR) Control chart.[32]

The XmR control chart is designed by first developing a listing of risk factors as independent variables, such as are identified in Table 9.5. The length of stay is the dependent variable for this linear regression model. The model is developed on only those live discharges that had no coded complications from the index hospitalization. Once a final length of stay prediction model is complete, the cases for a specified time interval (e.g. 1 year) are aligned in chronologic order. The total predicted days for each hospital are set equal to the total observed days. The observed days of hospitalization for each case is subtracted by the predicted days. The absolute difference is then determined between sequential cases, that is, |case 1 minus case 2|, |case 2-case 3|, |case 3-case 4|, etc. The average of absolute differences gives the moving average. Thus, if there were 50 operations of one type (e.g. colon resections) that were performed in 1 year in a hospital, there would be 49 absolute moving differences. To achieve an upper limit at 3-σ, the moving average is multiplied by 2.66, and this yields the upper limit for lengths of stay over the predicted value that defines the case as a RApoLOS outlier (Fig. 9.5).[33,34] Outlier cases are removed from the sequence and the upper limit is recomputed. The process is iteratively repeated until no outlier cases remain.

Thus, a rate of RApoLOS outliers can be determined by hospital and even by surgeon. Using patient samples from the National Inpatient Sample for the Healthcare Cost and Utilization Project, Table 9.8 identifies the rates of RApoLOS outliers by procedure and compares them with inpatient death rates.[35-38] Of interest, approximately 10–15% of RApoLOS outliers of each of these operative categories did not have coded complications identified in the discharge administrative abstract. The cost profile of the RApoLOS outliers without coded complications were similar to outliers with coded complications but were statistically much greater than costs of nonoutlier cases that had coded complications. It is concluded that RApoLOS outliers without coded complications have had the complicating event omitted from the discharge abstract.

There are advantages to using the RApoLOS outlier as a measure of severe complications rather than identifying the frequency of specific coded events. In our previous studies,[33,34] we have identified that the majority of coded complications do not result in any extension of hospitalization and are not associated with any significant increase in hospital cost. For example, in total knee replacement we have found a 29% rate of coded complications but only a 4.5% rate of RApoLOS outliers, in colon surgery a 41% rate of coded complications but a 7% rate of RApoLOS outliers, and in coronary artery bypass grafting a 66% rate of coded complications but only a 7.5% rate of RApoLOS. The identification of the RApoLOS appears to give a measure of severity to complications. It also has the advantage of being an objectively determined measure based on length of stay rather than events coded for the hospitalization.

There are limitations to using this methodology. The accuracy of risk adjustment is always a source of concern. As in the assessment of risk-adjusted mortality rates, the use of readily available clinical information at admission (e.g. laboratory data) will hopefully improve risk estimates. This methodology has been primarily applied to elective operations, since emergent cases will require accurate present on admission coding to determine which coded events are risk factors at admission, and which are complications from the subsequent inpatient stay. There also remain concerns about administrative and disposition issues of patients that could explain some components of the excess length of stay but should not be a major issue in elective surgical care. Finally, a question can certainly be raised about where the upper limit should be set to designate a given case as being an outlier or not. In Figure 9.5, the upper limit is illustrated at 3σ, 2.5σ, and 2σ. This will affect the number of outlier events that are

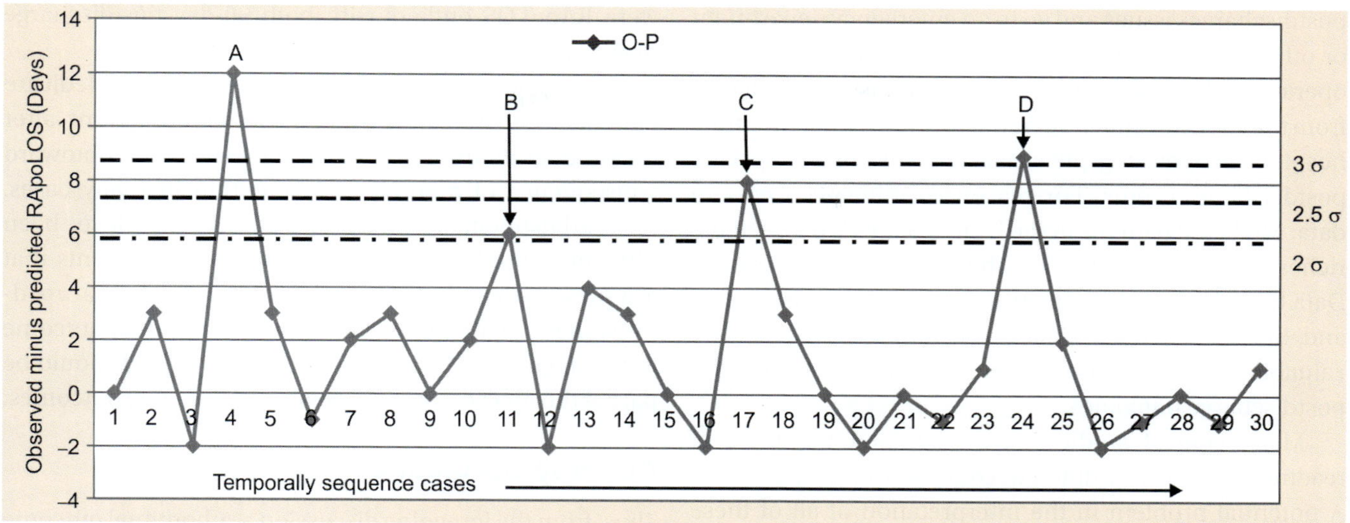

Fig. 9.5: A schematic representation of a moving average control chart, which illustrates the plot observed length of stay subtracted by predicted length of stay. The 3σ, 2.5σ, and 2σ upper limits are illustrated to identify outliers at each of threshold.

Table 9.8 Frequency of deaths, RApoLOS outliers, and overall adverse outcomes rates among studied surgical procedures.

Operative procedure	*Total patients*	*Inpatient deaths*	*RApoLOS outliers*	*Adverse outcomes*
Total knee replacement	160,482	206 (0.1%)	7,106 (4.4%)	7,312 (4.6%)
Total hip replacement	72,467	97 (0.1%)	2,987 (4.1%)	3,084 (4.3%)
Colorectal resection	54.321	542 (1.0%)	3,826 (7.0%)	4,368 (8.0%)
Carotid endarterectomy	43,700	126 (0.3%)	2,217 (5.1%)	2,343 (5.4%)
Aortic surgery	9,090	264 (2.9%)	721 (7.9%)	985 (10.8%)
Femoropopliteal bypass	14,543	161 (1.1%)	859 (5.9%)	1,020 (7.0%)
Hysterectomy	183,614	35 (0.02%)	4,965 (2.7%)	5,000 (2.7%)
Lung resection	12,182	336 (2.8%)	880 (7.2%)	1,216 (10.0%)
Coronary artery bypass grafting	53,750	1,037 (1.9%)	5,151 (9.6%)	6,188 (11.5%)

(RApoLOS: Risk-adjusted postoperative length of stay).

identified. It is evident that additional research needs to evaluate the RApoLOS. This early evidence is encouraging that it can be a more discriminating measure than mortality rates or complication frequencies.

Postdischarge Deaths and Readmissions

Events following discharge from the hospital need to be incorporated into evaluations of outcomes and quality assessments of care. Many complications of care may not be declared until after the patient has been discharged. Inpatient complications of care may be incompletely managed or the disposition of the patient for the weeks following discharge may be to a suboptimal circumstance with inadequate postdischarge care. The consequence may be readmission to the hospital and in some circumstances early postdischarge deaths.

The assessment of postdischarge events has been obscured by several issues. Should the period of evaluation be 30, 60, 90, or more days after discharge? The time interval varies depending upon the criteria used by the specific investigators. The quality of data to identify postdischarge events is inconsistent from country-to-country. Nationalized healthcare systems typically have central repositories of data that permit easier identification of readmissions and postdischarge deaths. In the United States, patient follow-up occurs in physician private offices and are not known to the hospital where the index inpatient care was delivered. Patients may have postdischarges issues and go to an emergency department or other physician different from the one performing the operation. Readmissions can occur in hospitals different from the site of the index operation without either the initial hospital or operating physician knowing of the specific postdischarge events. For reasons of difficult access to data, Medicare patients in the United States have been the richest source of information about postdischarge events. Data bases accumulated by the Veterans Administration[39] and by the American College of Surgeons[40] have been valuable sources of correlation of inpatient events with postdischarge outcomes.

Many clinical studies have examined the rates of readmission following different cohorts of surgical patients. A potential problem in the interpretation of all of these studies is that commonly readmissions are indexed to the date of the operation and not to the date of discharge. A consistent finding in these studies is that readmission is more likely in those patients who experienced complications during the index inpatient episode. However, if a complication of care extends the inpatient length of stay to 14, 17, or 21 total days, then the period of risk for being counted as a readmission is very brief if a 30-day postoperative window is used. A strong argument could be made that the operative event and not the discharge day should be used for the computation of readmissions, but to do so means that a 60- or 90-day window is most suitable to catch all of the readmission events linked to the index operation.

In a study of over 13 million Medicare inpatients in the United States, rates of readmission after acute hospitalization have been identified at 19% within 30 days of discharge and an aggregate of 34% within 90 days.[41] Surgery readmissions for all procedures was 16% at 30 days and were noted to be 10% for major hip/knee operations, 24% for vascular surgery, and 17% for major bowel operations.

In a study of over 2 million Medicare elective surgical patients, we identified the 90-day all-cause readmission rate to be 9%.[28] The inpatient mortality rate for this study was 0.54%, but the 90-day postdischarge death rate of 0.71%. In elective coronary artery surgery, there was a 15.5% readmission rate at 90 days postdischarge, a 2.4% inpatient mortality rate, and a 1.2% 90-day-postdischarge mortality rate. In elective colon surgery, there was a 14% 90-day readmission rate, a 2.7% inpatient mortality rate, and a 3% 90-day postdischarge mortality rate. An important observation in this study was the statistically significant association ($p < .0001$) of those patients who were RApoLOS outliers with both 90-day postdischarge deaths and readmissions.

The evidence that is principally derived from Medicare patients is that readmission is a common event after major operations and that it represents an untoward consequence of a surgical intervention in many cases. Risk adjustment to predict readmissions have been difficult to model and identification of those events that are preventable remains unclear.[42] It is likely that readmission is a significant measure of a suboptimal outcome in the majority of patients after operations and should be part of the metrics for the assessment of quality outcomes.

Adverse Surgical Outcome

Thus, from the foregoing discussion a suboptimal outcome following a surgical episode of care could be measured by any of a number of criteria. A unifying concept has been to identify the adverse surgical outcome (ASO). A definition that we have proposed for an ASO includes all inpatient and 90-day postdischarge deaths, all RApoLOS outliers, and all 90-day postdischarge readmissions. This definition avoids the problems of effective surveillance and the subjective determination of whether a complication of care has occurred. It would mean that minor events in the patient's convalescence that did not prolong hospitalization or result in a readmission would not be included. This measure can be objectively measured and eliminates the subjectivity of assignment of complications. In the absence of any component of the ASO, an episode of surgical care can be considered to be satisfactory. As will be seen in the subsequent discussion on economics, a unifying concept of an ASO becomes essential for the evaluation of the excess costs of care and for the development of alternative methods for payment reform.

ECONOMICS

Surgical economics is the description and analysis of the delivery and costs of providing surgical services. The economics of surgical care share most of the same features that are identified in healthcare economics, with perhaps the notable difference that costs in surgery are episodic and generally not recurring as is seen in chronic medical conditions, and that costs tend to be large in association with these episodic events. The overall large costs of surgical care are high professional costs, the requirements for specialized hospital or ambulatory surgical facilities for the provision of surgical care, and the expensive technology that has evolved in surgical care over recent decades. The technological evolution within surgical care is likely to be sustained and makes the prospects for more expensive care very likely.

The costs of healthcare in general and surgical care in specific have become major issues for the economies of the world. Whether expenditures are paid by public or private revenues, the costs of healthcare have grown faster than inflation in virtually all countries over the last 20 or more years, and methods to maintain the vast array of healthcare services at affordable costs have become a universal problem. Most efforts to restrain expenditures short of restricting access have largely failed to this point. In no country has the growth of healthcare costs been more dramatic than in the United States. Current expenditures are at 18% of gross domestic product (GDP)[43] and current estimates project this figure to continue to increase if current growth rates in cost are sustained. This progressive growth in the percentage of GDP in healthcare means than other goods and services are being displaced and other areas of personal or government expenditures are being redirected for the provision of medical care.

In Figure 9.6, the costs of care for commonly performed surgical procedures in the United States are illustrated.[44] The costs illustrated are only for the hospital component of care with no professional or postdischarge costs. These costs have been observed during and immediately following a major economic recession in the United States and worldwide. Projections would indicate that costs for surgical care will continue to grow both due to increased volume of care but also due to costs that are greater than prevailing inflation rates.

Multiple reasons explain the rapid growth in medical and surgical expenditures. First, there is a dysfunctional relationship between the consumer of care and the providers of care. Whether in a government-operated healthcare system or in a privately paid system, no direct financial relationship exists between the patient and the service provider. The interposition of the third-party payer in the form of government or private insurer means that for most care the patient wishes to have as much as the system will bear, and in the absence of policy restrictions the provider has no impediments for providing the services independent of their necessity. The moral hazard of this relationship has been vigorously debated.

A second consideration in the growth of expenditures is that an inelastic supply and demand relationship exists between the purchase of health services and the availability of services. In surgical care in particular, patients with acute and potentially life-threatening illness are not in a position to shop for the best price or the most efficient care. Patients with colon cancer, a perforated appendix, unstable angina, or an acutely ischemic lower extremity have an understandable demand for services at any cost and will not be inclined to negotiate prices or forego treatment because it is too expensive. Major illness preempts the market dynamics of supply and demand. In the United States this is illustrated by the observation that 10% of patients consume 65% of the annual healthcare expenditures (Table 9.9).[45] Huge costs in the extremely ill are clearly major drivers of overall surgical and medical expenditures.

Surgical economics are extremely complex and cannot be covered in its entirety in this brief discussion. The premise will be made that comparisons that are internal to the delivery system will identify heterogeneity in costs for the provision of similar episodes of surgical care, that is, some surgeons and hospitals are more cost-effective than others and that the differences in processes and performance can be a key to the identification of excess costs of care. Systematic comparative effectiveness and efficiency may be a method for reductions of cost without inappropriate restriction of services.

Appropriateness of Care

In the United States, much discussion has centered on the issue of inappropriate surgical care as a major issue

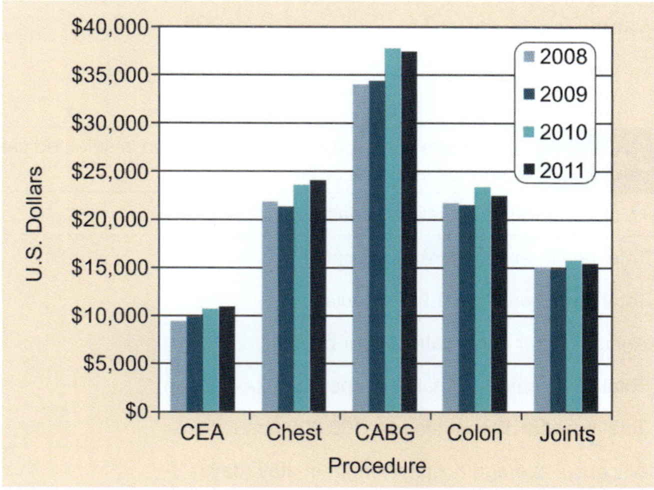

Fig. 9.6: Hospital costs for carotid endarterectomy (CEA), open chest operations (Chest), coronary artery bypass grafting (CABG), colon resection (Colon), and total joint replacement (Joints) for years 2008–2011 in the U.S.

in excess costs. Geographic studies have identified that the frequency of operations is quite heterogeneous in different areas of the country and that better health outcomes have not been the net result in areas of higher utilization.[46,47] The implication has been that inappropriate operations, for marginal indications and financial gain by health providers, are a driver of higher healthcare costs. A counter argument would be that low-volume areas of selected operations may actually be due to poor availability of necessary services. Although no one would argue that perverse incentives of more payments for more operations may well lead to inappropriate care, a comparison of US per capita utilization of services generally demonstrates little evidence of overutilization. Compared to other OECD (Organization for Economic Cooperation and Development) countries, the annual number of physician visits, acute hospital beds, annual hospital inpatient days, and average length of stay are at or below comparative norms (Table 9.10).[48] The utilization of imaging studies (computerized tomography and magnetic resonance imaging scans) does exceed international norms. Unfortunately, the utilization of specific surgical procedures is not reported for comparative purposes. However, the price for hospital and physician services is dramatically greater per unit of service than the comparator OECD reference countries.[49] These comparative data would implicate that it is not the overutilization of services but rather the price of individual services that accounts for the increased costs of care in the United States.

Table 9.9 Percentage of US healthcare costs that are spent on subsets of patients for the year 2009.

Population (%)	*Annual healthcare expenditures (%)*	*Mean expenditures/ patient ($)*
Top 1	21.4	87,570
Top 5	50	40,682
Top 10	65	26,767
Top 30	90	–
Top 50	97	–
Lower 50	3	236

Excess Costs of Adverse Surgical Outcomes

Major complications of inpatient surgical care have been consistently demonstrated to be a major economic burden in the delivery of healthcare. Complications in inpatient surgical care lead to reoperations, prolonged lengths of stay, readmissions to the hospital, and increased use of healthcare resources (e.g. antibiotics).[50] Many investigations have explored the increased economic costs that are attendant to SSIs, cardiac events, prolonged postoperative ileus, cardiac events, and the many other complications of major surgical procedures. Assessments of these excess costs commonly take gross averages of uncomplicated cases and subtract that cost from the total costs of the complicated patient to arrive at an estimate of excess costs. Not uncommonly, if the complication of interest is SSI, the full excess costs using such models will be attributable to that event when complications of postoperative surgical care may well occur in clusters and attribution of costs become a difficult proposition.[51] Assignment of average costs to a complication can also be more difficult to understand when complications of

Table 9.10 Healthcare resource costs and utilization in selected categories between the United States and the average for OECD reference countries for the year 2011.

Healthcare category (unit of measure)	*United States*	*OECD average*	*US/OECD ratio*
Total health expenditure ($ per capita)	$8,508	$3,322	2.6
Total physicians (per 1,000 population)	2.5	3.2	0.8
Annual doctor consultations (per capita)	4.1	6.6	0.6
Total acute care hospital beds (per 1000 population)	2.6	3.4	0.8
Total hospital discharges (per 100,000 population)	12,549	15,561	0.8
All cause, average hospital length-of-stay (days)	4.8	7.5	0.6
Magnetic resonance imaging examinations (per 1,000 population)	102.7	48.3	2.1
Computerized tomography examinations (per 1,000 population)	273.8	128.2	2.1

(OECD: Organization for Economic Cooperation and Development).

care occur across a wide spectrum of severity as has been discussed earlier.

To define the risk-adjusted costs of uncomplicated care, we have examined large populations of patients undergoing specific operations. We have chosen elective operations since clear identification of risk factors versus complications cannot be adequately defined with conventional studies of administrative data for emergency operations. First, patients who are live discharges with no coded complications and were not RApoLOS outliers are examined for total hospital cost. Hospital costs are estimated by taking the total billed charge from the hospitalization and multiplying it by the report cost-to-charge ratio for that facility. Because payments for care are not linked to the actual costs employed in the care of individual cases but are rather agreed upon prices by private or public payers, the cost-to-charge multiplier, while having some shortcomings, represents a more accurate representation of actual inpatient costs of care.

These total costs of care then become the dependent variable for each operation and a linear regression model is created using age, gender, and the generic risk factors that are chronic diseases potentially associated with increased cost (e.g. diabetes) as the independent variables. Because different hospitals in different regions of the United States have different costs of living, hospital dummy variables are included in the development of the linear prediction model so that coefficients for each risk factor are not inflated by local cost variation. Only statistically significant risk factors are included in final models. This final prediction model of hospital cost for each operation permits the calculation of a predicted cost for each patient that is adjusted to patient-specific preexisting conditions. Because all hospital effects have been removed from the predicted value from the risk model, the predicted value is then multiplied by the wage index for each hospital that adjusts for local cost of living differences.

The excess cost of each adverse outcome is then computed by taking those RApoLOS outliers for each procedure and subtracting the locally adjusted predicted cost for a routine case of comparable risk profile from the observed cost. The excess costs per RApoLOS for a panel of different surgical procedures are presented in Figure 9.7.[37] Of interest, when patients who are RApoLOS outliers but are without coded complications are evaluated, their excess costs are similar to those patients who are outliers with coded complications and are statistically different from the entire population of patients who were not outliers.

Similar calculation of excess costs of readmission following inpatient elective operations can be computed. Patients who are readmitted within 30, 60, or 90 days after discharge are compared with risk-adjusted similar patients who were not readmitted and the excess costs of readmission are identified. As has been noted earlier, the full costs of readmission will be obscured if the number of readmissions is linked to the date of the operation rather than the date of discharge especially if the reference period is only 30 days. The largest excess costs are identified among patients who are both RApoLOS outliers for the index hospitalization who are then readmitted to the hospital within 90 days of discharge (Fig. 9.8).[28] Excess costs for these patients approach 4–5 times the costs that would be predicted had the patients not been an RApoLOS or a 90-day postdischarge readmission.

Estimates of the excess costs of care usually have been for only the hospital component of total expenditures. Physician payments for both the inpatient and the postdischarge components of care are really only available through the Medicare database and are very difficult to extract completely. For surgical care, the physician component includes the operating surgeon, anesthesiology services, critical care services, and other consultants that may be employed both during and following the index hospitalization. Postdischarge physician costs are further compounded by differentiation of ancillary costs (i.e. pharmaceuticals, laboratory, and imaging studies) of care that may be to attributable to the surgical procedure or costs that may be part of the continuing care of preexisting

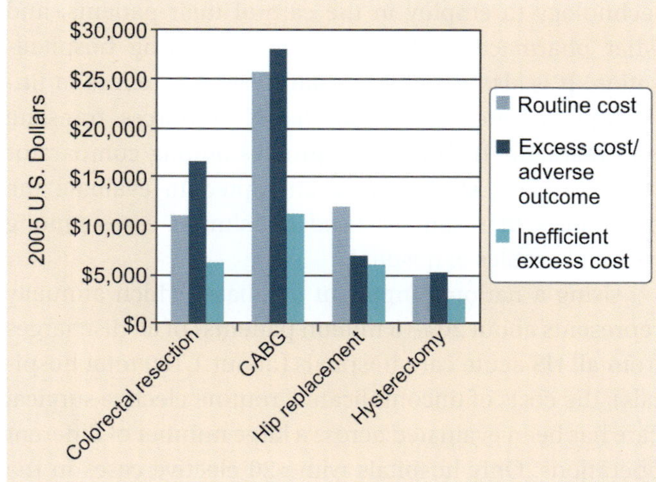

Fig. 9.7: Excess dollars spent for adverse outcomes and inefficient care for colorectal resections, coronary artery bypass grafting total hip replacement, and hysterectomy (2005 dollars).

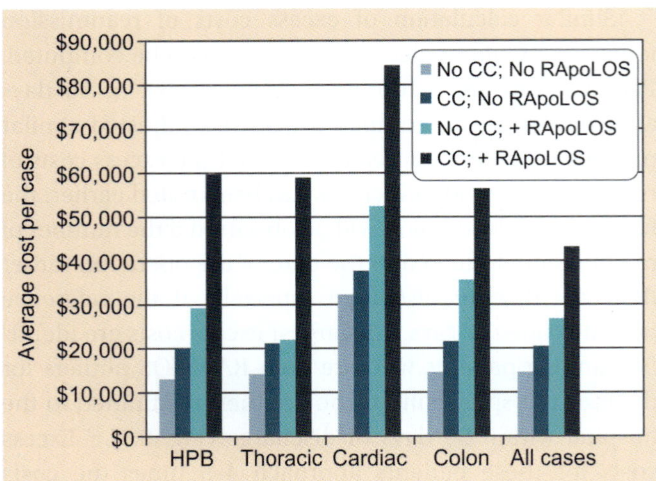

Fig. 9.8: Combined effects on increased costs of care by combining risk-adjusted postoperative length of stay outliers and readmission costs in hepatic–pancreatic–biliary operations, Open thoracic operations, cardiac operations, colon resections, and all procedures studied among 21 groups of Medicare surgical procedures (2010 dollars).

and unrelated medical conditions. True cost accounting of postdischarge costs will likely require prospective definition and not be easily extracted from administrative claims data.

Excess Costs of Inefficiency

It is generally recognized that there is marked heterogeneity in the utilization of resources for the care of surgical patients in different hospitals. Surgeons have different attitudes about when patients can be discharged, what technology to employ in the care of their patients, and what pharmaceuticals are employed during hospitalization. It is also recognized that these differences in utilization of different hospital-based resources translate into markedly different cost profiles among comparator hospitals. Few studies have attempted to evaluate the differences in resources used for similar cases among national profiles of hospital.

Using a national inpatient database, which annually represents about 20% (8 million patients) of all discharges from all US acute care hospitals (about 1,100 total hospitals), the costs of uncomplicated, routine elective surgical care has been evaluated across a large number of different operations. Only hospitals with >20 elective cases in the database for each operation of interest are included in this analysis. Those hospitals that have risk-adjusted adverse outcome rates (deaths + RApoLOS outliers) > 2.56 standard deviations ($p < .005$) from the mean of all hospitals are considered to have suboptimal outcomes and are removed from the data set.

Patients from remaining hospitals after removal of those with suboptimal outcomes were then used to develop a linear prediction model using only those live discharges that were not RApoLOS outliers. As before, hospital dummy variables were employed. Within the patients for each hospital in each surgical group, the predicted costs (adjusted for local wage indices) were subtracted from the observed to establish patient-level costs that were less than or exceeded prediction. Total excess costs were computed for each hospital, and those with costs exceeding 3.29 standard deviations ($p < 0.001$) were considered inefficient. There excess costs exceeding the risk-adjusted costs of the efficient hospitals are identified in Figure 9.7.

Obviously, the cut points for defining a hospital as inefficient are an arbitrary one and the limit employed in these studies may be too extreme. Even with a 3.29 standard deviation cut point, we have identified that approximately 15–18% of hospitals have excess costs for the uncomplicated routine surgical cases within each category. Even more impressive is to perform a scatter plot of adverse outcome rates against average costs of routine cases and to identify the large number of hospitals that have risk-adjusted costs less than the average but also have adverse outcome rates that are average or below average. Such comparative studies clearly indicate that considerable cost savings in elective surgical care can be achieved without compromising the quality of outcomes that are observed.

Other Surgical Cost Issues

Effectiveness and efficiency are the two macroscopic issues that define excess costs in healthcare. There are components within this larger picture that contribute to the issue. Many of these issues have complex social and political features that make objective assessment of their role in healthcare cost difficult to assess and even more difficult to manage. Each of the following requires some innovative solutions to enhance cost-effective care for the future.

Futile care for patients with medically nonrecoverable conditions is always discussed. The global aging of the population makes the issue of older patients with severe disease the center of this discussion. Of course, prospectively defining what is futile is very difficult, and the perspective of futile care has changed as the effectiveness of critical care in the intensive care unit and expanded treatments for advanced cancer and other illnesses has improved. The arguments about when and if care should be withheld or withdrawn for a severely ill patient frequently becomes an ethical issue that has little objective evidence to direct the debate. All clinicians have had the experience of an extremely ill surgical patient whose prospects for survival were remote who has completely recovered, and these anecdotal accounts further obscure the debate. A recent publication examined a 3-month experience in five ICUs. A total of 11% of patients ($n = 123$) were considered to be receiving futile care by one or more critical care specialist.[52] Of these patients, 84 died in the hospital, 20 died within 6 months after discharge, and the remainder survived in a severely compromised health condition. Futile days of cost were nearly four per patient at a cost of $4000 per day.

There is no question that large sums of money are spent on advanced illness with small prospects for patient recovery but the percentage of care that would meet the criteria of being futile remains undefined, in large part because the threshold for defining futile care has been difficult. The definition becomes obscure depending upon one's perspective of futile care at a societal level or futile care that involves a personal family member. Many families and many surgeons themselves are unwilling to accept any defined point of futility in care. Both the American Medical Association[53] and the American College of Surgeons[54] have issued statements about the responsibility of physicians to not provide care that is deemed to be futile, but no guidance is provided about the definition of when that limit has been reached. This will clearly be an area for debate in future years.

Medical malpractice: A major issue in the United States but one that has increased in importance in other countries is the cost of medical negligence and malpractice litigation. The public dissemination of advances and standards in the delivery of healthcare has increased expectations. When outcomes have not met these expectations, then patients may turn to the legal system for redress. Similarly, the use of new drugs and new medical devices that have not had years of evaluation may lead to suboptimal outcomes or unanticipated complications. The consequences of malpractice and product litigation are substantial annual costs of insurance for physicians, hospitals, and manufacturers. Surgeons particularly have been the focus of high malpractice costs, which are the consequences of higher rates of litigation than other medical specialties. A second cost of malpractice litigation has been defensive medical practices where excessive services are employed in patient care to avoid the appearance of inadequate care. Failure to employ specific diagnostics or specific imaging studies are commonly cited issues in legal claims. Failure of clinicians to adhere to published guidelines or recommendations is another increasing source of litigation and cost. Clinicians argue that expectations are excessive, and attorneys contend that patients are entitled to a "standard of care." Some jurisdictions have placed limitations on noneconomic damages (e.g. pain and suffering) in the litigation process. Others have argued that contingency fee arrangements should be limited. The full scope of the economic impact of medicolegal activity continues to be debated and potential solutions are being explored, albeit not with the speed that many surgeons would desire.

Medical education is an infrequently discussed issue in the overall costs of healthcare. In the United States, a medical degree ordinarily requires 8 years for completion after high school. The 4 years of dedicated medical school require acquisition of loans for most students to complete the process, with total education indebtedness commonly exceeding $200,000 at graduation. Current tuition and fees at US medical schools are profiled in Figure 9.9.[55] Postgraduate training extends the education process for another 5–7 years or more, and interest on the debt is rolled over into the principal during this extended training period. Substantial gross debt is thus accumulated at the time of graduation and places demand on professional income expectations when the post-graduate training period has been completed.

Another feature of cost in medical education has been the increased costs of postgraduate education. Traditionally, the postgraduate years of specialty training has had an apprenticeship structure where the young medical graduate would work with a surgeon or group of surgeons to learn surgical procedures. Postgraduate surgical education transitioned into being hospital based. The trainee would work long hours in return for the educational experience. Hospitals assumed the costs in the 1940s and 1950s by providing living accommodations and a modest stipend. During the 1960s stipends increased such that by the 1970s, postgraduate surgical trainees earned a salary commensurate with skilled labor, but again long hours (>80 h/week) and services for the hospital in the form of continuing care for inpatients, performance

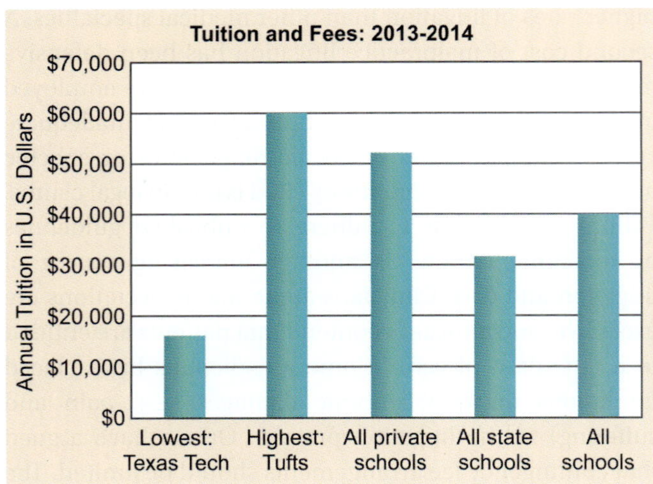

Fig. 9.9: Tuition and fees for 1 year of medical school in the United States (2013–2014) at the lowest tuition institution (Texas Tech), the highest (Tufts), the average for all private medical schools, the average for State medical schools (in-State residents), and the overall average for all medical schools reporting (n = 136).

of minor procedures on the ward, and assistance in the operating room were provided. Even in the United States, postgraduate costs became a direct expenditure to the federal government.

During the last 30 years, the increasing salary for postgraduate education has been accompanied by a reduction in strictly service-related activities without educational benefit, and excessive weekly and nighttime work hours for surgical trainees in particular have been progressively restricted. The result has been that postgraduate education has become a major cost to hospitals and governments while services provided by the trainee have declined. In addition, much of surgical postgraduate education and the majority of nonsurgical training have moved to the ambulatory, outpatient venue, which has a further diminished value to the hospital-based source of payment.

Technology: The last 30–40 years have seen dramatic developments in healthcare technology. More sophisticated but expensive drugs have emerged with remarkable therapeutic benefit. Biological therapies such as monoclonal antibodies have dramatically increased in number. Sophisticated imaging in the form of computerized tomography, magnetic resonance imaging, and positron-emission tomography have revolutionized diagnostic accuracy but at considerable economic cost. Minimally invasive surgical techniques and robotic consoles have provided an amazing technological input into traditional surgical management but have done so at spiraling costs and expensive training for surgeons and support personnel. The public has come to expect new technology, entrepreneurs have benefited from this profitable enterprise, and the cost of care has steadily increased. New technology including pharmaceutical development is viewed as the major driver in the increased costs of healthcare that exceed GDP growth. While technology has generally been associated with an overall reduction in costs in most industries, in healthcare technology results in a progressive increase in costs with alarming prospects for the future.[56] The Congressional Budget Office has identified accelerating technology costs as the major driver for the unsustainable increasing cost burden of healthcare in the United States.[57]

This rapid development has not been paralleled by objective methods for the assessment of cost-effectiveness of new technology. Many have argued that the law of diminishing returns has now been achieved in healthcare where spiraling costs have resulted in minimal or no added value over previously existing technology. All would generally agree that laparoscopic surgical methods and minimally invasive endovascular methods have been substantial improvements for the care of patients. But have single-port laparoscopic procedures or robotic techniques justified the increased costs over those methods that have been replaced? The debate over new technology will continue and hopefully better technology assessment will evolve. The rapid expansion of healthcare technology and its attendant increase in costs will be the source of considerable attention in the next decade and beyond.

INTEGRATION OF INFORMATICS, OUTCOMES, AND ECONOMICS

In the above discussion, it can be shown that informatics tools applied to large data sets of patient data can generate useful information about the outcomes and the costs of surgical care. It is likely that refinements in these informatics tools will permit better risk adjustment and more precise identification of outcomes and costs.

In Figure 9.10, a scatter plot of hospitals in the United States is presented that demonstrates outcome and cost outliers and serves as an example of the integration of informatics, outcomes, and costs. In our several studies, we have identified similar patterns of performance relative to suboptimal outcomes and costs. We have consistently identified that a reference group of hospitals (about 75%

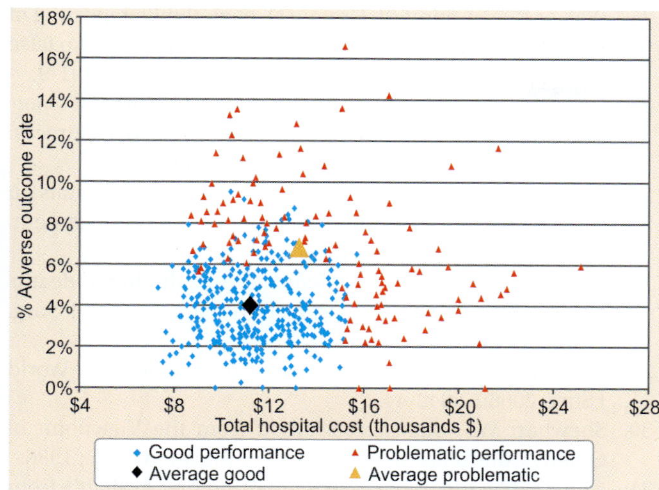

Fig. 9.10: This scatter plot illustrates the relationship among 453 hospitals for adverse outcome rates and the average costs of routine care in total knee replacement. (2005 dollars). With permission from Michael Pine and Associates, Chicago, IL, USA.

nationally) meets the performance criteria for both risk-adjusted outcomes and costs. The adjustment of the performance of all hospitals to that of the reference group results in a 25% reduction in attributable risk for adverse outcomes and nearly a 10% reduction in excess costs of care.

These analytic tools provide the basis for the design of a new surgical episode-based payment model. Using reference hospitals illustrated in Figure 9.10, the costs of routine care (those without an adverse outcome) and the frequency and the costs of adverse outcomes can be computed on a risk-adjusted basis. The risk-adjusted probability of an adverse event is multiplied by the excess costs of that adverse event to yield a surgical warranty, which is added to the routine costs of that case.[58] A prospective price for all services inclusive of postdischarge readmissions and all professional costs can be designed. An aggregated "bundled" payment can be analytically defined.[59] The episode-based pricing strategy will hopefully realign the incentives of care for hospitals and surgeons for improved outcomes and lesser costs.

SUMMARY

Progress in healthcare for the future must represent the convergence of informatics, outcomes, and economics. Informatics becomes the pathway to convert massive amounts of data into useful information. Not just information to guide scientific inquiry, but information to disseminate direction to practicing clinicians for better and more efficient care of patients, and information that will provide objective outcomes and accurate costs of care. The reality is that the spiraling costs of healthcare are unsustainable and that new models must drive the evaluation of cost-effective care for the future.

The emphasis on cost-effective care means that the objective measurement of outcomes and the avoidable costs of care will be integrated into a consolidated concept. New technology must be evaluated in terms of better outcomes and at what level of increased costs. Established methods of care require a more uniform application of methods demonstrated to optimize outcomes and reduce costs. Although many will criticize this approach as being a business model and that healthcare is more than a business, the reality is that the spiraling costs of healthcare are unsustainable. New models using informatics tools applied to large and detailed clinical databases must drive the evaluation of cost-effective care for the future.

FURTHER READING

1. Hanson CW: Healthcare Informatics. New York: McGraw-Hill; 2006.
2. Wager KA, Lee FW, Glaser JP: Healthcare Information Systems: A Practical Approach for Healthcare Management. San Francisco: Jossey-Bass; 2009.

REFERENCES

1. Leape LL, Brennan TA, Laird NM, et al. Incidence of adverse events and negligence in hospitalized patients. Results of the Harvard Medical Practice Study II. N Engl J Med. 1991;324:377-84.
2. Kamruzzaman J, Begg R, Sarker R. Overview of artificial neural networks and their applications in healthcare. In: Begg R, Kamaruzzaman J, Sarker R (Eds). Hershey, PA: Idea Group Publishing; 2006. Chapter 1. pp. 1-19.
3. Bennett CC, Hauser K. Artificial intelligence framework for simulating clinical decision-making: a Markov decision process approach. Artif Intell Med. 2013;57:9-19.
4. Brookes T. The top five free internet search engines, 2010. [online] Available from http://www.ehow.com/list_6518209_top-five-internet-search-engines.html. Accessed June 4, 2015.
5. US National Library of Medicine and National Institutes of Health. Pubmed. [online] Available from http://www.ncbi.nlm.nih.gov/pubmed. Accessed January 6, 2014.
6. Low AFH, Phillips AB, Ancker JS, et al. Financial effects of health information technology: a systematic review. Am J Manag Care. 2013;19:SP369-76.
7. Institute of Medicine of the National Academies. (2003). Key Capabilities of an Electronic Health Record. Washington, DC: The National Academic Press. [online] Available from http://books.nap.edu/openbook.php? record_id=10781. Accessed June 4, 2015.

8. Agency for Healthcare Research and Quality: HCUP methods series: The case for the POA indicator: update 2011, report #2011-05. [online] Available from http://www.hcup- us.ahrq.gov/reports/methods/2011_05.pdf. Accessed January 16, 2014.
9. Campbell EM, Sittig DF, Ash JS, et al. Types of unintended consequences related to computerized provider order entry. J Am Med Inform Assoc. 2006;13:547-56.
10. Stone WM, Smith BE, Shaft JD, et al. Impact of a computerized physician order-entry system. J Am Coll Surg. 2009; 208:960-9.
11. U.S. Food and Drug Administration. Radio Frequency Identification. [online] Available from http://www.fda.gov/Radiation-EmittingProducts/RadiationSafety/ElectromagneticCompatibilityEMC/ucm116647.htm. Accessed January 6, 2014.
12. Blumenthal D, Tavenner M. The "meaningful use" regulation for electronic health records. N Engl J Med. 2010; 363: 501-4.
13. Archer N, Fevrier-Thomas U, Lokker C, et al. Personal health records: a scoping review. J Am Med Inform Assoc. 2011;18:515-22.
14. National Health Information Network. [online] Available from http://www.healthit.gov/policy-researchers-implementers/nationwide-health-information-network-nwhin. Accessed October 30, 2013.
15. Adler-Milstein J, Bates DW, Jha AK. Operational health information exchanges show substantial growth, but long-term funding remains a concern. Health Aff. 2013;32: 1486-92.
16. Agency for Healthcare Research and Quality. Healthcare Cost and Utilization Project (HCUP). [online] Available from http://www.ahrq.gov/research/data/hcup/index.html. Accessed January 6, 2014.
17. Research Data Assistance Center-Centers for Medicare and Medicaid Services. Research Identifiable Files. [online] Available from http://www.resdac.org/cms-data/request/research-identifiable-files. Accessed January 6, 2014.
18. Fry DE. Fifty ways to cause surgical site infections. Surg Infect. 2011;12:497-500.
19. National Institute for Health and Care Excellence. Surgical site infection (QS49). [online] Available from http://guidance.nice.org.uk/QS49. Accessed January 7, 2014.
20. Pine M, Jordan HS, Elixhauser A, et al. Enhancement of claims data to improve risk adjustment of hospital mortality. JAMA. 2007;297:71-6.
21. Fry DE, Pine M, Jordan HS, et al. Combining administrative and clinical data to stratify surgical risk. Ann Surg. 2007; 246:875-85.
22. Bruce J, Russell EM, Mollison J, et al. The measurement and monitoring of surgical adverse events. Health Technol Assess. 2001;5:1-194.
23. Pearse RM, Moreno RP, Bauer P, et al. Mortality after surgery in Europe: a 7 day cohort study. Lancet. 2012;380:1059-65.
24. Symons NRA, Moorthy K, Almoudaris AM, et al. Mortality in high-risk emergency general surgical admissions. Brit J Surg. 2013;100:1318-25.
25. Walker K, Neuburger J, Groene O, et al. Public reporting of surgeon outcomes: low numbers of procedures lead to false complacency. Lancet. 2013; pii: S0140-6736(13):61491-9.
26. Henderson A, Henderson S. Provision of a surgeon's performance data for people considering elective surgery. Cochrane Database Syst Rev. 2010;(11):CD006327.
27. Dimick JB, Staiger DO, Birkmeyer JD. Ranking hospitals on surgical mortality: the importance of reliability adjustment. Health Serv Res. 2010;45:1614-29.
28. Fry DE, Pine M, Pine G. Medicare post-discharge deaths and readmissions following elective surgery. Am J Surg. 2014;207:326-30.
29. Sokol DK, Wilson J. What is a surgical complication? World J Surg. 2008;32:942-44.
30. Shewhart WA. Statistical Method from the Viewpoint of Quality Control. New York: Dover Publications, Inc.; 1986.
31. General Electric. What is six sigma? [online] Available from http://www.ge.com/en/company/companyinfo/quality/whatis.htm.
32. Lee K, McGreevey C. Using control charts to assess performance measurement data. J Qual Improv. 2002;28: 90-101.
33. Fry DE, Pine M, Jones BL, et al. Adverse outcomes in surgery: redefinition of post-operative complications. Am J Surg. 2009;197:479-84.
34. Fry DE, Pine M, Jones BL, et al. Control charts to identify adverse outcomes in elective colon resection. Am J Surg. 2012;203:392-6.
35. Pine M, Fry DE, Jones BL, et al. Controlling costs without compromising quality: paying hospitals for total knee replacement. Med Care. 2010;48:862-8.
36. Fry DE, Pine M, Jones BL, et al. Comparative effectiveness and efficiency in peripheral vascular surgery. Am J Surg. 2011;201:363-8.
37. Fry DE, Pine M, Jones BL, et al. The impact of ineffective and inefficient care on the excess costs of elective surgical procedures. J Am Coll Surg. 2011;212:779-86.
38. Fry DE, Pine M, Jones BL, et al Inefficiency is the major driver of excess costs in lung resection. J Thor Cardiovasc Surg. 2011;142:1418-22.
39. Mull HJ, Borzecki AM, Loveland S, et al. Detecting adverse events in surgery: comparing events detected by the Veterans Health Administration Surgical Quality Improvement Program and the Patient Safety Indicators. Am J Surg. 2013; pii: S0002-9610(13):00643-0.
40. Lucas DJ, Haider A, Haut E, et al. Assessing readmission after general, vascular, and thoracic surgery using ACS-NSQIP. Ann Surg. 2013;258(3):430-9.
41. Jencks SF, Williams MV, Coleman EA. Rehospitalizations among patients in the Medicare fee-for-service program. N Engl J Med. 2009;360:1418-28.
42. Kansagara D, Englander H, Salanitro A, et al. Risk prediction models for hospital readmission: a systematic review. JAMA. 2011;306:1688-98.
43. The World Bank: Health expenditure, total (% GDP). [online] Available from http://data.worldbank.org/indicator/SH.XPD.TOTL.ZS. Accessed June 4, 2015.

44. Agency for Healthcare Research and Quality. HCUPnet. [online] Available from http://hcupnet.ahrq.gov/Accessed January 16, 2014.
45. Cohen S, Yu W. (2012). The concentration and persistence in the level of health expenditures over time: estimates for the U.S. population, 2009–2010. Statistical Brief #392. November 2012. Rockville, MD: Agency for Healthcare Research and Quality. [online] Available from http://www.meps.ahrq.gov/mepsweb/data_files/publications/st392/stat392.pdf. Accessed December 15, 2013.
46. Song Y, Skinner JS, Bynum JPW, et al. Regional variations in diagnostic practices. N Engl J Med. 2010;363:45-53.
47. Mittler JN, Landon BE, Fisher ES, et al. Market variations in intensity of Medicare service use and beneficiary experiences with care. Health Serv Res. 2010;45:647-69.
48. Organization for Economic Cooperation and Development (OECD). OECD Health Data. [online] Available from http://www.oecd.org/health/health-systems/oecdhealthdata2013-frequentlyrequesteddata.htm. Accessed January 15, 2014.
49. Anderson GF, Squires DA. Measuring the U.S. health care system: a cross-national comparison. Issue Brief (Commonw Fund). 2010;90:1-10.
50. Zhan C, Miller MR. Excess length of stay, charges, and mortality attributable to medical injuries during hospitalization. JAMA. 2003;290:1868-74.

Additional references appear in the online version of this book.

10

Case Study: Laparoscopic Access to the Multiply Operated Abdomen

Jordan M Cloyd, Sherry M Wren

THE PROBLEM

The most commonly employed method for access to the abdomen for laparoscopy includes insertion of a Veress needle through the umbilicus, followed by the establishment of pneumoperitoneum and insertion of trocars. In patients with previous abdominal surgery, this blind approach may lead to unacceptably high rates of visceral and vascular injuries (Fig. 10.1).

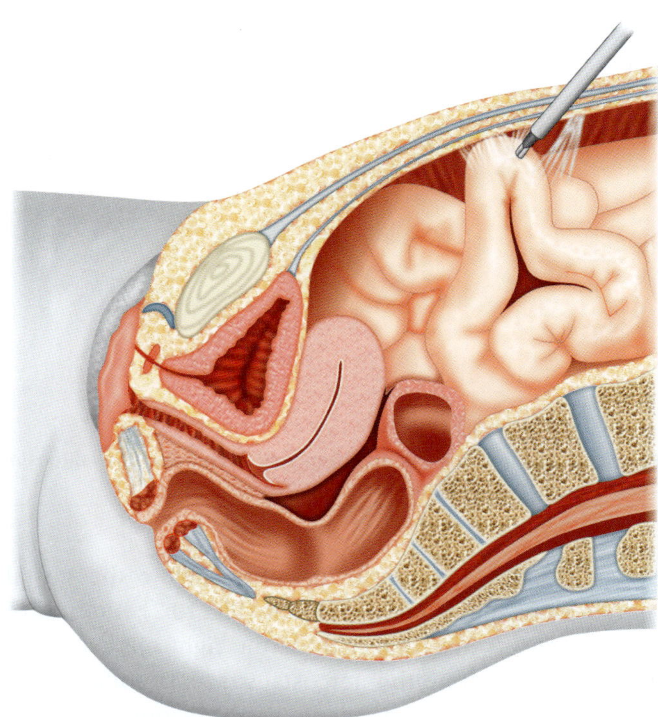

Fig. 10.1: An example of bowel injury during laparoscopic trocar placement related to scar tissue from prior surgery.

THE TYPICAL CASE

A 56-year-old woman with a history of hypertension, obesity, and chronic obstructive pulmonary disease presents for the evaluation of recurrent sigmoid diverticulitis. Her past surgical history includes a total abdominal hysterectomy and bilateral salpingo-oophorectomy via a lower midline incision 3 years ago and an open appendectomy via a McBurney's incision 32 years ago. In the past year, she has experienced three episodes of acute left lower quadrant abdominal pain, twice requiring hospitalization. Computed tomography demonstrated sigmoid diverticulitis. The most recent colonoscopy confirmed the presence of sigmoid diverticula without evidence of neoplasia. Given the chronicity of her symptoms, she is interested in undergoing elective sigmoidectomy. She has learned of the potential benefits of laparoscopy and wonders whether her operation could be performed by that method.

DIAGNOSTIC DILEMMAS

Laparoscopy offers several advantages compared to conventional open surgery, including decreased postoperative pain, earlier return to normal activities, reduced blood loss, and fewer postoperative complications such as wound infections and incisional hernias. However, complications associated with gaining abdominal access can be a serious cause of laparoscopy-associated morbidity. Patients with previous abdominal or pelvic operations are at higher risk of complications due to the presence of adhesions to the anterior abdominal wall. Although previous abdominal surgery does not preclude attempts at laparoscopic entry, the surgeon should be cognizant of previous operations, location of incisions, and any history of peritonitis. Knowledge of alternative methods of abdominal access is critical to the safety of laparoscopic surgery.

MANAGEMENT OPTIONS

Access techniques may be classified as either closed or open entry. In patients without previous epigastric surgery, one of the safest locations for closed entry is Palmer's point in the left upper quadrant. Using an orogastric tube to decompress the stomach, a Veress needle is inserted

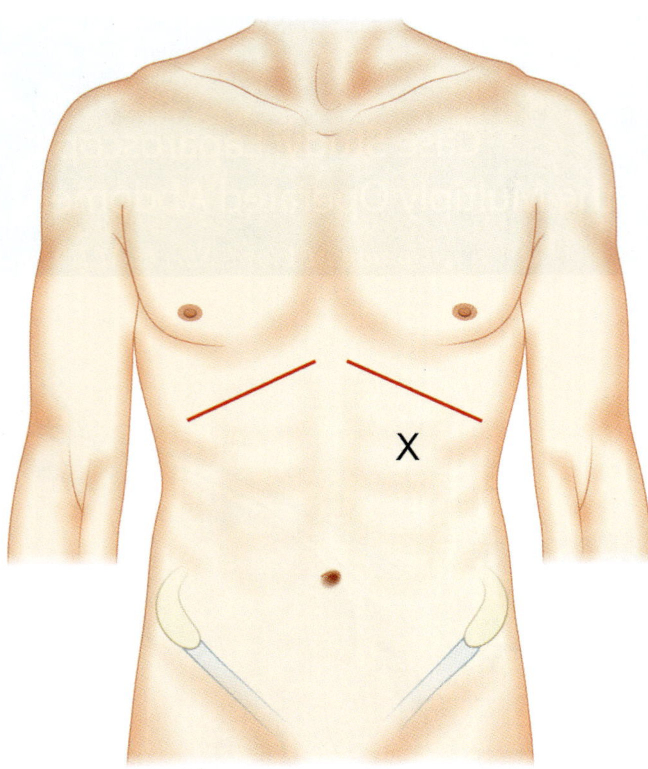

Fig. 10.2: Palmer's point is approximately 3 cm below the left costal margin in the midclavicular line.

percutaneously two finger breadths below the costal margin along the midclavicular line (Fig. 10.2). Alternative sites for Veress insertion include the right medial costal margin or the left ninth intercostal space. Umbilical stalk placement of the Veress needle is not recommended in patients with prior midline incisions. The intraperitoneal location should be confirmed with aspiration and/or the saline drop test. Close attention should be paid to the opening pressure. If elevated (>5 mm Hg), the Veress should promptly be removed and an alternative method of entry pursued.

After the establishment of pneumoperitoneum, the primary port can be inserted blindly along the Veress track or elsewhere on the abdomen. Alternatively, an optical trocar, which accommodates a zero degree laparoscope and allows for direct visualization of the planes of the abdominal wall during insertion, may be used.

Although they do not eliminate access-related morbidity, open-entry methods may be associated with fewer complications. The Hasson method entails exposing the fascia directly via a 2-cm skin incision and the insertion of a 10–12 mm blunt trocar under direct visualization. In some cases, the surgeon may elect to use a hand-assist port. Typically placed either in the midline or through a Pfannenstiel incision, a 7–9 cm minilaparotomy is made, any adhesions to the abdominal wall are cleared, and a hand-port device is placed under direct visualization. With any access technique, subsequent laparoscopic ports should be placed after insufflation and under direct visualization of the trocar entry. It is not uncommon to perform a limited adhesiolysis to allow for trocar placement near a previous incision.

Critical to any successful laparoscopic procedure is safe abdominal access. Knowledge of multiple entry methods and alternatives will allow the motivated surgeon to perform laparoscopic surgery safely even in the multiply operated abdomen. In this particular case, because there was scarring at the umbilicus from the previous hysterectomy, the patient was advised that Palmer's point would provide the safest initial entry site. A Veress needle technique was used, and access was safely established.

FURTHER READING

1. Ahmad G, O'Flynn H, Duffy JMN, et al. Laparoscopic entry techniques. Cochrane Database Syst Rev. 2012;2:CD006583.
2. Varma R, Gupta JK. Laparoscopic entry techniques: clinical guideline, national survey, and medicolegal ramifications. Surg Endosc. 2008;22:2686-97.
3. Vilos GA, Ternamian A, Dempster J, et al. The Society of Obstetricians and Gynaecologists of Canada. Laparoscopic entry: a review of techniques, technologies, and complications. J Obstet Gynaecol Can. 2007;29:433-65.

11

Case Study: Nutritional Support of the GI Fistula Patient

Jennifer R DeFazio, Irma Fleming, John C Alverdy

THE PROBLEM

A gastrointestinal (GI) fistula is defined as an abnormal physical connection between two epithelial surfaces (i.e., intestine, skin) that should otherwise remain separate. This term is most often used in reference to GI fistulas whereby the intestinal lumen is connected to the skin allowing discharge of its contents to the outside. This type of "enterocutaneous" fistula, referring to the intestine and skin, can cause major wound healing complications. Enterocutaneous fistulas are associated with appreciable morbidity and have mortality rates between 3% and 22%.[1,2] Small bowel fistulas account for most enterocutaneous fistulas, and those in the more proximal GI tract (i.e., stomach, pancreas, duodenum) are often the most devastating. These patients often develop electrolyte, protein, fat, and vitamin deficiencies together with dehydration and acid-base imbalance problems. These nutritional disturbances are present in 50–90% of patients and significantly influence the overall morbidity and mortality.[2]

Most proximal small bowel fistulas (75–85%) arise from previous trauma or surgical intervention due to iatrogenic bowel injury, infection or anastomotic leakage.[3] Operations for malignancy, inflammatory bowel disease (IBD), and adhesiolysis are the most common procedures that predispose to fistula formation.[1] Spontaneous small bowel fistulas are most likely to originate in patients with IBD (especially Crohn's disease), cancer, peptic ulcer disease, or pancreatitis.[1] Fistulas are classified as either low output (<500 mL/day) or high output (>500 mL/day). Anatomic location, length, and diameter of the fistula tract influence the output volume.[1] Many fistulas (especially those with low output) will spontaneously close with nonoperative treatment. Factors such as foreign bodies, prior radiation exposure, IBD, infection, neoplasms, an epithelialized fistula tract, a distal obstruction, sepsis, and steroids may preclude a spontaneous closure.[2]

THE TYPICAL CASE

A 36-year-old man with a known diagnosis of regional enteritis presents to the emergency department with nausea, vomiting, and abdominal distention. Upright abdominal X-rays demonstrate multiple air-fluid levels. The patient is admitted, nasogastric suction is implemented, and intravenous fluid support results in the reduction in tachycardia and a urine output of 50 mL/h. However, after 18 h of conservative management, the clinical obstruction is not improved and the patient undergoes laparotomy. A densely obstructed segment of distal ileum is identified and the patient undergoes small bowel resection with an end-to-end anastomosis.

All goes well until the 5th postoperative day, when the primarily closed midline incision demonstrates erythema and induration. The patient's temperature is 38.5° C. The wound is locally explored in the expectation of draining a wound infection, which is successfully done. Two days later, the patient has small bowel content draining from the fascia of the opened surgical incision. A computed tomography scan is performed, and an anastomotic leak is suspected based on inflammation at the anastomotic site with small air bubbles surrounding the area. There is no abscess or fluid in the abdomen, and the daily fistula output is <200 mL/24 h while the patient is nil by mouth. The patient is treated with total parenteral nutrition (TPN), aggressive wound care management, and antibiotics. Three weeks later the fistula spontaneously closes, and the wound shows signs of epithelialization.

DIAGNOSTIC DILEMMAS

The ultimate goals for the treatment of small bowel fistulas are complete closure and return of the patients to their baseline functional state. According to Polk,[3] a three-stage approach to fistula management starts with recognition of the disease process and stabilization of the patient. Treatment of sepsis and source control are the primary steps for stabilization. The rapid correction of fluid, electrolyte, and acid-base status must also be implemented during this early phase of treatment. In addition, nutrition should be begun as soon as possible. The next critical phase of treatment includes nutritional assessment and feeding access. Often this phase includes TPN and assessment of the bowel and fistula tract. Once the patient is stabilized and the nutritional goals are realized, the last phase includes definitive nutritional management.

MANAGEMENT OPTIONS

Parenteral nutrition has long been the foundation of nutritional support for patients with enterocutaneous fistulas. Its ability to decrease GI secretions by 30–50% was felt by many clinicians to be critical to the treatment of proximal and/or high output fistulas.[3,4] Total parenteral nutrition (TPN) can be used as the sole nutritional support, and numerous researchers have reported low mortality rates and high spontaneous closure rates with this approach.[3,5] However, TPN is not without important consequences such as morbidity due to central line insertion, catheter sepsis, and metabolic complications. Early enteral feeding in critically ill surgical patients has been proven to be beneficial throughout the recent literature. However, there are common contraindications such as intestinal discontinuity, insufficient usable bowel length, inability to achieve or maintain reliable enteral feeding access, intolerance of feeds, or dramatic increases in fistula output.[3] Transition to partial or total enteral feeding has been advocated in recent reports to prevent atrophy of GI mucosa as well as support the immunologic and hormonal functions of the gut and liver and decrease infectious complications.[6] Levy[6] et al. reported that up to 85% of enterocutaneous fistula patients may be able to transition to enteral nutrition exclusively. Enteral nutrition has also been shown to provide many of the benefits of TPN with as little as 20% of required calories.[7] Options for enteral access include nasojejunal or percutaneous gastrostomy/jejunostomy tube, feeding jejunostomy distal to fistula, or fistuloclysis (direct instillation of feeds into the distal limb of a fistula).[8] In 2004, Teubner et al.[8] reported the complete transition to enteral feeds via fistuloclysis in 11 or 12 fistula patients and also reported improved bowel caliber, thickness, and ability to hold sutures with enteral nutrition. Overall, enteral feeding has proved to have numerous benefits, minimizing the complications associated with parental feeding when tolerated in fistula patients; thus it is a preferred option when feasible.

Surgical management of fistulas is required when conservative measures fail. This policy often requires lengthy and planned operations with complete fistula tract excision, complete excision of the involved segment of bowel, and reconstructive surgery of the abdominal wall to achieve complete coverage of the peritoneum and its contents with an abdominal wall closure that is free of tension and with an excellent blood supply.

REFERENCES

1. Zinner MJ, Ashley SW. Abdominal abscess and enteric fistulae. In: Zinner M Jr, Ashley S (Eds.). Maingot's Abdominal Operations, 12th ed. New York:McGraw-Hill Companies, Inc; 2013.
2. Davis KG, Johnson EK. Controversies in the care of the enterocutaneous fistula. Surg Clin N Am. 2013;93:231-50.
3. Polk TM, Schwab CW. Metabolic and nutritional support of the neterocutaneous fistula patient: a three-phase approach. World J Surg. 2012;36:524-33.
4. Lloyd DA, Gabe SM, Windsor AC. Nutrition and management of enterocutaneous fistula. Br J Surg. 2006;93:1045-55.
5. MacFadyen BV, Dudrick SJ, Ruberg RI. Management of gastrointestinal fistula with parenteral hyperalimentation. Surgery. 1973;74(1):100-5.
6. Levy E, Fileux P, Cugnenc PH, et al. High output external fistulae of the small bowel: management with continuous enteral nutrition. Br J Surg. 1989;76:676-9.
7. Evenson AR, Fischer JE. Current management of enterocutaneous fistula. J Gastrointestinal Surg. 2006;10(3):455-64.
8. Teubner A, Morrison K, Rabishankar HR, et al. Fistuloclysis can successfully replace parenteral feeding in the nutritional support of patients with enterocutaneous fistula. Br J Surg. 2004;91(5):625-31.

12

Anesthesia and Pain Control

Philip M Hopkins, Dudley J Bush

Key Points

- To minimize anesthetic risk, the principles of optimization should be applied to the preoperative patient.
- When using general anesthesia, the anesthetist must determine for each patient the optimal technique for airway maintenance and ventilation and decide which combination of anesthetic agents to utilize.
- Local or regional anesthesia is a good alternative to general anesthesia in selected patients: systemic toxicity is their commonest complication.
- A pain service if appropriately utilized is an excellent resource not only to assist in the management of perioperative pain but also to manage patients with chronic pain conditions.

INTRODUCTION

Anesthesia and surgery share a symbiotic relationship. A limited array of minor surgical procedures and heroic more major procedures, for the purposes of saving life or relieving excruciating pain, have been practiced for several thousand years. It is only since the demonstration of anesthesia (and the recognition of the need for antisepsis), however, that surgery has flourished. Indeed, advances in surgical procedures have often followed advances in anesthesia. Conversely, advances in anesthetic techniques have often been driven by the need to accommodate proposed advances in surgery.

Just as the anesthesiologist needs a good grounding in the fundamentals of surgical practice, the surgeon requires an understanding of what the anesthesiologist does to his patient. The purpose of this chapter is therefore to outline the basic principles of anesthesia, which will include the rationale for choice of anesthetic techniques, the use of intraoperative monitoring, and relevant pharmacology of drugs used in anesthesia. We will also describe relevant aspects of perioperative care that are influenced by, or can themselves influence, the management of anesthesia. Special emphasis will be given to the management of pain.

We will begin from an historical perspective, as the development of anesthesia over the past 150 years provides a template upon which an understanding of modern anesthesia can be constructed.

HISTORY AND DEVELOPMENT OF GENERAL ANESTHESIA

The first successful public demonstration of anesthesia is generally credited to William Morton, a dental surgeon from Boston, Massachusetts who, in 1846, administered ether to render a patient insensible during the drainage of an abscess of the jaw. Previously, the best that could be offered to patients facing the daunting prospect of surgical treatment was to be stupefied with alcohol or extracts of plants such as the opium poppy or the mandrake.

Morton's discovery of etherization was indeed a landmark, and its news spread rapidly through North America and, by steamship, to Europe. The properties of ether led others to experiment with other vapors. In 1847, the anesthetic properties of chloroform were discovered by an Edinburgh obstetrician, James Young Simpson.

Ether and chloroform are volatile liquids administered by inhalation. They were the mainstay of anesthesia for over 100 years, and their modern derivatives are still used in the great majority of anesthetics. Ether and chloroform were so successful because they provided all the components of anesthesia. When ether is inhaled it provides, following a period of excitation, analgesia. As the concentration of ether rises in the body, the subject will lose consciousness and will subsequently become unresponsive to mild surgical stimuli. As the concentration of ether in the body rises further, responses to more noxious stimuli are obtunded. With exposure to still further increasing concentrations, profound muscular relaxation ensues. Anesthesia can be defined as a reversible state that provides the triad of unconsciousness, lack of response to noxious stimuli, and muscle relaxation.[1]

There were problems, however, with the use of both ether and chloroform. Induction of anesthesia with ether is technically difficult and prolonged. Its physical properties dictate that equilibration within the body is slow, and it is extremely irritating to the airway. This airway irritability leads to a high incidence of coughing and laryngeal spasm, the latter occasionally being intractable. The slow uptake leads to a prolonged period of excitation, and there are tales of patients who struggled so much that they could not be kept on the table. For the same reason that induction of anesthesia with ether is slow, recovery is prolonged. It was not unusual for patients to remain asleep for several days after major surgery when ether was used as the sole anesthetic. Despite these drawbacks, ether might still have a place in modern anesthesia if it were not for its highly explosive nature, especially in combination with oxygen. It was for this reason that operating theater environments were required to have the most stringent measures for the avoidance of spark production from static electricity.

Chloroform was preferred to ether by many practitioners because induction was smoother, as chloroform is less irritant to the airway. Induction and recovery, however, were still relatively slow. Chloroform is no longer used because it frequently provoked cardiac arrhythmia, which could be fatal. It also has an incidence of fatal hepatotoxicity of approximately 1:1000 administrations.

Many of the techniques developed by anesthetic pioneers to limit the undesirable effects of ether and chloroform are retained in modern anesthetic practice. In the late 19th century both the preanesthetic use of morphine (premedication) and the coadministration of nitrous oxide with the inhalational anesthetic were found to lead to a smoother and more rapid induction of anesthesia, a lower requirement for the inhalational anesthetic and subsequently a more rapid recovery. Morphine and nitrous oxide are still used frequently to contribute to the analgesic component of anesthesia.

The manufacture of barbituric acid in 1896 and the description of its hypnotic properties led to the realization that anesthesia might be produced by drugs administered parenterally. Efforts to manipulate the barbiturate ring to produce a drug with rapid onset and recovery eventually resulted in the production of the thiobarbiturate, thiopental, which was introduced into clinical practice in 1934. It was soon realized that thiopental, administered intravenously, produced a rapid and smooth induction of anesthesia and that anesthesia could be maintained by further doses of the drug. This technique became so popular, especially in the United States, that by the early 1940s it was the anesthetic agent of choice. Unfortunately, the marked cardiovascular depression caused by thiopental was not recognized until the United States was drawn into the conflict of the Second World War with the bombing of Pearl Harbor. In peacetime, surgical operations were restricted to the young and healthy, as older patients or those with coexisting medical disease often succumbed under anesthesia. At Pearl Harbor there was a large number of casualties requiring surgical treatment. In these shocked patients, the standard dose of thiopental used caused cardiovascular decompensation and death on the operating table for many of those who had survived the original trauma. Following this experience, thiopental became almost exclusively an intravenous induction agent, with volatile anesthetics being used for subsequent maintenance of anesthesia.

The introduction into clinical practice of the final group of drugs to provide a specific component to the triad of anesthesia also took place around the time of the Second World War. These drugs were the neuromuscular blocking agents. The first of these, curare, was an alkaloid from South America used as an arrow, or blowpipe dart, tip poison by the local hunters. The properties of curare had, in fact, been described in the early 19th century,[2] but it was not until 1942 that Griffiths and Jackson in Canada demonstrated the clinical usefulness of the reversible paralysis provided by curare.[3] Soon after this a synthetic compound, succinylcholine was introduced.[4,5] Succinylcholine with its rapidly produced profound paralysis and short duration of action became widely adopted as the drug of choice for facilitating tracheal intubation.

Although the introduction of the neuromuscular blocking drugs as the newest class of drugs in anesthesia occurred more than 60 years ago, anesthesia is inherently safer now than it was in 1950. Within the major classes of anesthetic drugs there are new variants with improved pharmacokinetic and pharmacodynamic profiles and fewer side effects. Apart from drug developments, many other areas of research have contributed greatly to the improved safety of anesthesia. These include major advances in our understanding of fundamental cardiovascular and respiratory physiology, advances in technology that have produced improvements in hardware for the

Table 12.1 A classification for timing of admission and operation. This classification, published in the first UK Confidential Enquiry into Perioperative Deaths (CEPOD),[6] is useful for defining the time constraints placed on preoperative optimization of the patient's concurrent medical problems and physiological status.

Admission	
Elective	At time consented between patient and surgical service
Urgent	Within 48 hours of consultation
Emergency	Immediately after consultation
Operation	
Emergency	Immediate operation, resuscitation simultaneous with surgical treatment (e.g. ruptured aortic aneurysm; head, chest and abdominal injuries); operation usually within 1 hour
Urgent	Delayed operation as soon as possible after resuscitation (e.g. intestinal obstruction, perforation, major fractures); operation usually within 24 hours
Scheduled	An early operation, but not immediately life saving (e.g. cancer, cardiovascular surgery); operation usually within 1–3 weeks
Elective	Operation at a time to suit both patient and surgeon (e.g. cholecystectomy, hernia, joint replacement)

delivery of anesthesia and, more importantly, huge advances in monitoring capabilities. We have also improved our ability to recognize, and manage appropriately, life-threatening complications such as anaphylaxis and malignant hyperthermia (MH).

PREOPERATIVE MANAGEMENT

Fitness for Anesthesia

We introduce this commonly used term principally to urge against its use. It is a term with little value. We can, in fact, anesthetize anyone, no matter how sick they may be and, with due care and attention from surgeon and anesthesiologist, the majority will survive. However, one of the founding principles of medicine is "first of all do no harm", and there is great scope for the anesthesiologist to do harm. The risk of doing so can be greatly reduced by treating or controlling any coexisting medical condition. Thus, we prefer that a *principle of optimization* be adopted. This principle can be defined as achieving the best state of health for the patient within the constraints of time imposed by the nature of the surgical pathology. It is useful for these purposes to classify surgical procedures according to the urgency of the pathology as described in the British Confidential Enquiries into Perioperative Death (Table 12.1).[6]

Management of Coexisting Medical Disease

The standard approach for the management of any medical or surgical case is followed: the patient history, clinical examination, and relevant investigations are obtained to make diagnoses, followed by appropriate treatment. It is worth remembering that >90% of medical diagnoses can be made on the basis of the patient's history, a further 4–6% from the clinical examination, and the remainder (i.e. a minority) from laboratory and radiological investigations.[7] The anesthetic history will, therefore, focus on eliciting a detailed past medical history and a thorough review of the body system symptomatology. Of particular value is to ascertain an indication of the functional reserve of the cardiovascular and respiratory systems. This evaluation can be done through enquiry of the patient's exercise tolerance and by noting what it is that limits their exercise capacity. The anesthesiologist will also want to know any previous problems that the patient may have had with anesthesia and also whether there is any family history of problems with anesthesia that may suggest a familiar disorder, such as pseudocholinesterase deficiency or MH. Details of concurrent medication and known drug allergies are also most important.

Physical examination is guided by the clinical history, but the anesthesiologist will always wish to exclude abnormal cardiovascular and respiratory signs. A record of the patient's blood pressure is essential.

There is no such thing as a *routine* preoperative investigation. Each investigation should be specifically indicated according to the criteria that either the chance of an abnormal finding is sufficiently high, or the importance of the result is so important, that they outweigh the discomfort and inconvenience to the patient and the cost of the test. Considerations for the advisability of various tests include the patient's age, sex, ethnic origin, their medical and drug history, the nature of the surgical pathology, and the nature of the operation itself (e.g. expected blood loss). Table 12.2, adapted from Roizen,[7] provides a guide to the more common investigations.

Table 12.2 A strategy for preoperative investigations. This scheme provides a rationale for ordering investigations before anesthesia and surgery. It should be applied only if a full medical history and clinical examination have been done.

Test	*CBC*	*Sickle test*	*Clotting*	*U&E*	*Glucose*	*LFT*	*CXR*	*ECG*	*Pregnancy test*
Patient Age									
Neonate	+								
≥40 years	F							M	
≥50 years	F							+	
≥70 years	+							+	
Ethnic origin									
Afro-Caribbean,	+*	+*							
Asian,									
Mediterranean									
Suspected preoperative condition									
Cardiovascular disease				+			+	+	
Respiratory disease							+	+	
Renal disease	+		±	+					
Diabetes mellitus				+	+			+	
Hepatic disease			+		+	+			
Anemia	+								
Bleeding disorder	+		+						
Malignancy	+		±				±		
Radiation therapy	+						±	±	
Possible pregnancy									+
Medications									
Diuretics				+					
Steroids				+	+				
Anticoagulants	+		+						
Surgical procedure associated with significant blood loss	+								

(+: obtain; ±: possibly obtain; F: obtain in females; M: obtain in males; +*: obtain if sickle status unknown).
Adapted from Roizen.[7]

Timing of Preoperative Anesthetic Assessment

Outpatient anesthetic assessment facilities provide the most cost-effective means of optimizing any newly diagnosed or inadequately treated medical conditions. With the aid of well-designed questionnaires (the future is online completion), such a facility can be successfully led by nurses, with a minority of patients requiring to be seen by an anesthesiologist.

The particular implications of some of the more important and/or common medical disorders encountered by the anesthesiologist will now be discussed.

Cardiovascular Disorders

Cardiovascular complications are probably the greatest cause of morbidity and mortality associated with anesthesia. This fact reflects the high incidence of cardiovascular disease, the physiologic demands of surgical operations, and the effects of anesthetic drugs on the cardiovascular system. There is good evidence that poorly controlled ventricular failure, ischemic heart disease (especially recent myocardial infarction), abnormal cardiac rhythm, and cardiac valve lesions are associated with an increased risk from anesthesia.[8] Consensus guidelines for the preoperative management of patients with cardiovascular disease

Table 12.3	Risk of major cardiac events according to type of operation.
1. *High risk (> 5%)*	
• Aortic surgery	
• Major vascular surgery	
• Peripheral vascular surgery	
2. *Intermediate risk (1–5%)*	
• Body cavity surgery	
• Carotid endarterectomy	
• Head and neck surgery	
• Orthopedic surgery	
• Prostate surgery	
3. *Low risk (< 1%)*	
• Endoscopic procedures	
• Superficial procedures	
• Cataract surgery	
• Breast surgery	
• Ambulatory surgery	

presenting for noncardiac surgery have been published in the United States and Europe.[9,10] In general, the degree of risk is related to:

1. The extent of end-organ damage
2. Cardiorespiratory functional capacity
3. The nature of the surgical procedure

For elective surgery, known cardiovascular conditions should in principle be optimally treated before operation. Elective surgery should not proceed within 30 days of myocardial infarction as the risk of reinfarction is markedly raised. When the extent of the cardiovascular pathology would ordinarily require surgical intervention, e.g. prosthetic valve replacement, carotid endarterectomy, coronary artery bypass grafting, this should always be prioritized ahead of medium or high-risk noncardiac surgery (Table 12.3). Before subjecting patients awaiting noncardiac surgery to coronary stenting, the implications of the poststent antiplatelet therapy for the proposed operation should be considered by surgeon, cardiologist, and anesthesiologist. Interim optimization of medical therapy to cover the surgical period may be the least risky approach.

There is a relatively poor evidential base to guide the perioperative management of patients who present preoperatively with raised blood pressure. This fact probably reflects the relatively recent understanding of hypertension as a generalized disease of the cardiovascular system in which the correlation of blood pressure readings with the degree of organ damage, and therefore symptoms and risk, is surprisingly weak.[11] An adverse effect of raised preoperative blood pressure on outcome after anesthesia would not surprise most anesthesiologists, who are familiar with the marked lability in blood pressure during anesthesia of such patients. However, until further evidence emerges, our recommendation for elective surgery is that operation be postponed for those with a systolic blood pressure of >180 mm Hg or a diastolic blood pressure >110 mm Hg (160 mm Hg or 100 mm Hg, respectively, in the presence of hypertensive organ damage, such as ischemic heart disease). Even discounting the potential reduction in risk of anesthesia, treatment of blood pressure greater than these levels is warranted in any case, as long-term health is improved.[12] It seems prudent, therefore, to establish such patients on antihypertensive medication prior to elective surgery.

Respiratory System

Chronic obstructive pulmonary disease (COPD), including asthma, is common. Many patients with asthma are usually symptom-free, and, in general, they provide little increased anesthetic risk so long as usual medication is continued up to the time of operation and care is taken effectively to obtund the response to airway instrumentation. Many symptomatic patients with COPD, however, are not on maximal medical therapy, and there is therefore the potential to improve their respiratory status preoperatively. It is important to apply the principle of optimization to these patients; otherwise, there is an increased risk of bronchospasm, pulmonary infection, and respiratory failure during and after anesthesia. Changes in airway reactivity persist for several weeks after an acute exacerbation of asthma or other forms of COPD. We recommend that operation is postponed, whenever feasible, for at least 3 weeks after such an acute episode.

Acute upper respiratory tract infections (URTI) are also common, especially in pediatric anesthetic practice. Again there is no hard evidence to guide the anesthesiologist as to when the symptoms are sufficient to caution against proceeding with any operation. Anesthesia does decrease airway mucus clearance and small airway closure, predisposing to chest infection. Anesthesia is also immunosuppressive, predisposing to secondary bacterial infection and also viral proliferation. There are rare instances of viral myocarditis leading to terminal myocardial failure in patients anesthetized during acute URTI. With these considerations it is probably unwise to anesthetize, for elective surgery, patients with the following acute symptoms: pyrexia, productive cough, nonclear nasal discharge, "flu-like" symptoms (malaise, myalgia, feeling generally unwell). Conversely, those patients with only a mild sore throat or coryza with a clear nasal discharge probably pose no added risk.

Diabetes Mellitus

Problems for the anesthesiologist are that diabetes is a multisystem disease and that blood glucose control will necessarily be disturbed by perioperative interventions. The major secondary effects of diabetes requiring consideration by the anesthesiologist are small and large blood vessel occlusive disease (especially ischemic heart disease), diabetic cardiomyopathy, autonomic neuropathy, gastric stasis, and renal impairment.

Hypoglycemia is potentially lethal within 5–10 minutes, and it is therefore safer to tend toward hyperglycemia (6–10 mmol/L) during the perioperative period, which is in fact the normal response to operative stress. Blood glucose control during the perioperative period is easier on a background of preoperative stability within the normal range. Glycemic status can be assessed by asking the patient about the quality of their blood sugar control at home, a random blood sugar analysis, and analysis of the glycosylated hemoglobin, which gives an indication of long-term blood sugar control. Patients with diabetes with poor control should have elective surgery postponed and be referred back to their diabetologist for optimization of their diabetic regimen.

Perioperatively, blood glucose control is disturbed by the period of fasting and by the stress response to surgery. Type-2 diabetics taking longer acting hypoglycemics should stop these the day before operation. Patients controlled on insulin require an individualized perioperative regimen that will depend on the nature of the operation and how quickly they can resume an oral intake. Several regimens for prescribing dextrose and insulin perioperatively have been described:

1. Give a reduced dose of the usual morning insulin and commence a dextrose infusion.
2. The Alberti regimen (GIK):[13] This is a 500-mL infusion containing 10% dextrose, 10 mmol potassium chloride, and 10–20 units of soluble insulin. The infusion is run at 100 mL/h.
3. Dextrose infusion and separate insulin infusion, the rate of which is determined according to a sliding scale whereby the insulin infusion rate is increased with increasing blood glucose concentrations.

The use of separate infusions with a sliding scale of insulin is the most flexible and is the most commonly used for major surgery and also for other operations in which resumption of oral intake may be delayed, but the key to the safe use of any of these techniques is regular blood glucose (and potassium) monitoring.

Anemia

Anemia is present in up to 75% of some surgical populations and is an independent predictor of adverse outcome in cardiac[14] and noncardiac surgery.[15] For elective surgery anemia should be corrected by treatment of the underlying cause where possible. Such correction is preferable to acute preoperative red blood cell transfusion, which itself is associated with increased perioperative adverse outcomes.

There is little consensus on acceptable hemoglobin levels during the perioperative period, but the following is a guide:

- >6 g/dL for compensated chronic anemia
- >8 g/dL for otherwise healthy patients in whom the expected blood loss is <500 mL
- >10 g/dL for patients with cardiorespiratory disease or with increased oxygen demand or for those in whom the expected blood loss at operation is >500 mL

Concurrent Medication

Anesthesia is probably the most extreme form of polypharmacy encountered routinely in medical practice. It is unusual for an anesthesiologist to administer fewer than three different drugs during the course of a procedure. The more usual number is between 5 and 10 drugs. None of these drugs is free of side effects. There is a huge potential for adverse drug interaction with the patient's concurrent medication. These interactions may be pharmacodynamic, involving desired or unwanted drug effects, or pharmacokinetic. The details of these interactions are beyond the scope of this chapter, but Table 12.4 lists drugs with implications for the anesthesiologist, giving an indication for the necessity of a detailed drug history.

Preoperative Fasting

Anesthesia causes a marked reduction in the tone of the gastroesophageal sphincter. Anesthetized patients are, therefore, at risk of regurgitation of stomach contents which might then be aspirated into the unprotected airway, leading to airway obstruction from solid material or aspiration pneumonitis. Either of these is potentially fatal.

Table 12.4 Drugs with implications for anesthesia. Concurrent medication with drugs in any of these categories may influence the choice of anesthetic technique or perioperative management. A detailed drug history is essential.

1. Antihypertensives, especially ACE inhibitors
2. Antiarrhythmics
3. Anticoagulants
4. Steroids
5. Antibiotics
6. Oral contraceptives
7. Monoamine oxidase inhibitors
8. Tricyclic and SSRI antidepressants
9. Levodopa
10. Sedatives and tranquillisers
11. Antidiabetic drugs
12. Drugs of abuse, including alcohol.

The risk of these complications can be avoided by ensuring that the stomach is empty by ordering an appropriate period of starvation. For adults this is usually 4 hours for clear fluids and 6 hours for other fluids and food. Gastric emptying is more rapid in children, who also tolerate starvation less well, and therefore a period of 2 hours for clear fluids and 4 hours for other fluids and food is appropriate for infants.

Gastric emptying is delayed by fear, anxiety, pain, trauma, opioid analgesics, pregnancy, obesity, and autonomic neuropathy (e.g. diabetes). When an empty stomach cannot be ensured, the anesthesiologist must take measures to protect the airway using a rapid sequence induction of anesthesia. This procedure involves intravenous induction, occlusion of the upper esophagus using manual compression over the cricoid cartilage, and intubation of the trachea using a cuffed tracheal tube.

Premedication

The following is a list of the possible uses of premedicants: anxiolysis, amnesia, antiemesis, analgesia, antisialogogues, antiarrhythmic (antivagal), antacid and aspiration prophylaxis, antihistamine (atopic patients or those with a history of allergy to anesthetic drugs), anesthesia sparing. The most common indication for premedication in general anesthetic practice is anxiolysis.

Preoperative Anxiety

It is important to attempt to reduce the level of anxiety in all patients.[16] Preoperatively, anxiety is associated with tachycardia, hypertension, dysrhythmias, and nausea. Unrelieved preoperative anxiety is associated with increased postoperative pain, increased postoperative nausea and vomiting, and prolonged hospitalization.

Treatment of anxiety may be pharmacological or nonpharmacological. A most effective nonpharmacological therapy for anxiety is a preoperative visit by the anesthesiologist. An opportunity for the anesthesiologist to explain to the patient what they will experience and to answer any questions from the patient is as effective as any drug treatment. However, some patients may still benefit from anxiolytic premedication. Oral anxiolytic premedication with benzodiazepines is efficacious. It is best to avoid drugs such as diazepam, which have active metabolites with long half-lives.

Anesthetic Preoperative Management for Emergency Surgery

The time constraints placed by emergency surgery invariably mean that there will be little opportunity to reduce the risk to the patient resulting from chronic medical disorders. The principle of optimization must still be applied, however, for the best results. In the context of emergency surgery this principle will involve resuscitation of the patient from the effects of the acute surgical pathology. Attention must be paid to achieve adequate oxygenation, to transfuse when necessary, to rehydrate the patient, and to correct electrolyte disturbances. All these measures will enable the patient to tolerate best the hemodynamic insults imposed by anesthesia.

ANESTHESIA TECHNIQUES

The anesthetic technique will be planned by the anesthesiologist on the basis of their preoperative assessment. Factors influencing the choice of technique include the physical characteristics and medical condition of the patient, the nature of the operation, and the preference of the anesthesiologist himself. Perhaps the most fundamental choice is that between a general anesthetic technique and regional or local anesthetic technique. There are only a few operations in which general anesthesia is mandatory but many situations in which a local or regional anesthetic technique might be recommended to the patient on the basis of a reduced risk or fewer side effects. There is, however, a misconception that local or regional anesthesia is always safer than general anesthesia. There are risks with any technique that uses large doses of local anesthetic and specific risks associated with individual techniques

Flowchart 12.1: Choice of anesthetic technique. The anesthesiologist must plan the choice of drugs to be used (for induction and maintenance of anesthesia), the methods of airway management, and ventilation of the lungs. These choices are interdependent, and the overall plan is based on the patient's physical characteristics, their medical problems, the surgical pathology, and the nature of the operation.

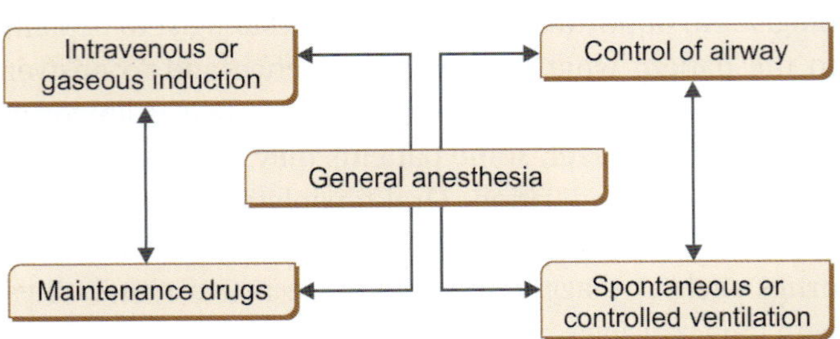

(*see* below). For some patients with ischemic heart disease, the anxiety of being awake (or sometimes even the thought of this) during their operation can provoke ischemia. This effect is especially dangerous when accompanied by hypotension, which frequently occurs during spinal or epidural anesthesia. The combination of general and regional anesthetic techniques is common, especially for major abdominal and thoracic procedures.

General Anesthetic Techniques

The anesthesiologist must decide what drugs to use, what method of airway maintenance to use, and whether ventilation is to be spontaneous or controlled. Each of these choices influences other aspects of choice of technique (Flowchart 12.1).

Airway Maintenance

A tracheal tube is used when ventilation is to be controlled in the paralyzed patient, e.g. abdominal, thoracic, or neurosurgery, when the surgical site precludes the safe use of an alternative less invasive airway device, e.g. maxillofacial or other head and neck surgery, or when protection of the lungs from aspiration of gastric contents is required, e.g. emergency surgery. In other circumstances the airway may be maintained using a manual chin lift or jaw thrust, with or without an oropharyngeal or nasopharyngeal airway, or, more commonly nowadays, using a laryngeal mask airway (Fig. 12.1).

Method of Ventilation

Controlled ventilation is required when profound paralysis is used to provide optimal surgical conditions, such as in body cavity surgery or where it is necessary to control closely the arterial partial pressure of CO_2, such as in neurosurgery. A prolonged operation is a relative indication for controlled ventilation.

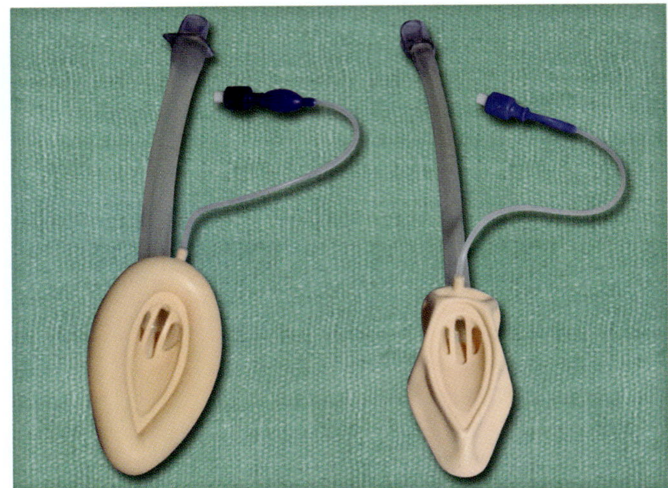

Fig. 12.1: The laryngeal mask airway. The laryngeal mask has proved a useful addition to methods of airway control. It is inserted through the mouth into the pharynx without the need for neuromuscular blockade, enabling "hands-free" maintenance of a clear airway. It does not provide protection against pulmonary aspiration of regurgitated stomach contents.

Choice of Anesthetic Drugs

There are over 40,000 different combinations of anesthetic drugs that can be used. Most anesthesiologists prefer to use an intravenous induction of anesthesia, although when intravenous access is difficult or not well tolerated (some children and adults with needle phobia) inhalational induction with modern volatile anesthetics is relatively quick and pleasant. An opioid analgesic is used invariably, unless a regional or local anesthetic technique is also used, and a neuromuscular blocking drug is used if paralysis is required. Anesthesia can be maintained with an inhalational anesthetic or with total intravenous anesthetic (TIVA). TIVA is facilitated by infusion pumps incorporating pharmacokinetic models that enable real-time estimation of plasma and effect-site concentration of the drug.

Local and Regional Anesthetic Techniques

Regional anesthesia is where local anesthetic drugs are injected proximal to the site of operation to block more than one nerve trunk supplying the relevant region. A local anesthetic technique is where local anesthetic drugs are injected directly into the operative field. The major complication common to all local and regional anesthetic techniques is systemic toxicity (*see* below). This effect can occur when an inappropriately large dose of local anesthetic is injected in the correct site, or when an appropriate dose is injected intravascularly. When any regional anesthetic or local anesthetic technique using large volumes of local anesthetic is employed, full resuscitation facilities must be available and a trained anesthetist must be present.

Some Common Regional Anesthetic Techniques

- *Spinal and epidural anesthesia.* Local anesthetic solution is placed around the nerves as they leave the spinal cord. In the spinal technique, a fine needle is used to perform a lumbar puncture and a small volume of local anesthetic is injected into the cerebrospinal fluid (CSF). In the epidural technique, a larger volume of local anesthetic is injected into the epidural space in which the nerves pass outside the dura. Both of these techniques block the sympathetic outflow from the spinal cord and cause hypotension, which may be profound when the block is extended over several dermatomal levels. Injection of an excessive dose of local anesthetic into the subarachnoid space (overdose of spinal technique or inadvertent dural puncture using standard volumes in the epidural technique) can cause unconsciousness as the local anesthetic drug reaches the brain via the CSF. Dural puncture can lead to a "spinal" headache caused by leakage of CSF. This symptom occurs in about 1% of spinal blocks and is related to the size of needle and the type of bevel used. Inadvertent dural puncture using a larger epidural needle produces a headache much more frequently. Many spinal headaches can be managed successfully with bed rest, simple analgesics and hydration. Where these simple measures fail, sealing of the dural hole by injection of the patient's own blood into the epidural space (epidural blood patch) is usually effective.
- *Upper limb techniques.*
  - Brachial plexus block. The nerves forming the divisions, cords, and roots of the brachial plexus are enclosed within a fascial sheath extending from the neck to the axilla. Injection of local anesthetics within this sheath has the potential to produce anesthesia of the upper limb. Successful identification of the brachial plexus has improved with the use of ultrasound-guided techniques.[17] There are three common approaches to the brachial plexus: in the neck (interscalene approach), the supraclavicular approach where the plexus crosses the first rib, and the axillary approach. The axillary approach is especially useful for operations on the palm of the hand requiring ulnar and median nerve block. The supraclavicular approach is ideal for procedures on the joints of the hand and carpus. There is a risk of pneumothorax with the supraclavicular approach, but in experienced hands this is minimal. The interscalene approach is suitable for anesthesia of the shoulder, upper arm, and elbow. It usually misses the ulnar nerve distribution and should, therefore, be combined with an axillary block when anesthesia for the medial aspect of the elbow is required. Interscalene block invariably produces a Horner's syndrome and phrenic nerve paralysis. Bilateral interscalene block is, therefore, contraindicated.
  - Intravenous regional anesthesia (Bier's block). This was described in 1908 by August Bier, who injected procaine intravenously below a tourniquet. In modern practice lidocaine or prilocaine 40 mL is injected into a vein of the exsanguinated forearm, and anesthesia is established within 5–10 minutes. Tourniquet discomfort can be limited using a double tourniquet technique, but great care must be taken to isolate the local anesthetic in the exsanguinated limb for a minimum period of 20 minutes. If the tourniquet is accidentally deflated before this time sufficient local anesthetic will remain in the venous system to cause acute systemic toxicity. After this period, sufficient local anesthetic will have dispersed from the veins into the tissues of the forearm and will remain bound to the tissues long enough for systemic toxicity to be avoided. The use of bupivacaine in intravenous regional anesthesia has been associated with several deaths due to its lower tissue affinity and its higher cardiac toxicity.
- *Lower limb techniques.* In addition to bilateral lower limb anesthesia provided by spinal or epidural techniques, unilateral regional anesthesia of the lower limb can be achieved using a combination of femoral and sciatic nerve blocks. The availability of high resolution portable ultrasound devices has increased their use.

DRUGS IN ANESTHESIA

Local Anesthetics

Local anesthetics block axonal conduction by inhibition of sodium channel conductance. The binding site on the sodium channel is accessed through the intracellular pore, and thus the drugs need to enter the axons before they can take effect. At normal body pH, local anesthetic drugs are bases with good lipid solubility, but in acidotic conditions the drug is heavily ionized and penetration of the lipid membrane of the axon is slow. If injected intravascularly local anesthetics will block other sodium channels, and a block of those in the brain and the heart is responsible for the major systemic side effects of these drugs. When the increase in plasma concentration of a local anesthetic is gradual, neurologic manifestations of toxicity always precede serious myocardial effects. Early features of systemic toxicity include paresthesia of the extremities, circumoral paresthesia (which may be described as numbness around the mouth or strange tastes in the mouth), and tinnitus. As the plasma concentration rises, the patient becomes drowsy, progressing to unconsciousness, and fitting. In the heart, the local anesthetics block conduction of the cardiac action potential and also have a negative inotropic effect. A large bolus dose of intravenous or intra-arterial local anesthetic will produce a sudden collapse with unconsciousness, fitting, and cardiac arrest. Resuscitation will often need to be prolonged if the patient is to survive. Intravenous lipid emulsion (Intralipid) rescue has been used to aid resuscitation.[18]

The key to avoiding systemic toxicity of local anesthetics is to avoid intravascular injection can best be done by use of ultrasound visualization and frequent pausing of injection to aspirate for blood. When local anesthetic solutions are injected into heavily vascularized tissues, such as the head and neck or the intercostal spaces, and when applied topically to mucous membranes, large dosing may result in sufficient systemic absorption of the drug to produce systemic symptoms. When these circumstances apply, the patient should be carefully monitored for early signs of toxicity. Local anesthetic solutions prepared with vasoconstrictors, such as epinephrine, can reduce the systemic absorption of the local anesthetic and thereby increase the safety margin of the drug.

Structurally, local anesthetic drugs are classified according to whether they have an ester or amide bond linking lipophilic and hydrophilic regions. Examples of ester local anesthetics include cocaine, procaine, tetracaine, and 2-chloroprocaine. Amide local anesthetics are now more commonly used than the esters. Commonly used examples of amide local anesthetics are lidocaine, prilocaine, bupivacaine, and ropivacaine.

Volatile Anesthetics

The currently available volatile anesthetic drugs are halogenated hydrocarbons (halothane—not now available in all countries) related to chloroform or halogenated ethers (isoflurane, sevoflurane, desflurane) related to ether. Compared with ether and chloroform, these drugs all have a rapid onset of anesthetic action and are eliminated rapidly, although clinically important differences in uptake and recovery do exist between the modern drugs. All the modern volatile anesthetics, but to varying degrees, cause vasodilation and myocardial depression, whereas some are more pungent to breathe than others. They all trigger MH in susceptible individuals (*see* below). The use of halothane has declined over fears of rare occurrences of severe hepatotoxicity, especially upon repeated exposure. Many anesthesiologists prefer volatile anesthetics to intravenous anesthetics for maintenance of anesthesia because, at equilibration, the partial pressure of the drug at the site of action will equal the partial pressure in the alveoli. Alveolar gas can be sampled and analyzed for the anesthetic partial pressure on a breath by breath basis. The anesthesiologist, therefore, does not need to be troubled by interpatient pharmacokinetic variability.

Intravenous Anesthetics

Thiopental is still used, but has been replaced for most cases by propofol. Both propofol and thiopental cause cardiovascular depression, but propofol affords a more rapid recovery, is associated with a lower incidence of anaphylactic reactions and is less likely to be associated with postoperative nausea and vomiting than thiopental. Etomidate is an alternative intravenous drug for induction of anesthesia. It has less cardiodepressant effects than thiopental or propofol but is reserved for elderly patients or those with established cardiovascular disease because induction is less smooth (hiccoughs and limb movements are frequent), it increases airway secretions, it causes pain on injection and also a high incidence of postoperative vomiting.

Opioid Analgesics

Morphine is still used as an intraoperative analgesic, but many anesthesiologists prefer the more specifically designed potent and shorter acting synthetic opioids. These include fentanyl, sufentanil, alfentanil, and the most recently introduced, remifentanil. These short acting potent opioids can provide profound intraoperative analgesia in the knowledge that their effects will wear off rapidly, allowing a predictable return to spontaneous ventilation. The offset of their action must be anticipated in the postoperative period and alternative methods of analgesia substituted when necessary.

Neuromuscular Blocking Drugs

Apart from curare, these drugs can be recognized from their names because they all end in -ium. The effects of long acting neuromuscular blockers (e.g. rocuronium) can persist beyond the duration of the reversal agent given at the end of the procedure. This was a well-recognized complication with the use of curare, and the event became known as recurarization. With the modern shorter acting drugs, e.g. atracurium and vecuronium, this problem is less likely to occur.

INTRAOPERATIVE MONITORING

As we have already mentioned, the development of monitoring equipment and standards for their use has been a major contributor to the improvement in anesthetic safety. Monitoring should be instituted before induction of anesthesia and maintained continuously into the postoperative period. The most important form of monitoring is the presence of an anesthetist throughout the conduct of the anesthetic. Every patient subjected to general anesthesia should be monitored by the use of the electrocardiogram, pulse oximetry, systemic blood pressure, and capnography. There is a substantial body of evidence to suggest that body temperature monitoring should be included in this list of minimal standards, especially for procedures lasting >30 minutes. Additional monitoring may be required when there is preexisting disease, when special techniques are used (e.g. planned hypotension), or according to the type of operation. For example direct intra-arterial and central venous pressure monitoring can provide useful information. Several "noninvasive" techniques for estimating cardiac output are available. Transesophageal echocardiography is now routine in cardiac surgery.

Several devices that use processed neurophysiological data to provide an indication of adequacy and depth of anesthesia have become available in recent years. Their purpose is principally to avoid patients becoming aware under anesthesia that involves neuromuscular block (*see* below), but there is also evidence to suggest that excessive depth of anesthesia may be associated with increased postoperative morbidity and mortality.[19] The main drawback of these devices is their cost.

In addition to monitoring the patient, essential functioning of the anesthetic machine should be monitored (Fig. 12.2). This monitoring includes maintenance of the oxygen supply and detection of leaks or disconnections in the breathing system.

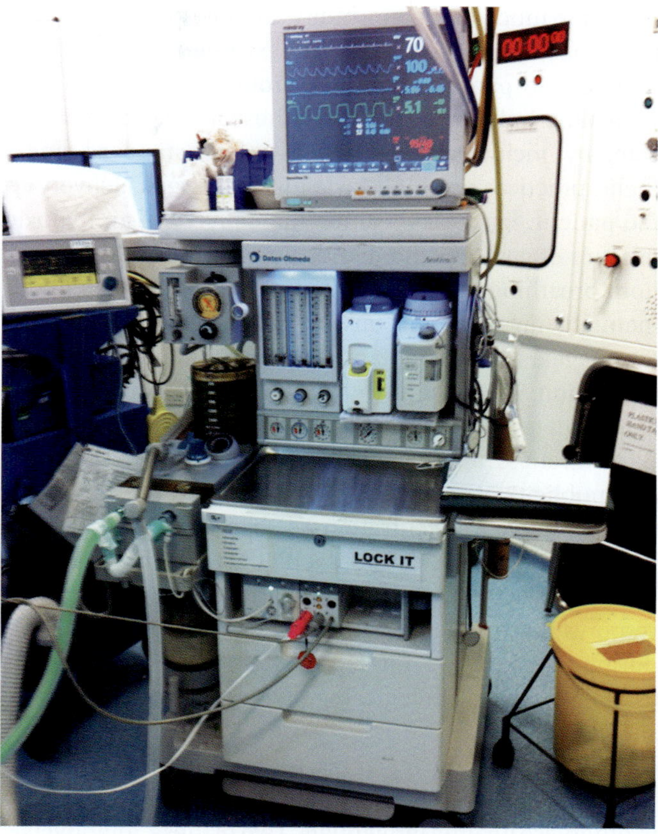

Fig. 12.2: A modern anesthetic machine. In addition to the delivery of gases and anesthetic vapors to the patient, this machine contains an integrated monitoring package, which includes monitors of patient vital signs and functioning of the breathing circuits, ventilator, and the machine itself. Application of such comprehensive monitoring (and appropriate interpretation of the information) is a crucial part of the safety of modern anesthesia.

ANESTHETIC MORBIDITY AND MORTALITY

It is difficult to differentiate the contribution of anesthesia from that of the surgical pathology in defining the risk of anesthesia *per se*. The risks of anesthesia increase with age and severity of comorbidities. The inherent risk of death from anesthesia is estimated to be 0.6–0.8 per 100,000, with approximately 47% of these deaths due to drug errors, 44% to adverse drug reactions, 3.6% involving obstetric anesthesia, 2.6% resulting from intubation problems in non-obstetric patients, and the remainder from other causes.[20]

Cardiovascular complications are the major cause of morbidity and mortality associated with anesthesia and surgery. Factors contributing to the cardiovascular complications are preexisting disease, metabolic derangement due to the surgical pathology, and the effects of the anesthetic drugs themselves.

While much of the morbidity and mortality associated with anesthesia is related to preexisting medical conditions of the patient, there are problems that can occur in healthy individuals. Some of these are avoidable. This category includes several areas of substandard anesthetic practice, resulting in failure of oxygen delivery to the patient. Examples include the delivery of an hypoxic mixture of gas, anesthetic machine failure or disconnection, breathing circuit disconnection or leak, inability to maintain an adequate airway (including unrecognized esophageal intubation), and failure to maintain adequate ventilation. The resulting hypoxia from any of these causes will result rapidly in brain damage or death.

Awareness under anesthesia has received considerable publicity in recent years. It is due to the failure to provide adequate concentrations of hypnotic drugs during the procedure. It is only a problem when the patient is paralyzed, as the nonparalyzed patient is able to move in response to stimulation. The true incidence of awareness during operations is not known, but it may be as high as 0.01%. Severe psychological sequelae may occur following such an episode.

Life-threatening reactions to anesthetic drugs are a rare but important cause of major morbidity and mortality in otherwise healthy individuals. Two of these, anaphylaxis and MH, are worthy of further mention.

Anaphylaxis

Allergic anaphylaxis is a systemic reaction caused by release of histamine and other mediators of the immune system. Drug-induced anaphylaxis is most commonly a classical type 1 hypersensitivity reaction involving IgE, but non-IgE reactions do occur. The clinical features of anaphylaxis are any combination of bronchospasm, hypotension, angioedema, and urticaria. Severe anaphylactic reactions require aggressive treatment with administration of oxygen, intravenous fluid loading, and epinephrine. Investigation of suspected anaphylaxis includes serial serum mast cell tryptase measurements (immediate, 1–2-h postevent and 24 hours), subsequent skin testing and, where available, drug-specific IgE assays. Skin testing is useful to identify the causative agent and assess cross-sensitivity with other drugs in the same therapeutic class. The drugs most commonly implicated in anaphylaxis are intravenous antibiotics and drugs used in anesthesia, principally neuromuscular blocking drugs. The incidence of allergy to chlorhexidine and patent blue is increasing, whereas latex allergy is less common with the reduced use of latex in medical devices and equipment.

Malignant Hyperthermia

Malignant hyperthermia is a pharmacogenetic disorder.[21] MH susceptible individuals carry one of several mutations in genes that code for proteins regulating intracellular calcium metabolism in skeletal muscle. Unless these people are exposed to one of the triggering agents (all volatile anesthetics and succinylcholine), they appear as normal healthy individuals. When the reaction is triggered under anesthesia, however, a devastating combination of hypermetabolism, muscle rigidity, and rhabdomyolysis occurs. The first cases reported in the 1960s were noted for the extreme rise in body temperature (hyperthermia), which was termed malignant because it invariably preceded death. Anesthesiologists are trained to recognize the earliest features of an MH reaction (excessive muscle rigidity following succinylcholine, hypercapnia, and tachycardia) and to institute treatment before the reaction progresses to an irreversible stage. Treatment involves the withdrawal of the triggering agent, hyperventilation with 100% oxygen, body cooling, correction of metabolic disturbances, and intravenous administration of dantrolene, which acts on the muscle to inhibit the progressive rise in intracellular calcium ion concentration. MH is an autosomal dominantly inherited disorder with an incidence of approximately 1:10,000 of the population. DNA-based confirmation of diagnosis is available when a familial mutation has been identified, but otherwise definitive diagnosis involves in vitro pharmacological contracture testing of excised muscle strips taken at open biopsy.

PAIN CONTROL

Physiology of Pain

Pain is defined as "an unpleasant sensory and emotional experience associated with actual or potential tissue damage or described in terms of such damage."[22] Postoperative pain is an example of acute pain, which is defined as pain of recent onset and usually limited duration. It is usually related to the duration and magnitude of the causal insult.[23] The perception of acute pain involves multiple interacting peripheral and central physical mechanisms together with individual psychological and environmental factors.

Peripheral Mechanisms

Tissue injury results in the release of chemical mediators (algogens) from damaged cells, leading to a local inflammatory response.[24] Some algogens, such as bradykinin,

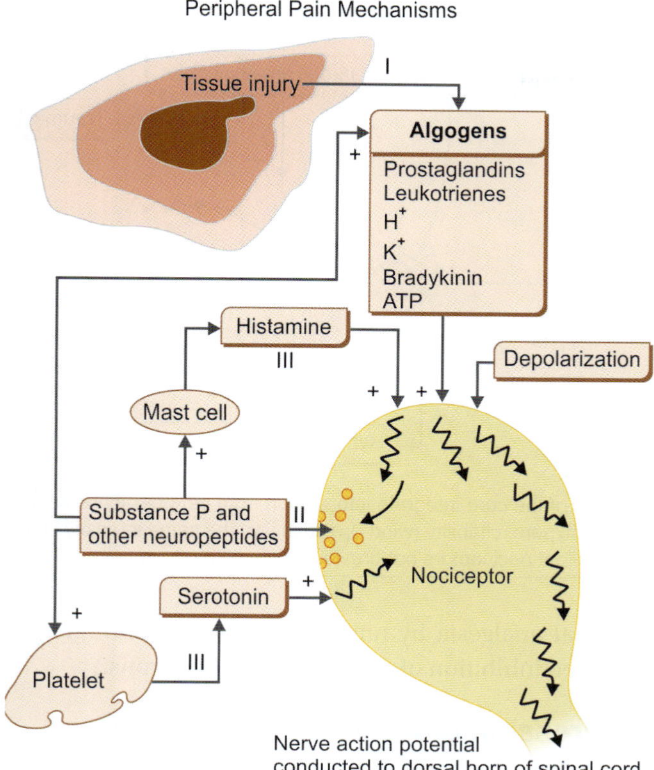

Fig. 12.3: Peripheral pain mechanisms. Tissue injury results in release of algogens (1) which trigger nociceptors to depolarize and release neuropeptides (2). This leads to further release of peripheral algogens (3) and further nociceptor activation.

potassium, protons, serotonin, and histamine, directly activate pain receptors (nociceptors), whereas others, including the prostaglandins (PGE_2 and PGE_1), nerve growth factor, leukotrienes, and the peptide, substance P, lower the discharge threshold of nociceptors, but do not directly trigger them[25] (Fig. 12.3).

Pain signaling afferent nerves include slow conduction velocity unmyelinated C fibers, which mediate diffuse dull pain, and a minority of larger diameter partially myelinated A-delta fibers, which are responsible for more immediate well-localized pain. There are several types of nociceptors, the most common being polymodal C fiber bare nerve endings but include receptors to heat, mechanical stimulus, protons, and potassium ions. Sodium channels are key modulators of neuronal activation and transmission in nociceptive nerve transmission, and there are discrete slow inactivating channels in nociceptive neurons. The sodium channel kinetics are modified in the nociceptive response resulting in neuronal hyperexcitability.[26] Activation of afferent nociceptive nerve fibers results in retrograde release of further peptide algogens from the nociceptor (substance P and calcitonin gene-related peptide), exacerbating the response. This positive feedback loop, termed neurogenic inflammation, also recruits populations of previously silent nociceptors and A-beta mechanoreceptor fibers to mediate pain. This process results in the clinically familiar state of primary hyperalgesia, an increased responsiveness to painful stimulus around the area of injury.

Central Mechanisms

Afferent nociceptive C and A-delta fibers synapse in the superficial layers of the dorsal horn of the spinal cord, primarily the substantia gelatinosa. Interneurons in this area receive input from multiple nociceptive and mechanoreceptor afferents and subsequently project to interneurons both at other spinal levels and in ascending nerve tracts. Dorsal horn interneurons also receive inhibitory input from descending nerve pathways (Figs. 12.4A and B). There is great potential for the processing and modification of nociceptive information as it passes through the dorsal horn.[27] From the dorsal horn, nociceptive traffic ascends in the spinothalamic and spinoreticular tracts of the spinal cord to thalamic, limbic, and eventually cortical structures.

Important neurotransmitters in the dorsal horn include peptides such as substance P, neurokinins, calcitonin gene-related peptide and cholecystokinin, and excitatory amino acids, principally glutamate and aspartate. Currently, there are few available analgesics based upon antagonists to these neurotransmitters, although ketamine has some utility. The substantia gelatinosa is rich in opioid receptors, which act to inhibit nociceptive impulse transmission, and this is a major site of action of opioid analgesics.

Central Sensitization

Repetitive noxious stimulation of the dorsal horn, such as tissue damage, results in a progressive escalation of the response of the interneuron cells to further stimulation. Low frequency stimulation of C fibers results in "wind-up", which is an exaggerated response to a stimulus, whereas higher frequencies produce long-term potentiation (LTP) in which the response outlasts the stimulus. Mechanisms involve activation of *N*-methyl D-aspartate (NMDA) receptors leading to calcium influx, activation of protein kinase pathways, and ultimately altered receptor activation and migration. The result is secondary hyperalgesia, in which pain is felt outside the original area of noxious

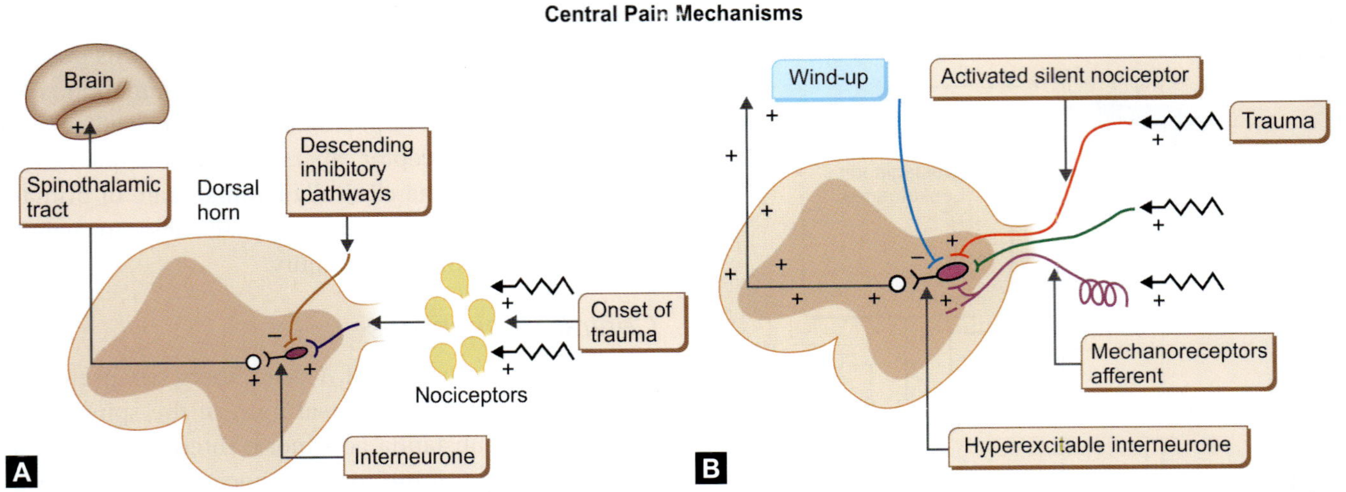

Central Pain Mechanisms

Figs. 12.4A and B: Central pain mechanisms. (A) Interneurons in the dorsal horn of the cord integrate information from peripheral nociceptors and descending inhibitory influences. (B) Prolonged noxious stimulation results in hyperexcitability (wind-up) such that the same intensity stimulus produces a larger response, including recruitment of mechanoreceptors and silent nociceptors not previously mediating pain.

stimulus, and allodynia, i.e. is pain in response to a normally innocuous stimulus such as light touch. Wind-up, LTP, and secondary hyperalgesia constitute central sensitization. Dorsal horn wind-up explains why pain is felt in a large area adjacent to a wound and why normally innocuous touch and movement is so painful (Figs. 12.4A and B).[28] Later, there are transcription changes in dorsal root ganglia cells resulting in expression of altered proteins, further enhancing the central sensitization.[29]

Activation of NMDA receptors by glutamate is pivotal in the mechanism of central sensitization and NMDA antagonists are potential novel analgesics, although the only clinically available agent is ketamine, an anesthetic agent that has psychomimetic side effects limiting its use. In animal models preemptive analgesia (analgesia given before noxious stimulus) will abort central sensitization in animal models, leading to a marked reduction in analgesic requirements. Preemptive analgesia has a more limited benefit in reducing pain in clinical practice: only epidural analgesia before lower limb amputation and colonic resection has demonstrated efficacy.[30]

Descending Inhibition

Higher centers can influence pain perception by means of the periaqueductal gray matter (PAG) in the upper brainstem, which contains high concentrations of opioid receptors and projects via the nucleus raphe magnus and dorsolateral funiculus to the dorsal horn of the spinal cord. The PAG receives input from the cortex, hypothalamus, and thalamus and is also a major site of action of opioid analgesics. Activation of the PAG from higher centers results in spinal analgesia by noradrenergic- and serotonergic-mediated inhibition of dorsal horn interneurons.

Progression of Acute to Chronic Pain

Chronic or persistent pain may follow noxious stimulation including surgical operations and often expresses neuropathic features. Risk factors include moderately severe pain before operation, repeat or prolonged operations, nerve injury, psychologic factors such as anxiety and tendency to catastrophize, poorly controlled postoperative pain, and postoperative chemo- or radiotherapy. Attention has been given to preventing postoperative persistent pain. There is evidence that epidural analgesia provided to manage pain after thoracotomy and open colonic resection reduces the likelihood of persistent pain, although there was no extra benefit from commencing the analgesia preemptively, before the incision. Reductions in postoperative pain have been demonstrated with wound infiltrations of local anesthesia following iliac bone graft harvest and with paravertebral block and gabapentin for mastectomy. Ensuring adequate postoperative analgesia is probably more important than giving it preemptively (Table 12.5).[30,31]

THERAPEUTIC OPTIONS FOR POSTOPERATIVE ANALGESIA

Assessment of Pain

Variability in clinical response means that pain relief therapy must be individualized. This is best done by use

Table 12.5 Incidence of chronic pain after various types of operation.

Type of surgery	*Incidence of severe chronic pain %*
Amputation of limb	5–10
Thoracotomy	10
Mastectomy	5–10
Inguinal hernia	2–4
CABG	5–10
Cesarean section	4

of repeat self-assessment to guide administration using a numerical or visual analog scale.[32] Scores of ≥70% represent severe pain, and reductions of 30% are clinically meaningful in many situations. Self-reporting of pain is not always possible at extremes of age or in patients with severe cognitive impairment. Assessment of static (rest) and dynamic (movement-related) pain is required to ensure that physical therapy and ambulation are possible. Serial observations of pain and side effects of analgesia (such as sedation) should be visually charted along with other physiologic variables to allow trends to be recognized[33] (Table 12.6).

Systemic Opioids

Systemic opioids remain the most commonly used analgesics after major surgical operations. They are usually given by the parenteral route as the oral route is unavailable. All full opioid agonists are equally effective, acting at specific opioid receptors in the central nervous system (CNS), some of which modulate pain transmission and some of which are involved in other processes. Currently available opioids are not specific for receptors in pain pathways and so can produce side effects. However, opioids remain useful because the therapeutic margin is adequate. There are interindividual pharmacokinetic differences and opioid receptor polymorphisms that may favor individual choice and flexible dosing of opioid.

The most serious adverse effect of strong opioid analgesia is central respiratory depression. As this effect is usually accompanied by progressive sedation, serial assessment of sedation is an early predictor of respiratory depression.[34] Opioids interfere with normal sleep mechanisms, producing episodic airway obstruction and consequent hypoxemia. Routine supplementary oxygen therapy is indicated while strong opioid analgesics are given. In an emergency, the respiratory depression (but also the analgesia) can be temporarily reversed by naloxone, a specific antagonist at the opioid receptor.

Table 12.6 Pain and sedation scoring systems. Pain and sedation are scored as part of regular postoperative monitoring and the results used to tailor therapy to individual needs.

Pain score (by patient directly)	*Definition*
0	No pain at rest or upon movement
1	No pain at rest, slight pain on movement
2	Slight pain at rest, moderate pain on movement
3	Moderate pain at rest, severe pain on movement
4	Severe pain at rest and on movement
Sedation score (by observer)	*Definition*
0	Alert
1	Mild
2	Moderate, frequently drowsy, easy to rouse
3	Severe, difficult to rouse
4	Asleep, but easy to awake

Opioid side effects include nausea, slowing of gastrointestinal motility and urinary retention. Recent work has also suggested that they may cause immunosuppression, although the clinical significance of this action is not clear especially after short-term administration. The nausea can be managed with appropriate antiemetics such as ondansetron, low-dose droperidol, and dexamethasone, but the other side effects are less easily mitigated. Development of psychologic dependence (addiction) is rare following postoperative opioid analgesia providing there is no previous history of substance abuse. Some opioids and their metabolites accumulate in renal or hepatic impairment, resulting in an increased risk of side effects unless doses are reduced.

Genetic Influences

Polymorphisms in genes that code for cytochrome P450 enzymes can cause major variation in the metabolism and thus the clinical effect of some opioids. CYP2D6 activity influences metabolism of codeine, tramadol and oxycodone. Ten percent of the populations are unable to convert codeine to active metabolites and experience no pain relief with this drug. There is less clinical variability in the clinical effect of oxycodone or tramadol.[35]

Morphine

Morphine is the commonest full opioid used after a major surgical operation because it is familiar and cheap. Opioid requirement is more closely related to age than body weight. Clinical analgesia requires that the plasma

Table 12.7 Features of other opioids used for postoperative analgesia.

Opioids.	*Features*
Oxycodone	A useful alternative to morphine in iv PCA, relatively safe in renal impairment.
Meperidine	Lower maximum analgesic ceiling and shorter action than morphine. Not safe in renal impairment because of the accumulation of the neurotoxic metabolite norpethidine. Not recommended for routine use.
Fentanyl	Highly lipid soluble potent synthetic opioid that can be used for postoperative analgesia by the iv route; PCA by nasal and iontophoresis assisted transdermal routes have been employed with inconclusive results. Relatively safe in renal impairment.
Buprenorphine	Highly lipid soluble partial agonist opioid that can be administered as a sublingual preparation. Relatively safe in renal impairment and less risk of respiratory depression.
Tramadol	Has weak opioid activity combined with central adrenergic activity offering analgesia with reduced opioid adverse effects.
Tapentodol	Similar to tramadol but more potent opioid properties.

morphine concentration is maintained above a threshold level, the minimum effective analgesic concentration (MEAC). This level can vary six-fold between individuals, so a flexible dosing regimen is required. Clinically active metabolites of morphine accumulate in renal impairment, so the drug is best avoided in this scenario. Morphine requirement tends to decrease with age in adults as CNS penetration is increased.

There are other clinically available opioids, although none is used as frequently as morphine (Table 12.7).

Patient-Controlled Opioid Analgesia

The traditional method of postoperative analgesia has been intermittent intramuscular or subcutaneous morphine given upon request. However, this technique has been largely supplanted by newer methods of delivery such as patient-controlled analgesia (PCA). PCA accommodates interindividual variations in plasma opioid MEAC to achieve more effective analgesia more safely, albeit with a larger overall opioid consumption. PCA uses a feedback loop in which opioid is titrated against residual pain by the patient directly, using small fixed doses of opioid from a programmable intravenous pump. Further requests within the predetermined lockout period are ignored rather than stored for delivery later (Fig. 12.5).

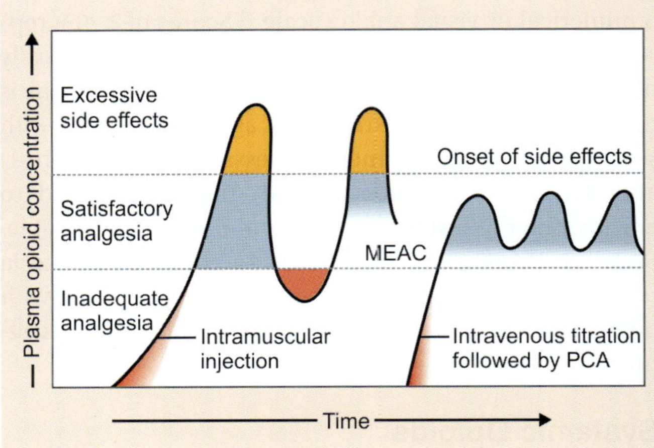

Fig. 12.5: Maintenance of analgesia with parenteral opioid. Patient-controlled analgesia (PCA) is able to maintain plasma opioid concentration closer to the minimum effective analgesic concentration (MEAC) resulting in improved analgesia and reduced side effects.

A potent opioid of rapid onset and intermediate duration of activity, such as morphine, is needed for effective PCA. Other opioids can be used, most usually oxycodone as it behaves similarly to morphine. Extensive experience with morphine has shown that for healthy adults a 1-mg bolus with a lockout period of 5 minutes is usually satisfactory, although parameters can be individualized. PCA is most successful after initial analgesia is established in the post-anesthesia care unit by nurse-administered titration.

PCA is relatively safe because the serious adverse effect of respiratory depression is reliably accompanied by progressive sedation and is related to the incremental accumulation of opioid. If the patient becomes sedated, further doses will not be initiated until plasma opioid concentration decreases and the patient is more alert. Nevertheless, serial recording of the adequacy of the pain relief and adverse effects such as sedation are still required, and protocols to facilitate this recording should be introduced when PCA is used. Operation of the device by a third party and the use of a continuous background infusion to prevent the patient waking in pain or the use of additional sedative drugs all compromise the inherent safety of the technique.

PCA is preferred to intermittent intramuscular analgesia by patients. In fact, patients rarely titrate themselves to complete analgesia, choosing instead to balance analgesia against side effects, predominantly nausea, and sedation.[36] PCA is ineffective in confused patients or young children because these individuals cannot satisfactorily complete the feedback loop.

PCA can be used by other routes: intranasal PCA is possible and is equally effective to the intravenous route. Subcutaneous PCA has been used, but the results are more variable, and an iontophoresis-enhanced transdermal fentanyl has been used but none has supplanted the intravenous route.

Ketamine, an NMDA antagonist, can be added to the PCA regimen and will decrease opioid requirement, improving analgesia and reducing nausea.

Nonsteroidal Anti-Inflammatory Agents and Oral Analgesia

The nonsteroidal anti-inflammatory drugs (NSAIDs) interfere with PG synthesis by inhibition of the enzyme cyclo-oxygenase (COX) acting in the peripheral tissues, together with some additional analgesic activity in the CNS. A subset, coxibs, are selective for COX-2, which is predominantly involved in pain and inflammation pathways and spare COX-1 found in other tissues, but coxibs have not proved able to reduce the main perioperative adverse effects of this group of drugs.

The NSAIDs produce important adverse effects through inhibition of the synthesis of PG, which is involved in homeostasis in many body systems. The adverse effects most relevant to postoperative analgesia include:

- Serious cardiovascular complications including myocardial infarction. This complication is seen with both nonselective agents and coxibs, and they should be avoided in patients with cardiovascular and cerebrovascular disease.
- A reversible inhibition of platelet aggregation, leading to an increased risk of perioperative bleeding in some circumstances.
- Acute renal failure by interference with PG-mediated renal vasodilation and a subsequent decrease in total renal blood flow. The renal failure is sometimes reversible; risk factors include increased age, previous renal impairment, and a major operation with associated hypotension and hypovolemia.
- Bronchospasm in some asthmatic individuals.
- Peptic ulceration is a well-known side effect of chronic NSAID therapy, but it is not usually seen within the duration of perioperative NSAID analgesia.

Nonsteroidal anti-inflammatory agents have a limited ceiling for analgesia and are inadequate as sole agents in severe pain. Combination of an NSAID with opioid-based PCA may result in improved quality of analgesia together with a reduction in the dose of opioid required, with reduced opioid side effects.[37]

Acetaminophen (paracetamol) is a nonopioid agent with a poorly understood mechanism of action that does not involve inhibition of PG synthesis. It is effective after a minor operation, and combination products containing acetaminophen and weak opioid are often used for less severe postoperative pain. The main adverse effect is hepatotoxicity in overdose.

Spinal Analgesia

Spinal analgesia involves the delivery of various drugs via the epidural or intrathecal route. Optimum results are achieved using a continuous infusion of a mixture of drugs with differing mechanisms of action including opioid, dilute local anesthetic, and alpha-2 agonists such as clonidine and dexmedetomidine because these agents are synergistic. The epidural route is usually used for postoperative analgesia by infusions as it is safer. Spinal analgesia provides the most effective analgesia currently available for severe postoperative pain.[38]

When local anesthetic is used, the epidural catheter must be sited close to the vertebral level innervating the site of operation. Potential complications of spinal local anesthetics include immobility from motor blockade and circulatory hypotension. The latter is a result of vasodilation and bradycardia from sympathetic blockade. The hypotension can be important in patients with preexisting hypovolemia, but it will respond to intravenous fluid challenge and vasoconstrictor agents, such as ephedrine; the bradycardia will respond to atropine. Bupivacaine is the most commonly used spinal local anesthetic because it combines a long duration of action with an absence of tachyphylaxis.

Opioids delivered by the intrathecal route produce high-quality analgesia by achieving high concentrations of drug at opioid receptors in the dorsal horn of the spinal cord. A fraction of the equivalent parenteral analgesic dose is usually adequate, so the incidence of systemic opioid side effects is reduced, although opioid induced respiratory depression remains a potential risk.

Spinal opioid usage can produce respiratory depression as a result of transport of opioid to the medullary respiratory center via the CSF. This effect can occur after a delay of up to 18 hours when morphine is used and is more likely in the elderly or if parenteral opioids or sedatives are given simultaneously. Monitoring of sedation and respiratory rate and the provision of supplementary oxygen are required for the safe use of a spinal opioid (as when using a systemic opioid).[39] Other complications of spinal opioid use include sedation, pruritus, urinary retention, and nausea. The most feared complication is epidural hematoma or infection, which can produce potentially devastating neurological injury albeit very rarely. It is important that those caring for this patient group act promptly if neurological deficit develops.

Clinical Use of Spinal Analgesia

Achieving optimum results from spinal analgesia demands skilled resources and requires serial observations of pain relief, dermatomal level of sensory block, volume status, blood pressure, sedation, and respiratory rate. The infusion rate of the local anesthetic and opioid must be carefully regulated to optimize the dermatomal block level so as to produce analgesia without excessive spinal nerve block, which increases hypotension and immobility. Because of the complexity the maximum benefit is achieved in a more aggressively monitored environment than the general ward. Patient-controlled epidural analgesia (PCEA) can be used with patient-initiated boluses analogous to intravenous PCA. PCEA produces improved analgesia, but it does not have the same inherent safety as intravenous PCA because respiratory depression as a result of a spinal opioid can be delayed; it does not offer the same safety margin, therefore.

There is evidence that continuous epidural analgesia with dilute local anesthetic and opioid can improve patient outcome compared with systemic opioid via PCA. After major upper abdominal or thoracic surgery epidural analgesia reduces the incidence of myocardial infarction, renal failure, and pulmonary dysfunction. Epidural analgesia hastens the return of gastrointestinal function following laparotomy (including colorectal procedures), when compared with systemic opioid analgesia.

Other Local Anesthetic Techniques

Thoracic paravertebral infusion of local anesthetic produces a similar effect to spinal analgesia in selected indications, producing profound but unilateral thoracic analgesia with fewer side effects; it is particularly useful after a thoracotomy and breast surgery. Transversus abdominus and rectus sheath blockade offers similar benefits for some abdominal operations. Other useful techniques with evidence of effectiveness include simple wound infiltration and infusions with local anesthetic, intra-articular local anesthetic after arthroscopy, and peripheral local anesthetic nerve blocks, such as brachial plexus blockade after orthopedic procedures.

These can all provide useful postoperative analgesia with minimal side effects for appropriate sites of operation. Usually, these techniques are not used alone, but they are combined with systemic analgesia as part of a multimodal analgesia technique.

Multimodal Analgesia

The combination of different analgesic techniques, including local anesthetic blocks, epidural analgesia together with NSAIDs, has been termed multimodal analgesia. The pain relief produced by drugs and techniques with complimentary mechanisms of action is superior to that resulting from individual medications. Multimodal analgesia when combined with more proactive rehabilitation after operation improves overall outcome and can shorten inpatient stay. This is the strategy of Fast-Track surgery and has been demonstrated to lead to earlier discharge in colorectal and joint replacement procedures.[40]

ROLE OF THE ANESTHESIOLOGIST IN PAIN MANAGEMENT

While oral analgesia may suffice for minor operative procedures, often parenteral analgesia is required, most usually by means of PCA, whereas in appropriate cases spinal analgesia offers real advantage. Anesthesiologists are uniquely placed to coordinate more complex acute pain management effectively because of their knowledge of analgesic pharmacology and perioperative physiology. Planning for effective postoperative analgesia needs to begin preoperatively and often comprises an integral part of the anesthetic technique, such as when an epidural catheter is sited perioperatively for postoperative use.

Most large hospitals now have an Acute Pain Service (APS) that usually comprises anesthesiologists and specialist nurses. The APS is responsible for developing safe local protocols for pain management, training, and certifying other medical and nursing staff in pain therapies, and will usually supervise more complex techniques, such as epidural infusions, or complex cases such as pain management in the illicit drug abuser. It has been demonstrated that the APS improves the effectiveness of pain management where it has been introduced.[41,42]

REFERENCES

1. Rees GJ, Gray TC. The anaesthetic triad. Br J Anaesth. 1950;22:83-86.
2. West R. Curare in man. Proc Roy Soc Med. 1932;25:1107.
3. Griffith HR, Jackson GE. The use of curare in general anesthesia. Anesthesiology. 1942;3:418-20.
4. Bovet D, Bovet-Nitti F, Guarino S. Proprieta farmachodinamiche di alcuni derivate della succinilcolina dotate di azione curarica. Rendiconti Istituto Superiore di Sanita (Roma). 1949;12:106-37.
5. Bourne JG, Collier HOJ, Summers GF. Succinylcholine (succinoylcholine). Muscle relaxant of short duration. Lancet. 1952;i:1225-9.
6. Buck N, Devlin HB, Lunn JN. The report of the confidential enquiry into perioperative deaths. Nuffield Provincial Hospitals Trust and The King Edward's Hospitals Fund for London. London, 1987.
7. Roizen MF. Preoperative patient evaluation—what's appropriate. ASA Annual Refresher Course lectures 1986;412.
8. Detsky AS, Abrams HB, Forbath N, et al. Cardiac assessment of patients undergoing non-cardiac surgery; a multifactorial clinical risk index. Arch Int Med. 1986;146: 2131-4.
9. Poldermans D, Bax JJ, Boersma E, et al. Guidelines for preoperative cardiac risk assessment and perioperative cardiac management in non-cardiac surgery: the Task Force for Preoperative Cardiac Risk Assessment and Perioperative Cardiac Management in Non-cardiac Surgery of the European Society of Cardiology (ESC) and endorsed by the European Society of Anaesthesiology (ESA). Eur J Anaesthesiol. 2010;27:92-137.
10. Fleisher LA, Beckman JA, Brown KA, et al. ACC/AHA 2007 guidelines on perioperative cardiovascular evaluation and care for noncardiac surgery: a report of the American College of Cardiology/American Heart Association Task Force on Practice Guidelines (writing committee to revise the 2002 guidelines on perioperative cardiovascular evaluation for noncardiac surgery). J Am Coll Cardiol. 2007;50: e159-e242.
11. Giles TD, Materson BJ, Cohn JN, et al. Definition and classification of hypertension: an update. J Clin Hypertens. 2009;11:611-4.
12. Mancia G, De Backer G, Dominiczak A, et al. 2007 Guidelines for the management of arterial hypertension. The Task Force for the Management of Arterial Hypertension of the European Society of Hypertension (ESH) and of the European Society of Cardiology (ESC). Eur Heart J. 2007;28: 1462-536.
13. Alberti KGMM. Diabetes and surgery. Anesthesiology. 1991;74:209-11.
14. Karkouti K, Wijeysundera D, Beattie W. Risk associated with preoperative anemia in cardiac surgery: a multicenter cohort study. Circulation. 2008;4:478-84.
15. Musallam K, Tamim H, Richards T, et al. Preoperative anaemia and postoperative outcomes in non-cardiac surgery: a retrospective cohort study. Lancet. 2011;9800:1396-407
16. McCleane GJ, Cooper R. The nature of preoperative anxiety. Anaesthesia. 1990;45:145-52.
17. Hopkins PM. Ultrasound guidance as a gold standard in regional anaesthesia. Br J Anaesth. 2007;98:299-301.
18. Picard J, Ward SC, Zumpe R, et al. Guidelines and the adoption of 'lipid rescue' therapy for local anaesthetic toxicity. Anaesthesia. 2009;64:122-5.
19. Kertai MD, Palanca BJ, Pal N, et al. Bispectral index monitoring, duration of bispectral index below 45, patient risk factors, and intermediate-term mortality after noncardiac surgery in the B-Unaware Trial. Anesthesiology. 2011; 114:545-56.
20. Gottschalk A, Van Aken H, Zenz M, et al. Is anesthesia dangerous? Dtsch Arztebl Int. 2011;108:469-74.
21. Hopkins PM. Malignant hyperthermia—pharmacology of triggering. Br J Anaesth. 2011;107:48-56.
22. Merskey H, Albe-Fessard DG, Bonica JJ. Pain terms: a list with definitions and notes on usage. Pain. 1979;6:249-52.
23. Ready LB, Edwards WT. Management of Acute Pain: A practical Guide. Taskforce on Acute Pain. Seattle, WA: IASP; 1992.
24. Wolf CJ, Ma Q. Nociceptors—noxious stimulus detectors. Neuron. 2007;55(3):353-64.
25. White FA, Wilson FM. Chemokines as pain mediators and modulators. Curr Opin Anesthesiol. 2008;21(5):580-5
26. Momin J, Wood JN. Sensory neuron voltage-gated sodium channels as analgesic drug targets. Curr Opin Neurobiol. 2008;18(4):383-8
27. Besson JM. The neurobiology of pain. Lancet. 1999;353: 1610-5.
28. Sandhuler J. Models and mechanisms of hyperalgesia and allodynia. Physiol Rev. 2009;89(2):707-58.
29. Ji RR, Gereau RWT, Malcangio M, et al. MAP kinase and pain. Brain Res Rev. 2009;60(1):135-48
30. Katz J, Clarke H. Preventative analgesia and beyond: current status, evidence and future directions. In: Macintyre PE, Walker SM (Eds). Clinical Pain Management: Acute Pain, 2nd edition. London: Hodder Arnold; 2008.
31. Macrae WA. Chronic post surgical pain. Br J Anaes. 2008; 101(1):77-86.
32. Valley MA. Pain measurement. In: Raj PP (Ed). Pain Medicine—A Comprehensive Review. St Louis: Mosby; 1995. pp. 36-46.
33. Breivik H, Borchgrevink PC, Allen SM, et al. Assessment of pain. Br J Anaes. 2008;101(1):17-24.
34. Villa H, Smith RA, Augustyniak MJ, et al. The efficacy and safety of pain management before and after implementation of hospital-wide pain management standards: is patient safety compromised by treatment based solely on numerical pain ratings? Anesth Analg. 2005;101(20): 474-80.
35. Stamer UM, Stuber F, Genetic factors in pain and it's treatment. Curr Opin Anesthesiol. 2007;20(5):478-84.
36. Hudcova J, McNichol W, Quah C, et al. Patient controlled opioid analgesia versus conventional opioid analgesia for post-operative pain. Cochrane Database Syst Rev. 2006(4): CDC003348.

37. Gajraj N, Joshi G. Role of cyclooxygenase-2 inhibitors in postoperative pain management. Anesthesiol Clin North America. 2005;23(1):49-72.
38. Nishimori M, Ballantyne JC, Low JH. Epidural Pain relief versus systemic opioid based analgesia for abdominal aortic surgery. Cochrane Database Syst Rev. 2006;3: CDC005059.
39. Horlocker TT, Burton AW, Connis RT, et al. Practice guidelines for the prevention, detection, and management of respiratory depression associated with neuraxial opioid administration. Anesthesiology. 2009;110(2):218-30.
40. White PF, Kehlet H, Neal JM. The role of the anesthesiologist in fast-track surgery: from multimodal analgesia to perioperative care. Anesth Analg. 2007;104(6):1380-96.
41. Counsell D, Macintyre PE, Breivik H. Organisation and role of acute pain services. In: Breivik H, Campbell WI, Nicholas MK (Eds). Acute Pain Management: Practice and Procedures. London: Hodder Arnold; 2008.
42. Macintyre PE, Schug SA, Scott DA, et al. Working Group of the Australian and New Zealand College of Anaesthetists and Faculty of Pain Medicine, Acute Pain Management: Scientific Evidence, 3rd edition ANZCA, FPM: Melbourne; 2010.

13

Principles of Endoscopy

David I Watson, John Chen, Adrian Chung, Paul Hollington

Key Points

- Flexible gastrointestinal endoscopy is an indispensable tool for gastrointestinal surgeons that encompasses both diagnosis and an increasingly more sophisticated range of interventions, including diagnosis and treatment of early and advanced cancers, and an expanding range of "incisionless" procedures.
- Flexible endoscopes are used for upper gastrointestinal endoscopy, endoscopic retrograde cholangiopancreatography (ERCP), colonoscopy, enteroscopy, and endoscopic ultrasound (EUS) procedures.
- Training is critical for safe and effective endoscopic practice. Integration of endoscopy training within surgical training programs and collaboration with gastroenterologists is important for safe practice.

GENERAL PRINCIPLES

The development of minimal access techniques for diagnosis and treatment in surgical practice has facilitated shorter hospital stays, quicker recovery, and reduced morbidity rates in many areas of surgical practice. At the same time, flexible gastrointestinal endoscopy has developed from a simple diagnostic tool to encompass an increasingly more sophisticated range of interventions, and this has blurred the boundary between gastroenterology and gastrointestinal surgery. Endoscopy is now an indispensable tool, as it enhances surgical planning across a wide spectrum of gastrointestinal disease. For the treatment of some diseases, endoscopy and surgical operations offer alternative treatment options. When gastrointestinal surgeons include endoscopy within their scope of practice and can offer both endoscopic and surgical options, they are well placed to consider the pros and cons of the competing procedures and then to recommend an appropriate option.

Flexible endoscopes are used for upper gastrointestinal endoscopy, endoscopic retrograde cholangiopancreatography (ERCP), colonoscopy, enteroscopy, and endoscopic ultrasound (EUS) procedures. Whereas in the past, endoscopes used a bundle of fiber optic fibers to transmit the image to an eyepiece, video endoscopes are now the current standard. Video endoscopes comprise a microchip camera and lens within the tip of the scope, and the image is transmitted electronically to a processing unit and displayed on a video monitor. Over recent decades, improved camera optics, high-definition video signals, magnification and narrow band imaging features have greatly improved the diagnostic utility of gastrointestinal endoscopes.

Gastrointestinal endoscopes have flexible shafts, which allow the endoscope to be maneuvered to access difficult cavities, although the flexibility of the instrument shaft can at times limit its usefulness as a therapeutic instrument. Hand piece design is similar for all types of endoscope and allows a single operator to steer and advance the tip of the instrument and simultaneously perform various procedures or functions (Fig. 13.1A). The tip of the endoscope is manipulated by two rotating levers (up/down and left/right) to achieve angulation, which allows it to be manipulated around bends to facilitate inspection of internal organs.

The end of the endoscope (Fig. 13.1B) contains a number of hollow channel outlets and an objective lens, in addition to one or more lenses at the end of fiber-optic channels, which provide illumination from a cold light source. One of the hollow channels allows gas to be insufflated, or water to be instilled for lens irrigation, as well as serving as a suction channel; these functions are controlled using two buttons on the hand piece. Another hollow channel allows the passage of instruments such as biopsy forceps, guidewires, snares, and other instrumentation. Some types of endoscope have a second instrument channel to facilitate various procedures. Most flexible endoscopes are end-viewing, although side-viewing duodenoscopes are used for ERCP

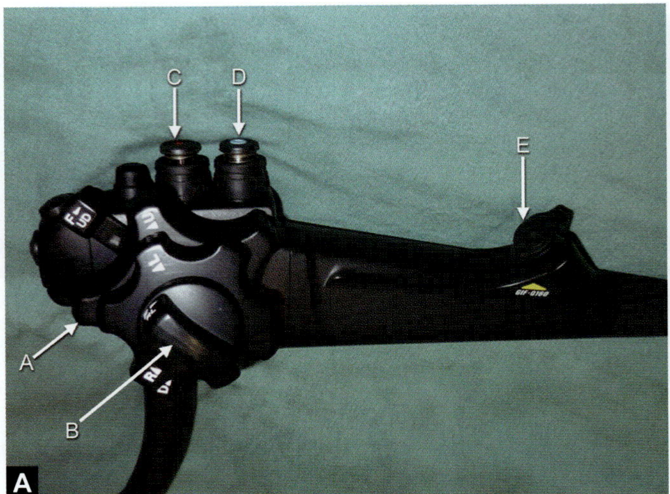

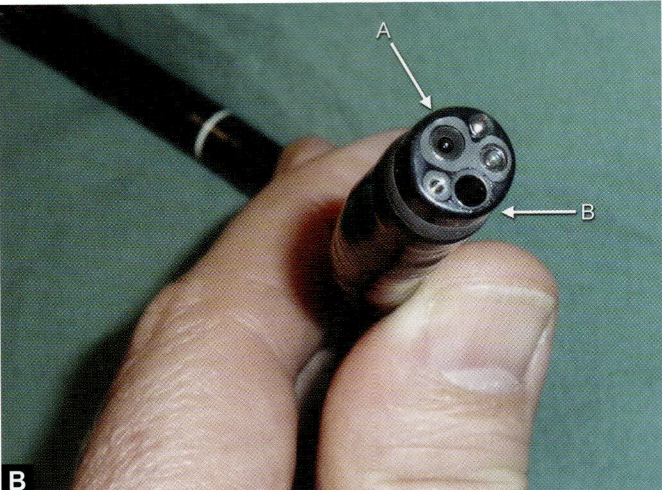

Figs. 13.1A and B: (A) Typical endoscope hand piece for upper gastrointestinal endoscopy (A= lever to deflect endoscope tip up vs. down, B = lever to deflect endoscope tip left vs. right, C = suction button, and D = insufflation/lens irrigation button, E = opening of instrument channel); (B) tip of endoscope for upper gastrointestinal endoscopy (A = camera lens and B = opening of instrument channel.

to allow viewing and cannulation of the ampulla of Vater, and EUS scopes also have an angled lens.

Many endoscopes allow image processing or manipulation to enhance the ability to detect subtle or indistinct pathology. Most endoscopes have four or five additional buttons on the hand piece, which can be used to select various imaging functions as well as providing the ability to perform additional functions such as freezing images or capturing and storing image data. Examples of image alteration include magnification, changing the depth of field, enhancing resolution or contrast, altering colors or utilizing specific wavelengths of light (narrow band imaging) to enhance vascular pattern visualization, or autofluorescence detection. Narrow band imaging is the most common image enhancement technology, and it is now standard within most of the latest model endoscopes. It uses a filter to limit the spectrum of light used for imaging to wavelengths of 440–460 nm (blue) and 540–560 nm (green). As these wavelengths are absorbed by hemoglobin, blood vessels appear dark, providing contrast which aids the identification of abnormal mucosal patterns and subtle pathologies.

In general, endoscopy procedures are performed under conscious sedation in an outpatient or day procedure setting. Occasionally, some patients will undergo procedures such as diagnostic gastroscopy without sedation, whereas a few patients require general anesthesia, for example, for prolonged therapeutic procedures or for airway protection when there is a high risk of aspiration. Anesthesia support is desirable when using sedation, although not always routinely available. Patients usually undergo endoscopy in the left lateral position, although other positions such as supine and prone are occasionally used, for example, ERCP in prone position and percutaneous endoscopic gastrostomy (PEG) in the supine position.

Training is critical for safe and effective practice. Various national bodies integrate endoscopy training within surgical training programs or work collaboratively with gastroenterology societies to ensure that agreed training and accreditation standards are met. In general, there are specific training requirements for each type of endoscopy practice, and in areas of niche practice such as the newer therapeutic applications.

UPPER GASTROINTESTINAL ENDOSCOPY

Diagnostic Endoscopy

Upper gastrointestinal endoscopy entails examination of the esophagus, stomach, and proximal duodenum using a flexible gastroscope. This is the preferred investigation when esophageal, gastric, or proximal duodenal pathology is suspected, and also facilitates a range of therapeutic interventions. The standard gastroscope is just >1 m in length and between 5 mm and 13 mm in diameter, depending on the purpose of the scope. Standard gastroscopes measure approximately 10 mm in diameter and are selected for most diagnostic and therapeutic purposes (Figs. 13.1A and B). Thinner endoscopes are used to navigate tight strictures, can be passed orally or transnasally, and are better tolerated in unsedated patients but have a narrower channel for instruments and poorer optics. Wider "therapeutic" gastroscopes contain either a wider instrument channel for the passage of larger diameter instrumentation or two instrument channels to allow simultaneous passage of instruments with suction, irrigation, and insufflation.

At upper gastrointestinal endoscopy the esophagus, stomach, and first and second parts of the duodenum are routinely inspected. With more effort the distal duodenum can also be inspected. When learning gastroscopy, the more difficult aspects of the procedure are intubation of the esophagus and passage of the endoscope through the pylorus. However, the maneuvers required reliably to complete the examination are usually rapidly mastered. Avoiding too much neck extension aids esophageal intubation, and minimizing gastric distension during the early parts of the procedures makes passage of the endoscope into the duodenum easier. The endoscope is best manipulated using a combination of up and down deflection of the endoscope tip with torque (rotation) of the endoscope shaft to change the direction of the tip, while at the same time advancing or withdrawing the endoscope.

Indications for diagnostic upper gastrointestinal endoscopy include investigation of upper abdominal pain, symptoms consistent with gastroesophageal reflux disease, or unexplained anemia, and also for follow-up of known pathologies such as Barrett's esophagus (Fig. 13.2A), peptic ulcer disease, and small benign tumors. Lesions can be diagnosed by visual appearances (Figs. 13.2B and C), or biopsies can be taken to clarify endoscopic appearances and aid with Barrett's esophagus surveillance. In surgical practice, upper gastrointestinal endoscopy also aids surgical planning prior to esophageal or gastric resection, as it defines the relationship between pathology and critical anatomical landmarks. Narrow band imaging and magnification aid visual identification of subtle pathology and are particularly helpful when undertaking surveillance endoscopy for patients with Barrett's esophagus. In general, patients are positioned in the left lateral position, although occasionally the supine position is used for some therapeutic procedures such as PEG, dilatation for achalasia, and esophageal stent placement.

Therapeutic Endoscopy

A range of therapeutic interventions are feasible at the time of endoscopy (Table 13.1). The scope of these procedures continues to expand and encroach on conventional surgical practice as new instrumentation is developed.

Dilatation

Perhaps the most common therapeutic intervention during endoscopy is dilatation. Typically, this is undertaken to expand a visible stricture, although some endoscopists perform empirical dilatation for patients presenting with dysphagia who have no visible lesion in the esophagus. Esophageal strictures are usually managed by passing a bougie. These tapered dilation devices can be passed blind, passed over a guidewire, or passed over a guidewire with fluoroscopy guidance. In general, blind unguided passage of a bougie should be avoided, as this is associated with a higher risk of esophageal perforation. If a guidewire can be placed across a stricture under direct vision, sometimes using a narrow diameter endoscope, then passage of a Savary-Gilliard type bougie over the wire is a safe approach. Bougie diameters generally range up to 18–20 mm. If multiple bougie changes are required or the endoscope cannot be passed through the stricture, that is, the lumen beyond the stricture cannot be visualized, then fluoroscopic guidance is the safest approach. Care should be taken when dilating very tight strictures or malignant strictures as the esophageal wall can be split, leading to perforation.

Balloon dilation devices that pass through the instrument channel of the endoscope are also available and provide an alternative option for dilatation of strictures when the lumen beyond a stricture cannot be visualized. These balloon dilators are also useful for dilation of pyloric and duodenal strictures related to peptic ulcer disease and anastomotic strictures after surgical procedures such as gastroenterostomy or gastric bypass. Balloons, which inflate to a diameter of up to 20 mm, are available.

Larger balloons, which inflate to diameters of 30 mm, 35 mm, and 40 mm, are used for dilatation of the gastroesophageal junction region in patients with achalasia. These devices do not fit within the instrument channel of the endoscope and so must be passed over a guidewire using fluoroscopy.

Hemostasis

Endoscopic methods for hemostasis have revolutionized the management of upper gastrointestinal hemorrhage. Before the early 1990s, most major acute hospitals would have seen operations for upper gastrointestinal bleeding on a daily basis. Now, such operations are seldom required, confirming the efficacy of endoscopic hemostasis in most patients with upper gastrointestinal bleeding.

Hemorrhage can be successfully controlled in most patients with bleeding peptic ulcers by injection of saline or saline/adrenaline solutions at bleeding sites and within the base of bleeding peptic ulcers, with or without the use of energy sources such as heater probes or argon plasma coagulation (APC) or endoscopically applied clips. Bleeding from esophageal varices has also become easier to deal with the development of banding techniques, which have largely superseded sclerotherapy.

Percutaneous Endoscopic Gastrostomy

In most patients requiring long-term enteral feeding tubes, percutaneous placement under endoscopic guidance provides a rapid, low-risk method for tube placement. Contraindications to this technique are the inability to pass an endoscope into the stomach (e.g., obstructing esophageal cancer) and previous upper abdominal surgery with adhesions that separate the anterior gastric wall from anterior abdominal wall during endoscopic inflation of the stomach. Radiological or surgical approaches are required when PEG placement is not feasible.

Stenting

Expandable metal stents can be placed across strictures in the esophagus, pylorus, and duodenum or used to seal leaks from the gastrointestinal tract. Multiple stents are marketed, but in general they can be classified as covered versus uncovered and removable versus permanent. Covered stents have a plastic layer built into the metal mesh, which minimizes tumor ingrowth or seals a hole in the gastrointestinal tract. Removable stents have a loop at either end that can be grasped and pulled into the endoscope to collapse the end of the stent, thereby allowing it to be pulled out through the esophagus. Once a stent is in place it starts to generate a fibrotic tissue reaction, where its open end presses against adjacent tissues, and this can progress to form a stricture. In general, even a removable stent can be difficult to remove beyond 3 months after placement. Occasionally, a stent can migrate through the wall of the gastrointestinal tract and enter an adjacent structure. In the esophagus, these problems can arise after a stent has been in place for >6–12 months, and this is fatal when erosion into the aorta or airway occurs.

Ablation of Barrett's Esophagus

The observation that destruction of the metaplastic columnar mucosa of Barrett's esophagus in the presence of an acid-free environment is followed by healing with a new squamous mucosa has led to techniques for ablation of Barrett's esophagus. Common endoscopic methods to achieve this include radiofrequency ablation (RFA),[1] photodynamic therapy (PDT),[2] and APC. Radiofrequency ablation is the newest technique, and it seems to provide more reproducible regression of Barrett's esophagus. Randomized trials have shown that both PDT and RFA ablation of high-grade dysplasia (HGD) reduce the short-term risk of subsequent cancer development, although longer term data are awaited.[3] There is currently no evidence to support ablation of nondysplastic Barrett's esophagus or Barrett's esophagus with low-grade dysplasia outside the context of clinical trials. Health economic studies suggest that ablation in individuals with Barrett's esophagus without HGD is unlikely to be cost-effective.

Mucosal Resection

Small pieces of esophageal or gastric mucosa (up to 20-mm diameter) can be excised using endoscopic mucosal resection (EMR). Two techniques are available—a lift and cut technique and a band and cut technique. The principle is to use suction to create a pseudopolyp within a cap placed on the end of the endoscope and then to use a snare with cautery to cut and remove this piece of mucosa, while leaving the underlying muscle intact. The banding technique (Duette EMR procedure, Cook Medical) is technically easier and probably safer to perform (Figs. 13.2D and E). It uses a tight rubber band to separate the mucosa from the muscle layer to create the pseudopolyp. Multiple resections can be undertaken at a single endoscopy, but care needs to be taken to avoid circumferential excision within the esophagus as this will lead to stricture formation. This technique is well suited to the removal of early stage visible lesions within Barrett's esophagus, and it provides tissue for diagnosis and staging. Sequential EMR excision of residual short segments of Barrett's esophagus can also be undertaken, and treatment of early intramucosal esophageal cancer confined to the mucosa (i.e., not invading the submucosa) can be curative. Larger lesions can sometimes be treated using endoscopic submucosal dissection (ESD), which entails excision of a larger area of mucosa as a single piece. However, the learning curve for this procedure is long, and expertise is not widely available outside Asian countries with a high incidence of esophageal and gastric cancer, for example, Japan. Complications of endoscopic resection include perforation, bleeding, and esophageal stricture, with greater risk following ESD.

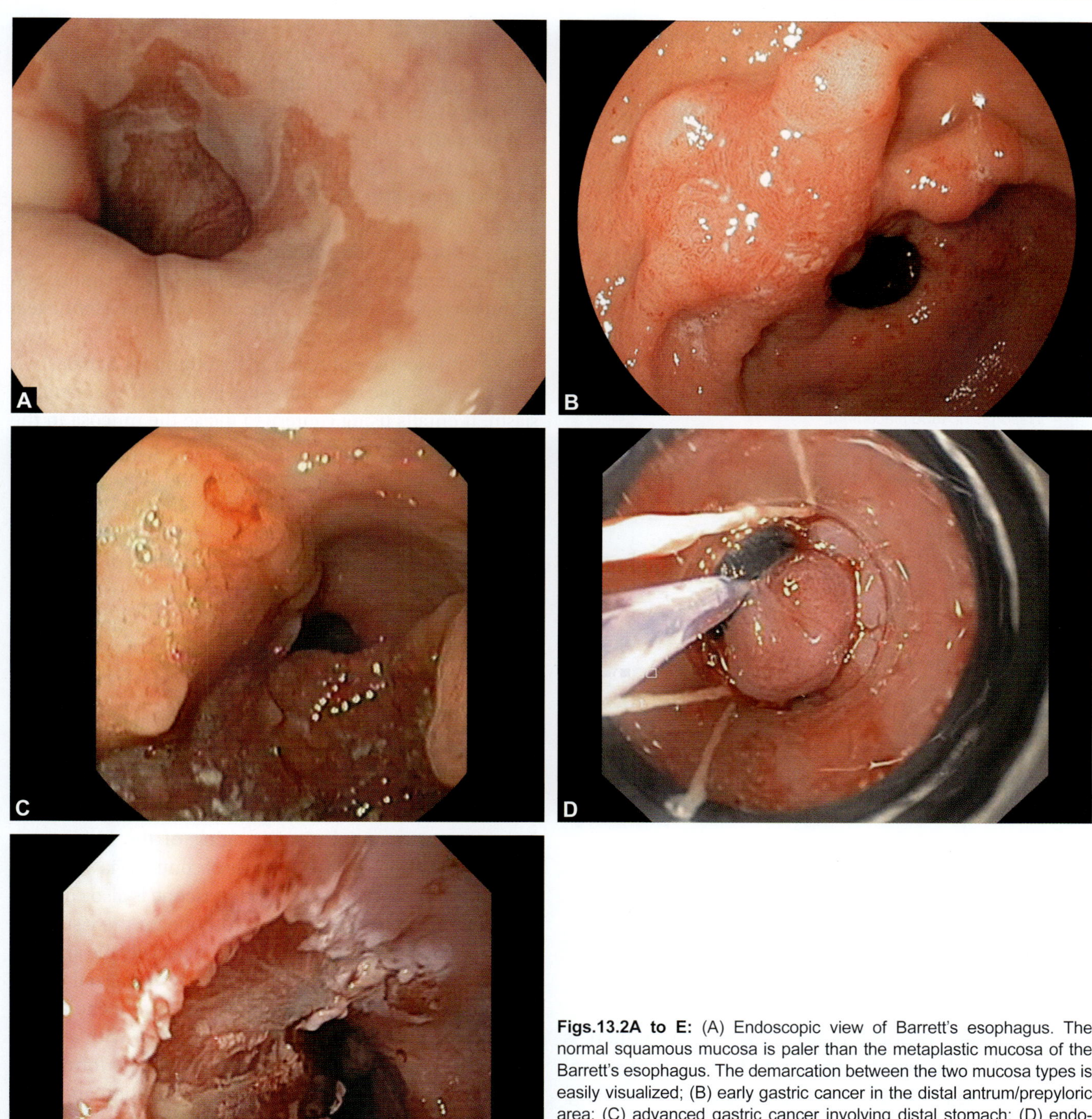

Figs.13.2A to E: (A) Endoscopic view of Barrett's esophagus. The normal squamous mucosa is paler than the metaplastic mucosa of the Barrett's esophagus. The demarcation between the two mucosa types is easily visualized; (B) early gastric cancer in the distal antrum/prepyloric area; (C) advanced gastric cancer involving distal stomach; (D) endoscopic mucosal resection using Duette system. A dysplastic area of Barrett's esophagus has been converted to a pseudopolyp after applying a "band" and is cut off using a snare; and (E) after endoscopic mucosal resection the cut mucosal edges are seen, and the exposed esophageal muscle is inspected to ensure that it is not bleeding or perforated.

Interventions for Esophageal Perforation

Endoscopically applied clips, originally designed for control of hemorrhage, can also be used to close perforations in the upper gastrointestinal tract. These devices work best when used to close small holes that arise iatrogenically during an endoscopic procedure, as the edges to be closed are fresh and major contamination beyond the gastrointestinal

Table 13.1	Therapeutic upper gastrointestinal endoscopy procedures.
• Dilatation of strictures	
– Bougie	
– Balloon	
• Hemostasis	
– Injection	
– Heater probe	
– Argon coagulation	
– Clipping	
• Feeding tube placement	
– Percutaneous endoscopic gastrostomy (PEG)	
– Percutaneous endoscopic jejunostomy (PEJ)	
– Nasogastric tube placement	
• Stenting	
– Esophageal	
– Pyloric	
– Duodenal	
• Ablation of Barrett's esophagus using an energy source	
– Radiofrequency ablation (RFA)	
– Argon plasma coagulation (APC)	
– Photodynamic therapy (PDT)	
• Mucosal resection	
– Endoscopic mucosal resection (EMR)	
– Endoscopic submucosal resection (ESD)	
• Closure of perforations	
– Endoscopic clips	
• Other complex procedures	
– Endoscopic fundoplication for gastroesophageal reflux	
– Treatment of achalasia	
• Pneumatic dilatation	
• Peroral endoscopic myotomy (POEM)	

tract is unlikely. This technique is less effective if there is appreciable delay occur between perforation and subsequent endoscopy, as the resultant induration, swelling, and friability that develop at the site of perforation limit the effectiveness of the clips. A newer-design "over the scope" clip is capable of closing larger defects and might be more suitable for larger holes or in patients in whom treatment delays have occurred.

Other Novel Procedures

In the late 1990s and early 2000s, a range of endoscopic treatments for gastroesophageal reflux were proposed. The earlier procedures created a narrowing at the gastroesophageal junction and were subsequently shown to be ineffective as they failed to create a flap valve, which was the essential step required for a successful antireflux procedure. More recent interest has been generated by procedures that attempt endoscopically to replicate a laparoscopic partial fundoplication. The EsophyX device (EndoGastric Solutions, Seattle) is the only device to reach market, but the medium term outcomes have been disappointing compared with laparoscopic fundoplication, and enthusiasm for endoscopic treatment of gastroesophageal reflux appears to be waning.[4]

An endoscopic approach to myotomy for achalasia—peroral endoscopic myotomy—has generated recent enthusiasm. It entails using cautery to incise the mucosa in the mid-esophagus, followed by creation of a submucosal tunnel in the distal esophageal wall and then division of the lower esophageal sphincter. Early reports demonstrate that this is an effective procedure, although longer term outcomes and safety outside a small number of centers of expertise remain uncertain.[5]

ENDOSCOPIC RETROGRADE CHOLANGIOPANCREATOGRAPHY

Endoscopic retrograde cholangiopancreatography is performed with a side-viewing duodenoscope (Fig. 13.3A) in conjunction with fluoroscopy for diagnostic investigation and therapeutic intervention of pancreatobiliary diseases. It incorporates radiological imaging of the biliary tree and/or pancreatic duct with the use of contrast via a catheter injection. The side-viewing duodenoscope is also complementary to the end-viewing gastroscope for the visualization of some parts of the duodenum, especially the ampulla and duodenal tumors, which are poorly visualized with a standard gastroscope. Endoscopic retrograde cholangiopancreatography may also be used together with a "baby scope" via its large-bore working channel to perform cholangioscopy as well as videoendoscopy of the pancreatic duct. With the more recent development and widespread use of magnetic resonance cholangiopancreatography (MRCP), ERCP is now mainly used for therapeutic intervention such as stenting of the bile or pancreatic ducts or extraction of calculi from the biliary tree.

Indications and Contraindications for ERCP

The most common indication is endoscopic retrograde cholangiography (ERC) for the investigation and intervention

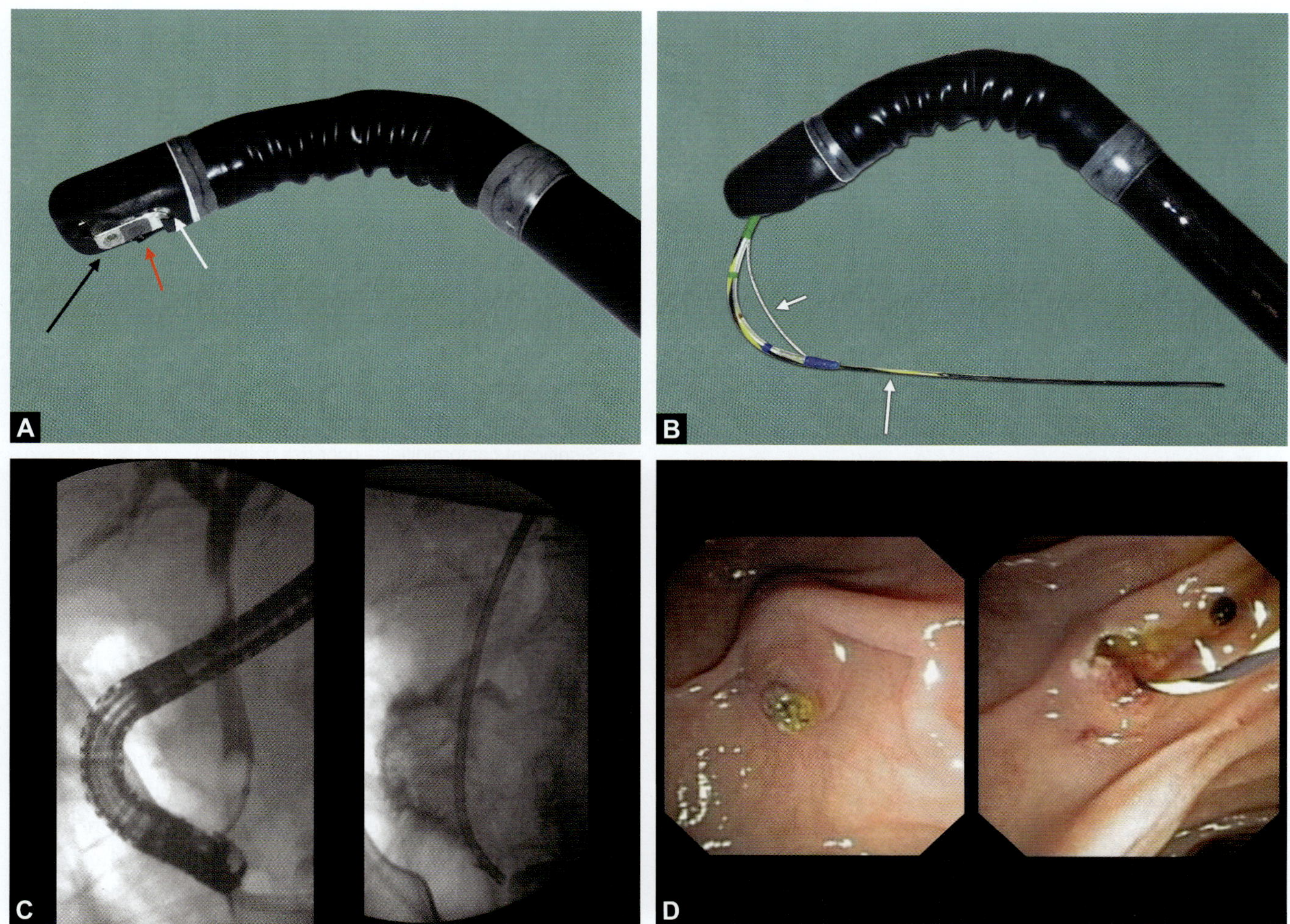

Figs. 13.3A to D: (A) Duodenoscope with side-viewing lens (black arrow), suction irrigation channel (red arrow), and working channel for cannulation and instrumentation (white arrow); (B) duodenoscope with sphincterotome (short arrow) inserted via working channel with guidewire (long arrow) in situ. The bowing of the sphincterotome allows for manipulation of the guidewire for optimal angulation and biliary cannulation; (C) Mirizzi's syndrome with stricture in the upper bile duct caused by stone and complete emptying of contrast after placement of a plastic stent across the narrowing; and (D) impacted ampullary stone, treated with papillotomy followed by sphincterotomy and subsequent extraction.

of biliary stone disease. Other indications include benign and malignant strictures of the biliary tree and bile leak from biliary or liver surgery or liver trauma (Table 13.2). Indications for endoscopic retrograde pancreatography (ERP) include evaluation of the ductal changes of chronic pancreatitis, extent of main duct intraductal papillary mucinous neoplasm involvement, and pancreatic stenting for pancreatic stricture, pancreatic leak, or pseudocyst. Endoscopic retrograde pancreatography with pancreatic sphincterotomy is also performed as a preventative treatment for recurrent pancreatitis secondary to sphincter of Oddi dysfunction or pancreas divisum.

Relative contraindications for ERCP include coagulopathy, hemodynamically unstable patients, previous gastrectomy where reconstruction renders endoscopic access to the duodenum difficult (e.g., Billroth II or total gastrectomy), gastric outlet obstruction, and esophageal stricture (Table 13.3).

Equipment, Sedation, Antibiotic Prophylaxis, and Positioning of Patients for ERCP

The endoscope used for ERCP is a side-viewing duodenoscope (*see* Fig. 13.3A), which can be used in patients aged ≥2–3 years. For younger patients a slimmer scope should be used. The standard side-viewing scope is about 13 mm in diameter and has a working channel that is 4.2 mm in diameter. This channel allows instrumentation including the insertion of a slim baby scope for cholangioscopy and pancreaticoscopy (i.e. visualization of bile duct and

Table 13.2 Clinical indications for ERCP.

Indications
Indications for endoscopic retrograde cholangiography (ERC)
• Gallstone disease
– Bile duct stones
– Biliary pancreatitis
– Mirizzi's syndrome
– Hepatolithiasis
• Benign biliary strictures
– Anastomotic stricture after liver transplantation
– Bile duct injury
– Primary sclerosing cholangitis
– Focal sclerosing cholangitis
– IgG4 cholangiopathy
• Malignant strictures
– Pancreatic carcinoma
– Cholangiocarcinoma
– Gallbladder carcinoma
– Portal lymph node metastases
– Metastatic liver disease
• Bile leak
– Post-cholecystectomy
– Post-liver resection
– Trauma
– After bile duct exploration
Indications for endoscopic retrograde pancreatography (ERP)
• Pancreatic duct leak
• Pancreatic pseudocyst
• Pancreatic duct stones
• Pancreatic duct stricture
• Pancreatitis secondary to pancreatic divisum
• Pancreatitis secondary to sphincter of Oddi dysfunction

pancreatic duct). This wide working channel also allows the introduction of a wide range of temporary or permanent biliary or pancreatic stents.

Endoscopic retrograde cholangiopancreatography is traditionally performed in the prone position with the patient resting on two pillows, one on the chest and the other one on the hip with the mouth turned to patient's right for endoscopic intubation. The prone position minimizes the risk of aspiration during the procedure. The pillows prevent compression of the stomach and duodenum to allow stomach and duodenal insufflation for visualization. Endoscopic retrograde cholangiopancreatography can be performed in other positions such as left lateral, swimmers, and supine. The side-viewing duodenoscope is designed for optimal visualization in the prone position. The prone position also provides better cholangiographic

Table 13.3 Contraindications to ERCP.

Contraindications
Anatomical factors
• Large duodenal diverticulum
• Duodenal stricture proximal to ampulla of Vater
• Previous surgery limiting access to the duodenum
– Billroth II gastrectomy
– Roux En Y biliary reconstruction
• Esophageal narrowing
– Esophageal stricture
– Inflated gastric band
Clinical factors
• Coagulopathy
• Jaundice secondary to hepatic dysfunction
• Significant comorbidities—poor risk patient

visualization of the hepatic bifurcation and pancreatic duct, compared with the lateral or swimmer's position. Unfortunately, if respiration is compromised the traditional prone position makes urgent endotracheal intubation difficult, and for this reason some units routinely intubate patients and perform the procedure under general anesthesia. In general, if the ERCP is anticipated to be difficult and lengthy, intubation and general anesthesia should be considered. For anticipated short procedures such as removal of a plastic stent, ERCP under sedation in the lateral position should be adequate. In general, when ERCP is performed in obese patients or patients with a history of illicit drug use, general anesthesia should be utilized.

There has been considerable debate about the use of prophylactic antibiotics. In general, procedures that are likely to require prolonged manipulation of the biliary tree, as well as those with potential to be followed by impaired bile flow, should be considered for prophylactic antibiotic cover. The antibiotics used should cover gram-negative bacilli and achieve high concentrations in bile, and they should be administered immediately before the procedure commences.[6]

Diagnostic ERCP

Before the widespread use of MRCP, ERCP was the standard technique for diagnosing biliary tract disease. Other modalities that have been used to evaluate the biliary tree include ultrasound, oral cholecystogram, intravenous cholangiogram, and hepatobiliary iminodiacetic acid (HIDA) scan. Magnetic resonance cholangiopancreatography has replaced ERCP as the main diagnostic tool for biliary and pancreatic duct imaging. Magnetic resonance cholangiopancreatography is particularly useful in circumstances where ERCP cannot be performed, especially when the bile duct and pancreatic are not accessible following previous Billroth II gastrectomy or Roux-en-Y biliary reconstruction, gastric outlet, or duodenal obstruction. Diagnostic ERCP is now mainly performed where MRI is contraindicated.

With the patient sedated or under general anesthesia, the side-viewing endoscope is introduced into the esophagus. As passage of the scope down the esophagus is blind, a history of dysphagia is a relative contraindication, and for patients with an esophageal stricture the stricture should be dilated with a minimum 15-mm diameter bougie before attempting to pass the side-viewing scope. Inflated gastric bands should also be completely deflated before ERCP. Once inside the stomach, a gastroscopy should be performed, knowing that the visualization with the side-viewing scope is limited. The pylorus is next intubated, and the first, second, and third parts of the duodenum are inspected. Adequate insufflation of the second part of duodenum is essential for safe cannulation of the ampulla of Vater. Poor visualization of the ampulla may be due to abdominal or tumor compression of the duodenum, leakage of insufflated gas, anatomical variation, or distortion due to previous operations.

The most common difficulty is probably related to selective cannulation of the desired duct (bile duct vs. pancreatic duct). This can arise from poor positioning, duodenal distortion, or location of the papilla inside a duodenal diverticulum. Occasionally, the main papilla is located in the third part of the duodenum. Marked respiratory excursion, duodenal peristalsis, or sphincter of Oddi spasm can add difficulty to cannulation. Both intravenous buscopan or glucagon can decrease duodenal peristalsis and sphincter of Oddi contraction to facilitate ductal cannulation.

The second common difficulty is failure to cannulate the biliary duct. The insertion of the bile duct into the common channel is more obtuse than the pancreatic duct. Hence, if cannulation is not directed in line with the bile duct, cannulation of the pancreatic duct is likely. Several manipulations can be performed in this setting to facilitate bile duct cannulation. These include the use of a sphincterotome to increase the angulation of the catheter (Fig. 13.3B) and a papillotome to incise the papilla to allow cannulation of the bile duct. Endoscopic ultrasound-guided nonanatomical cannulation of a dilated biliary tree has been described, especially in the setting of neoplasm when the distal bile duct has been destroyed or distorted.

The biliary tree can be cannulated either directly by a catheter or by initially passing a guidewire. The position of the guidewire or catheter can then be confirmed with fluoroscopy. If the guidewire is directed toward the patient's right side following cannulation, then it is likely to be in the biliary tree. On the contrary, if the guidewire veers toward the patient's left, it is likely that pancreatic duct has been cannulated. Initial slow contrast injection is necessary to confirm whether the desired duct is cannulated. Forceful injection of the pancreatic duct can lead to acute pancreatitis. Cholangiography will demonstrate left and right hepatic ducts as well as the cystic duct. The abnormalities to be defined on imaging include abnormal anatomical variation, the presence of strictures, the presence of filling defects, dilatation of the biliary tree, and the presence of a biliary leak. For pancreatography, it is important not to inject too much contrast as this can lead to pancreatitis.

Table 13.4 Complications of ERCP.

- Pancreatitis
- Perforation of duodenum or duodenal diverticulum
  - From sphincterotomy
  - From passage of guidewire
- Bleeding following sphincterotomy
- Infection
  - Cholangitis
  - Cholecystitis
  - Infection of pseudocyst
- Stent complications—poor position
- Jammed Dormia basket

Complications of ERCP

Endoscopic retrograde cholangiopancreatography is associated with a number of morbidities, as well as a small risk of mortality (Table 13.4). The most important is pancreatitis. This complication is more prevalent when ERCP is performed for patients with sphincter of Oddi dysfunction, when pancreatic sphincterotomy is performed, or after ampullectomy or inadvertent pancreatic duct contrast injection. Although most ERCP-induced pancreatitis is self-limiting, a small percentage of patients can develop severe pancreatitis leading to death. Duodenal perforation from difficult or diverticular intubation, papillotomy, or sphincterotomy is another serious complication, which is associated with an appreciable mortality risk if not recognized early. Bleeding from sphincterotomy can be acute or sometimes delayed by several days. Cholangitis, cholecystitis, jamming of a Dormia basket in the bile duct, and guidewire perforation of the biliary tree are other potential complications. Poor deployment of plastic or metal stents can result in poor biliary drainage, side branch, or cystic duct occlusion, as well as difficulty in retrieving temporary stents.

Specific Interventions and Indications

Choledocholithiasis and Mirizzi's Syndrome

Jaundice, deranged liver enzymes, pancreatitis, and cholangitis due to common bile duct (CBD) stones are by far the most common indication for therapeutic ERC. Stones in the CBD can be managed in several ways, depending on their number, size, or clinical circumstances. Common bile duct stones <1 cm in diameter can usually be extracted with a balloon or basket following biliary sphincterotomy. However, if the numbers of stones are either too many or too large, extraction of all the stones at the first procedure may not be possible, and excessive manipulation with a basket and/or balloon can result in trauma and edema to the biliary tree and ampulla. In this situation, it is best to pass a temporary biliary stent to overcome bile duct obstruction. A follow-up procedure can be performed about 8–10 weeks later when edema and swelling have subsided. Occasionally, it may take three to four sessions to clear the biliary tree. If it is anticipated that several sessions are required or the stones are unlikely to clear, despite repeated attempts, consideration should be given for laparoscopic exploration and extraction of stones. In patients with Mirizzi's syndrome (Fig. 13.3C), a decompressing temporary biliary stent should be placed and consideration should be given for surgical extraction of the stone at cholecystectomy.

Biliary Stricture

The most common biliary stricture causing obstructive jaundice is due to a pancreatic head tumor. Other causes include posttransplant anastomotic stricture, sphincter of Oddi dysfunction, primary and secondary biliary sclerosis, cholangiocarcinoma, gallbladder carcinoma, and extrahepatic perihilar lymphadenopathy. Biliary stricture can be treated with biliary dilatation and/or biliary stenting. The type of stent used depends on the circumstances. For palliation of jaundice due to a malignant stricture, a permanent covered or uncovered metal stent should be used. For benign strictures, a removable plastic or fully covered metal stent is used. Occasionally, multiple plastic stents are sequentially inserted over a period of 12 months to prevent premature recurrence of the stricture following their removal.

Rendezvous Technique for Failed Biliary Cannulation

When cannulation of the papilla cannot be safely achieved, the biliary tree can be accessed via a percutaneous radiological technique. The guidewire can then be passed down the biliary tree into the duodenum. This long guidewire can be retrieved via the duodenoscope, and the biliary tree can then be accessed. This "rendezvous technique" avoids the use of an external biliary drain when managing a biliary stricture.

Papillotomy and Sphincterotomy

When the ampulla of Vater cannot be cannulated, a papillotomy can be performed using "needle-knife" cauterization to access the bile duct. A direct incision is made into the papilla at 11 o'clock using needle cauterization of the biliary sphincter to access the bile duct. This maneuver is followed by biliary sphincterotomy (Fig. 13.3D). If cannulation fails after initial excessive manipulation and papillotomy, a repeat ERCP a few days later when edema settles may be successful. Biliary sphincterotomy using a bow sphincterotome (*see* Fig. 13.3B) is performed to allow extraction of bile duct stones, facilitate placement of biliary stents, or allow passage of a "baby" scope for cholangioscopy and biopsy of biliary strictures.

Biliary and Pancreatic Stenting

Stenting of the biliary tree is performed for biliary stricture or biliary leak. A biliary sphincterotomy is usually required before placement. Temporary plastic or removable metallic biliary stents are used for benign biliary strictures or malignant strictures before surgical resection. For bile leak from the biliary tree after liver resection, cholecystectomy, or liver trauma, sphincterotomy with or without insertion of a temporary 10Fr biliary stent usually suffices; in most instances, the leak resolves within 24–48 hours.

Biliary and Pancreatic Manometry

Sphincter of Oddi dysfunction may be suspected in patients with recurrent biliary type pain or recurrent acute pancreatitis associated with biliary or pancreatic dilatation or elevated liver function tests. In such cases, biliary and/or pancreatic manometry should be considered. If there is evidence of focal stenosis, which manifests as high sphincter of Oddi pressure, biliary and pancreatic sphincterotomy may be curative.

ENDOSCOPIC ULTRASOUND

Endoscopic ultrasound enables real-time high-resolution imaging of the gastrointestinal tract and adjacent extraluminal structures. This technique has an established role in the staging of upper gastrointestinal and pancreatobiliary malignancies and also facilitates tissue sampling to enhance diagnostic accuracy. Therapeutic applications of EUS include drainage procedures, coeliac plexus neurolysis, and, more recently, fiducial placement (radio-opaque marker) for guidance of radiotherapy and intra-tumoral injection of chemotherapy.[7]

Equipment

Radial and Linear Echoendoscopes

Echoendoscopes are modified oblique-viewing endoscopes with either a radial or curvilinear array ultrasound transducer at the tip. The transducers scan at frequencies of between 5 MHz and 20 MHz and a water-filled balloon may be placed over the tip to enhance acoustic coupling with the luminal mucosal surface.

The scanning plane of a radial echoendoscope lies perpendicular to the endoscope shaft (Fig. 13.4A), providing a 360° image in which the transducer is based at the center, similar to the slices seen on a CT scan. Earlier mechanical instruments had a rotating transducer at the scope tip. Newer electronic instruments have no moving parts, are more durable, and permit Doppler assessment to differentiate between ductal and vascular structures. The radial echoendoscope is most useful for assessment of submucosal lesions of the upper gastrointestinal tract and for staging of upper gastrointestinal malignancies.

Linear echoendoscopes scan in the same plane as the shaft of the endoscope and the images are similar to those obtained with transabdominal ultrasound (Fig. 13.4B). In the image, the transducer is seen at the top of the image above a 180° field of view. Alignment between the scope shaft and the ultrasound beam allows fine-needle aspiration (FNA) needles to be passed into lesions of interest under direct ultrasound guidance. The shaft of the linear instrument is also wider than the radial echoendoscope, permitting instrumentation through a larger (up to 3.8-mm diameter) instrument channel. Interpretation of images obtained with the linear echoendoscope is highly dependent on the orientation of the scope tip, and there is a steeper learning curve in comparison with the radial instrument. However, the linear echoendoscope can be used for almost any situation in which EUS is indicated and has the added benefit of facilitating FNA-guided tissue sampling and therapeutics.

Other specialized instruments include "blind" slim mechanical radial probes, which are passed over a guidewire. These can traverse the majority of malignant esophageal strictures. Mini-probes range from 2.0 mm to 2.6 mm in diameter and are fed through the instrument channel of the standard gastroscope. They scan at frequencies up to 30 MHz, allowing high-resolution imaging within the biliary tree or of superficial upper gastrointestinal malignancies. Endobronchial and anorectal echoendoscopes are also available.

FNA Needles

Fine-needle aspiration needles range in size between 25 G and 19 G. A stylet prevents contamination by normal gut mucosa as the needle is passed into the target lesion. Smaller 25 G needles are preferred for the acquisition of tissue from solid pancreatic lesions as larger needles increase the bloodiness of the sample. For aspiration of cysts and drainage procedures, the 19 G needle is appropriate. A 19 G Tru-Cut needle has been developed for the purpose of obtaining a core specimen, although this is difficult to use, particularly when the echoendoscope is angulated within the second part of the duodenum. Recently, developed FNA needles with a side opening and reverse bevel (ProCore needle, Cook Medical, Winston-Salem, NC) may enhance the acquisition of core biopsies.

EUS Technique

Endoscopic ultrasound procedures are performed predominantly in an outpatient setting with conscious sedation. Intramural lesions are assessed by passing the echoendoscope adjacent to the area of interest, then aspirating luminal air and inflating a water-filled balloon at the tip of the echoendoscope to facilitate contact with the area of interest. Water may at times be instilled into the gut lumen to improve the view, although one should be conscious of the risk of aspiration into the lungs, particularly during examination of the esophagus. The gut wall is depicted in five distinct layers that correspond to the superficial and deep mucosa, submucosa, muscularis propria, and adventitial or serosal layer (Fig. 13.4C).

Extraluminal structures are assessed by a "station" based approach (Table 13.5), which varies depending on whether the radial or linear instrument is used. For example, pancreatic examination with the linear instrument begins with the echoendoscope within the stomach, where

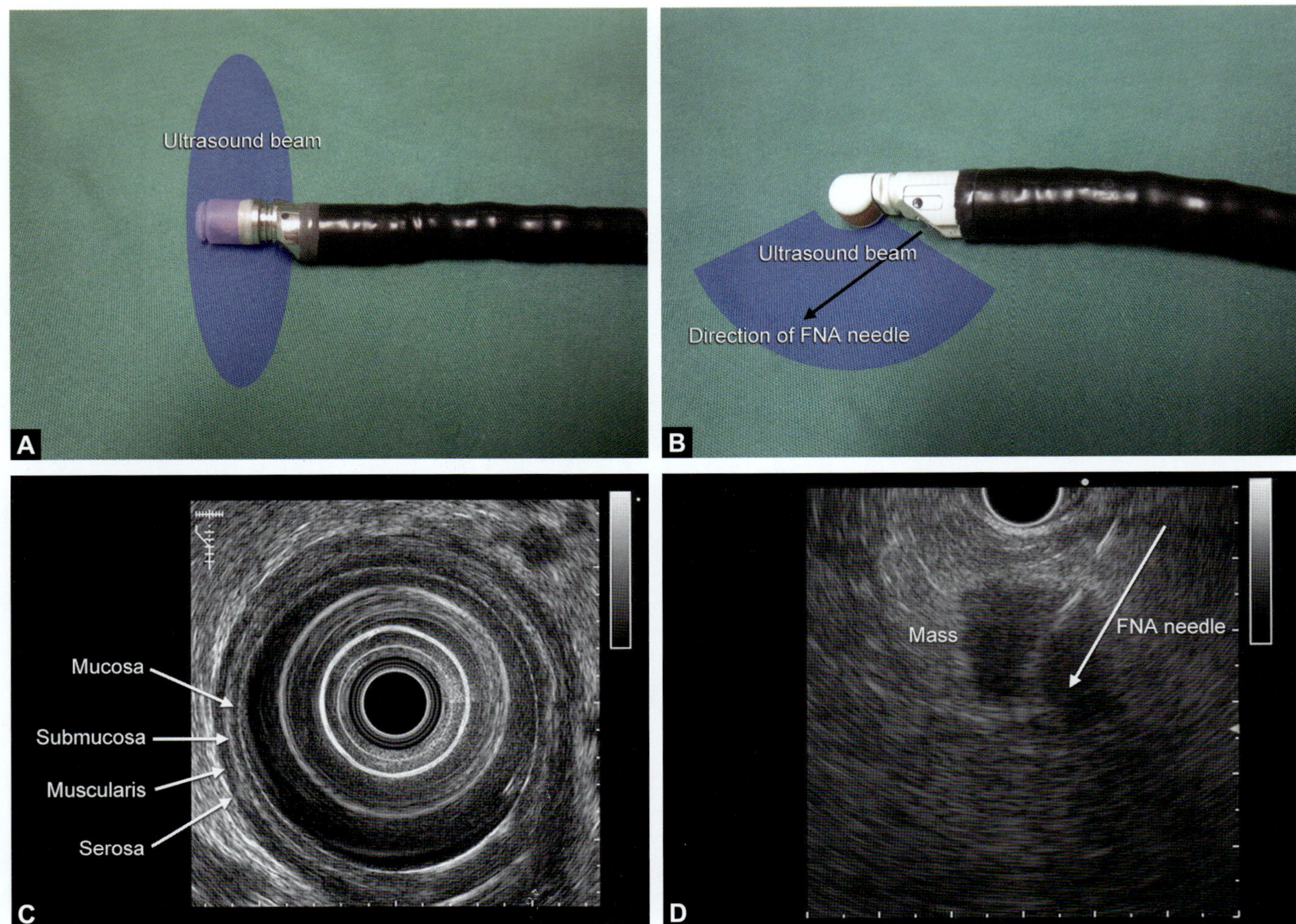

Figs. 13.4A to D: (A) Radial EUS image: The plane of scanning is perpendicular to the shaft of the echoendoscope; (B) linear EUS image: The plane of scanning is in line with the shaft of the echoendoscope. The path of the FNA needle is visible under ultrasound; (C) sonographic appearance of the gastric wall with the radial echoendoscope. The individual wall layers have characteristic hypoechoic (dark) and hyperechoic (bright) features; and (D) FNA of pancreatic lesion with the linear echoendoscope.

Table 13.5 A station-based approach to endoscopic ultrasound.

Station	*Region*	*Structures*
Esophagus	Posterior mediastinum	Heart, pleura, spine, great vessels, and posterior mediastinal lymph nodes
Stomach	Upper retroperitoneum	Abdominal aorta, celiac trunk, superior mesenteric artery and vein, splenic artery and vein, portal confluence, pancreatic body and tail, gallbladder, spleen, retroperitoneal lymph nodes, left kidney and adrenal gland, and left liver lobe
Duodenal bulb	Lower retroperitoneum	Pancreatic head, common bile duct, portal confluence, and gallbladder
Second part of duodenum	Lower retroperitoneum	Pancreatic uncinate, ampulla, and abdominal aorta

the celiac axis, pancreatic body, and tail are examined. The pancreatic head and CBD are best visualized from within the duodenal bulb, and the pancreatic uncinate process and the ampulla of Vater are best examined with the echoendoscope in the second part of the duodenum.

Endoscopic ultrasound fine-needle aspiration of extraluminal lesions is performed by passing the FNA needle through the gut wall under real-time ultrasound guidance (Fig. 13.4D).[8] Color Doppler aids avoidance of vascular structures within the needle path. Once the FNA needle lies within the target lesion, the stylet is withdrawn and the needle is passed back and forth, whereas the tip of the echoendoscope is subtly manipulated to simulate a "fanning motion". The needle is then withdrawn from the scope and the aspirated contents are expressed onto a slide or transport medium for further analysis. Several variables purporting to increase the diagnostic yield of EUS-FNA for solid masses have been assessed. The number of needle passes through the lesion (at least six for pancreatic masses and at least three for lymph nodes) and the presence of an on-site cytologist improve diagnostic yield, whereas the use of suction on the stylet during the procedure does not.

The complication rate of diagnostic EUS procedures is similar to that of standard endoscopic examinations. Care should be used when passing the oblique-viewing instrument through the oropharynx as the tip of the echoendoscope is longer and more rigid than a standard gastroscope. The overall complication rate for EUS-FNA procedures is 1–2%, including infection, hemorrhage, pancreatitis, and duodenal perforation. Infection is most likely with EUS-FNA of pancreatic cystic lesions, and prophylactic antibiotics are recommended when this is undertaken. Antibiotic prophylaxis is not necessary during other FNA procedures of solid lesions or lymph nodes.

EUS for the Diagnosis and Staging of Malignancies

Staging of luminal gastrointestinal malignancies is conventionally described according to the TNM classification, which allocates a grade to the depth of invasion (T), presence of locoregional lymph node metastases (N), and the presence of distant metastases (M). Although EUS is not used to determine M stage, it does facilitate assessment of T and N stages for gastrointestinal malignancies. When compared with conventional radiological imaging, EUS has superior accuracy for T and N staging in many cases. Fine-needle aspiration sampling of regional lymph nodes further improves diagnostic accuracy. Endoscopic ultrasound provides vital information, which may identify patients with unresectable disease and avoid an unnecessary operation, for example, if a pancreatic mass is seen to invade the superior mesenteric vein or if contralateral malignant mediastinal lymph nodes are found in a patient with pulmonary malignancy.

Esophageal, Gastric, and Rectal Cancer

Endoscopic ultrasound enables visualization of the gut wall in five distinct layers and is superior to CT, MRI, and PET for the locoregional staging of esophageal cancer, with a diagnostic accuracy of 80–90%.[9,10] Accurate locoregional staging is vital to determine whether patients will benefit from adjuvant chemotherapy. Endoscopic ultrasound is more sensitive than CT and positron emission tomography (PET) for the detection of malignant celiac lymphadenopathy, which indicates unresectable disease. The role of EUS in the assessment of superficial esophageal cancer is more controversial, and EMR should be considered for these lesions, as it better determines T staging for T1a versus T1b versus Ts lesions. Endoscopic ultrasound is particularly useful for identifying submucosal extension of cancer above or below the area of visible mucosal involvement.

In early gastric cancer, EUS is used to assess for submucosal invasion (T1b) and, if absent, the patient may proceed to endoscopic resection. Endoscopic ultrasound is superior to CT in the locoregional staging of established gastric cancer, although the distinction between T2 (invasion of muscularis propria) and T3 (invasion of serosa) staging is difficult. Patients with T2 disease or greater may benefit from a diagnostic laparoscopy to look for peritoneal disease. Endoscopic ultrasound is also useful for T staging of gastric lymphomas and for FNA full-thickness biopsy of the gastric wall if linitis plastica is suspected.

Endoscopic ultrasound is superior to CT and MRI for the T staging of rectal cancer and complementary to CT for N staging.[11] The accuracy of EUS in the detection of residual or recurrent gastrointestinal luminal malignancies following chemotherapy or radiotherapy is uncertain.

Submucosal Gastrointestinal Lesions

Submucosal lesions are a common incidental finding during gastroscopy. Endoscopic ultrasound identifies the layer of origin and can determine characteristic features such as anechogenicity of duplication cysts or hyperechogenicity within lipomas. Endoscopic ultrasound fine-needle aspiration may yield further information, including the presence of *c-kit*, which distinguishes benign leiomyomas from potentially malignant gastrointestinal stromal tumors (GISTs). Submucosal lesions within the colon can be assessed using the EUS mini-probe, fed through the instrument channel of the colonoscope.

Pancreatic Cancer and Cystic Neoplasms

Endoscopic ultrasound is considered complementary to CT and MRI in the locoregional staging of pancreatic cancer.[12] Staging sensitivity for lesions <3 cm in diameter is better with EUS, although there have been conflicting findings when comparing the accuracy of EUS with CT and MRI for the assessment of vascular invasion or nodal involvement.[13] Endoscopic ultrasound fine-needle aspiration of pancreatic cancer has high sensitivity and specificity and is preferred to percutaneous biopsies due to the risk of needle track seeding with the latter method. This technique allows differentiation of pancreatic adenocarcinoma, neuroendocrine tumors, and lymphomas, which guides the surgical approach or chemotherapeutic options if the malignancy is deemed unresectable. The addition of *k-ras* mutation analysis in the FNA specimen may increase the diagnostic yield.

Pancreatic cystic neoplasms may be benign, premalignant, or malignant, and the use of EUS is complementary with other imaging modalities in their assessment. Endoscopic ultrasound may be more sensitive for the detection of malignant features such as mural nodules. Cystic fluid sampling through EUS-FNA for carcinoembryonic antigen and *k-ras* aids in the diagnosis of mucinous cysts, which have definite malignant potential.[14]

Lung Cancer

Endoscopic ultrasound fine-needle aspiration is more sensitive than CT and PET for the detection of posterior mediastinal lymphadenopathy (aortopulmonary window, subcarinal and periesophageal stations) in nonsmall cell lung cancer, reducing the need for mediastinoscopy or thoracotomy by up to 50%. The left liver lobe and left adrenal gland—common sites of metastasis—can also be assessed.

Mediastinal Lymphadenopathy

Mediastinal lymphadenopathy may be due to infective and granulomatous disease, lymphoma, pulmonary malignancy, or metastatic disease. Bhutani et al.[15] described sonographic features of lymphadenopathy (size >1 cm, hypoechogenicity, distinct margins, and rounded contour), which collectively have 80% specificity for the diagnosis of malignancy but low sensitivity. Lymphadenopathy within the posterior mediastinum is accessible to EUS-FNA, whereas the anterior mediastinum is best seen with endobronchial ultrasound due to air interference within the trachea.[16]

EUS for Benign Disease

Biliary Stones

Endoscopic ultrasound is superior to transabdominal ultrasound and CT and comparable to MRCP for the assessment of suspected choledocholithiasis. Endoscopic ultrasound may be more sensitive for microlithiasis and gallstones <5 mm in diameter. When compared with the gold standard of ERCP, the sensitivity and specificity of EUS for gallstone disease have been reported to be 94% and 95%, respectively.[17] Endoscopic retrograde cholangiopancreatography is the preferred approach in patients with a high pretest probability of choledocholithiasis due to the ability to perform therapeutic intervention.

Benign Pancreatic Disease

Endoscopic ultrasound plays a complementary role to CT and MRI in the diagnosis of chronic pancreatitis, which may display characteristic sonographic features of hyperechoic stranding, hypoechoic lobularity, ductal thickening, and ductal calculi. Autoimmune pancreatitis may mimic pancreatic malignancy, and EUS-FNA aids diagnosis through the acquisition of tissue, which can be stained for the presence of IgG4.

Perianal Disease

Anal sphincter defects can be identified with EUS during the investigation of incontinence. Endoscopic ultrasound is complementary to MRI and evaluation under anesthesia for the assessment of perianal Crohn's disease.

Therapeutic Applications of EUS

EUS Fine-Needle Injection Therapy

Endoscopic ultrasound fine-needle injection (FNI) is used with a 22 G or 19 G FNA needle to target extraluminal structures under direct ultrasound guidance. Celiac plexus blockade in patients with pancreatic malignancy is achieved through the injection of a combination of bupivacaine and triamcinolone, and this technique is associated with high durability, a low complication rate, and a superior safety profile, compared with the CT-guided percutaneous approach. Celiac block is generally less effective in patients with chronic pancreatitis pain.

Endoscopic ultrasound fine-needle injection of ethanol has been reported for the ablation of pancreatic cysts, insulinomas, hepatic metastases, and GISTs. Intratumoral injection of paclitaxel and brachytherapy implants through EUS-FNI in patients with locally advanced pancreatic malignancy has also been described. Case series have reported EUS-guided injection of cyanoacrylate for the treatment of bleeding gastric varices, fiducial (radio-opaque marker) placement to guide stereotactic radiotherapy, and fine-needle tattoo injection of small pancreatic tumors prior to resection. With the exception of EUS-guided celiac plexus blockade, indications for EUS-FNI remain within the realm of clinical trials.

EUS-Guided Drainage Procedures

Endoscopic transmural drainage of symptomatic pancreatic pseudocysts has a high technical success rate and is a minimally invasive alternative to surgical or percutaneous approaches, although direct comparisons have not been reported. Endoscopic ultrasound enables precise guidance of the initial puncture site through the wall of the stomach or duodenum, avoiding nearby vascular structures. The transmural tract is dilated, and a single fully covered metal stent or multiple plastic double pigtail stents are passed to create a cystogastrostomy or cystenterostomy. Using a similar method, case reports have also described EUS-guided drainage of subphrenic, hepatic and pelvic abscesses, bilomas and, acute cholecystitis. In addition, EUS-guided ERCP and biliary decompression has been used as an alternative to operation when ERCP is not possible due to failed duct cannulation or surgically altered anatomy.

Contrast-Enhanced EUS and Tissue Elastography

Ultrasound contrast agents contain a suspension of microbubbles of heavy gases such as perfluorocarbons, which are injected intravenously. An ultrasound wave causes the gas microbubble to vibrate, sending a strong acoustic signal back to the ultrasound probe, depicted as a bright echo signal on the monitor. The vascularity of pancreatic lesions results in characteristic appearances when using contrast-enhanced EUS. Ductal adenocarcinomas demonstrate hypovascularity (dark) compared with normal pancreatic parenchyma, whereas inflammatory, microcystic, and neuroendocrine tumors are isovascular or hypervascular (bright).

Endoscopic ultrasound elastography incorporates software that estimates the degree of tissue axial strain created when compressed by ultrasound waves, indicative of tissue elasticity. The elasticity is portrayed as different colors superimposed on the EUS image. Reduced elasticity may be seen in adenocarcinomas and malignant lymph nodes. The use of the above two techniques is not yet widespread and requires further study.

COLONOSCOPY

Colonoscopy entails endoscopic examination of the large bowel using a colonoscope, for diagnosis and some therapeutic applications.

Equipment

Although the specifications of colonoscopes vary, in general, those designed for adult use have a working length of approximately 1,500 mm and diameter of around 13 mm. The distal 150 mm can be angulated to approximately 180° in all directions. The colonoscope also contains a channel for gas insufflation, lens irrigation, and suction, and a second channel for the passage of instruments such as snares. This channel is usually 3–4 mm in diameter and located below the objective lens to allow instruments to enter the field of view inferiorly. Some colonoscopes also have auxiliary channels, such as additional irrigation channels connecting to flushing pumps, or second instrument channels. Gas insufflation during colonoscopy using either normal air or carbon dioxide facilitates luminal views to maximize mucosal inspection. Carbon dioxide has the advantage of rapid reabsorption, which minimizes postprocedural bloating and discomfort.[18]

Anatomical considerations can result in difficultly in achieving a complete colonoscopic examination, and some colonoscopes have additional features designed to facilitate the passage of the instrument, such as the ability to vary the flexibility of the shaft during the examination. Other examples include a three-dimensional colonoscope guidance system, which allows visualization of the instrument configuration in real time to avoid loop formation, and double-balloon colonoscopes, which can be used to concertina the bowel over the instrument using a push-and-pull technique. This maneuver helps achieve more proximal penetration.

Indications and Risks

Colonoscopy is used to visualize the lumen of the rectum and colon and is usually also able to intubate the terminal ileum via the ileocecal valve to view the distal small bowel. Conditions affecting the colonic mucosa or the bowel wall can be visualized and biopsied for histopathological analysis, and extrinsic pathology affecting the bowel may sometimes be identified. Alternative investigations include the use of double-contrast barium enema, MRI colonography, or CT colonography, but these all have a lower sensitivity for the detection of subtle mucosal pathologies and very small neoplastic lesions, and they carry their own risks related to the requirement for bowel preparation and insufflation. In addition to facilitating tissue diagnosis via biopsy, colonoscopy has the additional advantage of being able to provide therapeutic intervention, such as

Table 13.6 Complications of colonoscopy.

• Bowel preparation issues
– Dehydration
– Electrolyte disturbance
– Renal failure
• Perforation
– Splitting/tearing of colon wall
– Rupture of a diverticulum
– Polypectomy injury
• Bleeding
• Vagal reflex bradycardia
• Ignition of flammable gases

polyp removal, stenting, or dilating strictures, or decompressing colonic pseudo-obstruction.

Whether a diagnostic or therapeutic procedure, colonoscopy is an invasive intervention and has a range of potential complications (Table 13.6).[19] The risks of the procedure, therefore, need to be weighed against the benefits for each individual patient. The sensitivity for detecting significant pathology is high, but specific complications such as perforation can be serious. Although ranges of perforation rates are quoted in publications, it can be assumed that a rate of 1 in 1,000 colonoscopies is accurate, although a proportion of these can be treated nonoperatively if the perforation is contained. Free perforation usually requires surgical intervention, and some of these patients require formation of a stoma, particularly if there has been a delay in recognition of the complication.

Mechanisms of perforation fall into the following three main categories: splitting or tearing of the bowel wall, rupture of a diverticulum, or thermomechanical injury related to polypectomy. Splitting of the bowel wall usually occurs due to overinflation or overstretching at flexures. The latter results from the bow-stringing effect of the relatively rigid colonoscope passing through the compliant but angulated flexure, whereas overinflation usually affects the cecum even when insufflation is occurring more distally. Colonic diverticula are pseudodiverticula comprising mucosa that has herniated through the muscularis propria and are, therefore, thin walled and easily traumatized. Perforation can result from insufflation at the neck of the diverticulum or from direct trauma from the end of the colonoscope, which is more likely in the setting of multiple large diverticula hindering identification of the true lumen. Polypectomy can result in an immediate full-thickness defect in the bowel wall, although more commonly perforation manifests after the colonoscopy due to a full-thickness burn with subsequent necrosis.

Bleeding can also complicate a therapeutic colonoscopy; it may necessitate transfusion or some form of intervention to control the bleed. The rate of this complication is generally reported to be <1 in 100 therapeutic procedures.[2] Many patients are on antiplatelet or anticoagulant therapies, and their management will be determined on an individual basis, taking relative risks into consideration. For example, anticoagulation for a high-risk condition will usually not require cessation prior to a diagnostic colonoscopy, particularly if the chance of detecting pathology requiring subsequent intervention is low.

Additional complications can result from bowel preparation before colonoscopy or from sedation during the procedure or recovery period. Bowel preparation can result in dehydration and electrolyte disturbance, leading to renal impairment or cardiac arrhythmia.[4] Although components of bowel preparation may involve dietary restrictions, enemas, or laxatives, the mainstay of preparation comprises ingestion of lavage solutions. Lavage is achieved either through a volume effect after consumption of solutions containing polyethylene glycol (which is not absorbed by the gut) or through the osmotic effect of smaller volume solutions such as preparations based on sodium phosphate. These preparations require intake of water in addition to the bowel preparation fluid, and they carry a higher risk of fluid and electrolyte imbalance than nonosmotic solutions.[20]

Vagal reflex bradycardia occurs occasionally due to colonic distension or traction, and this is treated by the administration of intravenous atropine. Deflation by removal of some gas should be performed, and care is taken not to overinflate with subsequent insufflation.

Mortality rates reported for colonoscopies vary but are usually considered to be in the order of 1 in 10,000 and related to perforation, bleeding, bowel preparation, or sedation.[2] The risk of transmissible infection at colonoscopy is extremely small, and most likely relates to failure of the sterilization process.[5] Ignition of inflammable gases such as methane when using diathermy has been reported, although the risk is extremely low. However, the use of mannitol bowel preparation should be avoided as this can increase the risk.

Procedure

Colonoscopy is usually performed in dedicated endoscopy suites, which can be situated in outpatient or inpatient settings. Higher risk patients may require the procedure to be performed in a hospital operating room with increased anesthetic support. Bowel preparation must be adequate to facilitate views of the entire mucosal surface. A number of classification systems have been developed to describe the success of preparation in order to aid interpretation of the findings and to modify practice if repeated procedures are indicated. Mucosal views can be augmented using syringe flushes via a portal accessing the irrigation/suction channel, and solutions reducing surface tension can be added to eliminate excessive bubbles. The use of irrigation pumps can improve the adequacy of bowel preparation further by allowing the use of higher volumes of flush with a higher pressure jet, but auxiliary irrigation channels are required.

Patient comfort is very important during colonoscopy. The procedure does have the potential to be very uncomfortable due to bowel wall stretch or overdistension, often resulting from looping during passage of the colonoscope or overinflation. Sedatives and/or analgesic medications are usually given to maintain comfort, but additional measures can be undertaken to limit the degree of discomfort, including changing the patient's position during the procedure to facilitate progress of the colonoscope, or having an assistant apply external abdominal pressure to prevent loop formation. In addition, the use of carbon dioxide insufflation gas, avoiding excessive insufflation volumes, and aspirating gas on withdrawal can all aid comfort. Sedation may be given by the endoscopist, an anesthetist or a third party such as a nurse, depending on the clinical scenario. Patients receiving sedation require monitoring of oxygen saturation, pulse and blood pressure during the procedure, and the subsequent period of recovery until specific discharge criteria are met. Recovery periods can vary considerably. Oxygen is given during the sedation period.

Before introducing the colonoscope, it is important to perform digital rectal examination. Not only does this facilitate subsequent passage of the instrument by lubricating the anal canal, but it ensures detection of anal pathology, which can be missed by the colonoscope, which provides poor views of the canal itself. Reduction of resistance in the distal bowel can facilitate easier passage of the instrument in the proximal colon, and it is useful to ensure that lubricant is reapplied to the shaft during the procedure. Advancement of the tip of the instrument may be hindered by shaft loop formation, and it is important to remove a loop by applying torque and withdrawing the shaft before resuming advancement. Torque steering applied by the hand holding the instrument shaft during advancement is used to negotiate bends and angulations, in addition to using the hand piece wheels for tip orientation, and intermittent suction may be required to concertina the bowel over the instrument and further facilitate progress.

Patients with stomas may require intubation via the stoma and/or the anal canal, and the procedure is usually commenced supine rather than in the standard left lateral position. The extent of the examination may require passage to the cecal pole or the terminal ileum depending on the clinical scenario. The location of the tip of the colonoscope is not always easily identifiable, due to looping, tortuosity, or redundancy, and confirmation of the proximal extent of the examination is obtained by looking for specific landmarks as the instrument is advanced. For example, angulation of the splenic and hepatic flexures is usually readily identifiable, with dark pigmentation visible transmurally corresponding to the spleen and liver, respectively. The sigmoid and transverse colon have characteristic appearances—the lumen of the transverse colon has a triangulated appearance due to the taeniae, whereas the sigmoid colon often has thicker mucosal folds due to relative hypertrophy of the muscularis propria. The ileocecal valve is situated on a cecal fold and usually has a characteristic prominent and yellowish appearance, often with a dimple in the center of the free edge. The appendiceal orifice and convergence of the taenia at the triradiate fold should also be visible within the cecum (Fig. 13.5A). Other important landmarks during colonoscopy may include prominent rectal submucosal veins and the carpet-like appearance of mucosal villi in the ileum (Fig. 13.5B).

When landmarks confirming cecal intubation are not identifiable, transillumination of the abdominal wall may be useful to confirm location of the instrument tip in the right lower quadrant, achieved by dimming the procedure room lighting and increasing the cold light source intensity. Progress may be hindered by the specific pathology encountered, sometimes necessitating additional investigations or repeat procedures, although reaching and identifying the pathology may be all that is required, particularly if bowel proximal to the impasse is to be subsequently removed at operation. Colonic spasm can increase the difficulty of colonoscopy, and administration of intravenous Buscopan may aid progress. Spasm relief occurs simultaneously with a reflex tachycardia, and the medication should be used with caution in patients with heart disease. Caution is also required in patients with

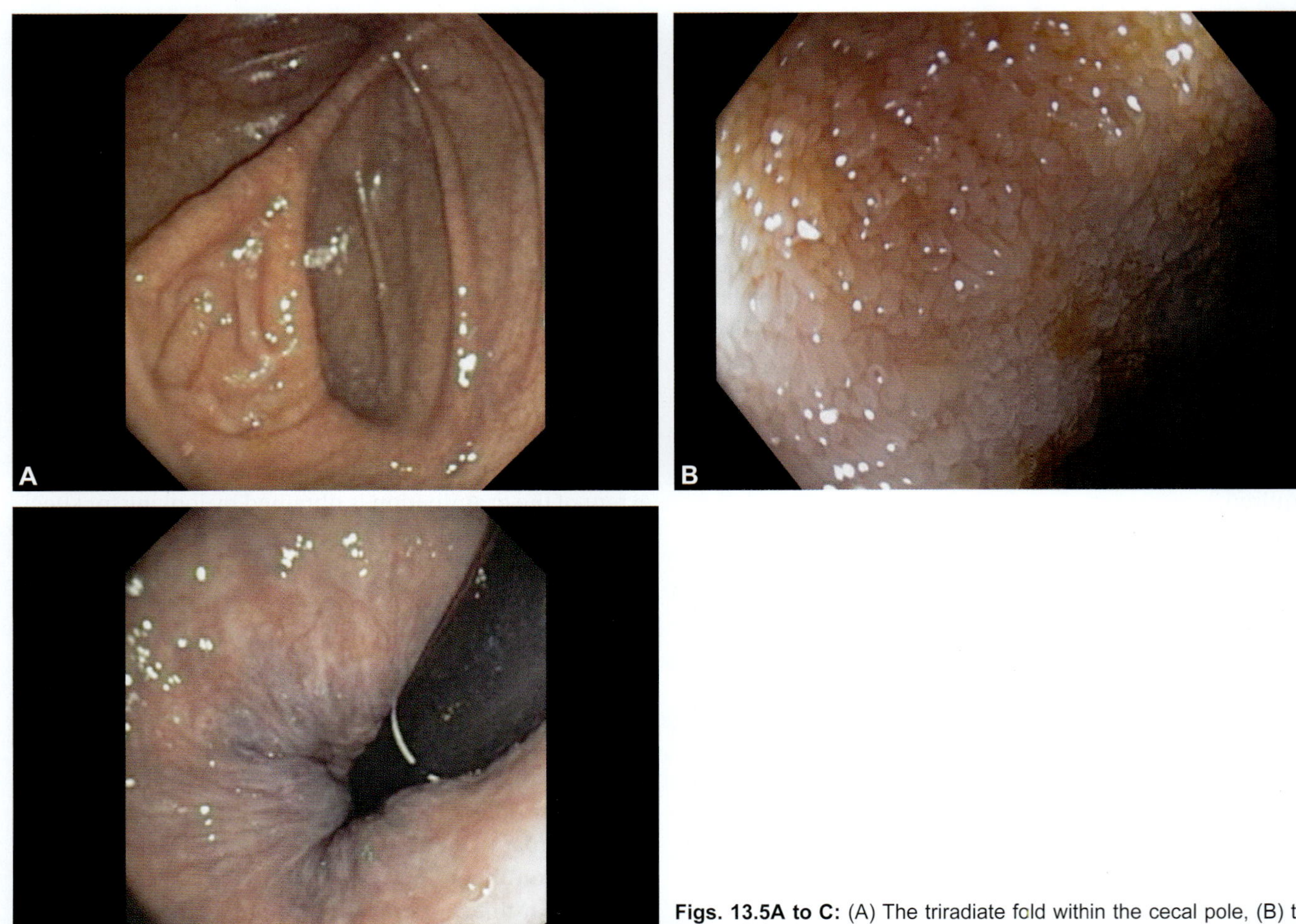

Figs. 13.5A to C: (A) The triradiate fold within the cecal pole, (B) the characteristic appearance of ileal mucosal villi, and (C) rectal retroflexion displaying internal hemorrhoids.

untreated narrow-angle glaucoma, who can experience eye symptoms as Buscopan can raise intraocular pressure.

Ileal intubation may be difficult but is usually most easily achieved by orientating the tip of the colonoscope via the application of torque so that the ileocecal valve is situated at the inferior aspect of the field of view and is close to the tip. The tip can then be steered downward while simultaneously insufflating to blow open the valve lips, and the instrument is then advanced while continuing to insufflate until it is well within the ileal lumen.

Mucosal views are often better achieved during withdrawal of the colonoscope after the proximal extent has been reached, and it is important to use torque steering to view behind mucosal folds. The time taken for withdrawal has been shown to correlate well with the identification of pathology, and short viewing times may miss important lesions. Retroflexion of the tip of the colonoscope should be performed to obtain good views of the anorectal junction, exclude low rectal pathology, and assess internal hemorrhoids. It is achieved by full application of both tip steering wheels at the junction of the lower and middle thirds of the rectum and torque steering once the tip is fully retroflexed (Fig. 13.5C).

Colonoscopic Procedures (Table 13.7)

Polypectomy

Colonoscopic polypectomy reduces the risk of subsequent colorectal cancer but is not without risk and can be technically challenging.[21] Small polyps may be resected using forceps with diathermy ("hot biopsy"), as this can be easier than snare application, but this approach carries a risk of incomplete resection of larger lesions. Alternatively, a cold-snare technique can be applied to small polyps to avoid the risk of diathermy-related perforation. Although endoscopy-specific electrosurgical generator units have inbuilt safety

Table 13.7 Therapeutic interventions at colonoscopy.

• Polyp removal
• Stricture treatment
– Stenting
– Dilatation
• Decompressing of pseudo-obstruction
• Hemostasis
– Clips
– Coagulation

features, which decrease the wattage output as tissue impedance rises due to desiccation during current flow, diathermy should always be used judiciously, with the lowest power setting applied for the shortest duration to perform the required task.

Identification of subtle or flat lesions before biopsy or removal may be aided using chromoendoscopy techniques. Dye such as dilute methylene blue is sprayed onto the mucosal surface via a catheter to enhance the mucosal pit pattern and help visualization of areas of abnormality. Narrow band imaging can achieve a similar effect.

Larger polyps require removal using a snare, and diathermy is utilized to ensure hemostasis and minimize the risk of recurrence. Pedunculated polyps can have quite substantial vessels within the stalk and require adjuvant measures to control hemostasis, such as the application of clips or endo-loops via the instrument channel. All polyp material should be retrieved and sent for histopathological analysis, but this can be difficult for polyps or fragments too large to be aspirated via the suction channel, and may require the use of retrieval nets inserted via the instrument channel. Polyp material that is retrieved by aspiration is collected in dedicated traps, allowing specimen isolation from varying locations in the bowel.

Endoscopic resection of sessile lesions should only be attempted if the lesion is of benign appearance or if it can be lifted with submucosal injection using a catheter with an advanceable needle.[6] Submucosal fluid can aid polypectomy and also minimizes the risk of damage to deeper layers of the bowel wall. Saline can be used for submucosal lifting, although it is rapidly absorbed. Colloid solution is an alternative, which remains in the submucosal plane for longer during polypectomy. Additional substances can be mixed with either saline or colloid, such as dilute adrenaline to minimize the immediate bleeding risk or methylene blue to allow better submucosal plane visualization on completion of polypectomy. Various snare types, shapes, and sizes are available for use depending on the characteristics of the polyp requiring removal. Methylene blue is not a permanent marker, but polypectomy sites are able to be permanently tattooed using a carbon particle solution for later identification in those polyps with a higher risk of recurrence, such as large lesions or those resected piecemeal.[22] The tattoo solution is injected into the submucosal plane and can also be used to mark the location of lesions referred for surgical resection, particularly if laparoscopic resection is to be considered (when localization of the pathology can be difficult intraoperatively). These lesions should be tattooed just beyond the distal margin of the lesion in three segments of the luminal circumference to avoid the tattoo being obscured by the mesentery; full-thickness injection should be avoided.

Other Procedures

Although polypectomy is the most common therapeutic application at colonoscopy, other therapeutic interventions include stricture dilatation or stenting. A catheter containing a hydrostatic balloon can be used to deliver a measured and controlled amount of radial pressure to benign strictures, facilitating dilatation. Stricture dilatation is associated with a risk of perforation, and strictures often require repeated procedures with incremental pressure increases to relieve symptoms.[23] Malignant strictures of the colon may be amenable to stenting with expandable metal stents, particularly those involving the left colon. Stents can be used in the palliative setting, or as a bridge to operation in patients presenting with colonic obstruction. Extrinsic compression tends to be less suitable for stenting due to problems with stent migration, and rectal lesions are not usually candidates for stenting because the distal end of the stent causes tenesmus if placed too low.

Additional therapeutic colonoscopy applications include banding of symptomatic internal hemorrhoids and argon beam coagulation of bleeding radiation proctitis.

REFERENCES

1. Hur C, Choi SE, Rubenstein JH, et al. The cost effectiveness of radiofrequency ablation for Barrett's esophagus. Gastroent. 2012;143:567-75.
2. Overholt BF, Lightdale CJ, Wang KK, et al. Photodynamic therapy with porfimer sodium for ablation of high-grade dysplasia in Barrett's esophagus: international, partially blinded, randomized phase III trial. Gastrointest Endosc. 2005;62:488-98.
3. Shaheen NJ, Sharma P, Overholt BF, et al. Radiofrequency ablation in Barrett's esophagus with dysplasia. N Engl J Med. 2009;360:2277-88.

4. Hoppo T, Immanuel A, Schuchert M, et al. Transoral incisionless fundoplication 2.0 procedure using EsophyX for gastroesophageal reflux disease. J Gastrointest Surg. 2010;14:1895-901.
5. Swanstrom LL, Kurian A, Dunst CM, et al. Long-term outcomes of an endoscopic myotomy for achalasia: the POEM procedure. Ann Surg. 2012;256:659-67.
6. Steinberg JP, Braun BI, Hellinger WC, et al. Trial to Reduce Antimicrobial Prophylaxis Errors (TRAPE) study group. Timing of antimicrobial prophylaxis and the risk of surgical site infections: results from the trial to reduce antimicrobial prophylaxis errors. Ann Surg. 2009;250:10-16.
7. Adler DG, Jacobson BC, Davila RE, et al. ASGE guideline: complications of EUS. Gastrointest Endosc. 2005;61:8-12.
8. Varadarajulu S, Fockens P, Hawes RH. Best practices in endoscopic ultrasound-guided fine-needle aspiration. Clin Gastroenterol Hepatol 2012;10:697-703.
9. Pouw RE, Heldoorn N, Herrero LA, et al. Do we still need EUS in the workup of patients with early esophageal neoplasia? A retrospective analysis of 131 cases. Gastrointest Endosc. 2011;73:662-8.
10. van Vliet EP, Heijenbrok-Kal MH, Hunink MG, et al. Staging investigations for oesophageal cancer: a meta-analysis. Br J Cancer. 2008;98:547-57.
11. Kwok H, Bissett IP, Hill GL. Preoperative staging of rectal cancer. Int J Colorectal Dis. 2000;15:9-20.
12. DeWitt J, Devereaux B, Chriswell M, et al. Comparison of endoscopic ultrasonography and multidetector computed tomography for detecting and staging pancreatic cancer. Ann Intern Med. 2004;141:753-63.
13. Soriano A, Castells A, Ayuso C, et al. Preoperative staging and tumor resectability assessment of pancreatic cancer: prospective study comparing endoscopic ultrasonography, helical computed tomography, magnetic resonance imaging, and angiography. Am J Gastroenterol. 2004;99:492-501.
14. Ogura T, Yamao K, Sawaki A, et al. Clinical impact of K-ras mutation analysis in EUS-guided FNA specimens from pancreatic masses. Gastrointest Endosc. 2012;75:769-74.
15. Bhutani MS, Hawes RH, Hoffman BJ. A comparison of the accuracy of echo features during endoscopic ultrasound (EUS) and EUS-guided fine-needle aspiration for diagnosis of malignant lymph node invasion. Gastrointest Endosc. 1997;45:474-9.
16. Larsen SS, Krasnik M, Vilmann P, et al. Endoscopic ultrasound guided biopsy of mediastinal lesions has a major impact on patient management. Thorax. 2002;57:98-103.
17. Tse F, Liu L, Barkun AN, et al. EUS: a meta-analysis of test performance in suspected choledocholithiasis. Gastrointest Endosc, 2008;67:235-44.
18. Wu JH. The role of carbon dioxide insufflation in colonoscopy: a systematic review and meta-analysis. *Endoscopy* 2012;44:128-36.
19. Fisher D, Maple JT, Ben-Menachem T, et al. Complications of colonoscopy. Gastrointest Endosc. 2011;74:745-52.
20. Belsey J, Epstein O, Heresbach D. Systematic review: adverse event reports for oral sodium phosphate and polyethylene glycol. Aliment Pharm Ther. 2009;29:15-28.
21 Tolliver KA, Rex DK. Colonoscopic polypectomy. Gastroenterol Clin N Am. 2008; 37:229-51.
22. Kethu SR, Banerjee S, Desilets D, et al. Endoscopic tattooing. Gastrointest Endosc. 2010;72:681-5.
23. Lohsiriwat V. Colonoscopic perforation: incidence, risk factors, management and outcome. World J Gastroenterol. 2010; 16:425-30.

14

Vascular Access

William S Havron III, Joshua Gierman, Roxie M Albrecht

Key Points

- Appropriate line placement technique and strict infection control in site maintenance are essential to prevent catheter-related bloodstream infections (CRBSIs).
- Adherence to technique is often ignored in the placement of peripheral intravenous (IV) catheters, but diligence is required in insertion to avoid complications.
- Appropriate indications and technique are requirements to optimize intraosseous catheter placement.
- Indications for peripherally inserted central catheters (PICCs) must be understood to limit their complications.
- As with all intravascular devices, arterial catheters require precise placement to prevent complications.

HISTORY OF VASCULAR ACCESS

The discovery of intravenous (IV) access has impacted on medicine and the care of patients in a fashion that very few advances have done. Intravenous access is ubiquitous in modern-day medicine. Access to the venous system is currently utilized in all aspects of care for phlebotomy, the infusion of medications and various solutions, and invasive monitoring. The state of IV access has only come to fruition in relatively recent times and is the result of ingenuity and innovation through experimentation conducted by numerous medical pioneers.

The earliest attempts at IV treatments were rooted in early interest in the transfusion of blood. At a time when the treatment of ailments still revolved around bloodletting, a select few attempted to transfuse the blood of one subject into another. The first known attempt of IV treatment occurred in 1492 when Pope Innocent VIII fell ill. The physician caring for him attempted to transfuse him with the blood of three boys. The IV transfusion was conducted by anastomosing the veins of the donors directly to the veins of the Pope. This effort resulted in the death of the Pope and all three boys. This ended IV therapy for over a century until Andreas Libavius revisited the notion in his work *Alchemia* in 1597. He proposed the transfusion of blood from one individual to another through interconnected cannulation devices made of silver. Although he wrote about this procedure, it is not documented that he actually performed it.[1]

In 1628, William Harvey described the circulatory system after completing numerous cadaveric dissections, a monumental step for IV therapy. Christopher Wren developed a system for IV infusions fashioned from the bladder of a pig and using a quill for the infusion cannula. His first attempt was in 1658 when he infused "a mixture of wine, ale, opium, and liver of antimony into a dog's veins."[1] The infusion was successful as the dog survived. The quill proved to be an ineffective IV device and led to the development of cannulation instruments made from silver.

The cholera outbreak in Europe led to the next major advance in infusion therapy. In 1831, Dr William Brooke O'Shaghnessy identified the extensive loss of volume associated with cholera and proposed the infusion of a saline-like solution for treatment.[2] Latta subsequently utilized a saline solution to treat the dehydration associated with the disease with good outcomes.[1,3] These events brought infusion therapy from the laboratory to clinical medicine.

In 1950, an anesthesiology resident at the Mayo Clinic developed a plastic infusion catheter using a system of covered polyvinyl needles, which led to "over-the-needle configuration."[1,4] This development serves as the basis of our current peripheral IVs.

Central venous access began in 1929 when a German surgical resident (Werner Forssmann) accessed his own antecubital vein with a 4 French ureteral catheter for a distance of 35 cm. With the catheter in place, he walked to the radiology department and obtained an X-ray, which revealed the tip of the catheter to be in his right atrium. For his unauthorized experiments, he was subsequently dismissed from his residency.[5] Working with Forssmann's technique, Andre Counard and Dickinson Richards applied it clinically in cardiovascular physiology.[5] For their advancements in central venous access, Forssmann, Counard, and Richards were awarded the Nobel Prize in medicine in 1956.

The application of central venous access was employed in clinical medicine as early as 1952 when Albaniac utilized subclavian vein venipuncture for resuscitation and blood transfusions in injured French soldiers. The technique of subclavian venous access was modified by Wilson.[5] By the late 1960s, subclavian catheters were routinely placed using the Seldinger technique.[5] Prior to this, central catheters were placed by passing the catheter through a trocar inserted into the subclavian vein. Further advancements in vascular access included tunneled lines, improved catheters, and the eventual application of ultrasound to aid in placement. Vascular access continues to improve through utilization of protocols to reduce central line infections and refined devices to improve patient safety.

PREPARATION: THE PATIENT AND THE PRACTITIONER

The incidence of CRBSI has prompted investigation of every aspect of IV lines including the preparation of the skin, technique for line placement, and the care of the indwelling line. Understanding the importance of practicing appropriate local skin preparation and the adherence to appropriate aseptic technique is essential in decreasing CRBSI-associated morbidity and increased hospital costs.

One of the most important risks for CRBSI is bacterial load of the skin at the site of insertion. Reducing this bacterial load is essential in the prevention of infection. Many different solutions have been used to cleanse the skin before the placement of lines. Traditionally, iodine-containing solutions and 70% alcohol were predominantly used. Recently, numerous studies have shown the superiority of chlorhexidine-based solutions in preventing infections associated with indwelling catheters.[6] A 2002 meta-analysis demonstrated a reduction in CRBSI by 50% when comparing chlorhexidine and iodine.[7] Further studies have documented the cost-effectiveness of chlorhexidine for skin preparation in line placement.

The studies of chlorhexidine have focused mostly on reduction in infection for central line placement, arterial line placement, and surgical site preparation. However, there is a paucity of data evaluating the use of chlorhexidine as skin preparation for placing peripheral IVs. Nevertheless, chlorhexidine has been extrapolated as the preferred agent based upon studies at the surgical site and in central line placement.

Preparation for the practitioner prior to line placement plays an integral role in prevention of infection. Extensive evidence exists showing the correlation between good hand hygiene by providers and the reduction in infectious risk to patients.[6] The Centers for Disease Control and Prevention guidelines for the prevention of intravascular catheter-related infections in 2002 strongly recommend handwashing before any IV catheter placement utilizing either antiseptic soap or alcohol-based solutions. The use of gloves does not preclude the need for handwashing.[8]

The use of aseptic technique by practitioners is important in infection control. For peripheral venous catheters, the use of clean, not sterile gloves, is acceptable as long as the insertion site is not touched by the practitioner after the skin has been cleaned; this is known as the "no touch" technique.[8] The increased infectious risk with central lines demands a higher level of asepsis. Raad and colleagues demonstrated a substantially reduced incidence of CRBSI when maximal sterile barrier precautions (sterile gloves, gowns, large drapes, surgical caps, and masks) were employed rather than standard precautions (sterile gloves and small drapes).[8,9] For arterial lines, the rate of CRBSI is comparable to temporary central lines and it requires the same level of sterile precautions for placement.[10]

Sometimes urgent access is required and skin preparation may not be optimal. However, if rapid access has been needed, those lines should be replaced by standard technique when feasible.

PERIPHERAL INTRAVENOUS ACCESS

Peripheral venous access is used primarily for fluid resuscitation, administration of antibiotics, chemotherapy, and other parenteral medications. Peripheral IV access is chosen for a limited duration. Placement of a peripheral IV catheter may seem a low-risk procedure, but it has risks for site infection. Thus, guidelines should be used in selecting the type of catheter, size, location, skin preparation, dressings, and duration of use or replacement. The use of steel needles has been largely replaced by devices made of various polymers that provide ease of insertion and less vein irritation. Catheter size ranges typically from 14 to 25 gauge and lengths of 0.75–2 inches (2–5 cm). The size depends on the clinical situation, size of patient, and size of vein. For routine fluid and medication administration, it is best to pick an accessible vein distally. Considerations in choosing the location in routine circumstances include the length of time the catheter will be in place, comfort to the patient, risk of unintentional removal, or trauma. Relative contraindications for peripheral site placement include severe edema, burns, injury to the extremity, cellulitis, previous lymph node dissection, and the ventral forearm veins as candidates for vascular access fistula placement. Typically clinicians will choose the veins of the nondominant dorsum of the hand as the first location for routine peripheral venous access. These are the easiest to visualize, but are more difficult to stabilize and are prone to vascular injury from infused solutions and medications. The most preferred site for catheterization is the basilic or cephalic veins of the forearm for comfort and stabilization of the catheter. In situations of trauma, shock, or emergencies, the basilic, median cubital, or cephalic veins in the antecubital fossa are options for large bore venous access. The veins of the dorsum of the foot or the saphenous vein of the lower leg can be used if the upper extremity veins are inaccessible. Insertion of cannulas in the feet can be painful and at more risk for infection and phlebitis, and should generally be avoided if possible. The external jugular is also a site for "peripheral" access. Placement in this location is facilitated by turning the patient's head to the contralateral side, placing the patient in the Trendelenburg position, and asking a cooperative patient to perform a Valsalva maneuver as the vein is cannulated, or alternatively by placement of a finger on the vein just superior to the clavicle to distend the vein.

There are several adjuncts to improve success of peripheral venous cannulation. These include warming the extremity, tapping or stroking the vein following tourniquet placement, and positioning the extremity dependent to the heart. Topical agents and infrared devices have also been developed to improve cannulation success. In one study, cannulation was achieved with fewer attempts following the application of 2% nitroglycerin ointment to the dorsum of the hand in emergency department patients, with minimal side effects.[11] Near-infrared imaging systems currently being marketed to help with phlebotomy and establishment of peripheral IV access, particularly in children, have not demonstrated convincing evidence in randomized controlled studies to improve the success rate of peripheral IV catheter placement.[12,13]

To manage the pain and discomfort of peripheral IV cannulation, especially in children, a number of agents are on the market. Two commonly used topical agents are Eutectic Mixture of Local Anesthetics (EMLA) cream (lidocaine 2.5% with prilocaine 2.5%; AstraZeneca, Wilmington, DE), Ametop gel (4% tetracaine; Smith & Nephew Healthcare Ltd, Hull, UK), and patches such as Synera (ZARS Pharma, Salt Lake City, UT, USA), and Rapydan (Eurocept Group, Trapgans 5, 1244 RL Ankeveen, The Netherlands) containing a mixture of 7% lidocaine and 7% tetracaine are placed on the site of cannulation 30–60 minutes prior to the attempt. For maximal skin absorption, EMLA is applied beneath an occlusive semipermeable dressing.[14] The prilocaine component of EMLA accentuates the formation of methemoglobin (MetHb) by a mechanism involving metabolism of prilocaine to o-toluidine and subsequent oxidation of hemoglobin to MetHb. It is recommended that EMLA should be avoided in neonates with a gestational age of <37 weeks and in infants under the age of 1 year who are receiving other methemoglobin-inducing agents such as acetaminophen, phenytoin, sulfonamides, and nitrates/nitrites.[15] Eutectic mixture of local anesthetics onset of action is 45–60 minutes with duration of 4 hours. The Synera delivery system, which is available in the United States, is a disposable patch and oxygen-activated system that uses heat to enhance drug absorption. It is recommended to place the patch 20–30 minutes prior to venous cannulation. Side effects of patch application in studies were limited to transient mild erythema and itching.[16] Needle-free pressurized delivery systems are also available that use compressed carbon dioxide or helium to allow local anesthetic to penetrate the epidermis or subcutaneous space. The J-Tip device (National Medical Products Inc., Irvine, CA) is a needle-free jet injection of 1% buffered lidocaine that has been shown to provide effectiveness in pain control and cost-benefit when compared to other local anesthetic strategies in peripheral cannulation in children.[17,18]

Once access has been achieved, the catheter should be stabilized by a semipermeable transparent dressing or commercial stabilizing device. Catheters should be flushed following intermittent injections of medications and with changes of infusions. Meta-analysis has shown that saline is as effective as heparin in maintaining patency, preventing phlebitis, and increasing duration in peripheral IV locks.[19]

The CDC recommends in adult patients that peripheral IVs be changed every 72–96 hours, regardless of function and location. However, Rickard and coworkers in 2012 published a large (3,283 patients, 5,907 catheters) multicenter randomized trial on the standard practice of changing peripheral IVs every 72–96 hours versus changing them as clinically indicated. Clinical indications for

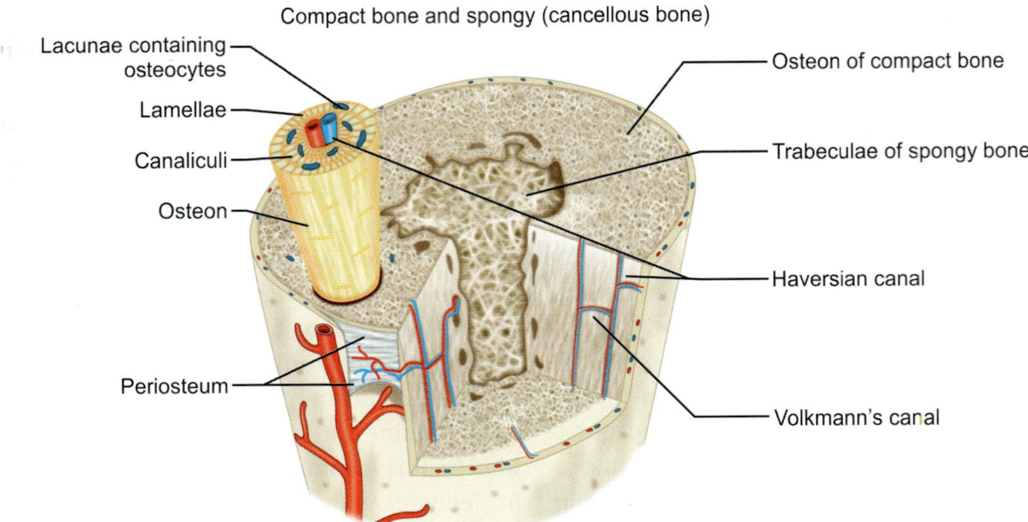

Fig. 14.1: Long bone diagram with Haversian and Volkmann canals.

changing peripheral IVs included phlebitis, suspected infection, infiltration, or occlusion. The primary outcome of the study was phlebitis at the IV site during use or 48 hours following removal. They found no difference in phlebitis, catheter occlusion, IV infiltration, infusion failure, CRBSI, all bloodstream infections, or mortality.[20] The CDC guidelines recommend clinically indicated replacement in children.[21,22] These recommendations do not apply to urgently-placed catheters or those placed at other facilities. Finally, catheter sites should be inspected for 48 hours after removal to detect postinfusion phlebitis.

INTRAOSSEOUS ACCESS

It is not uncommon for surgeons to be confronted with difficult IV access. Typically central lines are placed in these circumstances, but in the context of the acute resuscitation, this may not be feasible or advisable. In the emergency setting, an intraosseous line can provide reliable access.

The use of intraosseous access has increased in popularity. Previously utilized on very rare occasions in children, the emergence of several commercially-available products has led to an increase in its use. Intraosseous access is being utilized in both the prehospital and emergency in-hospital setting. Current intraosseous devices provide rapid and reliable access.

Drinker and colleagues reported intraosseous access in 1922. They hypothesized that access to the intraosseous space would provide a noncollapsible route to the venous system. They demonstrated that solutions infused into the intraosseous space gained rapid access to the circulation.[23,24] Following this work, the use of intraosseous access in the military setting was employed for wounded soldiers during World War II. With the advent of plastic IVs, intraosseous use declined.[24] In the 1980s, intraosseous access resurfaced in the pediatric population and was subsequently incorporated into the pediatric advanced life support (PALS) guidelines.[14] More recently, intraosseous access has been demonstrated to be safe and effective.[25,26] It represents a good option for the patient needing emergency resuscitation in whom reliable IV access is not attainable. Intraosseous access can be obtained rapidly and with a high rate of success. This route of administration can accommodate the infusions of fluids as well as various medications and is able to achieve flow rates acceptable for resuscitation and for contrast computed tomography (CT) studies. Physicians caring for emergency patients should understand how intraosseous infusion is accomplished and be familiar with intraosseous access techniques.

The intraosseous cavity consists of the medullary cavity and the cancellous bone. Infused solutions gain access to the venous circulation through vessels within the Haversian and Volkmann canals (Fig. 14.1). Various locations have been utilized for intraosseous access and vary depending on the device utilized. Sites used include the proximal tibia, distal tibia, proximal humerus, distal radius, distal femur, sternum, and calcaneus. The most common sites for access are the proximal tibia and proximal humerus, followed by the sternum. Intraosseous

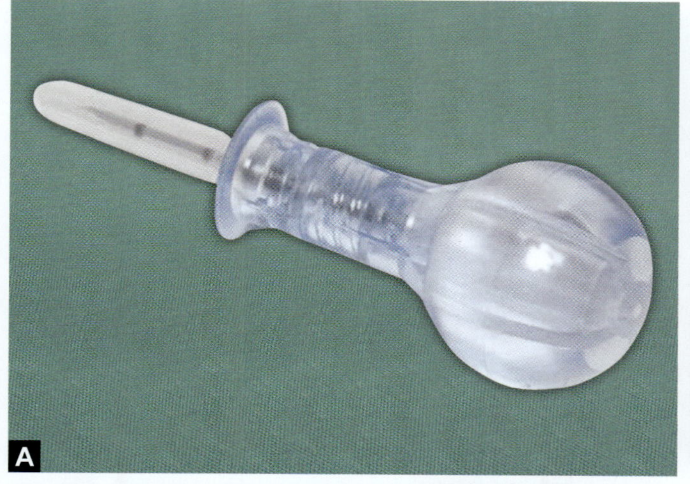

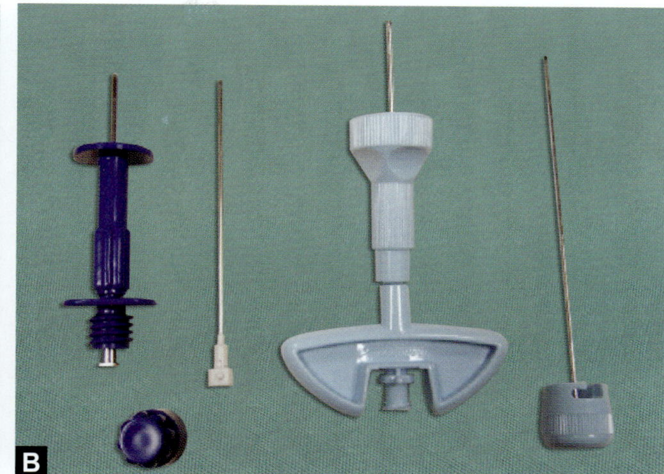

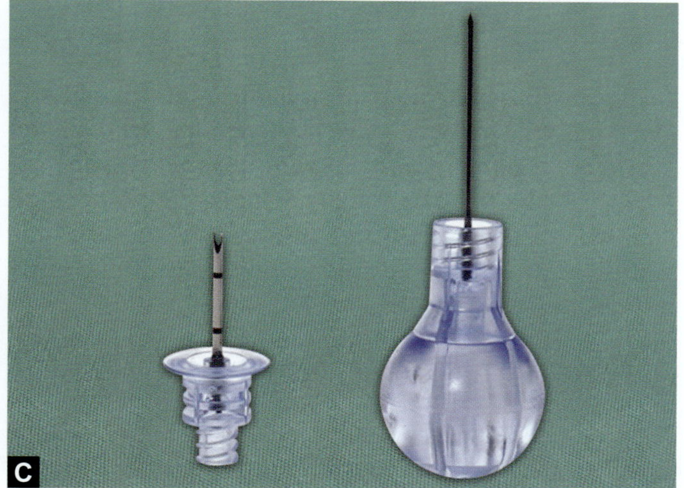

Figs. 14.2A to C: Intraosseous manual device.

access can be obtained with manual devices designed to push the access needle into the bone. These devices consist of an access needle with a central trocar. Once placed, the trocar is removed and the hollow access needle serves as the infusion port. These are more suited for the pediatric population as pediatric bones are softer and are easier to access manually than adult bones.

Multiple devices have been evaluated and found to be safe and have high first attempt success rates (Figs. 14.2A to C). Both drill-driven and impact-driven devices are available for use (Fig. 14.3). Locations of access are specific for the type of device. Currently, the most common locations for access in the adult population are the proximal tibia, just distal to the tibial tuberosity, and the proximal humerus. Both locations have been well studied, with the tibial placement being the most widely used. Ong and colleagues compared intraosseous access to the tibia and humerus using a single commercially available device. They showed that both access sites had high insertion success rates, with no significant difference in flow rates between the tibia and humerus and also that the flow rates in both locations were increased with the use of pressure infusion.[27]

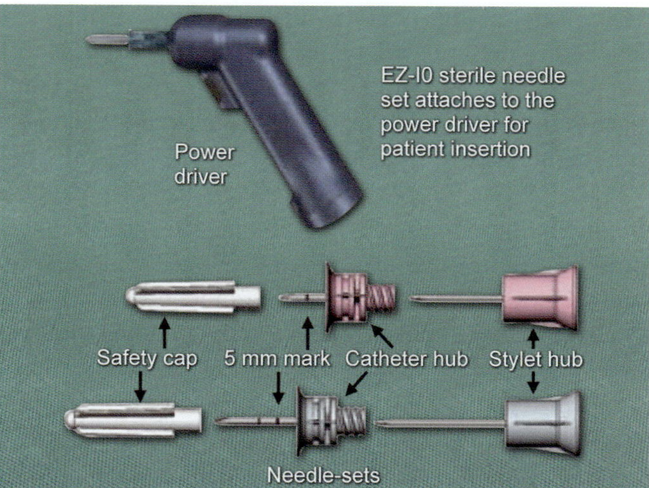

Fig. 14.3: Drill intraosseous device.

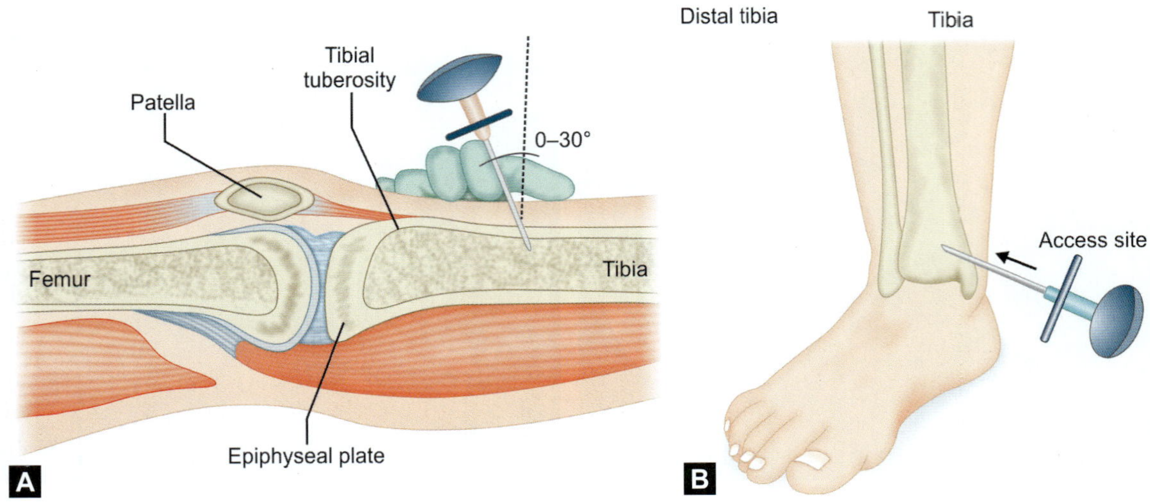

Figs. 14.4A and B: Proximal (A) and tibial (B) intraosseous devices.

Placement is relatively simple. Following skin preparation, the area is locally anesthetized. For proximal tibial insertion, the access site is two fingerbreadths below the tuberosity. Ideally, insertion will be directly between the two palpable borders of the tibia anteriorly (Figs. 14.4A and B). For the humerus, the location for placement is in the greater tuberosity (Figs. 14.5A to D). Care is taken to avoid placement of the device medial to this structure to avoid injury of nearby structures and to ensure optimal positioning. Once access has been obtained, the inner trocar portion is removed. The access port should be well seated in the bone and should not be movable with gentle pressure. The device is flushed with saline and if it flows easily and there is no evidence of extravasation, it is attached to the infusion, typically under pressure. Placement of all devices is similar; however, once in place, manufacturers of various devices recommend different steps prior to infusion.

Contraindications to intraosseous access include a fracture in the extremity of the targeted site, previous surgical operations with hardware in the bone for placement, infection (including cutaneous, subcutaneous, and osteomyelitis) at the proposed site or within the bone planned for access, extensive tissue loss, and local vascular compromise, recent failed intraosseous access in the same location, and inability to locate appropriate landmarks.[28] Depending on the device used for access, osteogenesis imperfecta, severe osteoporosis, and other bone diseases may also be contraindications.[28] The potential complications from the use of intraosseous access are uncommon but include local cellulitis, osteomyelitis, extravasation of infused substances, compartment syndrome, damage to surrounding neurovascular structures, fat emboli, and fractures. The authors have encountered a deltoid compartment syndrome from intraosseous access. Pneumothorax, mediastinitis, and injury to intrathoracic structures are complications from sternal access. Removal of the intraosseous device is advised as soon as alternative intravascular access has been achieved.

CENTRAL VENOUS ACCESS

Central venous access is exceedingly common among surgical patients. In the United States intensive care units, there are 15 million central venous catheter days each year.[29] Access to the central venous system is necessary for both short- and long-term needs. In this discussion, we will focus on temporary central venous access. Central line usage is frequent, and so are complications of placement and the need for care after placement. Understanding the relevant local anatomy and the procedure for line placement is essential to minimize the risks. Equally important is the understanding of various measures utilized in the daily care of lines and the importance of preventing complications associated with indwelling lines.

Indications for Central Access

Access to the central venous system affords the practitioner many benefits not available with peripheral access that can be essential to patient management. The indications for line placement are numerous, and the benefit of line placement should be weighed against the potential complications. Central access is routinely obtained in the intensive care setting for invasive monitoring. A central

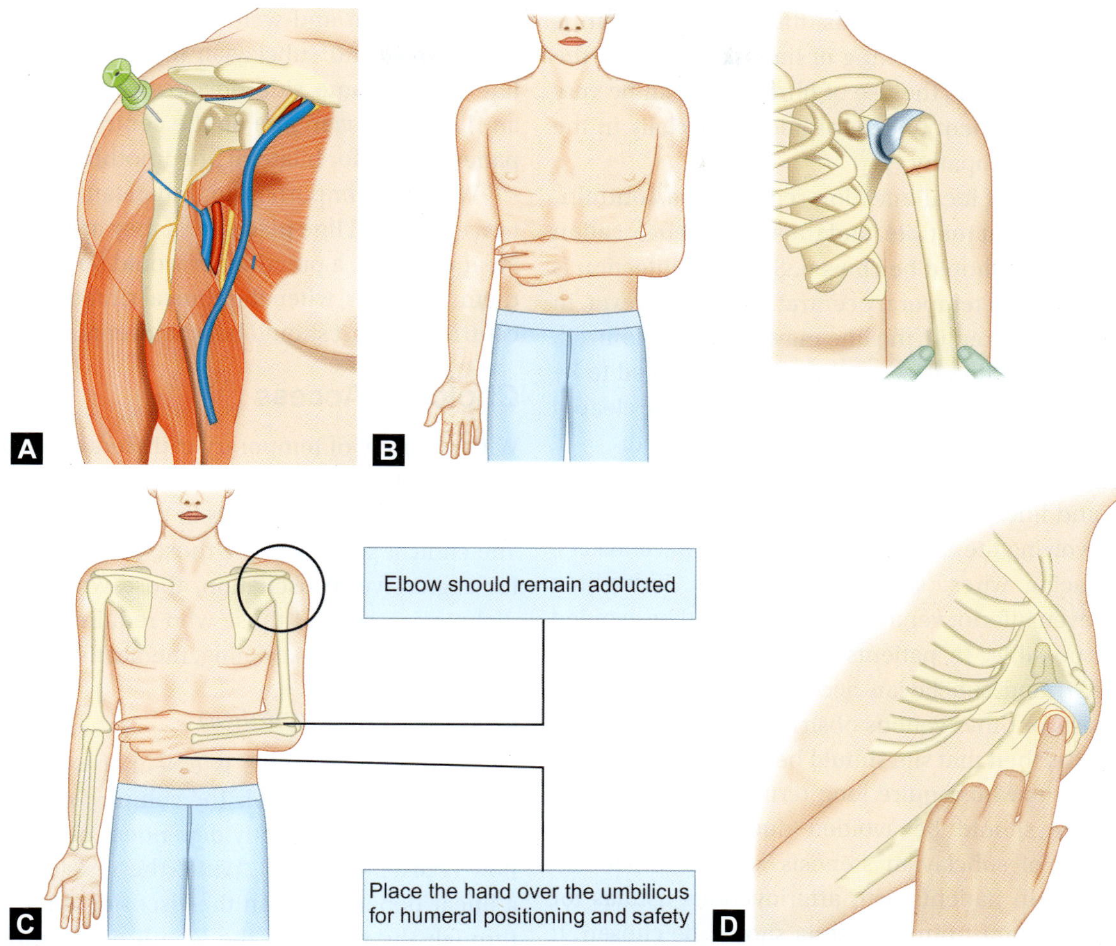

Figs. 14.5A to D: Placement of a humeral intraosseous device. (A to C) The shoulder is held adducted with the elbow flexed across the upper abdomen. The inset in B shows the greater tuberosity, which is chosen for insertion of the device well away from the shoulder joint (in blue) and the surgical neck of the humerus (black line). (D) A finger is placed over the chosen site on the greater tuberosity.

line with the tip located in the superior vena cava allows measurement of central venous pressure. Central access permits administration of numerous medicines that cannot be given through a peripheral line. Vasoactive medications like vasopressors and inotropes are given through central access due to the incidence of phlebitis when given peripherally. Likewise chemotherapy and parenteral nutrition are administered through central access. Hemodialysis and plasmapheresis are common indications for temporary central access. Inability to obtain peripheral access is often the indication for central line placement. In the setting of acute resuscitation, central access may often be indicated especially if large bore peripheral access is not attainable. Relative indications include the need for frequent blood sampling and patient comfort. Once the indication for line placement has been met, the line should be promptly removed.

Contraindications for Central Access

While there are clinical factors that may preclude central line placement in a particular location, there are no absolute contraindications to obtaining central access. Coagulopathy and thrombocytopenia are relative contraindications to line placement and are applicable to all locations for access. If the clinical scenario allows, attempts to correct the derangement should be made before proceeding with line placement. When placing central lines in individuals with coagulopathy, it is wise to choose a location in which the venipuncture site can be monitored for hematoma formation and direct pressure can be applied. In these situations, the internal jugular (IJ) and femoral veins should be chosen if possible. The location of the subclavian vein precludes application of direct pressure and is difficult to assess for hematoma and other bleeding complications. For these reasons, the subclavian vein is routinely avoided in the setting of line placement in the coagulopathic patient. The use of ultrasound can be very beneficial in placement of central lines, especially in the patient with coagulopathy.

The presence of local infection represents a contraindication to access at that site, and thus a different location for central access should be chosen. Systemic infection is less of an issue with temporary central access. However, in the setting of bacteremia, the line may become colonized, and once the infection is cleared the line may need to be removed. The systemic infection should always be cleared before any long-term indwelling devices are placed.

Patients with implanted medical devices should raise concern, and line placement should be sought at a location not involving these devices. Locations of pacemakers, internal pacing wires, subcutaneous ports, indwelling lines, and even inferior vena cava filters should be avoided whenever possible. In patients with superior vena cava syndrome, IJ and subclavian access should be avoided. If thrombosis or other venous obstructions are present at any given site, then that site should be avoided.

For patients who require long-term dialysis, the subclavian veins should be avoided due to the possible development of subclavian stenosis and its impact on future access. In patients with arteriovenous fistulas for access, sites distant from the fistula should be chosen. If additional access is needed in those patients who have indwelling tunneled catheters for hemodialysis, a distant site should also be utilized whenever possible.

Anatomic abnormalities and local trauma can be considered relative contraindications to central access in specific locations. In the setting of trauma, a variety of injury patterns can be considered relative contraindications for specific site selection. Whenever possible, extremities that require operative intervention, especially vascular repair, should be avoided. The presence of clavicular fractures is a relative contraindication to accessing the ipsilateral subclavian vein. In the setting of hepatic trauma or suspected inferior vena cava injury, the femoral sites should be avoided. Likewise, if intrathoracic great vessel injury is of concern, femoral access should be considered. In the setting of thoracic trauma, if central access is needed, an access site above as well as below the level of injury is desirable. In the setting of a known or suspected pneumothorax, accessing the ipsilateral subclavian or jugular vein is preferred, and accessing the contralateral IJ and subclavian is relatively contraindicated. With pneumothorax being a known and well-described complication associated with IJ and subclavian line placement, placing the line on the same side obviates this concern. However, an IJ or subclavian line on the contralateral side puts the patient at risk for bilateral pneumothoraces.

While it is important to understand the contraindications to central line placement, they are all relative. In the ideal situation, a practitioner would be able to avoid all of them. However, when the clinical situation dictates urgent central access, it should be whatever means possible.

Choice of Access

With a variety of temporary catheters available for use in the central venous system, the ultimate choice is dependent on the patient's needs in the current clinical setting. The clinical groupings are those who need central access for aggressive resuscitation, those who need temporary dialysis access, and those who require central access for monitoring, blood sampling, medications, etc.

Lines for Resuscitation

The correct line choice is essential when large volume resuscitation is the goal. The volume flow rate of a liquid through a tube is greatly dependent on the resistance to flow (Poiseuille's law). While the resistance to flow has a linear dependence on the viscosity of the fluid passing through the tube and the length of the tube itself (with higher flow rates being achieved with shorter catheter lengths and less viscous fluid), the radius is also important. The radius is the primary variable in calculating the resistance to flow. Simply put, a catheter with a larger diameter will achieve higher flow rates in large volume, rapid resuscitations (e.g. traumatic injury).

A variety of catheters can be used for the purpose of resuscitation. Typically, chosen are 9 Fr introducers and selected large caliber temporary lines. These lines allow for high flow rates and are ideal in the setting of high volume resuscitations (Fig. 14.6). The 9 Fr introducer can be a conduit through which one can place a pulmonary artery catheter for invasive monitoring. In addition, once the acute resuscitative needs have been addressed, a single- or double-lumen catheter designed to interface with the introducer itself can be placed through the lumen and locked in place (Fig. 14.7). This device permits additional ports. The use of large bore dialysis lines affords the immediate availability of multiple ports. These lines should be removed and replaced with conventional central lines once acute resuscitation is complete.

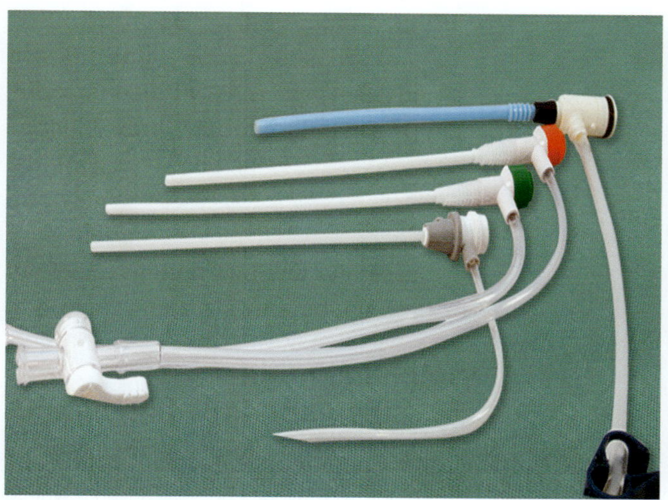

Fig. 14.6: Various size introducers.

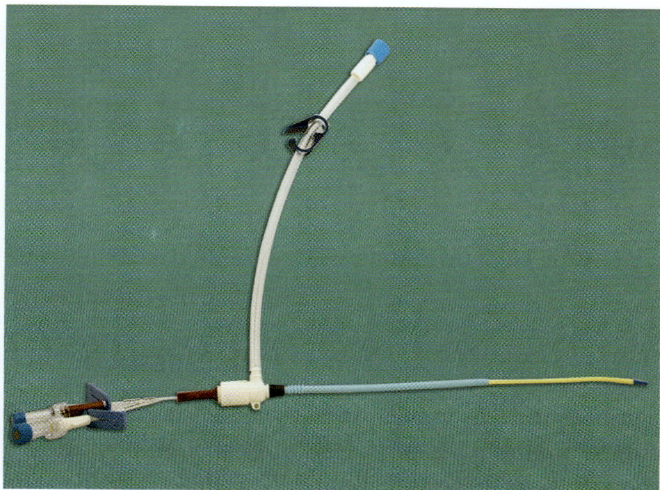

Fig. 14.7: Arrow introducer with single-lumen, double-lumen, triple-lumen inner cannulas.

Lines for Routine Central Access

Catheter selection will depend on the clinical need. A variety of central catheters exists ranging from single lumen central catheters to five lumen catheters with size ranging from 4 to 10 Fr. There is no difference in the incidence of CRBSI based on the number of access ports.[30,31] The use of multi-access port central catheters results in a decrease in the need for peripheral access.[30] Thus, the choice of line and number of ports should be individualized to patient needs.

Line selection can be an important consideration in control of CRBSI. Infectious complications of the central catheter will be influenced by catheters that are heparin-coated and antibiotic impregnated. The antibiotic-impregnated and heparin-coated catheters will reduce CRBSIs.[32] The use of antibiotic-impregnated central venous catheters is cost-effective.[33] Recent guidelines recommend the use of antimicrobial (chlorhexidine/silver sulfadiazine or minocycline/rifampin) impregnated catheters when catheter use is expected for longer than 5 days[34] (Fig. 14.8) Many institutions require antimicrobial-impregnated catheters for the prevention of CRBSI.

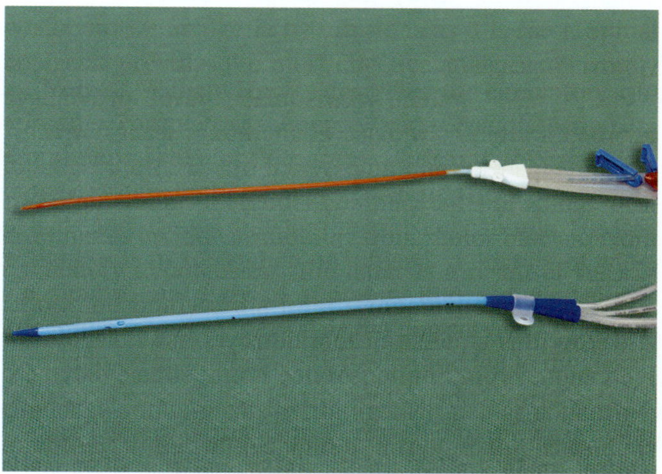

Fig. 14.8: Cook and Arrow triple-lumen catheters.

TEMPORARY DIALYSIS ACCESS

A temporary dialysis catheter is often necessary in critically ill patients with acute renal failure or those with end-stage renal disease as a short-term bridge to permanent dialysis access. A temporary dialysis catheter is placed using standard techniques, but there are special considerations.

The Quinton–Mahurkar catheter, which is a dual lumen catheter with staggered ports to prevent recirculation, is a typical dialysis catheter.[35] A triple lumen version with a smaller third port may be used for limited access. Catheter choice should be based on site selection, with a goal of positioning the tip in the superior vena cava at the cava-atrial junction. Because of the stiffness of temporary catheters, atrial placement should be avoided.[35,36] Femoral lines are longer and should be placed with the tip in the infrarenal inferior vena cava[36] (Fig. 14.9).

The Kidney Disease Outcome Quality Initiative (KDOQI) recommends the IJ vein for dialysis access. Although the internal jugular approach is not tolerated by patients as well as the subclavian approach, the risks of subclavian

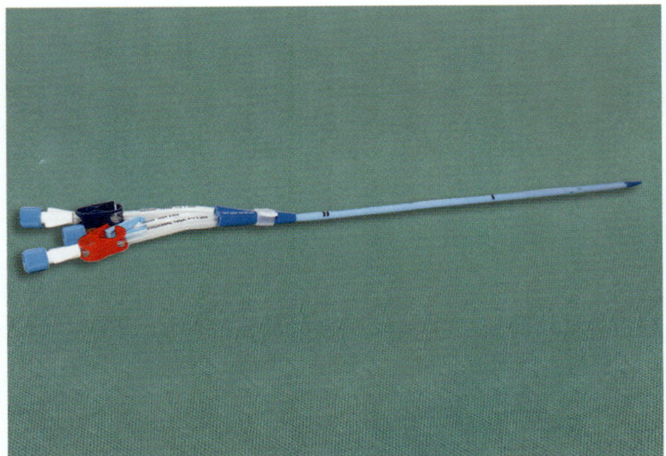

Fig. 14.9: Temporary dialysis catheter.

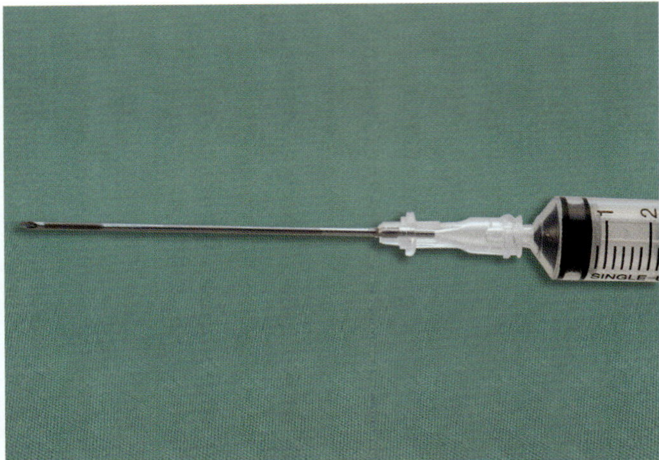

Fig. 14.10: Needle on syringe with alignment of bevel and syringe numbers.

vein stenosis and compromising long-term access in the ipsilateral limb justify this recommendation. Femoral access is associated with higher rates of infection and deep venous thrombophlebitis (DVT),[37-40] and is undesirable in obese patients and those who cannot receive DVT prophylaxis. Other factors affecting site choice include cervical collars, extremity injury, skin infections, soft tissue defects, and pre-existing DVT. The clinician must weigh the risks and benefits in choosing a site for the temporary dialysis catheter.

In most cases, temporary dialysis catheters are placed at the bedside. Patients with a history of multiple central lines or DVT involving the upper and lower extremity (or the jugular veins) should have an ultrasound evaluation of potential access veins. Some patients may even require fluoroscopy to place these lines successfully.

After placement, correct positioning should be confirmed by a chest X-ray for jugular and subclavian lines. Lines that are not in the correct position should be repositioned by a simple pull back, repositioned with fluoroscopy, or should be replaced in favor of a new access site. Catheters that raise suspicion for placement within the arterial system, or possibly with the tip outside of the venous system, require prompt further evaluation. Because of the larger size of these catheters, simply pulling a catheter that has been placed in the arterial system, extracirculatory mediastinum, or pleural space could lead to potentially catastrophic consequences. Contrast angiography or CT should be obtained accurately to determine catheter positioning. If a dialysis catheter is demonstrated to be intra-arterial or in an extravenous position, then surgical removal should be considered.

CENTRAL VENOUS ACCESS: TECHNIQUE AND SITES

The sites available for central venous access are the subclavian, IJ, and femoral veins. The access site may vary based on numerous factors. Body habitus, extremity restrictions, various indwelling medical devices, patient comfort, DVT, and other variables can all contribute to the decision of the selected site. Practitioners should be comfortable with the various location options, techniques for placement including ultrasound assistance, and the complications associated with each.

Temporary central venous catheters are all placed using a Seldinger technique, regardless of the access site. While the various anatomic and technical considerations are essential to safe and accurate cannulation of the desired vessel, the technical aspects of line placement remain constant. Informed consent of the patient is generally required. The patient is placed head-down to avoid air embolism. Skin preparation is done with chlorhexidine solution. Surgeons, assistants, and observers should wear caps, masks, gowns, and gloves. Infection control practices are paramount. The field is draped, exposing only the desired location. Local anesthetics are then used. Once the anatomic landmarks have been identified, the 18 gauge introducer needle attached to syringe is used to cannulate the desired vessel. The bevel of the needle should be oriented upward (Fig. 14.10). The syringe is constantly aspirated once the skin is punctured. If attempts to cannulate the vein are unsuccessful, the syringe should be withdrawn and air/debris/clot from the syringe evacuated before a second attempt. Lateral movement of the needle should

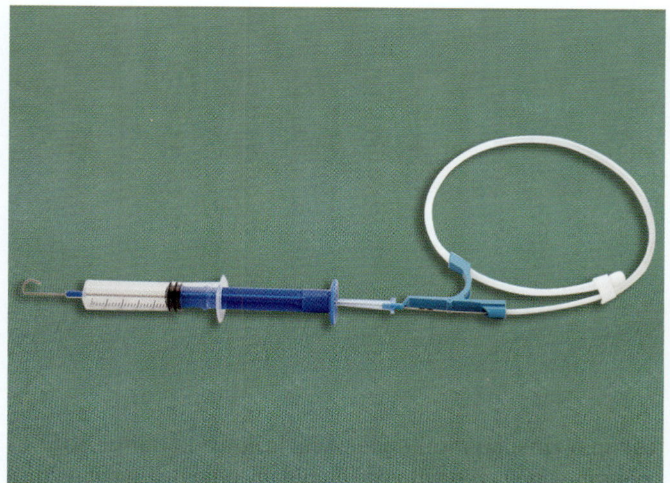
Fig. 14.11: Blue Raulerson syringe.

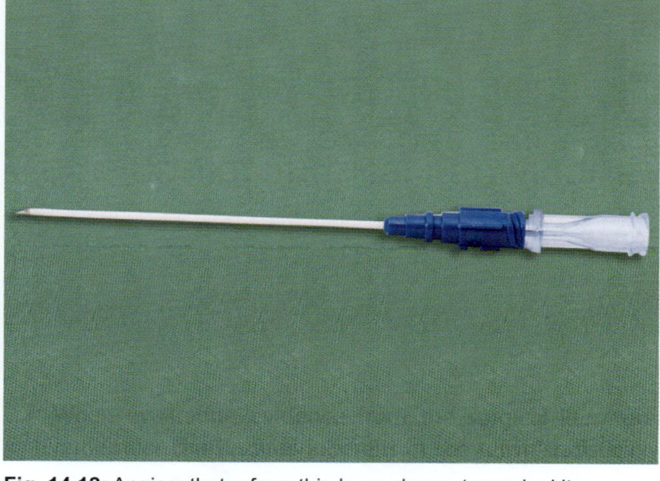
Fig. 14.12: Angiocatheter from thin layer chromatography kit.

be avoided during cannulation attempts as this may lacerate vascular structures. When the vein is cannulated and aspiration of blood is noted, the syringe is removed leaving the cannulation needle in place, and the needle orifice is digitally occluded to prevent air embolus. The backflow of blood is observed from the needle to ensure it is not pulsatile. The Seldinger wire is then threaded through the needle into the vessel lumen.

Several commercially available central line kits have a cannulating syringe that, when attached to the introducer 18 gauge needle, allows for wire placement through the body of the syringe itself and ultimately through the needle (Fig. 14.11). Also available in many central line kits is a smaller diameter cannulating needle with an angiocatheter (Fig. 14.12). Once blood is aspirated, the needle is minimally advanced to ensure that the angiocatheter has accessed the lumen and reaspiration ensures the location within the lumen. The angiocatheter is then advanced over the needle. The needle is removed, the hub of the angiocatheter is occluded, and the wire is advanced through the angiocatheter into the vessel lumen. The passage of the wire should be without resistance. Do not force the wire. If resistance is encountered, the wire should be removed and the vein is recannulated. If an ectopic position is noted on cardiac monitors during wire placement, the wire should be withdrawn until the ectopy ceases. Once the wire has been inserted, the needle and cannulating syringe or the angiocatheter is removed over the wire. Control of the wire is maintained throughout the procedure. A small skin incision is made at the cannulation site adjacent to the wire. The dilator is passed over the wire until the tip of the dilator is at skin level and the wire exits the distal end of the dilator. The dilator is used over the wire to enlarge the insertion site and subcutaneous tract (Figs. 14.13A to H). It is not necessary to insert the entire dilator to the hub as this can lead to vascular injury and complications. If the dilator does not pass freely over the wire, do not force it. If resistance is encountered, make sure the skin incision is adequate. If this is not the case, then withdraw the wire and recannulate the vein or attempt to thread the angiocatheter over the wire and then remove the wire. If the angiocatheter is still in the vessel, the wire can be replaced and dilation attempted again. Forcing a dilator when it will not move freely over the wire can cause the wire to kink and should not be done.

Once the tract has been dilated, the dilator is removed with the wire in place. The distal port of the central line is threaded over the wire. While the wire is held in position, the catheter is advanced from the tip at skin level over the wire, into the vein. During placement, make sure the other access ports are closed. With the line in place, the wire is removed. Once the line is in position, all ports should be aspirated and flushed. This should occur easily for all ports. If one or two of the ports do not aspirate blood, they may be against a vessel wall. Injection of a small volume of saline may be helpful, and aspiration is repeated. The line can be withdrawn in small increments while aspirating the nonfunctioning ports. If this is unsuccessful and if blood can be aspirated from the distal port, the wire can be reinserted and the line manipulated followed by reaspiration. If the distal port does not aspirate freely, do not replace the wire through the catheter as the tip may no longer be in the vessel.

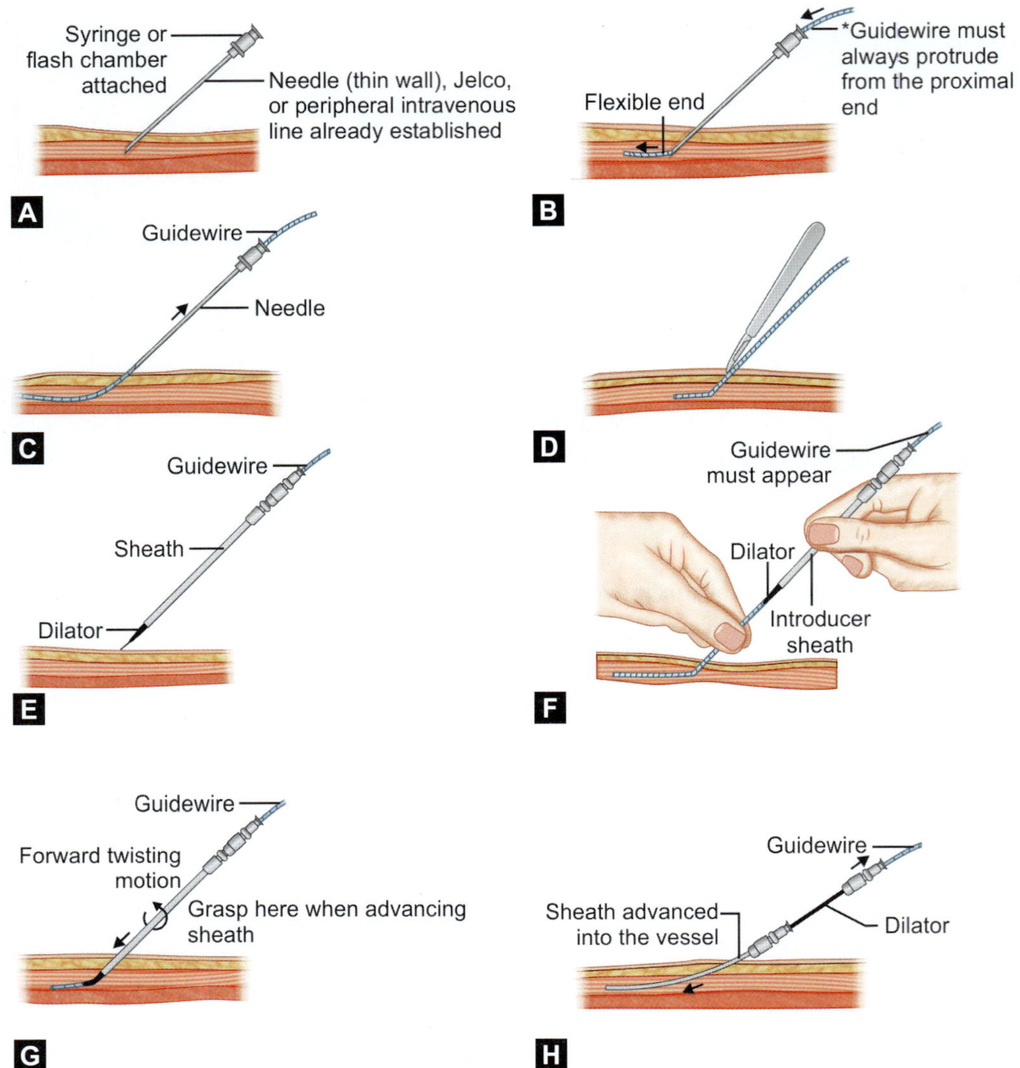

Figs. 14.13A to H: Technique for central venous cannulation. (A) The needle is inserted into the vein. (B and C) The flexible guidewire is advanced through it (B) before the needle is withdrawn. (D) A small skin incision is made next to the puncture site. (E) A dilator is passed over the guidewire for a short distance to enlarge the insertion site and subcutaneous track. (F and G) The dilator is removed, leaving the guidewire in place, and the introducer sheath is advanced over the wire into the vein. (H) The guidewire is then removed.

If the line is in place and one or more ports do not aspirate, there are several options, including a chest X-ray with further manipulation of the line, injection of contrast under fluoroscopy, or removal and reattempted placement. When the line is in place and functioning, it is sutured into position and an occlusive dressing is placed. A chest X-ray is obtained for jugular and subclavian lines, and once the position is confirmed, the line can be used. Femoral lines may be used immediately after placement if the ports can be aspirated and flushed with ease.

Optimal location of the catheter tip can be difficult to achieve. For lines placed in the superior vena cava, the ideal location of the catheter tip is at the atriocaval junction. In an average-sized male patient, IJ and subclavian lines placed from the right will reach the superior vena cave near the atriocaval junction at approximately 15–16 cm distance. The same lines placed from the left will reach the cava-atrial junction at approximately 20–21 cm distance. These distances will vary by patient height and body habitus. There are formulas for calculating distance from skin puncture to the atriocaval junction, which claim success rates of 97% for placing the catheter tip in the superior vena cava.[41] For femoral lines, the average distance from either common femoral vein to the iliac vein bifurcation is 20 cm. Ideal placement for the tip is in the inferior vena cava. For this reason, femoral lines can typically be inserted to the hub. For the femoral approach, catheters up to 30 cm in length are available.

Occasionally, a central line will need to be changed over a guidewire. These line changes should be reserved for malfunctioning catheters and should not be done for the prevention of infection or when infection is suspected or present. Changing a central line over the guidewire is conducted in the same manner as new line placement. The central line dressing is removed, the skin is prepared, and the area is appropriately draped. The distal port is identified and then flushed and aspirated. If the distal port cannot be aspirated, either the lumen or the line is no longer within the lumen of the vessel. Thus, if the distal port does not flush, the line change should be aborted and a new line placed in another location. Once it is confirmed that the distal port is patent, the wire can be fed down the distal port into the vessel. The indwelling line is removed over the wire, leaving the wire in place. The new central line can be placed over the wire into the vessel. Once at the desired depth, the wire is removed. All access ports on the new line are aspirated and flushed and the line is secured. Chest X-ray is required for verification of placement before use.

Internal Jugular Vein

Accessing the IJ vein is dependent on a comprehensive understanding of the relevant anatomy. The important landmarks utilized to cannulate the IJ vein are the angle of the mandible, the clavicle, the sternocleidomastoid muscle with identification of the sternal and clavicular muscle bodies, the sternal notch, and the external jugular vein. The patient is ideally positioned with the arms at the side and the neck is gently extended with the head turned slightly away toward the side opposite the planned site (Fig. 14.14). Patients are placed in a slight Trendelenburg position to enhance venous distention. The neck is then cleaned and draped. Because of infection control issues, the presence of a tracheostomy may make the jugular vein an undesirable site for access.

There are four common approaches to the jugular vein: the standard or anterior, central, posterior or lateral, and supraclavicular. Most clinicians are most comfortable with the anterior approach, but all are effective and with various patient anatomic variants, knowing all can be useful.

When using the anterior approach, the carotid pulse is palpated at the medial border of the sternocleidomastoid muscle at a point halfway between the sternal notch and the angle of the mandible. Using the thyroid cartilage as a landmark reference point is helpful to identify this location. At approximately the level of the cricoid cartilage, the needle is placed through the skin at the lateral border of the sternocleidomastoid muscle. The angle of entry is between 30° and 45°. While palpating the carotid pulse, the tip of the needle is aimed at the ipsilateral nipple as this guides the course of the needle into the IJ vein and not the artery. While aspirating the syringe, the needle is advanced until venous blood is obtained. Once the needle is in place, the wire can be inserted and the line is placed using the Seldinger technique.

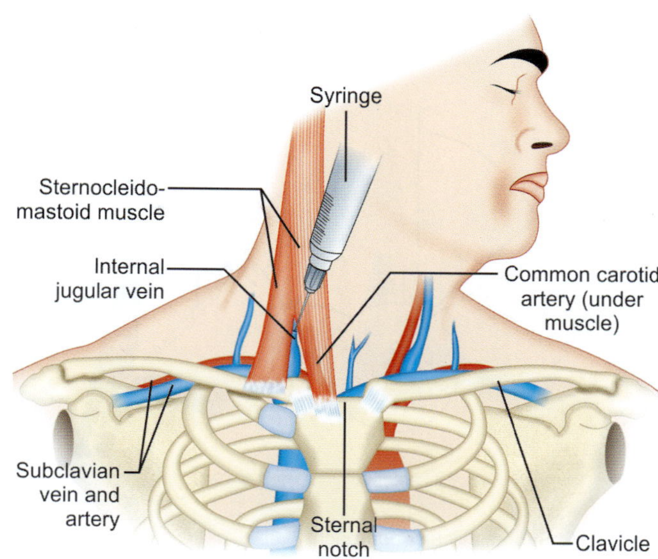

Fig. 14.14: Internal jugular anatomy and approaches.

The central approach uses the same major anatomic landmarks. In this approach, the sternocleidomastoid is palpated and the apex of the sternal and clavicular heads is identified as an entry site. The carotid artery is palpated for a reference point, the introducer needle pierces the skin at an angle of 30°–45° and the tip of the needle is directed toward the ipsilateral nipple. If the IJ is not found, the needle may need to be directed slightly more medially, always keeping in mind the location of the carotid artery.

The supraclavicular approach is very similar to the central approach. The sternal and clavicular bodies of the sternocleidomastoid are identified, and the medial aspect of both muscle bellies are traced to their insertion sites on the sternum and the clavicle. The IJ courses directly between these two muscle bellies, and thus an entry site several centimeters above the clavicle, directly between the

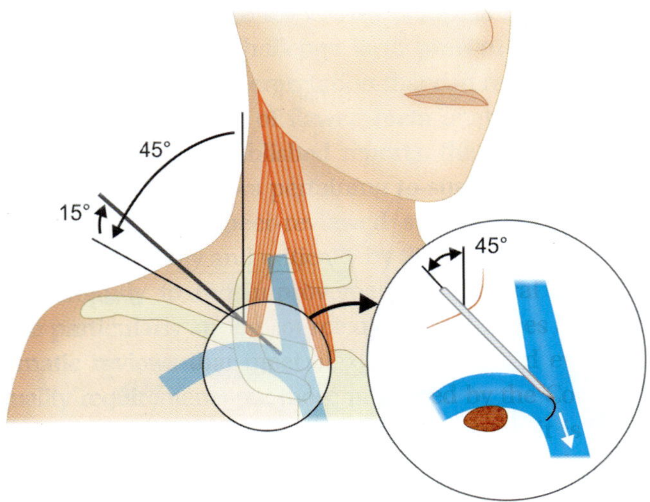

Fig. 14.15: Supraclavicular approach.

muscle bellies is identified (Fig. 14.15). An angle of entry close to 45° is typically used to lessen the risk of pneumothorax and the needle is directed toward the ipsilateral nipple.

When using the posterior or lateral approach, the lateral border of the sternocleidomastoid muscle is identified and the entry point is located just superior to the point at which the external jugular vein courses over the lateral border of the sternocleidomastoid. If the external jugular vein is not identifiable, the entry point can be found anatomically by using the origin of the muscle at the mastoid and its insertion site on the sternoclavicular joint. A point along the muscles course approximately one third of the length from its origin at the mastoid process can be used to locate the insertion site as well. Anatomically, this will be in a location more cranial to the muscle's bifurcation. Also, this site is at the level of the superior border of the thyroid cartilage. With this approach, the angle of entry will be closer to 30° and the needle will be directed toward the sternal or jugular notch. If this course is unsuccessful, the needle can be directed more cranially toward the contralateral sternoclavicular joint or more caudally toward the ipsilateral sternoclavicular joint.

With any approach to the IJ vein, the risk of carotid artery puncture exists. Severe injury can occur, but is uncommon. Hematoma with the potential for airway or vascular compromise, pseudoaneurysm formation, arteriovenous fistulas, and embolic stroke in patients with carotid atherosclerotic disease are potential complications. When the anatomy is difficult to identify or coagulopathy exists, a finder needle can be used to identify the jugular vein. The smaller gauge finder needle (typically 22 gauge) is used at the anatomic entry point. When successful, the needle can either be left in place as a road map for the larger 18 gauge introducer needle or removed after the location has been identified followed by cannulation.

While both sides allow for excellent central access, the straighter course of the right jugular vein to the superior vena cava makes for easier access. The left side, after joining with the subclavian vein to form the innominate vein, courses across the mediastinum before merging with right-sided structures to form the superior vena cava. This relatively tortuous course on the left can make central line placement more challenging.

Subclavian Vein

Many surgeons utilize the subclavian vein as the preferred access site. The subclavian anatomy is relatively consistent. The subclavian vein originates lateral to the first rib as the continuation of the axillary vein. It courses posterior to the clavicle and subsequently takes a posterior direction behind the sternoclavicular joint, where it joins the IJ vein. The vein parallels that of the subclavian artery and is located anterior and inferior to the artery. The vein is posterior to the clavicle and superficial to the pleura and pleural space (Fig. 14.16).

The clavicle and the sternal notch are the most important anatomic landmarks when approaching the subclavian vein. The subclavian vein can be accessed from a supraclavicular or, more commonly, an infraclavicular approach. From a technical standpoint, right-handed clinicians typically prefer accessing the right subclavian vein because of a lower pleural apex.

With a subclavian approach, the patient is positioned in slight Trendelenburg position and access may be facilitated by having an assistant pull the ipsilateral arm gently toward the feet. A small shoulder roll between the scapulae may be beneficial.[42,43] The surgeon performing the procedure will often stand at the level of the shoulder for an infraclavicular approach or above the shoulder for the supraclavicular approach.

For the infraclavicular approach, landmark identification begins with palpation of the clavicle and sternal notch. Access to the subclavian vein via the infraclavicular approach can be achieved through a medial, middle, or a lateral insertion point relative to the mid-clavicular line. The middle approach is considered to be the most common[44] (Fig. 14.17).

While it is important to anesthetize the skin and subcutaneous tissues at the insertion site, patient comfort

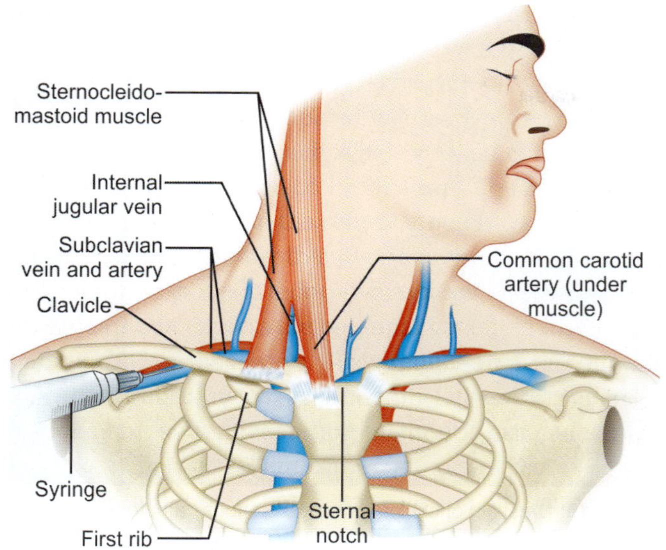

Fig. 14.16: Subclavian anatomy.

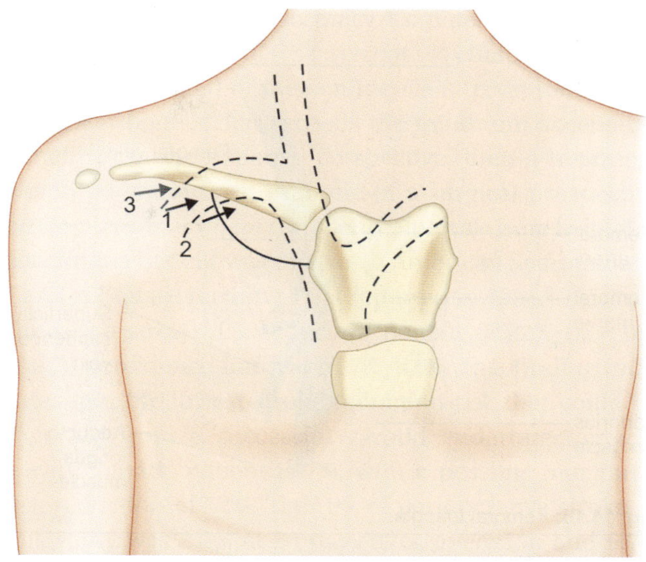

Fig. 14.17: Access points for subclavian vein. 1: Aubaniac (1952) and Wilson, et al. (1962); 2: Davidson, et al. (1963), Corwin and Moseley (1966), Morgil, et al. (1967); 3: Tofield (1969).

is often facilitated by injecting local anesthetic along the inferior aspect of the clavicle as well as slightly deep into the clavicle in the area of the clavipectoral fascia. For the middle approach, the mid-clavicular line is identified and is followed for several centimeters below the clavicle. This point will be 1–2 cm lateral to the bend in the clavicle. The introducer (18 gauge) needle with the bevel facing up is attached to a syringe is used to pierce the skin. Constant negative force should be applied to the syringe until blood is aspirated. The angle of the needle should be just off horizontal at 10°–15° initially. The needle should be directed toward the sternal notch. The trajectory should be coursing directly posterior to the clavicle. Gently bumping the clavicle with the needle and then "walking" it down the clavicle until the needle passes just underneath can help ensure that the trajectory is not too deep. Once under the clavicle, the needle trajectory should remain in the same horizontal plane. Some surgeons advocate applying external downward pressure on the needle by using the nonoperating hand to push in the skin and subcutaneous tissue overlying the needle, thus forcing the needle in a deeper plane. The vein will be typically accessed as the needle passes under the bend in the clavicle. The medial and lateral approaches are conducted in the same manner with the needle directed toward the sternal notch. For the lateral infraclavicular approach, the insertion site is lateral to the midclavicular line 2–3 cm below the clavicle. The needle is still oriented toward the sternal notch and courses under the bend in the clavicle. As the insertion site is more lateral and the target is unchanged, the course of the needle is more of a direct horizontal line in relation to the more cranial direction of the mid approach. The insertion site for the medial approach is 1–2 cm inferior to the medial third of the clavicle. Cannulation often requires a steeper angle of needle introduction to pass under the clavicle. With the needle still aimed toward the sternal notch, the trajectory is in a more cranial direction in comparison to the mid approach. Once the vein is cannulated, the wire is placed and the line is positioned using the Seldinger technique. Dilating the tract is more difficult with infraclavicular subclavian lines than it is with other central lines because of the dense clavipectoral fascia.

The supraclavicular approach to the subclavian vein is less common but can be useful. The insertion of the sternocleidomastoid muscle on the clavicle is the initial landmark identified. Once palpated, the insertion site for the supraclavicular stick is a centimeter above the clavicle just lateral to the sternocleidomastoid. The needle is aimed at the sternomanubrial junction or just inferior to the opposite nipple. The subclavian vein is superficial in this location.

Femoral Vein

The femoral vein is often considered the access site of last resort because of the perception of higher rates of infection and DVT than lines placed elsewhere. Recent studies have demonstrated that the infection rates between the three sites are comparable.[38,45,46] However, the risk of DVT favors not routinely using the femoral veins.[47] Femoral

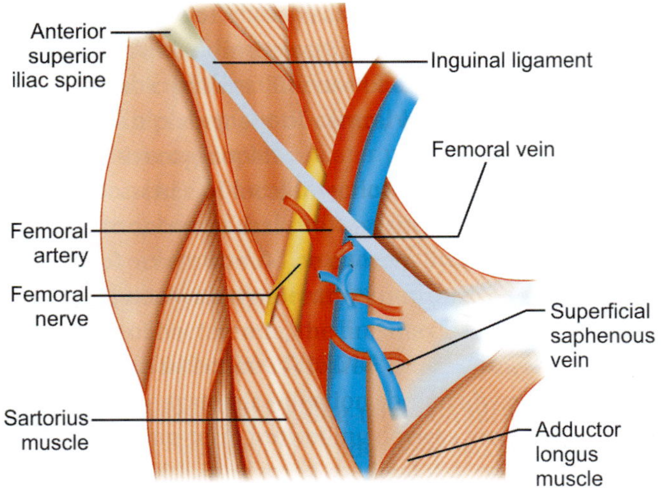

Fig. 14.18: Femoral triangle.

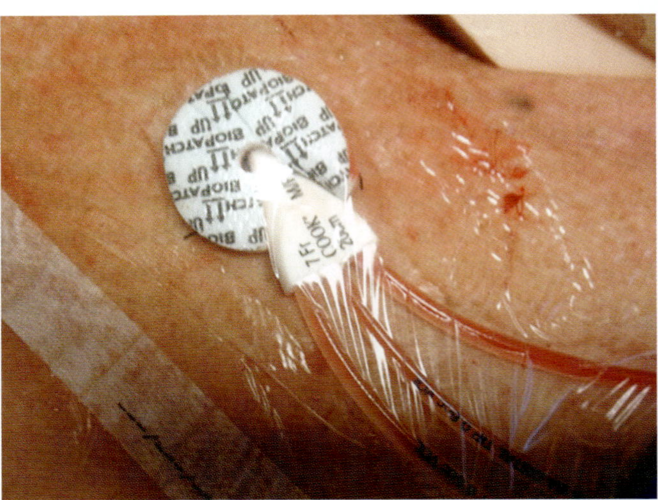

Fig. 14.19: Dressing of choice for central venous catheter site.

central lines are typically employed when there is an increased risk of complications such as bleeding from coagulopathy or when other locations are not available. Occasionally, the femoral site is utilized because of its relative ease when compared to other sites, especially in emergency circumstances.

The femoral vein lies within the femoral triangle in the proximal anterior thigh. The femoral triangle contains the femoral nerve laterally, femoral artery as the middle structure, and the femoral vein medially. The location of the femoral artery correlates with the midpoint between anterior superior iliac spine and pubic symphysis Identification of the two bony landmarks and palpation of the femoral artery are the key landmarks used to locate the femoral vein anatomically (Fig. 14.18).

Positioning of the patient for femoral access is accomplished in the supine position with the bed level. The targeted leg should be straight, slightly lateralized in an abducted position, and externally rotated. The location for skin puncture is directly medial to the arterial pulse and 1–2 cm below the inguinal ligament. The needle is advanced at an angle between 30° and 45° until blood is aspirated. A finder needle may be used to identify the location of the femoral vein in difficult situations.

CARE OF THE INDWELLING CENTRAL LINE

Once a central line has been placed, it is imperative that it be cared for properly in an effort to reduce the risk of infection and to prevent its unintended removal. The rate of CRBSIs can be significantly lowered when appropriate measures are taken to care for the indwelling line. The CDC guidelines for dressing and line care are summarized here.

Once the central line is placed, a sterile dressing should be applied. This dressing begins with the use of a chlorhexidine-impregnated sponge at the insertion site.[34] The routine use of chlorhexidine-impregnated sponges has been shown to reduce the incidence of CRBSIs.[48] Dressings can either be sterile gauze or a semipermeable, transparent, sterile dressing (Fig. 14.19). Gauze is used for local bloody drainage or diaphoresis. Gauze dressings are changed every 2 days, while the transparent dressings are changed every 7 days. Dressings are always changed any time they become soiled or disrupted. Skin care should be done daily with a chlorhexidine solution. Care should be taken to avoid submersing the central line and the insertion site in water.[34]

The dressings and surrounding areas should be inspected daily by the medical team, and the insertion site is inspected at the time of dressing changes. For new onset fever or local site tenderness, the dressing should be removed and the site inspected. Systemic prophylactic antibiotics are contraindicated at the time of placement or during the duration of the indwelling line. The use of an antibiotic and/or heparin lock is not indicated with short-term central venous access. Antibiotic ointment at the insertion site should be avoided except in hemodialysis lines.[34] The routine use of antibiotic-containing ointments has been associated with the development of fungal infections and increased bacterial resistance.[49,50]

When considering infection prevention, there is no role for the routine removal and replacement of indwelling central catheters, nor is it necessary to routinely change them over a guidewire. Central venous catheters should not be removed solely on the basis of fever. If catheter infection is suspected, then the catheter should be removed and replaced. In the setting of catheter infection or suspected infection, the line should not be changed over a guidewire. Guidewire exchanges should be reserved for the replacement of malfunctioning noninfected, nontunneled central lines.[34]

COMPLICATIONS OF CENTRAL VENOUS CATHETERS

Central venous catheterization has a complication rate of up to 15%.[51] Complications can be grouped into three main categories: technical, infectious, and thrombotic.

Technical

Technical complications associated with central line placement can range over a spectrum of severity. Arterial puncture is a common complication that occurs in up to 9.4% of IJ, 4.9% of subclavian, and 15% of femoral attempts.[51] Hematoma formation can occur at a frequency as high as 2% in IJ and subclavian approaches and as high as 4.4% in the femoral approach.[51] The documented incidence of pneumothorax is around 0.2% with IJ lines and 3.1% with the subclavian approach.[51] Other associated technical complications include tension pneumothorax, vascular injury, cardiac injury, arrhythmia, thoracic duct injury, tracheal injury, nerve injury, air embolism, catheter malposition, stroke, and loss of the wire during insertion. Fortunately, these complications are uncommon. Experience of the practitioner reduces complications and increases the probability of successful line placement.[52] The incidence of complications increases with the number of unsuccessful cannulation attempts.[51,53]

Infectious

Infectious complications, i.e. CRBSIs, continue to be the most common complication associated with central access. Each year in the United States, roughly 250,000 CRBSIs occur, with up to 62,000 associated patient deaths.[37] With aggressive infection control programs, improved catheter care, adherence to sterile technique during placement, and limiting the number of catheter days by removing catheters when they are no longer needed, the incidence of infection has decreased. As previously noted, CRBSIs occur with equal frequency regardless of the site of placement and underscores the need of aggressive prevention strategies.[37]

Thrombotic

Thrombotic complications associated with central catheters include catheter thrombosis, venous thromboembolism, and thrombophlebitis. Catheter occlusion can occur in up to one-third of central venous catheters, and is usually caused by development of a fibrin sheath or a thrombus plug at the tip of the catheter. Nonfunctioning ports can be treated with an infusion of a fibrinolytic agent, followed by flushing with heparinized saline.[54] If this maneuver is not successful or the line becomes repeatedly occluded, the line may need to be replaced.

Catheter-associated DVT is especially problematic in critically ill patients who cannot receive chemoprophylaxis, and in patients with femoral catheters. The rate of DVT in critically ill patients with a central venous catheter is 7.4%.[55] Rates of DVT with femoral catheters have been reported from 9% to 22%.[39,56] If a patient develops a catheter-related DVT, the line should be removed and anticoagulation started. If the patient has limited access options, the line can be left in place during anticoagulation.

Thrombophlebitis and septic thrombosis are diagnoses that should be suspected in patients with a thrombus associated with a catheter infection that does not demonstrate improvement of infectious signs with removal of the catheter. In catheters inserted through peripheral veins, expression of pus or purulence from the affected vein necessitates removal of the vein. In the absence of discharge, simple thrombophlebitis can be treated with antibiotics, elevation, and warm compresses. In cases of septic thrombosis of the larger central veins, excision is not a practical option. These patients should be treated with anticoagulation and antibiotics.[40] A Fogarty catheter thrombectomy can be considered for those who fail to improve with initial therapy.

PERIPHERALLY INSERTED CENTRAL CATHETERS

A PICC is the technique that was first reported in 1975.[57] The catheter may be a single- or multi-lumen polyurethane or silicone rubber catheter, which is 50–70 cm in length and between 3 Fr and 8 Fr in diameter. The catheter is inserted in an arm vein and is advanced centrally so that the tip lies in the superior vena cava or at the cavoatrial junction. Indications for placement of a PICC are similar to those of central venous catheters for acute and long-term settings including: poor peripheral IV access, central venous monitoring, frequent blood sampling, parenteral nutrition, long-term chemotherapy, long-term antibiotic therapy, and repeated administration of blood or blood products.

The most common insertion sites for PICCs are the veins in the antecubital fossa: cephalic, basilic, and median cubital veins. The basilic vein is preferred as it offers the largest diameter of upper extremity vessels and provides a less tortuous entry into the subclavian vein. The nondominant arm should be considered for ease of self-care following placement. Visualization of the access points of entry in the upper arm is usually aided by the use of ultrasound. Once intravascular, the catheter is advanced to a pre-measured length or an electromagnetic tracking system is used for optimal tip position in the superior vena cava or cavoatrial junction. A chest X-ray is obtained with conventional placement to establish appropriate tip position. As with all central venous catheter placements, appropriate site preparation and maximal barrier precautions should be followed. Once placed, the PICC is secured by an anchoring suture or a sutureless fixation device. Sterile, transparent, semipermeable, self-adhesive, polyurethane dressings should be used unless contraindications exist. Dressing changes should be done using aseptic techniques every 7–14 days or if the dressing becomes damp, loosened, no longer occlusive or adherent, soiled, or there is fluid accumulation beneath the dressing. Patients who are discharged home with PICCs undergo dressing changes in outpatient clinics by visiting nurses or are given explicit written and pictorial instructions for self-managed dressing changes, catheter care, and indications to notify healthcare professionals. PICCs may have an indwelling longevity for weeks-to-months with proper management. The use of PICCs in the hospital setting has grown steadily in an attempt to supplement high-risk traditional nontunneled, multiple-lumen central venous catheters for prolonged IV access and cost-effectiveness compared with other central venous catheters.[58-61]

Complications of PICC lines are similar to other central lines including dislodgment, malpositioning, catheter fracture, catheter occlusion, mechanical phlebitis, DVT, and CRBSI. Venous thrombosis has been attributed to the venipuncture, size of the catheter, the friction contact between the PICC and the inner lining of the vein due to the movement of the arm together with the obstruction to normal blood flow. Mural thrombus presents as swelling of the extremity distal to the point of the occlusion.[62] A systemic review and meta-analysis of the risk of venous thromboembolism associated with PICCs found an association with a higher risk of DVT than central venous catheters, especially in the critically ill or those with malignancy. The weighted frequency of PICC-related DVT was 13.9% in the critically ill patients and 6.7% in patients with cancer. However, despite the prevalence of DVT, pulmonary embolism is infrequent with PICCs. Clinicians should take into consideration the higher risk of thrombosis in patients who are critically ill or those with malignancy against the benefit of a PICC versus a conventional central line access device.

Intraluminal thrombus may form inside the catheter and result in inability to draw blood from the catheter due to partial or complete occlusion. Instillation of alteplase, a fibrinolytic agent, may be successful at resolving the occlusion and preventing removal of the catheter.[63] PICCs are considered a central line, and thus PICC line infections are included in data regarding CRBSI. Some evidence suggests that PICCs are associated with a lower risk of CRBSI than other devices,[64] and thus the use of PICCs in the acute care setting is a safe alternative to high-risk short-term central venous catheters.[65,66] Other studies have shown a higher risk of CRBSI with PICC versus standard central lines.[67,68] Chopra and colleagues performed a systematic review and meta-analysis of 23 unique studies involving 57,250 patients reporting the occurrence of CRBSI in patients with PICCs compared with conventional central lines.[69] They reported a 10-fold greater risk of CRBSI among hospitalized patients (5.2%) than among outpatients who received PICCs (0.5%). Additionally, hospitalized patients who underwent PICC placement experienced CRBSI rates that statistically paralleled those associated with conventional central catheters. Overall the unweighted incidence of PICC-related CRBSI among hospitalized patients was 5.2% (76 of 1473) versus 5.8% (76 of 1302) in those who received central lines. Rates of PICC-associated CRBSI relative to conventional central line CRBSI were similar for patients with cancer, those who were critically ill, and those requiring total parenteral nutrition. Outpatients experienced a lower percentage of CRBSI events with PICCs (0.5%) than with central lines (2.1%). The increased infection risk in the hospital setting must be considered when choosing a PICC over standard peripheral access.

ARTERIAL LINES

Arterial lines are commonly used in the care of the critically ill patients. They are utilized for continuous invasive blood pressure monitoring and frequent blood sampling including arterial blood gases. More recently, they have been employed with a variety of devices to follow stroke volume variation, cardiac output, and cardiac index. They are used in many different hospital settings including the emergency room, the care of critically ill patients in the intensive care unit, and in the operating room.

The indications for placing arterial lines are widely varied within the hospitalized patient population. They can be applied in the care of patients in shock, those individuals undergoing extensive operative procedures, traumatic brain injuries, unstable hemodynamic status, respiratory failure, the need for serial arterial blood gases, patients undergoing resuscitation, hypertensive crises, the use of vasoactive medications, and in the high-risk or elderly population.

Arterial line placement can be performed through a percutaneous approach or, less commonly, after cutdown. Locations for placement are varied, but the most common locations are in the radial artery, femoral artery, and the dorsalis pedis. Other sites have been utilized including the brachial artery, axillary artery, and the ulnar artery; however, these sites are discouraged for use.

The radial artery is the predominant site chosen for placement. The superficial nature of the artery as well as the collateral vascular supply distally makes the radial artery the ideal initial choice. The collateral circulation within the hand provides the optimal setting for monitoring through one arterial source, while minimizing the risk of distal ischemia. This premise is dependent on an intact palmer arch and adequate collateral flow. These features can be assessed before performing the procedure by completing an Allen's test. The Allen's test is done by digital compression of the patient's radial and ulnar arteries. With inflow occluded, the patient is asked to make a fist and then relax the hand. Once the hand is pale, the practitioner releases the inflow occlusion of the ulnar artery. If the palmar circulation is intact, there should be brisk return of flow to the hand despite continued occlusion of the radial artery.

Barone and colleagues[70] reviewed the utility of Allen's test and concluded that it should not be considered the standard of care when placing radial arterial lines because (1) the criteria for the test are not agreed upon, (2) the relevance of an equivocal result is unclear, (3) it does not accurately predict the development of hand ischemia, and (4) critically ill patients are unable to participate in the examination.[70] Given these factors, performing the test before placement of an arterial line does not ensure that the patient will not develop an ischemic complication, but it may provide useful information about perfusion to the hand.

To place a radial arterial line, the patient's wrist is gently extended (dorsiflexed) with the palm facing up. The skin is cleaned and draped. The goal should be a percutaneous approach, with cut downs reserved for emergency access needs. There are arterial line systems that are completely contained with the needle, wire, and catheter together and others with the components separate. The radial artery is palpated and the location for planned access is identified. Local anesthetic is used in conscious patients. Cannulation of the radial artery should be attempted distally toward the wrist, but then more proximally if unsuccessful. The entry into the skin and artery should be at an angle of 30°–60°, and the needle should be advanced until arterial flow is encountered. Once cannulation is completed, the wire should be advanced and the catheter is advanced over the wire using the Seldinger technique (Fig. 14.20). Typically, a 20 gauge catheter is utilized in adult patients. Once in place, the wire is withdrawn, the catheter is connected to the transducer, and the system is calibrated. The catheter is sutured into position, and a sterile dressing is applied.

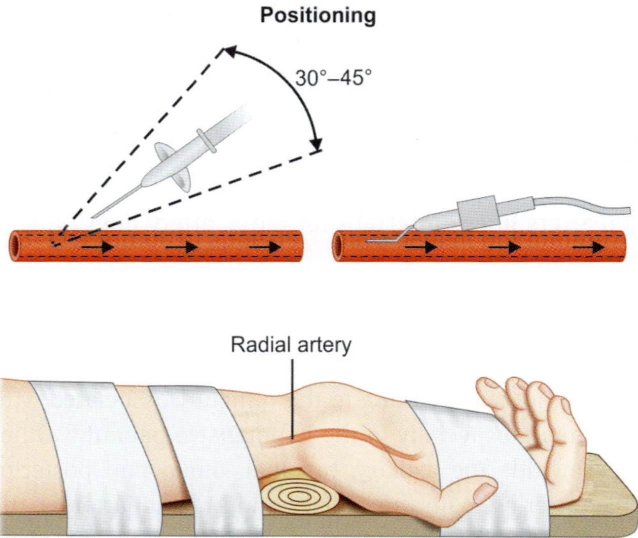

Fig. 14.20: Radial artery placement.

While complications of radial arterial line placement are uncommon, the hand should be inspected routinely for signs of ischemia and other complications. The main complications documented include permanent ischemic changes, temporary occlusion (thrombosis), sepsis, local infection, pseudoaneurysm, hematoma, and bleeding. The most common complication is temporary occlusion of the artery, with a documented occurrence rate between 1.5% and 35% depending on the source.[71] If evidence of a complication arises, the catheter should be removed and replaced elsewhere.

The easy accessibility of the femoral artery makes it an appealing choice for arterial cannulation. The femoral artery line is placed in similar fashion to the radial arterial line, although the system utilized typically requires cannulation of the femoral artery with a needle and syringe. The procedure begins by identifying a femoral pulse. The vein is medial to the arterial pulse. The area is widely cleaned and draped. Insertion of the needle should be approximately 1–2 cm below the inguinal ligament to avoid the retroperitoneal space (Fig. 14.21). Once cannulated, the syringe is removed, pulsatile flow is noted from the needle, and then a wire is placed through the needle. The remainder of the procedure is continued with placement of the catheter over the wire using the Seldinger technique. The catheter used for femoral lines is longer (12 cm) than the short catheter of other arterial lines. The complications associated with femoral artery lines are similar to those with radial line placement. It is important to note that bleeding after femoral placement can occur into the retroperitoneum and thus may not be readily identified. Another consideration with femoral arterial puncture is that atherosclerotic disease of the vessel poses a risk for embolic events distally. A meta-analysis evaluated the common complications associated with all arterial line placement showed that the mean incidence of permanent ischemic injury was 0.18% (3/1,664 patients) for femoral artery lines and 0.09% for radial artery lines (4/4217 patients).[71]

The dorsalis pedis artery has been utilized for arterial monitoring with very low complication rates; it is completed similarly to the radial artery line.[71] This location is often not selected due to the difficulty associated with placement, especially in the hypotensive patient.[71] Other sites include the axillary, brachial, ulnar, and posterior tibial arteries. With the axillary and brachial arteries, the concern for limited collateral circulation to the distal upper extremity should be considered, and use should be reserved in those patients in whom the radial and femoral sites are not available. With the ulnar artery often being the dominant supply to the hand, this artery is typically avoided.

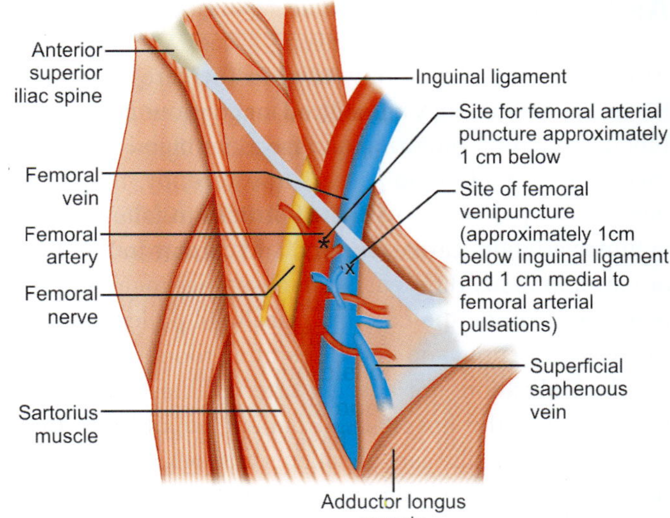

Fig. 14.21: Femoral arterial line position (below inguinal ligament).

The use of ultrasound in the placement of arterial lines has been advocated. A prospective randomized study evaluated the placement of radial arterial lines by blind palpation compared to placement with ultrasound guidance.[72] The ultrasound group had a shorter time required for placement, fewer attempts were needed, and fewer sites were required for placement. All results reached statistical significance. While not reporting complications, the data does appear to show the use of ultrasound to be beneficial in the placement of radial arterial lines. Further studies are needed to evaluate benefit in reduction in complications. Once arterial lines are in place, line care is conducted similarly to that of central venous lines.[71]

Arterial lines should be changed when the clinical scenario dictates. Eyer and colleagues showed in a randomized, prospective study that there is no difference in infection rates between scheduled arterial catheter changes and in those changed when needed.[73] Thus, the practitioner has to be vigilant daily for the development of complications.

ULTRASOUND GUIDANCE

Ultrasound scanning has been employed in all aspects of vascular access from peripheral IVs to image-guided cannulation for central access. While the landmark-based approach has been utilized for many years in the placement of central lines, the associated complication rate has many searching for a way to improve the technique. The use of ultrasound guidance was first documented in the 1980s, and since that time numerous studies have been conducted to evaluate its effectiveness.

Each year in the United States over 5 million central venous lines are placed, with an associated overall complication rate of approximately 15%.[51] Several well-conducted studies have demonstrated a reduction in complications as well as a higher rate of successful first attempts when ultrasound guidance is used, especially for placement in the IJ vein. This extensive body of literature has led to several organizations, including the American College of Surgeons, to release statements in support of ultrasound guidance for the placement of central venous catheters. The use of ultrasound guidance in the placement of central lines was advocated by the Agency for Healthcare Research and Quality in 2001, when they recommended the practice as one of the top 11 evidence-based practices that improve patient care and safety.[74]

Clinically, the use of ultrasound is most effective when cannulating the IJ vein; however, it is effective in all locations. Ultrasound scanning allows the practitioner to identify the anatomy, assess the patency of the venous structures, view the puncture of the vein, and wire placement. While ultrasound is a very helpful tool, it does not obviate the need for a comprehensive understanding of local anatomy or the proper technique for line placement.

The ultrasound probe can be used initially to identify the intended targeted vessel. Using the probe and the known anatomical landmarks, a practitioner can identify the location for line placement and determine if the intended vessel is appropriate. After the desired location has been prepared and draped, the ultrasound probe with sterile cover is placed over the intended access site and the area scanned. When the desired location has been identified, gentle compression of the probe against the skin will show the compressible nature of venous structures in contrast to their arterial counterparts. This maneuver is also important to ensure that the vein is patent and is appropriate for line placement. With the probe in place, the placement of the line is undertaken in the same routine fashion as previously discussed. With this technique, the introducer needle can be seen with the probe and can be guided toward the vein; cannulation of the vein can then be observed. Once the vein has been cannulated, the placement of the wire into the vein can also be seen and the wire can be tracked within the lumen of the vessel to ensure proper placement (Fig. 14.22). It is likely that ultrasound will be used with increasing frequency in the future for central and arterial line placement.

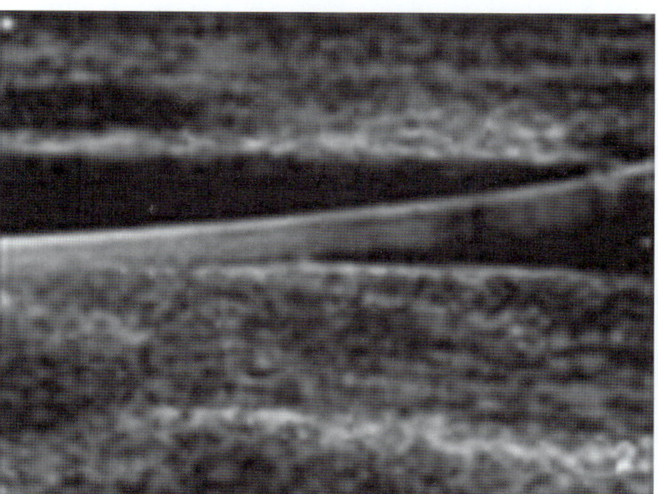

Fig. 14.22: Ultrasound with wire in vein.

REFERENCES

1. Rivera AM, Strauss KW, van Zundert A, et al. The history of peripheral intravenous catheters: how little plastic tubes revolutionized medicine. Acta Anaesth Belg. 2005;56:271-82.
2. O'Shaughnessy WB, et al. Proposal of a new method of treating the blue epidemic cholera by the injection of highly oxygenised salts into the venous system. Lancet. 1831;11:274-7.
3. Latta T. Injections in cholera. Lond Med Gazz. 1832;379-82.
4. Massa DJ, Lundy JS, Faulconer A Jr, et al. A plastic needle. Mayo Clinic Proc. 1950;25:413-5.
5. Michael V, Beheshti MD. A concise history of central venous access. Tech Vasc Interv Radiol. 2011;14(4):184-5.
6. Rodriguez-Paz JM, Pronovost P. Prevention of catheter related blood stream infections. Adv Surg. 2008;42:229-48.
7. Chaiyakonapruh N, Veenstra DL, Lipsky BA, et al. Chlorhexidine compound with povidone-iodine solution for vascular catheter site care: a meta-analysis. Ann Intern Med. 2002; 136(11):792-801.
8. O'Grady NP, Alexander M, Dellinger EP, et al. Guidelines for the prevention of intravascular catheter related infections. Clin Infect Dis. 2002;35(11):1281-1307.
9. Raad II, Hohn DC, Gilbreath BJ, et al. Prevention of central venous catheter related infections by using maximal sterile barrier precautions during insertion. Infect Control Hosp Epidemiol. 1994;15:231-8.
10. Kluger DM, Maki DG. The relative risk of intravascular device related bloodstream infections in adults. In: Abstracts of the 39th Interscience Conference on Antimicrobial Agents and Chemotherapy. San Francisco: American Society for Microbiology; 1999. p. 514.

11. Roberge RJ, Kelly M, Evans TC, et al. Facilitated intravenous access through local application of nitroglycerin ointment. Ann Emer Med. 1987;16(5):546–9.
12. De Graaff JC, Cuper NJ, Mungra AA, et al. Near-infrared light to aid peripheral intravenous cannulation in children: a cluster randomized clinical trial of three devices. Anaesthesia. 2013;68:835-45.
13. Yen K, Gorelick MH. New biomedical devices that use near-infrared technology to assist with phlebotomy and vascular access. Pediatr Emer Care. 2013;29:383-8.
14. Lycka BA. Medical indications for using a topical anesthetic. Persect Pain Manage.1991;1:9-12.
15. Package insert Copyright 1991, 2005, 2010 Astrazeneca Canada Inc.
16. Curry SE, Finkel JC. Use of the Synera™ patch for local anesthesia before vascular access procedures: a randomized, double-blind, placebo-controlled study. Pain Med. 2007;8(6):497-502.
17. Spanos S, Booth R, Koenig H, et al. Jet injection of 1% buffered lidocaine versus topical ELA-Max for anesthesia before peripheral intravenous catheterization in children: a randomized controlled trial. Pediatr Emer Care. 2008;24 (8):511-5.
18. Pershad J, Steinberg SC, Waters TM. Cost-effectiveness analysis of anesthetic agents during peripheral intravenous cannulation in the pediatric emergency department. Arch Pediatr Adolesc Med. 2008;162(10): 952-61.
19. Goode CJ, Titler M, Rakel D, et al. A meta-analysis of effects of heparin flush and saline flush: quality and cost implications. Nurs Res. 1991;40(6):324-30.
20. Rickard CM, Webster J, Wallis MC, et al. Routine versus clinically indicated replacement of peripheral intravenous catheters: a randomized controlled equivalence trial. Lancet. 2012;380:1066-074.
21. O'Grady NP, Alexander M, Burns LA, et al. Guidelines for the prevention of intravascular catheter-related infections. Clin Infect Dis. 2011;52:e162-93.
22. O'Grady NP, Alexander M, Dellinger EP, et al. Guidelines for the prevention of intravascular catheter-related infections. Infect Control Hosp Epidemiol. 2002;23:759-69.
23. Drinker CK, Drinker KR, Lund CCl. The circulation of the mammalian bone marrow. Am J Physiol. 1922;62(1):1-52.
24. Miller LJ. Intraosseous vascular access—state of the art: An essential emergency medical skill. [Online] Available from acls.mshpreps.com.
25. Leidel BA, Kirchhoff C, Braunstein V, et al. Comparison of two intraosseous access devices in adult patients under resuscitation in the emergency department: A prospective randomized study. Resuscitation. 2010;81(8):994-9.
26. Leidel BA, Kirchhoff C, Bogner V, et al. Comparison of intraosseous versus central venous access in adults under resuscitation in the emergency department with inaccessible peripheral veins. Resuscitation. 2012;83(1):40-5.
27. Ong ME, Chan YH, Oh JJ, et al. An observational, prospective study comparing tibial and humeral intraosseous access using the EZ-IO. Am J Emerg Med. 2009;27:8-15.
28. The consortium on intraosseous vascular access in healthcare practices: Recommendations for the use of intraosseous vascular access for emergent and non-emergent situations in various healthcare settings: a consensus paper. Crit Care Nurse. 2010;30(6):e1-7.
29. Mermel LA. Prevention of intravascular catheter related infections. Ann Intern Med. 2000;132:391-402.
30. Farkas JC, Liu N, Bleriot JP, et al. Single versus triple lumen central catheter related sepsis: A prospective randomized study in critically ill population. Am J Med. 1992;93(3):277-82.
31. Gil RT, Kruse JA, Thill-Baharozian MC, et al. Triple versus single lumen central catheters: A prospective study in a critically ill population. Arch Intern Med. 1989;149(5): 1139-43.
32. Veenstra DL, Saint S, Saha S, et al. Efficacy of antiseptic-impregnated central venous catheters in preventing catheter related bloodstream infections. JAMA. 1999;281(3):261-7.
33. Veenstra DL, Saint S, Sullivan SD. Cost effectiveness of antiseptic-impregnated central venous catheters for the prevention of catheter-related bloodstream infections. JAMA. 1999;282(6):554-60.
34. O'Grady NP, Alexander M, Burns LA, et al. Healthcare Infection Control Practices Advisory Committee (HICPAC): guidelines for the prevention of intravascular catheter related infections. Clin Infec Dis. 2011;52(9):e162-93.
35. Schwab SJ, Beathard G. The hemodialysis conundrum: hate living with them, but can't live without them. Kidney Int. 1999;56:1-17.
36. Duntley P, Siever J, Korwes ML, et al. Vascular erosion by central venous catheters. Chest. 1992;101(6):1633-8.
37. Lorente L, Henry C, Martín MM, et al. Central venous catheter-related infection in a prospective and observational study of 2595 catheters. Crit Care. 2005;9(6):R631-R635.
38. Marik PE, Flemmer M, Harrison W. The risk of catheter related bloodstream infections with femoral venous catheters as compared to subclavian and internal jugular venous catheters: A systematic review of the literature and meta-analysis. Crit Care Med. 2012;40(8):2479-85.
39. Trottier SJ, Veremakis C, O'Brien J, et al. Femoral deep vein thrombosis with central venous catheterization: Results from a prospective randomized trial. Crit Care Med. 1995;23: 52-9.
40. Stein JM, Pruitt BA Jr. Suppurative thrombophlebitis a lethal iatrogenic disease. N Engl J Med. 1970;282:1452-5.
41. Lum P. A new formula based measurement guide to optimal positioning of central venous catheters. JAVA. 2004;9(2): 80-85.
42. Boyd R, Saxe A, Phillips E. Effect of patient positioning upon success in placing central venous catheters. Am J Surg. 1996;172(4):380-2.
43. Jesseph JM, Conces DJ Jr, Augustyn GT. Patient positioning for subclavian vein catheterization. Arch Surg. 1987; 122(10):1207.
44. Tan BK, Hong SW, Huang MH, et al. Anatomic basis of safe percutaneous subclavian venous catheterization. J Trauma. 2000;48(1):82-6.

45. Parienti JJ, Thirion M, Mégarbane B, et al. Members of the cathedia study group: femoral versus jugular venous catheterization and the risk of nosocomial events in adults requiring acute renal replacement therapy: A randomized controlled trial. JAMA. 2008;299(20):2413.
46. Deshpande KS, Hatem C, Ulrich HL, et al. The incidence of infectious complications of central venous catheters at the subclavian, internal jugular, and femoral sites in an intensive care unit population. Crit Care Med. 2005;33(1):13-20.
47. Meredith JW, Young JS, O'Neil EA, et al. Femoral catheters and deep venous thrombosis: a prospective evaluation with venous duplex sonography. J Trauma. 1993;35(2):187-90.
48. Timsit JF, Schwebel C, Bouadma L, et al. Dressing Study Group: Chlorhexadine-impregnated sponges and less frequent dressing changes for prevention of catheter related infections in critically ill adults. JAMA. 2009;301(12):1231-41.
49. Flowers RH 3rd, Schwenzer KJ, Kopel RF, et al. Efficacy of an attachable subcutaneous cuff for the prevention of intravascular catheter-related infections: a randomized controlled trial. JAMA. 1989;261(6):878-83.
50. Zakrzewska-Bode A, Muytjens HL, Liem KD, et al. Mupirocin resistance in coagulase—negative Staphylococci after topical prophylaxis for the reduction of colonization of central venous catheters. J Hosp Infect. 1995;31(3):189-93.

Additional references appear in the online version of this book.

15

Diagnostic and Interventional Radiology

Charles R Hickam, Fred A Mettler Jr

Key Points

- When reading a radiograph, it is necessary to note the projection and patient position and to check the patient's name and the time and date of the study. It is important systematically to review all the structures seen on the film and to make comparisons to previous films when available.
- Plain films may be diagnostic, but, if not, they may suggest that further diagnostic studies are needed to clarify an abnormality seen on the plain films.
- Ultrasonography is a very technician-dependent study. It is a relatively inexpensive noninvasive study, which is useful to diagnose some common conditions such as cholelithiasis, cholecystitis, and an abdominal aortic aneurysm. It is also useful to evaluate retroperitoneal pathology.
- Computed tomography (CT) scans use 10–100 times more radiation than a plain film. Most CT studies utilize a contrast agent to improve the diagnostic capabilities of the study.
- Magnetic resonance imaging (MRI) does not use ionizing radiation. An MR study provides exquisite images of the central nervous system and stationary soft tissue. Blood flow may also be evaluated by using MR angiographic techniques.
- Nuclear medicine studies are valuable for the diagnosis of a pulmonary embolus, cholecystitis and the identification of biliary leaks and to differentiated neonatal hepatitis from biliary atresia. They may also be helpful in localizing the site of gastrointestinal bleeding and to identify a site of infection.
- Interventional techniques area an alternative to open surgical techniques that allow for less-invasive therapies in many areas of the body.

INTRODUCTION

Radiology plays an important role in the diagnosis and treatment of surgical patients. In the current milieu of medical care, selection of the diagnostic or therapeutic study that will provide the necessary information safely and most cost-effectively is an important issue. The purpose of this chapter is to provide a broad overview of diagnostic and interventional radiologic studies commonly requested by surgeons and the most appropriate use of each of these studies.[1]

The chapter also reviews specific clinical entities critical to the management of a surgical patient and percutaneous interventions that are used as an adjunctive or alternative to a surgical procedure. Vascular diagnostic and interventional procedures may be performed by vascular surgeons, interventional radiologists or cardiologists, and these vascular procedures are discussed in other relevant chapters and books.[2]

IMAGING MODALITIES

Plain X-Ray Examinations

Regular X-rays (plain X-rays, also sometimes called conventional radiographs) account for about 75% of imaging examinations. The historical imaging receptor was a film/screen combination. Newer systems are called computed radiography or digital radiography. Once either type of image is stored in the computer, it can be displayed on a monitor for interpretation or transmitted to remote locations for viewing. Use of contrast agents permits visualization of anatomic structures that are not normally seen. If imaging is done with standard format, the blood vessels appear white. Contrast agents instilled orally, rectally, or retrograde into the ureter or bladder incur little or no risk unless aspiration or perforation occurs. With the intravenously or intra-arterially administered agents, a small but real risk of contrast reaction exists. This is something to be considered before ordering a contrast-enhanced CT scan. About 5% of patients will experience an immediate mild reaction, such as a metallic taste or a feeling of warmth; some experience nausea and vomiting, wheeze, or get hives as a result of these contrast agents. Because contrast agents also can reduce renal function, they should not generally be used in patients with compromised renal function (eGFR < 50–60 mL/min). A small number (about 1 in 1,000) of patients have a severe reaction to intravascular contrast. This may be a vasovagal reaction, laryngeal edema, severe hypotension, an anaphylactic-type reaction, or cardiac arrest. The risk of death from a study using intravenously administered contrast agents is between 1 in 40,000 and 1 in 100,000.

Fluoroscopy

Fluoroscopy uses a standard X-ray tube and captures multiple sequential images on an image intensifier; it then displays them on a monitor or stores them electronically. Images are usually obtained at 7–30 frames per second. The X-ray tube can operate in a continuous manner or in a pulsed mode (with the latter resulting in much less radiation dose to the patient and operator). The field of view also has an effect on dose, with a smaller field of view resulting in a higher patient dose. Fluoroscopes can result in very high patient doses and skin injuries (Fig. 15.1). It is imperative for the operator to be aware of the radiation dose, especially during the course of difficult interventional cases.

Computed Tomography

Computed tomography is accomplished by passing a rotating fan beam of X-rays through the patient and measuring the transmission at thousands of points. Most modern scanners not only have the helical motion but also have multiple rows of detectors and can obtain over 100 image data slices at once. The appearance of tissues on CT scan depends to some extent on the computer manipulation, but in general the basic four densities on CT images are the same as those in plain X-rays: air is black, fat is dark gray, soft tissue is light gray, and bone or calcium and contrast agents are white. The greater sensitivity of CT compared with plain X-rays allows areas of tiny punctate calcification to be seen.

Contrast agents, frequently used in CT scans, are usually the same water-soluble oral, rectal, or intravenous iodinated agents used in other imaging studies. Intravenous contrast agents are common, being used in probably 75% of all CT studies, and obviously carry the risk of contrast reactions discussed previously. Rapid acquisition of images allows the intravenously administered contrast to be displayed and images acquired in arterial (CT angiography), venous or delayed phases with only a single injection. The appeal of CT is that a large number of structures are visualized simultaneously, which quickly allows identification of macroscopic pathology.

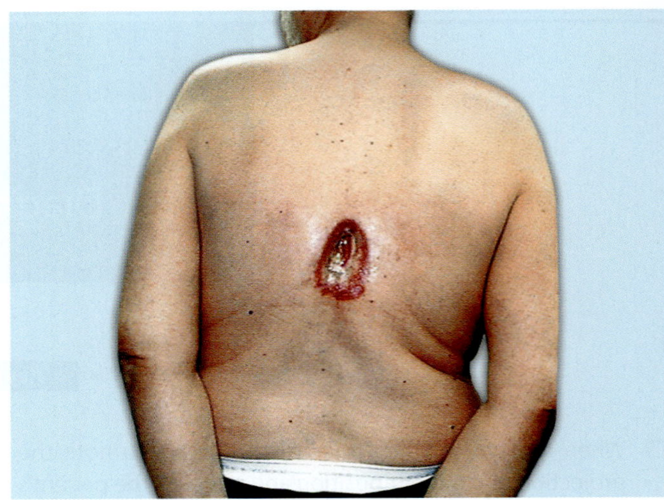

Fig. 15.1: Radiation skin burn with necrosis and ulceration 12 months after a prolonged cardiac interventional procedure.

Ultrasound

Ultrasound examination uses high-frequency sound waves to make images. The image is made by sending high-frequency sound into the patient and assessing the magnitude and time of returning echoes. Echoes are the result of interfaces or changes in elasticity. Typically, a cyst has few if any echoes, because it is mostly water. Tissues such as liver and spleen give a picture with rather homogeneous small echoes due to the fibrous interstitial tissue. High-intensity echoes are caused by calcification, fat, and air.

The technology of ultrasound is attractive because it does not use ionizing radiation, and the machines are relatively inexpensive. For these reasons, ultrasound has found widespread use in obstetrics, line placement in intensive care units and in emergency rooms. Real-time ultrasound allows the images to be seen in sequential frames just as in a movie. This capability has proved popular for imaging rapidly moving structures, such as the heart, and for image-guided needle biopsy. In addition to using echoes to generate images, the ultrasound equipment can analyze the returning echo frequencies. This Doppler analysis allows identification of moving blood as well as its direction and velocity.

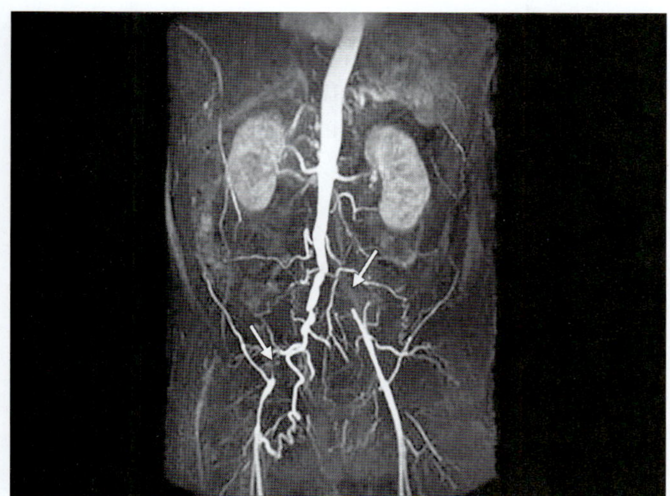

Fig. 15.2: Magnetic resonance arteriogram of the abdominal and pelvic vessels. The aorta and both kidneys are clearly visualized. There is a complete obstruction of the left common iliac and right common femoral arteries (arrows) with distal flow through to collateral vessels.

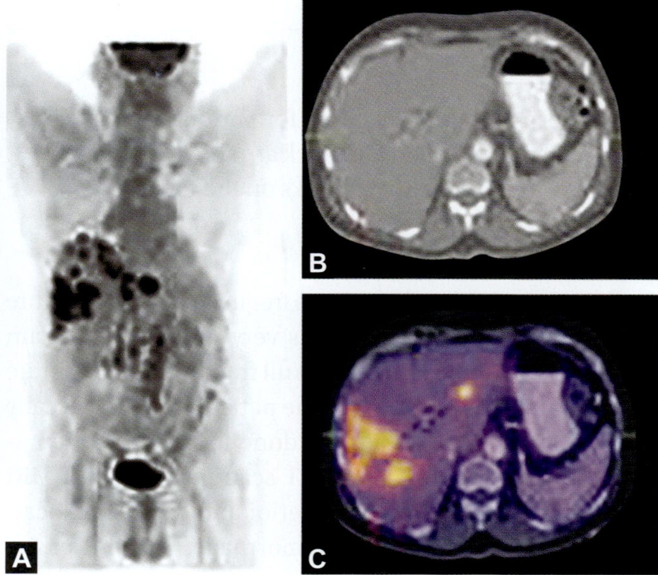

Figs. 15.3A to C: Positron emission tomography computed tomography (PET/CT) hybrid imaging. (A) Coronal PET nuclear medicine image and (B) computed tomography data can be coregistered to provide a single image (C) combining both functional and anatomical information. In this case the patient has colon cancer with hepatic metastases that were not easily seen on the CT scan alone.

Nuclear Medicine

Nuclear medicine images are made by giving the patient a short-lived radioactive material. The most commonly used radionuclides decay rapidly and have half-lives of only minutes or hours. Most materials administered are not detectable a day or so after administration. With the attachment of a radionuclide (such as technetium-99 m) to specific carrier compounds, location of the radioactivity can be imaged and measured in a chosen organ or tissue, such as the thyroid, bone, lung, heart, abscess, or tumor. A major advantage of nuclear medicine is its ability to obtain an image of physiologic function.[3]

Magnetic Resonance Imaging

Magnetic resonance imaging generates images by applying a varying magnetic field to the body. Although many MRI techniques exist, the two basic types of images are T1 and T2. T1 images show fat as a white or bright signal, whereas water [or cerebrospinal fluid (CSF)] is dark. On a T2 image, fat is dark and blood, edema, and CSF appear white. Unfortunately, calcium and bone are difficult to see on MR images. What people think are the (white) bones is really visualization of fat in the marrow. Computer manipulation of MR images allows slices similar to those of CT orientation to be used. An intravenous contrast agent (gadolinium) is often used in conjunction with MRI. Serious patient reactions are very rare with this agent, although nephrogenic systemic fibrosis has occasionally been reported in patients with severely impaired renal function (eGFR < 30 mL/min).

The primary advantages of MRI are that it obtains exquisite images of the central nervous system and stationary soft tissues (such as the knee joint). It also does not use ionizing radiation. Recent developments and shorter imaging times have allowed images of the heart and blood vessels to be generated without the need to inject anything into the patient.[2] MR angiography (MRA) can be used to provide excellent anatomic detail of vascular disease process (Fig. 15.2). Disadvantages of MRI have been artifacts due to patient motion, inability to bring ferrous objects near the magnet and cost.

Hybrid Imaging

Increases in computer power and advances in equipment manufacturing have allowed data imaging sets from various modalities to be combined and the images coregistered. The most popular use of this has been integration of positron emission tomography functional nuclear medicine data with computed tomography anatomical data (PET/CT) (Figs. 15.3A to C). This currently has wide use in the imaging of cancer.[3] Other forms of hybrid imaging exist, including PET combined with MRI.

HEAD AND NECK

Imaging

Suggested imaging procedures for various clinical situations involving the head and neck are shown in Table 15.1. There are also excellent textbooks on the topic.[4,5]

Head Trauma

Skull X-rays are ordered much too frequently. A skull fracture without loss of consciousness is very rare. Serious brain injury may be found without a skull fracture. If a moderate or severe injury is present and the patient is neurologically unstable, a CT scan should be done to exclude a hematoma. It is preferable to do a CT scan instead of an MRI examination because of the superior ability of CT to localize skull fractures and fresh hemorrhage. It also is easier to manage an unstable patient in a CT scanner than in an MRI machine. Air within the cranial vault is almost always the result of trauma and is easily seen on CT. If the patient is neurologically stable, an MR scan is preferable to look for parenchymal shearing injuries.

Intracranial Hemorrhage

If the presence of acute intracranial hemorrhage is suspected, the study of choice is a CT scan done without intravenous contrast. The scan is done without contrast because acute hemorrhage appears to be white on a CT scan. Subdural hematomas are seen as crescent-shaped abnormalities between the brain and the skull. They can cross suture lines, but they do not cross the tentorium or falx. For epidural (extradural) hematomas, the major differential point from an imaging viewpoint is that they are lenticular rather than crescentic and tend not to cross suture lines of the skull. Epidural hematomas are associated with temporal bone fractures that have resulted in a tear of the middle meningeal artery.

Transient Ischemic Attack (TIA) and Stroke

In the acute setting, the initial test of choice is a CT scan to differentiate an ischemic event from a hemorrhagic one. A second CT scan can be obtained in 24–72 hours if the diagnosis is in doubt, but an MRI is more sensitive in identifying early ischemic damage and may establish the cause of the TIA. A stroke may be ischemic or associated with hemorrhage. An acute hemorrhagic stroke is most easily visualized on a noncontrasted CT scan. A purely ischemic acute stroke is difficult to visualize on a CT scan unless mass effect is present. An acute ischemic stroke is very easy to see on an MRI study, because the edema (increased water) can be identified as a bright area on diffusion-weighted images.

Intracranial Aneurysm and Arteriovenous Malformations

The best initial way to visualize intracranial aneurysms is with CT or MRI. In a setting of acute headache and suspected acute intracranial bleeding, a noncontrasted CT study should be done. If the noncontrasted CT is negative, it is followed by a contrasted CT. In the acute setting, CT or MRI angiogram is usually performed. For patients who have a long history of headache, or a familial history of aneurysms, a noninvasive MR angiogram is probably the procedure of choice. Aneurysms and AVMs may be treated with surgically or transarterial placement of coils or other substance to fill the cavity.

Primary Brain Tumors and Metastases

A variety of brain tumors are found. The study of choice is a CT or MRI scan with and without intravenous contrast. The more edema and the more enhancement after administration of intravenous contrast, the more malignant the lesion is likely to be. The examination with the best resolution for the pituitary region is MRI. Metastatic disease is best identified using MRI with intravenous gadolinium. A contrasted CT scan can be used, but it is not as sensitive as MRI. Most metastases enhance with contrast agents.

Head and Neck Cancer

Although many head and neck cancers are detected clinically or by endoscopy, full evaluation and staging involves assessment of local tumor extension, nodal spread, and evaluation of pulmonary metastases. The diagnostic workup usually includes a contrasted CT scanning; however, optimal staging also includes flourine-18 fluorodeoxyglucose (^{18}F-FDG) hybrid PET/CT scanning. While CT scanning or MRI can easily identify enlarged nodes, these nodes may be reactive especially in patients with poor dental hygiene. In addition, CT cannot detect malignancy in normal size nodes. Occasionally, cervical adenopathy is present without an obvious primary malignancy and in these cases percutaneous lymph node biopsy is often performed as described below.

Table 15.1 Suggested initial imaging modalities for head and neck problems.

Clinical problem	*Initial imaging study*
Skull fracture	CT scan including bone windows
Major head trauma	CT (neurologically unstable); MRI (neurologically stable)
Mild head trauma	Observe; CT (if persistent headache)
Acute hemorrhage	Noncontrasted CT
Intracerebral aneurysm or arteriovenous malformations	MRI
Aneurysm (chronic history)	MR angiogram or CT angiogram
Transient ischemic attack	Noncontrasted CT, MRI if vertebrobasilar findings; consider carotid ultrasonography if bruit present
Acute stroke(suspected hemorrhagic)	Noncontrasted CT
(suspected nonhemorrhagic)	MRI
Cranial neuropathy	MRI with and without contrast
Tumor or metastases	MRI
Carotid/vertebral dissection (ipsilateral Horner's or unilateral headache)	CT angiogram of head and neck
Abscess	Contrasted CT or MRI
Preoperative for cranial surgery	Contrast angiography
Seizure(new onset or poor therapeutic response)	MRI
(new onset post traumatic)	CT or MRI
(febrile or alcohol withdrawal without neurologic deficit)	Imaging not indicated
Focal neurologic deficit	MRI or CT without contrast
Vision loss(adult sudden or proptosis)	MRI with and without contrast
(head injury)	CT
(child acute or progressive) or proptosis	MRI
Ophthalmoplegia	MRI with and without contrast
Unexplained confusion or altered level of consciousness	MRI or CT without contrast
Neuroendocrine [e.g., hyperthyroidism (high TSH), Cushing's syndrome (high ACTH)], hyperprolactinemia, acromegaly, precocious puberty, etc.)	MRI with and without contrast
Facial fracture	Plain X-ray, CT for complicated cases
Carotid bruit	Duplex ultrasound
Epiglottitis	Lateral soft tissue X-ray of neck
Foreign body	Plain X-ray if calcified or metallic (fish bones not visible)
Retropharyngeal abscess	Lateral soft tissue X-ray of the neck; if positive, CT to determine extent
Lymphadenopathy , nontender, single or multiple (or no decrease in size over 4 weeks)	CT with IV contrast (preferred) or MRI without contrast
Solitary neck mass (febrile patient)	CT with IV contrast
Pulsatile neck mass	CT with IV contrast
Solitary or multiple neck masses (child)	US or CT with IV contrast
Thyroid nodule (palpable)	Fine needle aspiration (possibly with ultrasound guidance)

(CNS: Central nervous system; CT: Computed tomography; MRI: Magnetic resonance imaging; SPECT: Single-photon emission computed tomography).

Source: Adapted with permission from Mettler FA. Essentials of Radiology, 3rd edition. Philadelphia, PA: Elsevier/Saunders; 2014.

Retropharyngeal Abscess

Retropharyngeal abscess is a cause of upper airway obstruction as well as a cause of dysphagia. The soft tissue lateral X-ray is the initial imaging procedure of choice, usually showing prevertebral soft tissue swelling. Air may or may not be within these swollen soft tissues. An intravenously contrasted CT scan is often of great value to help discern the lateral and inferior margins of the abscess and the location of the great vessels of the neck as well as extension inferiorly into the mediastinum or laterally into the region of the carotid artery and jugular vein.

Thyroid

Thyroid nodules are very common in the general population, occurring in up to 50–60% of autopsies among elderly patients. The vast majority of nodules are benign and are often found incidentally on CT or ultrasound examinations, causing a lot of anxiety among patients. Ultrasound can differentiate a cystic from solid thyroid lesion and is commonly used to direct fine-needle aspiration according to consensus guidelines.[6]

Parathyroid

The most common parathyroid problem requiring imaging is hypercalcemia secondary to a parathyroid adenoma or to hyperplasia. Because adenomas can be very difficult to locate at operation, a nuclear medicine scan using radioactive compounds that accumulate in the thyroid or parathyroid is used. Hybrid imaging with single-photon emission computed tomography and regular CT (SPECT/CT) images are very accurate in localizing the adenomas.

Percutaneous Needle Biopsy of the Neck

Thyroid biopsy is typically performed using ultrasound-guided 23–25 gauge fine-needle aspiration or nonaspiration capillary technique. There are a number of sonographic features of a thyroid nodule that tend toward malignancy including microcalcifications (70% predictive value), marked lesion hypoechogenicity relative to strap muscles, poorly defined margins, greater AP dimension and vascularity within the nodule.[7] Lymph node biopsies are performed with fine-needle technique but also with an additional 18-gauge core biopsy to evaluate nodal architecture. Lymph node biopsies in the neck are typically done to evaluate enlarged nodes in patients with a mouth, pharyngeal or laryngeal cancer. Ultrasound also can be used to guide percutaneous laser or ethanol ablation of selected malignant cervical nodes.

CHEST

Imaging

Suggested initial imaging procedures for various clinical situations involving the heart and lungs are shown in Tables 15.2 and 15.3. There are also excellent textbooks on the topics.[8-12]

Pneumothorax

If there is mediastinal shift or depression of the hemidiaphragm with displacement of the heart and trachea away from the side with the pneumothorax, the patient has a potentially lethal tension pneumothorax. One cm of space lateral to the lung constitutes a pneumothorax of about 10%; 5 cm of space between the lateral chest wall and the lung margin constitutes a pneumothorax of about 30%. Air tends to collect in the highest position in the pleural space, and therefore it can be difficult to appreciate a small or moderate-sized pneumothorax on a frontal chest radiograph of a patient who is supine. When a chest tube is properly placed, connected to a vacuum and unobstructed, a persistent pneumothorax raises the possibility of a bronchopleural fistula. Another consideration is an anterior pneumothorax with a posteriorly placed chest tube.

Pleural Effusion

A pleural effusion seen on a routine upright chest radiograph usually contains at least 100 mL. The most typical location is in the most dependent portion of the pleural space; therefore, pleural effusions are best seen on upright chest radiographs. The appearances of larger effusions vary according to patient position. On an upright film there is increasing basilar density and loss of definition of the hemidiaphragm. If a patient is supine, the effusion will be layered in the posterior pleural space, which results in a relative increased density or whiteness of the affected hemithorax compared with the normal side. A decubitus film with the suspect side facing downwards is often helpful. Massive pleural effusions are often malignant. When there is a moderate or large pleural fluid collection with pneumonia, an empyema or malignancy should be suspected.

Table 15.2 Suggested initial imaging for cardiovascular problems.

Clinical problem	*Imaging study*
Most cardiac problems	Initial posteroanterior and lateral chest radiography
Congestive heart failure (new or worse)	Chest radiography and ejection fraction; wall motion evaluation by nuclear medicine or echocardiography
Congestive heart failure (chronic)	Chest radiography
Hypertension (suspected essential)	No imaging indicated
Hypertension (suspected renal artery stenosis)	Nuclear medicine captopril renogram or magnetic resonance or CT angiogram
Left ventricular ejection fraction	Gated nuclear medicine blood pool study or echocardiography
Chest pain or shortness of breath (suspected	Chest X-ray and CT angiogram pulmonary embolism)
Shortness of breath (suspected cardiac origin)	Chest X-ray and echocardiography
Blunt chest trauma (suspect aortic injury)	Chext X-ray, CT angiogram
Acute chest pain	
(suspected myocardial infarction)	Electrocardiography, chest radiography, and coronary angiography (suspect aortic dis-section) Chext X-ray, CT angiogram
(nonspecific low probability of coronary disease)	Electrocardiography, chest X-ray
Chronic chest pain	
(low probability of coronary disease)	Chest X-ray
(moderate probability of coronary disease)	Chest X-ray, echocardiography or nuclear medicine cardiac perfusion scan
(high probability of coronary disease)	Nuclear medicine cardiac perfusion scan or coronary angiogram
Coronary ischemia	Electrocardiography; if negative, then stress electrocardiogram, nuclear medicine, myo-cardial perfusion study, or stress echocardiogram; if positive, then coronary angiogram
Endocarditis	Echocardiography
Valvular disease	Echocardiography
Pericardial effusion	Echocardiography
Constrictive pericarditis	Echocardiography, if equivocal, then CT
Aortic trauma	CT with contrast
Thoracic aortic dissection	CT with IV contrast or transesophageal ultrasonography
Abdominal aortic aneurysm (symptomatic)	CT with IV contrast;
(asymptomatic)	Ultrasonography for screening. Ultrasound or non-contrast CT for follow-up
Deep venous thrombosis	Duplex ultrasonography
Sudden painful cold leg	CT angiogram or MR angiogram
Carotid bruit	Duplex ultrasonography; if high-grade stenosis, then contrast angiography
Claudication	Doppler ultrasonography of lower extremity

(CT: Computed tomography).

Source: Adapted with permission from Mettler FA. Essentials of Radiology, 3rd edition. Philadelphia, PA: Elsevier/Saunders; 2014.

Percutaneous Chest Tubes

Chest tubes are placed in the pleural space either percutaneously or surgically to evacuate pneumothoraces (Figs. 15.4A and B), hemorrhage, empyemas, chylothorax, and recurrent or persistent effusions.[13-15] Historically rigid large-bore catheters were utilized, but more recently there is a trend toward smaller and softer catheters. The soft catheters are an acceptable alternative to stiff pleural tubes. Large bore catheters are typically > 14 Fr. Patients on mechanical ventilation with barotrauma or with hemithorax are best managed with large bore tubes, but most patients with pleurodesis, complicated parapneumonic effusions and most pneumothoraces are effectively managed with small bore catheters. Injection of tissue plasminogen activator (tPA) or deoxyribonuclease (DNase) is a useful adjunct for the treatment of multiloculated complex pleural fluid collections. After pulmonary resection there is controversy whether there is a significant difference in duration of pneumothorax or duration of hospital stay if the chest tube is placed to suction or water seal. Some authors recommend that water seal be used after a brief period of suction.

Table 15.3 Suggested initial imaging procedures for various chest problems.

Clinical problem	*Imaging study*
Pneumonia (diagnosed clinically)	Chest X-ray (confirmatory)
(immunocompromised patient with negative chest X-ray)	CT without contrast
Trauma	Chest X-ray, CT
Chest pain, acute (low probability of CAD)	Chest X-ray (additional studies depend on suspected cause) Chest pain, chronic (low-to-intermediate probability of CAD)Chest X-ray (possibly US or NM cardiac stress test)
Chest pain, chronic (high probability of CAD)	NM or US cardiac stress test or coronary angiogram)
Shortness of breath (severe or long duration or in adult age	Chest X-ray. 40 years or older)
(negative chest X-ray, pulmonary origin suspected)	Chest CT (high resolution)
Hypertension (uncomplicated)	No imaging needed
(moderate or severe)	Initial chest X-ray
Asthma (suspected superimposed disease or resistant to therapy)	Chest X-ray
Interstitial lung disease	Chest X-ray, pulmonary function studies
Immunosuppressed patient (with fever, cough, or dyspnea)	Chest X-ray
Foreign body	Inspiration/expiration chest X-ray
Aspiration pneumonia	Chest X-ray
Mediastinal mass	Contrasted CT
Solitary pulmonary nodule	CT without contrast (high resolution). If indeterminate FDG PET/CT.
Lung tumor or lung metastases screening)	Chest X-ray and CT
Pleural mass or fluid	CT
Localization of pleural effusion for thoracentesis	Stethoscope, ultrasound
Suspected pneumothorax	Chest X-ray (expiration view as well)
Hemoptysis	Chest X-ray, CT with IV contrast
Pulmonary embolism	Chest X-ray, and CT angiogram or nuclear medicine lung scan
Coronary ischemia	Stress ECG, stress nuclear medicine (myocardial perfusion scan) or stress echocardiogram, coronary angiogram
Aortic aneurysm	CT without and with IV contrast or transesophageal ultrasound
Aortic tear	CT without and with IV contrast or CT angiogram
Aortic dissection	CT with IV contrast or transesophageal ultrasound
Preoperative or admission of patient	Chest X-ray not indicated unless acute or chronic cardiopulmonary disease
Intensive care unit patient	Chest X-ray upon admission, transfer and clinical indication only

(CAD: Coronary artery disease; COPD: Chronic obstructive pulmonary disease; CHF: Congestive heart failure; CT: Computed tomography; US: Ultrasound; NM: Nuclear medicine; ECG: Electrocardiogram; PA: Posteroanterior; FDG PET/CT: Fluorodeoxyglucose positron emission tomography/computed tomography).

Source: Adapted with permission from Mettler FA. Essentials of Radiology, 3rd edition. Philadelphia, PA: Elsevier/Saunders; 2014.

Lung Trauma

Pulmonary contusions are common after lung trauma, occur without rib fractures, and are seen within hours of an accident. Contusions are seen radiographically as ill-defined pulmonary parenchymal opacities caused by hemorrhage and edema. Uncomplicated contusions resolve within 4–5 days. Pulmonary hematomas are caused by bleeding as a result of shearing injuries of the lung parenchyma. These can present as nodules or masses and may cavitate. These lesions often take weeks to resolve.

Pulmonary Nodules

Pulmonary nodules are usually detected incidentally on a chest X-ray or CT scan. A solitary pulmonary nodule may be due to a granuloma or lung cancer, but other etiologies include a single metastatic lesion, septic embolus, arteriovenous malformation, hamartoma, or even a small area of rounded atelectasis. If it is well defined and round, it is much more likely to be benign than if it is irregular or indistinct in its margins. Calcification that is very dense or within a nodule suggests that it is most likely a granuloma.

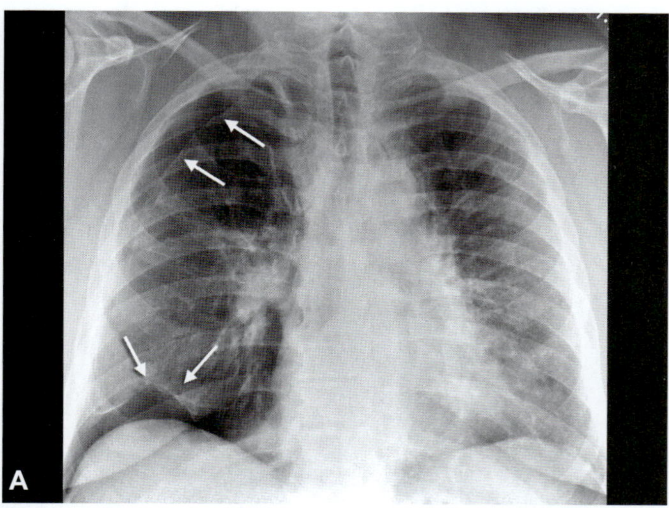

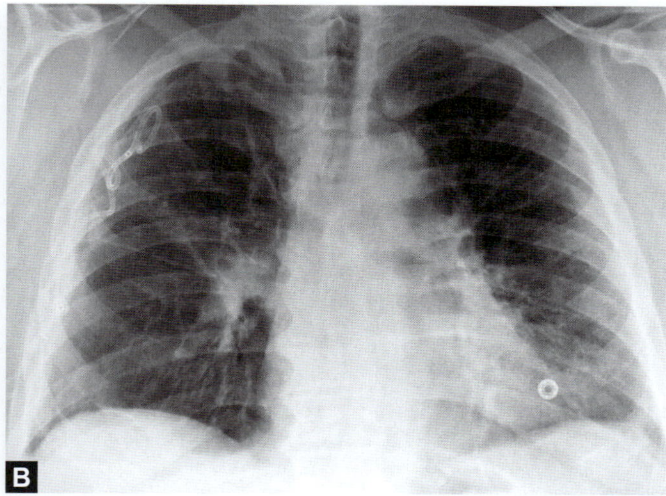

Figs. 15.4A and B: Pneumothorax. (A) A moderate persistent pneumothorax is seen at the right lung apex and base (arrows). (B) After insertion of a small bore pleural tube the pneumothorax is significantly reduced.

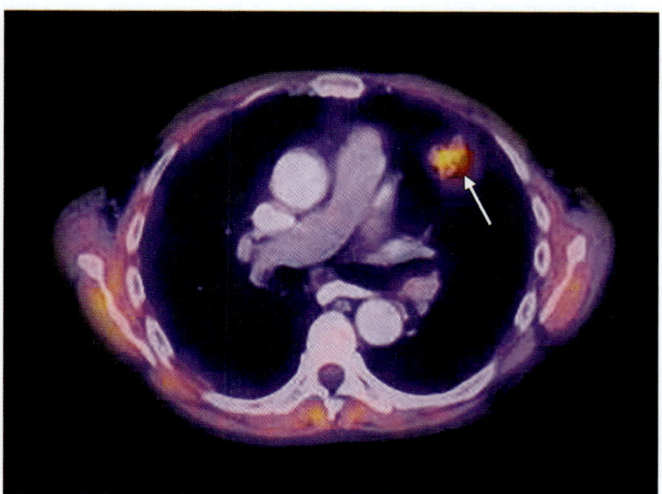

Fig. 15.5: Lung cancer. A computed tomography (CT) scan demonstrated a small mass in the left lung. A fluorine-18 fluorodeoxyglucose positron emission tomography computed tomography (PET/CT) scan shows the lesion (arrow) to be very metabolically active raising high suspicion of a malignancy. An active infection is also possible.

The calcification, however, should be centrally located in the nodule. If calcification is eccentrically located in a nodule a neoplasm should be considered.

A nodule that has remained unchanged in size for 2 years can be considered benign. Stability for a period of 1 year is not enough, because slow-growing tumors may not change appreciably in a 12-month interval.[16] Fluorine-18 fluorodeoxyglucose PET/CT scans are used to help determine whether a nodule or mass is benign or malignant (Fig. 15.5). This test is usually performed when a fine-needle aspiration is impractical or the patient has a known cancer and a new lung or mediastinal mass. The radioactive tracer used is FDG. Malignant lesions have a high metabolism, and most will actively accumulate the tracer.

Lung Cancer

Chest CT is frequently used to find or characterize pulmonary nodules or masses that are suggestive of neoplasm[7] and to look for metastatic pulmonary nodules. Analysis of the CT scan should include not only the location and size of the pulmonary lesion, but also whether it has pleural or chest wall involvement and whether there is hilar or mediastinal adenopathy. The accuracy of CT in determining chest wall invasion is about 50%, but invasion is suggested by pleural thickening, contact of > 3 cm between the pleura and the tumor, obtuse angles between the tumor and pleura, or increased density of the extrapleural fat. A pleural effusion usually indicates a poor prognosis since lung cancers commonly metastasize to the opposite lung, liver, bones, brain, and adrenal glands. A chest CT performed in a patient who has suspected lung cancer should be continued through the liver and adrenal glands.

Whether to screen for lung cancer is a common question. Many years ago, it was clear that annual chest X-rays did little or nothing to reduce mortality from lung cancer, even in smokers. By the time lesions were clearly identified, they were advanced enough for many to have metastasized. Recent research using periodic low-dose CT for lung cancer screening of current (30+ pack years or former smokers (quit < 15 years) and who were age 55–74

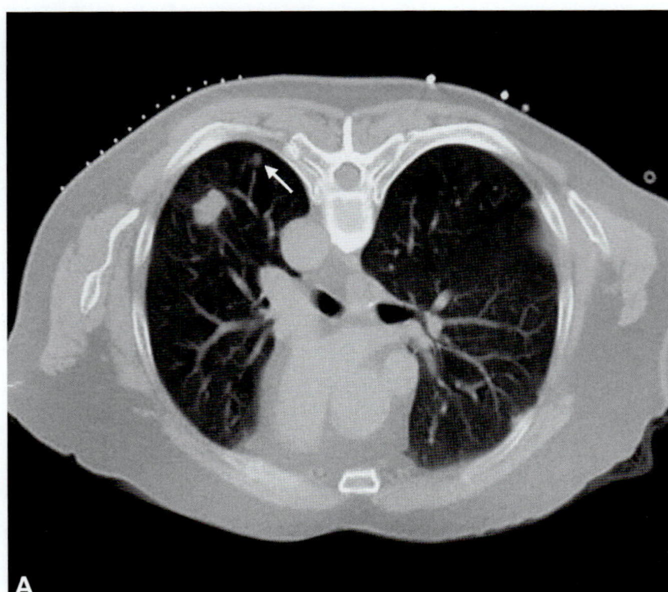

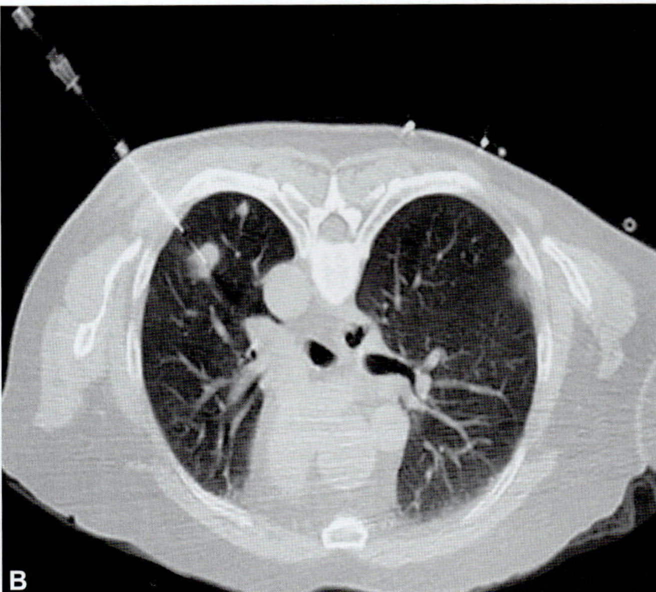

Figs. 15.6A and B: Percutaneous lung needle biopsy. (A) A prone computed tomography (CT) scan reveals a 1.5 cm lung mass and a tiny nodule (arrow) posteriorly in the left lung. (B) A needle biopsy of the mass is being performed using CT guidance. The other nodule was too small to reliably biopsy and if that were the only lesion the patient would have had a follow-up CT in a few months.

indicates that CT screening may confer a 20% reduction in lung cancer mortality. Guidance from the American Society for Clinical Oncology is as follows:

1. For smokers and former smokers ages 55–74 who have smoked for 30 pack-years or more and either continue to smoke or have quit within the past 15 years, annual screening with low-dose computed tomography (LDCT) should be offered over both annual screening with chest radiograph or no screening, but only in settings that can deliver the comprehensive care.
2. For individuals who have accumulated fewer than 30 pack-years of smoking, are either younger than 55 or older than 74, or who quit smoking > 15 years ago, as well as for individuals with severe comorbidities that would preclude potentially curative treatment and/or limit life expectancy, CT screening should not be performed.

Percutaneous Needle Biopsy of the Chest

Percutaneous needle biopsy of various chest lesions is readily accomplished utilizing fluoroscopic, CT or CT-fluoroscopy guidance (Figs. 15.6A and B). The techniques used are typically either fine-needle aspiration biopsy or core biopsy. Fine-needle aspiration biopsy is usually done with a coaxial technique, using an outer 17–19 gauge needle and an inner cutting or Chiba needle. Biopsies can be done on large pulmonary parenchymal masses, small nodules, pleural masses or even "ground glass" infiltrates. With large masses, care must be taken to avoid the center of the lesion that often may be necrotic and may not yield a diagnosis. Accuracy rates for large masses is often 90% or greater. Accuracy rates for diagnosis of small (< 1 cm) pulmonary nodules is reported to be about 50–75% and has a higher complication rate than larger pulmonary lesions. Accuracy rates for diagnosis of "ground glass" opacities are about 80%.

The most frequent complication is pneumothorax. The reported rate of pneumothorax rate varies widely but usually is reported to be between 15% and 30%. Thoracostomy tubes are needed to treat about one-fifth of the cases. Biopsy of smaller lesions is associated with up to a 50% pneumothorax rate. Larger coaxial needle size (18-gauge or greater) is associated with about a 50% higher pneumothorax rate as compared to thinner needles. Reported pneumothorax rate with core biopsy is up to 60%, with about one-third requiring a chest tube. Risk factors for pneumothorax include presence of COPD, the absence of a history of ipsilateral surgery, small lesion size, long needle path (> 4 cm), repeated pleural puncture and when the needle is inserted less perpendicular to the pleura. If a pneumothorax occurs during the procedure, a chest tube insertion may be avoided by manual aspiration before the needle is removed.[17,18]

The second most common complication is pulmonary, with reported frequencies ranging between 5% and 30%. The lower figure is based on hemoptysis and the higher figure is based on opacity seen around the biopsy site after

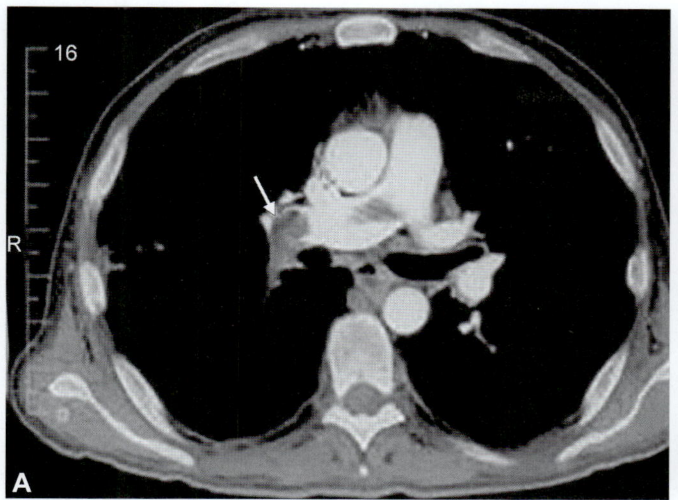

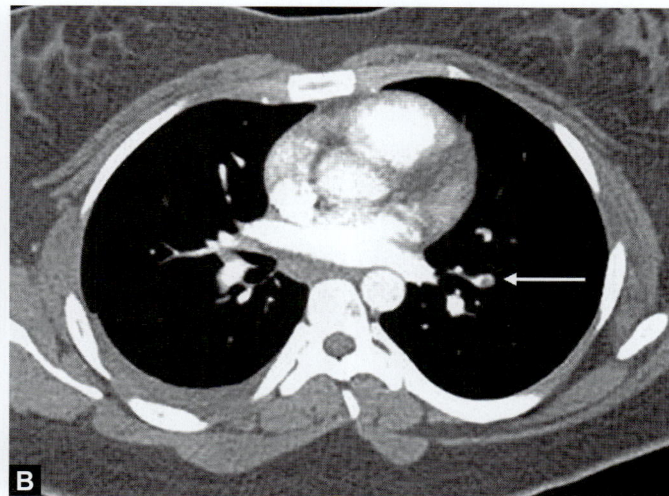

Figs. 15.7A and B: Pulmonary emboli. (A) A contrast-enhanced computed tomography (CT) scan of the chest shows a large clot (arrow) obstructing the right main pulmonary artery. (B) A small pulmonary embolism (arrow) is also seen on the left.

the procedure. As with pneumothorax, small lesion size, COPD and long biopsy path are associated with higher risk. Bleeding seen as opacity around the biopsy site is usually self-limited; however, if there is cough with hemoptysis the procedure is typically terminated.

Other complications include air embolism and tumor seeding, but these are extremely rare. Air embolism, which can be fatal, is reported in < 0.1% of procedures and probably results from placement of the needle in the pulmonary vein. Tumor seeding of the pleura or chest wall is reported in about 0.05% of lung biopsies but up to 4% with mesotheliomas.

Pulmonary Embolism (PE)

The chest X-ray findings in a patient with PE are relatively nonspecific, and the major reason for ordering a chest X-ray is to exclude other causes of the patient's symptoms. Occasionally a small pleural effusion, atelectasis, or an elevated hemidiaphragm may be present. If infarction of a portion of the lung is a result of the embolism, a peripheral wedge-shaped infiltrate may be noted. Historically a nuclear medicine ventilation/perfusion (V/Q) lung scan was the procedure of choice, but currently CT pulmonary angiography is the preferred initial imaging study for suspected pulmonary embolus (except for young females) (Figs. 15.7A and B). Computed tomography pulmonary angiography combined with ultrasound or D-dimer is the most effective algorithm.[19] With the current generation CT scanners, coverage of the entire chest in high resolution can be achieved in one short breath hold lasting a few seconds. Some difficulties with spiral CT protocols are the need for very precise timing of the contrast bolus to produce a diagnostic examination, and the clinical quandary presented by the detection of small peripheral emboli in normal persons or patients with minor symptoms. Incidental emboli are found in 1–5 % of the patients and many of these patients have malignancies. Incidental emboli are even more common in very old patients. Thus, the question of overdiagnosis of pulmonary emboli by CT angiography has been raised. If nuclear medicine scans or CT scans are equivocal and if a patient has positive tests for deep venous thrombosis, and clinical suspicion is high, the individual usually is treated.

BREAST

Imaging

Mammography is complementary to physical examination, and each can detect an appreciable number of tumors not found by the other. The primary purpose of mammography is to detect small breast cancers and, by so doing, to improve survival. Mammograms are often referred to as "screening" or "diagnostic/workup". The latter have special views and often use magnified images.

Ultrasound examination is often used as an adjunct to mammography to determine whether a lesion is solid or cystic and to localize a lesion for needle biopsy. Ultrasound can be a useful adjunctive method but should not be relied on as a screening method for breast cancer. Computed tomography scanning is not indicated for examination of the breast. Magnetic resonance imaging is occasionally used in selected patients.[20]

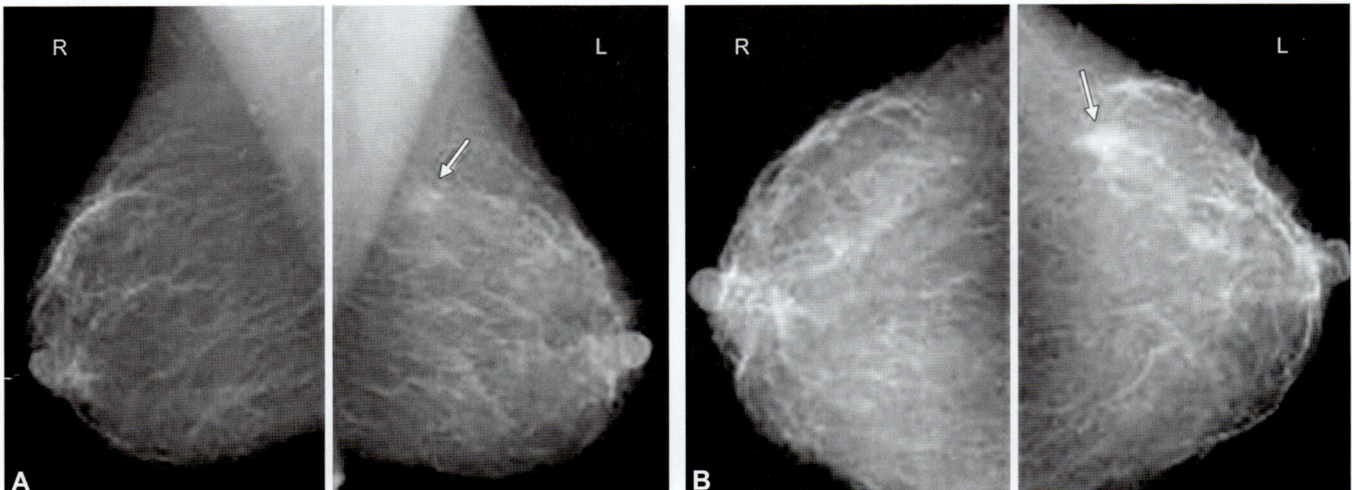

Figs. 15.8A and B: Breast cancer. Axillary oblique views (A) and craniocaudal views (B) of the right and left breast show an asymmetrical density (arrows) in the upper outer aspect of the left breast. Any asymmetrical density should raise suspicion of a neoplasm.

Computer-aided-detection (CAD) programs are built into modern digital mammography equipment and are commonly used to analyze the digital breast images for suspicious areas; they alert the radiologist to findings that may have been missed on initial image inspection. Literature remains divided on whether use of CAD increases early cancer detection rate; however, the use of the system increases the number of breast biopsies and false positive examinations.

Investigation and Biopsy of Breast Lesion

Once a suspicious lesion is identified on both craniocaudal and axillary oblique views (Figs. 15.8A and B), further investigation usually ensues in the form of a "diagnostic" magnified mammogram and an ultrasound examination or a biopsy. If the suspicious lesion is not palpable, a stereotactic needle biopsy or needle localization can be performed. In the X-ray stereotactic procedure, the patient is placed face down on a table with the breast suspended, and images are taken with coordinates. These coordinates are entered into a computer, and a core-biopsy gun is fired, taking a core sample of the lesion for pathologic analysis. Biopsy can also be done with ultrasound or MRI guidance (Figs. 15.9A and B). The needle localization procedure is done for nonpalpable lesions immediately before operation for excision or lumpectomy (Figs. 15.10A to D). A thin needle is inserted until it is shown that the end of the needle is either at or slightly past the lesion. At this point, a small amount of blue dye is injected, and a thin, hooked wire is passed through the needle. The needle is withdrawn, leaving the wire in place. The surgeon then removes the tissue near the end of the hooked wire. The biopsy specimen is X-rayed to make sure that the lesion of interest has been removed. The lymph node drainage of a breast cancer can be very variable. As a result, before operation for a known breast cancer, many surgeons will want the patient to have a nuclear medicine procedure to localize the sentinel node. A small amount of radioactive substance is injected near the lesion site, and then the radioactivity migrates to the nearest draining lymph node. This node can be marked or localized at operation, and in theory it is the node that is most likely to contain metastases.

Breast Cancer Screening

Breast cancer screening methods may include clinical breast examination (performed by a trained healthcare professional) and mammography. Breast self-examination is not recommended as a screening tool. Much discussion over the last decade has concerned the indications for screening mammography. Current guidelines are shown in Table 15.4. Ultrasound examination of the breast should not be considered to be a primary screening tool, because it cannot differentiate carcinomas from fibroadenomas or other benign solid lesions. It is most helpful in the initial workup of a young woman with a palpable lesion. Magnetic resonance imaging is used for screening in selected women who have a high risk (20–25% or greater) of breast cancer, those with an inherited gene mutation (BRCA1 or BRCA2), chest radiotherapy under the age of 30, or a personal history of lobular or ductal carcinoma in situ.

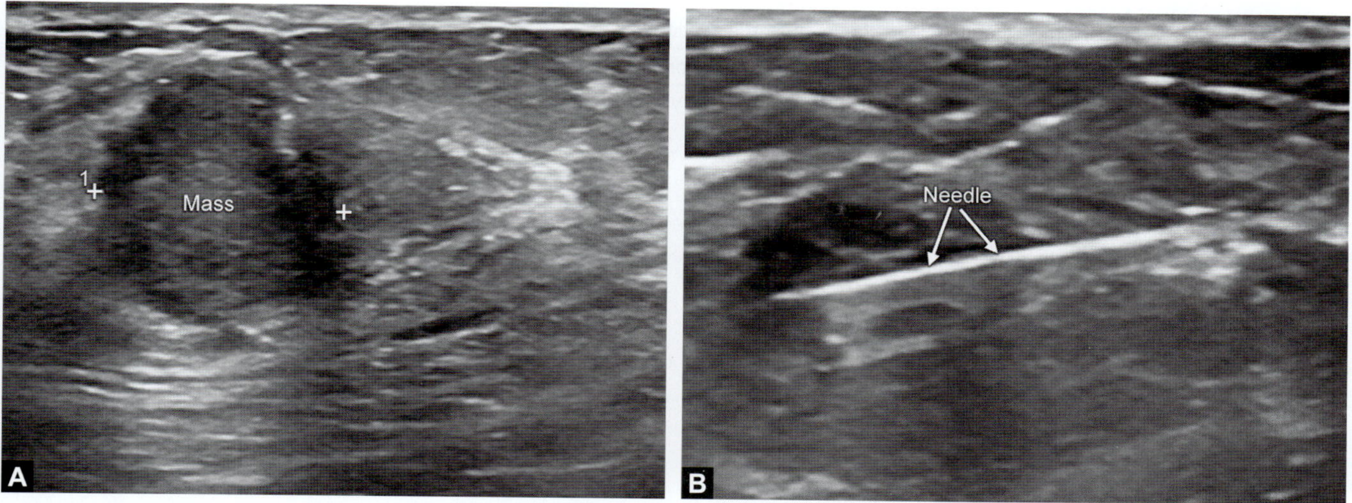

Figs. 15.9A and B: Ultrasound guided needle biopsy of breast cancer. (A) An ultrasound image shows a hypoechoic lesion with some central echoes indicating a mass rather than a cyst. (B) Another ultrasound image showing a core biopsy needle (arrows) in the lesion.

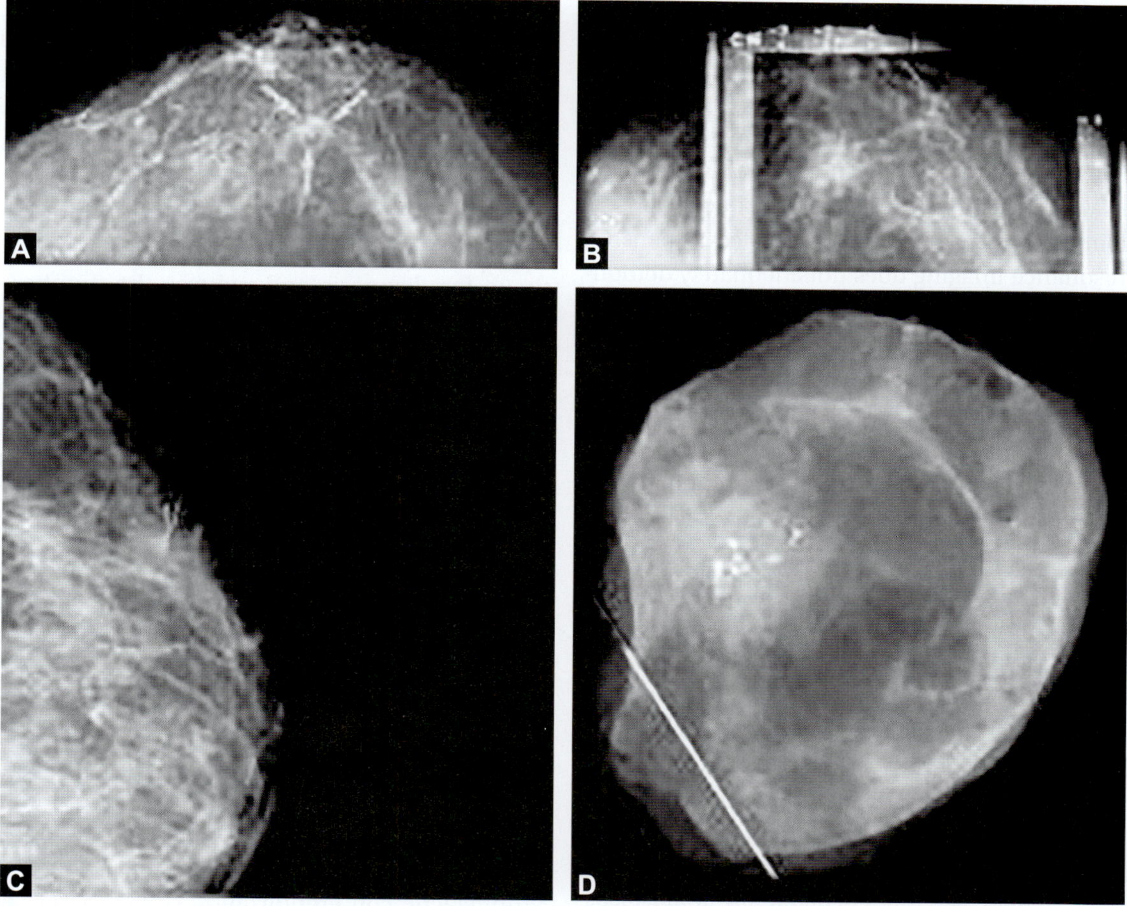

Figs. 15.10A to D: Localization and biopsy of a breast cancer. (A) A group of suspicious calcifications (arrows) is seen on a craniocaudal view of the left breast. (B) Needle localization is first performed by repeating the mammogram in the same projection but with an overlying grid that has coordinates. A needle is then inserted straight down at the appropriate coordinates. A lateral view of the breast is obtained, and when it is clear that the tip of the needle is in the right location, a hooked wire is inserted through the needle, and the needle is withdrawn (C). The patient is then taken to the operating room, and the specimen of concern at the end of the wire is removed. A magnified specimen X-ray is then obtained (D) to ensure that the suspicious calcifications have been removed.

Table 15.4 Breast cancer screening guidelines for various organizations as of 2015.

	American Cancer Society	*National Cancer Institute*	*U.S. Preventive Services Task Force*
Mammography	Age 40–44 annually personal choice Age 45–54 annually > Age 55 every 2 years	Every 1–2 years beginning age 40	Every 2 years ages 50–74
Clinical breast exam			
(age 20–39)	Every 3 years	No recommendation	Not enough evidence
(age 40 and greater)	Every year	No recommendation	Not enough evidence

GASTROINTESTINAL SYSTEM

Imaging

Suggested initial imaging procedures for various clinical situations involving the abdomen and pelvis are shown in Table 15.5. The reader is also referred to recent textbooks on the topic.[21,22]

Liver

Focal Liver Lesions

Currently MRI appears to be a little more sensitive and specific in the diagnosis of focal liver lesions than CT. It also allows multiplanar imaging. However, CT is distinctly better than MRI at demonstrating extrahepatic lesions as part of a comprehensive evaluation and is less expensive. Magnetic resonance imaging does not adequately demonstrate diffuse hepatic disease except for hepatic iron overload. The current standard MRI examination of the liver includes diffusion, T1-weighted, T2-weighted, and contrast-enhanced sequences. In general, T1 images are better for anatomic detail, while lesions are more conspicuous on T2 images. Gadolinium is used with dynamic scanning techniques to maximize detection and characterization of liver lesions.

Metastases are the most common malignant masses in the liver. They may be solid, necrotic, cystic or calcified, and avascular or hypervascular. Metastatic disease must be considered in the differential diagnosis of virtually all hepatic masses. Most metastases on CT are seen as low-density masses in the portal venous phase of contrast enhancement. Cavernous hemangiomas are the most common benign liver lesion and are found in about 7% of the population. Up to 10% of people have multiple hemangiomas, which can be mistaken for metastases. The lesions are more common in women and are usually < 5 cm in diameter. On CT there is a well-defined hypodense mass on unenhanced scans. The characteristic pattern of enhancement with a contrast bolus is nodular enhancement from the periphery. On delayed images the lesion becomes isodense or hyperdense compared with normal liver. On MRI hemangiomas have a "light bulb" bright T2 signal and a similar contrast enhancement pattern. Atypical hemangiomas can be evaluated with a nuclear medicine red blood cell study or MRI.

Liver Biopsy and Drainage

Ultrasonographically visible liver masses near the dome that move appreciably during respiration or abut the capsule can be biopsied in real time. CT is preferred for deep lesions such as para-aortic nodes or mediastinal masses, for lesions not seen by ultrasonography and for difficult access cases. Fine-needle biopsy with or without aspiration provides a cellular sample that can be stained. The presence of a cytopathologist during the biopsy slightly prolongs procedure time, but ensures adequate tissue for diagnosis and reduces the number of repeat biopsies. Core biopsy samples contain tissue structure and are sent for histologic diagnosis. A percutaneous transjugular approach for nonfocal liver disease is often selected for patients with uncorrectable coagulopathy, ascites, thrombocytopenia, obesity, and poor pulmonary function.

Pyogenic liver abscesses can be treated either with percutaneous catheter drainage or percutaneous needle aspiration (18 gauge trocar needle) in combination with systemic antibiotics (Figs. 15.11A to C). Treatment with aspiration may require multiple attempts but may be as effective as continuous catheter drainage.[23]

Liver Tumor Chemoembolization and Ablation

Documentation of portal vein patency and a detailed diagnostic angiogram are essential before treatment. Prophylactic coil embolization of nontarget vessels may be necessary if there is unfavorable anatomy to prevent inadvertent ischemia. Prophylactic antibiotics before and after treatment reduce the risk of postembolization abscess formation. A percutaneous transcatheter infusion of a combination of a long lasting contrast agent, an

Table 15.5 Suggested initial imaging study to order for various abdominal problems.

Clinical problem	*Imaging study*
Gastroesophageal reflux	
Mild or transient symptoms	Medical therapy
Severe or persistent symptoms	Endoscopy with biopsy
Esophageal obstruction	Barium swallow
Esophageal tear	Gastrografin swallow
Bowel perforation or free air	Upright chest and supine abdominal plain radiograph; supine and left lateral decubitus, if patient is unable to stand
Hematemesis	Endoscopy (less preferred, contrast UGI series)
Gastric or duodenal ulcer	Test for Helicobacter pylori; if medical therapy fails, endoscopy or double contrast upper GI series
Trauma, blunt or penetrating	Chext X-ray, supine/upright abdomen and CT with IV contrast
Abdominal aortic aneurysm	Supine and lateral abdomen, then ultrasound or CT with IV contrast
Pancreatic mass or inflammation	CT or MRI
Pancreatic pseudocyst follow-up	CT or ultrasound
Acute abdominal pain with fever (? abscess)	CT with IV contrast
Liver lesion	
(incidental non-cystic found on ultrasound)	MRI or CT with and without IV
(suspect metastases) MRI or CT with and without IV contrast	MRI or CT with and without IV
Acute cholecystitis	Ultrasound
Chronic cholelithiasis	Right upper quadrant ultrasound
Common duct obstruction	Right upper quadrant ultrasound
Jaundice	
(painful)	Ultrasound or CT with and without IV contrast
(painless, suspect biliary obstruction)	CT with and without IV contrast
(painless, suspect liver)	Ultrasound
Suspected bile leak	Nuclear medicine hepatobiliary study
Small bowel stricture or polyp	CT enterography
Intestinal obstruction	Supine and upright radiograph of abdomen as an initial study, followed by those listed below
Esophagus or stomach obstruction	UGI and small bowel series or endoscopy
Small bowel obstruction	CT with IV contrast
Distal small bowel or colon obstruction	Barium enema
Crohn's disease	CT with IV contrast or CT enterography
Right upper quadrant pain	Ultrasound or nuclear medicine hepatobiliary scan (□ ? Murphy's sign, fever)
Right lower quadrant pain	Ultrasound, if female <45 years; CT, if suspect inflammatory process
Appendicitis	
(adults)	CT
(children)	Ultrasound
Suspected pelvic abscess	CT with IV contrast or ultrasound
Ulcerative colitis	Colonoscopy; if incomplete or unavailable, barium enema
Ischemic colitis	CT with IV contrast
Suspected renal or ureteral stone	Noncontrast CT
Uterine or ovarian pathology	Ultrasound
Abdominal tumor	CT with IV contrast
Colon cancer	Colonoscopy; if incomplete double contrast barium enema
Acute diverticulitis (LLQ pain)	CT with IV contrast
Rectal bleeding (obvious)	
(dark red)	Esophagogastroduodenoscopy; if not available, UGI series
(bright red)	Colonoscopy
Positive fecal occult blood test	
(older than 40 years)	Colonoscopy
(younger than 40 years with GI symptoms)	Helicobacter pylori test, therapeutic trial; if fails, endoscopy or UGI series

(CT: Computed tomography; MRCP: Magnetic resonance cholangiopancreatography; GI: Gastrointestinal; UGI: Upper gastrointestinal).
Source: Adapted with permission from Mettler FA. Essentials of Radiology, 3rd edition. Philadelphia, PA: Elsevier/Saunders; 2014.

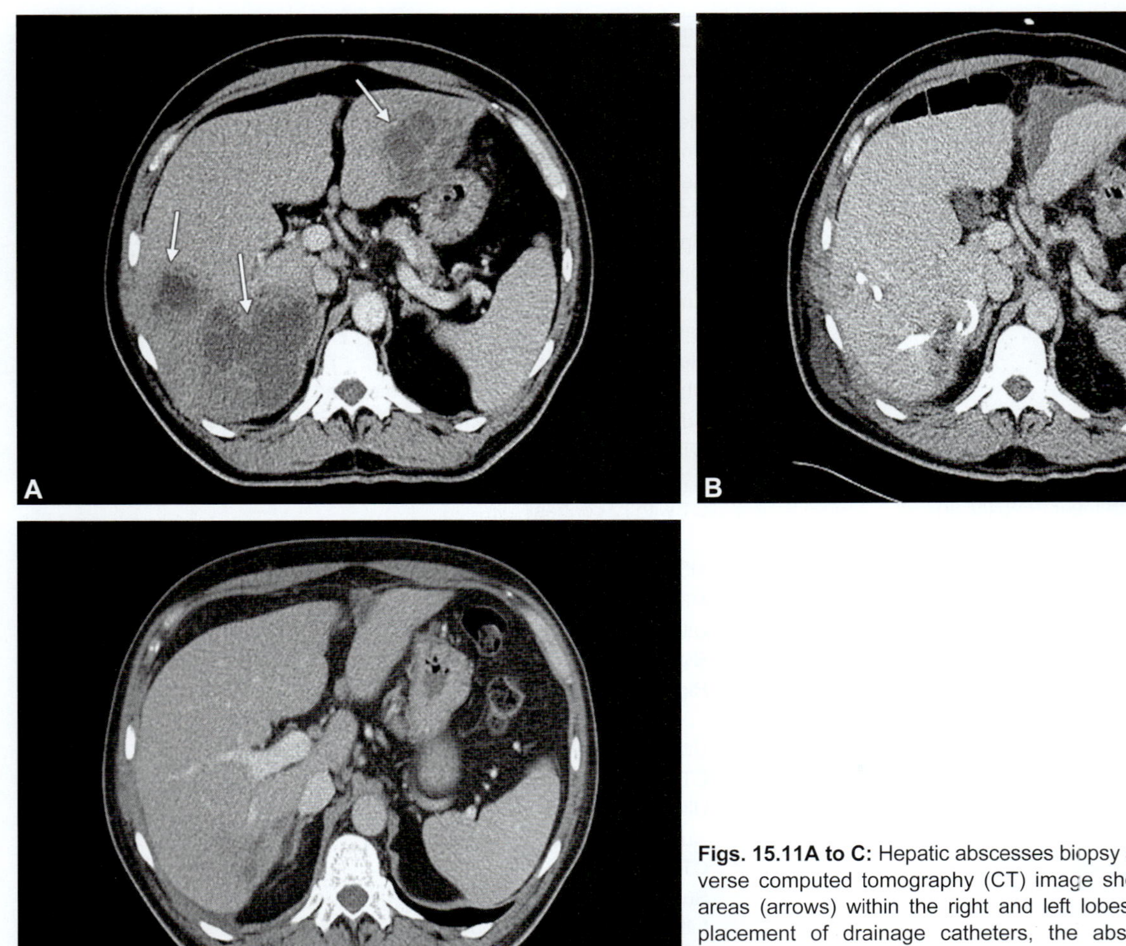

Figs. 15.11A to C: Hepatic abscesses biopsy and drainage. (A) A transverse computed tomography (CT) image shows multiple low density areas (arrows) within the right and left lobes. (B) After percutaneous placement of drainage catheters, the abscesses are significantly resolved. (C) Three weeks later the CT scan shows almost complete resolution.

appropriate chemotherapeutic agent, and an embolic agent is a relatively effective treatment for unresectable hepatic malignancies. Occluding arterial inflow with embolic particles delays washout of the chemotherapy drug and may increase contact time with the tumor. Lipiodol is taken up by hepatocellular carcinoma and serves as a marker of viable tumor on CT images. Postembolization syndrome with fever, chills, and nausea following treatment may be severe. Tumors < 3 cm in size in a favorable location can be treated ethanol injection under real-time ultrasound imaging.

In addition to embolization, hepatic neoplasms can be treated by percutaneous thermal ablation. With the radiofrequency ablation (RFA) or microwave method a needle-like probe is introduced percutaneously into the tumor, a current is delivered and heat is generated at the tip using an alternating current delivered through a 14–21 gauge needle that is electrically insulated except for the terminal 1–3 cm. The cryoablation probe uses liquid nitrogen or argon gas to freeze the tissue. Thermal ablation is used to treat unresectable hepatomas (HCC) in early cirrhosis and colorectal liver metastases. Most treatments for HCC can be done under conscious sedation, but extensive liver metastases may require general anesthesia. Following thermal ablation, for inoperable colorectal metastases the 5-year survival rate is about 30% and for HCC it is 40–50%. Limitations include the volume of tissue that can be treated (up to 4–5 cm in diameter) or 3–5 tumors.[24] Some authors feel that hepatic resection is superior to percutaneous ablation for tumors > 3 cm in diameter.

Gallbladder

Cholecystitis

In spite of the fact that nuclear medicine hepatobiliary imaging is slightly more specific in the diagnosis of acute

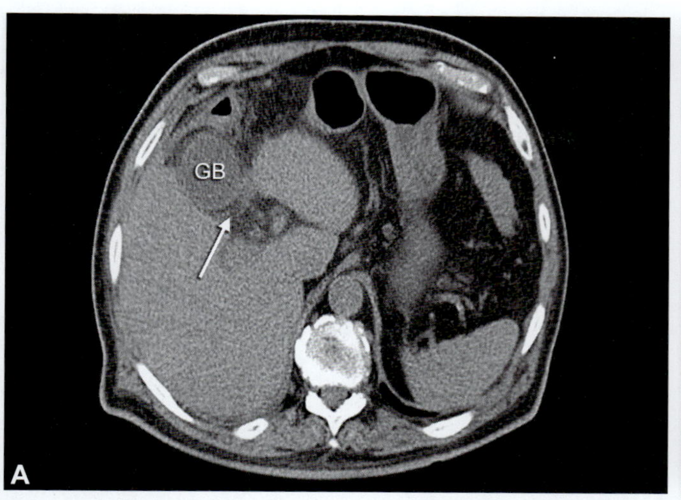

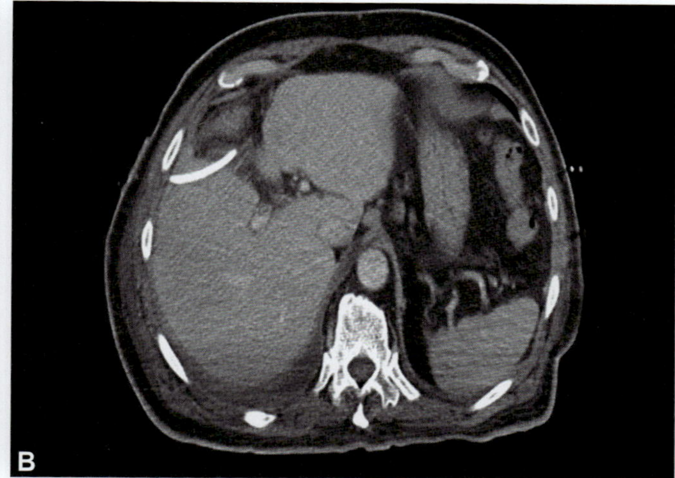

Figs. 15.12A and B: Percutaneous cholecystostomy. (A) A computed tomography scan in a severely debilitated febrile patient shows a thick walled gallbladder and surrounding edema (arrow). (B) Transthoracic transhepatic placement of a drainage tube stabilized the patient.

cholecystitis, ultrasonography is often the imaging study of choice. Ultrasound detects 95% of all gallstones. The ultrasound diagnosis of acute cholecystitis requires the presence of cholelithiasis and a positive ultrasonographic Murphy sign. This sign is present when transducer pressure over the gallbladder causes pain, but it can be falsely negative in emphysematous, gangrenous or perforated cholecystitis. Other less specific findings include a dilated gallbladder, gallbladder wall thickening, and pericholecystic fluid.

Failure to visualize the gallbladder when a nuclear medicine hepatobiliary study is carried out to 4 hours has a very high specificity for acute cholecystitis. In chronic cholecystitis, the gallbladder fills with activity, but later than normal. The nuclear medicine hepatobiliary examination has a 95% accuracy rate for detecting acute cholecystitis.

Cholecystostomy

Management of most biliary abnormalities is now performed via laparoscopic or endoscopic methods. There remain, however, some indications for percutaneous procedures. Percutaneous cholecystostomy may be performed at the bedside under ultrasonographic guidance in critically ill patients who have a distended thick-walled gallbladder, spiking fevers and no other identifiable etiology (Figs. 15.12A and B). Prophylactic antibiotics are required before manipulation to prevent bacteremia. The catheter should be left in place for 4–6 weeks to allow a tract to form and prevent intraperitoneal bile leakage when the tube is removed. Gallbladder aspiration is as effective as catheter drainage for the treatment of acalculous cholecystitis.

Biliary Obstruction

Benign biliary obstruction may be a consequence of common bile duct stones or an iatrogenic injury in otherwise healthy patients. In most patients dilated bile ducts are imaged using ultrasound, CT or MR cholangiogram (Figs. 15.13A to C). A fluoroscopic cholangiogram performed through an existing T-tube, endoscopic retrograde cholangiopancreatography or a percutaneous transhepatic approach can define the nature of the obstruction. Although operation is usually the treatment of choice, in high-risk patients strictures may be dilated with balloons, with or without stent placement. Strictures tend to recur and repeated dilatation may be necessary.

Malignant biliary obstruction may be treated initially by percutaneous transhepatic drainage. Internal-external drainage catheters placed from a percutaneous transhepatic approach allow access to the biliary system and can be exchanged over a guidewire to maintain patency. Self-expanding metallic and plastic endoprostheses can be placed percutaneously or endoscopically for palliation in patients who have a short life expectancy. Endoscopic or percutaneous access to endoprostheses obstructed by debris and tumor in growth allows further intervention, with varying degrees of success.

Spleen

The spleen is the most commonly traumatized solid organ. Findings range from contusion to frank organ fracture. Although surgeons usually try to manage these injuries conservatively, splenic rupture may be noted even a week

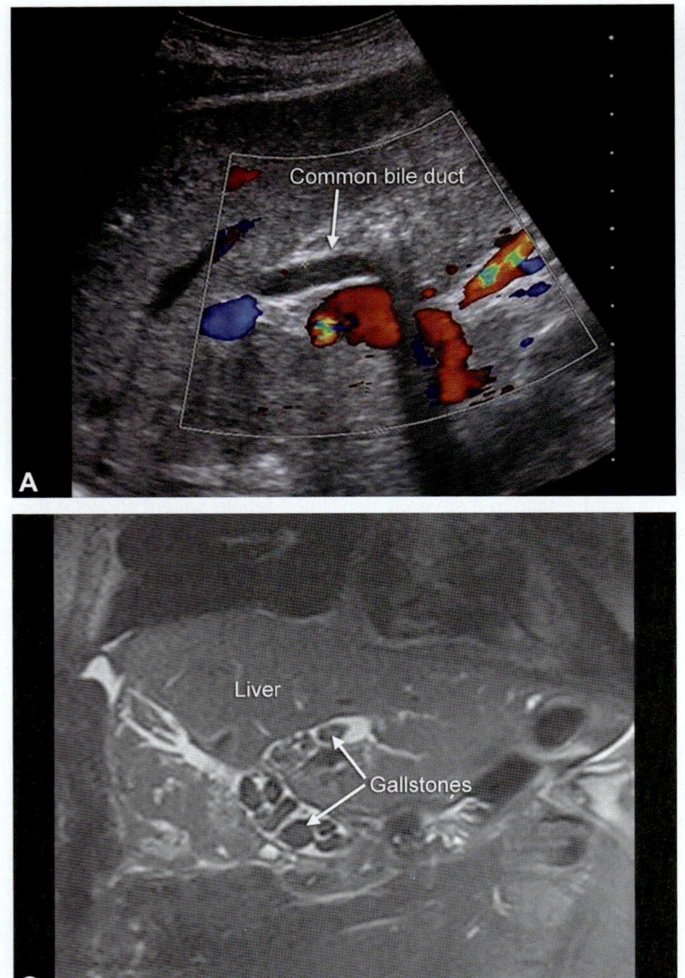

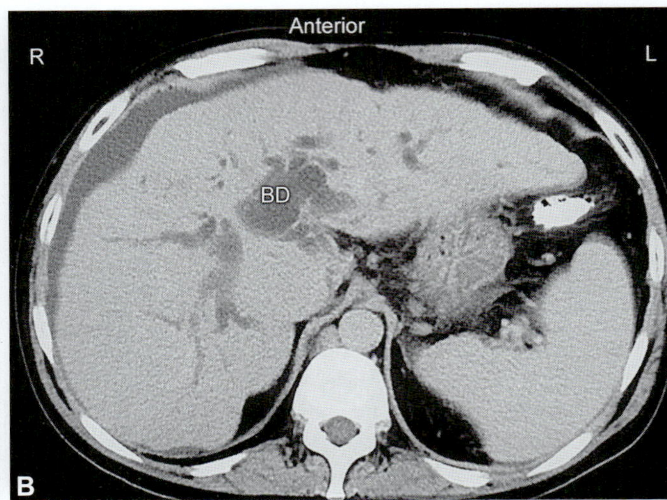

Figs. 15.13A to C: Biliary dilatation. (A) Color Doppler ultrasound. In addition to displaying anatomy, ultrasound can analyze blood flow direction and velocity. In this longitudinal image of the liver, the red is blood in the portal vein flowing toward the transducer (located on the anterior aspect of the abdomen) and the blue represents blood flowing away from the transducer. The common bile duct is prominent and has no color. (B) A computed tomography scan shows multiple low-density dilated bile ducts centrally in the liver. (C) In a different patient, a magnetic resonance cholangiopancreatography shows a dilated biliary system containing multiple large gallstones (arrows).

to 10 days after the initial injury. A CT scan is the test of choice. Hemorrhage and hematoma usually appear as areas of lower density than the spleen. Round or irregular dark areas represent intrasplenic hematomas or lacerations, and abnormal crescentic areas at the edge of the spleen represent subcapsular hematomas. Post-traumatic splenic bleeding can often be managed with embolization. In addition to being identifiable as trauma, focal splenic lesions can easily be seen on a CT scan. These can be due to splenic abscesses, infarcts, tumors, and occasionally cysts. The sensitivity of CT for detection of these is high, but the specificity is poor, and often the clinical history is necessary to narrow the differential diagnosis. The complication rate of splenic percutaneous biopsy is low and similar to that of other abdominal organs.

Pancreas

The diagnosis of pancreatitis is clinical, but imaging is used to determine prognosis and identify complications. Computed tomography is normal in onethird of cases of acute pancreatitis. The CT findings of pancreatitis include pancreatic enlargement, decreased density due to edema, intrapancreatic fluid collections, and blurring of gland margins caused by inflammation. Peripancreatic CT findings include peripancreatic fluid collections and stranding densities, and thickening of retroperitoneal fat and fascial planes. Necrosis of the gland results in liquefaction of the tissue, evidenced by loss of normal enhancement on a dynamic contrast-enhanced CT.

Pancreatic drainage is usually done for pseudocyst, abscess or necrosis (Figs. 15.14A and B). Drainage can be done endoscopically, percutaneously, or surgically. Both endoscopic and percutaneous drainage are available for drainage of pancreatic abscesses. Drainage of uncomplicated pseudocysts is most often performed endoscopically or surgically. Indications for drainage are presence of symptoms, enlargement of cyst, complications including hemorrhage, rupture, and suspicion of malignancy.

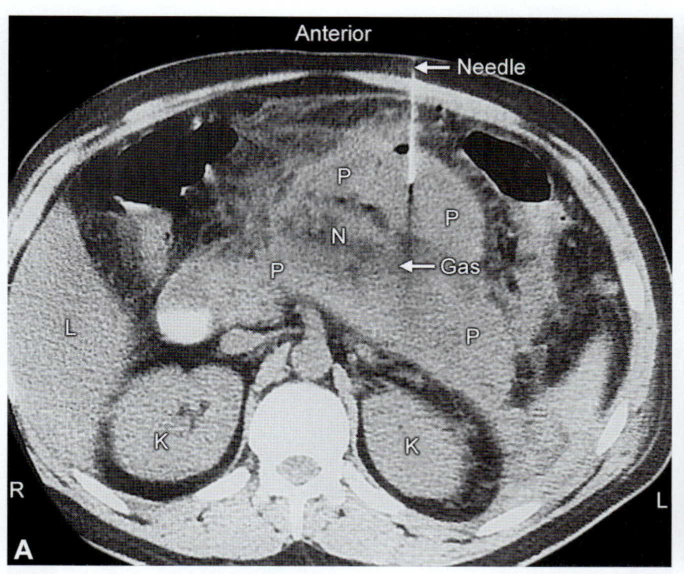

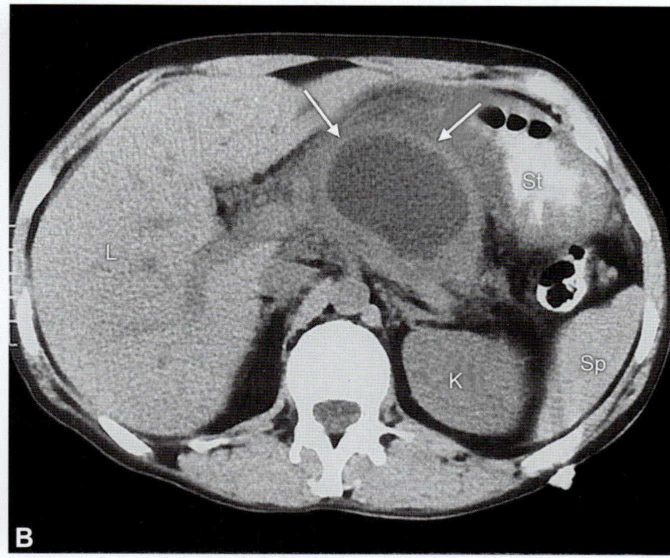

Figs. 15.14A and B: Complications of pancreatitis. (A) A transverse computed tomography (CT) scan in a patient with pancreatitis and a persistent fever shows a very enlarged pancreas (P); a low-density area within it represents necrosis of the pancreas. Also noted is a small gas bubble due to the formation of a pancreatic abscess. A needle has been inserted under CT guidance to obtain material for culture and to place a percutaneous drain. (B) In a second, patient who is a chronic alcoholic, the CT scan demonstrates a well-defined low-density area within the pancreas (arrows). This represents a pancreatic pseudocyst.

Percutaneous drainage is indicated for poor risk patients, for immature cysts and infected pseudocysts.[25] Endoscopic pseudocyst drainage is preferred for mature pseudocysts with a distinct capsule abutting the stomach.

Pancreatic ductal adenocarcinoma accounts for 95% of the malignant tumors of the pancreas. The tumor may be detected by dynamic, thin-section, contrasted CT as a low density mass, most frequently in the head of the pancreas. Tumors in the head or uncinate process (60–70% of cases) may be quite small and can encroach on the bile duct, causing jaundice. Tumors in the body and tail develop without symptoms until they are large. Secondary signs of pancreatic cancer on CT include atrophy of the distal gland, smooth dilatation of the pancreatic duct and dilatation of both the bile duct and main pancreatic duct ("double duct" sign). Biopsy may be needed to differentiate a pancreatic neoplasm from focal pancreatitis in difficult cases.

Small and Large Intestine

Enterostomy Tubes

Nasogastric tubes are appropriate for feeding of 30 days or less. Long-term support for head and neck malignancies or neurologic conditions requires percutaneous gastrostomy (PEG) and gastrojejunostomy feeding tubes that are placed under fluoroscopy, using standard over-the-wire technique and insufflation of the stomach (Figs. 15.15A to E). A CT scan is often obtained prior to the procedure to assess anatomy. The procedure can have a significant rate (2–6%) of major complications (including death 0.3%, peritonitis or hemorrhage 1–2%) and minor complications of about 10%. Complication rates are typically higher in patients with malignancies. Approximately 5–15% of patients will have post procedure pneumoperitoneum that is often benign but about 10% patients with pneumoperitoneum will require emergent surgical intervention.[26] Small bowel access is necessary for patients who are unable to tolerate gastric feedings. Manipulation through the pylorus and beyond the ligament of Treitz with a catheter and wire combination allows proper jejunal placement for enteral feedings. Direct percutaneous jejunostomy is also possible. Feedings can be started 6 hours after placement. Flushing the catheter with tap water following each feeding assists in long-term patency.

Colonic Obstruction Versus Colonic Paralytic Ileus

The key to the differentiation of colonic obstruction and paralytic ileus on a plain abdominal film is whether there is dilatation of the cecum. The cecum is the most dilated portion of the colon in large bowel obstruction, irrespective of the site. If the transverse colon is more dilated than the cecum, a diagnosis of ileus should be considered. An abnormally distended transverse colon (> 6 cm diameter) is suggestive of megacolon. A toxic megacolon can result from ulcerative colitis, Crohn's disease or infectious causes.

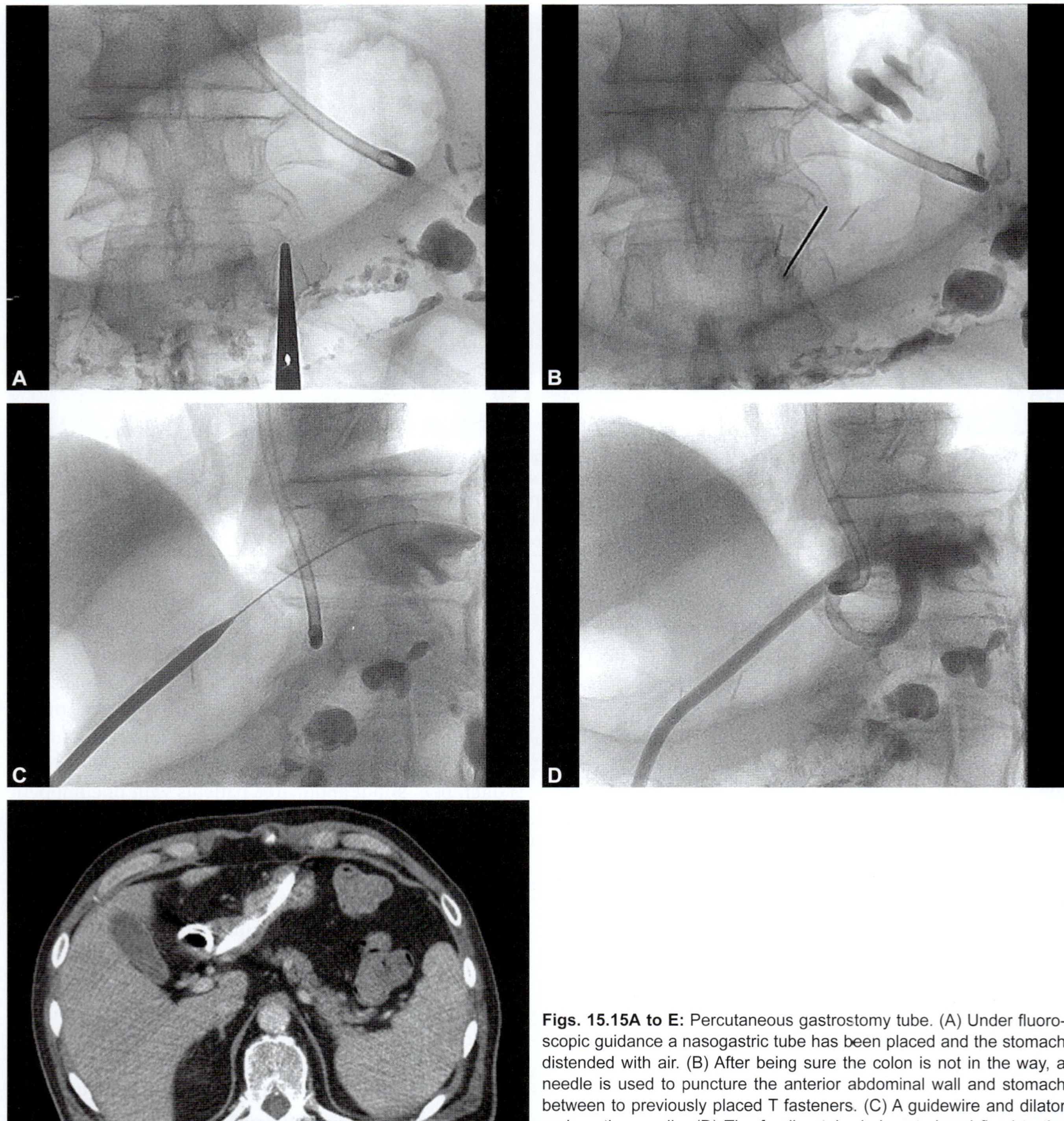

Figs. 15.15A to E: Percutaneous gastrostomy tube. (A) Under fluoroscopic guidance a nasogastric tube has been placed and the stomach distended with air. (B) After being sure the colon is not in the way, a needle is used to puncture the anterior abdominal wall and stomach between to previously placed T fasteners. (C) A guidewire and dilator replace the needle. (D) The feeding tube is inserted and fixed to the abdominal wall. (E) Transverse computed tomography scan shows the tube within the gastric lumen.

Acute colonic distension (cecum > 9 cm diameter) is associated with an increased risk of perforation. Patients with a chronically distended colon have only a small risk of perforation. Chronic distension may be a result of chronic laxative abuse, neuromuscular disorders (including diabetes mellitus), psychogenic problems or metabolic problems (electrolyte imbalance, hypothyroidism, morphine derivatives).

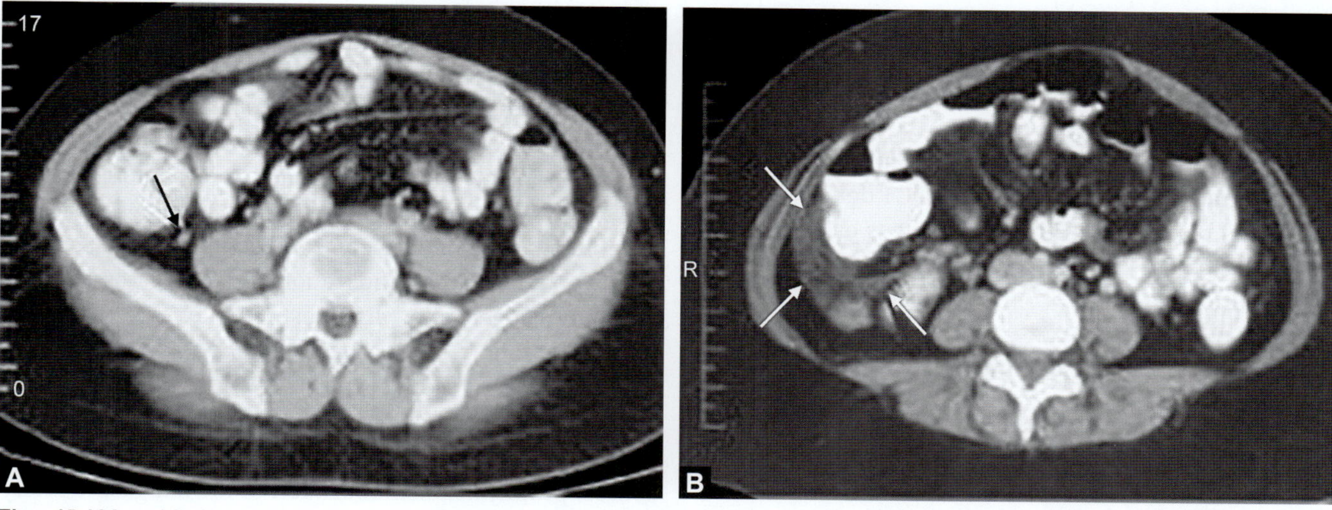

Figs. 15.16A and B: Normal appendix and appendicitis. (A)The appendix can be seen on this computed tomography (CT) scan image where it joins the cecum (arrow). (B) In a patient with mild appendicitis, the CT scan shows stranding due to edema (arrows) in the tissues surrounding the cecum.

A sigmoid volvulus is about three times more common than a cecal volvulus. A sigmoid volvulus is seen on the plain abdominal film as a massively dilated loop of colon that looks like an inverted U projecting up out of the pelvis toward the right upper quadrant. Air is usually seen in the proximal colon. With a cecal volvulus, there is a dilated loop of colon pointing towards the left upper quadrant and there is usually associated small bowel dilatation. If clinically indicated, the diagnostic study of choice for both these conditions is a barium enema.

Appendicitis

Ultrasound scanning of the appendix is an accurate method for diagnosing appendicitis. The normal appendix may not be visualized or may appear < 6 mm thick. The wall should be no > 3 mm thick. When the appendix is identified, pressure is applied with the transducer. If the lumen can be obliterated by pressure, the appendix is normal. The diagnostic finding in appendicitis is a noncompressible, sausage-shaped, blind-ending pouch that has inflamed and rigid walls. If ultrasound is nondiagnostic, CT is indicated. Identification of an appendicolith suggests appendicitis. In experienced hands the overall accuracy of ultrasound is about 90%. Due to lack of qualified staff and often lacking availability of ultrasound after hours, CT scanning has become the most common diagnostic test (Figs. 15.16A and B). CT scanning also has the advantage of being easily interpretable and finding other potential causes of the patient' symptoms. With CT, early appendicitis can be recognized by diameter > 7 mm, wall thickening, and edema surrounding the appendix. After rupture an abscess can be localized and characterized for potential percutaneous drainage.

Diverticulitis

Computed tomography is excellent for demonstrating diverticulitis, including paracolic inflammation and abscess. In this setting, the pericolic fat is increased in density. The colonic wall is thickened, and the pericolic abscess appears as a soft tissue or fluid density mass. Computed tomography is also useful for demonstrating the complications of diverticulitis, which include bowel obstruction and fistula formation. Sinus tracts may lead to larger abscess cavities in the peritoneal or retroperitoneal compartments.

Abdominal and Pelvic Abscess

The pelvis is the most common site for abscess formation. Plain film findings of abscess include a soft tissue mass, a collection of extraluminal gas, viscus displacement, localized or generalized ileus, elevation of the diaphragm, pleural effusion, and pulmonary basilar changes. A focal collection of extraluminal gas is the most specific sign of abscess, but is uncommon.

Computed tomography signs of an abscess include a peripherally enhancing loculated fluid collection, often with internal debris and air-fluid levels. The walls of the fluid collection are often thick and irregular. Gas within the fluid collection is strong evidence of an abscess. Fascia adjacent to the abscess is thickened, while surrounding the abscess may be increased in density and contains soft tissue strands due to inflammation. Oral and rectal contrasts are sometimes needed to differentiate unopacified loops of bowel from abscess collections. CT is the imaging method of choice when a periappendiceal abscess is suspected. A periappendiceal phlegmon is seen as an indurated soft tissue mass with a CT density > 20 HU. A liquefied mass < 20 HU in CT density is evidence of an abscess. Abscesses > 3 cm generally require surgical or catheter drainage.

Percutaneous Fluid Drainage

CT is the modality of choice for diagnosing abdominal abscess and fluid collections. It allows access to small or deep collections such as pelvic and psoas abscesses. Subphrenic, perihepatic and loculated collections are better visualized with ultrasound. Low pelvic abscesses can be treated with CT-guided transgluteal or ultrasound-guided transrectal or transvaginal drainage. Needle aspiration can be used for diagnosis and to confirm the necessity of drainage. Prophylactic antibiotics are given before drainage to prevent bacteremia. The over-the-wire (Seldinger) technique is used routinely for access, and locking-loop catheters are placed to decrease the risk of inadvertent early removal. Multiple catheters may be required for complete drainage of loculated fluid. Responsible patients may be discharged with tubes in place and followed up as outpatients. Catheters are removed when drainage decreases to < 20 mL/day and an imaging study shows no residual fluid or fistula tract.

Trauma

CT is the imaging method of choice for blunt abdominal trauma. Liver, spleen and renal injuries are easily identified with contrastenhanced CT. A laceration is seen as an irregular cleft through the parenchyma with associated intra-abdominal or periorgan blood. Fractures are lacerations that extend from one surface of an organ to another. Subcapsular hematomas are seen as peripheral low-density lenticular-shaped masses that displace parenchyma inward. Hematomas appear as irregular low-density areas within the parenchyma. CT examination is limited in the detection of bowel injuries. Pneumoperitoneum is a rare, but specific finding. Fluid around the root of the mesentery, in the leaves of the mesentery and adjacent to a bowel loop, as well as irregular bowel wall thickening, suggests the possibility of bowel or mesenteric injury.

Gastrointestinal Hemorrhage

Therapeutic angiography may be indicated for patients who have marked gastrointestinal hemorrhage. The bleeding rate required for visualization is 0.5–1.0 mL/min. The celiac axis, superior mesenteric, and inferior mesenteric arteries are selected for completeness. A transcatheter infusion of vasopressin may help to control bleeding. Pharmacologic failure may require embolization of feeding vessels with Gelfoam pledgets after vasoconstriction effects have worn off. Embolization is associated with a risk of bowel infarction, which requires subsequent resection when the patient becomes more stable. If an upper gastrointestinal bleed is documented by endoscopy without an angiographic source, prophylactic embolization of the left gastric artery may be considered.

Bowel Ischemia

Bowel ischemia is a clinically difficult diagnosis. The appearance is often similar to that of mechanical bowel obstruction. CT scanning is often performed for abdominal pain or suspected obstruction. If ischemia is high on the list of clinical suspicion, CT scan without and with intravenous contrast is indicated (Figs. 15.17A and B). Abnormal renal function due to dehydration may preclude use of intravenous contrast material in a number of patients. Many CT findings are nonspecific including bowel wall thickening, dilated bowel loops, ileus, and thumb-printing of the mucosa.

Acute mesenteric ischemia is typically due to arterial thromboembolic disease and low-flow states. CT findings include segmental bowel wall thickening, bowel dilatation, enhancement abnormalities (increased bowel wall density on noncontrasted CT scan or lack of enhancement with intravenous contrast), intravascular thrombus, pneumatosis, portal venous gas, and ascites.[27] Mesenteric venous ischemia and thrombus is less frequent. Patients with acute venous thrombosis often present with midabdominal pain out of proportion to clinical findings. Chronic thrombosis is often an incidental finding seen in patients with cirrhosis, portal hypertension, and varices. The CT diagnosis is made by visualization of thrombus seen as a low density structure within the vein.[28]

Colorectal Cancer

A debate is ongoing as to whether colonoscopy, barium enema, or CT virtual colonoscopy is the appropriate

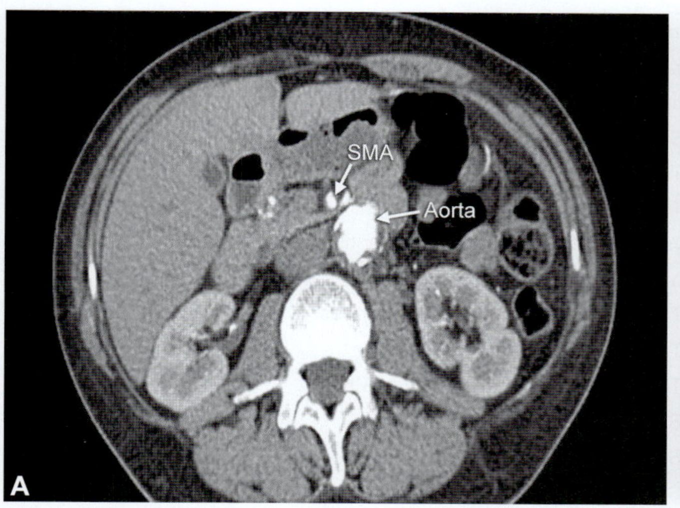

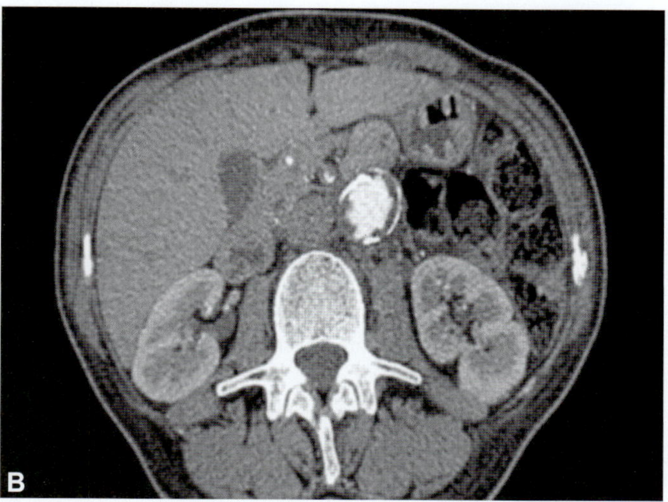

Figs. 15.17A and B: Superior mesenteric artery (SMA) occlusion. (A) A transverse image from a computed tomography angiogram shows arterial contrast in an atherosclerotic aorta and SMA (arrow). (B) Another image from a study several days later shows that there has been occlusion.

method of workup or screening. Barium enema is relatively inexpensive compared with colonoscopy, and it has about the same accuracy rate. The advantage of colonoscopy is that if a lesion is identified, a biopsy can be performed immediately. Screening for polyps and colon cancer is commonly done by a fecal guaiac occult blood test (gFOBT) and sigmoidoscopy. An FOBT has a high incidence of false-positive results from a diet high in red meat or peroxide-containing vegetables (e.g., broccoli, turnips, cauliflower). A new type of fecal occult blood test called a fecal immunochemical test (FIT or iFOBT) is superior to the guaiac text. Sigmoidoscopy provides only very limited visualization of the colon. After a positive FOBT, colonoscopy is usually performed. If colonoscopy is not available or if there is inadequate visualization of the entire colon, a double-contrast barium enema may be performed.

The recommendations for colorectal cancer screening vary among organizations. For persons older than 50 years who are at average risk, the American College of Physicians (ACP) recommends optical colonoscopy or flexible sigmoidoscopy. High-risk patients should be screened beginning at age 40 or 10 years younger than the age at which the youngest affected relative was diagnosed with colorectal cancer. High-risk patients are recommended to have only optical colonoscopy. Screening is not recommended for most patients over 75 years old or who have a life expectancy of < 10 years. For persons with positive screening test results of any type, optical colonoscopy should be used. The recommended interval for screening average risk patients is generally 10 years for optical colonoscopy, 5 years for double-contrast barium enema, CT colonoscopy and flexible sigmoidoscopy and annually for gFOBT or iFOBT. While the American Cancer Society and the American College of Radiology recommend use of CT colonoscopy for screening, the ACP guidelines do not recommend CT colonoscopy and the U.S. Preventative Services Task Force (USPSTF) found that there was insufficient evidence to assess the benefits and harms of this procedure.

CT scanning is usually done to assess the extent of disease locally and in lymph nodes and the liver. Accuracy for detection of lymph node metastases is poor (~60%). If the nodes are enlarged, they probably have tumor within them, but nodes can be of normal size and still contain tumor. A CT scan with intravenous contrast of the liver often will show multiple low-density metastases.[18] F-FDG PET/CT scans are currently being used to look for distant metastases or in those with suspected recurrence of colon cancer.

GENITOURINARY TRACT

Imaging

Suggested initial imaging procedures for various clinical situations involving the genitourinary system are shown in Table 15.6, and the reader is referred to an excellent textbook on the topic.[29]

Table 15.6 Suggested initial imaging studies for common clinical genitourinary problems.

Clinical problem	*Imaging study*
Acute onset flank pain. Suspected ureteral calculus	Noncontrasted CT
Recurrent nephrolithiasis	US with plain X-ray or low-dose CT
Hematuria (painless)	CT urogram
Acute pyelonephritis in a complicated patient	CT with and without IV contrast
Recurrent urinary tract infection	Cystoscopy. CT if nonresponding or high risk patient
Cystitis (uncomplicated in a female)	No imaging
Abscess	CT with and without intravenous contrast
Renal trauma with suspicion of multisystem injury	CT with intravenous contrast
Suspected renal mass	CT with and without IV contrast or MRI
Renal failure	US
Hydronephrosis	US
Obstructive voiding symptoms	US kidneys and bladder
Bladder rupture	Cystogram or CT cystogram
Urethral obstruction or tear	Retrograde urethrogram
Bladder cancer	Cystoscopy, CT with intravenous contrast for regional and distant disease
Suspected renovascular hypertension	CT angiogram, MR angiogram, Captopril renogram or Doppler US
Acute onset scrotal pain. Suspected testicular torsion	Doppler US
Testicular or scrotal mass or trauma	Doppler US
Testicular malignancy	US (CT for metastases)
Pelvic mass (female)	US
Pelvic pain (female)	US
Cervical cancer (screening or <2 cm)	No imaging
(2 cm or greater)	MRI with and without contrast
Ovarian cancer (screening)	Not recommended for general population.
Ovarian cancer (high risk or symptoms)	US
Endometrial cancer (low grade)	No imaging
(high grade)	MRI or CT
Uterine fibroids (initial, enlarging, painful, or bleeding)	Pelvic US
Prostate cancer	PSA measurement and biopsy (not imaging), nuclear medicine bone scan (to exclude osseous metastases)
Acute pelvic pain (female reproductive age group)	US
Vaginal bleeding	US

(CT: Computed tomography; PSA: Prostate-specific antigen; US: Ultrasound; MRI: Magnetic resonance imaging).
Source: Adapted with permission from Mettler FA. Essentials of Radiology, 3rd edition. Philadelphia, PA: Elsevier/Saunders; 2014.

Kidney

Urinary Obstruction and Nephrostomy

Obstruction from urinary tract stones, extrinsic compression or invasion of the ureter by pelvic, abdominal or urothelial tumors is treated by antegrade percutaneous nephrostomy if a retrograde approach is unsuccessful. Ultrasound guidance is appropriate if there is hydronephrosis and the patient is not obese. Fluoroscopy, with or without contrast, is used more frequently when access for stone removal is requested. Percutaneous urinary diversion allows healing of a ureteral fistula or surgical anastomosis. In chronically obstructed systems, residual function can be assessed following drainage. A nephrostomy catheter or a guidewire placed through the renal pelvis into the bladder provides access to the collecting system for interventional procedures such as stone removal, internal stenting, retrieval of stent fragments, stricture dilatation under fluoroscopic guidance, nephroscopic operation, and brush biopsy.

Percutaneous nephrostomy procedures are quite safe with reported mortality rates of 0.04%, and the incidence

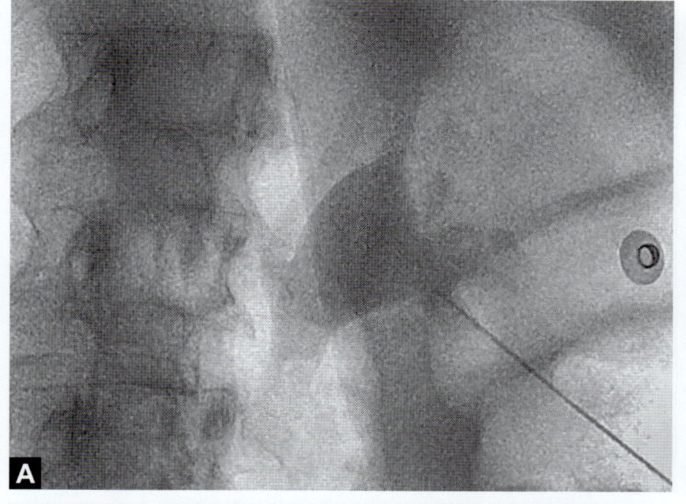

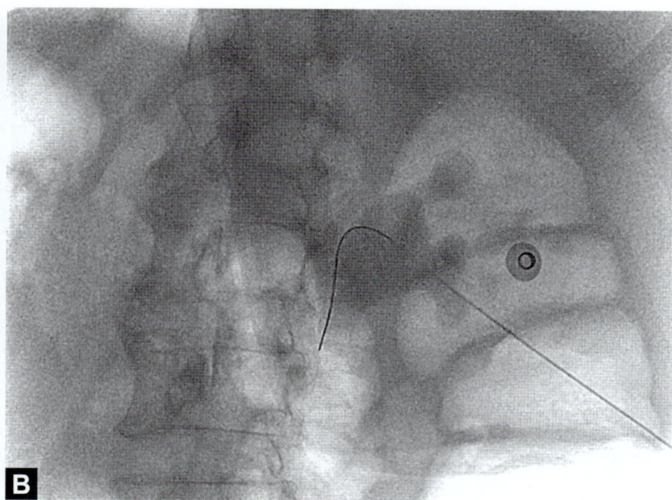

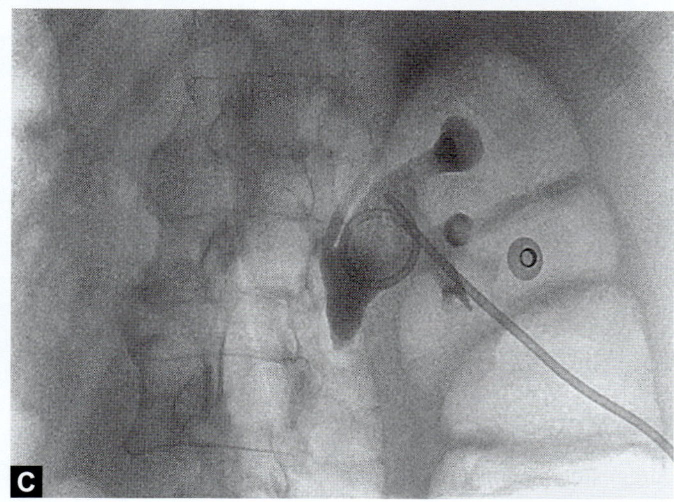

Figs. 15.18A to C: Percutaneous nephrostomy. (A) Under fluoroscopic guidance a needle is inserted into a posterior renal calyx. (B) A guidewire is put through the needle and the needle is withdrawn. (C) Following serial dilitations, a drainage catheter has been placed over the wire and the wire then removed.

of important complications is about 5%. The procedure is performed with a puncture below the 11th rib and via a posterolateral approach into a single posterior calyx (Figs. 15.18A to C). Contrast is instilled via a catheter over the wire while avoiding overdistension of the collecting system.[30] After tract dilatation a self-retaining drainage catheter is placed. Due to limitations of shock wave lithotripsy and ureteroscopy, percutaneous nephrolithotomy is used for large and complex renal stones.[31] The procedure, however, is the most morbid of minimally invasive surgical procedures for stone removal. Recent miniaturization advances have allowed lithotomy to be done through 16–20 gauge tracts.

Urinoma

Postoperative, post-transplant, and post-trauma urinomas that cause symptoms resulting from a mass effect or infection require drainage. Real-time ultrasound guidance decreases the risk of complications during placement, but difficult approaches require CT imaging. Treatment of the underlying problem generally results in spontaneous resolution of the urinoma.

Tumor Biopsy, Embolization, and Ablation

Previously with percutaneous biopsy of renal tumors, there had been concern about safety and accuracy. With more recent experience, the risk of tumor seeding appears almost negligible, and serious bleeding is unusual and almost always self-limited. Needle core biopsy with or without fine-needle aspiration provides an accurate diagnosis about 90% of the time.[32]

Management of renal tumors has changed over the last decade particularly with nephron-sparing treatment options including partial nephrectomy, thermal and cryoablation (Figs. 15.19A and B). In spite of this radical nephrectomy remains the most common procedure.

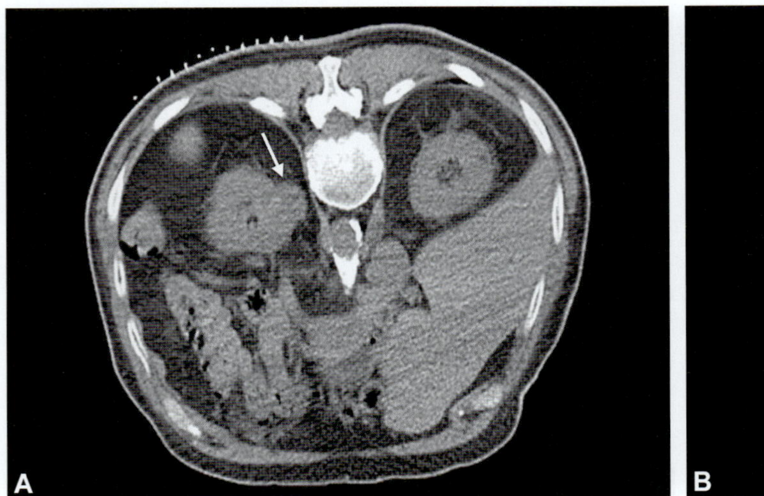

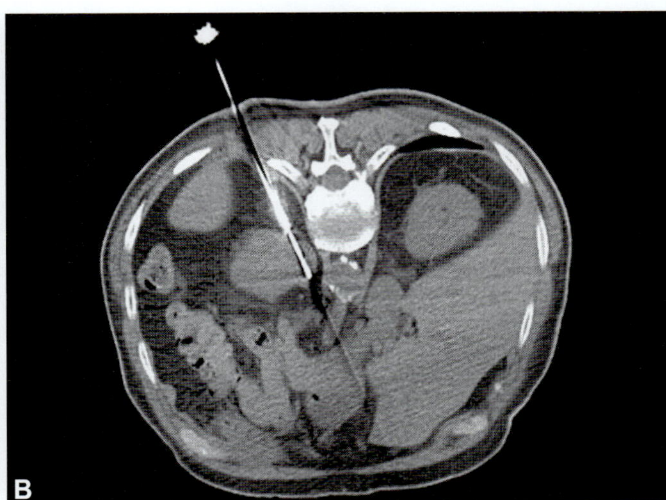

Figs. 15.19A and B: Cryoablation of renal cell carcinoma. (A) A prone transverse noncontrasted CT image shows a left renal mass (arrow). (B) A cryoablation probe has been inserted through the mass.

Arterial embolization of renal cancer has been used preoperatively or for pain palliation. While there is some debate, transcatheter ethanol, Gelfoam or coil ablation of a highly vascular renal cell carcinoma immediately before resection can decrease operative blood loss. Other than reduction of blood loss there appears to be no benefit in terms of other complications or survival.[33] Symptoms (lumbar pain, fever, nausea, hypertension, and hematuria) become severe if nephrectomy is delayed > 1 day.

As with hepatic neoplasms, renal cancers can be treated with percutaneous, or less commonly, endoscopic radiofrequency (RFA) and cryoablation. These procedures are best done with small (< 4 cm) exophytic tumors in patients who are not ideal surgical candidates and have a need for nephron sparing treatment. Successful treatment is less likely as the tumor becomes larger or more central. Most tumors require one or more overlapping ablations with the probes. Cryoablation is the most evaluated probe ablative technique, and 10-year cancer specific survival rates of 80% have been reported. Based on relatively short follow-up studies, the complication and survival results with RFA and cryoablation appear comparable.[34]

Uterus

Treatment of symptomatic uterine fibroids may be done by hysterectomy, myomectomy or uterine artery embolization. Uterine artery embolization (UAE) is less invasive, does not require general anesthesia, and has a shorter hospital stay. UAE is contraindicated in women with current genitourinary infection or malignancy, and there is a postembolization risk of major complication requiring emergency hysterectomy. Embolization has been shown to reduce or eliminate symptoms in about 75% of patients, although younger women appear to have a higher treatment failure rate than women over 40. Repeat embolization is needed in about 10% of women, and about 2–3% will still require hysterectomy or myomectomy.[35,36]

MUSCULOSKELETAL SYSTEM

Imaging

Suggested initial imaging procedures for various clinical situations involving the musculoskeletal system are shown in Table 15.7. The reader is also referred to textbooks on the topic.[37-40]

Percutaneous Bone Biopsy

Percutaneous core bone biopsy may be done to exclude a malignant lesion or occasionally for infection. CT guidance allows safe approach into small otherwise inaccessible lesions while avoiding damage to important structures (Figs. 15.20A and B). Usually 3–4 cores are obtained targeting the most aggressive appearing portion of the lesion, sampling multiple portions when the lesion is large and avoiding necrotic areas. Major complications are rare; minor complications are reported to be postbiopsy fever (1%), pain (16%), bruising (16%), and swelling (10%). Reported diagnostic yield and accuracy are reported to range from about 70–95%. Lower success rates are reported for intraosseous lesions with no extraosseous component, sclerotic lesions, benign and low-grade neoplasms, lesions of soft tissue origin as well as lesions in and around the spine.[41,42]

Table 15.7 Suggested initial imaging studies of choice for various musculoskeletal problems.

Clinical problem	*Imaging study*
Fracture (acute or follow-up)	Plain X-ray
Cervical spine trauma	CT [however if low risk by NEXUS or CCR criteria imaging usually not appropriate]
Thoracic/lumbar spine trauma	Plain X-ray or CT (spinal fracture at one level indicates risk of spinal fractures elsewhere)
Stress fracture	Plain X-ray (if negative consider nuclear medicine bone scan)
Metastases	Nuclear medicine bone scan, plain X-ray in area of pain
Osteomyelitis	Plain X-ray; if negative, then MRI or nuclear medicine three-phase bone scan
Neck pain (chronic)	Plain X-ray (if negative and neurologic signs/symptoms do MRI)
Low back pain	Bed rest (for several weeks)
Without radiculopathy	Imaging not indicated
With radiculopathy	Noncontrasted CT or MRI
Prior lumbar surgery	MRI without contrast
Surgical or intervention candidate	MRI without contrast
Suspicion of cancer, infection	MRI or bone scan
immunosuppression	MRI without contrast
Monoarticular joint pain	Plain X-ray, if conservative therapy fails, then MRI
Shoulder acute pain	Plain X-ray
Shoulder acute pain (postsurgical repair)	MRI
Shoulder persistent pain (negative X-ray) MRI	
Elbow chronic pain	Plain X-ray (if negative and suspect osteochondral, tendon, ligament injury, do MRI)
Hip suspected avascular necrosis	Plain X-ray (if negative or equivocal, do MRI)
Hip trauma	Plain X-ray, if negative and suspicion persists, do MRI
Knee pain (non-traumatic)	Plain X-ray (if negative or effusion, do MRI)
Knee acute trauma (focal tenderness or	
effusion or inability to bear weight	Plain X-ray (if fracture, do CT; if negative, do MRI)
Knee replacement (routine follow-up)	Plain X-ray
Pain after knee replacement	Plain X-ray and aspiration (if negative, do nuclear medicine infection scan)
Knee replacement (suspected loosening)	Plain X-ray (if negative for infection, do CT)

(CT: Computed tomography; MRI: Magnetic resonance imaging; US: Ultrasound).
Source: Adapted with permission from Mettler FA. Essentials of Radiology, 3rd edition. Philadelphia, PA: Elsevier/Saunders; 2014.

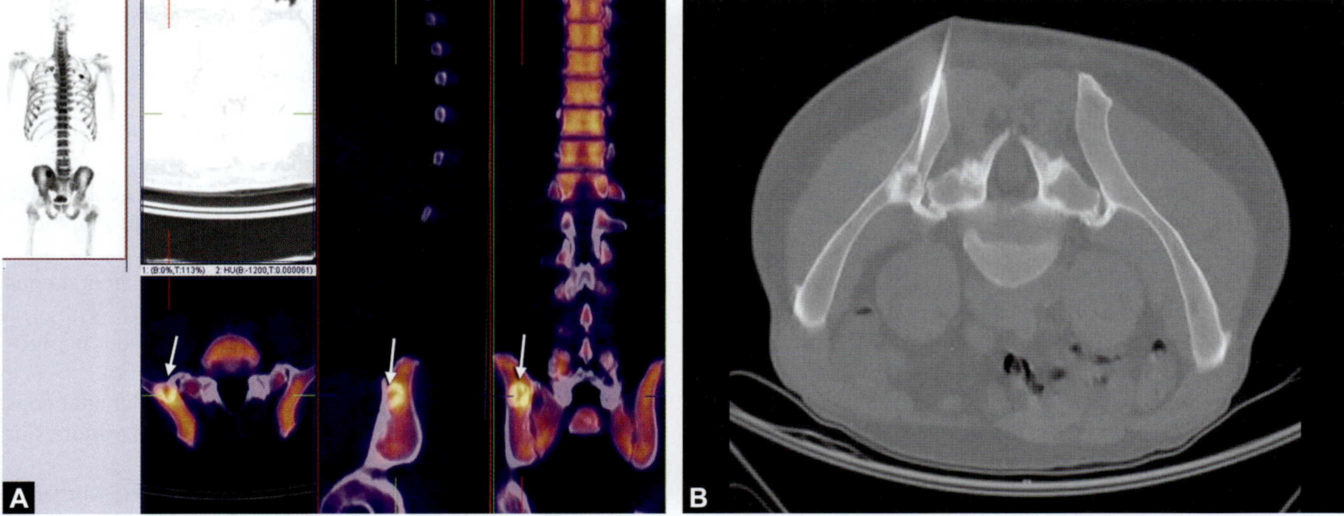

Figs. 15.20A and B: Percutaneous bone biopsy. (A) Images from a hybrid positron emission computed tomography/computed tomography (PET/CT) bone scan show a metabolically active lesion in the right ilium (arrows). (B) A prone CT image shows the bone biopsy needle approaching the lesion.

Arthrography

It is common to evaluate the status of cartilage and joint tears with either MRI or occasionally ultrasound. Arthrography may be performed when there are complex clinical questions particularly postoperatively. Historically, arthrography was performed with fluoroscopic guidance and imaging, but more recently it is performed with ultrasound, MRI, and less commonly CT. Dilute contrast is used. For MRI it is gadolinium and for CT the contrast may be iodinated material or less commonly air. Accuracy varies according to the pathology. MR arthrography has slightly better accuracy (about 95%) for rotator cuff or labral tears than does either ultrasound or MRI (both about 85–90%). There is an extensive literature on MR arthrography of joints including the shoulder, elbow, wrist, hip, knee, and ankle.[43-45]

REFERENCES

1. Mettler FA. Essentials of Radiology, 3rd edition. Philadelphia, PA: Elsevier/Saunders; 2014.
2. Valji K. The Practice of Interventional Radiology. Philadelphia, PA: Elsevier/Saunders; 2012.
3. Mettler FA, Guiberteau MJ. Essentials of Nuclear Medicine Imaging, 6th edition. Philadelphia: WB Saunders; 2013.
4. Som PH, Curtin HD. Head and Neck Imaging, 5th edition. Philadelphia, PA: Mosby; 2011.
5. Yousem DM, Zimmerman RD, Grossman RI. Neuroradiology: The Requisites, 3rd edition. Philadelphia, PA: Mosby; 2010.
6. Cooper DS, Doherty GM, Haugen BR, et al. for American Thyroid Association Guidelines Taskforce on Thyroid Nodules and Differentiated Thyroid Cancer. Revised American Thyroid Association management guidelines for patients with thyroid nodules and differentiated thyroid cancer. Thyroid. 2009;19(11);1167-214.
7. Titton RL, Gervais DA, Boland GW, et al. Sonography and sonographically guided fine-needle aspiration biopsy of the thyroid gland: Indications and techniques, pearls and pitfalls. Am. J. Roentgenol. 2003;181:267-71.
8. Ho V, Reddy GP. Cardiovascular Imaging. Philadelphia, PA: Elsevier/Saunders; 2011.
9. Manning WJ, Pennell DJ. Cardiovascular Magnetic Resonance, 2nd edition. Philadelphia, PA: Elsevier/Saunders; 2010.
10. Hansell DM, Lynch DA, McAdams P, et al. Imaging of Diseases of the Chest, 5th edition. Philadelphia, PA: Mosby; 2010.
11. Goodman LR, Felson's Principles of Chest Roentgenology, 3rd edition. Philadelphia, PA: Saunders; 2006.
12. Naidich DP, Webb R, Muller NL, et al. Computed Tomography and Magnetic Resonance Imaging of the Thorax, 4rd edition. Philadelphia, PA: Lippincott Williams & Wilkins; 2007.
13. Mahmood K, Wahidi MM. Straightening out chest tubes: what size, what type and when. Clin Chest Med. 2013;34(1):63-71.
14. Light RW. Pleural controversy: optimal chest tube size for drainage. Respirology. 2011;16(2):244-8.
15. Cooke DT, David EA. Large-bore and small bore chest tubes; types, function and placement. Thorac Surg Clin. 2013;23(1):17-24.
16. MacMahon H, Austin JHM, Gamsu G, et al. Guidelines for management of small pulmonary nodules detected on CT scans; a statement from the Fleischner Society. Radiology. 2005;237(2):395-400.
17. Wallace MJ, Krishnamurthy S, Broemeling LD, et al. CT-guided percutaneous fine-needle aspiration biopsy of small pulmonary lesions. Radiology. 2002;225(3):823-8.
18. Wu CC, Maher MM, Shepard JA. Complications of CT-guided percutaneous needle biopsy of the chest: prevention and management. Am J Roentgenol. 2011;196(6):W678-82.
19. Raymakers AJ, Mayo J, Marra CA, et al. Diagnostic strategies incorporating CT angiography for pulmonary embolism: a systematic review of cost-effectiveness analyses. J Thorac Imaging. 2014;29(4):209-16.
20. Kopans D. Breast Imaging, 3rd edition. Philadelphia, PA: Lippincott Williams & Wilkins; 2006.
21. Federle MP, Jeffrey RB, Woodward PJ, et al. Diagnostic Imaging Abdomen, 2nd edition. Salt Lake City: Amirsys; 2010.
22. Gore RM, Levine MS. Textbook of Gastrointestinal Radiology, 3rd edition. Philadelphia, PA: WB Saunders; 2008.
23. Lee SH, Tomlinson C, Temple M, et al. Imaging-guided percutaneous needle aspiration or catheter drainage of neonatal liver abscesses: 14-year experience. Am J Roentgenol. 2008;190(3):616-22.
24. Gillams AR. The use of radiofrequency in cancer. Br J Cancer. 2005;92(10):1825-9.
25. Pitchumoni CS, Agarwal N, Pancreatic pseudocysts. When and how should drainage be performed ? Gasteroenterol Clin North Am. 1999;28(3):615-39.
26. Covarrubias DA, O'Conner OJ, McDermott S, et al. Radiologic percutaneous gsastrostomy: review of potential complications and approach to managing the unexpected outcome. Am J Roentgenol. 2013;200(4):921-31.
27. Schieda N, Fasih N, Shabana W. Triphasic CT in the diagnosis of acute mesenteric ischemia. Eur Radiol. 2013;23(7):1891-900.
28. Singal AK, Kamath PS, Tefferi A. Mesenteric venous thrombosis. Mayo Clinic Proc. 2013;88(3):285-94.
29. Dunnick NR, Sandler CM, Newhouse JH, et al. Textbook of Uroradiology, 4th edition. Philadelphia, PA: Lippincott Williams & Wilkins; 2007.
30. Zangoria RJ, Dyer RB. Do's and don'ts of percutaneous nephrostomy. Acad Radiology. 1999;6(6):370-7.
31. Antonelli JA, Pearle MS. Advances in percutaneous nephrolithotomy. Urol Clin North Am. 2013;40(1):99-113.
32. Volpe A, Finelli A, Gill IS, et al. Rationale for percutaneous biopsy and histologic characterization of renal tumors. Eur Urol. 2012;62(3):491-504.
33. May M, Brookman-Amissah S, Pflanz S, et al. Pre-operative renal arterial embolization does not provide survival benefit in patients with radical nephrectomy for renal cell carcinoma. Br J Radiol. 2009;82(981):724-31.

34. Venkatesan AM, Wood BJ, Gervais DA. Percutaneous ablation in the kidney. Radiology. 2011;261(2):375-91.
35. Goodwin SC, Spies JB, Worthington-Kirsch R, et al. Uterine artery embolization for treatment of leiomyomata: long-term outcomes from the FIBROID registry. Obstet Gynecol. 2008;111(1);22-33.
36. Scheuring-Muenkler C, Koesters C, Powerski MJ, et al. Clinical long-term outcome after uterine artery embolization; sustained symptom control and improvement of quality of life. J Vasc Inter Radiol. 2013;24(6):765-71.
37. El-Khoury GY, Bennett L, Stanley M. Essentials in Musculoskeletal Imaging. Philadelphia, PA: WB Saunders; 2003.
38. Helms CA, Major NM, Anderson M, et al. Musculoskeletal MRI, 2nd edition. Philadelphia, PA: Saunders Elsevier; 2008.
39. Resnick D. Bone and Joint Imaging, 3rd edition. Philadelphia, PA: WB Saunders; 2005.
40. Rogers LF. Radiology of Skeletal Trauma, 3rd edition. Philadelphia, PA: WB Saunders; 2002.
41. Huang AJ, Halpern EF, Rosenthal DI. Incidence of delayed complications following percutaneous CT-guided biopsy of bone and soft tissue lesions of the spine and extremities; a 2-year prospective study and analysis of risk factors. Skelet Radiol. 2013;42(1):61-8.
42. Omura MC, Motamedi K, UyBico S, et al. Revisiting CT-guided percutaneous core needle biopsy of musculoskeletal lesions: contributors to biopsy success. Am J Roentgenol. 2011;197(2):456-61.
43. Rhee RB, Chan KK, Lieu JG, et al. MR and CT arthrography of the shoulder. Semin Musculoskelet Radiol. 2012; 16(1):3-14.
44. Llopis E, Fernandez E, Cerezal L. MR and CT arthrography of the hip. Semin Musculoskelet Radiol. 2012;16(1):42-6.
45. Fritz J, Fishman EK, Small KM, et al. MDCT arthrography of the shoulder with datasets of isotropic resolution; indications, technique and applications. Am J Roentgenol. 2012; 198(3):635-46.

16

Principles of Oncology

Thomas N Wang, Kirby I Bland

Key Points

- Cancer epidemiology demonstrates that regional variation in the incidence of a particular malignancy is associated with genetic and environmental factors. Identifying specific variations in cancer incidence provides clues for potential methods of eliminating associated cancer determinants or risk factors.
- Cancer cells acquire six biological capabilities necessary for carcinogenesis: proliferative signaling, evading growth suppressors, resisting cell death, enabling replicative immortality, inducing angiogenesis, and activating invasion and metastasis. These hallmarks of cancer constitute an organizing principle for understanding oncogenesis and provide a framework for future treatment algorithms.
- Staging of cancers allows for effective communication among cancer specialists and enables accurate comparison of outcome and survival between groups.
- Surgery, radiation therapy, and chemotherapy are powerful modalities for the treatment of cancer, used separately or in combination. The treatment algorithm for any individual patient with cancer is dependent on the cell of origin and its tumor biology.

INTRODUCTION

In the late nineteenth century, William Stewart Halsted first used the term *radical mastectomy* to describe an aggressive surgical procedure for the treatment of breast cancer. He derived the word *radical* from the Latin word *radix*, which means "root." Halsted believed that it was necessary to excavate the buried roots of cancer in the body by removing all structures touched by the primary tumor or by its lymphatic connections. Therefore, extirpation of breast cancer required the complete en bloc excision of the skin, both pectoral muscles, the clavicle, and the lymph nodes of the axilla and the neck:[1] an operation that also conveyed the modern English meaning of the word *radical*, as the procedure was both aggressive and extreme.

Although Halsted was not the first surgeon to perform the radical mastectomy, his understanding of the observations of earlier pioneers of surgery paved the way for the development of modern-day oncologic principles. He demonstrated that the natural history of breast cancer progression was local tumor growth followed by spread to regional lymph nodes before advancing to distant sites. By halting the locoregional progression of breast cancer with radical mastectomy, he prevented early breast cancers from developing into advanced stage disease. However, his results also exhibited the limitations of operative resection because of its inability to cure more advanced cancer. Patients with lymph node-positive breast cancer or distant metastases gained no benefit in survival. Therefore, his radical approach to treatment of breast cancer was only successful in treating patients with nonaggressive, early stage disease who did not need a radical operation, and it failed in treating patients with aggressive, late-stage disease.[1]

Operative excision remains the pivotal modality in the curative and palliative treatment for patients with solid tumors. Few cancers with the exception of hematologic malignancies are cured without surgical therapy. However, the limitations of surgery have confounded and exasperated physicians for centuries. Even well-selected patients who undergo technically perfect surgical oncology procedures often succumb to recurrent disease and cancer-related deaths years after treatment. As demonstrated by Halsted, increasingly aggressive and radical operations have not resulted in better outcomes. Yet, the development of the Halsted radical mastectomy was necessary for the better understanding of the natural history of breast cancer progression and the importance of considering tumor biology in the treatment of cancer patients.

Why surgical therapy fails in the treatment of cancer is because cancer is a genetic disease. Neoplasia occurs through specific alterations in the genome leading to the expression of capabilities for cancer cell survival. Although Halsted taught us the importance of pursuing cancer beyond what we could visualize with the removal of potential sites of advanced disease, surgical cure is limited by the inability to treat the genetic process of oncogenesis. Oncogenesis begins at the molecular level as a normal cell is transformed into a malignant cell through a multistep process conferring capabilities or hallmarks unique to cancer cells. This chapter will review the molecular mechanisms underlying the six hallmarks of cancer and how oncologists have exploited these mechanisms to treat cancer. In addition, it will review the multidisciplinary approaches to cancer treatment and the importance of cancer staging in determining a treatment plan. As molecular characteristics of cancer cells are utilized clinically, molecular biology will influence the surgical care of cancer patients. The function of surgical oncology is to improve therapeutic decision making and to provide optimal surgical intervention through better understanding of molecular biology in oncologic processes.

EPIDEMIOLOGY

According to estimates from the International Agency for Research on Cancer (IARC), in 2008 there were 12.7 million new cancer cases worldwide, of which 5.6 million occurred in economically developed countries and 7.1 million in economically developing countries. Approximately 7.6 million deaths are attributable to cancer each year worldwide (about 21,000 cancer deaths a day), 2.8 million in developed countries and 4.8 million in developing countries. As a comparison, cancer has overtaken heart disease as the top cause of death in the developed world since at least 2004, and cancer deaths will take over as the number killer worldwide by the end of the next decade. By 2030, the estimated number of new cancer cases is expected to grow to 21.4 million and cancer deaths to 13.2 million with the aging of the population and the reduction in childhood mortality.[2]

The true figures for cancer incidence and mortality could be even higher than the above estimates as developing countries adopt Western lifestyles such as tobacco smoking, high fat diets, low fiber diets, physical inactivity and safer reproductive practices. Cancers related to these factors, such as lung, colorectal and breast, are increasing in economically transitioning countries and will continue to do so unless preventive measures are utilized. Table 16.1 provides the estimated numbers of total new cancer cases and deaths in 2008 by United Nations designated areas. In economically developed countries, the three most commonly diagnosed cancers were prostate, lung, and colorectal among men, and breast, colorectal and lung among women. In developing countries, the three most commonly diagnosed cancers were lung, stomach and liver in men, and breast, cervix and lung in women (Fig. 16.1).[3]

Factors that contribute to regional differences in the types of cancer presentation or cancer outcome include regional variations in the prevalence of risk factors, availability and quality of cancer screening and treatment, and population age structure (Fig. 16.2). In 2008, the leading cancers in developing countries were related to infection: stomach and liver in men and cervix and stomach in women. The incidence of infection-related cancers is three times higher in developing countries than developed countries, with stomach being the most common worldwide followed by liver and uterine cervix. Infectious agents that cause certain cancers, such as hepatitis B virus (HBV) in hepatocellular carcinoma, *Helicobacter pylori* in stomach cancer, and human papillomavirus (HPV) in cervical cancer, could be prevented through vaccines, antibiotics, improved sanitation, and education programs. By contrast, cancers related to unhealthy practices such as tobacco use, heavy alcohol consumption, and obesity are most effectively prevented by patient education to encourage healthy behavior modifications. Screening has been proved effective in reducing mortality for breast, cervical, and colorectal in developed countries and must be instituted in economically developing countries.[2]

MOLECULAR BASIS OF CANCER

Cancer is a disease that evolves through dynamic changes in the genome. It is a multistep process of cellular transformation driven by the acquisition of genetic alterations and resulting in a malignant derivative of the normal cell of origin. Analyses of pathologic specimens of different tumor types have revealed intermediary stages of transformation as normal cells evolve progressively into invasive cancer cells via a series of premalignant states. With each stage of progression toward malignancy, the transformed cell acquires a succession of genetic changes, which confer additional growth advantages.

The most commonly described sequence of carcinogenesis with its attendant molecular genetic alterations is elucidated in colorectal cancer (Flowchart 16.1). Initially

Table 16.1 Estimated number of new cancer cases and deaths by world area (GLOBOCAN 2008, excludes nonmelanoma skin cancer).

	Cases			Deaths		
	Male	*Female*	*Overall*	*Male*	*Female*	*Overall*
Eastern Africa	100,800	120,200	221,100	85,400	88,300	173,700
Middle Africa	29,500	37,400	66,900	25,600	27,600	53,200
Northern Africa	81,500	82,900	164,400	65,400	55,400	120,800
Southern Africa	40,600	38,600	79,200	29,300	25,500	54,800
Western Africa	72,500	111,600	184,100	61,300	78,000	139,300
Eastern Asia	2,135,300	1,585,400	3,720,700	1,511,800	928,600	2,440,400
South-Central Asia	651,100	772,000	1,423,100	496,800	483,200	979,900
South-Eastern Asia	336,700	388,800	725,600	258,600	242,400	501,000
Western Asia	118,500	104,800	223,300	86,700	64,400	151,200
Caribbean	42,800	36,500	79,300	26,300	21,500	47,800
Central America	84,000	92,600	176,600	52,500	55,800	108,300
Northern America	831,800	772,100	1,603,900	332,500	305,900	638,300
South America	318,000	332,100	650,100	200,600	185,300	385,900
Central and Eastern Europe	494,600	490,600	985,200	351,700	283,000	634,800
Northern Europe	248,400	231,800	480,200	126,400	116,300	242,700
Southern Europe	398,800	315,000	713,900	225,000	155,500	380,500
Western Europe	569,600	464,700	1,034,300	258,900	204,900	463,800
Australia/New Zealand	70,300	56,700	127,000	27,600	21,400	49,100
Melanesia	3,300	3,700	7,000	2,600	2,500	5,100
Micronesia	300	400	700	200	200	400
Polynesia	600	600	1,100	300	200	600

(Reproduced with permission from American Cancer Society.[3])

proposed by Vogelstein, the multistep process for colorectal cancer was deduced from the prevalence of mutations in normal mucosa, small-to-large adenomas, in situ carcinomas, and finally invasive colorectal cancers.[4] The first step in the process is the loss of the *APC* gene. The hyperproliferative epithelium then undergoes a series of mutations that allow it to proliferate. These include activation of oncogenes (such as *ras*, *fos*, and *myc*) and DNA hypomethylation, which confers genetic instability, allowing for the accumulation of more mutations.[5] The hyperproliferative epithelium progresses from a small adenoma to a large adenoma as mutations are acquired. Late in the process, loss of the DCC (deleted in colon cancer) gene, and mutation or loss of *p53* results in the invasive carcinoma stage.[6]

The number of genes known to be involved in tumorigenesis is growing at an exponential rate as cancer researchers continue to add layers of complexity to a scientific literature that is already too complex. However, understanding the process of carcinogenesis may be simplified by developing a conceptual understanding of a small number of underlying principles that govern the transformation of normal cells into malignant cancers. Through their observations in tumor biology, Hanahan and Weinberg proposed an organizing principle that provides a solid foundation for understanding the biology of cancer, which is absolutely essential for all oncologists and cancer researchers.[7] The six hallmarks of cancer—sustaining proliferative signaling, evading growth suppressors, resisting cell death, enabling replicative immortality, inducing angiogenesis, and activating invasion and metastasis—are distinctive and complementary capabilities acquired by tumor cells that enable growth and metastatic dissemination (Fig. 16.3).

Sustaining Proliferative Signaling

Normal tissues regulate the ability of cells to undergo DNA synthesis and enter the cell cycle for cell growth and division by the production and release of growth-promoting signals. These mitogenic signals ensure normal cell number

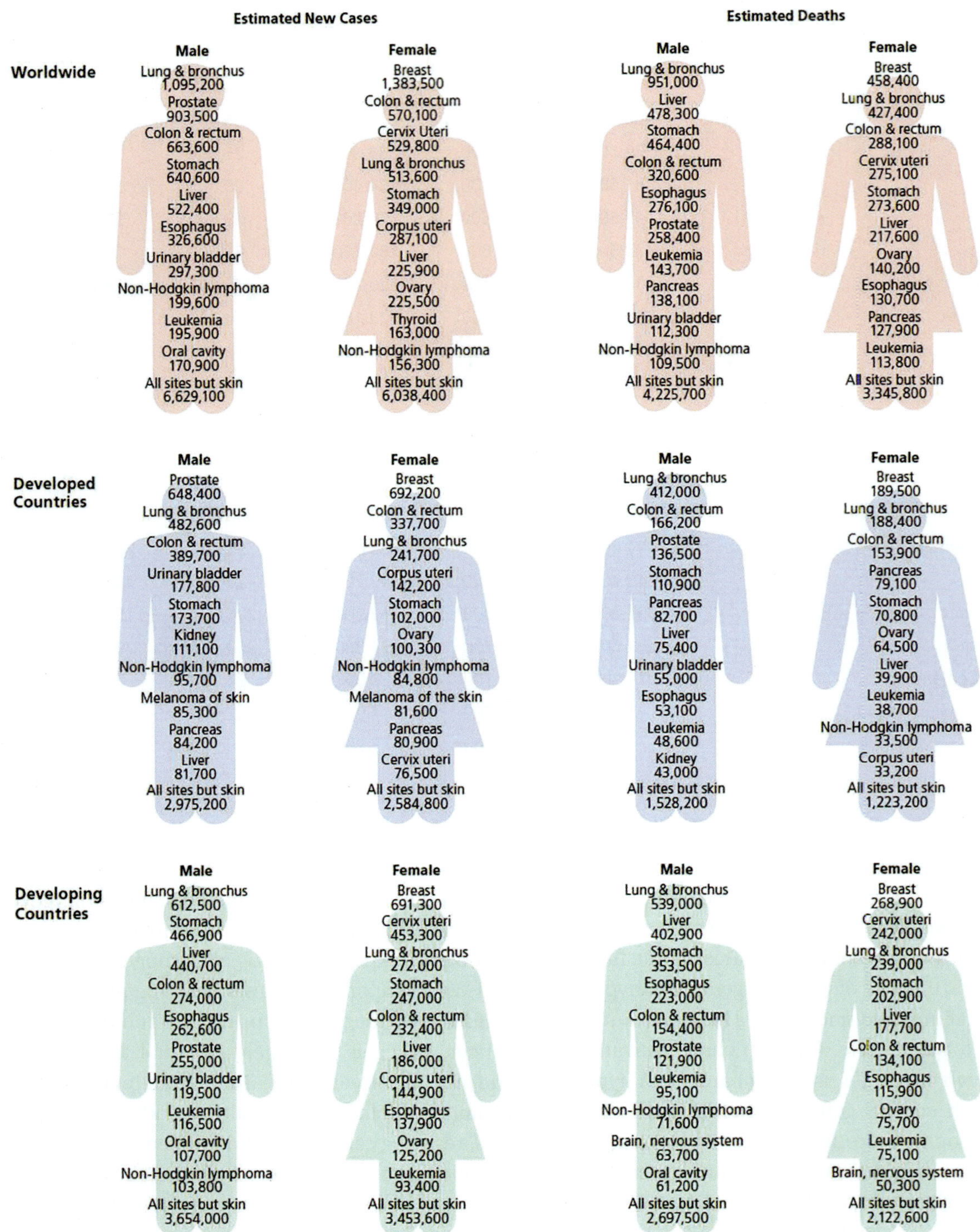

Fig. 16.1: Estimated new cancer cases and deaths worldwide for leading cancer sites by level of economic development (GLOBOCAN, 2008). (Reproduced with permission from American Cancer Society.[3])

and maintain normal tissue architecture and function. Cancer cells are able to deregulate these signals, resulting in autonomous growth and cell division by multiple mechanisms.[8,9] Cancer cells may produce growth factor ligands themselves, thereby developing autocrine proliferative stimulation. Receptor signaling can also become hyper-responsive through the elevation of the number of cancer cell growth receptors expressed on its cell surface.

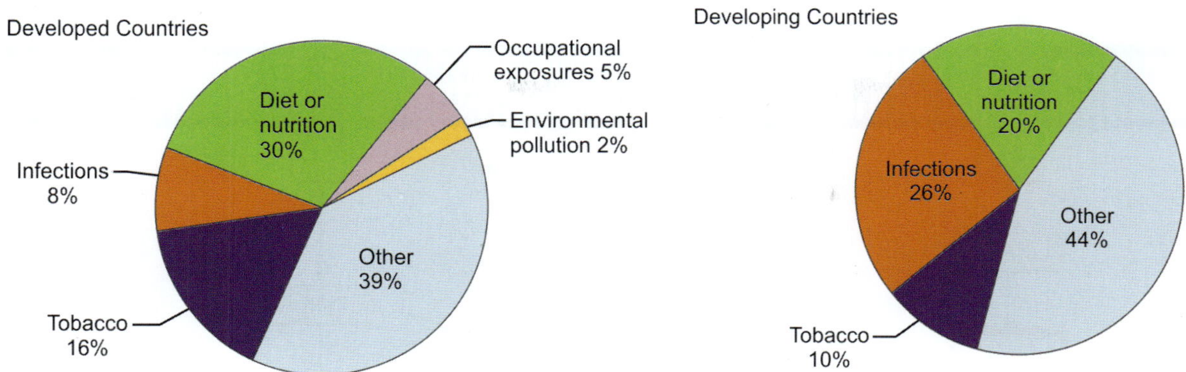

Fig. 16.2: Proportion of cancer causes by major risk factors and level of economic development (GLOBOCAN, 2008). (Reproduced with permission from American Cancer Society.[3])

Flowchart 16.1: Vogelstein's proposed model of the sequence of carcinogenesis with the genetic mutations elucidated in colon cancer.

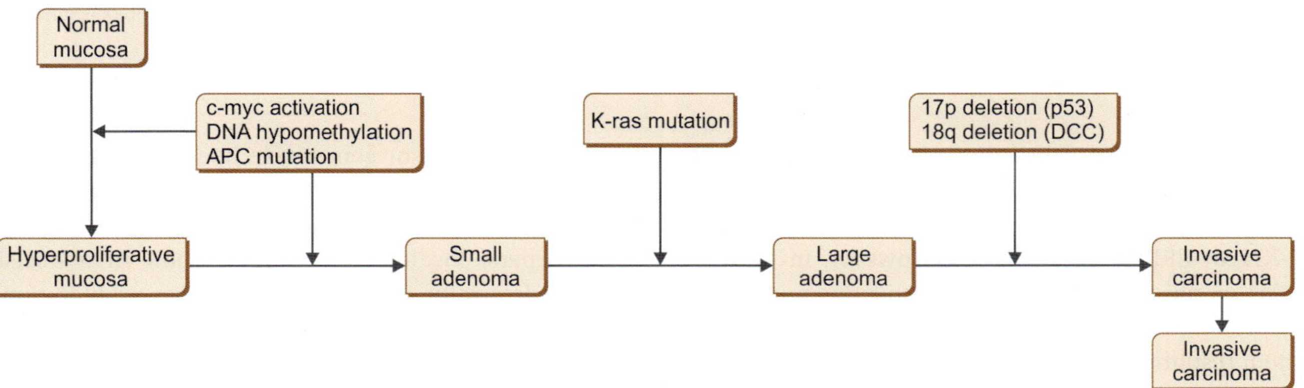

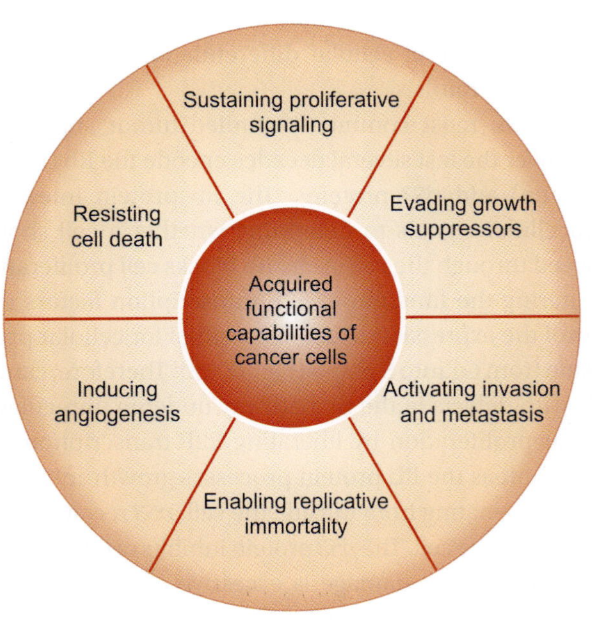

Fig. 16.3: Six hallmarks of cancer. Redrawn from Hanahan D, Weinberg RA.[7]

Cancer cells may alternatively stimulate surrounding normal stromal cells to produce growth factors, resulting in paracrine proliferative stimulation.[10,11] In some tumors, the cooperating stromal cells may themselves depart from their normal development in order to sustain the growth of the cancer cells. Even inflammatory cells attracted to sites of neoplasia may enhance (rather than eliminate) tumor growth potential. In addition, cancer cell growth receptor structure may be altered, resulting in ligand-independent activation of intracellular tyrosine kinase domains, which emit signals through a myriad of intracellular signaling pathways that upregulates cell cycle proteins.

Growth factor independence may also result from constitutive activation of downstream components from the receptor, completely obviating the need for ligand-mediated receptor activation. One example of this process is the mutated form of the B-Raf protein that is found in over 40% of human melanomas and is the most common somatic mutation in this disease. B-Raf is a serine/threonine kinase and a component of the RAS-RAF-MEK-MAPK pathway (Fig. 16.4), which is activated in many

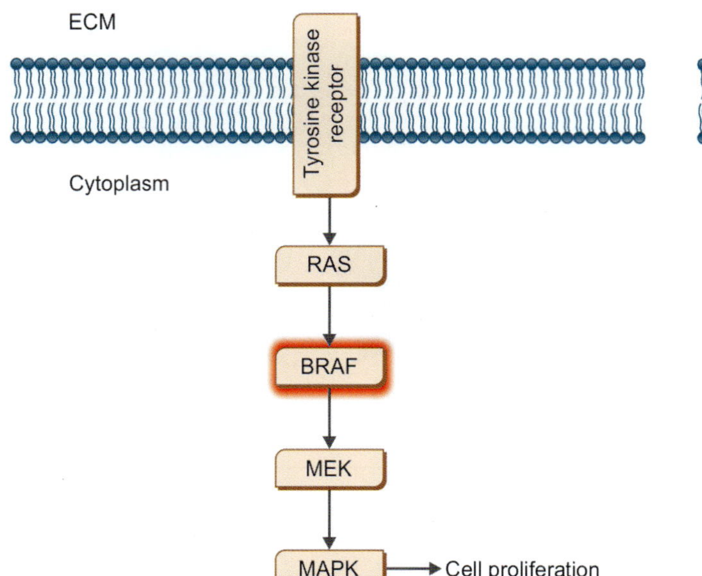

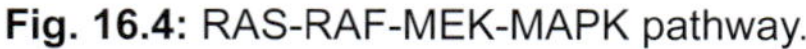
Fig. 16.4: RAS-RAF-MEK-MAPK pathway.

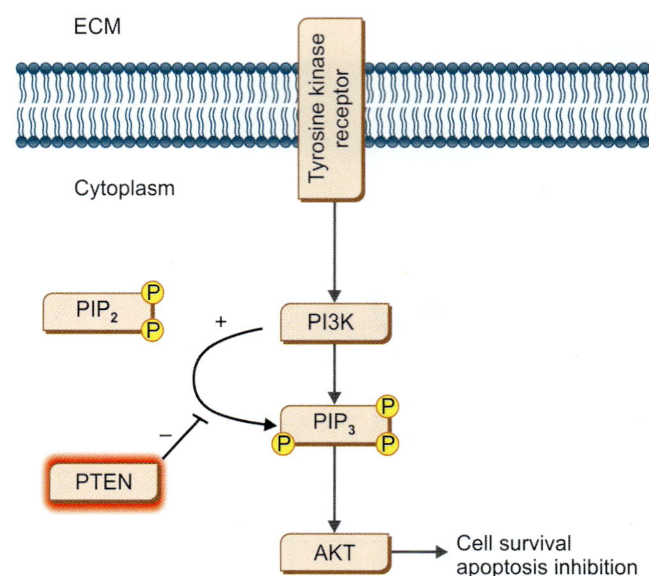

Fig. 16.5: PTEN/PI3K/AKT pathway.

cancers. In normal cells, the RAS to mitogen-activating protein (MAP)-kinase pathway occurs only with stimulation through the binding of the tyrosine kinase receptor (c-KIT or ERBB4) by its ligand. However, in melanoma cells that possess a B-Raf with an activating mutation, the RAF to MAP kinase pathway remains constitutively activated, resulting in continued cell growth and cell proliferation, completely independent of its receptor status.[12]

Defects in the normal cell growth feedback loops are also capable of enhancing proliferative signaling. For example, phosphatase and tensin homolog (PTEN), a tumor suppressor gene product, normally functions to inhibit PI3 kinase (PI3K) activation of AKT, a serine/threonine kinase that induces a variety of responses including increased cell growth and proliferation. PTEN inhibits the transformation of PI3K to its final product phosphatidylinositol (3,4,5) triphosphate (PIP_3), which activates AKT (*see* Fig. 16.5). Inactivation of PTEN amplifies PI3K signaling and promotes tumor cell growth. PTEN expression is often lost by promoter methylation in many human tumors, including melanoma.[13]

Evading Growth Suppressors

In addition to activating positive stimuli for cellular proliferation through cell growth signaling, tumor cells must also have the ability to evade cellular mechanisms that negatively regulate cellular proliferation. Tumor suppressor genes play an important role in limiting cell growth and proliferation in normal cells. Similar to PTEN, dozens of tumor suppressor genes have been discovered by the observation of their characteristic inactivation in human or animal cancers. The tumor suppressors operate as gatekeepers, located at a branch point in a decision tree to determine whether cells undergo proliferation or senescence. Tumor suppressors block proliferation by two distinct mechanisms: (1) cells may be forced into their quiescent phase (G_0) from which they may be able to reemerge on some future occasion when extracellular signals permit or (2) cells may be induced to enter into a permanent state of cellular differentiation and never be able to enter mitosis.

The two most commonly studied tumor suppressor genes over the last several decades encode the Rb (retinoblastoma) and *p53* proteins. The Rb protein integrates extracellular signals to determine whether a cell should proceed through the cell cycle. Rb blocks cell proliferation by altering the function of E2F transcription factors that control the expression of genes essential for cellular progression from G1 into S phase (Fig. 16.6).[14] Therefore, cancer cells with defects in the Rb pathway undergo unregulated cellular proliferation by liberating E2F transcription factors. Whereas the Rb protein processes growth-inhibitory signals originating from outside the cell, *p53* receives input from within the cell. The *p53* protein inhibits cell cycle progression if genome damage is excessive or metabolites of DNA synthesis are at suboptimal levels. In addition, if cellular systems develop irreparable damage, *p53* can trigger apoptosis, or programmed cell death. Various human

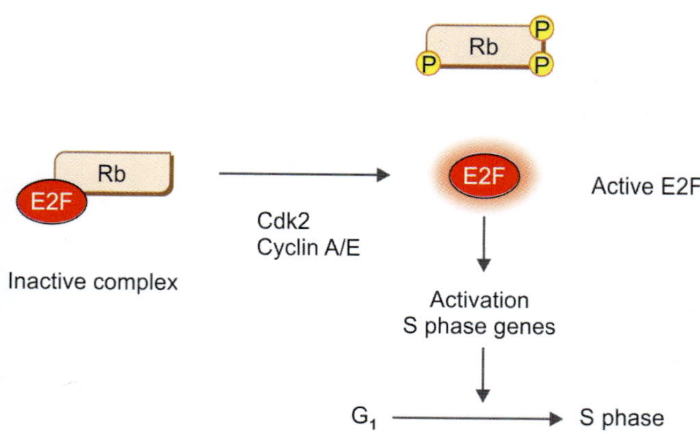

Fig. 16.6: Rb inhibits cell cycle progression by altering function of E2F transcription factor. Cdk2, cyclin-dependent kinase 2.

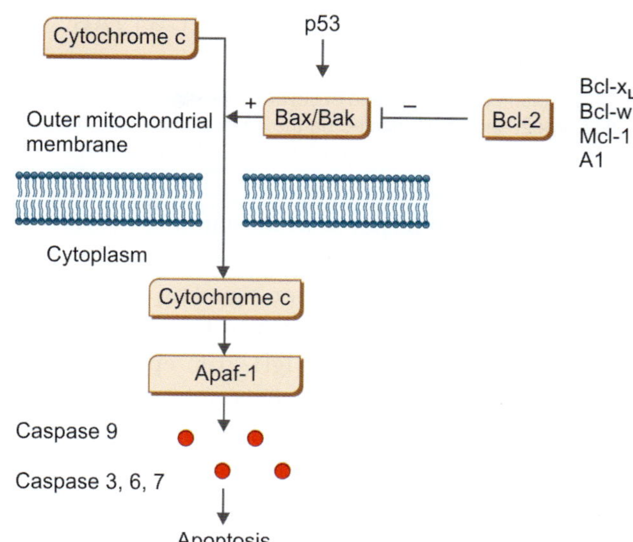

Fig. 16.7: Bax and Bak disrupt the mitochondrial outer membrane releasing the proapoptotic signaling protein, cytochrome c. Bcl-2 family of regulatory proteins inhibit apoptosis by suppressing Bax and Bak.

tumor cells possess loss-of-function mutations of the *p53* gene, often seen in the progression to an invasive phenotype during carcinogenesis. Interestingly, *p53* null mice usually develop normally until later in life when they acquire leukemias and sarcomas, suggesting the importance of redundant mechanisms that may constrain inappropriate replication of cells lacking a key growth suppressor.[15]

Recent studies have elucidated the mechanisms underlying contact inhibition, a mode of growth control that is abrogated during tumorigenesis. Normal cells grown in two-dimensional culture yield confluent cell monolayers, as contact inhibition suppresses further cell proliferation. On the contrary, in tumor cells, contact inhibition is abolished, and cells continue to proliferate after reaching a confluent monolayer, growing on top of one another in multiple layers. One mechanism of contact inhibition involves the cytoplasmic product of the *NF2* gene, Merlin. Merlin strengthens cell-to-cell attachments by coupling cell-surface adhesion molecule, E-cadherin, to a transmembrane tyrosine kinase receptor, EGF. In addition, Merlin sequesters growth factor receptors, limiting their ability to activate growth signaling.[16] The *NF2* gene is a tumor suppressor whose loss of function results in the development of neurofibromatosis in humans. A second mechanism of contact inhibition involves the LKB1 epithelial polarity protein necessary for the maintenance of tissue integrity. LKB1 is another tumor suppressor gene that inhibits the mitogenic effects of the powerful Myc oncogene. Loss of function of LKB1 results in the destabilization of the epithelium, and the epithelial cells become susceptible to Myc-induced tumor cell transformation.[17] These two mechanisms and others play an important role in maintaining normal tissue architecture and epithelial integrity through suppressing proliferative signals. Compromising these mechanisms is necessary for the development of unregulated cell growth in tumorigenesis.

Resisting Cell Death

Programmed cell death, or apoptosis, serves as the ultimate barrier to cancer development by preventing further proliferation of an abnormal cell. Therefore, attenuating the mechanisms that activate apoptosis is paramount for tumorigenesis to occur. Activation of apoptosis is controlled by the balance of pro- and antiapoptotic members of the Bcl-2 family of regulatory proteins.[18] Bcl-2, along with its closest relatives Bcl-x_L, Bcl-w, Mcl-1, and A1, is an inhibitor of apoptosis. These proteins suppress two proapoptotic triggering proteins, Bax and Bak, which are embedded in the mitochondrial outer membrane. In the absence of inhibition by the antiapoptotic regulatory proteins, Bax and Bak disrupt the integrity of the outer mitochondrial membrane, causing the release of proapoptotic signaling protein, cytochrome c. The released cytochrome c activates, in turn, a cascade of caspases that act via their proteolytic activities to induce the multiple cellular changes associated with the apoptosis (Fig. 16.7).

Apoptosis is triggered by physiologic stresses that cancer cells experience during tumorigenesis including elevated levels of oncogene signaling and DNA damage associated with hyperproliferation.[18] Most notable is a DNA-damage sensor that functions via the *p53* tumor suppressor;[19] *p53* induces apoptosis by upregulating

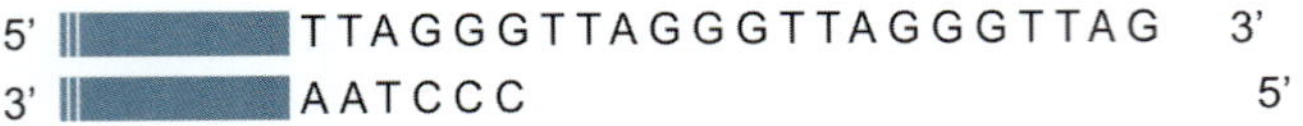

Fig. 16.8: Telomere is composed of several thousand tandem hexanucleotide repeat segments located on the ends of chromosomes. With each cell division, the telomere shortens by 50–100 base pairs.

expression of Bax in response to substantial levels of DNA damage and other chromosomal abnormalities. Alternatively, insufficient survival factor signaling (for instance inadequate levels of interleukin-3 in lymphocytes or of insulin-like growth factor 1/2 [Igf1/2] in epithelial cells) can elicit apoptosis through a BH3-only protein called Bim. In addition, hyperactive signaling by certain oncoproteins, such as Myc, leads to cell death unless counterbalanced by anti-apoptotic factors, suggesting that the overexpression of specific oncogenes is also a trigger for apoptosis.[19]

Tumor cells have evolved a variety of strategies to limit or circumvent the diversity of apoptosis-inducing signals that they encounter during carcinogenesis. Defects in the control pathway of apoptosis or inappropriate production of apoptosis suppressing proteins result in failure of abnormal cells to die when they should and contribute to the induction of cancer. Probably the most common strategy employed by tumor cells is the loss of *p53* tumor suppressor function, which eliminates this critical damage sensor from the apoptosis-inducing mechanism. Alternatively, tumors may achieve similar ends by increasing expression of antiapoptotic regulators (Bcl-2 or Bcl-x_L) or by downregulating proapoptotic factors (Bax or Bak). The multiplicity of apoptosis-avoiding mechanisms presumably reflects the diversity of apoptosis-inducing signals that cancer cell populations encounter during their evolution to the malignant state.

Enabling Replicative Immortality

Unlike normal cells, cancer cells possess the capacity for unlimited replication by overcoming two crucial anticancer defense barriers: senescence and crisis/apoptosis. Normal cells can only undergo a finite number of cell divisions before they enter into a nonproliferative but viable phase termed senescence. Through the disabling of tumor suppressor genes such as *p53* and Rb, tumor cells may circumvent senescence and continue multiplying for additional generations before reaching a crisis phase, in which the great majority of cells in the population die. Infrequently, rare variant cells emerge from the crisis phase and exhibit the ability of unlimited replicative potential.[20]

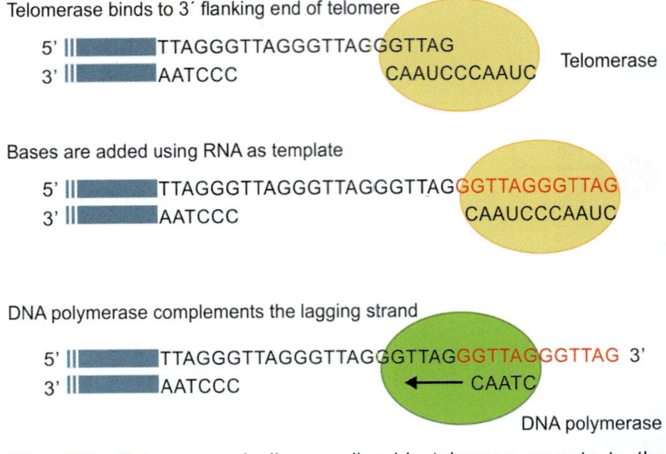

Fig. 16.9: Telomerase (yellow oval) adds telomere repeats to the 3' ends of DNA in immortalized cells to permit unlimited cell division.

This transition to unlimited replication is termed immortalization, a trait possessed by all cancer cells and attributed to their ability to avoid telomeric DNA shortening.

The length of telomeric DNA in a cell dictates how many successive generations of growth and division are possible. The telomere is composed of several thousand tandem hexanucleotide (a six base pair sequence element) repeat segments located on the ends of chromosomes (Fig. 16.8). With each cell division, the telomere shortens by 50–100 base pairs. This progressive shortening is attributed to the inability of DNA polymerase to completely replicate the 3' ends of chromosomal DNA during the S phase. The shortening of the telomeres continues until they are unable to protect the ends of chromosomal DNA from end-to-end chromosomal fusions, a process that generates unstable dicentric chromosomes and karyotypic disarray, resulting in the cell entering the crisis phase and apoptosis.[21]

Immortalized cells avoid telomeric shortening by upregulating the expression of telomerase enzyme, a specialized DNA polymerase, which adds telomere repeat segments to the ends of telomeric DNA (Fig. 16.9). By extending telomeric DNA, telomerase activity results in cells that are resistant to the induction of apoptosis through end-to-end chromosomal fusions. Therefore, maintenance of telomere length above a critical threshold permits unlimited cell division. Although telomerase is absent in normal human cells, it is present in over 90% of immortalized cells in culture and is highly expressed in human cancer cells. By expressing telomerase, cancer cells are able to overcome the barriers of senescence and crisis/apoptosis. Conversely, suppressing telomerase activity by gene knockout experiments in animal studies and by inhibitors of the telomerase enzyme will activate these barriers to cell proliferation.[22]

Inducing Angiogenesis

Vascular supply of nutrients and oxygen is necessary for tissue growth and survival, obligating all cells to reside within 100 mm of a capillary blood vessel. During embryogenesis, the formation of blood vessel involves the development of new endothelial cells and formation into tubes (termed vasculogenesis) and the sprouting of new vessels from existing ones (termed angiogenesis). After completion of tissue formation, further new blood vessel growth is strictly regulated, and in the adult tissues occurs only transiently during the female reproductive cycling and wound healing. In contrast, incipient neoplasias acquire the ability of angiogenesis by turning on an "angiogenic switch," causing the formation of new vessels from existing normally quiescent vessels in order to sustain tumor growth.[23]

Counteractive factors that induce or oppose angiogenesis determine the status of the angiogenic switch in both normal physiologic and pathologic states. Signaling proteins that bind to stimulatory or inhibitory vascular endothelial cell surface receptors regulate the formation of new blood vessels. The most commonly studied signaling protein of angiogenesis is vascular endothelial growth factor-A (VEGF-A). The VEGF-A gene encodes a ligand that can bind to three different transmembrane tyrosine kinase receptors (VEGFR1-3) found on vascular endothelial cells, thereby stimulating the formation of new blood vessel growth. The VEGF-A gene expression can be upregulated by hypoxia during normal physiologic development of blood vessels (e.g. wound healing) and by oncogene signaling during tumorigenesis. Thrombospondin-1 (TSP-1) is another angiogenic signaling protein that can evoke both suppressive and stimulatory effects on new blood vessel growth depending on the levels of TSP-1 and its effects on extracellular matrix degrading proteases.[24] More recently, evidence suggests that it may inhibit angiogenesis through direct effects on endothelial cell migration, proliferation, survival, and apoptosis and by antagonizing VEGF-A activity.[25]

Over the last decade, many investigators have demonstrated that tumors exhibit diverse patterns of neovascularization regulated by both the cancer cells and the surrounding stromal microenvironment. For instance, ductal pancreatic adenocarcinomas appear hypovascularized with stromal "deserts" that are largely avascular,

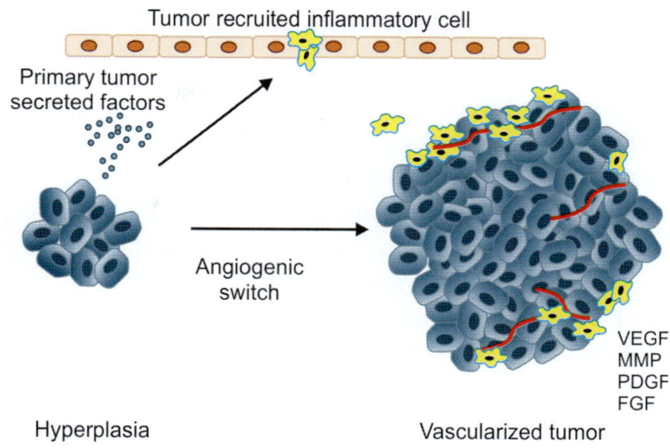

Fig. 16.10: The angiogenic switch. Recruitment of bone marrow-derived cells such as macrophages promotes angiogenesis at the periphery of some tumors by the upregulation of angiogenic factors (VEGF: Vascular endothelial growth factor; MMP: Matrix metalloproteinases; PDGF: Platelet derived growth factor; FGF: Fibroblast growth factor).

whereas other cancers such as pancreatic neuroendocrine carcinomas and renal cell carcinomas are densely vascularized. The variation in vascularity appears to be related to the differences and complexity of tumor angiogenesis regulation. In some tumors, dominant oncogenes, such as *Ras* and *Myc*, can upregulate the expression of angiogenic factors as well as increase proliferative signaling. In other malignancies, immune inflammatory cells within the tumor stroma may drive angiogenesis by producing inductive or inhibitory signaling proteins. These bone marrow-derived cells of the innate immune system such as macrophages, neutrophils, mast cells, and myeloid progenitor cells assemble at the periphery of the tumors in order to regulate ongoing tumor growth through the control of angiogenic switch (Fig. 16.10).[26,27]

Understanding the mechanism of endogenous inhibitors of angiogenesis, including TSP-1, elucidates the importance of inhibitory signals of angiogenesis as a barrier to carcinogenesis. Deletion of genes encoding several endogenous angiogenesis inhibitors in mouse models results in the enhancement of tumor growth, whereas tumor growth is severely impaired by increasing the levels of endogenous angiogenesis inhibitors.[28] The first angiogenesis inhibitor to attain clinical approval was bevacizumab, which inhibits VEGF-A by forming a protein complex with VEGF-A that is incapable of binding with its receptor (VEGFR). By exploiting the knowledge about the mechanisms of endogenous inhibitors of angiogenesis, various clinical and preclinical compounds are being developed to target this important hallmark of cancer.

Activating Invasion and Metastasis

Eventually in carcinogenesis, most human primary cancers well develop pioneer cells, which invade adjacent tissues and travel to distant sites. These distant settlements of tumor cells, or metastases, comprise the final stage of cancer progression and are the cause of 90% of cancer deaths. Cancer invasion and metastasis is a multistage process depicted as a sequence of discrete steps termed the invasion-metastasis cascade (Fig. 16.11). The cascade reflects a succession of cellular changes, which begins with (1) cancer cell invasion of surrounding tissues, followed by (2) intravasation into nearby blood and lymphatic vessels. The malignant cells then (3) transit through the lymphatic and hematogenous systems, (4) escape from the lumina of the vessels into the parenchyma of distant tissues (extravasation), (5) form micrometastases, and finally (6) grow into macroscopic tumors, termed colonization.[29]

Typically, the hallmark of invasion and metastasis begins with carcinoma cells developing alterations in their shape and their attachment to other cells and the extracellular matrix. Adhesion molecules such as E-cadherin form tight junctions with neighboring cells and the extracellular matrix during normal tissue development, maintaining the quiescence of the cells within epithelial cell sheets. Highly aggressive carcinoma cells alter the expression of cell–cell and cell–matrix adhesion molecules by the downregulation or mutational inactivation of the E-cadherin gene. Conversely, many tumor cells will potentiate the upregulation of adhesion molecules normally associated with cell migration during embryogenesis and inflammation. N-cadherin, another adhesion molecule normally expressed in migrating neurons and mesenchymal cells during organogenesis, is upregulated in many invasive carcinoma cells.[30]

Various investigators have observed that cancer cells can acquire other attributes coopted from processes involved in embryogenesis that enable invasion and metastasis. This developmental regulatory program is referred to as the "epithelial-mesenchymal transition" (EMT) and describes the means by which transformed epithelial cells can acquire the abilities to invade, to resist apoptosis, and to disseminate.[7] By activating a set of EMT-inducing transcription factors, including Snail, Slug, Twist, and Zeb1/2, malignant cells evoke the traits implicated in the processes of invasion and metastasis including loss of cellular adhesion, conversion from polygonal to spindle shape morphology, expression of matrix-degrading enzymes, increased motility, and resistance to apoptosis.[31]

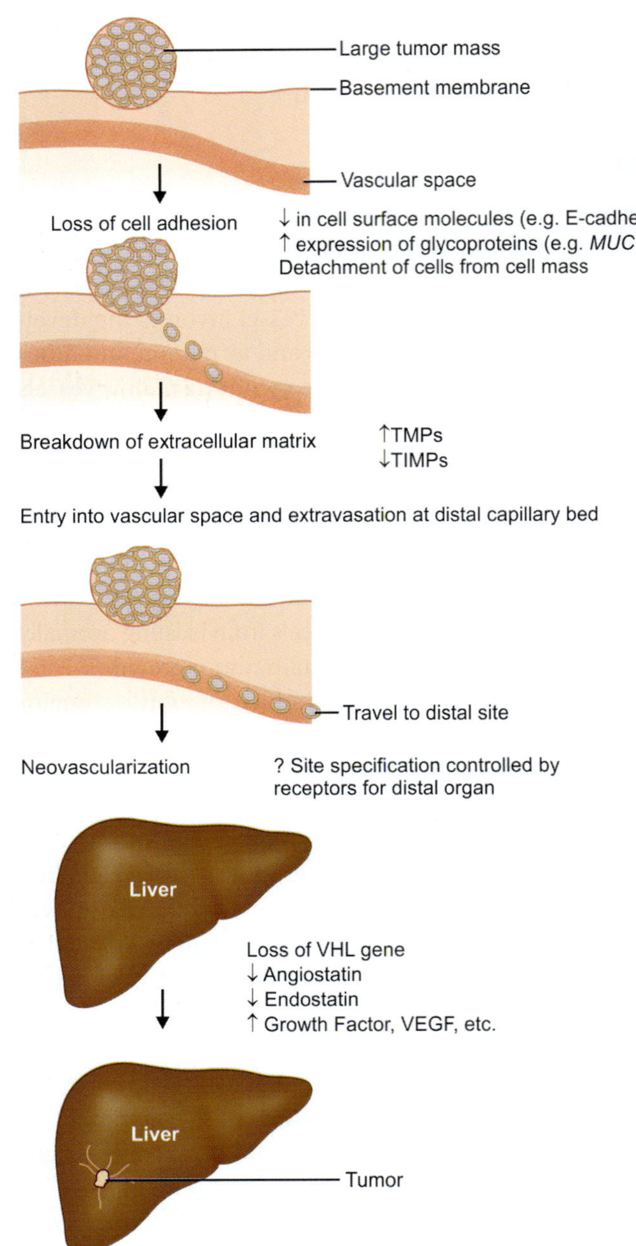

Fig. 16.11: Development of metastases—This requires that a tumor cell is capable of detaching from the tumor mass, degrading the extracellular matrix, invading into the vascular space, extravasating at a distal capillary bed and neovascularization. The tumor cell secretes factors that have an effect on surrounding cells (e.g. a variety of growth factors that cause proliferation of endothelial cells). (TIMPs: Tissue inhibitors of matrix metalloproteinases; VEGF: Vascular endothelial growth factor; TMPs: Metalloproteinases; VHL: Von-Hippel Lindau).

Interaction of cancer cells with adjacent tumor-associated stromal cells also plays an important role in activating the EMT-inducing transcription factors, and this crosstalk between cells is integral to the invasion-metastasis cascade. Cancer cells at the periphery of carcinomas adjacent to stromal cells undergo an EMT, suggesting that these cells receive heterotypic stimuli that are distinct from cancer cells located in the center of a tumor.[32] By recruiting adjacent host immune system cells, cancer cells can also promote local invasion and dissemination. Macrophages at the tumor periphery of many malignant tumors supply matrix-degrading enzymes such as metalloproteinases and cysteine cathepsin proteases so that tumor cells do not need to provide their own degrading enzymes.[33] Tumor-infiltrating inflammatory cells have also been shown to induce and sustain tumor angiogenesis, to stimulate cancer cell proliferation, and to evade immune destruction.[27]

Colonization of distant tissue microenvironment by disseminated tumor cells may be the most complex and poorly understood aspect of carcinogenesis. Most disseminated tumor cells are poorly adapted to the foreign tissue microenvironment and may need to develop multiple enabling programs in order to thrive. Tissue-specific colonization programs may even originate from metastatic cells, which return back to the primary tumor. Distant migrating micrometastases may modify the invasive and metastatic phenotypes of the primary tumor cells by altering the genetic expression of enabling programs.[34] Therefore, colonization is dependent upon cell-biological systems involving critical stromal support cells to create a permissive tumor microenvironment for cancer progression.

Although cancers can recur locally after apparently adequate treatment and affect survival of the patient, most patients die from metastatic disease. More than a century ago, Stephen Paget discovered the nonrandom pattern of visceral metastasis suggesting that certain tumor cells (the seed) had a specific affinity for the microenvironment of certain organs (the soil). Metastases only resulted when the seed and soil were compatible. There are few effective therapies for the treatment of solid tumor metastases. Much current work is focused on the process by which a cancer cell acquires the ability to metastasize. However, clinical metastasis depends also on multiple interactions between metastatic cells and the microenvironment of specific organs. Therefore, future therapy of metastasis will also need to target the microenvironmental factors that are favorable for the growth and survival of metastatic cells.

PRINCIPLES OF CANCER MANAGEMENT

When discussing the staging of malignant disease, the terms "early" and "late" cancer are often used, yet these terms are indistinct. To remedy this difficulty, a uniform system to classify cancers has been developed by the American Joint Committee on Cancer (AJCC) and the Union Internationale Contre le Cancer (UICC) that allows physicians to categorize tumors globally in a consistent manner. This classification system allows effective communication between surgeons and accurate comparison of outcome and survival data between groups.

The AJCC-UICC staging system is based on the premise that as tumor size increases, the risk of nodal metastases increases until, finally, distant metastases occur. Patients can be staged on:

- Clinical criteria (c)
- Pathologic specimens (p)
- After treatment (r)
- At autopsy (a)

The appropriate subscript should be used when staging patients. The AJCC-UICC staging system is based on:

- Tumor size (T)
- Nodal status (N)
- Presence or absence of distal metastases (M)

For some tumors, grade (G) is also important. The TNM system is then subcategorized into numbers based on increasing size (T_{0-4}), nodal involvement (N_{0-2}), and the presence or absence of metastatic disease (M_{0-1}). The subscript "x" is used if tumor size or the presence of regional or metastatic disease cannot be accurately determined.

The final element is then divided into four stages based on TNM criteria.

As extent of disease is one of the most important prognostic factors for outcome, and stage is based on the extent of disease, staging of tumors is one of the most important prognostic indicators of outcome. Accurate staging of the patient aids the physician in treatment planning, gives an indication of prognosis, and allows evaluation and comparisons of treatments. Certain caveats should be remembered when using this staging system:

- Whenever accurate classification according to TNM is not possible, the lowest number should be used.
- If multiple synchronous lesions are identified within an organ, the lesion with the highest T value dictates the stage.
- Stage 0 denotes noninvasive disease, and stage 4 usually indicates the presence of metastases.

TUMOR MARKERS

Although tumor markers were initially proposed as a method for screening patients for cancer, they are most often used for diagnosis, prognosis, and detection of recurrence. Table 16.2 identifies the common serum tumor markers used in oncologic surgery.

Table 16. 2 Serum tumor markers used in surgical oncology. An application score of 1 indicates used for screening, 2 indicates used for diagnosis, 3 indicates used for prognosis, and 4 indicates used for monitoring course and therapeutic responses.

Tumor site	*Approved and unapproved tumor biomarker*	*Antigen source*	*Application score*
Alimentary tract (stomach, pancreas, colorectum)	CEA*	Oncofetal epithelium	2,3,4
	CA 19–9	Mucin-type glycoprotein	2,3,4
	CA 50, CA 195, CA 72–4, TAG 72	Mucin-type glycoprotein	4
Prostate	Prostate-specific antigen*	Prostate glycoprotein, serine protease	1,2,3,4
	Prostate acid phosphatase*	Prostate cellular protein	3,4
Liver (hepatocellular adenocarcinoma)	AFP*	Carrier protein liver cell	1,2,3,4
	CEA*	Hepatocellular oncofetal epithelium	(?3),4
Ovary	CA 125*	Glycoprotein, surface protein of ovarian cell	(?2),3,4
	Placental alkaline phosphatase (Regan isozyme)	Heat-stable acid phosphatase of placental origin	(?2),4
	β-HCG (embryonal teratoblastoma)	Urinary HCG peptide	2,4
Breast	CEA*	Oncofetal epithelium of neoplasm	4
	CA 15–3	Similar antigen from milk fat globules and membranes of breast cancer metastasis	3,(?4)
	CAM 26, M29	Antigenic high-molecular-weight glycoprotein (mucin)	Unknown
	CA27.29, MCA		
Testis (germ cell origin)	AFP*	Serum carrier protein testicular cell (malignant teratoblastoma)	2,3,4
	β-HCG (embryonal teratoblastoma)	Malignant teratoblastoma carrier protein	2,3,4
	Lactate dehydrogenase* and placental alkaline phosphatase* (seminoma)	Heat-stable phosphatase and dehydrogenase, seminoma origin	3,4
Thyroid	Thyroglobulin*	Thyroid hormone inversely correlates with thyroid-stimulating hormone	1,(?3),4
	Calcitonin* (medullary cancer)	Parafollicular C cell of thyroid	1–4
	NSE (medullary cancer)	Glycolytic isoenzyme specific to parafollicular C cell	4
Lung	NSE (SCCL)	Isoenzyme with specific antigenicity to SCCL	4
	CK-BB (SCCL)	Creatine kinase brain isoenzyme	?2
Neuroendocrine			
Carcinoid	5-Hydroxyindoleacetic acid*	Peptide urinary metabolite of indoleacetic acid	2,(?3,?4)
Neuroblastoma	NSE	Isoenzyme with antigenicity to neuroendocrine neural blastogenic cells	4
Pancreas	Insulin	Non-β islet cell of the pancreas	1,2,4
Stomach	Gastrin	G cell gastric antrum	1,2,3,4
Pituitary	Adrenocorticotropic hormone	Anterior pituitary hormone	1,2,3,4
Bone	Alkaline phosphatase	Heat-stable phosphatase with bone fraction specificity	2,3,4
Head and neck	Squamous cell carcinoma	Squamous cell antigenicity	3,4
Trophoblastic	HCG (hydatidiform mole, invasive mole and choriocarcinoma)	Urinary and serum marker of gestational trophoblasts	2,3,4
Myeloma	Bence Jones immunoglobulins*	Urinary light chain IgG protein	2,3

(AFP: α-fetoprotein; CEA: Carcinoembryonic antigen; HCG: Human chorionic gonadotropin; NSE: Neuron-specific enolase; SCCL: Small cell carcinoma of the lung). Asterisk (*) shows markers approved by the US Food and Drug Administration.

Table 16. 3 Surgical strategies used in the management of solid tumors.

Type of surgery	*Rationale*	*Examples*
Biopsy	Removal of tissue/organ for diagnosis or staging.	Lymph node biopsy for diagnosis or staging of patient disease, e.g. lymphoma, sentinel node biopsy for melanoma micrometasis
Preventive	Removal of organ at risk in hereditary cancer syndromes	Proctocolectomy in hereditary colon cancer; thyroidectomy in multiple endocrine neoplasia II syndrome
Primary (definitive)	Definitive therapy of primary tumor and regional site(s) of disease	Segmental mastectomy, colon resection
	Organization of therapeutic strategies with other oncology and medical disciplines	Radiation oncology, medical oncology, pediatric oncology, endocrinology consultation
Cytoreductive	Reduction of tumor volume of primary, regional or metastatic foci to enhance responsiveness to adjuvant modalities	Ovarian carcinoma, lymphoma (Burkitt's lymphoma)
Palliative	Enhance organ function	Bypass and resection of colon cancer obstruction
	Relieve symptoms of progressive disease	"Toilet" mastectomy
	Diminish risk of immediate death	Gastrectomy for hemorrhage from carcinoma
	Enhance quality of life	Brain metastasis from melanoma with neurologic symptoms
Metastatic disease	Curative intent—staging determines solitary focus of metastasis	Colorectal hepatic metastasis, soft tissue or bone sarcoma metastatic to lung
	Noncurative intent—operative cure unlikely, palliation achieved only with resection of metastases	Regional lymph node dissection for skin or vascular fixation of melanoma or squamous carcinoma

Tumor markers currently play an important role in the management of patients with cancer. A few have been used as screening tools in certain populations at risk (e.g. prostate-specific antigen or PSA in older men). However, most tumor markers are currently being used to determine response to treatment and to detect recurrent disease in an asymptomatic patient. Although some heterogeneity occurs with each tumor marker and its associated malignancy, tumor markers provide clinically useful information when positive, and may be incorporated into the management and monitoring of cancer patients.

SURGICAL PRINCIPLES

The surgeon plays an important role in the diagnosis, clinical assessment, and treatment of patients with cancer. In all cases, the patient should be properly assessed to ensure that the benefit of the surgical procedure outweighs the risk of surgical intervention. Knowledge of the functional reserve and regenerative capacity of an organ is also important, for example in the evaluation of a patient with hepatocellular carcinoma for possible resection. For a patient undergoing an oncologic surgical procedure, it is imperative that the surgeon understands the pattern and route of tumor dissemination. This information aids the surgeon during the operative procedure, and the knowledge gained from accurate operative staging can profoundly affect prognosis and treatment decisions. For example, ovarian carcinoma is notorious for peritoneal seeding and metastatic implantation along the diaphragm. Laparotomy for this disease would be incomplete without close examination of the retrocolic gutters and the diaphragmatic recesses; an improper surgical evaluation can lead to misdiagnosis, understaging and inadequate treatment. The two most important concepts in surgical oncology are:

- An understanding of the biology of the disease
- Proper patient selection

The oncologic surgeon is responsible for the diagnosis of the primary tumor as well as the clinical assessment and proper therapy of the patient. Table 16.3 depicts the principal roles of the surgeon in the management of solid tumors. The oncologic surgeon plays a critical role in the diagnosis and therapy of solid tumors as well as in the evaluation for cancer recurrence. Flowchart 16.2 depicts the algorithm for the management of cancer patients commonly utilized at comprehensive cancer centers.

BIOPSY

Surgeons are often called upon to provide tissue for a pathologic diagnosis of a cancer. Tissue diagnosis of a mass can be based on a few cells in an aspiration cytology specimen or the entire mass from an excisional biopsy. It

Flowchart 16.2: Principal roles of the surgical oncologist for the management of solid tumors. (CEA: Carcinoembryonic antigen).

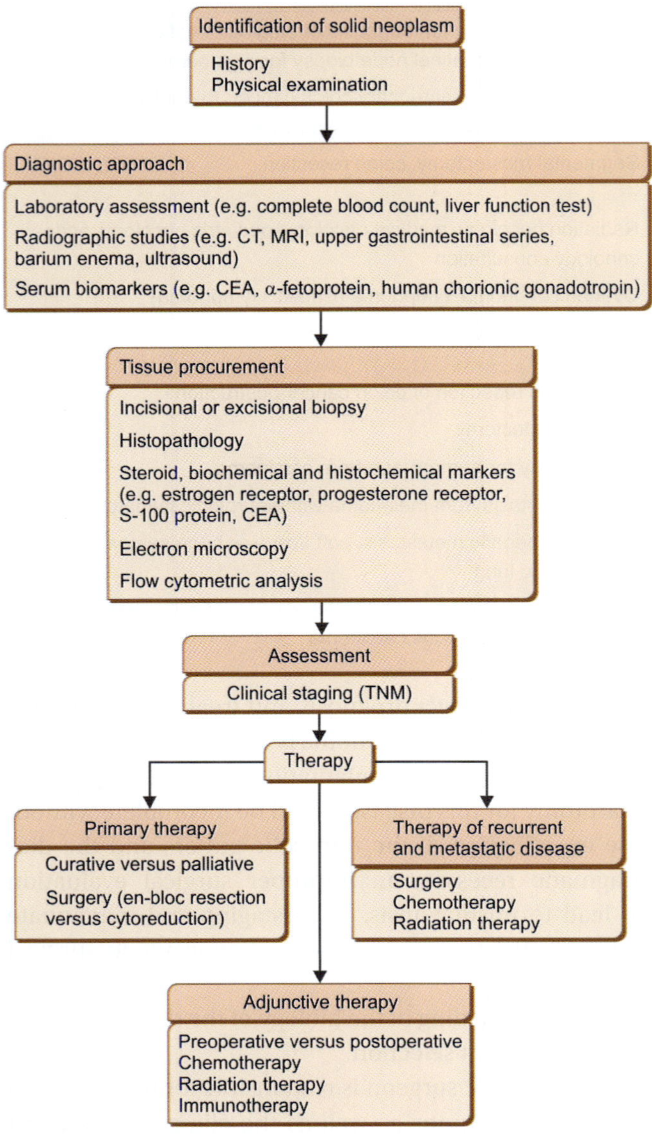

Source: Adapted with permission from Chung MA, Bland KI. Principles of oncology. In: Corson JD, Williamson R (Eds.). Surgery. New York: Mosby; 2001.

is important that several principles are adhered to because an improper biopsy can at best lead to an inconclusive diagnosis and at worst convert a locally curable lesion into a disseminated one.

The first principle is to determine the nature of the biopsy, assuming that one is indeed necessary. If surgical management will not be altered, a biopsy should not be performed because all biopsies carry some, albeit relatively low, risk of morbidity. The limitations of information that can be gained from the biopsy must be known. For example, even in the most experienced hands, it is sometimes difficult to interpret the cells obtained from an aspiration biopsy.

With incisional biopsies the biopsy tract must subsequently be included in the resection because the tumor has been violated. This principle is particularly important for limb sarcomas, as improper planning may vitiate the best incision for the definitive procedure (Figs. 16.12A and B). It is unclear whether seeding of the tract can occur with needle aspirations, but care should be taken with large-core biopsies. Special care is required to prevent dissemination of tumor cells while performing the biopsy. If an intraoperative biopsy is being carried out, the surrounding tissue should be protected; this is particularly important for ovarian biopsies because spillage during the procedure may result in peritoneal seeding. Hemostasis must be achieved because postoperative hematomas in the incisional biopsy bed may contaminate the surrounding field. For excisional biopsies, the specimen must be correctly orientated. This procedure is especially important in breast lesions, for which the excisional biopsy may be the definitive surgical procedure.

Handling of the biopsy material is important. Sufficient material should be obtained, because special stains may be required in difficult cases. Histochemical stains can be used for tumor differentiation and diagnosis. Immunohistochemistry can be very sensitive for detecting the presence or absence of specific proteins in histologic material and has greatly added to the information gained from pathologic specimens. The most commonly used immunohistochemical markers used in diagnostic pathology are listed in Table 16.4. The use of immunohistologic stains greatly aids the pathologist in differentiating tumors of unclear etiology.

Finally, knowledge of the differential diagnosis is important because some diagnostic tests cannot be performed on material that has been fixed in formalin (e.g. markers for lymphoma require frozen tissue).

PREVENTIVE SURGERY AND SCREENING PROGRAMS

The role of surgery in the management of cancer patients is summarized in Table 16.3. Increased understanding of hereditary cancers can identify individuals who are at increased risk of developing cancer. Operative resection can sometimes be appropriate as a preventive measure for colorectal cancer, breast cancer, and thyroid cancer.

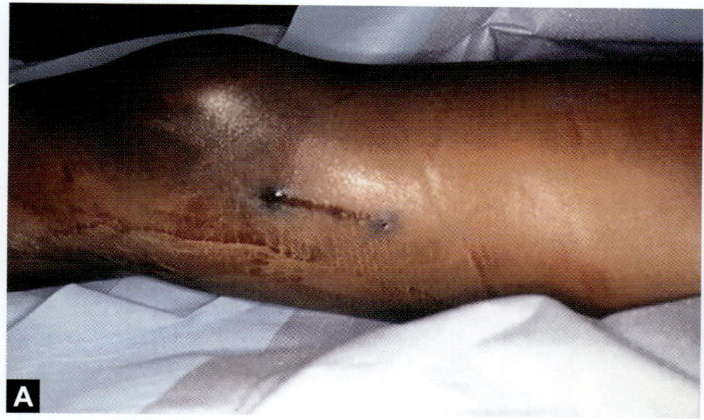

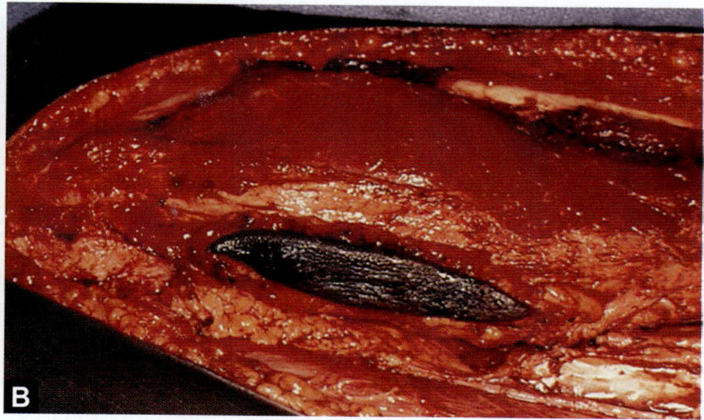

Figs. 16.12A and B: Technique for biopsying extremity lesions. It is important to orient incisions properly when performing incisional biopsies. (A) Scar from a longitudinal incisional biopsy overlying a soft tissue mass. In this extremity sarcoma, the site of the longitudinal excision placed at the time of the incisional biopsy can be easily excised with the final surgical procedure. An incorrectly placed horizontal excision would have required the excision of more normal tissue and jeopardized function of the leg. (B) The soft tissue mass, along with the biopsy scar and tract, are excised in continuity at the time of the surgical extirpation.
Courtesy: Richard M Terek, MD, Department of Orthopedics, Brown University, USA.

In these circumstances, the entire organ at risk should generally be removed to abolish the cancer risk completely. If the entire organ cannot be removed, or if the morbidity would be excessive, then the remnant has to be continually kept under surveillance (e.g. the rectal cuff after subtotal colectomy for familial adenomatous polyposis).

Aside from their role in hereditary cancer syndromes, surgeons play an important role in cancer screening programs. Screening of populations at risk for malignancy can allow detection of disease at either a premalignant or an early stage, which enables complete surgical resection and cure. Currently, there are screening programs for breast, colorectal, cervical, and prostate cancer in the USA and Europe; and for gastric, esophageal, and hepatic cancers in Asia.

For a screening program to be successful, the screened condition has to be prevalent within the population at risk. One example of a successful screening program and the advent of surgical resection for prevention of disease is gastric cancer screening in Japan.

Although the incidence of stomach cancer is on the decline in the USA and Europe, it continues to have a high incidence in Japan. When diagnosed at an early stage, gastric carcinoma has a 5-year survival rate in excess of 90%. When diagnosed at a more advanced stage, the outcome is very poor (5-year survival <20%). As a result of the high incidence of this malignancy in Japan, a gastric screening program has been practiced there since the 1960s and consists of indirect radiographic imaging of the stomach in six views. Since the introduction of mass screening in the 1960s, the age-adjusted death rate from stomach cancer has been on a downward decline. By 1985, >5 million Japanese had been screened and over 6,000 new cases of gastric cancer had been diagnosed, of which >50% were early-stage gastric cancers. When the outcome of patients with gastric cancer diagnosed through a screening program versus those detected by symptoms were compared (i.e. screened vs nonscreened), the curative resectability and 5-year survival rates were significantly better in the screened group (90.5% and 86.2%, respectively, for the screened group, 66.7% and 61% for the nonscreened group).[35]

Other desirable features of a screening test are that it should be cheap and safe, with a high sensitivity and specificity.

SURGICAL OPERATIONS WITH CURATIVE INTENT

Surgical resection remains the mainstay in the treatment of solid tumor malignancies, with approximately 75% of patients undergoing operation with a curative intent. Whenever feasible, an en bloc resection of the tumor should be attempted. Adhesions between the tumor and surrounding normal tissue should be assumed to be malignant and, if possible, be removed intact with the specimen. Violation of the tumor may lead to spillage and recurrence of local disease. Every attempt must be made to obtain margins that are microscopically free of tumor cells. In many cancers, simple extirpation of the neoplasm with microscopic free margins is curative. The easiest time to remove a malignancy is during the first surgical procedure.

Table 16.4 Commonly used immunohistological markers of diagnostic value in oncologic pathology.

Antigen marker	*Organ or tissue source*	*Marker purpose*
Carcinoembryonic antigen	Alimentary tract (stomach, small bowel, liver, pancreas)	Identifies oncofetal antigen in primary, metastatic and recurrent adenocarcinoma
	Colorectum	Identifies oncofetal antigen in primary, metastatic and recurrent adenocarcinoma
	Breast	Nonspecific for metastatic adenocarcinoma
	Pulmonary	Differentiates adenocarcinoma (+) versus mesothelioma (–)
S-100 protein	Skin	Evidence of antigen protein marker in selective tissue
	Cartilage	
	Soft tissue	
Lymphoid		
LeuMI	Hematopoietic, lymphatic	Identifies Reed–Sternberg cells in T cell lymphoma (Hodgkin's disease)
Ber-H2	Hematopoietic, lymphatic	Analogous to Ki-1 Reed–Sternberg cell of Hodgkin's disease
L-26	Hematopoietic, lymphatic	Pan-B cell marker
UCHL1	Hematopoietic, lymphatic	Pan-T cell marker
Leukocyte common antigen	Hematopoietic, lymphatic	Pan-lymphoid marker
Peptide hormones	Stomach, G cell	Gastrin
	Pancreas (non-β islet cell)	Insulin
	Thyroid, parafollicular cell	Calcitonin
	Pituitary (anterior lobe)	Adrenocorticotropic hormone
Steroidal hormone	Breast	Estrogen-progesterone receptor
	Prostate	Androgen receptor
	Germ cell malignancies	
β-Human chorionic gonadotropin	Ovary	Identifies ovarian trophoblastic disease
		Identifies ovarian carcinoma
		Identifies embryonal carcinoma
CA 125	Ovary	Identifies ovarian carcinoma tumor volume
α-Fetoprotein	Ovary	Identifies endodermal sinus tumor
	Testis	Identifies nonseminoma tumors (embryonal carcinoma, teratocarcinoma, yolk-sac tumor and nonseminoma combinations)
Human placental lactogen	Placenta/uterus	Identifies nontrophoblastic nongonadal tumor
Organ specific		
Prostate-specific antigen	Prostate	Produced by organ-specific epithelium of prostate
Thyroid follicular	Thyroid follicle	Differentiates follicular versus nonfollicular cells of thyroid and nonthyroid tissues
GCDFP-15 (breast)	Apocrine epithelium, breast epithelium	Differentiates apocrine and breast tissue from surrounding epithelium
Muscle differentiation		
Smooth musculature	Smooth muscle	With desmin, differentiates smooth versus striated muscle tissues
Skeletal musculature	Striated muscle	
Myoglobin	Striated muscle	
MyoD1 gene	Striated muscle	
Intermediate filaments		
Desmin	Muscle	Differentiates muscle
Neurofilaments	Nerve	Neural differentiation
Vimentin	Mesoderm	Identifies mesenchymal cells
Glial fibrillary	Glial stroma	Acid protein marker of glial differentiation
Keratin	Epithelium	Epithelial differentiation

Although surgical operation remains the mainstay in the locoregional treatment of solid tumors, there is a general trend away from the use of radical procedures to treat cancer. This change in treatment philosophy has arisen from three factors:

- A better understanding of the biology of tumor metastasis
- Increased use of multimodality treatment, particularly the use of radiation to treat local and regional disease
- Detection of cancers at an earlier stage and smaller tumor size.

The surgical treatments of malignant melanoma and breast cancer are good examples of this trend toward conservatism. Historically, it was recommended that a 4–5 cm margin should be excised around a melanoma to decrease local recurrence. However, this recommendation has now been changed, based on the results of a multi-institutional randomized trial of melanomas of intermediate thickness (1–4 mm) that showed no difference in local recurrence or survival for patients treated with 2-cm versus 4-cm surgical margins.[36]

Similarly, the routine use of modified radical mastectomy to treat breast cancer has been altered to include the use of breast conservation (lumpectomy, axillary dissection, and adjuvant breast radiation) for most cases.[37]

It is important that the oncologic surgeon be cognizant of the different approaches to the management of the cancer patient; not only may the timing of the surgical procedure be altered but also additional surgical techniques may be required during the surgical procedure. For example, if postoperative radiation is a consideration, radiographic surgical clips that cause minimal radiographic distortion can be used to aid in delineating the site at risk for recurrent disease. Loops of small bowel can be excluded from the pelvis by retroverting the uterus, creating an omental flap, or inserting a polyglactin 90 mesh (Vicryl).

CYTOREDUCTIVE OPERATIONS

Cytoreductive operations are used for selected malignancies that are known to respond to chemotherapy or radiation. The rationale for this approach to cancer therapy is that the minimum of residual tumor bulk may improve the sensitivity to chemotherapy or irradiation. Cytoreduction has been used successfully for advanced ovarian carcinoma and Burkitt's lymphoma. For stages III and IV ovarian carcinoma, this treatment approach may result in a statistically significant lengthened duration of progression-free and overall survival.[38]

PALLIATIVE OPERATIONS

Patients for palliative operations have to be selected carefully to ensure that the benefits of the procedure outweigh its morbidity. Under these circumstances, the patient has to be symptomatic. Palliative surgery can be used to:

- Relieve symptoms or for pain control (e.g. "toilet" mastectomy for breast carcinoma)
- Decrease the morbidity associated with the primary neoplasm (e.g. gastrectomy for herald gastrointestinal hemorrhage related to advanced gastric carcinoma)
- Extirpate lesions that affect the function of a vital organ or structure (e.g. pulmonary carcinoma obstructing a bronchus).

OPERATIONS FOR METASTATIC DISEASE

A growing body of evidence suggests that for selected cancers, operations can be carried out to treat metastatic disease with a curative intent. When considering surgical therapy of metastases, there should be a limited quantity of metastatic disease, preferably limited to one organ, and evidence that the metastatic deposit can be adequately resected without jeopardizing the function of the organ. In addition, the morbidity and mortality rate associated with the resection must be acceptable.

Three factors govern outcome after surgical resection for metastatic disease: the number of metastases, the tumor doubling time, and the primary histology. Surgery for metastatic disease is most frequently performed for hepatic metastases from a colorectal primary tumor and for pulmonary metastases from a sarcoma. However, the best long-term survival rates following hepatic resection are seen with neuroendocrine tumors, reflecting the importance of the primary histology.

Hepatic Resection

No prospective randomized trials have evaluated surgical resection of colorectal metastases to the liver. Nonetheless, it appears there is a survival benefit for the surgical resection of liver metastases in carefully selected patients. Scheele and colleagues[39] reviewed the natural history of 1,209 patients who had hepatic metastases from colorectal carcinoma:

- There were no 5-year survivors for patients who were deemed unresectable; the median survival after diagnosis of hepatic metastases was 6.9 months.

Table 16. 5 Outcome of patients who have hepatic metastases from colorectal carcinoma treated with curative hepatic resection

Series	Number	Time period	5-year survival rate (%)	10-year survival rate (%)
Memorial Sloan-Kettering	612	1985–1994	NS	17
Johns Hopkins Hospital	226	1984–1992	40	26
University of Toronto	423	1992–2002	47	28
University of Erlangen and Nuremberg, Erlangen, Germany	350	1960–1992	39	24
University of the Sacred Heart, Rome, Italy	251	1992–2007	39	24

- Similarly, there were no 5-year survivors for patients who had resectable disease, but did not undergo a hepatic resection, and the median survival for this group of patients was 14.2 months.
- For patients who underwent a curative resection of their metastatic hepatic disease, the 5-year and 10-year survival rates were 40% and 27%, respectively, and the median survival was 26 months.
- Patients who had a noncurative hepatic resection (i.e. residual cancer after surgery) experienced a median survival similar to the group who had resectable disease but did not undergo resection.

Table 16.5 summarizes some of the recent data on outcome for patients with hepatic metastases who undergo a curative resection. The 5-year survival rate for those with a curative resection ranges from 25% to 35%.

In most series, it is rare for patients who are disease-free at 5 years to develop recurrent disease. The most important prognostic factors for a favorable outcome after liver resection for colorectal metastases are the ability to achieve a tumor-free margin and the absence of extrahepatic disease. There are some patients who benefit from repeat hepatic resections for colorectal metastases. The Repeat Hepatic Metastases Registry,[40] which has registered 170 patients from 20 institutions, reports a 5-year survival rate of 32% after repeat hepatic resection. It is important to recognize that most patients with colorectal metastases to the liver are not candidates for surgical resection. However, for the minority who do qualify, hepatic resection offers the opportunity of a cure.

Hepatic resections for metastases from a primary neuroendocrine malignancy offer an opportunity for palliation as well as a cure. The most common neuroendocrine primary is a carcinoid, and liver metastases from this primary are associated with the symptoms of carcinoid syndrome, which can be debilitating. As this malignancy can be indolent, it is not surprising that there are 5- and 10-year survivors even if the hepatic resection has not been curative. In a series from the Mayo Clinic of patients hepatic resection for metastatic neuroendocrine carcinomas,[41] the 4-year survival rate was 73% and symptomatic relief was achieved in 90% of patients, with a mean duration of palliation of 19.3 months.

Pulmonary Resection

Although pulmonary resections have been performed for lung metastases from a variety of primary tumors, lung resections (or lung metastasectomies) are most frequently performed for sarcomatous metastases. Pulmonic metastasectomies allow the surgeon to remove more than one metastatic deposit, with a margin of normal tissue, while preserving lung function. The 5-year survival rate after lung resection for metastases from a primary sarcoma ranges from 25% to 40%. The largest series of patients who have undergone surgical treatment of lung metastases from sarcoma is reported by the European Organization for Research and Treatment of Cancer—Soft Tissue and Bone Sarcoma Group.[42] In this series, the 5-year survival rate was 35%. The factors associated with a good prognosis after resection included:

- A disease-free interval of longer than 2.5 years duration between diagnosis and development of metastasis
- Tumor-free margins at lung resection
- Age under 40 years
- Primary tumor with a low tumor grade.

RADIATION ONCOLOGY

Radiation can be used:

- For definitive cancer management (e.g. head and neck cancers)
- As an adjunct to surgical management (e.g. breast cancer)
- As part of an interdisciplinary approach to cancer (e.g. sarcomas).

The type of radiation used clinically can be divided into brachytherapy, when the radiation source is close to the target, and teletherapy, as in external beam radiation.

Regardless of the source of radiation, the dose that the patient receives is governed by the inverse square law—that is, there is a rapid decrease in radiation received as one moves away from the source. The absorbed radiation dose is measured in grays (Gy) and is the amount of energy per unit mass absorbed (1 Gy = 1 joule/kg).

Most patients with solid tumors receive radiotherapy externally (external beam radiation). This type of therapy is usually well tolerated by patients and is often given in daily fractions over a 4- to 6-week period. The role of external beam radiation has been evaluated in a variety of solid tumors and shown to decrease the local recurrence rate. For example, the use of adjuvant external beam radiation after curative surgery has been shown to decrease the local recurrence rate by 50% in both invasive and noninvasive breast cancer. As radiotherapy is a local treatment, its use has little impact on systemic disease and overall survival.

One of the disadvantages of external beam radiotherapy is that the dose that can be delivered to the target area is limited by the toxicity to the surrounding organs. This problem can be partially overcome by the use of brachytherapy, which can deliver a large dose of radiation to a small surface area without the limitation of radiation-induced changes in the skin. In a prospective randomized trial to evaluate the use of radiotherapy as an adjuvant treatment for sarcomas, it was found that the addition of brachytherapy decreased the local recurrence rate from 14% to 4% with no effect on overall survival.[43] The benefit of brachytherapy for local control was most marked for high-grade sarcomas, and a follow-up trial to evaluate the role of radiotherapy for low-grade sarcomas confirmed these observations.[44]

Effects of Radiation

Radiation has two effects on the cell:

- It directly causes DNA cross-linking which, if unrepaired, may prevent the cell from proliferating.
- In the presence of oxygen, it produces oxygen-free radicals that also affect the cell.

For radiation to have an effect on the cell, the cell has to proliferate. Therefore, regions of the body with a high proliferative index, such as the bone marrow, oral mucosa and gastrointestinal tract, are very sensitive to radiation. These characteristics can be exploited by the radiotherapist. As cells that are in the mitotic phase are more sensitive to the effects of radiation, the use of chemotherapy agents that can synchronize cells into a specific stage of the cell cycle results in more damage to the tumor cells. Also, increasing oxygen delivery to the tumor enhances cell killing, and this has been exploited by using hyperbaric oxygen and preoperative radiotherapy.

Radiotherapy as an Adjunct to Surgery

Radiotherapy can be delivered either pre- or postoperatively (or sometimes both). Clinical trials are now in place to determine that modality of therapy should be used first. There are advantages to both schemes. Preoperative (neoadjuvant) radiotherapy may result in tumor size reduction and organ preservation, may sterilize tumor cells that are distant from the primary lesion, and may allow for a tumor-free margin. Theoretically, because the tumor bed has not been violated, the blood supply and oxygen delivery to the tumor cells should remain intact. For rectal lesions, the presence of the tumor in a place decreases the likelihood that the small bowel will be in the radiated field, in contrast to an abdominoperineal resection procedure.

Advocates for postoperative (adjuvant) radiotherapy point out that radiation results in inflammation and may result in a more difficult surgical dissection. This problem can be minimized by waiting 4–6 weeks after the completion of radiotherapy before performing the definitive operative procedure. Postoperative radiotherapy allows accurate pathologic staging of the tumor and better patient selection for adjunct treatments, and there is no delay in the surgical extirpation of the tumor.

Adverse Effects of Radiotherapy

There are early and late adverse effects of radiotherapy:

- The acute effect is marked by inflammation in normally proliferating or renewing tissues, such as the skin, bladder, gastrointestinal tract, and bone marrow, which are the most sensitive to radiation injury.
- Delayed effects of radiation are secondary to vasculitis and ischemia and are characterized by tissue necrosis, fibrosis, fistula formation, nonhealing ulcers, and spinal cord ischemia.

Two special adverse effects of radiation should be mentioned. Radiotherapy can cause mutations in normal cells, which can result in:

1. Mutations in the germ line (hereditary defects)
2. Mutations in somatic cells, and hence tumor formation (e.g. sarcoma in the postirradiated breast).

CHEMOTHERAPY FOR CANCER

Chemotherapy remains a mainstay in the fight against cancer. There are four ways that chemotherapy can be used for treating cancer:

- Primary treatment for certain malignancies (e.g. leukemia and lymphomas)
- Induction therapy for advanced disease (e.g. inflammatory breast cancer)
- Adjuvant therapy to prevent the development of metastatic disease in patients at increased risk
- A radiosensitizer (e.g. for head and neck malignancies).

Combination versus Single-agent Therapy

The use of chemotherapeutic drugs, and the success in treating cancer with these agents, is based on a few principles. With very few exceptions (i.e. choriocarcinoma and Burkitt's lymphoma), combination drug therapy should be used. Single-agent chemotherapy is rarely effective because of the Goldie-Coldman hypothesis,[45] which states that the rate at which tumor cells develop chemoresistance is a function of the intrinsic genetic instability of the tumor. Even if this rate is as low as 10^{-6}, in a mass of l-cm diameter that contains 10^9 cells there would be at least one resistant clone. This tumor mass would initially give a partial or complete response to chemotherapy, but then recur as the resistant clone increased in number. Therefore, it is imperative to use a combination of drugs with different toxicities and modes of action, and to eradicate all tumor cells. Chemotherapy should be given at the maximal tolerated dose and with the shortest time interval to maximize "tumor cell kill".

Chemotherapy and Growth Fraction

The response of tumors to chemotherapy is affected by tumor growth biology. In humans, the growth fraction of a mass is not constant and once a certain size is attained, the growth fraction decreases. On average, growth fraction peaks when the tumor is approximately 37% of its maximal size. This is the rationale for the use of chemotherapy in the adjuvant setting and for the use of cytoreductive surgery when tumor load is, theoretically, at a minimum.

Chemoresistance

There are two types of chemoresistance:[46]

- Intrinsic resistance occurs when the cell acquires a generic defense mechanism and becomes resistant to a host of chemotherapeutic agents—the multidrug resistance (MDR) phenotype is an example of this and results from an increase in cellular P-glycoprotein, which regulates the transport of toxins out of the cell.
- Extrinsic resistance is the development of a mutation to a specific step in the pathway used by a specific agent.

Chemotherapeutic agents commonly used and their mode of action are summarized in Table 16.6.[47]

Drug Trials

There are three phases to drug testing in humans. In phase I trials, the objective is identification of a maximal tolerated

Table 16.6 Classes of chemotherapeutic agents and their modes of action.

Class	*Example*	*Mode of action*
Antimetabolites	Antifolates: MTX, 5FU	Inhibit steps in one carbon metabolism for purine synthesis—MTX inhibits dihydrofolate reductase, 5FU inhibits thymidylate synthetase
	Purine analogs: 6-mercaptopurine	Inhibit de novo purine synthesis
Antibiotics	Bleomycin	Causes breaks in DNA
	Doxorubicin	Interferes with topoisomerase II and causes DNA breaks
	Mitomycin C	Crosslinks DNA
Platinum analogs	Cisplatin	Binds to DNA and forms DNA adducts
Alkylating agents	Melphalan, chlorambucil, cyclophosphamide	Binds to DNA and forms DNA adducts
Vinca alkaloids	Vincristine, vinorelbine	Binds to tubulin causing mitotic arrest
	Paclitaxel	Binds to microtubules
	Etoposide	Interferes with topoisomerase II and inhibits nucleoside transport
Topoisomerase inhibitors	Camptothecin	Inhibits topoisomerase I and unraveling of DNA before replication fork
Acridine dyes	Amsacrine	Intercalates DNA causing DNA breaks
Retinoids	Retinol	? Causes differentiation of malignant cell

(5-FU: 5-fluorouracil; MTX: Methotrexate).

dose (MTD) for the drug and its associated toxicities. The starting dose for the drug is usually 1/10 the lethal dose in 10% of mice (LD_{10}), and the dosage is rapidly increased. In a Phase I trial, a therapeutic effect is not required. Once the MTD and side effects of an agent have been determined, a Phase II trial is conducted to ascertain clinical efficacy. If successful, a phase III trial can be designed, the objective of which is to determine if the new agent is better than current treatments.

IMMUNOTHERAPY FOR CANCER

A cancer develops when there is an imbalance between the cancer cell and the host's immune system. Immunotherapy can be used to augment the host's immune system to eradicate cancer cells.[47] This can be done in a nonspecific manner by the delivery of cytokines that stimulate the T_H1 arm of the immune system and results in lysis of cancer cells. Alternatively, vectors can be designed to deliver known TAAs that would then result in the production of T cells, which would target any cell expressing the tumor antigen, including the cancer cell. This type of targeting has been hampered by difficulty in identifying suitable TAAs that are expressed on the cell surface and are immunogeneic.

Nonspecific Immunotherapy

Initial work on augmenting the immune response against cancers was nonspecific. Bacillus Calmette-Guerin (BCG), a known immunostimulant, has been used in the treatment of melanoma, breast, colon and bladder carcinomas. The rationale is that because tumors have tumor antigens that are foreign to the immune system and BCG is an immunostimulant, BCG administration would increase the immune response to the tumor antigens. This works best if BCG is in the immediate vicinity of the tumor antigen. Therefore, it is not surprising that the best responses were obtained with intravesical therapy of bladder carcinoma and in-transit metastases for melanoma.

Interleukin-2 and IL-12 are cytokines that are critical modulators of the T_H1 arm of the immune system.[47] Clinical trials have been designed using these cytokines to treat cancer. Although the results have been very encouraging, the use of cytokines as biologic modifiers has been hampered by the large doses required with systemic administration and by the associated side effects (pulmonary capillary leakage with IL-2 and septic shock with IL-12).

More Specific Immunotherapy

Recent work has focused on more specific techniques to augment the immune system. It is known that the immune system can recognize tumor antigens, and it has been hypothesized that increasing the delivery of tumor antigens will increase the immune response. Tumor cells can be removed from patients, irradiated and readministered to the patient. As mentioned earlier, lymphocytes that recognize tumor antigens can be found infiltrating the tumor bed. These tumor-infiltrating lymphocytes can be removed once the tumor has been excised, proliferated in vitro and readministered to the patient. Such therapies, however, are expensive, time consuming and limited to a few facilities that can process the tumor tissue. With the advent of molecular techniques to clone tumor antigens, viral vectors that secrete tumor antigens have been designed and irradiated cancer cells can be engineered to secrete cytokines.[48] Vectors such as BCG can also be designed to express tumor antigens and to secrete cytokines simultaneously to maximize the immune response to the tumor antigen. In this manner, the immune response can be directed against tumor antigens and therefore tumor cells.

Monoclonal Antibodies

Monoclonal antibodies that are specific for known tumor antigens can be easily generated. The results from clinical trials using this type of approach are now being reported. Recently, a monoclonal antibody targeting the cytotoxic T-lymphocyte antigen-4 (CTLA-4) has gained success in the treatment of melanoma, significantly improving the survival rates of patient with metastatic melanoma for the first time.[49] This drug, named ipilimumab (Yervoy), blocks the CTLA-4 inhitory signal produced by antigen presenting cells such as dendritic cells and induces an immune response that persists after the completion of treatment. The success of ipilimumab emphasizes the need to further investigate immune modulating targets in the future.

Future Developments in Immumotherapy

As knowledge increases about how the immune system recognizes tumor antigens and how tumors evade the immune system, the methods used to design immunotherapeutic agents will become more sophisticated. This will probably involve the use of costimulatory molecules, the use of synthetic peptides carrying immunogenic epitopes and a combination of the different mediators that are deemed crucial in the immune response. It is conceivable that in the future vaccines will be generated not only for use in cancer therapy, but also for cancer prevention.[48]

GENE THERAPY FOR CANCER

Cancer treatment has traditionally focused on organ involvement, with radiotherapy and operations used for local and regional disease and chemotherapy targeted at metastatic disease. With increasing knowledge about the molecular events that are involved in carcinogenesis, attempts are now being made to target cancer treatment at the molecular and cellular levels. Since 1990, when the first attempt at replacing a single gene defect was made, the number of gene therapy trials has exploded. In 1999 there were more than 100 trials in place, and over 50% were targeted for cancer patients.[50]

Either the cancer cell or the host immune system can be manipulated by gene therapy. Gene therapy can be used to alter tumor cell sensitivity to specific drugs, to introduce tumor suppressor activity in instances where it is absent or to inactivate oncogenic proteins.

As many of the steps involved in carcinogenesis have been identified, the absence of an essential controlling protein in the cell cycle can be replaced or, conversely, abnormal expression of an oncogene can be corrected. For example, *p53* is a crucial protein for cell cycle regulation and programed cell death (apoptosis). In cell culture, the replacement of normal *p53* protein results in loss of the malignant phenotype. Gene therapy can target the replacement of *p53* expression. Abnormal expression of an oncogene can be neutralized with antisense DNA that binds to the mRNA of the abnormal protein and prevents its expression.

Other than targeting proteins involved in carcinogenesis, gene therapy can be used to target a drug effect by inserting a suicide gene. Thymidine kinase is an enzyme that converts nontoxic nucleoside analogs, such as ganciclovir, into phosphorylated compounds that act as chain terminators and kill dividing cells. Vectors can be used to deliver this enzyme to cancer cells, resulting in their demise when ganciclovir is administered.

Another pool of gene therapy is the delivery of enzymes to hematopoietic cells that confer drug resistance, as this would facilitate further dose escalation of chemotherapeutic regimens.

Gene therapy can be used to alter the host's immune response to the tumor cell. One example of this approach is the introduction of specific genes, such as cytokines or co-stimulatory molecules that increase the immunogenicity of tumor antigens. Alternatively, tumor-infiltrating lymphocytes can be obtained from the patient's tumor, modified to enhance their cytotoxic capability, expanded in vitro and reintroduced into the patient.

Vectors

The vectors used to deliver genes to cells can be divided into viral and nonviral agents. Viruses allow integration of foreign DNA into the cellular genome. The host cell then expresses the foreign DNA as if it were its own. The most popular viruses used for gene therapy are the retroviruses (adenovirus, herpes simplex virus and adeno-associated virus), which have been used in more than 50% of the clinical trials to date. However, there are some problems with using viruses as vectors:[51]

- It is difficult to target which cells viruses will infect, and this is particularly important if a gene is being replaced.
- The efficiency of DNA transfer is <1% with viral vectors and, because viruses trigger the immune response, the amount of virus that can be given is limited.
- There is a real, albeit unproved, concern that because DNA integration is a random event, it is possible that using viruses to deliver DNA may result in integration of this foreign DNA near an oncogene or tumor suppressor gene, resulting in cancer formation.

Nonviral modes of delivering foreign genes include vectors such as BCG, liposomes and naked DNA. Bacillus Calmette-Guerin can be used as a biologic modifier for cancer therapy if it is altered to express cytokines and tumor antigens. Foreign DNA can be packaged in liposomes that have lipid-rich membranes, allowing delivery of DNA into the nucleus. This DNA is then expressed by the cell. Alternatively, naked DNA can be physically placed in the nucleus using a shotgun technique. The last two techniques are currently being developed, but to date have been very inefficient.

MOLECULARLY TARGETED THERAPY FOR CANCER

The advancement of systemic therapy for cancer necessitates the understanding of biologic systems present in the cancer cell microenvironment. Over the last several decades, clinicians have been inundated with a multitude of molecularly targeted therapeutic agents. Targeted therapy prevents the progression of cancer by inhibiting

Table 16.7 Classes of molecularly targeted therapies and their modes of action.

Hallmark targeted	*Example*	*Mode of action*
Sustaining proliferative signaling	Imatinib mesylate	Inhibits tyrosine kinase phosphorylation in abl, c-kit, and PDGF-R
	Erlotinib	Inhibits EGFR tyrosine kinase in metastatic non-small cell lung cancer and pancreatic cancer
	Cetuximab, Panitumumab	Monoclonal antibody inhibit EGFR in colon cancer and non-small cell lung cancer
	Trastuzumab	Inhibits HER2/neu receptor in breast cancer
	Vemurafenib, Dabrafenib	Interrupts BRAF/MEK/MAPK pathway in cells with V600E BRAF mutation
Evading growth suppressers	Everolimus	Inhibits mTOR downstream signaling of tumor cell growth
Resisting cell death	Bortezomib	Induces apoptosis by inhibiting proteasome degradation of pro-apoptotic proteins, e.g. *p53*
	Obatoclax, Navitoclax, Gossypol	Inhibits Bcl-2
Enabling replicative immortality	Imetelstat	Short-chain nucleic acid molecule inhibits telomerase activity
Inducing angiogenesis	Bevacizumab	Anti-VEGF monoclonal antibody
	Apatinib	Inhibits VEGF receptor 2
Activating invasion and metastasis	c-MET	Inhibits HGF receptor activity in cell motility and invasion

(abl: Abelson proto-oncogene; PDGF-R: Platelet-derived growth factor receptor; EGFR: Epidermal growth factor receptor; HER2: Human epidermal growth factor receptor 2; VEGF: Vascular endothelial growth factor; mTOR: Mammalian target of rapamycin).

specific molecules needed for carcinogenesis and metastasis instead of interfering with all rapidly dividing cells. Therefore, targeted cancer therapies are also less harmful to normal cells, unlike traditional chemotherapy. At the forefront of targeted therapies, the development of various tyrosine kinase inhibitors has completely changed the outcome of previously fatal malignancies. Both chronic myelogenous leukemia and gastrointestinal stromal tumors are now successfully treated diseases due to the drug imatinib mesylate. Other drugs have also been successful in inhibiting the other hallmarks of cancer, as summarized in Table 16.7.[52]

The development of targeted therapies has also demanded that clinicians are more aware of the molecular basis of cancer in order to successfully treat individual patients. These novel anti-cancer agents often target specific proteins within a key hallmark of cancer. Knowledge of the patient's stage of cancer progression and mechanism of carcinogenesis is necessary to effectively treat each individual. The strategy for cancer treatment will require an understanding of the carcinogenic pathway of that particular patient's disease. For instance, treating a cancer patient with bevacizumab, an anti-VEGF monoclonal antibody, requires that the clinician is cognizant that the angiogenesis pathway is enabled by the patient's cancer. Similarly, utilizing a BRAF inhibitor, such as vemurafenib, may not be effective in treating a melanoma patient whose tumor does not have a specific BRAF mutation. In addition, successful treatment of cancer patients in the future may require targeting multiple carcinogenesis pathways. The ability of a tumor cell to develop resistance to chemotherapy may be due to its systematic acquisition of multiple hallmarks of cancer during its tranformation from a normal cell to a malignant cell. Therefore, targeting one hallmark of a patient's cancer would not be effective in preventing disease progression as another hallmark gains importance. Also, different cells within the tumor population may have acquired different hallmarks; therefore, co-targeting multiple components of different hallmarks may be the best strategy.

FUTURE HORIZONS CONCERNING CANCER

Over the past three decades we have witnessed tremendous strides in the understanding of cancer at the molecular level. Knowledge of the six hallmarks of cancer provides a framework for the clinician to comprehend the molecular complexities of carcinogenesis. Understanding the biological capabilities acquired by malignant cells will be important to the clinician, as the division between basic science and clinical medicine becomes obscured. Evidence for this already exists as we have seen a burgeoning of molecularly targeted therapies designed against specific capabilities of cancer cells with their concomitant improvement in treatment efficacy.

Despite the success of molecularly targeted drug therapies, we have also witnessed resistance to effective treatment as tumor cells can develop redundant pathways to evade cell death. For example, cancer cells, in response to potent angiogenesis inhibitors, may reduce their dependence on angiogenesis and shift to tumor invasion and metastasis. The initially hypoxic tumor cell, now devoid of its own vascularity, utilizes the suurounding stromal proteases to invade the normal tissue vasculature. Evidence of this is seen in glioblastoma patients treated with antiangiogenic therapies. Shortly after treatment these patients developed extensive tumor metastases. Therefore, future cancer therapies must incorporate the targeting of multiple hallmarks of cancer in order to prevent the adaptation of other capabilities. The application of this concept will result in further successes in cancer treatment.

Finally, in the near future, we will see the individualization of cancer therapy with the development of designer drugs, which target specific attributes of the cancer cell. Essential to the evolution of the hallmarks of cancer is genome instability, which generates the genetic mutations that permit acquisition of these capabilities. Therefore, the explosion of knowledge gained from the completion of the Human Genome Project has been critical in understanding the genetic influences on cancer. Comprehension of the genetic factors will be paramount for the clinician in identifying patients with hereditary syndromes who are at risk for cancer, and in selecting those who need further testing, counseling, and treatment. The future will see a point when the replacement of individual genetic defects will prevent the final stage of carcinogenesis. The impact of gene therapy will change how we manage patients with cancer.

As our understanding of the spectrum of what makes a cancer cell malignant becomes more sophisticated, an organizing principle is needed to determine the best treatment approach. Halsted's theory of a stepwise progression of cancer from primary disease to lymphatic metastasis to distant spread provided us with a model to predict the boundaries of this disease. He inspired future surgical oncologists to question the reason behind the ineffectiveness of surgery in curing advanced disease. Although Halsted may not have been correct in assuming that he could halt the spread of cancer through more radical surgery, his vision of cancer being a stepwise progression was accurate. Oncogenesis occurs through the sequential acquisition of genetic abnormalities that confer capabilities or hallmarks unique to a cancer cell. The organizing principle of the hallmarks of cancer provides a logical approach to understanding the molecular mechanisms of carcinogenesis and offers a framework for the development of future treatment algorithms.

REFERENCES

1. Osborne MP. William Stewart Halsted: his life and contributions to surgery. Lancet Oncol. 2007;8:256-65.
2. Ferlay J, Shin HR, Bray F, et al. GLOBOCAN 2008, Cancer Incidence and Mortality Worldwide: IARC Cancer Base No.10 [Internet]. Lyon, France: International Agency for Research on Cancer. 2010; Available from http://globocan.iarc.fr. [Accessed on Sep 17, 2014].
3. American Cancer Society. Global Cancer Facts & Figures 2nd Edition. Atlanta: American Cancer Society; 2011.
4. Fearon ER, Vogelstein B. A genetic model for colorectal tumorigenesis. Cell. 1990;61:759-67.
5. Lengauer C, Kinzler KW, Vogelstein B. DNA methylation and genetic instability in colorectal cancer cells. Proc Natl Acad Sci USA. 1997;94:2545-50.
6. Takanishi DM Jr, Angriman I, Yaremko ML, et al. Chromosome 17p allelic loss in colorectal carcinoma. Clinical significance. Arch Surg. 1995;130:585-9.
7. Hanahan D, Weinberg RA. Hallmarks of cancer: the next generation. Cell. 2011;144:646-74.
8. Lemmon MA, Schlessinger J. Cell signaling by receptor tyrosine kinases. Cell. 2010;141:1117-34.
9. Witsch E, Sela M, Yarden Y. Roles for growth factors in cancer progression. Physiology. 2010;25:85-101.
10. Cheng N, Chytil A, Shyr Y, et al. Transforming growth factor-beta signaling-deficient fibroblasts enhance hepatocyte growth factor signaling in mammary carcinoma cells to promote scattering and invasion. Mol Cancer Res. 2008;6:1521-33.
11. Bhowmick NA, Nelson EG, Moses HL. Stromal fibroblasts in cancer initiation and progression. Nature. 2004;432:332-7.
12. Davies MA, Samuels Y. Analysis of the genome to personalize therapy for melanoma. Oncogene. 2010;29:5545-55.
13. Jiang BH, Liu LZ. PI3K/PTEN signaling in angiogenesis and tumorigenesis. Adv Cancer Res. 2009;102:19-65.
14. Burkart DL, Sage J. Cellular mechanisms of tumour suppression by the retinoblastoma gene. Nat Rev Cancer. 2008;8:671-82.
15. Sherr CJ, McCormick F. The RB and p53 pathways in cancer. Cancer Cell. 2002;2:103-22.
16. Curto M, Cole BK, Lalemand K, et al. Contact-dependent inhibition of EGFR signaling by Nf2/Merlin. J Cell Biol. 2007;177:893-903.
17. Partanen EB, Nieminen AI, Klefstrom J. 3D view to tumor suppression: Lkb1, polarity and the arrest of oncogenic c-Myc. Cell Cycle. 2009;8:716-24.
18. Adams JM, Cory S. The Bcl-2 apoptotic switch in cancer development and therapy. Oncogene. 2007;26:1324-37.
19. Junttila MR, Evan GI. p53—a Jack of all trades but master of none. Nat Rev Cancer. 2009;9:821-9.

20. Hayflick L. Mortality and immortality at the cellular level: a review. Biochemistry. 1997;62:1180-90.
21. Blasco MA. Telomeres and human disease; ageing, cancer and beyond. Nat Rev Genet. 2005;6:611-22.
22. Greenberg RA, Chin L, Femino A, et al. Short dysfunctional telomeres impair tumorigenesis in the INK4aD cancer-prone mouse. Cell. 1999;97:515-25.
23. Hanahan D, Folkman J. Patterns and emerging mechanisms of the angiogenic switch during tumorigenesis. Cell. 1996;86:353-64.
24. Qian X, Wang TN, Rothman VL, et al. Thrombospondin-1 modulates angiogenesis in vitro by up-regulation of matrix metalloproteinase-9 in endothelial cells. Exp Cell Res. 1997;15:403-12.
25. Kazerounian S, Yee KO, Lawler J. Thrombospondins in cancer. Cell Mol Life Sci. 2008;65:700-12.
26. Baeriswyl V, Christofori G. The angiogenic switch in carcinogenesis. Semin Cancer Biol. 2009;19:329-37.
27. Qian BZ, Pollard JW. Macrophage diversity enhances tumor progression and metastasis. Cell. 2010;141:39-51.
28. Nyberg P, Xie L, Kalluri R. Endogenous inhibitors of angiogenesis. Cancer Res. 2005;65:3967-79.
29. Talmadge JE, Fidler IJ. AACR centennial series: the biology of cancer metastasis: historical perspective. Cancer Res. 2010;70:5649-69.
30. Cavallaro U, Christofori G. Cell adhesion and signaling by cadherins and Ig-CAMs in cancer. Nat Rev Cancer. 2004;4:118-32.
31. Micalizzi DS, Farabaugh SM, Ford HL. Epithelial-mesenchymal transition in cancer: parallels between normal development and tumor progression. J Mammary Gland Biol Neoplasia. 2010;15:117-34.
32. Hlubek F, Brabletz T, Budczies J, et al. Heterogeneous expression of Wnt/beta-catenin target genes within colorectal cancer. In J Cancer. 2007;121:1941-8.
33. Kessenbrock K, Plaks V, Werb Z. Matrix metalloproteinases: regulators of the tumor microenvironment. Cell. 2010; 141:52-67.
34. Kim MY, Oskarsson T, Acharyya S, et al. Tumor self-seeding by circulating cancer cells. Cell. 2009;139:1315-26.
35. Hanazaki K, Sodeyama H, Wakabayashi M, et al. Surgical treatment of gastric cancer detected by mass screening. Hepatogastroenterology. 1997;44:1126-32.
36. Balch CM, Urist MM, Karakousis CP, et al. Efficacy of 2 cm surgical margins for intermediate-thickness melanomas (1 to 4 mm). Results of a multi-institutional randomized surgical trial. Ann Surg. 1993;218:262-9.
37. Fisher B, Anderson S, Redmond CK, et al. Reanalysis and results after 12 years of follow-up in a randomized clinical trial comparing total mastectomy with lumpectomy with or without irradiation in the treatment of breast cancer. N Engl J Med. 1995;333:1456-61.
38. Van der Burg ME, van Lent M, Buyse M, et al. The effect of debulking surgery after induction chemotherapy on the prognosis in advanced epithelial ovarian cancer. N Engl J Med. 1995;332:629-34.
39. Scheele J, Stangl R, Allendorf-Hofmann A. Hepatic metastases from colorectal carcinoma: impact of surgical resection on the natural history. Br J Surg. 1990;77:1241-6.
40. Fernandez-Trigo V, Shamsa F, Sugarbaker PH. Repeat liver resections from colorectal metastasis. Repeat hepatic metastases registry. Surgery. 1995;117:296-304.
41. Chen H, Hardacre JM, Uzar A, et al. Isolated liver metastases from neuroendocrine tumors: does resection prolong survival? J Am Coli Surg. 1998;187:88-92.
42. van Geel AN, Pastorino U, Jauch KW, et al. Surgical treatment of lung metastases: The European Organization for Research and Treatment of Cancer Soft Tissue and Bone Sarcoma Group study of 255 patients. Cancer. 1996;77: 675-82.
43. Brennan MF, Hilaris B, Shiu MH, et al. Local recurrence in adult soft-tissue sarcoma. A randomized trial of brachytherapy. Arch Surg. 1987;122:1289-93.
44. Pisters PW, Harrison LB, Woodruff JM, et al. A prospective randomized trial of adjuvant brachytherapy in the management of low-grade soft tissue sarcomas of the extremity and superficial trunk. J Clin Oncol. 1994;12:1150-5.
45. Goldie JH, Coldman AJ. A mathematical model for relating the drug sensitivity of tumors to their spontaneous mutation rate. Cancer Treat Rep. 1979;63:1727-33.
46. Baguley BC. Multiple drug resistance mechanisms in cancer. Mol Biotechnol. 2010;46:308-16.
47. DeVita VT. Chemotherapy agents. In: Devita VT, Hellman S, Rosenberg SA (Eds.). Cancer. Principles and practice of oncology, 9th ed. Philadelphia: JB Lippincott; 2010: 360–460.
48. Rosenberg SA, Robbins PF, Restifo NP. Cancer immunotherapy. In: Devita VT, Hellman S, Rosenberg SA (Eds.). Cancer. Principles and practice of oncology, 9th ed. Philadelphia: JB Lippincott; 2010: 332-44.
49. Delyon J, Maio M, Lebbe C. The ipilimumab lesson in melanoma: achieving long-term survival. Semin Oncol. 2015;42:387-401.
50. Pazarentzos E, Mazarakis ND. Anticancer gene transfer for cancer gene therapy. Adv Exp Med Biol. 2014;818:255-80.

Additional references can be found in the online version of this book.

17

Geographic Factors Influencing Surgical Practice

Glenn W Geelhoed, Daniel S Vryhof

Key Points

- The epidemiology of surgical diseases varies in different parts of the world. Social, topographic, geographic, and climatic conditions are responsible for some of these differences.
- In developing countries, many patients present with very advanced surgical disease.
- In the tropics, trauma, infectious diseases, tumors, and disorders of the gastrointestinal tract make up the bulk of surgical practice.
- Ultrasonography has proved to be a valuable diagnostic tool in developing countries because of its wide applicability to many clinical problems and its ease of use.
- As a result of limited resources in developing countries, most operative procedures are carried out using regional or local anesthetic techniques if possible.
- Neglected tropical diseases are a major disease burden in developing countries and may require surgical participation in diagnosis and in the management of related complications.
- Inaccessibility to care remains the biggest challenge facing developing and low-income countries.

INTRODUCTION

Geography is the scientific description of the physical features of what is our planet, and, as it is ever changing—glaciers calve, mountains lift up, rivers widen—we human inhabitants and curious explorers try to learn about our home and how to adapt to the changing circumstances of our environment. One of the ways we have sought to adapt to our environment is to improve our fitness for inhabiting it by controlling illness and congenital or acquired defects in form and function. The most immediate of these healing arts is surgery. This chapter explores the intersection of geography and surgery.

Surgery and its evolving techniques constitute a profession that continues to keep pace not just with the demands of the privileged populations fortunate enough to live in the more bountiful geographic parts of earth, but to spread the benefits of the healing arts over all populations inhabiting it, even the parts we least understand. There may be many counterintuitive things to be learned by the exploration of the earth and its diverse ecologic niches and the people who inhabit each. We can easily misunderstand not only the geography of these foreign environments, but also the people who inhabit them, and the diseases that they experience.

They are, after all, not at all *like* us—they *are* us.

THE IMPORTANCE OF PLACE

Human health and illness "take place". Place influences many of the conditions that result in health or illness. Indeed, place-related health factors may be the primary determinants of outcome. Geography is one of the factors in the matrix of the environment in which human and other beings are embedded, especially at the "extremes". Geography may be the principal cofactor in climatic determinants, or central to other environmental factors such as air, water, sunlight, soils, and food sources. It may also be an ancillary factor in economic, political, and socioanthropologic features. The complex of these features may limit the ability of individuals and societies to adapt as they seek optimal living conditions and health-preserving environments. And the limits to adaptation are those that coerce an individual or society to seek help in healthcare for mitigation of illness or for health enhancement.

Medicine, surgery, and public health are among the disciplines that have evolved to assist in health preservation or restoration. Access to such services can be empowering for individuals and whole societies whose health and illness "take place" even if there may be greater mobility in modern populations. Access to care becomes critical when it is not easily available, and, curiously, geographers have been the ones to define for each continent "the pole of inaccessibility," the place to which one cannot gain access, or at least not easily. This geographic term will be extended for our purposes to represent inaccessibility that is the result of political, economic, and cultural barriers. "Inaccessibility" then becomes more widely distributed globally than at only the poles of geographic extremity.

When we consider surgical services, these "poles of inaccessibility" are areas where "place" has failed to support the population. They are often formed around the fulcrum of economics, such that a defined group of diseases have become known as "diseases of poverty". These diseases are more often found in the poles of inaccessibility and are characterized by late presentation of advanced disease that otherwise might be preventable in populations with better access to health and healthcare. When people generalize about "Third World" patterns of illness and the constrained resources with which they might be addressed, they often focus on those afflicted as the beginning and the end of the problem, neglecting the role of place in the disease.

The First-World advances in healthcare, so dramatically exhibited in immunizations and resulting in the near disappearance of some communicable diseases, or in the surgical repair or replacement of many organs, are as out of reach by contemporary developing world populations as completely as if they were embedded in medieval or even prehistoric times. Awareness of such truly life-saving care elsewhere leads to even greater frustration and desperation in those suffering curable illness.

MORTALITY AND MORBIDITY

Mortality is the loss of years from life. It is the result of lethal encounters with infectious or traumatic illnesses in younger ages or predominantly degenerative or malignant diseases in older life years. The familiar causes of loss of human life on planet earth are easy to extract from the bills of mortality, including DAMMM—Diarrhea dehydration, Acute respiratory infections, Malaria, Measles and Malnutrition (Fig. 17.1). DAMMM represents the top five causes of death, still, on this planet, and often occur to those under five, resulting in large losses of human potential. For many of these acute illnesses that cause or contribute to death, we seek cures, available if not always accessible.

Morbidity is the loss of life from years. The illnesses so described are not so much lethal as chronic and disabling, resulting in a large "burden" in prolonged life years in both individual and populations measured by "disability adjusted life years" (DALYs). In addition to the degenerative diseases of older populations in the developed world—cardiovascular, neurologic or malignant, and osteoarthritic—those in the developing world experience neglected tropical diseases.[1] This cumulative "burden of disease" decreases life potential. We seek to mitigate such disability limitations. For these diseases of high morbidity, we seek not so much to cure, the objective for diseases of high mortality, but to control, limiting the disability burden of disease.

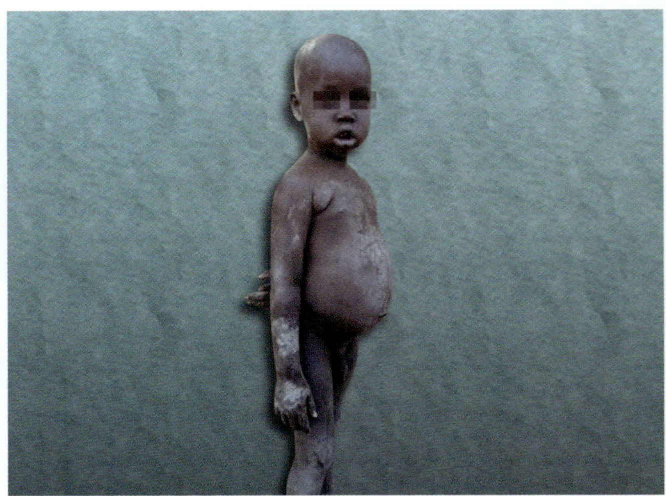

Fig. 17.1: Malnutrition in the form of Kwashiorkor is seen in this child. This condition is commonly seen with associated parasitic infections in these children.

But again, healthcare designed for the cure and control of mortality and morbidity works only if it is accessible. Healthcare practitioners must grapple across the multiple barriers of geography, economics, political, and socioanthropologic factors that limit uptake of medical and surgical care as much, and for some even more than, our biologically limited abilities in disease control for a great many illnesses and people affected by them. Such healthcare access requires more than a fundamental understanding of the pathophysiology of the illnesses. For many of the world's populations, there are more cultural barriers to access to care than there are medical ones.

POVERTY AND DISEASE

Poverty is perhaps the best predictor of a person's health. Poverty comes with a litany of contributing factors that predispose a person to disease. These include crowded living conditions, unsafe water, inadequate sanitation, disproportionate occupation as sex workers, malnutrition,

Table 17.1 The leading causes of death in rank order from 1 through 10 for the world population, high-income, and low-income countries.

Causes of Death	*World Population*	*Highest Income Countries*	*Lowest Income Countries*
Ischemic heart disease	1	1	5
Stroke	2	2	4
Chronic lung disease	3	5	
Lower respiratory tract infection	4	6	1
Pulmonary cancers	5	3	
HIV/AIDS	6		2
Diarrheal disease	7		3
Diabetes mellitus	8	8	
Road injury	9		
Hypertensive heart disease	10	9	
Colon/rectal cancers		7	
Dementia diseases		4	
Breast cancer		10	
Malaria			6
Preterm birth complications			7
Tuberculosis			8
Birth asphyxia and birth trauma			9
Protein/calorie malnutrition			10

Source: World Health Organization. http://www.who.int/mediacentre/factsheets/fs310/en/. Accessed January 5, 2014.

and poor access to healthcare. Poverty and disease go hand in hand because they synergize. Conditions of poverty predispose people to disease. Disease is costly and destroys productivity, bringing people into poverty and trapping them there. Table 17.1 illustrates the differences in causes of death among high-income and low-income countries of the world.

The poor carry a hugely disproportionate amount of treatable disease and they are the least prepared or equipped to fight it. The three biggest poverty-related diseases are acquired immunodeficiency syndrome (AIDS), malaria, and tuberculosis.[2] Developing countries account for 95%, 98%, and 90% of the prevalence of these diseases, respectively. Practitioners, no matter where they serve, must know the extent of poverty present in the population to be served, and they must be able to diagnose and treat the specific diseases that accompany poverty in the area.

For example, inadequate sanitation and poor water management bring parasitic diseases such as malaria, diarrheal diseases, and schistosomiasis. According to the United Nations Children's Fund (UNICEF), contaminated water causes the deaths of over 3,000 children every day. These types of parasitic diseases can increase the risk of human immunodeficiency virus (HIV) transmission as well.[3] Malnutrition does as well. It increases the rates of HIV infection, as well as other diseases, by interfering with the system of immune response. Malnutrition can also increase the rate of transmission of HIV from mother to child.[4] And further, high levels of pollution, in urban areas and in areas with high exposure to indoor cooking fires, put residents at high-risk for asthma and other respiratory infections.

Neglected tropical diseases (NTDs) are another huge source of morbidity in the developing world. They are called "neglected" because they receive a disproportionately small amount of funding for research and treatment than do other tropical diseases. Neglected tropical diseases include soil-transmitted helminthic parasites, African trypanosomiasis, Chagas disease, leishmaniasis, lymphatic filariasis, guinea worm, onchocerciasis, schistosomiasis, and trichomoniasis. These diseases are very common among the poor and in the developing world (Fig. 17.2), but they remain "neglected" because they do not result in large numbers of fatalities compared to, e.g. malaria, respiratory infections, or HIV.

In addition, it should be noted that NTDs and non-neglected diseases are often comorbid with each other.

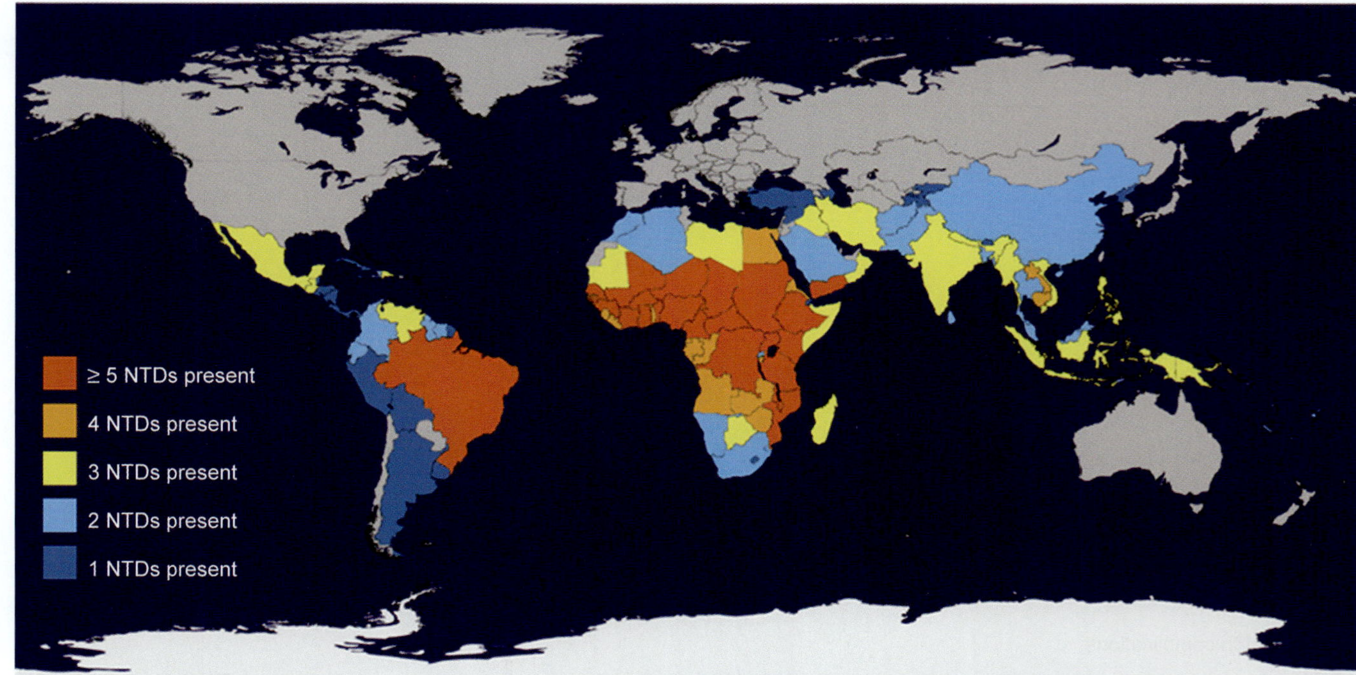

Fig. 17.2: The distribution of the neglected tropical diseases by countries of the world.
Source: http://www.cdc.gov/globalhealth/ntd/diseases/index.html.

One disease can make the other disease worse or, at least, increase the likelihood of infection. Neglected tropical diseases also account for a large amount of lost DALYs. Even if the disease is not deadly, it can rob people and populations of productivity, deprive children of healthy development and school attendance, and cause a great deal of suffering and misery.

POPULATION DYNAMICS

Populations in the Third World tend to be younger due to higher rates of mortality as well as higher birth rates. The higher death rates seen in developing countries can be caused by a number of factors ranging from disease prevalence and lack of available healthcare to political instability and conflict. The birth rate of a country is often inversely related to its level of wealth and development. Higher income countries, where the life expectancy is longer and the average level of formal education received is higher, are associated with lower birth rates. Low-income countries with low levels of education are associated with high birth rates. There are also cultural and religious factors that affect birth rates.

Being aware of the age distribution in the country is the first clue to understanding what types of surgical problems will most likely be encountered. Trends in population dynamics can be visualized through the use of population pyramids.[5] There are four main classes of pyramids that describe the stages by which countries generally develop. The first stage is very wide at the base, indicating a high birth rate, and curves up to a very sharp point, indicating a high death rate and a short life expectancy. Countries with this type of age distribution have a low median age. As the life expectancy of a country rises slightly and the death rate declines, the middle of the pyramid expands. This represents stage two in development. These countries have a higher percentage of people between the ages of 15 years and 65 years.

Stage three involves a continued increase in life expectancy and decline in death rate as well as a declining birth rate. In the course of population development, the pyramids may have lost their triangle shape as a greater percentage of the populace is surviving to old age, but the base is still the widest point indicating large numbers of people in their youth. This stage of development is marked by the end of population growth, "ZPG" or Zero Population Growth.

Stage four happens when the birth rate actually falls low enough that the population pyramid becomes top heavy. This is often combined with a low death rate and high life expectancy. These types of pyramids are being seen in some developed countries of Europe and in Japan.

Whereas a country in stage one or two may have problems with an abundance of children and uneducated youth to support, countries in stage four are beginning to struggle to support an aging population that is no longer in its productive years but still has a long time to live.

A country's development usually progresses from stage one to stage four, and health needs and societal issues can be predicted as a reflection of these demographics. Countries in stages one and two have high rates of morbidity and mortality from infectious disease. Their healthcare delivery infrastructure is probably underdeveloped and ineffective. They are supporting a large population of children with a moderate number of working age people. By stage four, the population has shifted to an older median age. The largest healthcare problems become related to old age and degenerative disease, and to paying to support a larger percentage of retirees in the population. In both stages one and four, a squeeze is being put on the working population.

POPULATION DISTRIBUTION

Besides a changing age distribution occurring with development, the geographic distribution within the developing world is changing. Relatively speaking, people in the developing world (and the entire world in general) are moving from rural areas into cities. This migration results in some interesting epidemiological changes. With a move from a rural setting to the city come changes in lifestyle and diet that are associated with an increase in obesity and all of its associated health problems as well as metabolic diseases like diabetes and cardiovascular disease.[6-8] Such diseases of affluence and lesser physical activity are not the only diseases seen to be on the increase. As urban populations quickly expand in the developing world, crowded unsanitary conditions outstrip the health and sanitation infrastructure in place, leaving the cities vulnerable to epidemics of communicable disease.

An interesting example is the spread of dengue fever in urban areas.[9] Unplanned urban expansion leads to water management and hygiene problems. *Aedes* mosquitoes that transmit dengue thrive in the dirty water of city slums. This can be contrasted with the *Anopheles* mosquitoes that transmit malaria that prefer clean water for breeding. What is being seen is that people growing up in urban areas do not develop as much resistance to malaria as their rural counterparts because the *Anopheles* mosquitoes do not breed well in the dirty city water. When such urban dwellers do get malaria, they are more susceptible to its deadly complications. High concentrations of both people and disease vectors result in high levels of dengue fever as well as rising levels of cerebral malaria.[10,11]

Places in urban Africa are unique in that they represent the intersection between first and third world health problems. As a surgeon, you may find yourself going straight from a strictly Third-World procedure like a sigmoid volvulus repair to a strictly First-World procedure like an appendectomy. In cities of the developing world, there is an overlapping intersection of wealth, poverty, and geography that allows horses and zebras to run together.

Urban Africa is not the only example of such an intersection. In the sense that illnesses and surgical care "take place," they do so because they are very much part of an interaction with people who identify themselves with characteristic homelands. These people are physiologically adapted to the environments in which they live—from Eskimos to desert nomads to rainforest pygmies to altitude-born Montagnards—and this may have some genetic basis in their metabolic adaptations over a long period of accommodation. Examples are easy to list, from agriculture to achieve food security, architecture to secure shelter, and even clothing and costuming for advantages in various climatic and social conditions.

There may be as many, and often more, anthropological reasons for the uptake of healthcare practices than for medical ones. The truth of this statement is ever more apparent in the management of large-scale public health problems like HIV/AIDS or the emergence of multidrug-resistant tuberculosis in marginalized societies. The critical role of culture in disease patterns and their control was apparent already to the father of anatomic pathology, Rudolph Virchow, when he wrote: "Whenever mass disease occurs, it is a result of disturbance of human culture".[12]

SEEING PEOPLE AND PLACE

The point of these descriptions of reality is that poverty creates a perfect storm of disease. Living in poverty often entails malnutrition, which increases susceptibility to parasites and vice versa. Parasites increase the risk of HIV infection. Human immunodeficiency virus increases the risk of tuberculosis infection (the number one cause of death by infectious disease worldwide). Any of these diseases can by itself push a person or a family into poverty. And the cycle continues, perhaps generation to generation.

Breaking the cycle in an effort to achieve health and productivity is made even more difficult by a tragic lack of available healthcare. People are forced to live with the burden of untreated disease far longer than their counterparts in the developed world. Their diseases and surgical needs are not cured and ever more productivity is lost. But this is the factor that doctors are best equipped to reverse. If effective and equitable healthcare can be available to the poorest people of the developing world, the seemingly never-ending cycle of poverty-disease-poverty can be broken.

It begins with seeing people and place. A good clinician treats patients. A great physician cares for people, individually and collectively, in their environmental, social, and political context. Many of those people are probably unlike the practitioner in many ways—language, other components of culture, nutrition, and religion. And often the patients and the problems they carry are "foreign" to the practitioner who learned the healing arts in a quite different environment.

It begins with sensitivity. Although practitioners have learned that a patient should never be identified by the disease (the crude reductionism of referring to the "gall bladder in bed five"), they may be less reluctant to identify a patient by socioeconomic status, often referring to them collectively as "the poor". Relying on and reinforcing the stereotypes of the "haves" and "have nots," the giver and the receiver, the caregiver and the care recipient, the rich West and the resource-poor Third World, limits the practitioner's ability to fully grasp the healing possibilities of the situation. Being labeled "poor" should not be the fundamental characteristic of any one because it limits options, ignores what the patient and the culture bring to the situation, and prevents practitioners from fully seeing both people and place.

DELIVERY OF SURGICAL CARE: IMPROVISATION AND INGENUITY

Often in developed-world care practices, futile care is expended on patient problems simply because it is available. Even though a cure is improbable or impossible, and the patient's morbidity symptoms are extended, perhaps worsened, the "technological imperative" prevails: "We have it, and you are going to get it, whether or not it works to resolve your problem." The developing world rarely has such an option. Practitioners who treat late-stage disease advanced at its first presentation must employ a method that is rare in the developed world: rationing care according to the greatest good for the largest number.

One of the benefits of working along with and learning from the local clinicians who have had a long history of coping with shortages in supplies and skills is learning their improvisations. They make care possible by applying principles, not necessarily along with all the plumbing of modern surgical care products and features. Those used to working in the limited healthcare environment of developing countries live by the aphorism "We have no money; therefore we must think". Improvisation and ingenuity rule the day.

Surgeons who practice in developing countries or remote areas must often deal with inadequate infrastructural support. Public infrastructure affects the availability and transport of supplies and equipment, the time required to reach medical services in emergency conditions and the transfer of information or advice.

Climatic conditions that involve extremes of temperature and humidity often influence surgical care and decision-making. The tropics display contrasting rainy and dry seasons with relatively high average temperatures all year, whereas circumpolar and high-altitude regions are bitterly cold for long periods. Attention must therefore be paid to providing acceptable working conditions and protecting supplies and equipment from temperature fluctuations, humidity, mold, dust, dryness, and insect infestation. Climate control (cooling and/or heating), refrigeration, dehumidifiers, equipment covers, and other strategies for dealing with adverse conditions are often lacking and must be instituted as finances allow.

The water supply may be unreliable. Cisterns, wells, and pumps from rivers or ponds serve as primary or supplementary water sources. In developing countries, Western-world back-up generators may serve either as the sole source of electricity or as a supplement to inconsistently available public power.

A steam autoclave (powered by electricity, gas, wood, coal, or kerosene) is preferred for sterilizing instrument sets. Since disposable gowns and drapes are prohibitively expensive, linens used for operations are sterilized using a steam autoclave. Soaking solutions sterilize scissors, blades, and needles without the dulling or rusting of steam autoclaving. Boiling of instruments may be suboptimal but is commonly the only method available for sterilization of instruments. If available, small ethylene oxide ampoule systems allow repeated sterilization of rubber and plastic tubes, catheters, drains, electrical cords, and instruments such as diathermy pencils and power drills.

Anesthetic options depend upon patient factors, the procedure, availability of drugs and trained personnel, and monitoring capability. Pulse oximeters are durable, relatively affordable, and enhance the safety of anesthesia by monitoring of oxygenation and prompt identification of problems. Surgeons in developing countries are quite comfortable using regional or spinal anesthetics for most elective operations below the diaphragm, the upper limbs, and even head-neck procedures. Use of general anesthesia necessitates additional equipment and personnel and so the surgeon is often forced to consider alternatives. Ketamine is a neuroleptic agent that provides dissociative anesthesia and is used extensively in developing countries because of its effectiveness, availability, relatively low cost, and presumed safety. Airway monitoring is mandatory.[13]

Emergency intra-abdominal procedures often present an anesthetic challenge for surgeons in developing countries. Spinal anesthetic can be used for emergency procedures below the diaphragm, but hypovolemia must be corrected before anesthesia to avoid hypotension. A general anesthetic with a controlled airway is always the preferred choice if appropriate equipment, agents, and personnel are available.

The availability of operating room equipment will influence what can be done in the operating room and will challenge the ingenuity of the surgeon for improvisation. Operating room essentials include a suitable operating room table, a lighting system, suction, and instruments. Nonessential but useful equipment are electrocautery, a fiberoptic headlight, and retractor systems.

With respect to operating room equipment and supplies, a standard principle that applies invariably is the reuse of everything considered single-use and disposable in the developed world. Due to product liability concerns and claims of patient safety, rather good equipment is consigned to disposal in the developed world, making a larger market for consumption. It is true that the reuse of such items as electrocautery units, suction tips and tubing, and various surgical instruments designed for one-clip firing and then disposal requires special care (thorough cleaning and sterilizing) to make it safe for repeat service. But this simply illustrates the inevitable difference between a labor-intensive economy and a materials-intensive economy. The medical features of such distinction are probably a more easily understandable and justifiable extension of these economic realities than many others.

As an example, in some areas of the world, rubber surgical gloves are too precious for a single use. They can be washed and hung out to dry and prepared for resterilization and reuse (Fig. 17.3). The hot steam of a pressure cooker neutralizes any possibility of transmission of communicable disease agents, but it can degrade some of the equipment so resterilized. When the items are torn or otherwise unfit for their usual intended purpose, the ingenious "entropy industries" of Third World economies (the "breaking down" of "found parts" to reduce them to some other less organized function they might still perform) takes over and the no longer usable surgical gloves may reappear as surgical drains, flutter valves, or patches in repair of surgical sheets or gowns. In remote missions, even laparotomy pads are wrung out, washed, and autoclaved to see a much prolonged service use than their First World fate of incineration.

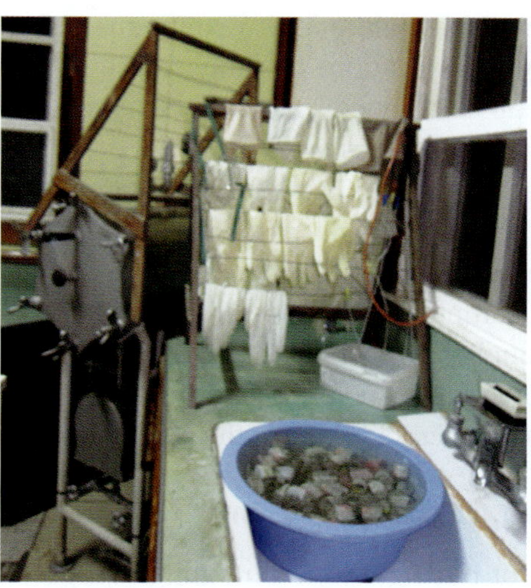

Fig. 17.3: Surgical gloves in North Luzon in the Philippines are hung out to dry after washing and then will be rewrapped and sterilized in a pressure cooker.

In addition to extending the usable life of various items to be recycled, there may be substitutions for others in short supply or which are prohibitively expensive at the point of purchase. Such substitutions might include the use of monofilament nylon fishing line of various pound-test strengths in substitute for nonabsorbable suture. Locally available honey is a good substitute for more expensive purpose-made topical antiseptic treatments, such as in burn dressings or in chronic ulcer debridement. Plastic food storage bags serve as inexpensive barrier protection gloves when handling dressings, examining wounds, and performing digital rectal examinations. For centuries, surgeons in remote parts of the world have used worn sheets and cloth for bandages, and towels as laparotomy pads. "Re-rod" of concrete re-enforcement supplies can be used as external framework for orthopedic traction suspension. Used bags or bottles of intravenous fluids can be reconstituted with reverse osmosis water and the desired quantities of salts and sugars mixed in. Ultraviolet light irradiation can sterilize the solutions in the translucent containers, particularly in the high-intensity radiation of high-altitude environments. Improvisation, ingenuity, organization, frugality, reuse of "disposable" equipment and encouraging local manufacture can improve the supply system.

Some of the political/cultural aspects of current medical practice actually assist in making available cast-off or redundant supplies for reuse in remote medical mission settings. Outdated or discarded but unused sterile supplies from First World health economies can be collected and can supply the developing world when hospitals and clinicians make the scavenging effort.

Imaging, Endoscopy, and Laparoscopy

The cost of buying and maintaining equipment, as well as the need for well-trained personnel, has limited access to sophisticated radiologic equipment in most developing countries to a few university centers. However, ultrasonography has been widely used because of its relatively low cost and the relative ease for training personnel in its use. It is particularly helpful in obstetrics and general surgery. Ultrasonography is most useful in the diagnosis of ascites, abdominal masses, and the differentiation of cystic and solid masses.

Flexible endoscopy is being used with increasing frequency, even in more remote geographic areas. Initial cost and maintenance limit the universal availability of the valuable diagnostic tool.

In most developing countries, there has been increased use of laparoscopy as a diagnostic tool, particularly in the management of patients who have acute abdominal pain.[14] Often this procedure is carried out in these regions using nondisposable equipment and locally crafted dissectors. Creative surgeons in India have been able to decrease the instrument cost to US$1.20 per patient.[15] Worldwide, experience suggests that laparoscopy is especially helpful in the management of patients who have gynecologic disorders. This technology will undoubtedly gain broader acceptance in developing countries when issues such as equipment cost, maintenance and repair charges, and training of the surgical team become standardized.[16]

Personnel

The surgeon in a remote or developing region has the enormous responsibility not only to provide care for his or her patients, but also to identify appropriate individuals to participate in the healthcare delivery team. Physicians, nurses, and technicians often need to be recruited, educated, trained in the nuances of the locale and motivated to practice quality healthcare in a less than ideal setting. These same challenges obviously apply to anesthesiology personnel: a striking example exists in Malawi, where there is one physician anesthesiologist for the entire nation.

In most tropical hospitals, the surgeon often bears the burden of creating the appropriate environment among these individuals of varied training so that each member of the team feels that he or she plays a vital role in providing the very best surgical care. Key in developing a viable surgical service is a small group identity that emphasizes each member's responsibility, value, and importance.

Laboratory Services

Most clinical laboratories in developing countries have limited resources and abilities, so physicians need to monitor laboratory functions carefully. Although most laboratories now have the ability to screen for HIV, most do not have the ability to carry out what most surgeons in developed countries would consider as routine analyses such as electrolytes, liver function tests, coagulation studies, blood cultures, and arterial blood gases. Despite the prevalence of hepatitis, screening tests are not uniformly available.

Although most surgeons in developed countries take the information gleaned from intraoperative frozen sections for granted, this technology is generally not available in most developing countries. Unless specimens are processed locally, the turnaround time for histopathologic reports can be measured in months in many regions, and so the surgeon has to make important decisions without the benefit of this information.

Transfusions in the tropics often involve on-the-spot donor recruitment and immediate transfusion and as such the transfusion service typically functions as a blood typing and collection station. The blood bank is heavily used by obstetrics units as a result of multiparity, short intervals between parturition, poor nutrition, and peripartum hemorrhage. Motor vehicle trauma victims are another major user. Children may have chronic or acute anemia of nutritional, hemolytic, hemoglobinopathic, or unknown origin and often require transfusion. Local customs and beliefs can inhibit blood donation, and to establish and maintain a blood bank in such areas is difficult and often impossible. "Walking" blood banks, in which volunteers in an institution, organization, or community are typed, can provide an emergency supply.

There are few alternatives since hemoglobin substitutes and volume expanders other than crystalloid solutions are not usually available. Autotransfusion has been promoted, but is infrequently practiced in most tropical medical centers. Patients who have a ruptured ectopic pregnancy, vascular injuries, and splenic or hepatic injuries without bowel contamination are the most appropriate candidates for simultaneous autotransfusion. Modern autotransfusion systems are impractical because of the initial expense, high cost of disposable components, and infrequency of use with attendant unfamiliarity. Galley pot collection and gauze sieving of blood in the peritoneal cavity with retransfusion have been performed in developing world hospitals with varying results, enthusiasm, and recommendations.

For some elective procedures in which there is an anticipated transfusion requirement, patients can donate one unit of blood at weekly intervals for 2 or 3 weeks before their operation and take hematinics, maintain a well-balanced diet in the interim and then receive their own banked blood at the time of operation. This delayed autotransfusion has only limited application, because most transfusion requirements occur in emergencies or in debilitated patients.

DELIVERY OF SURGICAL CARE: DIAGNOSIS AND TREATMENT

It is important to note the differences in presentation of morbidity in the Third World. In general, diseases and surgical cases are going to present at a much later stage. Patients who have been living with ever-present disease their whole lives are less likely, or are unable, to seek care until the situation becomes truly dire. This is a wide-ranging problem for multiple reasons. In the case of many diseases, e.g. typhoid or kala-azar, the window for therapeutic intervention may have passed. The same goes for malignancies that, if diagnosed earlier, could have been better treated. Sophisticated evaluation of disease is usually scarce in a developing world setting, but when the disease has progressed longer, it often presents with more distinctive symptoms.

General Surgery

Developing countries have many of the same surgical problems that are encountered in Western Europe and the United States. However, delay in seeking care results in the surgical condition being far more advanced than would ordinarily be encountered. Groin hernias are commonly quite enormous and are a major challenge (Fig. 17.4). The

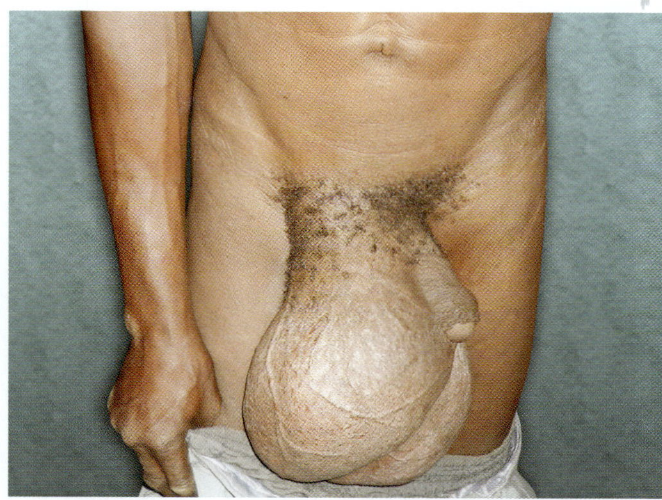

Fig. 17.4: A large and neglected hernia case from Ghana where the "lost domain" of bowel contents requires peritoneal air insufflation before repair can be undertaken.

"loss of domain" from chronic large groin hernias pose problems of increased abdominal pressure and limited diaphragmatic excursion, and may require a strategy of pneumoperitoneum preoperatively to permit surgical reduction. Incarceration and strangulation of groin hernias is common and requires surgical repair.

A procedure that is common in certain parts of the developing world is the removal of goiters. Goiters are common due to the dietary deficiency of iodine. Iodine replacement therapy may be effective. Large goiters will not resolve with iodine replacement therapy. In these cases, the patient will have trouble breathing or swallowing and removal of the goiter may be necessary (Fig. 17.5).

Cutaneous infections and soft tissue abscesses are frequent in developing countries. Protein-calorie malnutrition and associated diseases (e.g. HIV infection) are associated with the increased frequency and severity of these infections. *Staphylococcus aureus* is a common pathogen for abscesses of the skin, subcutaneous tissue, pyomyositis, osteomyelitis, and pyarthrosis. Multiple abscesses are common. These infections commonly involve the hands and feet, with delays in treatment often resulting in deformities and loss of function. Treatment remains complete surgical drainage and debridement. Antibiotics are in short supply and are principally used for short courses to limit consequences of bacteremia.

Abdominal problems that require operative intervention can be classified as infectious, congenital, vascular, inflammatory, or neoplastic. Changing demographics and patterns of day-to-day life, including dietary changes, may

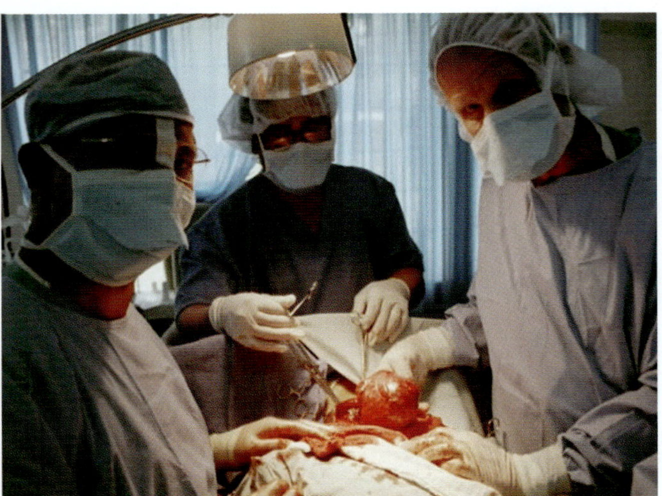

Fig. 17.5: Thyroidectomy is a frequent operation for relief of airway compressing goiter in the iodine deficiency areas of Mindanao (Philippines).

be responsible for an evolving pattern of disease in the tropics that require abdominal procedures. For reasons that are not clear, appendicitis is more prevalent than it was 20 years ago. Appendiceal perforation, strangulated bowel (caused by intestinal obstruction, hernia, volvulus), and perforation of duodenal ulcers are leading causes of secondary bacterial peritonitis and carry a high mortality rate from delays in seeking medical care. *Helicobacter pylori* infection is a common cause of peptic ulcers and makes perforated peptic ulcers a continued indication for abdominal operation.

Sigmoid volvulus is reported as a frequent cause of intestinal obstruction in areas of Africa. Typical symptoms of intestinal obstruction are observed and delays in seeking care yield a high rate of perforation or strangulation. Endoscopic management can be attempted, but operation may be required if there is any suspicion of strangulated or ischemic bowel or if the nonoperative approach is unsuccessful. Resection at laparotomy usually requires colostomy. Not infrequently a loop of small bowel is caught up in a twist of the sigmoid colon mesentery, producing a concomitant closed loop obstruction and strangulation of the small bowel, the so-called compound volvulus or ileosigmoid knotting. An additional small bowel resection and reanastomosis must be performed in this case.

Unusual infectious causes for laparotomy are encountered. Typhoid perforation of the ileum is a particularly challenging problem. Intestinal perforations due to cytomegalovirus are seen in patients with advanced HIV disease. Amebic liver abscesses sometime rupture into the peritoneal cavity or into the pleural space, and necrotizing amebic colitis can mimic ischemic colitis or a toxic megacolon.[17]

Benign biliary tract issues are less common in developing countries. Infrequent in Africa, cholelithiasis is ubiquitous in parts of South America and biliary stone diseases, including hepatolithiasis, is of enormous clinical importance throughout Asia. Both calculous and acalculous cholecystitis appear to be increasing in the tropics and in desert countries. Tropical climates may have cholangitis and an association of cholangiocarcinoma with several orally ingested parasites, including *Ascaris lumbricoides*, *Clonorchis sinensis*, and *Opisthorchis* sp. Ultrasound availability has increased diagnostic accuracy of biliary tract disease.[18]

Vascular procedures tend to be performed for trauma and rarely for atherosclerosis. The increased use of tobacco and the potential for an increased life expectancy with better preventive strategies in developing countries will likely lead to increased occlusive peripheral vascular disease in the future.

Trauma

Trauma operations are also much needed in the developing world. There is a high incidence of traffic-accident-related injuries as well as burns. Motor vehicle accidents (MVAs) are common in overcrowded cities where traffic laws are nonexistent or unenforced. The situation is worse when large numbers of pedestrians, bicyclists, and even livestock compete for use of narrow, unmaintained roads. Also, most cooking in the developing world is done over fires, often made using charcoal or paraffin-based burners. Cooking accidents and house fires are not uncommon. Residual contractures and hypertrophic scarring are often disabling in survivors of acute burns.

Something that should be noted about trauma surgery in the developing world is that in many places the infrastructure is not in place to get patients to the hospital in time for the necessary intervention (Fig. 17.6). With MVAs, burns, or violent injuries like gunshot or machete wounds, there may be a high volume of cases that result in over 50% of available hospital beds being occupied by trauma patients. In addition to the high morbidity and mortality rates associated with blunt and penetrating trauma, a patient's disability and the impact on the family or community unit can be overwhelming. A formidable challenge for the delivery of trauma care in the Third World is the development of prehospital management

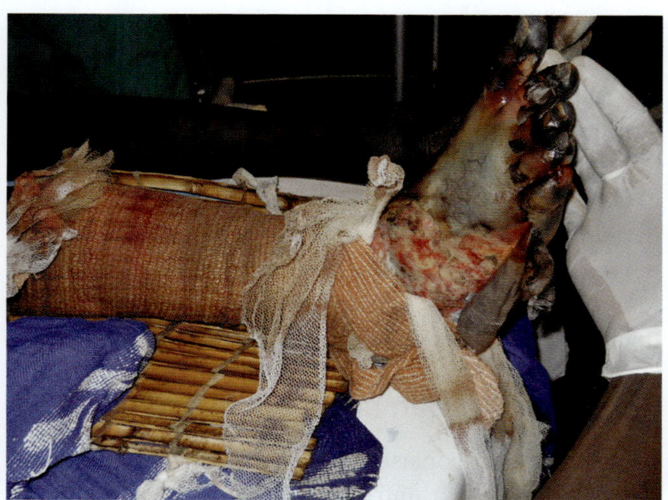

Fig. 17.6: Gangrene of the lower extremity resulted after 6 weeks of traditional splinting for an open fracture following a motor bike accident in Bor, South Sudan.

and transportation, and training of hospital personnel in the basics of trauma resuscitation and management.

Surgeons practicing in the tropics and other developing countries have the challenge of managing patients with bites from wild animals, snakes, spiders, scorpions, insects, and other humans. The problems and sequelae of human bites are often underappreciated and may be mismanaged by the uninitiated and inexperienced surgeon. Wounds from bites require local cleansing and debridement. All should be left open for secondary wound closure. Many bite wounds do not present until after infection is present. Antibiotics to cover human mouth anaerobes (penicillin) or *Pasteurella* sp. (ampicillin) for dog/cat bites may be necessary if infection occurs.

Poisonous snake bites vary in incidence and type by topography and location. The treating physician must consider both the local and systemic manifestations of a poisonous snake bite. Antivenom treatment is essential and can be life-saving. A concern in extremity snake bites is compartment syndrome, which may require incision and fasciotomy. Scorpion stings and spider bites present problems of severe local lesions (scorpion) or ulcers with ischemic necrosis (brown recluse spiders). Systemic hypersensitivity reactions with bronchospasm and hypotension (bees and wasps) or generalized muscle spasms (black widow spiders) are also issues.

Oncology

While communicable diseases have had a predominant role in deaths in Third World and low-income countries, cancers have been identified with increasing frequency. Increased tobacco use, environmental and occupational exposures to carcinogens, and, interestingly, diet and obesity have emerged as variables that are increasing the incidence of cancers in the developing world.[19] Infection-associated cancers including hepatocellular carcinoma from Hepatitis B and C, *Helicobacter* infections resulting in gastric carcinoma, and human papillomavirus infections resulting in cervical carcinoma are important causes in these countries. Burkitt's lymphoma is probably the best recognized infectious cancer in its association with the EB virus of the human herpes viruses. An increased incidence of Kaposi's sarcoma is being seen in association with HIV infections. Cancers in the Third World are commonly far advanced compared to those seen in high-income countries. As has been identified, only 5% of global cancer funding will be received by the 70% of cancer cases in the developing world.[20] Thus, the challenge for the surgeon in these countries will be to provide oncology care within the limits of available funding and to prioritize cancer care with the many other emergent surgical needs that are encountered.

Obstetrics and Gynecology

The tropical obstetrician routinely faces problems related to a lack of antenatal care, obstructed labor, eclampsia, peripartum hemorrhage, ruptured ectopic gestation, and infertility. Most deliveries are performed in the patient's home with traditional birth attendants or older women supervising the delivery. Young age at first pregnancy, dietary deficiencies, and small stature increase the incidence of cephalopelvic disproportion. Suboptimal predelivery care combined with prolonged and difficult labor and delivery lead to an increased chance of infection, fetal, and maternal deaths. Prolonged, difficult labor and delivery can also produce ischemia of the genital canal and adjacent tissues with eventual pressure necrosis and creation of an obstetric fistula. These fistulas between the bladder or rectum and the vagina, if unrepaired, leave a painful condition that is hygienically unacceptable secondary to infection and urinary/rectal incontinence. Affected women are often ostracized from families and communities as unclean. This problem is common in some developing countries because of a tendency for young, often malnourished and underdeveloped girls to marry or become pregnant.[21] The majority of vesico- and rectovaginal fistulas can be repaired through a vaginal approach using local tissues.

Orthopedics

Musculoskeletal problems are ubiquitous in Third World countries. Trauma is a leading cause for acute orthopedic services, but neglected fractures also become a source of disability and disfigurement that need scarce management skills (*see* Fig. 17.6). Orthopedic trauma and related osteomyelitis patients occupy a large number of hospital beds in a typical tropical surgical ward. Congenital (e.g. talipes equinovarus) and developmental conditions (e.g. rickets) are common. Bacterial (e.g. osteomyelitis/pyarthrosis), and viral infections (poliomyelitis) result in morbidity and functional impairment. African populations have acute bone, chest, and abdominal crises, and avascular necrosis of the hip is sickle cell disease. Sustained and strenuous labor activities result in joint degenerative diseases.

Urology

Urologic problems may be congenital, infectious, obstructive, or neoplastic. Undescended testes, hypospadias, posterior urethral valves, and torsion of the testis are congenital anatomic problems. The diagnosis of torsion of the testis in a male who has a tender scrotum and testis can be excluded only by direct observation at surgery. The incidence of nephroureterolithiasis is relatively uncommon among sub-Saharan Africans, but stone-related disorders are frequent in the Sudan and Yemen. Since endoscopic and ultrasonic techniques are often not available in the tropics, open operation is often the only option.

Lower tract obstruction in older men generally results from benign prostatic hypertrophy, prostatic carcinoma, or urethral stricture, secondary to previous gonococcal urethritis. Benign prostatic hypertrophy is treated by prostatectomy, usually open rather than transurethral. Urethral stricture can be managed by repeated bougienage, suprapubic tube cystostomy, direct vision internal urethrotomy, or urethroplasty.

Patients in the tropics who have genitourinary malignancies often present with advanced disease. The more subtle signs of hematuria or masses are often ignored until urinary function is markedly compromised or a mass grows to such a size that it becomes noticeable by all. Cancers of the kidneys, bladder, prostate, and penis (squamous cell carcinoma) are generally seen at an advanced nonoperative stage. Infestation by *Schistosoma haematobium* may produce granulomas of the ureters and bladder and result in bleeding, obstructive uropathy, pyelonephritis, or carcinoma of the bladder.

Fournier's gangrene is not infrequent as a polymicrobial disease of the male genitalia. The onset is sudden and painful, often in the dependent scrotum, and is accompanied by fever and toxemia. There is a partial or full-thickness slough of the scrotum that may progress to exposure of the testes before healthcare is sought. In addition to appropriate antimicrobial therapy with penicillin, aggressive debridement is usually essential. Management may occasionally include the need for split-thickness skin grafts or even rotation of flaps.

Ear, Nose, Throat, and Dental Surgery

Foreign bodies, neoplasms, infections, allergic conditions, maxillofacial trauma, and congenital anomalies are all seen in a tropical surgical practice. Tuberculous cervical adenitis, Ludwig's angina, dental abscesses, and otitis media with or without mastoiditis are common infections of the head and neck. Tracheostomy is often necessary for croup or laryngotracheobronchitis as a complication of measles. Cancrum oris (or noma) is a polymicrobial infection of mouth that is quite destructive and leads to oronasocutaneous fistulas and ankylosis of the temporomandibular joint. Debridement of nonviable tissue, penicillin and metronidazole, and nutritional support are considered the treatment for cancrum oris. Complex orofacial deformities are common results.

Plastic Surgery

One of the more challenging aspects of surgical practice in the tropics relates to management of large infected and neglected wounds. This problem is intensified by the lack of adequate equipment and supplies. Keloid and hypertrophic scars, which are characteristic of patients of African descent, represent both functional and cosmetic problems. In Third World societies where manual labor plays a major role, burns and other injuries require prompt treatment to avoid fibrosis and contractures.

Cleft lip with or without a palatal defect is a common congenital abnormality (Fig. 17.7). There are marked geographical differences in the incidence of cleft lip/palate, which occurs at a high frequency in the Philippines and a low frequency in sub-Saharan Africa. Scarce resources and limited expertise often prevent timely intervention.

Neurosurgery

Optimal care of patients who have neurosurgical disorders, whether traumatic, infectious, vascular, congenital, or neoplastic, requires imaging technologies. The limited availability of CT and MRI results in neurosurgery care being limited to a relatively small number of centers. Neurosurgical practice in the tropics focuses largely on the management of head trauma. Without imaging technology, the decision to intervene operatively for a head injury victim is often based on clinical suspicion of an epidural or subdural hematoma. These patients have a "diagnostic" cranial exploration through burr holes, with drainage if an epidural or subdural hematoma is found. Patients who have open depressed skull fractures require operative management for debridement, hemostasis, elevation of the depressed fragments, and closure and coverage of the dura mater.

Traumatic injury to the spine is particularly devastating because of both the acute and chronic care issues associated with these injuries. Motor vehicle accidents are a common cause. Acute phase management is challenging to avoid pulmonary, genitourinary, and septic complications. Spinal cord injury rehabilitation programs are almost nonexistent in developing countries, and spinal cord injuries pose genuine problems to avoid longer-term problems of urinary or decubitus ulcer-related sepsis.

Tuberculous spondylitis (Pott's disease) is not an uncommon cause of paralysis. If the patient presents acutely within a few days of onset of paralysis or if the patient deteriorates neurologically while on antituberculous therapy, exploration and drainage of the paraspinous abscess is warranted.

Pediatric Surgery

The problems of congenital anomalies in newborns are compounded by the stigma associated with imperforate anus, abdominal wall defects, and neural tube defects. Parents may avoid healthcare or operation because of a lack of appreciation that such conditions can be satisfactorily managed. Hirschsprung's disease, urinary tract abnormalities, and pediatric tumors are often detected after the child has been named and officially recognized as a family or clan member, so surgical help is usually sought.

Intussusception is the leading cause of intestinal obstruction in children aged between 3 months and 2 years. Hydrostatic reduction is not routinely used because of the uncertainty of adequate reduction and the scarcity of fluoroscopic units. Delayed operative reduction is the usual management and a nonviable intussusception results in increased morbidity and deaths.

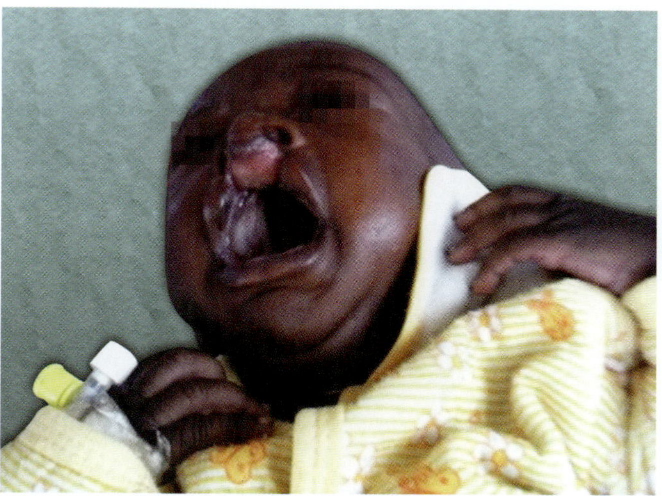

Fig. 17.7: Cleft lip and palate are often not seen until very advanced age because of the absence of facilities or surgeons to repair them.

Cardiothoracic Surgery

Cardiac operations, whether for valvular disorders or atherosclerotic heart disease, require personnel and equipment that may only exist within a limited number of centers within an entire country. Rheumatic fever with resultant valvular problems, congestive failure, congenital heart diseases, endomyocardial fibrosis and other cardiomyopathies (e.g. Chagas' heart disease) and the pericardial problems of constriction (tuberculosis) and effusion (pyopericardium) are the major problems that face the cardiologist and cardiac surgeon. Although uncommon in Africa, the incidence of coronary artery disease, conduction abnormalities, and aneurysm formation is increasing in the Pacific with Westernization and increased prevalent tobacco use.

The noncardiac thoracic surgeon deals primarily with tuberculosis, thoracic empyema (especially after measles), hemoptysis, bronchiectasis and lung abscess. Lung cancer is expected to increase as smoking increases.

Ophthalmology

Of all preventable blindness worldwide, 80% occurs in patients who live in developing countries. In these regions, blindness often results from trauma, trachoma, onchocerciasis, corneal scarring, xerophthalmia (dryness resulting from vitamin A deficiency), and cataracts. Unusual eye-associated infections are encountered (Fig. 17.8). Cataracts are a leading cause of blinding and the number is steadily increasing. Access to ophthalmologists is severely limited and eye treatment centers are as infrequent as cardiac

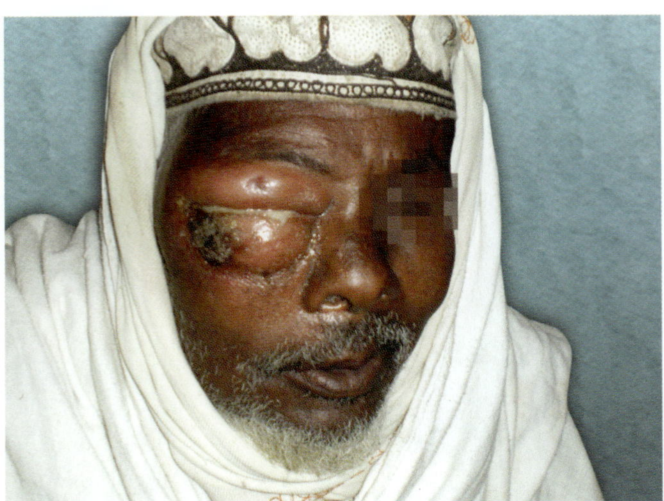

Fig. 17.8: A case of periorbital anthrax in a goat herder in Ethiopia.

centers. Thus, most people who have treatable eye diseases do not see an ophthalmic surgeon.

Special Conditions: Tropical Infectious Diseases

Endemic infectious diseases constitute a small portion of the clinical workload for the surgeon in tropical areas. In tropical areas unique infections are encountered, or infections known to Western world surgeons may be encountered with a greater clinical prevalence. The surgeon working in tropical areas should be familiar with these diseases.

Bacterial Infections

Typhoid fever is caused by ingestion of the *Salmonella enterica subspecies enterica*. Hemorrhage from and perforation of ileal ulcers are potentially fatal complications of typhoid fever. Perforation that results in secondary bacterial peritonitis may occur after prolonged periods of fever, catabolism, undernutrition, and immunosuppression.

Management requires volume resuscitation, initiation of diuresis, antibiotics followed by operative intervention, and source control of the perforation. Ileal ulcers are typically antimesenteric in position and usually within 2 feet (0.6 m) of the ileocecal valve. Multiple perforations require segmental resection with retention of the ileocecal valve if possible. Mortality rates may approach 30% in many developing countries. Typhoid outbreaks indicate fecal-oral transmission and require efforts at education for disease prevention.

Tetanus: Even with government-sponsored modern immunization programs, many people in the tropics remain unprotected from tetanus (*Clostridium tetani*). Neonatal tetanus remains a lethal and common problem in many areas. Antenatal immunization for mothers along with education about umbilical cord care, circumcision, and facial markings can alleviate these unnecessary neonatal deaths. Without previous immunization and appropriate wound care, even trivial injuries are potentially lethal.

Initial treatment for all patients who have tetanus includes thorough wound debridement. A large and neglected limb wound may require amputation, and tetanus secondary to a septic abortion may necessitate a hysterectomy. Active and passive immunization should accompany debridement as the initial treatment for the unimmunized patient. In the absence of intensive care units and ventilators, the management choices for patients who have severe tetanus include sedation without control of the airway; sedation with control of the airway (oro- or nasotracheal tube, tracheostomy) without paralysis; and sedation with control of the airway, paralysis, and manual or mechanical ventilation.

For each option, competent individual nursing care for monitoring, suctioning, and turning the patient is essential. Most deaths from tetanus result from asphyxia, aspiration, or pneumonia. A tube gastrostomy is often used to provide for the increased nutritional needs of these patients.

Leprosy (Hansen's disease): This is a chronic infection caused by *Mycobacterium leprae*. Patients who have leprosy may require operative intervention to prevent or treat complications of the feet, hands, and eyes. Ulcers of the feet with or without accompanying osteomyelitis of the underlying bones demand treatment with bed rest, debridement, antibiotics, adequate footwear, and a change of lifestyle, with rest intervals off the feet and daily foot care and surveillance. Tendon transfers can improve the pinch or intrinsic muscle function of a hand or counter a drop-foot gait, and thereby enhance limb function and rehabilitation. Occasionally a transtibial amputation is necessary for ulcers.

The eyes of patients with Hansen's disease deserve special attention. With facial nerve damage, the orbicularis oculi muscles become paretic and the lids do not close completely (lagophthalmos), which leads to corneal exposure, desiccation, and irritation. An insensitive cornea can become irreversibly damaged. Timely tarsorrhaphy or a temporalis muscle transplant procedure can preserve vision.

Tuberculosis: Infection with *Mycobacterium tuberculosis* has demonstrated some decline in worldwide incidence, but it remains a significant public health issue in tropical

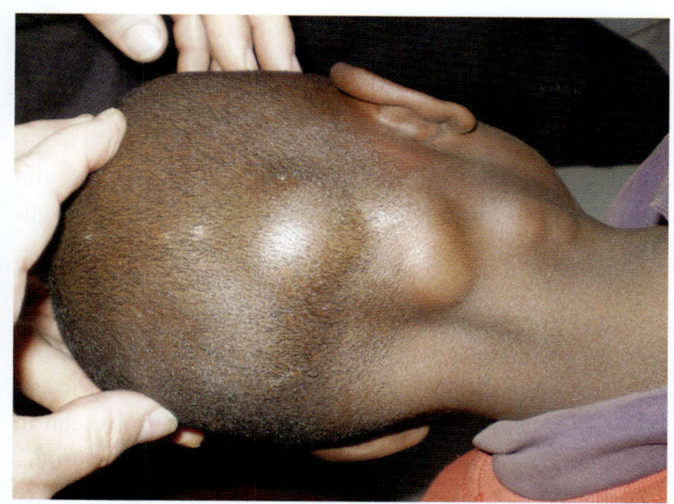

Fig. 17.9: Posterior cervical and occipital lymph nodes are illustrated in a patient with extrapulmonary tuberculosis. The child was treated with the multidrug directly observed therapy system.

climates and in developing countries.[22] Tuberculosis is associated with drug resistance, the HIV epidemic, outmoded methods of treatment, and noncompliance with therapy. Sub-Saharan Africa and Southeast Asia are the areas with the highest prevalence and estimated annual risk for tuberculosis.

This ubiquitous disease with protean manifestations remains a scourge among economically deprived, overcrowded, and underfed populations. Pulmonary tuberculosis with cavities, empyema, and destroyed lung remains the primary presentation of *M. tuberculosis* infection. Tuberculous adenitis, abdominal and hepatic tuberculosis, Pott's disease with or without neurologic deficit, urinary tuberculosis, and tuberculous arthritis are important differential diagnoses for the surgeon to consider for patients who have failure to thrive, masses or fever (Fig. 17.9). Gastrointestinal tuberculosis and tuberculous peritonitis must be considered along with neoplasms in patients who have weight loss, ascites, and an abdominal mass. Even tuberculosis of the skin and breast may masquerade as carcinoma. A renewed challenge in the current era of HIV infection and drug-resistant organism is Pott's disease.

A diagnosis of pulmonary tuberculosis depends upon the symptoms, radiologic signs, and positive organism identification. Smears for acid-fast organisms are the bacteriologic standard. Culture capability for diagnosis, subgrouping, and drug sensitivity testing is not usually available.

Multiple drug chemotherapy is the primary treatment and treatment is focused upon whether the patient has latent or active disease.[23] The surgeon obtains material for diagnosis (e.g. by bronchoscopy, lymph node biopsy) and treats complications. Tube thoracostomy is used to treat pneumothorax, empyema, and pyopneumothorax. Elective resections are used for bronchostenosis, bronchiectasis, destroyed lung, giant emphysematous bullae, resistant organisms, and recalcitrant patients who have sputum-positive, localized open cavities. Pericardiectomy may be required for patients who have constrictive pericarditis. Emergency thoracotomy with lobectomy or pneumonectomy is required for cases of life-threatening hemoptysis, a not unusual sequel of smoldering inflammation. The Eloesser flap permits open drainage of a residual pleural space without the need of a chest tube chronically.

Buruli ulcers are a skin and soft tissue infection from *Mycobacterium ulcerans*, a slow-growing mycobacterium that produces a toxin (mycolactone) responsible for its clinical manifestations. These ulcers are seen across Africa, Southeast Asia, and Australia. The toxin causes necrosis of the dermis, subcutaneous fat, and deep fascia, and creates a painless ulcer without adenopathy. Smears of curettings of the undermined edges of the ulcer reveal acid-fast bacilli. Treatment consists of debridement, local temperature elevation (as with a goose-neck lamp), and split-thickness skin grafting. Rifampin (rifampicin) may promote healing of preulcerative lesions, but is not effective for established lesions.[24]

Viruses

Viral infections in tropical and Third World countries are numerous. Only a limited number of them can be realistically discussed within this chapter and only those of particular surgical significance will be addressed.

Chronic hepatitis infection: Hepatitis B virus (HBV) and hepatitis C virus (HCV) are major issues as blood-borne pathogens (*see* Chapter 7, "Infection, Inflammation, and Antibiotics"). They are significant in Third World and tropical environments because of high prevalence rates. The end result of chronic infection commonly is hepatic cirrhosis and hepatocellular carcinoma. The highest rates of HBV are in sub-Saharan Africa with 5–10% of the adult population having chronic infection.[25] Hepatocellular carcinoma is common but resources to care for these patients are limited. Efforts are continuing to vaccinate all newborns for HBV.

Hepatitis C virus is also common in North Africa and Central/East Asia. Globally, over 130 million people have chronic HCV infection.[26] A significant number of chronic infections will lead to hepatic cirrhosis and hepatocellular carcinoma. Access to diagnosis and effective treatment represents a major problem in developing countries. No vaccine for HCV is available.

Human immunodeficiency infection (*see* Chapter 7, "Infection, Inflammation, and Antibiotics") has been an international disease that is most prevalent in sub-Saharan Africa.[27] The advanced stage of HIV infection (AIDS) results in severe immunosuppression with patients developing opportunistic infections or neoplasms as the result. Complications of HIV disease are the main reasons for surgical involvement in the treatment of these patients. While no cure has been developed for this infection, effective antiretroviral therapy is available. Only about one-third of patients in low-income countries are being treated for HIV infection. No vaccine has been proven effective for the prevention of HIV infection.

An issue of considerable concern with HBV, HCV, and HIV infections for the surgeon is occupational risk of these infections when performing operative procedures. Developing countries have high prevalence rates of these infections, and it is likely that multiple patients will be encountered that have one or more of these blood-borne infections. All surgeons should be vaccinated for HBV. The prevention of HCV and HIV infection is the avoidance of percutaneous injury and blood exposure during operations. Double-gloving and face shields should be used. Any percutaneous or skin exposure event should promptly be managed by skin cleansing of the site with an antiseptic solution. The best prevention is a constant awareness of sharp instruments in the operating room to avoid injury.

Other Viruses: Many other viruses are of concern in developing countries. Human herpes viruses are associated with Burkitt's lymphoma and Kaposi's sarcoma. Human papillomavirus is the putative agent of cervical carcinoma. Rabies continues to be an issue in these countries. Recent outbreaks of viral hemorrhagic fever virus infections have called particular attention to Ebola virus, but in the Third World there are an abundance of different viruses associated with hemorrhagic fever. The hemorrhagic fever viruses are fulminate diseases with a rapid onset of a systemic inflammatory response and attendant coagulopathy. Not only are they major disease issues for the Third World, but in an era of transcontinental transportation they may appear anywhere. At present, only supportive care can be provided for these infections since no specific antiviral treatment is available.

Mycoses

The topography, temperature, and humidity of the tropics present an ideal milieu for the growth of fungi, and deep mycotic infections occur throughout the tropics. Of the many mycotic infections that can be encountered, the clinically important mycoses include mycetoma, aspergillus granuloma, phycomycosis, histoplasmosis, and chromoblastomycosis.

Mycetoma of the foot (Madura foot) is a clinically recognized disease with swelling, draining sinuses, and discharge of granules. These infections can be subgrouped into actinomycetoma, which is actually a bacterial infection with *Actinomyces* sp. The eumycetoma is caused by fungi.[28] The disease is most common in semidesert zones where foot trauma results in wounds that are contaminated with the responsible pathogen. Surgical debridement is often necessary for successful treatment. Severe cases may require amputation. Actinomycetoma can be treated with penicillin. Eumycetoma is medically treated with azole compounds. The clinical dilemma in Third World settings is the inability to get reliable culture results to differentiate the responsible pathogen.

Parasitic Diseases

Guinea worm disease or dracunculiasis is transmitted by drinking water contaminated with tiny crustaceans that contain immature forms of the parasite *Dracunculus medinensis*.[29] One year later, adult female worms up to 1 m long emerge through the skin, usually of the lower limb, which produces an abscess. The patient may be incapacitated for months but infections are infrequently fatal. Surgical removal of the worm is commonly employed, but care must be taken to not break the parasite during the process because of adverse tissue reactions that follow. No chemotherapy is available and the host does not develop an immune response from infection. A global campaign to eradicate dracunculiasis by improving access to clean water is currently reducing the number of cases to a very small number.

Schistosomiasis (bilharzia) is an infection of over 200 million people in the world. Infection occurs after skin contact with the *Schistosoma* sp. in contaminated fresh water.[30] The pathogen migrates systemically into the veins of different tissues. Eggs are produced by the parasite and a robust inflammatory response of the host provokes tissue damage. Portal hypertension, pulmonary hypertension, and fibrotic complications of the urinary tract are the more common clinical manifestations of chronic disease.

Intestinal polyps are associated with schistosomiasis and may require removal either by operation or colonoscopy because of bleeding. There is an association between urinary schistosomiasis and carcinoma of the bladder. Effective treatment for this disease is with praziquantel, and steroids may be added to blunt the inflammatory response. Surgical care may be required in these patients to manage bleeding varices and gastrointestinal polyps, large fibromas of the lung and urinary tract, and stricture disease or malignancies of the urinary tract.

Hydatid, or echinococcal, cysts occur from ingestion of the eggs of the tapeworm *Echinococcus* sp.[31] The eggs hatch into larval cestodes, which then penetrate the intestinal wall and disseminate. This leads to the formation of cysts most commonly in the liver but also in the lung, and occasionally elsewhere. Patients usually develop pressure symptoms from the large cyst. Operative evacuation of the cyst has been the treatment of choice for most patients who have hydatid cysts. Hypertonic saline solution or 0.1% cetrimide is injected into the cyst prior to evacuation. The operative goal is removal of the cyst contents and lining without fluid leakage, which causes a potential toxic or anaphylactic reaction. Spillage of cyst contents or the lining of the cyst may result in recurrent cyst formation. Albendazole and mebendazole therapy have been used for smaller hydatid cysts and may be employed as adjunctive therapy in patients with large cysts.

Trypanosomiasis is caused by the *Trypanosoma* sp. parasites. There are two very different diseases caused by these parasites; hence, they are divided by their geographical occurrence as African trypanosomiasis and American trypanosomiasis.

African trypanosomiasis is caused by *Trypanosoma brucei* and is found only in Africa. It is commonly known as "sleeping sickness". It is transmitted by the bite of the tsetse fly. The parasite enters the circulation and eventually infects the blood-brain barrier. The chronic disease leads over 1–2 years to neurological symptoms and somnolence. Death usually occurs without treatment within 3 years from infection. Pentamidine is the first-line treatment, with other options being used but with limited availability.[32]

American trypanosomiasis is caused by *Trypanosoma cruzi* infection.[33] It is found principally in Central and South America. Infection is transmitted by the triatomine bug, although it is a blood-borne pathogen and has been associated with transmission from transfusion and vertical transmission to infants. There is an acute phase to the infection with parasites identifiable in blood, which

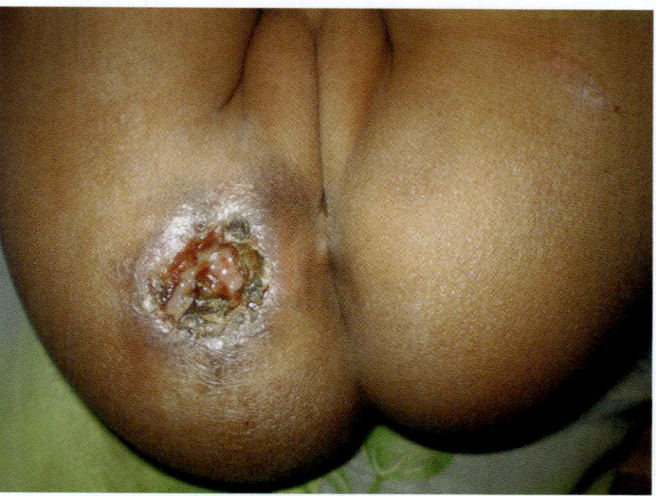

Fig. 17.10: Cutaneous leishmaniasis is a result of the trypanosomes of *Leishmania* sp. that may ulcerate the skin as shown. The cutaneous form for disfiguring but typically does not involve the viscera. Visceral leishmaniasis is commonly a lethal infection.

evolves into a chronic phase where the parasite is totally intracellular. Muscle cells appear to be the major cell target with poor cardiac contractility, heart conduction problems, and megaesophagus/megacolon in the gastrointestinal tract. Nifurtimox and benznidazole are used for treatment, but both are considered investigational in the United States. Medical treatment does not reverse the cardiac and megaesophagus/megacolon abnormalities once they are present. Surgical approaches are used for achalasia and megacolon.

Leishmaniasis is transmitted by sandfly bites and is caused by several *Leishmania* species of parasites. The infection has a cutaneous and a visceral form. The cutaneous disease results in painful skin ulcerations (Fig. 17.10). The visceral form of the disease may involve the liver, spleen, or bone marrow and is commonly fatal without treatment. Pentavalent antimonial compounds are the traditional treatment. Recently liposomal amphotericin is used for visceral leishmaniasis. Other drugs are being explored.[34]

Filariasis is transmitted to humans by insect bite vectors. The disease is caused by the nematode order *Filariidae*.[35] These are clinically grouped as cutaneous, lymphatic, and body-cavity infections. The estimated prevalence of these disabling infections is 1,50,000 people.

Cutaneous filariasis (onchocerciasis) is caused by *Onchocerca volvulus*. The disease is primary a dermatitis infection. Biopsy of infected areas of the iliac crest or scapular areas is the only role for surgeons in the care of

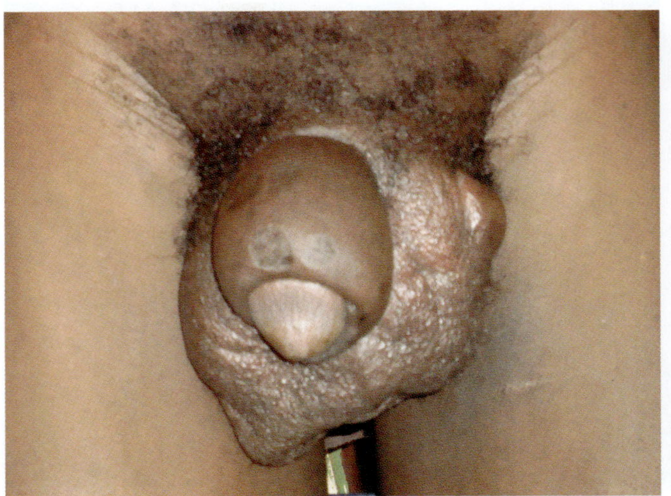

Fig. 17.11: Filariasis can give lymphedema of the genitalia by parasitic lymphatic obstruction.

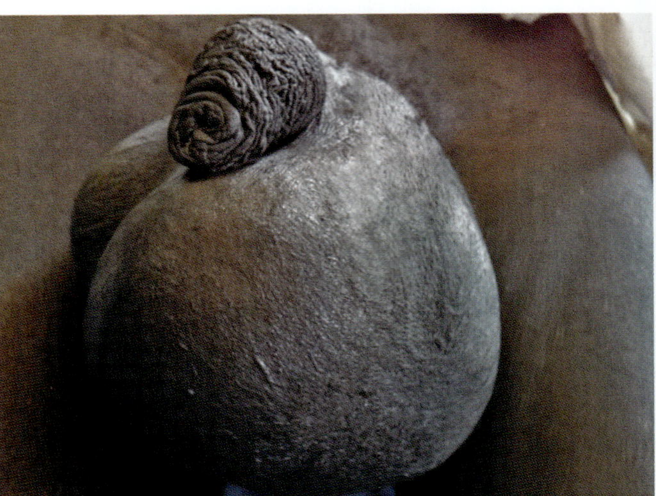

Fig. 17.12: Hydrocele is a marker of filariasis as if often correlated with the parasitic burden.

these patients. Ivermectin prevents proliferation of the organism. The organism persists through the short course of its natural life and is removed slowly, preventing the filaricidal reaction that occurs if too much antigen is released at once (a problem with older filaricides).

Lymphatic filariasis (elephantiasis) is transmitted by mosquitos and is caused by the nematodes of *Wuchereria bancrofti, Brugia malayi,* and *Brugia timori*. These infections are the most common of the filarial diseases, and the parasites sequester in the lymphatics of the genital areas and the extremities (Fig. 17.11). Lymphedema, hydroceles, and clinical elephantiasis are the consequences. Diethylcarbamazine and other agents are used for systemic treatment. Scrotal elephantiasis can be treated by excision of redundant tissue and placement of the testes in upper thigh adductor pockets or in a newly constructed scrotum. Large hydroceles may benefit from surgical repair (Fig. 17.12). For elephantiasis that is refractory to all conservative measures, excision of involved skin and lymphedematous subcutaneous tissues to the investing fascia of the muscle followed by skin grafts may be employed. There are many surgical variations on this basic theme, all of which are associated with morbid complications.

Body-cavity filariasis is due to *Mansonella perstans*. These insect-bite transmitted parasites reside in serous body cavities, mesentery, and the retroperitoneum. Most of these infections remain asymptomatic. A minority are associated with angioedema, arthralgia, fever, and other systemic symptoms. Antiparasitic treatments have not been demonstrated to be effective, and uncertainty remains about the need for the treatment of most cases.

Ascariasis: The fecal-oral transmitted infection caused by the helminth *Ascaris lumbricoides* is thought to infect over one billion people of the world.[36] Abdominal discomfort, distention, and nausea are common symptoms. The bulk of intestinal worms will cause intestinal obstruction that requires laparotomy. Options during laparotomy include milking the worm mass bolus into the cecum and right colon, enterotomy with manual worm removal and decompression, or rarely resection of involved bowel. Ascariasis is also reported to cause volvulus, intussusception, appendicitis, intestinal perforation, granulomatous peritonitis, pancreatitis, biliary obstruction, pyogenic cholangitis, acute cholecystitis, and perforation of the bile ducts. Considering the prevalence of this ubiquitous parasite, the actual number of patients who warrant operative intervention is extremely small.

Special Conditions: Polar Medicine

"Poles of inaccessibility" include, of course, the poles—the extreme margins of the globe in Arctic and Antarctic, which are characterized by extreme variation in light and other irradiations, and temperature extremes. The massive residuals of the last ice age remain, even if retreating in size, and can be many kilometers thick from all the snow that has fallen over millennia. Ice cores may give a calendar of earth's climate history, and an account of certain artificial or natural events that have occurred in the deep archives of these records—such as spores from faraway biomes and the advent of certain nondegradable man-made elements such as plasticizers and fluorocarbons.

The poles are unique for another reason. Green plants in the tropics produce oxygen, but the organic detritus is also oxidizing. That, along with the slash-and-burn practices of forest clearing, may result in net zero oxygen production. The consumption of combustibles subtracts from the positive oxygen production of photosynthesis. Much of the oxygen repletion of earth's atmosphere must come, therefore, from the sea and the upper layers of the oceans where the phytoplankton live. That air circulates globally, bringing the necessary elements of life around the entire planet. That atmospheric circulation occurs nowhere as violently as it does at the poles where the mass of cold polar air sinks rapidly owing to its increased density. On reaching the icy surface of the flat Antarctic shield, there is little in the way of structure to impede it (there are no trees or buildings to dissipate the force of the falling air) and these katabatic winds reach high velocities, sweeping most loose objects before them.

Although the massive Antarctic ice continent imprisons a lot of the globe's fresh water, the continent is officially a desert. Less than 10 inches of precipitation fall per year from the cold arid air near the poles. Almost all of that has remained there minus the quantity that has sublimated or "calved" off the edges of the ice sheet as glaciers push to the Antarctic Ocean.

Cold-Ice-Wind-Desert: This harsh environment is not lifeless, but it has only a few vegetations consisting of moss and algae with their long lives and short growing seasons, putting the poles among the more fragile of earth's plant ecosystems. Well-insulated aquatic birds and penguins abound, with cetacean mammals, also insulated by thick blubber layers. All are subsisting on the same base of the food chain in the crustacean ocean krill.

For human visitors (there really are no "inhabitants"—people subsist in resupplied research stations dependent upon the outside temperate world), there are many dangers to exposure in this climate. One is obvious in that exposed skin would freeze in a very short time given the winter time ambient temperatures of minus 40–50° (it is hardly necessary to add C or F since they are nearly equivalent at this extreme). This danger is compounded by the wind-chill factor if the katabatic winds are also factored in. In winter, there is a near absence of sunlight for periods of several months with implications for temperatures and other effects of light, e.g. human mood swings (the SAD Syndrome—Seasonal Affective Disorder) and vitamin D deficit (usually requiring concentrations up through the food chain of fat soluble vitamins or otherwise synthetically replaced).

In the other extreme of summer at the poles, other problems present themselves. Sunlight is constant and circadian rhythm is lost with disturbances in human sleep patterns and affect as well. Combined with the sense of isolation in a massive, disorienting, often featureless wilderness of hostile extreme conditions, some Arctic hunter-gatherers or explorers have succumbed to psychotic breaks. They have been known to strip off clothing and expire due to exposure in a syndrome with the Eskimo name "Piblotek". A more common condition of very painful sun exposure is the burned retina of snow blindness. Prevention requires a means of filtering out the highly intense irradiation with pinhole apertures or smoked glass.

An ironic combination of burns can occur in exposed skin at polar conditions—frostbite and sunburn. An even more exposed and delicate environmental interface is the tracheobronchial and alveolar membrane. The desiccated air can dry out mucous membranes and chilled air can freeze the unprotected membranes, especially at higher respiratory rates as with exertion. Heat loss from the body can be rapid in such environments, even given completely adequate skin-protective clothing, if tachypnea is accelerating heat loss.

Special Conditions: High Altitude

Many of the problems seen with exposure in polar environments are also common to high altitude physiology. They can be further compounded by diminished atmospheric pressures and the hypoxia of diminished partial pressures of rarified atmospheric oxygen, often when greater oxygen consumption is called upon in climbing. Snow and ice and frigid air may be common as well as the additional high exposure from steep inclines and angles of attack in ascent, and, especially, descent.

No one "lives" above 7,000 m elevation; it is a very hostile environment for habitation. If one is keen on visiting for whatever purpose, this is done not in a steady state of equilibrium but by borrowing heavily from the reserves of energy stores and compensatory mechanisms. The glycolysis of hypoxia is skewed and oxyhemoglobin dissociation is shifted during hyperventilation. Higher ventilation rates are needed to compensate for low atmospheric oxygen (FiO_2). The increased ventilation rate results in alkalinization of the blood.

Another consequence is the rapid desiccation of the mucous membranes of the tracheobronchial tree. When this occurs, an almost diphtheria-like membrane crusts the respiratory passages and when it sloughs it is difficult to clear. A characteristic hacking cough is common in these conditions and is so characteristic of Everest trek summiteers that it has acquired the name of the "Khumbu cough". Climbers in some instances have been incapacitated by breaking ribs in intense fits of coughing to clear these respiratory tract plugs. On at least several occasions in my own experience and in the literature confirming this experience, a Heimlich maneuver has been required to help clear the airway obstruction of the dried mucosal membrane occluding the upper airway.

Another hazard that is not frequently reported is unexpected sunburn on the palate and inner nares. With nostrils flared and open-mouthed deep breathing, a climber can experience a burn from the sunlight glare reflecting right off the glacier being climbed. The ulceration from daytime exposure may give problems in eating, compounding the decreased appetite generally experienced at altitudes sufficient to give relative hypoxia.

Even extensive exertion short of technical climbing—such as trekking to Everest base camp—can produce annoying minor disabilities that are magnified as the altitude increases. Putting a glove back on once removed becomes a very major undertaking, or getting anything back into a backpack. The closing of a zipper can take concentrated effort. Loss of coordination is particularly critical in footing, often most problematic on descent, when the anticipation of the next movements toward summiting is behind one and an almost lackadaisical carelessness can set in. Because judgment impairments are common in hypoxia, and as the implications of modification are more difficult to see without the third order thinking often missing due to the single-minded push during exhaustion, climbers should adhere to a well-thought-out plan.

As passengers traveling in a commercial jetliner, we can be sitting comfortably as the outside temperature may be recorded as -40 degrees (either F or C!) and with a headwind of 100 knots at an altitude of 8,000 m. We may be told "we are crossing the atmospheric jet stream". If one is sitting uncomfortably at the identical altitude on any of the fourteen of Earth's 8,000-m peaks, it is the same jet stream we might be exposed to without benefit of a pressurized temperature-controlled airliner cabin. The calculation of that same wind speed and atmospheric temperature leads to a daunting determination of the wind-chill!

Under conditions approaching such extremes, even minor irritants grow into major problems. An annoying toothache may get worse as a signal of an expanding air pocket trapped in a maxillary sinus or a filled dental cavity as the atmospheric pressure decreases with ascent. These are the kinds of individual problems that can occur at altitude that might be self-manageable.

The more sinister problems of acute mountain sickness (AMS), high altitude pulmonary edema (HAPE), and high altitude cerebral edema (HACE) require help in both personnel and devices for rescue and descent. Acute mountain sickness is characterized by headache, nausea, loss of strength, and well-being. Those afflicted are robbed of strength for exertion and AMS can culminate in vomiting and dehydration. It is often the product of rapid ascent, and accommodation is sometimes reached by a rest day allowing for further acclimatization. Acetazolamide (Diamox) has been recommended for prevention to shift the oxyhemoglobin dissociation curve with this carbonic anhydrase inhibitor. I have not used it prophylactically, reserving it instead for the early onset of AMS, while modifying my rate of ascent. Not everyone with the sniffles is a victim of AMS, which is almost always over-diagnosed as HAPE because of acute awareness of the latter condition, which can be lethal.

High altitude pulmonary edema is diagnosed by the characteristic decrease in peripheral breath sounds and rales in the bases of the lungs. Late stages exhibit frothy pink sputum, anxiety, and breathlessness. High altitude cerebral edema is an acute emergency, requiring immediate repressurization and evacuation to a more accommodating altitude. The edemas in both cases of HAPE and HACE are hypoxia-induced, and almost all require corticosteroids in membrane-stabilizing doses and an increase in oxygen tension. This might be affected by the use of a pressure suit such as a Gamow bag or administration of supplemental bottled oxygen.

Both emergencies require evacuation for stabilization. There is a conundrum in this as well, since the very high altitudes at which such emergencies might occur are also at the extreme limits of the lift that can be expected for helicopter rescues. Often evacuation is a very rough overland trip of the same precipitous trek the climber has come up. Intensive nursing care is required, hardly conducive to a rock-face recovery.

A simple means to detect early changes and to head off some of the altitude problems has been the widespread use of pulse oximetry to measure oxygen saturation. A slowed rate of ascent is indicated by any precipitous decrease in O_2 saturations that suggests the need for a slower rate of ascent. Oximetry readings can indicate that acclimatization has occurred and that it is safe to proceed.

Operating at altitude should happen only in emergency temporizing procedures, and can involve such useful devices as insertion of chest tubes or airway clearing through tracheostomy or endoscopic lavage. For most practical purposes, the rule of thumb will be rapid evacuation to a lower altitude to a more advantageous facility. Rather than attempting any definitive care on the precarious mountain slope, a "scoop and run" response is best and could include external stabilization of fractures or Gamow bag and O_2 administration.

If an environment is available to attempt an operation, simple "cold sterilization" or immersion for a period of time in antiseptic of iodine or another antimicrobial solution may be adequate for surface sterilization of solid steel surgical tools. Other items may require heat and pressure sterilization. It is important to recognize that the statement reads "sterilization" and not "boiling". While most vegetative organisms would be killed by a period of immersion at the temperature water boils at sea level, a practitioner, when conducting surgical clinics in the Himalayas, must remember that if water boils at 80°C at that level of altitude, this is hardly an adequate temperature for killing spores that might transmit disease. Several atmospheres of pressure must be added to make for a much higher temperature for adequate steam sterilization.

Unfortunately, political and social factors continue to complicate delivery of medical care to these extreme environments. Practitioners have long had to do considerable explaining when checking in some of the drugs and devices that go into the cargo hold of aircraft when traveling to remote areas. It has long been impossible to carry narcotic or anesthetic agents in passenger compartments. And since the 2013 Boston Marathon bombing incident, it is difficult to transport even such a utilitarian device as a pressure cooker.

Special Conditions: Diving and Decompression

At most geographic points at sea level, we humans are subject to one atmospheric pressure and one G of gravitational pull. For most of us, the only time we experience higher than atmospheric pressure is when we leave the air environment and descend through the denser medium of water. We might seem to escape that gravitational pull by submersion in neutral buoyancy, but we are under considerably more pressure in the water than in the atmosphere. The higher density of seawater is apparent when we effectively double the weight of the entire column of earth's atmosphere bearing down on us at the surface of the sea within 5 m under its surface. The deeper we go, the less time we have at those depths. This is because increased pressure effectively decreases the volume of air contained in the limited capacity of scuba tanks. It is not just a matter of capacity for compressed gas in the tank, but also for the gases compressed within us as the explorers of such depths, since there are physiologic consequences of such pressure changes.

In the first few meters of descent, a diver can identify problems of any body cavities with entrapped gases such as the middle ear. If one cannot rapidly clear the Eustachian tube and add air by Valsalva maneuver to increasingly pressurize the middle ear, the water pressure might continuously depress the tympanic membrane to the point of an implosion. The equilibration of pressures across such a mobile membrane is easier than that for fixed cavities such as in the cranial sinuses, teeth or parts of the gastrointestinal tract. "Clearing" this imbalance by equilibrating pressures as one descends is relatively easy at the beginning of the dive. What is often less apparent during the ascent, at the time that air supplies are running low and there is a push to get to the surface, is that these same processes must occur in reverse, as the compressed gases inside the body expand on ascent from the depths.

While under pressure, the amount of gas in solution in body fluids such as blood increases. If one is at depth for an extended period, these increased gas tensions in the blood are themselves problematic and may cause confusion and enrapture of the "nitrogen narcosis". Unless special gas breathing mixtures displacing some of the nitrogen with an inert gas such as helium are employed, breathing compressed regular air will result in a large amount of nitrogen dissolved in the bloodstream. Even without evidence of such "raptures of the deep" disturbance with "safe limits" of nitrogen in the blood at depth, on ascent, particularly if rapid, the dissolved gases "bubble out" and obstruct small arteriole blood flow in the condition referred to as the "bends". A slow ascent is necessary to degas the bloodstream along with "hang time" at a depth of about one additional atmosphere.

In addition to the danger from compressed gases in the bloodstream is the danger of rapidly expanding air in the lung during ascent. To prevent this, a nearly constant "air leak" of bubbles should be continuous on ascent to decompress the expanding lungful of air. Failing to do so, and in a rapidly distending lung, the lung might rupture, particularly if there were any congenital or acquired defects such as an emphysematous bleb. The result would be a pneumothorax and the accumulated air in the pleural space would likewise expand, but it would not be able to escape the chest cavity. As it expands, it would collapse the lung still further and might even shift the mediastinum over to the opposite side compromising the function of the lung on the unaffected side. This tension pneumothorax compromises not only ventilation but venous return to the heart, and constitutes an emergency that is relieved only by allowing the air trapped under tension to escape—a thoracostomy by needle or chest tube.

Similar compression/decompression disruption of viscera can happen from underwater explosions in which the compressive shock wave travels through the water with considerably more force than it would from the same dissipation in compressible air. The hydraulic fluid wave can rupture viscera through which it passes.

The extremes of pressure—from the hyperbaric submarine exposures to the less than half atmospheric air pressures of high altitude mountaineering—have been the limits of the extreme conditions faced by human beings. The shifts in such pressures were only as rapid as ascent from ocean depths to the surface or up to mountain altitudes. But aerospace travel, with its high rates of speed and very large and much faster pressure shifts, has led to considerable equilibration discomfort ranging from distressing to major organ damage in sudden decompression and blast injuries. Mountain altitude and ocean depth are no longer the limits to pressure/decompression injuries.

Addressing Inaccessibility

A principal barrier to surgical care that makes for very late presentation of nearly all illnesses seen in the developing world is inaccessibility to healthcare. The patient may have ignorance as to the condition from which he or she suffers, and that ignorance might even be shared by the primary caregivers if and when the problem can be brought to whatever primary medical attention exists, usually at some large remove from where the patient lives. This means that the patient must travel precisely at the time of the growing disability to attain access, and from that point be referred again to someone who might be equipped to address the problem. It would be a far more efficient system if the care could come to where the patients live, obviating the requirement for them to travel to find it, when they might not even be aware of a need to seek out help or that there is anything that can be done for their problem.

This is the rationale behind the concept of mobile surgical missions. Mobile surgical vehicles bring specialized care to the people most afflicted, a "workaround" for the problems of geographic inaccessibility. The vehicle brings care to the patient in the milieu in which the patient lives, carrying the equipment and expertise to the primary care clinic into which it might "dock". The practitioners can at the same time work to indigenize the skills by teaching the local healthcare workers about the surgical conditions that might be electively repaired. Regular visits to the community bring residents not only the awareness of the problem but its fixability and the means by which this might be done. In other words, hope.

Deployment of mobile surgical vehicles brings care to the people afflicted rather than expecting them to know enough to make their way to achieve care on their own, often into environments that might be quite foreign to them. When such mobile surgical care has been done, the isolated people in remote rural areas have been quite receptive to their new access to healthcare. Patient preparation and permission for surgical problems that might be repaired on an elective basis are obtained for a scheduled interval visit by the primary care unit. Then the specialized vehicle can come to "dock" with their primary care unit for days or weeks, delivering the needed care and "working around' inaccessibility.

The problem of access then becomes a problem of logistics: shifting the focus and energy from somehow getting the patient to a fixed center for care to, instead, getting a somewhat cumbersome unit to the field site where it can access the patient population. If such a unit were carried in a road-based vehicle, it could soon become apparent that the areas where it might be needed are often isolated from any recognizable "road". But accommodations can and have been made. In the interior of Ecuador, the vehicle to deliver surgical care is designed to accommodate the narrow Andean Mountain roads and rocky overhangs and still navigate successfully for reaching the patient care sites. In the region of South Sudan, the roads are rudimentary in almost all sites where such care would be needed. Indeed, at the time such a mobile surgical unit was proposed in the new nation-state of the Republic of South Sudan, the whole country possessed <20 km of paved roadway. But rugged off-road vehicles such as those used in military operations with appropriate clearances and suspensions have made it possible to deliver such surgical care units over even primitive conditions of roadways, often navigating by global positioning system and performing stream crossings by fording small rivers.

Access to some areas will be seasonal, such as in the high mountain passes of the Himalayas or Andes. The drivers refer to the road surface as "black top" (crushed rock and gravel) or "white top" (the frozen snow and ice of the long winter) in the province of Himachal, in Himalayan India, with each condition presenting its own set of hazards. High snow pack often interrupts delivery when the passes are closed for many months each winter, but the drivers welcome the harder surfaces of the frozen surface when the stability is greater than during the annual snowmelt that carries a high hazard of avalanche.

Along the equatorial beltline of the globe, the perpetual equinox is accompanied by only two major seasonal changes—the wet and the dry. Assuming the rudimentary roads are navigable in the dry season half of the year, such roadways are inundated during the rainy season, particularly in the floodplains of two of the greatest river systems—the Nile and the Amazon. There is no way that a wheeled vehicle can get to remote sites during the rainy season in South Sudan when the largest wetland on earth, the Great Sudd, is under ≥2 m of the overflow along the Nile river floodplain. Facts will have to be faced. Neither the patients moving to a fixed site nor the caregivers dependent upon dry land vehicles to access them are mobile during the extended period of the annual inundation.

But there is a solution, even an opportunity. The high water of the rainy season provides access to people and sites along the largest navigable rivers on earth through the simple conversion of floating the same mobile vehicle on a barge to make stops along the high water ports. This method of care delivery has been used on the Amazon and lake-based primary care sites, such as Lake Victoria, and is proposed for the Volta, Nile and Congo rivers.

An important feature of the mobile surgical care concept is the container in which the personnel and equipment can be set up to care for the patients. Such container-clinics often contain their own generators, solar, wind, and/or petrol-powered. Fuel and water storage and filtration systems are used while needed for sustained practice until resupply, often when moving on to another docking site. The propulsion system for the platform can be in the form of a tractor-trailer, railroad car, cargo aircraft, or tugboat. And they can be interchangeable independent leasable units.

The mobile surgical mission concept has been successfully implemented in a number of places. An extended experience in mobile surgical practice in which the authors have participated was under the combined leadership of Drs Edgar Rodas and Edgar B Rodas Jr, and the Cinterandes Foundation. This organization has performed over 6,550 surgical procedures over 25 years in Ecuador in both remote and inner urban settings. The total experience has exhibited a surgical mortality of zero, a surgical infection rate of less than 1.0% and morbidity less than contemporary, and comparable inpatient urban hospitalization experience. The patients are returned to their home environment immediately in which recovery has been dramatically enhanced. At the same time as the surgical clinics are being held, the medical screening clinics, instructional sessions, public health outreaches, and the maternal and child care clinics have constituted a rising tide, which has lifted all aspects of community health through the periodic visits of the mobile surgical unit.

Almost none of the patients so treated could have found their way into a modern urban hospital center or afforded the care potentially denied to them but made more accessible over both the geographic and economic barriers breached by the mobile surgical practice. This model in blanketing all regions of a single South American nation with four distinctive geographic zones—the Amazon jungle, the Andes Mountains, the Pacific Coastal Plains and the Galapagos littoral—have all been made accessible through the mobile surgical vehicle that has also incorporated the features of telemedicine back to urban hospital centers and Ministries of Health for follow-up care and consultation.

CONCLUSION

The single factor of low income can mire those so afflicted into a high-risk population in terms of nutritional status, educational, employment, and life prospects. Poverty is also the most common factor in several acquired illness patterns such as the water-borne illnesses or soil transmitted helminths, birth rates, and infant mortality. Poverty and disease pattern, as well as life potential, are interdependently linked in the dismal science of resource-constrained environments, both as cause and effect. Despite a wide variety of methods tried to cover the expenses of healthcare, the resources brought to bear on health-related problems vary widely over many parts of the world. Usually some combination of public or private payment for needed services accounts for the scarcity of skilled modern health-care in almost all areas of the developing world. It is an ironic but easily understood free-market fact that the regions of the world with the highest disease burden are most often the same regions that attract the fewest healthcare practitioners.

The authors have partnered with Cinterandes Foundation in combination with Mission to Heal to extend the successful experience of mobile surgical unit principles.[37] Their hope is to internationalize this model to multiple other sites in the developing world, to bridge still further barriers geographic and otherwise, and to provide greater access to care, even at the alleged African "pole of inaccessibility."

SUGGESTED READING

1. Geelhoed GW. Mission to Heal: Sharing Medical Knowledge at Africa's Pole of Inaccessibility. Austin, TX: Greenleaf Book Group; 2014.
2. Snowden, Frank M. Emerging and reemerging diseases: a historical perspective. Immunol Rev. 2008;225:9.
3. Soper, Nathaniel J. Editor-in chief, Cohen Recardo V., Aun, Frederico, Geelhoed, Glenn W. editors. Problems in General Surgery: Surgical Tropical Diseases. Philadelphia, PA: Lippincott Williams and Wilkins. Vol 18, number 4. December 2001.
4. Tarpley, John L, and Meier, Donald E. Geographic features of surgical practice. In: Williamson R, Corson JD. Surgery. St. Louis: C.V. Mosby Co.; 2000. Ch. 14.

REFERENCES

1. Hotez, PJ. Forgotten People, Forgotten Diseases: The Neglected Tropical Diseases and Their Impact on Global Health and Development, 2nd edition. Washington, DC: ASM Press; 2013.
2. Barter DM. Tuberculosis and poverty: the contribution of patient costs in sub-Saharan Africa—a systematic review. BMC Public Health. 2012;12:980.
3. Harms G, Feldmeier H. HIV infection and tropical parasitic diseases—deleterious interactions in both directions? Trop Med Int Health. 2002;7:479-88.
4. Piwoz EG, Preble EA. HIV/AIDS and Nutrition: A Review of the Literature and Recommendations for Nutritional Care and Support in Sub-Saharan Africa (PDF). Washington DC: Academy for Educational Development;2000. p. PN-ACK-673.
5. United Nations Department of Economics and Social Affairs: World population prospects: the 2012 revision. Available from http://esa.un.org/unpd/wpp/Demographic-Profiles/index.shtm#. [Accessed January 8, 2015].
6. Hernández AV, Pasupuleti V, Deshpande A. Effect of rural-to-urban within-country migration on cardiovascular risk factors in low- and middle-income countries: a systematic review. Heart. 2012;98:185-94.
7. Adeboye B. Obesity and its health impact in Africa: a systematic review. Cardiovasc J Africa. 2012;23:512-521.
8. Vorster HH. The emergence of cardiovascular disease during urbanisation of Africans. Public Health Nutr. 2002;5: 239-43.
9. Tantawichien T. Dengue fever and dengue haemorrhagic fever in adolescents and adults. Paediatr Int Child Health. 2012;32(Suppl 1):22-7.
10. De Silva PM, Marshall JM. Factors contributing to urban malaria transmission in sub-Saharan Africa: a systematic review. J Trop Med. 2012;2012:819563. doi: 10.1155/2012/819563. Epub October 18, 2012.
11. Qi Q, Guerra CA, Moyes CL, et al. The effects of urbanization on global *Plasmodium vivax* malaria transmission. Malar J. 2012;11:403. doi: 10.1186/1475-2875-11-403.
12. Geelhoed GW. Plagues and pestilences in history: a model for the current AIDS pandemic. Panetics. 2000;9:1.
13. Meier DE, OlaOlorun DA, Nkor SK, et al. Ketamine: a safe and effective anesthetic agent for children in the developing world. Pediatr Surg Int. 1996;11:370-3.
14. Ogbonna BC, Obekpa PO, Momoh JT, et al. Laparoscopy in developing countries in the management of patients with an acute abdomen. Br J Surg. 1992;79:964-6.
15. Udwadia TE, Udwadia RT, Menon K, et al. Laparoscopic surgery in the developing world: an overview of the Indian scene. Int Surg. 1995;90:371-5.
16. Raiga J, Kasia JM, Canis M, et al. Introduction of gynecologic endoscopic surgery in an African setting. Int J Gynaecol Obstet. 1994;46:261-4.
17. Holcombe C. Surgical emergencies in tropical gastroenterology. Gut. 1995;36:9-11.
18. Rana SS, Bhasin DK, Nanda M, et al. Parasitic infestations of the biliary tract. Curr Gastroenterol Rep. 2007;9:156-64.
19. Vineis P, Wild CP. Global cancer patterns: causes and prevention. Lancet. 2014;383:549-57.
20. Edge J, Buccimazza I, Cubasch H, et al. The challenges of managing breast cancer in the developing world—a perspective from sub-Saharan Africa. S Afr Med J. 2014;104:377-9.
21. Creang AA, Genadry RR. Obstetric fistulas: a clinical review. Int J Gynecol Obstet. 2007;99 (Suppl 1):S40-S47.
22. World Health Organization: Global tuberculosis report (2014). Available from http://www.who.int/tb/publications/global_report/en/. [Accessed December 15, 2014].
23. Centers for Disease Control: Tuberculosis Treatment. Available from http://www.cdc.gov/tb/topic/treatment/default.htm. [Accessed December 15, 2014].
24. Hoover AZ. Buruli ulcer. Available from http://emedicine.medscape.com/article/1104891-overview. [Accessed December 15, 2014].
25. World Health Organization: Hepatitis B. Available from http://www.who.int/mediacentre/factsheets/fs204/en/. [Accessed December 15, 2014].
26. World Health Organization. Hepatitis C. Available from http://www.who.int/mediacentre/factsheets/fs164/en/. [Accessed December 15, 2014].
27. World Health Organization. HIV/AIDS. Available from http://www.who.int/mediacentre/factsheets/fs360/en/. [Accessed December 15, 2014].
28. Ahmed AA, van de Sande WW, Fahal A, et al. Management of mycetoma: major challenge in tropical mycoses with limited international recognition. Curr Opin Infect Dis. 2007; 20:146-51.

29. Centers for Disease Control: Dracunculiasis. Available from http://www.cdc.gov/parasites/guineaworm/. [Accessed December 15, 2014].
30. Ahmed SH. (2014). Schistosomiasis treatment and management. Available from http://emedicine.medscape.com/article/228392-overview [Accessed December 15, 2014].
31. Dandan IS. (2014). Hydatid cysts treatment and management. Available from http://emedicine.medscape.com/article/178648-treatment. [Accessed December 15, 2014].
32. Centers for Disease Control: Parasites-African Trypanosomiasis. Available from http://www.cdc.gov/parasites/sleepingsickness/. [Accessed December 15, 2014].
33. Centers for Disease Control. American Trypanosomiasis. Available from http://www.cdc.gov/parasites/chagas/. [Accessed December 15, 2014].
34. den Boer M, Argaw D, Jannin J, et al. Leishmaniasis impact and treatment access. Clin Microbiol Infect. 2011;17:1471-7.
35. Knopp S, Steinmann P, Hatz C, et al. Nematode infections: filariasis. Infect Dis Clin North Am. 2012; 26:359-81.
36. Dold C, Holland CV. Ascaris and ascariasis. Microbes Infect. 2011;13:632-7.
37. CinterAndes: Mobile Surgery. Available from http://www.cinterandes.org/index.php/en/. [Accessed January 8, 2015].

18

Surgical Management of the Elderly

Konstantinos G Lasithiotakis, Ioannis E Petrakis

Key Points

- Care of the elderly surgical patient is influenced by the physiologic changes that accompany normal aging.
- Geriatric care aims at achieving maximum functional capacity, independence and comfort, and minimum caregiver stress.
- The three goals in geriatric surgical management are to maintain and maximize life span and independent function, reduce disabilities, suffering and pain, and enhance quality and dignity of life.
- Elective procedures can be performed successfully even in frail, high-risk patients if time is provided to optimize the patient's medical status.
- An integrated multidisciplinary approach is the key to a successful outcome and should be implemented as early as possible.

INTRODUCTION

Geriatric surgery is a newly described branch of medicine that studies the surgical diseases of older adults. The term comes from the Greek γέρος (*geros*) meaning "old man" and ιατρός (*iatros*) meaning "healer." Geriatric surgery assesses the effect of various physical, mental, and social changes in people undergoing surgical treatment in order to optimize surgical outcomes through better selection of the patient, better selection of the treatment and individualized targeted interventions. Geriatric surgery is multidisciplinary in that the medical conditions of elderly surgical patients overlap with several fields such as gerontology, internal medicine, family medicine, psychology, psychiatry, and rehabilitation. Geriatric surgeons coordinate a treatment plan with the involvement of several disciplines in order to optimize surgical outcomes. Geriatric surgery, like surgical oncology, is not organ- or system oriented but it is discipline oriented. In this setting, geriatric surgery is called to put individual settings and rules for elderly patients presenting with disease that may demand surgical intervention.

POPULATION AGING AND DISEASE BURDEN

The world is reaching a demographic milestone characterized by an expansion of older age groups and simultaneous decline of the proportion of younger persons, more pronounced in the developed industrialized countries. In 1950, just 8% of the world population was aged 60 years or over. In 2011, the percentage of individuals over 60 years in the developed regions of the world was 26.5%, and it is going to reach 41.2% by 2050. Driven by falling fertility rates and remarkable increases in life expectancy, population aging will continue, even accelerate (Table 18.1). A different perspective on population aging is gained by examining the number of additional years that someone

Table 18.1 Distribution of the age of the population of the world 2011, 2050, and 2100.

	Population in 2011			*Population in 2050*			*Population in 2100*		
	0–25	25–59	60+	0–25	25–59	60+	0–25	25–59	60+
More developed regions	29.1	48.9	26.5	27.6	40.5	41.2	28.2	39.3	44.7
Less developed regions	47.2	19.8	9.8	35.0	44.8	23.7	30.3	42.4	34.5

Source: Population Division of the Department of Economic and Social Affairs of the United Nations Secretariat (2011). World Population Prospects: The 2010 Revision. New York: United Nations.

Table 18.2 Life expectancy at birth.

	Calendar year		
	2005–2010	*2045–2050*	*2095–2100*
World	67.9	75.6	81.1
Africa	55.2	68.2	77.1
Europe	75.4	81.7	87.4
Asia	69	76.7	81.8
N. America	78.2	83.2	88.4
Oceania	76.6	82.5	86.7

Data from Population Division of the Department of Economic and Social Affairs of the United Nations Secretariat (2011). World Population Prospects: The 2010 Revision. New York: United Nations.

Table 18.3 Life expectancy at 60 years of age.

WHO region	*Male (years)*	*Female (years)*
World	18	21
Europe	21	24
America	21	24
Western Pacific	19	22
South-East Asia	15	18
Africa	14	16

Data from World Health statistics (2011). Geneva: World health Organization; 2011.

who has already reached the age of 60 might expect to live (Tables 18.2 and 18.3). This is a more meaningful measure of longevity of the elderly than total life expectancy at birth, which is influenced for example by perinatal and early life deaths.

The total burden of disease faced by older people is a combination of both premature death and poor health experienced during life. In the elderly, the biggest causes of disease are, in order of importance, ischemic heart disease, visual disorders, dementia, cancers and stroke and chronic obstructive pulmonary disease.[1] Cancer is primarily a disease of older people, with incidence rates increasing with age for most types of cancer. More than 60% of cancers are diagnosed in people aged 65 and over, and more than a third are diagnosed in patients aged 75 and over. Prostate cancer accounts for more than one in four cases of cancer diagnosed in older men. Other common cancers for men in this age group are lung and bowel cancer. Over a third of cases diagnosed in elderly women are breast cancers; lung and bowel cancers account for approximately 10% each. The highest incidence rate for cancer is in the +75 age group, in whom the rates have increased by approximately 30% between 1975 and 2010.[2] Approximately 40% of all-listed surgical procedures in the United States refer to patients older than 65 years old

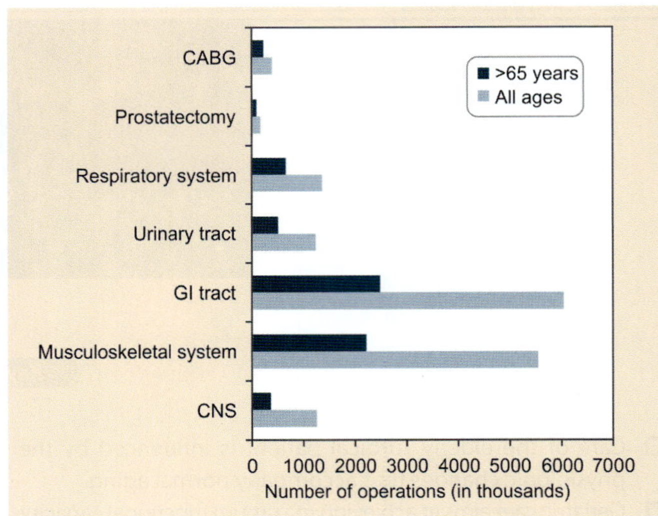

Fig. 18.1: Number of all-listed procedures for discharges from short-stay hospitals, by procedure category and age: United States, 2010. (CABG: Coronary artery bypass grafting; GI tract: Gastrointestinal tract operations; CNS: Central nervous system operations).
Data from CDC/NCHS National Hospital Discharge Survey, 2010.

(Fig. 18.1). The phenomenon of population aging is expected to impact on the workload for several surgical specialties. Specialties such as general surgery, cardiothoracic, urologic, vascular, and orthopedic surgery will experience a steady increase in workload, whereas other specialties such as obstetrics and pediatrics are going to decrease.

THEORIES OF AGING

Aging of the cell, cellular *senescence*, is a phenomenon characterized by limited ability to divide. Senescence is inevitable in normal cells, and it is determined by the number of times the cells divide rather than the age of the cell per se. The *telomeres,* which are protecting protein structures at the end of chromosomes, represent the "molecular clock" or the counting mechanism of cell division. The average length of telomeres diminishes with aging of cells, whereas the inhibition of telomere shortening makes them immortal. The exact mechanisms of molecular causes of aging have not been elucidated so far, although there has been much speculation.

Modern biological theories of aging comprise two main categories: programmed and damage theories. Programmed theories suggest that aging is a process that follows a certain timetable and is the continuation of human growth and development. Programmed theories are mainly associated with the sequential activation and inactivation of certain genes, hormone activity (IGF signaling, neuroendocrine system), and immune system decline leading to vulnerability to disease and thus death.[3] Indeed, abnormal immune response has been linked with several diseases such as Alzheimer's, cardiovascular disease and cancer, all of which are common in the elderly. Damage or error theories consider environmental damage to various levels as the cause of aging. Damage to proteins due to cross-linking, superoxide, and other free radicals plus damage to all macromolecular components of the cell and the accumulation of genetic mutations cause cells to deteriorate, malfunction, and eventually die. Simple wearing out of vital parts of cells and tissues from repeated use leads to aging and death. This theory agrees with the finding that the greater an organism's rate of basal energy consumption, the shorter its life span, as well as with the observation that caloric restriction in animal models markedly extends their life span.[3]

AGING AND SUCCESSFUL AGING

Aging can be defined as the "progressive decrease in functional ability of the organism over time." Common characteristics of aging in humans are the increased probability for death, the increased susceptibility to disease, the decreased homeostasis, and the progressive decrease of functional capacity. There is no general agreement on the age at which a person becomes old. However, in most developed countries the age of 65, roughly equivalent to retirement age, is said to be the lowest cutoff point for old age. Based on studies regarding physical activity, functional independence and youthfulness of the cerebral arteries, an alternative cutoff point of 75 years has been recently suggested. For this reason, a discrimination between early elderly (65–75 years) and late elderly (> 75 years) would be reasonable.[4] *Biological (physiological) age*, which is age in terms of physiological capacity, is not necessarily synonymous with calendar age. The assessment of the biological age of the patient is pivotal in geriatric surgery and will be discussed in detail below. Successful aging refers to the minimal functional deterioration with age, and it has three components: (a) low probability of disease, (b) high cognitive and physical function capacity, and (c) active engagement with life. Adaptation and emotional well-being are the cornerstones of successful aging. Subjective quality of life (QoL) is considered by the elderly to be more important than the absence of disease and other subjective measures of physical and mental health. Six dimensions of successful aging have been suggested: (1) no physical disability over the age of 75 as rated by a physician; (2) good subjective health assessment (i.e. good self-ratings of one's health); (3) length of undisabled life; (4) good mental health; (5) objective social support; and (6) self-rated life satisfaction in eight domains (marriage, income-related work, children, friendship and social contacts, hobbies, community service activities, religion, and recreation/sports). The concept of successful aging is of great value not only to designate a group of clearly optimal surgical candidates but also to guide the decision making in their management.[5,6]

PHYSIOLOGY OF AGING

Changes in Cardiovascular Physiology

With increasing aging there is a loss of myocytes of the ventricles and a decrease in pacemaker cells of the sinus. Afterload, which represents peripheral vascular resistance, increases as a result or progressive of sclerosis of the blood vessels. Vascular smooth muscle becomes less responsive to β-adrenergic stimulus even though the overall levels of plasma catecholamines increase. This phenomenon contributes to increased afterload of the elderly with stress. Reduced aortic compliance results in higher variability of stroke volume with changes of cardiac function. This change is reversible through regular aerobic exercise. Increased stiffness of the myocardium decreases diastolic left ventricular filling, and this may lead to earlier hypotension if venous return (preload) is reduced. Many conditions of the elderly, such as depleted intravascular volume and the use of nitrates or diuretics, may reduce preload. The response to volume depletion, is also hampered in the elderly because of the reduced compliance of the left ventricle and its decreased responsiveness to β-adrenergic stimulus. The overall effect is an intolerance of the elderly to volume depletion. Another characteristic cardiovascular change of the elderly is postprandial hypotension, which may predispose to fall, syncope, and cardiovascular events. Impaired diastolic left ventricular filling depends on left atrial contraction. Therefore, patients with atrial fibrillation (AF) may experience a reduction in cardiac output. The maximal heart rate during exercise diminishes appreciably with age. Diastolic dysfunction is another prevalent physiological cardiological change of the elderly; it is attributed to reduced relaxation of the left ventricle and the presence of several cardiac conditions. The results of this change is that a large proportion of elderly patients, possibly as many as 50%, may have congestive heart failure (CHF; reduced cardiac output) with normal left ventricular function (i.e. with LVEF >50%).[7] The best surrogate marker of cardiovascular reserve is the maximal cardiac output, which is the cardiac output multiplied by heart rate at peak exercise. Besides age-related physiological changes in the cardiovascular system, there are several diseases with a high prevalence in the elderly such as coronary artery disease, mitral and aortic regurgitation, aortic stenosis and AF. Among conduction disorders, second-degree atrioventricular (AV) block, left bundle branch block and pace rhythm are associated with new coronary events in the elderly, unlike AV block, left atrial hemiblock and right bundle branch block.

Changes in Respiratory Physiology

Physiological changes of the respiratory system include morphological changes similar to those observed with mild emphysema associated with loss of the elasticity of the lung. The chest wall becomes less elastic with age, sternopleural articulations become calcified and musculoskeletal disorders such as kyphosis contribute to higher demands from the respiratory muscles, which themselves exhibit decreased capacity due to aging. Even more important is the responsiveness of breathing control in the elderly. Therefore, older patients often fail to increase their ventilation in response to stressors such as atelectasis, heart failure, and hypovolemia. Forced vital capacity (FVC) decreases with age by an annual amount that reaches approximately 30 mL/year, and the decrease is greater in men than in women. The ratio between forced expiratory volume in one second (FEV_1) and FVC also decreases with age, whereas total lung capacity and functional residual capacity changes are not physiologically important. Arterial oxygenation (PaO_2) decreases with age; a frequently used formula for estimating PaO_2 is 100–AGE/3. Interestingly, the PaO_2 decrease is higher when studied in the recumbent than the upright position.[8] Accordingly, the alveolar arterial grade ($P(a\text{-}a)O_2$) increases [approximate formula: AGE/(4 + 4)]. All these physiological changes underscore the fact that elderly surgical patients have lost most of their respiratory reserve and they may not tolerate surgical stress, pain, and bed rest. Moreover, they may not respond appropriately to major respiratory changes, and they may develop respiratory failure while they seem comfortable, without either tachypnea or tachycardia. For this reason, an increased index of suspicion is needed, with frequent measurement of oxygen saturation (SpO_2) and arterial blood gas analysis in order to allow early detection and appropriate management of respiratory complications in the postoperative period.

Changes in Gastrointestinal System

Swallowing abnormalities are very common in the elderly. Most of them are attributed to oral disorders (mastication, first phase of swallowing), dysfunction of the upper esophageal constrictor and esophageal motor dysfunction (reduced peristalsis, delayed emptying, prominent tertiary peristalsis). Healthy elderly people need more swallows in order to deliver the same amount of food to the esophagus, and they are more likely susceptible than younger subjects to inspiration and prolonged coughing after multiple swallowing. Presbyesophagus is characterized by dysphagia and aperistalsis due to degenerative motor function in the elderly, but the contribution of aging to this condition is not clear. Visceral pain threshold in the elderly is markedly higher compared with younger subjects. Gastroduodenal secretion of acid decreases with age, which explains the increased incidence of *Helicobacter pylori* infection in patients over 60 years (which exceeds 75%). Similarly, reduced secretion of intrinsic factor makes pernicious anemia commoner in the elderly. Motor function changes of the stomach and small bowel with aging are clinically unimportant, and intestinal absorption is largely unaffected. Both hepatic mass and blood flow are reduced approximately by half after 65 years of age, but liver cell function is well preserved during aging. Hepatic clearance of drugs in the elderly is reduced by 10–50%, and this may lead to extremely high serum levels of drugs metabolized by the liver. The regenerative capacity of liver is not affected, however. Exocrine function of the pancreas does not change in the elderly, whereas a 10% decrease in β-cell function every decade has been shown in healthy subjects.[9] Although colonic transit time does not increase with age, constipation is one of the most common gastrointestinal complaints, mainly being perceived as excessive straining with defecation. This change has been attributed to various factors such as inappropriate increase of anal sphincter tone during defecation, neuromuscular degeneration, and the use of various medications. In particular, neuropsychiatric agents such as anticholinergic antidepressants and neuroleptics are associated with a high incidence of constipation and laxative usage. Pelvic outlet obstruction describes a group of mechanical disorders of the anorectum leading to constipation or incontinence, especially in older women. Multiparity does not account for the decrease in rectoanal pressures with age, unless there is a rectal prolapse.

Changes in Musculoskeletal System

A progressive loss of bone is observed during aging coupled with decreased osteoblast activity, increased osteoclast activity and hormonal changes. These changes lead to increased bone fragility. Bone mass is measured by dual-energy X-ray absorptiometry. A T score >1 is considered normal, –1 to –2.5 is osteopenia, and scores <–2.5 are consistent with osteoporosis. Dual-energy X-ray absorptiometry scanning does not assess bone quality or volume. FRAX (fracture risk assessment tool) is a tool to predict the risk of fracture taking into account various factors such as smoking and family history.[10] Measures that can be taken to decrease bone loss include lifestyle modifications, calcium and vitamin D supplementation, smoking, and alcohol cessation. Vitamin D deficiency in the elderly is due to decreased intestinal absorption and decreased production from the skin. Vitamin D supplementation in the elderly appears to reduce the risk of fall and vertebral fractures. Bisphosphonates decrease osteoclast activity and reduce bone loss, but their long term use is associated with marked suppression of remodeling that itself can lead to fractures. Gastrointestinal complaints and ulceration are common side effects of these medications. Calcitonin inhibits the osteoclasts. Selective estrogen receptors modulators such as raloxifene may increase the risk for stroke and thromboembolism. Parathyroid analogs are not cost-effective, have many injection-site side effects and may cause hypocalcemia.

Similar to bone, peak muscular mass is reached at about 30 years of age. The rate of decrease reaches 10% for every decade after the age of 50. This change predisposes the elderly to muscle strains after intense body activity, which are painful and may not recover completely. To decrease the risk of injury, balanced intensity and fatigue along with warming up the muscle is suggested. Regular weight-bearing exercise improves long-term function, body mass, and strength. Tendons become stiffer and less compliant in the elderly, predisposing to tendinopathy and ready tendon rupture, especially after cortisol injection, which produces additional collagen thinning. Changes in articular cartilage composition result in decreased water content and increased stiffness of the tissue. Aging of the cartilage is a different process from osteoarthritis, but it may predispose to it. Aging of the intervertebral disc accounts for the back pain that is often reported by the elderly. The collagen ratio of both the peripheral and central parts of the disc increases with aging, leading to stiffness and back pain; it may also result in disc herniation and spinal stenosis.

Changes in Renal Function

Aging is associated with glomerular sclerosis leading to a decrease of glomerular filtration rate (GFR) by 1 mL/min/year for every year after 40 years of age. This change is responsible for postoperative renal morbidity. However, plasma creatinine levels remain the same. In patients with normal creatinine levels (<1.3 mg/dL), a simple formula to calculate creatinine clearance and GFR is the Cockroft–Gault formula. Normal values of serum creatinine do not represent a normal GFR, however. Care should be taken to adjust the dosage of drugs excreted from the kidney to the GFR value. However, low GFR in the elderly does not necessarily imply renal disease. Both low extracellular fluid volume (postural hypotension, rapid weak pulse, low urine sodium despite "normal intake" and in the absence of diuretics) and malnutrition [malnutrition universal screening test (MUST) scale, low albumin, very low blood urea nitrogen (BUN) and BUN: Cr ratio <10] should be checked in all elderly patients with a low GFR. The ascending limb of Henle's loop progressively loses its capacity to reabsorb sodium, and this change is a major cause of dehydration and hyponatremia in the elderly. Low levels of aldosterone resulting from reduced renal production from kidneys may render them susceptible to higher levels of plasma potassium. This effect may be enhanced and become life-threatening with the use of spironolactone and acetyl cholinesterase (ACE) inhibitors. Because of the decreased capacity for alkaline excretion in elderly individuals with reduced GFR, the administration of lactate Ringers solution may greatly increase serum levels of bicarbonate (to which lactate is metabolized). Poor water conservation in the elderly is a result of the aforementioned changes and diminishing perception of thirst, but it is not mediated by serum antidiuretic hormone. Therefore, when oral hydration is prescribed for elderly patients, one must always bear in mind the fact that they are unlikely to drink the suggested amount of water.[11]

PREOPERATIVE EVALUATION

Before any elective operation in an elderly patient, three main issues have to be addressed:

1. What is the indication for operation?
2. What is the expected outcome of the surgical therapy in terms of QoL, physical independence, and cognitive impairment?
3. What is the informed preference of the patient (i.e. after having an informed discussion about therapeutic alternatives)?

Table 18.4	Preoperative evaluation of the geriatric patient checklist.
In addition to standard history and physical examination and laboratory tests:	
•	Assess cognitive ability and mental capacity of the patient to understand the treatment option
•	Set treatment goals taking into account preservation of functionality and quality of life
•	Discuss with the patient and his environment the patient's wishes, expectations after presenting all indicated treatment modalities. Discuss the possibility of needing assistance after operation
•	Perform a comprehensive geriatric assessment of the patient including indexes of cognitive function, nutritional status, independence in daily activities and instrumental daily activities, depression, polypharmacy, drug interactions, social support
•	Perform preoperative cardiac evaluation
•	Take accurate medication history, consider perioperative adjustments, and drug interactions

Most elderly surgical patients would not undergo even a low-risk treatment if marked functional or cognitive impairment was a likely outcome[12] (Table 18.4).

RISK–BENEFIT ASSESSMENT FOR OPERATION

For young patients, the usual goal of surgical therapy is cure of the underlying condition. From a technical point of view, there is no difference between resecting a tumor in an elderly patient or a young patient. On the other hand, the tolerance and the response of the elderly to trauma is greatly different and depends mainly on the frailty of the patient. Elderly patients attach greater importance to outcomes such as relief of symptoms and improvements in QoL. Arriving at an appropriate treatment decision with the elderly surgical patient is therefore typically more complicated. It requires a thorough assessment of:

- Treatment goals of the individual
- Therapeutic options
- Risks related to these options
- Natural history of the surgical condition.

Fit elderly patients may very appropriately choose to undergo a major surgical resection (e.g. for cure of a malignancy). By contrast, outcomes such as cure and extending life expectancy are likely to be less important for patients who face considerable risks from a major procedure. Limited surgical procedures and nonsurgical alternatives must be considered carefully for such patients in order to achieve goals such as relief of pain and other symptoms. Elective procedures can often be conducted with a low risk, even in frail patients, provided the surgeon has time to optimize the patient's condition. Early referral for elective care and an active approach to surgical problems are appropriate not only for the fit elderly patient, but for the frail and compromised individual as well.[13] The hazards of a procedure conducted as an emergency are much greater than when the surgical problem can be dealt with electively, and the difference can be especially marked in the elderly. Therefore, avoiding a future surgical emergency may be a very relevant consideration in determining the most appropriate approach to an elective problem. Similarly, for some patients with malignancy or an abdominal crisis, an appreciable operative mortality rate may be acceptable if the alternative to operation is early death.[14]

The risks associated with a major surgical procedure may be modest and entirely reasonable in an elderly patient who has maintained high levels of physical, social, and intellectual activity lifelong. Similarly, morbidity and mortality are very low following even major elective procedures in the "young" elderly (aged 65–74 years), especially when concomitant illnesses are absent or well controlled. By contrast, risks are greater in "middle" and "oldest" old patients, and the frail institutionalized patient with restricted mobility and multiple medical problems may face unacceptable risks from even minor interventions.

The nature and extent of the surgical procedure are important determinants of risk. Procedures that can be carried out under local anesthesia, such as inguinal hernia repair, are typically limited in extent and are accompanied by a near-zero mortality regardless of age and other factors.

A very important step is to evaluate whether the disease represents a threat to the patient's health or function within their remaining lifetime. The term "competing risks" describes how a number of diseases may compete to threaten the patient's life. It is well documented that both caregivers and health professionals underestimate the older person's willingness to undergo treatment. Furthermore, older people in general want to know about their diagnosis and prognosis. The vast majority of elderly patients want as much information as possible about their malignant disease. Decision making in geriatric surgery requires that the surgeon has sufficient knowledge about the remaining life expectancy of the patient, the anticipated natural progress of the cancer disease, and the operative risks for the individual patient.[15] It has been shown that after major abdominal operations most elderly patients will experience protracted disability at 6 months, and their physical and mental functioning may never return to preoperative levels. One should always keep in mind the old principle of medicine, "ωφελέειν ή μη βλάπτειν" (first do not harm), when balancing the risk of surgical operations in the elderly population. Is the patient more likely to die from worsening of his comorbid disease (competing risk) after operation than from an unoperated cancer or a hernia in the long term? This is the key question when balancing the risk-benefit of surgery in the elderly, and it is the most difficult one to answer. Sometimes it is better to discourage a patient from undergoing a high-risk operation that might potentially be lifesaving.

FRAILTY AND COMPREHENSIVE GERIATRIC ASSESSMENT

Many elderly patients, even those with a major comorbidity or disability, will have excellent outcomes even after major surgical operations. The identification of this important subgroup remains a great challenge in geriatric surgery. Common preoperative risk assessment tools such as American Society of Anesthesiologists (ASA) score and Lee cardiac index have many limitations in that they focus on a specific organ or system (Lee) or they depend on the subjective evaluation of a physician (ASA).

Functional reserve is defined as the difference between basal and maximum function of the organ, and it represents the ability of the organism to overcome stress or disease. The functional reserves decrease gradually during late adulthood, and they are markedly reduced in patients over 65 years (Fig. 18.2). The decrease of the functional reserves is a central concept of the principles of geriatric surgery (Tables 18.5 and 18.6). Comprehensive geriatric assessment (CGA) represents a multidimensional and multidisciplinary evaluation of the functional reserves. It is essentially a systematic approach to collecting data on the medical, psychological, social, and functional status of elderly patients. Comprehensive geriatric assessment has been extensively used in the field of gerontology,

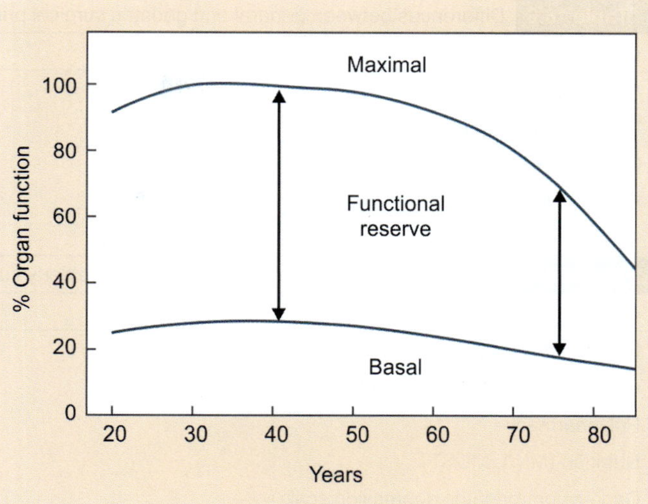

Fig. 18.2: Functional reserve is the difference between maximal and basal functions, and it is decreased with aging.
Source: Muravchick S. Preoperative assessment of the elderly patient. Anesthesiol Clin North Am. 2000;18(1):71-89.

Table 18.5 Principles of geriatric surgery.

Nonspecific or subtle clinical presentation of disease in combination with social factors in the elderly leads to delayed diagnosis
Reduced functional reserve as a result of aging and comorbidity: a. Render the elderly patients vulnerable to surgical stress and to surgical complications b. Result in poor outcomes of emergency operations in the elderly due to inability for a preoperative preparation and selection
Age per se is not a contraindication for any surgical operation

and its use, together with strong long-term management, improves survival and function in older persons.[16] In operative surgery, there is mounting evidence that CGA is a valuable tool in helping to make decisions about the suitability of elderly cancer patients for surgical intervention by predicting postoperative morbidity (Table 18.7). Information obtained through CGA is invaluable not only because it allows for better selection of patients, but mainly because it may lead to improvement of the provided surgical care through targeted interventions. From this point of view, CGA should be seen as a tool that optimizes surgical management and not as a means to exclude patients from operative treatment.[17]

Frailty is the main output measure of CGA. It characterizes patients with complex and challenging medical problems and a higher susceptibility to adverse outcomes, such as institutionalization. Frailty can be thought of as a decreased physiological reserve across multiple organ systems. It is defined as a condition or syndrome that

Table 18.6 Differences between general and geriatric surgical principles.

General surgery	*Geriatric surgery*
Aim: To cure the disease	Aim: To cure if possible/take care always
Investigation and diagnosis is important	Investigation as per the wishes and convenience of elders
Curative/extensive surgery	Curative/palliative surgery
Preserve life at any cost	Preserve functional capacity

Table 18.7 Main approaches on assessing frailty in the elderly surgical patients.

Comprehensive geriatric assessment	*Frailty phenotype*
Physical dependence (ADL, IADL)	*Shrinkage*: Unintentional weight loss >10 past year
Comorbidity (Charlson, cumulative illness rating)	*Weakness*: Decreased grip strength
Polypharmacy	*Exhaustion*: Self-reported poor energy and endurance
Nutrition (MNA, MUST)	*Low physical activity*: Low weekly energy expenditure
Depression (geriatric depression scale)	*Slowness*: Slow walking
Cognitive impairment (MMSE)	
Social support	

(ADL: Activities of daily life; IADL: Instrumental activities of daily life; MNA: Mini-nutritional assessment test; MUST: Malnutrition universal screening tool; MMSE: Mini-mental status examination).

results from a multisystem reduction in reserve capacity to the extent that a number of physiological systems are close to or pass the threshold for symptomatic clinical failure. Several methods of determining frailty have been reported, and there is no consensus on which one is best for use in the surgical population. However, two main definitions based on clusters of components are found in the literature: a physical phenotype of frailty, based on five measurable items of functional impairments, and a multidomain phenotype, based on the accumulation of identified deficits revealed by the CGA (Table 18.8). The physical phenotype considers disability and comorbidities such as dementia as distinct entities and therefore outcomes of the frailty syndrome, whereas comorbidity and disability can be components of the multidomain phenotype. The analytic nature of the multidomain phenotype possibly allows for better identification of targets for intervention. The CGA-based stratification has been shown to predict independently postoperative morbidity and mortality as well as prolonged hospitalization (Table 18.7).[18]

Comorbidity

The extent of comorbidity increases with age, and increasing comorbidity may substantially affect morbidity and mortality in older adults undergoing operation. In oncological patients, comorbidity is inversely related to overall survival independent of cancer stage. It increases both the risk of dying from other reasons than cancer and the toxicity of chemotherapy, and it is a major factor in discontinuation of treatment. In surgical patients, comorbidity increases significantly postoperative morbidity and mortality rates. Several indices have been proposed to quantify comorbidity in the elderly. The Charlson Comorbidity Index (CCI) is the most extensively studied of these. It is a weighted index that takes into account the number and severity of comorbid conditions. The CCI is a list of 19 conditions, each of which is assigned a weighting (1–6) (Table 18.9). Weightings reflect the ability of each condition to predict 1-year mortality. The CCI is the sum of the weightings for all conditions observed in a patient. Higher scores indicate greater comorbidity. Other comorbidity assessment tools include the Cumulative Illness Rating Scale (CIRS), which addresses all relevant physiological systems rather than being based on specific diagnoses.[19]

Physical Disability

Because physical disability and handicap cover a very wide and fundamental concern in health, a great number of scales designed to measure physical disability and daily function have been reported in the literature. The most widely used ADL (activities of daily life) scales are the Katz scale and the Barthel index. These scales have been developed to study the effects of disease and treatment in elderly and chronically ill patients. They quantify the degree of independence in bathing, dressing, using the

Table 18.8 Prospective studies in the effect of geriatric assessment before surgery.

First author/year	*N*	*Age (min, mean)*	*Disease*	*Type of geriatric assessment*	*Result*
Lasithiotakis et al. (2013)[51]	57	>65	Uncomplicated biliary disease—laparoscopic cholecystectomy	CGA (IADL, polypharmacy, ADL, MMSE, MUST, CCI)	Preoperative CGA may predicts postoperative complications and prolonged postoperative hospital stay
Pope et al. (2006)[52]	460	>65	Breast/gastrointestinal/genitourinary cancer	PACE (Satariano's modified index of comorbidities, Folstein MMS, ADL, IADL, geriatric depression scale, BFI, ECOG-PS, ASA)	PACE was associated with postoperative complications
Harari et al. (2007)[53]	83	>65	Orthopedic/ gastrointestinal/ urology/other	Screened through 18 risk factors → referral for broad assessment by a team (geriatrician, nurse specialist, occupational therapist, physiotherapist, social worker)	Improved postoperative outcomes in orthopedic patients (complications, length of stay)
Makary et al. (2010)[54]	594	>65	Wide range of operations, 57% abdominal, 58% for cancer	Shrinking Weakness (grip strength) Exhaustion Low activity Slowed walking speed	Frailty independently predicts postoperative complications, length of stay, and discharge to a skilled or assisted-living facility in older surgical patients and enhances conventional risk models.
Kristjanson et al. (2009)[55]	178	>70	Colorectal cancer surgery	PADL, IADL, CIRS, Polypharmacy, MNA, MMSE, GDS	CGA can identify frail patients at high risk for severe complication

(IADL: Instrumental activities of daily life; ADL: Activities of daily life; MMSE: Mini-mental status examination; MUST: Malnutrition universal screening tool; CCI: Charlson comorbidity index; CGA: Comprehensive geriatric assessment; PACE: Preoperative assessment of cancer in the elderly; BFI: Brief fatigue inventory; ECOG-PS: Eastern cooperative oncology group performance status; ASA: American society of anesthesiology score; CIRS: Cumulative illness rating scale; GDS: Geriatric depression scale; PADL: Personal activities of daily life).

Table 18.9 Charlson comorbidity index scoring.

Score	*Condition*
1	Myocardial infarction (history, not ECG changes only)
	Congestive heart failure
	Peripheral vascular disease (including aneurysm ≥ 6 cm
	Cerebrovascular disease: CVA with mild or no residua or TIA
	Dementia
	Chronic pulmonary disease
	Connective tissue disease
	Peptic ulcer disease
	Mild liver disease (without portal hypertension, includes chronic hepatitis)
	Diabetes without end organ disease (excludes diet-controlled alone)
2	Hemiplegia
	Moderated or severe renal disease
	Diabetes with end-organ damage (retinopathy, neuropathy, nephropathy or brittle diabetes)
	Tumor without metastases (exclude if >5 years from diagnosis)
	Leukemia (acute or chronic)
	Lymphoma
	Moderate or severe liver disease
3	Metastatic solid tumor
6	AIDS (nit just HIV positive)

For each decade >40 years of age, a score of 1 is added to the abode score.
(ECG: Electrocardiogram; CVA: Cerebrovascular accident; TIA: Transient ischemic attack; AIDS, acquired immunodeficiency syndrome, HIV: Human immunodeficiency virus).

Table 18.10 Parameters used to assess independence in physical activity.

Activities of daily life (Katz scale—ADL)	*Instrumental activities of daily life (Lawton Brody—IADL)*
Bathing	Ability to use telephone
Clothing	Shopping
Using toilet	Food preparation
Transfer from bed and to bed unassisted	Housekeeping
Urinary and/or stool incontinence	Laundry
Feeding	Mode of transportation
	Responsibility for own medications
	Ability to handle finances

Source: For details on how to use these scales refer to McDowell I.[20]
(ADL: Activities of daily life; IADL: Instrumental activities of daily life).

toilet, moving around the house, and eating—topics that Katz selected to represent "primary biological functions." These scales are concerned with more severe levels of disability mainly in institutionalized and elderly patients (Table 18.10). Lawton and Brody in 1969 extended the ADL concept to include problems more commonly experienced by those living in the community. Such problems were associated with limitation in activities such as mobility in the community, shopping, cooking, and managing money, all of which were termed instrumental activities of daily life (IADL). Therefore, IADL are more complex than ADL. They have been developed for use in the community care of the elderly, stressing the need to restore patients to meaningful social roles. Therefore, IADL scales are commonly used in the general elderly population who are less than severely handicapped.

Cognitive Assessment

Measures of mental status constitute a large part of clinical geriatrics because of their sharp increase with age and their impact on functional independence and successful aging. Problems of cognition form a wide spectrum ranging from mild decline in recall and memory and concentration to dementia, which is the most extreme form of cognitive deterioration. Dementia is difficult to measure. Since it involves a decline from a previously higher level of function, its measure is dynamic rather than static. Moreover, symptoms of dementia mimic other reversible conditions such as intoxication, depression, delirium, hypothyroidism, hyperparathyroidism, or cerebral infarction that must be excluded before dementia is diagnosed. A common condition among surgical patients is delirium, which is associated with alterations in the level of consciousness that lead to confusion and inability to focus and concentrate. The Mini-Mental State Examination (MMSE) has been the most widely used tool for assessing cognitive impairment. However, its use in the last years has declined due to significant copyright restrictions; newer, freely available tools such as the Saint Louis University Mental Status (SLUMS) (Table 18.11) have become popular. The MMSE was designed to give a practical clinical assessment of change in cognitive status in geriatric inpatients. It covers the person's orientation to time and place, recall ability, short-term memory, and mathematical ability. It may be used as a screening test for cognitive loss or as a brief bedside cognitive assessment. It cannot be used to diagnose dementia. The Short Portable Mental Status Questionnaire (SPMSQ) is a brief and simpler tool that can be also used to detect relatively severe levels of cognitive impairment.

Depression—Social Reserves

"Depression" covers a wide range of states, from feeling sad, helpless, or demoralized to grief, poor self-esteem or a major depressive episode. In surgical practice, depression is associated with worse outcomes due to noncompliance with treatment and rehabilitation. Major depression may lead even to suicide. Since depression is a very common and well-studied disease in the geriatric population, depression scales are among the best established in the literature. The Geriatric Depression Scale (GDS) is a screening test for depression in elderly people, a self-rating scale intended primarily for clinical applications (Table 18.12).

"Social support and reserve" is generally defined in terms of the availability of people whom the individual trusts, on whom he can rely, and who make him feel cared for and valued as a person. It embraces patients' living arrangements, particularly where and with whom they live (e.g. alone in an isolated house, in a busy apartment

Table 18.11 VAMC SLUMS examination.

VAMC SLUMS EXAMINATION

Questions about this assessment tool? E-mail aging@slu.edu

Name________________________ Age____________

Is the patient alert?____________ Level of education______________

Score	Item
__/1	❶ 1. What day of the week is it?
__/1	❶ 2. What is the year?
__/1	❶ 3. What state are we in?
	4. Please remember these five objects. I will ask you what they are later. Apple Pen Tie House Car
__/3	5. You have $100 and you go to the store and buy a dozen apples for $3 and a tricycle for $20. ❶ How much did you spend? ❷ How much do you have left?
__/3	6. Please name as many animals as you can in one minute. ⓪ 0-4 animals ❶ 5-9 animals ❷ 10-14 animals ❸ 15+ animals
__/5	7. What were the five objects I asked you to remember? 1 point for each one correct.
__/2	8. I am going to give you a series of numbers and I would like you to give them to me backwards. For example, if I say 42, you would say 24. ⓪ 87 ❶ 648 ❶ 8537
__/4	9. This is a clock face. Please put in the hour markers and the time at ten minutes to eleven o'clock. ❷ Hour markers okay ❷ Time correct
__/2	❶ 10. Please place an X in the triangle. ❶ Which of the above figures is largest?
__/8	11. I am going to tell you a story. Please listen carefully because afterwards, I'm going to ask you some questions about it. Jill was a very successful stockbroker. She made a lot of money on the stock market. She then met Jack, a devastatingly handsome man. She married him and had three children. They lived in Chicago. She then stopped work and stayed at home to bring up her children. When they were teenagers, she went back to work. She and Jack lived happily ever after. ❷ What was the female's name? ❷ What work did she do? ❷ When did she go back to work? ❷ What state did she live in?

______ TOTAL SCORE

SCORING		
High School Education		Less than High School Education
27-30	Normal	25-30
21-26	Mild Neurocognitive Disorder	20-24
1-20	Dementia	1-19

CLINICIAN'S SIGNATURE ______ DATE ______ TIME ______

SH Tariq, N Tumosa, JT Chibnall, HM Perry III, and JE Morley. The Saint Louis University Mental Status (SLUMS) Examination for detecting mild cognitive impairment and dementia is more sensitive than the Mini-Mental Status Examination (MMSE) - A pilot study. *Am J Geriatr Psych* 14:900-10, 2006.

Table 18.12 Geriatric depression assessment scale (examples of questions used to assess the risk for depression in the elderly).

Circle the answer that best describes how you felt over the past week:		
Are you basically satisfied with your life?	Yes	**No**
Do you often get bored?	**Yes**	No
Do you prefer to stay at home, rather than going out and doing things?	**Yes**	No
Do you feel full of energy?	Yes	**No**
Do you think that most people are better off than you are?	**Yes**	No

Bold answers are score with 1. A total score >4 (out of 15 question of the full test) indicates depression.

Table 18.13	Parameters assessed in the evaluation of social support.
Frequency and nature of social contacts (e.g. friends and senior citizens' groups):	
Family visits	
Marital status	
Religious or spiritual participation	
Driving and availability of other forms of transportation	
Caregivers and support systems available to the patient (e.g. church, senior citizens' groups, friends, neighbors)	
The ability of family members to help the patient (e.g. their employment status, their health, traveling time to the patient's home).	
The quality of the relationship of the patient with his family members and their attitude toward the patient (availability and willingness to help)	
Current and past hobbies	
Economic difficulties due to retirement, a fixed income, or death of a spouse or partner are discussed	

building), accessibility of their residence (e.g. upstairs or a hill), and what modes of transportation are available to them. Accessibility to healthcare and a pharmacy are important resources. Ideally, a home visit should provide critical information on, for example, the state of food in the refrigerator and daily activities from the condition of the bathroom. The number of rooms, number and type of phones, and the condition of plumbing and heating systems and air-conditioning are also determined, as is the availability of elevators and stairs. Having patients describe a typical day provides valuable information. Meaningful information that should be obtained from the patients is presented in Table 18.13. Several standardized scales to measure social support have been developed, but they have not validated so far in geriatric surgical patients.[20]

DIFFERENCES IN DISEASE PRESENTATION IN THE ELDERLY

The presentation of disease in elderly patients may be atypical, lacking customary clinical features. Several surgical conditions may be disguised by nonspecific geriatric syndromes and will rapidly improve if the precipitating factors are appropriately treated. Elderly patients tend to attribute early symptoms and signs to other coexisting diseases or aging itself, and they go to hospital only when the disease is advanced. Additionally, they may overuse analgesics, which mask early symptoms of serious surgical disease. This phenomenon causes appreciable delay in diagnosis and is associated with a worse overall outcome of the treatment. For example, acute mesenteric ischemia may be indicated only by acute confusion without abdominal pain or tenderness. The pain of appendicitis tends to begin low down in the abdomen but may be diffuse from the outset. Bacteremia, for example from infection of the biliary or urinary tracts, may present without fever but with mental confusion, decrease in functional status and vague malaise. Heart failure may be manifested as nocturnal agitation due to orthopnea, and edema in bedridden patients should be sought in the sacral region rather than the lower limbs.

The aged patient is less likely to mention any coexisting illness because they have a general tendency to minimize or illness (considering it an inevitable consequence of old age) or because a limitation in mobility (e.g. due to arthritic pain) has masked symptoms of underlying pathology. The latter is not uncommon. For example, if a patient does not exert himself or herself very much, then functional reserve of a particular organ system will not frequently be challenged. Therefore, a patient with underlying ischemic heart disease may never complain of angina or dyspnea.

Informed Consent

The patient, the consenting family member, or the legal guardian should be informed about the procedure and any potential complications or disabilities. Decisional capacity is a prerequisite for providing informed consent or refusal that is legally and ethically valid. A patient need not have the same level of awareness at all times to provide legally adequate informed consent. For instance, there may be windows of lucidity between episodes of increased confusion in the evening (sundowning). In most cases, the care team makes the proper judgment regarding decisional capacity. Formal mental status testing may help determine whether a patient should be considered capable of making this type of decision. If a patient is considered unable to provide informed consent, the first alternative is any specific written document or empowerment executed when the patient was capable of choosing and intending to direct their future care.

Drug History—Polypharmacy

Drug history: The drug history should be recorded, and a copy should be given to patients or their caregiver. It should contain:

- Drugs used
- Dose
- Dosing schedule
- Prescriber
- Reason for prescribing the drugs
- Precise nature of any drug allergies

All drugs used should be recorded: topical drugs (which may be absorbed systemically), over-the-counter drugs (which can have serious consequences if overused and may interact with prescription drugs), dietary supplements, and medicinal herb preparations (because many can interact adversely with prescription drugs). Either the patients or a family member should be asked to bring in all of the above drugs and supplements at the initial visit and periodically thereafter. Clinicians can make sure that patients have the prescribed drugs, but possession of these drugs does not guarantee adherence. Counting the number of tablets in each vial during the first and subsequent visits may be necessary. If someone other than a patient administers the drugs, that person is interviewed. Patients should be asked to demonstrate their ability to read labels (often printed in small type), open containers (especially the child-resistant type), and recognize drugs. Patients should be advised not to put their drugs into one container.

Polypharmacy and Drug Interactions

Elderly people tend to be on a number of different medications, which means there is an increased risk of a potential interaction with the agents used for the anesthetic. However, current long-term medications should usually be continued throughout the hospital stay. It is often difficult to ascertain exactly which medications are being taken, especially in cases of acute admission to hospital. Drugs may be inadvertently stopped, patients themselves may stop taking medication or they may be confused as to what drug they are taking. Alcohol and tobacco are the drugs most commonly stopped abruptly on admission to hospital, often with deleterious results. It may be necessary to obtain exact details of current medications and social habits from a relative or from the patient's general practitioner. Therefore, a thorough pharmacological history is necessary to establish whether the patient is on any drugs that could complicate the anesthetic procedure. A decision to either discontinue the therapy (if appropriate) or substitute it with an alternative drug will prevent such complications. Some examples of certain medicines that would have to be temporarily stopped or substituted include the following: anticoagulants, which should be discontinued before operation, and diuretics such as furosemide, which should be stopped the night before (to prevent a diuretic-induced volume depletion and hypokalemia during operation). However, warfarin should be replaced with heparin, which enables operations to be safely carried out only a few hours after its discontinuation because of its shorter half-life. Other medicines may need to be continued perioperatively. This is especially true for antihypertensive treatment (such as β-blockers and ACE inhibitors), as an adequate blood pressure control is essential in reducing the risk of perioperative ischemia. Withdrawal of such medications may have a detrimental effect on blood pressure and heart rate and increase perioperative morbidity and mortality.

Cardiovascular Evaluation

A practice guideline for perioperative cardiovascular evaluation for noncardiac surgery is proposed by the American College of Cardiology and American Heart Association Task Force.[21] Patients are assessed with a stepwise approach according to the clinical predictors, the risk of the proposed operation and the functional capacity.

The major clinical predictors are unstable coronary syndromes, decompensated CHF, significant arrhythmias, and severe valvular disease. Intermediate clinical predictors are mild angina pectoris, prior myocardial infarction, compensated or prior CHF, and diabetes mellitus. Minor clinical predictors are advanced age, abnormal ECG findings, rhythms other than sinus, low functional capacity, history of stroke, and uncontrolled systemic hypertension.

The assessment of functional capacity can be based on energy expenditure. Activities requiring one to four metabolic equivalents (METs) include eating, dressing, using the bathroom, walking indoors, walking one to two blocks on level ground, and doing light housework. Activities requiring 4–10 METs include climbing stairs or walking up a hill; running a short distance; scrubbing floors or moving furniture; and recreational activities, such as golf, bowling, dancing, and playing tennis. Self-reported exercise tolerance has been shown to be useful for helping to predict in-hospital perioperative risk, even when using relatively simple and familiar measures.

Surgical procedures are also classified as high risk, intermediate risk, or low risk. High-risk procedures include major emergency operations, aortic and other major vascular procedures, peripheral vascular procedures, and anticipated prolonged procedures associated with large fluid shifts or blood loss. Intermediate-risk surgical procedures include carotid endarterectomy, head and neck procedures, intraperitoneal and intrathoracic procedures, orthopedic surgery, and prostate surgery. Low-risk surgical procedures include endoscopic procedures, skin and breast operations, cataract surgery, and superficial procedures.

If an emergency operation is needed, the patient's risk stratification and management is assessed afterward. If the operation is urgent or elective and if the patient has had coronary revascularization within 5 years and has had no recurrent symptoms or signs, then the patient may be taken to the operating room. If the patient has recurrent symptoms or signs but has had a recent coronary evaluation, such as an angiogram or stress test, with a favorable result, then the operation is performed. If the patient has unfavorable results during coronary evaluation or if a change in symptoms occurs, then the following four clinical predictors are considered. If the patient has major clinical predictors, consider performing coronary angiography or delaying the operation.

1. For high-risk patients who are not candidates for coronary revascularization, the surgeon may wish to either (1) delay the upcoming operation if the patient's overall status can be improved or (2) cancel the operation if the risk posed by the patient's surgical condition is lower than the patient's cardiac risk.
2. The use of coronary revascularization as a preventive step to reduce cardiac risk before noncardiac surgery has not been studied prospectively. A large retrospective analysis suggests that any decrease in risk produced by having coronary artery bypass graft surgery before having noncardiac surgery was offset by the risk posed by the angiography and coronary artery bypass grafting.
3. The clinician deciding whether to refer the intermediate- or high-risk patient for revascularization must weigh the added risks posed by angiography and coronary artery bypass grafting (or percutaneous transluminal coronary angioplasty or stent procedure) against the potential reduction in short-term (perioperative) and long-term risk. Some patients have an independent need for coronary bypass. In these patients, the planned noncardiac operation may lead to investigation into coronary revascularization with a goal of reducing long-term morbidity and mortality. Whether the patient is a candidate for coronary revascularization should therefore be determined based on the same clinical grounds that govern the need for coronary revascularization in the nonoperative setting. An individualized approach that weighs patient preferences, the urgency of the upcoming operation and the urgency of the patient's coronary status is recommended.
4. When the clinical predictors are intermediate, minor or absent, decisions regarding the operation and further testing depend on the risk of the procedure and the capacity patient's functional noninvasive tests available for further risk stratification include those that assess left ventricular function (radionuclide angiography), cardiac ischemia (exercise or pharmacologic stress testing and ambulatory electrocardiographic monitoring), or both (dobutamine stress echocardiography).

Exercise stress testing cannot be performed in a substantial proportion of patients who are undergoing vascular surgery (30–70%) or in patients with diseases that impair walking ability.

Dipyridamole-thallium imaging and dobutamine stress echocardiography (especially if the results are negative) provide useful information on stratification for patients having vascular surgery who are deemed to be at intermediate risk on clinical evaluation.

Although not well studied, very elderly persons can have presbycardia (decreased function of cardiac muscle) and silent coronary artery disease even in the absence of cardiac risk factors. Consider noninvasive testing if a very stressful operation is planned.

Perioperative β-blocker therapy has been shown to reduce long-term (6-month) mortality rates, with few adverse effects. Thus, the perioperative use of atenolol is recommended in patients with coronary artery disease or risk factors for coronary artery disease unless the patient has a major contraindication such as asthma. A study by Siddiqui and colleagues demonstrated that perioperative β-blocker therapy was underused in patients with risk factors for coronary artery disease, despite evidence that its use in appropriate cases decreases mortality.

Because of the lack of controlled evidence, no recommendations can be made either for or against the use of other medical therapies, such as digitalis, nitrates, or calcium-channel antagonists. Therapy with these drugs should be continued or started based on the same criteria that would apply in the nonoperative setting.

Hypertension

If the initial evaluation indicates mild or moderate hypertension and no associated metabolic or cardiovascular abnormalities, there is no reason to delay the operation. Antihypertension medications should be continued during the perioperative period; however, a diastolic blood pressure of 110 mm Hg or higher requires preoperative control. Importantly, β-blockers and clonidine should not be withdrawn because of a potential rebound in heart rate and blood pressure. In the postoperative period, acute elevations in blood pressure are common. Labile blood pressures, sometimes with marked hypotension, can occur in hypertensive patients. Occasionally, uncontrolled pain, ischemia, fluid overload, emergence excitement, electrolyte abnormalities, anxiety, or a distended bladder can cause hypertension. As much as 30% of postoperative hypertension is idiopathic and resolves within 3 hours. When secondary causes are not responsible for the rise in the blood pressure, treatment should be considered with calcium channel antagonists, β-blockers, and drugs that block both α- and β-adrenergic receptors. Hydralazine, a potent vasodilator, should be avoided in patients with hypertensive hypertrophic cardiomyopathy because the diastolic filling can be compromised by reflex tachycardia from rapid vasodilatation.[22]

COMMON PERIOPERATIVE ISSUES IN THE ELDERLY

Respiratory System

All anesthetics (with some exceptions such as nitrous oxide) depress the respiratory centers and have a marked effect on gas exchange. As a result, one of the many responsibilities of the anesthetist is that of the patient's airway and respiratory system. Pulmonary disease increases the risk of postoperative complications, accounting for 40% of postoperative complications and 20% of deaths. Age-related changes, such as increased closing volumes and decreased expiratory flow rates, predispose older persons to pulmonary complications. Interventions such as preoperative smoking cessation, antimicrobial therapy for bronchitis, perioperative bronchodilator therapy, optimization of therapy for uncompensated right heart failure, inhalation of humidified gas, postural drainage, and chest physiotherapy can reduce pulmonary complications, lower mortality, and shorten hospital stays. Pulmonary function testing is indicated in patients considered for lung resection. Abnormalities suggesting an increased risk of postoperative pulmonary complications include a vital capacity of < 50% of predicted, a forced expiratory volume in one second of < 2 L or < 50% predicted, and the presence of substantial hypoxemia or hypercapnia.

Postoperatively, an age-associated weakness of the intercostals and accessory muscles of respiration will reduce the ability of the patient to cough forcibly. However, they should be encouraged to do so in order to remove secretions and prevent consolidation. Atelectasis and chest infections are more common in the elderly due to degeneration of the respiratory epithelium and a resultant ineffective mucociliary action (further compounded if the patient has a history of smoking, which is common in the older population). A combination of the residual effects of anesthesia, prolonged effect of neuromuscular blocking agents and postoperative pain can all contribute to these respiratory complications. However, problems can be reduced if it is remembered that the perioperative opioid dose required for an elderly patient is much less than that required in a younger adult. Complications with the respiratory system often present postoperatively, and steps should be taken to reduce the likelihood of such occurrences by a combination of appropriate and adequate analgesia, early mobilization and supplemental oxygen for at least 12 hours postoperatively or for a number of days should pulse oximetry indicate.

Early resumption of sitting and standing will minimize the decrease in functional residual capacity and closure of small airways that occur in the supine position. Effective postoperative analgesia is essential to facilitate mobilization and to minimize changes in vital capacity and functional residual capacity. Parenteral narcotics have been associated with more frequent respiratory disturbances following operation, and epidural techniques and nonnarcotic analgesics may therefore be particularly valuable in the elderly patient.[4] Because of a loss of elastic lung recoil and other factors, the lung volume at which small airway closure begins to occur is larger in older subjects, promoting atelectasis and resulting in ventilation–perfusion mismatch and impaired gas exchange. These consequences emphasize the importance of resuming an upright posture and expanding lung volumes postoperatively. Measures such as incentive spirometry, positive pressure breathing and regular breathing exercises may complement the basic measures of pain management and mobilization. Supplemental oxygen may be useful for blunting the lowest values of oxygen saturation and the associated increases in heart rate in the early postoperative period.[50] It does not alter the underlying mechanisms responsible, however, and should be used with some rationale since it may present an additional minor barrier to mobility and self-care.

Preoperative strategies for preventing postoperative pulmonary complications include preoperative optimization of pulmonary function in patients whose COPD and asthma is poorly controlled, smoking cessation, preoperative intensive inspiratory muscle training and selective pulmonary function tests.[23]

Neuropsychiatric Disorders

Delirium, dementia, and depression are the common important syndromes to consider. The major manifestation of delirium is an abrupt change in cognition and consciousness. In hospitalized elderly persons with delirium lasting >1 week, the likelihood is that severe cognitive impairment, sleep pattern disturbance, and mood lability will be worse compared to those with delirium of shorter duration. New-onset visual hallucinations in elderly patients are more suggestive of delirium than of a new psychiatric disorder. Delirium occurs after general surgery in 10–15% of patients, after orthopedic surgery in 28–61% of patients, and after cataract surgery in 1–3% of patients; it is associated with higher rates of morbidity and poor outcome. The length of stay in the hospital for a patient with delirium is increased by 60%, and their rate for nursing home placement is five times higher. Intraoperative factors include the type of operation, hypoperfusion, and anesthetic drugs. Several studies have found no difference in the effects of general, epidural, or spinal anesthesia on postoperative delirium rates if medications are controlled for in the analysis. Intraoperative meperidine use increases the risk of delirium by two to seven times that of other opioids. Intraoperative use of barbiturates and long-acting benzodiazepines also increases the risk of postoperative delirium. Postoperative factors associated with delirium include hypoxia and hypocapnia.[24]

The rate of postoperative delirium decreases from 61% to 48% when geriatric assessment is performed both preoperatively and postoperatively and when appropriate interventions are implemented. Perioperative interventions should focus on thrombosis prophylaxis, oxygen therapy, prevention and treatment of perioperative hypotension, and prompt identification and treatment of postoperative complications. Improving orientation by placing clocks, calendars, and appropriate lighting; decreasing sensory overload; providing reassurance; and using personal hearing aids and eyeglasses are some of the nonpharmacologic interventions for delirium. Intubated patients should have access to communication via word boards and paper and pencil.

When alcohol abuse is suspected, the patient should be questioned about symptoms or signs of physiologic dependence and any organ damage. Withdrawal from alcohol or benzodiazepines should be considered in delirium that occurs within 24–72 hours of hospitalization. Prophylactic treatment for anticipated alcohol withdrawal should include thiamine and short-acting benzodiazepines. Elective surgery should be delayed until the risk of delirium tremens has abated. Patients with Parkinson disease require special attention during the perioperative period. Withholding medications in patients who are unable to take anything by mouth can aggravate symptoms. Patients may experience hypoxia from stiffening of chest wall muscles, transfer dysphagia, and worsened tremor (which can cause increased pain at the operative site). If possible, a weighted feeding tube can be used to administer the medication at appropriate times. Patients who take levodopa may develop orthostatic hypotension, nightmares, hallucinations, and, occasionally, delirium, all of which may be worsened by an anesthetic and operation. Anticholinergic drugs, such as trihexyphenidyl, are used alone in the early stages of treatment and later to supplement levodopa. Adverse effects may include dry mouth, urinary retention, constipation, confusion, delirium, and impaired thermoregulation due to decreased sweating. Meperidine and propoxyphene should be avoided in elderly persons because of the accumulation of toxic metabolites and the potential severe reaction.

Of all patients admitted for repair of hip fractures, 15% have dementia. However, older patients may easily enter into a state of confusion following stresses such as infection or dehydration, which are potentially reversible. Simple steps such as adequate fluid maintenance and prophylactic antibiotic treatment prove to be useful in reducing the incidence of such states postoperatively. Depression is common among older patients in general and can be exacerbated by any acute illness or hospitalization.[25]

Thromboembolic Disease

The Fifth American College of Chest Physicians Consensus Conference on Antithrombic Therapy recommends the following for older surgical patients:

General surgery without clinical risk factors for thrombosis[26]: Elastic stockings or intermittent pneumatic compression (IPC) is recommended during the operation and throughout the postoperative period or low-dose unfractionated heparin (LDUH) should be given 2 hours before and every 12 hours after the operation.

General surgery with any clinical risk factors, such as prolonged immobilization or paralysis, obesity, varicose veins, CHF, or pelvic or leg fractures: Low molecular weight heparin (LMWH) or LDUH should be given every 8 hours. If the patient is also prone to bleeding or infection, IPC can be used instead.

General surgery with multiple clinical risk factors or with a history of previous deep vein thrombosis, malignancy, stroke, spinal cord injury, or a hip fracture: LDUH or LMWH combined with IPC should be used; for very high-risk patients, perioperative warfarin is an alternative.

Total hip replacement: Postoperative LMWH should be given every 12 hours, low-intensity warfarin therapy (to keep international normalized ratio of 2–3) should be initiated preoperatively or immediately postoperatively.

Total knee replacement: Postoperative LMWH should be given every 12 hours. Intermittent pneumatic compression is the most effective nonpharmacologic regimen and is comparable to LMWH.

Hip fracture repair: Fixed-dose LMWH or low-intensity warfarin should be started preoperatively.

Thermoregulation

Anesthesia impairs the thermoregulatory response (which would ordinarily bring about vasoconstriction and shivering) due to its inhibition of autonomic function. An immobile, peripherally dilated patient in a cold theatre is thus at risk of becoming hypothermic unless preventive measures are taken. This risk is much greater in an elderly patient, even under normal circumstances, because older people are generally not able to regulate their temperature as well and their basal metabolic rate is lower (they produce heat more slowly). Adverse effects of perioperative hypothermia are associated with cardiac arrhythmias, reduced cardiac output, altered oxyhemoglobin dissociation and vasoconstriction, and ultimately decreased tissue oxygenation, impaired coagulation and platelet function (thus increasing the risk of blood loss intraoperatively), prolongation of drug effects, immune dysfunction, and resultant increased risk of infection. Steps to prevent hypothermia, which can be carried out in the pre-, intra- and postoperative setting for major procedures, include preoperative skin preparation and postoperative cleansing using warmed solutions, conservation of heat using active air warming systems, minimizing exposed surfaces, warming intravenous fluids and blood products, using humidified gases and forced-air warming, warming the operating room until the patient is covered, wrapping the patient up with blankets and covering the head if possible.

Regional versus General Anesthesia

A regional anesthetic confers a smaller risk of postoperative hypoxemia as it avoids the negative respiratory effects of a general anesthetic such decreased pulmonary function and gas exchange. However, the changes in the healthy aged respiratory system alone are not sufficient to warrant a different form of anesthetic.

A high regional blockade could impair respiratory muscle function, leading to difficulty in mechanical respiration. Additionally, since there is a reduction in upper airway tone in the elderly, there is an increased risk of airway obstruction (particularly during sleep). Should a regional anesthetic be administered, the anesthetist must be aware of this risk, especially if sedation has been given. Furthermore, the practicalities of a regional anesthetic may not be feasible in a confused elderly patient with impaired cognitive function. Regardless of the regional technique, failure to achieve or maintain the required anesthesia can occur on occasion and necessitate general anesthesia. A combination of major regional and general anesthesia is used increasingly in an attempt to achieve the advantages of each. Placement of a catheter in the epidural space allows titration of local anesthetics to achieve the desired level of block during the surgical procedure together with postoperative administration of local anesthetics and/or narcotics for analgesia.

Local Anesthesia

The use of local anesthesia for surgical procedures has increased considerably in recent years as methods for minimizing postoperative pain and length of stay have been explored. Operations using local anesthesia, such as elective inguinal hernia repair, are typically limited in extent, but are accompanied by a near zero mortality. Satisfaction among motivated and cooperative patients is high, and early discharge is facilitated by effective pain management.

The clearance of lidocaine (lignocaine) and bupivacaine is reduced in the elderly, who are probably more prone to cardiac dysrhythmias and therefore to the cardiotoxicity of local anesthetic drugs, especially bupivacaine. Care should be taken in deciding upon the amount of local anesthetic used in the elderly patient and in avoiding an inadvertent vascular injection.

PAIN MANAGEMENT

Optimal management combines pharmacologic and other techniques. Simple psychological preparation, instruction and reassurance have been shown to reduce postoperative narcotic use and shorten length of stay and should be a routine element of a pain management plan.[27]

Patient-controlled analgesia: Patient-controlled analgesia (PCA) using intravenous opioid administration has gained widespread acceptance as its effectiveness and patient satisfaction have become apparent, especially when compared with traditional, intramuscular, nurse-administered opioids.[27]

The major side effects are those of systemic opioid administration. Patients with cognitive impairments, whether acute or longstanding, may be unable to master the technique of PCA and therefore receive inadequate or excessive analgesia.

Bolus or continuous epidural administration: Bolus or continuous epidural administration of opioids or local anesthetics for patients undergoing major abdominal, pelvic, and thoracic procedures has received considerable attention in recent years. Continuous epidural analgesia has been shown to reduce the incidence of postoperative deep venous thrombosis in some settings, to improve respiratory function, and to minimize ileus following abdominal procedures. Respiratory depression is, however, more severe in the elderly than in younger patients and may occur as a result of absorption of opioids into the bloodstream or cephalad migration in the cerebrospinal fluid, depending upon the lipid solubility of the specific opioid. Urinary retention may accompany epidural administration of both opioids and local anesthetics. Epidural local anesthesia may also cause motor and sympathetic blockade. However, in the elderly patient who is confused following major surgery, epidural opioid administration may achieve more reliable anesthesia than patient-controlled intravenous administration.

Nonsteroidal anti-inflammatory drugs (NSAIDs): The role of NSAIDs in postoperative analgesia is broadening, particularly as an adjunct to narcotics. By reducing the quantity of narcotics required to achieve effective analgesia, adverse effects are minimized as well. NSAIDs have both peripheral and central effects and can be given parenterally, orally or as a suppository. The risk of NSAID-induced gastritis and clinically important bleeding appears to be low. NSAIDs should be used with caution in elderly surgical patients, especially those who have hypovolemic states and those known to have renal dysfunction.[28]

NUTRITION

Nutritional screening has been defined as "a process to identify an individual who is malnourished or who is at risk for malnutrition to determine if a detailed nutrition assessment is indicated." It should be carried out within 24 hours of admission to an acute care center. The goal of nutritional assessment is to identify any specific nutrition risk(s) and determine the presence of definite malnutrition. The assessment may lead to recommendations for improving nutritional status, for example by changing the diet or giving enteral nutrition (EN) or parenteral nutrition (PN), or merely a recommendation to repeat the screening in due course. Nutritional assessment has been defined as "a comprehensive approach to diagnosing nutrition problems that uses a combination of the following: medical, nutrition, and medication histories; physical examination; anthropometric measurements; and laboratory data." It provides a logical basis for nutritional intervention (Table 18.14).

In designing a nutritional program, it should be remembered that most sick elderly patients require at least 1.0–1.2 g protein/kg per day and 20–30 kcal/kg per day of nonprotein energy, depending on the severity of the disease, the degree of current inflammation/catabolism, the physical activity level and the need for and time course of rehabilitation. Although current literature review suggests that slightly higher protein amounts (1.5 g/kg per day) are warranted in the malnourished elderly to improve nitrogen balance and restore lean body mass, studies specifically addressing protein supply by parenteral route are still lacking. Nevertheless, in acutely hospitalized older patients energy intake is rarely sufficient to cover the basal energy expenditure. Many older people also suffer from specific micronutrient deficiencies, which should be corrected by supplementation.

Experts define malnutrition as "an acute, subacute, or chronic state of nutrition, in which varying degrees of over nutrition or under nutrition with or without inflammatory activity have led to a change in body composition and diminished function." Parameters used to diagnose malnutrition in the screening and assessment processes

Table 18.14 Mini-nutritional assessment screening tool.

Screening questions	*Scoring*
Has food intake declined over the past three months due to loss of appetite, digestive problems, chewing, or swallowing difficulties?	0 = Severe decrease in food intake 1 = Moderate decrease in food intake 2 = No decrease in food intake
Involuntary weight loss during the last 3 months?	0 = Weight loss > 3 kg or > 6.6 pounds 1 = Does not know 2 = Weight loss 1–3 kg or 2.2–6.6 pounds 3 = No weight loss
Mobility?	0 = Bed or chair bound 1 = Able to get out of bed/chair, but does not go out 2 = Goes out
Has the patient suffered psychological stress or acute disease in the past 3 months?	0 = Yes 2 = No
Neuropsychological problems?	0 = Severe dementia or depression 1 = Mild dementia 2 = No psychological problems
Body mass index (BMI)? (weight in kg/height in m)	0 = BMI < 19 1 = BMI 19 to < 21 2 = BMI 21 to < 23 3 = BMI 23 or greater
If unable to obtain BMI: Calf circumference (CC) in cm	0 = CC < 31 3 = CC 31 or greater
Screening score (max. 14 points) 12–14 points: normal nutritional status 8–11 points: at risk of malnutrition 0–7 points: malnourished	

reflect both nutrition intake and severity and duration of disease. These factors may lead to changes in body habitus and metabolic alterations associated with poor outcome. An International Consensus Guideline Committee has proposed an approach to diagnosing malnutrition in adults based on etiology, thus integrating the present understanding of inflammatory responses to disease and trauma. The Committee proposed the following nutritional diagnoses: (1) starvation-related malnutrition, which is chronic starvation without inflammation, (2) chronic disease-related malnutrition, where inflammation is chronic and of mild to moderate degree, and (3) acute disease or injury-related malnutrition, where inflammation is acute and severe.

Institution of PN in older subjects generates the same medical and ethical problems as EN and so the same questions should be asked:

- Does the patient suffer from a condition that is likely to benefit from PN?
- Will PN improve outcome and/or accelerate recovery?
- If the patient suffers from an incurable disease, can QoL and well-being still be maintained or improved by PN?
- Does the anticipated benefit of nutritional support outweigh the potential risks?
- Does PN accord with the expressed or presumed will of the patient, or in the case of incompetent patients, of his/her legal representative?
- Are there sufficient resources available to manage PN properly?
- If long-term PN implies a different living situation (e.g. institution vs. home), will the patient derive benefit from it?

Parenteral nutrition is a safe and effective therapeutic procedure provided that it is managed by an experienced team. Age per se is not a reason to exclude patients from PN. Parenteral nutrition may allow adequate nutrition in patients who cannot meet their nutritional requirements via the enteral route, and should be limited to situations in which EN is contraindicated or poorly tolerated. Parenteral nutrition support should be instituted in the older person facing a period of starvation of > 3 days when oral nutrition or EN is impossible, and when oral nutrition or EN has been or is likely to be insufficient for > 7–10 days.

Pharmacological sedation or physical restraining of the patient to make PN possible is not justified. Although PN is a useful method of nutritional support in malnourished patients, unlike EN and oral nutritional supplements it a much less often justified in geriatric patients. Insulin resistance leading to a lower glucose utilization and hyperglycemia, together with impairment of cardiac and renal functions, are the most relevant features. They may warrant the use of formulae with higher lipid content providing up to 50% of total energy intake. Deficiencies in vitamins, trace elements, and minerals should be suspected in older subjects. The effect of nutritional support on restoration of depleted body cell mass is lower in elderly patients than in younger subjects; however, the oxidation capacity for lipid emulsions is not negatively influenced by age. Both the central and peripheral routes can be used for PN in geriatric patients, but the osmolarity of peripheral fluids should not exceed 850 mOsmol/L.

Although PN can improve nutritional status in older as well as younger adults, active physical rehabilitation is essential for muscle gain. Peripheral or central venous access for fluid and electrolyte replacement is mandatory in emergencies and in situations where strict fluid balance is required. The subcutaneous route is possible for fluid administration in order to correct mild to moderate dehydration but not to meet other nutrient requirements. Parenteral nutrition can support improvement of functional status, although the margin of improvement is lower than in younger patients, and it can reduce mortality and morbidity rates. However, as PN has more complications than EN, the oral and enteral route should be used whenever possible. There are no specific complications of PN in geriatric patients, but problems tend to be more frequent due to associated comorbidities. Parenteral nutrition and parenteral hydration should be considered as medical treatments rather than as basic care. Both require intravenous cannulation and a physician's prescription. Their use should therefore be balanced against a realistic chance of improvement in the general condition.[29–32]

ELECTIVE VERSUS EMERGENCY REFERRALS

Referrals for a surgical opinion in the frail nursing home patient are often not sought until the problem has become urgent or complications have arisen. The added clinical complexity and the acute physiologic stress in this situation results in much greater risks and poorer outcomes following emergency than elective operations.[33]

An active approach to surgical consultations should be adopted for nursing home patients and the frail elderly, as problems can often be managed safely and effectively on an elective basis and their evolution into more hazardous emergency problems forestalled. The care of nursing home patients and the frail elderly in general is more challenging in many respects than that of younger and fitter patients. It should be undertaken by surgeons who are interested and knowledgeable about the specific issues that arise and are prepared to:

- Deal with the complexities imposed by comorbidities, cognitive impairments, and do not resuscitate status.
- Carefully assess risk before operation and "survivability" in the face of complications.
- Educate their colleagues, and patients and their families, about current operative and other approaches to surgical problems.

The involvement of a geriatric consultation team has been shown to be effective in improving the survival and functional status of elderly patients admitted to hospital with acute medical problems who have moderate to severe impairments, affecting their physical, cognitive, social functioning and ability to conduct activities of daily living.

Another study of such patients showed that care in a special unit designed to assist them to maintain or achieve independence in self-care improved their ability to look after themselves and reduced the likelihood of discharge to a long-term care institution.[34]

It remains to be established whether a combined consultation service involving physicians, surgeons, anesthesiologists, and other experts would improve outcomes for frail elderly surgical patients.

SPECIFIC SURGICAL PROBLEMS

Geriatric Trauma

Elderly patients are less likely to sustain serious injury than their younger counterparts, but they are at higher risk of death following trauma. The most common causes of death after injury are falls, car accidents, and burns. Falls are very common in the elderly, accounting for approximately half of deaths due to injury. Even minor injuries in this age group can cause major complications because of the reduced functional reserves and the multiple medications, especially anticoagulants. Maintenance of the airway patency is challenging due to dentition, small oral aperture, and cervical arthritis. Chest injuries and rib fractures are common in the elderly but are less well tolerated and may progress to respiratory deficiency. Normal blood pressure in the chronic hypertensive patient and normal heart rate in the case of β2-blockers may falsely indicate normovolemia. Additionally chronic use of diuretics is usually associated with depleted intravascular volume and electrolytes disturbances that may be either the cause of injury or factors that complicate it. Neurological examination of the patient can be also problematic due to the possibility of pre-existing neurological and cognitive deficits. Primary management of the injured patient should follow the advanced trauma life support protocol and the rule ABCDE (airway, breathing, circulation, deficit, environment)[35]:

When evaluating an injured elderly patient always consider the possibility of *abuse*. Physical findings suggesting abuse include the following:

1. Multiple contusions in various stages of healing or in unusual parts that are difficult to reach (i.e. back, genitals)
2. Periorbital ecchymoses and nasal injuries
3. Oral injury
4. Unusual alopecia pattern
5. Fractures in unusual sites for elderly (i.e. other than hip, humerus, vertebrae)
6. Multiple burns in various sites and in different stages of healing
7. The caregiver or husband does not want to leave the patient alone despite our insistence or when he/she does not appear to the hospital at all or he/she does not let the patient describe the accident or the patient and/or the caregiver is unexplainably fearful
8. The injury pattern does not agree with the referred mechanism of injury. In the case of suspected or diagnosed abuse, it is necessary to inform police and social services, depending on the legislature of each country, so as to protect the patient from his abusive environment.

Breast Cancer

More than half of new breast cancers are diagnosed in patients older than 65 years. Colloid and papillary carcinoma, which has more favorable prognosis, is more common in the elderly but still represent only 10% of the total. On the other hand, inflammatory and myeloid cancer is less common in the elderly women. Older patients are more likely to have breast cancer with estrogen receptor (ER) and progesterone receptor expression, with or without HER2 overexpression. HER2-positive tumors decrease from 22% among women younger than 40 years to 10% in women 70 years or older. Tumor size and nodal involvement increase with age, at least partly explained by delayed diagnosis in older women. Screening for breast cancer reduces mortality, especially in ages 50–69 years, but there is evidence from several studies that its benefit may extend to age 70 or greater.

Total mastectomy in the elderly is associated with a low mortality of $<1\%$ and an overall morbidity of $<10\%$. In patients with severe comorbidities, mastectomy with local anesthesia or nerve block may be considered and may offer adequate local control of the disease. Contraindications to breast-conserving surgery are the same as in younger patients, but elderly patients may prefer this type of treatment. Postoperative radiotherapy has a major impact on local recurrence but probably a lower effect on overall survival. For patients >70 years lumpectomy plus tamoxifen is a rationale treatment for small, ER-positive breast cancers. Issues regarding access and transport of the patient for postoperative radiotherapy may influence the treatment schedule; partial breast irradiation (5 days) or intraoperative radiotherapy (IORT) can be attractive modalities in selected patients. When considering omitting postoperative RT after conservative operations, one should take into account that most recurrences occur within 5 years of operation and that radiation therapy is well tolerated by elderly patients.

Failure to identify the sentinel node may be higher in the elderly as well as the incidence of postoperative lymphedema. For patients with clinical axillary metastasis, lymph node dissection is the treatment of choice. In frail women with major comorbidity, tamoxifen or an aromatase inhibitor may appropriate primary treatment for receptor-positive breast cancer. For the rare case of a frail patient with a receptor-negative tumor, wide resection alone may be the appropriate treatment. If the life expectancy is longer than 5 years, adjuvant chemotherapy may be considered. However, in patients over 70 years, death due to non-breast cancer causes is higher in all stages of the disease except for those with distant metastasis.[36,37]

Pressure Sores

Prolonged pressure in an elderly patient with limited mobility results in compromised oxygenation of soft tissues, ischemia and tissue necrosis. External pressure lasting >2 hours leads to irreversible tissue damage. The severity of such damage ranges from ulceration to infection and exposure of bones. Most pressure sores occur during the first 14 days in hospital and correlate with the acute phase of the illness. Moisture of the surrounding area and incontinence, not rough repositioning of the patient, contribute to pressure sore formation. Patient-related factors include malnutrition and edema. Common positions on the bed may worsen bed sores. The semirecumbent position with the head of the bed elevated causes high shearing forces on the soft tissues because they hold by friction the patient from sliding down. The Braden scale for predicting pressure sore risk is a useful nursing tool that takes into account all these risk factors. The first step in assessing a bed sore is careful history and physical examination to determine risk factors. Secondly, the stage of the sore is classified as follows:

- Stage I: Skin intact but erythematous for >1 hour after relief of pressure.
- Stage II: Blistering or other lesions in the dermis with or without infection.
- Stage III: Subcutaneous destruction extending into muscle, with or without infection.
- Stage IV: Involvement of bone or joint with or without infection.
- Suspected deep tissue injury: Purple- or maroon-localized area of discolored intact skin or blood-filled blister due to damage of underlying soft tissue from pressure or/and shear.
- Unstageable: Full-thickness tissue loss in which the base of the ulcer is covered by slough and/or eschar in the wound bed.

A careful distinction should be made between osteitis (often observed in stage IV pressure ulcers) and osteomyelitis. Osteitis is an inflammation of the most superficial necrotic aspect of the exposed bone that is colonized by skin flora. This condition can be tolerated very well by the immunocompetent patient for long periods. Osteomyelitis is infection of the bone requiring bone biopsy and culture for definite diagnosis. Clinical suspicion of osteomyelitis should be raised in the presence of pus that is not controlled by adequate surgical debridement and/or signs of systemic sepsis. Bone scans and MRI are commonly used to diagnose osteomyelitis underlying pressure sores and can be particularly useful in the case of complex sores associated with perianal fistulas, or bone abscesses. Infections of the soft tissue are usually polymicrobial. *Staphylococci* and *Streptococci* are the most common organisms cultured from infected ulcers followed by *E. coli*, *Proteus*, *Bacteroides*, and *Pseudomonas*. Deep tissue cultures give better sensitivity results than swab cultures. Involvement of an infectious disease specialists is necessary in the case of sepsis due to pressure sores and osteomyelitis.

Management of pressure sores should address four parameters: reduction of pressure, surgical debridement, treatment of infection, and optimization of the nutrition of the patient.[38]

Pressure reduction involves frequent (every 1–2 hours) turning of the patient, use of specific air mattresses, and use of pads or pillows under the lower legs to prevent heel ulcers. Pharmacological or surgical treatment of contractures and spasticity may alleviate pressure from certain body parts. Urinary catheters and, in rarer cases, colostomy may be necessary for the treatment of large, contaminated, persisting pressure sores. Nursing care is of the utmost importance in keeping the area clean and dry and reducing shearing forces during turning and transport. Wound debridement may be mechanical or chemical. Sharp excision demands careful recognition of necrotic tissue. Usually the extent of necrosis is larger than that of the superficial skin, but bleeding during debridement is an indication of overzealous surgery. Chemical debridement may include a group of agents commercially available (proteolytics, collagenases, etc.). Necrotic infected tissue demands surgical debridement, however. Heel sores seldom need surgical debridement as opposed to local care with dressings and antibiotics (to maintain as much tissue as possible). After debridement, regular care with packing materials and frequent assessment for infection or necrosis should be maintained. Negative pressure therapy (vacuum-assisted device) may accelerate healing. Surgical treatment of pressure sores should be considered when the precipitating factors have been managed and after careful consideration of the risk-benefit ratio. Complex flap closure may be used, but the recurrence rate reaches 40% regardless of operative and postoperative management.[39]

Colorectal Cancer

The incidence of colorectal cancer increases progressively with age and is approximately 20 times higher in patients over 65 years old, reaching an annual incidence of 300 cases per 100,000. Adenomatous polyps are found in half the elderly patients in Western countries, whereas large polyps (>1 cm) are present in 1 of 6 patients. Older patients present with advanced unresectable colorectal cancer more often than their younger counterparts. Colorectal cancer screening provides the diagnosis in approximately half the older group of patients. Fecal occult blood test has twice the positive predictive value in the elderly. Colonoscopy offers the potential to both detect and remove suspicious lesions, but since it cannot easily be undertaken without sedation there is a potential for cardiopulmonary complications. Present guidelines regarding colorectal cancer screening state that for individuals over 75 years the benefit of screening is questionable, and it is not recommended after the age of 85 years.

Several studies have shown that the results of colorectal operations in the elderly are poorer than those in a younger cohort. The main reasons are the higher prevalence of coexisting illness and the higher rate of emergency operations. In general, mortality after elective colorectal operations in the elderly is low (<5%), but it increases sharply to 20–30% in the emergency setting. Postoperative morbidity is also higher in the elderly, although the long-term survival for each stage is equivalent between younger and older patients. Mechanical bowel preparation exposes the older patient to the risk of renal failure and should be used cautiously if at all. For low rectal tumors in elderly patients with very limited life expectancy or severe comorbidity, local treatments are well tolerated even if they are not curative; they include transanal microscopic microsurgery, ablation, and radiation. Elderly patients with compromised sphincter function may become incontinent, however, after lower anterior resection. Acute colonic obstruction due to cancer is a common surgical emergency in the elderly. Colonic stents seem to be promising in decompressing colonic obstruction due to advanced tumors, avoiding emergency operation and allowing preoperative preparation. Laparoscopic surgery is as beneficial in this group as it is in younger patients. Elderly patients are less likely to receive adjuvant treatment because of a greater perceived risk of toxicity, which is not necessarily substantiated.[40,41]

Upper Gastrointestinal Cancer

Esophageal cancer is diagnosed more often in patients over 65 years. Reports on the outcome of esophagectomy in elderly patients have been controversial. In general, postoperative morbidity rates may reach as high as 50%, with a mortality rate of up to 20% in patients over 80 years old. However, these data are mainly retrospective and subject to major selection bias. Results from high-volume specialized centers show comparable morbidity, mortality, and survival rates after esophagectomy for cancer to those in younger patients. Among population-based data, age, comorbidity, and operation in a low-volume hospital are independent predictors of postoperative mortality. Thus, centralization of these operations in high-volume tertiary hospitals seems rational. Palliative resections are associated with very high mortality rates (>20%) and should be avoided whenever possible; chemotherapy, radiation therapy, and endoscopic stenting are safer options.[42,43]

Gastric cancer is the second commonest cause of cancer-related death worldwide. More than half the new cases are diagnosed in patients over 65 years of age. The overall decrease in incidence of gastric cancer has been reported mostly among the elderly, who develop distal gastric cancer more often than younger patients. Gastric adenocarcinomas are more often well differentiated but are associated with higher rate of multiplicity and metastasis. Elderly compromised patients are less likely to receive a total gastrectomy for cancer, but this is not necessarily associated with a poorer oncological outcome. Therefore, gastric resections and radical lymphadenectomies should be taken into account the frailty of the patient. In large population-based studies, postoperative mortality ranges well below 10%, and age alone does not represent an independent risk factor for postoperative death in elderly patients. However, postoperative morbidity and mortality rates are higher in older patients, especially those over 80 years of age. Both overall survival and improvement of QoL are achieved following curative resections. The role of preoperative and adjuvant therapy in the elderly patient with gastric cancer has not been addressed by specific studies, but many older patients will benefit from multimodality therapy.[44]

Abdominal Wall Hernias

Repair of abdominal wall hernias represent the most common surgical procedure in the elderly patient. Most of them are groin hernias, 10% are incisional and <5% are femoral hernias. One or two of every 100 individuals will develop inguinal hernia every year in Western populations, but only 1 out 10 hernia repairs in the elderly are emergency operations. Older patients have direct inguinal hernia (up to 50%) and sliding hernia more often than the young. Through self-neglect, inguinal hernias may attain an extremely large size in the elderly and contain a large part of the abdominal viscera, the reduction of which into the peritoneal cavity may compromise respiratory function and increase the intra-abdominal pressure.

Although surgical repair is the definitive treatment for abdominal wall hernias, watchful waiting has emerged in recent years as an attractive option for asymptomatic or minimally symptomatic hernias. Nearly one third of such patients will eventually become symptomatic and require operations, but the low rate of emergency operations (<2%) is not associated with increased mortality. An important consideration for the conservative treatment of hernias is the fact that with longer follow-up an even larger proportion of patients will demand operation, and their declining general health in the interim must increase the operative risk. Nevertheless, for the very compromised elderly patient with mildly symptomatic or asymptomatic hernia, a watchful waiting strategy seems justified. Patients managed nonoperatively should be told how to avoid increased intra-abdominal pressure (i.e. due to constipation, chronic cough, and lifestyle) and when to seek immediate medical attention (i.e. symptoms of incarceration or strangulation). Femoral hernias and small incisional hernias are at higher risk of strangulation and should therefore be operated.

Elective hernia repair can safely be performed in the elderly population under local or regional anesthesia, this being associated with lower postoperative pain and shorter hospitalization.[45] Careful patient selection is necessary, however. Patients with dementia, marked anxiety or psychiatric disease are not good candidates for local or regional anesthesia because of inability to cooperate during the operation. Excessive use of sedation, especially in patients with respiratory disease, may lead to respiratory insufficiency. Very obese patients and those with large or scrotal hernias cannot easily undergo hernioplasty under local anesthesia. Tension-free repair with prosthetic mesh reduces postoperative pain and virtually eliminates recurrence. Laparoscopic techniques in appropriately trained hands may offer patients lower postoperative pain, shorter postoperative stay and better cosmetic results. The value of minimally invasive techniques in the setting of abdominal wall hernias remains to be fully elucidated.[46]

Cholecystitis

Gallstone disease is the commonest indication for operation in the elderly. The prevalence of gallstones in the general population is <20%, but it increases progressively with age to exceed 50% in those over the age of 65 years. Fewer than 2% of asymptomatic patients per year will become symptomatic and require cholecystectomy. These patients may not report typical symptoms of gallstones until the onset of a severe or potentially lethal complication of the disease such as empyema of the gallbladder. Nevertheless, in the absence of adequate prospective evidence to support the opposite, elective cholecystectomy for asymptomatic biliary stones is not generally recommended.[47]

Older patients are more likely to require emergency cholecystectomy due to the higher rate of severe and complicated gallstone disease in the elderly such as choledocholithiasis, acute cholecystitis, emphysematous cholecystitis, gallbladder perforation, empyema, acute cholangitis, and gallstone pancreatitis. Up to one third of patients 50–60 years old undergoing cholecystectomy have bile duct stones. For patients 70–80 years old, this rate exceeds 50%. Older patients undergoing laparoscopic cholecystectomy, whether in the emergency or elective setting, have higher rates of postoperative morbidity, mortality, and conversion than those who are younger. Fit elderly people with uncomplicated symptomatic gallstone disease are excellent candidates for laparoscopic cholecystectomy. On the other hand, frail patients develop more postoperative complications, have longer postoperative stay, and higher postoperative pain compared with their fitter counterparts.[48,49]

Gallstone disease should enter the differential diagnosis of any abdominal pain or unexplained sepsis in the frail elderly patient. For patients with acute cholecystitis who do not consent to operation or cannot tolerate general anesthesia, percutaneous cholecystostomy or even open cholecystostomy under local anesthesia are good alternatives in the presence of fever and a tender mass.[50] For patients with symptomatic gallstones who are not candidates for surgery, the available alternatives are pharmacologic dissolution with agents such as ursodeoxycholic acid and extracorporeal shock wave lithotripsy. These methods, however, are hampered by their low efficacy and cost-effectiveness.

REFERENCES

1. Good health adds life to years. Global brief for World Health Day 2012. Printed by the WHO Document Production Services, Geneva, Switzerland; 2012.
2. Cancer Incidence by age. Available from http://www.cancerresearchuk.org/cancer-info/cancerstats/incidence/age/. [Accessed May 10, 2013].
3. Jin K. Modern biological theories of aging. Aging Dis. 2010; 1(2):72-4.
4. Bowen RL, Atwood CS. Living and dying for sex. A theory of aging based on the modulation of cell cycle signaling by reproductive hormones. Gerontology. 2004;50(5):265-90.
5. Depp C, Vahia IV, Jeste D. Successful aging: focus on cognitive and emotional health. Annu Rev Clin Psychol. 2010;6: 527-50.
6. Rowe JW, Kahn RL. Successful aging. Gerontologist. 1997; 37(4):433-40.

7. Aronow W FW. Chapter 50: Physiologic changes in cardiac function with aging. In: Rosenthal R ZM, Katlic M (Eds). Principles and Practice of Geriatric Surgery, 2nd edition. New York: Springer; 2013. pp. 621-7.
8. Campbell E. Chapter 47: Physiological changes in respiratory function. In: Rosenthal R ZM, Katlic M (Eds). Principles and Practice of Geriatric Surgery. New York: Springer; 2013. pp. 596-603.
9. Brown N LJ, Zenilman M. Chapter 58: Age related changes in the gastrointestinal tract. In: Rosenthal RA, Zenilman ME, Katlic MR (Eds). Principles and Practice of Geriatric Surgery. New York: Springer; 2013. pp 711-9.
10. Fujiwara S, Nakamura T, Orimo H, et al. Development and application of a Japanese model of the WHO fracture risk assessment tool (FRAX). Osteoporos Int. 2008;19(4):429-35.
11. Minaker K. Chapter 24: Common clinical sequelae of aging. In: Goldman LSA (Ed). Goldman's Cecil Medicine, 24th edition. Philadelphia: Elsevier Mosby; 2011.
12. Fried TR, Bradley EH, Towle VR, et al. Understanding the treatment preferences of seriously ill patients. N Engl J Med. 2002;346(14):1061-6.
13. Zenilman ME. Surgery in the nursing home patient. Surg Clin North Am. 1994;74(1):63-77.
14. Walsh TH. Audit of outcome of major surgery in the elderly. Br J Surg. 1996;83(1):92-7.
15. van Leeuwen BL, Kristjansson SR, Audisio RA. Should specialized oncogeriatric surgeons operate older unfit cancer patients? Eur J Surg Oncol. 2010;36(Suppl 1):S18-22.
16. Stuck AE, Siu AL, Wieland GD, et al. Comprehensive geriatric assessment: a meta-analysis of controlled trials. Lancet. 1993;342(8878):1032-6.
17. Pasetto LM, Lise M, Monfardini S. Preoperative assessment of elderly cancer patients. Crit Rev Oncol Hematol. 2007;64(1):10-8.
18. Partridge JS, Harari D, Dhesi JK. Frailty in the older surgical patient: a review. Age Ageing. 2012;41(2):142-7.
19. Zekry D, Loures Valle BH, Lardi C, et al. Geriatrics index of comorbidity was the most accurate predictor of death in geriatric hospital among six comorbidity scores. J Clin Epidemiol. 2010;63(9):1036-44.
20. McDowell I. Social health. In: McDowell I (Ed). Measuring Health: A Guide to Rating Scales and Questionnaires, 3rd edition. New York: Oxford University Press; 2006. pp. 150-61.
21. Fleisher LA, Beckman JA, Brown KA, et al. ACC/AHA 2007 Guidelines on Perioperative Cardiovascular Evaluation and Care for Noncardiac Surgery: Executive Summary: A Report of the American College of Cardiology/American Heart Association Task Force on Practice Guidelines (Writing Committee to Revise the 2002 Guidelines on Perioperative Cardiovascular Evaluation for Noncardiac Surgery) Developed in Collaboration With the American Society of Echocardiography, American Society of Nuclear Cardiology, Heart Rhythm Society, Society of Cardiovascular Anesthesiologists, Society for Cardiovascular Angiography and Interventions, Society for Vascular Medicine and Biology, and Society for Vascular Surgery. J Am Coll Cardiol. 2007; 50(17):1707-32.
22. Lien SF, Bisognano JD. Perioperative hypertension: defining at-risk patients and their management. Curr Hypertens Rep. 2012;14(5):432-41.
23. Chow WB, Rosenthal RA, Merkow RP, et al. Optimal preoperative assessment of the geriatric surgical patient: a best practices guideline from the American College of Surgeons National Surgical Quality Improvement Program and the American Geriatrics Society. J Am Coll Surg. 2012;215(4): 453-66.
24. Demeure MJ, Fain MJ. The elderly surgical patient and postoperative delirium. J Am Coll Surg. 2006;203(5):752-7.
25. Cicerchia M, Ceci M, Locatelli C, et al. Geriatric syndromes in peri-operative elderly cancer patients. Surg Oncol. 2010; 19(3):131-9.
26. Hirsh J, Dalen J, Guyatt G. The sixth (2000) ACCP guidelines for antithrombotic therapy for prevention and treatment of thrombosis. American College of Chest Physicians. Chest. 2001;119(1 Suppl):1S-2S.
27. Egbert AM, Parks LH, Short LM, et al. Randomized trial of postoperative patient-controlled analgesia vs intramuscular narcotics in frail elderly men. Arch Intern Med. 1990; 150(9):1897-903.
28. Bettelli G. Anaesthesia for the elderly outpatient: preoperative assessment and evaluation, anaesthetic technique and postoperative pain management. Curr Opin Anaesthesiol. 2010;23(6):726-31.
29. McMahon MM, Nystrom E, Braunschweig C, et al. A.S.P.E.N. clinical guidelines: nutrition support of adult patients with hyperglycemia. JPEN J Parenter Enteral Nutr. 2013;37(1): 23-36.
30. Mueller C, Compher C, Ellen DM. A.S.P.E.N. clinical guidelines: nutrition screening, assessment, and intervention in adults. JPEN J Parenter Enteral Nutr. 2011;35(1):16-24.
31. Sobotka L, Schneider SM, Berner YN, et al. ESPEN guidelines on parenteral nutrition: geriatrics. Clin Nutr. 2009; 28(4):461-6.
32. Volkert D, Berner YN, Berry E, et al. ESPEN guidelines on enteral nutrition: geriatrics. Clin Nutr. 2006;25(2):330-60.
33. Zenilman ME, Bender JS, Magnuson TH, et al. General surgical care in the nursing home patient: results of a dedicated geriatric surgery consult service. J Am Coll Surg. 1996;183(4):361-70.
34. Landefeld CS, Palmer RM, Kresevic DM, et al. A randomized trial of care in a hospital medical unit especially designed to improve the functional outcomes of acutely ill older patients. N Engl J Med. 1995;332(20):1338-44.
35. American College of Surgeons. Chapter 10: Extremes of age. In: ATLS: Advanced Trauma Life Support Program for Doctors, 9th edition. Chicago: American College of Surgeons; 2012. pp. 247-58.
36. Petrakis IE, Paraskakis S. Breast cancer in the elderly. Arch Gerontol Geriatr. 2010;50(2):179-84.
37. Biganzoli L, Wildiers H, Oakman C, et al. Management of elderly patients with breast cancer: updated recommendations of the International Society of Geriatric Oncology (SIOG) and European Society of Breast Cancer Specialists (EUSOMA). Lancet Oncol. 2012;13(4):e148-60.

38. Bluestein D, Alemu Y, Avrahami I, et al. Influence of microcalcifications on vulnerable plaque mechanics using FSI modeling. J Biomech. 2008;41(5):1111-8.
39. Reddy M, Gill SS, Rochon PA. Preventing pressure ulcers: a systematic review. JAMA. 2006;296(8):974-84.
40. Papamichael D, Audisio R, Horiot JC, et al. Treatment of the elderly colorectal cancer patient: SIOG expert recommendations. Ann Oncol. 2009;20(1):5-16.
41. Audisio RA, Papamichael D. Treatment of colorectal cancer in older patients. Nat Rev Gastroenterol Hepatol. 2012;9(12):716-25.
42. Cijs TM, Verhoef C, Steyerberg EW, et al. Outcome of esophagectomy for cancer in elderly patients. Ann Thorac Surg. 2010;90(3):900-7.
43. Chang AC, Lee JS. Resection for esophageal cancer in the elderly. Thorac Surg Clin. 2009;19(3):333-43.
44. Saif MW, Makrilia N, Zalonis A, et al. Gastric cancer in the elderly: an overview. Eur J Surg Oncol. 2010;36(8):709-17.
45. Kurzer M, Kark A, Hussain ST. Day-case inguinal hernia repair in the elderly: a surgical priority. Hernia. 2009;13(2):131-6.
46. Simons MP, Aufenacker T, Bay-Nielsen M, et al. European Hernia Society guidelines on the treatment of inguinal hernia in adult patients. Hernia. 2009;13(4):343-403.
47. Overby DW, Apelgren KN, Richardson W, et al. SAGES guidelines for the clinical application of laparoscopic biliary tract surgery. Surg Endosc. 2010;24(10):2368-86.
48. Lasithiotakis K, Petrakis J, Venianaki M, et al. Frailty predicts outcome of elective laparoscopic cholecystectomy in geriatric patients. Surg Endosc. 2013;27(4):1144-50.
49. Kuy S, Sosa JA, Roman SA, et al. Age matters: a study of clinical and economic outcomes following cholecystectomy in elderly Americans. Am J Surg. 2011;201(6):789-96.
50. Li M, Li N, Ji W, et al. Percutaneous cholecystostomy is a definitive treatment for acute cholecystitis in elderly high-risk patients. Am Surg. 2013;79(5):524-7.

Additional references can be found in the online version of this book.

19

Surgical Management of Children and Neonates

Stig Sømme, Jacob C Langer

Key Points

- Physiologic considerations are important in neonatal and pediatric surgery.
- Pediatric surgical conditions can be organized by age: newborns, infants, toddlers, preschool and school age, and adolescents.
- Pediatric trauma is the leading cause of death after infancy and the leading preventable health problem in children.

INTRODUCTION

Pediatric general and thoracic surgery is now approaching the century mark since its origin. This historic beginning has generally been attributed to Dr William Ladd, a Boston surgeon. After witnessing the scope and severity of injury sustained by the children of Halifax after a munitions ship exploded in the harbor in 1914, Ladd returned to Boston to focus the remainder of his career exclusively on the surgical care of children. The specialty of pediatric surgery is characterized by an intimate overlap with adult general and thoracic surgery as well as with pediatric medicine.[1] The first formal association of pediatric surgeons was established in 1947, when the Surgical Section of the American Academy of Pediatrics (AAP) was established. Around that time, general surgeons or urologists performed most operations on infants and children in both children's and adult general hospitals, and the operative morbidity and mortality rates were high.[2]

Pediatric surgery has since established itself as an independent pediatric and surgical subspecialty in many countries. It has professional relationships with both pediatric as well as surgical professional associations; within the United States, it sponsors its own training process approved by the American College of Graduate Medical Education (ACGME); it has its own specialty board of qualification and certification under the American Board of Surgery (ABS); and it has its own journals, multiple specialty-specific textbooks, and independent surgical organizations. As the specialty of pediatric surgery has matured, the outcomes for the surgical care of children have improved dramatically as a result of improved and more advanced surgical techniques, parenteral nutrition, specialized neonatal and pediatric intensive care units (ICUs), and pediatric anesthesia.[2]

In this chapter, we discuss important aspects of the pediatric surgical patient, with a focus on neonates, infants, and small children. Adolescent patients are in many ways similar to adult patients, and will not be the focus of this chapter.

PHYSIOLOGIC CONSIDERATIONS

Neonates are commonly classified based on their gestational age and weight. A "term" infant is born between 37 and 42 postmenstrual weeks of gestational age. A preterm infant is generally defined as one born before 37 weeks, and often has specific needs and clinical concerns. The level of prematurity greatly affects outcomes and risks for these infants, ranging from the extremely premature but viable 24-week neonate with birth weights approaching 500 g, to near term neonates with normal birth weights born at 36 weeks. The level of prematurity also influences anticipated surgical needs. Common surgical procedures in preterm infants include inguinal hernia repair, drainage or resection for necrotizing enterocolitis (NEC), ligation of patent ductus arteriosus, and procedures to obtain intravenous (IV) access. On the other hand, full-term neonates are more likely to require operative treatment for congenital anomalies, and older infants and children are more likely to develop tumors, sustain trauma, and develop intussusception and inflammatory conditions such as appendicitis.

Fluids/Electrolytes

The fraction of water in the body changes greatly from birth to the end of the first year. At birth, water makes up about 75% of the weight of a term baby. Most notably during the first week of life, but also in the following months, total body water slowly falls from 75% to 60% of total body weight. Likewise, extracellular fluid makes up 45% of total body weight at birth and then falls to 20% by the end of the first year. The kidneys in newborns, and especially premature infants, do not have the same ability to concentrate urine when compared to those of older children and adults. Thus, accurate fluid management is vitally important in the infant. A newborn will not produce much urine during the first few days of life. Consequently, potassium is generally not added to the IV fluids until urine production increases, after which the daily requirement is about 2 mEq/kg.

Newborns who cannot receive enteral nutrition will need parenteral IV fluids and total parenteral nutrition (TPN). Maintenance IV fluids in the newborn are administered at 70 mL/kg/day for the first day of life. The initial fluid is 10% dextrose (D10) without any electrolytes, due to the tendency for neonates to develop hypoglycemia. Over the next few days, as urine production increases, the rate is slowly increased to 100 mL/kg/day and sodium is added, usually in a 0.2% D10 solution. The sodium requirement of a full-term infant is 2 mEq/kg/day.

Many surgical neonates have excessive fluid loss from exposed bowel (gastroschisis, ruptured omphalocele), intra-abdominal inflammation (NEC), or gastric losses from a nasogastric tube (intestinal atresia, bowel resection, gastroschisis); it is critical to increase the fluid administration with a correct replacement fluid to avoid dehydration and acid-base abnormalities.

Acid–Base Status

Metabolic alkalosis is usually the result of loss of gastric secretions, and is often associated with respiratory compensation resulting in hypoventilation. Infants with a gastric outlet obstruction are particularly prone to gastric losses, and these can result in metabolic acidosis. These losses must be replaced with normal saline and potassium, or the infant will quickly become dehydrated and develop electrolyte abnormalities.

Children with a bowel obstruction will also require replacement fluids to maintain fluid volume homeostasis, but metabolic acidosis is usually not seen because of concurrent bicarbonate losses from the small intestine.

Metabolic acidosis is generally secondary to lactic acidosis as a result of poor tissue perfusion. It is corrected by dealing with the underlying problem, commonly sepsis, chemical inflammation (in meconium peritonitis), hypovolemia, or anemia. Metabolic acidosis can also be secondary to intestinal ischemia from mid-gut volvulus, strangulated hernia, or NEC. Fluid resuscitation must be addressed quickly in these cases before considering operation.

Respiratory acid–base abnormalities are often seen in neonates with congenital diaphragmatic hernia (CDH) or congenital lobar emphysema and in premature infants with respiratory distress syndrome and chronic lung disease of prematurity. Management of respiratory acid–base abnormalities ranges from supplemental O2 or continuous positive airway pressure, to conventional mechanical ventilation and high-frequency oscillatory ventilation. In the most extreme cases, extracorporeal membrane oxygenation (ECMO) can be used to rest the lungs until the underlying problem improves. The use of ECMO in infants with CDH is variable, but is most effective for children with severe pulmonary hypertension in the absence of critical pulmonary hypoplasia.

Nutrition

The nutritional needs of a growing child are important to consider in pre- and postoperative care. The nutritional needs of older children are not very different from those of adults. Infants, on the other hand, are more precarious in their nutritional needs because of their rapidly developing bodies and brains. Although strong data to guide clinical practice in regards to when to start TPN are lacking, the principle that guides practice is that a child should not be without adequate nutrition for more than a few days. This rule of thumb stems from observations that a child's developing body and brain are more sensitive to a decrease in caloric intake than the typical adult patient.

Enteral Nutrition

Breast milk is the preferred enteral nutrition in the neonate. However, there are excellent infant formulas that can replace breast milk if it is not available. Mothers of neonates must be well supported and encouraged in the use of breast pumps if desired. For infants in whom enteral nutrition is delayed due to a surgical condition, colostrum and breast milk can be stored and used when nutrition is introduced. In many centers, breast milk banks have been developed to provide donated breast milk to neonates for whom the mother's milk is not available.

Predigested or partially predigested formulas and medium-chain triglycerides are often used for infants with malabsorption, short intestinal length, or an ileostomy. These formulas can help improve absorption and permit weaning from parenteral nutrition. Finally, many infants with intestinal failure are dependent on continuous enteral feeding as part of a bowel rehabilitation program. Placement of a gastrostomy tube often facilitates transfer from the neonatal intensive care unit (NICU) and ultimately discharge from the hospital. If a pediatric patient can be nutritionally supported using the gastrointestinal tract, then this is the preferred mode of nutrition delivery.

Infants and children with many surgical conditions may have difficulty gaining weight. For example, infants with CDH will often require a higher caloric intake due to their increased work of breathing, children with cystic fibrosis have increased nutritional requirements due to pancreatic insufficiency and their pulmonary disease, and children with gastroschisis and NEC may have poor nutrient absorption due to mucosal injury. It is important to make sure that patients with conditions requiring additional nutritional support achieve normal growth. A common postoperative intervention in infants is to fortify the breast milk or formula to increase its caloric density. The caloric density of breast milk and standard infant formula is 20 kcal/oz or 70 kcal/100 mL. This caloric density can be increased by up to 30% to help with weight gain.

In older children with inflammatory bowel disease (IBD) or weight loss related to critical illness, nasogastric-feeding tubes (NG) can be used to add enteral nutrition at night. Another option, particularly if caloric supplementation is required on a long-term basis, is a surgically placed gastrostomy or gastrojejunostomy tube.

Parenteral Nutrition

Parenteral nutrition is delivered intravenously. Although nutrition can be delivered through peripheral veins, there is a limit to how many calories can be supplied this way. Central venous catheters (CVCs) can be used to deliver more concentrated dextrose solutions without causing harm to the vein. Central venous catheters are essential when caring for infants and children who cannot tolerate enteral nutrition. Central venous catheters can be placed peripherally as a peripherally inserted central venous catheter (PICC), most commonly in the antecubital fossa.

The CVC can be tunneled under the skin for a distance before it enters into a vein; these catheters are cuffed to secure them in a subcutaneous location. The cuff is made of Dacron, a polyester product that creates a dense fibrotic scar to the surrounding tissue. This fibrosis secures the catheter and also prevents bacteria from migrating along the tract and into the tissue and bloodstream. Nontunneled catheters and PICC lines are more commonly used in older children, but use of PICC lines and nontunneled catheters in infants is on the rise.

Obtaining IV access in the premature small infant can be a challenge. Surgically placed lines are often necessary. These are commonly placed in the internal jugular vein with a cut down on to the vein and tunneled to an exit site on the anterior chest. This technique can be used in premature infants with a weight of only 500 g. In larger infants, it is possible to place the catheter in the external jugular vein, the subclavian vein, or the saphenous vein in the groin.

Implantable ports are commonly placed in children with oncologic conditions; these are less commonly used for parenteral nutrition only. The procedure is similar to the placement of a tunneled CVC.

Total parenteral nutrition is currently utilized extensively in the NICU and the pediatric surgical service in general. Prior to the advent of TPN, several surgical conditions in children that currently treated with high rates of survival would have been fatal. Examples of conditions in which most patients need TPN are gastroschisis, small bowel atresia, diaphragmatic hernia, and NEC.

TPN was developed in the 1960s and 1970s, with much of the initial work investigated by Dudrick and colleagues.[3] These studies supported administering a hypertonic glucose solution in order to achieve a positive nitrogen balance. Since then proteins and fats began to be routinely administered intravenously. The administration of lipids is important for infants to obtain essential fatty acids and the building blocks necessary for nerve myelination and development of the nervous system.

Infants with short intestinal length or intestinal failure for other reasons often require prolonged TPN use. Multiple complications are associated with TPN use, the most serious of which is liver failure from TPN-induced cholestasis. Also known as TPN-associated liver disease, this feared complication is commonly associated with bloodstream infections (bacteremia). Bacteremia related to indwelling CVCs is important for several reasons. Central venous catheter-associated bloodstream infections contribute to TPN-induced liver disease, and if the CVC is removed it can become increasingly difficult to obtain access in the future. Soy-based IV lipids (e.g. intralipid) have also been identified as possibly contributing to the development of cholestasis. Thus, there is an increased interest in finding alternatives to the soy-based lipids. A fish oil based solution (Omegaven) has gained popularity because of reports documenting reversal of TPN-induced liver disease with the administration of this omega-3 fatty acid solution. Another IV fat solution, SMOF (soy, medium fatty acids, omega-3, fish oil), is currently under investigation in a randomized trial comparing it to standard soy-based formula. The proponents of SMOF state that it has a balanced omega-6 to omega 3 ratio and provides all the essential fatty acids. A pure soy-based IV fat solution has a much higher level of omega-6, which could contribute to a proinflammatory state.

Another approach to reduce the risk of TPN-induced liver disease has been to reduce the amount of soy-based lipids administered. The normal amount of lipids administered is 3 g/kg/day. Recently several centers have started reducing this to 1 g/kg/day and even 1 g/kg/day only 3 days a week to avoid TPN-induced liver disease. One concern in regards to reducing fatty acid intake is that insufficient amounts of essential fatty acids may cause a deficiency and as a result affect development of the nervous system.[4]

Possibly the most important measure to avoid liver disease is to give trophic enteral feeds. Enteral feeds stimulate bile production and gallbladder emptying, which is felt to be protective in preventing TPN-associated liver disease. Additionally, they prevent atrophy of the intestinal tract and thereby avoid the translocation of gut flora. Current and ongoing investigations are likely to change the way in which TPN lipids are administered in the future.

During TPN therapy it is important to monitor patients closely: electrolytes, glucose, calcium, phosphorus, and magnesium should be measured twice weekly. A complete blood count, in addition to transaminases, bilirubin, and creatinine, should be measured at the beginning of therapy and every 2 weeks for the duration of TPN administration. Accurate fluid intake and output should be measured. In patients on long-term TPN or in whom TPN is administered at home, less frequent blood tests may be required if the laboratory values remain stable.

Recently there has been a shortage of trace elements. Such shortages predominantly affect patients on long-term TPN and can lead to unusual deficiencies in single trace elements.

Biometric data should be collected to ensure proper weight gain and growth. In infants, 100–200 g of weight gain per week is expected. Weight, height, and head circumference in infants are plotted in the percentile diagram, adjusted for prematurity, and followed over time.

Hemodynamics

The two most common forms of shock seen in children are hypovolemic shock and septic shock.

Neonates and infants normally have a lower baseline blood pressure than adults, and often shock does not lower the blood pressure any further. This finding is most pronounced in the premature infant. In contrast to adults, who develop tachycardia in response to shock, neonates become bradycardic and develop lactic acidosis. Lactic acidosis is a result of inadequate end-organ perfusion from bradycardia, decreased venous return, and subsequently decreased cardiac output.

The physiologic response to shock in older children is similar to that of adults, except that children have an even greater ability to compensate than adults and may lose 45% of circulating blood volume before there is a decrease in blood pressure. After this degree of hypovolemia develops, even a small amount of additional intravascular fluid loss may cause complete circulatory collapse. Subtle signs such as decreased pulse pressure and tachycardia can easily be overlooked in a patient in pain but can be an important warning sign of imminent cardiovascular collapse.

Hypovolemic shock is the result of an inadequate circulating blood volume from the loss of intravascular and extracellular fluid. Common causes include bleeding, which leads to decreased intravascular volume, and protracted diarrhea or vomiting, which leads to loss of extracellular fluid as a result of dehydration and electrolyte imbalances.

The most important goal in treating hypovolemic shock is to correct the source of intravascular fluid loss. Crystalloids are administered to correct IV fluid loss and blood is administered if indicated. In neonates, the hematocrit should be kept above 45% to optimize end-organ perfusion. Pharmacologic support is less commonly needed for hypovolemic shock, since correction of the intravascular volume loss often quickly improves physiologic parameters.

Hospitals should establish a massive transfusion protocol to be used if there is suspicion or evidence of major blood loss. This protocol includes fresh frozen plasma, platelets, and rhesus-negative, type O, packed red blood cells administered in a ratio of 1:1:1. Platelets and plasma are usually given after the transfusion of 40 mL/kg of crystalloids and 20 mL/kg of packed red blood cells.

The trauma patient with acute blood loss should be admitted to the surgical service. Resuscitation must be started in the emergency department before the patient is moved to the radiology department for additional imaging, to the operating room, or to the ICU.

The most common cause of septic shock is gram-negative septicemia. The source of the gram-negative bacteria can be the intestinal tract, the urinary tract, or the respiratory tract. Neonates also commonly develop shock due to gram-positive sepsis from CVC-related infection. In septic shock the decrease in the circulating blood volume is secondary to the effect of endotoxins on the capillary bed. The endotoxin increases capillary permeability, which results in pooling of fluid in the tissue.

The treatment of septic shock is initially focused on the administration of IV fluids. Crystalloids, normal saline, or lactated Ringer's are the standard solutions used for resuscitation. In patients with capillary leak or with a low albumin (<2.0 g/dL), colloids may be used to help keep the fluid intravascular. The most commonly used colloid is albumin, which is a human plasma product and carries a small risk of transferring blood-borne infections. It is important to send blood cultures and start IV broad-spectrum antibiotics when septic shock is suspected.

It is often necessary to start inotropic therapy if ongoing evidence of inadequate end-organ perfusion is present after normalization of central venous pressure with IV fluid expansion, and correction of the hematocrit with transfusion of blood products. The pharmacologic agents most commonly used are dopamine, epinephrine, norepinephrine, and vasopressin.

Surgical Conditions According to Age

Table 19.1 shows the most common surgical diseases seen in children, according to the age group in which each condition is most often seen.

Many conditions can also be seen across a broad range of ages. However, there is benefit in emphasizing the age window in which the majority of cases present in order to assist the clinician in arriving at a differential diagnosis in an individual patient.

Table 19.1 Most important pediatric surgical diagnoses by age group.

Age group / Diagnosis
Neonate
Intestinal obstruction (atresias, meconium obstruction, Hirschsprung's disease)
Anorectal malformations
Abdominal wall defects (omphalocele, gastroschisis)
Congenital diaphragmatic hernia
Developmental lung anomalies (CPAM, pulmonary sequestration)
Necrotizing enterocolitis
Infant
Hirschsprung's disease
Hypertrophic pyloric stenosis
Intussusception
Malrotation
Inguinal hernia
Undescended testis
Choledochal cyst and biliary atresia
Toddler
Appendicitis
Meckel's diverticulum with bleeding or obstruction
Inguinal hernia and hydrocele
Wilms' tumor and neuroblastoma
Non-accidental trauma
Preschool and school age
Appendicitis
Inguinal hernia
Umbilical hernia
Trauma
Adolescent
Appendicitis
Cholelithiasis and cholecystitis
Inflammatory bowel disease
Pectus excavatum and carinatum

SURGICAL PROBLEMS OF THE NEWBORN

Prenatal Diagnosis

Many congenital anomalies are suspected and easily identified prenatally, but others are more difficult to identify [e.g. esophageal atresia (EA) with tracheoesophageal fistula (TEF), malrotation, and anorectal malformations]. As increasing numbers of women worldwide have access to prenatal care and undergo a routine scan around 20 weeks' gestation, many congenital anomalies are detected early, which has reduced the incidence of surgical emergencies resulting from undetected anomalies and improved the outcomes for these anomalies. In addition, early detection can allow time for a prenatal consultation with a pediatric surgeon. The goal of this consultation is to provide the family with information, form accurate expectations, and develop a comprehensive plan for delivery with the foremost goal of reducing the risk and avoiding the consequences of a neonatal surgical emergency. In some cases, this process may require a change in the mode (i.e. cesarean section), location (i.e. perinatal center vs. community hospital), or timing (i.e. preterm) of delivery. In rare cases, there may also be an indication for in utero surgical intervention, which should only be done in specialized centers with a multidisciplinary fetal intervention program.

In neonates born with an undiagnosed surgical condition, it is important to provide safe transfer to an institution with a high-level NICU and pediatric surgical support. It is optimal to have a specialized neonatal transport team experienced in the transfer of NICU patients responsible for the transfer.

Preliminary Assessment and Resuscitation

The initial assessment of a newborn with a suspected surgical problem is very important, as a thorough examination and simple X-rays are usually all that is required to provide a diagnosis. Intravenous access can often be obtained through the umbilical vein, and if arterial access is needed the umbilical artery can be used. Additional peripheral IV lines and/or PICCs can be placed as needed. If IV access is required for a long duration, several weeks to months, the pediatric surgeon can place a tunneled CVC. Nasogastric or orogastric drainage tubes should be placed when appropriate.

Neonates with a surgical condition should be administered a standard 10% dextrose solution at a maintenance rate of 60 mL/kg per 24 hours. Additional fluid requirements are provided with normal saline solution. Potassium is not provided until urine is produced. Electrolytes must be checked frequently because of the potential for serious electrolyte abnormalities in patients with fluid loss from intestinal obstruction or exposed organs.

Vitamin K should be administered as an intramuscular injection in preparation for operation.

Neonates, in particular premature infants, are prone to become hypothermic. Heat loss can be prevented with the use of incubators, heat-lamps, or simply swaddling the neonate in warm blankets. Keeping the newborn dry is also important in preventing heat loss. In infants with gastroschisis or bladder/cloacal exstrophy, the lower part of the body can be placed in a plastic bag to reduce evaporative heat loss.

Neonatal Surgical Conditions

Most surgical conditions diagnosed in the neonatal period are the result of congenital anomalies. Most of these conditions are rare, with a frequency of 1 in 2,500 births for gastroschisis, to 1 in 5,000–10,000 births for Hirschsprung's disease, intestinal atresia, duodenal atresia, anorectal malformations, TEF, EA, cystic pulmonary airway malformations (CPAMs), and CDH. These conditions should be cared for by subspecialty-trained pediatric surgeons, usually in a dedicated children's hospital or pediatric unit with an NICU.

The most common abdominal wall defect is gastroschisis, which is characterized by a defect to the right of the umbilical cord through which most or all of the intestine protrudes (Fig. 19.1A). Most cases are now suspected prenatally because of elevation of the maternal α-feto protein, and can be accurately diagnosed with ultrasound scanning. Gastroschisis is typically not associated with chromosomal or other anomalies, except for intestinal atresia that occurs in 10–15% of patients. Because the newborn with gastroschisis typically has all of its intestine outside the abdominal cavity, IV fluid resuscitation and adequate temperature control are important since the evaporative losses from the exposed bowel are considerable.

After inspection of the intestine by a pediatric surgeon, the intestine is reduced back into the abdomen either primarily or with the assistance of a spring-loaded silo (Figs. 19.1B and C). The fascia is either closed with sutures or left to close by secondary intention, an approach that works very well due to the ability of an umbilical ring to contract circumferentially. An infant with gastroschisis has a median stay of 5 weeks in the hospital due to intestinal dysmotility, and during this time the infant is dependent on TPN. In countries in which TPN is not readily available, survival is dismal. However, in most developed countries the survival is over 90%.

Omphalocele (also called exomphalos) is an abdominal wall defect that is characterized by failure of the viscera to return to the abdominal cavity from the umbilical cord at 12 weeks' gestation, leaving a sac over the herniated viscera (Fig. 19.2). Omphalocele differs from gastroschisis in a number of ways. The abdominal wall defect can be of various sizes, and the viscera are covered by a sac consisting of Wharton's jelly. Occasionally, the sac is ruptured, making the distinction between omphalocele and gastroschisis more difficult. Omphalocele has a high incidence of associated anomalies and chromosomal anomalies. This condition is frequently diagnosed prenatally and warrants a thorough investigation of the fetus, which includes amniocentesis, fetal echocardiogram, and a detailed ultrasound scan. If available, fetal MRI may be of great help to identify additional anomalies. Small omphaloceles can be closed primarily with excellent outcomes, but large

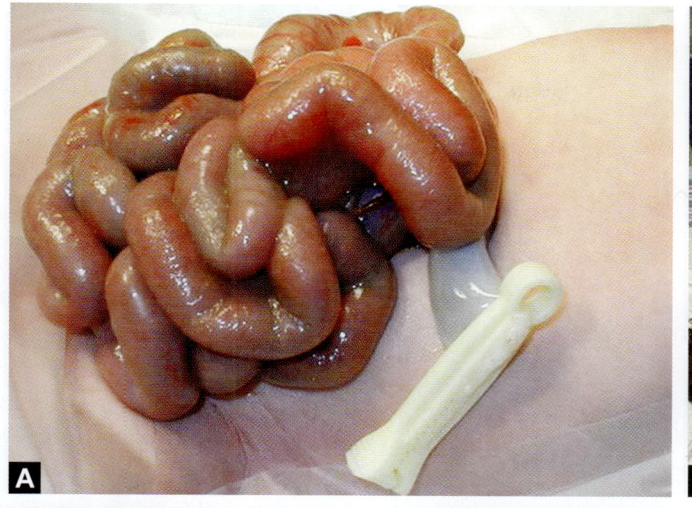

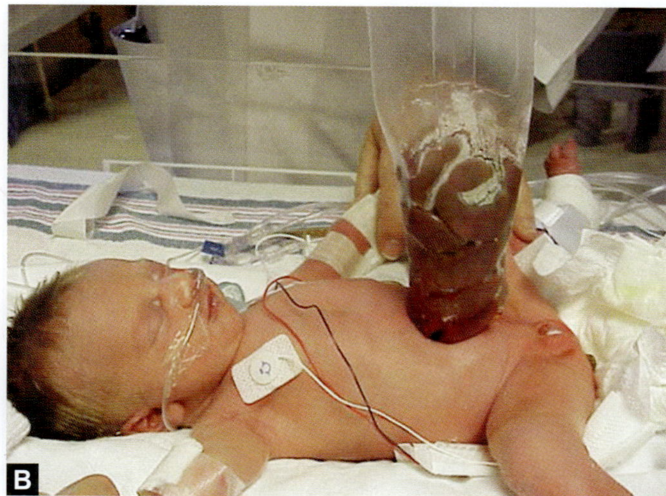

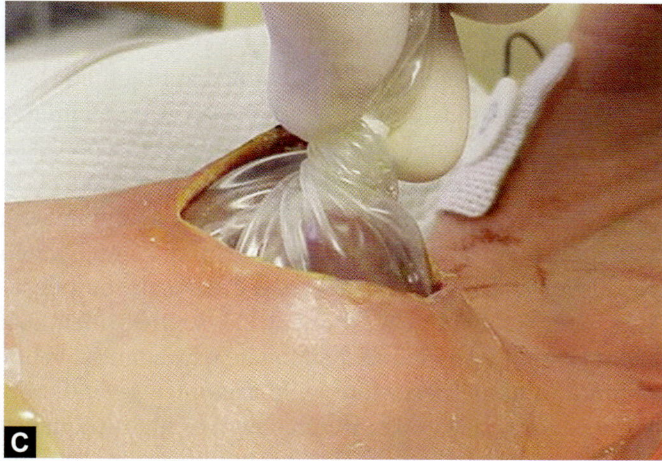

Figs. 19.1A to C: (A) Infant with gastroschisis. (B) Placement of a preformed silo. (C) After gradual reduction of the viscera, the fascial defect can be closed surgically or a dressing can be placed and the defect allowed to close by secondary intention.

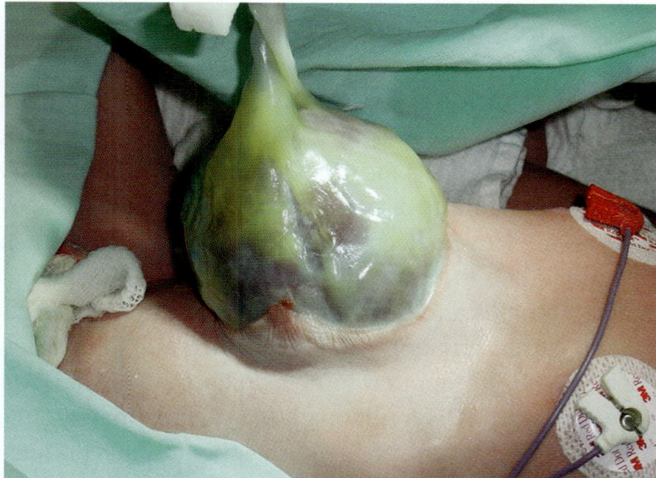

Fig. 19.2: Infant with omphalocele.

defects must often be closed in a staged fashion. Long-term outcome for children with omphalocele is usually determined by the presence and severity of associated structural and chromosomal anomalies.[5]

Esophageal atresia, with or without TEF, is a congenital anomaly characterized by a blind-ending esophageal pouch. Most commonly this occurs with a TEF connecting the end of the distal esophagus to the back of the trachea just above the carina (85%). This condition is often associated with a spectrum of other anomalies known as the VACTERL syndrome (vertebral anomalies, anorectal malformations, cardiac anomalies, tracheoesophageal malformations, renal anomalies, and limb anomalies). Esophageal atresia with a distal TEF is usually repaired in the first day or two of life. About 10% of EAs consist of pure EA without a fistula. These infants often have a long gap between the blind-ending pouch and the distal esophagus, which makes it impossible to connect the two ends primarily. Management is therefore expectant, with initial placement of a gastrostomy feeding tube. Since the esophagus grows disproportionately to the rest of the body, the gap becomes shorter over time, and a primary repair can usually be accomplished within 3 months. If the gap remains too long for an anastomosis, a variety of other

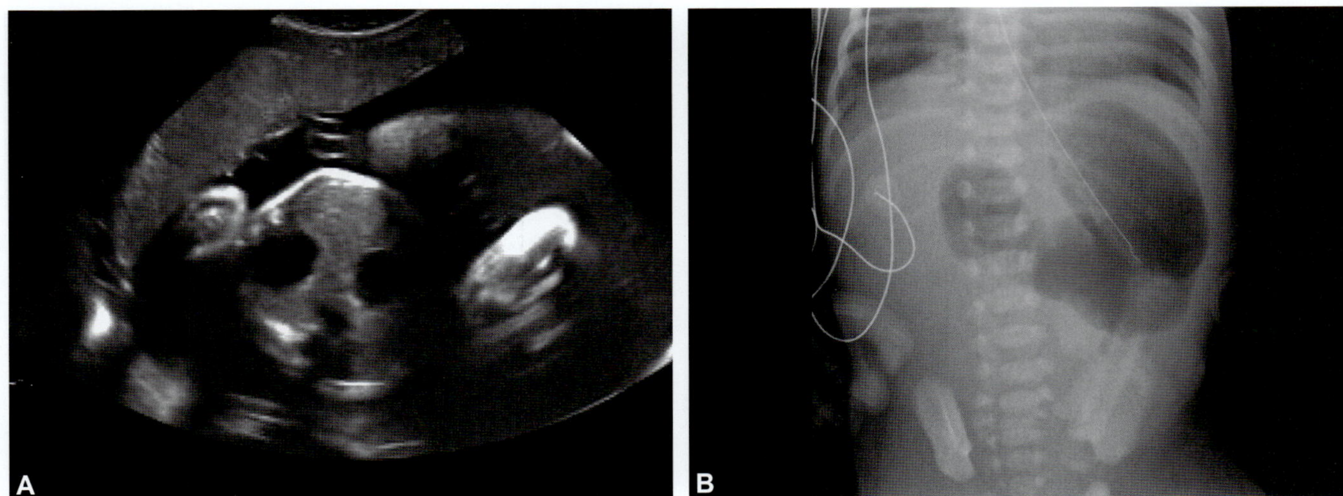

Figs. 19.3A and B: Typical "double bubble" seen in children with duodenal atresia. (A) On prenatal ultrasound. (B) On postnatal abdominal X-ray.

techniques have been described, including sequential elongation of the esophageal ends and replacement of the esophagus with stomach or colon.[6,7]

Duodenal atresia consists of an obstruction in the second portion of the duodenum, probably due to failure of recanalization during early embryonic life. Prenatally polyhydramnios is almost always present, and prenatal US demonstrates a "double bubble" (Fig. 19.3A), which is pathognomonic for duodenal atresia. Duodenal atresia is associated with trisomy 21 in one third of cases and with congenital heart disease in 25% of cases, so prenatal diagnosis should stimulate karyotype analysis and fetal echocardiography. Postnatally a "double bubble" can be seen on plain abdominal X-ray (Fig. 19.3B), and contrast studies are usually not necessary. Duodenal atresia does not require an urgent operation, since it is easy to keep the stomach and first portion of the duodenum decompressed with a nasogastric or orogastric tube. Surgical repair is usually done in the first few days of life and consists of either a duodenoduodenostomy or a duodenojejunostomy.

Intestinal atresia can affect the proximal intestine, the distal small intestine, or the colon. Most cases are spontaneous, but there are reports of familial cases. Intestinal atresia is also associated with cystic fibrosis and gastroschisis. The surgical repair usually consists of an end-to-end anastomosis between the two ends of intestine, and often a tapering enteroplasty is necessary because of the huge discrepancy in diameter between the two ends. Occasionally, a diverting stoma is needed.

Congenital diaphragmatic hernia is commonly diagnosed prenatally. Eighty-five percent of patients have a left-sided posterolateral defect of the diaphragm through the foramen of Bochdalek. Congenital diaphragmatic hernia is a condition with highly variable severity. All infants with CDH have some degree of pulmonary hypoplasia, and the degree of hypoplasia is predictive of survival. In addition to pulmonary hypoplasia, many children with CDH develop severe pulmonary hypertension, which results in right-to-left shunting and cardiac decompensation, with resultant death in many cases. The principle of management is to maintain adequate oxygenation, ventilation and tissue perfusion while minimizing ventilator-induced lung injury.[8] Techniques such as high-frequency oscillation, inhaled nitric oxide, inotropic support, and the judicious use of prostaglandins are used to accomplish this goal. Extracorporeal membrane oxygenation is sometimes needed for the most severely affected infants. Surgical repair of the defect is delayed until the child has been stabilized and pulmonary artery pressure is subsystemic. It can take 2–3 weeks for the reactivity of the pulmonary vasculature to improve sufficiently to allow for a safe surgical repair. Large defects often require a prosthetic patch or muscle flap to bridge the gap between the diaphragmatic remnants and the chest wall, while smaller defects can be closed primarily. The recurrence rate after patch repair has been reported to be as high as 15%.[9] Survival in infants with CDH traditionally was approximately 50%, but since the advent of "gentle ventilation" techniques survival has improved to 75–80% in many centers. However, this improvement in survival has been accompanied by an increase in morbidity, including respiratory, nutritional musculoskeletal, and neurological issues.[10] Thus, long-term multidisciplinary follow-up after CDH repair is important.

Congenital lung cysts are often diagnosed prenatally on ultrasound scanning. The cysts are classified into congenital cystic airway malformation (CCAM) and pulmonary sequestration. Congenital cystic airway malformations can be further classified based on the size of the cysts in the lesion (micro- vs macrocystic lesions, or type 1–5 using the Stocker classification), and sequestrations are often classified based on the location (extra- vs intrapulmonary sequestrations). Cystic pulmonary airway malformation is a newer term used that incorporates the full spectrum of cystic lung lesions. The term "hybrid lesion" is often used to describe lesions that have features of both CCAM and sequestration, usually consisting of a cystic lung mass with a systemic feeding vessel typical of pulmonary sequestration. Bronchial atresia is a term used to describe a possible etiology for hyperinflation of a lobe or a segment, but may be difficult to identify on imaging. More commonly, bronchial atresia is identified by a pathologist after resection of the CPAM.

Prenatally, a CCAM will often undergo exponential growth between 20 and 28 weeks, but in approximately 70% of fetuses, the lesion will then decrease in size and will be asymptomatic at birth.[11] In the other 30%, the lesion will not decrease in size, or may increase and cause hydrops and fetal demise. A CCAM volume ration (CVR) >1.6 is predictive of hydrops with loss of the fetus. In these cases, fetal intervention, consisting of thoracoamniotic shunting for macrocystic lesions or fetal lobectomy for microcystic lesions, may be beneficial.[12] It has recently been shown that maternal systemic steroid treatment with dexamethasone will in most cases stop and reverse the growth of the CCAM.[13] Fetal intervention is therefore rarely necessary.

After birth, newborns with prenatally diagnosed lung cysts should undergo a thorough physical and radiological evaluation with emphasis on the airway and lungs. If the infant does not exhibit respiratory distress after a period of observation, it is reasonable to discharge the infant. Often the chest X-ray is completely normal, but this does not mean that the CCAM or sequestration is no longer present. At 3 months of age, a CT scan is obtained to evaluate and characterize the lesion. Cystic pulmonary airway malformations are often not resected until after 3 months of age, since they are rarely symptomatic early in life. Because of a lack of strong evidence dictating routine resection for congenital lung cysts, the evidence for resection versus expectant management must be reviewed in detail with the family before a decision is made to remove the cystic lung lesion. In most cases, a lobectomy is required, and this can usually be accomplished safely using a thoracoscopic approach.

Intra-abdominal cysts are also seen commonly prenatally. The most common cause in a female fetus is an ovarian cyst. In both genders, the cysts can also include mesenteric cysts, intestinal duplication cysts, and less commonly cysts from the biliary system, liver and pancreas. After birth, a repeat US will usually provide an accurate diagnosis. Ovarian cysts that are <4 cm in diameter can safely be observed, and most will resolve on their own over time. Simple ovarian cysts >4 cm in diameter are at higher risk of torsion, and should be aspirated percutaneously. Ovarian cysts that recur after aspiration should be resected. Complex ovarian cysts may have undergone torsion prenatally or may be teratomas. Although some authors advocate an expectant approach to these cysts, most prefer early resection. Nonovarian neonatal abdominal cysts can also be managed with a period of observation and repeat ultrasound studies, but should be resected if they do not decrease in size or if they become symptomatic. Most cysts can be resected using laparoscopic-assisted techniques.

Necrotizing enterocolitis is an inflammatory condition primarily affecting neonates who are premature and small for gestational age, although it can also be found in full-term infants. A related variant consisting of isolated ileal perforation also primarily affects premature infants. In its mildest form, NEC can present with symptoms of feeding intolerance, abdominal distension, and localized pneumatosis intestinalis on abdominal X-ray. This form of NEC can be treated with a course of bowel rest and antibiotics before feeding is restarted. Necrotizing enterocolitis can also involve more extensive areas of the intestine, which causes severe systemic symptoms, with thrombocytopenia, coagulopathy, septic shock, and intestinal perforation. It is therefore recommended to follow patients with NEC with serial abdominal X-rays to look for evidence of free intra-abdominal air, portal venous gas, and loops of intestine that appear to be fixed in one position. More recently, ultrasound has been used in patients with NEC to look for evidence of decreased or absent perfusion to segments of intestine. Indications for surgical intervention include bowel perforation and continued sepsis despite medical therapy. Surgical options include exploratory laparotomy, or placement of an intraperitoneal drain under local anesthesia. The latter procedure is primarily used for premature infants under 1,500 g with intestinal perforation, and it is associated with similar outcomes in this group of children.[14]

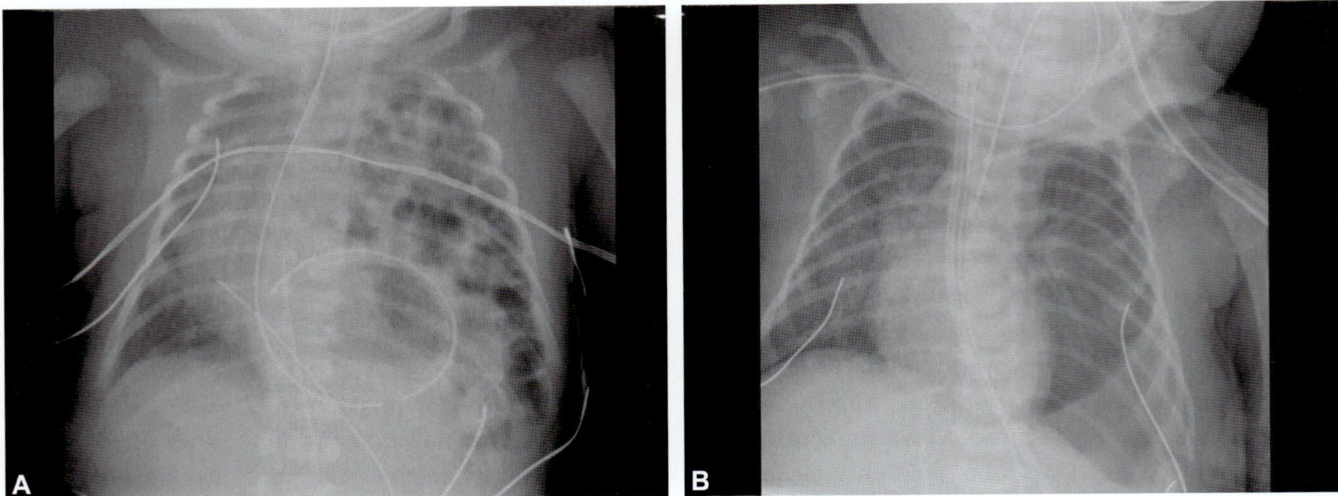

Figs. 19.4A and B: Diaphragmatic hernia (Bochdalek hernia), left side. (A) Before repair; (B) After repair.

If a laparotomy is done, the ischemic intestine should be resected and a proximal diverting stoma created. In isolated ileal perforation and cases of NEC with localized disease and minimal systemic sepsis, it is reasonable to consider resection or repair of perforation with primary anastomosis and no stoma.

In recent years an increasing number of neonatal surgical operations have been described using minimal access techniques, including laparoscopic and thoracoscopic approaches, or using an umbilical incision which leaves an almost invisible scar.[15,16]

SURGICAL CONDITIONS IN INFANTS

Several congenital anomalies may present in the first year of life, after the neonatal period, including small and initially asymptomatic CDH, CPAMs, rotation abnormalities, and Hirschsprung's disease. There are also a number of common surgical conditions that characteristically present in the first year of life, including hypertrophic pyloric stenosis, intussusception, and inguinal hernia.

Congenital diaphragmatic hernia can present outside the neonatal period. Late-presenting CDH is usually diagnosed incidentally on a chest X-ray done for other reasons, but can present with intestinal obstruction because of herniation of intestine into the chest (Figs. 19.4A and B).

Rotation abnormalities include a spectrum of disorders characterized by lack of normal intestinal rotation or incomplete rotation. Although many of these children are asymptomatic, some have a narrow-based mesentery which put them at risk of mid-gut volvulus, which can cause intestinal ischemia or necrosis if uncorrected. This is a true surgical emergency, and therefore early diagnosis and operation (detorsion of the mid-gut and a Ladd procedure, which places the intestines into a position of nonrotation) is imperative. Since the abdominal X-ray may be unhelpful in these children, an urgent upper contrast study must be done in any child who presents with bilious vomiting. If the ligament of Treitz is abnormally situated, laparotomy should be done emergently. Ultrasound scan can also be helpful in demonstrating abnormal orientation of the superior mesenteric artery and vein or a "whirlpool" sign on Doppler imaging. The management of the asymptomatic child with a rotation abnormality is controversial, and laparoscopy can be useful in determining the length of the mesenteric base and the need for a Ladd procedure.[17]

Hirschsprung's disease[18] is a condition characterized by the absence of intestinal ganglion cells in the rectum and colon. It is rarely diagnosed prenatally; approximately 50% of patients present with distal intestinal obstruction in the first month of life. Diagnosis is now common in the neonatal period because of the ease and accuracy of suction rectal biopsies and the heightened level of suspicion among neonatologists. However, many infants present after the neonatal period, usually with a picture of chronic constipation, and often associated with failure to thrive. Most infants can undergo a primary "pull-through" procedure in which the aganglionic bowel is resected and the normally innervated bowel is anastomosed just above the anal sphincter. In most cases, this procedure can be done using a transanal or laparoscopic technique (Fig. 19.5). A staged approach with a temporary stoma may be necessary in the older child with severe constipation for an extended period who has developed a massively and chronically

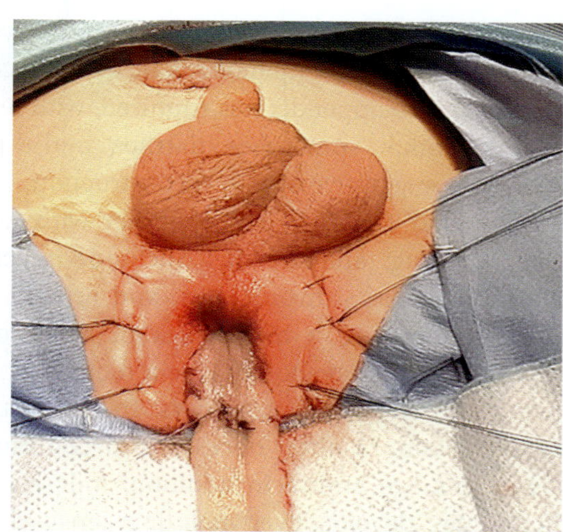

Fig. 19.5: Transanal pull-through procedure for Hirschsprung's disease. The stitch marks the biopsy site used to identify normally innervated colon.

dilated large intestine proximal to the aganglionic colon. A temporary stoma may also be necessary in children with neonatal cecal perforation, severe enterocolitis, suspected total colonic aganglionosis, and in settings without reliable pathology support. Long-term outcomes in patients with Hirschsprung's disease are excellent, although many children will have problems with persistent obstructive symptoms, soiling, or enterocolitis over the first 5–10 years of life.[18]

Hypertrophic pyloric stenosis is a surgically correctable condition characterized by gastric outlet obstruction from a hypertrophic pylorus, which occurs in approximately 1:400 infants. Pyloric stenosis affects boys three to four times more often than girls. The most common presentation is a first-born child between the ages of 3–6 weeks who presents with projectile, nonbilious vomiting. Because of the recurrent vomiting of gastric contents, the electrolytes can become quite deranged leading to hypokalemic hypochloremic alkalosis. It is important to provide fluid resuscitation with normal saline and potassium in order to correct the electrolyte abnormalities preoperatively. It may take >24 hours to correct the electrolyte abnormalities in an infant who has been vomiting for several days.

Pyloric stenosis is surgically corrected with a Ramstedt pyloromyotomy, which can be performed laparoscopically, through an umbilical incision or through a right upper quadrant incision. It is not uncommon that general surgeons in rural settings perform this operation, although the complication rate has been shown to be higher among general surgeons who do a small volume of pyloromyotomies.[20]

After the pyloromyotomy has been performed it is safe to feed the infant. However, it may take a few days before intake is adequate, and postoperative vomiting is common. If the vomiting persists for >3–5 days, there is concern that the pyloromyotomy was inadequate and it may need to be redone. This complication is seen in approximately 1% of patients. Perforation after pyloromyotomy is even rarer, but if unrecognized can be a potentially fatal complication.

Intussusception is most commonly seen between 3 and 12 months of age. However, intussusception can occur up to 4 or 5 years of age, particularly if there is a pathological lead point such as a polyp, inverted Meckel's diverticulum, or tumor. Intussusception is most commonly seen in the ileocecal area of the intestine. The diagnosis is suspected based on a history of intermittent severe abdominal pain, vomiting, or current-jelly stools, and is confirmed by ultrasound scan or contrast enema. A barium or air enema reduction, performed most often by a pediatric radiologist, can reduce the intussusception and has become the standard of care. In some cases multiple attempts at radiological reduction are necessary. About 25% of patients will need surgical management, either because of unsuccessful attempts at radiological reduction or because of perforation or multiple recurrences. Ten percent of the patients requiring surgical management will have a lead-point.[21]

Inguinal hernia is common in infants and young children. Most inguinal hernias in children are indirect and result from a patent processus vaginalis. The incidence is highest in the first 2 years of life. About 5% of children will develop an inguinal hernia, and it is five times more common in boys than girls. Premature infants have a much higher incidence of inguinal hernias. Infants born prior to 32 weeks or with a birth weight <1,000 g, have a 20% chance of developing an inguinal hernia.

Inguinal hernias more commonly affect the right side (65%) than the left side (20%) and bilateral inguinal hernias occur in 15% of patients. The most serious complication is incarceration, which occurs in up to 30% of infants with a hernia, and is associated with a 10% risk of testicular atrophy.[22] For this reason, repair should be done expeditiously in infants with a new diagnosis of inguinal hernia.[23] If a hernia does become incarcerated, it can usually be reduced by an experienced pediatric surgeon and repaired within 48–72 hours after the edema has subsided. Surgical correction can be performed under spinal anesthesia, but is more commonly performed under general anesthesia in children. A caudal or ilioinguinal block is often performed in children <2 years of age, to provide pain relief after the operation.

Inguinal hernia repair is the most common operation performed in children. Studies indicate that outcomes are slightly better when a pediatric surgeon performs the operation compared to a general surgeon, although general surgeons who carry out a high number of cases have similar outcomes to pediatric surgeons.[24]

Hydroceles are very common, and are also caused by a patent processus vaginalis that contains fluid rather than intestine. In some cases, the processus vaginalis closes, trapping the fluid in the scrotum or along the spermatic cord (noncommunicating hydrocele). Over time the fluid becomes reabsorbed, and therefore surgical intervention is unnecessary. Noncommunicating hydroceles are associated with a history of slow decrease in size with no daily fluctuation in size and inability to reduce the fluid on examination. In general, hydroceles should not be operated on until at least 2 years of age, and only then if there is no decrease in size. The diagnosis of communicating hydrocele can be made if the hydrocele is not resolving by age of 2 years, and should be repaired electively to avoid the possibility of bowel coming through the patent processus sometime in the future.

SURGICAL CONDITIONS IN THE TODDLER

Toddlers (ages 1–3 years) may develop all of the surgical conditions discussed in the infant category, but do not develop hypertrophic pyloric stenosis.

Appendicitis is occasionally seen in children <4 years. Most children (70%) with appendicitis in this age group will present after the appendix has ruptured, with fevers, abdominal distention, sometimes diarrhea, and a plain abdominal X-ray suggestive of a bowel obstruction.

The differential diagnosis for a toddler with fevers, distention, vomiting, and diarrhea includes infectious gastroenteritis, Meckel's diverticulitis, and urinary tract infection, and therefore a high index of suspicion is necessary. These children should have a rectal examination, which may detect a pelvic abscess. The use of ultrasound and CT scan is often necessary to confirm the diagnosis in this age group. In addition, toddlers with appendicitis may develop overwhelming sepsis due to the fact that the omentum is less capable of walling off the pus in a child with free perforation.[25]

Lower gastrointestinal bleeding due to Meckel's diverticulum can occur at any age, but is most common in the toddler age group. The bleeding is due to ulceration in the ileal mucosa secondary to acid secretion from ectopic gastric mucosa in the diverticulum. There is usually a "sentinel" bleed that stops, followed by painless massive bright red blood per rectum, often with a need for transfusion. The diagnosis is made by a technetium nuclear scan, in which the tracer is concentrated in the ectopic gastric mucosa in the lower abdomen (Figs. 19.6A and B). The sensitivity of the scan can be increased by pretreatment with an H-2 blocker. In addition, occasionally an intestinal duplication cyst will have ectopic gastric mucosa and can present in the same way; the Meckel's scan will be positive in those cases as well. The treatment of Meckel's diverticulum is excision, which in most cases

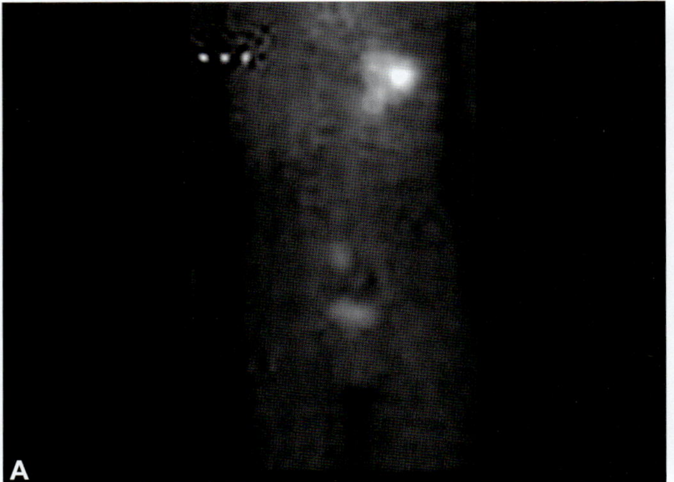

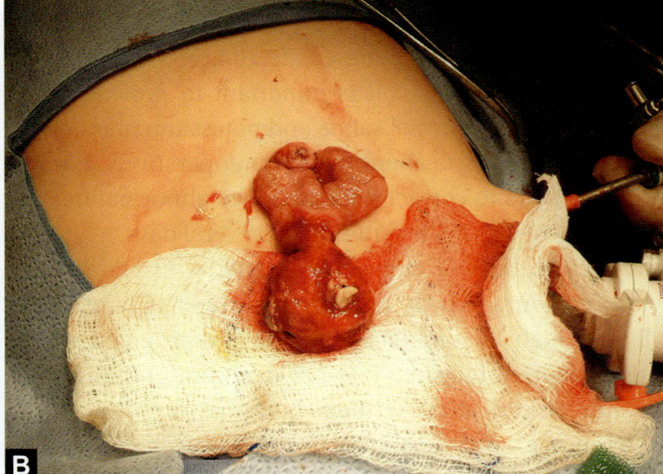

Figs. 19.6A and B: Meckel's diverticulum. (A) Radionuclide scan shows a "hot" spot in the lower abdomen; (B) At the time of surgery.

can be done laparoscopically. In a child with a classical history and a negative nuclear scan, it is appropriate to perform laparoscopy, and in most cases a Meckel's diverticulum will be found despite the negative scan.

The two most common pediatric solid tumors (excluding brain tumors) are Wilms' tumor and neuroblastoma. These can develop at any age, including prenatally, but most commonly present in toddlers. The most common presentation is an asymptomatic abdominal mass, which is often extremely large at the time it is noticed by the parents. Management depends on the stage at the time of diagnosis, but usually involves a combination of surgical resection, chemotherapy, and radiation.

SURGICAL CONDITIONS IN PRESCHOOL AND SCHOOL AGE

Children in the ages from 3 years to 6 years have many of the same surgical issues as toddlers and older children. In this age group, appendicitis and inguinal hernias are the most common surgical conditions that require intervention. In addition, trauma is commonly seen in this age group.

Umbilical hernias are usually present at birth, and are most common in the African population. In 95% of cases, the hernia will resolve on its own over time, and this can take up to 8–10 years. The risk of incarceration of an umbilical hernia during childhood is remote, and repair in the first year or second year of life is associated with a higher rate of recurrence. Therefore, most pediatric surgeons will not repair an umbilical hernia until the child is 4–5 years of age, assuming that it is not decreasing in size at that time.

SURGICAL CONDITIONS IN ADOLESCENTS

Adolescents have overall few surgical needs. Appendicitis, trauma, and inguinal hernia are the most common surgical conditions encountered in this age group. Inflammatory bowel disease is also seen in this age group.

Appendicitis is the most common surgical condition encountered in hospitalized children. Appendicitis can often be accurately diagnosed by a detailed history, physical examination, and laboratory investigations [primarily white blood cell (WBC) count with differential, and urinalysis]. A number of appendicitis scores have been developed that have been validated in children.[26] However, in recent decades most children also receive diagnostic imaging in an attempt to make the diagnosis more accurately and prevent negative operations. In addition to looking for the specific findings of appendicitis, imaging can be helpful in identifying other pathology that may masquerade as appendicitis, such as ovarian cysts or torsion, IBD, omental torsion, and enlarged mesenteric lymph nodes ("mesenteric adenitis"). In skilled hands, ultrasonography can be quite accurate in diagnosing appendicitis, but sometimes the scan cannot visualize the appendix, particularly in obese children. Computerized tomography has also been extensively studied in children, and has been found to be very accurate. However, recent recognition of the long-term adverse effects of ionizing radiation from CT has pushed most clinicians to use other methods.

The surgical treatment of appendicitis is appendectomy, which can be performed through an open incision in the right lower quadrant or laparoscopically. The advantage of laparoscopic appendectomy is a decreased risk of developing a superficial wound infection and decreased length of stay.[27] There are conflicting data in the surgical literature in regards to cost for open versus laparoscopic appendectomy. The equipment cost is higher for laparoscopic appendectomy, but since many studies have shown a shorter length of stay and decreased wound infection, the equipment cost may be outweighed by the decreased cost associated with decreased length of stay, and decreased readmissions and visits related to wound infections. A recent Cochrane review including studies with adult and pediatric patients found a slightly increased risk of intra-abdominal infections after laparoscopic appendectomy.[28]

Patients with nonperforated appendicitis should receive perioperative prophylactic antibiotics. Patients with perforated appendicitis should receive preoperative antibiotics plus a 5- to 7-day course of postoperative antibiotics. The antibiotic choice should provide coverage for gram-negative bacteria, anaerobes, and enterococcus; many combinations of antibiotic that have been shown to be effective. Once the patient has become afebrile and the WBC has normalized, the child can be discharged. The importance of additional antibiotic treatment with oral antibiotics in this setting is unclear. If the WBC remains elevated, the fever persists, and/or the patient is not doing well clinically by day 5–7, repeat imaging should be done to look for an intra-abdominal abscess. If there is an abscess that is accessible, it is reasonable to attempt image-guided drainage.

For children with perforated appendicitis and a long history of disease consistent with appendicitis, who have an established abscess or phlegmon, it is often safest to drain the abscess if possible, and place a PICC line for antibiotic treatment. The duration of treatment is primarily determined by clinical progression, but it is common to treat empirically for 10–14 days. For some patients with persistent symptoms and incompletely drained collections, the use of tissue plasminogen activator through the drain has been shown to be safe and may accelerate resolution.[29] There is controversy regarding whether an interval appendectomy should be performed following nonoperative treatment of an appendiceal abscess or phlegmon. The risk of the operation must be weighed against the risk of recurrent appendicitis.[30]

Inflammatory bowel disease (IBD) affects adolescents more commonly than any other age group. It is uncommon for children < 10 years of age to develop IBD, and the incidence increases appreciably in children over 15 years.

Crohn's disease (CD) can affect any portion of the gastrointestinal tract, and is characterized by transmural inflammation that ultimately results in fibrosis and stricture formation. The most commonly affected part of the intestine is the terminal ileum, where it typically causes obstructive symptoms and occasionally leads to perforation and fistula formation. Ulcerative colitis (UC), on the other hand, is limited to the colonic mucosa, and most often results in bloody diarrhea rather than obstructive symptoms. However, 10% of children with CD have disease limited to the colon, and 10% of patients presenting with colitis have features of both UC and CD, and are therefore categorized as "indeterminate colitis" or "inflammatory bowel disease-undetermined (IBD-U)".

IBD is usually managed medically, initially with a combination of high-dose steroids, anti-inflammatory salicylic acid derivatives, antibiotics, and most recently anti-TNFα antibodies. If medical treatment fails to result in remission, or a complication develops, surgical treatment becomes necessary.

The operation of choice for UC is total proctocolectomy with ileoanal J-pouch reconstruction. This procedure can be done laparoscopically and can often be performed in two stages with colectomy, pouch formation and loop ileostomy as the first stage and ileostomy closure as the second stage. A three-stage approach, with subtotal colectomy and ileostomy as the first stage, proctectomy and loop ileostomy as the second stage, and ileostomy closure as the third stage should be used for children on high-dose chronic steroids, those with malnutrition, those with indeterminate colitis, and the very young child in whom the probability of the colitis being due to CD is much higher than in the older child.

Patients with CD will often need operation for symptoms of ileal obstruction. The most common operation is an ileocecectomy with primary anastomosis, which can be performed using a laparoscopic-assisted approach in most cases. Patients with more proximal small bowel disease will usually need segmental resection. If there is extensive small bowel involvement at multiple sites, strictureplasty should be performed, since there is no benefit to achieve free margins. The need for reoperation approaches 35% at 10 years and 45% at 15 years. Patients with colonic CD that is unresponsive to medical therapy require colectomy. If the rectum is relatively disease-free, an ileoproctostomy can be created, but the recurrence rate is very high and quality of life tends to be poor. If the rectum is involved with CD the best option is usually an end-ileostomy. Some surgeons have done J-pouch reconstruction for CD, but most surgeons believe that CD is a contraindication to this operation. On the other hand, children with IBD-U can have a pouch created, although there is probably a higher risk of pouch failure due to severe pouchitis in these patients.

Children with CD often develop severe perianal disease, either as the initial presenting symptom or after a diagnosis of CD has already been made. Although benign crypt-related abscesses and fistulae are common in the infant age group, it is important to consider and pursue the diagnosis of CD in any child older than 2 years of age who presents with a perianal abscess or fistula. The surgical management of perianal CD includes drainage of abscesses and placement of a seton to provide ongoing drainage. Medical therapy includes the use of antibiotics such as metronidazole, and the use of anti-TNF drugs. For those children in whom the disease cannot be controlled medically, a loop ileostomy or occasionally a total proctocolectomy is sometimes necessary.

Pectus excavatum (Fig. 19.7) and pectus carinatum are both common forms of chest wall deformity that are often referred to pediatric surgeons. They are often present since early childhood, but usually worsen at the time of puberty. There is considerable controversy regarding the physiological consequences of pectus excavatum, but in most cases the main reason to consider surgical correction is the cosmetic appearance of the chest. The traditional operation was described by Ravitch and involves resection of the involved costal cartilages and transverse sternotomy to bring the lower sternum into a more normal position. More recently Nuss described a less invasive technique in which a bar is placed behind the sternum

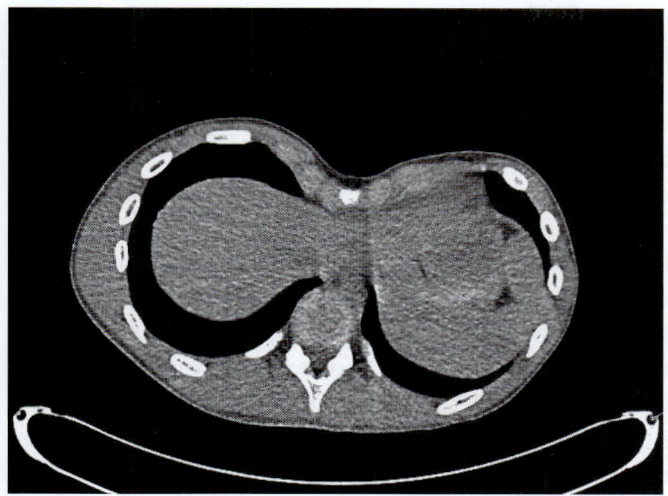

Fig. 19.7: CT scan chest of patient with pectus excavatum.

under thoracoscopic visualization and left in place for several years. Although most surgeons are now using the Nuss procedure, there is still controversy regarding which is the better operation.[31]

Pectus carinatum is not associated with any physiological abnormalities, but is often a major cosmetic problem for adolescents. The Ravitch procedure can be used to repair this defect, but in recent years excellent results have been reported using bracing without need for surgical correction.[32]

PEDIATRIC TRAUMA

Trauma is the leading cause of death after infancy in children and it is the leading preventable health problem in children.

The most common causes of injury-related deaths are:

- Motor vehicle crashes
- Submersion injuries
- Homicide
- Suicide
- Non-accidental trauma
- Fire

There are over 11,000 injury related deaths in children <20 years annually in the United States. The long-term disability resulting from these injuries is estimated to be more than three times the mortality rate and is primarily the result of brain injury. Pediatric trauma results in a very high number of emergency department visits and in over 300,000 hospitalizations yearly.

There are nearly 2,000 confirmed deaths from non-accidental injury yearly in the United States and about 6 million children are mistreated and harmed yearly. Child abuse almost exclusively affects young children <4–5 years, children who are not able to protect themselves. It is likely that there are many child abuse cases unaccounted for every year, and it is important to have a high level of suspicion for child abuse when seeing a young pediatric trauma patient.

Annual lifetime cost of injuries to children in the United States is in the order of several hundred million dollars.

In developing countries, where access to healthcare often is limited, pediatric trauma has an even greater impact on individuals, many will not receive adequate care and the number of deaths from accidents is often not well recorded. In developing countries, there is also less emphasis on and resources available for preventive care. Lack of car seats for children, seat belts, bicycle helmets, and designated sidewalks, as well as unsafe road conditions contribute to a high rate of trauma and trauma-related deaths.

Risk of trauma also varies when comparing genders and age groups. Boys have a tenfold increased risk of death from risk-taking behavior when compared to girls. As mentioned previously, infants and toddlers are at highest risk of child abuse resulting in death or permanent disability.

Pediatric trauma patients may be best served in a designated trauma center, and added pediatric qualifications may further improve outcomes.[33,34] The initial evaluation of a pediatric trauma patient should take place in the emergency department, ideally in a designated trauma bay. A trauma activation system greatly improves the response time for the trauma team, and this in turn reduces the time it takes to complete a trauma workup.

The American College of Surgeons designates pediatric trauma centers as part of its trauma center accreditation process. Pediatric trauma centers have on their staff board-certified pediatric surgeons and neurosurgeons, in addition to a pediatric ICU, immediate access to X-ray, CT scan imaging, and laboratory results.

Certain types of injuries are more common in children and will be discussed below.

Head Trauma

Seventy-five percent of pediatric trauma deaths are from head injuries. A pediatric Glasgow Coma Scale (GCS) assessment should be made upon initial evaluation; if the GCS is 8 or less the child should be intubated to secure the airway. Children with a GCS <15 should undergo a CT scan of the head. Approximately 9% will have CT findings when presenting with a GCS of <15. Although only 1% of children with a GCS of 13–15 will need surgical interventions, imaging is important in identifying those in need of an intervention and can dictate increased monitoring, and possibly follow-up imaging.

The most common traumatic head injuries are: skull fracture, epidural hemorrhage, subdural hematoma, and subarachnoid bleeding. In addition, diffuse axonal injury is more common in children than in adults. It is often characterized by minimal or no findings on CT with a profoundly depressed level of consciousness.

All head trauma with associated CT findings should be managed by neurosurgery. Key aspects in managing head trauma are:

- Intracranial pressure monitoring to assure adequate perfusion pressure to the brain
- Seizure prophylaxis with antiseizure medication
- Temperature regulation or induced hypothermia
- Hypertonic saline to maintain a normal or high normal serum sodium

Thoracic Trauma

After head trauma, thoracic trauma is the second leading cause of death in pediatric trauma patients. The most common causes of thoracic trauma are motor vehicle accidents, pedestrian versus motor vehicle accidents, bicycle accidents, and falls.

Children have a more compliant chest wall than adults and more force is therefore transmitted to internal chest organs. Children are at greater risk for tension pneumothorax and have less of an ability to compensate by increasing heart rate in the setting of hypovolemia.

About 80% of chest trauma in children is from blunt trauma. Penetrating chest trauma is more common in adolescents and can make up a greater portion of trauma in inner-city environments where gun violence is common.

Abdominal Trauma

Most abdominal trauma in children is from blunt injury, which accounts for over 90% of injuries to the abdomen. Fortunately most patients with solid organ injuries do not require surgical intervention. These injuries are best diagnosed with a contrast CT scan. The CT scan allows for grading of injury to the solid organs and thus the injury can be managed according to a protocol.

The most commonly affected organs are spleen, liver, kidneys, and pancreas. Spleen and liver injuries rarely require surgical intervention.[35] The general rule of thumb for laparotomy in pediatric splenic and liver injury is a requirement for replacement of >50% of the blood volume.[19] Pancreatic duct disruption is sometimes seen and may require distal pancreatectomy, stent placement, or drainage of pancreatic pseudocyst. This injury can be seen in combination with a chance fracture of upper lumbar spine (L1-2) and duodenal hematoma. The mechanism for this injury is quite often a lap seat belt. Duodenal hematoma is best managed by placement of a feeding tube distal to the duodenal obstruction and then expectant management until there is evidence that there is no longer obstruction of the duodenum. The obstruction can take one to several weeks to resolve. Sometimes, an additional nasogastric tube has to be placed to drain secretions from the stomach.

Orthopedic Trauma

Children will commonly sustain fractures during accidents. As part of the trauma evaluation, a complete orthopedic surgical evaluation should be performed if there is suspicion for fractures, and an orthopedic surgeon should be consulted if there is suspicion or evidence of a fracture.

REFERENCES

1. Ziegler MM. The history of pediatric surgery in the United States. In: Operative Pediatric Surgery, Ziegler MM, Azizkhan RG, Weber TR (Eds). New York, NY: McGraw-Hill Companies; 2003. pp. 3-11.
2. Koop CE. A perspective on the early days of pediatric surgery. J Ped Surg. 1998;33(7):953-60.
3. Wilmore DW, Dudrick SJ. Growth and development of an infant receiving all nutrients exclusively by vein. JAMA. 1984;203(10):860-64.
4. Diamond IR, Pencharz PB, Feldman BM, et al. Novel lipid-based approaches to pediatric intestinal failure-associated liver disease. Arch Pediatr Adolesc Med. 2012(166):473-8.
5. Christison-Lagay ER, Langer JC. Neonatal abdominal wall defects. Semin Fetal Neonatal Med. 2011;16:164-72.
6. Nasr A, Langer JC. Mechanical traction techniques for long-gap esophageal atresia: a critical appraisal. Eur J Pediatr Surg. 2013;23:191-97.
7. Loukogeorgakis SP, Pierro A. Replacement surgery for esophageal atresia. Eur J Pediatr Surg. 2013;23:182-90.
8. Chiu PPL, Langer JC. Surgical conditions of the diaphragm: posterior diaphragmatic hernias in infants. Thorac Surg Clin. 2009;19:451-61.
9. Jacelewicz T, Chiang M, Oliveira C, et al. Late surgical outcomes among congenital diaphragmatic hernia (CDH) patients: why long-term follow-up with surgeons is recommended. J Pediatr Surg. 2013;48:935-41.

10. Chiu P, Sauer C, Mihailovic A, et al. The price of success in the management of congenital diaphragmatic hernia: is improved survival accompanied by an increase in long-term morbidity? J Pediatr Surg. 2006;41:888-92.
11. Miller JA, Corteville JE, Langer JC. Congenital cystic adenomatoid malformation in the fetus: natural history and predictors of outcome. J Pediatr Surg. 1996;31:805-8.
12. Adzick NS. Management of fetal lung lesions. Clin Perinatol. 2009;36(2):363-76.
13. Tsao K, Hawgood S, Vu L, et al. Resolution of hydrops fetalis in congenital cystic adenomatoid malformation after prenatal steroid therapy. J Pediatr Surg. 2003;38(3):508-10.
14. Moss RL, Dimmitt RA, Barnhart DC, et al. Laparotomy versus peritoneal drainage for necrotizing enterocolitis and perforation. N Engl J Med. 2006;354:2225-34.
15. Suri M, Langer JC. Circumumbilical vs transverse abdominal incision for neonatal abdominal surgery. J Pediatr Surg. 2011;46:1076-80.
16. Blinman T, Ponsky T. Pediatric minimally invasive surgery: laparoscopy and thoracoscopy in children. Pediatrics. 2012;130(3):539-49.
17. Hsiao M, Langer JC. Value of laparoscopy in children with a suspected rotation abnormality on imaging. J Pediatr Surg. 2011;46(7):1347-52.
18. Langer JC. Hirschsprung's disease. Curr Opin Pediatr. 2013;25(3):368-74.
19. Davies DA, Pearl RH, Ein SH, et al. Management of blunt splenic injury in children: evolution of the non-operative approach. J Pediatr Surg. 2009;44:1005-8.
20. Langer JC, To T. Does pediatric surgical specialty training affect outcome after Ramstedt pyloromyotomy? A population-based study. Pediatrics. 2004;113:1342-7.
21. Somme S, To T, Langer JC. Factors determining the need for operative reduction in children with intussusception: a population-based study. J Pediatr Surg. 2006;41(5):1014.
22. Walc L, Bass J, Rubin S, et al. Testicular fate after incarcerated hernia repair and/or orchiopexy performed in patients under 6 months of age. J Pediatr Surg. 1995;8:1195-7.
23. Zamakhshary M, To T, Guan J, et al. Risk of incarceration of inguinal hernia among infants and young children awaiting elective surgery. CMAJ. 2008;179:1001-5.
24. Bohrenstein SH, To T, Wajja A, et al. Effect of subspecialty training and volume on outcome after pediatric inguinal hernia repair. J Pediatr Surg. 2005;40:75-80.
25. Aziz O, Athanasiou T, Tekkis PP, et al. Laparoscopic versus open appendectomy in children: a meta-analysis. Ann Surg. 2006;243:17-27.
26. Goldman RD, Carter S, Stephens D, et al. Prospective validation of the pediatric appendicitis score. J Pediatr. 2008;153:278-82.
27. Kahn MN, Fayyad T, Cecil TD, et al. Laparoscopic versus open appendectomy: the risk of postoperative infectious complications. JSLS. 2007;11(3):363-7.
28. Sauerland S, Jaschinski T, Neugebauer EAM. Laparoscopic versus open surgery for suspected appendicitis. Cochrane Database Syst Rev. 2010;(10):CD001546. DOI: 10.1002/14651858.CD001546.pub3
29. Shawyer AC, Amaral JGPV, Langer JC. The role of tissue plasminogen activator in the management of complex intra-abdominal abscesses in children. J Pediatr Surg. 2012;47:1380-84.
30. Hall NJ, Jones CE, Eaton S, et al. Is interval appendicectomy justified after successful nonoperative treatment of an appendix mass in children? A systematic review. J Pediatr Surg. 2011;46:767-71.
31. Nasr A, Fecteau A, Wales PW. Comparison of the Nuss and the Ravitch procedure for pectus excavatum repair: a meta-analysis. J Pediatr Surg. 2010;45:880-86.
32. Martinez-Ferro M, Fraire C, Bernard S. Dynamic compression system for treatment of pectus carinatum. Semin Pediatr Surg. 2008;17:194-200.
33. Oyetunji TA, Haider AH, Downing SR, et al. Treatment outcomes of injured children at adult level trauma centers: are there benefits from added specialized care? Am J Surg. 2011;201(4):445-9.
34. Matsushima K, Schaefer EW, Won EJ, et al. Injured adolescents, not just large children: difference in care and outcome between adult and pediatric trauma centers. Am Surg. 2013;79:267-73.
35. Stylianos S. Outcomes from pediatric solid organ injury: role of standardized care guidelines. Curr Opin Pediatr. 2005;17:402-6.

Case Study: Preventable Complications During Central Venous Access 20

James M Goff Jr

THE PROBLEM

Misplaced access wires and arterial cannulation during central venous access are challenging problems and their management requires careful consideration of the anatomic location of the complication and the clinical condition of the patient. Both complications can be managed with endovascular or open surgical techniques. Attention to wire access/control and immediate recognition of inadvertent intra-arterial access are critical to avoid these complications.

THE TYPICAL CASE

Case 1—Misplaced Access Wire

A 68-year-old man presented to the emergency department with acute respiratory failure caused by congestive heart failure. The emergency medicine physician, who reported that the patient was very uncooperative during the procedure, placed a right internal jugular vein central venous triple lumen catheter under ultrasound guidance. The patient was admitted to the medical intensive care unit (MICU) and postprocedure chest X-ray (CXR) demonstrated the triple lumen catheter to be in good position (Fig. 20.1).

On hospital day 2, the patient became agitated and pulled out his triple lumen catheter. CXR was obtained and demonstrated a wire at the junction of the right jugular and subclavian veins (Fig. 20.2).

A CT scan of the chest and abdomen was performed and confirmed the wire origin as described and through the right heart into the inferior vena cava (Figs. 20.3 and 20.4). Vascular surgery was consulted and an abdominal X-ray was obtained and confirmed the location of the wire with the wire terminus in the left internal iliac vein (Fig. 20.5). The patient was taken to the endovascular suite and under local anesthesia through a percutaneous left femoral vein access, the wire was engaged and moved into the left external iliac vein and removed with a gooseneck snare.

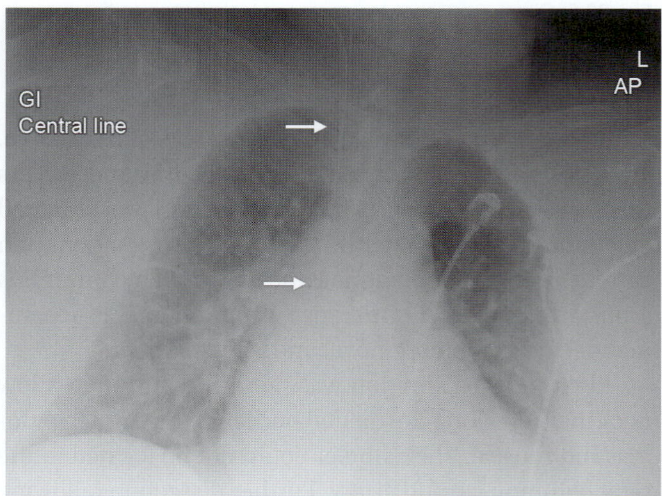

Fig. 20.1: Central venous access (wire likely retained in catheter at this time).

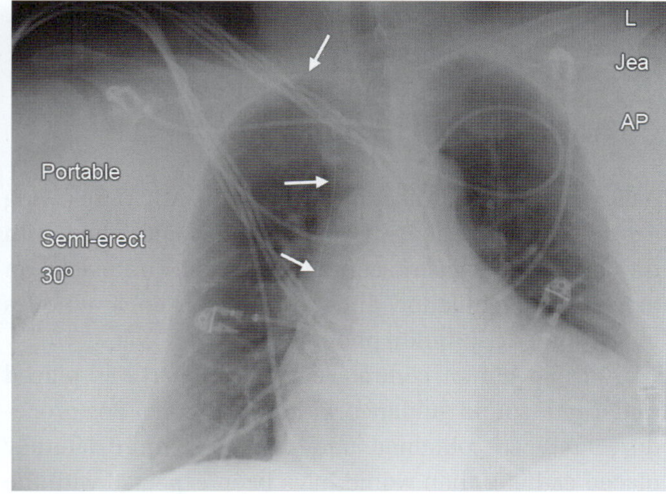

Fig. 20.2: Wire at right jugular—subclavian vein junction and through the right heart.

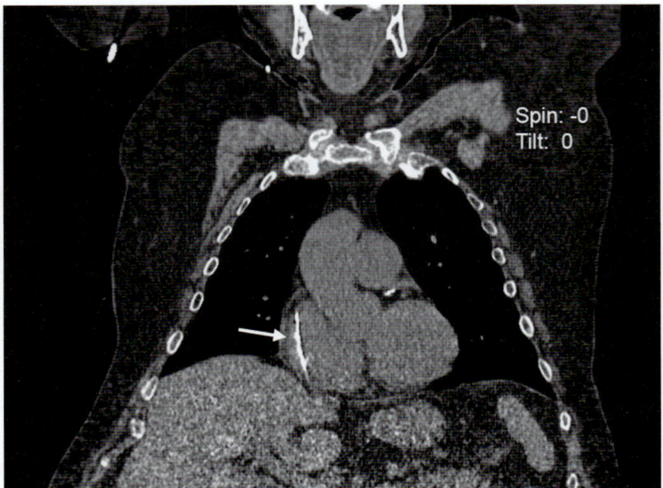

Fig. 20.3: Wire in right heart.

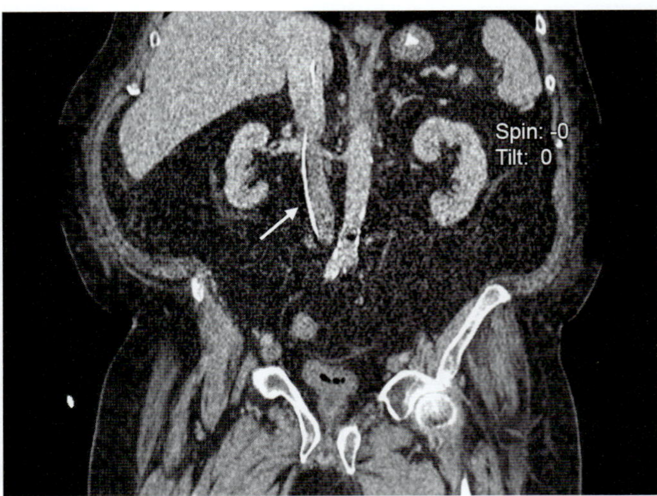

Fig. 20.4: Wire in the inferior vena cava.

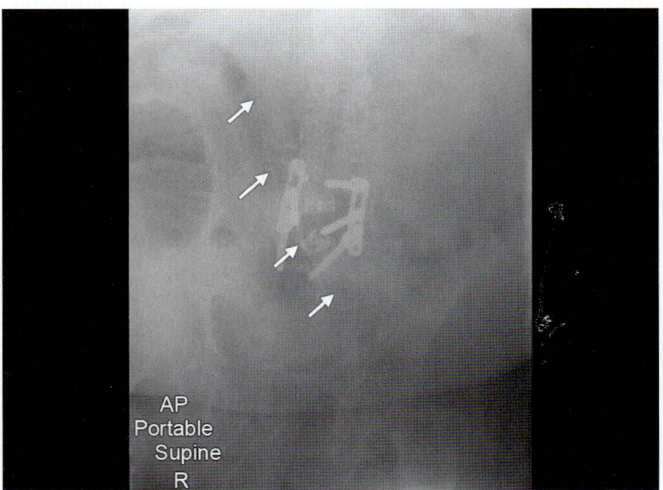

Fig. 20.5: J tip wire terminus in the left internal iliac vein.

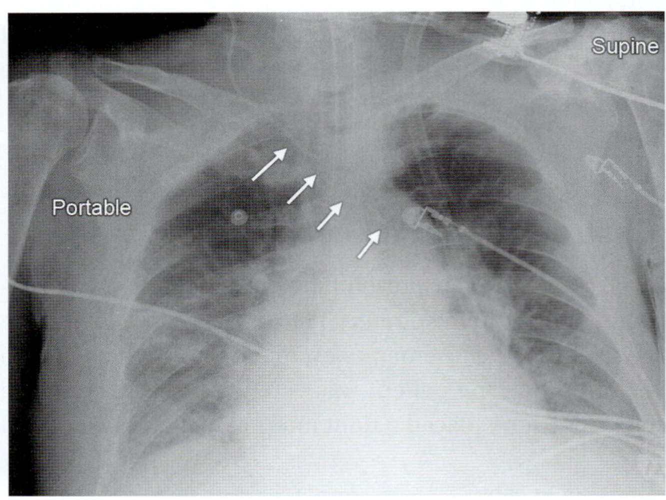

Fig. 20.6: Chest X-ray showing course of triple lumen catheter.

Case 2—Arterial Cannulation

A 65-year-old man was transferred to the MICU following a respiratory arrest. He was emergently intubated with the aspiration of gastric contents, sedated, and placed on mechanical ventilation and broad-spectrum antibiotics for presumed aspiration pneumonia.

A triple lumen central venous catheter was placed under ultrasound guidance without difficulty. Postprocedure CXR was obtained and showed a more laterally placed catheter than would have been expected with the catheter tip in the aortic arch (Fig. 20.6). Two hours after catheter placement, confirmation of the catheter position prior to use was requested by the nurse at the bedside. The CXR was reviewed and a misplaced arterial access was suspected. A carotid duplex ultrasound was obtained and showed the catheter in the proximal right common carotid artery with hematoma and questionable thrombus around the catheter. Operative exploration was recommended for catheter removal and arterial repair.

Right neck exploration was performed through a low neck incision along the medial border of the sternocleidomastoid muscle. The catheter could not be located in the right common carotid artery. Further dissection following the course of the catheter demonstrated the catheter to enter the subclavian artery just distal to the origin of the

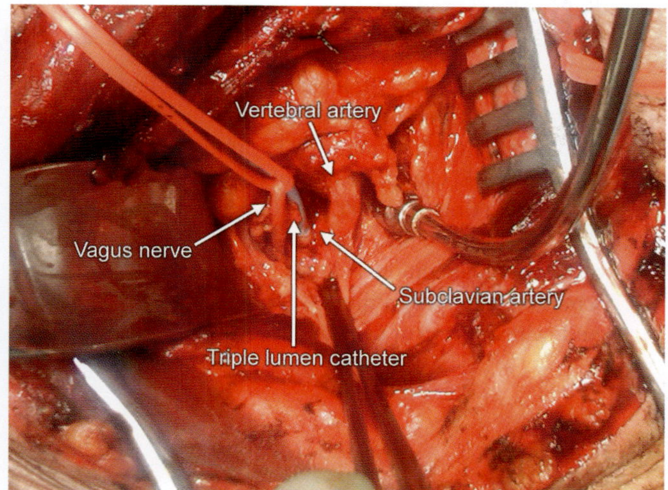

Fig. 20.7: Triple lumen catheter in the subclavian artery.

vertebral artery (Fig. 20.7). The subclavian artery was mobilized and a purse string suture was placed into the artery around the catheter entry site. The catheter was removed and the suture was secured. At the completion of the operative procedure, a left internal jugular vein central venous access was placed under ultrasound guidance. The patient was returned to the MICU for further medical management.

DIAGNOSTIC DILEMMAS

Central venous catheter placement is a common procedure performed by a wide variety of providers in multiple clinical specialties. Appropriate placement of a central venous catheter requires knowledge of anatomic landmarks (for either internal jugular vein or subclavian vein access), use of ultrasound to differentiate venous from arterial structures, and confirmation that central venous access has occurred.

Central venous catheter placement into the internal jugular vein is facilitated by the use of ultrasound. The vein is usually identified at the base of the neck or more cephalad, and it is distinguished from the artery by lack of pulsation and compressibility. Once identified, Seldinger technique is used to place an entry needle under direct ultrasound visualization. Placing the patient in Trendelenburg position can assist placement. Confusion can occur in identifying the internal jugular vein if the ultrasound probe is placed laterally to the sternocleidomastoid muscle and other vascular structures are identified or if compression is not used to differentiate between the artery and the vein.

Immediately following catheter placement, confirmation of correct location is essential. All access wires must be removed. Early identification of arterial misplacement occurs when removing the guidewire with a return of pulsatile arterial blood. Arterial placement can also be identified during aspiration and flushing of the catheter. Finally, concern for a retained wire or arterial access should occur if there is difficulty infusing through the catheter. Completion CXR is essential to confirm proper central venous access placement.

MANAGEMENT OPTIONS

Retained guidewires with central venous access is an avoidable complication. The most common factor leading to this complication is inattention or distraction of the operator during the procedure. Fortunately, most retained guidewires can be removed percutaneously by an experienced interventional radiologist or endovascular surgeon.

Early identification of a misplaced arterial access, particularly from a neck approach, can be managed with removal of the catheter and manual compression assuming that the arterial puncture site is accessible (above the clavicle) and that the catheter diameter is small. Removal of the catheter typically occurs immediately following placement when arterial cannulation is suspected from pulsatile blood or identified on an immediate postprocedure CXR, which demonstrates the catheter in an incorrect location. Care must be taken with this approach, as large hematomas can occur and there is a risk for stroke with carotid artery compression.

Late identification of an arterial catheterization requires a thoughtful and individualized patient care plan depending on the diameter of the catheter/sheath involved, the presumed site of arterial injury, and the treatment options available. If the anatomy is unclear, duplex imaging can be helpful to identify the course of the catheter, its entry point into the artery, and any associated hematoma or intra-arterial thrombus. Regardless of the approach, it is critical to leave the catheter/sheath in place within the artery until there is a definitive treatment plan.

Experienced operators in endovascular techniques have used a variety of techniques including closure devices and covered stents to close arterial puncture sites, typically those involving the subclavian artery. Recently, closure devices have also been used to repair carotid arteries following inadvertent arterial cannulation. Endovascular techniques by experienced surgeons are most attractive and best employed where vascular control is difficult (below or behind the clavicle). Additionally, operators must be prepared to immediately perform open operative arterial repair if these techniques fail.

Surgical repair allows for proximal and distal vascular control of the injury site and direct inspection of the arterial injury. Surgical repair should be considered for all patients in whom endovascular repair is not an option, the catheter has been in an artery for a prolonged period of time, or the catheter/sheath size is large.

FURTHER READING

1. Bechara CF, Barshes NR, Pisimisis G, et al. Management of inadvertent carotid artery sheath insertion during central venous catheter placement. JAMA Surg. 2013;148:1063-66.
2. Kusminsky RE. Complications of central venous catheterization. J Am Coll Surg. 2007;204:681-96.
3. McGee DC, Gould MK. Preventing complications of central venous catheterization. N Engl J Med. 2003;348:1123-33.
4. Schummer W, Schummer C, Graser E, et al. Loss of the guidewire: mishap or blunder. Br J Anaesth. 2002;88:144-6.

Case Study: 21
Preparation of the Elderly Patient for Elective Surgery

Seth Waits, Michael J Englesbe

THE PROBLEM

Each year 5 million Americans over the age of 65 have inpatient surgery. Older patients are at increased risk of poor surgical outcomes, demonstrating higher rates of postoperative complications, longer lengths of stay, more utilization of skilled nursing facilities, increased mortality, and higher costs when compared with younger patients undergoing similar procedures.[1] In addition, these older patients are expected to drive a 47% increase in surgical procedures through 2020.[1,2] Within this context, efforts to improve postoperative outcomes will have tremendous importance as our highest-risk surgical population continues to expand.

THE TYPICAL CASE

A 67-year-old man is being evaluated for an elective colostomy takedown. Two years ago, during an episode of diverticulitis, he underwent a laparotomy for sigmoid colectomy and colostomy. He has a medical history significant for obesity, chronic obstructive pulmonary disease (COPD), and poorly controlled type-2 diabetes mellitus. He appears moderately frail. Although proceeding very slowly, he is able to get out of a chair and onto the exam table by himself. He lives alone and completes all of his own activities of daily living. Preoperative labs show a modestly decreased serum albumin but are otherwise within normal limits. His EKG and chest X-ray are normal. His forced expiratory volume 1 is 65% of predicted.

DIAGNOSTIC DILEMMAS

This patient will be guided through the informed consent process based on the surgeon's perspective of the risks and benefits of surgery. The surgeon must consider both procedure- and patient-specific factors as they decide whether to recommend surgery. Standard risk-assessment variables such as diabetes, coronary artery disease, and hypertension are common and provide inadequate discrimination between older patients. This diagnostic dilemma is managed by the surgeon through a subjective assessment of the patient's vigor and physiologic reserve, sometimes referred to as the "eyeball test." Although inherently subjective, this assessment can be informed by objective measures of risk. These measures include functional assessments and preoperative imaging. Most importantly, novel risk assessment tools should focus on remediable surgical risk.

Frailty Assessment

Frailty is defined as "the biologic syndrome of decreased reserve and resistance to stressors, resulting from cumulative declines across multiple physiologic systems, and causing vulnerability to adverse outcomes."[3] Although best described as a facet of aging, frailty is also understood to play a role in susceptibility and natural history of a wide range of chronic illnesses. A clinical frailty assessment takes 30 minutes and provides a useful 0–5 point scale. When compared to their nonfrail counterparts, frail patients have inferior surgical outcomes and require special attention to informed consent, preparation for surgery, and postoperative care protocols.[4] Even simpler than a formal frailty assessment are single functional assessment measures such as the timed up-and-go test or a timed walking test. Like frailty, these tests help identify older patients who are at high risk of poor outcome following surgery. In addition to physical characteristics, assessment of cognitive capacity and risk factors for postoperative delirium should also be considered.[5]

Morphomic Assessment

Almost all patients who undergo major surgery have preoperative cross-sectional imaging. As radiologists and surgeons review the cross-sectional images, they often focus on the primary area of disease, inadvertently missing the vast amounts of additional data. Insights into a patient's overall health, degree of physiologic reserve, and ability to tolerate and recover from surgery can be characterized by considering factors such as core muscle size, muscle density, and aortic calcification. As can be appreciated in the

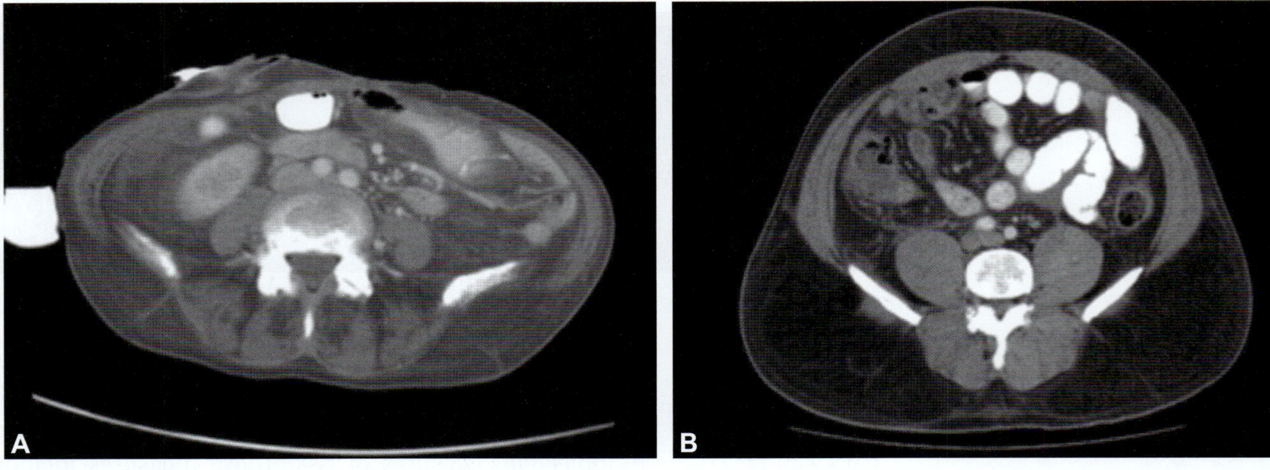

Figs. 21.1A and B: The power of analytic morphomics: Two patients have a similar conventional risk evaluation (diabetes, coronary artery disease, chronic obstructive pulmonary disease, and case complexity) but have distinct physical characteristics evident upon cross-sectional imaging.

CT scans displayed in Figures 21.1A and B, two patients may have similar conventional risk evaluations (diabetes, coronary artery disease, COPD, and case complexity) but have distinct physical characteristics evident in cross-sectional imaging. The patient on the right has large, dense trunk muscles, no tissue swelling, no vascular calcification, and high bone density. Based on these differences, morphomic assessment will demonstrate that the patient on the right is at much lower risk of postoperative morbidity and mortality.

MANAGEMENT OPTIONS

Risk assessment of older patients should focus on recognizing potentially remediable surgical risk. After identification of patients through functional assessment or preoperative imaging, at-risk patients should undergo preoperative training, sometimes referred to as "prehabilitation." Prehabilitation programs should focus on patient-centered care, education, exercise, nutrition, smoking cessation, and healthcare empowerment. For example, a patient with preoperative deconditioning can be managed with a prehabilitation exercise regimen. Significant work needs to be done to identify optimal patient-specific exercise regimens, but it is true that relatively simple home-based regimens offer a significant opportunity to improve outcomes. It is not apparent if outcome improvements are related to actual physiologic change or to patient engagement in their care. Nonetheless, it is clear that patients demonstrate enthusiasm and motivation to participate in perioperative exercise regimens in the setting of elective surgery. Institutional investment in prehabilitation programs can yield significant improvements in surgical outcomes for older patients. Further, these programs yield a significant return on investment by reducing complications, length of stay, and costs for older surgical patients.

An effective prehabilitation program should include a robust education on postoperative expectations. Following surgery, the management of the multiple drugs being taken by the elderly and, similarly, managing the issues of pain and delirium can be extremely challenging. Collaboration with geriatricians and physical therapy specialists is critical during the postoperative hospital stay, while care planning and coordination are important to assure a smooth transition of care to the outpatient setting. Walking and specific strength training can be continued immediately following surgery, at a slower, less intense level. Continuation of the prehabilitation program will foster continuity and empower patients to participate in the care.

REFERENCES

1. Etzioni DA, Liu JH, Maggard MA, et al. The aging population and its impact on the surgery workforce. Ann Surg. 2003;238(2):170-7.
2. Etzioni DA, Liu JH, O'Connell JB, et al. Elderly patients in surgical workloads: a population-based analysis. Am Surg. 2003;69(11):961-5.
3. Fried LP, Tangen CM, Walston J, et al. Frailty in older adults: evidence for a phenotype. J Gerontol A Biol Sci Med Sci. 2001;56(3):M146-56.
4. Makary MA, Segev DL, Pronovost PJ, et al. Frailty as a predictor of surgical outcomes in older patients. J Am Coll Surg. 2010;210(6):901-8.
5. Chow WB, Rosenthal RA, Merkow RP, et al. Optimal preoperative assessment of the geriatric surgical patient: a best practices guideline from the American College of Surgeons National Surgical Quality Improvement Program and the American Geriatrics Society. J Am Coll Surg. 2012;215(4):453-66.

22

Case Study: Management of the Severe Pulmonary Contusion

Daniel Lollar, Gregory J Jurkovich

THE PROBLEM

Blunt trauma to the chest is common. Mechanisms include direct trauma and sudden deceleration injuries of internal organs, typically due to motor vehicle collisions or falls from heights. Most blunt forces are absorbed by the chest wall, resulting in soft tissue injury and rib fractures. Further potential for injury to underlying lung parenchyma, blunt cardiac trauma, and great vessel injury must always be suspected. Lung parenchymal injury can be sharp (lacerations due to broken rib fragments causing pneumo/hemothorax) or blunt (pulmonary contusion). While pulmonary contusions are rarely an immediately life-threatening injury, they can cause progressive and potentially severe hypoxia, and the management can be complex and difficult.

THE TYPICAL CASE

A 22-year-old man was brought in by ambulance to the emergency department after a single-vehicle collision. According to the emergency medical service, the patient was the unrestrained driver of a car traveling at an unknown speed that lost control and crashed into a pole. The patient smelled of alcohol and was obtunded with a score on the Glasgow Coma Scale of 12. He had been hemodynamically stable throughout transport but vomited en route and was now intubated. In the emergency department, the patient maintained O_2 saturations of 92–95% on 1.0 FiO_2, and had coarse breath sounds on the right. A chest X-ray showed an obvious right upper lobe opacity without hemopneumothorax. He remained hemodynamically stable and was sent to the computed tomography (CT) scanner. Scans revealed a grade II liver laceration and nondisplaced fractures of ribs 5 and 6 with opacification of the bilateral upper lobes, worse on the right. The patient was admitted to the intensive care unit (ICU) for observation and ventilator care. Resuscitation continued with crystalloid titrated to urine output. On hospital day 2, a chest X-ray demonstrated worsening opacification of the right lung and new opacification of the left upper lobe. The patient was still ventilated. On hospital day 4, he spiked a temperature to 39.2°C and was started empirically on ceftriaxone. Bronchoscopy revealed two corn kernels and mucus without purulence; lavage specimen grew methicillin-sensitive *Staphylococcus aureus*. The patient was treated with antibiotics for 8 days, being extubated on day 6, and discharged to an acute rehabilitation facility on day 11.

DIAGNOSTIC DILEMMAS

After the Advanced Trauma Life Support primary survey had shown hemodynamic normality, one of the first questions to arise in this case is what imaging was needed to complete the secondary survey. A chest X-ray was necessary as an adjunct to the primary survey. In a hemodynamically stable (normal) patient with an appropriate mechanism, most traumatologists would proceed to a chest CT to look for associated injuries. Recent data have tried to clarify which patients require additional imaging, indicating that chest CT can be limited to those with more than one of the following: over age 60, major mechanism of injury [fall > 20 feet (6 m), MVC > 40 mph], chest pain, intoxication, altered mental status, distracting injury, or tenderness on examination.[1]

In addition to pulmonary contusion, a concern about aspiration must also be entertained in patients with altered mental status and consistent imaging. Typically, pulmonary contusions will not be visible until 6 hours after injury.[2] Aspiration, however, may be visible on initial imaging. Confirmation of aspiration includes gastric contents seen during intubation or if emesis has been witnessed. Aspiration should be diagnosed and treated with early bronchoscopy. In the setting of evolving pulmonary contusion, aspiration is associated with increased inflammation in animal models.[3] The timing of bronchoscopy, the role of bronchoalveolar lavage, and the choice of antibiotics pending definitive cultures are all diagnostic challenges in this setting.

MANAGEMENT OPTIONS

A severely injured patient with pulmonary contusions presents a resuscitative dilemma. Data from animal models suggest that aggressive fluid resuscitation increases the size of contusion and decreases oxygen exchange.[4] However, patients in hemorrhagic shock should be globally resuscitated to reverse any end-organ ischemia, and have the causative injury managed irrespective of their pulmonary injury. Clinical staff should aim to resuscitate the patient to the point of reversing end-organ ischemia without overloading him. Volume status should be meticulously monitored by whatever method is readily available. While invasive monitoring (Swan-Ganz catheter) has fallen out of favor in most surgical ICUs, the value of central venous pressure measurement is unchallenged. Newer adjuncts include transesophageal ultrasound to measure cardiac chamber size as a surrogate for volume status, and peripheral pulse contour-based hemodynamic monitoring to assess cardiac output.[5]

Despite older literature suggesting improvement with routine early mechanical ventilation, data since the mid-1970s[6] have indicated that intubation and mechanical ventilation should be used selectively for patients who progress to respiratory failure.

Additionally, evidence is accumulating that pressure support mode via either mask or artificial airway is associated with improved outcomes.[7] In severe unilateral pulmonary contusion in which there is a significant difference in compliance, one should consider independent lung ventilation. Inverse ratio ventilation and high-frequency oscillation have been found to improve oxygenation but not outcome in cases refractory to pressure support modes.

Although beyond the scope of this chapter, rib fixation should be considered in patients with severe pulmonary contusion associated with a marked flail chest.

FURTHER READING

1. Cohn SM, DuBose JJ. Pulmonary contusion: an update on recent advances in clinical management. World J Surg. 2010;34:1959-70.
2. Raghavendran K, Notter RH, Davidson BA, et al. Lung contusion: inflammatory mechanisms and interaction with other injuries. Shock. 2009;32(2):122-30.
3. Simon B, Ebert J, Bokhari F, et al. Management of pulmonary contusion and flail chest: an Eastern Association for the Surgery of Trauma practice management guideline. J Trauma Acute Care Surg. 2012;73:S351-61.

REFERENCES

1. Rodriguez RM, Anglin D, Langdorf MI, et al. NEXUS chest: validation of a decision instrument for selective chest imaging in blunt trauma. JAMA Surg. 2013;148:940-46.
2. Reynolds JH, Jones H. Thoracic trauma. In: Adam A et al. (Eds.). Grainger and Allison's Diagnostic Radiology, ed. 6. 2015; Edinburgh: Churchill Livingstone.
3. Raghavendran K, Davidson BA, Huebschmann JC, et al. Superimposed gastric aspiration increases the severity of inflammation and permeability injury in a rat model of lung contusion. J Surg Res. 2009;155:273-82.
4. Fulton RL, Peter ET. Physiologic effects of fluid therapy after pulmonary contusion. Am J Surg. 1973;126:773-7.
5. Thiele RH, Bartels K, Gan TJ. Cardiac output monitoring: a contemporary assessment and review. Crit Care Med. 2015; 43(1):177-85.
6. Trinkle JK, Richardson JD, Franz JL, et al. Management of flail chest without mechanical ventilation. Ann Thorac Surg. 1975;19:355-63.
7. Shackford SR, Virgillio RW, Peters RM, et al. Selective use of ventilator therapy in flail chest injury. J Thorac Cardiovasc Surg. 1981;81:194-201.

23 Assessment and Monitoring in Critical Illness

Jean-Louis Vincent

Key Points

- Effective treatment of the critically ill surgical patient requires timely and accurate assessment of biochemical and physiological abnormalities.
- The ABCDE algorithm of airway, breathing, circulation, disability, and exposure should always be followed in the initial assessment of the critically ill patient.
- The sequential organ failure assessment (SOFA) and other assessment scores are important for monitoring progress of care but also in the evaluation of severity of critical illness.
- Effective hemodynamic support and oxygenation of the patient are the mainstays in the management of these patients.
- Renal, metabolic, and neurologic support continue to be important in the overall management of the critically ill patient.

"There is no more difficult art to acquire than the art of observation"—William Osler.

Unlike the situation for most groups of patients, the critically ill patient is at high risk of sudden deterioration and death. As such, history taking and clinical assessment, vital components of routine medical practice, must be more rapid and specifically directed than in other situations so as not to delay immediate resuscitation and stabilization. Clearly, initial assessment of the critically ill patient will depend on the presenting features and focus on likely diagnoses. Clinical assessment is complemented by a range of biochemical, hematologic, immunologic, pathologic, and radiologic tests as well as various monitoring devices and techniques providing additional data to assist decision making at the bedside. Once urgent treatment(s) has been started, continued monitoring of the patient's condition, and response to therapy will provide vitally important information to provide diagnostic and prognostic insight and to guide future therapeutic choices.

In this chapter, we discuss the most important elements of initial assessment and monitoring of the key organ systems in critically ill patients. We do not discuss specific aspects of management, as these are covered in subsequent chapters.

ASSESSMENT

Even in the urgency of critical illness, careful clinical assessment is crucial. The word "assess" is derived from the Latin verb "assidere" meaning "to sit by," suggesting careful observation without intervention. Nevertheless, in the critically ill patient, initial assessment is often conducted almost simultaneously with the start of treatment, and therapeutic interventions are adjusted as a result of continuing assessment or monitoring. In the critically ill patient, some aspects of clinical assessment may not be as appropriate or as immediately important as in other clinical situations; for example, in a sedated, paralyzed, and mechanically ventilated intensive care unit (ICU) patient, clinical assessment will focus more on skin turgor and cardiac rates and rhythm than on respiratory signs or mental status.

Assessment will also vary according to the location and presentation of the patient. For example, a patient being admitted to the ICU after having already been stabilized in the emergency room will require a shorter period of initial assessment but a more detailed focus on "second-phase" monitoring, concentrating more on the (dys)function of individual organs.

The key aspects of initial clinical assessment in a critically ill patient can be considered using the ABCDE algorithm: airway, breathing, circulation, disability, and exposure.[1,2]

Airway

The most important initial assessment of the airway is to ensure that it is clear and free of any form or degree of obstruction, including as a result of edema, a foreign body, or direct traumatic injury. Importantly, patients with a depressed level of consciousness may be unable to maintain their airway.

Breathing

Once it has been established that the airway is clear, the patient's rate and quality of respiration should be assessed. Presence of dyspnea or tachypnea can be easily noted in the spontaneously breathing patient. Asymmetric chest movement and/or breath sounds on auscultation can indicate pneumothorax or endotracheal tube malposition. Dullness or hyperresonance on chest percussion suggests specific pathologies, e.g. hemothorax or pneumothorax, respectively. Pulse oximetry can provide an indication of adequate oxygenation, but it can be unreliable, especially in critically ill patients with reduced peripheral circulation due to vasoconstriction, e.g. in shock.[3] Arterial blood gases provide a more accurate indication of arterial oxygenation as well as giving additional information on arterial carbon dioxide ($Paco_2$) pressure, which can help differentiate causes of respiratory failure and guide therapy.

Circulation

Important aspects of initial circulatory assessment include pulse rate, rhythm, and volume determined by palpation and/or auscultation. Blood pressure should be measured noninvasively or via an arterial line if the patient is hemodynamically unstable, although the degree of hypotension may not reflect the severity of the shock, especially in patients who have a history of chronic hypertension. The clinical signs of circulatory shock generally reflect the resultant poor perfusion and include (1) cold, clammy skin with cyanosis and reduced capillary refill, (2) decreased urine output to <0.5 mL/kg/h, and (3) disorientation and confusion because of decreased cerebral perfusion.[4] Although still a research tool at present, observation of the microcirculation using orthogonal polarization spectral or sidestream darkfield imaging may be helpful in the initial assessment of the severity of shock[5]; further clinical studies are needed to confirm its precise role in these patients. Blood lactate levels also provide important additional information about the presence of shock (*see* later). Increasingly too, echocardiography is being used as part of the initial assessment of critically ill patients to help identify and differentiate cardiac causes of shock.[4]

Table 23.1 The Glasgow Coma Scale.[6] The final score is the sum of all the points and can be considered either as a global total score or in terms of its three component scores, e.g. E1 V2 M3.

Category	*Points*
Eye opening	
Spontaneous	4
To speech	3
To pain	2
None	1
Best verbal response	
Oriented	5
Confused but coherent	4
Inappropriate and muddled	3
Incomprehensible	2
None	1
Best motor response	
Obeys commands fully	6
Localizes to pain	5
Withdraws from painful stimulus	4
Flexor response to painful stimulus	3
Extensor response to painful stimulus	2
No response	1

Disability

The degree of disability essentially refers to the neurological status and is assessed primarily using the Glasgow Coma Scale (GCS) score (Table 23.1).[6] In the sedated critically ill patient, the GCS is difficult to assess reliably: one should use the "assumed" GCS, i.e. the GCS that the patient would have in the absence of sedation and/or anesthesia (this can only be evaluated before and/or after that period, or sometimes based on imaging techniques). Obviously, an anesthetized patient may be transiently comatose without having neurological failure.

Exposure

Exposure refers to anything that may provide useful insight into the patient's condition and includes relevant elements

Table 23.2 The SOFA score.[10]

Score points	*1*	*2*	*3*	*4*
Respiration				
PaO_2/FiO_2	< 400	< 300	< 200 with respiratory support	< 100 with respiratory support
Cardiovascular				
Hypotension*	MAP < 70 mm Hg	Dopamine ≤ 5 or dobutamine in any dose	Dopamine > 5 or epinephrine ≤ 0.1 or norepinephrine ≤ 0.1	Dopamine > 15 or epinephrine > 0.1 or norepinephrine > 0.1
Liver				
Bilirubin mg/dL	1.2–1.9	2.0–5.9	6.0–11.9	> 12.0
Renal				
Creatinine mg/dL	1.2–1.9	2.0–3.4	3.5–4.9	5.0
or urine output			or < 500 mL/24h	or < 200 mL/24h
Coagulation				
Platelets × $10^3/mm^3$	< 150	< 100	< 50	< 25
Central nervous system				
Glasgow coma scale	13–14	10–12	6–9	< 6

*Adrenergic agents administered for at least 1 h (doses are given in μg/kg/min)

of history (e.g. history of depression, medication history, and possible overdose or intoxication) and examination (e.g. body temperature to indicate fever or hypothermia, signs of trauma, bleeding, skin rashes, and needle marks).

Severity Scores

As part of the initial assessment of most ICU patients, an outcome prediction score, such as the Acute Physiology and Chronic Health Evaluation II score[7] or the Simplified Acute Physiology System (SAPS) II score,[8] is calculated, although these tools were not designed for individual prognostication but rather to predict the risk of death of groups of ICU patients.[9]

Of greater value in individual patients are the organ dysfunction scores, which assess the degree of individual and global organ dysfunction. Perhaps the most widely used score is the SOFA, developed in 1994 during a consensus conference[10] (Table 23.2). Using variables regularly measured in all ICUs, the function of six-organ systems (respiratory, cardiovascular, renal, hepatic, central nervous, and coagulation) is scored from 0 (normal function) to 4 (most abnormal), giving a possible score of 0–24 (Table 23.2). A total score > 15 is correlated with mortality rates of > 90%,[11] and the total SOFA thus provides an indication of likely prognosis. An increasing number of individual organ failures is also associated with increased mortality,[11] but more importantly provides a useful indication of which organs are likely to need immediate supportive therapy. Repeated calculation of the SOFA score can provide an indication of changes in organ function over time and give valuable prognostic information.

MONITORING

Monitoring of the critically ill patient has two main functions: (1) to help understand what is going on in the presence of a life-threatening emergency of which the etiology is unclear and (2) to prevent a life-threatening emergency from developing (Fig. 23.1). Once the initial assessment is complete and initial therapies have been started, monitoring thus becomes important to provide further information for diagnostic and prognostic purposes and to determine the response to treatment. The word "monitor" is derived from the Latin word "monere" meaning to warn or remind, and monitoring must be considered as an alert system and aid to decision making; it is not a therapy in itself, and the impact of any monitoring device on outcomes will depend on the availability of effective therapies to correct abnormal parameters and correct interpretation and application of the monitoring data.

For the purposes of this chapter, we separate as much as possible the different monitoring systems according to the organ system being observed; although in the real-life situation, it is the combination of elements from all the

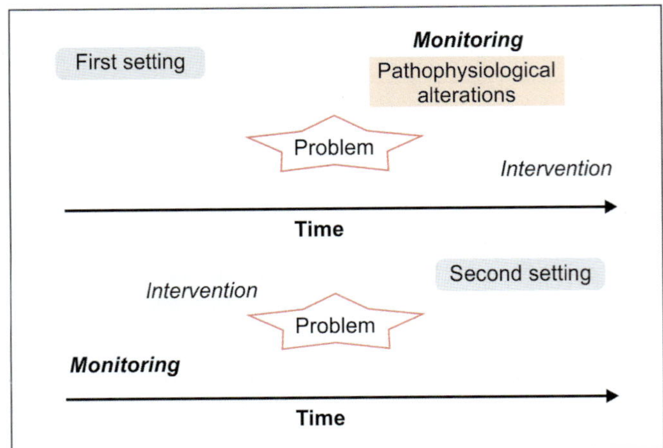

Fig. 23.1: Monitoring of the critically ill patient has two main functions: the first is to help understand what is going on in the presence of a life-threatening emergency of which the etiology is unclear (e.g. a patient with persistent hypotension, but the reason is not known); the second is to prevent a life-threatening emergency from developing (e.g. in the anesthetic room, monitoring is often used to optimize fluid status).

monitors together with findings from repeated clinical assessment that provide the physician with the global picture needed to start or adjust therapy.

Cardiovascular and Hemodynamic Monitoring

Electrocardiogram

The electrocardiogram (ECG) is one of the best-known pieces of monitoring equipment, providing useful information not only on cardiac rhythm and rate and cardiac ischemia but also on electrolyte imbalance and toxic effects of certain drugs. Continuous ECG monitoring, generally using three or five bipolar leads, is widely used in ICU patients, especially when they are hemodynamically unstable and at risk of significant arrhythmia.

Blood Pressure

Blood pressure monitoring is again standard in all critically ill patients. Most such patients will, at least until stabilized, require continuous arterial pressure monitoring, which has generally been conducted invasively via an arterial line. This line is usually inserted in the femoral or radial arteries, but the axillary and dorsalis pedis arteries can also be used. The arterial lines can also be used for repeated arterial blood sampling, notably for blood gas analysis. The risk of major complications associated with arterial line insertion is <1%, but complications include pseudoaneurysm formation, distal ischemia, and sepsis.[12] Noninvasive continuous blood pressure monitors using various methods including finger-cuff or oscillometric devices have been developed, although they may be reliable in clinically stable patients and some have demonstrated good accuracy in certain groups of patients[13]; in critically ill patients, they have generally shown poor agreement with intra-arterial measures[14] and are not currently recommended in hemodynamically unstable patients. Noninvasive measures of mean arterial pressure rather than of systolic blood pressure may correlate better with invasive measures.[15]

Central Venous Pressure

The central venous pressure (CVP) is measured via a venous catheter inserted into the external jugular, internal jugular, subclavian, or femoral veins and positioned with the tip of the catheter in the superior vena cava near its junction with the right atrium. More than 15% of patients will have a complication associated with central venous catheterization, most commonly mechanical, infectious, or thrombotic in nature.[16] Complications can be limited by careful selection of insertion site, sterile insertion technique, and use of ultrasound-guided insertion. Central venous catheters can also be inserted via a peripheral access, the so-called peripherally inserted central catheter.

Once inserted, the CVP is monitored continuously using a pressure transducer. The CVP directly reflects right atrial pressure and, indirectly, right ventricular end-diastolic pressure, thus providing an indication of right heart function and right ventricular preload. The CVP is influenced by intravascular volume, venous tone, and cardiac contractility. It has been widely used to assess volume status, although this approach is too simplistic. The Surviving Sepsis Campaign guidelines recommend targeting a CVP of 8–12 mm Hg for the initial resuscitation of septic patients, largely because of the relatively simple nature of this measure.[17] The CVP may have limitations as an indicator of fluid responsiveness, especially when values are elevated,[18] but a positive response to fluid loading is more likely when the values are low.[17] As with all monitoring equipment, users should be aware of its limitations: the CVP can be affected by various factors that are relatively frequent in ICU patients, including tricuspid valve disease, right ventricular compliance, and reduced left ventricular function.[19] An increase in intrathoracic pressure related to decreased lung compliance or positive end-expiratory pressure can also increase the CVP. Importantly, although CVP monitoring requires placement of a central line, this line has other uses in critically

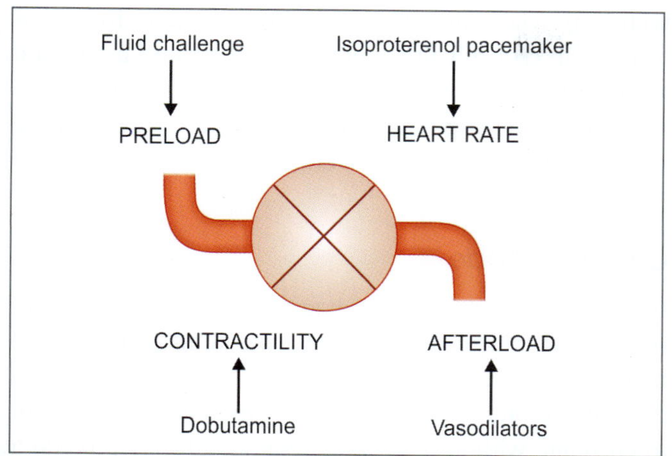

Fig. 23.2: Schematic drawing of the four determinants of cardiac output and potential interventions to increase cardiac output based on these factors.

Box 23.1 Available techniques for cardiac output monitoring.

Invasive
Thermodilution (pulmonary artery catheter)
Less-invasive
Dye dilution*
Transpulmonary dilution (thermodilution, lithium dilution)
Arterial waveform analysis (from invasive pressure tracing)
Transesophageal Doppler
Noninvasive
Cardiac Doppler (echocardiography)
Suprasternal aortic Doppler
Arterial waveform analysis (from non-invasive tracing)
Partial CO_2 rebreathing
Bioimpedance/bioreactance

*Almost abandoned.

ill patients, such as for administration of large infusions of fluids and drugs irritant to smaller peripheral veins, and it can provide a point of access for venous blood sampling, thus avoiding repeated venipuncture.

Cardiac Output

The cardiac output is the volume of blood pumped by the heart over one minute and provides an indication of global perfusion. Cardiac output is the product of the heart rate and the stroke volume, which is itself dependent on the contractility, the preload, and the afterload (Fig. 23.2)[20]; correct interpretation of cardiac output must, therefore, include an evaluation of each component. Cardiac output varies considerably among patients and in the same patient over time.

There are many different methods of estimating cardiac output, varying in degrees of invasiveness and accuracy, and each has specific limitations and advantages (Box 23.1). No method is available that can directly measure cardiac output: all use estimations. The choice of monitoring device will depend not only on local availability and skills but also on the reason for monitoring in a specific patient and the severity of their disease.

The pulmonary artery catheter (PAC), a multilumen catheter with a balloon tip that enables it to be floated through the right heart into the pulmonary artery, has been widely used to measure cardiac output over the years. Complications associated with PAC insertion and use are uncommon if users are experienced and well trained, but correct interpretation and application of the data obtained are crucial if PAC insertion is to prove beneficial.[21] The main advantage of PA catheterization over other less invasive monitoring devices is that it can be used simultaneously to measure other variables that are important in the hemodynamically unstable critically ill patient, including pulmonary artery occlusion pressure, right- and left-sided cardiac filling pressures, and mixed venous oxygen saturation (SvO_2).[21] The PAC is typically inserted via the jugular or subclavian vein. Using the PAC, the cardiac output can be measured by the thermodilution technique, in which boluses of ice-cold fluid are injected through the PAC into the right atrium and changes in temperature are monitored in the pulmonary artery. Using a thermal filament or coil that warms blood in the superior vena cava and a thermistor to measure changes in blood temperature at the PAC tip, cardiac output can be monitored almost continuously, although as the displayed results are averaged over a period of some 10 minutes, the displayed value may not be reliable in very unstable patients.[22] In recent years, with increased availability of less invasive techniques to estimated cardiac output, PAC use has decreased and routine PAC insertion is not recommended for moderate- or low-risk patients, but it can still be useful in severely or critically ill patients or high-risk surgical patients in whom knowledge of the multiple simultaneous parameters that can be obtained using this device can help guide the most appropriate therapy.[21,23]

There are several approaches that can be used to estimate cardiac output less invasively than by PAC insertion, including techniques that use thermodilution or indicator dilution but via a peripheral arterial catheter, and devices that estimate cardiac output from the arterial pressure waveform (*see* recent review).[22] Echocardiography is increasingly used in the evaluation of the critically ill patient, and in addition to providing important diagnostic information, it can be used to estimate cardiac output. Echo-Doppler techniques provide reasonable estimates of cardiac output compared to PAC-derived values, but cannot generally be used to provide continuous monitoring, require training, and are operator dependent. Transesophageal monitoring may be particularly useful in the intraoperative or immediate postoperative setting, as patients generally have an endotracheal tube in situ and are still anesthetized or sedated, enabling good images to be obtained over a longer period of time. In such settings, esophageal Doppler use for monitoring flow-related hemodynamic variables and optimizing fluid replacement has been shown to reduce postoperative complications, need for ICU admission, and length of hospital stay.[24] Today's newer, thinner probes for transesophageal echo-Doppler assessment can be left in place and provide a continuous visualization of the cardiac chambers in the ICU.

Bioimpedance, bioreactance, and carbon dioxide rebreathing techniques have also been proposed for the noninvasive monitoring of cardiac output, but these techniques are less reliable. Further study is needed to define their place in the surgical and critically ill patient population.

Oxygenation and Respiratory Monitoring

Although hemodynamic parameters, such as blood pressure and cardiac output, are widely used to monitor adequacy of tissue perfusion, they may not offer reliable indications of tissue oxygenation, especially in conditions of shock in which oxygen transport and metabolism are disturbed. Other measures of tissue oxygenation are, therefore, of use.

Pulse Oximetry

Pulse oximetry uses a finger or ear probe to estimate the relative concentrations of oxygenated and deoxygenated hemoglobin in the tissue and thus provides an indication of arterial oxygenation (SpO_2). Pulse oximeters cannot distinguish between carboxyhemoglobin or methemoglobin and oxyhemoglobin, so may overestimate oxygenation in some patients. Similarly, nail polish or skin pigmentation can potentially influence readings. Pulse oximeters have reasonable accuracy and precision in the higher range of SaO_2 values, but these qualities decrease in hypoxemia, and in patients with very low cardiac output measurements, it become less reliable.[25,26] Pulse oximetry can provide an early warning sign of likely hypoxemia indicating the need for arterial gas analysis, but is not itself associated with improved outcomes in routine postoperative monitoring.[27] In critically ill patients with shock and peripheral vasoconstriction, it may be difficult to obtain a signal. Forehead sensors using reflectance technology may be more reliable and less sensitive to peripheral vasoconstriction in such patients.[28]

Carbon Dioxide

$Paco_2$ is important in the diagnosis and monitoring of respiratory failure. It is usually measured from arterial blood gases and can be monitored continuously if an arterial catheter is in situ. Venous blood gas values seem to correlate with arterial blood gases and may provide a useful initial indication of acid–base status.[29] Less invasive techniques are also available. End-tidal CO_2 ($etCO_2$), which represents the CO_2 present in the exhaled gases at the end of expiration, fairly accurately reflects arterial CO_2 if there is no ventilation-perfusion mismatch, and it can be measured using volumetric capnography or colorimetric detectors that are attached directly to the endotracheal tube.[26,30] Transcutaneous Pco_2 ($PtcCO_2$) devices, usually placed on the earlobe, measure tissue CO_2, which is slightly higher than arterial CO_2. Studies have suggested that this technique can provide acceptable assessments of $Paco_2$ in various groups of critically ill patients, but regular recalibration and membrane change is required and further study is needed to accurately define its role in respiratory monitoring.[26]

SvO_2

SvO_2 reflects the balance between oxygen consumption (VO_2) and delivery (DO_2) and thus provides an indication of the global adequacy of tissue oxygenation. It is measured by a PAC and reflects the level of venous oxygenation in the whole body. The oxygen saturation in the superior vena cava ($ScvO_2$), measured using a central venous catheter and thus reflecting the venous oxygenation of the upper part of the body,[31] can be used as a surrogate for SvO_2 if the patient does not have a PAC in situ, but the two values are not interchangeable. $ScvO_2$ is usually slightly less than SvO_2, but in patients with shock, particularly in sepsis, redistribution of blood away from the hepatosplanchnic vascular system toward the cerebral and coronary circulations results in $ScvO_2$ levels that are slightly higher than SvO_2. In critically ill patients, however, changes in $ScvO_2$ generally parallel changes in SvO_2 so that the absolute difference between the two parameters may not be so important.[31] SvO_2 in

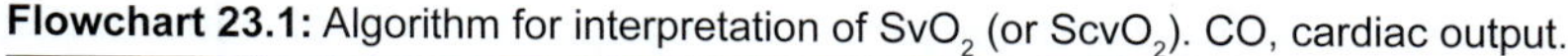

Flowchart 23.1: Algorithm for interpretation of SvO_2 (or $ScvO_2$). CO, cardiac output.

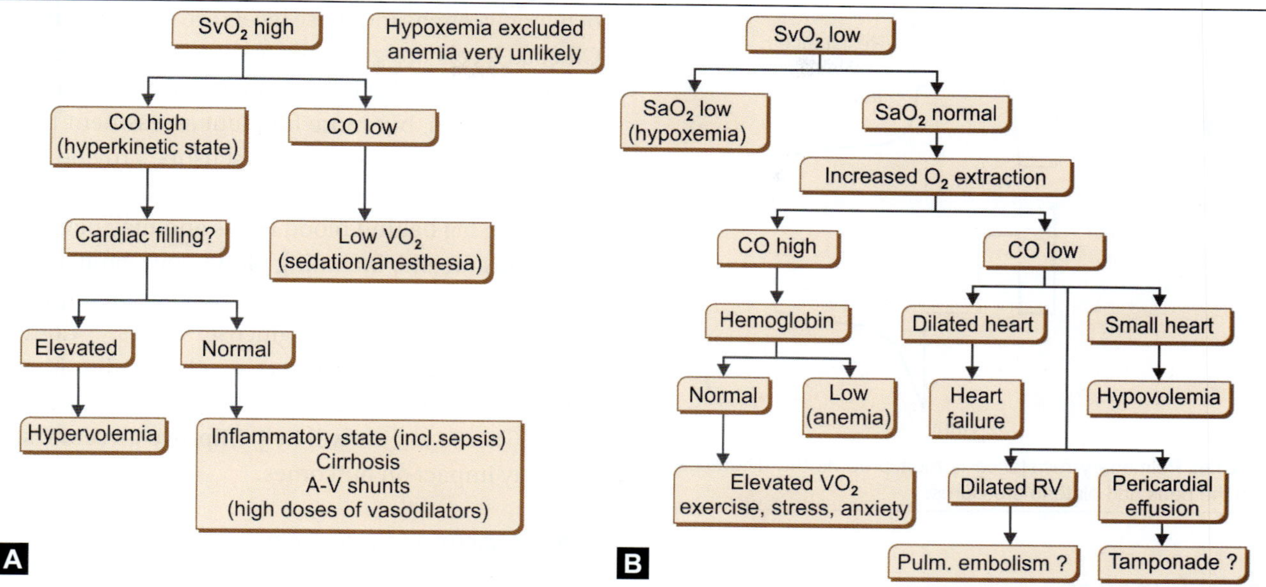

combination with other measurements, such as cardiac output and arterial oxygen saturation, can provide useful diagnostic information. Flowchart 23.1 provides an algorithm for interpretation of SvO_2 (or $ScvO_2$).

Blood Lactate Levels

Blood lactate levels are increased in patients with anaerobic metabolism and thus reflect tissue hypoxia. Increased blood lactate levels are associated with increased morbidity and mortality, and therapy guided to reduce lactate levels may be associated with improved outcomes in critically ill patients.[32,33] The normal value is close to 1 mEq/L (0.7–1.3 mEq/L), so that even a slight increase to around 1.5 mEq/L may be pathological. When blood lactate levels are increased, it is important to know in which direction they are trending (Fig. 23.3), because an isolated value provides limited information; repeated measurements must be thus obtained to follow the time course. Some speak about assessment of "lactate clearance," but this is a misnomer: lactate levels represent the balance between production and elimination (or clearance) and both are altered in acute circulatory failure. In patients with elevated lactate levels, a study by Jansen and colleagues showed that targeting a 20% decrease in lactate over 2 hours is a reasonable target.[32]

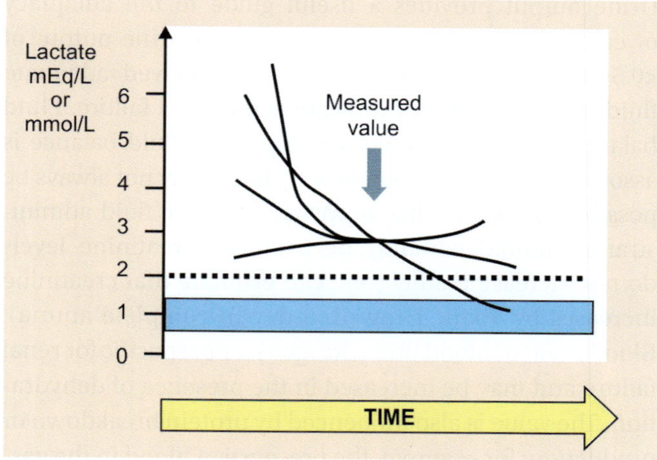

Fig. 23.3: An isolated blood lactate level provides limited information, but the trend in lactate from repeated measures gives an indication of whether the patient's status is improving or worsening. The shaded area represents normal range.

Respiratory Mechanics

Various measures can be used to monitor respiratory function in critically ill patients, including airway pressures, lung volumes, work of breathing, and capnometry, but a detailed review of these techniques is beyond the scope of this chapter; the reader is referred to recent reviews on this subject.[26,34] Measures of respiratory mechanics provide useful information regarding lung function and help optimize ventilator settings. Thoracopulmonary compliance is the change in volume for a given change in pressure and is obtained by dividing the tidal volume by the pressure difference associated with the lung inflation. The airway resistance (related to bronchospasm) is evaluated by the difference between peak and plateau pressures (Fig. 23.4).

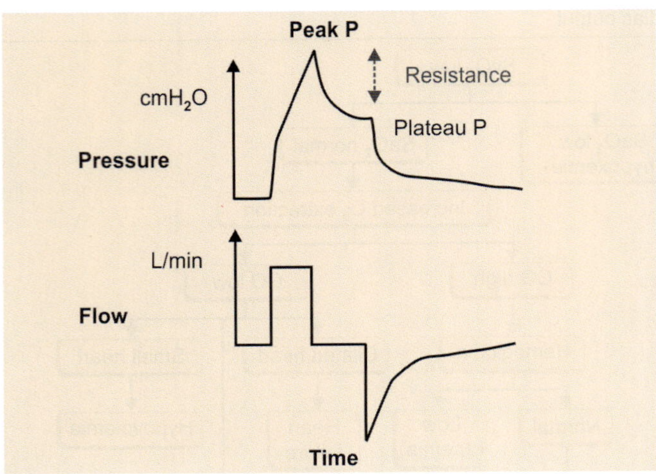

Fig. 23.4: Pulmonary resistance is measured as the difference between the peak and plateau pressures.

Renal Function

Urine output provides a useful guide to the adequacy of cardiac output and renal function. A urine output of <0.5 mL/kg/h in patients who have received adequate fluid resuscitation may indicate acute renal failure. Fluid balance should be monitored. A positive fluid balance is associated with worse outcomes,[35] but it may not always be possible to prevent this; however, excessive fluid administration should certainly be avoided. Creatinine levels do not increase readily (one can estimate that creatinine increases by about 1 mg/dL a day in complete anuria). Blood urea (or blood urea nitrogen) is not specific for renal failure and may be increased in the presence of dehydration. The value is also influenced by protein breakdown or production; for example, the presence of blood in the gastrointestinal tract may increase urea levels without renal failure. Modest alterations in renal function may be documented by the use of new biomarkers, such as neutrophil gelatinase-associated lipocalin (NGAL) or cystatin C[36] or a panel of markers.[37]

Metabolic Function

Various aspects of metabolic function can be monitored in critically ill patients, but most, e.g. protein and energy delivery, refer to established critical illness. Glycemia is, however, an important parameter that should be measured and monitored early, because careful control of blood glucose levels is associated with improved outcomes: some professional societies now recommend target blood glucose levels of between 140 and 180 mg/dL,[38] but modern software enables levels to be kept < 150 mg/dL without risk of hypoglycemia, and these levels are probably preferable. Glucose levels are generally assessed intermittently from venous or arterial blood samples analyzed using point-of-care devices, but more frequent assessment may be of value. Subcutaneous glucose sensors provide readings every few minutes but monitor interstitial fluid glucose, which can lag behind blood levels and may be influenced by various factors, including blood flow, capillary permeability, and presence of edema, making them potentially less reliable than blood glucose values.[39] Continuous intravascular glucose sensors are being developed that will allow for real-time continuous blood glucose monitoring. These systems will help improve glycemic stability and may impact on outcomes.

Neurological Function

Critically ill patients are at risk of neurological dysfunction and deterioration from both primary and secondary neurologic insults. Most critically ill patients will not need complex neuromonitoring techniques, but intracranial pressure, cerebral perfusion pressure, cerebral blood flow, jugular venous bulb oximetry, electroencephalography, and evoked potentials may be necessary in some individuals, and choice of monitoring device must be made based on presenting features and likely disease processes.[40] Direct assessment of cell metabolism with brain PO_2 ($PbrO_2$) or microdialysis techniques is also possible.

CONCLUSION AND FUTURE PERSPECTIVES

Appropriate and adequate assessment and monitoring of the critically ill patient are essential, but it is the correct interpretation of the monitored values and the administration of effective therapies that will actually affect a patient's chances of survival. The number and types of devices available for monitoring in the critically ill patient are vast, and we have tried to focus on the key global areas rather than on specific techniques or equipment. Clearly all patients are different and monitoring needs to be carefully and thoughtfully applied on an individual basis. Not all patients, for example, will need neurological monitoring or detailed evaluation of respiratory mechanics, but in most patients, several variables will need to be monitored to obtain the best possible picture of ongoing status and response to treatment. Individual static values are important as baselines, but trends in values over time in general provide more valuable information than any absolute value. The future will increasingly see noninvasive techniques taking precedence over invasive techniques, but these latter still currently have an important role in hemodynamically unstable patients with complex problems. Automated systems and decision support software will assist in interpretation of the multiple monitoring systems present on our patients. Monitoring of biomarkers for various diseases, such as sepsis and acute renal dysfunction, will be used, as these markers are validated and biomarker-guided treatment is shown to be of benefit. Monitoring of the microcirculation will also likely become more important, as techniques to improve regional tissue oxygenation and perfusion are shown to be effective. Finally, and perhaps most importantly, no monitoring technique or device can improve outcomes alone: the data obtained from the monitors is just a guide to help make informed decisions about the most effective management approach in the individual patient.

REFERENCES

1. Robertson LC, Al-Haddad M. Recognizing the critically ill patient. Anaesthesia Intensive Care Med. 2013;14:11-4.
2. Thim T, Krarup NH, Grove EL, et al. Initial assessment and treatment with the airway, breathing, circulation, disability, exposure (ABCDE) approach. Int J Gen Med. 2012;5:117-21.
3. Jubran A. Pulse oximetry. Crit Care. 1999;3:R11-R17.
4. Vincent JL, De Backer D. Circulatory shock. N Engl J Med. 2013;369:1726-34.
5. De Backer D, Hollenberg S, Boerma C, et al. How to evaluate the microcirculation: report of a round table conference. Crit Care. 2007;11:R101.
6. Teasdale G, Jennett B. Assessment of coma and impaired consciousness. A practical scale. Lancet. 1974;2:81-4.
7. Knaus WA, Draper EA, Wagner DP, et al. APACHE II: A severity of disease classification system. Crit Care Med. 1985;13: 818-29.
8. Le Gall J-R, Lemeshow S, Saulnier F. A new simplified acute physiology score (SAPS II) based on a European/North American multicenter study. JAMA. 1993;270:2957-63.
9. Vincent JL, Moreno R. Clinical review: scoring systems in the critically ill. Crit Care. 2010;14:207.
10. Vincent JL, Moreno R, Takala J, et al. The SOFA (Sepsis-related Organ Failure Assessment) score to describe organ dysfunction/failure. On behalf of the Working Group on Sepsis-Related Problems of the European Society of Intensive Care Medicine. Intensive Care Med. 1996;22:707-10.
11. Vincent JL, de Mendonca A, Cantraine F, et al. Use of the SOFA score to assess the incidence of organ dysfunction/failure in intensive care units: results of a multicenter, prospective study. Working group on "sepsis-related problems" of the European Society of Intensive Care Medicine. Crit Care Med. 1998;26:1793-800.
12. Scheer B, Perel A, Pfeiffer UJ, et al. Clinical review: complications and risk factors of peripheral arterial catheters used for haemodynamic monitoring in anaesthesia and intensive care medicine. Crit Care. 2002;6:199-204.
13. Jagadeesh AM, Singh NG, Mahankali S. A comparison of a continuous noninvasive arterial pressure (CNAP) monitor with an invasive arterial blood pressure monitor in the cardiac surgical ICU. Ann Card Anaesth. 2012;15:180-84.
14. Hohn A, Defosse JM, Becker S, et al. Non-invasive continuous arterial pressure monitoring with Nexfin does not sufficiently replace invasive measurements in critically ill patients. Br J Anaesth. 2013;111:178-84.
15. Lehman LW, Saeed M, Talmor D, et al. Methods of blood pressure measurement in the ICU. Crit Care Med. 2013;41: 34-40.
16. McGee DC, Gould MK. Preventing complications of central venous catheterization. N Engl J Med. 2003;348:1123-33.
17. Dellinger RP, Levy MM, Rhodes A, et al. Surviving sepsis campaign: international guidelines for management of severe sepsis and septic shock: 2012. Crit Care Med. 2013;41: 580-637.
18. Marik PE, Baram M, Vahid B. Does central venous pressure predict fluid responsiveness? A systematic review of the literature and the tale of seven mares. Chest. 2008;134:172-8.
19. Smith T, Grounds RM, Rhodes A. Central venous pressure: uses and limitations. In: Vincent JL (Ed). Functional Hemodynamic Monitoring. Heidelberg: Springer; 2005. pp. 99-110.
20. Vincent JL. Understanding cardiac output. Crit Care. 2008; 12:74.
21. Vincent JL. The pulmonary artery catheter. J Clin Monit Comput. 2012;26:341-5.
22. Vincent JL, Rhodes A, Perel A, et al. Clinical review: update on hemodynamic monitoring—a consensus of 16. Crit Care. 2011;15:229.
23. American Society of Anesthesiologists Task Force on Pulmonary Artery Catheterization. Practice guidelines for pulmonary artery catheterization: an updated report. Anesthesiology. 2003;99:988-1014.
24. Abbas SM, Hill AG. Systematic review of the literature for the use of oesophageal Doppler monitor for fluid replacement in major abdominal surgery. Anaesthesia. 2008;63:44-51.
25. Jubran A. Pulse oximetry. Intensive Care Med. 2004;30: 2017-20.
26. Brochard L, Martin GS, Blanch L, et al. Clinical review: Respiratory monitoring in the ICU—a consensus of 16. Crit Care. 2012;16:219.
27. Pedersen T, Moller AM, Hovhannisyan K. Pulse oximetry for perioperative monitoring. Cochrane Database Syst Rev. 2009;CD002013.
28. Nesseler N, Frenel JV, Launey Y, et al. Pulse oximetry and high-dose vasopressors: a comparison between forehead reflectance and finger transmission sensors. Intensive Care Med. 2012;38:1718-22.
29. Treger R, Pirouz S, Kamangar N, et al. Agreement between central venous and arterial blood gas measurements in the intensive care unit. Clin J Am Soc Nephrol. 2010;5:390-94.

30. Donald MJ, Paterson B. End tidal carbon dioxide monitoring in prehospital and retrieval medicine: a review. Emerg Med J. 2006;23:728-30.
31. Reinhart K, Kuhn HJ, Hartog C, et al. Continuous central venous and pulmonary artery oxygen saturation monitoring in the critically ill. Intensive Care Med. 2004;30:1572-8.
32. Jansen TC, van Bommel J, Schoonderbeek FJ, et al. Early lactate-guided therapy in intensive care unit patients: a multicenter, open-label, randomized controlled trial. Am J Respir Crit Care Med. 2010;182:752-61.
33. Bakker J, Nijsten MW, Jansen TC. Clinical use of lactate monitoring in critically ill patients. Ann Intensive Care. 2013;3:12.
34. Grinnan DC, Truwit JD. Clinical review: respiratory mechanics in spontaneous and assisted ventilation. Crit Care. 2005;9:472-84.
35. Vincent JL, Sakr Y, Sprung CL, et al. Sepsis in European intensive care units: results of the SOAP study. Crit Care Med. 2006;34:344-53.
36. Prowle JR, Liu YL, Licari E, et al. Oliguria as predictive biomarker of acute kidney injury in critically ill patients. Crit Care. 2011;15:R72.
37. Kashani K, Al-Khafaji A, Ardiles T, et al. Discovery and validation of cell cycle arrest biomarkers in human acute kidney injury. Crit Care. 2013;17:R25.
38. Kavanagh BP, McCowen KC. Clinical practice. Glycemic control in the ICU. N Engl J Med. 2010;363:2540-6.
39. Van Herpe T, Mesotten D. Blood glucose measurements in critically ill patients. J Diabetes Sci Technol. 2012;6:22-8.
40. Stocchetti N, Roux PL, Vespa P, et al. Clinical review: Neuromonitoring—an update. Crit Care. 2013;17:201.

24

Shock

Christine Cocanour, Ian Brown

Key Points

- Shock is the clinical manifestation of perfusion that is inadequate to meet the metabolic demands of the cell.
- The diagnosis of shock is based on clinical, hemodynamic, and biochemical findings.
- Shock is the result of four potential and not necessarily exclusive pathophysiologic mechanisms: hypovolemic (blood or tissue fluid loss), cardiogenic (acute cardiac pump failure), obstructive (pulmonary embolism, cardiac tamponade or, tension pneumothorax), and distributive (severe sepsis, release of inflammatory mediators or spinal cord injury).
- The goals for the initial management of shock are the same regardless of its etiology—maintain oxygenation, restore vascular volume, and tissue perfusion. Management will differ depending upon the cause of shock. The important components of shock resuscitation are summarized in the VIP rule: Ventilate (oxygen administration), Infuse (fluid resuscitation), and Pump (administration of vasoactive agents).[1]

INTRODUCTION

"Shock is the manifestation of the rude unhinging of the machinery of life" (Samuel V Gross, 1872).[2]

Our understanding of the pathophysiology of shock and the disease processes that result in shock has evolved since Gross' observation in 1872. Shock is the clinical syndrome that results from inadequate tissue perfusion. Shock occurs when oxygen delivery is insufficient to meet the metabolic demands of tissues, with cellular dysfunction being the result. The cellular injury that results induces both structural and functional changes, which further compromise perfusion leading to more cellular injury. If this vicious cycle is not promptly interrupted, the initial reversible cellular injury will progress to organ dysfunction and death. Early, adequate treatment of shock is essential to survival.

Shock is a clinical state of acute circulatory failure that results from four potential and not necessarily exclusive pathophysiologic mechanisms.[3] The first, hypovolemic, is a decrease in venous return from either internal or external fluid loss. The second, cardiogenic, is due to pump failure and can occur as a result of a loss of contractility from acute myocardial infarct, end-stage cardiomyopathy, advanced valvular heart disease, or from cardiac dysrhythmias. The third, obstructive, results from mechanical impediment to circulation such as pericardial tamponade, pulmonary embolus, or tension pneumothorax. The fourth, distributive, is loss of vascular tone that results in maldistribution of blood flow and may be the consequence of sepsis, anaphylaxis, or spinal cord injury. The features of each mechanism of shock may overlap, and in some cases a patient may have two or more mechanisms at play. For example, a trauma patient may have hypovolemic shock from blood loss, obstructive shock from tension pneumothorax, and distributive shock from a spinal cord injury. Figure 24.1 shows a schematic of the four basic pathophysiologic types of shock.

EPIDEMIOLOGY

Up to one-third of patients admitted to an intensive care unit (ICU) are in shock.[3] Shock can also be categorized according to the underlying cause as hemorrhagic, anaphylactic, septic, or due to spinal cord injury. Hypovolemia is the most common cause of shock seen in surgical critical care. In the trauma or postoperative patient, hemorrhage must be considered as the cause of shock until proven otherwise. Additional sources of fluid loss include gastrointestinal losses, losses from invasive devices (thoracostomy tubes and peritoneal drains), or massive gastrointestinal fluid sequestration seen with bowel obstruction. Intravascular fluid may leak into the interstitium secondary to

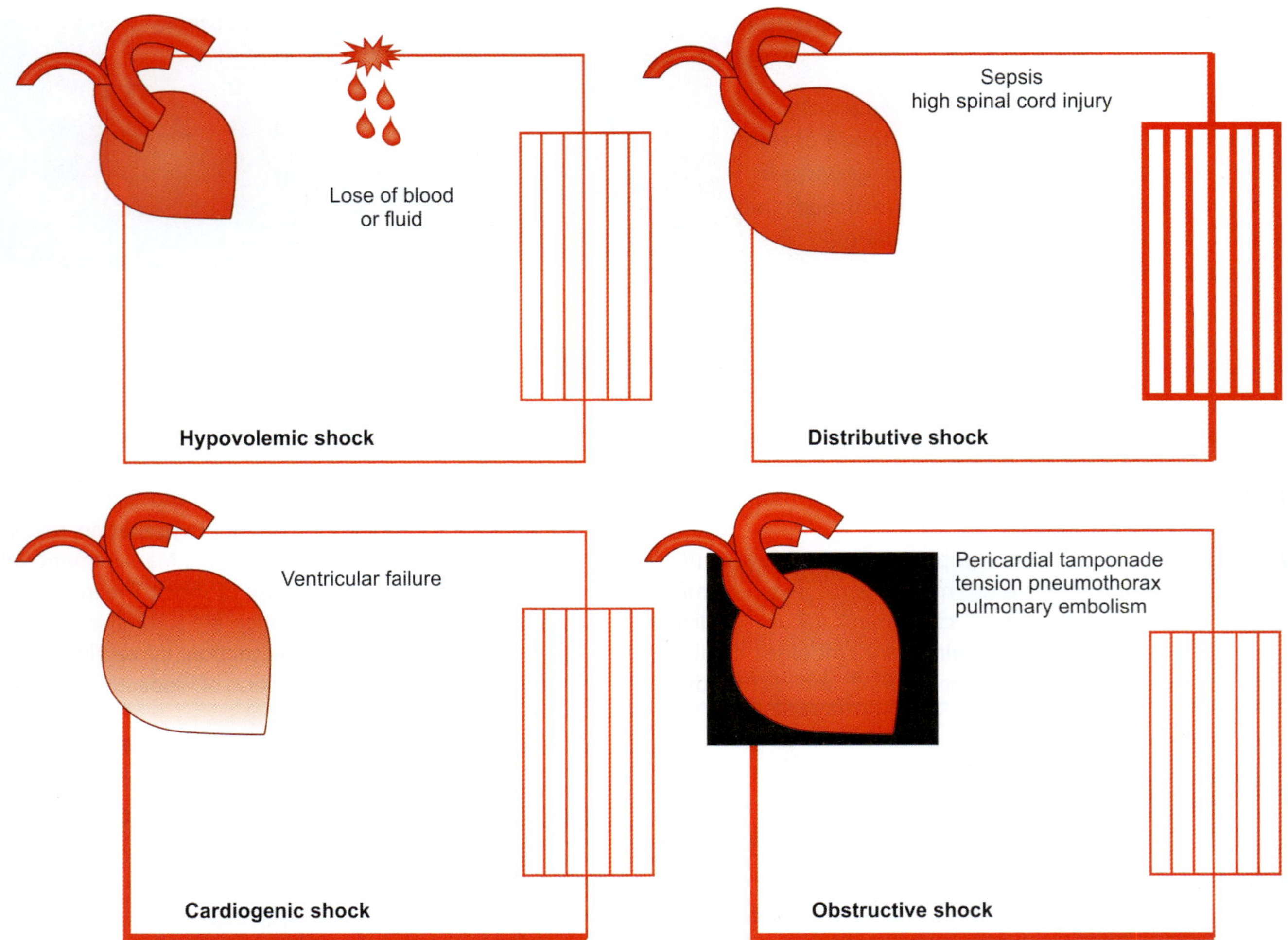

Fig. 24.1: The cardiovascular system has three components: blood, a medium to deliver oxygen and nutrients and remove waste; a pump, the heart; and vessels to deliver the blood and allow delivery of oxygen and nutrients and remove waste. Shock represents a functional failure of one of those three components. Depicted are the four basic types of shock: distributive (failure of vasculature), hypovolemic (loss of blood or fluid), cardiogenic (pump failure), and obstructive (heart or vessels are blocked).

decreased plasma oncotic pressure, increased hydrostatic pressure, or increased vascular permeability from inflammation.

Septic shock is the most common cause of shock in all ICU populations. In a study of 1,679 European ICU patients, septic shock was the most frequent cause of shock (62%), followed by cardiogenic shock (CS) (17%) and hypovolemia (16%).[4] It is the most severe manifestation of sepsis, with reported case-fatality rates ranging from 40% to 50% but reaching as high as 80%.[3]

Traumatic shock, which differs from hemorrhagic shock, is a distributive form of shock. It results from the combination of blood loss, soft tissue, and bony injury that leads to the activation of inflammatory cells and the release of circulating factors such as cytokines and intracellular molecules that modulate the immune response. The inflammatory mediators that are released in response to trauma are similar to those released in sepsis, as are the signaling pathways.

Cardiogenic shock has been most commonly studied in patients with acute myocardial infarction (MI). Its incidence in this population has remained constant at 6–9% over the past several decades.[3] In a multinational study of patients who developed CS, the in-hospital case-fatality rate was 59.4%.[3]

PATHOPHYSIOLOGY

Numerous mechanisms are at play in maintaining homeostasis both in the setting of normal physiology and in the setting of shock. These mechanisms primarily govern intravascular volume, cardiac function, and vasodilation.

An important early compensatory mechanism to preserve homeostasis is activation of the adrenergic system with release of catecholamines. This endocrine action has three main effects: peripheral vasoconstriction, increased cardiac output (CO), and volume expansion. Catecholamines cause peripheral vasoconstriction to increase blood pressure and venular constriction to increase blood return to the heart (i.e. preload). Arteriolar constriction occurs mainly in the systemic vascular beds, such as skeletal muscle and intestines, in an attempt to preserve blood flow to the vital organs (heart, brain). It is done through stimulation of α-1 receptors expressed by arterial smooth muscle cells of the peripheral vascular system. Catecholamines increase CO through tachycardia and increased cardiac contractility. This action is mediated through β-2 receptors on cardiomyocytes. Epinephrine (adrenaline), along with cortisol and glucagon, increases glucose concentration in the extracellular space, which draws water out of the cells by osmotic forces and expands the interstitial volume.

Another critical mechanism for hormonal regulation of homeostasis is the renin–angiotensin system. When activated, it contributes to peripheral vasoconstriction. In the setting of reduced renal blood flow, juxtaglomerular cells within the kidneys secrete renin into the circulation. Renin converts angiotensinogen released by the liver to angiotensin I. Angiotensin I is then converted to angiotensin II by angiotensin-converting enzyme in the lungs. Angiotensin II causes vasoconstriction, which in turn increases blood pressure. Angiotensin II also stimulates the secretion of aldosterone from the adrenal cortex. Aldosterone increases renal reabsorption of sodium and water, which helps preserve intravascular volume (i.e. preload).

Vasopressin stimulates receptors responsible for peripheral vasoconstriction as well as increased CO and oxygen delivery in the setting of hypotension. Arginine vasopressin receptor (AVPR1A) is responsible for vasoconstriction and is expressed on vascular smooth muscle, hepatocytes, and platelets. Stimulation of the AVPR1A receptor also induces nitric oxide production in coronary vessels and pulmonary vessels, which augments CO and systemic oxygen delivery. Stimulation of AVPR1B by vasopressin also releases adrenocorticotropic hormone. Sepsis can result in downregulation of the receptor AVPR1A. AVPR2 (V2 receptor) is expressed in the renal collecting duct. AVPR2 stimulation increases retention of water. Signaling activates adenylate cyclase and the resulting cyclic AMP signals for the movement of aquaporin-2 water channels from cytoplasm to the apical membrane of collecting duct cells. AVPR2 receptor stimulation also increases release of von Willebrand factor, von Willebrand factor multimers, and thus the risk of clotting. Stimulation of AVPR2 is therefore the mechanism for increased coagulation in response to desmopressin.

Sepsis is a unique situation in which a systemic response to infection alters normal homeostasis and physiology. In the setting of a localized injury or infection, the response of the body is directed at containing the insult. Classically, the response is described by the four components: rubor, dolor, calor, and tumor. Initially, the injury is recognized through pattern recognition of tissue injury or pathogenic organisms.[5] Toll-like receptors bind to lipids, nucleic acids, and bacterial components such as flagellin, setting off signaling cascades similar to those of inflammatory cytokines such as interleukin 1 (IL-1). Pathogens and necrotic tissue also undergo phagocytosis by local resident antigen presenting cells, which then results in the production of chemokines and migration to local lymph nodes for presentation to and activation of T and B cells of the adaptive immune system. Chemokines released by both local antigen presenting cells and vascular endothelial cells then work to recruit innate effector cells such as neutrophils to the site of injury. Vascular flow changes to increase blood flow to injured tissue beds for delivery of necessary proteins and effector cells. Inducible nitric oxide synthase leads to increased nitric oxide production, which together with histamine release from resident mast cells and basophils leads to subsequent arteriolar vasodilation. Capillary beds open. This phenomenon leads to relative stasis of flow within the capillary beds and venules. Venule endothelial cells change to allow increased vascular permeability. This action is driven by factors such as histamine, bradykinin, leukotrienes, substance P, and many other classes of chemical mediators. Histamine and other factors activate intracellular signaling pathways within endothelial cells that lead to phosphorylation of contractile and cytoskeletal proteins, such as myosin. Cytokines such as IL-1, tumor necrosis factor (TNF), and interferon-γ (IFN-γ) also induce structural reorganization of the endothelial cell cytoskeleton. Together, these agents lead to increased intercellular space to allow proteins and cells to enter the interstitium. Endothelial cells express E-selectin, P-selectin, CD31, VCAM-1, and ICAM-1 on their cell surfaces to facilitate margination, rolling, and adhesion of effector cells to endothelium. Increased vascular permeability leads to increased interstitial oncotic pressure and

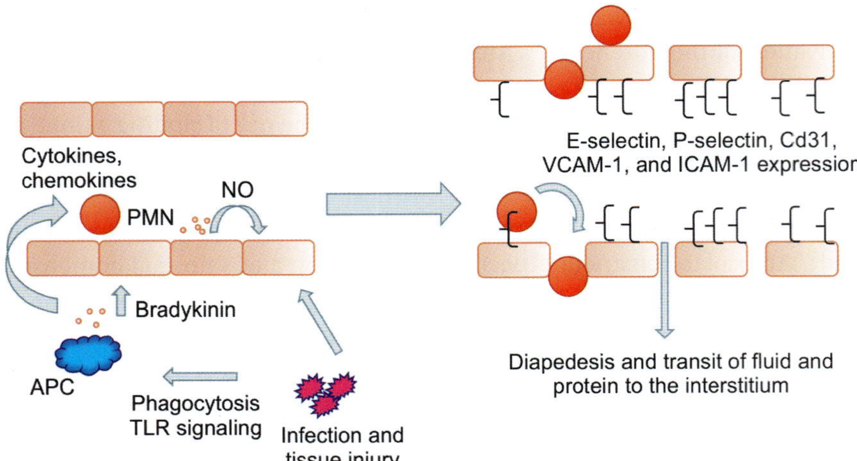

Fig. 24.2: Injury and inflammation elicit signals that vasodilate arterioles and increase vascular permeability of venules. The resulting loss of intravascular fluid together with increased vascular bed volume results in hypovolemia and shock in the setting of sepsis.

loss of intravascular volume. The coagulation pathway then intersects with the immune response as clotting factors engage extravascular tissue factor. Neutrophils either engulf pathogens or interact with platelets to form aggregates such as neutrophil extracellular traps to contain infection (Fig. 24.2).[6]

In a local injury or infection, such a response leads to a relatively small redistribution of volume from the intravascular to extravascular compartment. However, injury and infection at times elicit systemic inflammation, termed *systemic inflammatory response syndrome (SIRS)* in injury or sepsis in the setting of infection. The mechanisms that shift a response from local to systemic are unclear but may be related to quantity and quality of tissue injury and the nature of the infectious pathogen including factors such as endotoxin and exotoxin production. When such a response occurs systemically, the resulting fluid shift from the intravascular to extravascular space leads to a distributive shock. Septic shock can cause appreciable organ injury. The mechanism is likely to be multifactorial and may be due to combined effects of hypoperfusion, reperfusion, and inflammation. Additionally, the mechanisms of homeostasis become altered. Sepsis initially increases serum vasopressin levels 20- to 200-fold. After the initial release, levels then rapidly decline as stored vasopressin is depleted. Production and release of new vasopressin may also remain impaired after this initial depletion. The Vasopressin and Septic Shock Trial (VASST) demonstrated low vasopressin levels for up to 7 days after the onset of sepsis.[7]

An interesting but incompletely understood aspect of the distributive shock of sepsis is the loss of serum proteins such as albumin. The total body albumin pool measures about 3.5–5.0 g/kg of body mass. Approximately 40% of this is present in the plasma compartment, while the rest is present in extravascular compartments. Approximately 2 g/kg or 120–145 g of albumin transits daily into the extravascular space in a 70 kg person. According to Starling's theory, the rate of albumin transit to the extravascular space depends on the permeability of the wall and hydrostatic and oncotic pressures on either side of the wall.[8] Some albumin transport is passive and some is active by way of transport receptors such as albondin.[9,10]

Bound albumin enters vesicles within the endothelial cell and is discharged on the interstitial side within 15 seconds. Most of the extravascular albumin returns to the circulation by lymphatic drainage. Albumin also enters the gastrointestinal tract (about 1 g each day) where its digestion releases amino acids, which may be reabsorbed. Urinary loss in a healthy person is usually no more than 10–20 mg/day. A 70 kg person degrades approximately 14 g of albumin each day. Albumin is broken down in large part within muscle and skin but also within liver, kidneys, and other organs.

Critical illness alters the generation, distribution, and degradation of albumin. Trauma and sepsis reduce albumin mRNA levels.[11] This is part of the acute-phase reaction mediated by cytokines, mainly IL-6 and TNF-α.[12,13] Sepsis also alters distribution by increasing capillary leakage.[14] The mediators of this leakage are numerous, some of which are still being discovered; those currently known include endotoxin, cytokines such as TNF-α and IL-6a, arachidonic acid metabolites such as leukotrienes and prostaglandins, complement components C3a and C5a, vasoactive peptides such as bradykinin and histamine, and chemokines such as macrophage inflammatory protein 1α.

Transcapillary albumin transit increases by up to 300% in patients with septic shock. The lymph has a low albumin concentration, however, suggesting sequestration or degradation of extravascular albumin. In sepsis and in critical illness, serum albumin concentration decreases early in the course of disease and does not increase again until the recovery phase of the illness. The function of circulating albumin in septic shock is not fully understood. A low serum albumin concentration in critical illness is associated with a poor outcome.[15] However, studies of critically ill patients have shown that correcting hypoalbuminemia has no impact on outcome.[16,17]

Albumin administration does appear to be beneficial for burn patients. In the first 24 h, there is increased capillary permeability and transcapillary fluid shift. After 24 h, administration of albumin in profoundly hypoalbuminemic patients promotes the reabsorption of edema.[18] The Guidelines of the Consensus Conference in Paris have stated that albumin is not necessary for burns covering <15% of the body surface, but is essential from the start of the treatment for patients with >50% burns.[19]

RECOGNITION OF SHOCK

Early recognition of shock is essential for improving outcome. The diagnosis of shock is based on clinical, hemodynamic, and biochemical findings. Clinical signs of shock typically include arterial hypotension and evidence of altered tissue perfusion. Visible signs of shock are seen in three clinical windows: the skin, the kidneys, and the brain.[1] Cutaneously, shock is manifested by cyanosis; pale, cold, and clammy skin; and by slow capillary refill. The kidneys decrease urine output to <0.5 mL/kg/h. Neurologically, shock manifests as altered mentation with confusion, disorientation, and obtundation.

Although the presence of arterial hypotension is considered a sign of shock, hypotension is not a prerequisite for the diagnosis of shock. Compensatory mechanisms may preserve blood pressure with vasoconstriction in the presence of compromised tissue perfusion.[3] The patient who is chronically hypertensive may actually be hypotensive with what would be considered a normal blood pressure. A recent consensus conference recommended that arterial hypotension be defined as systolic blood pressure (SBP) of <90 mm Hg, or mean arterial pressure (MAP) of <65 mm Hg, or a decrease of >40 mm Hg from baseline.[3]

The normal blood lactate is <1 mEq/L, and in shock lactate levels are typically >2 mEq/L. The increase in blood lactate levels indicates abnormal cellular function. It may be due to increased production, decreased clearance, or a combination of the two. In tissue hypoxia, whether global or localized, lactate is overproduced and underutilized as a result of impaired mitochondrial oxidation. Even if systemic oxygen delivery (DO_2) is not low enough to cause generalized hypoxia, microcirculatory dysfunction can cause regional tissue hypoxia and hyperlactatemia.[20] The amount of lactate produced by anaerobic glycolysis is an indirect marker of oxygen debt, tissue hypoperfusion, and the severity of hemorrhagic shock. It has been used as a diagnostic parameter and prognostic marker of hemorrhagic shock since the 1960s.[21] In distributive shock, the pathophysiology of elevated lactate is more complex and may involve increased glycolysis and inhibition of pyruvate dehydrogenase. Hyperlactatemia resulting from aerobic glycolysis is activated in response to stress through epinephrine-dependent stimulation of the β2-adrenoceptor. Inflammation also drives aerobic glycolysis through cytokine-dependent stimulation of cellular glucose uptake.[20]

In trauma patients, base deficit is a useful measurement and has been correlated with transfusion requirements within the first 24 hours, and with the risk of post-traumatic organ failure or death.[21] In patients with injuries and associated alcohol consumption, base deficit may be a better predictor than lactate as alcohol can increase the level of lactate in the blood.[21]

DIFFERENTIAL DIAGNOSIS

Once the presence of shock is recognized, the underlying mechanisms responsible for shock—hypovolemia, distributive, cardiogenic, and obstructive—must be identified. History and clinical examination will often provide the diagnosis. A history of trauma would suggest hemorrhagic shock, chest pain, CS, and infection sepsis. But many patients are not straightforward. A patient in septic shock may have chronic heart failure and a trauma patient may have both hemorrhagic shock and neurogenic shock. Hemodynamic measurements are often needed to better characterize the type of shock when patients present with either complex situations or major comorbidities.

Cardiac output is usually elevated in distributive shock, while it is decreased in the other three types of shock.

Table 24.1 Types of shock and the expected hemodynamic changes and findings with echocardiography.

Type of shock	*Cardiac output*	*SvO_2*	*CVP*	*Echo findings*
Distributive	Normal or high	Normal or high	Low	Normal cardiac chambers and preserved contractility
Hypovolemic	Low	Low	Low	Small cardiac chambers with normal or high contractility
Cardiogenic	Low	Low	High	Large ventricles, poor contractility
Obstructive	Low	Low	High	Pericardial effusion, dilated inferior vena cava, and small ventricles with tamponade; dilated right ventricle and small left ventricle with pulmonary embolism or pneumothorax

(SvO_2: Mixed venous oxygen saturation; CVP: Central venous pressure).

Hypovolemic shock is associated with low blood pressure and low intravascular volume, while these are elevated in CS. Obstructive shock will often have an elevated central venous pressure (CVP) but cardiac findings will differ based on etiology (Table 24.1). Static variables such as CVP, stroke volume, CO, or pulmonary artery occlusion pressure (PAOP) should always be interpreted in the context of other measurements and findings. Outside of grossly deranged values, a single deranged value is insufficient to conclude that the parameter is too high, too low, or appropriate for any particular patient.

Evaluation of the CO, cardiac function, and preload is essential and can be obtained using various techniques. Point of care echocardiography is a useful and expedient tool for determining the type of shock and may help guide management in the ICU (*see* Table 24.1).[22,23] It is now proposed as the first-line evaluation modality.[1] The information can be obtained rapidly by bedside physicians with minimal echocardiographic training. Numerous focused echocardiographic examinations have been detailed, but all focus on cardiac and inferior vena cava (IVC) evaluations.[23] These protocols assess for pericardial effusion and tamponade, left ventricular (LV) contractility, right ventricular (RV) strain, and cardiac valvular assessment. Evaluation of the IVC assesses its size and collapsibility. Additional information can be obtained from thoracic ultrasound by specifically looking for the evidence of pneumothorax, pleural effusion, or pulmonary edema.

INITIAL APPROACH TO THE PATIENT IN SHOCK

The initial approach to every patient in shock is the same. Hemodynamic support to supply tissues with adequate oxygen is essential to the reversal of shock and prevention of further organ dysfunction and potential organ failure. Resuscitation must begin immediately, while investigations are carried out to identify the type and source of shock. A useful mnemonic is the VIP rule: ventilate, infuse, and pump.[1]

Administration of oxygen should be started immediately. If peripheral vasoconstriction is marked, pulse oximetry may be inaccurate or unobtainable. Placement of an arterial line can facilitate monitoring blood pressure, but also for monitoring arterial blood gases. For patients with severe dyspnea, hypoxemia, or persistent or worsening acidemia, intubation and mechanical ventilation should be performed expeditiously. Noninvasive ventilation is fraught with risk and potential technical failure, leading to cardiac arrest and death. Endotracheal intubation has the added advantage of reducing the oxygen demand of respiratory muscles and decreasing LV afterload by increasing intrathoracic pressure. However, intubation may unmask unsuspected hypovolemia. Patients who are hypovolemic may experience a sudden drop in blood pressure with intubation and mechanical ventilation.

Fluid administration is a major component of shock resuscitation. It aims to restore intravascular volume, increasing CO, and improving microvascular perfusion. But often, hemodynamic resuscitation requires a complex strategy of careful monitoring. Venous return is in equilibrium with CO through sympathetically mediated responses that regulate venous capacitance, arterial constriction, and cardiac contractility. Depending upon the type of shock, adjuncts to fluid administration such as catecholamine infusions may need to be considered to augment cardiac contraction and venous return.

Fluid Resuscitation

Although the use of asanguinous fluid resuscitation was described over 200 years ago, the ideal resuscitation fluid does not yet exist. Resuscitation fluids are broadly categorized into colloid and crystalloid. Proponents of colloid argue that they will remain intravascular longer than crystalloid, resulting in lower volumes needed for resuscitation. Proponents of crystalloid argue that they are inexpensive, widely available, and are established as a resuscitation fluid.

Normal saline has been one of the most commonly used crystalloid solutions for shock resuscitation. However, infusion of large volumes of saline results in hyperchloremic metabolic acidosis. This metabolic acidosis is associated with both immune and renal dysfunction. In an attempt to avoid fluid overload, hypertonic saline solutions have been used, particularly in patients with traumatic brain injury. However, both short- and long-term outcomes have not been significantly affected.[24]

"Balanced" or "physiologic" salt solutions are crystalloid solutions that attempt chemically to approximate extracellular fluid and are variations of the original Hartmann's or Ringer's solutions. They may contain lactate, acetate, gluconate, or malate. The use of these solutions for initial resuscitation in trauma or in postoperative patients has been shown to be safe and associated with a significant decrease in the rate of major complications including a lower incidence of postoperative infection, renal replacement therapy, and metabolic acidosis.[24] These solutions are increasingly being recommended as first-line resuscitation fluids for patients undergoing surgical operation and trauma resuscitation.[24]

Human albumin in saline (4–5%) is considered the reference colloidal solution. The Saline versus Albumin Fluid Evaluation (SAFE) study, which was a blinded, randomized control trial of albumin and saline, showed no significant difference in death or development of new organ failure between the two arms.[25] However, subgroup analysis showed that in patients with traumatic brain injury, the use of albumin was associated with a significant risk of death at 2 years. This outcome was attributed to an increase in intracranial pressure, particularly in the first week after injury. Patients with shock from sepsis, however, had an associated decrease in the adjusted risk of death at 28 days when resuscitated with albumin.

Because of the high cost and limited availability of albumin, semisynthetic colloids have been developed. They have a shorter duration of effect than albumin and are actively metabolized and excreted. Initially considered safe in limited amounts, hydroxyethyl starch solutions have recently been associated with increased rates of acute kidney injury and increased renal replacement therapy in ICU patients and are no longer recommended for shock resuscitation.[24]

The selection and use of resuscitation fluids is largely determined by the clinician's preference, which is influenced by institutional protocols, cost, and availability. Guidelines have been developed for specific disease states using low level evidence and expert opinion. The type of fluid used for resuscitation should be determined by the fluid that is lost and carefully monitored as excessive volume expansion is dangerous and can result in organ dysfunction.

Drugs

Vasoactive Agents

Venous return equilibrates with CO through sympathetically mediated regulation of venous capacitance, arterial conduction, and myocardial contractility. Fluid resuscitation may require augmentation by vasopressor agents to treat shock. In patients in whom hypotension is severe or persists despite adequate fluid administration, the use of vasopressors is indicated. Vasoactive agents are often needed in cardiogenic and distributive types of shock. When hypovolemia is the cause of shock, it must be corrected quickly. But if hypotension from hypovolemia is severe and prolonged, a vasopressor may be considered temporarily to augment blood pressure. Fluid resuscitation should be ongoing with the goal of discontinuation of the vasopressor as soon as possible after decreased tissue perfusion is corrected.

Vasopressors

Adrenergic agonists have rapid onset of action, short half-life, and are easily adjusted. Beta-adrenergic stimulation increases blood flow through increasing heart rate and contractility, which also increases the risk of myocardial ischemia. Alpha-adrenergic stimulation increases vascular tone and blood pressure but can also decrease CO and impair tissue perfusion, especially in the hepatosplanchnic region. Norepinephrine (noradrenaline) is considered the vasopressor of choice.[1] It has predominantly α-adrenergic properties but has enough β-adrenergic effects to maintain CO.

Dopamine has predominantly β-adrenergic effects at low doses and α-adrenergic effects at high doses, but is a relatively weak agent. Dopamine at 3 μg/kg/min may selectively dilate the hepatosplanchnic and renal circulations, but studies have not shown a protective effect on renal function.[1] Dopaminergic stimulation may also cause immunosuppression through its effect on the hypothalamic-pituitary system via a reduction in the release of prolactin.[1] In randomized, controlled trials, dopamine had shown no advantage over norepinephrine as a first-line treatment for shock and was associated with increased risk of dysrhythmias and death at 28 days for patients with CS and higher rates of death for those patients with septic shock.[1]

Epinephrine (adrenaline) has predominantly β-adrenergic at low doses and α-adrenergic effects at high doses. Its use is associated with increased rates of dysrhythmia, decreased splanchnic blood flow, and an increase in blood lactate levels.[1] It is usually considered a second-line agent.[1]

Vasopressin is a potent endogenous hormone primarily responsible for regulating plasma osmolality and volume. Vasopressin deficiency can develop in hyperkinetic forms of distributive shock. In the VASST, low-dose vasopressin used as an adjunct to norepinephrine was found to be safe, and it may have had a survival benefit in patients with less severe forms of shock and in those who also received glucocorticoids.[7] Doses should be no higher than 0.04 units/min and used only in those with a high CO.

Inotropic Agents

Dobutamine is the inotropic agent of choice. With primarily β-adrenergic activity, it improves CO. It has limited effects on arterial pressure, but in hypovolemic patients it may decrease blood pressure and in patients with myocardial dysfunction it may result in an increased blood pressure. Doses should be titrated to achieve adequate tissue perfusion rather than supranormal, predetermined levels. In patients with septic shock, dobutamine may improve capillary perfusion, independent of its systemic effects.[1] Doses in excess of 20 μg/kg/min have little benefit.

Phosphodiesterase type 3 (PDE3) inhibitors such as milrinone have both inotropic and vasodilatory properties. Through inhibition of the enzyme that breaks down cyclic adenosine monophosphate (cAMP), the increased intracellular concentration of cAMP in the heart increases cardiac inotropy, chronotropy, and dromotropy. In vascular smooth muscle, it promotes relaxation. At normal therapeutic doses, PDE3 inhibitors tend to have a greater vascular effect than cardiac effect, thus lowering the arterial pressure in the presence of increased CO. Phosphodiesterase type 3 inhibitors may be useful in patients whose β-adrenergic receptors are downregulated or in patients who have recently been treated with beta blockers.[1]

Mechanical Support

Although intra-aortic balloon pump (IABP) counter-pulsation has been recommended in past AHA guidelines as a Class I recommendation for the treatment of CS complicating acute MI, a randomized, prospective trial showed that IABP did not significantly reduce 30-day mortality. Current guidelines recommend that IABP or alternative LV devices be considered in patients with CS who do not quickly stabilize with pharmacologic therapy.[26]

Venoarterial extracorporeal membrane oxygenation (ECMO) may be used as a temporary lifesaving measure in patients with reversible CS or as a bridge to heart transplantation. It has also been successfully used for pediatric patients with severe septic shock, and was recently suggested as a valuable therapeutic option for adults with severe septic shock plus refractory cardiac and hemodynamic failure.[27]

GOALS OF SHOCK RESUSCITATION

End points of resuscitation are difficult to define. Hemodynamic measurements for the determination of the type of shock and the adequacy of resuscitation are the same. Classic teaching emphasized normalization of heart rate, blood pressure and urine output. However, occult hypoperfusion may persist despite normalization of these parameters. Continued organ dysfunction raises concern for ongoing shock, yet underlying disease may be the cause of derangement rather than hypoperfusion.

Arterial Pressure

Blood pressure must be individualized for all patients. In trauma patients with hemorrhagic shock, European guidelines recommend targeting a SBP of 80–90 mm Hg until major bleeding has been stopped in the initial phase and in the absence of brain injury.[21] In trauma patients with hemorrhagic shock and severe traumatic brain injury, the guidelines recommend maintaining a MAP >80 mm Hg.[21] In CS, guidelines no longer recommend a target blood pressure.[3] In the setting of CS, maintaining increased arterial pressures will increase systemic vascular resistance, which can in turn have the negative consequences of decreased stroke volume and CO. A MAP of around 65 mm Hg is considered sufficient in most patients with septic shock, although in patients with a history of hypertension, a higher MAP is associated with a lower risk of acute kidney injury.[3] Placement of an arterial catheter allows continuous monitoring as well as providing access for regular blood gas and laboratory analysis.

Advanced hemodynamic monitoring may not be needed in patients who rapidly respond to the initial therapy based on clinical examination and echocardiography. In cases of severe shock or in patients with complex conditions or comorbidities, advanced hemodynamic monitoring may be useful for both diagnosis and guiding therapy. Continuous or semicontinuous measurements of CO and/or mixed venous oxygen saturation (SvO_2) are particularly useful; however, no single variable should be used for either the diagnosis or management of shock. Frequent re-evaluation is key to providing appropriate management.

SvO_2/$ScvO_2$

Mixed venous oxygen saturation can provide valuable information about the balance between oxygen transport and utilization. During normal metabolism, DO_2 far exceeds consumption (VO_2), making VO_2 independent of DO_2 over a wide range of values. With either decreased DO_2 or increased VO_2, there is increased oxygen extraction from blood, which results in decreased oxygen saturation of venous hemoglobin as it leaves the tissue. Oxygen saturation is measured using a catheter-based fiberoptic reflective spectroscopy in either the pulmonary artery (SvO_2) or superior vena cava ($ScvO_2$). A normal value does not necessarily indicate that all tissues have adequate oxygenation as this is a pooled venous value, but a low SvO_2 (<65%) is highly suggestive of tissue hypoperfusion.[28]

Measuring SvO_2 requires placement of a pulmonary artery catheter, while $ScvO_2$ requires placement of a central line. Rivers and coworkers showed that mortality was improved by increasing $ScvO_2$ to >70% early in the course of sepsis (early goal-directed therapy).[29] Two recent multicenter randomized controlled trials, the ProCESS and the ARISE trials, failed to reproduce these results, although both had overall lower mortality and higher mean baseline $ScvO_2$ values compared to the Rivers et al. study.[29-31]

A high $ScvO_2$ value is of little help when lactate levels are high as it cannot tell if oxygen transport is adequate but there is still local hypoperfusion. The venoarterial carbon dioxide difference (pCO_2 gap) has been suggested as another measurement to identify patients who remain under-resuscitated. It measures the difference in the partial pressure of CO_2 (pCO_2) between mixed or central venous blood and arterial blood. Values of >6 mm Hg suggest an insufficient blood flow to tissues, even when the $ScvO_2$ is >70%.[3]

Preload

When tissue perfusion appears inadequate, the correct therapeutic option must be selected. Preload, cardiac contractility and afterload are all important determinants of CO and oxygen delivery. Intravascular volume is the primary determinant of cardiac filling pressure or preload.

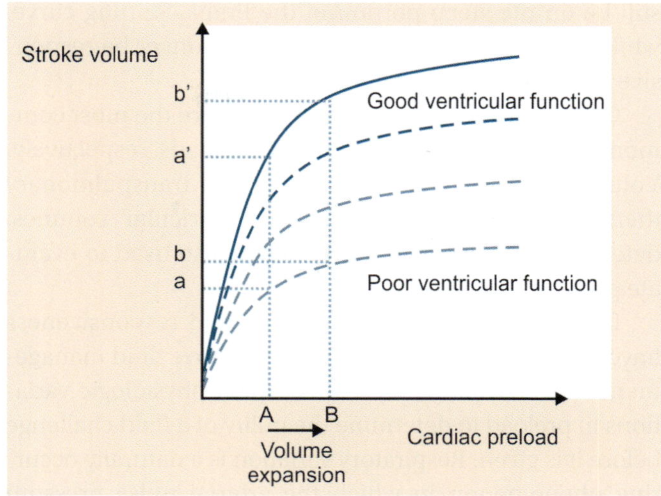

Fig. 24.3: The relationship between stroke volume and cardiac preload depends upon the ventricular function. This set of Frank–Starling curve explains why the effects of a volume expansion (increase in cardiac preload from A to B) can induce effects on stroke volume of small (from a to b) or of large (from a' to b') magnitude. It is also the reason why the effects of volume expansion cannot be predicted from a static value of cardiac preload (A). Contractility is dynamic and requires frequent re-evaluation. Over a period of time, one patient may have many different curves during resuscitation for shock.

Preload relates directly to stroke volume and therefore both CO and tissue perfusion as seen visually in the Frank–Starling curve (Fig. 24.3). The slope is not constant, but as preload increases, additional increases in filling pressures produce incrementally less augmentation of stroke volume to the point that further increases in preload do not produce any further increase in stroke volume or may even cause a decrease in stroke volume. Therefore, volume expansion is of maximal benefit when the heart is functioning on the steep portion of the Frank–Starling curve and is of minimal benefit or may even be deleterious when the heart has higher filling pressures.

The slope and position of the Frank–Starling curve are also dependent upon cardiac function. Underlying cardiac disease, acute cardiomyopathy, changes in intrathoracic pressure (positive end-expiratory pressure [PEEP]), or vasoactive medications will alter the curve. It is, therefore, important to know whether stroke volume will respond to volume expansion. Static measures such as CVP or PAOP have traditionally been used to assess preload. Outside of grossly deranged values, a single value does not allow you to know if the measurement is too high, too low, or just right for any particular patient. Because of intrapatient and interpatient variability, a single value is impossible to interpret. For example, a patient may have a high CVP but still be on the steep portion of the Frank–Starling curve, while a patient with a low CVP may no longer be responsive to preload augmentation.

Central venous pressure and PAOP are the most commonly used estimates of RV and LV preloads, respectively. Volumetric parameters as measured by transpulmonary thermodilution and end-diastolic ventricular volumes, determined by echocardiography are also used to evaluate preload.

Dynamic measures of assessing fluid responsiveness have been proposed in an effort to improve fluid management. These dynamic measures exploit physiologic variations in preload to determine the utility of a fluid challenge before it is given. Respiratory variation is a naturally occurring phenomenon in which the arterial pulse pressure falls during inspiration and rises during expiration due to changes in intrathoracic pressure secondary to negative pressure ventilation (spontaneous breathing). With mechanical ventilation, the same phenomenon occurs, but in reverse, with arterial pressure rising during inspiration and falling during expiration due to positive pressure ventilation. During a positive pressure breath, RV filling has been shown to decrease by 20–70%, leading to a decrease in stroke volume that is amplified by an increasing degree of hypovolemia.[3] Variability in preload is more pronounced when the heart is functioning on the steep portion of the Frank–Starling curve, such that increased variability corresponds to preload responsiveness. Different dynamic measures are available and can be assessed at the bedside by standard and minimally invasive hemodynamic monitoring systems. The most commonly used techniques are pulse pressure variation (PPV) and stroke volume variation (SVV), passive leg raise (PLR), and evaluating respiratory variation in the IVC diameter. The predictability of dynamic measures of volume responsiveness has been studied extensively in critically ill patients.[28] PPV-, SVV-, and PLR-induced changes are all highly accurate in predicting an increase in CO in response to volume expansion.[28]

Importantly, any single measure of preload should be evaluated in context with other measurements. All of the different measures of preload have limitations. Numerous studies have reported the inability of both the CVP and PAOP to predict a change in CO in response to volume expansion.[28] Central venous pressure remains inaccurate even when trended in response to volume expansion.[28] Pulse pressure variation and SVV are proven to be good predictors of fluid responsiveness in sedated, mechanically ventilated patients without spontaneous breathing and in normal sinus rhythm (anesthetized patients). However, measurement of PPV had no predictive value in the subgroup of patients with spontaneous breathing.[3]

Optimal fluid management will improve patient outcomes. Both hypovolemia and hypervolemia are detrimental. Consensus guidelines recommend that fluid resuscitation should be started immediately upon recognition of the shock state.[1,3] Commonly used preload measures (CVP, PAOP, end-diastolic volume) should not be used alone to guide fluid resuscitation, nor should a specific ventricular filling pressure or volume be targeted. Dynamic measures of fluid responsiveness are favored over static measures when conditions are applicable.

Because shock is characterized by oxygen demand that exceeds supply, it was thought that repayment of oxygen debt would be signaled by reaching the point that oxygen extraction would become independent of oxygen delivery. Shoemaker and colleagues observed that survivors of shock more often achieved supranormal levels of DO_2 (>600 mL/min/m^2) as compared to nonsurvivors.[32] Unfortunately, randomized, controlled trials of resuscitation to supranormal physiology showed that this was not beneficial and appeared detrimental. The increased volume expansion that was required increased risk of pulmonary edema, intestinal ischemia, and abdominal compartment syndrome.[33,34]

StO_2

Tissue hemoglobin saturation (StO_2) may be measured using near infrared spectroscopy. It provides a continuous, noninvasive measurement of oxygen supply-demand dynamics through measurement of tissue perfusion of either subcutaneous or skeletal muscle. Tissue hemoglobin saturation is a measure of the microvasculature and is primarily indicative of the venous oxyhemoglobin concentration. Its estimation is of the local tissue rather than of the systemic condition. It has correlated favorably with base deficit and DO_2 in traumatic shock, but its utility in sepsis is unclear.[28]

Lactic Acid

Both elevation and failure to normalize lactate concentrations are highly predictive of adverse outcomes for critically ill patients in shock.[28] Lactate levels >2 mEq/L (mmol/L) are usually considered indicative of shock, but values >1.5 m mol/L in patients with septic shock are associated with increased mortality.[3] An early decrease in blood lactate levels may indicate a resolution of global

Table 24.2 Clinical and physiologic response to hemorrhage.

Hemorrhage severity	*Class I*	*Class II*	*Class III*	*Class IV*
Blood loss (mL)	<750	750–1,500	1,500–2,000	>2,000
% Circulating volume	15	15–30	30–40	>40
Pulse rate (per minute)	<100	>100	>120	>140
Blood pressure	Normal	Normal	Decreased	Decreased
Pulse pressure (mm Hg)	Normal	Decreased	Decreased	Decreased
Respiratory rate (per minute)	14–20	20–30	30–40	>40
Urine output (mL/hour)	>30	20–30	5–15	Negligible
Mental status	Slightly anxious	Mildly anxious	Anxious, confused	Lethargic

Values are estimated for a 70 kg adult.

Source: Adapted from American College of Surgeons/Advanced Trauma Life Support[35]

tissue hypoxia and is associated with a decreased mortality rate.[3] In patients with hemorrhagic shock, survival was 100% in those who had normalization of lactate levels with 24 hours. It dropped to 77.8% at 48 hours and to 13.6% for those patients in whom lactate levels were >2 m mol/L for >48 hours.[21]

Consensus guidelines for monitoring of patients with shock have recommended serial measurements of lactate and/or base deficit to evaluate not only the outcome and prognosis but also to guide therapy. European guidelines recommend obtaining both parameters in trauma.[21]

SPECIFIC SHOCK STATES

Hemorrhagic Shock

Shock in a trauma patient is presumed to be hemorrhagic until proven otherwise. The clinical and physiologic response to hemorrhage has been classified according to the amount of blood loss (Table 24.2). Loss of up to 15% of the circulating volume produces little noticeable response. Loss of up to 30% of the circulating volume may result in mild tachycardia, tachypnea, and anxiety. With 30-40% of blood loss, the patient becomes hypotensive, markedly tachycardic, and confused. When >40% of the blood volume has been lost, it is immediately life threatening with hypotension unresponsive to initial fluid resuscitation and coma.

Young, healthy patients are better able to compensate blood loss and may manifest fewer clinical symptoms. These patients maintain a near normal blood pressure until precipitous cardiac collapse ensues. Older patients are less able to tolerate hemorrhage due to underlying atherosclerotic vascular disease, diminished cardiac compliance, inability to elevate the heart rate or cardiac contractility in response to hemorrhage, and the overall decline in physiologic reserve. Drugs such as beta blockers may block the compensatory response to hemorrhage. Patients on anticoagulants or antiplatelet agents may suffer increased blood loss.

Multiple sites have potential for hemorrhage, but the areas that can potentially cause hypotension and shock are limited. Active bleeding from extremity wounds or scalp lacerations can result in significant hemorrhage, especially if near large arteries or veins. Persistent bleeding from smaller vessels can cause shock, if left untreated. Soft tissue hematomas can harbor an appreciable blood loss, especially in elderly patients whose skin has lost its elasticity due to aging. However, before concluding that these sites are the cause of shock, intracavitary hemorrhage must be excluded. The chest, abdomen, and pelvis are each capable of enough blood loss to cause death. Physical examination will offer clues to the site of hemorrhage. Decreased breath sounds, abdominal pain, or pelvic instability may raise suspicion of intracavitary or retroperitoneal hemorrhage. The abdomen may contain several liters of blood before altering the physical signs. Chest X-ray can be used quickly to rule out a major hemothorax. FAST (focused abdominal sonography for trauma) exam or diagnostic peritoneal aspiration can be used to quickly identify intraperitoneal blood. The pattern of pelvic fracture on X-ray may raise suspicion for potential massive blood loss.

The priorities in patients with hemorrhagic shock are to secure the airway, support breathing and ventilation, control the source of hemorrhage, and resuscitate with early administration of blood products while limiting the amount of crystalloid solution. Patients who transiently respond to fluid or blood administration with an increase in hemodynamic parameters, but again become hypotensive, must be presumed to be actively bleeding. These patients often have injuries that require operative intervention. Patients who have had marked blood loss, but in whom hemorrhage has stopped, will respond appropriately to resuscitative efforts.

Patients with uncontrolled hemorrhage are at risk to develop the "bloody, vicious cycle" of acidosis, hypothermia and coagulopathy. Damage control resuscitation was developed to treat intravascular volume deficits, the acute coagulopathy of trauma, preserve oxygen-carrying capacity, repair the endothelium, and prevent dilutional coagulopathy. It is defined as the early administration of blood products in a balanced ratio (1:1:1 for FFP:platelets:RBCs), prevention and immediate correction of coagulopathy, and minimization of crystalloid fluids.[36] This blood product ratio is the closest approximation to reconstituted whole blood. Damage control resuscitation principles have been associated with improved outcomes compared with more traditional transfusion practices including decreased transfusion amounts, fewer inflammatory complications, and improved survival. The Pragmatic, Randomized Optimal Platelet and Plasma Ratio (PROPPR) trial that was designed to compare the effectiveness and safety of a 1:1:1 transfusion ratio with a 1:1:2 transfusion ratio in trauma patients showed no significant differences in mortality at 24 hours and 30 days between the two groups. However, more patients in the 1:1:1 group achieved homeostasis and fewer died from exsanguination within 24 hours.[36] Despite more plasma and platelets, there was no difference in inflammatory-mediated complications such as acute respiratory distress syndrome, multiple organ failure, infection, venous thromboembolism, and sepsis.

The use of tranexamic acid (TXA) remains controversial.[37] The CRASH-2 trial was a large international randomized, placebo-controlled trial in trauma patients that found TXA was associated with a 1.5% reduction in 28-day all-cause mortality in adult trauma patients with signs of bleeding.[38] Its benefit was greatest in the most severe shock group, with a 28-day all-cause mortality of 30.6% for TXA group versus 35.1% for placebo group [relative risk (RR), 0.87; 99% confidence interval (CI) 0.76–0.99] and when given early. When given ≤1 hour from injury, TXA was associated with the greatest reduction in deaths from bleeding (5.3% vs. 7.7%; RR, 0.68; 95% CI, 0.57Y0.82; *P* <0.0001). Tranexamic acid given between 1 and 3 hours after injury also reduced the risk of death caused by bleeding (4.8% vs.6.1%; RR, 0.79; 95% CI, 0.64Y0.97; *P* = 0.03), but when given after 3 hours of injury it was associated with an increased risk of death.(4.4% vs.3.1%; RR, 1.44; 95% CI, 1.12Y1.84; *P* = 0.004). Napolitano and co-authors suggested that the rational approach for TXA use in trauma was to give to adult trauma patients with severe hemorrhagic shock (SBP ≤75 mm Hg), with known predictors of fibrinolysis, or with known fibrinolysis by thromboelastography (LY30 >3%) and only administer TXA <3 hours from the time of injury.[39] Tranexamic acid is given as 1 g intravenously over 10 minutes, then 1 g intravenously over 8 hours.

Neurogenic Shock

Neurogenic shock is a distributive form of shock that occurs following injury to the cervical or high thoracic spinal cord. Most often due to vertebral fracture, spinal cord injury can also result from penetrating injury to the spinal cord or even an epidural hematoma that impinges on the cord but is not accompanied by fracture. Characterized by hypotension and bradycardia, the cause of neurogenic shock is attributed to loss of supraspinal control of the sympathetic nervous system, which results in loss of vasomotor tone and pooling of blood in the periphery. The sympathetic fibers to the heart exit the spinal cord at the T1–T4 level, so that injuries at or above this level result in decreased myocardial contractility and heart rate. Parasympathetic outflow is carried by the vagus nerve, which originates in the medulla. Therefore, a cervical or high thoracic spinal cord injury may completely transect spinal, cardiac and vasomotor sympathetic fibers from above while the parasympathetic fibers remain intact.[40] Bradycardia is less problematic when the injury is in the upper thoracic spinal cord or is less severe, as cardiac sympathetic neurons remain under brainstem control, leaving vagal and sympathetic influences more in balance.[41] Both hypotension and bradycardia may be present for up to 5 weeks after injury.

The initial treatment of hypotension is with fluid. However, once it is determined that there are no other causes responsible for shock, vasopressors must be considered as an adjunct. Hypotension in patients with acute spinal cord injury leads to decreased cord perfusion and the potential for further ischemic cord injury. Maintaining a MAP ≥85 mm Hg for 5 to 7 days after injury is recommended. The choice of vasopressor will depend upon the level of injury. Alpha-receptor agonists result in peripheral vasoconstriction and elevation of blood pressure. Beta-receptor agonists increase cardiac contractility and heart rate. Cervical and upper thoracic cord injuries down to T6 warrant a vasopressor with both inotropic and chronotropic as well as vasoconstrictive properties. Dopamine and norepinephrine, which have both $\alpha 1$ and $\beta 1$ receptor effects, are reasonable choices. For lower thoracic lesions and lumbar injuries, phenylephrine is a good choice if a peripheral vasoconstrictor is needed.[42] Bradycardia can further contribute to secondary cord injury. Scheduled oral albuterol is recommended for patients with cervical and high thoracic spinal cord injury to prevent symptomatic bradycardia, although some patients may require placement of a pacemaker.[43] Bradycardia generally resolves within 2–5 weeks of the injury.

Cardiogenic Shock

Cardiogenic shock is end organ hypoperfusion due to cardiac failure. The definition of CS includes hemodynamic parameters: persistent hypotension (SBP 80–90 mm Hg or MAP 30 mm Hg lower than baseline) with severe reduction in cardiac index and adequate or elevated filling pressures.[44] Diagnosis is usually confirmed with echocardiography. Myocardial infarction (MI) with LV failure is the most common cause of CS. Complications of MI, especially mechanical complications such as ventricular septal rupture or papillary muscle rupture can cause CS. However, any cause of acute, severe LV or RV dysfunction may lead to CS. Acute myopericarditis and cardiomyopathy may both present with ST elevation, release of cardiac markers, and shock in the absence of serious coronary artery disease. Acute valvular regurgitation, typically caused by endocarditis or chordal rupture due to trauma or degenerative disease, may also cause CS. Risk factors for development of CS in the context of MI include anterior MI, hypertension, diabetes mellitus, multivessel coronary artery disease, prior MI or angina, prior diagnosis of heart failure, ST elevation myocardial infarction (STEMI), and left bundle branch block (LBBB).

Myocardial injury causes systolic and diastolic dysfunction. A decrease in CO leads to a decrease in systemic and coronary perfusion. This process exacerbates ischemia and causes cell death in the infarct border zone. Inadequate systemic perfusion triggers reflex vasoconstriction, which is usually insufficient. Systemic inflammation may play a role in limiting the peripheral vascular compensatory response and may contribute to myocardial dysfunction. Whether inflammation plays a causal role or is only an epiphenomenon remains unclear. Revascularization leads to relief of ischemia. It has not been possible to demonstrate an increase in CO or left ventricular ejection fraction as the mechanism of benefit of revascularization; however, revascularization does significantly increase the likelihood of survival with good quality of life.[44]

Antithrombotic therapy with aspirin and heparin, routinely recommended for MI, should be given for CS. Clopidogrel may be deferred until it is known whether operation is needed or whether revascularization can be accomplished using percutaneous coronary intervention when indicated. Negative inotropes and vasodilators (including nitroglycerin) should be avoided. Arterial oxygenation and near-normal pH should be maintained to minimize ischemia. Intensive insulin therapy improves survival in hyperglycemic critically ill patients and is recommended for use in complicated MI. Echocardiography is often used for assessment and monitoring. Pharmacologic support includes inotropic and vasopressor agents in the lowest possible doses to maintain coronary and systemic perfusion until shock resolves. Although inotropes are necessary to treat cardiac failure, they also increase myocardial oxygen demand in the myocardium where supply is already limited. In the past, intra-aortic balloon counterpulsation has been the mainstay of treatment for cardiac failure. However, in a prospective, randomized controlled trial, Thiele and colleagues showed no difference in 30-day mortality between the use of IABP and the best available medical therapy when early revascularization was planned.[45] Early revascularization in patients with CS shows a clear survival advantage, whether performed percutaneously or surgically. Thrombolytic therapy is less effective, but is indicated when percutaneous coronary intervention is impossible or if MI and CS onset were within 3 hours.

Septic Shock

Septic shock is a vasodilatory form of shock that occurs from the body's inflammatory response to infection. Multidisciplinary consensus has established definitions for the response that occurs.[46,47] The SIRS occurs as a response to a wide variety of physiologic insults including infection, and is defined as the presence of two or more of the following conditions: temperature >38°C or <36°C, pulse rate >90 beats/min, respiratory rate >20 breaths/min or $PaCO_2$ <32 mm Hg, white blood cell count >12,000/mm^3 or <4,000/mm^3, or >10% immature (band) forms. Sepsis is defined as the systemic inflammatory response to infection. Severe sepsis occurs when sepsis is complicated by acute organ dysfunction. Septic shock is a subset of severe sepsis and occurs when sepsis is complicated by hypotension that is refractory to fluid resuscitation or by hyperlactatemia. Table 24.3 shows the diagnostic criteria for sepsis from the 2001 International Sepsis Definitions Conference.[47]

Table 24.3 Diagnostic criteria for sepsis, severe sepsis, and septic shock in adults.

Sepsis (documented or suspected infection plus ≥1 of the following)
General variables
• Fever (core temperature, >38.3°C)
• Hypothermia (core temperature, <36°C)
• Elevated heart rate (>90 beats/min or >2 SD above the upper limit of the normal range for age)
• Tachypnea
• Altered mental status
• Substantial edema or positive fluid balance (>20 mL/kg of body weight over a 24-h period)
• Hyperglycemia [plasma glucose, >120 mg/dL (6.7 mmol/L)] in the absence of diabetes
Inflammatory variables
• Leukocytosis (white cell count, >12,000/mm^3)
• Leukopenia (white cell count, <4,000/mm^3)
• Normal white cell count with >10% immature forms
• Elevated plasma C-reactive protein (>2 SD above the upper limit of the normal range)
• Elevated plasma procalcitonin (>2 SD above the upper limit of the normal range)
Hemodynamic variables
• Arterial hypotension (systolic pressure, <90 mm Hg; MAP, <70 mm Hg; or decrease in systolic pressure of >40 mm Hg in adults or to >2 SD below the lower limit of the normal range for age)
• Elevated mixed venous oxygen saturation (>70%)
• Elevated cardiac index (>3.5 L/min/m^2)
Organ dysfunction variables
• Arterial hypoxemia (ratio of the partial pressure of arterial oxygen to the fraction of inspired oxygen, <300)
• Acute oliguria (urine output, <0.5 mL/kg/h or 45 mL/h for at least 2 h)
• Increase in creatinine level of >0.5 mg/dL (>44 µmol/L)
• Coagulation abnormalities (international normalized ratio, >1.5; or activated partial-thromboplastin time, >60 s)
• Paralytic ileus (absence of bowel sounds)
• Thrombocytopenia (platelet count, <100,000/mm^3)
• Hyperbilirubinemia [plasma total bilirubin, >4 mg/dL (68 µmol/L)]
Tissue perfusion variables
• Hyperlactatemia (lactate, >1 mmol/L)
• Decreased capillary refill or mottling
Severe sepsis (sepsis plus organ dysfunction)
Septic shock [sepsis plus either hypotension (refractory to intravenous fluids) or hyperlactatemia]

(SD: Standard deviation; MAP: Mean arterial pressure).

The Surviving Sepsis Campaign's clinical guidelines for the management of severe sepsis and septic shock are organized into two "bundles" of care: the initial management bundle that should be accomplished within 6 hours of the patient's presentation and an ICU management bundle.[48] Important points from the initial management bundle are shown in Table 24.4. The implementation of these bundles is associated with improved outcome.[49,50]

The principles of the initial management bundle are to begin resuscitation and begin diagnosis and treatment of the infection. Resuscitation involves use of intravenous fluids and vasopressors as necessary. The initial management of infection requires deciding on a probable diagnosis, obtaining cultures, initiating appropriate and timely empirical antibiotics, and obtaining source control. The choice of empirical antibiotics depends upon the suspected source of infection, the patient's setting (hospital, nursing home, etc.), previous recent exposure to antibiotics and the local microbial susceptibility patterns. Because inappropriate or delayed antibiotic treatment is associated with increased mortality, antibiotics must be started as early as possible and cover all potential pathogens. After

Table 24.4 Important points from guidelines for the initial treatment of severe sepsis and septic shock.

Resuscitation
• Begin goal-directed resuscitation during first 6 h after recognition of sepsis using crystalloid as the initial fluid and consider the addition of albumin
• Begin initial fluid challenge in patients with tissue hypoperfusion and suspected hypovolemia, to achieve ≥30 mL of crystalloids per kilogram of body weight
• Continue fluid-challenge technique as long as there is hemodynamic improvement
• Avoid hetastarch formulations
• Use norepinephrine as the first-choice vasopressor to maintain a MAP of ≥65 mm Hg
• Use epinephrine when an additional agent is needed to maintain adequate blood pressure
• Add vasopressin (at a dose of 0.03 units/min) with weaning of norepinephrine, if tolerated
• Avoid the use of dopamine except in carefully selected patients (e.g. patients with a low risk of arrhythmias and either known marked LV systolic dysfunction or low heart rate)
• Infuse dobutamine or add it to vasopressor therapy in the presence of myocardial dysfunction (e.g. elevated cardiac filling pressures or low cardiac output) or ongoing hypoperfusion despite adequate intravascular volume and MAP
• Avoid the use of intravenous hydrocortisone if adequate fluid resuscitation and vasopressor therapy restore hemodynamic stability; if hydrocortisone is used, administer at a dose of 200 mg per day
• Target a hemoglobin level of 7–9 g/dL in patients without hypoperfusion, critical coronary artery disease or myocardial ischemia, or acute hemorrhage
Infection control
• Obtain blood cultures before antibiotic therapy is administered
• Perform imaging studies promptly to confirm source of infection
• Administer broad-spectrum antibiotic therapy within 1 h after diagnosis of either severe sepsis or septic shock
• Reassess antibiotic therapy daily for de-escalation when appropriate
• Perform source control with attention to risks and benefits of the chosen method within 12 h after diagnosis

Adapted from Dellinger RP et al.[48]

the first 6 hours, the guidelines focus on monitoring and support of organ function, avoidance of complications, and de-escalation of antibiotics when appropriate. The only immunomodulatory therapy that is currently suggested is a short course of hydrocortisone (200 mg to 300 mg per day for up to 7 days or until vasopressor support is no longer required) for patients with refractory septic shock. Although recommended by a meta-analysis, there are conflicting results.[51]

Based on the underlying pathophysiology of sepsis, treatments attempting to interrupt the initial cytokine cascade or to interfere with dysregulated coagulation have been tested and all have been disappointing. Only activated protein C gained regulatory approval and was later withdrawn from the market due to post-approval concern about its safety and efficacy. The use of statins has been proposed to reduce the incidence or improve the outcome of sepsis and severe infection through numerous observational studies, yet no randomized, controlled trials have confirmed this finding.[51]

Obstructive Shock

Mechanical obstruction of the circulation by impeding venous return to the heart or preventing cardiac filling is termed obstructive shock. Tension pneumothorax, cardiac tamponade, and pulmonary embolism are the most common causes. Tension pneumothorax manifests with diminished breath sounds over one hemithorax, hyperresonance to percussion, jugular venous distension, and shift of mediastinal structures to the unaffected side. Unfortunately not all of these clinical signs may be evident on physical examination if other injuries exist. Jugular venous distension may not be present if hypovolemia from other injuries is present. A tension pneumothorax should be a clinical diagnosis, and placement of thoracostomy tube should be done prior to obtaining a chest X-ray. If the chest X-ray is obtained because diagnostic signs have been missed, the typical findings include deviation of the mediastinal structures, depression of the hemidiaphragm, and hypo-opacification with absent lung markings. For the multiply-injured patient with hypotension, the placement of bilateral chest tubes may be both diagnostic and therapeutic. In these circumstances, obtaining a chest X-ray is both unnecessary and potentially a waste of resources.

Cardiac tamponade results from accumulation of fluid within the pericardium. In trauma patients, it most commonly occurs with penetrating injury. Echocardiography can quickly diagnose the presence of fluid and tamponade and is part of the FAST exam. Patients who present with tamponade and circulatory collapse require immediate pericardial decompression through a left anterolateral thoracotomy. Patients in whom the amount of pericardial fluid has not accumulated to the point of causing hemodynamic compromise can undergo additional studies. Pericardial fluid can be seen on computed tomography, or if not seen well with transthoracic echocardiographic windows, transesophageal echocardiography may be diagnostic.

Traumatic Shock

Shock in trauma patients is most commonly hypovolemic from blood loss, but there is also a distributive form of shock that is seen in trauma patients. Traumatic shock results from soft tissue and bony injury that activates inflammatory cells and the release of circulating factors such as cytokines and intracellular molecules that modulate the immune response. Mild-to-moderate blood loss can magnify this response. The inflammatory mediators that are released in response to tissue injury (damage-associated molecular patterns, i.e. ribonucleic acid, uric acid, and high mobility group box 1) are recognized by many of the same cellular receptors and activate similar signaling pathways that recognize bacterial products elaborated in sepsis (pathogen-associated molecular patterns) such as lipopolysaccharide.[52,53] The pattern recognition receptors include the toll-like receptor family of proteins. Therapy for traumatic shock focuses on the correction of the elements driving the inflammatory reaction and restoring perfusion and supportive care to avoid further complications.

REFERENCES

1. Vincent JL, De Backer D. Circulatory shock. N Eng J Med. 2013;369:1726-34.
2. Gross S. A System of Surgery: Pathologic, Diagnostic, Therapeutic and Operative. Philadelphia: Lea and Febiger; 1872.
3. Cecconi M, De Backer D, Antonelli M, et al. Consensus on circulatory shock and hemodynamic monitoring. Task force of the European Society of Intensive Care Medicine. Intensive Care Med. 2014;40:1795-815.
4. De Backer D, Biston P, Devriendt J, et al. Comparison of dopamine and norepinephrine in the treatment of shock. N Eng J Med. 2010;362:779-89.
5. Akira S, Uematsu S, Takeuchi O. Pathogen recognition and innate immunity. Cell. 2006;124:783-801.
6. Brinkmann V, Reichard U, Goosmann C, et al. Neutrophil extracellular traps kill bacteria. Science. 2004;303:1532-5.
7. Russell JA, Walley KR, Singer J, Gordon AC, et al. Vasopressin versus norepinephrine infusion in patients with septic shock. N Engl J Med. 2008;358:877-87.
8. Ganong WF. Dynamics of blood and lymph flow. In: Review of Medical Physiology, 17th edition. Connecticut: Appleton and Lange; 1995. pp. 525-41.
9. Schnitzer JE, Carley WW, Palade GE. Specific albumin binding to microvascular endothelium in culture. Am J Physiol. 1988;254:H425-37.
10. Schnitzer JE, Oh P. Albondin-mediated capillary permeability to albumin. Differential role of receptors in endothelial transcytosis and endocytosis of native and modified albumins. J Biol Chem. 1994;269:6072-82.
11. Moshage HJ, Janssen J, Franssen JH, et al. Study of the molecular mechanism of decreased liver synthesis of albumin in inflammation. J Clin Invest. 1987;79:1635-41.
12. Perlmutter DH, Dinarello CA, Punsal PI, Colten HR. Cachectin/tumor necrosis factor regulates hepatic acute-phase gene expression. J Clin Invest. 1986;78:1349-54.
13. Castell JV, Gomez-Lechon MJ, David M, et al. Acute-phase response of human hepatocytes: regulation of acute-phase protein synthesis by interleukin-6. Hepatology. 1990;12:1179-86.
14. Fleck A, Hawker F, Wallace PI, et al. Increased vascular permeability: a major cause of hypoalbuminaemia in disease and injury. Lancet. 1985;1:781-4.
15. Murray MJ, Marsh HM, Wochos DN, et al. Nutritional assessment of intensive-care unit patients. Mayo Clin Proc. 1988;63:1106-15.
16. Stockwell MA, Soni N, Riley B. Colloid solutions in the critically ill. A randomised comparison of albumin and polygeline 1. Outcome and duration of stay in the intensive care unit. Anaesthesia. 1992;47:3-6.
17. Stockwell MA, Scott A, Day A, et al. Colloid solutions in the critically ill. A randomised comparison of albumin and polygeline 2. Serum albumin concentration and the incidences of pulmonary oedema and acute renal failure. Anaesthesia. 1992;47:7-9.
18. Manelli JC. [Is albumin administration useful in critical care for burnt patients?]. Ann Fr Anesth Reanim. 1996;15:507-13.
19. Sanchez R. [Role of albumins in burnt patients: its efficacy during intensive care. Addendum to the expert guidelines of the Consensus Conference, Paris, December 15th, 1995]. Ann Fr Anesth Reanim. 1996;15:1124-9.
20. Kraut JA, Madias NE. Lactic acidosis. N Engl J Med. 2014;371:2309-19.
21. Spahn DR, Bouillon B, Cerny V, et al. Management of bleeding and coagulopathy following major trauma: an updated European guideline. Crit Care. 2013 Apr 19;17:R76.

22. Beaulieu Y, Marik PE. Bedside ultrasonography in the ICU: part 1. Chest. 2005;128:881-95.
23. Seif D, Perera P, Mailhot T, et al. Bedside ultrasound in resuscitation and the rapid ultrasound in shock protocol. Crit Care Res Pract. 2012;2012:503254.
24. Myburgh JA, Mythen MG. Resuscitation fluids. N Engl J Med. 2013;369:2462-3.
25. The SAFE Study Investigators. A comparison of albumin and saline for fluid resuscitation in the intensive care unit. N Engl J Med. 2004;350:2247-56.
26. American College of Emergency Physicians; Society for Cardiovascular Angiography and Interventions, O'Gara PT, Kushner FG, Ascheim DD, et al. ACCF/AHA guideline for the management of ST-elevation myocardial infarction: a report of the American College of Cardiology Foundation/American Heart Association Task Force on Practice Guidelines. J Am Coll Cardiol. 2013;61:e78-140.
27. Bréchot N, Luyt CE, Schmidt M, et al. Venoarterial extracorporeal membrane oxygenation support for refractory cardiovascular dysfunction during severe bacterial septic shock. Crit Care Med. 2013;41:1616-26.
28. Pieracci FM, Biffl WL, Moore EE. Current concepts in resuscitation. J Intensive Care Med. 2012;27:79-96.
29. Rivers E, Nguyen B, Havstad S, et al. Early goal-directed therapy in the treatment of severe sepsis and septic shock. N Eng J Med. 2001;345:1368-77.
30. Pro CI, Yealy DM, Kellum JA, et al. A randomized trial of protocol-based care for early septic shock. N Eng J Med. 2014;370:1683-93.
31. The ARISE Investigators and the ANZICS Clinical Trials Group: Goal-directed resuscitation for patients with early septic shock. N Eng J Med. 2014;371:1496-506.
32. Bland RD, Shoemaker WC, Abraham E, et al. Hemodynamic and oxygen transport patterns in surviving and nonsurviving postoperative patients. Crit Care Med. 1985;13(2): 85-90.
33. McKinley BA, Kozar RA, Cocanour CS, et al. Normal versus supranormal oxygen delivery goals in shock resuscitation: the response is the same. J Trauma. 2002;53:825-32.
34. Balogh Z, McKinley BA, Cocanour CS, et al. Supranormal trauma resuscitation causes more cases of abdominal compartment syndrome. Arch Surg. 2003;138:637-42.
35. American College of Surgeons Committee on Trauma. Advanced Trauma Life Support ATLS Student Course Manual, 9th Ed. Chicago, IL: American College of Surgeons; 2012.
36. Holcomb JB, Tilley BC, Baraniuk S, et al. Transfusion of plasma, platelets, and red blood cells in a 1:1:1 vs a 1:1:2 ratio and mortality in patients with severe trauma: the PROPPR randomized clinical trial. JAMA. 2015;313:471-82.
37. Valle EJ, Allen CJ, Van Haren RM, et al. Do all trauma patients benefit from tranexamic acid? J Trauma Acute Care Surg. 2014;76:1373-8.
38. CRASH-2 trial collaborators, Shakur H, Roberts I, Bautista R, et al. Effects of tranexamic acid on death, vascular occlusive events, and blood transfusion in trauma patients with significant haemorrhage (CRASH-2): a randomised, placebo-controlled trial. Lancet. 2010;376(9734):23Y32.
39. Napolitano LM, Cohen MJ, Cotton BA, et al. Tranexamic acid in trauma: how should we use it? J Trauma Acute Care Surg. 2013;74:1575-86.
40. Bilello JF, Davis JW, Cunningham MA, et al. Cervical spinal cord injury and the need for cardiovascular intervention. Arch Surg. 2003;138:1127-9.
41. Furlan JC, Fehlings MG, Shannon P, et al. Descending vasomotor pathways in humans: correlation between axonal preservation and cardiovascular dysfunction after spinal cord injury. J Neurotrauma. 2003;20:1351-63.
42. Ploumis A, Yadlapalli N, Fehlings MG, et al. A systematic review of the evidence supporting a role for vasopressor support in acute SCI. Spinal Cord. 2010;48:356-62.
43. Evans CH, Duby JJ, Berry AJ, et al. Enteral albuterol decreases the need for chronotropic agents in patients with cervical spinal cord injury-induced bradycardia. J Trauma Acute Care Surg. 2014;76:297-301.
44. Reynolds HR, Hochman JS. Cardiogenic shock: current concepts and improving outcomes. Circulation. 2008;117:686-97.
45. Thiele H, Zeymer U, Neumann FJ, et al. Intra-aortic balloon support for myocardial infarction with cardiogenic shock. N Engl J Med. 2012;367:1287-96.
46. Bone RC, Sibbald WJ, Sprung CL. The ACCP-SCCM Consensus Conference on sepsis and organ failure. Chest. 1992; 101:1481-3.
47. Levy MM, Fink MP, Marshall JC, et al. 2001 SCCM/ESICM/ACCP/ATS/SIS International Sepsis Definitions Conference. Crit Care Med. 2003;31:1250-6.
48. Dellinger RP, Levy MM, Rhodes A, et al. Surviving Sepsis Campaign: international guidelines for management of severe sepsis and septic shock: 2012. Crit Care Med. 2013;41:580-637.
49. Levy MM, Dellinger RP, Townsend SR, et al. The Surviving Sepsis Campaign: results of an international guideline-based performance improvement program targeting severe sepsis. Crit Care Med. 2010;38:367-74.
50. Ferrer R, Artigas A, Levy MM, et al. Improvement in process of care and outcome after a multicenter severe sepsis educational program in Spain. JAMA. 2008;299:2294-303.

Additional references appear in the online version of this book.

25

Nutritional Support

Marco Braga

Key Points

- Postoperative catabolism must be reduced by feeding the patient.
- Nutritional status must be assessed before operation.
- Severely malnourished patients should receive perioperative nutrition.
- Enteral route is the first choice in surgical patients.
- Energy and protein requirements should be covered.
- Pharmaconutrition modulates inflammatory/immune response after operation.
- Immunonutrition improves short-term outcome following gastrointestinal (GI) cancer surgery.
- Postoperative interruption of oral feeding is generally unnecessary.

STRESS RESPONSE TO SURGERY

After operation, proinflammatory cytokines activate the stress response via the hypothalamus that stimulates release of pituitary hormones. Adrenocorticotropin causes the release of cortisol, glucagon, and catecholamines. Cortisol is a catabolic glucocorticoid hormone that mobilizes energy stores and promotes gluconeogenesis in the liver, leading to increased insulin resistance. Hyperglycemia has been associated with reduced wound healing, and with increases in postoperative infection and overall morbidity. During and soon after operation high blood cortisol levels increase protein breakdown, which then exceeds protein synthesis.[1] The result is catabolism of muscle proteins to provide substrates for gluconeogenesis (Fig. 25.1).

The two-phase hypermetabolic response to injury described by Cuthbertson[2] can be summarized in an initial *ebb phase*, occurring within several hours of the injury and lasting for 2–3 days, and a *flow phase* lasting for days to weeks depending on injury severity. The ebb phase consists of a reduction in cardiac output, oxygen consumption, basal metabolic rate, and glucose tolerance. Conversely, the flow phase is characterized by an increase in cardiac output, respiratory rate, oxygen consumption, and skeletal muscle catabolism with consequent negative nitrogen balance. Although the simple two-phase model may not completely reflect the complex metabolic postinjury response, the association between severe injury and hypermetabolism still represents a cornerstone in surgical care. Major surgery, critical illness and sepsis, and traumatic and burn injuries all induce elevations in the metabolic rate in an attempt to restore homeostasis. Although initially beneficial, the exaggerated and prolonged inflammatory, metabolic, and catabolic responses induce sharp alterations in the immune response, increase clinical complications, delay recovery and increase mortality (Table 25.1). Severe injuries induce a hypercatabolic response that, along with a heightened inflammatory response, leads to organ failure.

The attenuation of the hypermetabolic response through nutritional and pharmacologic interventions results in improved patient outcomes. Moreover, proteolysis and muscle catabolism can be reduced by feeding the patient continuously following a traumatic injury (Fig. 25.2).

METABOLIC INTERVENTIONS

Injured patients require fluid resuscitation to prevent hypoperfusion. A simple and reliable indicator of volume status is urinary output (target value: 0.5 mL/kg/h for adults and 1 mL/kg/h for children). Pulmonary edema and cardiac dysfunction can result from excess fluid administration and hypervolemia. Due to the increased caloric and protein requirements, early initiation of nutritional support is also necessary. Nutritional supplementation is needed to counteract dietary deficiencies, to support healing and

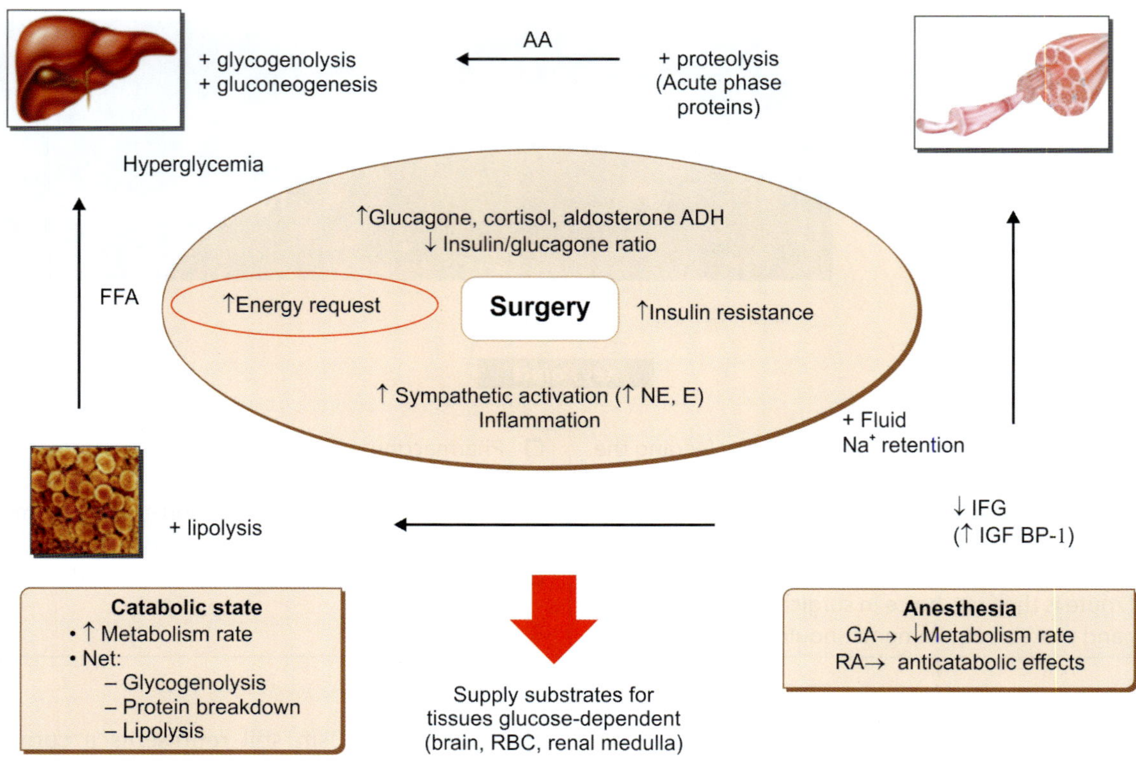

Fig. 25.1: Postsurgery metabolic response.

Table 25.1 Impact of surgical trauma on the immune response.

Surgical trauma	
Specific immunity	*Nonspecific immunity*
↓ T and B proliferation/function	↑ Leukocytes, monocytes
↓ CD4/CD8	↑ Macrophages
↓ NK activity	↑ Acute phase proteins
↓ Production IL-2, IL-3, IFNγ	↑ PGE_2, LCT, TBX
↓ IL-2r	↓ PMN function (chemotaxis, phagocytosis, killing)
↓ Immunoglobulins	↑ Neopterin
	↑ Oxygen free radicals
	↑ Adhesion molecules
	↓ Fibroblasts, collagen

recovery, and to reduce the effects of muscle catabolism, which is the major contributor to adverse outcomes after operation or other trauma.

Muscle proteolysis causes the release of glutamine and alanine, which are required for protein synthesis and also play a key role for supporting hepatic gluconeogenesis. Alanine and ammonia are derived from glutamine in the gut and are converted to urea. To limit protein catabolism and the excessive release of these amino acids, an adequate nitrogen and energy supplementation is required.

For prompt recovery from operation or injury, adequate availability of glucose, amino acids, lipids, and micronutrients is needed. Therefore, artificial nutrition should be started early to enable coverage of nutritional targets. The enteral route should be preferred because it preserves gut mucosa structure and function, including the complex immune network (Flowchart 25.1). In the absence of enteral feeding splanchnic blood flow is diminished, leading to mucosal atrophy, bacterial proliferation, and translocation with a higher risk of developing systemic infections and sepsis (Table 25.2).

Besides nutritional supplementation, other metabolic interventions can contribute to preventing muscle catabolism. Insulin is one of the most important anabolic hormones, promoting glycogenesis and glucose uptake into muscles and fat. However, during the response to surgical stress the amount of insulin secreted does not adequately meet the increased needs. Moreover, cells become resistant to the insulin secreted. The degree of inadequate insulin secretion and peripheral tissue resistance is closely related to the magnitude of the operation.[3] Both low insulin production and insulin resistance contribute to a net catabolic state and hyperglycemia.

Clinically, this process plays a major role in favoring the occurrence of postoperative complications, mainly

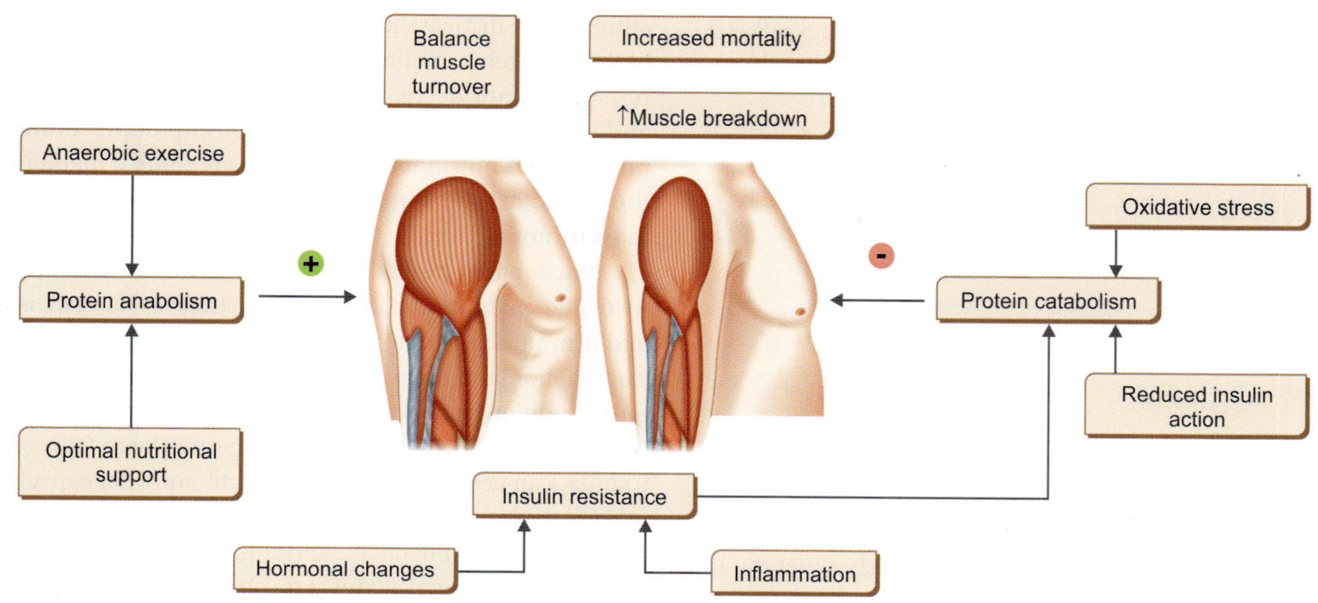

Fig. 25.2: Effect of nutritional support on protein catabolism and insulin resistance.

Flowchart 25.1: Gut immune system network. The intestine is the organ with the highest number of immune competent cells. It interacts and processes thousands of food and bacterial antigens.

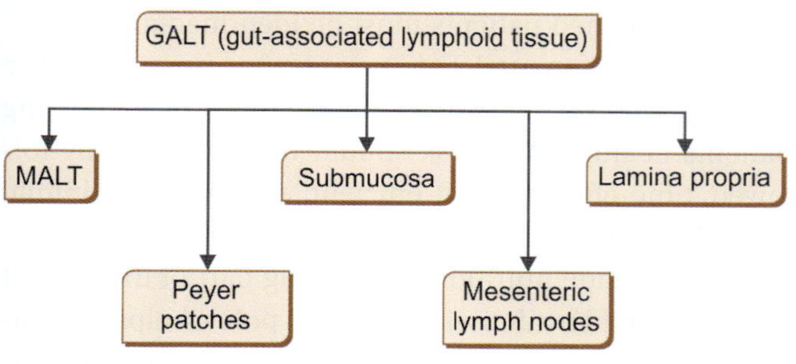

Table 25.2	Pathogenesis of gut microbial translocation.
1.	Morphofunctional alteration of the gut barrier
2.	Qualitative and quantitative alteration of the microflora
3.	Failure of local and systemic immune response

Clinical consequences of microbial translocation may occur when at least two of the above factors are present.

infections. A substantial reduction in insulin sensitivity is associated with a marked increase in the risk of both major complications and severe infections postoperatively. Clinical trials found that intensive insulin therapy significantly decreased the incidence of infections and sepsis, improved organ function, reduced insulin resistance, and reversed the post-traumatic catabolic state. Undoubtedly, euglycemia decreases morbidity and healing time in the postoperative patient. The poor control of blood sugar level can result in increased morbidity and mortality in all patients, regardless of the presence of baseline diabetes. Detrimental effects of hyperglycemia on nervous, immune, respiratory, and renal systems translate to hyperinflammation, increased infectious complication rate, prolonged length of hospital stay, and high mortality rate.[4] On the other hand, low blood sugar is equally dangerous. Hypoglycemia adversely affects the circulatory and both the autonomic and central nervous systems.

Tight glycemic control is a key factor for rapid wound healing and prompt patient recovery. The widespread adoption of protocols aiming at tight glycemic control by intensive insulin administration reduces both insulin resistance and hyperglycemia, and it has been also associated with a reduced complication rate and improved outcome parameters in injured and postoperative patients.[4] Although most physicians agree that maintenance of normoglycemia is beneficial, controversy persists regarding the best target for blood glucose levels and insulin therapy. A range between 5.5 and 8.0 mmol/L should reduce the risk due to hyperglycemia and avoid hypoglycemia episodes.

Early ambulation and prompt rehabilitation still remain very important goals in patients undergoing all types of operation. Exercise rehabilitation programs can be safely implemented in the early postoperative period: tailored pre-exercise evaluation as well as a close monitoring during exercise is mandatory. Exercise exerts positive effects on lean body mass, resting energy expenditure, muscle strength, range of motion, thermoregulation, and quality of life.

Table 25.3 Nutritional screening tools in acute hospitalized patients.

Screening tool	Evidence	Patients
NRS-2002	I	Medical and surgical
SGA	I	Medical and surgical
MST	II	Oncology
MUST	II	Medical and surgical
NST/BAPEN	II	Acute, surgical
Simple, two-part	II	Acute, surgical
NRS	III	Medical and surgical

NUTRITIONAL ASSESSMENT

The presence of malnutrition has been shown to increase morbidity and mortality rates, diminish function and mobility, decrease quality of life, increase frequency and length of hospital admissions, and lead to higher healthcare costs.[5] Malnutrition includes not only undernutrition conditions, like classical marasmus or kwashiorkor, but also the increasingly frequent conditions of overweight and obesity. In the last decades, several definitions of malnutrition have been proposed. A comprehensive definition is any alteration in the physiology, composition or function of the organism attributable to diet, or disease state that adversely affects outcome. Many screening tools have been developed to standardize the criteria for identifying undernourished patients (Table 25.3).

The Subjective Global Assessment is widely employed, easy to implement, and can predict patients "at risk" for malnutrition.[6] It relies on elements of patient history and physical examination more than on biochemical markers or anthropomorphic data. More recently, the Nutrition Risk Score (NRS-2002) has been derived.[7] Weight loss, body mass index, and food intake history data are coupled with information on diagnosis and severity of illness. NRS-2002 is a good predictor of the occurrence of length of hospital stay, postoperative mortality, and overall morbidity in acute care and GI surgical patients.[8] NRS-2002 does not include serum albumin, which is a reliable predictor of postoperative outcome. In fact, patients with low serum albumin have been noted to have increased length of stay, increased risk of infection, and increased mortality.[9] However, for patients stressed by inflammation or infection albumin is considered a "negative acute phase protein", decreasing in response to acute stress.

C-reactive protein (CRP), transferrin, prealbumin, and retinol binding protein have also been used along with albumin as surrogate markers of nutritional status. None of these proteins are linked directly to energy and protein reserve. All are decreased in acute inflammatory states, and while there is an indirect relationship between these proteins and nutritional status, they are more a marker of the catabolic state of the host and the resultant lean body mass turnover.

Functional status and anthropometric indexes can help to define malnutrition. Changes in triceps fat thickness and arm muscle circumference can be noted on physical examination and measured objectively. However, edematous condition can alter anthropometric parameters, while acute disease processes, such as congestive heart failure or trauma, can acutely affect grip strength and vital capacity, making these measurements inaccurate.

Simple, cost-effective, and time-efficient strategies to assess nutritional status are often not implemented preoperatively. Despite overwhelming acceptance by surgeons that appropriate nutritional status is associated with a low postoperative complication rate, only a minority of clinicians routinely screen patients preoperatively for nutritional risk.

Malnourished patients must be identified and appropriately supplemented before and after operation. The ideal method for diagnosing malnutrition or identifying patients at nutritional risk should be simple, easily followed, time-efficient, cost-efficient, and provide minimal disruption to the proposed surgical plan. Some institutions have made nutritional screening part of the patient data collected on admission, and this policy helps to identify those patients who would benefit from the intervention by the nutritional support team. Unfortunately, these teams of experts are not readily available at some or even most institutions and are seldom utilized in outpatient or ambulatory setting to identify patients at risk for malnutrition prior to elective general surgery.

Provided that a cancer patient is not severely malnourished, operation should not be delayed. Conversely, if the patient is severely malnourished, the outcomes can be improved if nutritional repletion is planned preoperatively and operation consequently delayed.[10] In deciding how long to spend in repleting a patient, it must be remembered that severe malnutrition usually occurs over several days/weeks, so its complete reversal requires a long time. Data suggest that nutrition given preoperatively for at least 1 week improves outcomes in severely malnourished patients with an unintentional weight loss >15% of body weight. Durations of <1 week failed to demonstrate favorable results.[11] There are no objective data to say when repletion occurs, but trends in prealbumin seem to be the most frequently employed parameter in clinical practice. Certainly, the conversion from a stressed, catabolic state to an anabolic state will result in increases in prealbumin as well as other negative acute phase proteins.

Postoperatively nutritional parameters should be assessed, taking into account that the acute stress response not only has a profound influence on biomarkers, but it also impacts on protein catabolism. Increased metabolic rate and protein turnover demand a greater energy and protein intake. Since patient outcome results from the interactions between the extent of pre-existing malnutrition, the magnitude of injury, and the degree and duration of hypermetabolism, several techniques to quantify the degree of stress have been studied, including measurement of the metabolic rate, assessing the nitrogen losses versus nitrogen intake, the level of serum cytokines, and finally, sequential measurements of serum protein levels. IL-6 high levels can switch hepatic protein synthesis from constitutive to acute phase protein production, causing elevations in serum fibronectin, CRP, and $\alpha 1$ acid glycoprotein while albumin and prealbumin synthesis falls. There are a number of ways to assess the adequate protein and targeted energy delivery, from simple equations to complex algorithms. However, in critically ill or stressed patients, the best way to evaluate and measure appropriate energy delivery remains indirect calorimetry.[12]

ROUTE OF ADMINISTRATION FOR NUTRITIONAL SUPPORT

The operative "insult" itself causes systemic inflammation, immune suppression, and metabolic changes resulting in hypermetabolism. The inability to maintain adequate nutrient delivery during these hypercatabolic conditions makes the patient susceptible to major nutrient deficiencies, which increase the risk of infection, organ failure, and mortality. When patients are unable to cover both energy and protein requirements by eating, the use of specialized nutrition support through parenteral and/or enteral route is necessary to provide the required amount of nutrients.

Use of parenteral nutrition (PN) as first choice in patients undergoing elective operation has been promoted in the past by evidence in the literature. However, the supposed ability of PN to reduce postoperative complications has relied on studies with poor methodologic quality scores. Conversely, in recent studies with higher methodologic scores PN was associated with significantly greater postoperative infection rates than standard therapy.[13] These data question the role of PN in supporting patients undergoing elective operation. Three nutritional options can be evaluated for any patient undergoing elective operation: oral feeding, enteral nutrition (EN), and PN. Perioperative care demands early intake of energy and proteins as a major aim. Regular hospital food should be the first choice for nutrition in most postoperative patients, but it is essential to monitor and record the adequacy of such intake. In patients taking an inadequate amount of regular food, sip feeds can be recommended. For those who are unable to take orally sufficient amounts of food to meet basal needs, artificial nutrition should be given, EN being the first option (Table 25.4). A standard polymeric diet should be used in most cases. Several randomized trials on postoperative enteral feeding showed a significant reduction of postoperative morbidity, particularly infectious complications, even if patients received a low energy intake in the first few days.

Table 25.4 Advantages of postoperative enteral feeding over parenteral nutrition.

Early postoperative enteral feeding: advantages over parenteral nutrition
• Improves gut barrier function
• Reduces hypermetabolic response after trauma
• Enhances immune response (local and systemic)
• Lower risk of hyperglycemia/electrolytes abnormalities
• Earlier recovery of gut motility
• Enhances gut mucosa oxygen tension
• Lower costs

A large multicenter study suggested that in malnourished patients postoperative early enteral feeding should be preferred to PN.[14] In fact, surgical patients fed enterally had an improved outcome compared with patients treated parenterally, and the nutrition-related health costs are substantially reduced when the enteral route is used. Additional benefits on postoperative outcome were reported in malnourished patients with GI cancer when a diet enriched with specific substrates was given perioperatively.[15]

In cases of prolonged GI dysfunction, PN should be given until enteral function returns. When using the parenteral route, too little or too much salt and water must be avoided and glycemia should be tightly monitored. Standard prescriptions should give about 25 kcal/kg/day, with 30–40% of energy derived from fat. Nitrogen intake of

Table 25.5 Micronutrients daily requirements in adults when given parenterally.

Vitamin	*Requirement*
Thiamin (B1)	6 mg
Riboflavin (B2)	3.6 mg
Niacin (B3)	40 mg
Folic acid	600 mcg
Pantothenic acid	15 mg
Pyridoxine (B6)	6 mg
Cyanocobalamin (B12)	5 mcg
Biotin	60 mcg
Ascorbic acid (C)	200 mg
Vitamin A	3,300 IU
Vitamin D	200 IU
Vitamin E	10 IU
Vitamin K	150 mcg
Trace element	*Standard intake*
Chromium	10–15 mcg
Copper	0.3–0.5 mg
Iron	1.0–1.2 mg
Manganese	50–100 mcg
Selenium	60–100 mcg
Zinc	2.5–5 mg
Molybdenum	20 mcg
Iodine	130 mcg
Fluoride	1 mg

0.15–0.2 g/kg/day is usually adequate. The recommended amounts of mineral and micronutrients should also be supplied (Table 25.5).

Absolute contraindications to enteral feeding and thus mandatory indications for PN include intestinal obstruction, intestinal ischemia, and acute peritonitis. Relative contraindications include high-output fistulas, severe malabsorption, severe shock with impaired splanchnic perfusion, and fulminant sepsis.[16] In each of these circumstances, use of enteral feeding should be individualized on a case-by-case basis. Inadvertent reasons leading to use of PN, however, may result because of the delays in initiation of EN. In patients with GI anastomoses, surgeons are reluctant to start enteral feeding early; therefore, the parenteral route is often used. In these patients, changing institutional strategies, implementing nurse-driven protocols, and challenging traditional practices will result in more successful delivery of EN.

When patients undergoing elective operation develop a relative intolerance to enteral feeding, should supplemental PN be added to reach both energy and protein targets? A meta-analysis showed that while there was significantly greater cost with the addition of supplemental PN, there was no corresponding improvement in infection rate, hospital length of stay, or duration of mechanical ventilation.[17] The results of the EPANIC (Early Parenteral Nutrition in Critical Illness) study, which include 90% of elective surgery patients, showed no advantage from supplemental PN added during the first week of hospitalization over hypocaloric EN. Patients were significantly more likely to be discharged alive from the ICU if they were randomized to late initiation of PN, compared to those in whom PN was initiated earlier.[18] The main criticism of the EPANIC study was that patients experienced only moderate surgical stress and therefore they were not really candidates for supplemental specialized artificial nutrition therapy. In fact, the average ICU length of stay was about 3 days, so few patients in either group were actually exposed to PN. Moreover, a high parenteral glucose load was given.

Different results were found in high-risk medical ICU patients receiving EN.[19] Experimental group patients had supplemental PN added after 3 days if they were receiving <60% of measured energy requirements by EN alone. Controls continued to receive EN alone for a week, regardless of caloric delivery. Patients randomized to PN supplementation had a reduction in both new infections and duration of mechanical ventilation as well as a shorter hospital length of stay. However, being a study on medical ICU patients, its applicability to elective surgery patients could be limited.

Delivery of energy intentionally restricted to 80% or less of caloric requirements (permissive underfeeding) has been a strategy in certain clinical situations. In nonobese critically ill patients, the use of permissive enteral underfeeding was associated with a worse outcome, whereas in the obese critically ill patients permissive underfeeding is an important strategy to reduce fat mass, maintaining lean body mass if protein provision meets or exceeds requirements. A meta-analysis showed that permissive parenteral underfeeding in various surgical populations reduced infection by 40% and hospital length of stay by a factor of 2.49 compared to patients randomized to full caloric provision at goal.[20] Permissive underfeeding should not be applied in severely malnourished cancer patients receiving preoperative PN. In fact, there is no rationale for this strategy in patients who have not yet undergone the physiologic stress of the surgical procedure. In early postoperative patients in whom full EN is not yet feasible, permissive underfeeding might result in improved insulin sensitivity and potentially in better postoperative outcome.[21]

PERIOPERATIVE NUTRITION

Preoperative nutrition therapy is designed to prepare the patient metabolically for the insult of the surgical operation, not to make up for months of deteriorating nutritional status. Patients who may benefit from nutrition support will not be appropriately identified if a well-defined assessment of nutritional status is not performed preoperatively. Most operations for cancer, especially those of the upper GI tract, are associated with a high nutritional risk. Issues to address are the severity of the surgical insult, the patient's current nutritional status, and the possibility of anatomic alterations that may predispose to nutritional risk. The severity of the insult is often difficult to quantify. Esophageal, pancreatic, and complex hepatobiliary operations carry an appreciable postoperative morbidity. The stratification method should also consider procedures with high rates of infectious complications and prolonged hospitalization. These factors should be taken into account when the clinician evaluates the potential benefits of perioperative nutrition support. Key components for the appropriate identification of patients at nutritional risk include dietary history, recent weight loss, body fat, muscle mass, presence of fluid accumulation, and grip strength.[22] In a patient identified at high risk from a nutritional status assessment, the elective operation should be delayed until appropriate intervention is undertaken. The goal of nutritional support is optimal preparation of the patient from a metabolic standpoint for the impending surgical insult and not to achieve a well-nourished state.

The appropriate duration and measures used to assure sufficient delivery of nutrition therapy remain difficult to determine. In the case of benign conditions, the delay can be as long as is needed to reduce the risk. In malignant conditions, the therapy should be relatively short due to the concern for progression of disease and the malnutrition-related characteristics of the underlying malignant condition. In these cases, the clinician desires the quickest approach to realizing some of the benefits of nutrition support without inappropriately delaying the intervention. With regard to shorter intervals of nutrition support, some concepts can be extrapolated from the multiple randomized controlled trials comparing immunonutrition to standard controls in respect of the days of nutrition support that are required to positively impact outcome. Collectively, these data suggest that many of the benefits of nutrition support can be obtained in as little as 5–7 days.

Innovations in preoperative nutrition therapy have been developed to minimize periods of fasting, reduce insulin resistance postoperatively, and preserve muscle function. The type of nutritional support delivered is largely dictated by the patient's ability to meet caloric and protein needs and tolerance of oral intake. Patients tolerating >80% of the caloric goal should receive counseling only, while patients who take from 60% to 80% should receive oral nutritional supplements. Patients taking <60% should be given artificial support, employing the enteral route in the first instance. Patients with contraindications to enteral support who are determined to be at nutritional risk should be given PN at least 7 days before operation.

Providing access to the upper GI tract at operation and closely monitoring resuscitative measures in its early aftermath help to prepare the patient for postoperative EN. The possibility of gaining direct access to intraperitoneal structures gives the operating surgeon a valuable opportunity to establish appropriate nutrition in the postoperative period. It is common practice in several operations including esophagectomy and pancreatoduodenectomy to place a feeding jejunostomy at the time, thereby anticipating a low energy and protein intake during the first postoperative week and limiting the associated problems. When defined protocols have been followed, early EN has been well tolerated, with energy and protein requirements covered by postoperative day 4 in the vast majority of patients.[23]

Increasing efforts to eliminate surgical dogma have resulted in more aggressive attempts to feed those patients soon after operation even in the presence of GI anastomoses. The Enhanced Recovery After Surgery (ERAS) pathway is a multimodal strategy aiming to minimize the surgical stress and to improve postoperative functional recovery. Compared with traditional perioperative care, the ERAS program represents a fundamental shift in the process of care. While traditional surgical management is characterized by a state of insulin resistance, the ERAS pathway allows the patient to maintain insulin sensitivity throughout the perioperative phase by implementing multiple interventions, such as preoperative carbohydrate loading, minimally invasive surgery, pain control without long-acting opioids, early oral feeding, and mobilization. Reducing the fasting period both before and after operation is a major determinant in the ERAS protocol, so patients are encouraged to start oral diet on the same day or the day after operation, according to the type of surgical procedure. This approach could restrict the indications for postoperative artificial nutrition, whether enteral

Table 25.6 Interactions between nutritional substrates and gut immune system.

Nutrient	*Target*	*Effect*	*Mechanism*
LC fatty acids	T cells	Migration to Peyer patches	Increased adhesion molecules
Omega-6 fatty acids	T cells	Lower immune response	Eicosanoids modulation
Omega-3 fatty acids	Macrophages	Lower inflammatory response	Reduced proinflammatory cytokines
Docosahexaenoic acid	Monocytes	Increased antigen presentation	Increased MHC class II
Eicosapentaenoic acid	Monocytes	Reduced antigen presentation	Reduced MHC class II
Glutamine	T cells	Higher T-cell response	Higher Th2 cytokines
Arginine	Monocytes	Increased phagocytosis and killing	Higher oxygen radicals and TNF α
Zinc	GALT	Increased lymphopoiesis	Reduced T-cell apoptosis
Carotenoids	T cells	Antioxidant anti-inflammatory	Higher IL-4
Vitamin A	GALT	Increased NK-cell activity	Higher Th2 and IgA
Selenium, Vitamin E	GALT	Reduced lipid peroxidation	Higher glutathione

or parenteral. The application of the ERAS program in patients undergoing colorectal surgery has been shown to reduce care time by >30% and to reduce postoperative complications by up to 50%.[24]

Relevant issues in postoperative nutrition are timing and tolerance of enteral support. Multiple factors contribute to the delay in initiation of postoperative EN, such as fear of aspiration, inadequate resuscitation, concern for the integrity of a fresh anastomosis, and the attitude that early nutritional support will result in little impact on outcome.[25] Surgical dogma has long suggested that enteral feeding in the setting of a fresh anastomosis should be withheld until there is return of GI function. Concerns are twofold: reduced motility associated with operative manipulation and a higher risk of anastomotic complications. These concerns often result in the delayed initiation of enteral support by several days. A recent randomized controlled trial by Barlow and colleagues examined early feeding via jejunostomy tubes in patients undergoing hepatobiliary, gastrectomy, esophagectomy, and pancreatectomy procedures and demonstrated reduced infectious complications and length of stay, as well as good tolerance in patients who were fed early.[26] To elucidate the potential harmful impact of early enteral feeding in patients with gut anastomoses, Lewis and associates performed a meta-analysis involving 1,173 patients. It was shown that early enteral feeding was not associated with a higher anastomotic dehiscence rate, while a trend toward reduction of both length of stay and mortality was found.[21] Recent large experiences with early oral feeding in patients who underwent colorectal resections clearly support the fact that prolonged postoperative fasting does not favor anastomotic healing.[24]

PHARMACONUTRITION

Among the proposed strategies to reduce postoperative infections and its related costs, artificial nutrition is recognized as an important part of patient care. Recently, the main focus of clinical nutrition has moved from simply covering energy and nitrogen requirements (*nutritional support*) to the new concept of supplementing selected nutritional substrates, mainly arginine, glutamine, and omega-3 fatty acids, because of their specific pharmacological effects (*nutritional therapy*). The main target of these new diets is not solely to provide energy and nitrogen, but to modulate inflammatory postinjury response and to counteract postoperative immune impairment, which may per se increase patient susceptibility to infectious complications. This framework suggested that nutrients be studied as pharmacological agents administered in physiologic and supraphysiologic doses (Table 25.6). To identify the best combination of substrates and their optimal dose remains a very difficult task.

Conflicting results have been published on the effects of single substrates on infection and morbidity rates, length of hospital stay, and other outcome parameters. Potential explanations for discrepancies include variable effects of each substrate depending on dose, nutrient interactions, and heterogeneity of patients with different metabolic and catabolic conditions. Similarly, an individual's genome may influence metabolic requirements and immune response.

Glutamine

Glutamine is the most abundant free amino acid in the bloodstream under normal circumstances. Under

Table 25.7 Glutamine supplementation. Randomized controlled trials in elective surgery.

RCT	Patients	Nutritional status	Glutamine dipeptide dose (g/kg/day)	Morbidity (glutamine vs control)	LOS (glutamine vs control)
Lin (2002)[46]	48	Undefined	0.42	No difference	No data
Exner (2003)[47]	45	Undefined	0.5	No difference	Similar
Klek (2005)[48]	105	Well-nourished	0.4	No difference	Reduced
Yao (2005)[49]	40	Undefined	0.5	No difference	Reduced
Jo (2006)[50]	60	Well-nourished, malnourished	0.3	No difference	Similar
Oguz (2007)[51]	109	Undefined	1	Reduced	Reduced
Engel (2009)[52]	78	Undefined	0.74	No difference	Similar
Fan (2009)[53]	40	Undefined	0.2	No difference	Similar
Gianotti et al.[30]	428	Well-nourished	0.4	No difference	Similar
Marton (2010)[54]	55	Well-nourished, malnourished	0.5	No difference	Similar
Lu (2011)[55]	50	Undefined	0.45	Reduced	No data

conditions of critical illness or with GI disorders, glutamine levels may not be adequate to meet demands and becomes conditionally essential.[27] Although alanine and glutamine constitute only 7% of normal muscle protein, they account for 60–70% of the amino acids released into the circulation by stressed or septic muscle cells. Glutamine is central to cellular energy, cell proliferation, renal acid–base regulation, and nitrogen and carbon metabolism.[28] Within the intestine, glutamine is particularly important as the preferred fuel source by enterocytes and for the vast mass of immune cells within the gut-associated lymphoid tissue, where up to 50% of available glutamine is metabolized following enteral feeding. Once activated, immune cells such as lymphocytes and macrophages utilize increased quantities of glutamine for energy, in addition to glucose.

The route and dose of glutamine administration should be considered carefully, since enteral glutamine is rapidly metabolized by the splanchnic bed at low doses and may not reach the portal vein. The effectiveness of glutamine supplements in PN among critically ill patient subgroups is still undetermined, but its use has been recommended in ICU patients.[16] There are several reasons to assume a clinical efficacy of glutamine supplementation in surgical patients, mainly its proven metabolic, immunologic, and pharmacologic effects and the increased demand and tissue consumption of glutamine following operation.[28] Previous randomized controlled trials and meta-analyses suggested a positive effect of intravenous glutamine dipeptide on both postoperative morbidity and length of hospital stay in patients undergoing major elective operations[29] (Table 25.7).

However, most of the trials have suffered from certain drawbacks: (i) the sample size was not calculated and the number of randomized patients per group was low, with potential statistical underpower; (ii) parenteral glutamine dipeptide was added to total PN even if the large majority of patients had normal nutritional status; (iii) patients included were often nonhomogeneous for primary disease (cancer and benign disease together), type of operation (vascular, abdominal, urogenital), and baseline nutritional status; and (iv) the dose of glutamine dipeptide ranged widely. For these reasons, firm conclusions are difficult to draw, and the results should be considered more in terms of generating a hypothesis than as providing strong clinical evidence. A recent multicenter RCT carried out in 428 GI cancer patients showed that parenteral glutamine supplementation did not significantly affect relevant outcome measures.[30] Glutamine supplementation did increase the plasma pool, suggesting that postoperative utilization and consumption of glutamine was not increased differently from ICU patients. Interestingly, plasma glutamine remained stable after operation in control patients not receiving glutamine supplementation. This fact could be due to constant flux of glutamine from muscle or alternatively could reflect a lack of increased glutamine consumption by other tissues.[30]

Recently, a large randomized trial showed no advantage in patients receiving glutamine added to PN, compared to controls receiving PN alone.[31] Based on these recent negative studies, supplemental parenteral glutamine cannot be recommended.

Glutamine supplementation should be tested in malnourished patients who represent cohorts with high glutamine demand and/or potential baseline deficits. Both the length of preoperative treatment and the amount of glutamine still represent unsolved issues, the aim being to obtain adequate tissue and plasma levels at the time of operation.

Arginine

Arginine is a dibasic conditionally essential amino acid. De novo biosynthesis of arginine utilizes citrulline as a precursor, and citrulline is provided by glutamine metabolism in the intestine. Arginine levels increase collagen synthesis and also regulates lymphocyte function, especially T-cell,[32] stimulating lymphocyte proliferation through increased expression of surface T-cell receptors and cytokines. Arginine is the substrate for two myeloid cell enzymes that are upregulated during immune activation: inducible nitric oxide synthase (iNOS) and arginase.[32] Inducible nitric oxide synthase produces nitric oxide (NO), an important cell signaling molecule that regulates vasodilation of blood vessels and vascular permeability. As an active antimicrobial compound within intra- and extracellular compartments, NO is also directly bactericidal and is utilized by leukocytes and macrophages to destroy microbial pathogens.

Recent findings suggest that the type of response generated, Th1 or Th2, is influenced by the nature of injury. Trauma and major surgery patients appear to generate Th2 responses, whereas septic patients appear to generate Th1 responses. Clinical data suggest that septic patients, but not trauma or elective surgery patients, may have elevated circulating NO levels, supporting the case for specific Th1 versus Th2 responses in specific injury. In general, most ICU patient and elective surgery populations may benefit from arginine supplementation. However, current recommendation does not suggest arginine supplementation in patients with septic shock because of the potential harm induced by excessive NO production. For the same reason, hemodynamically unstable patients should not receive additional arginine or enteral formulas in general.

Omega-3 Fatty Acids

Omega-3 fatty acids have potent anti-inflammatory properties mediated through incorporation in membrane structure, where they compete with omega-6 fatty acids in the form of arachidonic acid, as well as suppression of proinflammatory transcription factors and modulation of eicosanoid production. Omega-3 fatty acids are isolated from cold water fish species, flax seed, and canola oil and are used for their proposed anti-inflammatory properties. During cellular stress or damage, fatty acids are released from the membranes by phospholipases and are converted by cyclooxygenase and lipoxygenase enzymes into powerful secondary messenger hormones, eicosanoids. Eicosanoids derived from omega-6 fatty acids promote 2- and 4-series eicosanoids, such as prostaglandin E2, prostaglandin A2, and leukotriene B4, which are highly proinflammatory. Omega-3 fatty acids promote the less inflammatory eicosanoids of the 3- and 5-series, such as prostaglandin E3 and leukotriene B5. Due to the competitive effects between omega-6 and omega-3 fatty acids, the recommended ratio is 2:1–4:1 (omega-6:/omega-3).[33] These effects may play an important role in suppressing the generalized inflammatory response and subsequent immunosuppression and capillary leakage after major surgery. Resolvins and protectins are novel omega-3 fatty acid products derived from eicosapentaenoic acid and docosahexaenoic acid following neutrophil–endothelial interactions. These lipid mediators play a key role in the resolution of inflammation and promotion of wound healing.

Nucleotides

Nucleotides are small-molecular-weight compounds found in all cells that are used to synthesize RNA and DNA. During rapid cell growth and proliferation, nucleotides can become limiting if de novo synthesis and scavenging pathways do not compensate. Under normal conditions, pancreatic enzymes digest dietary RNA from plant and animal food sources and recover approximately 2–5% of ingested RNA. Supplementing nucleotides can reduce the necessity of de novo synthesis. Low nucleotide availability can have deleterious effects on immune function, since effective adaptive mediated immune responses require rapid cell proliferation. No clinical studies have examined the effect of nucleotides alone in critically ill patients; rather, nucleotides have been added with other nutrition support compounds, including glutamine, arginine, and omega-3 fatty acids. There are currently no recommendations for the use of nucleotides in critically ill patients.

Immunonutrition (Arginine + Omega-3 Fatty Acids + Nucleotides)

Most of the randomized controlled trials performed so far in elective surgical patients have tested a combination of arginine, omega-3 fatty acids, and nucleotides, commonly defined as immunonutrition. Immunonutrition has been associated with modulation of inflammatory response, enhancement of cell-mediated immune response, and

Table 25.8 Systematic reviews and meta-analyses carried out on the effectiveness of immunonutrition in surgery.

Author	RCTs	Control group	Patients	Short-term outcome	Patients who benefit
Marik and Zaloga[38]	21	Standard EN	1,908	Lower morbidity Shorter LOS	Malnourished Well-nourished
Cerantola et al.[37]	21	Standard EN	2,730	Lower morbidity Shorter LOS	Upper GI Lower GI
Drover et al.[39]	35	Standard EN	3,445	Lower morbidity Shorter LOS	GI and non-GI Upper/Lower GI
Marimuthu (2012)[56]	26	Standard EN	2,496	Lower morbidity Shorter LOS	GI cancer

upregulation of gut function parameters in the early postoperative period. In particular, perioperative immunonutrition was associated with better operative small bowel and colon microperfusion, as measured by laser Doppler flowmetry system. Moreover, in the first postoperative days higher circulating levels of nitric oxide, better intestinal mucosa oxygen metabolism measured by intestinal tonometry, and lower plasma levels of intestinal isoenzyme of alkaline phosphatase (which is released in the peritoneal fluid and plasma after intestinal hypoxic insult) were found in patients who were given perioperative immunonutrition.[34] These findings support the concept that the better gut microperfusion in patients receiving immunonutrition translates into a better gut oxygen tension, delivery, and utilization. It should be stressed that an intraoperative deficiency of both blood flow and oxygenation of the gut could impair the healing of anastomoses and could promote translocation of endotoxins and bacteria from the gut to systemic blood.

Prospective, randomized, double-blind clinical trials have demonstrated that patients fed before and after elective major GI surgery with immunonutrition had a significant reduction of both postoperative infections and length of hospital stay when compared to patients fed with a standard enteral formula.[35] Interestingly, preoperative administration of immunoenhancing diets reduced postoperative infection rate also in a series of well-nourished GI cancer patients.[36] Accordingly, European Guidelines state that perioperative immunonutrition is effective regardless of the baseline nutritional status of the patients.[10] However, several trials differed in terms of patient groups, nutritional formulas and protocols for immunonutrition administration, while control groups received various treatments such as standard enteral formula, PN, or no nutritional support. Therefore, systematic reviews and meta-analyses have been carried out to clarify further the clinical relevance of perioperative immunonutrition with a good selection of trials included in the analysis, resulting in low data heterogeneity and homogeneous control groups receiving an isoenergetic, isonitrogenous standard enteral formula (Table 25.8). Studies comparing enteral immunonutrition with total PN have been excluded. In these cases, the better outcome found in the immunonutrition group could be explained not only by the properties of specific substrates given but also by the different route of nutrients administration.

Meta-analyses conducted by Cerantola et al.[37] and Marik and Zaloga[38] have shown that perioperative immunonutrition significantly reduces overall morbidity rate, particularly postoperative infectious complications and length of stay in both upper and lower GI surgery. These benefits occurred regardless of baseline nutritional status, although they were more pronounced in malnourished patients. Drover et al.[39] performed the largest systematic review on perioperative administration of arginine-supplemented diets, showing significant outcome benefits in both upper GI and lower GI surgery and in non-GI surgery (mostly head and neck). The best clinical results were obtained when arginine and omega-3 fatty acids were given together, in line with previous studies showing no benefit from arginine supplementation alone in head and neck cancer patients[40] or from omega-3 fatty acid supplementation alone in patients undergoing esophagogastric cancer surgery.[41] It could be that arginine and omega-3 fatty acids act synergistically to modulate both immune and inflammatory postoperative response and consequently to improve short-term postoperative outcome.

Arginine deficiency after surgical stress was reported >30 years ago, although the underlying mechanisms have remained unknown for years. An early postoperative increase in myeloid-derived cells expressing arginase 1 that deplete arginine has been recently reported.[42] Coupled with a poor arginine intake, this process could

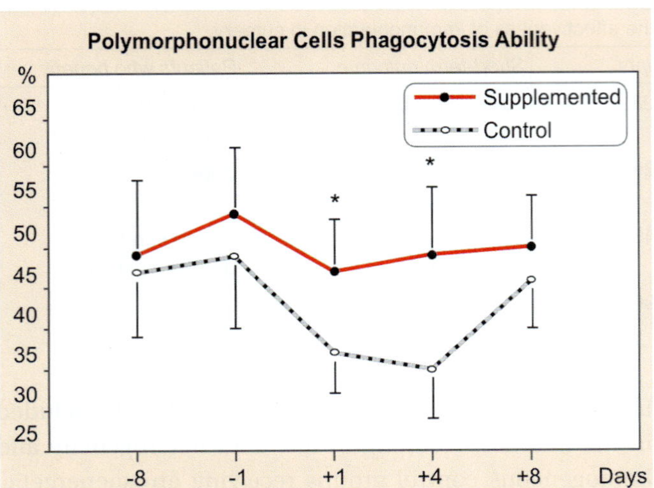

Fig. 25.3: Phagocytosis ability in patients receiving perioperative immunonutrition (supplemented) and perioperative standard diet (control). Perioperative treatment started 7 days before surgery and was prolonged for 7 days after surgery. *p = 0.001.

lead to an arginine-deficiency state and consequently to a suppression of T-lymphocyte function. Arginine supplementation can overcome this deficiency, while omega-3 fatty acids supplementation can blunt upregulation of myeloid-derived cells and decrease arginase 1 expression.[43]

Starting immunonutrition before operation is a key point for improving immune parameters in the early postoperative period (Fig. 25.3). When immunonutrition was started after operation, the improvements in phagocytosis ability, lymphocyte mitogenesis, and cytokine profiles took many days to develop.[34] This finding supports the hypothesis that the amount of substrates given in the first days after operation is not sufficient to reach adequate tissue and plasma concentrations. In fact, it takes some days for immune-enhancing nutrients to become incorporated into the host tissues and alter inflammatory mediators and fatty acid profiles. Since the impairment of the host defense mechanisms occurs immediately after operation, immunonutrients should be given before operation to obtain adequate levels at the time of surgical stress.

The high cost of these new nutritional products could be considered a major drawback for their routine use. However, economic analyses carried out by "blind" economists on data gathered from randomized clinical trials showed that perioperative immunonutrition led to a substantial saving in healthcare resources consumed.[44] In fact, the saving due to the reduction in postoperative infectious complications by perioperative immunonutrition more than offsets the higher cost of the supplemental diet.

According to literature data, the appropriate candidates for immunonutrition are all patients undergoing elective major surgery who are at high risk of developing postoperative infectious complications, regardless of their baseline nutritional status. However, postoperative infection risk is continuously changing according to new advances in perioperative care and surgery. In the last years, mini-invasive surgery and ERAS multimodal protocols are gaining popularity among surgeons, and both have been associated with lower postoperative infection rates and shorter hospital stay after colorectal surgery.[24,45,57,58] Since the vast majority of trials showing the effectiveness of immunonutrition have been carried out in patients who underwent open surgery with traditional perioperative care, it would be interesting to investigate whether the ERAS pathway can alter nutritional and pharmaconutritional policies for minimal invasive surgery.

Future research should investigate molecular signaling pathways and should better elucidate specific mechanisms of action and possible other interactions between immune-enhancing substrates. Moreover, dose–response studies should clarify the optimal dose of substrates required to maximize benefits in surgical patients.

CONCLUSION

The trauma of a surgical operation itself causes systemic inflammation, immune suppression, and metabolic changes resulting in hypermetabolism. The inability to maintain adequate nutrient delivery during these hypercatabolic conditions makes the patient susceptible to major nutrient deficiencies, which may increase the risk for infection, organ failure, and mortality. For those patients who are unable to meet both energy and protein requirements orally, artificial nutrition should be given, EN being the first option. In undernourished patients, perioperative nutrition significantly reduces the postoperative morbidity rate, and benefits can be obtained when nutrition support lasts at least 5–7 days. Nevertheless, large gaps have been observed between what the evidence suggests and what is seen in actual clinical practice. Lack of nutritional assessment in high-risk surgical patients, low utilization of artificial nutrition in patients nil by mouth for >7 days, and long periods of time in which hospitalized surgical patients are receiving no nutrition intake have all been reported.

In the last decade, the field of specialized nutrition has progressed in knowledge and complexity, moving from the simple coverage of micro/macronutrients requirements to proper metabolic support, particularly for immune and inflammatory response modulation. This new approach, called pharmaconutrition or nutritional therapy, is supported by several randomized trials, and meta-analyses clearly showing relevant benefits in postoperative short-term outcome.

REFERENCES

1. Gore DC, Jahoor F, Wolfe RR, et al. Acute response of human muscle protein to catabolic hormones. Ann Surg. 1993;218:679-84.
2. Cuthbertson DP. Post-shock metabolic response (Arris-Gale Lecture to the Royal College of Surgeons of England). Lancet. 1942;239:433-7.
3. Thorell A, Nygren J, Ljungqvist O. Insulin resistance: a marker of surgical stress. Curr Opin Clin Nutr Metab Care. 1999;2:69-78.
4. Van den Berghe G, Wouters P, Weekers F, et al. Intensive insulin therapy in the critically ill patients. N Engl J Med. 2001;345:1359-1367.
5. Covinsky KE. Malnutrition and bad outcomes. J Gen Intern Med. 2002;12:956-7.
6. Detsky AS, Mclaughlin JR, Baker JP, et al. What is subjective global assessment of nutritional status? JPEN. 1987;11: 8-13.
7. Kondrup J, Rasmussen HH, Hamberg O, et al. Nutritional risk screening (NRS-2002): a new method based on an analysis of controlled clinical trial. Clin Nutr. 2003;22: 321-36.
8. Scheisser M, Muller S, Kirchoff P, et al. Assessment of a novel screening score for nutrition risk in predicting complications in gastrointestinal surgery. Clin Nutr. 2008;27:570-641.
9. Daley J, Khuri SF, Oprian C, et al. Risk adjustment of the postoperative morbidity rate for the comparative assessment of the quality of surgical care: results of the National Veterans Affairs Surgical Risk Study. J Am Coll Surg. 1997;185:328-40.
10. Weimann A, Braga M, Harsanyi L, et al. ESPEN guidelines on enteral nutrition: surgery including organ transplantation. Clin Nutr. 2006;25:224-44.
11. Veterans Affairs Total Parenteral Nutrition Cooperative Study Group. Perioperative TPN in surgical patients. N Engl J Med. 1991;325:525-32.
12. McClave SA, McClain CJ, Snider HL. Should indirect calorimetry be used as part of nutritional assessment? J Clin Gastroenterol. 2001;33:14-19.
13. Braunschweig CL, Levy P, Sheean PM, et al. Enteral compared with parenteral nutrition: a meta-analysis. Am J Clin Nutr. 2001;74:534-42.
14. Bozzetti F, Braga M, Gianotti L, et al. Postoperative enteral vs. parenteral nutrition in malnourished patients with gastrointestinal cancer: a randomised multicentre trial. Lancet. 2001;358:1487-92.
15. Braga M, Gianotti L, Nespoli L, et al. Nutritional approach in malnourished surgical patients: a prospective randomized trial. Arch Surg. 2002;137:174-80.
16. Braga M, Ljungqvist O, Soeters P, et al. ESPEN guidelines on parenteral nutrition: surgery. Clin Nutr. 2009;28:378-86.
17. Heyland DK, Dhaliwal R, Drover JW, et al. Canadian Critical Care Clinical Practice Guidelines Committee. Canadian clinical practice guidelines for nutrition support in mechanically ventilated, critically ill adult patients. JPEN. 2003;27:355-73.
18. Casaer MP, Mesotten D, Hermans G, et al. Early versus late parenteral nutrition in critically ill adults. N Engl J Med. 2011;365:506-17.
19. Heidegger CP, Berger MM, Thibault R, et al. Supplemental parenteral nutrition in critically ill patients. Lancet. 2013;370:1072-7.
20. Jiang H, Sun MW, Hefright B, et al. Efficacy of hypocaloric parenteral nutrition for surgical patients: a systematic review and meta-analysis. Clin Nutr. 2011;30:730-7.
21. Lewis SJ, Andersen HK, Thomas S. Early enteral nutrition within 24 h of intestinal surgery versus later commencement of feeding: a systematic review and meta-analysis. J Gastrointest Surg. 2009;13:569-75.
22. Jensen GL, Bistrian B, Roubenoff R, et al. Malnutrition syndromes: a conundrum vs continuum. JPEN. 2009;33:710-14.
23. Braga M, Gianotti L, Gentilini O, et al Early gut feeding after digestive surgery. Results of a nine-year experience. Clin Nutr. 2002;21:59-65.
24. Varadhan KK, Neal KR, Dejong CH, et al. The enhanced recovery after surgery (ERAS) pathway for patients undergoing major elective open colorectal surgery: a meta-analysis of randomized controlled trials. Clin Nutr. 2010;29:434-40.
25. Drover JW, Cahill NE, Kutsogiannis J, et al. Nutrition therapy for the critically ill surgical patient: we need to do better! JPEN. 2010;34:644-52.
26. Barlow R, Price P, Reid TD, et al. Prospective multicentre randomised controlled trial of early enteral nutrition for patients undergoing major upper gastrointestinal surgical resection. Clin Nutr. 2011;30:560-6.
27. Lacey JM, Wilmore DW. Is glutamine a conditionally essential amino acid? Nutr Rev. 1990;48:297-309.
28. Wilmore DW. The effect of glutamine supplementation in patients following elective surgery and accidental injury. J Nutr. 2001;131:2543S-9S.
29. Zheng YM, Li F, Zhang MM, et al. Glutamine dipeptide for parenteral nutrition in abdominal surgery: a meta-analysis of randomized controlled trials. World J Gastroenterol. 2006;12:7537-41.
30. Gianotti L, Braga M, Biffi R, et al. GlutamItaly Research Group of the Italian Society of Parenteral, and Enteral Nutrition. Perioperative intravenous glutamine supplementation in major abdominal surgery for cancer: a randomized multicenter trial. Ann Surg. 2009;250:684-90.
31. Heyland D, Muscedere J, Wischmeyer PE, et al. A randomized trial of glutamine and antioxidants in critically ill patients. N Engl J Med. 2013;368:1489-97.
32. Morris SM. Recent advances in arginine metabolism. Curr Opin Clin Nutr Metab Care. 2004;7:45-51.
33. Calder PC. Rationale and use of n-3 fatty acids in artificial nutrition. Proc Nutr Soc. 2010;69:565-73.

34. Braga M, Gianotti L, Cestari A, et al. Gut function and immune and inflammatory responses in patients perioperatively fed with supplemented enteral formulas. Arch Surg. 1996;131:1257-65.
35. Braga M, Gianotti L, Radaelli G, et al. Perioperative immunonutrition in patients undergoing cancer surgery: results of a randomized double-blind phase 3 trial. Arch Surg. 1999;134:428-33.
36. Gianotti L, Braga M, Nespoli L, et al. A randomized controlled trial on pre-operative oral supplementation with a specialized diet in patients with gastrointestinal cancer. Gastroenterology. 2002;122:1763-70.
37. Cerantola Y, Hubner M, Grass F, et al. Immunonutrition in gastrointestinal surgery. Br J Surg. 2011;98:37-48.
38. Marik PE, Zaloga GP. Immunonutrition in high-risk surgical patients: a systematic review and analysis of the literature. JPEN. 2010;34:378-86.
39. Drover JW, Dhaliwal R, Weitzel L, et al. Perioperative use of arginine-supplemented diets: a systematic review of the evidence. J Am Coll Surg. 2011; 212:385-99.
40. van Bokhorst-De Van Der Schueren MA, Quak JJ, Kulk DJ, et al. Effect of perioperative nutrition, with and without arginine supplementation, on nutritional status, immune function, postoperative morbidity, and survival in severely malnourished head and neck cancer patients. Am J Clin Nutr. 2001; 73:323-32.
41. Sultan J, Griffin SM, Di Franco F, et al. Randomized clinical trial of omega-3 fatty acid-supplemented enteral nutrition vs. standard enteral nutrition in patients undergoing oesophagogastric cancer surgery. Br J Surg. 2012;99:346-55.
42. Popovic PJ, Zeh HJ, Ochoa JB. Arginine and immunity. J Nutr. 2007;137:1681S-5S.
43. Bansal V, Syres KM, Makarenkova V, et al. Interaction between fatty acids and arginine metabolism: implications for the design of immune-enhancing diets. JPEN. 2005; 29:S75-S80.
44. Braga M, Gianotti L, Vignali A, et al. Hospital resources consumed for surgical morbidity: effects of preoperative arginine and omega-3 fatty acid supplementation on costs. Nutrition. 2005;21:1078-86.
45. Braga M, Vignali A, Gianotti L, et al. Laparoscopic versus open colorectal surgery. A randomized trial on short term outcome. Ann Surg. 2002;236:759-67.
46. Lin MT, Kung SP, Yeh SL, et al. The effect of glutamine-supplemented total parenteral nutrition on nitrogen economy depends on severity of disease in surgical patients. Clin Nutr. 2002;21:213-8.
47. Exner R, Tamandl D, Goetzinger P, et al. Perioperative GLY-GLN infusion diminishes the surgery-induced period of immunosuppression: accelerated restoration of the lipopolysaccharide-stimulated tumor necrosis factor-alpha response. Ann Surg. 2003;237:110-5.
48. Klek S, Kulig J, Szczepanik AM, et al. The clinical value of parenteral immunonutrition in surgical patients. Acta Chir Belg. 2005;105:175-9.
49. Yao GX, Xue XB, Jiang ZM, et al. Effect of perioperative parenteral glutamine-dipeptide supplementation on plasma endotoxin level, plasma endotoxin inactivation capacity and clinical outcome. Clin Nutr. 2005;24:510-5.
50. Jo S, Choi SH, Heo JS, et al. Missing effect of glutamine supplementation on the surgical outcome after pancreaticoduodenectomy for periampullary tumours: a prospective, randomized, double-blind, controlled clinical trial. World J Surg. 2006;30:1974-82.

Additional references appear in the online version of this book.

26

Pulmonary Support

Philip S Barie, Jared Huston, Mia Talmor

Key Points

- Respiratory complications are common after surgical operations, multiple trauma, and severe sepsis. Their prevention and management require a sound knowledge of normal lung function and its mechanisms of control, as well as the pathophysiology of disease. At-risk patients should be identified on admission (or beforehand, for elective surgery) and monitored continuously for development of complications.
- Preoperative assessment of lung function includes clinical evaluation, chest radiography (CXR), electrocardiography (ECG), blood gas analysis, spirometry before and after bronchodilator therapy, and potentially split-lung function studies.
- Factors that contribute to postoperative respiratory insufficiency include inhalational anesthetic agents, postoperative pain, narcotic analgesics, and chest/upper abdominal incisions.
- Acute lung injury (ALI) and acute respiratory distress syndrome (ARDS) comprise a range of pulmonary injuries characterized by the acute onset of hypoxia and decreased lung compliance in the absence of left ventricular failure.
- Nosocomial pneumonia remains commonplace, difficult to diagnose, and is associated with high rates of morbidity and mortality.
- Specific measures including ventilator support are needed to prevent or treat the various causes of respiratory insufficiency in surgical patients including atelectasis, aspiration pneumonitis, nosocomial pneumonia, and ARDS.
- Noninvasive ventilation may avoid intubation or reintubation for awake, cooperative patients with marginal oxygenation or ventilation.
- Modern mechanical ventilators provide several modes of ventilation, with the goals of improved gas exchange, better patient comfort, and rapid liberation from the ventilator.
- Unconventional or adjunctive methods of ventilatory support include independent lung ventilation, extracorporeal membrane oxygenation (ECMO), high-frequency ventilation (HFV), inhaled nitric oxide (iNO), and prone positioning (PP).
- Sedation should be used judiciously, monitored regularly to titrate effect and avoid oversedation, and withdrawn transiently each day during a "sedation holiday" to assess readiness for liberation from mechanical ventilation.
- Adherence to a "ventilator bundle" decreases the length of mechanical ventilation and the incidence of ventilator-associated pneumonia (VAP).

INTRODUCTION

Major operations nearly always affect lung function. The direct effects of thoracic surgical operations are obvious, but there are typical indirect effects of anesthetics and analgesics. Respiratory complications are also associated commonly with the nonoperative management of complex problems such as severe pancreatitis or multiple injuries. A major pulmonary complication can be life-threatening, even with prompt recognition and management; some can be anticipated and possibly prevented. Comprehensive knowledge of normal pulmonary physiology is essential to appreciate the impact of operative interventions on the respiratory system and to enable effective prophylaxis and therapy.

NORMAL PULMONARY PHYSIOLOGY

Lung Structure and Mechanics

Inhaled gas is warmed and humidified in the upper airway (the naso-oropharynx and trachea). Particulate matter is filtered for eventual expulsion by coughing or expectoration to prevent lower airway exposure. The lower airway is a branching series of airways that decrease progressively in size as they increase in number, resulting in a tremendous increase in available surface area for gas exchange.

The upper airway and the major divisions of the lower airway comprise the anatomic dead space (V_D), which comprises about 2 mL/kg body weight in an adult. The

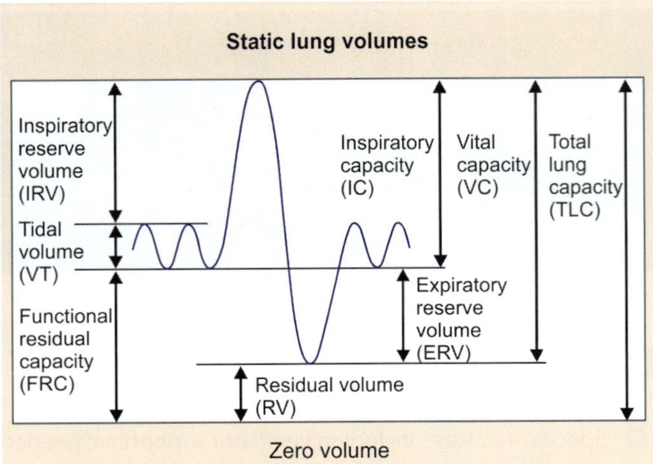

Fig. 26.1: Static lung volumes. The curve indicates the lung volumes that can be measured by simple spirometry (i.e. VT, IRV, ERV, IC, and VC). The RV cannot be measured by spirometry, and therefore it is impossible to measure FRC or TLC without using more sophisticated methods than spirometry.

Source: Adapted with permission from Nunn JF. Nunn's Applied Respiratory Physiology, 4th edition. Butterworth–Heinemann. 1993. pp. 2.

cartilaginous major airways (trachea and mainstem, lobar, segmental, and subsegmental bronchi) decrease in size from a mean diameter of 18 mm to 1 mm. These connect with the membranous bronchi, including the bronchioles and terminal bronchioles. The respiratory bronchioles, alveolar ducts, and alveolar sacs are the most distal.

Familiarity with the standard definitions of lung volumes and capacities is necessary to understand lung inflation and deflation (Fig. 26.1). There are classically four lung volumes:

- Tidal volume (V_T)
- Inspiratory reserve volume (IRV)
- Expiratory reserve volume (ERV)
- Residual volume (RV).

Combinations of these volumes form four capacities. All four lung volumes together constitute total lung capacity (TLC). The IRV, V_T, and ERV together form the vital capacity (VC). The ERV and RV form the functional residual capacity (FRC), the volume of gas in the lungs at normal end-expiration. The closing capacity (CC), which is the RV in normal individuals, is the lung volume at which small airways close, inhibiting the further flow of gas. Spirometry measures V_T and gas flow rates over time. As maximal exhalation does not empty the lungs completely, specialized techniques (e.g. helium dilution, nitrogen washout, and body plethysmography) are needed to measure any lung volume that includes RV (i.e. TLC, FRC, and RV itself).

Respiratory Responses in the Maintenance of Homeostasis

Aside from gas exchange, respiratory responses play other major roles to maintain acid-base homeostasis. The concept of respiratory control of acid-base balance can be misleading because cellular respiration does not play a primary role. Short-term regulation of acid-base balance is largely a function of feedback mechanisms that govern ventilation. Afferent and efferent impulses from medullary respiratory centers participate as well as mechanoreceptors in the chest wall, diaphragm, and pulmonary parenchyma, but the principal regulatory systems are the chemoreceptors in the aortic arch and carotid body.

Excretion of carbon dioxide (CO_2) is the principal mechanism by which the lung maintains normal pH. Gas exchange is regulated by the duration of red blood cell (RBC) transcapillary transit time and the diffusion characteristics of oxygen (O_2) and CO_2 across the alveolarcapillary membrane, as well as by matching of the distribution of alveolar ventilation (V_A) and perfusion (Q). Diffusion abnormalities or the development of V_A/Q inequality (mismatching) may impair CO_2 excretion in pulmonary disease or injury.

Regulation of Normal Ventilation

Neural mechanisms regulate rhythmic inhalation and exhalation. Neurons found in both the dorsal and ventral medulla are responsible for the integration of neural and chemical stimulation and the stimulation of respiratory muscles are distinct from the hydrogen ion (H^+) chemoreceptors:[1,2]

- Dorsal respiratory neurons regulate neural and chemical signals, and principally affect inspiration
- Ventral respiratory neurons regulate both inspiratory and expiratory activity.

Many of the ventral neurons project to the thoracic spinal cord to innervate the intercostal and abdominal musculature, whereas the dorsal motor neurons coalesce in the phrenic nerves. Other neurons located in the rostral pons inhibit the firing of the medullary neurons, acting as a physiologic filter to produce smooth regular ventilatory activity.[2] Central excitatory and inhibitory neurons receive afferent impulses from mechanoreceptors in the chest wall and lung.[3]

Mechanoreceptor Influences

Chest wall mechanoreceptors consist of tendon receptors in the diaphragm and intercostal muscles that are principally inhibitory, but these have little effect compared with that of the pulmonary mechanoreceptors. Muscle spindles, which are abundant in the intercostal muscles, maintain V_T in the presence of decreased chest wall motion, thereby opposing the action of the tendon receptors.

At least three kinds of intrapulmonary receptors modify ventilation via vagal afferents:[4]

- Irritant receptors located in the airway epithelium from the trachea to the distal respiratory bronchioles respond to local irritants or mechanical deformation of the tracheobronchial tree, producing bronchoconstriction and hyperventilation
- Pulmonary stretch receptors, present in airway smooth muscle, enhance the bronchodilation that occurs with lung expansion, and act with irritant receptors to regulate airway diameter during breathing
- Juxtacapillary receptors are located in the interstitial space of the alveolar wall and are stimulated by interstitial edema or fibrosis;[3,5] their activity may explain tachypnea with pulmonary edema.

Pulmonary and chest wall mechanoreceptors interact to increase the activity of expiratory muscles during lung inflation and so reduce end-expiratory lung volume to normal. Afferent signals from these receptors are processed in the brainstem to adjust both respiratory frequency and V_T and so minimize energy expenditure.

Stimulation of almost any afferent somatic nerve, especially pain fibers, results in a reflex increase in minute ventilation (V_E). Increased body temperature is also a potent stimulus of hypothalamic receptors. Hypothalamic efferents are transmitted directly to excitatory neurons, which produces an increase in V_E independent of the increase in CO_2 production caused by hyperthermia.

Physiology of Chemoreceptor Activity

Adjustments of ventilation and circulation in response to alterations in partial pressure of oxygen (PO_2), partial pressure of carbon dioxide (PCO_2), and pH are mediated by two distinct chemoreceptor systems.[6] Central chemoreceptors respond to changes in cerebrospinal fluid [H+] concentration and are primarily responsible for:

- Determining resting V_E
- Ventilatory and circulatory adjustments during hypercapnia and chronic disturbances of acid–base balance.[7]

Centrally, there are two distinct CO_2-sensitive chemoreceptor types, one of which is protected by the blood-brain barrier. Both central types of chemoreceptors are affected rapidly by diffusible molecular CO_2. However, the brain, owing to the blood–brain barrier, is affected slowly by changes in $[H^+]$ or $[HCO_3^-]$. Consequently, central chemoreceptors respond differently to acidosis resulting from hypercapnia or from organic acids such as lactic acidosis.[8] Increases in arterial PCO_2 ($paCO_2$) produce linear increases in V_E, which are influenced predominantly by central chemoreceptor drive.[9] The two central CO_2 chemoreceptor mechanisms may counteract. For example, central chemoreceptors can suppress peripheral chemoreceptor responses by suppressing autonomic efferents. Therefore, there may be no response in mild hypoxia.

Peripheral chemoreceptors respond to changes in arterial PO_2 (PaO_2) rather than O_2 content (CaO_2). Stimulation of peripheral chemoreceptors is entirely responsible for increased V_E produced by hypoxia and for some of the increase caused by hypercapnia.[8] Carotid body chemoreceptors are probably more important than those in the aortic body.[6,10] The carotid body receives sympathetic and parasympathetic efferent stimulations. Afferent impulses to the brainstem as well as inhibitory efferents are transmitted in the carotid sinus nerve. The effects of increased $PaCO_2$ and, to a lesser extent, decreased pH on carotid body activity are greater during hypoxia than hyperoxia, which accounts for the synergistic effects of hypoxia and hypercapnia on ventilatory drive. This synergism may be mediated by a peripheral chemoreceptor influence on central chemosensitivity (enhanced during hypercapnia),[11] which may serve to counteract the direct depressant effect of hypoxia on respiratory motor neurons. Additionally, carotid body stimulation of brainstem excitatory neurons may increase V_E by mechanisms unrelated to ventilatory rate.

Gas Exchange

After alveoli are ventilated with fresh gas, O_2 and CO_2 are exchanged by diffusion. Diffusion is inversely proportional to membrane thickness and depends also on the solubility and molecular weight of the gas. Higher solubility allows CO_2 to diffuse 20 times faster than O_2. The alveolar PO_2 (P_aO_2) is approximately 105 mm Hg (14.0 kPa), whereas the venous O_2 tension (PvO_2) is 40 mm Hg (5.3 kPa), which creates a diffusion gradient for O_2 across the alveolar-capillary membrane. Pulmonary arteriolar PCO_2 is 46 mm Hg (6.1 kPa), equilibrating to an end-capillary PCO_2 of approximately 40 mm Hg (5.3 kPa).

The lung has a large reserve before diffusion becomes impaired. Mean pulmonary capillary transit time is approximately 0.5 seconds. The diffusion equilibrium for

O_2 occurs within 0.25 second and CO_2 reaches equilibrium even faster. Diffusion limitation can be demonstrated when:

- Transit time is decreased (e.g. exercise, increased perfusion)
- The diffusion gradient is narrower (e.g. high altitude) and
- Functional membrane area is lost (e.g. after lung resection, in fibroproliferative disease).

Interference with diffusion exaggerates the differences among the alveolar and arterial PO_2 and PCO_2, but abnormalities of gas exchange caused purely by abnormalities of diffusion or ventilation are rare. Rather, V_A/Q mismatching is the major culprit.

The distribution of V is not uniform, even in normal lung.[12,13] Pleural pressure (P_{pl}) in the upright position is further below atmospheric pressure at the apex than at the base of the lung. Consequently, transpulmonary pressure (P_t) [alveolar pressure (P_{alv}) - P_{pl}] is greater at the base of the lung; alveoli at the apex are generally more expanded. However, the distribution of inspired gas is not determined passively by anatomy. Regional variations in lung compliance caused by normal airway elasticity or inflammation, bronchial hyper-reactivity, mechanical airway obstruction, or pulmonary edema can influence the distribution of V.[13] The particular lung volume from which an inspiration is begun is also important. Within the range of normal V_T, alveoli are ventilated better at the bottom than at the top of the lung.[12] At very low lung volumes near RV, P_{pl} at the dependent portion of the lung exceeds airway pressure (P_{aw}), which results in atelectasis. During a breath taken at or near RV, such as during ALI/ARDS (which decrease FRC), gas entering the lungs is distributed preferentially to nondependent areas.

Distribution of pulmonary Q is complex compared to the distribution of V_A.[12] Blood flow is influenced by gravity, which provides a gradient of increasing blood pressure and perfusion towards the lung bases (or dorsal lung in supine patients) that is greater than the distribution gradient of ventilation. The distribution of Q is also influenced by pulmonary blood volume, right ventricular output, mean pulmonary artery pressure (P_{pa}), pulmonary vascular resistance, and lung volume (physiologic dilation of extra-alveolar capillaries keeps vascular resistance low at higher lung volumes). The application of positive-pressure ventilation, particularly positive end-expiratory pressure (PEEP), accentuates redistribution of Q towards the most gravity-dependent portion of the lung because Q ceases when alveolar pressure (P_A) exceeds perfusion pressure in nondependent lung.[12]

The lung can be divided into three zones in terms of pressure relationships. In zone I lung, P_A always exceeds Ppa_{syst}; therefore, the lung is not perfused and all ventilation to the lung is V_D. In zone II lung, P_{alv} is intermediate between Ppa_{syst}; and Ppa_{diast}; and therefore, perfusion is intermittent and variable. In zone III (dependent) lung, Ppa_{diast} always exceeds P_{alv}, and perfusion is continuous, but shunt (Qs/Qt), i.e. perfusion of nonventilated lung, may occur because many alveoli are atelectatic or flooded and hence cannot be ventilated: Qs = pulmonary blood flow to areas of shunt, Qt = pulmonary blood flow.

Other than gravity, vascular responses mediated by both local and extrapulmonary mechanisms are the most important determinants of pulmonary perfusion distribution. Both alveolar hypoxia and arteriolar hypoxemia (SaO_2<80%) cause pulmonary vasoconstriction.[14] Hypoxemia (oxygen saturation or SaO_2) results in chemoreceptor-mediated vasoconstriction via adrenergic efferent pathways.[15] Acidosis also causes vasoconstriction and enhances the pressor effect of hypoxia, effects that are attenuated by alkalosis.

Efficient gas exchange depends upon V_A/Q matching within the lung. Abnormalities may develop of V, Q, or both. Inequality of V_A/Q is the most common cause of hypoxemia in people with lung disease or injury.[12,16] The major factor in determining SaO_2 is the V_A:Q ratio, not the absolute quantity of each; even if V_A/Q distribution is abnormal, arterial blood gases are little affected if they remain matched. The normal V_A:Q in the whole lung is about 0.85, with the low V_A/Q areas in the lung base compensating for the higher ratios in the relatively nonperfused apex. In disease, V_D as well as Qs/Qt may develop. Matching of V_A/Q is maintained better in the supine position because gravity-induced differences of perfusion are attenuated; there is little or no zone I lung when the normal lung is supine, but ARDS can cause V_A/Q mismatching even in supine lung, which may be ameliorated transiently by placing the patient prone. Also, hypoxic vasoconstriction is the most potent mechanism for normalizing an abnormal V_A:Q.[14] Drugs that abolish hypoxic vasoconstriction (e.g. pulmonary vasodilators such as nitroglycerin and nitroprusside) may worsen P_AO_2 when given to a patient who has ARDS.

Oxygen and Carbon Dioxide Transport

Oxygen is transported in the blood in two forms:

- The small amount of dissolved O_2 carried in physical solution
- That bound to hemoglobin (Hb) (oxyhemoglobin, O_2Hb).

The CaO_2 is the sum of these two components. Oxygen delivery (DO_2), the amount of O_2 transported to the tissues per minute, is the product of perfusion and CaO_2. The amount of dissolved O_2 in the blood is a function of PaO_2 representing 0.003 mL O_2/100 mL blood for each mm Hg PO_2 (approximately 1% of CaO_2). Hemoglobin carries 1.34 mL O_2/g when saturated fully. The total amount of O_2Hb is determined by SaO_2 and Hb concentration. Under normal conditions, O_2Hb averages 19.6 mL O_2/100 mL blood.

The SaO_2 can be related to PaO_2 through the O_2Hb dissociation curve (Figs. 26.2A to C). At high PaO_2, the curve becomes flat; as a result, there is a progressively marginal increase in SaO_2 and therefore CaO_2, as PaO_2 increases. When SaO_2 is >95%, increases in PaO_2 have little effect on CaO_2. Conversely, at SaO_2 values of 20–80%, the curve is steep and small changes in PaO_2 have a large effect on SaO_2. This phenomenon is advantageous because only a small gradient is needed to offload O_2 from Hb. In the hypoxemic patient, CaO_2 and therefore Do_2 can be seriously compromised by a small decrease in PaO_2. Conversely, small amounts of supplemental O_2 can cause substantial improvement if ventilatory mechanics and V_A/Q matching are preserved.

Red blood cells generate 2,3-diphosphoglycerate (2,3-DPG), which lowers the affinity of Hb for O_2, thereby favoring offloading of O_2 to the tissue. A deficiency of 2,3-DPG, as occurs invariably in banked blood, causes a left shift of the O_2Hb dissociation curve. The P_{50} is that PO_2 needed to achieve an SaO_2 of 50%, so serving as a marker of the position of the curve. The normal P_{50} corresponds to a PO_2 of 26.6 mm Hg (3.54 kPa). A left shift of the curve (secondary to a low 2,3-DPG concentration, alkalosis, or hypothermia) is a marker of increased affinity of Hb for O_2 and impaired O_2 offloading. A right shift (secondary to hyperthermia or acidosis) indicates that O_2Hb affinity is decreased.

Carbon dioxide is carried in the blood in three forms:

- Dissolved CO_2, which is 20 times more soluble than O_2, accounts for only 5% of CO_2 in arterial blood
- Most of the CO_2 is carried as $[HCO_3^-]$ formed from the dissociation of carbonic acid (H_2CO_3)
- Carbamino compounds, which are formed from the combination of CO_2 with the terminal amino group of some blood proteins (only a small portion of CO_2 in blood).

Reduced Hb has approximately 3.5 times the ability to combine with CO_2, as O_2Hb; therefore, more CO_2 can be carried in venous blood at any given PCO_2. The observation that arterial blood at any given PCO_2 has a smaller CO_2 content than venous blood at the same PCO_2 is called the Haldane effect.[12] This physiologic observation is important for understanding CO_2 exchange.

The Haldane effect occurs because of the relationship between the Hb molecule and the $[H^+]$ generated by the conversion of CO_2 into $[HCO_3^-]$. Hydrogen ions generated by $[HCO_3^-]$ synthesis are buffered almost exclusively by binding to Hb. Deoxygenation of Hb favors binding of $[H^+]$ because reduced Hb is a weaker acid than O_2Hb. As a result of this proton binding, at any PCO_2 more $[HCO_3^-]$ is present in blood and therefore its CO_2 content is greater when Hb is reduced. Direct CO_2 binding to Hb is also facilitated in deoxygenated rather than oxygenated blood. The net result of the Haldane effect is to permit vast quantities of CO_2 to be transported in venous blood while minimizing changes in venous pH and PCO_2 compared with those in arterial blood.

PULMONARY FAILURE AND DYSFUNCTION

Pathophysiology

Anesthesia, the anatomic location of the operative procedure, and pre-existing conditions all impact upon postoperative ventilatory function by altering respiratory muscle function and disrupting lung mechanics. An understanding of these processes requires knowledge of lung mechanics and how operative procedures and anesthesia alter these mechanics, often resulting in postoperative pulmonary complications.

Lung Volumes

The relationship of CC (closing capacity) to functional residual capacity (FRC) forms a basis for pathophysiologic ventilatory changes postoperatively (Figs. 26.2A to C). Normally, FRC is greater than CC. During a tidal breath, the small airways remain open throughout inhalation and exhalation. If CC is greater than FRC, a tidal breath may open small airways partially or not at all, which results in atelectasis and mismatched V_A/Q.

Thoracic and abdominal procedures cause restrictive lung function abnormalities. All of the lung volumes are reduced. The VC and FRC can be reduced as much as 50–70% during the first 24 hours after surgical operations (Table 26.1).[17] These changes occur shortly after anesthesia induction and can last as long as 14 days postoperatively.

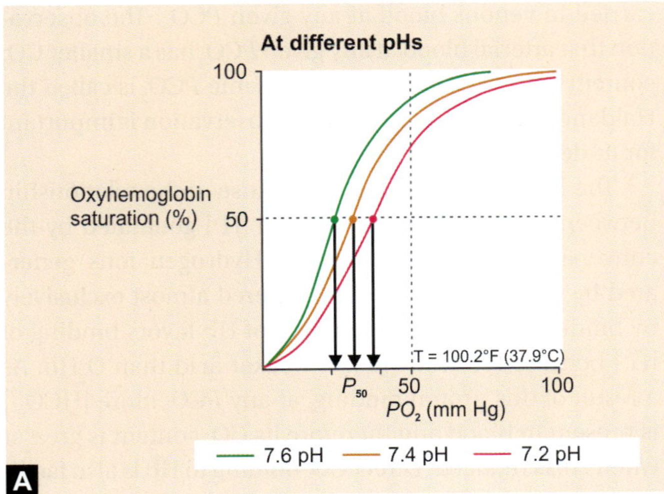

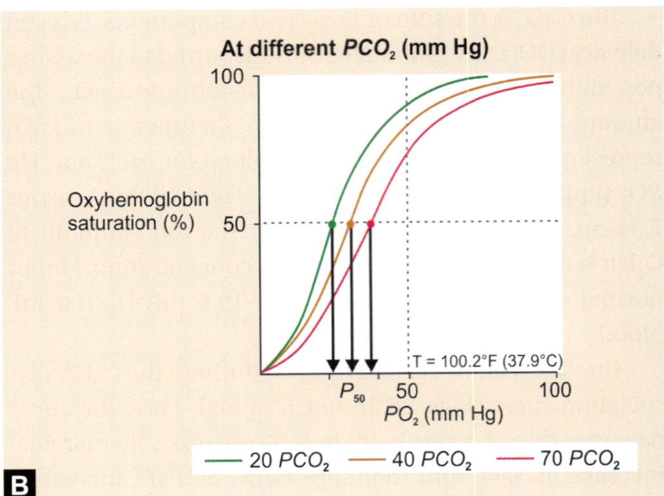

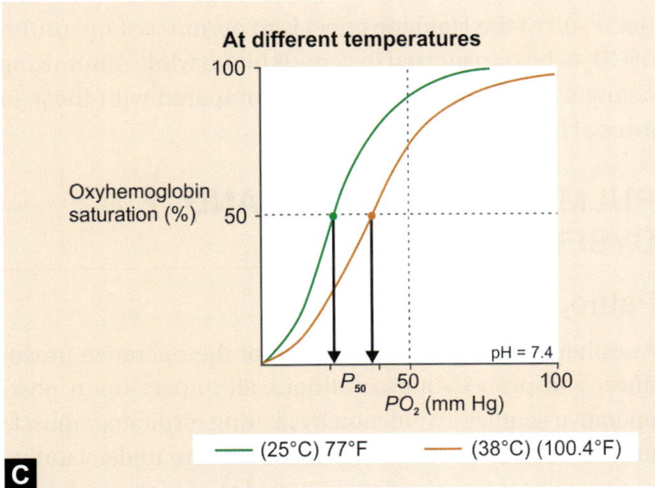

Figs. 26.2A to C: Effects of varying pH, partial pressure of carbon dioxide (PCO_2), and temperature on oxyhemoglobin dissociation.
Source: Adapted with permission from Weibel ER. The pathway for oxygen. Harvard University Press; 1984. p. 149. Copyright 1984 by the President and Fellows of Harvard College.

Table 26.1 Postoperative functional residual capacity (percentage of preoperative values) according to site of incision.

Site of incision	*Postoperative day*			
	1	3	5	7
Upper abdomen	71	81	90	90
Lower abdomen	88	115	101	102
Extremity	97	103	108	96
Chest	83	85	93	88
Sternotomy	59	58	65	NA

Source: Data from Miller CL, Martin JL. Changes in lung function following anesthesia and surgery. In: Breslow MJ, Miller CF, Rogers M, (Eds). Perioperative Management. St Louis: Mosby; 1990. Pp. 194-212.
(NA: Data not available).

General anesthesia itself is not causative, as similar abnormalities may be seen in patients under epidural anesthesia. Pain and muscle splinting contribute to the reduced lung volumes, but effective pain control does not immediately restore lung volumes to preoperative levels.

Effects of Anesthesia on Ventilatory Function

General anesthesia predisposes to upper airway obstruction, impairs protective reflexes against aspiration, and depresses mucociliary clearance mechanisms. The FRC decreases after induction,[18] but remains stable for the duration of the anesthetic. Virtually all anesthetic agents share this property, which is caused by changes in both chest wall conformation and motion regardless of whether there is neuromuscular blockade. Anesthetics also decrease diaphragmatic tone at end-exhalation, decreasing thoracic volume further.[19] Atelectasis begins to develop in dependent portions of lung within 10 minutes of induction.[20]

Breathing at lower lung volumes increases the elastic recoil of the lung and decreases lung compliance,[20] but healthy nonparalyzed patients can compensate for this and the partial airway obstruction (smaller lumen than the native trachea) caused by the endotracheal tube, and can maintain V_E by increasing the work of breathing.

The alveolar–arterial O_2 gradient ($D[A\text{-}a]O_2$) decreases in direct proportion to decreased FRC in anesthetized subjects[21] because of intrapulmonary shunting and perfusion of low V_A/Q areas. The phenomenon is accentuated in elderly patients and by pre-existing lung disease. Inhibition of hypoxic vasoconstriction by inhalational agents is the primary mechanism of V_A/Q mismatching under anesthesia.[22] The degree of atelectasis also correlates with Qs/Qt in anesthetized patients. All halogenated anesthetic agents impair normal responses to hypoxemia and hypercapnia by depressing carotid body chemoreceptors,[23] and they impair the peripheral chemoreceptor-mediated ventilatory response to acidemia.[24]

Atelectasis, decreased FRC, and increased $D[A\text{-}a]O_2$ persist in the postoperative period only in patients who have undergone general anesthesia for a thoracic or abdominal procedure (Table 26.1).[17] Diaphragm dysfunction, rather than the persistent effects of anesthetic or the restrictive effects of incisional pain, is most important in the pathogenesis of prolonged abnormalities. Diaphragm dysfunction is not abolished by epidural fentanyl[25] and the response to phrenic nerve stimulation is normal.[26]

Postoperative Lung, Chest Wall, and Diaphragm Dysfunction

Cough and mucociliary transport protect the lungs and airway from environmental and infectious agents. Endotracheal intubation itself suppresses airway reflexes, which increases the risk of respiratory infection. During the induction of general anesthesia in supine patients, cephalad diaphragm displacement accounts for a loss of 350–750 mL of thoracic volume. Intravenous anesthetics (except ketamine) depress diaphragmatic tonic activity and volatile anesthetics depress synaptic transmission, affecting the intercostal muscles preferentially. The loss of respiratory muscle tone mediated by inhibitory phrenic nerve efferents rapidly results in atelectasis. At 1 and 24 hours postoperatively, 90% and 50% of the anesthetic-induced atelectasis is still present, respectively.

Coughing is inhibited because of pain and narcotic use. Respiratory muscle dysfunction reduces the expulsive force and effectiveness of the cough. Mucociliary clearance is reduced for 2–6 days following general anesthesia because of:

- Ciliary damage from dry anesthetic gases
- Increased mucus viscosity
- Reduced clearance from atelectatic areas.

Epidural local anesthetics ablate the inhibitory signals from visceral sympathetic receptors, but prolonged recumbency and sedation mean that epidural analgesia does not prevent atelectasis completely. In contrast, epidural narcotics ameliorate pain, but do not affect phrenic nerve function, although ventilation is depressed centrally.

After cardiac operations, late postoperative atelectasis is not explained solely by diaphragm dysfunction. Variables associated with atelectasis include the number of saphenous vein grafts, use of internal mammary grafts, the length of cardiac bypass time, entering of the pleural space, hypothermia, and ischemia of alveolar epithelium, which results in decreased surfactant production.

Perfusion of the pulmonary circulation with potassium cardioplegia solution may cause atelectasis as a result of cytotoxicity. Phrenic nerve paralysis (caused by topical cooling used for cardioplegia)[27] develops in about 10% of patients who undergo cardiothoracic operations.

In routine thoracic operations, reduced surfactant activity can result from mechanical compression of the lung and accumulation of lung water. Changes in pulmonary function after thoracotomy may last as long as 3 weeks.[16] In addition to loss of functional lung tissue, chest wall compliance decreases as much as 75%. Hypoventilation and respiratory acidosis can persist into the first postoperative day. These changes are exacerbated by opioid analgesics. Hypoxemia can last up to 10 days. The deliberate intraoperative collapse of one lung to facilitate exposure is unique to lung and mediastinal operations. Although hypoxic vasoconstriction minimizes any increase in Qs/Qt, the lung must be inflated periodically during operations to prevent atelectasis. There is no difference in VC or peak flow in patients who undergo sternotomy compared with those who have a formal posterolateral thoracotomy. After 4–7 days, the sternotomy patient recovers more rapidly than the thoracotomy patient.[16]

During and immediately after pneumonectomy, the mediastinum shifts toward the evacuated hemithorax and the remaining lung distends. Distention of the remaining lung, movement of the diaphragm, and the production of connective tissue to fill the evacuated thoracic space resulted in a reduction of thoracic volume until it was realized that the mediastinum can be kept in place (neutral position) until fibrosis occurs.

After abdominal operations, the patient adapts to a pattern of breathing with little abdominal volume change and increased rib cage excursion. The accessory muscles of ventilation assume increased importance. Contraction of abdominal muscles is prominent in exhalation, but its importance in generating V_T is not known. The shift from using the diaphragm to intercostal muscles is accompanied by redistribution of V and less inspiratory gas delivery to the lower lobes. Abdominal muscle activity during exhalation decreases the FRC. The CC is reached during a tidal breath. The net result is atelectasis.

Diagnosis and Monitoring

Acute respiratory failure often develops precipitously, so it can be difficult to separate, at least temporally, diagnostic procedures from the initial therapy. The spectrum of presenting illness is variable and underlying illness such as an acute exacerbation of chronic obstructive pulmonary disease (COPD) or pre-existing therapy (e.g. mechanical ventilation) can influence the presentation.

The physical examination provides valuable information. Inspection identifies cyanosis, chest wall excursion and use of accessory muscles, dyspnea,[28] and respiratory rate. Palpation of the suprasternal notch confirms a midline trachea (it is deviated in tension pneumothorax). Percussion dullness may identify a pleural effusion or parenchymal consolidation.

Auscultation is especially important. Symmetry of breath sounds and rales or rhonchi should be detectable, although chest auscultation is challenging in a patient who is obtunded yet phonating (e.g. moaning in pain), markedly tachypneic, too anxious to cooperate (common in hypoxemia), on a mechanical ventilator, or amidst the din of an intensive care unit.

Laboratory studies to diagnose pulmonary dysfunction consist of:

- Serum electrolytes and arterial or mixed venous blood gases
- Screening tests for the presence of thrombosis (e.g. blood tests, Doppler ultrasound)
- Radiologic studies—CXR and computed tomography (CT)
- Scintigraphy (now used seldom)
- Bronchoscopy
- Microbiologic cultures and antibiotic susceptibility testing
- Pleural fluid chemistry and culture.

Not every test is necessary for every patient. Electrolyte concentrations may help to identify patients who have metabolic muscular failure (e.g. hypocalcemia, hypokalemia, hypomagnesemia, and hypophosphatemia); $[HCO_3^-]$ may help determine the chronicity of respiratory acidosis. Arterial blood gas determination identifies hypoxemia, hypo- or hypercapnia, and arterial pH, and estimates the SaO_2. Most patients who have early respiratory failure have acute respiratory alkalosis because of their increased respiratory drive, which may be sufficient for brief periods to overcome hypoxemia. The nonintubated hypoxemic patient who is normocapnic, PaO_2:F_IO_2 <300 on any fractional inspired oxygen (F_IO_2), may fail precipitously.

If the reasonable assumption is made that the pH–PCO_2 relationship is linear across the typical range of pH seen clinically (7.25–7.55), each 10 mm Hg change in $PaCO_2$ accounts for 0.08 pH units. Therefore, any pH that is lower or higher than that accounted for by the $PaCO_2$ represents the metabolic rather than the respiratory component. It is believed that a spontaneously ventilating patient cannot overcompensate for an acid–base disorder (i.e. a patient who has a primary respiratory alkalosis and metabolic compensation cannot have an arterial pH <7.40). However, this rule cannot be relied upon in a mechanically ventilated patient. Mixed venous blood gases can be used to calculate VO_2 or Qs/Qt or to assess circulatory function in low-flow states or acute respiratory failure with critical hypoxemia. Normally, PvO_2 is 40 mm Hg (5.3 kPa) and Svo_2 is approximately 70%. If Pvo_2 is <35 mm Hg (<4.7 kPa), there is either insufficient F_IO_2, increased VO_2, or perfusion is critically low (decreased DO_2). If PvO_2 is <30 mm Hg (<4.0 kPa), anaerobic metabolism supervenes.

Chest radiography is the other mainstay of pulmonary diagnosis, but is overused.[29] Screening by CXR of asymptomatic preoperative patients has a low yield. For diagnosis in acute respiratory failure, anteroposterior portable CXR is often obtained (Fig. 26.3). The major limitations are that:

- About 20% of lung parenchyma is obscured by the heart or diaphragms
- The CXR can be normal with pulmonary dysfunction (e.g. pulmonary embolism, V_A/Q mismatch)
- Chest radiographs in seriously ill patients are seldom pristine
- One abnormality can often obscure another (e.g. pleural effusion overlying pneumonia, pneumonia complicating ARDS).[30]

Computed tomographic scans may be necessary for precise diagnosis (Figs. 26.4 to 26.12).[31,32] Helical (spiral) CT scans, which provide continuous volumetric data acquisition as the patient moves through the gantry, have short acquisition times, improved vascular imaging, and provide better enhancement of parenchymal organs. They also require lower doses of intravenous contrast material to complete the study.[31]

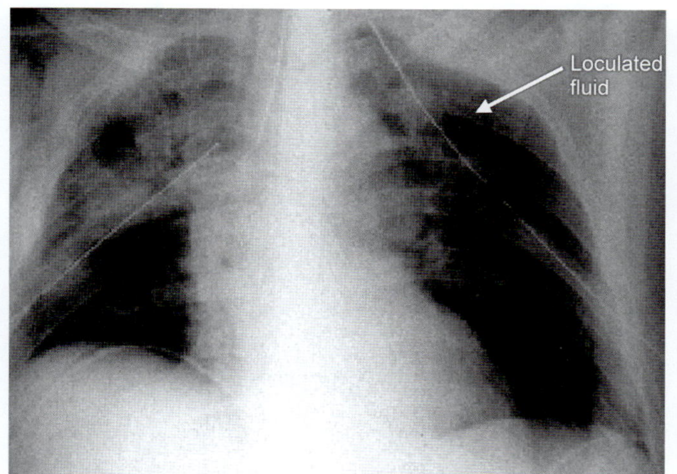

Fig. 26.3: Portable anteroposterior chest radiograph of a multiply injured patient. The radiograph demonstrates bilateral thoracostomy tubes. The lungs have re-expanded, but there is discernible loculated fluid at the apex of the left lung. This sign suggests injury to the thoracic aorta. There are also bilateral pulmonary contusions.

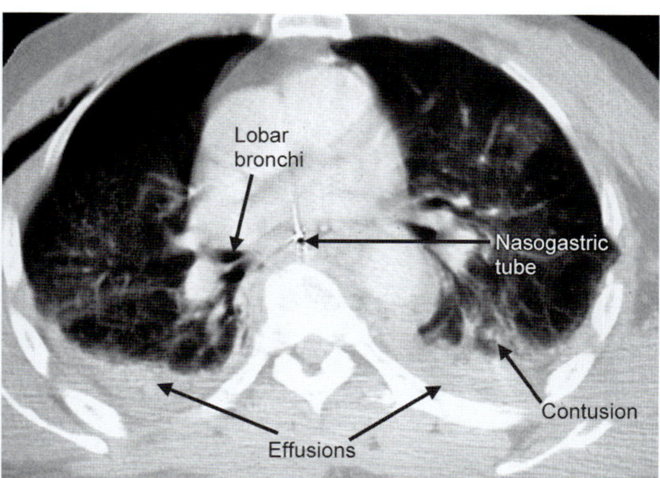

Fig. 26.4: Conventional computed tomographic scan of the chest of the patient shown in Figure 26.3. This demonstrates numerous pathologic findings. Transverse lucencies in both lung hila are lobar bronchi. The small circular lucency surrounded by streak artifact just anterior to the vertebral body is a nasogastric tube. In both hemithoraces, pneumothorax (more prominent on the patient's right), parenchymal contusion (more prominent on the left), and effusion (bilateral) are visible from ventral to dorsal.

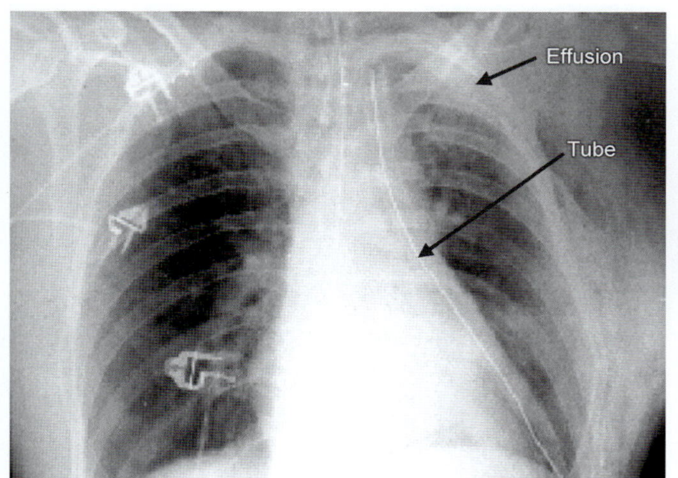

Fig. 26.5: Multiple trauma patient. This anteroposterior portable chest radiograph shows a left thoracostomy tube in place for apparently successful drainage of a hemopneumothorax. Complete expansion of the left lung was impeded by a loculated effusion at the apex.

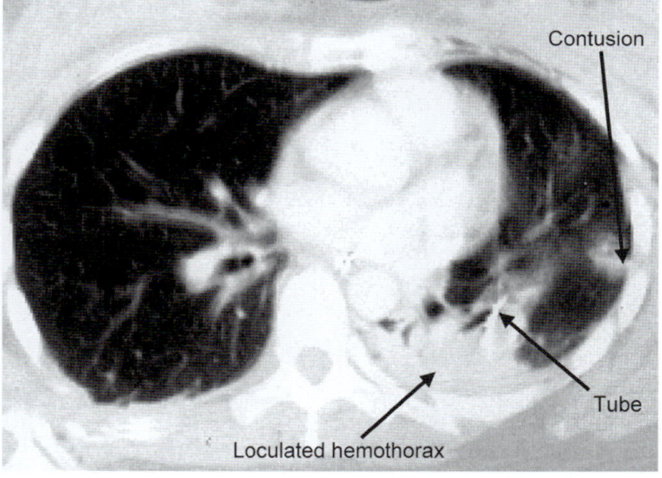

Fig. 26.6: Helical computed tomographic scan to evaluate the findings shown in Figure 26.5. A large pulmonary contusion and residual loculated hemothorax can be seen. The crescent-shaped artifact adjacent to the contusion on the left is the thoracostomy tube. Conventional single-view anteroposterior portable chest radiographs do not visualize approximately 20% of the lung parenchyma.

Pleural Effusion

Pleural effusion is common after operation and may represent a sympathetic response to acute inflammation below the diaphragm, congestive heart failure, iatrogenic fluid overload, traumatic hemothorax, or pneumonia (Figs. 26.7 to 26.12). The presence and magnitude of pleural effusions are often appreciated best by CT.

In cases of fluid overload, patients may be treated successfully with diuretics or observation alone.[33] Thoracentesis can be both diagnostic and therapeutic; tube thoracostomy may be indicated for a large effusion, the unstable patient (especially with refractory hypoxemia),[34] a recurrent effusion, or hemothorax. Following drainage of an effusion, the CXR may have improved diagnostic yield. An exudative effusion is associated with infection,

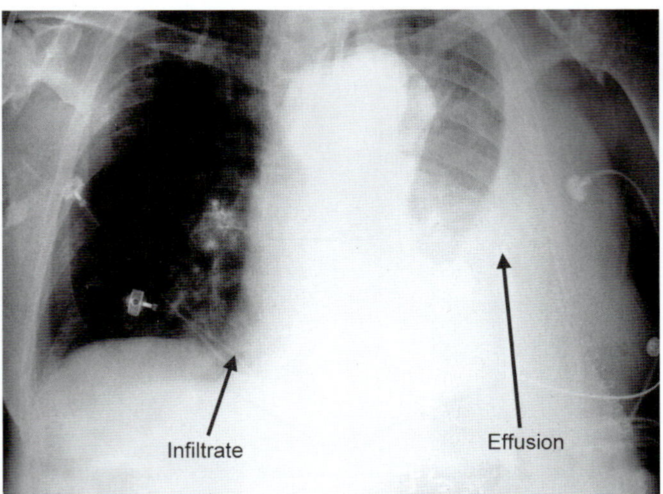

Fig. 26.7: Post-repair of a type III thoracic aortic dissection through a left thoracoabdominal incision to reconstruct several abdominal visceral vessels. A large left pleural effusion obscures much of the left hemothorax and there is a suggestion of a right middle lobe infiltrate.

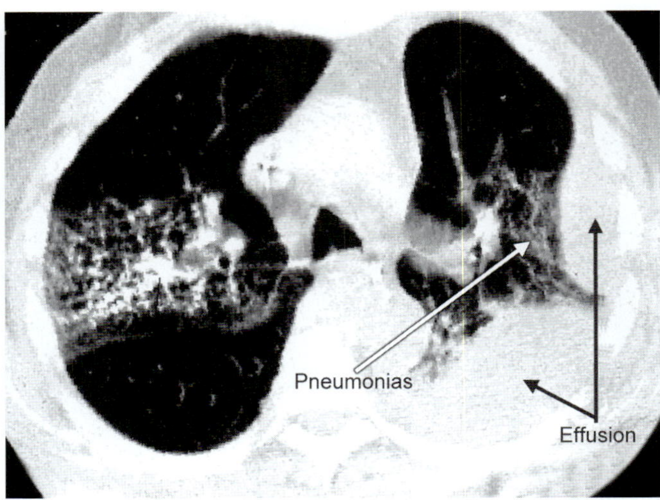

Fig. 26.8: Helical computed tomographic scan of the patient shown in Figure 26.7. This shows bilateral pneumonias as well as a multiloculated left pleural effusion. There is substantial entrapment on the left. This proved to be empyema complicating Gram-negative pneumonia. The large right lower lobe pneumonia is not apparent on the portable anteroposterior chest radiograph shown in Figure 26.7.

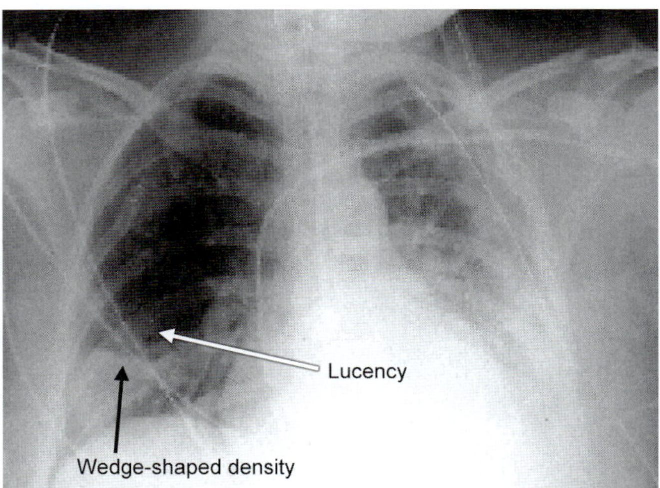

Fig. 26.9: Persistent sepsis following phlebectomy for suppurative thrombophlebitis. The left hemithorax shows almost completely obscured lung parenchyma of the left lower lobe despite drainage of a pleural effusion by thoracostomy. Also noted is a discrete wedge-shaped density just above the right costophrenic angle, which has a suggestion of cavitation reminiscent of necrotizing pneumonia (the lucency adjacent to the density at its superomedial border).

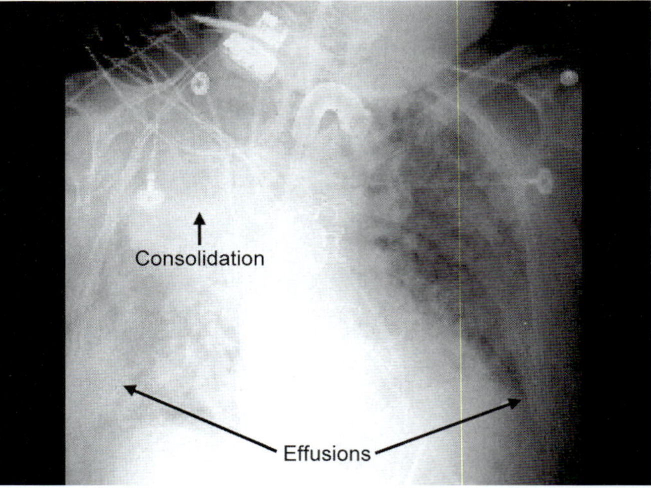

Fig. 26.10: Patient who has chronic obstructive pulmonary disease secondary to smoking and amiodarone-induced pulmonary fibrosis and superimposed acute respiratory distress syndrome following emergency surgery. In addition, the patient appears, by portable chest radiograph, to have bilateral pleural effusions and dense consolidation of the right upper lobe.

but numerous classification schemes have precluded a consensus definition.[35]

Nosocomial Pneumonia

Nosocomial pneumonia develops >72 hours after hospitalization.[36,37] Pneumonia that becomes manifest before this is community-acquired, which has important implications for diagnosis and therapy, because the pathogens differ and multidrug-resistant organisms are less likely.[38] Pneumonia is relevant to surgical practice because it is nearly as common as surgical site infection, yet is probably overdiagnosed.

A diagnosis of nosocomial pneumonia poses both clinical and microbiologic challenges, especially in ventilator-dependent patients in whom the incidence of pneumonia may be as high as 1–3% per day.[36] Neither routine sputum

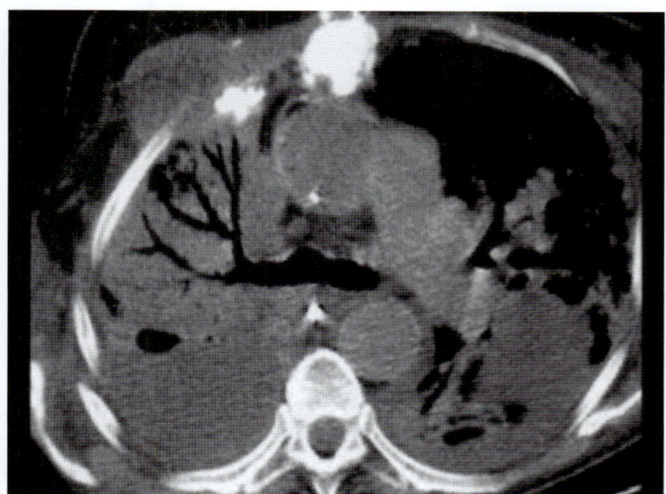

Fig. 26.11: Helical computed tomographic scan of the patient shown in Figure 26.10. Extensive organization of the right upper lobe is apparent from the branching air bronchogram. At the distal portion of the middle of the three branching bronchi is an area of cavitation that is not evident on the chest radiograph. Directly ventral is a large loculated right pleural effusion that may be infected.

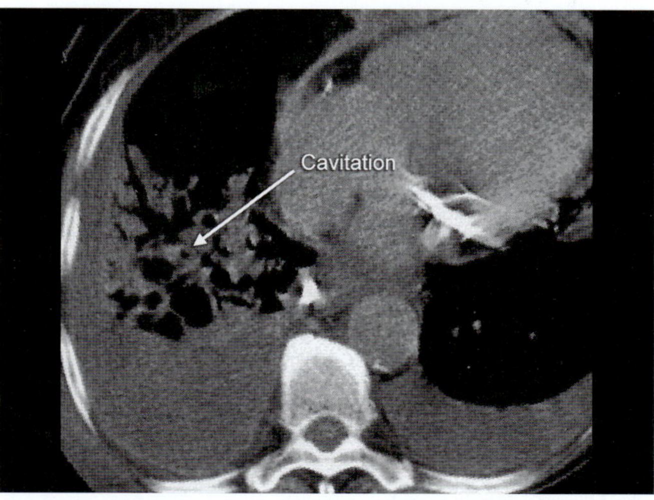

Fig. 26.12: Another image from the same study shown in Figure 26.11. This reveals an extensive cavitating process of the right upper lobe consistent with necrotizing pneumonia. The extent of the bilateral pleural effusions, not apparent in Figure 26.11, can be seen here.

aspirates[39] nor portable CXR[40] have diagnostic specificity. Sputum collected via a conventional suction catheter is unreliable because such specimens are often contaminated with upper airway flora, or by pathogens sequestered in the glycocalyx biofilm that accumulates in the lumens of artificial airways. The pharynx and airway tube (if present) are colonized rapidly during hospitalization with potential respiratory tract pathogens. Potential pathogens are believed to gain access to the lower respiratory tract after aspiration of pharyngeal (or gastric) secretions.

The classic findings of fever, purulent sputum, leukocytosis, and a new pulmonary infiltrate on CXR are caused by pneumonia in fewer than 50% of cases.[41] In particular, most cases of aspiration of gastric contents result only in chemical pneumonitis, which does not culminate in bacterial pneumonia. It is especially difficult to diagnose pneumonia in the presence of acute respiratory failure;[38] estimates from bronchoscopic surveillance data suggest that bacterial pneumonia complicates 20–65% of cases of ARDS.[42]

Overdiagnosis results in an overuse of antibiotic therapy, which is expensive, potentially morbid (myriad antibiotic-related complications), and promotes the emergence of resistant pathogens.[43,44] The consequences of prolonged ventilator dependence, prolonged duration of hospital stay, and increased mortality rate are well documented.[45,46]

Sputum sample acquisition so as to avoid contamination has been advocated, but remains controversial; collection may be facilitated by fiberoptic bronchoscopy with or without bronchoalveolar lavage (BAL). The protected-specimen brush has a sensitivity of 70–90%. Quantitative bacteriology showing 10^4 colony-forming units (CFU)/mL is a consensus indicator of invasive infection.[47] Bronchoalveolar lavage increases the overall accuracy of bronchoscopic diagnosis by increasing the specificity.[48-50] Either the protected specimen brush test or BAL can be carried out with no need for bronchoscopy. Unfortunately, validation of the diagnosis does not appear to improve outcome,[51] perhaps because the need for bronchoscopy delays therapy when time is of the essence.[52]

New Definitions

Frustration over the diagnosis of nosocomial pneumonia has prompted the US Centers for Disease Control and Prevention (CDC) to proffer new definitions. The frustrations include the confusion caused by a lack of consensus definitions for healthcare-associated pneumonia, hospital-acquired pneumonia, VAP, and the lack of sensitivity and specificity of existing definitions of VAP. Moreover, extant definitions include a CXR component, despite the fact that CXR is unreliable for the diagnosis of VAP.[40] Acknowledged also is that pneumonia is not the only pulmonary complication that may afflict the mechanically ventilated patient.

Newly defined conditions include ventilator-associated conditions and ventilator-associated events (Tables 26.2 to 26.6). Ventilator-associated pneumonia is classified as possible or probable under the new definitions. The new

Table 26.2 Ventilator-associated events (VAE) surveillance algorithm.

Ventilator-associated condition (VAC)
After a period of stability or improvement on the ventilator, the patient has at least one of the following indicators of worsening oxygenation:
1. Increase in daily minimum* F_IO_2 of ≥0.20 (20 points) over the daily minimum F_IO_2 in the baseline period, sustained for ≥2 calendar days
2. Increase in daily minimum* PEEP values of ≥3 cm H_2O over the daily minimum PEEP in the baseline period†, sustained for ≥2 calendar days
*Daily minimum defined by lowest value of F_IO_2 or PEEP during a calendar day that is maintained for at least 1 hour.
†Daily minimum PEEP values of 0–5 cm H_2O are considered equivalent for the purposes of VAE surveillance.
On or after calendar day 3 of mechanical ventilation and within 2 calendar days before or after the onset of worsening oxygenation, the patient meets both of the following criteria:
1. Temperature >38°C or <36°C, OR white blood cell count ≥12,000 cells/mm³ or ≤4,000 cells/mm³ AND
2. A new antimicrobial agent(s) is started, and is continued for ≥4 calendar days
Infection-related ventilator-associated complication (IVAC)
On or after calendar day 3 of mechanical ventilation and within 2 calendar days before or after the onset of worsening oxygenation, ONE of the following criteria is met:
1. Purulent respiratory secretions (from one or more specimen collections and defined as for possible VAP) AND one of the following:
• Positive culture of endotracheal aspirate*, ≥10^5 CFU/mL or equivalent semi-quantitative result
• Positive culture of bronchoalveolar lavage*, ≥10^4 CFU/mL or equivalent semi-quantitative result
• Positive culture of lung tissue, ≥10^4 CFU/g or equivalent semi-quantitative result
• Positive culture of protected specimen brush*, ≥10^3 CFU/mL or equivalent semi-quantitative result*
2. One of the following (without requirement for purulent respiratory secretions):
• Positive pleural fluid culture (where specimen was obtained during thoracentesis or initial placement of chest tube and NOT from an indwelling chest tube)
• Positive lung histopathology
• Positive diagnostic test for *Legionella* spp.
• Positive diagnostic test on respiratory secretions for influenza virus, respiratory syncytial virus, adenovirus, parainfluenza virus, rhinovirus, human metapneumovirus, coronavirus
On or after calendar day 3 of mechanical ventilation and within 2 calendar days before or after the onset of worsening oxygenation, ONE of the following criteria is met:
1. Purulent respiratory secretions (from one or more specimen collections)
• Defined as secretions from the lungs, bronchi, or trachea that contain >25 neutrophils and <10 squamous epithelial cells per low power field (lpf, × 100)
• If the laboratory reports semi-quantitative results, those results must correspond to the above quantitative thresholds
2. Positive culture (qualitative, semi-quantitative, or quantitative) of sputum*, endotracheal aspirate*, bronchoalveolar lavage*, lung tissue, or protected specimen brushing*
*Excludes the following:
• Normal respiratory/oral flora, mixed respiratory/oral flora, or equivalent
• *Candida* species or yeast not otherwise specified
• Coagulase-negative *Staphylococcus* species
• *Enterococcus* species
Possible ventilator-associated pneumonia (see Table 26.5)
Probable ventilator-associated pneumonia (see Table 26.6)
Patient has a baseline period of stability or improvement on the ventilator, defined by ≥2 calendar days of stable or decreasing daily minimum* F_IO_2 or PEEP values. The baseline period is defined as the 2 calendar days immediately preceding the first day of increased daily minimum PEEP or F_IO_2. Information is in the public domain.
*Daily minimum defined by lowest value of FiO_2 or PEEP during a calendar day that is maintained for at least 1 hour.
FiO_2, fractional inspired oxygen; PEEP, positive end-expiratory pressure; CFU, colony-forming unit.

Table 26.3 Ventilator-associated condition (VAC).

After a period of stability or improvement on the ventilator, the patient has at least one of the following indicators of worsening oxygenation:
1. Increase in daily minimum* F_IO_2 of ≥0.20 (20 points) over the daily minimum F_IO_2 in the baseline period, sustained for ≥2 calendar days
2. Increase in daily minimum* PEEP values of ≥3 cm H_2O over the daily minimum PEEP in the baseline period†, sustained for ≥2 calendar days

Daily minimum PEEP values of 0–5 cm H_2O are considered equivalent for the purposes of VAE surveillance.
Patient has a baseline period of stability or improvement on the ventilator, defined by ≥2 calendar days of stable or decreasing daily minimum* F_IO_2 or PEEP values. The baseline period is defined as the 2 calendar days immediately preceding the first day of increased daily minimum PEEP or F_IO_2.
*Daily minimum defined by lowest value of F_IO_2 or PEEP during a calendar day that is maintained for at least 1 hour.
FiO_2: Fractional inspired oxygen; PEEP: Positive end-expiratory pressure; VAE: Ventilator-associated events.

Table 26.5 Possible ventilator-associated pneumonia (VAP).

Patient meets criteria for VAC and IVAC
On or after calendar day 3 of mechanical ventilation and within 2 calendar days before or after the onset of worsening oxygenation, ONE of the following criteria is met:
1. Purulent respiratory secretions (from one or more specimen collections)
• Defined as secretions from the lungs, bronchi, or trachea that contain >25 neutrophils and <10 squamous epithelial cells per low power field [lpf, × 100]
• If the laboratory reports semi-quantitative results, those results must be equivalent to the above quantitative thresholds OR
2. Positive culture (qualitative, semi-quantitative, or quantitative) of sputum, endotracheal aspirate, bronchoalveolar lavage, lung tissue, or protected specimen brushing
Excludes the following:
• Normal respiratory/oral flora, mixed respiratory/oral flora, or equivalent
• *Candida* species or yeast not otherwise specified
• Coagulase-negative *Staphylococcus* species
• *Enterococcus* species

(VAC: Ventilator-associated complication; IVAC: Infection-related ventilator-associated complication).

definitions are detailed and cumbersome, and the reader is directed elsewhere if in-depth knowledge is required. It is unclear whether this terminology will ever be adopted

Table 26.4 Infection-related Ventilator-Associated Complication (IVAC).

Patient meets criteria for VAC
On or after calendar day 3 of mechanical ventilation and within 2 calendar days before or after the onset of worsening oxygenation, the patient meets both the criteria as follows:
1. Temperature >38 °C or <36°C, OR white blood cell count ≥12,000 cells/mm³ or ≤4,000 cells/mm³ AND
2. A new antimicrobial agent(s) is started, and is continued for ≥4 calendar days

(VAC: Ventilator-associated complication).

Table 26.6 Probable ventilator-associated pneumonia (VAP).

Patient meets criteria for VAC and IVAC
On or after calendar day 3 of mechanical ventilation and within 2 calendar days before or after the onset of worsening oxygenation, ONE of the following criteria is met:
1. Purulent respiratory secretions (from one or more specimen collections and defined as for possible VAP) AND one of the following:
• Positive culture of endotracheal aspirate, ≥10⁵ CFU/mL or equivalent semi-quantitative result
• Positive culture of bronchoalveolar lavage, ≥10⁴ CFU/mL or equivalent semi-quantitative result
• Positive culture of lung tissue, ≥10⁴ CFU/g or equivalent semi-quantitative result
• Positive culture of protected specimen brush, ≥10³ CFU/mL or equivalent semi-quantitative result
*Same organism exclusions as noted for possible VAP, OR
2. One of the following (without requirement for purulent respiratory secretions):
• Positive pleural fluid culture (where specimen was obtained during thoracentesis or initial placement of chest tube and NOT from an indwelling chest tube)
• Positive lung histopathology
• Positive diagnostic test for *Legionella* spp.
• Positive diagnostic test on respiratory secretions for influenza virus, respiratory syncytial virus, adenovirus, parainfluenza virus, rhinovirus, human metapneumovirus, and coronavirus

(VAC: Ventilator-associated complication; IVAC: Infection-related ventilator-associated complication; CFU: Colony forming unit).

for routine clinical use, or will remain just a construct for epidemiologic reporting to the National Healthcare Safety Network (NHSN) of CDC. An initial analysis of utility for classification of critically ill surgical patients suggests the new classification system to be inaccurate and of minimal usefulness.[53]

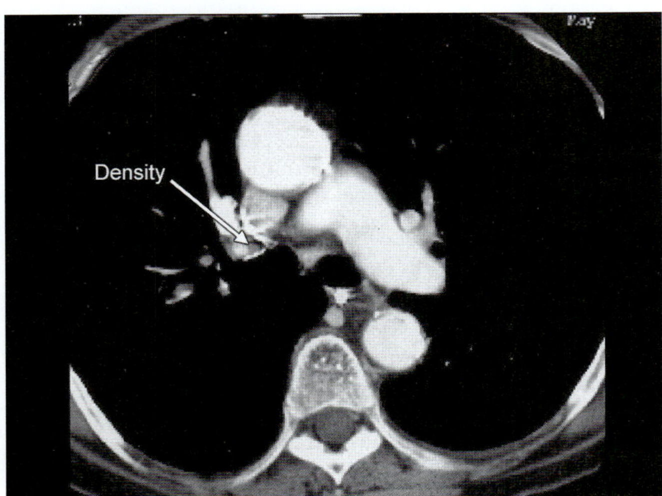

Fig. 26.13: Helical computed tomographic scan with intravenous contrast performed in a patient with suspected pulmonary embolism. A complex heterogeneous density is present in the right main pulmonary artery, consistent with pulmonary embolism.

Venous Thromboembolic Disease

Deep venous thrombosis and pulmonary embolism (or venous thromboembolic disease, VTE) are often occult and can produce sudden, catastrophic deterioration. The clinical risk, combined with the high-frequency and notoriously unreliable physical findings, means that diagnostic tests are carried out frequently. Doppler ultrasound is utilized most frequently for diagnosis of lower extremity venous thrombosis, although accuracy is low for clot in infrageniculate (below-knee) or pelvic veins.[54] Helical CT has supplanted pulmonary arteriography for the diagnosis of pulmonary embolism among patients able to receive intravenous contrast. Helical CT is excellent for visualizing thrombus in central pulmonary arteries (sensitivity and specificity, both 94%) (Fig. 26.13),[55] but it has lower sensitivity for the identification of small subsegmental clots. However, the Prospective Investigation of Pulmonary Embolism Diagnosis (PIOPED) study indicated that only 6% of patients have isolated distal emboli.[56]

Thrombus is detected in as many as 12% of patients despite the use of prophylaxis. An inexpensive whole blood D-dimer assay has high specificity and may be used to exclude VTE in patients in combination with a normal lower extremity ultrasound study, although surgical procedures may activate coagulation sufficiently to cause the assay to be positive for several days after operation.

Ventilation/perfusion scans are no longer a mainstay of pulmonary embolism diagnosis. The PIOPED study indicated that "low probability" scans had a 14% positive predicted value for the diagnosis[56] and high-probability scans had a positive predictive value of nearly 80%. However, when the CXR is abnormal, matching defects on the CXR and the perfusion scan are problematic. Scans in intensive care unit patients are therefore impractical.

PRINCIPLES OF MECHANICAL VENTILATION

A mechanical ventilator converts energy into work that augments or replaces the patient's own work of breathing.[57] Usually, the ventilator only provides assistance. Optimal ventilator management is tailored to individual ventilatory mechanics. The amount of pressure necessary to increase lung volume is crucial. Flow, pressure, and volume interact to define resistance and compliance. Compliance may decrease in conditions such as ALI/ARDS, whereas resistance may change as a result of bronchospasm or an obstructed endotracheal tube.

Ventilator function is therefore determined by the:

- Input (power transmission and conversion)
- Control paradigm (mode)
- Output (flow pattern, transpulmonary pressure, and volume).

Ventilators may be regulated by means of pressure, volume, flow, or time.[57] The choice of ventilator mode depends upon the underlying disease, physiologic reserve, and potential complications. Pressure or flow constitutes the controller in most circumstances. "Volume" ventilators actually measure and control flow and derive a calculated volume for display purposes. A flow-controlled ventilator supplies gas until a predetermined volume is delivered, regardless of the pressure necessary. Barotrauma may occur if compliance is low. A pressure-controlled ventilator delivers gas until a predetermined pressure is reached, after which gas flow ceases. Hypoventilation may occur if resistance is high or compliance is low.

Once the control variable has been determined, the ventilatory cycle can be considered. The most common variables that define a cycle are time and pressure:

- With time-triggering, the ventilator initiates breaths at a set frequency regardless of the patient's efforts
- With pressure-triggering, the patient's inspiratory effort is sensed and the breath is delivered in response to a predetermined decrement in airway pressure.

A flow trigger is more sensitive than a pressure trigger, even when the pressure trigger is maximally sensitive [i.e. 1 cm H_2O (98 Pa)], hence the work of breathing is minimized. Once provided with the desired V_T, peak inspiratory flow rate and flow waveform, modern flow-controlled ventilators adjust inspiratory time (T_I) automatically within narrow boundaries that approximate the normal T_I:expiratory time (T_E) ratio of approximately 1:3. Over-riding this relatively constant ratio (i.e. to provide inverse-ratio ventilation [IRV]) requires shifting to a pressure-controlled mode.

The clinician defines:

- Fractional inspired oxygen
- Sensitivity to patient demand
- Mode of output—options chosen frequently include a volume-preset mode, a pressure-preset mode, synchronized intermittent mandatory ventilation (SIMV), and pressure support ventilation (PSV).

In volume-preset mode, output is defined by inspiratory gas flow, V_T, the machine rate, and a timing variable (sometimes set indirectly through the choice of the flow characteristic). Each machine breath is therefore of fixed V_T regardless of the patient's effort.

In pressure-preset mode, V_T, and inspiratory flow vary with the impedance of the system and the patient's effort. Patient effort defines V_T if compliance and resistance are constant. Increased impedance can result in decreased V_E, hypoxemia, and hypercapnia, but the patient is not at risk of barotrauma or ventilator-associated lung injury (VILI).

During SIMV, a specified frequency of volume-preset breaths is delivered; the patient breathes spontaneously between machine breaths. The ventilator senses inspiratory effort before delivering the breath and will not ventilate during spontaneous exhalation, hence the synchronization.

A popular use of PSV is as an adjunct to weaning, either alone or combined with SIMV. In PSV mode, a target pressure is applied to the airway, which augments respiratory muscle inflation pressure.[58] Inspiratory flow then declines progressively to a threshold, at which time exhalation begins. It is believed that PSV offers the patient autonomy over inspiratory flow, V_T, and T_I.

Peak and plateau airway pressures are crucial parameters for the clinician to manage for patients on the ventilator. The ARDSnet trial examined conventional mechanical ventilation of patients with ALI/ARDS with a V_T of 10 mL/kg versus V_T of 6 mL/kg, and found a significant improvement in oxygenation, a decrease in VILI, and decreased mortality related to ALI/ARDS.[59] Subsequent investigation has demonstrated that low-V_T ventilation is also beneficial during routine mechanical ventilation for general anesthesia administered to moderate-to-high-risk abdominal surgery.[60] Tidal volumes as low as 4 mL/kg may be used to maintain the P_{plat} at <30 cm H_2O to minimize barotrauma (or "volutrauma").

BAROTRAUMA

Some presentations of barotrauma are subtle, whereas others cause acute profound derangements of homeostasis. Overt manifestations include pneumomediastinum, pneumopericardium, subcutaneous emphysema, pneumoperitoneum and pneumoretroperitoneum, systemic air embolism, pneumothorax, and bronchopleural fistula.

Alveolar rupture is usually the cause. For example, air that originates from a tracheostomy or a pharyngeal mucosal laceration can dissect into the mediastinum. Extrapulmonary air can also originate from the lung after blunt or penetrating chest trauma, minor procedures on the upper torso (e.g. needle lung biopsy, central venous catheter insertion), or esophageal perforation. Mediastinitis caused by gas-forming organisms can be confused radiographically with barotrauma.

Pneumomediastinum is the most frequent manifestation of barotrauma, followed by pneumothorax, and subcutaneous emphysema. Tension pneumothorax and systemic air embolism can be immediately life-threatening, whereas there is minimal risk from subcutaneous emphysema and pneumoperitoneum *per se*. The clinical presentation of patients who have pneumothorax can range from an asymptomatic radiographic finding to the agitation, respiratory distress, and hypotension of a tension pneumothorax. Clinical settings that are associated with a high risk of developing a pneumothorax include ventilation at high lung volumes (>12 mL/kg), use of PEEP >15 cm H_2O (1.5 kPa), high peak [>50 cm H_2O (4.9 kPa)] or plateau [>35 cm H_2O (3.5 kPa)] airway pressures, later-onset ARDS, and severe obstructive airways disease (COPD or asthma).

Elevated peak airway pressure used to be the consensus mechanism of barotrauma. Possible extrinsic causes of high peak airway pressure include a high peak inspiratory flow rate, high intrinsic or extrinsic airway resistance, and a small airway. Intrinsic causes of high peak airway pressure include bronchospasm, secretions, edema fluid, and any cause of airway narrowing. High pleural or transpulmonary pressures may be caused by coughing, shivering, seizures, agitation, splinting from chest wall pain, pneumothorax or pleural effusion, ascites, abdominal packs or binding, or the Trendelenburg position.

Increasing credence is now given to alveolar overdistention rather than high airway pressure in the pathogenesis of barotrauma. The likelihood of pneumothorax can be reduced by using smaller V_T (~6 mL/kg) and avoiding hyperventilation. If barotrauma develops, it is most important to manage the underlying illness. Reduction of PEEP, V_T, and V_E to the lowest possible levels is important and permissive hypercapnia (pH >7.20, $PaCO_2$ <80 mm Hg) should be considered. "Prophylactic" chest tubes are not mandatory in patients at risk or for those who have pneumomediastinum alone. However, any pneumothorax that develops on positive pressure ventilation should be decompressed to ensure that it will not recur because of the risk of tension pneumothorax.

VENTILATOR-ASSOCIATED LUNG INJURY

Acute lung injury and ARDS affect the lungs heterogeneously. The distribution of edema fluid, ventilated versus flooded alveoli, and consequently V_A/Q matching vary among gas exchange units. Moreover, the lung manifests a brisk local and systemic inflammatory response when injured or when ventilated mechanically. The ARDSnet trial[59] demonstrated improved outcomes from ALI/ARDS after ventilation with lower V_T and V_E, resulting in lower airway pressures, less overdistention of recruitable alveoli, less shear stress on lung tissue, and lower mortality despite the paradox that most patients with ALI/ARDS do not die from an inability to oxygenate or ventilate. Rather, most such patients die in association with the multiple organ dysfunction syndrome, which has been linked closely with a rampant systemic inflammatory response. If less ventilation is better, it is hypothesized that more ventilation may be injurious, or indeed provocative to the lung, leading to the concept of ventilator-associated lung injury (VALI).[61]

VALI occurs from excessive mechanical stress to the lung, either from excessive V_T or excessive airway pressure. Mechanical ventilation induces a pulmonary and systemic cytokine response, which can be minimized by limiting overdistention and phasic recruitment/derecruitment of lung. Experimental and clinical data demonstrate that the mechanism of VALI is the proinflammatory response in the lung and the periphery, and that the response and injury are attenuated by lung protective ventilation strategies.

ALTERNATIVES TO CONVENTIONAL MECHANICAL VENTILATION

In some circumstances, conventional mechanical ventilator modalities may be unnecessary or even inadequate to the task (e.g. refractory hypoxemia or too-high airway pressures). Whereas modern ventilators allow modification of flow rate and flow patterns to accomplish adequate, safe mechanical ventilation while minimizing deleterious effects, consideration should be given as to whether the patient's oxygenation and ventilation can be maintained noninvasively.

Noninvasive Ventilation

Ventilatory support delivered without establishing an endotracheal airway is "noninvasive ventilation" (NIV). Current technique utilizes positive pressure ventilation delivered through a nasal or face mask, and its usage is expanding in the management of acute and chronic respiratory failure and potentially for some patients with heart failure. Putative benefits of NIV are numerous, owing to avoidance of the complications of endotracheal intubation. Noninvasive ventilation preserves swallowing, feeding, speech, cough, and physiologic air warming and humidification by the naso-oropharynx. Nonintubated patients communicate more effectively, require less sedation, and are more comfortable. In addition, patients are often able to continue with standard oral nutrition. Noninvasive ventilation eliminates complications such as trauma with tube insertion, mucosal ulceration, aspiration, infection (e.g. pneumonia, sinusitis), and dysphagia after extubation.

In a randomized, prospective trial of 48 patients with acute hypoxemic respiratory insufficiency following pulmonary resection, Auriant and colleagues compared standard mechanical ventilation with nasal mask NIV.[62] The need for postoperative reintubation and mortality were reduced in patients receiving NIV as a part of respiratory support. Similarly, Squadrone and co-workers randomized 209 patients with respiratory failure in the postanesthesia care unit after major abdominal surgery to oxygen alone, or with continuous positive airway pressure (CPAP) by mask.[63] Patients who received oxygen plus CPAP had a significantly lower intubation rate, and also lower rates of pneumonia, infection, and sepsis.

Crucial to successful NIV is an awake, cooperative, spontaneously breathing patient. Airway, electrocardiographic, or hemodynamic instability argues against the use of NIV. An additional requirement is an intact cough reflex and ability to clear secretions, the absence of which is a common reason for failure of NIV. Relative contraindications include the inability to fit and seal the mask adequately, inability to cough with prompting, or inability to remove the mask in the event of emesis. A hypothetical contraindication is recent gastrointestinal surgery with aerophagia and gut distention. If pressures used to ventilate the patient are kept <30 mm Hg, the closing pressure of the lower esophageal sphincter should not be exceeded, and aerophagia should be avoided. Morbid obesity is also a relative contraindication owing to increased airway pressure requirements arising from body habitus and the weight of the chest wall and abdominal viscera while the patient is supine.

The most common complication of NIV is focal skin necrosis, which is most common over the bridge of the nose but may also occur over the zygoma. The incidence is 7–10% among patients receiving full-face mask NIV. Other complications (incidences, 1–2% each) include gastric distention, aspiration, and pneumothorax. Conceptual concerns with gastric distention are subsequent vomiting, aspiration, and pneumonia. Conjunctivitis may develop secondary to air leaks near the eyes in about 2% of patients. The most serious complication is failure to recognize when NIV is not providing a patient with adequate ventilation, oxygenation, or airway patency. Delayed placement of an artificial airway, or failure of placement thereof, may cause continued deterioration or death.

Pressure-Controlled Ventilation

Pressure-controlled ventilation (PCV) is a pressure-limited, time-cycled mode that is controlled completely by the ventilator, without patient participation. Inspiratory P_{aw} increases early in the respiratory cycle, and is maintained at that specified P_{aw} throughout the remainder of the inspiratory phase. In PCV, inspiratory flow decreases exponentially during lung inflation in order to keep P_{aw} at the preselected value. The primary disadvantage of PCV is the tendency for inflation volumes to vary with changes in the mechanical properties of the lungs. When a constant peak inflation P_{aw} is reached, the inflation volume decreases as airway resistance increases or lung compliance decreases.

Inverse-Ratio Ventilation

Inverse-ratio ventilation is a combination of PCV (hence, PC–IRV) with a prolonged T_I. One way to increase T_I is to decrease the inspiratory flow rate; the T_I:T_E ratio from the usual 1:3–4 to 2:1 (up to 4:1). Benefits of IRV include improved oxygenation and the prevention of atelectasis. On occasion, the early use of PC–IRV can facilitate tapering of F_IO_2 and decrease PEEP and peak inspiratory P_{aw}. Detrimental during PC–IRV is potential stacking of breaths (auto-PEEP) because T_E is so short, with high P_{aw}, hyperinflation and volutrauma, CO_2 retention, decreased $\dot{Q}$ from impaired venous return, and metabolic acidosis.

Airway Pressure Release Ventilation

Airway pressure release ventilation (APRV), which has been available since the mid-1990s but is still not used universally, allows for the unloading during exhalation of any positive pressure provided during inhalation, in order to facilitate the egress of the tidal breath. Release of airway pressure from an elevated baseline simulates exhalation. Technically, APRV is time-triggered, pressure-limited, time-cycled mechanical ventilation. Conceptualizing APRV as CPAP with regular, brief, intermittent releases of P_{aw} may facilitate understanding. It can augment V_E in the patient breathing spontaneously, or provide full support to the apneic patient. Advantages of APRV include lower peak P_{aw}, lower P_{pl}, lower V_E, minimal effect on $\dot{Q}$, and improved $\dot{V}A/\dot{Q}$ matching. The mode may facilitate spontaneous breathing by the patient. Sedation requirements may be decreased, and neuromuscular blockade should be able to be avoided. Disadvantages of APRV include the pressure-limited control of ventilation, increased effects of airway and circuit resistance on ventilation, decreased transpulmonary pressure (P_L), and potential interference with spontaneous ventilation. Facilitated exhalation may make APRV beneficial in patients with bronchospasm or reactive airways disease. This mode of ventilation can be used as a weaning modality. Although increasingly popular, and anecdotal evidence suggests that it may be beneficial,[64] the advantage of APRV over other modes of ventilation is unproved.

The terminology of APRV differs somewhat from other modes of mechanical ventilation. Four important terms include pressure high (P_{high}), pressure low (P_{low}), time high (T_{high}), and time low (T_{low}). The P_{high} term describes the baseline P_{aw} (the higher of the two pressures), alternatively called CPAP, inflating pressure, or the $P1$ pressure. The P_{low} term describes the P_{aw} resulting from the release of pressure (alternatively called PEEP, release pressure, or the $P2$ pressure). The T_{high} time refers to the time during which P_{high} is maintained ($T1$), whereas T_{low} refers to the duration of time when airway pressure is released ($T2$). Mean airway pressure can be calculated from the equation:

$$\frac{(\text{P1} \times \text{T1}) + (\text{P2} \times \text{T2})}{\text{T2} + \text{T1}}$$

Application of APRV to the patient must be individualized. Initial settings are deduced partly from the result of conventional mechanical ventilation, which should be attempted initially for most patients. The plateau airway pressure (P_{plat}) from conventional ventilation (if not >35 cm H_2O) is converted to P_{high}, aiming for a V_E of 2–3 L/min (lower than with conventional ventilation). The P_{low} is set initially at 0 cm H_2O. The setting for T_{high} is a minimum of 4 seconds, and T_{low} is set at approximately 0.8 second (0.5–1.0 s). Spontaneous breathing is permitted. Rarely, a higher P_{high} (40–45 cm H_2O) is needed for patients with low compliance (e.g. morbid obesity, abdominal distention, and ARDS). For all patients, T_{high} is lengthened progressively to 12–15 seconds, usually in 1–2 second increments, as lung mechanics improve. Longer T_{high} prevents the cyclical opening and closing of small airways that is believed to be a cause of VILI. The T_{low} parameter is optimized when expiratory flow decreases to 25–50% of peak expiratory flow.

Clinical improvement may not occur until 8–16 hours after transitioning to APRV (also with IRV). After improvement, weaning from APRV is guided by general principles of weaning. Weaning from APRV is accomplished primarily by manipulation of P_{high} and T_{high}. High pressure is decreased in increments of 2–3 cm H_2O down to about 15 cm H_2O, and T_{high} is lengthened progressively to 12–15 seconds, usually in 1–2 second increments. Minute ventilation must be monitored carefully for signs of hypoventilation during the transition. The goal is to switch the patient to pure CPAP of 6–12 cm H_2O, at which point the patient may be extubated, all conditions permitting.

Some confusion arises with similar modes of ventilation. Other than that it is usually used noninvasively, bi-level positive airway pressure (BiPAP) differs from APRV only in the timing of T_{high} and T_{low}; the latter is longer in BiPAP.

ADJUNCTIVE AND RESCUE MODALITIES

Heliox

Helium has lower density than O_2 or N_2. Substituting helium for N_2 reduces the density and thus viscosity of the gas in direct proportion to the amount of helium admixed. Breathing heliox (the concentration in clinical use ranges from 80:20 to 60:40) results in more laminar flow, reduced airway resistance, and reduced work of breathing. Heliox may be useful in clinical situations where resistance to airflow is high, including asthma, acute exacerbations of chronic bronchitis or COPD, other causes of bronchospasm, and upper airway obstruction with stridor. Breathing heliox is well tolerated, without notable adverse effects. Disadvantages include high cost and limited utility when a high F_IO_2 is required. Ventilators must also be recalibrated when heliox is delivered by ventilator rather than face mask (the usual route), to ensure that the flow of gas is measured correctly.

Permissive Hypercapnia

Permissive hypercapnia may develop when the lungs are ventilated with a low V_T, permitting $PaCO_2$ to increase. Permissive hypercapnia aims to avoid hyperinflation-induced VILI by limiting P_{plat} (as a surrogate of static alveolar pressure) to approximately 30–35 cm H_2O while allowing $PaCO_2$ to increase in the absence of any contraindications. Contraindications and adverse effects include cerebral edema or high intracranial pressure, convulsions, depressed cardiac function, arrhythmias, increased pulmonary vascular resistance, tachypnea, increased work of breathing, dyspnea, respiratory distress, headache, sweating, and biochemical disturbances related to acidosis. Permissive hypercapnia may be utilized up to physiologic limits (i.e. $PaCO_2$ up to 80 mm Hg, arterial pH as low as 7.20). The absolute level of $PaCO_2$ and the permissible degree of acidosis is debated, as there is concern of alveolar derecruitment and possible worsening of V_A/Q mismatching, as well as potential adverse effects on the central nervous, cardiovascular, and renal systems.

Prone Positioning

Prone positioning, most commonly using a specialty bed, is a modality that improves oxygenation by decreasing V_A/Q mismatching. [65] Positive-pressure ventilation exacerbates mismatching by creating zone I conditions in nondependent lung, especially in supine patients. Ventilated lung segments that tend to be in nondependent portions of lung, and perfused lung segments (and higher pulmonary vascular pressures and hence, lung edema) that tend to be in dependent portions of lung are inverted by PP, and newly-dependent well-ventilated lung segments are well perfused for several hours until the effects of gravity and positive airway pressure restore the previous conditions, at which time the patient may be returned to the supine position. Drainage of secretions may also be facilitated in the prone position. The cycle may be repeated several times. Several trials have shown improvement in PaO_2:FiO_2 and mortality when PP is used to treat ARDS.[66,67] Complications with PP include pressure sores, increased need for sedation, facial edema, and difficulty maintaining airway patency or restoring it if compromised when the patient is inverted.[67]

Inhalation Therapy—Nitric Oxide and Epoprostenol

Inhaled nitric oxide is a selective pulmonary vasodilator that acts on the alveolar endothelium to produce regional vasodilation in well-ventilated lung units. Nitric oxide at a dose of 40 PPM improves V_A/Q mismatching, hypoxemia, and pulmonary hypertension in patients with ALI/ARDS. By contrast, systemic vasodilators cause pulmonary vasodilation in nonventilated lung, thereby abrogating hypoxic vasoconstriction and exacerbating V_A/Q inequality and hypoxemia. Nitric oxide is also a bronchodilator and has beneficial anti-inflammatory properties for lung transplant patients. After inhalation, it diffuses rapidly into the bloodstream, where it is metabolized rapidly and excreted via the urine, minimizing systemic effects. Several randomized trials suggest that iNO• may improve oxygenation for up to 72 hours, but neither increased survival nor a shorter duration of mechanical ventilation was observed. Also, rebound pulmonary hypertension has been reported with cessation of therapy.

Epoprostenol (also known as prostacyclin or PGI_2) has vasodilator, antiproliferative, antithrombotic, anti-inflammatory, and antimitogenic properties, the former of which is most germane hereto. Prostacyclin performs its function through a paracrine signaling cascade that activates G protein-coupled receptors on platelets and endothelial cells. This, in turn, signals adenylyl cyclase to produce cyclic adenosine monophosphate (cAMP), which activates protein kinase A (PKA). Protein kinase A then continues the cascade by phosphorylating the myosin light chain and inhibiting myosin light-chain kinase, which leads to smooth muscle relaxation and vasodilation.

Nine prospective randomized controlled trials have been published for iNO•, reporting on changes in oxygenation or clinical outcomes.[68] Seven reports of aerosolized epoprostenol (aEPO) were examined for changes in oxygenation. [68] Based on available data, the use of either iNO or aEPO is safe to use in patients with ALI or ARDS to improve oxygenation transiently. No differences have been observed in survival, ventilator-free days, or attenuation in disease severity. Therefore, neither iNO• nor epoprostenol is recommended currently for rescue therapy of ALI/ARDS.

High-Frequency Ventilation

High-frequency ventilation has been used with success for respiratory failure in neonates and children. This modality achieves low mean P_{aw} at low V_T (often smaller than V_D) and a high-frequency respiratory rate (2.5–30 Hz) to achieve ventilation while preventing alveolar overdistention. This mode is conceptually attractive, as it achieves many of the goals of lung-protective ventilation. High-frequency ventilation is used most often to support complex thoracic surgical procedures (e.g. one-lung or split-lung ventilation), or to facilitate fiberoptic bronchoscopy or healing of bronchopleural fistulae. In a single randomized trial, HFV was ineffective for adult patients with severe ARDS who have failed conventional ventilation.[69]

Independent Lung Ventilation

Acute lung injury is recognized to be heterogeneous within a lung, but also may be heterogeneous between lungs (e.g. aspiration pneumonitis confined to one lung). The left lung is smaller than the right in human beings. Moreover, when lung injury is asymmetric, differences in compliance exist between the lungs. Consequently, conventional mechanical ventilation delivers a larger V_T to the more compliant lung, which may cause overdistention and VILI. Additionally, overdistention disrupts blood flow through alveolar vessels, diverting flow to the underventilated lung, worsening V_A/Q mismatch. Independent lung ventilation (ILV) has been described to ventilate the more-diseased lung while avoiding overdistention of the more-normal lung.

Using a dual-lumen endotracheal tube with a bifurcated tip such that each mainstem bronchus can be intubated separately, gas can be delivered using two ventilators, dedicated one to each lung. Typically, the V_T is set equal for both lungs, but this may be irrational both anatomically and physiologically, as the left lung is usually smaller than the right, and higher airway pressure may be anticipated in the more-injured lung. Alternatively, ventilator settings may be adjusted to produce equal P_{plat} in both lungs. The ventilators may be managed independently, and the lungs may be monitored independently by pressure measurements, compliance calculations, and capnography.

Independent lung ventilation is used seldom. Modern ventilators and lung-protective ventilation strategies have obviated many of the difficulties that made ILV attractive when described initially in the 1970s. The dual-lumen endotracheal tube is challenging to place and keep positioned. Patients require heavy sedation and oftentimes neuromuscular blockade. Combinations of ILV with newer modes of ventilation have not been described.

Extracorporeal Membrane Oxygenation

Extracorporeal membrane oxygenation provides oxygenation of blood and CO_2 removal via an extracorporeal circuit by the application of intermediate-term cardiopulmonary bypass for the treatment of potentially reversible cardiac or pulmonary failure for patients of any age. If successful, sufficient gas exchange permits reduced support of positive-pressure ventilation or even extubation, thereby lowering the incidence of VILI, VAP, and other complications associated with mechanical ventilation. The original logic of ECMO for severe respiratory failure is that marginal patients may be rescued if their lungs are allowed to rest and heal rather than endure the morbidity of mechanical ventilation, high F_IO_2, and high P_{aw} that might otherwise be required, but ECMO is not available in all centers. Extracorporeal membrane oxygenation has been considered for treatment of severe ARDS affecting adult patients when all other treatment options have failed, but advocates argue that earlier use is appropriate and could improve outcomes.

Over the years, ECMO therapy has undergone substantial changes in indications, technique, and materials. Technical progress has been made in the pumps, oxygenators, and coating of artificial surfaces, leading to greater biocompatibility and a lower rate of procedure-related complications. Injury of the thoracic aorta, even if contained, is a contraindication to ECMO use. The potential of new inline pumps in combination with a decreasing incidence of procedure-related complications may lead to a re-evaluation of the role of ECMO in the early therapy of ARDS.

EVALUATION OF RESPIRATORY FAILURE

Hypoxemia

There are many possible causes of hypoxemia. The FiO_2 may be too low. Ventilator malfunction or inappropriate settings must be excluded. There may be a gas leak or a disconnection from the patient. Hypoventilation may occur as a result of diminished drive related to fatigue, medications, or neurologic injury. Artifact related to a sensor malfunction must also be considered.

Increased V_A/Q inequality may result from progressive disease or hypovolemia. Airway-related causes of hypoventilation include bronchospasm, mechanical obstruction, intrinsic PEEP, or frequent suctioning. Pulmonary vasodilators abolish hypoxic vasoconstriction and can worsen Qs/Qt. Other causes of Qs/Qt include atelectasis, pneumothorax, pulmonary edema, pulmonary parenchymal hemorrhage, and pneumonia.

Low DO_2 may result from decreased perfusion, hemoglobin concentration, or SaO_2. Hemodialysis can cause hypoxemia for several reasons and pulmonary embolism must be considered. Initial management is to increase the F_IO_2 to 1.0 while ventilating the patient by hand. Ventilator settings and the function of sensors should be confirmed.

Bilateral ventilation and a possible tension pneumothorax are shown by auscultation. Direct laryngoscopy is used to confirm that the airway tube is properly positioned. A portable CXR should be performed and end-tidal CO_2 ($P_{ET}CO_2$) determined.

Hypocapnia or Hypercapnia

Normally, $PaCO_2$ is higher than $P_{ET}CO_2$ by 1 mm Hg so capnography is reliable as a continuous measure. Hypocapnia is a clue to the etiology of hypoxemia and $P_{ET}CO_2$ provides useful information itself as follows:

- Loss of the capnograph signal indicates disconnection from the ventilator and hypocapnia excludes the presence of hypoventilation
- Sudden increases in $P_{ET}CO_2$ can be caused by increased perfusion, the release of a tourniquet, or sodium bicarbonate therapy
- Gradual increases in $P_{ET}CO_2$ can be caused by hypoventilation or increased CO_2 production from catabolism
- Sudden decreases in $P_{ET}CO_2$ may be caused by hyperventilation, decreased perfusion, pulmonary or air embolism, obstruction of the airway, or a gas leak
- Gradual increases in $P_{ET}CO_2$ may be caused by decreased VO_2 or decreased pulmonary perfusion
- Undetectable $P_{ET}CO_2$ from the onset reflects esophageal intubation.

Acute respiratory alkalosis has many causes. Excessive V_E often results from inappropriate ventilator settings. Pain, discomfort, or agitation should be considered, and occasionally the optimal treatment may be extubation. Some patients who have brain injuries manifest central neurogenic hyperventilation. Patients who have metabolic acidosis hyperventilate to correct arterial pH.

Acute respiratory acidosis also has many causes, including inadequate V_E from inappropriate ventilator settings. Oversedation, excessive analgesia, or an acute change in mental status should also be considered. Patients, who have metabolic alkalosis, hypoventilate to correct arterial pH. The usual causes of metabolic alkalosis in patients who have had a surgical operation are hypokalemia, loss of gastrointestinal fluids, and diuretics.

ACUTE RESPIRATORY DISTRESS SYNDROME

The spectrum of injury in ARDS is broad and the injuries are heterogeneous. Not every patient has severe disease or progresses to the chronic fibroproliferative form of the syndrome.[70] As a result of this variability, the diagnosis is usually based upon clinical criteria, but the enormous variation of definitions used in the literature makes comparisons difficult among the studies.

Diagnostic criteria for ARDS have been updated by recent consensus.[71] The consensus criteria require (1) an onset within 1 week of a known clinical insult or new or worsening respiratory symptoms; (2) bilateral CXR opacities not explained by effusions, atelectasis, or nodularity; (3) respiratory failure not explained by cardiac failure or fluid overload (echocardiography is needed to exclude hydrostatic edema); and (4) a specified degree of hypoxemia (Table 26.7). Criteria reflecting decreased lung compliance and pulmonary wedge pressure measurements have been supplanted. Using the Berlin definition, stages of mild, moderate, and severe ARDS were associated with increased mortality (27%, 95% confidence interval [CI] 24–30%; 32%, 95% CI 29–34%; and 45%, 95% CI 42–48%, respectively; P <0.001) and increased median duration of mechanical ventilation in survivors (5 d, interquartile range [IQR] 2–11 d; 7 d, IQR 4–14 d; and 9 d, IQR 5–17 d, respectively; P <0.001). However, the Berlin consensus definition had poor predictive validity for mortality, with an area under the receiver-operating characteristic curve of 0.577 (95% CI, 0.561–0.593).

The lung injury score (LIS) (Table 26.8)[72] is one of several scores that describe pulmonary injury reproducibly and accurately. Radiographic, oxygenation, ventilation, and compliance criteria are summed and divided by the number of components assessed. A score >2.5 points defines ARDS, whereas a score of <2.5 reflects congestive heart failure and less severe forms of ALI. The LIS can be manipulated by therapy, specifically the use of PEEP, but PEEP also improves oxygenation, so it does not matter whether the calculation is made before or after instituting PEEP. Both the consensus conference definition and the LIS have a positive predictive value of >90% for the diagnosis of ARDS.

The development of ARDS is rarely subtle. The patient should have a clearly defined clinical risk factor and is

Table 26.7 Oxygenation criteria for the 2012 Berlin consensus conference definition of acute respiratory distress syndrome (ARDS).

Degree of hypoxemia	*PaO_2:FiO_2*	*PEEP or CPAP level*
Mild	200–<300	>5 cm H_2O
Moderate	100–<200	>5 cm H_2O
Severe	<100	>5 cm H_2O

Source: Adapted with permission from The ARDS Definition Task Force. Acute respiratory distress syndrome. The Berlin definition. JAMA. 2012;2526-33.

(*PaO_2*: Arterial partial pressure of oxygen; *FiO_2*: Fractional inspired oxygen; PEEP: Positive end-expiratory pressure; CPAP: Continuous positive airway pressure).

Table 26.8 Lung injury score for diagnosis of acute respiratory distress syndrome.

Parameter	*Points*
Chest Radiograph	
No infiltrate	0
One quadrant	1
Two quadrants	2
Three quadrants	3
Four quadrants	4
Hypoxemia: PaO_2:FiO_2	
>300	0
225–299	1
175–224	2
100–174	3
<100	4
Positive end-expiratory pressure (cm H_2O)	
<5	0
6–8	1
9–11	2
12–14	3
>15	4
Static compliance (mL/cm H_2O)	
>80	0
60–79	1
40–59	2
20–39	3
<19	4
Lung Injury Score (LIS) is obtained by dividing the sum of the points scored by the number of components used and ARDS is defined as LIS >2.5.	

Source: Adapted with permission from Murray JF, Matthay MA, Luce JM, et al. An expanded definition of the adult respiratory distress syndrome. Am Rev Respir Dis. 1988;138:720-6.

(*PaO_2*: Arterial partial pressure of oxygen; *FiO_2*: Fractional inspired oxygen; ARDS: Acute respiratory distress syndrome).

almost always in respiratory distress if not overt respiratory failure. Tachypnea is often the first sign, particularly with spontaneous ventilation. Hypoxemia may precede clinically apparent pulmonary edema, but treatment to reduce edema (diuretics, ultrafiltration) may not improve the hypoxemia.

The radiographic lesion of ARDS is a typical "ground glass" infiltrate that is coalescent and diffuse. Derangements in gas exchange may occur without radiologic changes. As the injury progresses, dyspnea develops as interstitial edema progresses to alveolar flooding, resulting in atelectasis and decreased FRC.

Decreasing PaO_2 or increasing $D(A-a)O_2$ are not good markers of lung injury in ARDS. In the setting of Qs/Qt, decreased PvO_2 can lower PaO_2 subsequently because there is direct mixing of venous with arterial blood through areas of shunt. Oxygen extraction from ventilated alveoli is already maximal and cannot compensate. A low Pvo_2 may result from low PaO_2, low hemoglobin concentration, low perfusion, or increased VO_2. This heterogeneity, reflective of underlying disease or injury, is a crucial issue because death of ARDS patients usually results from multiple organ dysfunction syndrome rather than respiratory failure.

PREVENTION OF RESPIRATORY FAILURE

Preoperative Preparation and Assessment

Many patients who develop acute respiratory failure in the perioperative period do so because of catastrophic illness rather than intrinsic pulmonary disease. Preoperative testing is of no value or impossible in an emergency situation. However, preoperative assessment of pulmonary function is of value for patients who have a history of lung disease or those for whom pulmonary resection is contemplated.[73]

The criteria for increased risk of pulmonary morbidity after thoracotomy are well established, but not for patients who have other types of operations. Operability for pulmonary resection is assessed by evaluation of:

- Baseline pulmonary function
- The contribution of the tissue proposed for resection to overall pulmonary function (by split-function studies) or pulmonary vascular studies, as pulmonary resection can sometimes precipitate cor pulmonale.

Preoperative assessment of the candidate for nonthoracic operations should focus on identification of chronic airway obstruction, possible preoperative therapy to minimize risk, and the choice of operative incision in the case of laparotomy. Outcomes may be improved if operation is performed under regional rather than general anesthesia.[74] However, few data suggest that outcome is improved by optimizing pulmonary function before elective procedures.

Information of value from the history includes the frequency and intensity of bronchospasm, previous asthma therapy (including previous hospitalizations and corticosteroid use), and previous mechanical ventilation. The smoking history should be quantitated. Nutritional status, concomitant heart disease, and current therapy (including O_2 use) should be documented, as should recent changes in cough or sputum production suggestive of infection.

Physical examination findings are often absent. Use of accessory muscles, a "barrel" chest and cyanosis are uncommon except in advanced emphysema. Chest auscultation of a patient who has asthma may be normal between episodes. Evidence of right ventricular failure (peripheral edema, prominent right ventricular impulse, loud or widely split P_2 heart sound, and neck vein distention) should be sought specifically.

A preoperative CXR may be of value for patients who have symptoms of airway obstruction. Radiographic clues to airway obstruction include depression of the right hemidiaphragm at or below the seventh rib anteriorly on a conventional posteroanterior view, a cardiac silhouette that has a transverse dimension <11.5 cm, and a retrosternal air space (i.e. the space between posterior edge of the sternum and cardiac silhouette on a lateral CXR) measuring >4.4 cm. Important airflow obstruction may be associated with a normal CXR. Hyperlucency and increased bronchial markings are not valuable as indicators of chronic lung disease.[75]

Most laboratory studies are of little predictive benefit, although the blood urea nitrogen and serum albumin concentrations have been incorporated into a risk prediction model for postoperative respiratory failure derived from male patients who received care in the US Veterans Affairs (VA) Healthcare System (Table 26.9).[76] This model is simple to apply and may be useful for identification of the patient at risk, although the single most powerful predictor in the model is open abdominal aortic aneurysm repair (an operation that is now performed seldom), and it has not been validated for female patients. Chronic obstructive pulmonary disease is a modest predictor. In COPD, elevated $[HCO_3^-]$ suggests chronic respiratory acidosis. Polycythemia may suggest chronic hypoxemia. A PaO_2 of <60 mm Hg (8.0 kPa) on room air correlates with pulmonary hypertension and a $PaCO_2$ >45 mm Hg (>6.0 kPa)

Table 26.9 Multifactorial risk index for predicting postoperative respiratory failure in men undergoing major noncardiac surgery.

Preoperative predictor		*Point value*
Type of surgery		
Open abdominal aortic aneurysm		27
Thoracic		21
Neurosurgery		14
Upper abdominal		14
Peripheral vascular		14
Emergency surgery		11
Serum albumin concentration <3 g/L		9
Blood urea nitrogen concentration (>30 mg/dL)		8
Partial or full dependency		7
History of chronic obstructive pulmonary disease		6
Age		
>70 years		6
60–69 years		4
Risk stratum	Point values	Probability of postoperative respiratory failure
1	<10	0.5%
2	11–19	2.2%
3	20–27	5.0%
4	28–40	11.6%
5	>40	30.5%

Source: Adapted from Arozullah AM, Daloy J, Henderson WG, et al. Multifactorial risk index for predicting postoperative respiratory failure in men undergoing major noncardiac surgery. Ann Surg. 2000;232:242-53.

is associated with increased perioperative morbidity.[77] Electrocardiography may reveal pulmonary hypertension (right axis deviation, right ventricular hypertrophy, and right atrial enlargement). Supraventricular tachycardia is common during acute exacerbations of COPD and also in stable patients postoperatively.[78] Such arrhythmias in patients who have COPD reflect a poor prognosis.[79]

Spirometry before and after bronchodilators is simple and safe to carry out. The forced expiratory volume in one second (FEV_1) and forced vital capacity (FVC) usually provide sufficient information for clinical decision making. Dyspnea occurs when FEV_1 is <2 L, whereas an FEV_1 <50% of the predicted value predicts exertional dyspnea. In COPD, FVC decreases less than the FEV_1, which results in an FEV_1:FVC <0.8.[80] Spirometric abnormalities correlate with the incidence of postoperative atelectasis and pneumonia, particularly if:

- FEV_1 is <1.2 L or <70% of that predicted
- FVC is <1.7 L or <70% of that predicted or
- FEV_1:FVC is <0.65.[81,82]

If spirometric parameters improve by >15% after bronchodilators, therapy should be instituted perioperatively. If pulmonary resection is contemplated, abnormal spirometry may be followed by split-lung function studies (bronchospirometry, radionuclide imaging with ^{133}Xe ^{99m}Tc). An FEV_1 value from the contralateral lung >800 mL is required to proceed with pneumonectomy.[83] For abdominal operations, there is no indication for studies other than spirometry and arterial blood gas analysis.

Chronic bronchodilator therapy should be continued. Patients who have COPD may benefit from preoperative oral antibiotics if they have bronchitis and purulent sputum, but expectorants and mucolytic agents are useless and may actually promote bronchospasm.[84] Cessation of cigarette smoking is important for all patients who smoke >10 cigarettes per day.[85] Even short-term abstinence (48 hours):

- Decreases the carboxyhemoglobin level to that of a nonsmoker
- Abolishes the cardiovascular effects of nicotine
- Improves mucosal ciliary function.

Sputum volume decreases after 1–2 weeks of abstinence and spirometry improves after about 6 weeks.

Prevention of Specific Abnormalities

Aspiration can be minimized by meticulous clinical care. Nasogastric tubes, if present, should be left in place for the minimum time needed. Medications that cause obtundation should be given sparingly. The head of the bed is kept 30° elevated at all times unless contraindicated or hemodynamic measurements are being taken.[43,46] Tube cuff leaks must be reported and corrected promptly, by reintubation if necessary. All patients who have had a translaryngeal airway for >7 days should have a swallowing evaluation before oral feeding is attempted because the incidence of glottic dysfunction is high. If a feeding tube has not been implanted surgically into the stomach or duodenum, enteral feedings may be administered postpylorically by a soft nasoduodenal tube, or via the stomach with the aid of a prokinetic agent (i.e. erythromycin) if high gastric residuals are detected via diligent regular monitoring.

Nosocomial pneumonia is linked with aspiration,[86] so prevention of aspiration is germane in preventing pneumonia. In addition, early extubation using a fast-track weaning protocol is beneficial[87] because of the association between pneumonia and prolonged intubation. Systemic antibiotic use should be minimized.[43,44] The use of closed-system airway suction catheters may also be beneficial. Selective digestive decontamination with topical and oral antibiotics is controversial, but the addition of topical 0.12% chlorhexidine mouthwash applied to buccal mucosa (as part of a "ventilator bundle") is effective to reduce the risk of VAP, i.e. head-of-bed up 30° insofar as possible, daily sedation holiday/assessment for liberation from ventilator, VTE prophylaxis, prophylaxis against gastric stress-related gastric mucosal hemorrhage with a histamine H_2 receptor antagonist, or proton-pump inhibitor.[88]

Prevention of VTE is essential but complex.[54,89] Prophylaxis may be directed at deep venous thrombosis or pulmonary embolism. Virtually any patient who undergoes a general anesthetic of >30 minutes duration has an increased risk of developing VTE. The highest risk exists in someone who has had a previous episode of VTE, but other inherently high-risk situations include cancer operations, major pelvic operations, orthopedic operations on the pelvis or lower limbs, multiple injuries associated with prolonged immobility (especially neurologic injuries or combined neurologic and orthopedic injuries) and obesity.[90,91] Prophylaxis of postoperative VTE must be tailored to risk; for example, continuation for 4 weeks following abdominal cancer operations is now recommended.[90]

Early ambulation is important for everyone and is sufficient for patients having minor operations.[90,91] For patients at moderate risk (>40 years of age, general anesthesia, and no high-risk factors), sequential compression devices or subcutaneous unfractionated heparin are sufficient. For patients at high risk, mechanical compression and a subcutaneous heparinoid or fondaparinux have been combined, although the synergistic benefit is debatable. Low-dose warfarin is a consideration for high-risk patients, but has largely been supplanted by the subcutaneous low-molecular-weight heparins (LMWH), which are effective for prophylaxis[90,91] (and therapy) and may be associated with a slightly lower risk of bleeding complications as compared to subcutaneous unfractionated heparin.[92] The association between spinal hematoma and epidural catheter use in patients who receive LMWH contraindicates these agents for patients who are receiving epidural analgesia, and for 12 hours before and after catheter insertion and removal.

Interruption of the vena cava with a "filter" placed percutaneously is very expensive and may trade a decreased risk of early pulmonary embolism for an increased risk of developing recurrent deep venous thrombosis later.[93] Vena cava filters have been advocated prophylactically for some high-risk patients (e.g. trauma and spinal cord injury patients), but cost-effectiveness has not been demonstrated. A clear indication for filter placement is documented VTE in a patient who cannot receive heparin (e.g. as a result of a recent neurosurgical operation, active gastrointestinal bleeding, or heparin-associated thrombocytopenia).

Only a few measures are of documented benefit in reducing the risk of developing ARDS.[94-96] Prevention of aspiration is germane, as are measures to reduce the risk of nosocomial infection.[97] Rapid, effective resuscitation, and operative control of primary sources of infection or bleeding from injuries is intuitive. Early long bone fracture stabilization is beneficial.[98] Blood transfusion should be minimized, and avoided unless absolutely necessary.[99]

MANAGEMENT OF RESPIRATORY FAILURE

Atelectasis

Atelectasis is the most common cause of early postoperative fever[100] and can therefore cause morbidity (e.g. tachycardia, increased Vo_2, and catabolism) as well as pulmonary dysfunction. Noninvasive measures for treatment (e.g. incentive spirometry, chest physical therapy) should initially be tried. Bronchoscopy may be considered for patients who do not respond or who have inspissated secretions. Therapeutic bronchoscopic aspiration can relieve airway obstruction quickly if there is complete atelectasis of a lung or lobe. There is generally no benefit to fever suppression in the absence of any cardiovascular embarrassment; indeed, there may be harm.[101]

Aspiration

If the pH of the aspirated material is <2.5, lung injury is instantaneous. There is therefore no benefit to lavage with $NaHCO_3$ or immediate bronchoscopy if there is no sign of mechanical obstruction caused by particulate matter, although surveillance sputum cultures are indicated to identify progression to bacterial infection. For the same reason, antibiotics are not indicated initially for what proves to be only a sterile chemical pneumonitis in more than two-thirds of cases. The clinician needs to be resolute in the decision to withhold antibiotics because aspiration pneumonitis produces a systemic cytokine-mediated inflammatory response characterized by fever, leukocytosis, and a fluid requirement that can be indistinguishable from bacterial sepsis. Hypoxemia is treated with O_2 and mechanical ventilation if necessary.

Nosocomial Pneumonia

Difficulties in diagnosis mean that empiric therapy is often necessary.[38] *Staphylococcus aureus* and *Pseudomonas aeruginosa* are the two most common pathogens, but most enteric gram-negative bacilli can cause pneumonia.[102] In nonaspiration pneumonia, the presence and importance of anaerobic flora is unclear. They are seldom cultured (perhaps because of the high $F\text{io}_2$ in the airway) and the likely anaerobic organisms present are nonpathogenic mouth flora. Most clinicians administer antibiotics for nosocomial pneumonia to cover *S. aureus* and *P. aeruginosa*, including possible resistant strains, but do not include antianaerobic coverage.

The mortality rate of nosocomial pneumonia is high (25% for staphylococcal pneumonia, 35% for Gram-negative pneumonia, 70% for *P. aeruginosa* pneumonia). It appears to be higher if empiric therapy is not started promptly.[52] However, as many patients are proved not to have pneumonia ultimately, selective withholding of antibiotics with careful clinical evaluation,[50] de-escalation to a more narrow-spectrum agent once antibiotic susceptibilities are known, or discontinuation once the cultures prove negative have been advocated.[103] There are several possible antibiotic choices, including beta-lactam/beta-lactamase combination drugs (often with an aminoglycoside), third- or fourth-generation cephalosporins, fluoroquinolones, and carbapenems. Antibiotic choice is predicated upon local susceptibility patterns. Global increases in bacterial resistance[104] may mandate consideration of an aminoglycoside or polymyxin as empiric Gram-negative therapy against a possible multidrug-resistant or carbapenemase-resistant organism.[104,105] Some authorities routinely treat *P. aeruginosa* and Enterobacteriaceae with two drugs, including an aminoglycoside, but there is no evidence of benefit, and aminoglycosides do increase substantially the risk of acute kidney injury.[106] Inhaled antibiotics are unsubstantiated but are administered sometimes as rescue therapy.[107] Duration of therapy for nosocomial pneumonia remains somewhat unclear, although recent data indicate that shorter courses of therapy (e.g. 7–8 days) are as effective as longer regimens (e.g. 14 days).[108]

Venous Thromboembolic Disease

Anticoagulation with intravenous heparin followed by a period of warfarin therapy has been the traditional treatment, but numerous alternatives exist, including LMWH therapy and oral direct Factor Xa or Factor IIa inhibitors.[109] Low-molecular-weight heparin along with vitamin K antagonists and ambulation have revolutionized the treatment of VTE in the acute phase. In general, VTE patients require 3 months of treatment with anticoagulants, with options including LMWH, vitamin K antagonists, or a direct inhibitor. After this time, decisions for further treatment are based on balancing the risk of VTE recurrence, determined by etiology of the VTE (transient risk factors, unprovoked or tumor-associated), against the risk of major hemorrhage from treatment. Better prediction tools for major hemorrhage are needed.

A severe case of pulmonary embolism may also require O_2, mechanical ventilation, pharmacologic right heart afterload reduction therapy, and management of supraventricular tachyarrhythmias. Rarely, thrombolytic therapy is needed to treat pulmonary embolism if oxygenation and hemodynamics cannot be supported. Thrombolytic therapy carries a dangerous risk of bleeding in the first 10–14 days postoperatively and hence should be used cautiously in the postoperative patient.

Acute Respiratory Distress Syndrome

Acute respiratory distress syndrome is the stereotypical response of the lung to injury.[96] The incidence varies depending upon the precipitant, but ranges from 1.5 to 5.3/100,000 population per year.[96] Some precipitants affect the pulmonary parenchyma directly, whereas others reflect the pulmonary response to a systemic insult. The strongest associations between ARDS and individual risk factors exist for:

- Sepsis (approximately 40% of all cases)
- Major trauma

- Multiple transfusions (>10 units of RBC concentrates)
- Aspiration of gastric contents
- Pulmonary contusion
- Multiple fractures
- Acute pancreatitis
- Smoke inhalation.[96]

Whatever the causal relationship, the result is the same: pulmonary edema despite low or normal pulmonary microvascular pressures, hypoxemia caused by intrapulmonary *Qs/Qt*, alveolar flooding, and markedly decreased lung compliance. Shunt develops from loss of functional alveoli because of surfactant loss, atelectasis, and alveolar flooding. Hypoxic vasoconstriction decreases perfusion to underventilated alveoli in an attempt to restore abnormal V_A/Q. In compensation, substantial diversion of perfusion to areas with better V_A/Q matching can result in overperfusion of "normal" units relative to ventilation, paradoxically causing poor V_A/Q matching.

Simultaneously, a proinflammatory response is activated. Neutrophils adhere to pulmonary capillary endothelium and are activated, which results in endothelial injury, increased permeability, and microthrombosis.[102] Microembolization of particulate debris occurs if hepatic reticuloendothelial host defenses are impaired or as a consequence of fibrin deposition in coagulopathy. This process results in increased areas of lung that are ventilated but not perfused. This V_D, expressed as a fraction of V_T (V_D/V_T), is normally about 0.3. Therefore, in normal ventilation, approximately 30% of each breath fills V_D, most of which (about 2 mL/kg) is the anatomic V_D of the large airways. In ARDS, *Vd*/*Vt* can increase to 0.7–0.8. The increased *Vd*/*Vt* results in a geometric increase in the work of breathing and rapid ventilatory failure.

Microvascular injury leads eventually to:

- Pulmonary hypertension
- Loss of hypoxic vasoconstriction
- Further derangements in *Va*/*Q* matching.

Although pulmonary edema is the hallmark of ARDS, gas exchange abnormalities often do not correlate with the degree of edema. Alterations in lung mechanics tend to be marked in comparison to those characteristic of hydrostatic edema. Peribronchial edema can cause bronchoconstriction and humoral mediators (especially leukotrienes) have direct effects on airway tone. Increased airway reactivity can persist long afterwards in survivors.

Positive End-Expiratory Pressure Therapy

Mechanical ventilation with supplemental O_2 and high levels of PEEP has been the mainstay of therapy for ARDS for nearly 50 years.[110] Increased FRC results from PEEP by alveolar recruitment. As FRC rises above CC, a greater percentage of perfused lung is ventilated, which yields a decreased *Qs*/*Qt* fraction. Oxygenation can usually be supported, but the associated morbidity—barotrauma (pneumothorax or pneumomediastinum, with a reported incidence of about 5%), reduced perfusion,[111] difficulty in supporting renal function, and pneumonia–is commonplace.

Therapy with PEEP may cause substantial decreases in perfusion that must be avoided[111] as there is no advantage if DO_2 is reduced. Decreased preload results in decreased venous return because of increased intrathoracic pressure. Cardiac contractility is impaired as a result of altered ventricular septal mechanics and anatomy, pulmonary hypertension, and increased right heart afterload. The intraventricular septum shifts towards the left ventricle to decrease left ventricular volume.

As PEEP causes cardiac and pulmonary morbidity, and prolonged exposure to FiO_2 >0.6 is itself toxic to the lung, algorithms have been employed to "optimize" PEEP and minimize the potential for barotrauma and O_2 toxicity.[94] No method has proved to be superior. The therapeutic end-point should be achievement of adequate oxygenation—PaO_2 >60 mm Hg (>8.0 kPa; 90% SaO_2 with a normal saturation curve)—on Fio_2 of <0.6 without a reduction in perfusion. The only therapeutic modalities that are proved to be of benefit are low-V_T ventilation with PEEP, periodic PP to support restoration of *V*/*Q* matching, and restrictive fluid administration.[94,112,113]

Patient–Ventilator Dyssynchrony

If a mechanically ventilated patient has difficulty oxygenating or ventilating, there may be a problem that is intrinsic to the patient, ventilator, or patient–ventilator interface (i.e. the artificial airway). The entire system must be evaluated. Dyssynchrony or "fighting the ventilator" is a problem when some ventilatory drive is preserved. Active exhalation superimposed on the machine breath causes peak airway pressure to increase precipitously. Initially, ventilation by hand with pure O_2 is indicated, while the machine backup rate and inspiratory gas flow are increased (up to 1.5 L/s). A change in trigger mode may help (e.g. from assist-control ventilation to SIMV). If manual ventilation relieves the problem, the source is probably the ventilator. Ventilator-related causes include gas leaks, inadequate FiO_2, and excessive work of breathing.

These patients require sedation that is monitored closely and titrated for effect to the minimal effective degree [e.g. a score of 0 or -1 on the Richmond Agitation

Sedation Scale (Table 26.10)],[114,115] ideally with propofol or dexmedetomidine rather than a benzodiazepine, with or without an opioid (e.g. fentanyl or hydromorphone as needed for pain) or rarely neuromuscular blockade.[116,117] Each similar episode requires thorough consideration because reflexive sedation of the hypoxemic patient may be disastrous. Other causes of agitation must be considered, including pain, hypoxemia, pneumothorax, and delirium. Other potential causes of sudden respiratory distress include migration or obstruction of the endotracheal tube, bronchospasm, acute pulmonary edema, pulmonary embolism, and intrinsic PEEP. Sudden alterations in body posture, hypoxemia caused by drugs (vasodilators, lipid solutions), and abdominal distention (e.g. abdominal compartment syndrome) may play a role in selected patients.

Difficult-to-Liberate Patients

Respiratory drive may be depressed by structural damage, sleep deprivation, oversedation, or metabolic alkalosis. Patients may have phrenic nerve or neuromuscular disorders. Decreased muscle strength may follow chronic hyperinflation, malnutrition, acidosis, mineral and electrolyte disorders (especially hypophosphatemia), renal failure, and disuse. Increased ventilatory requirements may be caused by increased CO_2 production, increased *Vd* or inappropriately increased drive. Increased work of breathing, which is now quantifiable, may also lead to failure to liberate from the ventilator.[118]

A favorable outcome is predicted by:

- PaO_2 >60 mm Hg (>8.0 kPa) on FiO_2 <0.35
- $D(A\text{-}a)O_2$ <350 mm Hg (<46.6 kPa) and
- PaO_2:FiO_2 >200.

Additional predictors include:

- Vital capacity >10 mL/kg
- A negative inspiratory force <–25 cm H_2O (<2.5 kPa)
- V_E <10 L/min
- Maximum voluntary ventilation higher than twice the resting V_E.

The latter four predictors are effort-related and therefore less reliable.

Methods for discontinuing mechanical ventilation include abrupt discontinuation, trials of spontaneous breathing (T-piece trials or CPAP), SIMV, and PSV. The last two modalities are often combined. Advocates of SIMV emphasize a limited need for sedation, normalized V_A/Q, decreased VO_2, and reduced fatigue. Proponents of PSV emphasize increased patient comfort derived from control over each breath, but if the patient cannot initiate each cycle, hypoventilation may ensue. Use of PSV can decrease the work of breathing, but neither method is superior.

Table 26.10 Richmond Agitation-Sedation Scale (RASS).

Score term description
+4 Combative. Overtly combative, violent, immediate danger to staff
+3 Very agitated. Pulls or removes tube(s) or catheter(s); aggressive
+2 Agitated. Frequent nonpurposeful movement, fights ventilator
+1 Restless. Anxious but movements not aggressive; vigorous
0 Alert and calm
–1 Drowsy. Not fully alert, but has sustained awakening (eye-opening/eye contact) to voice (>10 s)
–2 Light sedation. Awakens briefly with eye contact to voice (<10 s)
–3 Moderate sedation. Movement or eye opening to voice (but no eye contact)
–4 Deep sedation. No response to voice, but movement or eye opening to physical stimulation
–5 Unarousable. No response to voice or physical stimulation
Procedure for RASS Assessment
1. Observe patient
• Patient is alert, restless, or agitated (score 0 to +4)
2. If not alert, state patient's name and say to open eyes and look at speaker
• Patient awakens with sustained eye opening and eye contact (score –1)
• Patient awakens with eye opening and eye contact, but not sustained (score –2)
• Patient has any movement in response to voice but no eye contact (score –3)
3. When no response to verbal stimulation, stimulate patient by shaking shoulder or sternal rub
• Patient has any movement to physical stimulation (score –4)
• Patient has no response to any stimulation (score –5)

Source: Adapted from Sessler CN, Gosnell M, Grap MJ, et al. The Richmond Agitation-Sedation Scale: Validity and reliability in adult intensive care patients. Am J Respir Crit Care Med. 2002;166:1338-44.

Once the patient has been weaned, extubation may still fail. The incidence of extubation failure (need for reintubation within 7 days) is approximately 4% in patients who have had an operation. However, the morbidity rate in patients who fail is approximately 50%. Laryngeal incompetence and aspiration is a potential problem even after short-term intubation. Laryngeal edema is a relatively common cause of upper airway obstruction (7% incidence after 36 hours of intubation). The gag reflex does not predict the risk of aspiration, with both false-negative and false-positive predictions. Now used most commonly to assess readiness to liberate from the ventilator is the rapid shallow breathing index ("Tobin index"), which is simply the ratio of respiratory frequency to V_T (f/V_T). In a prospective study of several indicators, the f/V_T was the best predictor of successful weaning, with a sensitivity of 0.97 and specificity of 0.64.[119]

Tracheostomy

In the context of acute respiratory failure, there remains no consensus as to the appropriate timing of tracheostomy for the patient who has failed to liberate from the ventilator.[120,121] Neither is there consensus as to whether tracheostomy prevents or reduces the incidence of pneumonia or other complications of prolonged endotracheal intubation. Arguably, tracheostomy reduces patient discomfort compared with translaryngeal intubation, reduces work of breathing owing to the decreased resistance occasioned by the shorter tube, and may make for easier bedside pulmonary toilet. Tracheostomy is also usually necessary for placement of a convalescent ventilator-dependent patient in a long-term care facility.

As to whether percutaneous or open tracheostomy is preferable, 15 prospective, randomized-controlled trials involving nearly 1,000 patients were reviewed.[122] Pooled odds ratios (OR) revealed statistically significant results against percutaneous tracheostomy only for the complication of decannulation/obstruction (OR 2.79, 95% CI 1.29–6.03). There were significantly fewer complications for percutaneous tracheostomy with respect to surgical site infection (0.37, 0.22–0.62) and unfavorable scarring (0.44, 0.23–0.83). There were no differences for complications of false passage (2.70, 0.89–8.22), minor hemorrhage (1.09, 0.61–1.97), major hemorrhage (0.60, 0.28–1.26), subglottic stenosis (0.59, 0.27–1.29), or death (0.70, 0.24–2.01), although there was a trend to lower overall complication rates (0.75, 0.56–1.00) for percutaneous tracheostomy. Operative time was shorter for percutaneous tracheostomy by a mean of 4.6 minutes, and cost was less by approximately USD 456.

REFERENCES

1. Dempsey JA, Forster HV. Mediation of ventilatory adaptations. Physiol Rev. 1982;62:262-346.
2. Mitchell RA, Berger AJ. Neural regulation of respiration. Am Rev Respir Dis. 1975;111:206-24.
3. Widdicombe JG, Fillenz M. Receptors of the lungs and airways. In: Neil E (Ed). Handbook of Sensory Physiology: Enteroceptors. New York: Springer–Verlag; 1972. Pp. 80-98.
4. Cherniack NS. The regulation of ventilation. In: Fishman AP (Ed). Pulmonary Diseases and Disorders. New York: McGraw–Hill; 1980. Pp. 317-29.
5. Anthionisen NR, Cherniack NS. Ventilatory control in lung disease. In: Hornbein TF (Ed). Regulation of Breathing, vol. 2. New York: Marcel Dekker; 1981. Pp. 965-1004.
6. Neil E, Howe A. Arterial chemoreceptors. In: Neil E (Ed). Handbook of Sensory Physiology: Enteroceptors. New York: Springer–Verlag; 1972. Pp. 47-79.
7. Leusen I. Regulation of cerebrospinal fluid composition with reference to breathing. Physiol Rev. 1972;52:1-56.
8. O'Regan RG, Majcherczyk S. Role of peripheral chemoreceptors and central chemosensitivity in the regulation of respiration and circulation. J Exp Biol. 1982;100:23-40.
9. Dempsey JA, Forster HV, Ledhill N, et al. Effects of moderate hypoxemia or hypocapnia on CSF [H^+] and ventilation in man. J Appl Physiol. 1975;38:665-74.
10. Whipp BJ, Wasserman K. Carotid bodies and ventilatory control dynamics in man. Fed Proc. 1980;29:2668-73.
11. Pokorski M, Lahiri S. Aortic and carotid chemoreceptor responses to metabolic acidosis in the cat. Am J Physiol. 1983;244:R652-8.
12. West JB. Ventilation/blood flow and gas exchange. Oxford: Blackwell Scientific; 1977.
13. Milic–Emili J, Henderson JA. Dolovich MB, et al. Regional distribution of inspired gas in the lung. J Appl Physiol. 1966;21:749-59.
14. Fishman AP. Hypoxia and the pulmonary circulation: how and where it acts. Circ Res. 1976;38:221-31.
15. Olson NC, Robinson NE, Anderson DL, et al. Effect of carotid body hypoxia and/or hypercapnia on pulmonary vascular resistance. Proc Soc Exp Biol Med. 1982;170:188-93.
16. Schumacher PT, Rhodes GR, Newell JC, et al. Ventilation–perfusion imbalance after head trauma. Am Rev Respir Dis. 1979;119:33-43.
17. Miller CL, Martin JL. Changes in lung function following anesthesia and surgery. In: Breslow MJ, Miller CF, Rogers M, (Eds). Perioperative Management. St Louis: Mosby; 1990. Pp. 194-212.
18. Dueck R, Prutow RJ, Davies NJ, et al. The lung volume at which shunting occurs with inhalation anesthesia. Anesthesiology. 1988;69:854-61.
19. Froese AB, Brian AC. Effects of anesthesia and paralysis on diaphragmatic mechanics in man. Anesthesiology. 1974; 41:242-55.
20. Brismar B, Hedenstierna G, Lundquist H, et al. Pulmonary densities during anesthesia with muscular relaxation—a proposal of atelectasis. Anesthesiology. 1985;62:422-8.
21. Hewelett AM, Hulands GH, Nunn JF, et al. Functional residual capacity during anaesthesia. III. Artificial ventilation. Br J Anaesth. 1974;46:495-503.
22. Benumof JL, Wahrenbrock EA. Local effects of anaesthetics on regional hypoxic pulmonary vasoconstriction. Anesthesiology. 1975;43:525-32.
23. Knill RL, Gelb AW. Ventilatory responses to hypoxia and hypercapnia during halothane sedation and anesthesia in man. Anesthesiology. 1978;49:244-51.
24. Knill RL, Clement JL. Ventilatory responses to acute metabolic acidemia in humans awake, sedated, and anesthetized with halothane. Anesthesiology. 1985;62:745-53.

25. Simonneau G, Vivien A, Sartene A, et al. Diaphragm function induced by upper abdominal surgery: role of postoperative pain. Am Rev Respir Dis. 1983;128:899-903.
26. Dureuil B, Viires N, Cantineau JP, et al. Diaphragmatic contractility after upper abdominal surgery. J Appl Physiol. 1986;61:1775-80.
27. Dureuil B, Viires N, Pariente R, et al. Effects of phrenic nerve cooling on diaphragmatic function. J Appl Physiol. 1987;63:1763-9.
28. Wasserman K, Casaburi R. Dyspnea: physiological and pathophysiological mechanisms. Ann Rev Med. 1988:39:503-15.
29. Fong Y, Whalen GF, Hariri RH, et al. Utility of daily chest radiographs in the surgical intensive care unit: a prospective study. Arch Surg. 1995;130:764-8.
30. Henschke CL, Yankelevitz DF, Wand A, et al. Accuracy and efficacy of chest radiography in the intensive care unit. Radiol Clin North Am. 1996;34:21-31.
31. Van Rossum AB, Pattynama PM, Mallens WM, et al. Can helical CT replace scintigraphy in the diagnostic process in suspected pulmonary embolism? A retrospective-prospective cohort study focusing on total diagnostic yield. Eur Radiol. 1998;8:90-6.
32. Silverman PM, Cooper CJ, Weltman DI, et al. Helical CT: practical considerations and potential pitfalls. Radiographics. 1995;15:25-36.
33. Mattison LE, Coppage L, Alderman DF, et al. Pleural effusions in the medical ICU: prevalence, causes, and clinical implications. Chest. 1997;111:1018-23.
34. Talmor M, Hydo L, Gershenwald J, et al. Beneficial effects of chest tube drainage of pleural effusion in acute respiratory failure refractory to positive end-expiratory pressure ventilation. Surgery. 1998;123:137-43.
35. Heffner JE, Brown LK, Barbieri CA. Diagnostic value of tests that discriminate between exudative and transudative pleural effusions. Chest. 1997;111:970-80.
36. Pieracci FM, Barie PS. Strategies in the prevention and management of ventilator-associated pneumonia. Am Surg. 2007;73:419-32.
37. Ottosen J, Evans H. Pneumonia: Challenges in the definition, diagnosis, and management of disease. Surg Clin North Am. 2014;94:1305-17.
38. Wunderink RG. Ventilator-associated pneumonia. Failure to respond to antibiotic therapy. Clin Chest Med. 1995;16:173-93.
39. George DL. Epidemiology of nosocomial pneumonia in intensive care unit patients. Clin Chest Med. 1995;16:29-44.
40. Winer-Muram HT, Rubin SA, Ellis JV, et al. Pneumonia and ARDS in patients receiving mechanical ventilation: diagnostic accuracy of chest radiography. Radiology. 1993;188:479-95.
41. Meduri GU, Mauldin GL, Wunderink RG, et al. Causes of fever and pulmonary densities in patients with clinical manifestations of ventilator-associated pneumonia. Chest. 1994;106:1221-35.
42. Sutherland KR, Steinberg KP, Maunder RJ, et al. Pulmonary infection during the acute respiratory distress syndrome. Am J Respir Crit Care Med. 1995;152:550-6.
43. Kollef MH. Ventilator-associated pneumonia. A multivariate analysis. JAMA. 1993;270:1965-70.
44. Kollef MH. Antibiotic use and antibiotic resistance in the intensive care unit: are we curing or creating disease? Heart Lung. 1994;23:363-7.
45. Kollef MH, Sharpless L, Vlasnik J, et al. The impact of nosocomial infections on patient outcomes following cardiac surgery. Chest. 1997;112:666-75.
46. Kollef MH, Wragge T, Pasque C. Determinants of mortality and multiorgan dysfunction in cardiac surgery patients requiring prolonged mechanical ventilation. Chest. 1995;107:1395-401.
47. Souweine B, Veber B, Bedos JP. Diagnostic accuracy of protected specimen brush and bronchoalveolar lavage in nosocomial pneumonia: impact of previous antimicrobial treatments. Crit Care Med. 1998;26:236-44.
48. Timsit JF, Misset B, Azoulay E, et al. Usefulness of airway visualization in the diagnosis of nosocomial pneumonia in ventilated patients. Chest. 1996;110:172-9.
49. Croce MA, Fabian TC, Shaw B, et al. Analysis of charges associated with diagnosis of nosocomial pneumonia: can routine bronchoscopy be justified? J Trauma. 1994;37:721-7.
50. Croce MA, Fabian TC, Schurr MJ, et al. Using bronchoalveolar lavage to distinguish nosocomial pneumonia from systemic inflammatory response syndrome: a prospective analysis. J Trauma. 1995;39:1134-9.

Additional references appear in the online version of this book.

27

Cardiac Assessment and Support of the Surgical Patient

Nancy Parks, Ashley Morgan, Thomas Frohlich, Alden H Harken

Key Points

- The assessment and management of cardiac risk is an important preoperative objective to prevent avoidable complications of surgical care.
- Cardiac dysfunction is generally due to mechanical obstruction of flow from arterial narrowing of the coronary arteries or due to acute thrombotic events within the coronary circulation that lead to acute myocardial infarction.
- Meaningful preoperative assessment for cardiac risk prior to noncardiac surgery requires functional and objective clinical assessment before more sophisticated ventricular testing is deemed necessary.
- Elective low-risk operations without overt signs of unstable angina or acute cardiac syndrome do not require additional cardiac evaluation.
- Intermediate and high-risk noncardiac surgical patients may proceed to operations if reasonable exercise tolerance can be established, although beta-blockers and/or statins may be of benefit depending in part upon prior use by the patient.
- In general, noncardiac surgical patients with clinical evidence of acute cardiac syndrome should have a detailed cardiac evaluation and therapeutic intervention unless the urgency of the noncardiac indications for operation exceeds those of the patient's cardiac condition.

INTRODUCTION

Traditionally, physicians have examined and tested patients for indicators of increased surgical risk. This "prognostic testing" provides an estimate of the potential for adverse events following surgical intervention. Much more practical and useful is "predictive testing," which identifies patients who will benefit if the test leads to a specific, available intervention.[1] In no area has this predictive testing been more extensively employed than in the evaluation of cardiac disease for the patient undergoing major surgical procedures.

An equally important distinction is to identify an intervention that is ordinarily indicated as opposed to a therapy or procedure that is required exclusively by virtue of the planned operation. Interestingly, recent recognition of these distinctions has transformed preoperative planning into a vastly more practical and constructive process. Appropriately, we begin with a history and physical examination. In that the heart is a likely source of postoperative complications, a specific analysis of the patient's exercise capacity can be more sensitive than a lot of expensive and inconvenient "cardiology clearance" evaluations/tests.

The myocardium is subject to two major causes of dangerous vascular dysfunction: (1) an imbalance of coronary oxygen delivery relative to cardiomyocyte oxygen demand secondary to mechanical coronary artery atherosclerotic obstruction (which is typically chronic); and (2) thrombotic occlusion of a coronary artery associated with surgically induced hypercoagulability over an "unstable," but nonobstructive, coronary artery plaque (which is always acute). Additional issues that may be problematic and sources of potential dysfunction in the preoperative surgical patient are cardiomyopathy, rhythm disturbances, and increasingly the presence of previously unrecognized valvular heart disease. The potential for these dysfunctions is present before major operation and their recognition becomes the goal of preoperative cardiac assessment.

Surgical operations provoke both physical and psychological stress. Surgeons are obligated to balance the anticipated surgical benefit with an assessment of operative risk. But both the benefits and the risks are estimates. The purposes of this chapter are to review and refine the "risk" side of this equation.

PATHOGENESIS OF CARDIAC DYSFUNCTION

The heart is a sphere of muscle that for effective function must fill with blood during diastole and expel blood during systole (Fig. 27.1). Age and disease typically compromise both of these functions such that the increasing stiffness of the ventricles (reduced diastolic compliance) slows ventricular filling and microfibrosis of the ventricles reduces systolic contractility (ejection fraction). Systolic and diastolic dysfunctions are now appreciated as independent and separable components of myocardial dysfunction. The consequence of lost ventricular contractility is the development of cardiac hypertrophy with thickening of the ventricular walls (Fig. 27.2). A young, healthy compliant ventricle should fill completely during diastole in 130–200 ms.[1] As the heart rate increases, however, there is less time for complete ventricular filling. Thus, the "rule of thumb" is that patients can increase cardiac output by increasing heart rate up to 220 beats per minute (bpm) minus their age. Similarly, the increasing filling pressure (preload) of both ventricles infuses additional volume (end diastolic volume) such that stroke volume increases (Frank–Starling's law) up to a point, but excessive filling leads to an overdistended ventricle that does not contract effectively (Fig. 27.3).

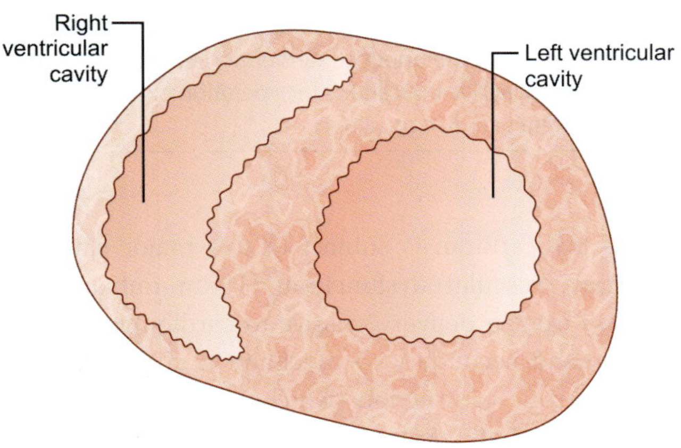

Fig. 27.1: Cross section through the heart at the level of the ventricular cavities.

Both systolic and diastolic dysfunctions are presumed to be related to microcardiomyocyte ischemia, leading to replacement of contractile fibers with fibroblasts. The aging and diseased heart muscle is gradually replaced with microscar. Displacement of functioning cardiac muscle by scar tissue results in impaired contraction and relaxation of the ventricles. This is a slow chronic process, and the patient will report progressive shortness of breath, fatigue, and exercise-induced chest pain. The "classic" inducers of symptomatic myocardial ischemia are acute exertion, acute anger or emotional upset, or a large meal. In obtaining the patient's history, these symptoms are elicited as having a slowly progressive and chronic pattern. For the purpose of this discussion, the definition of "unstable angina" is any change in the "pattern" of angina in the prior 6 weeks.[2,3]

The more ominous and less predictable manifestation of chronic heart disease is the acute thrombotic occlusion of a coronary artery. This event is associated with the acute chest pain, dyspnea, and other symptoms of a "heart attack" event that occurs without exertion. However, with general anesthesia, intensive care analgesic management, and aggressive sedation strategies in the postoperative period, the chest pain, and other related symptoms of myocardial infarction are masked. If the affected cardiac muscle,

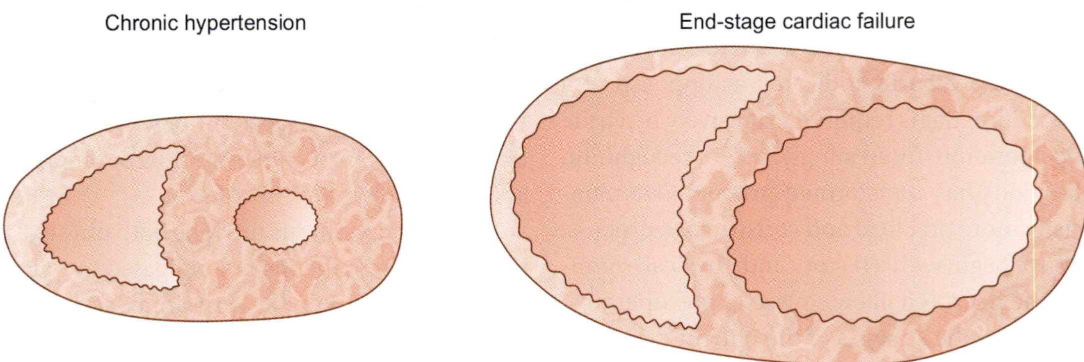

Fig. 27.2: Changes seen in the cross-sectional morphology of the chambers of the heart as a result of pathologic processes.

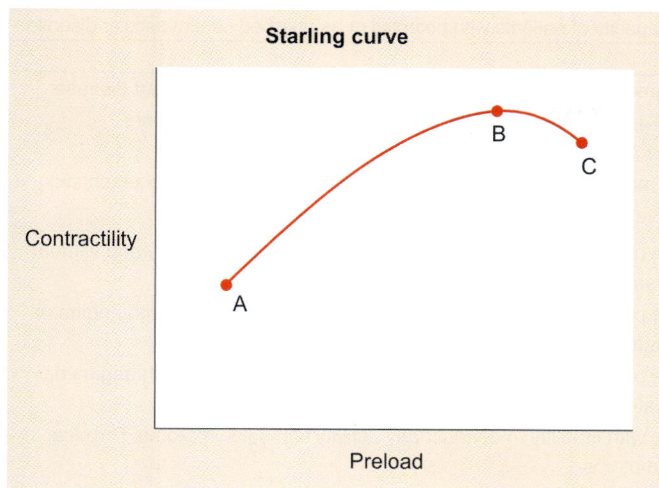

Fig. 27.3: Starling curve relating preload to contractility. As preload increases from point A to point B, contractility increases. Preload from point B to point C results in decreased contractility.

which is distal to the thrombotic occlusion, involves as much as 25% of the ventricular muscle mass, the mortality rate may exceed 50%. A smaller mass of acutely ischemic heart typically presents as ventricular hyperexcitability or ectopy [premature ventricular contractions (PVCs), ventricular tachycardia, and ventricular fibrillation]. Ischemic heart muscle is electrically unstable. Thus, PVCs may be interpreted to reflect ischemia whether this occurs while the patient is resting in the intensive care unit (ICU) or is induced during the exercise stress test.

Predictably, the chronic progressive angina due to regional exercise-induced myocardial ischemia correlates anatomically with stenotic lesions identified by coronary angiography. Unfortunately, and more frighteningly, "unstable coronary artery plaque" may appear pretty innocuous angiographically.[4]

PREOPERATIVE CARDIAC EVALUATION

History and Physical Examination

Assessment of risk begins with the history interview. This discussion focuses and refines treatments and, equally importantly, promotes the health literacy of the patients. Filtering the information acquired by internet-savvy patients not only enhances trust, but there is also persuasive evidence that patients who understand their disease and participate actively in their treatment have better outcomes.[5]

The traditional history still remains valid in making queries about chest pain with exertion, chest fullness, arm and jaw numbness, shortness of breath or fatigue with exertion, and palpitations. Dizziness and light headedness may be identified. Past histories of prior cardiac surgery, coronary angiography, or percutaneous coronary interventions are clearly important. Diabetes, hypertension, hypercholesterolemia, tobacco use, and family history or disease of the heart or peripheral vascular tree are important. The physical examination may identify evidence of arrhythmias, gallop rhythms, murmurs, or pulmonary rales. Dependent edema may reflect mild congestive failure and the peripheral vascular examination may indicate the presence of vascular disease that makes coronary involvement likely.

Functional Capacity and Objective Assessment

With the initial history and physical examination, the patient's functional capacity and objective assessment can be made. The patients can then be categorized into a Functional Class using the classification system from the New York Heart Association. The functional capacity of the patient has now been further refined with the addition of objective assessment (Table 27.1).

Recommendations for preoperative studies are commonly linked to the patient's Functional Class and to the presence of patient-specific risk factors. Any one of these active cardiac conditions requires additional evaluation and management: (1) unstable coronary syndromes including severe angina and a recent (<30 days) myocardial infarction, (2) decompensated or recent onset of heart failure, (3) significant arrhythmias including atrioventricular block and supraventricular tachycardia, and (4) severe valvular disease. Additional clinical risk factors for consideration are history of ischemic heart disease, history of congestive heart failure, history of cerebrovascular disease, preoperative treatment with insulin, and chronic renal failure (creatinine ≥ 2.0 mg/dL or 200 μmol/L). Patients without any of these risk factors are identified as having a <0.5% risk of a major cardiac event following a high-risk operation, while those with three or more risk factors will have >10% risk of a major cardiac event.

The presence of these clinical risk factors is then assessed in the context of the surgical risk that is to be undertaken.[6] High-risk operations are those operations with ≥5% risk of cardiac death or nonfatal myocardial infarction and include major aortic or peripheral vascular surgery. Intermediate-risk operations are those with an estimated risk of 1–5% for cardiac events and include

Table 27.1 The New York Heart Association classification of functional capacity of patients with potential or established cardiovascular disease.

Classification of functional capacity	*Definitions*
No heart disease	Healthy cardiac assessment without evidence or predisposition for active heart disease
No heart disease: predisposing etiologic factors	No cardiac disease is evident but with a history of family or personal risk factors (i.e. hypertension, hypercholesterolemia)
No heart disease: unexplained manifestations	Signs or symptoms that may be referable to heart disease but without current documentation
American Heart Association: classification	All patients with objective evidence of cardiovascular disease
Class I	Cardiovascular disease present but without any limitations of physical activity and without symptoms of cardiac disease with ordinary activity
Class II	Cardiovascular disease present but with slight limitation of physical activity with angina or other symptoms associated with ordinary activity
Class III	Cardiovascular disease present with marked limitation of physical activity with angina or other symptoms associated with modest activity
Class IV	Cardiovascular disease with inability to conduct any activity without symptoms. Physical activity exacerbates symptoms

major abdominal and thoracic operations. Low risk is considered endoscopy, superficial operations, and ambulatory procedures in which cardiac risk is considered <1%. The presence of three of the previously cited clinical risk factors in major vascular surgery should result in consideration for cardiac testing if it will change management. Intermediate-risk operations with three risk factors may not require additional testing if heart rate control has been achieved preoperatively. High-risk and intermediate-risk operations with one or two risk factors may similarly be considered for noninvasive testing if heart rate control is not achieved. No cardiac testing is recommended for low-risk procedures regardless of the presence of risk factors, and high- and intermediate-risk operations should proceed if no risk factors are identified.

Chest X-Ray and Electrocardiogram

The chest X-ray and the electrocardiogram (EKG, ECG) become first-order assessments of the cardiac risk of the noncardiac surgical patient after the physical examination. Chest X-ray is commonly done, especially in patients over 50 years of age, as a general screening evaluation for cardiopulmonary disease. It may identify cardiomegaly or calcific changes of vascular structures and is commonly performed for all Functional Class II or higher patients undergoing operations of high or intermediate risk. Chest X-ray is particularly useful in obese patients in whom the increased body mass compromises the details of the physical examination.

The American College of Cardiology/American Heart Association (ACC/AHA) guidelines generally recommend not only the use of a 12-lead EKG based upon the Functional Class of the patient but also take into consideration the risk of the operation for having cardiac complications. Thus, Functional Class I patients undergoing high-risk operations, and Functional Class II patients undergoing high- or intermediate-risk operations (especially if clinical risk factors are present) are all recommended to have a 12-lead preoperative EKG. Current practice indicates a 12-lead EKG for all operations entailing a general or spinal anesthetic in Functional Class III or IV patients regardless of any risk factors.

Exercise Stress Testing

An ACC/AHA task force published a comprehensive analysis of exercise stress testing as a tool to assess myocardial ischemia and functional capacity. This examination of published studies of high-risk patients prior to major vascular surgery demonstrated a disappointing lack of sensitivity in identifying obstructive coronary artery disease (CAD). About 50% of patients with a single stenotic lesion that compromised 70% of the coronary artery diameter had exercise stress tests with a "normal" result. For patients with three major coronary arteries involved, the sensitivity was better at 86%; but the specificity remained a fairly random event at 53%.[6] Preoperative exercise stress testing is generally recommended for patients with evidence of active cardiac conditions. Active cardiac conditions would include angina or recent myocardial infarction, clinical evidence of congestive heart failure, EKG evidence of arrhythmias, or evidence of valvular heart disease.

The conduct of an exercise stress test is a standard protocol. A 12-lead EKG is continuously monitored as the patient walks on a treadmill. The Bruce protocol is commonly employed,[7] although variations in the speed and slope of the treadmill can also be employed in an exercise stress test. Initially, the patient walks leisurely at a 1.7 miles per hour (2.7 km/h) speed on a 10% incline. In every 3 minutes, the incline is elevated by an additional 2%, and the treadmill speed is increased by about 1 mile per hour (1.6 km/h). Thus, the first several stages of a Bruce protocol are easily achieved by most patients. Yet, stage I of the Bruce protocol is equivalent to a little less than 4 metabolic equivalents (METs). One MET equals 3.5 mL O_2 consumed per kg body weight per minute—or the amount of oxygen consumed in a sedentary activity. The ACC/AHA equate walking a short distance with stage I on the Bruce protocol (or a little less than 4 METs), and climbing two flights of stairs equals 6 METs or stage II. By history, if a patient can manage 4 METs without chest pain, they do not need a preoperative stress test.[1,6]

Many of these conclusions are extrapolated from life table analyses assuming that surgical stress is equivalent to the accelerated stress of aging. In these studies, exercise capacity is more sensitive than noninvasive tests of CAD.[8] In a large group of medically treated patients with CAD, the 12% participants who could only manage stage I on a Bruce protocol suffered a 5% annual mortality rate while the 34% of participants who could achieve stage III enjoyed a 99% annual survival.

Since exercise tolerance has been proven to predict postoperative outcomes, surgeons can take advantage of it to assess patients in a way that is cost-effective. A verbal assessment of the patient's self-reported exercise tolerance, in which the patient estimates the distance that can be walked or the flights of stairs that can be climbed, will be as effective as more expensive and invasive testing. This finding was documented in a report from the University of Washington[9] in which 600 patients undergoing major surgery were found to have twice the rate of postoperative complication (20% vs. 10%, $p < 0.001$) if they were unable to walk four blocks or climb two flights of stairs during their preoperative interview.

A simple way to make the self-reported exercise tolerance more objective is directly to observe the patient performing a stair-climbing test. Many studies have verified this test as an assessment tool, especially in the field of lung resection for cancer. For many years, surgical resection has been the only curative option for patients with early-stage lung cancer. Due to the incidence of coexistent chronic obstructive pulmonary disease and cardiovascular disease, patients with lung cancer often have limited cardiopulmonary reserve even at rest. In order to decide preoperatively which of these physiologically impaired patients have the capacity to recover and benefit from thoracic surgery, pulmonary function tests and formal exercise tolerance tests are performed. This testing is both impractical and expensive, so some surgeons have adapted the pragmatic approach of watching patients climb stairs as part of a preoperative risk assessment.

Beginning in the 1960s, thoracic surgeons first reported the utility of preoperative stair climbing as a predictor of mortality following pneumonectomy. The execution is simple: a patient climbs several flights of stairs (studies use between two and five flights) at his/her own pace and records the number of flights climbed. This test has the advantages of being inexpensive and noninvasive. Not only does it reflect cardiac and pulmonary reserve, stair climbing also indicates less objective but equally important surgical variables such as motivation and psychological resilience. The results of this test correlate closely with pulmonary function and exercise tolerance tests. This relationship, which seems intuitive, has been validated in several studies in which the ability to climb stairs has been correlated with variables such as maximal oxygen uptake and forced expiratory volume in 1 s (FEV_1). In 1987, Bolton et al.[10] compared results of the stair-climbing test with standard pulmonary function tests in 70 patients. They found that the ability to climb three flights of stairs was 90% accurate at predicting an FEV_1 of >1.7 L. Pollock et al.[11] performed maximal oxygen uptake analysis on 31 patients while climbing stairs and reported that, like cardiopulmonary exercise testing, stair climbing accurately assessed both maximal minute ventilation and oxygen consumption (VO_2).

Stair climbing also correlates with postoperative mortality rates. In 1968, Van Nostrand et al.[12] reported that postpneumonectomy mortality was higher in patients who were unable to climb two flights of stairs. In 2001, Girish[13] similarly noted that among patients undergoing thoracic or abdominal surgery, who were unable to climb two flights of stairs before operation, 82% had a postoperative complication. For patients who could not negotiate a single flight, complications increased to 89%. Girish also found a trend in shorter length of postoperative hospital stay for patients who could climb more stairs. In 2007, Brunelli et al.[14] investigated the relationship between stair climbing and complications after lung resection in 640 patients and reported that mortality rate was 13 times higher and complications twice as common in patients who could climb <12 m than in those who could climb >22 m. In a subsequent study by Nicolić et al.[15] on 536 patients who underwent thoracic surgery, a 4% decrease in finger oximetry while climbing two flights of stairs before operation predicted a doubling of perioperative complications.

The American College of Chest Physicians[16] now includes stair climbing in their guidelines prior to lung resection by citing evidence that patients being considered for pneumonectomy who can walk less than one flight of stairs are at increased risk for perioperative death and cardiopulmonary complications, and should be considered for alternative therapies or nonstandard resections.

Obviously this test has its limitations. There are multiple reasons for inability to climb stairs that are not related to cardiac fitness. A patient might have perfect coronary arteries but debilitating neuromuscular disease, or any number of other impairments of ambulation. Stair climbing cannot completely replace formal cardiac evaluation for all patients. But it does provide a logical method of risk stratification for those patients who can successfully climb a minimum of two flights of stairs.

The stair-climbing test is an inexpensive and practical tool. Multiple authors[1] have developed tables relating common activities to METs and oxygen consumption (VO_2). Thus, a comprehensive historical analysis of the patient may obviate the need for the formal exercise test. In this regard, Bassuk et al.[17] have proposed a useful calibration metric. This group defines "mild exercise" as any activity during which you can sing, and "moderate exercise" as any activity during which you can only talk. In summary, if a patient can climb more than one flight of stairs without chest pain prior to moderate risk noncardiac and even vascular surgery, then that patient does not need an exercise tolerance test.

Ventricular Function Testing

The left ventricle is not a perfect sphere. Thus, calculations derived from a single axis M-mode or even a two-dimensional EKG can be problematic. Radionuclide angiography or gated blood pool imaging is intuitively likely to be more accurate. The patient receives an intravenous injection of technetium-99 (pertechnetate) tagged to his/her own red blood cells. When the patient's heart is scanned for low-level γ radiation, the radiation detected at end systole is related to the radiation emitted at end diastole. This equals ejection fraction. This is a logical conclusion since the γ-rays emit from the entire volume of blood in the left ventricle and are not calculated from any assumed geometric form based upon one or more echo-derived dimensions. The radiation derived from a single beat is not sufficient for reliable calculations, so sequential end systolic and end diastolic counts are "gated" from an EKG. This measure produces a MUlti-GAted scan. A healthy ventricle at rest ejects about 60% of its end diastolic volume (EF = 60%) with each beat. In patients with normal exercise capacity (two flights of stairs), ventriculography will rarely yield information that modifies perioperative strategy, and ventriculography is not recommended in patients prior to low- or moderate-risk operations.[1]

Practical Preoperative Risk Assessment

It is an oversimplification to assume that a single preoperative test might accurately assess the combination of cardiopulmonary fortitude, muscle strength, psychological resiliency, and "vitality" essential to weathering the stress of a major surgical procedure; but, when it comes to convenience, practicality, expense and reliability, "climbing a flight of stairs" compares very favorably with the other available tests.

Snowden et al.[18] subjected 389 patients to cardiorespiratory exercise testing prior to hepatobiliary surgery. Anaerobic threshold was the most robust predictor of postoperative mortality ($p = 0.003$), while age did not have statistical significance. Similarly, Prentis et al.[19] performed submaximal cardiopulmonary exercise testing on 185 patients prior to both open and endovascular aortic aneurysm repair. Again, anaerobic threshold was predictive of both the length of time in the ICU ($p = 0.002$) and the duration of hospital stay ($p = 0.0001$). Interestingly, it may even be possible to "train" for a surgical operation with a preconditioning program. Angevaren and coinvestigators[20] examined the Cochrane database of 11 studies relating physical activity to enhanced fitness as a strategy to improve cognitive function. Perhaps predictably, exercise interventions ("training") did increase maximum oxygen intake, which did coincide with improved cognitive function in the intervention group. The concept of surgical preconditioning or prehabilitation deserves considerably more study.

Evolving assessment of perioperative risk has benefited by substantial evidence-based attention since a 1996 update of the initial ACC/AHA guidelines for perioperative cardiovascular evaluation in noncardiac surgery was published.[6] The surgeon and patient must balance the anticipated benefits of operation with the estimated "risks." An update on this algorithm was published by an ACC/AHA task force and published in 2009.[21] Many sophisticated tests of physical status and cardiac function are now available. However, unless the results of a test are going to change the planned surgical therapy, there is questionable reason to obtain them.

Rohde et al.[22] studied 570 patients prior to major noncardiac surgery and identified that systolic dysfunction was only "marginally" associated with postoperative myocardial infarction and cardiogenic pulmonary edema. Similarly, a meta-analysis of eight studies assessing preoperative resting left ventricular function by radionuclide angiography derived a sensitivity of only 43% and a positive predictive value of only 13% for perioperative cardiac mortality.[23] Perhaps surprisingly, even resting left ventricular function was not identified as a consistent predictor of perioperative cardiac ischemic events.[24]

Why do we always obtain a resting 12-lead EKG, especially in geriatric patients, prior to surgery? Liu et al.[25] reviewed the 12-lead tracing in 515 elderly patients before elective and even urgent noncardiac surgery. Interestingly, three quarters of these patients did exhibit a baseline EKG abnormality and 3.7% died. The most likely causes of death were sepsis, multiorgan failure, bowel perforation, stroke, and respiratory failure. Cardiac causes were not among the top five causes of death.

A similar conclusion was derived by Schein and coinvestigators,[26] who randomly assigned elderly persons to a "testing" or "no-testing" group prior to 19,557 cataract operations. The latter group did not obtain resting EKGs in the absence of symptoms. These patients did experience 3.13% perioperative events (mostly, hypertension and bradycardia); but, the incidence was not predicted by preoperative testing. These authors concluded that "routine medical testing" did not measurably increase the safety of surgery.[26] It is increasingly apparent that when preoperative testing does not change what we do or does not influence perioperative outcomes, then we should stop the "testing."

SAFER SURGERY: PERIOPERATIVE PHARMACEUTICALS

Beta-blockers

Intuitively, slowing down the heart rate makes sense. About 80% of coronary perfusion occurs during diastole, so prolongation of diastole should increase coronary perfusion with a concurrent increase in myocardial oxygen delivery. A longer interval of diastolic filling should increase stroke volume. This hemodynamic improvement should be associated with a decrease in ischemic cardiac dysrhythmias and a resultant reduction in sympathetic tone.[27] Atherosclerosis is a systemic disease typically involving the coronary arteries early in its systemic progression. Thus, any patient who experiences claudication or transient ischemic attacks may be assumed to have concurrent CAD. Preoperative preparation of high-risk patients with low-dose beta-blockers (preferably for at least 2 weeks) is persuasively supported by many excellent studies.[28,29]

A Dutch study[29] collected 1,351 vascular patients (already high risk) and, by history alone, identified 846 of them with additional cardio-specific risk factors (very high risk). All of these patients were then screened with dobutamine stress echocardiography, and 173 of them exhibited inducible ventricular wall motion abnormalities (very, very high-risk patients). The Dutch investigators then tried to recruit these 173 patients into a prospective trial of surgery either with perioperative beta-blocker protection or "standard" perioperative care. Sixty-one patients refused, while 50 patients randomly received perioperative beta-blockers and 53 did not. The reported results were conclusive as only two patients in the beta-blocker group (3.4%) suffered the primary endpoints of death or nonfatal myocardial infarction, while 34% of the "standard" therapy patients did. Critical review of the data collection in this study has cast a shadow on some of the specifics, but many other groups[30] have derived similar recommendations that encourage perioperative beta-blocker protection in high- or even moderate-risk general and vascular surgical patients.

Because nonfatal myocardial infarction and cardiac deaths are uncommon outcomes in general surgery, the Peri-Operative ISchemic Evaluation (POISE) study investigators[31] did the power calculation and concluded that their study would require a very large number of patients to identify outcome differences for "low-risk" general surgical patients with and without perioperative beta-blockade protection. The POISE group gathered 8,351 patients from 190 hospitals in 23 countries. The logistics of this massive undertaking necessitated a very simple protocol. They wanted an adequate dose of beta-blocker to make a physiological difference, so they chose four to eight times the recommended dose of an extended-release beta-blocker, and their protocol permitted provision of this large dose to any patient with a heart rate of >60 bpm. Even using this ambitious strategy, beta-blockers proved protective in medium- and high-risk surgical patients. The authors also demonstrated that a large extended-release dose of beta-blocker given to low-risk patients with a heart rate of

60 bpm can occasionally provoke bradycardia, hypotension, and stroke. Fortunately, the ACC/AHA document evaluated this study and endorsed the perioperative protection with beta-blockers in high-risk patients, but cautioned that:

> "...routine administration of higher dose long acting metoprolol in beta blocker naïve patients on the day of surgery and in the absence of dose titration is associated with an increased mortality."[20]

Electrocardiographic evidence of myocardial ischemia is relatively common during surgical procedures performed on patients with untreated or treated hypertension.[32] Multiple smaller studies, while not achieving statistical significance, have reported less frequent intraoperative cardiac ischemia in patients with diabetes,[33] hypertension,[32] and advanced age[34] when protected with perioperative beta-blockade. In the case of any patient for whom the surgeon is worried about perioperative myocardial ischemia, it is easy to justify the judicious use of short- to medium-acting beta-blockers titrated to a heart rate of 70–90 bpm.

Recommendations on the perioperative use of beta-blockers are as follows:

1. When a surgical patient presents on beta-blocker drugs, the drugs should be continued.
2. When a high index of concern exists about perioperative myocardial ischemia, especially in a vascular surgical patient, then it is more likely than not that beta-blockers will be of benefit.
3. Optimal initiation of beta-blockers is 1–2 weeks prior to operation, targeting a heart rate of 70–90 bpm and monitoring to avoid hypotension and bradycardia.
4. Although a 2-week course is optimal, 2 days is better than 2 hours, which is generally considered to be better than no beta-blockers at all.
5. Although it is not completely accurate to extrapolate from nonsurgical studies of patients following a myocardial infarction, Cucherat[35] has collected 17 trials using beta-blockers in patients following a myocardial infarction. This investigator calculated that for every beta-blocker-induced reduction in a heart rate of 10 bpm, in the absence of hypotension, patients accrued a relative reduction in cardiac death of 30%.
6. Large doses of extended-release beta-blockers in drug-naïve, low-risk patients are contraindicated.

Statin Drugs

The use of statins (3-hydroxy-3 methylglutaryl coenzyme A or HMG-CoA reductase inhibitors) as perioperative protection against cardiovascular events is evolving. The HMG-CoA reductase is the rate-limiting step in cholesterol synthesis. Cholesterol is an obligate building block of cell membranes, and accordingly makes the use of a cholesterol synthesis inhibitor potentially deleterious. But statins also increase expression of low-density lipoprotein (LDL) receptors, thus increasing the clearance of circulating LDL cholesterol. Almost half a century ago, the Framingham study first associated high cholesterol with atherosclerotic cardiovascular disease. Over 75% of cholesterol is synthesized de novo in the liver, and only 20% is from dietary sources. Thus, endogenous production has been the focus of efforts at cholesterol control with pharmacologic agents. A decade ago, Law et al. reviewed several hundred trials targeting cholesterol[36] and concluded that a reduction in circulating LDL cholesterol of as little as 1.8 mm/L conferred a 60% reduction in ischemic heart disease and a 17% decrease in stroke.

Additional benefits of statin drug use other than cholesterol reduction have been reported. After adjusting for all other cancer risk factors, Poynter et al.[37] reported a 47% reduction in the relative risk of colorectal cancer associated with the use of statins. Inflammation has a common association with atherogenesis, neoplasia, and the human stress response. Albert et al.[38] have reported that statins blunt the inflammatory response.

Retrospective studies by Pan et al.[39] and Ouattara et al.[40] have both reported dose-dependent reduction in adverse cardiovascular outcomes with statins in coronary artery bypass strategy. Biccard[41] has reported the benefits of statins in vascular surgery and has emphasized that statins should not be stopped in the preoperative period. Statins appear to provide benefit both for patients with neoplastic disease and patients with cardiac disease. Patients who will benefit from beta-blockers are likely to be a similar population to those who will derive an advantage from statins. Like beta-blockers, optimal benefit is achieved from statins when they are taken at least 2 weeks before operation. Importantly, patients who have been on statin drugs before operation should not have them stopped.

PRACTICAL OPERATIVE PLANNING

The Stable Elective Patient

When the practical and focused history and physical examination have been accomplished, and the patient has been given a functional and objective assessment of cardiac risk (*see* Table 27.1), the stable elective patient should be managed by the algorithm in Flowchart 27.1:

Flowchart 27.1: The algorithm for management of the patient undergoing elective noncardiac surgery. (MET: Metabolic equivalent).

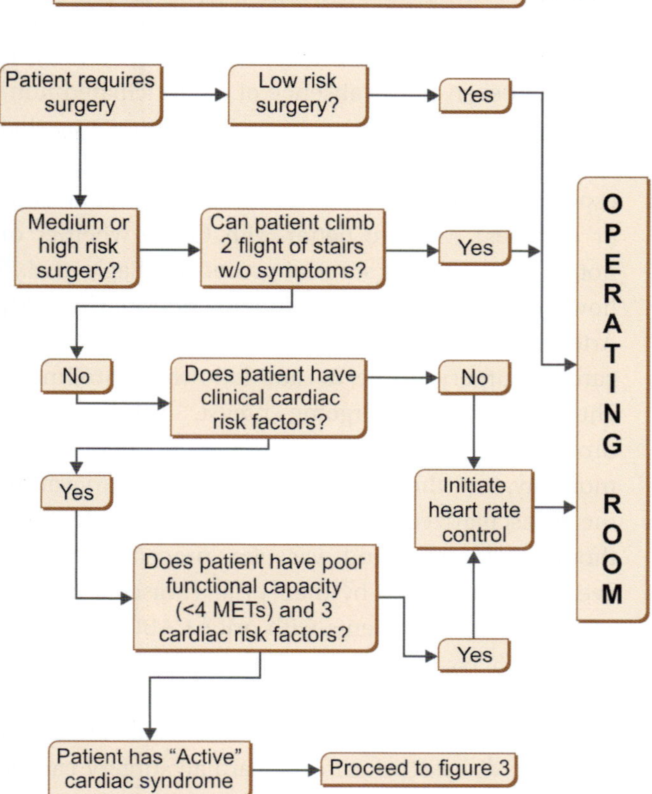

Flowchart 27.2: The algorithm for management of the patient undergoing urgent noncardiac surgery. (CAD: Coronary artery disease).

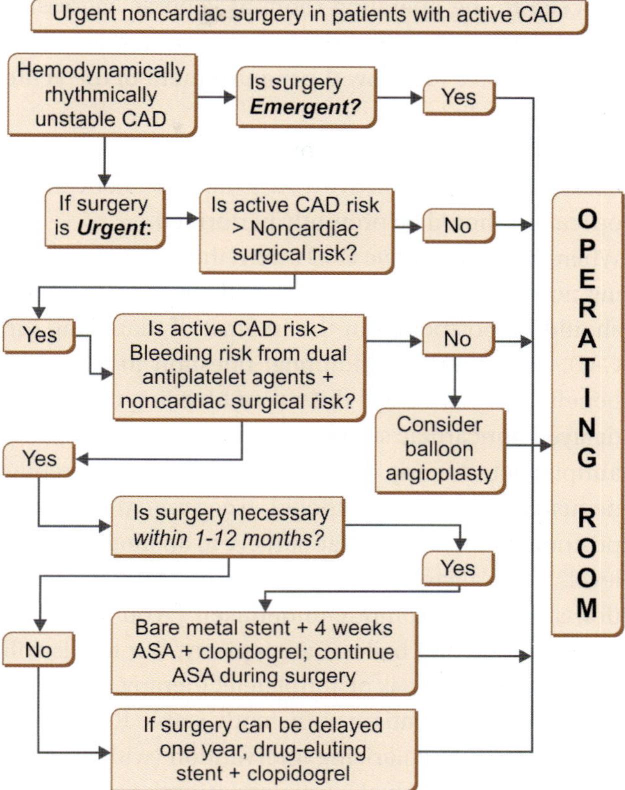

1. If the patient is scheduled for low-risk surgery, then the operation should proceed when scheduled without additional cardiac assessment.
2. If the patient is scheduled for medium- or high-risk surgery and can climb two flights of stairs without symptoms, then operation can proceed without additional cardiac evaluation. Consideration should be given to beta-blockers and statin drugs based upon current clinical criteria and whether these patients have been taking the drugs preoperatively.
3. If the patient cannot climb two flights of stairs without symptoms, but has no clinical cardiac risk factors, then operation should proceed with due consideration for the use of beta-blockers or statins.
4. If the patient has poor exercise capacity (<4 METs) and several cardiac risk factors, then proceed to operation after activating strategies for making it safer, as noted above.
5. If the patient exhibits symptoms and/or signs of an "active" cardiac syndrome, then proceed with preoperative assessment detailed in the algorithm as shown in Flowchart 27.2.

URGENT NONCARDIAC SURGERY IN A PATIENT WITH AN "ACTIVE CARDIAC SYNDROME"

Aggressive resuscitation of the hemodynamically unstable patient must be considered the highest priority. Goal-directed therapy (GDT) is based upon the logically sequential resuscitative steps: (1) volume repletion to an optimal central venous pressure, (2) cardiotonic agents to enhance pump function, and (3) transfusion to increase oxygen-carrying capacity and systemic oxygen delivery. This resuscitative strategy was initially proposed and validated as early (<6 hours) therapy for severe sepsis and septic shock.[42] More recently, this GDT algorithm has been prospectively randomized in patients following a major operation and has been confirmed as reducing postoperative complications.[43]

Following evidence-based strategies of initial resuscitation,[42,43] the management of an unstable patient requiring urgent noncardiac surgery should follow the algorithm depicted in Flowchart 27.2.

1. When surgical intervention is urgent, then in the case of hemodynamically or rhythmically unstable patient, proceed to the operating room as soon as aggressive resuscitation is accomplished. Extensive cardiac evaluation will have to follow the management of the acute surgical condition.
2. When the risks of postponing noncardiac surgery exceed the risks of active CAD, then the noncardiac operation should be promptly performed.
3. When the risks of active CAD *exceed* the risks of postponing noncardiac surgery, then the operative intervention should be postponed in the interest of managing the CAD. An important additional question in this risk–benefit analysis is "will the risk of bleeding during the delayed noncardiac surgery in a patient receiving dual antiplatelet therapy (mandatory following percutaneous coronary interventions) *exaggerate* the risks of postponing the noncardiac surgery to an unacceptable level? If the answer is yes, then the noncardiac operation should be promptly undertaken." You may consider temporizing balloon angioplasty, but this is still likely to incur the risk of antiplatelet therapy.
4. If you deem the patient sufficiently stable to undergo a coronary revascularizing intervention (with obligate postintervention dual antiplatelet/anticoagulation), then you should consider cardiac catheterization. The 2005 percutaneous coronary intervention guidelines[44] recommend clopidogrel 75 mg daily for at least 1 month following implantation of a bare metal stent. If the risk of bleeding during operation with dual antiplatelet therapy is too great and the noncardiac procedure cannot be postponed for a month, then it should proceed. The early experience with noncardiac surgical procedures soon (<6 weeks) following coronary stenting was so frightening that few surgeons have risked reliving that experience. Kaluza et al.[45] proceeded with noncardiac surgery in 40 patients in <6 weeks following placement of a bare metal stent. These investigations reported 7 myocardial infarctions (presumably secondary to stent thrombosis), 11 major bleeding events, and 8 postoperative deaths.

   Optimal dual antiplatelet therapy following placement of a bare metal stent is at least 3 months. If noncardiac surgery becomes mandatory prior to that period, clopidogrel may be discontinued (if surgically advisable) 5 days prior to operation, but aspirin may be continued perioperatively.
5. If noncardiac surgery can be safely postponed for 1 year, then the algorithm in Flowchart 27.1 is appropriate. At this time, it is important to consider whether coronary revascularization [percutaneous coronary intervention vs. coronary artery bypass grafting (CABG)] is indicated even in the absence of an anticipated noncardiac operation. The evidence is accumulating that specific cohorts of patients (two- and three-vessel CAD, especially with depressed ventricular function and/or diabetes) will fare better with CABG whether or not they anticipate a surgical procedure. Eagle et al.,[46] however, followed 3,368 patients in the Coronary Artery Surgery Study database who underwent noncardiac surgery in the decade following enrollment. These patients undergoing breast, orthopedic, or urological procedures suffered a <1% perioperative mortality, and there was no difference in survival for the revascularized patients. The patients undergoing thoracoabdominal and vascular procedures, however, were protected by their prior revascularization. Mortality rate in patients with prior CABG was lower (1.7% vs. 3.3%; $p = 0.03$), as was nonfatal myocardial infarction (0.8% vs. 2.7%; $p = 0.002$).

In summary, preoperative assessment of the patient with cardiac disease prior to noncardiac surgery can be effective in directing perioperative management and reducing the risk of cardiac-associated complications during the postoperative period. Functional assessments of cardiac disease become very effective in defining which patients may need more detailed preoperative evaluations and which may require specific therapeutic interventions.

REFERENCES

1. Smith R, Ng V, Twomey P, et al. Preoperative testing, planning and stratification. Elements of contemporary practice. In: Jurkovich GJ, Napolitano LM, Pearce WH, Pemberton JH, Soper NJ (Eds). ACS Surgery Online. New York, NY: WebMD; 2012.
2. Deckers JW. Classification of myocardial infarction and unstable angina: a reassessment. Int J Cardiol. 2013;167(6):2387-90.
3. Stone PH, Thompson B, Zaret BL, et al. Factors associated with failure of medical therapy in patients with unstable angina and non-Q wave myocardial infarction. A TIMI-IIIB database study. Eur Heart J. 1999;20(15):1084-93.
4. Sharifi M, Frohlich TG, Silverman IM. Myocardial infarction with angiographically normal coronary arteries. Chest. 1995;107:36-40.

5. Rudd RE. Improving Americans' health literacy. N Engl J Med. 2010;363:2283-5.
6. Eagle KA, Berger PB, Calkins H, et al. ACC/AHA guideline update for perioperative vascular evaluation for noncardiac surgery—executive summary: a report of the American College of Cardiology/American Heart Association Task Force on Practice Guidelines (Committee to Update the 1996 Guidelines on Perioperative Cardiovascular Evaluation for Noncardiac Surgery). J Am Coll Cardiol. 2002;39:542-3.
7. Bruce RA, Lovejoy FW Jr, Pearson R, et al. Normal respiratory and circulatory pathways of adaptation in exercise. J Clin Invest. 1949;28:1423-30.
8. Hlatky MA, Boineau RE, Higginbotham MB, et al. A brief self-administered questionnaire to determine functional capacity (the Duke Activity Status Index). Am J Cardiol. 1989;64:651-4.
9. Reilly DF, McNeely MJ, Doerner D, et al. Self-reported exercise tolerance and the risk of serious perioperative complications. Arch Intern Med. 1999;159:2185-92.
10. Bolton JW, Weiman DS, Haynes JL, et al. Stair climbing as an indicator of pulmonary function. Chest. 1987;92(5):783-8.
11. Pollock M, Cousar J, Martinez F, Celli B. Comparison of stair climbing to cycle ergometry in patients with chronic airflow obstruction (CAO). Chest. 1989;96(Suppl):231.
12. Van Nostrand D, Kjelsberg MO, Humphrey EW. Preresectional evaluation of risk from pneumonectomy. Surg Gynecol Obstet. 1968;127:306-12.
13. Girish M, Trayner E, Dammann O, et al. Symptom-limited stair climbing as a predictor of postoperative cardiopulmonary complications after high-risk surgery. Chest. 2001; 120(4):1147-51.
14. Brunelli A, Refai M, Xiumé F, et al. Performance at symptom-limited stair-climbing test is associated with increased cardiopulmonary complications, mortality, and costs after major lung resection. Ann Thorac Surg. 2008;86:240-7; discussion 247-8.
15. Nicolić I, Majerić-Kogler V, Plavec D, et al. Stairs climbing test with pulse oximetry as predictor of early postoperative complications in functionally impaired patients with lung cancer and elective lung surgery: prospective trial of consecutive series of patients. Croat Med J. 2008;49:50-7.
16. Brunelli A, Kim AW, Berger KI, et al. Physiologic evaluation of the patient with lung cancer being considered for resectional surgery: diagnosis and management of lung cancer, 3rd ed: American College of Chest Physicians evidence-based clinical practice guidelines. Chest. 2013;143(5 Suppl):e166S-90S.
17. Bassuk SS, Church TS, Manson JE. Why exercise works magic. Sci Am. 2013;309(2):74-9.
18. Snowden CP, Prentis J, Jacques B, et al. Cardiorespiratory fitness predicts mortality and hospital length of stay after major elective surgery in older people. Ann Surg. 2013; 257(6):999-1004.
19. Prentis JM, Trenell MI, Jones DJ, et al. Submaximal exercise testing predicts perioperative hospitalization after aortic aneurysm repair. J Vasc Surg. 2012;56(6):1564-70.
20. Young J, Angevaren M, Rusted J, et al. Aerobic exercise to improve cognitive function in older people without known cognitive impairment. Cochrane Database Syst Rev. 2015;4:CD005381.
21. Fleisher LA, Beckman JA, Brown KA, et al. 2009 ACCF/AHA focused update on perioperative beta blockade incorporated into the ACC/AHA 2007 guidelines on perioperative cardiovascular evaluation and care for noncardiac surgery: a report of the American college of cardiology foundation/ American heart association task force on practice guidelines. Circulation 2009;120:e169-276.
22. Rohde LE, Polanczyk CA, Goldman L, et al. Usefulness of transthoracic echocardiography as a tool for risk stratification of patients undergoing major noncardiac surgery. Am J Cardiol. 2001;87:505-9.
23. Kertai MD, Boersma E, Bax JJ, et al. A meta-analysis comparing the prognostic accuracy of six diagnostic tests for predicting perioperative cardiac risk in patients undergoing major vascular surgery. Heart. 2003;89:1327-34.
24. Fleisher LA, Barash PG. Preoperative cardiac evaluation for noncardiac surgery: a functional approach. Anesth Analg. 1992;74:586-9.
25. Liu LL, Dzankic S, Leung JM. Preoperative electrocardiogram abnormalities do not predict postoperative cardiac complications in geriatric surgical patients. J Am Geriatr Soc. 2002;50:1186-91.
26. Schein OD, Katz J, Bass EB, et al. The value or routine preoperative medical testing before cataract surgery. Study of Medical Testing for Cataract Surgery. N Engl J Med. 2000;342:168-75.
27. Dawood MM, Gutpa DK, Southern J, et al. Pathology of fatal perioperative myocardial infarction: implications regarding pathophysiology and prevention. Int J Cardiol. 1996;57:37-44.
28. Poldermans D, Boersma E. Beta-blocker therapy in noncardiac surgery. N Engl J Med. 2005; 353:412-4.
29. Poldermans D, Boersma E, Bax JJ, et al. The effect of bisoprolol on perioperative mortality and myocardial infarction in high-risk patients undergoing vascular surgery. Dutch Echocardiographic Cardiac Risk Evaluation Applying Stress Echocardiography Study Group. N Engl J Med. 1999;341: 1789-94.
30. Mangano DT, Layug EL, Wallace A, et al. Effect of atenolol on mortality and cardiovascular morbidity after noncardiac surgery. Multicenter Study of Perioperative Ischemia Research Group. N Engl J Med. 1996;335:1713-20.
31. POISE Study Group, Devereaux PJ, Yang H, et al. Effects of extended-release metoprolol succinate in patients undergoing non-cardiac surgery (POISE trial): a randomised controlled trial. Lancet. 2008;371(9627):1839-47.
32. Stone JG, Foëx P, Sear JW, et al. Risk of myocardial ischaemia during anaesthesia in treated and untreated hypertensive patients. Br J Anaesth. 1988;61:675-9.
33. Juul AB, Wetterslev J, Gluud C, et al. Effect of perioperative beta blockade in patients with diabetes undergoing major noncardiac surgery: randomised placebo controlled, blinded multicentre trial. BMJ. 2006;332:1482.

34. Zaugg M, Tagliente T, Lucchinetti E, et al. Beneficial effects from beta-adrenergic blockade in elderly patients undergoing noncardiac surgery. Anesthesiology. 1999;91:1674-86.
35. Cucherat M. Quantitative relationship between resting heart rate reduction and magnitude of clinical benefits in post-myocardial infarction: a meta-regression of randomized clinical trials. Eur Heart J. 2007;28:3012-9.
36. Law MR, Wald NJ, Rudnicka AR. Quantifying effect of statins on low density lipoprotein cholesterol, ischaemic heart disease and stroke: systematic review and meta-analysis. BMJ. 2003;326:1423.
37. Poynter JN, Gruber SB, Higgins PD, et al. Statins and the risk of colorectal cancer. N Engl J Med. 2005;352:2184-92.
38. Albert MA, Danielson E, Rifai N, et al. Effect of statin therapy on C-reactive protein levels: the pravastatin inflammation/CRP evaluation (PRINCE): a randomized trial and cohort study. JAMA. 2001;286:64-70.
39. Pan W, Pintar T, Anton J, et al. Statins are associated with a reduced incidence of perioperative mortality after coronary artery bypass surgery. Circulation. 2004;110(11 Suppl 1): II45-9.
40. Ouattara A, Benhaoua H, Le Manach Y, et al. Perioperative statin therapy is associated with a significant and dose-dependent reduction of adverse cardiovascular outcomes after coronary artery bypass surgery. J Cardiothorac Vasc Anesth. 2009;23:633-8.
41. Biccard BM. A peri-operative statin update for noncardiac surgery. Part II: statin therapy for vascular surgery and peri-operative statin trial design. Anaesthesia. 2008;63: 162-71.
42. Rivers E, Nguyen B, Havstad S, et al. Early goal-directed therapy in the treatment of severe sepsis and septic shock. N Engl J Med. 2001;345:1368-77.
43. Pearse R, Dawson D, Fawcett J, et al. Early goal-directed therapy after major surgery reduces complications and duration of hospital stay. A randomised, controlled trial [ISRCTN38797445]. Crit Care. 2005;9(6):R687-93.
44. Smith SC Jr, Teldman TE, Hirshfeld JW Jr, et al. ACC/AHA/SCAI 2005 guideline update for percutaneous coronary intervention: a report of the American College of Cardiology/American Heart Association Task Force on Practice Guidelines (ACC/AHA/SCAI Writing Committee to Update the 2001 Guidelines for Percutaneous Coronary Intervention). J Am Coll Cardiol. 2006;47:e1-121.
45. Kaluza GL, Joseph J, Lee JL, et al. Catastrophic outcomes of noncardiac surgery soon after coronary stenting. J Am Coll Cardiol. 2000;35(5):1288-94.
46. Eagle KA, Rihal CS, Mickel MC, et al. Cardiac risk of noncardiac surgery: influence of coronary disease and type of surgery in 3368 operations. CASS Investigators and University of Michigan Heart Care Program. Coronary Artery Surgery Study. Circulation. 1997;96:1882-7.

28

Acute Kidney Injury

Jan De Waele, Eric Hoste

Key Points

- The kidney is crucial for regulation of salt, water, and acid–base homeostasis.
- Acute kidney injury (AKI) is a multifactorial and heterogeneous condition. Acute kidney injury may be due to hypovolemia and poor kidney perfusion, inflammation or toxic injury to tubular cells of the kidney, or mechanical obstruction of the urine outflow system. Differentiation of the cause is critical for management of AKI.
- The current definition of AKI is sensitive, as less severe AKI also affects outcome and includes three severity grades. It is based on either a period of decreased urinary output or an increase in serum creatinine (SCR).
- There is no specific therapy for prevention or treatment of AKI. Prevention of AKI in surgical patients requires an understanding of those variables likely to cause the problem. Early detection and directed therapy are essential. Prevention and prompt management of hypovolemia, restricted use of nephrotoxic antibiotics, and avoidance of intravenous contrast agents are all essential.
- Indications for renal replacement therapy (RRT) for AKI include volume overload in case of oliguria, hyperkalemia, and severe acidosis. There are no hard data on the exact timing for initiation of RRT or the modality that is preferred. In severely ill patients, most physicians commence RRT early with a continuous RRT (CRRT) modality.

INTRODUCTION

Renal function is a complex assembly of physiologic processes that regulate the composition of body fluids. The principal function of the kidney is clearance of water-soluble toxins by filtration. In addition, the kidney plays a crucial role in regulation of the composition of extracellular fluid and maintains optimal osmolality, electrolyte composition, and acid-base status. The kidneys are also an integral part of the endocrine system, functioning both as effector organs that respond to hormones and as a regulator of other organs through the release of hormones.

Dysfunction of the kidney has been identified as a lethal condition for a long time. One of the earliest descriptions of renal function impairment in medical literature was by William Heberden in 1802. "Ischuria renalis" was defined by the very specific definition of "a total suppression" of urine output. A much more sensitive definition was used during World War I to describe "trench or war nephritis," a condition with a probable postviral etiology and characterized by proteinuria. Later during World War II, rhabdomyolysis-induced kidney dysfunction was defined by anuria. In the modern era, small decreases in glomerular filtration rate (GFR) can be detected more easily, and acute renal failure was introduced to describe the situation in which the kidney did not function adequately. Since the early days of medical descriptions of kidney dysfunction, different definitions have been used, ranging from very sensitive to very specific.[1]

DEFINITION

The terminology "acute kidney injury" (AKI) has been introduced recently to replace the previously widely used term "acute renal failure" that was first introduced in 1951. In contrast to "failure," "injury" indicates that less severe decreases of GFR are also important.

Conceptually, AKI is a continuum of different disease states, ranging from an at-risk situation up to extensive damage requiring renal replacement therapy (RRT). It is an abrupt reduction of kidney function characterized by an increase in creatinine concentration and/or a reduction in urinary output.[2] Acute kidney injury covers both acute dysfunction and acute structural damage to the kidney, or a combination of the two.

In 2002, the international consensus conference of the Acute Dialysis Quality Initiative (ADQI) proposed the RIFLE (Risk, Injury, and Failure; Loss; End-stage kidney disease) classification of AKI, based on SCR changes and urinary output.[3] This classification system has since been updated twice: first by the Acute Kidney Injury Network (AKIN) and recently by the Kidney Disease: Improving Global Outcomes (KDIGO).[2,4]

Patients are categorized to have either normal kidney function, stage 1 or risk, stage 2 or injury, or stage 3 or failure based on either SCR or urine output criteria (Table 28.1). Patients who are treated with RRT are classified as stage 3 AKI, irrespective of SCR concentration, or urine output. In addition to these severity stages, the original RIFLE classification also included loss and end-stage kidney disease for patients who were treated with RRT for 4 weeks and 3 months, respectively.

Cellular damage to the kidney can be quantified using newer biomarkers such as neutrophil gelatinase-associated lipocalin (NGAL) or the combination of tissue inhibitor of metalloproteinases-2 (TIMP-2) and insulin-like growth factor-binding protein-7 (IGFBP-7).[5,6] This measure allows detection of subclinical AKI, defined as biomarker positive AKI while SCR is not increased, although the clinical relevance remains unclear at this stage.[7]

Table 28.1 Kidney Disease: Improving Global Outcomes (KDIGO) definitions and classification of acute kidney injury.[4]

Definition			
• Any of the following criteria			
• Increase in SCR by ≥0.3 mg/dL (<26.5 μmol/L) within 48 hours			
• Increase in SCR to ≥1.5 times baseline, which is known or presumed to have occurred within the prior 7 days			
• Urine volume <0.5 mL/kg/h for 6 hours			
Staging			
	Diagnostic criterion		
Stage	*Absolute change in SCR*	*Relative change in SCR*	*Urinary output*
1	Increase ≥ 0.3 mg/dL (<26.5 μmol/L) within 48 hours	1.5–1.9 times baseline	<0.5 mL/kg/h for 6–12 hours
2		2.0–2.9 times baseline	<0.5 mL/kg/h for >12 hours
3	Increase to >4 mg/dL (353.6 μmol/L)	3.0 times baseline OR Initiation of RRT	<0.3 mL/kg/h for >24 hours OR Anuria for >12 hours

(RRT: Renal replacement therapy; SCR: Serum creatinine).

EPIDEMIOLOGY

Risk Factors for Development of AKI

Acute kidney injury is most often a consequence of another underlying disease (Fig. 28.1). In the large international multicenter BEST Kidney study, sepsis was indicated as the most prevalent underlying cause for AKI, followed by major surgery, cardiogenic shock, hypovolemia, drug-induced causes, hepatorenal syndrome, and obstruction.[8] Acute kidney injury occurred also more often in medical patients than surgical patients. Older patients and men also appeared to be at greater risk for developing AKI,[9] although in other settings such as cardiac surgery women are at greater risk for AKI.[10] Many of the risk factors for chronic kidney disease (CKD) (e.g. diabetes, African descent, and hypertension) have also been identified in AKI. However, this association may be confounded by the fact that CKD itself is a risk factor for AKI.

Incidence of AKI

The incidence of AKI depends on the definitions used, and historical data are often difficult to compare, as the definitions have been variable across studies that have investigated incidence.[11] The introduction of the RIFLE/AKIN/KDIGO classification has, however, led to a more consistent reporting of AKI, although differences in applying these new definitions remain.

AKI in the Intensive Care Unit

Acute kidney injury occurs in approximately one-third of intensive care unit (ICU) patients in the first 48 hours of their stay.[12,13] The reported incidence of AKI defined by the AKIN diagnostic and staging system during the whole ICU stay varies between 10.8% and 78.2% of ICU patients.[14,15] This large variation can be explained not only by the specific case mix studied but also by the duration of the study period (48 hours to whole ICU stay) and how the RIFLE or AKIN definitions are applied: full criteria, or a version without urine output or with variant urine output criteria, or with variant baseline SCR estimates.[16] The largest retrospective studies in general ICU patients studied during the whole ICU stay report an AKI incidence (defined by AKIN or RIFLE classification) of 35.4–67%.[17] Acute kidney injury severity staging by the AKIN/RIFLE allows early identification of patients at risk for progression to more severe AKI. In one study, 55% of patients who developed the least severe state of AKI according to the RIFLE classification progressed to more severe AKI.[18]

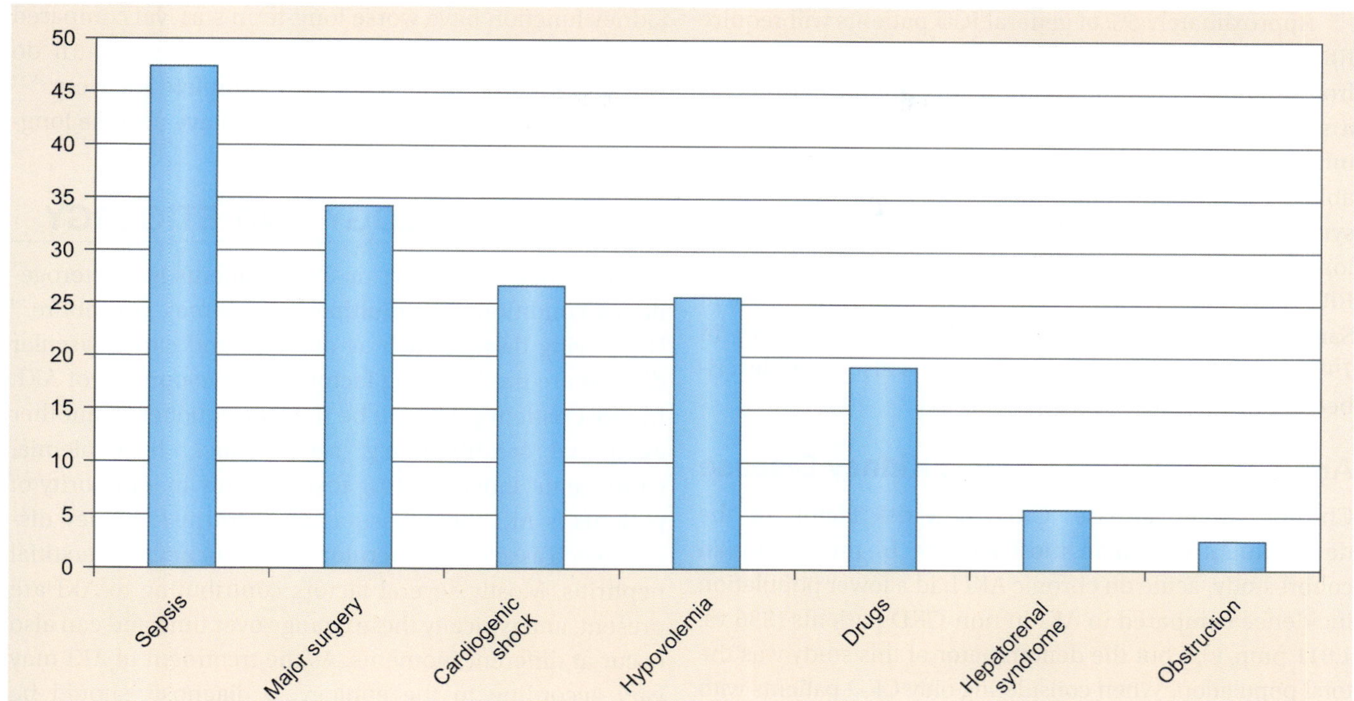

Fig. 28.1: Contributing underlying diseases associated with acute kidney injury.
Source: Data from Uchino S, Kellum JA, Bellomo R, et al. Acute renal failure in critically ill patients: a multinational, multicenter study. JAMA. 2005;294:813-8.

Community-Acquired AKI and Hospitalized Non-ICU Patients

Data on the incidence of community-acquired AKI are relatively scarce, and most come from developed countries. In recent years, some large laboratory-based studies have been published on the epidemiology of AKI. Although these data will identify all patients in whom a blood sample for SCR was analyzed, the true incidence of community AKI will still be underestimated. Less severe cases, e.g. as in outpatients with severe gastroenteritis or, at the other end of the spectrum, in terminal patients who are given palliative care, will not be included in these databases.

The incidence of less severe AKI has also increased over the years. In a series of two studies in 1979 and 1996, Nash and colleagues found that hospital-acquired AKI increased from 4.9% to 7.2% in the same institution in the United States.[19,20] Recent data illustrate that AKI is among the most prevalent of diseases. Uchino found an incidence of 18% in a sample of 20,126 hospitalized patients in Australia, when AKI was defined by the RIFLE classification (using only SCR criteria). In 2003, the population incidence of AKI in the Grampian region of Scotland defined by the RIFLE classification was 2,147 patients per million population per year (pmp/y).[21] This was still lower than the incidence reported in a study in a Northern California cohort of Kaiser Permanente beneficiaries in the period 1996 to 2003.[9,19] Here, the incidence of AKI showed an increase from 3,227 pmp/y in 1996–1997 to as high as 5,224 pmp/y in 2002–2003. This figure is comparable and even higher than the estimates for the incidence of sepsis in the United States, which range from 2,404 to 3,000 pmp/y.[22,23]

Requirement for Renal Replacement Therapy

Many studies that report on epidemiology of severe AKI use the need for renal replacement therapy (RRT) as a convenient way of counting cases. Although this may seem to be an objective criterion on first glance, it is in fact highly subjective since there are no agreed criteria for initiation of RRT. Over the years, criteria for initiation of RRT have shifted from "rescue" therapy for treatment of life-threatening uremic complications, such as pulmonary edema, uremic encephalopathy, or pericarditis (i.e. renal replacement), to a therapy that is initiated earlier in the course of AKI in order to facilitate other therapies such as parenteral nutrition (i.e. renal support).

Approximately 5% of general ICU patients will require RRT,[8,24,25] but due to case mix, this may vary from 2% to 20% from one institution to another. This proportion reflects a population incidence of 110–295 patients per million inhabitants per year,[9,21,25-27] an incidence that is comparable to that of acute lung injury, acute respiratory distress syndrome (ARDS), and severe sepsis.[28,29] Data from developed countries indicate that there is an increasing use of RRT for AKI. In the United States, the Nationwide Inpatient Sample Database observed an increase from 40 pmp/y in 1988 to 270 pmp/y in 2002,[27] which has also been described in other studies.[9,30]

AKI in Patients with Chronic Kidney Disease

Chronic kidney disease (CKD) is a risk factor for the development of AKI in most studies. In the Grampian cohort study, acute on chronic AKI had a lower population incidence compared to AKI in non-CKD patients (336 vs. 1,811 pmp/y),[21] but the denominator of this study was the total population. When considering only CKD patients with an estimated glomerular filtration rate (eGFR) <30 mL/min/1.73 m^2, the incidence of AKI in a cohort of Canadian patients was as high as 44.9%.[31] Also, more severe CKD was associated with greater odds for AKI requiring RRT (odds ratio for CKD stage 3 was 2, increasing to 40 for CKD stage 5).[32]

Mortality

Both severe AKI (defined by the need for RRT) and less severe AKI stages are associated with increased mortality.[16,33] There is even a clear stepwise relationship between increasing AKI severity grades and short in-hospital mortality. Of course, patients with more severe AKI are more likely to have more severe underlying disease and other organ dysfunction with subsequent impact on mortality. However, even when corrected for other determinants in multivariate analysis, there is an association between increasing AKI severity and mortality.[16] Not only short-term (in-hospital) outcome but also long-term mortality is affected by AKI. In a meta-analysis that included studies with different AKI definitions, AKI patients had a risk ratio (RR) of 2.3 compared to non-AKI patients for long-term mortality (8.9 deaths/100 person-year vs. 4.3 deaths/100 person-year).

Increasing AKI stages are associated with a stepwise decreased survival in up to 10-year follow-up.[34-36] Kidney-related factors that modulate this long-term mortality in AKI patients are increasing severity of AKI, recovery of kidney function, and CKD. Patients who do not recover kidney function have worse long-term survival compared to patients who partially recover, and they in turn do worse compared to patients with complete recovery.[36,37] Finally, patients with CKD before AKI have a worse long-term survival.[34,38]

PATHOPHYSIOLOGY AND ETIOLOGY

Acute kidney injury in critically ill patients is a heterogeneous condition, and multiple factors may contribute.[39] Underlying disease such as diabetes and cardiovascular disease are predisposing factors for development of AKI. In most patients, AKI will be the consequence of another extrarenal condition, e.g. septic shock, hypovolemia, cardiogenic shock, or drug toxicity. Only in a minority of patients is AKI the consequence of intrinsic kidney disease, such as acute glomerulonephritis or acute interstitial nephritis. Mostly several factors contributing to AKI are present, and typically these change over time and can also occur at different moments. As the treatment of AKI may vary according to the etiology, a diagnosis should be established as soon as possible.

The most used classification of AKI discriminates between prerenal, renal, and postrenal etiologies of AKI. Prerenal AKI is caused by a reduction in renal perfusion, and there is no structural abnormality.[40] In renal or intrinsic AKI, the kidney itself is affected, and structural kidney abnormalities as acute tubular necrosis or acute interstitial nephritis are present. In postrenal AKI, an obstruction of the urine outflow tract is the cause.

Biochemical indicators in urine and blood, together with clinical signs and directed imaging techniques (e.g. ultrasound scan), can help to differentiate prerenal, intrinsic renal, and postrenal disease.[41]

The difference between prerenal and intrinsic renal disease is often not so clear. It is uncertain whether prerenal AKI is a pure functional condition, and not associated with any damage to the kidney. Especially in the critically ill, multiple confounders may be present, some of them actually caused by attempts to treat the condition. Diuretic use, for example, can mimic intrinsic renal disease in patients whose AKI is in fact prerenal.

Prerenal AKI

Prerenal AKI affects about 50–60% of patients with AKI. It is a functional form of AKI that is by definition caused by inadequate blood flow to the kidneys, while the kidneys themselves are structurally normal.[42] Usually it is rapidly reversible when the underlying cause such as hypovolemia or low cardiac output is corrected. In some patients, abnormalities of the renal vasculature, such as renal artery stenosis, may also play a role.

Prerenal AKI has also been named volume-responsive AKI. While all volume-responsive AKIs by definition are a form of prerenal AKI, not each episode of prerenal AKI may be volume responsive. Typically, patients with cardiogenic shock are not always volume-responsive, though kidney function may improve when cardiac function improves.[43] There is also much debate on the role of fluid resuscitation and the impact of volume overload as a cause of AKI. In common causes of prerenal AKI such as in distributive shock or perioperative hypovolemia, inappropriate fluid resuscitation may in fact contribute to development of AKI through intra-abdominal hypertension (IAH) and increased venous outflow pressure.[44]

If this prerenal AKI state lasts long enough, hypoperfusion of the kidney may lead to real damage to the kidney, i.e. ischemia and acute tubular necrosis. The outer medullary region is especially at risk for these changes because, as a consequence of the particular renal vasculature, oxygen supply in this region of the kidney is limited while energy demands are high. However, it was demonstrated in an animal model of sepsis that renal blood flow, including blood flow in the medullary region of the kidney, is not decreased. Also, the vasoconstrictor noradrenaline did not decrease renal blood flow, but in fact increased renal blood flow.[45] An impaired microcirculation in the kidney due to inflammation may provide another explanation for the occurrence for prerenal AKI in this setting.[46]

It is uncertain when exactly a patient progresses from prerenal AKI to intrinsic renal AKI; only biopsy could answer this question. For obvious reasons, however, this is not done in routine clinical practice.

Intrinsic AKI

When there is associated damage to the kidneys, the patient classifies as having intrinsic renal disease. In contrast to prerenal AKI, this condition is not rapidly reversible and accounts for 30–40% of AKI.

Postrenal AKI

Postrenal AKI is the least frequent type, estimated at <10%. An obstruction of the urinary flow may be induced by obstruction at any level of the genitourinary tract. In patients with an indwelling urinary catheter, catheter blockage is a common cause of acute anuria and should readily be excluded.

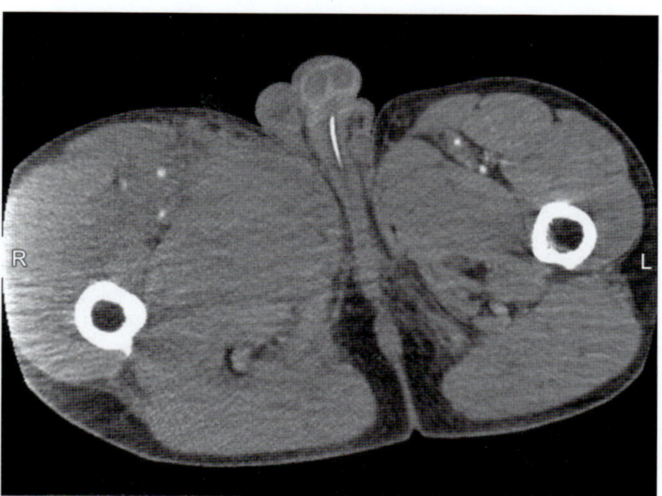

Fig. 28.2: An abdominal computed tomography scan of a trauma patient who fell from a height and was diagnosed with pelvic and multiple lower limb fractures. Severe contusion of the surrounding tissue was noted. Maximal creatinine phosphokinase level was 148,000; the patient became anuric despite fluid loading and required renal replacement therapy because of rhabdomyolysis.

SPECIFIC CAUSES OF AKI IN CRITICALLY ILL PATIENTS

Hemoglobinuria and Rhabdomyolysis

Hemoglobinuria is the consequence of hemolysis, e.g. after incompatible blood transfusion, and is rarely encountered if adequate precautions are taken. Patients develop acute hypotension, fever and a coagulopathy and produce discolored urine before becoming anuric.

Rhabdomyolysis, or release of myoglobin from muscles, develops following a wide range of events, but a principal mechanism among surgical patients is ischemia/reperfusion injury of skeletal muscles.[47] This injury can be caused by direct damage to the muscle, as observed in trauma patients or in patients who have been immobilized for a prolonged period of time (also intraoperatively) (Fig. 28.2).[48] Vascular ischemia can also lead to rhabdomyolysis. This ischemia/reperfusion phenomenon leads to inflammation and localized edema, which in turn may lead to elevated intracompartmental pressures that exacerbate ischemia and muscle necrosis.

Other causes of rhabdomyolysis include:

- Electrical injury in which a high voltage passes through muscle
- Myositis as, e.g., observed in necrotizing infections
- Neuromuscular blockade
- Statin therapy

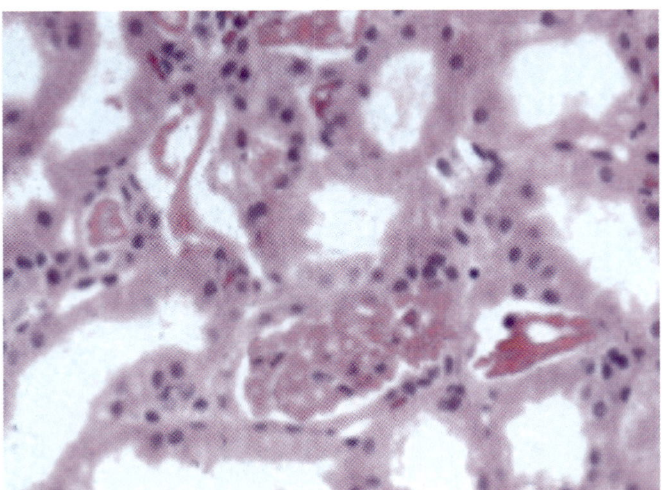

Fig. 28.3: Myoglobinuric renal failure. Renal biopsy of a patient who had rhabdomyolysis and myoglobinuria. Coarse eosinophilic casts of myoglobin are evident in the tubular lumen. Patients who deteriorate to develop acute kidney injury have more tubular cell damage than shown here. *Courtesy*: Donald C Houghton.

The magnitude of rhabdomyolysis is proportional to the elevation in serum creatinine phosphokinase (CPK). Clinical reviews show that patients who develop AKI associated with myoglobinuria generally have a serum CPK level exceeding 5,000 U/L, and in severe cases of rhabdomyolysis patients have CPK levels exceeding 100,000 U/L. Patients who are at high risk due to their clinical circumstances and who develop oliguria with a dark and heme-positive urine need immediate therapy.

Several mechanisms are hypothesized in myoglobin and hemoglobin-associated AKI as follows:[49]

- Tubular obstruction by the heme or myoglobin molecules (Fig. 28.3)
- Tubular cell toxicity by free radical oxygen species and inflammatory mediators
- Vasoconstriction of afferent arterioles by release of vasoactive agents: platelet activating factor, endothelin and prostaglandins are among those identified in experimental models of myoglobinuria

Hypovolemic or distributive shock often coexists in patients who have rhabdomyolysis (trauma, perioperative patients, prolonged muscle compression, and ischemia).

Intra-abdominal Hypertension

Patients develop IAH when the intra-abdominal pressure (IAP) exceeds 12 mm Hg; kidney function can be affected at levels >12 mm Hg, but clinical signs and symptoms may be subtle at this stage. The clinical conditions associated with the development of sufficient abdominal distension to produce IAH include:

- Fluid, blood or ascites filling the peritoneal cavity
- Hemorrhage into the retroperitoneum
- Bowel wall edema
- Intraluminal distension of the bowel with fluid or air
- Decreased compliance of the abdominal wall.

Abdominal compartment syndrome (ACS) is defined as an IAP of 20 mm Hg or higher, and new organ dysfunction develops as a consequence.[50] All organ systems may be affected, but apart from AKI, hypotension and respiratory insufficiency are the most common organ dysfunctions. Increased IAP may also affect neurological function as well as gastrointestinal and hepatic function.

A diagnosis of IAH is confirmed by IAP measurement, which can be measured using bladder pressures; measuring the abdominal girth or changes thereof is notoriously unreliable. The bladder pressure is measured by filling the bladder with a maximum of 25 mL sterile saline; several kits for measuring the IAP are commercially available. The zero reference for measurements is the midaxillary line; IAP is measured in the supine position with spontaneous muscle activity absent.[51]

Intra-abdominal hypertension has been identified as an independent risk factor for AKI in ICU patients; the kidney has also been coined the canary of IAH, as oliguria is often one of the first manifestations observed. Intra-abdominal hypertension has several effects on the kidney: it reduces arterial inflow, but outflow is also affected and probably one of the important contributors; also, hormonal changes may affect kidney function.[44] If IAP increases further, anuria may develop and other organ system dysfunctions will be present (Fig. 28.4).

In recent years, fluid resuscitation—and most importantly over-resuscitation—has been identified as an important cause of IAH.[52] Although surgical decompression remains the treatment of choice for overt ACS, several nonoperative management options are available. Targets for intervention include extraluminal and intraluminal collections and abdominal wall compliance. One of the simplest interventions to reduce IAP is paracentesis when peritoneal fluid is present; it has been found to avoid decompressive laparotomy in a considerable number of patients. Other treatment options include nasogastric suctioning, enemas, or the administration of neuromuscular blocking agents.[50]

Prevention of IAH is equally important, and in some patients prophylactic open abdomen management is necessary to prevent IAH and ACS. Typical conditions

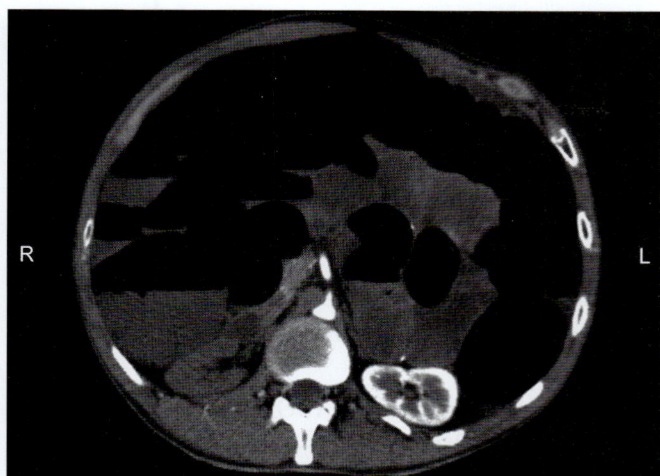

Fig. 28.4: Computed tomographic scan from a patient presenting with multiple organ failure due to abdominal compartment syndrome from intestinal obstruction. Intra-abdominal pressure was 45 mm Hg, and the perfusion of the left kidney was absent; the abdomen was decompressed and renal perfusion was restored.

include ruptured aortic aneurysm surgery, damage control laparotomy in trauma patients and operations for severe intra-abdominal infections.

Drug-Induced AKI

Drugs may affect kidney function in many ways; mechanisms include direct toxicity, formation of casts in the glomeruli, decreased renal blood flow, and interstitial nephritis. A list of drugs often associated with AKI is presented in Table 28.2.

Table 28.2 Selected drugs associated with acute kidney injury in surgical patients.

Immunosuppressant drugs
• Cyclosporin
• Tacrolimus
Chemotherapy
• Cisplatinum
• Methotrexate
• Rituximab
Antibiotics
• Aminoglycosides
• Penicillins
• Cephalosporins
• Rifampicin
Antifungals
• Amphotericin B
NSAIDs
Diuretics
• Frusemide
ACE inhibitors

Contrast-Associated AKI

As many patients are exposed to iodinated radiocontrast (i.e. for coronary angiography), this is one of the most prevalent causes of AKI. The etiology of contrast toxicity is incompletely understood. Similar to rhabdomyolysis, iodinated radiocontrast induces an inflammatory response with generation of free radical oxygen species that exert direct tubular toxicity and vasoconstriction, leading to decrease renal blood flow. Especially in severe ill patients, it is likely that contrast exposure is not the sole factor for development of AKI. For instance, severe sepsis, and other nephrotoxins such as aminoglycosides, may also contribute to AKI. Therefore, we advocate the use of the term contrast-associated AKI rather than contrast-induced AKI.

Contrast-associated AKI (CA-AKI) is associated with increased mortality and morbidity rates[53] and occurs in 5% of coronary angiography patients, up to 20% in patients who undergo emergency coronary angioplasty or in ICU patients who are undergoing a contrast-enhanced computed tomographic (CT) scan.[54,55]

Risk Factors for CA-AKI

Patients who have CKD (eGFR < 60 mL/min), AKI, diabetes, or vascular disease are at higher risk for CA-AKI. Also, patients who are treated with diuretics, NSAIDs, and metformin, or patients who are fluid-depleted are at increased risk.

Cardiorenal Syndrome

There is an important interaction between the heart and kidneys, and cardiorenal syndrome (CRS) is a condition characterized by cardiac and renal failure. In 2008, ADQI proposed a consensus definition for CRS and recognized five distinct types with different pathogeneses (Table 28.3).[56]

The pathophysiology of CRS is complex and differs according to the type of CRS. Cardiorenal syndrome type 1 occurs in 25% of patients with acute decompensated heart failure as a consequence of altered hemodynamics. Type 2 is the more rapid progression of CKD in the setting of chronic heart failure and is predominantly the consequence of accelerated apoptosis and fibrosis. In type 3 CRS, salt and water overload, uremia, and neurohumoral

Table 28.3	Classification of cardiorenal syndromes (CRS).
Type 1 CRS: Acute heart failure leads to acute kidney injury	
Type 2 CRS: Chronic heart failure leads to chronic kidney disease	
Type 3 CRS or acute renocardiac syndrome: Acute kidney injury leads to acute cardiac conditions such as arrhythmias or heart failure	
Type 4 CRS or chronic renocardiac syndrome: Chronic kidney disease contributes to chronic cardiac dysfunction	
Type 5 CRS, or secondary CRS, is a condition where both the kidney and heart are affected by a systemic disorder such as in sepsis or systemic lupus erythematosus	

Table 28.4	2007 IAC criteria for hepatorenal syndrome.[57]
• Cirrhosis with ascites	
• Serum creatinine > 1.5 mg/dL	
• No improvement of serum creatinine (decrease to a level ≤1.5 mg/dL) after at least 2 days of diuretic withdrawal and volume expansion with albumin. The recommended dose of albumin is 1 g/kg of body weight per day up to a maximum of 100 g/day	
• Absence of shock	
• No current or recent treatment with nephrotoxic drugs	
• Absence of parenchymal kidney disease	

dysregulation lead to acute cardiac dysfunction. Cardiac myocyte dysfunction and fibrosis in type 4 CRS lead to so-called CKD cardiomyopathy. Finally, in type 5 an acute and overwhelming condition such as severe sepsis leads to abnormal immune signaling, cellular toxicity, and enzyme activation, resulting in microcirculatory dysfunction and organ injury.

The categorization of CRS types helps to understand the different pathophysiologic mechanisms for CRS, and ultimately will help in finding specific therapies. As there is no specific therapy for CRS subtypes, the therapy of CRS is that of the underlying causative condition.

Hepatorenal Syndrome

Hepatorenal syndrome (HRS) refers to the occurrence of kidney injury in end-stage cirrhotic patients and occurs in up to 40% of cirrhotic patients within 5 years of diagnosis. Hepatorenal syndrome can be classified according to the clinical course. In type 1 HRS, patients have a rapid decrease in renal function with doubling of SCR within 2 weeks, and in type 2 HRS that (which typically occurs in chronic ascites) patients have a moderate decrease in kidney function. Hepatorenal syndrome carries a grim prognosis unless patients undergo liver transplantation soon after diagnosis: median survival for patients with untreated type 1 HRS can be as little as 2 weeks. According to the latest criteria of the International Ascites Club (Table 28.4), excluding another cause of AKI (e.g. shock or infection) is important. This fact makes it quite often difficult to establish the diagnosis of HRS in ICU patients.[57] Insights in HRS are evolving, and many patients with AKI or CKD may not be diagnosed with HRS. The ADQI group proposed using the term "hepatorenal disorders" to cover the whole spectrum of kidney disease in cirrhotic patients, thus incorporating HRS into this broader concept.[58]

Differentiating hepatorenal disorders from classical AKI can be challenging, and type 1 HRS should be considered a subtype of AKI when the ADQI AKI criteria are used. Hepatorenal syndrome is caused by renal vasoconstriction due to splanchnic arterial vasodilatation.

Prevention of hypoperfusion is of course essential in all forms of AKI, but it can be particularly challenging in patients with chronic liver disease. Hemodynamic monitoring can be used as a guide, but the presence of ascites may increase IAP and affect preload evaluation: central venous pressure will be higher in IAH, and stroke volume variation and pulse pressure variation (PPV) thresholds are affected: IAH patients typically have higher PPV thresholds. Also, passive leg raising can be affected with an IAP of 16 mm Hg identified as a cutoff for false-negative passive leg raising. Treatment of type 1 HRS consists of fluid resuscitation with albumin at a dose of 1 g/kg/d up to 100 g/d for 48 hours, then continued at 20–40 g/d in responders and always in combination with a vasopressor (the preferred agent is terlipressin but norepinephrine as an alternative). The target is to increase the blood pressure by 10 mm Hg or achieve a mean arterial pressure of at least 70 mm Hg. Vasopressin-analogues should be used with caution, as they can cause ischemia. Transjugular portosystemic shunt is the preferred treatment of type 2 HRS patients who have ascites and need repeated paracentesis. Renal replacement therapy in type 1 HRS patients should be reserved for liver transplant candidates, as the prognosis is very poor.

DIAGNOSIS

Diagnosis of AKI

Acute changes in the GFR result in a drop in urinary output and an increase in waste products that are normally cleared by the kidney. Although oliguria may be easy to diagnose in patients with indwelling urinary catheters, it may be difficult to estimate the exact urinary output in patients who do not have a bladder catheter. Increased

SCR concentration is, therefore, often used as a biomarker of AKI in the surgical patient. An important limitation is that various parameters affect SCR and urea concentration such as age, muscle mass nutrition, gender, and acute events, e.g. a gastrointestinal bleed or trauma. For instance, in patients who are severely ill and catabolic, SCR production decreases and SCR concentration is falsely low. Therefore, single measurements of SCR concentration may be misleading, and an increase of SCR is used for the definition and staging of AKI (*see* Fig. 28.1).

The gold standard for measuring the GFR is the inulin clearance, but this is rarely used in the critically ill. Several formulas are available as well to estimate the GFR (eGFR), and all of them are based on the SCR.[59] The Cockcroft-Gault formula requires age, weight, and gender to be entered in the formula and has proved to be unreliable in recent reports. The Modified Diet in Renal Disease formula is more adequate in chronic outpatients, but again proves inaccurate in critically ill patients. An alternative is the measured urinary creatinine clearance rather than the estimated GFR, which requires a complete urine collection over a timed interval. The creatinine concentration is calculated according to the following formula:

Creatinine clearance = (urine volume × urine concentration)/[serum creatinine concentration × duration of urine collection (min)]

The principal error in creatinine clearance calculations is related to an incomplete urine collection; the longer the collection interval, the smaller the error.

Diagnostic Approach in the Patient with AKI

Acute kidney injury as such is rarely the sole admission diagnosis, and mostly AKI is related to another event, e.g. infection, trauma, or surgery. As a first step, relevant medical history should be examined for the presence or risk factors and, if the patient is taking medications, potential nephrotoxic drugs should be identified and when possible stopped. Clinical examination should be focused primarily on identifying the underlying disease; symptoms directly related to AKI are rarely the primary reason for admission to the ICU.

Technical examinations may play a role, although adding harm to the kidney should be avoided. Ultrasound can rule out obstructive causes of AKI quite easily.

Contrast-enhanced CT scan should be used cautiously; if a diagnosis can be established without administration of contrast, a noncontrast-enhanced CT scan should be preferred. Magnetic resonance imaging may also be a worthy alternative. Laboratory investigations will allow diagnosis of typical complications of AKI such as hyperkalemia and acidosis.

Kidney biopsies are rarely needed. Most often empirical therapy can be initiated when a presumptive diagnosis has been made; biopsies are generally reserved for unresponsive cases when an uncommon form of intrinsic AKI, such as vasculitis, glomerulonephritis, or interstitial nephritis, is suspected.

Classical markers of AKI include SCR and urea. These parameters are measures of the filter capacity of the kidney or GFR. Cystatin C is an alternative filtration marker for creatinine that is less dependent on muscle mass. New biomarkers such as NGAL or the Nephrocheck (a combination of urinary TIMP-2 and IGFBP-7) indicate kidney damage, and may detect AKI before SCR or Cystatin C.[6,53]

PREVENTION OF AKI

General Recommendations

As in any other disease in the critically ill, prevention is better than treatment. Most ICU patients are at risk of AKI, so physicians should be aware of this fact and act accordingly. The first and most obvious target to prevent the development of AKI is maintaining adequate kidney perfusion. If there is a continued loss of intravascular volume, e.g. in traumatic hemorrhagic shock, controlling the bleeding source is essential, and fluid should be restricted until the bleeding has been controlled so as to limit systemic inflammation. In most other situations, hypovolemia should be corrected by immediate fluid administration, preferably guided by some form of hemodynamic monitoring, depending on experience and local protocols.

The choice of fluids is an ongoing controversy. Clinical studies found harm for starch-based colloids when patients were randomized to either receive starches or crystalloid solutions.[60-62] Further, crystalloid solutions with high sodium and chloride concentration such as NaCl 0.9% are also associated with decreased kidney perfusion, AKI, RRT, and even mortality.[63,64] Therefore, crystalloid solutions such as Ringer's lactate or Plasma-Lyte are preferred. When hemoglobin levels fall <7 g/dL, blood should be administered.

In case of fluid-unresponsive hypotension, vasoactive drugs may be required to maintain renal perfusion; norepinephrine (noradrenaline) is preferred over dopamine, as it is associated with fewer complications.[65,66] In some patients, inotropes may be required to increase cardiac output; again appropriate hemodynamic monitoring may be of great help to guide therapy.

The use of renal-dose dopamine—once standard practice in many units—is no longer advised, as studies could not demonstrate any benefit in prevention or treatment of AKI.[67] Also, furosemide does not prevent AKI despite the fact that this is often administered in the hope that "jump-starting" the kidney would prevent AKI.[67] The role of diuretics is limited to managing fluid balance and avoiding fluid overload.

In patients with IAH (see above), several nonsurgical options are available to reduce IAP, with percutaneous drainage of peritoneal fluid collections as the most obvious and readily available option. Also, removal of intraluminal contents by using nasogastric or rectal tubes may be helpful.

Avoiding extra harm from therapy or diagnostic investigations is crucial. Nephrotoxic agents should be removed or replaced when possible. In some cases, this policy may not be desirable. For example, when a patient is infected with multidrug resistant organisms, there may be less harm from antibiotic treatment than from continued septic shock due to inadequate antibiotic therapy. Contrast nephropathy should be prevented: for any administration of contrast agents, the necessity of the examination should be considered, and this holds especially true in patients at risk of AKI.

Rhabdomyolysis

Prevention of AKI in patients with hemoglobinuria or increased myoglobin concentration requires an early diagnosis. These conditions are typically associated with a number of clinical situations in which the clinician should have a high level of suspicion. Patients who develop rhabdomyolysis are frequently hypovolemic, and an intravenous infusion of isotonic saline solution has the dual advantage of restoring intravascular volume and producing physiologic changes that cause a diuresis.[68] In addition, alkalinization of the urine and mannitol is often used, although the evidence for these strategies is weak. It is hypothesized that alkalinization of the urine is beneficial for patients with iron-containing proteins in their urine. An increased urine pH permits greater solubility of the filtered hemoglobin and myoglobin and results in reduced toxicity of the filtered myoglobin proteins in the nephron's tubules. The alkalization of urine is accomplished by administration of sodium bicarbonate, which in some cases is required in large amounts to increase the urine pH to >6.0. The forced alkaline diuresis is usually required for <48 hours, by which time the rhabdomyolysis has abated.

Mannitol can be used to induce an osmotic diuresis, and it may also scavenge the detrimental effects of free radical oxygen species. Complications of this treatment include fluid overload, hypernatremia and alkalemia. When patients effectively become anuric, treatment should be stopped.

Sustained or increasing CPK levels should prompt consideration of interventions to control the myoglobin-producing muscle, including debridement or amputation. Finally, breakdown of muscles also results in release of intracellular potassium and hyperkalemia, which may be life-threatening especially when the patient develops AKI. Patients should, therefore, be monitored for signs of hyperkalemia, and potassium concentration should be monitored regularly.

Contrast-Associated AKI

Especially in at-risk patients, one should always consider avoiding iodinated contrast. When contrast-enhanced radiography is clearly indicated, the lowest possible dose of contrast should be administered; also, the modern low or iso-osmolar contrast agents should be used. Ideally, NSAIDs, metformin, and diuretics are stopped one day beforehand. Fluid depletion should also be corrected.[4,69]

In patients who are at risk, intravenous volume expansion is recommended, either by administering 1 L of saline (NaCl 0.9%) 12 hours before, and 1 L 12 hours after contrast administration, or by a bicarbonate solution (846 mL Glucose 5% + 154 mL of 1000 mEg/L $NaHCO_3$) at a rate of 3 m/kg for 1 hour before contrast administration, and 1 mL/kg per hour for 6 hours after contrast administration.[70]

There is controversy on the efficacy of N-acetylcysteine (NAC) for prevention of CA-AKI. As it is cheap and has few side effects, oral NAC (not intravenous!) is still suggested in patients who are at increased risk for developing CA-AKI. Fenoldopam and theophylline have also been also evaluated, but are not recommended at present.[4,69,71,72]

Contrast can be removed by hemodialysis. Although one study demonstrated a benefit of hemofiltration, alternative factors could explain these findings, and others could not confirm them. In a meta-analysis, hemodialysis and hemofiltration were not beneficial and can therefore not be recommended for prevention of CA-AKI.

TREATMENT OF AKI

Therapeutic options—in terms of treatment of AKI itself—are limited, so management is aimed at preventing further injury to the kidney and treating metabolic complications. There is no pharmacological therapy available for AKI as such. Treatment of the disease leading to AKI is the most obvious starting point.

Following the onset of AKI, patients develop complications and physiologic dysfunction that are proportional to the accumulation of toxic factors normally excreted in the urine. Uremic patients are lethargic and develop delirium, coma, and seizures. Uremic pruritus can be distressing.

Coagulopathy may develop in patients who have AKI, and bleeding can be a life-threatening complication. Defects in platelet function have been identified, including impaired platelet adhesion to the endothelium. The clinical manifestations of defective platelet function are bruising, epistaxis, blood loss from gastrointestinal mucosal injury, and surgical wound bleeding. Administration of desmopressin will improve the coagulopathy in most uremic patients.

The strategies used in prevention of AKI also apply to patients who have developed AKI, especially at the lower grades where recuperation of renal function is still considered possible. Maintaining kidney perfusion through fluid administration and vasoactive drugs (when required) is the most important aspect of therapy.

Treatment of AKI Complications

Hyperkalemia

Hyperkalemia is a potentially lethal complication of AKI that can have a rapid onset. Serum potassium levels >6 mEq/L are associated with changes in the electrocardiogram and are associated with increased risk for cardiac arrhythmias and cardiac arrest. Hyperkalemia should be an immediate concern for surgeons treating patients with AKI. Circumstances in which the risk for rapidly developing hyperkalemia is increased are massive lysis of cells (usually related to injury or infection) and reperfusion of skeletal muscle or bowel after a prolonged (>2 hours) ischemia. Electrocardiographic evidence of toxic hyperkalemia includes a peaked T wave, prolonged PR interval, and a junctional rhythm.

Treatment is aimed at both reducing the potassium concentration in the blood and removing the potassium from the body. Calcium therapy is indicated to reverse the decreased membrane excitability: an intravenous infusion of 10 mL 10% calcium gluconate provides a temporary protection (lasting 30–60 minutes) against the harmful effects of hyperkalemia.

An infusion of insulin that drives potassium into the cells, combined with a glucose load, will reduce the potassium concentration for up to 4–6 hours. More controversial is the administration of intravenous sodium bicarbonate. In theory, this also transiently decreases serum potassium because increasing extracellular pH shifts potassium into the cell. However, not all studies could confirm this action. Nebulized or intravenous β-2 adrenergic agents can also be used to lower potassium concentrations.

Although the above strategies will temporarily decrease the concentrations of potassium, they will not reduce the total amount of potassium in the patient. For this, additional strategies are required. The cation exchange resin sodium polystyrene sulfonate administered into the gastrointestinal tract binds potassium and has the sustained effect of reducing total body potassium content. However, this effect is moderate, and it will only commence several hours after administration. Patients who have undergone abdominal surgery should not be treated with these agents, given the risk of intestinal necrosis. Loop diuretics may help eliminate potassium through the urine. Hemodialysis is the definitive management of hyperkalemia due to its ability rapidly to reduce serum potassium levels, and it should be considered in all patients with therapy-resistant hyperkalemia.

Hypervolemia

Fluid overload and pulmonary edema are common conditions in surgical patients who develop AKI. The large volumes of fluid infused to resuscitate these patients and to prevent AKI are retained in patients who remain oliguric. Anasarca, ascites, pulmonary edema, and pleural effusions occur frequently in the perioperative setting. Excessive retention of interstitial fluid in patients with AKI may cause organ dysfunction, particularly in the lungs where pulmonary edema causes respiratory insufficiency. All the various methods of RRT (*see* below) are well suited for achieving a negative fluid balance, but hemodynamic consequences may differ according to the method used. In the recovery phase of AKI, diuretics may be used to manage the fluid balance in patients. Continuous infusion of diuretics is preferred over intermittent administration.

Table 28.5 A comparison of the types of renal replacement therapy for acute renal failure.

Type	Complexity	Efficiency	Cost	Anticoagulant therapy	Extracellular fluid	Use in hypotension volume control	Filtrate (l/day)	Urea clearance (ml/min)
Peritoneal dialysis	Low	Moderate	Moderate	No	Moderate	Yes	12.0	8.5
Intermittent hemodialysis	Moderate	Low	Low	Yes	Intermittent	No	—	—
Continuous arteriovenous hemofiltration	Moderate	Low and variable	Moderate	Yes	Good	No	14.4	10.0
Continuous arteriovenous hemodialysis with filtration	High	Moderate and variable	High	Yes	Good	Variable	14.4	26.7
Continuous venovenous hemofiltration	Moderate	High	Moderate	Yes	Good	Yes	24.0	16.7
Continuous venovenous hemodialysis with filtration	High	High	High	Yes	Good	Yes	19.2	30.0

Acidosis

As the kidneys are crucial for elimination of protons and acid–base homeostasis, metabolic acidosis may occur in patients with severe AKI. Less severe metabolic acidosis can be corrected by infusion of sodium bicarbonate. As this therapy is complicated by volume overload, intracellular acidosis, and rebound alkalosis, it is only indicated when pH is <7.15. Metabolic acids can very elegantly be removed by hemodialysis. Therefore, in AKI patients, metabolic acidosis is often an indication for initiation of RRT.

Drug Dosing in AKI Patients

Many of the drugs used in critically ill surgical patients are—at least partly—eliminated from the body by the kidneys, and thus require dose adaptation when renal function deteriorates. For drugs in which the end effect can be monitored clinically, this is not too much of a problem; for antibiotics, for example, underdosing may occur when package insert dosing is used, most notably because other pharmacokinetic parameters such as protein binding and volume of distribution may also have changed. In these circumstances, therapeutic drug monitoring may be advisable. Loading doses should not be different from patient with normal renal function.

RENAL REPLACEMENT THERAPY

When kidney function deteriorates and recovery is not to be expected in the next hours or days and toxic metabolites accumulate, RRT may be indicated. Important advances have been made regarding the role and techniques used, but for many issues such as timing, intensity, duration, or exact technique, there is no clear consensus; studies could not demonstrate superiority for any one approach. Renal replacement therapy practices are often determined by local experience and available hardware.

RRT Methods

Once a decision has been made to start RRT, several methods are available to replace renal function when a patient develops AKI (Table 28.5).

Clearance of urea and other toxic metabolites is a principal goal, as well as correction of acidosis, hyperkalemia, and other electrolyte abnormalities. In addition, RRT is often required to remove excess fluid infused perioperatively or during resuscitation.

There are two main categories of RRT method:

1. Hemodialysis and hemofiltration, alone or in combination and applied in an intermittent or continuous mode
2. Peritoneal dialysis.

The basic principles of hemodialysis and hemofiltration are different. Each of these has specific advantages and requirements, which may influence the choice for a specific RRT method in the individual ICU patient.

Hemodialysis

In hemodialysis, anticoagulated blood flows through an extracorporeal circuit, where it is exposed, through a semipermeable membrane, to a solution of dialysis fluid with a variable composition that has been selected according to the needs of the patient (Fig. 28.5). The dialysate flows in the opposite direction to blood. Solutes such as urea,

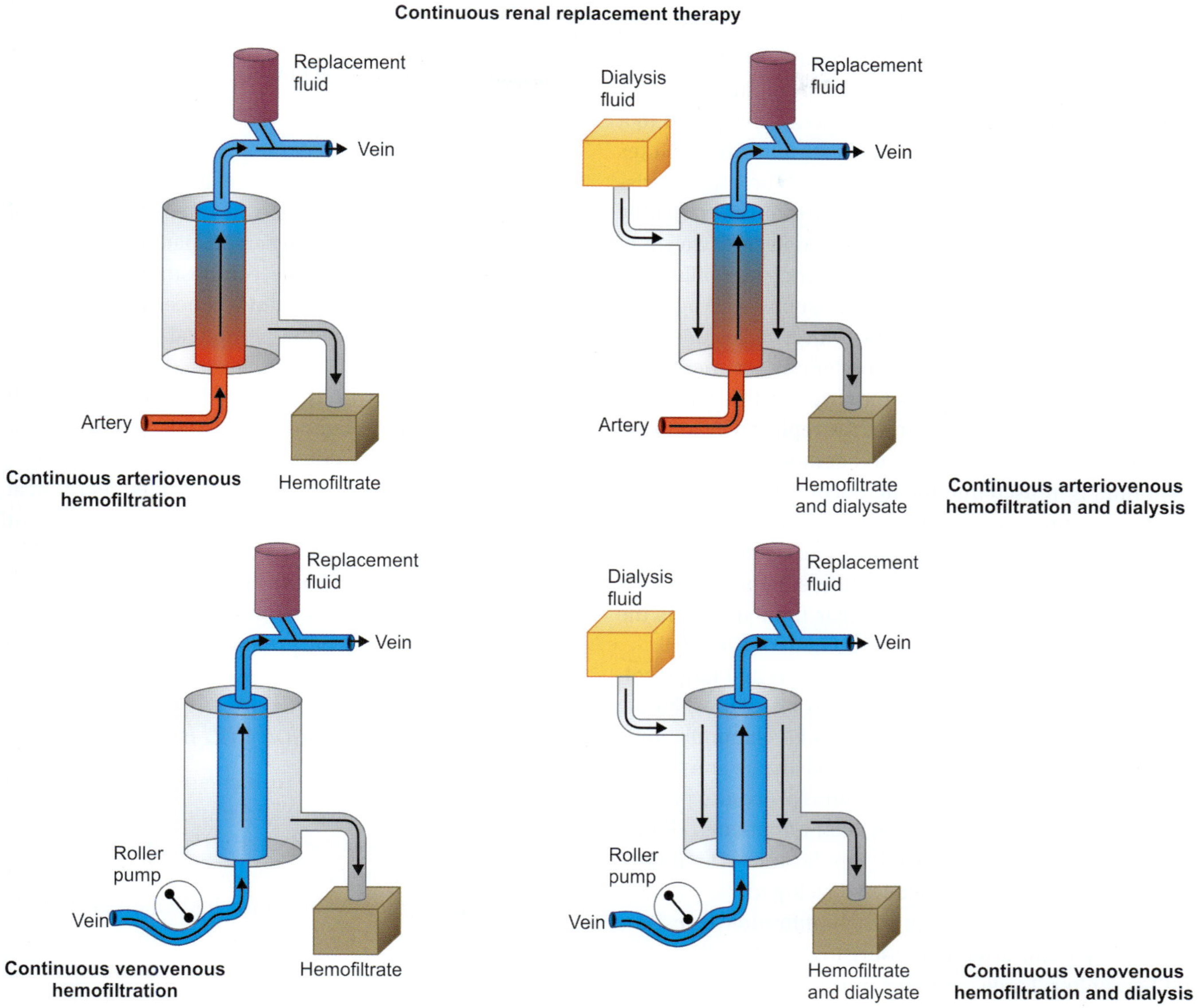

Continuous renal replacement therapy

Fig. 28.5: Continuous arteriovenous hemofiltration (CAVH) depends upon mean arterial pressure to generate a filtrate across the membrane. Continuous replacement fluid infusion is required. There is increased clearance with CAVH with a countercurrent of dialysis fluid. Continuous venovenous hemofiltration (CVVH) and CVVH with dialysis are similar to the processes described above except that a roller pump produces the filtration pressure in the blood instead of the patient's mean arterial pressure.

creatinine, and electrolytes diffuse from the blood to the dialysate in proportion to the difference in concentration. Therefore, to reduce hyperkalemia, the dialysate selected contains a lower concentration or no potassium. Diffusion is the principal mechanism of transmembrane transport, and therefore large electrolytes, such as phosphate ions, are cleared less efficiently than small molecules, such as urea.

One advantage of hemodialysis is its efficiency; large volumes of fluid can be removed, and plasma solute concentrations can be adjusted quickly. The principal disadvantage is hemodynamic instability, especially when short treatment periods (e.g. 4 hours) are used to remove a large volume of water. Hypotension is frequent during hemodialysis, and critically ill patients may compensate poorly for the shift of blood into the extracorporeal circuit.

Hemodialysis can be intermittent or continuous; in the latter case, it is most often combined with hemofiltration. Hemodialysis with hemofiltration or hemodiafiltration adds a countercurrent of dialysis fluid to the hemofilter. This additional design component improves the clearance of smaller solutes, which adds substantially to the effectiveness of hemofiltration alone.

Hemofiltration

Hemofiltration is an alternative technique for RRT (Table 28.5). The basic mechanism involves pumping anticoagulated blood through a circuit in which it is exposed to a highly permeable membrane by which fluid and solutes are filtered from the plasma. The permeability characteristics of filters used in hemofiltration vary, but most readily permit filtration of solutes that have a molecular weight of up to 20 kDa. Large solute clearance during hemofiltration enables removal of larger molecules such as myoglobin, insulin, heparin, and some drugs, which makes this form of RRT more efficient than hemodialysis for these purposes.[68] During continuous hemofiltration the volume of filtrate is large, and most of it must be replaced by infusion of a replacement fluid of selected composition. Replacement fluid is infused into the hemoconcentrated blood at the distal or proximal part of the filter, as it is returned to the patient. A net loss of body fluid can be accomplished by infusion of less fluid than was filtered. This fact allows for very easy control of intravascular fluid status, as the infusion can be adapted at every moment during RRT.

A major advantage of hemofiltration is that larger solutes can be effectively removed from circulating blood. It is also a method of RRT that causes less hemodynamic instability. It is a slower method for plasma clearance and is therefore used mostly as a continuous process to provide sufficient clearance to meet the need of patients. Hemofiltration methods have proved popular for ICU patients, and several techniques have been developed.[68]

Continuous arteriovenous hemofiltration uses the patient's systemic arterial pressure to drive blood through the hemofilter. Large cannulas in the femoral artery and vein are commonly used for this technique. The method's efficiency at filtration is proportional to the systemic arterial pressure, and hypotensive patients have limited capacity to filter. Slower flows through the hemofilter increase the risks of blood clots and occluded flow.

Continuous venovenous hemofiltration is accomplished by adding a pump to the circuit, which generates the flow and pressure in the hemofilter that accomplishes filtration. This circuit eliminates the need for arterial access, and venous access is often by a single catheter with a double lumen. Furthermore, it is a method that can work in hypotensive patients; because the pump controls the filtration pressure, high rates of filtration can be accomplished.

A recently introduced technique is a form of hemodialysis that is more adapted to the needs of the critically ill patient. Slow Low Efficiency Daily Dialysis sessions will take between 6 and 12 hours and are more efficient than short-term dialysis as well as better tolerated, particularly from a hemodynamic point of view.

Peritoneal Dialysis

The use of fluid exchanges to infuse and drain fluid from the peritoneal cavity has been an effective method of renal replacement for many years in patients who have CKD. Variation in the osmotic composition of the fluid allows a positive or negative fluid balance. The technique is simple to accomplish if the peritoneal cavity tolerates the fluid exchanges.

Peritoneal dialysis (PD) is rarely used in critically ill patients, however.[73] Hemodialysis and hemofiltration have emerged as more efficient techniques, and experience with PD in severely ill patients is limited. Peritoneal dialysis has been a favored method of renal replacement in small children and newborns with ARF because vascular access is not required.[74] If resources are limited or the need for dialysis is overwhelming (such as after a disaster), peritoneal dialysis may be preferred because it can be performed with simple equipment.

Choice of Dialysis Method and Intensity

It is intellectually attractive to increase the dose of the dialysis to increase efficiency and improve outcome. For a long time, it was assumed that a higher dose of RRT would benefit the patient, but randomized studies could not demonstrate an advantage for higher intensity RRT schemes.[4,75,76]

Similarly, CRRT has not been proven superior to intermittent strategies.[77] Continuous RRT is better hemodynamic-tolerated and is therefore recommended in hemodynamically unstable patients. Also, osmotic shifts are less pronounced in CRRT compared to intermittent RRT, which makes them the preferred modality in patients with cerebral edema, such as in traumatic brain injury or hepatic encephalopathy.[4]

Indications

There are no agreed indications for starting RRT in critically ill patients. The decision to initiate RRT may be primarily based on volume status, acidosis, and hyperkalemia. In addition, the serum concentrations of creatinine and urea and the presence of hyperphosphatemia, hypercalcemia, and hypermagnesemia may add to the decision to initiate RRT.[4,78]

Anticoagulation in RRT

The use of an external circuit requires some degree of anticoagulation, and this may predispose the patient to bleeding. In some patients, the use of anticoagulants may be formally contraindicated, e.g. postoperative or trauma patients at high risk of bleeding. In intermittent RRT, heparin (unfractionated or low-molecular-weight heparin) is mostly used to anticoagulate the patient. Coagulation should be monitored on a regular basis when continuous methods are used. When systemic anticoagulation is not possible, regional anticoagulation of the dialysis circuit can be accomplished with citrate infusion. Citrate chelates calcium, an essential electrolyte for coagulation. The citrate-calcium complex is in part removed by RRT, but in part will go back to the patient. There, citrate is converted to bicarbonate not only in the liver but also in other cells, which may limit its use in patients with severe liver dysfunction. To correct for the loss of calcium, a continuous infusion of calcium titrated on regular measurements of ionized calcium is crucial.[4]

Timing of RRT

The optimal timing for initiation of RRT remains unclear. Traditionally, RRT was postponed until the patient developed uremic toxicity. However, several studies suggest that early "prophylactic" hemodialysis is beneficial, although other studies do not support this finding.[10] The factors that influence the timing of renal replacement extend beyond renal function and control of azotemia. For example, better control of acidosis, fluid overload, and electrolyte composition and early institution of full nutritional support may all be possible, thereby benefiting the patient.[4]

Nutrition in RRT

As in other ICU patients, nutrition is an important component of the care delivered to support surgical patients who develop AKI. Enteral nutrition is to be preferred over parenteral nutrition. There is no evidence that AKI patients or patients receiving RRT require special formulations for enteral nutrition.[79,80] Fluid overload may be a problem in an anuric patient, however, and RRT may be required to avoid fluid accumulation.

Drug Dosing During RRT

Many medications are partially eliminated by the kidneys, so when AKI develops the dosage of these medications should be adjusted. But when RRT is started, drugs may also be eliminated via RRT. This process will be determined by antimicrobial, RRT, and patient characteristics such as the molecular weight of the drug, hydrophilic properties, protein binding, the membrane used, or the distribution volume. For many drugs such as antibiotics, it may be essential to monitor drug levels when the end effect cannot be assessed clinically.

REFERENCES

1. Hoste EA, Kellum JA. Acute kidney injury: epidemiology and diagnostic criteria. Curr Opin Crit Care. 2006;12:531-7.
2. Mehta RL, Kellum JA, Shah SV, et al. Acute Kidney Injury Network: report of an initiative to improve outcomes in acute kidney injury. Crit Care. 2007;11:R31.
3. Bellomo R, Ronco C, Kellum JA, et al. Acute renal failure—definition, outcome measures, animal models, fluid therapy and information technology needs: the Second International Consensus Conference of the Acute Dialysis Quality Initiative (ADQI) Group. Crit Care. 2004;8:R204-12.
4. Kidney Disease: Improving Global Outcomes (KDIGO) Acute Kidney Injury Work Group. KDIGO clinical practice guideline for acute kidney injury. Kidney Int. 2012;2:1-138.
5. Haase M, Bellomo R, Devarajan P, et al. Accuracy of neutrophil gelatinase-associated lipocalin (NGAL) in diagnosis and prognosis in acute kidney injury: a systematic review and meta-analysis. Am J Kidney Dis. 2009;54:1012-24.
6. Kashani K, Al-Khafaji A, Ardiles T, et al. Discovery and validation of cell cycle arrest biomarkers in human acute kidney injury. Crit Care. 2013;17:R25.
7. Ronco C, Kellum JA, Haase M. Subclinical AKI is still AKI. Crit Care. 2012;16:313.
8. Uchino S, Kellum JA, Bellomo R, et al. Acute renal failure in critically ill patients: a multinational, multicenter study. JAMA. 2005;294:813-8.
9. Hsu CY, McCulloch CE, Fan D, et al. Community-based incidence of acute renal failure. Kidney Int. 2007;72:208-12.
10. Thakar CV, Liangos O, Yared JP, et al. ARF after open-heart surgery: influence of gender and race. Am J Kidney Dis. 2003;41:742-51.
11. Kellum JA, Levin N, Bouman C, et al. Developing a consensus classification system for acute renal failure. Curr Opin Crit Care. 2002;8:509-14.
12. Joannidis M, Metnitz B, Bauer P, et al. Acute kidney injury in critically ill patients classified by AKIN versus RIFLE using the SAPS 3 database. Intensive Care Med. 2009;35:1692-702.
13. Bagshaw SM, George C, Dinu I, et al. A multi-centre evaluation of the RIFLE criteria for early acute kidney injury in critically ill patients. Nephrol Dial Transplant. 2008;23:1203-10.
14. Cruz DN, Bolgan I, Perazella MA, et al. North East Italian Prospective Hospital Renal Outcome Survey on Acute Kidney Injury (NEiPHROS-AKI): targeting the problem with the RIFLE Criteria. Clin J Am Soc Nephrol. (2007);2:418-25.

15. Lin CY, Chen YC, Tsai FC, et al. RIFLE classification is predictive of short-term prognosis in critically ill patients with acute renal failure supported by extracorporeal membrane oxygenation. Nephrol Dial Transplant. 2006;21:2867-73.
16. Hoste EA, Schurgers M. Epidemiology of acute kidney injury: how big is the problem? Crit Care Med. 2008;36:S146-51.
17. Ostermann M, Chang RW. Acute kidney injury in the intensive care unit according to RIFLE. Crit Care Med. 2007; 35:1837-43.
18. Hoste EA, Clermont G, Kersten A, et al. RIFLE criteria for acute kidney injury are associated with hospital mortality in critically ill patients: a cohort analysis. Crit Care. 2006;10:R73.
19. Hou SH, Bushinsky DA, Wish JB, et al. Hospital-acquired renal insufficiency: a prospective study. Am J Med. 1983; 74:243-8.
20. Nash K, Hafeez A, Hou S. Hospital-acquired renal insufficiency. Am J Kidney Dis. 2002;39:930-6.
21. Ali T, Khan I, Simpson W, et al. Incidence and outcomes in acute kidney injury: a comprehensive population-based study. J Am Soc Nephrol. 2007;18:1292-8.
22. Angus D, Wax R. Epidemiology of sepsis: an update. Crit Care Med. 2001;29:S109 -16.
23. Martin GS, Mannino DM, Eaton S, et al. The epidemiology of sepsis in the United States from 1979 through 2000. N Engl J Med. (2003);348:1546-54.
24. Metnitz PG, Krenn CG, Steltzer H, et al. Effect of acute renal failure requiring renal replacement therapy on outcome in critically ill patients. Crit Care Med. 2002;30:2051-8.
25. Bagshaw SM, Laupland KB, Doig CJ, et al. Prognosis for long-term survival and renal recovery in critically ill patients with severe acute renal failure: a population-based study. Crit Care. 2005;9:R700-9.
26. Prescott GJ, Metcalfe W, Baharani J, et al. A prospective national study of acute renal failure treated with RRT: incidence, aetiology and outcomes. Nephrol Dial Transplant. (2007);22:2513-9.
27. Waikar SS, Curhan GC, Wald R, et al. Declining mortality in patients with acute renal failure, 1988 to 2002. J Am Soc Nephrol. 2006;17:1143-50.
28. Goss CH, Brower RG, Hudson LD, et al. Incidence of acute lung injury in the United States. Crit Care Med. 2003; 31:1607-11.
29. Harrison D, Welch C, Eddleston J. The epidemiology of severe sepsis in England, Wales and Northern Ireland, 1996 to 2004: secondary analysis of a high quality clinical database, the ICNARC Case Mix Programme Database. Critical Care. 2006;10:R42.
30. Ali T, Tachibana A, Khan I, et al. The changing pattern of referral in acute kidney injury. QJM. 2011;104:497-503.
31. Lafrance JP, Djurdjev O, Levin A. Incidence and outcomes of acute kidney injury in a referred chronic kidney disease cohort. Nephrol Dial Transplant. 2010;25:2203-9.
32. Hsu CY, Ordonez JD, Chertow GM, et al. The risk of acute renal failure in patients with chronic kidney disease. Kidney Int. 2008;74:101-7.
33. Ricci Z, Cruz D, Ronco C. The RIFLE criteria and mortality in acute kidney injury: A systematic review. Kidney Int. 2008; 73:538-46.
34. Lafrance JP, Miller DR. Acute kidney injury associates with increased long-term mortality. J Am Soc Nephrol. 2010; 21:345-52.
35. Bihorac A, Yavas S, Subbiah S, et al. Long-term risk of mortality and acute kidney injury during hospitalization after major surgery. Ann Surg. 2009;249:851-8.
36. Hobson CE, Yavas S, Segal MS, et al. Acute kidney injury is associated with increased long-term mortality after cardiothoracic surgery. Circulation. 2009;119:2444-53.
37. Schiffl H, Fischer R. Five-year outcomes of severe acute kidney injury requiring renal replacement therapy. Nephrol Dial Transplant. 2008;23:2235-41.
38. Triverio PA, Martin PY, Romand J, et al. Long-term prognosis after acute kidney injury requiring renal replacement therapy. Nephrol Dial Transplant. 2009;24:2186-9.
39. Lameire N. The pathophysiology of acute renal failure. Crit Care Clin. 2005;21:197-210.
40. Payen D, Legrand M. Can we identify prerenal physiology and does it matter? Contrib Nephrol. 2011;174:22-32.
41. Singer E, Elger A, Elitok S, et al. Urinary neutrophil gelatinase-associated lipocalin distinguishes pre-renal from intrinsic renal failure and predicts outcomes. Kidney Int. 2011;80:405-14.
42. Macedo E, Mehta RL. Prerenal failure: from old concepts to new paradigms. Curr Opin Crit Care. 2009;15:467-73.
43. Vincent JL, De Backer D. ICU nephrology: the implications of cardiovascular alterations in the acutely ill. Kidney Int. 2012;81:1060-6.
44. De Waele JJ, De Laet I, Kirkpatrick AW, et al. Intra-abdominal hypertension and abdominal compartment syndrome. Am J Kidney Dis. 2011;57:159-69.
45. Peng ZY, Critchley LA, Joynt GM, et al. Effects of norepinephrine during intra-abdominal hypertension on renal blood flow in bacteremic dogs. Crit Care Med. 2008;36:834-41.
46. Le Dorze M, Legrand M, Payen D, et al. The role of the microcirculation in acute kidney injury. Curr Opin Crit Care. 2009; 15:503-8.
47. Zimmerman JL, Shen MC. Rhabdomyolysis. Chest. 2013; 144:1058-65.
48. Malinoski DJ, Slater MS, Mullins RJ. Crush injury and rhabdomyolysis. Crit Care Clin. 2004;20:171-92.
49. Holt SG, Moore KP. Pathogenesis and treatment of renal dysfunction in rhabdomyolysis. Intensive Care Med. 2001; 27:803-11.
50. Kirkpatrick AW, Roberts DJ, De Waele J, et al. Intra-abdominal hypertension and the abdominal compartment syndrome: updated consensus definitions and clinical practice guidelines from the World Society of the Abdominal Compartment Syndrome. Intensive Care Med. 2013;39:1190-206.

Additional references appear in the online version of this book.

Case Study: 29

Source Control in the Management of Intra-abdominal Infection

John MA Bohnen

THE PROBLEM

The source of an abdominal infection, usually a leak from the gut, must be controlled for the patient to survive, recover from the infection, and avoid early and long-term complications.[1] Source control denotes the removal of contaminants from the abdomen and prevention of further contamination. This may be as simple as removing an inflamed appendix, or more challenging and prone to failure, such as managing a recurrent duodenal perforation. When further contamination cannot be stopped for technical or patient safety reasons, proximal diversion or percutaneous or operative drainage externalizes contaminants, which may enable sufficient recovery for subsequent definitive operation, e.g. tube drainage followed by sigmoid resection and anastomosis.

THE TYPICAL CASE

A 60-year-old man underwent a laparoscopic right hemicolectomy for colonic carcinoma. After recovering well initially with resumption of solid intake orally, on the third day after operation he developed tachycardia, tachypnea, nausea, mild upper abdominal discomfort mainly at the port sites, and low-grade fever. Abdominal examination revealed tenderness mainly at the port sites, aggravated by coughing. The abdomen was distended, and auscultation revealed diminished but present bowel sounds. Chest examination revealed bronchial breathing, reduced air entry, and dullness in the right lower thorax posteriorly.

Chest X-ray and computed tomography (CT) scan of the abdomen and chest showed right lower lobe consolidation consistent with atelectasis and a moderate amount of free air and fluid in the peritoneal cavity.

DIAGNOSTIC DILEMMAS

The diagnosis of abdominal infection and the need to control the source of infection may be obvious in some situations, such as in a previous healthy person with a sudden gut perforation. Other conditions such as aging, neurological impairment, therapy with immunosuppressive drugs, and recent abdominal operation, as in our patient, may mask the signs of abdominal infection and make the diagnosis difficult to achieve.

A patient should recover within 2–3 days of an abdominal operation, especially when done laparoscopically. Delayed recovery should arouse suspicion.[2] Mild, nonspecific, and nonlocalizing signs after an open procedure are more difficult to interpret, since open laparotomy normally produces the signs of peritonitis for 2 or 3 days.

Maybe nothing serious is happening to this patient. Free air and mild abdominal pain may be present normally 3 days after a colon resection. Shortness of breath and atelectasis may be associated with pneumonia, pulmonary embolism, or other conditions that do not require an abdominal procedure. To open or laparoscope the abdomen and find no leak or infection may aggravate the problem.

But if he does have an abdominal infection, such as from a leaking anastomosis or unexpected intestinal injury, he will probably die if the leak is not controlled. The only way to find an abdominal source with certainty is to reoperate to explore the abdomen.

Diagnostic imaging with CT scan is accurate but not foolproof.[1] A CT scan is more helpful if radio-opaque contrast is administered orally and per rectum to look for a leak from the gut. If no extravasation of contrast is seen, the surgeon may wait a few hours and avoid an "unnecessary" operation if the patient improves, with a plan to operate if the patient deteriorates. However, the longer the surgeon waits on an uncontrolled source of infection, the more likely the patient will experience avoidable morbidity or death.

In situations of uncertainty, aggressive diagnostic and therapeutic intervention is essential. If time permits and the patient is not critically ill, CT scan with oral and rectal

Table 29.1 Examples of source control.

Source	*Control*
Localized abscess	Percutaneous or operative drainage
Perforated duodenal ulcer	Omental patch
Perforated gastric ulcer	Resection, with anastomosis; patch
Ischemic and/or perforated small intestine	Resection, primary anastomosis
Perforated appendix	Resection
Perforated colonic diverticulitis	Resection, proximal colostomy, rectal closure; subsequent re-anastomosis
Anastomotic breakdown	Exteriorization of the two ends

contrast will probably identify a source of intra-abdominal infection and point to the need to control it surgically or with tube drainage. For the patient deteriorating rapidly or in whom diagnostic imaging is not feasible, urgent abdominal exploration is indicated. The decision making becomes more challenging when the clinical and radiographic findings suggest but do not confirm ongoing contamination.

MANAGEMENT OPTIONS

The surgeon and radiologist viewed this patient's CT scan with contrast and found no leak from the gastrointestinal tract. The surgeon was unsure of what to do. Four hours later, the patient's blood pressure dropped suddenly, requiring fluids and inotropic agents. Because of this deterioration, the surgeon took the patient to the operating room immediately, opened the abdomen through a midline incision, and found fecal contamination from an unsuspected small bowel injury, perhaps from a cautery burn or retraction injury. The surgeon resected the segment of small bowel and did a primary anastomosis, saving the patient from progression of infection and death.

Methods to achieve source control depend on the underlying condition (e.g. cancer), anatomy, and location in the intestinal tract and peritoneal cavity. Some examples appear in Table 29.1.

REFERENCES

1. Solomkin JS, Mazuski JE, Bradley JS, et al. Diagnosis and management of complicated intra-abdominal infection in adults and children: Guidelines by the Surgical Infection Society and the Infectious Diseases Society of America. Clin Infect Dis. 2010;50:133-64.
2. Pusajo JF, Bumaschny E, Doglio GR, et al. Postoperative intra-abdominal sepsis requiring reoperation. Value of a predictive index. Arch Surg. 1993;128:218-23.

Case Study: 30
Use of Furosemide in the Postoperative Oliguric Patient

H Gill Cryer

THE PROBLEM

Oliguria is a relatively common problem during the immediate postoperative period in patients undergoing complex and often emergency procedures. Because oliguria is an early sign of impending acute renal failure and because the causes of acute renal failure are varied, it is important to ascertain the underlying cause and correct it if possible. Diuretics such as furosemide are often employed in this situation but remain controversial, because it is difficult to show that they alter outcome in acute renal failure. Furosemide clearly is of no benefit once renal failure is fully established, but is likely to be valuable during the early stages of renal failure before there is tubular cell damage. Moreover, furosemide is clearly harmful if given to volume-depleted patients and should be reserved for the patient who has failed volume loading and evidence of volume overload. In this situation, furosemide can be useful in establishing urine output, which can delay and potentially avoid dialysis.

THE TYPICAL CASE

A 50-year-old woman with a chronic enterocutaneous fistula after a sigmoidectomy and Hartmann's procedure for perforated diverticulitis 6 months ago was seen in the emergency department with fever, abdominal pain, lethargy, and expanding redness of the skin around her fistula site. On physical examination her temperature was 39° C, heart rate 115 beats per minute, and blood pressure 90/60 mm Hg. Her mucous membranes were moist, her lungs were clear, her pulse was bounding and rapid, and her abdomen was tender with erythema around a chronic fistula site that was draining obvious pus. Intravenous fluids were begun, and broad-spectrum antibiotics were ordered. A computed tomography scan showed a large intra-abdominal abscess with what appeared to be a dehisced Hartman's pouch and no extravasation of oral contrast. The patient was treated for sepsis and under percutaneous drainage of the intra-abdominal abscess by interventional radiology. Her sepsis resolved over the next several days, but she continued to have purulent drainage. A Gastrografin enema demonstrated a dehisced rectal stump communicating with the abdominal wound. In addition, she had a subcutaneous fistula from the stoma to the abdominal wound. She underwent bowel preparation and a semielective operation. Laparotomy revealed a long rectal stump pouch with breakdown of the suture line. The stump was dissected back to healthy rectum and resected. The colostomy was taken down, and an end-to-end anastomosis was performed between the descending colon and the rectum with a proximal diverting loop ileostomy. The wounds were all left open. At the end of the operation, the anesthesiologist said that the patient had not made any urine during the last hour despite 2 units of blood and several liters of crystalloid and colloid infusion. The patient had been given pressor drugs intermittently for hypotension during the operation but was off pressors at the end. The bladder was empty and the Foley balloon was palpable within the bladder. The left ureter was not seen during the dissection but was not thought to be injured.

In the recovery room, the Foley catheter was irrigated and found to be patent. The patient's skin was warm. Blood tests showed a hematocrit of 30 and a creatinine of 1.7 compared to a preoperative creatinine of 1.2. A chest X-ray showed mild pulmonary edema, and an electrocardiogram showed only sinus tachycardia with a heart rate of 110. Blood pressure was 110/80 mm Hg off pressors. Central venous pressure was 11 cm H_2O. She had received 4 L normal saline, 2 units of colloid (PlasmaLyte), and 2 units of blood over the 4 hours of her operation, and the estimated blood loss was 500 mL. She was given an additional 500 mL bolus of normal saline with no effect, followed by a 100 mg bolus and continuous intravenous furosemide infusion at 100 mg/h. The patient began to make urine approximately 30 minutes later. Her creatinine peaked at 2.2 (units) and decreased to 1.2 over the ensuing 48 hours. She diuresed satisfactorily, and fluid balance became negative on postoperative day 5. She was discharged from the hospital on postoperative day 8 with normal creatinine and urine output.

DIAGNOSTIC DILEMMAS

Oliguria (urine output <0.5 mL/kg per hour) is one of the first signs of renal dysfunction and is common during and immediately after complex operative procedures. It is important to identify the cause. According to conventional wisdom, the most common cause of oliguria in the postoperative patient is prerenal. In actuality, it is usually a complex mixture of hemodynamic, inflammatory, and direct toxic injury to the renal tubule added on to varying degrees of pre-existing renal dysfunction, which overcome normal homeostatic mechanisms to preserve glomerular filtration. Patients undergoing complex operations are often on multiple medications that can impair glomerular blood flow. They have often had recent imaging with nephrotoxic agents, they may be relatively dehydrated from bowel preparation, or they may have a systemic inflammatory response from inflammatory disease. During the operation itself, the patient often has periods of decreased cardiac output and hypotension as well as episodes of cytokine release from ischemia reperfusion injury and/or dissection of inflamed or infected areas. Occasionally, the cause of oliguria is postrenal and the Foley catheter should always be irrigated to make sure that it is not occluded.

MANAGEMENT OPTIONS

The pathogenesis of acute renal failure is time-related and usually progresses as follows. Decreased renal perfusion results in ischemia. Homeostatic mechanisms are initiated to preserve renal perfusion. The most important of these is a local rise in angiotensin II, which dilates preglomerular arterioles secondary to prostaglandin E2 production and constricts postglomerular vessels by a direct effect to maintain transglomerular filtration pressure. If the ischemic insult is severe, these homeostatic mechanisms are overcome and rapid cellular damage occurs. However, if the initial insult is mild, oliguria results with a time lag before cellular damage. Because furosemide will not work once cellular damage has occurred and can cause harm in the face of hypovolemia, it is not considered a frontline treatment of oliguria. Furosemide is a loop diuretic with a primary site of action in the thick ascending loop of Henle, so it must reach the proximal tubule via the vasa recta in order to be effective. If glomerular blood flow is decreased by hypovolemia and afferent arteriolar vasoconstriction, the drug will not get to its site of action. Therefore, once postrenal obstruction has been ruled out, the next step in the treatment of postoperative oliguria is to optimize hemodynamic status. Measures should include intravenous volume expansion, usually with boluses of crystalloid, increasing cardiac contractility with inotropes, optimizing heart rate, treating arrhythmias, and potentially decreasing afterload with vasodilators if the patient is vasoconstricted once volume had been repleted. Additionally, any drugs that could reduce glomerular filtration or systemic blood pressure should be discontinued if possible. If optimization of hemodynamic status does not result in increased urine output, then a trial of furosemide should be initiated. Since glomerular filtration rate is decreased and furosemide action is dependent on being filtered at the glomerulus to reach its target site of action, the preferred method of administration is by 100 mg bolus followed by a continuous intravenous infusion at 100 mg/h. In addition to promoting diuresis of salt and water in the volume-repleted patient, furosemide has potential benefits by inducing afferent arteriolar dilation via prostaglandin release and reducing oxygen consumption and energy expenditure in already vulnerable renal tubular cells. While no study has definitively shown that the use of furosemide improves mortality after the development of acute renal failure, the drug has been shown to promote or convert oliguric renal failure to nonoliguric renal failure. While this conversion may make fluid management easier, it does not necessarily mean that renal replacement therapy can be avoided. However, the use of furosemide in the postoperative oliguric patient once hemodynamic factors have been mitigated may theoretically prevent progression to acute renal failure. Unfortunately, this hypothesis has never been proven. If furosemide does not induce urine flow, then consideration should be given to early dialysis. Although the usual indications for dialysis are hypervolemia, hyperkalemia, and metabolic acidosis, there is convincing evidence that beginning dialysis early, before high elevations of blood urea nitrogen and creatinine occur, improves outcome. For this reason, we may never know if the use of furosemide is truly beneficial in the oliguric patient, but it remains a well-accepted step in the management of postoperative oliguria.

FURTHER READING

1. Coppolino G, Presta P, Saturno G. Acute kidney injury in patients undergoing cardiac surgery. J Nephrol. 2013;26:32-40.
2. Gandhi A, Husain M, Salhiyyah K, et al. Does perioperative furosemide usage reduce the need for renal replacement therapy in cardiac surgery patients? Interact Cardiovasc Thorac Surg. 2012;15:750-5.

Section 2

Trauma

***Section Editor:** John D Corson*

Parts

31

Initial Trauma Evaluation and Resuscitation

Kristen C Sihler, Brad M Cushing, Paul J Schenarts

Key Points

- A systematic approach to the initial assessment of trauma patients is essential to minimize the risk of preventable death and disability. This approach is laid out in the Advanced Trauma Life Support (ATLS) course (American College of Surgeons).
- Airway, breathing, circulation, disability, and exposure are the ABCDE first priorities of the initial assessment of the trauma patient.
- A primary survey to detect life-threatening states is followed by a secondary survey, which systematically evaluates all areas of the body. These surveys are repeated as necessary during the resuscitation.
- Diagnostic and therapeutic interventions specific to each suspected or defined injury are prioritized and promptly provided.
- The most common cause of preventable early death is undetected internal hemorrhage in the chest, abdomen, or pelvis.

PREHOSPITAL CARE

The key to successful resuscitation of trauma patients is an organized, highly reliable trauma system. This pre-established system will expedite transport of the patient to the most appropriate, but not necessarily the nearest, facility.

Definitive care for the severely injured patient cannot usually be provided in the prehospital setting. Cessation of internal bleeding, evacuation of an intracranial hematoma, and similar life- or limb-saving interventions require rapid operative intervention by a highly specialized and coordinated team using resources generally found only within a hospital setting. The primary task of prehospital care is to move patients rapidly to where they can obtain the definitive treatment they need. Field treatment is limited to interventions that must be undertaken to get patients to the hospital alive and to avoid additional deterioration, such as airway management and tourniquet application. Time is the enemy of the trauma patient, and there must be no delay from injury to definitive care that results from excess time at the scene. This principle has prompted the phrases "scoop and run" or in the setting of helicopter use, "swoop and scoop." Many emergency medical services (EMS) quality management programs monitor trauma scene times and continuously strive to reduce them.

The process by which patients are rapidly delivered to definitive care is driven by field assessment. Injury pattern and severity are identified and used to determine the level of care that will be necessary. Accurate matching of patients' need and available resources is a difficult task. Several field triage tools are available to assist with this process. They vary in subtle ways but essentially use physiologic criteria (blood pressure, pulse, respiratory, and neurologic status), identifiable anatomic injury (e.g. proximal long bone fracture, amputation), and the mechanism of the injury (e.g. fall from a substantial height, ejection from a motor vehicle) to predict injury severity and the need for high-level care. The triage algorithm (Flowchart 31.1) produced and recommended by the Centers for Disease Control and Prevention (CDC)[1] has been validated by several studies.[2,3] Once a patient has been assessed using these tools, provider judgment and region-specific triage and transport protocols direct patients by land or air to the needed and available level of care: trauma center, nontrauma center, pediatric or brain injury specialty center.

Field assessment and treatment are conducted by the approach espoused by the ATLS[4] and the Pre-Hospital Trauma Life Support[5] courses. The initial focus is on airway management and control because absence of an airway can be deadly within minutes. Additionally, inadequate ventilation and oxygenation resulting from a compromised

Flowchart 31.1: Triage decision scheme. Guidelines for field triage of injured patients—United States 2011 (CDC).

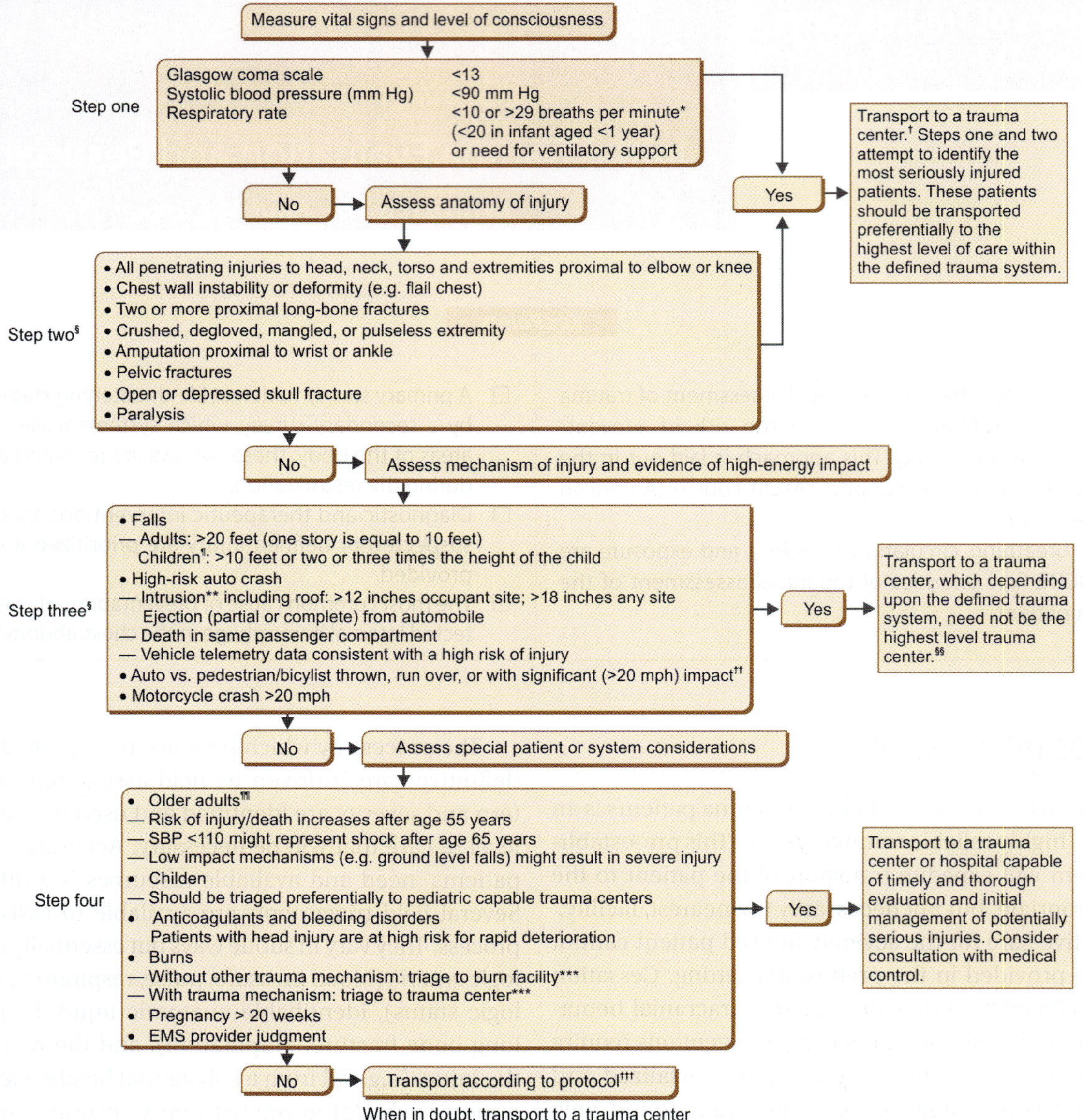

(EMS: Emergency medical services).

*The upper limit of respiratory rate in infants is >29 breaths per minute to maintain a higher level of overtriage for infants.

†Trauma centers are designated Level I-IV. A Level I center has the greatest amount of resources and personnel for care of the injured patient and provides regional leadership in education, research, and prevention programs. A Level II facility offers similar resources to a Level I facility, possibly differing only in continuous availability of certain subspecialties or sufficient prevention, education, and research activities for Level I designation; Level II facilities are not required to be resident or fellow education centers. A Level III center is capable of assessment, resuscitation, and emergency surgery, with severely injured patients being transferred to a Level I or II facility. A Level IV trauma center is capable of providing 24-hour physician coverage, resuscitation, and stabilization to injured patients before transfer to a facility that provides a higher level of trauma care.

§Any injury noted in Step two or mechanism identified in Step three triggers a "yes" response.

¶Age <15 years.

**Intrusion refers to interior compartment intrusion, as opposed to deformation which refers to exterior damage.

††Includes pedestrians or bicyclists thrown or run over by a motor vehicle or those with estimated impact >20 mph with a motor vehicle.

§§Local or regional protocols should be used to determine the most appropriate level of trauma center within the defined trauma system; need not be the highest-level trauma center.

¶¶Age >55 years.

***Patients with both burns and concomitant trauma for whom the burn injury poses the greatest risk for morbidity and mortality should be transferred to a burn center. If the nonburn trauma presents a greater immediate risk, the patient may be stabilized in a trauma center and then transferred to a burn center.

†††Patients who do not meet any of the triage criteria in Steps one through four should be transported to the most appropriate medical facility as outlined in local EMS protocols.

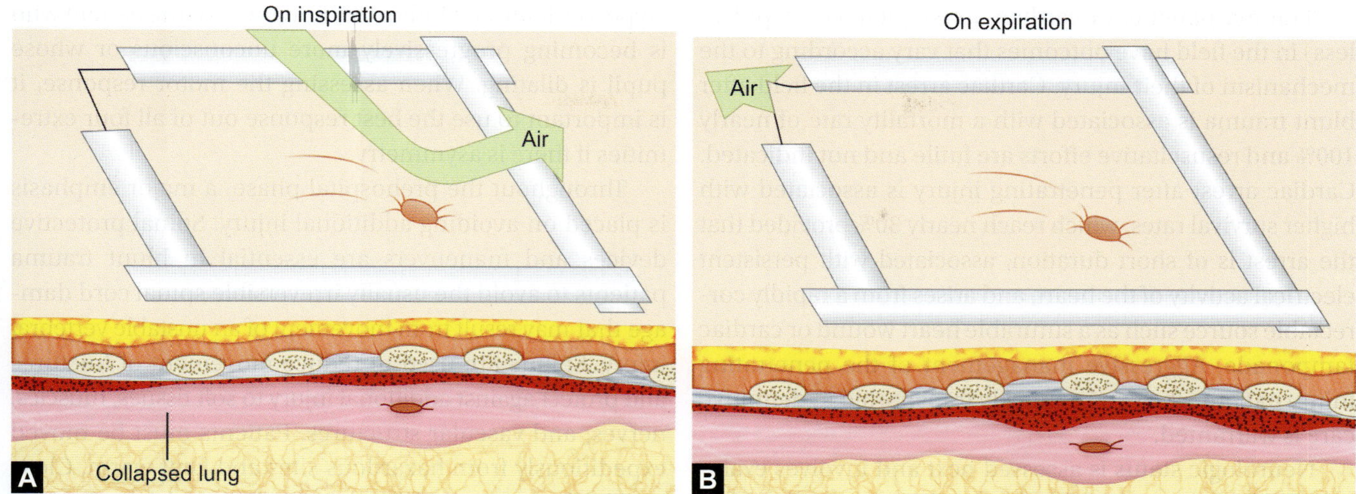

Figs. 31.1A and B: Treatment of sucking chest wound. On inspiration, the dressing seals the wound, preventing the entry of air; on expiration, trapped air is able to escape through the untapped section of the dressing.

airway clearly exacerbate the tissue injury seen with shock and trauma. Candidates for aggressive airway management are:

- Patients who cannot protect their airway as a result of decreased consciousness from brain injury or substance intoxication
- Patients whose airway is compromised from direct or surrounding injury or excessive bloody secretions.

Airway management options and techniques are described in more detail below but essentially include positioning, mechanical airways, translaryngeal intubation and surgical airways (e.g. cricothyroidotomy). Prehospital endotracheal intubation remains controversial, with some studies showing benefit and some showing harm. The risk:benefit ratio must be evaluated within the context of local factors.[6-9]

When the airway is secure, attention is turned to the assessment of breathing and maintenance of adequate oxygenation and ventilation. Provision of supplemental oxygen is adequate treatment for many patients, but those who have inadequate ventilatory drive or respiratory compromise from a pneumothorax, flail chest, or sucking chest wound must be identified and treated. Decompression for tension pneumothorax can be performed in the field with a hollow needle or a needle and one-way valve system. A chest tube is generally reserved for the hospital setting. A flail chest exists when ribs are broken in more than one place and move inward on inspiration, thus reducing the inspired tidal volume. Flail chests and pneumothoraces are frequently seen together and the pneumothorax may enlarge markedly if positive pressure is used to compensate for the flail. The field provider must be wary of this and closely monitor the respiratory status after intubation. A sucking chest wound most commonly results from a penetrating injury. Treatment involves coverage of the wound with a three-sided occlusive dressing (Figs. 31.1A and B). Accumulated air can escape, but no further air can be sucked into the chest on inspiration.

After the airway and breathing have been secured, the cardiovascular status of the patient is assessed. If the patient's blood pressure is low, then shock clearly exists. The shock state, however, can be present without hypotension. Peripheral perfusion and mental status should be assessed routinely to identify early shock. Agitation can be an early sign of shock. Correctable sources of shock in the field are external hemorrhage, cardiac arrhythmias and tension pneumothorax. Cardiac tamponade is rare, particularly with blunt trauma. External bleeding should be stopped by direct pressure. A tourniquet should be used for extremity vascular injury not controlled by direct pressure. Field tourniquet use is associated with improved survival compared to application of a tourniquet in the emergency department, especially if the tourniquet is applied before the onset of shock.[10] Cardiac arrhythmias should be identified and corrected by the algorithms outlined in the American Heart Association Guidelines.[11] Transport should not be delayed for insertion of an intravenous catheter. Administration of intravenous fluids in the urban setting has not been shown to provide a survival advantage.[12,13] Recently, prehospital use of tranexamic acid (an antifibrinolytic agent) in the setting of severe trauma has shown promise for improving survival.[14]

Trauma patients in cardiac arrest (defined as pulseless) in the field have outcomes that vary according to the mechanism of their injury. Cardiac arrest in the field after blunt trauma is associated with a mortality rate of nearly 100% and resuscitative efforts are futile and not indicated. Cardiac arrest after penetrating injury is associated with higher survival rates, which reach nearly 30% provided that the arrest is of short duration, associated with persistent electrical activity of the heart, and arises from a rapidly correctable source such as a suturable heart wound or cardiac tamponade. Aggressive management of the penetrating injury patient who can be quickly transported to definitive care is warranted.

Neurologic status is assessed next and involves evaluation of both brain and spinal cord function. The level of consciousness and brain injury is graded according to the Glasgow coma scale (GCS) (Table 31.1). This scale correlates with the severity of brain injury[15] and is widely used. It is essential to identify patients with rapidly progressive or focal neurologic symptoms (e.g. unilateral dilated pupil, asymmetry in motor function). Those with focal findings are likely to have intracranial hematomas, particularly epidural and subdural hematomas, and can have good neurologic outcomes if these lesions are rapidly evacuated. Routine hyperventilation of unconscious patients is not indicated because it is associated with decreased brain perfusion and worse outcomes.[16]

Table 31.1 Glasgow coma scale (GCS).

A. Eye opening	
Spontaneous	4
To voice	3
To pain	2
None	1
B. Verbal response	
Oriented	5
Confused	4
Inappropriate words	3
Incomprehensible sounds	2
None	1
C. Motor response	
Obeys commands	6
Localizes pain	5
Withdraws (pain)	4
Flexion (pain)	3
Extension (pain)	2
None	1
Total GCS points (A + B + C)	

Hyperventilation is indicated, however, for the patient who is becoming progressively more unconscious or whose pupil is dilating. When assessing the motor response, it is important to use the best response out of all four extremities if there is asymmetry.

Throughout the prehospital phase, a major emphasis is placed on avoiding additional injury. Spinal protective devices and maneuvers are essential in blunt trauma patients to avoid the usually irreversible spinal cord damage that may result from movement of an unstable vertebral injury. Splints are used to reduce movement of fractures and protect against additional injury to soft tissues, muscles, nerves, and vascular structures. Patients must be moved expeditiously from hazardous sites and kept warm. Close monitoring of vital signs is key to recognizing systemic deterioration. Electrocardiograms (EKGs), oxygen saturation, blood pressure, peripheral perfusion, and level of consciousness should also be monitored.

HOSPITAL CARE

Preparation and Organization for Hospital Resuscitation

Using the established trauma and EMS communication system, the receiving facility is able to obtain information about the nature and severity of the patient's injuries. Well-organized hospitals have trauma team activation systems that use field data to mobilize personnel and resources specific to the patient or patients arriving. These same hospitals have planned well in advance for trauma patient care by organizing their personnel and accumulating the necessary material resources. In the United States (US), hospitals have been guided in this task by a document entitled *Resources for Optimal Care of the Injured Patient*[17] produced and updated routinely by the American College of Surgeons Committee on Trauma (ACS-COT). Hospitals that have fewer resources have developed systems to assess and stabilize patients expeditiously and rapidly transport them to higher-level facilities capable of care for complex patients.

Resuscitation and Evaluation: The ATLS Approach

Overseeing and conducting the resuscitation and evaluation of the multi-trauma patient is a highly complex task requiring the ability to evaluate and treat multiple life-threatening conditions while directing the activities of the other personnel present to assist. The ACS-COT, through the ATLS course, has developed and taught a systematic approach, which is used around the world. The "primary survey" is conducted first to identify and treat life-threatening injuries. "Adjuncts" such as monitoring systems, urinary catheters and gastric tubes, and radiographs are used to assist in this process. When the life-threatening injuries have been dealt with, a "secondary survey" is conducted to identify and develop treatment regimens for additional injuries. Many trauma care providers also employ a third review ("tertiary survey"), which is conducted later in the hospitalization process to reduce the incidence of missed injuries. Such missed injuries are not usually life-threatening but may cause morbidity and prolong hospitalization. This systematic approach and the treatments of the more life-threatening injuries are discussed later.

The Primary Survey

The mnemonic "ABCDE" is used to remember the priorities of the primary survey:

- A—airway
- B—breathing
- C—circulation (including insertion of intravenous catheters)
- D—disability
- E—exposure and environmental control.

Each step of the survey logically proceeds to the next so that the most life-threatening conditions are identified and treated before advancing to the next step. This regimented approach is used when the resuscitation team is small (i.e. a physician and nurse). When multiple providers are available, the assessment proceeds by the same ABCDE approach, but numerous assessments and interventions can take place simultaneously.

The adjuncts that accompany the primary survey include EKG monitoring, blood pressure and oxygen saturation monitoring, the use of supplemental oxygen, and drawing of blood for laboratory evaluation. Continuous monitoring is essential to detect systemic deterioration and response to intervention. A gastric tube and Foley catheter should be inserted for patients noted to have marked physiologic derangement or to be at risk of deterioration from injuries identified in the primary survey. If deterioration ensues, it is also essential to go through the ABCDEs again to ensure that nothing is overlooked. The previously secured airway may be dislodged or new hypotension may arise from a pneumothorax that has developed on the side opposite the chest tube inserted for the initial pneumothorax. Throughout resuscitation, and especially during the primary survey, the person directing the effort must always recognize when further resources are required to care for the patient. Failure to recognize needs at the appropriate time results in delays in summoning a key consultant or initiating transfer to a higher level of care.

Airway Management

Airway management is the first priority when confronted with a multiple-injured patient, and failure to effectively manage the airway is a frequent cause of preventable death in trauma patients. Patients with obvious airway obstruction or coma have their airway actively addressed. Three types of patients may have their airway needs overlooked until there is severe compromise and greater difficulty with airway establishment:

- The first type are those patients who look stable initially but who are slowly deteriorating physiologically and neurologically. Their airway problems occur when they are no longer in the highly monitored and equipped resuscitation area—such trauma patients have been known to die in the radiology suite.
- The second type are trauma patients who have no initial airway or breathing problem but have circulatory instability that does not reverse rapidly with resuscitation.
- The third type are those patients who are agitated or combative—the tendency is to sedate these patients to conduct the assessment, particularly the radiologic assessment. The sedation may be sufficient to cause loss of the airway and spontaneous ventilation.

Partial or complete airway obstruction is most commonly caused by occlusion of the posterior pharynx by the tongue or lax musculature. Although this can be easily overcome with simple maneuvers, the addition of food, vomitus, blood, and injured tissues may make this a formidable task. Signs of airway obstruction include agitation, obtundation, cyanosis, load snoring, gurgling, or stridor. Swelling, laceration, or penetration in the neck should prompt a comprehensive assessment and a low threshold for definitive airway establishment.

Airway Maneuvers

The easiest airway opening maneuvers are the chin lift (Fig. 31.2), jaw thrust (Fig. 31.3), and chin lift/head tilt. The chin lift/head tilt maneuver has no role in the multiple-injured patient because it may exacerbate a spinal cord injury. A comparison of the aforementioned methods of

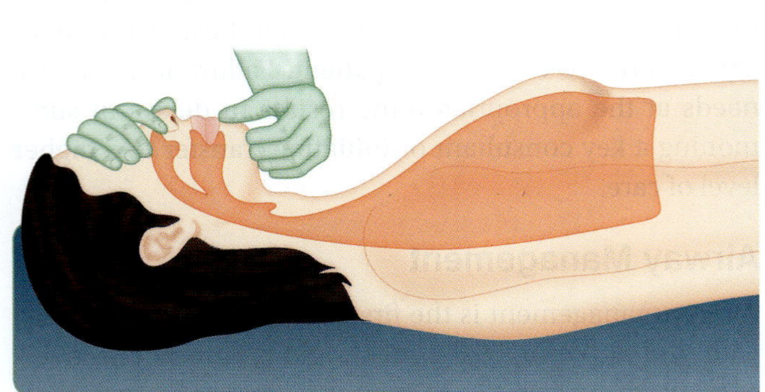

Fig. 31.2: Chin-lift maneuver. The tips of the fingers are placed beneath the patient's chin and the jaw is lifted anteriorly while the mouth is opened by drawing down on the lower lip with the thumb of the same hand.

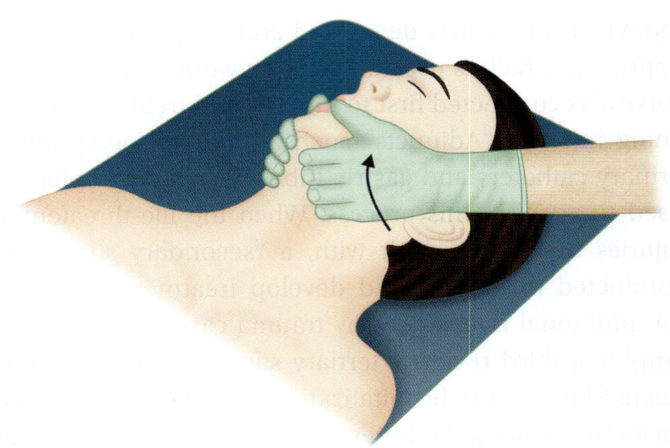

Fig. 31.3: Jaw-thrust maneuver. Two hands are placed on the mandibular rami and pushed anteriorly, so opening the airway.

opening airways in 120 anesthetized patients concluded that the chin lift was the easiest to perform and produced the greatest airway patency.[18]

Artificial Airways

Once the need for an airway has been recognized and established with the aforementioned maneuvers, further measures for airway support may be needed. Two easily inserted artificial airways may be used:

- The nasopharyngeal airway, which is used in awake or semiconscious patients, is inserted by advancing the airway into the nostril and directing it toward the nasal pharynx.
- The oropharyngeal airway, which is used in unconscious patients, may be inserted in two ways in adults—the first way is to insert it into the oral cavity in an inverted orientation, rotate it 180° and then advance it so that the distal end of the airway is lying in the hypopharynx; an alternative method is to place the airway with the assistance of a tongue blade and simply advance it to the proper location (this method is used in pediatric patients to avoid injury to the palate, which may occur with the inverted maneuver).

Each artificial airway is intended to prevent obstruction of the posterior pharynx by the tongue.

Endotracheal Intubation: In critically ill patients, particularly in the setting of brain injury, endotracheal intubation is often warranted. The presence of a cuffed tube in the trachea is considered a definitive airway. Although this is often successfully performed in the field or at transferring hospitals, malposition of the tube must always be considered. Endotracheal intubation can be accomplished by the nasal or oral route. Nasotracheal intubation is a blind technique that is contraindicated in patients who are apneic and those who have midface or basilar skull fractures. Patients who need to remain intubated beyond the emergency department may have fewer complications with orotracheal intubation.[19] Orotracheal intubation can be carried out without risk of cervical spine injury provided that in-line stabilization is maintained. There is no need for cervical spine radiographs before emergent intubation.

The most difficult steps in orotracheal intubation are clearing the airway and visualization of the vocal cords by laryngoscopy. Once the vocal cords are visualized, the endotracheal tube is passed directly between the cords into the trachea. Proper location is suggested by the presence of equal bilateral breath sounds and no borborygmi in the epigastric area. Confirm placement by capnography and tube position by a chest radiograph. Be aware that the chest X-ray (CXR) may look similar with both a tracheal and esophageal tube placement.

Airway Adjuncts

In patients who have a difficult airway, adjuncts such as a laryngeal mask airway (LMA), gum elastic bougie (GEB), fiberoptic scope, and video laryngoscopy may help achieve an endotracheal airway. The difficult airway should be anticipated. Look for a small mouth, pronounced overbite, or facial trauma. Facial hair may make preoxygenation difficult, providing less time to achieve intubation. The LMA does not provide a definitive airway but can buy time for additional skilled help to arrive. In addition, intubating LMAs allows for a cuffed endotracheal tube to be inserted through the LMA, thus providing a definitive airway. The GEB can be used when the vocal cords cannot be seen with direct laryngoscopy. It is passed blindly with the angled tip pointing anteriorly. The user will feel it track along the anterior tracheal rings if it is in the correct place. The endotracheal tube is then inserted over the GEB. Video laryngoscopy is a slightly different technique than direct laryngoscopy, but the technique is associated with better glottic visualization and may result in less cervical spine movement than direct laryngoscopy.[19a,19b] All facilities should have a plan for dealing with difficult airways that includes easily accessible airway adjuncts.

Surgical Airway

The inability to intubate the trachea in the absence of another way to oxygenate and ventilate the patient is the indication for a surgical airway. The two types of surgical airways appropriate for the trauma patient are cricothyroidotomy and tracheostomy.

Needle cricothyroidotomy is performed by inserting a 14-gauge intravenous cannula into the cricothyroid membrane. The end of the cannula is then connected to an oxygen source of at least 15 L/min (345 kPa), with either a Y-connector or a side hole cut in the tubing. Intermittent insufflation is achieved by intermittently placing the thumb over the hole. This technique provides adequate oxygenation for 30–45 minutes but does not provide very effective ventilation and CO_2 will accumulate.

Formal surgical cricothyroidotomy is performed by making a skin incision over the cricothyroid membrane, identifying this membrane, incising the membrane, inserting the blunt end of the scalpel, and rotating it 90°, thereby opening the space. Following this, an endotracheal tube or tracheostomy tube is inserted into the airway.

Emergency tracheostomy, though very rarely required, can be lifesaving, particularly in individuals who cannot be intubated because of facial injuries and who require adequate ventilation and oxygenation not achievable through a cricothyroidotomy. Rapid performance of this maneuver requires substantial surgical skill. An incision is made midway between the suprasternal notch and the superior thyroid notch in an avascular plane between the strap muscles that are retracted laterally, a tracheal hook is placed beneath the thyroid cartilage, the pretracheal fascia is opened, and a large blunt clamp is used to mobilize the tracheal isthmus cephalad. This displays the second, third, and fourth tracheal rings in most patients. An incision across the second or third ring and the use of a dilator will enable insertion of tracheostomy tube. A conventional endotracheal tube can be used temporarily if a tracheostomy tube is not available. It is difficult to secure and so should be changed out for a conventional tracheostomy tube when circumstances permit. Until then, a member of the team may need to hold the tube in place. In non-trauma situations, percutaneous tracheostomy has been advocated as an emergency airway maneuver, but doubts remain about the ability to perform it in the trauma patient without hyperextending the neck, so it is not currently recommended by the ACS-COT.

Clearly, the most frequent definitive airway management method used in the hospital setting is orotracheal intubation. Use of the other methods, particularly the surgical airway, is relatively rare. A tracheal tube and the paralytic agents administered to permit its passage clearly render the victim unable to give historic information or to complete a neurologic examination. Whenever possible, pertinent information as well as essential components of the neurologic examination should be obtained prior to intubation. Once an airway has been established, it is important to keep it in place until it is electively removed. Unintentional removal can be minimized by solidly securing the airway, dedicating a member of the team to monitor airway status, and sedating and securing the patient well.

Breathing

Once the airway is secure, the next priority is to evaluate and manage breathing. Evaluation should encompass oxygenation, ventilation, and work and mechanics of breathing. Most patients who require an airway need assistance with ventilation. This is accomplished with bag-valve ventilation for short periods and a mechanical ventilator for longer periods. Caution should be used with bag-valve ventilation to ensure that hyperventilation or hypoventilation does not occur, as this worsens mortality.[20] It is easy to inadvertently hyperventilate a patient when the provider's adrenaline is pumping. Adequate oxygenation and ventilation should be confirmed by checking arterial blood gases and constantly monitoring oxygen saturation. Ventilation can also be constantly assessed using end-tidal carbon dioxide monitoring if available. Many trauma patients have a metabolic acidosis caused by poor perfusion and their pH is preserved through high minute ventilation that eliminates carbon dioxide. This physiologic compensation needs to be taken into account when prescribing tidal and minute volume for assisted ventilation.

Conditions that inhibit effective ventilation are diagnosed and treated at this stage in the resuscitation. These include flail chest, pneumothorax, tension pneumothorax, hemothorax, and pain from fractured ribs. Transdiaphragmatic herniation of abdominal contents can also impede adequate ventilation.

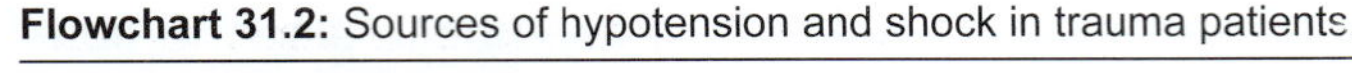

Flowchart 31.2: Sources of hypotension and shock in trauma patients.

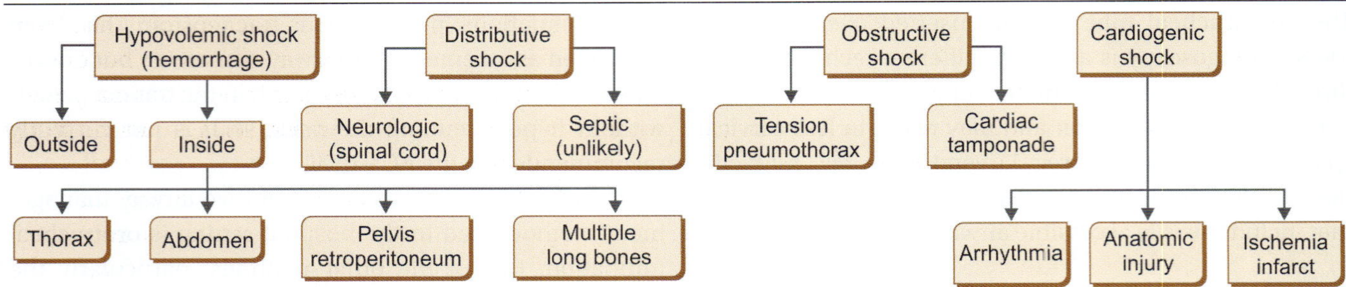

Circulation

Evaluation of the circulatory status begins with determination of systemic blood pressure, pulse, general appearance of the skin, and cardiac rhythm on EKG monitoring.

Generally, the carotid pulse is palpable at a systolic blood pressure of 60 mm Hg (7.8 kPa), the femoral pulse at 70 mm Hg (9.3 kPa), and radial pulse at 80 mm Hg (10.6 kPa).

Although hypovolemia secondary to hemorrhage is the most likely etiology of shock in the injured patient, other causes must always be considered. Flowchart 31.2 depicts the possible causes of shock in the trauma patient. It is very useful to mentally revisit this algorithm every time a patient becomes hypotensive during resuscitation. A cardiogenic source for shock is unusual, especially in the young trauma patient, but is clearly more common in the elderly. Elderly patients may have a precipitating cardiac event as the proximate cause of their trauma.

The cardiogenic causes of shock include myocardial ischemia or infarction, an arrhythmia, or an actual anatomic cardiac injury such as valvular disruption resulting from a direct blow to the heart.

The "obstructive" category includes tension pneumothorax and cardiac tamponade. Cardiac tamponade occurs with some frequency in penetrating chest trauma but is very rare in blunt trauma. Pericardiocentesis is, therefore, rarely indicated in blunt trauma and should not be carried out early in the assessment and management of hypotension.

The primary source of "distributive" shock in the trauma patient is spinal cord injury at the cervical level. This can be recognized by the accompanying warm and flushed periphery as well as by the lack of tachycardia.

Hemorrhage occurs either inside or outside the body. Blood loss from the scalp or facial fracture can be marked. Internal blood loss is typically from one or more of four locations as depicted in Flowchart 31.2. Chest and pelvic radiographs and abdominal ultrasonograms enable identification of other sites as the source of shock. Hypotension does not result from brain injury alone, and it is important that other explanations for the low blood pressure should be sought.[21]

Restoration of circulatory volume begins with placement of vascular access, which may be accomplished in several ways depending upon the patient's age and nature of injury. There are also several categories of fluid for resuscitation that may be used.

Vascular Access

Two large-bore intravenous catheters are established, typically in the antecubital veins. Percutaneous femoral vein catheterization is quick and safe. A saphenous vein cut down is indicated if vascular access cannot otherwise be accomplished secondary to vascular collapse and can be carried out at the groin or ankle level. Central venous catheter placement in the subclavian or internal jugular veins may be needed if there is the possibility of an inferior vena cava injury. Femoral vein cannulation in this scenario would not be helpful as infused fluids would pour out from the injury site. Access to the internal jugular vein is often compromised by the presence of a cervical collar and so frequently is a suboptimal choice. In children < 6 years, intraosseous infusion by cannulation of the medullary sinusoids of the tibia has been shown to be a successful means of intravenous access and is preferable to a central venous catheter.[22] In adults, intraosseous infusion is possible via the proximal tibia, proximal humerus, or sternum.

Types of Intravenous Fluids

The type of fluid used for expanding the intravascular space has been debated for many years.[23] Current management involves crystalloid initially but early utilization of blood and blood products.

Isotonic crystalloid solutions: The use of these solutions is based on the fact that during shock, fluid is lost from both the intravascular and interstitial spaces of the extracellular compartment.[24,25] Its use is standard in most hospitals in the US and is recommended in the American College of Surgeons ATLS Course.[4] Fluid resuscitation with isotonic crystalloid solutions begins with a 1000-mL bolus in adults or 20 mL/kg bolus in children. The rate of administration is then adjusted to the physiologic response. Intravenous fluids should be warmed to prevent iatrogenic hypothermia. Normal saline or Plasmalyte/Normosol may be used with blood product administration. Lactated Ringers should not be used with blood products as the preservative in the blood product chelates the calcium in lactated Ringers. Infusion of large volumes of crystalloid may cause a dilutional coagulopathy. Large volumes of normal saline will result in a hyperchloremic metabolic acidosis.

Colloid solutions: Colloid solutions do not have a role in the initial resuscitation of the trauma patient. Hydroxyethyl starch has been shown to worsen outcomes in some settings and should not be used.[26]

Hypertonic crystalloid solutions: Hypertonic crystalloid solutions have long been shown to be effective in the treatment of shock induced by hemorrhage[27-29] and have also been shown to be beneficial in the setting of closed head injury.[30] These solutions are thought to increase the extracellular compartment volume as a result of movement of fluid from the intracellular compartment.[31] In addition, these fluids also increase myocardial contractility, a property that is unrelated to volume expansion.[32]

Blood products: The purpose of transfusing blood is to expand the intravascular space while maintaining oxygen delivery. When time allows, fully cross-matched blood should be used. However, this may take up to an hour to obtain from the blood bank. For situations in which blood is needed quickly, type-specific blood can usually be available in several minutes. If the patient's condition is immediately life-threatening, it is appropriate to use type O, Rh-negative blood. Rh-positive blood can be used for males and females who are not of child-bearing age. When >10 units of packed red blood cells are going to be required in a 24-hour period, a massive transfusion protocol should be used. This massive transfusion protocol should provide at least 1 unit of fresh frozen plasma for every 2 units of packed red blood cells, cryoprecipitate for fibrinogen levels <150 mg/dL, and a dose of platelets for every 5–6 units of packed red cells.[33,34]

Therapeutic Endpoints

The work by Bickel et al.[13] reporting improved survival rates in an urban setting for hypotensive patients who had penetrating abdominal trauma and who were not given transfusion fluids has challenged current doctrine regarding therapeutic endpoints for resuscitation of shock following injury. It is now practice in many centers to limit crystalloid infusion and not resuscitate to a normotensive therapeutic endpoint. If the systolic blood pressure is >70 mm Hg (9.3 kPa), it is acceptable to proceed promptly to definitive repair of the cause of bleeding. The rationale for this approach is that replacement of intravascular volume and normotension encourages continued hemorrhage. While this strategy may be beneficial in the setting of urban penetrating injury, it is unclear whether it is effective in blunt trauma or when long transport times are involved. In addition, it may be detrimental in brain injury as it has been demonstrated that hypotension doubles the mortality rate by creating a secondary ischemic injury.[21]

Disability (Brief Neurologic Evaluation)

Brain injury is the leading cause of death after traumatic injury.[35] Early identification of injury to both the brain and the spinal cord is essential. The performance of a brief neurologic examination limited to determination of the level of consciousness, pupillary size, movement of extremities, and calculation of the GCS score will help identify neurologic injuries so that measures to prevent secondary injury can be undertaken. In addition, this provides a baseline for monitoring improvement or deterioration.

Special attention should be paid to identifying focal findings such as unilateral pupil dilatation or a motor finding that varies between the right and the left. These findings are associated with a higher incidence of brain injuries requiring operative intervention (i.e. subdural and epidural hematomas). Operations in this population can result in good neurologic outcomes if performed in a timely manner. Whenever possible, this brief neurologic examination should be conducted before medically paralyzing a trauma patient.

Exposure and Environmental Control

The last part of the primary survey is complete exposure of the patient. This facilitates identification of occult injuries. Care should be exercised during exposure to avoid inducing an iatrogenic injury by pulling clothes off the patient. Cutting off garments is, therefore, the preferred method for gaining exposure. Once disrobed, all patients, particularly pediatric patients, must be kept warm. Hypothermia has been shown to increase fluid requirements and independently increases the acute mortality rate after major traumatic injury.[36]

The Secondary Survey

The secondary survey begins by obtaining a focused history. Information about events related to the injury such as mechanism, velocity, injury to others, vital signs, and level of consciousness during transport and environmental factors should be obtained. Prehospital medical personnel are able to provide this information and their input should be sought. Additional information such as medical and operative history, current medications, allergies, and risk factors for alcoholism should also be sought. This may involve interviewing family members or contact with a primary physician for a patient who cannot provide a reliable history. The rest of the secondary survey consists of a careful systematic examination of the entire body. The airway, breathing, circulation, and neurologic status must be frequently monitored while performing this examination. Any alteration in the ABCDEs requires immediate attention before continuing with the secondary survey.

The head is examined for signs of injury such as lacerations, ecchymosis, and depressions. Visual acuity, pupillary size, and extraocular movements are all evaluated. The tympanic membranes are examined for the presence of hemotympanum or cerebrospinal fluid. The midface and jaw are examined for evidence of fractures. Mandible fractures are one of the most frequently missed injuries, so attention should be directed to a thorough examination of this structure. Likewise, the interior of the mouth is evaluated for broken teeth, occlusion, lacerations, and fractures. The anterior portion of the cervical collar should be removed with head stabilization to permit a full examination of the mandible and facilitate neck examination. The anterior and posterior aspects of the neck are next evaluated to determine the presence of injury. Special attention is paid to midline posterior pain or tenderness over the spine because these symptoms and signs guide subsequent evaluation of the cervical spine.

The full chest is examined externally as in the primary survey. The abdomen, perineum and rectum, and back are examined next. The abdominal examination should include a close look to note areas of contusion and abrasion as evidence of underlying injury. Particular attention should be directed at spotting a lap and shoulder belt mark. The lap portion of the mark should be across the pelvic bones. If it is across the soft portion of the abdomen, the patient is at risk for hollow viscus injury. A lap belt without a shoulder belt puts the patient at risk for a hyperflexion fracture of the lumbar spine, in addition to a hollow viscus injury. Seat belt marks may be very subtle initially. Attention should also be paid to entrance and exit sites as well as to the presence of subcutaneous missiles in the patient with a penetrating injury. Abdominal examination often cannot reliably exclude intra-abdominal injury, particularly if the level of consciousness is disturbed or broken bones focus the senses of the conscious patient. Failure to pursue a more aggressive assessment of the abdomen with repeat examinations or the diagnostic studies outlined later will result in unacceptable mortality and morbidity rates from delayed diagnosis or missed injury.

The pelvis should be palpated for tenderness in the awake patient, but there is no role for vigorous compression to assess stability in any patient before a pelvic radiograph has been obtained. The risks associated with this maneuver are dislodgment of clot in disrupted vessels and increased bleeding. The examination of a fractured pelvis should not be repeated without good clinical reason. All patients with suspected pelvic fractures need a rectal examination and, if applicable, a vaginal examination to look for penetration of fracture fragments into these areas. Blood or palpable fractures on either of these examinations means the pelvic fracture should be considered an open fracture and treated with prompt washout and antibiotics.

The musculoskeletal and nervous systems are then evaluated and neurologic status is compared with that obtained as part of the primary survey. Finally, the patient is rolled, while maintaining precautions against spinal cord injury, and the back is examined and the spine palpated.

Once the primary and secondary surveys have been completed, the person directing the resuscitation and assessment develops a prioritized problem list and outlines a further evaluation and treatment approach to:

- Rule out suspected injuries
- Better define noted injuries
- Provide ongoing monitoring and support
- Provide definitive treatment for identified injuries.

Diagnosis

Laboratory and imaging modalities are essential adjuncts to the complete assessment and management of trauma patients. The approach employed for a given patient is guided by findings noted in the primary and secondary surveys but is also guided by the quality and availability of modalities at the practitioner's institution. Technology, particularly imaging technology, is rapidly evolving. This requires that a provider stays up to date with imaging progress as it applies to the evaluation of trauma patients.

Laboratory Evaluation

Most centers have a panel of laboratory tests that are run as a routine or protocol for the severely injured patient. This protocol approach has been adopted to ensure that studies are not missed and to allow the resuscitation team to focus on the complex patient. A typical battery of tests would include hematology, chemistry, and coagulation profiles; urinalysis; blood gases; blood-alcohol level; toxicology screen; and blood type and screen. A more selective approach to laboratory evaluation may be considered with less severely injured patients.

Admission hemoglobin, hematocrit, and platelet count are important to establish a baseline. However, the hemoglobin and hematocrit can still be normal despite marked bleeding. A prothrombin time and partial thromboplastin time can be eliminated in selected patients—those who are definitively known not to be on anticoagulation, those without significant brain injury, and those who have not received significant crystalloid or any blood products prior to arrival at the trauma center. A serum bicarbonate should be included with the admission electrolyte panel to enable calculation of the base deficit. This base deficit, as well as serum lactate, provides a global assessment of oxygen debt—the amount of shock-induced anaerobic metabolism that a patient has experienced. A large base deficit or elevated lactate is associated with a poorer outcome, and reversal of the oxygen debt is a useful endpoint of resuscitation.

Serum creatine kinase and serum myoglobin should be measured to assess muscle damage and circulating pigment load in patients who have had a crush injury or who have been pinned down in one position for prolonged periods. There is no role for creatine phosphokinase isoenzymes in the routine evaluation of possible blunt cardiac injury because they do not correlate with anatomic injury or the other sequelae of blunt injury.[37] Isoenzymes can be obtained if a diagnosis of cardiac ischemia is being considered. Ethanol levels may help explain an altered mental status and screen for patients who may benefit from substance abuse counseling or alert caregivers to the need for prophylaxis for delirium tremens. Brief interventions in trauma centers for patients who were drinking at the time of their injury have been shown to reduce trauma recidivism.[38]

Imaging Modalities

Brain and skull injury: A computed tomogram (CT) scan is currently a test of choice to evaluate brain and skull injury. Nearly all operable injuries can be readily visualized on a noncontrast scan. Parenchymal and extraparenchymal lesions and skull fracture anatomy are evident.

A focal neurologic injury not explained by spinal or peripheral injury and a GCS score < 15 are accepted indications for a brain CT scan. The role of CT scanning in the population that has a GCS score of 15 with previous loss of consciousness and lack of objective focal neurologic findings is more debatable. The incidence of CT-demonstrated lesions is 5–7%, and <1% of patients need operative intervention. Proponents of routine scanning in this population claim that the small groups that need intervention receive it in a timely manner and that discharge is facilitated for the patients with normal scans. A significant blow to the head even without loss of consciousness in a patient on anticoagulation should prompt consideration for a CT scan even with a normal neurologic examination.

Hemodynamically unstable patients who require emergent operative intervention for hemorrhage should have the brain CT scan deferred if they have a nonfocal neurologic examination. The scan can usually be obtained after the operation or the neurosurgeon may elect to monitor the intracranial pressure intraoperatively if the operation will be a lengthy procedure. Hemodynamically unstable patients with focal neurologic findings (single dilated pupil or decreased movement on one side relative to the other) have a high incidence of operable epidural and subdural hematomas that need to be drained at the same time as the operation for bleeding. The decision to delay surgery in a patient with surgical bleeding in order to obtain a brain CT scan is a difficult one that should be made in conjunction with the neurosurgeon and based on the stability of the patient and the patient's response to early resuscitative efforts.

Facial fractures: Plain radiographs or a CT scan can be used to diagnose and define facial fractures, but a CT scan is clearly superior, and many advocate elimination of plain radiographs for other than assessment of the mandible. An axial CT scan is sufficient for most fractures, but coronal cuts are useful to better define orbital injury, particularly to the orbital floor. A panorex radiograph of the mandible demonstrates pathology well but requires a stable and cooperative patient who is able to sit up. The indications for facial bone evaluation include:

- Malocclusion
- Palpable bony fracture
- Crepitance or tenderness
- Restricted eye movement

- Abnormal maxillary–mandibular occlusion
- Penetrating injuries
- Severe soft tissue injury with swelling that precludes bone palpation.

The modern CT scanner can construct three-dimensional images of the bony anatomy to guide reconstruction.

Cervical spine injury: Patients with diffuse blunt trauma are considered to have cervical spine injury until fully evaluated. Most arrive at the hospital on a long backboard with a hard cervical collar in place. Injury is ruled out and the spine cleared by a combination of history, examination, and imaging studies. Evidence-based practice guidelines exist to guide the clearance process.[39] Patients with neurologic findings potentially attributable to the spinal cord are left in the hard collar and further evaluations are carried out. Patients without spinal cord findings are initially divided into those who can provide a reliable history and examination and those who are unreliable. A patient is deemed reliable if, in the judgment of the examining physician, he or she is able to concentrate and accurately report pain in the neck and tenderness on neck examination. Mind-altering medications, alcohol, brain injury, distracting injury (an injury that makes the patient unable to focus at the time of explanation, e.g. painful broken hand), intellectual disability, dementia, and a psychiatric disorder generally reduce the ability of the examiner to obtain a reliable examination.

If a patient is reliable, reports no pain, has no tenderness on examination, no evidence of fracture elsewhere in the spine, and is able to move the neck through its full range of motion without discomfort, the incidence of injury is so low that the neck is considered to be clear and the collar is removed. If the reliable patient has any of these findings, a CT scan of the neck should be obtained. Only if no CT scan is available, should plain radiographs of the neck be obtained. If no fracture or subluxation is noted and the patient continues to have a positive cervical spine examination, the last lesion that should be ruled out is an unstable pure ligamentous injury. This is evaluated with lateral radiographic views of the neck in flexion and extension or by magnetic resonance imaging (MRI). If flexion–extension views are inadequate, the patient with ongoing symptoms requires MRI. If either of these tests is adequate and does not show evidence of injury, the collar can be removed.

In patients with altered sensorium from any etiology, a cervical spine CT scan should be obtained. If no fracture or other pathology is noted, the literature remains divided on the correct course of action. Magnetic resonance imaging is one option for evaluation for unstable ligamentous injury but should be done within 72 hours of injury for highest accuracy.[40] However, the risks of taking an obtunded patient for MRI are real as is the risk of pressure ulcers if the collar remains in place. The other option is to remove the cervical collar on the basis of the negative CT scan, but a large series of MRI in obtunded patients showed a 1.1% incidence of ligamentous injury.[41] The Eastern Association for the Surgery of Trauma has declined to make a recommendation as to the appropriate treatment of the obtunded patient with a negative cervical spine CT scan.[39]

Cervical spine pathology can occur with penetrating injury, primarily gunshot wounds. These injuries result from a direct hit on the spine and are generally mechanically stable. A cervical collar can be placed on patients with penetrating neck wounds and offer the theoretic advantage of reducing bone fragment movement and additional injury. The collar, however, makes injury less evident and reduces the ability to monitor bleeding or swelling that may compromise the airway. Collar use for penetrating neck injury is currently unclear. It is clear that cervical collars and full radiologic evaluation are not indicated for penetrating head injury. In one study of 215 patients with gunshot wounds to the head, none had cervical pathology.[42]

Pelvic fracture and hemorrhage: An anteroposterior (AP) plain radiographic view of the pelvis should be obtained early in the assessment of patients who:

- Are hemodynamically unstable
- Claim to have pelvic pain or tenderness
- Are unable to provide a reliable examination.

If a fracture is noted, it can be better defined by a pelvic CT scan, which also provides information about associated bleeding. If contrast is injected into the bladder, or delayed images are obtained after contrast reaches the bladder, the CT scan can also provide information about bladder injury.

Bleeding from pelvic vessels disrupted with the pelvic fracture can be marked and cause death. Hemodynamic instability and evidence of a possible pelvic fracture should prompt application of a pelvic binder during the initial evaluation. Patients with pelvic fractures and hemodynamic instability not due to other sources of bleeding should be considered candidates for angiographic embolization. Patients with evidence of intravenous contrast extravasation in the pelvis or other signs of ongoing bleeding should also be considered for embolization. If embolization is not promptly available or does not correct the bleeding (as may occur with venous disruption), laparotomy with pelvic packing is another option for hemorrhage control in the hemodynamically unstable patient.[43]

Thoracic injury: The evaluation of thoracic injury has changed. Plain radiographs of the chest are still recommended by ATLS as an adjunct to the secondary survey, but other modalities have come into play. Bedside ultrasonography can reliably detect hemodynamically significant pneumothoraces, and CT angiography is now sufficient assessment for aortic injuries, obviating the need in most cases for dedicated aortic angiography.

Although the CXR does not reliably predict the detailed trajectory of a bullet or other missile, it does demonstrate most of the induced pathology and enables determination of transmediastinal injury. The diaphragmatic disruptions that cause early physiologic compromise can be seen, but the admission CXR misses approximately 50% of total diaphragm injuries, especially those from stab wounds. Findings associated with an increased incidence of mediastinal injury can also be noted and prompt the more definitive studies.

Increased use of CT scanning for the evaluation of an abdominal injury has increased recognition of chest pathology and led to the realization that a CT scan provides much greater resolution of pathology above the diaphragm. A CT scan demonstrates lung contusions, pneumothoraces, and hemothoraces, with increased sensitivity over chest radiographs.[44]

Diaphragm injury: Multiple noninvasive imaging modalities have been used in an attempt to diagnose diaphragmatic injury when disruption is not grossly evident on the initial CXR. To date, it is not clear which modality has the best sensitivity and specificity. Upper gastrointestinal series and barium enemas may reveal stomach or intestine in the pleural cavity as might CT scans, which may also reveal actual discontinuity of the diaphragmatic muscle. An ultrasound study can also show muscle disruption, but it is unclear how often this finding is evident in patients with known injury. Experience with MRI has been reported and may prove to be the best way to noninvasively assess the diaphragm, but its utility in potentially unstable patients remains to be elucidated.[45] Thoracoscopy and laparoscopy, though invasive, provide an accurate assessment of the diaphragm and are less invasive than thoracotomy or laparotomy. Small diaphragmatic wounds can also be repaired by thoracoscopic approaches.

Aortic disruption: Aortic injury is infrequent, but it is associated with mortality rates as high as 90% if the diagnosis is not made and the injury goes untreated. Patients succumb from free rupture of the vessel and exsanguination. This injury must be suspected in all patients who are subjected to large decelerating forces. The AP upright CXR can be used as a screen to select those patients who should have more definitive diagnostic tests, but up to 7% of patients with aortic disruption have a normal CXR.[46] A hemodynamically unstable patient with evidence of aortic injury on CXR and a positive Focused Assessment with Sonography for Trauma (FAST) study is likely unstable from the intra-abdominal injury. The first incision in the operating room in this case is a midline laparotomy incision. Aortic disruption, sufficient to cause vital sign changes, usually causes catastrophic cardiovascular collapse, rather than mere instability.

Table 31.2 Chest radiograph findings associated with aortic injury.

Mediastinal findings
Obliteration of aortic knob contour
Widened mediastinum (>8 cm) on upright radiograph
Loss of perivertebral pleural stripe
Depression of left main stem bronchus
Fractures
Upper ribs, especially first rib
Scapula
Sternum
Multiple left ribs
Other findings
Deviation of nasogastric tube
Trachea shifted to right
Apical pleural hematoma (capping), especially on left
Large left hemothorax

Table 31.2 lists the findings on the CXR that are associated with a higher incidence of aortic injury. The widened mediastinum is the finding most frequently seen with injury. The presence of a distinct aortic knob is the finding most reliably associated with an uninjured aorta. Patients with the findings listed in Table 31.3 as well as those with a normal chest radiograph, but severe high-speed deceleration as their mechanism of injury and extra-thoracic injuries such as severe pelvic fractures, should undergo additional diagnostic evaluation. Previously, the gold standard for making the diagnosis of aortic disruption was a thoracic angiogram. Most institutions now rely on CT angiography as their sole diagnostic test.[47,48]

Thoracic and lumbar spine injury: Approximately 2–3% of blunt trauma patients have thoracolumbar spine injuries.

Table 31.3 Risk factors for abdominal injury.

Mechanism of injury
For example, motor vehicle driver (steering wheel)
Findings on physical examination
Tenderness of the abdomen or lower chest
Abrasions or contusions on abdomen (including lap seat belt mark, especially if above the pelvic brim)
Hypotension on admission or at the accident scene or during transport
Laboratory findings
Admission base deficit (serum bicarbonate <21)
Gross hematuria
Radiographic findings
Lower rib fractures
Hemo- or pneumothorax
Lung contusion
Pelvic fracture
Lumbar or thoracic spine fracture

The majority of fractures involve vertebral bodies T11–L2. A CT scan of the thoracic and lumbar spine should be obtained in patients with back pain, lower extremity neurologic findings or cervical spine injury, and for those for whom adequate clinical examination is impossible. Plain radiographs are acceptable if CT scans are not available. Several retrospective studies and one combined retrospective and prospective study[49] have demonstrated that as many as 40% of alert patients with a thoracolumbar spine fracture do not complain of back pain, nor have tenderness on examination.

A fracture in one area of the spine mandates imaging of the entire spine.[50]

Abdominal injury: Penetrating injury: The patient who is hemodynamically unstable from a penetrating abdominal injury does not need additional evaluation of the abdomen before laparotomy. These patients should have a CXR to ensure that there is no concomitant chest injury if there is any possibility that the wounding agent(s) entered the chest. Hemodynamically stable patients with gunshot wounds to the abdomen may also be taken directly to the operating room for a laparotomy without additional investigation if it is clear that the bullet has entered the peritoneal cavity or they have positive peritoneal signs. If the bullet trajectory based on entrance and exit wounds in the stable patient is not clearly through the peritoneal cavity or the bullet may have hit the spine and the patient has a relatively benign examination, AP and lateral plain radiographs of the abdomen and pelvis may be obtained. They may demonstrate that the bullet is clearly in the peritoneal cavity or show findings such as free air and so prompt laparotomy is required. They may also suggest that the missile has not entered the peritoneal cavity and prompt further evaluation of that possibility with a CT scan or laparoscopy. Observation is seldom used for gunshot wounds that penetrate the peritoneal cavity, but successful nonoperative management of wounds that are seen by a CT scan to clearly involve only the liver has been reported.[51]

Unlike bullet wounds to the abdomen, which have a high incidence of intraperitoneal organ injury, knife wounds in the stable patient are associated with intraperitoneal injury, requiring operation in only 50% of cases. Routine laparotomy in this population results in too high incidence of nontherapeutic intervention. In addition, the cost and morbidity of the laparotomy does not quantify its routine use. Several options are available to identify those who have a higher risk of injury. These include observation, local anterior abdominal wound exploration to rule out peritoneal penetration, ultrasonography, triple contrast computed tomography, and laparoscopy. Diagnostic peritoneal lavage (DPL) is used less frequently than in the past. A detailed explanation of the relative advantages and disadvantages as well as sensitivities and specificities of each of these approaches is beyond the scope of this chapter and readers are referred to Chapter 40, "Abdominal, Urologic and Perineal Injuries".

Studies[52,53] have demonstrated that the routine intravenous pyelogram (IVP) provides little data that affect management and so make a good case for selective or no preoperative IVPs. Kidney function can be assessed intraoperatively in the exceedingly small number of patients with renal injury and where a decision about the approach to the injury would be modified with knowledge of the functional state of the contralateral kidney.

Blunt abdominal injury: Blunt trauma patients who present with ongoing hemodynamic instability with no extra-abdominal source for the instability should undergo an emergent laparotomy. The abdomen should be confirmed as the source of bleeding by ultrasonography or, less commonly, DPL.

Patients with blunt trauma to the torso and who are hemodynamically stable on presentation or who are easily resuscitated to stability should undergo abdominal evaluation beyond physical examination if they have abdominal tenderness or are unable to provide a reliable examination. Patients who are stable or stabilized, have no tenderness on a reliable physical examination, but have other risk factors for abdominal injury, should also be more fully evaluated. Factors associated with abdominal injury risk in this population are listed in Table 31.3 and include admission hypotension, base deficit, hematuria, pelvic fracture, lumbar or thoracic fractures, abdominal wall contusion, abrasion or seat belt marks, and a CXR that reveals lower rib fractures, hemothorax, pneumothorax, or lung contusion.

Several diagnostic options are available to supplement the initial physical examination. These include admission with frequent re-examination, DPL, computed tomography, and ultrasonography. Re-examination requires considerable personnel resources and a cooperative, reliable patient with no signs of possible injury. Computed tomography is the most commonly used diagnostic test, especially in a patient with equivocal findings on physical examination, neurologic injury, or multiple extra-abdominal injuries.[54]

Diagnostic peritoneal lavage: Diagnostic peritoneal lavage involves the insertion of a catheter through the anterior abdominal wall into the peritoneal cavity. Peritoneal contents are aspirated and the test is considered positive if intestinal contents or 10 mL of gross blood are returned. If neither of these criteria are met, 1 L of isotonic lavage solution is instilled, returned, and sent for analysis. The lavage is considered positive if there are >100,000 red blood cells/mm^3 or >500 white blood cells/mm^3 in the analyzed fluid or a Gram stain of the fluid reveals bacteria. Its use has declined markedly. Practitioners should be wary of using this test without adequate experience.

Abdominal computed tomography: Computed tomography has steadily gained favor as the diagnostic modality of choice for the stable trauma patient and this trend will continue. Scanners are more widely available and are now frequently installed in close proximity to the trauma resuscitation areas. They are increasingly faster, of higher resolution, and are being used more frequently for evaluating other body areas in the trauma patient. A CT scan is less invasive than DPL, evaluates both the peritoneal cavity and the retroperitoneum, and allows nonoperative management of many solid organ injuries. Like DPL, an abdominal CT scan is least sensitive for the identification of hollow viscus injury. Although some institutions report higher rates, the usual rate for successful identification of intestinal injury is approximately 50%. The incidence of intestinal injury from blunt trauma is, however, very low, but because of the concern about missed injuries, many institutions admit patients with abdominal symptoms and a negative CT scan for serial abdominal examinations.

Ultrasonography: FAST has largely replaced DPL for rapid assessment of the unstable patient. The objective of FAST is to identify intraperitoneal fluid as a marker of abdominal injury. In addition, the heart is examined for pericardial fluid and the lungs are examined for a pneumothorax. When used to identify intra-abdominal fluid, FAST is 73–88% sensitive, 98–100% specific, and 96–98% accurate.[54] Similar results are obtained by radiologists, surgeons, and emergency medicine physicians. However, up to 25% of abdominal injuries noted on a CT scan are not associated with free peritoneal fluid.[55] The clinical importance of these potentially missed injuries is yet to be documented.

FAST is a noninvasive technique that can be conducted in 4–5 minutes in the trauma resuscitation room without patient transport. Its use is limited in obese patients and those with marked subcutaneous emphysema because of poor image resolution. Like DPL and computed tomography, it is limited in its ability to detect hollow viscus injury. It can also assess the thorax for pneumothorax.

Flowchart 31.3 depicts how FAST can be used in both the hypotensive and stable trauma patients. The repeat FAST study for stable trauma patients is designed to pick up some of the patients with organ injury and no or minimal initial peritoneal fluid, who go on to bleed and accumulate more fluid. Use of FAST as a screening tool for computed tomography and as a replacement for DPL in stable trauma patients has been shown to safely reduce resource use.[56]

TRANSFER TO DEFINITIVE CARE

Most trauma patients transported to a hospital can be adequately cared for at that facility. There are, however, patients whose needs exceed available resources. These patients should be transferred to higher echelons of care as safely and rapidly as possible. Delay in transfer results from failure to identify the need for transfer early in the evaluation and resuscitation process and from excessive diagnostic testing. Recognition of the need for transfer can be facilitated by development of institution-specific clinical criteria that prompt transfer. The transfer process should be invoked as soon as the criteria are met. Using this approach, the time delay associated with having each specialist evaluate each patient and render an opinion on whether the injuries can be managed locally is avoided. Table 31.4 lists the type of patients who might be considered for transfer.

Once the decision is made to transfer a patient, the only diagnostic testing that should be undertaken is that

Flowchart 31.3: Focused assessment with sonography for trauma (FAST). Actions triggered by study results. (DPL: Diagnostic peritoneal lavage).

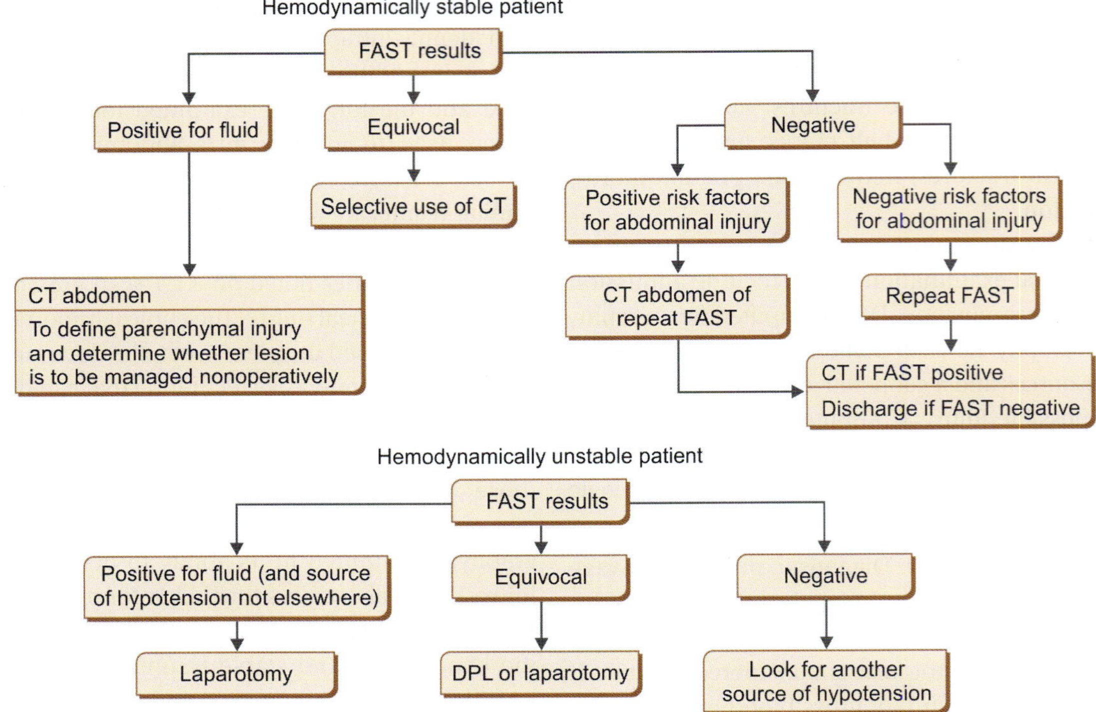

which identifies conditions that need to be addressed before transfer. Usually, this is only a CXR to rule out a pneumothorax and ensure endotracheal tube position. The one exception to this is in the hemodynamically unstable patient. The source of hypotension may need to be determined and potentially corrected to enable safe transfer. The decision whether to transfer or stabilize locally is a difficult one. It depends upon the degree of instability, the source of instability, local resources, the duration of transport, and the level of care available during transport. This decision making ideally should involve the surgeons both locally and at the trauma center. Safe transfer may require a laparotomy and splenectomy or some similar procedure at the local hospital prior to transfer.

Examples of diagnostic tests that should not be performed at the local hospital if the decision to transfer has been made include a CT scan of the brain or abdomen, DPL in the stable patient, and an angiogram.

Transport to definitive care, whether by land or air, invariably exposes the patient and providers to a more difficult care environment if any clinical conditions deteriorate. To reduce the possibility of untoward events en route, the transport team should be properly staffed, trained, and equipped, and the patient and all lines and tubes must be adequately secured. As endotracheal

Table 31.4	Criteria for consideration of transfer from level III centers to level I or II centers.
•	Carotid or vertebral artery injury
•	Torn thoracic aorta or great vessel
•	Cardiac rupture
•	Bilateral pulmonary contusions with a Pao_2:Fio_2 ratio <200
•	Major abdominal vascular injury
•	Grade IV or V liver injuries requiring transfusion of >6 U of red blood cells in 6 hours
•	Unstable pelvic fracture requiring transfusion of >6 U of red blood cells in 6 hours
•	Fracture or dislocation with loss of distal pulses
•	Penetrating injuries or open fracture of the skull
•	Glasgow coma scale score <14 or lateralizing neurologic signs (if no neurosurgical consultation is available)
•	Spinal fracture or spinal cord deficit
•	Complex pelvic/acetabulum fracture
•	More than two unilateral rib fractures or bilateral rib fractures with pulmonary contusion (if no critical care consultation is available)
•	Significant torso injury with advanced comorbid disease (such as coronary artery disease, chronic obstructive pulmonary disease, type 1 diabetes mellitus, or immunosuppression)

Source: Reproduced with permission from The Committee on Trauma. Resources for Optimal Care of the Injured Patient. Chicago: American College of Surgeons; 2014.

intubation is so difficult en route, any patient with brain injury or airway compromise and the potential to deteriorate should be intubated prior to departure and adequately sedated with short-acting agents. Transfer summaries should be provided to the receiving center prior to or with the patient, and the original radiographs should accompany the patient.

REFERENCES

1. Sasser SM, Hunt RC, Faul M, et al. Guidelines for field triage of injured patients: recommendations of the National Expert Panel on Field Triage, 2011. MMWR Recomm Rep. 2012;61(RR-1):1-20.
2. National Association of EMS Physicians; American College of Surgeons-Committee on Trauma. Field triage of the injured patient. Prehosp Emerg Care. 2011;15(4):541.
3. Faul M, Wald MM, Sullivent EE, et al. Large cost savings realized from the 2006 Field Triage Guideline: reduction in overtriage in U.S. trauma centers. Prehosp Emerg Care. 2012;16(2): 222-9
4. Advanced Trauma Life Support. Chicago: American College of Surgeons; 2012.
5. Pre-Hospital Trauma Life Support, 7th edition. Akron, Ohio: Emergency Training; 2010.
6. American College of Emergency Physicians; American College of Surgeons Committee on Trauma; National Association of EMS Physicians. Drug-assisted intubation in the prehospital setting. J Am Coll Surg. 2005;201(4):585.
7. American College of Emergency Physicians. Drug-assisted intubation in the prehospital setting. Ann Emerg Med. 2005; 46(2):214.
8. American College of Emergency Physicians. Drug-assisted intubation in the prehospital setting. Policy statement. Ann Emerg Med. 2011;58(1):113-4.
9. Wang HE, Davis DP, O'Connor RE, et al. Drug-assisted intubation in the prehospital setting (resource document to NAEMSP position statement). Prehosp Emerg Care. 2006; 10(2):261-71.
10. Kragh JF, Walters TJ, Baer DG, et al. Survival with emergency tourniquet use to stop bleeding in major limb trauma. Ann Surg. 2009;249:1Y7.
11. 2010 American Heart Association Guidelines for Cardiopulmonary Resuscitation and Emergency Cardiovascular Care Science. Circulation. 2010;122(19, suppl 3).
12. Lewis FR Jr. Prehospital intravenous fluid therapy: physiologic computer modelling. J Trauma. 1986;26:804.
13. Bickell WH, Wall MJ, Pepe PE, et al. Immediate versus delayed fluid resuscitation for hypotensive patients with penetrating torso injuries. N Engl J Med. 1994;331:1105.
14. CRASH-2 trial collaborators Effects of tranexamic acid on death, vascular occlusive events, and blood transfusion in trauma patients with significant haemorrhage (CRASH-2): a randomised, placebo-controlled trial. Lancet. 2010;376 (9734):23-32.
15. Kung WM, Tsai SH, Chiu WT, et al. Correlation between Glasgow coma score components and survival in patients with traumatic brain injury. Injury. 2011;42(9):940-4.
16. Guidelines for the Management of Severe Traumatic Brain Injury, 3rd edition. New York: Brain Trauma Foundation; 2007.
17. The Committee on Trauma. Resources for Optimal Care of the Injured Patient. Chicago: American College of Surgeons; 2014.
18. Guildner CW. Resuscitation—opening the airway: a comparative study of techniques for opening an airway obstructed by the tongue. J Am Coll Emerg Phys. 1976;5:588.
19. Holzapfel L, Chevret S, Madinier G, et al. Influence of long-term oro- or nasotracheal intubation on nosocomial maxillary sinusitis and pneumonia: results of a prospective, randomized, clinical trial. Crit Care Med. 1993;21(8): 1132-8.

19a. Paolini JB, Donati F, Drolet P. Review article: video-laryngoscopy: another tool for difficult intubation or a new paradigm in airway management? Can J Anaesth. 2013;60(2):184-91.

19b. Kill C, Risse J, Wallot P, et al. Videolaryngoscopy with glidescope reduces cervical spine movement in patients with unsecured cervical spine. J Emerg Med. 2013;44(4):750-6.

20. Dumont TM, Visioni AJ, Rughani AI, et al. Inappropriate prehospital ventilation in severe traumatic brain injury increases in-hospital mortality. J Neurotrauma. 2010;27(7): 1233-41.
21. Chestnut RM, Marshall LF, Klauber MR, et al. The role of secondary brain injury in determining outcome from severe head injury. J Trauma. 1993;34:216.
22. Sawyer RW, Bodai BI, Blaisdell FW, et al. The current status of intraosseous infusion. J Am Coll Surg. 1994;179:353.
23. Pollack CV. Prehospital fluid resuscitation of the trauma patient—an update on the controversies. Emerg Med Clin North Am. 1993;11:6l.
24. Shires GT, Canizaro PC. Fluid resuscitation in the severely injured. Surg Clin North Am. 1973;53:1341.
25. Shires GT, Cunningham JN, Backer CR, et al. Alterations in cellular membrane function during hemorrhagic shock in primates. Ann Surg. 1972;176:288.
26. Perner A, Haase N, Guttormesen AB, et al. Hydroxyethyl starch 130/0.42 versus Ringer's acetate in severe sepsis. N Engl J Med. 2012;367(2):124-34.
27. Velasco IT, Pontieri V, Rocha M, et al. Hyperosmotic NaCl and severe hemorrhagic shock. Am J Physiol. 1980; 239:H664.
28. Baue AE, Tragus ET, Parkins WM. A comparison of isotonic and hypertonic solutions on blood flow and oxygen consumption in the initial treatment of hemorrhagic shock. J Trauma. 1967;7:743.
29. Walsh JC, Zhuang J, Shackford SR. A comparison of hypertonic to isotonic fluid in the resuscitation of brain injury and hemorrhagic shock. J Surg Res. 1991;50:284.
30. Shackford SR, Bourguignon PR, Wald SL, et al. Hypertonic saline resuscitation of patients with head injury: a prospective, randomized clinical trial. J Trauma. 1998;44:50.

31. Nerlich M, Gunther R, Demling RH. Resuscitation from hemorrhagic shock with hypertonic saline or lactated Ringer's (effect on the pulmonary and systemic microcirculations). Circ Shock. 1983;10:179.
32. Wildenthal K, Mierzwiak DS, Mitchell JH. Acute effects of increased serum osmolality on left ventricular performance. Am J Physiol. 1969;216:898.
33. Sihler KC, Napolitano LM. Massive transfusion: new insights. Chest. 2009;136(6):1654-67.
34. Spahn DR, Bouillon B, Cerny V, et al. Management of bleeding and coagulopathy following major trauma: an updated European guideline. Crit Care. 2013;17:R76.
35. Shackford SR, Mackersie RC, Holbrook TL, et al. The epidemiology of traumatic death: a population based analysis. Arch Surg. 1993;128:571.
36. Gentilello LM, Jurkovich GJ, Stark MS, et al. Is hypothermia in the victim of major trauma protective or harmful?—a randomized, prospective study. Ann Surg. 1997;226:439.
37. Mattox KL, Flint KM, Carrico CJ, et al. Blunt cardiac injury. J Trauma. 1992;33:649.
38. Gentilello LM, Rivara FP, Donovan DM, et al. Alcohol interventions in a trauma center as a means of reducing the risk of injury recurrence. Ann Surg. 1999;230(4):473-80.
39. Como JJ, Diaz JJ, Dunham CM, et al. Practice management guidelines for identification of cervical spine injuries following trauma: update from the Eastern Association for the Surgery of Trauma practice management guidelines committee. J Trauma. 2009;67(3):651-9.
40. D'Alise MD, Benzel EC, Hart BL. Magnetic resonance imaging evaluation of the cervical spine in the comatose or obtunded trauma patient. J Neurosurg. 1999;91:54-59.
41. Hogan GJ, Mirvis SE, Shanmuganathan K, et al. Exclusion of unstable cervical spine injury in obtunded patients with blunt trauma: is MR imaging needed when multi-detector row CT findings are normal? Radiology. 2005;237:106-13.
42. Kaups KL, Davis JW. Patients with gunshot wounds to the head do not require cervical spine immobilization and evaluation. J Trauma. 1998;44:865-7.
43. Cullinane DC, Schiller HJ, Zielinski MD, et al. Eastern Association for the Surgery of Trauma practice management guidelines for hemorrhage in pelvic fracture—update and systematic review. J Trauma. 2011;71(6):1850-68.
44. Wagner RB, Jamieson PM. Pulmonary contusion. Evaluation and classification by computed tomography. Surg Clin North Am. 1989;69:31.
45. Boulanger BR, Mirvis SE, Rodriquez A. Magnetic resonance imaging in traumatic diaphragmatic rupture: case reports. J Trauma. 1992;32:89.
46. Fabian TC, Richardson JD, Croce MA, et al. Prospective study of blunt aortic injury: multicenter trial of the American Association for the Surgery of Trauma. J Trauma. 1997; 42:374.
47. Nagy K., Fabian T, Rodman G, et al. Guidelines for the diagnosis and management of blunt aortic injury: an EAST Practice Management Guidelines Work Group. J Trauma. 2000;48(6):1128-43.
48. Demetriades D, Velmahos GC, Scalea TM, et al. Diagnosis and treatment of blunt thoracic aortic injuries: changing perspectives. J Trauma. 2008;64(6):1415-8.
49. Frankl H, Rozycki GS, Ochsner M, et al. Indications for obtaining thoracic and lumbar spine radiographs. J Trauma. 1994;37:673.
50. Sixta S, Moore FO, Ditillo MF, et al. Screening for thoracolumbar spinal injuries in blunt trauma: an Eastern Association for the Surgery of Trauma practice management guideline. J Trauma. 2012;73(5 suppl 4):S326-32.

Additional references appear in the online version of this book.

32

Initial Surgical Care of the Trauma Patient

Thomas M Scalea, James V O'Connor

Key Points

- The most common indication for emergency surgery is hemorrhage.
- Surgeons should be familiar with various operative approaches to the chest and abdomen, and techniques for control of major vessels in the neck, arm, groin, and leg.
- Surgical incisions should provide optimal exposure and allow for extension for additional exposure, if required.
- Thoracic injuries most often require an anterolateral thoracotomy, unilateral or bilateral "clamshell", or a sternotomy.
- Abdominal injuries should be approached through a midline incision.
- In stable patients, angiography and arterial embolization techniques may obviate the need for an open operation, but these techniques should not be used in patients with continued hemorrhage and subclinical or clinical shock.
- Damage control is a strategy that controls life-threatening hemorrhage and is followed by resuscitation and definitive operation when the patient is more stable.

INTRODUCTION

Initial operative management of injured patients involves a stepwise process designed to identify immediately life-threatening injuries first, followed by those that potentially place the patient's life in danger. The goal is to provide the patient the best chance of survival with the least morbidity.

GENERAL TRAUMA PRINCIPLES

The incision should be chosen carefully. Occasionally, a patient has an operation to treat a specific injury, and the incision can expose a limited area. More often, injured patients are explored both to establish a diagnosis and to provide treatment. These patients are often critically ill and may be hypotensive. In these cases, the most versatile incision gives the surgeon the greatest number of options to deal with whatever is encountered. Incisions must provide adequate exposure of all potential areas of injury. It is unwise to make a small incision in order to obtain a better cosmetic result.

Blood and clots should be evacuated. The area should be packed to achieve temporary hemostasis. Any bleeding can be temporarily controlled with pressure, giving the anesthesiologist time to replenish the cardiac preload with blood and fluids and the surgeon time to ascertain the immediately life-threatening injuries.

Temporary hemostasis can be achieved in one of several ways as discussed below:

- Bleeding from solid organs (the liver, spleen, or even the lung) can be controlled by direct hand compression, packing with laparotomy pads, or both.
- Bleeding from major blood vessels, the aorta, vena cava or heart can be minimized with direct pressure, either with a finger, a sponge stick, or the fist.

Inexperienced surgeons often attempt to repair all injuries rapidly without allowing time for the anesthesiologist to transfuse the patient. This is not ideal for the hypovolemic and unstable patient and may lead to an irreversible situation that might have been prevented.

Once bleeding is controlled and the patient is partially resuscitated, a rapid but thorough search determines the full nature of the injuries. Major vascular injuries have the highest priority.

Control of Bleeding

Bleeding from solid viscera or mesenteric vessels has the next highest priority, followed by repair of injuries resulting in major contamination from the gastrointestinal tract. Afterward, a more leisurely search can be undertaken for other injuries such as ureteral, bladder, or esophageal injuries.

Despite a seemingly adequate incision, exposure may remain difficult. Injuries at the thoracic outlet or deep

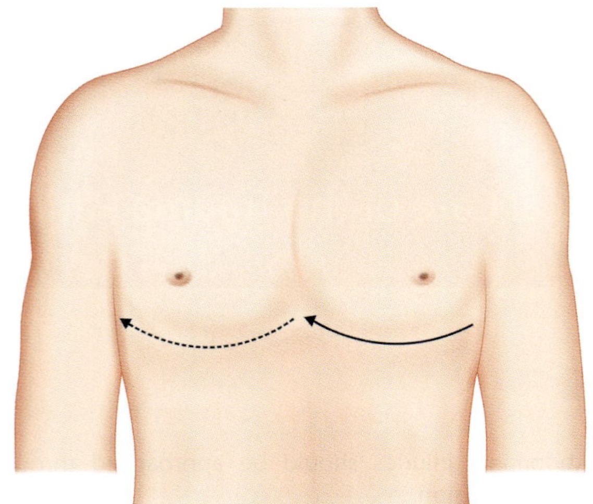

Fig. 32.1: Left anterolateral thoracotomy showing transthoracic extension.

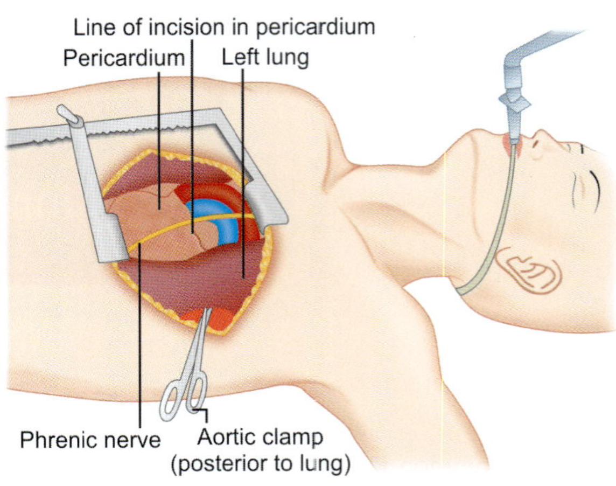

Fig. 32.2: Thoracic contents exposed through an anterolateral left thoracotomy.

within the pelvis can be difficult to visualize from a standard thoracic or abdominal incision. Virtually, any incision can be extended to increase exposure. It may, on occasion, be necessary to make a separate counterincision and to approach the injury from a different vantage point.

CHEST TRAUMA

Three alternative incisions are used for exposure within the thorax. These are as follows:

- Anterolateral thoracotomy
- Posterolateral thoracotomy
- Median sternotomy

Each of these incisions has both advantages and limitations.

Anterolateral Thoracotomy

An anterolateral thoracotomy carried out with the patient supine provides good exposure to the hemithorax. It can be placed anywhere from the third to the eighth intercostal space. When used for blind exploration, the fifth intercostal space is most often selected. A left-anterolateral thoracotomy is usually selected for emergency department thoracotomies.

An anterolateral thoracotomy provides good exposure of the pulmonary parenchyma and the pulmonary hilum. Extension across the sternum may be required for optimal exposure of any cardiac injury (Fig. 32.1). Anterolateral thoracotomies do not provide good exposure to the posterior mediastinum for descending aortic, esophageal or distal tracheal injuries.

Technique

Rotating the chest 20° on the operative side and fully extending the ipsilateral arm provide optimal exposure. A curvilinear incision is made from the lateral sternum to the axilla along the line of a rib. The subcutaneous tissue and muscles are divided with the cautery to minimize bleeding. The chest is entered along the superior aspect of the rib to avoid damage to the intercostal vasculature.

When this technique is used for an emergency department thoracotomy (for indications *see* Chapter 39, "Thoracic Trauma"), the following may happen:

- The chest is opened and the left lung observed to ensure it is moving during ventilation.
- The patient is given several cycles of cardiac massage, even with the pericardium closed, in order to perfuse the coronary arteries.
- The pericardium is then opened longitudinally anterior to the phrenic nerve (Fig. 32.2)—up to the takeoff of the aorta and pulmonary artery.
- Open cardiac massage is performed using a two-handed technique, timing the compressions to give sufficient time for the cardiac chambers to fill.
- Two-handed cardiac massage together with resuscitation and defibrillation should be continued until cardiac activity returns or the patient is declared dead—some surgeons recommend aortic cross-clamping as an initial step.

Extending the Incision

An anterolateral thoracotomy extended across the sternum to the contralateral chest (a clamshell thoracotomy)

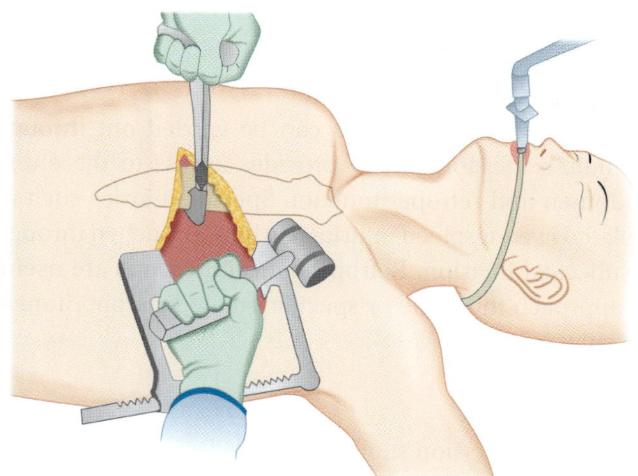

Fig. 32.3: Using a Lebsche knife to extend a left anterolateral thoracotomy to the right thorax.

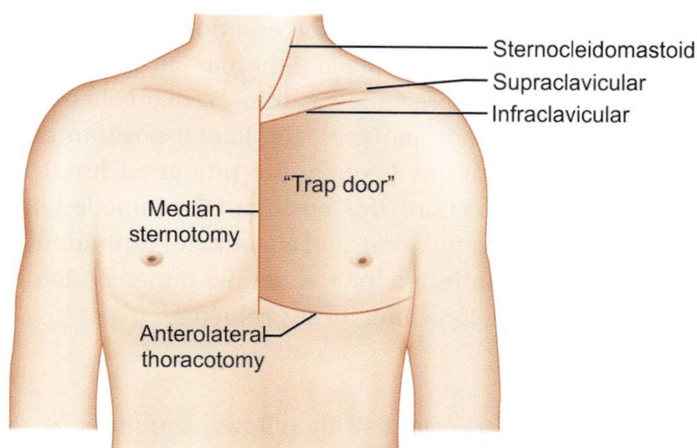

Fig. 32.4: Site of median sternotomy and incisions to increase exposure.

exposes all organs in the thorax and is easily performed using a Lebsche knife (Fig. 32.3). The internal mammary arteries are always divided, and must be clamped.

Median Sternotomy

A median sternotomy affords excellent access to the anterior mediastinum and is the incision of choice for approaching the heart, particularly in stable patients. It provides exposure to the aortic arch, the innominate, left common carotid and the right subclavian arteries. The authors believe that the proximal left subclavian artery can also be approached relatively easily via a sternotomy. The hilum of either lung can also be approached by opening the pleura. A sternotomy affords poor exposure of the periphery of the lung and the posterior mediastinum.

Sternotomies are best performed using an oscillating saw. The equipment must be available. It is more time consuming than a thoracotomy, so is not appropriate for patients near cardiac arrest.

Technique

A midline incision is made from the suprasternal notch to the xiphoid. Blunt finger dissection behind the manubrium and the xiphoid process frees anterior mediastinal structures. Ventilation should be suspended while the sternum is being divided. The innominate vein should be freed from the sternum before the sternal retractor is fully spread.

If necessary, the pericardium is split into the midline up to the aortic root. The caudal portion of the pericardium can be teed off, increasing the exposure to the heart. The pericardial edges can be tacked to the skin with a few sutures. Anterior mediastinal fat and the thymus can be dissected free giving access to the proximal great vessels. The pleura on either side can be opened widely providing access to the pulmonary hila.

Before closing, one must inspect the internal mammary arteries and ensure that there is no injury. Bleeding from bone edges at the sternum can generally be controlled with bone wax.

Extending the Incision

Additional incisions can be used to increase the exposure (Fig. 32.4). Supraclavicular extension involves making an incision along the clavicle. The sternoclavicular ligament can be divided and the proximal one-third or one half of the clavicle can be resected. This measure gives excellent exposure to the proximal subclavian or distal innominate arteries. Incisions along the anterior border of the sternocleidomastoid muscle provide exposure to the proximal and midportion of the common carotid artery.

Posterolateral Thoracotomy

A posterolateral thoracotomy is an excellent approach to the lung and posterior mediastinal structures. It is the incision of choice for the posterior mediastinal vasculature such as the aorta. The selection of right versus left posterolateral thoracotomy should be made depending upon the level of the injury. Upper mediastinal structures, such as the trachea and the upper esophagus, are best approached from the right. The distal esophagus is better approached from the left.

Posterolateral thoracotomies are not versatile as they do not provide any access to the anterior mediastinum. In addition, they involve placing the patient in a lateral position, which can precipitate cardiovascular collapse in severely hypovolemic patients. The lateral position also places one hemithorax (usually the uninjured lung) in the dependent position. This position may impede both oxygenation and ventilation, and encourages aspiration of blood into the unaffected lung. A double-lumen endotracheal tube may help to limit these problems.

Technique

Support can be provided with pillows, sandbags, or a "beanbag." Flexion of the bottom leg, with pillow support for the uppermost knee, avoids nerve compression. An axillary roll protects the neurovascular structures of the axilla.

The skin incision starts two finger breadths below the nipple in men and at the fourth intercostal space in women (Fig. 32.5). The latissimus dorsi and the serratus anterior muscles are divided and the scapula is lifted. The first rib is identified by the insertion of the scalenus anterior muscle. The intercostal space to be entered is selected. The chest is then explored.

Extending the Incision

There is virtually no way to extend a posterolateral thoracotomy if exposure is inadequate; it is best to repair injuries that are amenable via the posterolateral approach and make a counterincision to repair additional injuries. In patients who are critically ill, the chest wall can be packed or temporarily closed, and the patient turned supine. When the injuries are controlled, the patient can be repositioned and the chest can be closed.

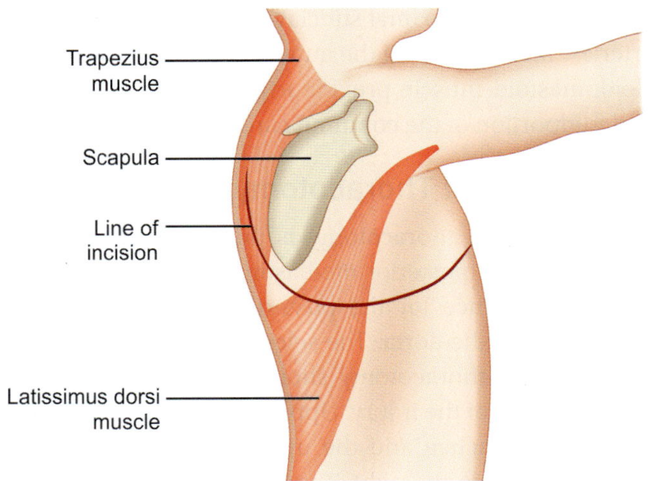

Fig. 32.5: Posterolateral thoracotomy.

ABDOMINAL TRAUMA

Choice of Incision

All abdominal explorations can be carried out through a midline incision, which provides access to the entire abdomen and retroperitoneum. Specific injuries such as isolated liver or spleen injuries can be approached through a subcostal incision. Retroperitoneal incisions are useful to approach the spine or specific isolated retroperitoneal vascular injuries.

Technique

The midline incision should be made from the xiphoid to the pubis. If there is concern for a pelvic vascular injury, protecting some space above the pubis allows for subcutaneous tunneling if a femoral–femoral bypass is required. Exposure to the spleen is increased by mobilizing the lateral retroperitoneal attachments. Exposure to the liver is increased by dividing the falciform and triangular ligaments, taking care to avoid damage to the phrenic and hepatic veins, and inferior vena cava. When all ligamentous structures have been divided, the right lobe of the liver can be elevated into the wound. The duodenum can be exposed by performing a Kocher maneuver, which also gives access to the head of the pancreas. The duodenum should be fully Kocherized to avoid missing subtle injuries.

The intraoperative surgical approach for a retroperitoneal hematoma is based on location (Fig. 32.6):

- Zone I (central) hematomas should always be explored.
- Zone II (lateral) hematomas should be explored after penetrating injury. Small injuries diagnosed on a preoperative computed tomogram scan can be observed. Expanding or pulsatile hematomas, known renal vascular injury, or massive urinary leaks prompt exploration after blunt trauma.
- Zone III (pelvic) hematomas should be explored if they are due to penetrating injury.

The "Mattox maneuver" (medial visceral rotation) involves medial rotation of the left kidney, pancreas, spleen, and descending colon. It provides exposure to the entire aorta and the left-sided pelvic vascular structures, kidney and ureter. The maneuver is performed by incising the lateral peritoneal reflection at the avascular white line of Toldt from the level of the distal sigmoid colon to the splenic flexure. The splenorenal and splenophrenic ligaments are divided, allowing mobilization of the spleen and the pancreas. The abdominal contents are then rotated medially, sweeping the retroperitoneal structures

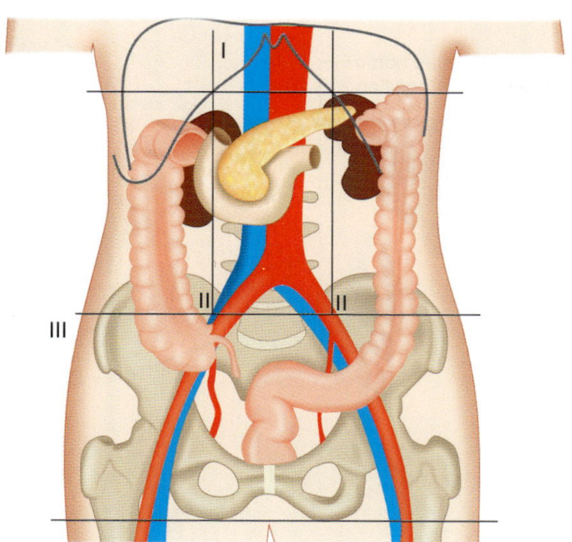

Fig. 32.6: Zones of the retroperitoneum: zone I, central; zone II, lateral; zone III, pelvic.

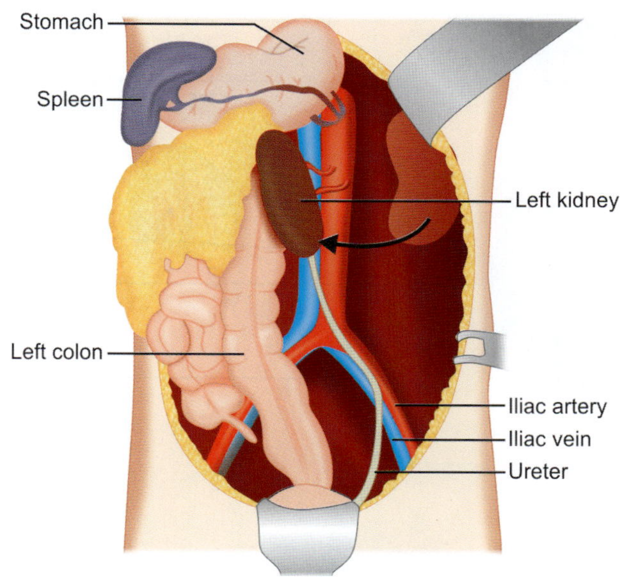

Fig. 32.7: The Mattox maneuver. A left-sided medial visceral rotation is done to provide exposure of the retroperitoneal structures.

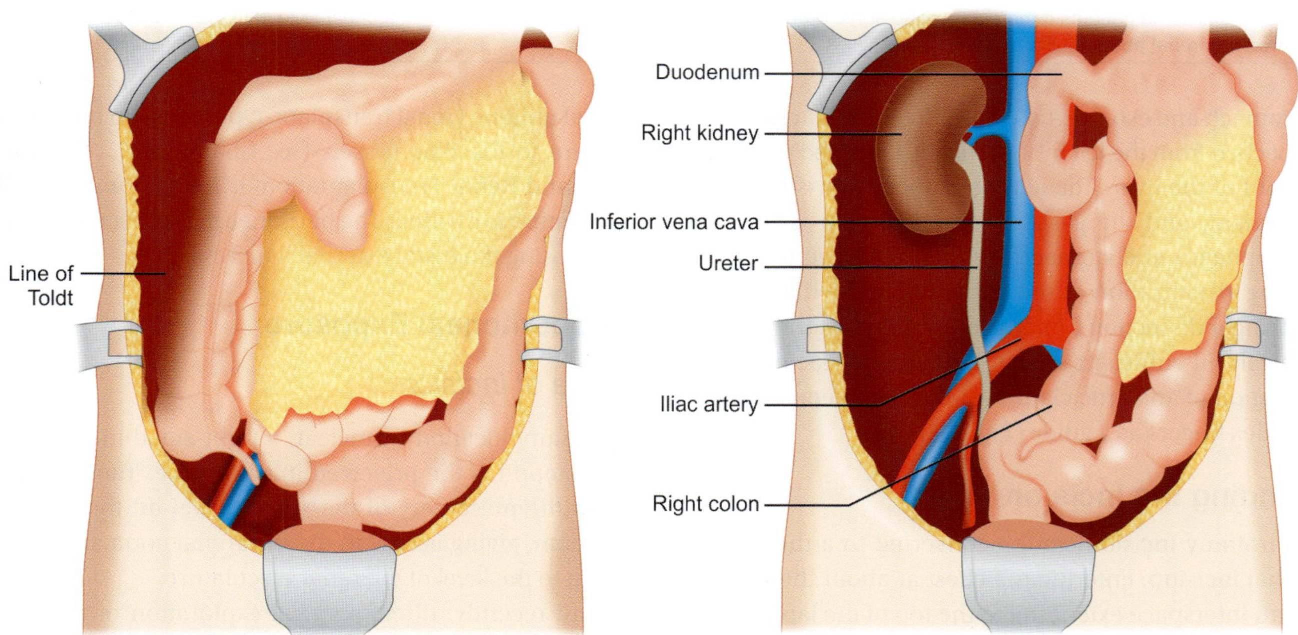

Fig. 32.8: The Cattell maneuver. A right-sided medial visceral rotation for exposure of the retroperitoneal structures.

posteriorly. Alternatively, the kidney may be left in place and the rest of the viscera rotated medially. If the kidney is mobilized, it is important to protect the ureter (Fig. 32.7).

The "Cattell maneuver" (right-sided medial visceral rotation) involves incision of the lateral peritoneal reflections of the ascending colon from the level of the cecum to the hepatic flexure. The duodenum is Kocherized and the head of the pancreas is mobilized. As on the left, the kidney may be mobilized or left in situ. This exposes the inferior vena cava and the pelvic vasculature. The infrarenal aorta can be exposed through this incision along with the vena cava (Fig. 32.8).

Access to the supraceliac aorta can be performed using an extended "Mattox maneuver" completely mobilizing

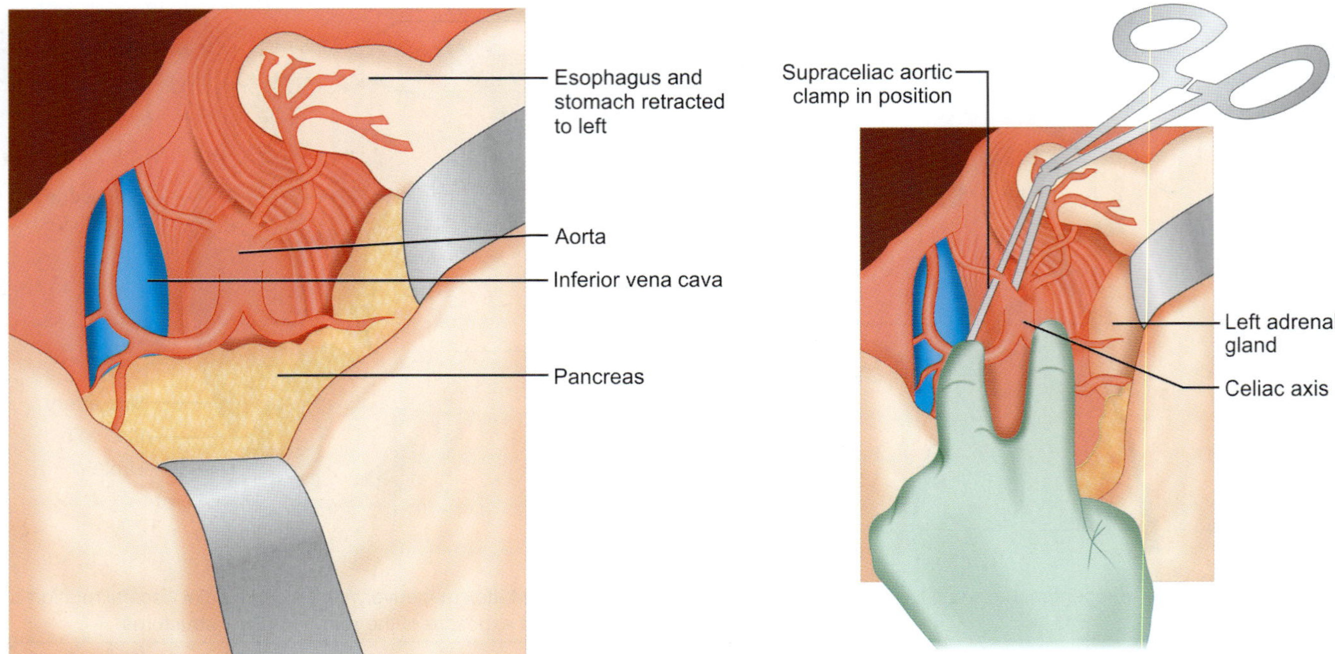

Fig. 32.9: Proximal aortic control. With a supraceliac aortic clamp, aortic control can be achieved quickly with minimal dissection. It works well for abdominal trauma patients if the supraceliac aortic area is not the site of injury. It is also an ideal technique to gain initial vascular control of a ruptured infrarenal abdominal aortic aneurysm.

the stomach and esophagus. Alternatively, this area can be approached from the left by incising the left-sided triangular ligament of the liver. The left lobe of the liver is retracted to the right, and the gastrohepatic ligament is divided. The esophagus and stomach are then retracted to the left allowing visualization of the right crus of the diaphragm. Blunt finger dissection from the medial and lateral aspects will clean off sufficient adventitial tissue to facilitate the application of an aortic clamp using the surgeon's middle and index fingers as a guide (Fig. 32.9).

Extending the Incision

A laparotomy incision can be converted to a thoracoabdominal incision, entering the chest at about the sixth or seventh interspace extending to the top of the laparotomy incision. The diaphragm is divided in a circumferential fashion leaving approximately 2.5 cm of diaphragm available for closure. This minimizes damage to the phrenic nerve. Through this incision on the right, the whole of the retrohepatic inferior vena cava can be approached laterally by retracting the liver anteriorly. On the left side, the supraceliac aorta can be explored.

Counterincisions over the femoral vessels may increase exposure to the retroperitoneal vessels. The inguinal ligament can be divided and repaired later, if necessary. In addition, a lateral oblique (renal transplant-type) incision increases exposure to the iliac vessels (*see* Chapter 117, "Dialysis Access and Renal Transplantation"). The abdominal wall musculature is divided. The peritoneum is reflected medially exposing the distal external iliac vessels.

Retroperitoneal Exposure

Choice of Incision

If the injury location is unclear, a right-sided medial visceral rotation is the preferred initial choice. The surgeon can lift the mesentery of the small bowel off the retroperitoneum, giving access to the infrarenal aorta and vena cava up to the level of the renal vasculature.

Until recently, direct surgical exploration of a pelvic retroperitoneal hematoma was thought to be unwise. Unroofing the hematoma, particularly from the abdomen, releases venous tamponade and produces torrential hemorrhage. As pelvic fracture bleeding is usually from the small tributaries of the hypogastric arteries, identifying specific bleeding points is difficult. Therefore, bony reduction, using an external fixator, and/or angiographic embolization was thought to be wiser.

More recently, extraperitoneal pelvic packing has become popular. First popularized in Europe, it is now widely used in North American trauma centers.[1,2] Extraperitoneal pelvic packing keeps the pelvic retroperitoneum separated from the abdominal cavity (*see* Chapter 41, "Pelvic, Lumbar and Thoracic Spine and Spinal Cord Injuries," for further discussion).

Techniques

In general, it is wise to control the aorta before directly exploring either side of the retroperitoneal vasculature. In patients who are in profound shock, the arteries are often intensely vasospastic. Positively, identifying the aorta before addressing the pelvic vasculature ensures that the surgeon does not make a mistake in identifying the bifurcation of the common iliac artery for the bifurcation of the aorta. A useful anatomic landmark is the sacral promontory. The aortic bifurcation is generally just cephalad.

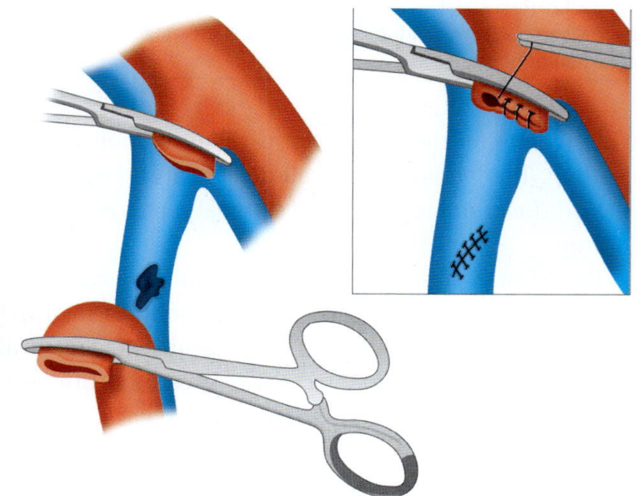

Fig. 32.10: Iliac artery is divided to facilitate exposure of the iliac vein. The artery can then be oversewn as shown or more ideally repaired after the venous injury is controlled.

Bleeding from the retroperitoneal veins is often quite impressive. The veins do not develop spasm when injured; therefore, they continue to bleed, even if the patient is in deep shock. It is often necessary to mobilize the artery off the vein in order to expose the venous structures directly, as they are generally located behind the arteries. The hypogastric vein can be particularly problematic. Occasionally, it is necessary to divide a hypogastric artery to obtain good exposure of the vein. Once the venous injury is repaired or ligated, the artery can be reconstructed or it can be ligated as well (Fig. 32.10).

The retroperitoneal vasculature can be explored via a "hockey stick" incision, made over the lower quadrant of the abdomen. The muscles are divided and the abdominal contents swept medially. This leads the surgeon directly down onto the retroperitoneal vasculature. The ureter should be identified and protected. The vascular structures can be controlled and injuries can be repaired.

Extraperitoneal pelvic packing can be performed via a midline incision or a Pfannenstiel incision (Fig. 32.11). The muscles are split and the retroperitoneal hematoma is entered. The hematoma can be evacuated and the retroperitoneum is packed. The group from Denver Colorado advocates precise packing utilizing three laparotomy pads on either side of the bladder.[3] Others simply use an adequate number of packs as required to stop the hemorrhage. If combined with a laparotomy, a Pfannenstiel incision may be preferable as it does not communicate directly with the incision used for the laparotomy.

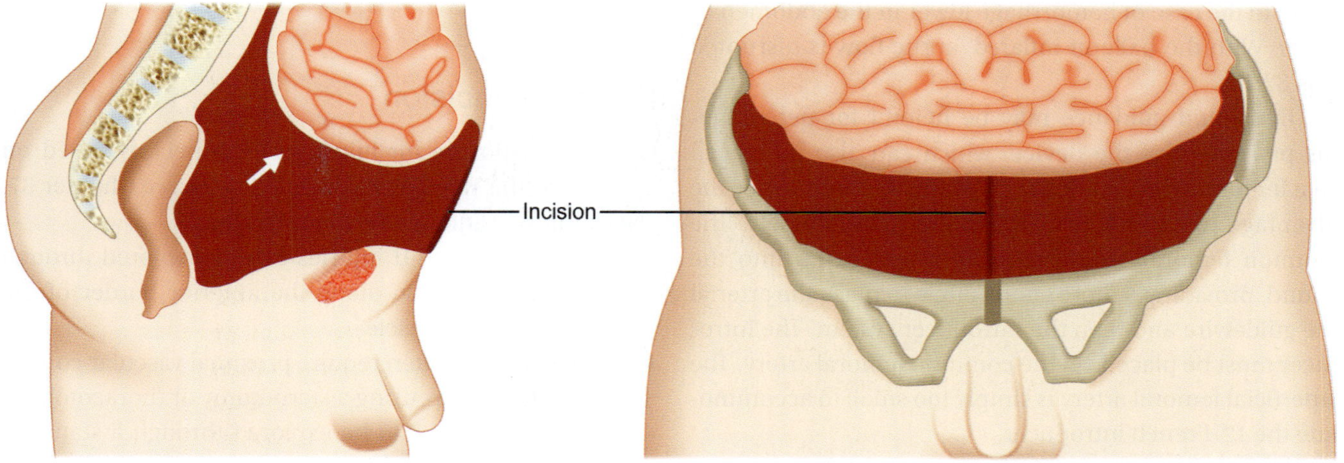

Fig. 32.11: Preperitoneal pelvic packing performed via a midline incision. A Pfannenstiel incision can also be used.

Temporary Aortic Control

Aortic occlusion can be very helpful in trauma patients in profound hemorrhagic shock, preserving flow to the most essential organs in the body, the heart and the brain. As a temporizing measure, it can be lifesaving.

Clamping the aorta at the diaphragm requires aortic dissection at the level of the diaphragm. In trauma patients, this often involves dissection around the area injured, such as the liver, or the more central retroperitoneal vasculature. This causes risks releasing any tamponade that may have formed, and/or directly dislodging clots. An alternative is to open the left chest and occlude the aorta within the thorax, allowing the surgeon to dissect in planes, distant from the injury. However, this requires opening a body cavity that was not injured. As this must be performed rapidly, there can be substantial blood loss from the chest wall musculature. In addition, the patient will lose heat through this newly opened body cavity. Finally, hemorrhage control may not be ideal, as the clamp is placed proximal to the injury, the injury may still bleed via collateral blood flow.

Recently, a technique has been developed to allow intraluminal aortic occlusion. This is termed resuscitative endovascular balloon occlusion of the aorta (REBOA). An occlusive balloon is positioned into the aorta via a femoral artery. A standard femoral arterial line is placed, and an Amplatz extra-stiff guidewire is inserted through the catheter. The catheter is removed and a 12-French introducer system is placed over the guidewire. The guidewire is left in place and a balloon-tipped catheter inserted over the guidewire. The catheter can be positioned in the distal thoracic aorta in the case of upper abdominal hemorrhage, in the lower abdominal aorta, or just above the aortic bifurcation in the case of hemorrhage lower in the abdomen or pelvis. With the balloon inflated, aortic flow is disrupted (Fig. 32.12).

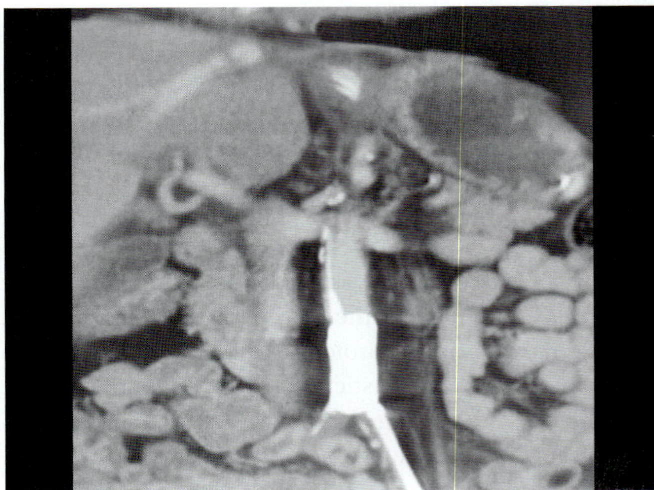

Fig. 32.12: Resuscitative endovascular balloon occlusion of the aorta. The balloon positioned in the lower aorta provides inflow occlusion for pelvic hemorrhage.

Ultrasound guidance may be helpful for percutaneous placement of the device, which can also be placed via a femoral artery cutdown. The latter technique has the advantage of directly visualizing the blood vessels. The common femoral arteries can be retracted up into the wound, providing a more gentle angle to place the arterial line guidewire and then the introducer system. The introducer must be placed via the common femoral artery. The superficial femoral artery is simply too small to accommodate the 12-French introducer.

The REBOA can provide time to transport the patient to the operating room, or as a temporary stabilizing effort to allow time for definitive transcatheter embolization of bleeding. The large arterial wall defect caused by placing the introducer mandates direct surgical repair of the arteriotomy.

The REBOA has been studied on animals with good results.[4,5] A recent series describes six patients in which the REBOA was used.[6] It was successfully placed in all six patients. In four patients, it was used as a bridge to angiographic embolization. There were no vascular complications.

The technology is being miniaturized. Now, 6- and 7-French introducer systems are being developed. This should make percutaneous placement far easier. In addition, the arterial femoral artery wall defect will then be small enough that direct surgical repair should not be necessary.

NECK TRAUMA

Choice of Incision

Operative exposure for injuries of the neck is based on location of the wound (zones I, II, or III; *see* Chapter 37, "Neck Injury") and hemodynamic status.

- Virtually all zone II injuries can be explored through a standard incision along the anterior border of the sternomastoid muscle.
- Zone I injuries often require proximal vascular control within the thorax using a sternotomy or thoracotomy.
- Zone III injuries can be explored through a standard sternocleidomastoid incision, but distal vascular control is difficult.

For zone I or zone III injuries, percutaneous balloons can provide temporary proximal vascular control limiting blood loss or the need for extensive incisions. The sternocleidomastoid incision gives access to the neurovascular bundle as well as to the trachea and esophagus. The esophagus is a more left-sided structure, so a left-sided incision is best to treat an isolated esophageal injury.

A collar incision may also be useful in some patients such as those with an anterior injury or if both sides of the neck must be explored, particularly after transcervical injuries. It gives better access to anterior mediastinal structures such as the trachea. Alternatively, the sternocleidomastoid incision can be curved across the anterior of the neck to expose both sides at any level.

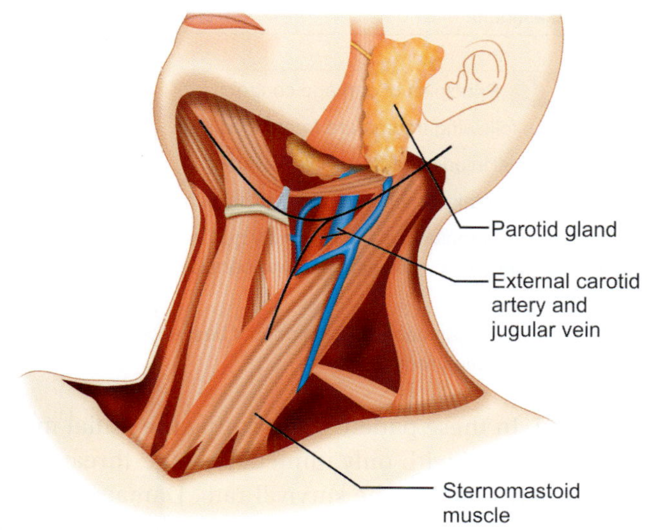

Fig. 32.13: Superficial neck anatomy.

Technique

The sternocleidomastoid incision is made along the anterior border of the sternocleidomastoid muscle, which is then retracted laterally (Fig. 32.13). The facial vein is a constant landmark and can be sacrificed to aid the exposure of the carotid sheath (Fig. 32.14). The carotid sheath is opened, and the jugular vein and carotid artery are isolated, avoiding damage to the vagus and recurrent laryngeal nerves. All vascular structures can be fully examined. The esophagus is located posterior and medial just anterior to the spine. A nasogastric (NG) tube may help in localizing the esophagus. The blood supply to the esophagus runs longitudinally, so the esophagus can be circumferentially dissected and the entire esophagus exposed from one side. Tracheal injuries are more problematic because the blood supply is segmental and enters posterolaterally. Circumferential mobilization of the trachea must, therefore, be avoided.

A collar incision is generally performed approximately 2–3 finger breadths above the suprasternal notch and extends across the neck from one sternocleidomastoid muscle to the other. Skin and subcutaneous tissue flaps can be raised, greatly increasing the exposure. Strap muscles can then be divided as necessary to give access to the trachea and other mediastinal structures.

Extending the Incision

The sternocleidomastoid incision gives good visualization of zone II of the neck. It can be combined with a sternotomy or supraclavicular incision increasing exposure for

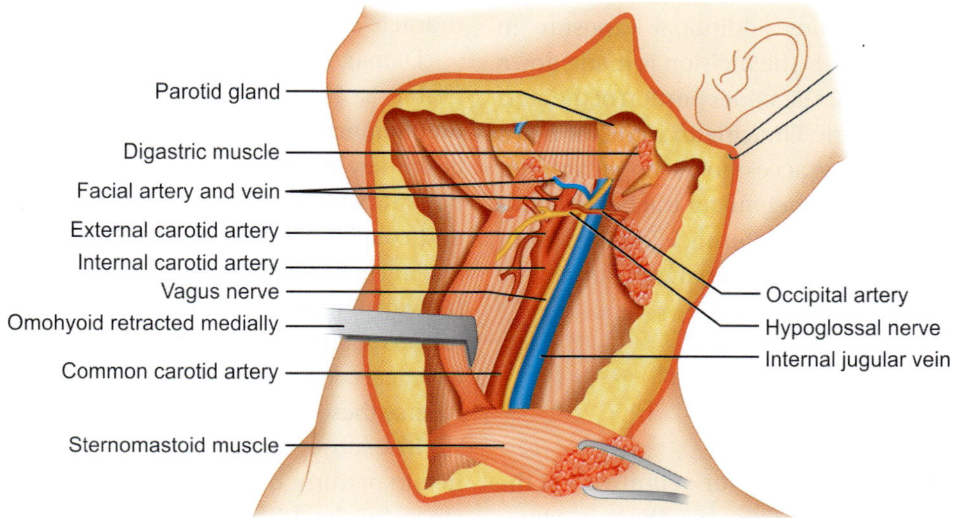

Fig. 32.14: Deep neck anatomy.

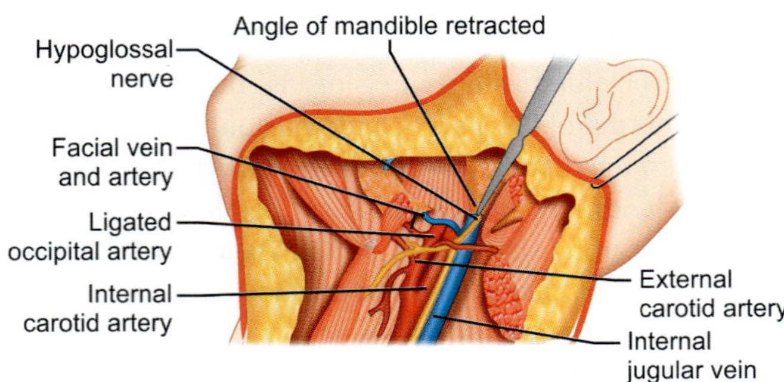

Fig. 32.15: Exposure of distal internal carotid artery. A step-wise technique for exposure of the internal carotid artery obviates the need for mandibular subluxation.

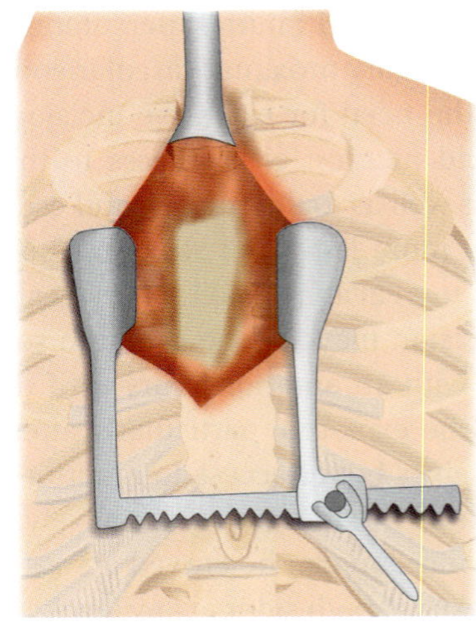

Fig. 32.16: A partial sternotomy provides excellent exposure for the upper mediastinum.

zone I injuries. Upper esophageal injuries within zone I can often be repaired through a neck incision because the esophagus can be fully mobilized. A collar incision can be combined with a sternotomy to increase exposure to the superior portion of the anterior mediastinum.

Exposure of the distal internal carotid artery can be problematic (Fig. 32.15). Mandibular subluxation and posterior osteotomy have been used, but these maneuvers are time consuming and can be associated with temporomandibular joint dysfunction or other complications. A posterolateral approach adapted from a radical neck dissection can be helpful. The sternomastoid muscle is divided, and the omohyoid muscle is retracted medially. The posterior belly of the digastric is divided, followed by the division of the remainder of the muscles in the base of the skull. The angle of the mandible can be retracted with a bone hook and, if necessary, the tail of the parotid gland can be amputated. This approach provides good access to the internal carotid artery within zone III of the neck.

A partial sternotomy gains additional exposure in zone I of the neck (Fig. 32.16). The incision is made down just below the angle of Louis. The upper portion of the sternum is then split. A pediatric Finochietto retractor helps spread the sternum, providing access to the upper anterior mediastinum. This can be very helpful for tracheal injuries that cannot be approached via a sternocleidomastoid or collar incision. It also provides additional exposure to the upper mediastinal blood vessels.

DAMAGE CONTROL

Introduction

In most cases, injuries can be cared for definitively at the time when they are identified. However, there is a subgroup of patients for whom alternative strategies may be helpful. In these patients, truncating the initial management to deal with only immediately life-threatening injuries may increase the survival rate. Damage control was first described for penetrating abdominal trauma.[7] It is now commonly used for blunt and penetrating injuries in the chest as well as for bony injuries and vascular and thoracic emergencies.

Table 32.1 Principles of damage control.
Early deaths following trauma are from blood loss
Gastrointestinal injuries cause problems later
Every maneuver takes more time than a clinician estimates
If one waits until problems manifest, it may be too late to correct them
Further surgery usually compounds hypothermia, coagulopathy, and acidosis
Repayment of oxygen debt is a high priority best accomplished outside the operating room

Damage control is based on a number of principles (Table 32.1). The first and most important principle is that hemorrhage control trumps all other concerns. Time is the key element in decision making when caring for patients with complex and multiple injuries. Hypothermia and coagulopathy occur after large volume transfusions, leading to further blood loss. The best strategy is prevention (i.e. keeping patients warm, so limiting shock and transfusion requirements). By the time the patient has developed a clinical coagulopathy or severe hypothermia, the ability to reverse these physiologic derangements is limited.

In a subset of patients, initial therapy should be modified to perform only life-threatening hemorrhage control. Once the hemorrhage is controlled, the patient should be taken to the intensive care unit where physiologic derangements can be corrected. When the patient has achieved adequate homeostasis, secondary issues such as gastrointestinal injuries, fractures, and soft tissue injuries can be assessed in a sequence that makes sense and does not subject the patient to additional risk.

Nomenclature

In 1908, a technique was described for temporary control of hepatic bleeding.[8] As the incidence of high-velocity penetrating trauma escalated, surgeons began truncating the initial operative procedure.[9,10] In the early 1990s, Rotondo et al. first coined the term "damage control," which is now used most frequently to describe the technique.[7]

Damage control is now accepted as a part of standard therapy for patients with life-threatening exsanguinating injuries. However, using this technique when not indicated increases intra-abdominal or intrathoracic complications.[11] If patients are severely hypotensive, acidotic, hypothermic, and coagulopathic before applying the technique, it is unlikely that any maneuver will result in increased survival rates.

Patient Selection

A number of clinical factors are important in the selection of patients. Some of these are as follows:

- Severe metabolic acidosis (pH < 7.3) or base deficit (pH > 10)
- Hypothermia [temperature < 95°F (35°C)]
- Coagulopathy

We generally attempt to keep total resuscitation and operative time to <90 minutes. When we approach 10 units of transfused blood, we consider the use of damage control. Any patient with marked hypotension has almost certainly lost 40% of total circulating blood volume.[12] It is wise to use damage control in these patients. In addition, at the time of exploration, if the abdomen or chest is full of blood, there has been massive blood loss. If the situation cannot be corrected immediately, damage control should be used. If damage control is used late, rebleeding necessitating immediate return to the operating room becomes more common. A review of the results of damage control in 200 patients over a period of 7 years showed that 36% died before re-exploration.[10] All of these patients died from acute cardiovascular insufficiency soon after admission to the intensive care unit. Over 17% of those who survived required emergency re-exploration for bleeding. Of these patients, only 24% survived. This figure contrasted with a 67% survival rate for all patients undergoing reoperation and a 77% survival rate for patients undergoing planned re-exploration.

Technique

Damage control is divided into five discrete phases:

- Phase 1: resuscitation and evaluation
- Phase 2: initial damage control operation
- Phase 3: secondary resuscitation
- Phase 4: definitive surgery
- Phase 5: long-term reconstruction

Phase 1

The initial evaluation of damage control in patients should be brief. Transportation should be rapid and designed to deliver the patient to the closest center to provide the level of care required. Occasionally, circumstances may require transport to a local hospital where the patient can have temporary control of blood loss. The patient can then be transferred to a higher-level center to receive definitive care.

Phase I should be directed toward identifying potential injuries. There is no role for the diagnosis of organ-specific injury. This will be identified at the time of surgery. Patients should be cross-matched for a large volume of red blood cells, and the blood bank should be alerted. Resuscitation and transportation must occur simultaneously. The resuscitation fluid of choice is blood, and liberal use of O-negative blood in the initial care is acceptable.

A chest X-ray can be done rapidly and can provide invaluable information. Hemothoraces can be identified that are not apparent on physical examination. Foreign bodies can be seen, and it is possible to determine whether the major vascular structures are at risk. A plain X-ray of the abdomen can reveal foreign bodies. Diagnostic peritoneal lavage or bedside ultrasonography can reveal intraperitoneal bleeding. Ultrasonography can also identify pneumono- or hemothoraces. X-rays should be developed and reviewed as the patient is being transferred to the operating room.

High-volume crystalloid resuscitation with a target of normalizing blood pressure dilutes clotting factors, displaces the hemostatic clot that often forms on injured arteries when the patient develops hypotension and creates repeating cycles of hemorrhage. Coagulopathy and hypothermia occur early, worsening the picture. Large-volume crystalloid infusion also activates the inflammatory cascade, likely worsening the outcome.[13] It is wise to target a blood pressure of approximately 80–90 mm Hg until surgical hemostasis is obtained. The use of crystalloid should be minimized and loss of circulating blood volume should be replaced with liberal use of blood, fresh frozen plasma, and platelets. The optimal ratio of plasma to red cells has not yet been determined. Some advocate a 1:1 ratio, while others believe 1:2 or 1:3 as efficacious.[14,15] Developing a massive transfusion policy specific to each institution helps ensure that blood and plasma are given in the desired ratio.

Phase 2

The goal of phase 2 is to identify immediately life-threatening injuries and control major blood loss. In addition, obvious gastrointestinal contamination should be rapidly controlled. Lastly, the clinician must identify all areas at high risk for injury. Perhaps the most important part of phase 2 is to identify the patient for whom damage control is necessary. Once the decision is made, all efforts are directed at completing this phase of the patient's care as quickly as possible.

A number of techniques are available to help limit time spent in the operating room. Some are as follows:

- Only vital vessels, aorta, or iliac arteries should be repaired.
- Expendable organs should be resected, not salvaged.
- Gastrointestinal contamination should be controlled with staplers or a temporary rapid, continuous single-layer suture repair.
- The bowel can be resected and the mesenteric bleeding can be controlled—no thought should be given to reconstruction at this time.
- Bladder injuries should be closed in a single layer and ureteral injuries either ligated or treated with external drainage using red rubber catheters.
- Nonanatomic resection of solid organs effectively controls blood loss.
- Occasionally, patients are too unstable to tolerate arterial reconstruction of even essential arteries—in these cases, temporary intraluminal shunts can be lifesaving; virtually any conduit can act as a temporary stent.

Commercial stents are available for small blood vessels. A chest tube used with Rummel tourniquets is an acceptable shunt for large vessels. Even the superior mesenteric artery has been successfully managed by the use of a temporary intraluminal shunt.[16] All veins other than the superior mesenteric vein, suprarenal inferior vena cava, and superior vena cava can be ligated.

Once the major hemorrhage has been arrested and any gastrointestinal contamination controlled, the next step is packing and temporary closure. Prolonged surgery will almost always result in worsening acidosis, hypothermia, and coagulopathy. It is essential, however, to be sure that all surgical bleeding is controlled. Nothing will aggravate the coagulopathy more than ongoing hemorrhage. Therefore, perivascular hematomas must be explored to avoid missing a major vascular injury that may become symptomatic in the early postoperative period.

Nonsurgical bleeding is generally controlled by packing. Packs should be inserted to produce local tamponade. The patient's own tissues can assist in producing tamponade. The diaphragm can be used to produce local pressure to arrest nonsurgical liver bleeding. In this case, packs should be inserted over the dome of the liver first, and gentle pressure can then be produced by packing under the liver. The goal should be to produce sufficient pressure to stop venous blood loss. The pelvis can be packed in a similar fashion using the bony pelvis as a buttress. Topical hemostatic agents can be used with the packs to promote hemostasis. Fibrin glue is excellent. Commercially available hemostatic dressings are also an option. Finally, tamponade can be produced by temporary organ closure. Deep venous bleeding from the liver can be controlled by packs or omentum and the liver capsule and parenchyma are closed over the packs or omentum to help increase the tamponade effect.

The "Bogata bag" is a 3-L saline bag that is cut open. The sterile portion can be placed onto the abdominal or thoracic organs and the opened intravenous fluid bag is rapidly sutured to the skin (Fig. 32.17). Most clinicians now use a vacuum dressing, either a commercially available product or a homemade one using a plastic drape, gauze, suction drains, or NG tubes.

Phase 3

The secondary resuscitation portion of the patient's care often lasts 12–24 hours. The goal is to return the patient to homeostasis as reliably as possible.

Commonly followed vital signs often dangerously underestimate the degree of physiologic derangement.[17] Patients seemingly stable can have a substantial oxygen debt. In general, blood and intravenous fluids are used to support peripheral oxygen delivery with a target of clearing lactate to normal, which has been correlated with the prevention of organ failure.[18] Although base deficit is a useful measure of depth of shock in the emergency department, this relationship is no longer intact following

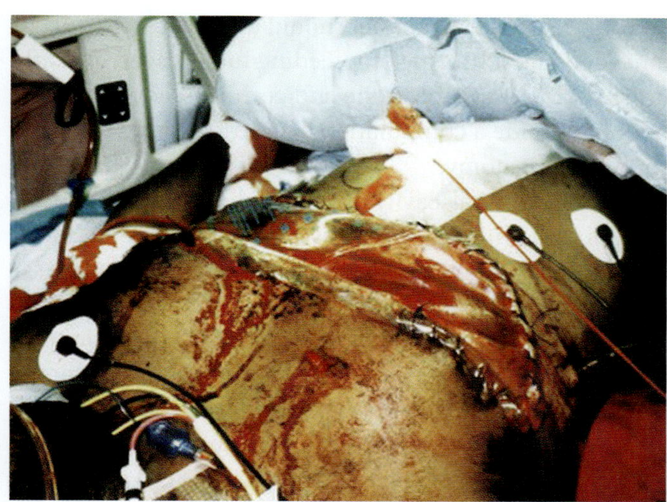

Fig. 32.17: Bogata bag used to close a bilateral thoracotomy.

initial resuscitation. If base deficit or anion gap are used as a substitute for lactate, therapy may be misdirected as much as 50% of the time.[19]

Correcting hypothermia is equally important. Maneuvers such as ambient warming and use of the "Level I" warmer help prevent the development of hypothermia. Despite this, many patients will be hypothermic at the time of intensive care unit admission. Warming intravenous fluids and NG lavage with warm fluid should be employed. Ventilatory circuits can also be warmed. Care should be taken not to use excessively warm temperatures in any internal body cavity. Ambient rewarming, using devices such as the Bair Hugger is also useful. For moderate-to-severe hypothermia, a continuous arteriovenous rewarming technique, first described by Gentilello et al., can be used.[20] This circuit uses the commercially available Level 1 rewarmer and has been reported to increase the core temperature by as much as 1°F/h (0.6°C). Newer devices designed to cool patients after cardiac arrest can be used to perform central warming. In extreme cases, patients can be rapidly warmed on cardiac bypass.

Treatment of coagulopathy helps limit ongoing nonsurgical blood loss. As it mostly takes some time to report back laboratory values, the coagulopathy status must be assessed using clinical judgment. Fresh frozen plasma and platelet packs should be given empirically to normalize the coagulation status.

Angiography can be extremely helpful to control ongoing blood loss, especially for vessels that are not easily surgically accessible. Transcatheter embolization allows nonoperative hemostasis and thus prevents the need for an early return to the operating room to control bleeding.

Table 32.2 Symptoms of abdominal compartment syndrome.

System	*Symptoms*
Cardiac	Decreased venous return, decreased cardiac output, decreased left ventricular stroke work, hypotension
Respiratory	Diaphragmatic displacement, increased peak airway pressures, increased upper quadrant mismatch, hypoxia, hypercarbia
Visceral function	Decreased blood flow, oliguria, gastrointestinal ischemia, hepatic ischemia

Deep central liver injuries are ideal for angiography. Even hepatic vein injuries have been successfully treated using percutaneous techniques.[21] Deep pelvic bleeding, lumbar arterial injuries, and injuries around the head and body of the pancreas are often temporarily controllable with packing followed by definitive embolization. Finally, if missiles have passed close to great vessels, diagnostic angiography can demonstrate arterial pseudoaneurysms or intimal injuries, enabling decisions about therapy.

Abdominal compartment syndrome: Intra-abdominal hypertension during the secondary resuscitation phase develops as the metabolic insult is reversed, and ongoing capillary leak worsens gastrointestinal edema. Nonsurgical bleeding may also continue despite packing until the coagulopathy has been corrected. These factors, plus a relatively tight abdominal closure, can produce intra-abdominal hypertension leading to abdominal compartment syndrome (ACS).

The symptoms of ACS are nonspecific (Table 32.2). Low cardiac output may be ascribed to shock and fluid requirements. Hypoxia and elevated pulmonary pressures may be blamed on shock and reperfusion or mechanical chest injury. Clinicians may forget to consider ACS as an etiology for failure to resuscitate. On physical examination, a patient with a tense, distended abdomen with elevated airway pressures, oliguria and poor cardiovascular function should make clinicians suspect ACS.

Intra-abdominal pressure can be directly measured using a urinary bladder catheter. With the patient in a supine position, 100–200 mL of sterile saline are injected into the bladder. The tubing of the urinary catheter bag is clamped distal to the culture aspiration port. A large-bore needle and tubing attached to a stopcock are then connected to a water manometer or a pressure transducer through the culture aspiration point. The top of the pubis serves as the zero point. Normally, intra-abdominal pressure is approximately zero. Abdominal pressure above 25 mm Hg is usually physiologically important.[22] By the time intra-abdominal pressure reaches 35–40 mm Hg, decompression is almost always warranted, though a lower threshold may be appropriate in patients with poor pulmonary function. The rate of increase in intra-abdominal pressure may be as important as the absolute number.[23] Acute increases as small as 5–10 mm Hg can produce an ACS. Patients with physiology consistent with ACS are probably best decompressed even with a marginal elevated bladder pressure.

If the diagnosis of ACS is made, prompt release is indicated to prevent ongoing shock and multiple organ failure. A comparison of patients treated with a primary mesh closure, who then needed decompression for ACS, and those treated with primary fascial closure showed that the mortality rate and incidence of acute respiratory and renal failure in the patients treated primarily with mesh were significantly lower.[24]

Diagnoses other than ACS must also be considered. Ongoing bleeding can require an unplanned re-exploration. In general, if patients are normothermic but require ongoing transfusion of >1–2 units/h or >15 units/h postoperatively, real thought must be given to re-exploration. Failure of lactate to return to normal—if cardiovascular performance is adequate—generally indicates a missed injury and ongoing blood loss, poorly controlled contamination, or an unrecognized gastrointestinal injury producing early sepsis, bowel infarction, or gas gangrene.

Phase 4

Once the patient has been returned to homeostasis, plans should be made for re-exploration and unpacking. In general, adequate homeostasis involves achieving normothermia [temperature >96.8°F (36°C)]; reversal of the coagulopathy (prothrombin time <15 s and platelet count >75,000) and optimal cardiovascular and respiratory performance. The serum lactate should be within normal limits or clearing. Unpacking is an elective procedure and should allow mobilization of whatever resources necessary to do that safely.

The first step during surgery is to unpack the patient. It is important to have an accurate estimate of the number of laparotomy pads placed in the patient at the time of the initial operation. This information should have been recorded in the operative note as well as in the operating room log book (but is notoriously unreliable). The patient should then be re-explored taking care to look for missed injuries. In particular, the areas of the pelvic vasculature, the pancreas, duodenum, and the area around the gastroesophageal junction should be carefully examined for subtle injuries.

The gastrointestinal tract should then be reconstructed if needed and a transpyloric feeding tube placed for early nutrition. A nasal tube is one choice. More secure surgical options include a combination of gastric–jejunal tube or a simple jejunostomy.

The abdominal cavity is irrigated, drains are placed as indicated and the incision is closed by a simple fascial closure. If fascial closure is not possible, a vacuum dressing is placed over the wound.

Occasionally, patients bleed sufficiently at reoperation and once again require temporary packing. Those patients should then be repacked and taken to the intensive care unit. Thought must be given to an alternative means of hemostasis such as angiography.

Although many patients do continue to improve, postoperative complications are common. Organ failure, such as respiratory or renal failure, may be a consequence of the magnitude of the original trauma as well as the therapeutic techniques used. Abdominal sepsis is common, as are wound and pulmonary infections. A myriad of gastrointestinal complications such as fistula formation have likewise been reported. Overall, abdominal sepsis occurs in approximately 20% of patients and respiratory failure in 10% of patients; other complications are far less common.

Phase 5

If primary fascial closure is not possible at the time of the initial re-exploration, it is often possible to get the fascia closed over the first ensuing week or so. Careful attention to fluid therapy is essential. Commercially available vacuum dressings may limit edema by removing intra-abdominal fluid and/or limiting inflammation.

There are a number of commercially available devices that both limit fascial retraction and help mobilize fascia to the midline by providing continuous tension on the fascia. A piece of mesh or Gore-Tex can be used and tightened every 1–2 days. When the fascia edges are relatively close to one another, the device or mesh can be removed and the fascia closed primarily. If done carefully, rates of primary fascial closure have been reported to approach 80–90%.[26] If a fascial closure is not possible, delayed abdominal closure must be planned. Various methods exist such as planned ventral hernia with a skin graft or mobilizing skin flaps to cover the viscera.

Hepatic Injuries

Damage control is most commonly used for severe liver injuries. The size of the liver, particularly the right lobe, can make controlling blood loss challenging. The triple blood supply of the liver (hepatic arterial, portal venous, and hepatic venous) increases the complexity of hemostasis. Although bleeding may have stopped spontaneously at the time of laparotomy or require minimal intervention in 50% of patients, over half of the deaths may be due to bleeding.[27]

Damage control is attractive for hepatic injuries. Therapy for liver injury such as resectional debridement or finger fracture results in oozing from the cut liver surface that can be difficult to control. In addition, bleeding from two of the three vascular beds (hepatic and portal venous) may be effectively controlled by packing. The location of the liver in the right upper quadrant makes packing attractive. The diaphragm can be used to exert pressure on the bleeding liver. Packs placed below and lateral to the injured segment can provide sufficient tamponade to control venous bleeding with minimal risk of causing ACS.

As angiography has been used more liberally in patients with liver injuries, the complication rate has increased. A recent series described major hepatic necrosis occurring in >40% of patients after hepatic embolization.[28] Hepatic ischemia is likely produced by the embolization, combined with ischemia from direct vascular injury and portal venous compression from packing of the liver. If major hepatic necrosis occurs, early formal right hepatic lobectomy is the best treatment choice.[29]

The original reports described removal of the packs through stab wounds in the flank.[30] Gauze packing was used for hemostasis and was exteriorized and removed under sedation at the bedside. Blind removal of packing may result in blood loss that goes undetected for some time. In addition, the opportunity to re-examine the liver and debride nonviable tissue justifies the risk of repeat laparotomy.

Early series on hepatic packing showed variable results. In those series, packing was sometimes used early, but often used when patients were reoperated for bleeding at the second or even third laparotomy. Survival rates varied between 50% and 80%, and infectious complications were common. However, packs were often left in for a longer period of time, up to 10 days (*see* Chapter 40, "Abdominal, Urologic and Perineal Injuries," for additional information).[31-33]

Nonhepatic Abdominal Injuries

The anatomic relationships within the pelvis make deep pelvic venous bleeding amenable to packing. All appreciable arterial bleeding must be controlled surgically. Packing for arterial injuries is doomed to failure. Bleeding areas in resection beds of the liver or spleen are amenable to packing. "Ooze" from the retroperitoneal dissection after a Mattox or Cattell maneuver in patients with coagulopathies may also be controllable with the use of packing or hemostatic dressings. Perioperative angiography may be used to identify lumbar arterial hemorrhage or bleeding points off ligated short gastric or renal arteries, often amenable to percutaneous embolization techniques.

Aortic or iliac arterial injuries are controllable with temporary intraluminal shunting, an attractive alternative to ligation and extra-anatomic bypass. Although iliac artery ligation may not always produce lower-extremity ischemia, it is preferable to maintain flow with a shunt. If selected, extra-anatomic bypass can be performed at the time of unpacking when the patient is stable and no longer hypothermic and coagulopathic.

There are sparse data concerning the use of damage control techniques for abdominal injuries where the liver was not involved. Stone's 1983 publication included a number of patients with both blunt and penetrating injuries that did not involve the liver.[34] The survival rate was significantly better when an abbreviated laparotomy was performed. In 1988, the group from King's County Hospital provided the first series of patients in whom damage control was used for such injuries.[9] Out of 11 patients, three patients died in the early perioperative period from irreversible hemorrhagic shock and acute organ failure. However, eight survived to undergo reoperation requiring a myriad of gastrointestinal reconstructive procedures.

Other Injuries

Chest

Occasionally, patients with thoracic injuries are amenable to damage control techniques. The thoracic cavity can be packed to control bleeding from the lung edges or the mediastinum.

Extremities

Damage control can also be used in serious extremity injuries such as patients with multitrauma and bony injuries. Temporary external fixation provides the advantages of rigid skeletal fixation and allows early mobilization of patients, decreasing pulmonary complications. External fixation is rapid and involves little blood loss. Patients can be returned to the operating room for conversion to standard permanent fracture fixation when stable.[35]

The appropriate timing of orthopedic and vascular repairs depends on a variety of factors including the type of injury and the availability of resources. Optimal results are obtained when there is a close collaboration with the trauma and vascular surgical teams. Temporary intraluminal shunting for arterial injuries is one option for taking care of patients with bony and vascular injuries. The shunt provides distal flow to the extremity while the patient undergoes fracture fixation, whether external or internal. Once the bone is rigidly stabilized, a more permanent vascular reconstruction can be performed. Often this reconstruction occurs in the same setting, but can occur later in patients with a multiplicity of injuries. Another option is to complete the vascular repair prior to the surgical treatment of the orthopedic injury.

Lastly, damage control techniques using packing may be appropriate for devastating extremity injuries.[36] Surgical bleeding is treated with venous ligation and arterial reconstruction or shunting, as appropriate. Muscle bleeders, difficult to control if deep in the wound, may be amenable to treatment with temporary packing and embolization.

REFERENCES

1. Ertel W, Keel M, Eid K, et al. Control of severe hemorrhage using c-clamp and pelvic packing in multiply injured patients with pelvic ring disruption. J Ortho Trauma. 2001; 15;7:468-74.
2. Colthren CC, Osborn PM, Moore EE. Preperitoneal packing for hemodynamically unstable pelvic fractures: a paradigm shift. J Trauma. 2007;62:834-9.
3. Burlew CC, Moore EE, Smith WR, et al. Preperitoneal pelvic packing/external fixation with secondary angioembolization: optimal care for life threatening hemorrhage from unstable pelvic fractures. J Am Coll Surg. 2011;212:628-35.
4. White JM, Cannon JW, Stannard A, et al. Endovascular balloon occlusion of the aorta is superior to resuscitative thoracotomy with aortic clamping in a porcine model of hemorrhagic shock. Surgery. 2011;150:400-9.
5. Markov NP, Percival TJ, Morrison JJ, et al. Physiologic tolerance of descending thoracic aortic balloon occlusion in a swine model of hemorrhagic shock. Surgery. 2013;153:848-56.
6. Brenner ML, Moore LJ, DuBose JJ, et al. A clinical series of resuscitative endovascular balloon occlusion of the aorta for hemorrhage control and resuscitation. J Trauma Acute Care Surg. 2013;75:506-10.
7. Rotondo MF, Schwab CW, McGonigal MD, et al. Damage control: an approach for improved survival in exsanguinating penetrating abdominal injury. J Trauma. 1993;35:375-83.
8. Pringle JH. Notes on the arrest of hepatic hemorrhage due to trauma. Ann Surg. 1908;48:541-9.
9. Talbert S, Trooskin SZ, Scalea TM, et al. Packing and reexploration for patients with nonhepatic injury. J Trauma. 1992;33:1-5.
10. Burch JM, Ortiz VB, Richardson RJ, et al. Abbreviated laparotomy and planned reoperation for critically injured patients. Ann Surg. 1992;215:476-84.
11. Guillermo H, Friese R, O'Keefe T, et al. Damage control laparotomy: a vital tool overused. J Trauma. 2010;60:53-9.
12. American College of Surgeons, Committee on Trauma. Advanced life support Course, Student Manual. Chicago, IL: American College of Surgeons; 1993.
13. Alam HB, Stanton K, Koustova E, et al. Effect of different resuscitative strategies in neutrophil activation in a swine model of hemorrhagic shock. Resuscitation. 2004;60:91-9.
14. Holcomb JB, Wade CE, Michalek JE. Increased plasma and platelet to red blood cell ration improves outcome in 466 massively transfused civilian trauma patients. Ann Surg. 2008;248:447-58.
15. Scalea TM, Bochicchio K, Lumpkins K, et al. Early aggressive use of fresh frozen plasma does not improve outcome in critically injured trauma patients. Ann Surg. 2008;248: 578-84.
16. Reilly PM, Rotondo MF, Carpenter JP, et al. Temporary vascular continuity during damage control intraluminal shunting for proximal superior mesenteric artery injury. J Trauma. 1995;39:757-60.
17. Scalea TM, Holman M, Fuortes M, et al. Central venous oxygen saturation: an early, accurate measurement of volume during hemorrhage. J Trauma. 1988;28:725-32.
18. Abramson D, Scalea TM, Hitchcock R, et al. Lactate clearance and survival following injury. J Trauma. 1993;35: 584-9.
19. Baron BJ, Scalea TM. Acute blood loss. Emerg Med Clin North Am. 1996;14:35-54.
20. Gentilello LM, Cobean RA, Offner PJ. Continuous arteriovenous rewarming: rapid renewal of hypothermia in critically ill patients. J Trauma. 1992;32:316-27.
21. Denton JR, Moore EE, Coldwell DM. Multimodality treatment for grade V hepatic injuries: perihepatic packing, arterial embolization, and venous stenting. J Trauma. 1997;42: 964-8.
22. Ridings PC, Bloomfield GL, Blocher CR, et al. Cardiopulmonary effects of raised intra-abdominal pressure before and after intravascular volume expansion. J Trauma. 1995; 39:1071-5.
23. Cooper C, Scalea TM. Abdominal compartment syndrome. In: Cameron JL (Ed). Current Surgical Therapy, 6th edition. St. Louis, MO: Mosby; 1998. pp. 937-44.
24. Simon RJ, Cirincione E, Ivatury RR, et al. Intra-abdominal hypertension in patients with catastrophic abdominal trauma: the benefit of prophylaxis and aggressive control. Crit Care Med. 1994;22:A72.
25. Rotondo MF, Zonies DH. The damage control sequence and underlying logic. Surg Clin North Am. 1997;77:761-77.
26. Miller PR, Meridith JW, Johnson JC, et al. Prospective evaluation of vacuum assisted fascial closure after open abdomen: planned ventral hernia rate is substantially reduced. Ann Surg. 2004;239:608-14.
27. Walt AJ. The mythology of hepatic trauma—or Babel revisited. Am J Surg. 1978;135:12-8.

28. Dabbs D, Stein DM, Scalea TM. Major hepatic necrosis: a common complication after angioembolization for treatment of high grade liver injuries. J Trauma. 2009;66:621-9.
29. Dabbs D, Stein DM, Philosophe B, et al. Treatment of major hepatic necrosis: lobectomy versus serial debridements. J Trauma. 2010;69:562-7.
30. Feliciano DV, Mattox KL, Jordan GL. Intra-abdominal packing for control of hepatic hemorrhage: a reappraisal. J Trauma. 1981;21:285-90.
31. Feliciano DV, Mattox KL, Burch JM, et al. Packing for control of hepatic hemorrhage. J Trauma. 1986;26:738-90.
32. Baracco-Gandolfo V, Vidarte O, Baracco-Miller V, et al. Prolonged closed liver packing in severe hepatic trauma: experience with 36 patients. J Trauma. 1986;26:754-6.
33. Ivatury RR, Nallathambi M, Gunduz Y, et al. Liver packing for uncontrolled hemorrhage: a reappraisal. J Trauma. 1986; 26:744-51.
34. Stone HH, Strom PR, Mullins RJ. Management of the major coagulopathy with onset during laparotomy. Ann Surg. 1983;177:532-5.
35. Scalea TM, Boswell SA, Scott JD, et al. External fixation as a bridge to intramedullary nailing for patients with multiple injuries and with femur fractures: Damage control orthopedics. J Trauma. 2000;48:613-21.
36. Henry SM, Tornetta P, Scalea TM. Damage control for the mangled pelvis and extremity. Surg Clin North Am. 1997; 77:879-95.

33

Military Surgery

David H Zonies

Key Points

- Military surgery differs from civilian surgical practice in terms of wounding mechanisms, wound patterns, resources allocation, and the continuum of care.
- Polytrauma due to blast and fragment injury is more likely in combat than in civilian trauma.
- Military trauma care is governed by doctrines of simple expedient surgical maneuvers and staged definitive care as patients move back from the combat zone to more resource intense and safer environments.
- Advances in en-route care have expanded the scope, practice, and timing of combat casualty care.

INTRODUCTION

Military or war surgery has made significant advances in the past decade of conflict. The combined experiences in Iraq and Afghanistan have transformed military surgery to a world-class system of surgical care. Yet, some tenets have remained unchanged over the past 75 years of conflict. The following quote in the prologue of the third edition of the "Emergency War Surgery Handbook," delivered by Dr Michael DeBakey after World War II, remains germane today:

"All the circumstances of war surgery thus do violence to civilian concepts of traumatic surgery. The equality of organizational and professional management is the first basic difference. The second is the time lag introduced by the military necessity of evacuation. The third is the necessity for constant movement of the wounded [service member], and the fourth—treatment by a number of different surgeons at different places instead of by a single surgeon in one place—is inherent in the third. These are all undesirable factors, and on the surface they seem to militate against good surgical care. Indeed, when the overall circumstances of warfare are added to them, they appear to make more ideal surgical treatment impossible. Yet this was not true in the war we have just finished fighting, nor need it ever be true. Short cuts and measures of expediency are infrequently necessary in military surgery, but compromises with surgical adequacy are not."[1]

The role of the military surgeon is not only to operate on the individual patient, but also to make every attempt at returning the patient back to his/her unit to fight. Military surgery may be defined as a development within the art and science of surgery, which is designed to carry out a specialized, essential, and highly significant mission under the adverse conditions of war. The mission of military surgery differs from civilian sector surgery in that it is performed on a mass production basis in what may amount to severely limited circumstances. Stated in another way, the military surgeon does what must be done rather than what could be done to casualties before either returning them to their units or rendering them transportable to the next higher echelon of medical care. To achieve these objectives, the military surgical care system depends upon an organized prehospital treatment and medical evacuation system and utilizes somewhat different and successively staged techniques to treat the penetrating, perforating, and blast injuries of the battlefield.[2]

Military surgery operates within the framework of a staged systematic approach to care. It extends beyond technical expertise and is based on a treatment chain providing through echelons of care. Such echelons are capable of providing surgical care of increasing sophistication. At each stage, the goal is to either return the wounded combatant to duty or evacuate them to the next higher echelon.

- Military surgery is practiced in an austere, resource-limited, and often dangerous environments.
- Mechanisms of injury are often opposite of civilian patterns; penetrating and blast injuries outweigh traditional blunt mechanisms observed in civilian trauma.

AN ORGANIZED APPROACH TO CARE

Until the most recent conflicts, war surgery was performed by surgeons who spent little time actually practicing combat surgery. Surgeons were either stationed at large military treatment facilities practicing general surgery or civilian trauma surgery. When surgeons were activated to war in the early 1990s, the Government Accounting Office reported that the military was incapable of providing "adequate, timely medical support during contingencies and problems with the planning and execution of these efforts." As a result of this and other such condemning reported shortfalls in medical readiness, the Department of Defense developed a joint trauma system. Such an organized system of trauma care was based on the civilian experience as outlined by the American College of Surgeons Committee on Trauma.[3] National population-based registry data demonstrated a consistent 15–20% mortality reduction in developed trauma systems. No such system existed in the military and it was desperately needed.

Immediately following September 11, 2001, the Joint Theater Trauma System was established to organize combat casualty care. Programmatic initiatives included formal predeployment training for nontrauma surgeons and the development of clinical practice guidelines. Such guidelines were derived from civilian evidence when available, based on the success of the Eastern Association for the Surgery of Trauma guidelines. When military-specific guidance was required, novel adaptation from available evidence was used in combination with subject matter expertise. There have been >35 clinical guidelines developed (Table 33.1).[4] A performance improvement program was co-developed for each guideline, so compliance and outcome could be monitored.

The success of the Joint Trauma System initiatives for battlefield care was reported in 2009.[5] When compared with a 4.3% national mortality observed in the national trauma databank, less than 23,000 matched cohort patients in the Joint Trauma Registry demonstrated a 5.2% death rate after battlefield hospital admission. Once a patient enters the military hospital system outside of the war zone, the mortality rate falls to <5%. Such organized efforts have led to the lowest mortality ever observed in the history of armed conflict.

THE ENVIRONMENT AND ECHELONS OF CARE

Military medicine, and specifically war surgery, is a supporting component of the fighting force. Priority for logistical support goes to the war fighters. Therefore, the medical system is organized by echelons, with only a small portion of the medical support being forwarded and with the higher echelon in the rear having most hospitals.[6] The magnitude of forward deployed surgical support, especially in short intense wars of sudden onset, will be seen as inadequate by civilian standards. The equipment and personnel available must be used in the most efficient fashion—to treat the most critically wounded that are likely to survive if appropriately treated.

Since World War I, it has been common to establish small surgical field hospitals as far forward on the battlefield as is reasonably safe, whose sole function is to operate on those at risk of dying in the near term. Their distinguishing characteristic is mobility, which comes at the expense of the sophistication and complexity of their surgical capability. Such forward surgical teams (FSTs) are staffed with 2–4 surgeons and are supplied to perform up to 30 major operations (e.g. thoracotomies and laparotomies to control hemorrhage and contamination, massive extremity trauma) over a 24–72-hour period (Figs. 33.1A and B). As most casualties die on the battlefield of exsanguinating hemorrhage, only 5–10% of the total casualty population are candidates for care by an FST.

Table 33.1 Examples of military clinical practice guidelines.

Amputation management	Blunt abdominal trauma	Cervical spine injury
Compartment syndrome	Acute burn care	Fresh whole blood transfusion
Fungal wound management	Urologic trauma	Neurosurgical management
Wartime vascular injury	Unexploded ordinance	Pelvic fracture care
Ocular and adnexal injuries	Damage control resuscitation	Catastrophic injury

Source: US Department of Army. (2013). JTTS Clinical Practice Guidelines. [online] Available from http://www.usaisr.amedd.army.mil/clinical_practice_guidelines.html. [Accessed June 1, 2013].

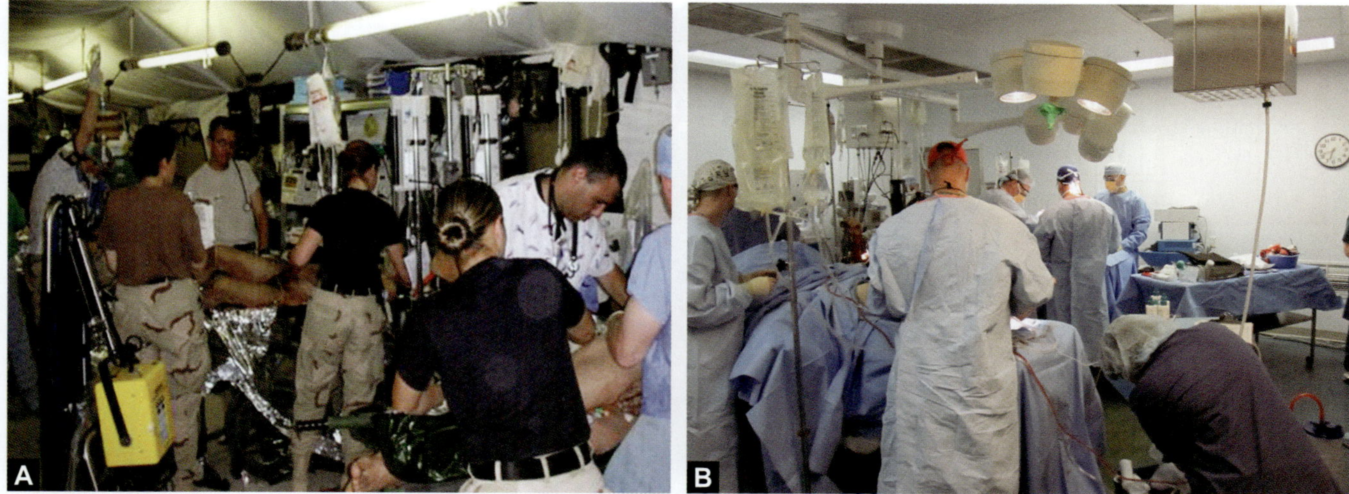

Figs. 33.1A and B: (A) The forward surgical team. Multiple trauma resuscitations may occur simultaneously. Up to 30 operations may be performed in a 72-hour period. However, there is limited holding capacity and patients must transfer to higher echelons of care. (B) Mass casualty surgery. Multiple operations may occur simultaneously in a single operating theater. Here, two major operations are occurring simultaneously during a mass casualty period.

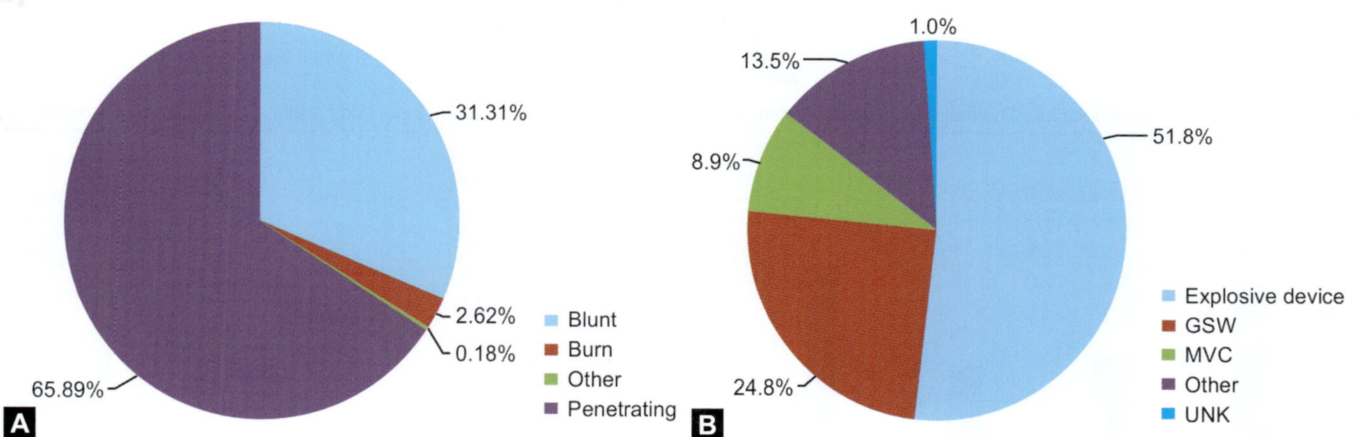

Figs. 33.2A and B: (A) Mechanism of injury in combat casualties. Over 60% of wounds are penetrating in nature, a significant departure from typical civilian casualty care. (B) Modern wounding patterns in combat casualties. More than half of wounding patterns include explosive devices followed by gunshot wounds. (GSW: Gunshot wound; MVC: Motor vehicle casualty; UNK: Unknown).

Most of these casualties have orthopedic, soft tissue, or head and facial wounds that require appreciable subspecialty care. Based on improved body armor, only about 5–10% of patients now sustain a thoracoabdominal injury requiring intervention. Survival after life-saving surgery at the FST depends upon the quality of evacuation to the higher echelons of care.

NATURE OF COMBAT INJURIES

Penetrating missiles cause the overwhelming majority of casualties in battle. The basic mechanisms of injury—penetrating, blast, blunt, and thermal—are similar to those found in civilian life. What is different is the relative prevalence of the mechanisms (Figs. 33.2A and B).

The anatomic distribution of wounds sustained by combat injury is described in Figure 33.3. Although blunt trauma is most common among civilians, trauma inflicted in land warfare is overwhelmingly penetrating. Data compiled from the Department of Defense records for World War II, the Korean War, the Vietnam War, and the wars in Iraq and Afghanistan indicate that penetrating missiles were the mechanism of injury in about 90% of all battle casualties (Fig. 33.4).[2]

"Blast" injury has been the most dominant injury mechanism in recent years. A perception arises from

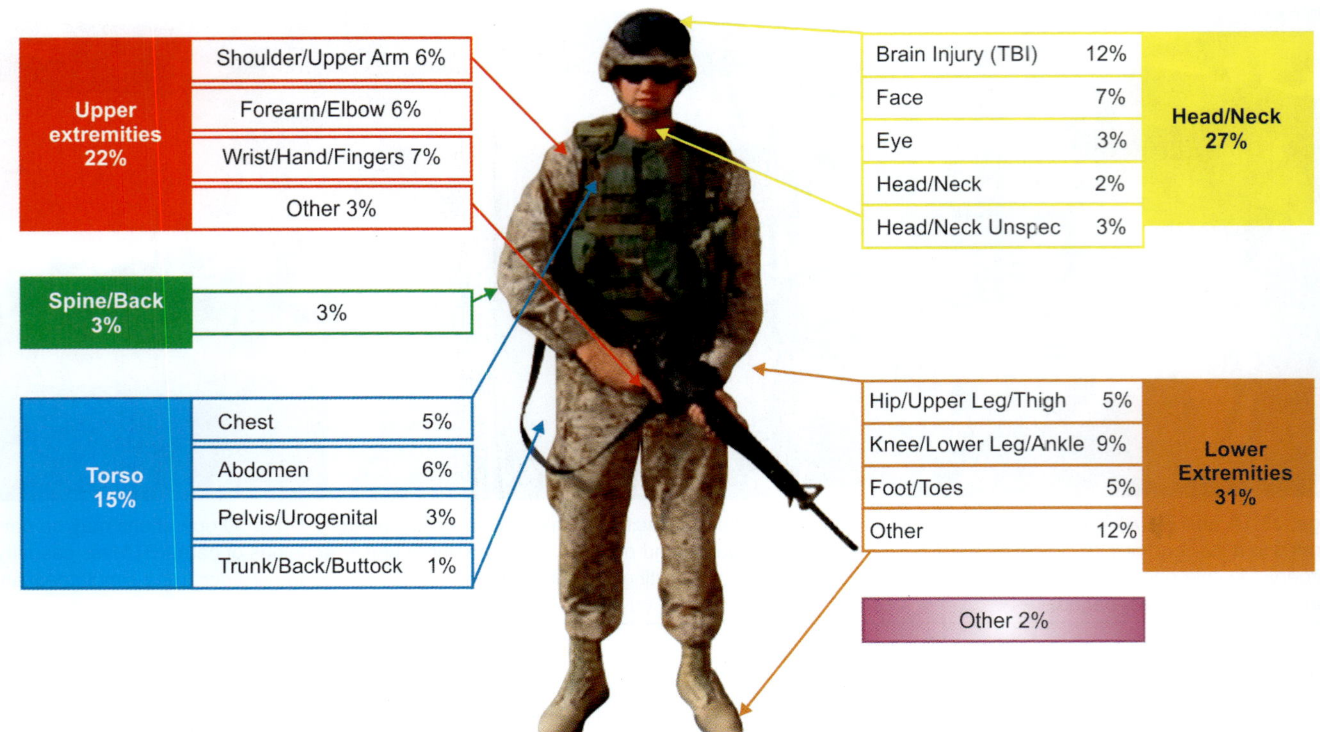

Fig. 33.3: Anatomic wound location. The majority of wounds affect the extremities due to improved personal body armor. (TBI: Traumatic brain injury).

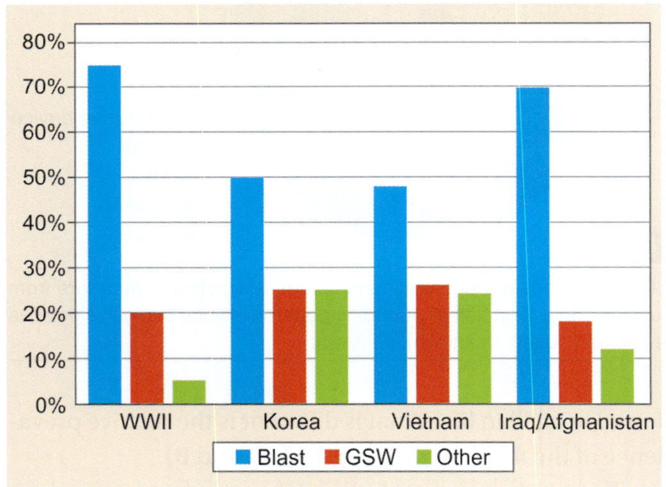

Fig. 33.4: Mechanism of injury by conflict. Blast injury remains the predominant mechanism of injury during combat. Similarities between World War II and today are stunning. (WWII: World War II; GSW: Gunshot wound). *Source*: Burris DG, FitzHarris JB, Holcomb JB (Eds). Emergency War Surgery, 3rd edition. Washington, DC: Borden Institute; 2004.

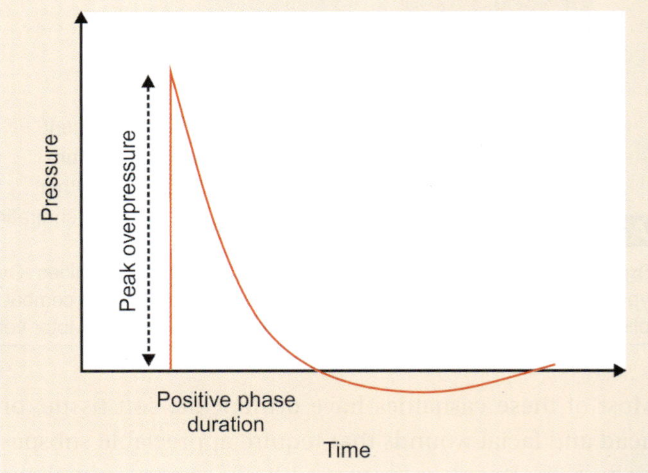

Fig. 33.5: Mechanism of blast injury. Initial effect of blast is a rapid overpressurization in the vicinity. This may result in rupture of hollow structures (e.g. tympanic space, gastrointestinal tract, lungs). This is followed by rapid decay and vacuum, ultimately returning to baseline atmospheric pressure.

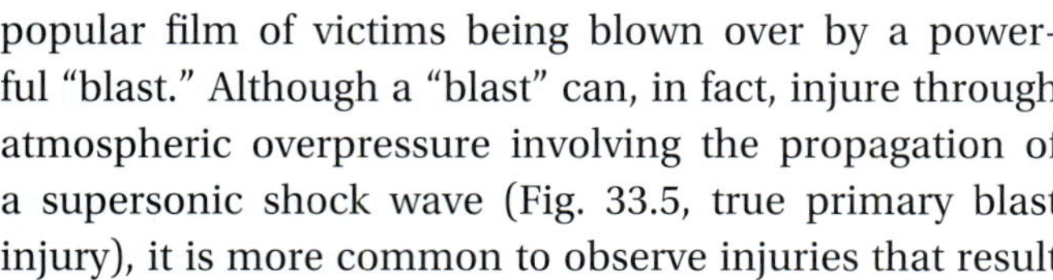

popular film of victims being blown over by a powerful "blast." Although a "blast" can, in fact, injure through atmospheric overpressure involving the propagation of a supersonic shock wave (Fig. 33.5, true primary blast injury), it is more common to observe injuries that result from a secondary blast. Secondary blast injury involves the generation of projectiles that cause penetrating injury to the victim. In a tertiary blast, the victim is thrown against a solid object resulting in blunt trauma (also known as translational blast injury). The latter effect arises from

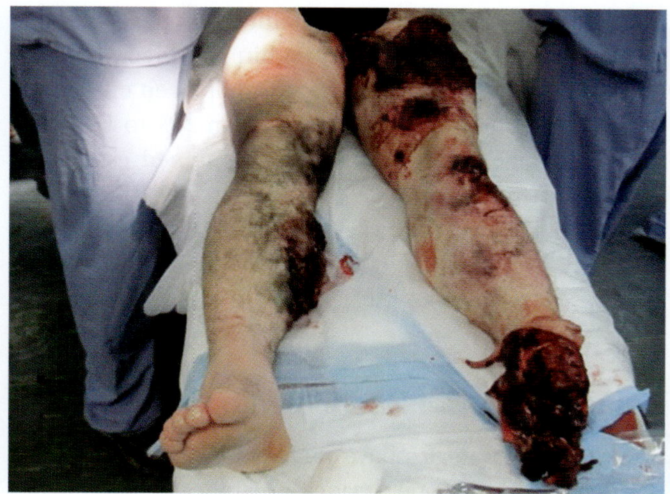

Fig. 33.6: Traumatic amputation. Foot amputation after stepping on an antipersonnel improvised explosive device. High-velocity projectiles and debris must be removed, and exposure of the fascial planes to just below the knee was required to obtain source control in this patient.

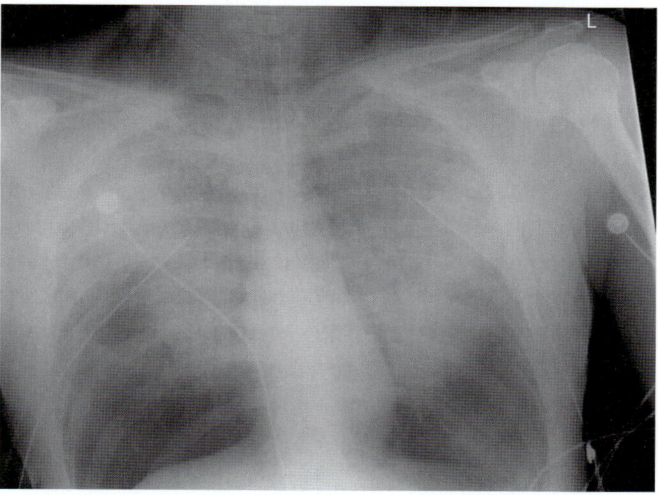

Fig. 33.7: Blast lung. Overpressurization during a primary blast injury resulted in this patient developing severe hypoxic failure. The characteristic butterfly appearance can be demonstrated here. This patient ultimately required extracorporeal lung support for severe, refractory acute respiratory distress syndrome.

the "blast wind"—the mass of air displaced by the explosion—which may obtain a transient velocity as high as 200 km/h.[7,8] This phenomenon is especially apparent when an extremity is amputated by the detonation of a buried antipersonnel mine (Fig. 33.6).

Much of the damage is done by penetrating missiles that arise secondarily from the ground, the soldier's boot, and even their foot. The secondary missiles, in conjunction with the blast wind, are responsible for the gross mutilation that is characteristic of such injuries. Not surprisingly, the term "mutilating blast injury" has been applied to the situation when the body or a substantial part of it disintegrates.

Primary blast injury—injury due to overpressure from a blast wave—is distinctly uncommon in surviving casualties except in the form of perforated tympanic membranes or "blast lung injury" (Fig. 33.7). Victims in close proximity to an explosion can be expected to sustain thermal injury in addition to being wounded by penetrating missiles and translational blast injury. When the victim is a crewmember of an armored vehicle, thermal injury results from secondary explosion, and fires arising from the vehicle's ammunition and fuel. Great efforts have been made to incorporate fire suppression systems within such vehicles to minimize burn casualties.

Blunt trauma, the mechanism responsible for most civilian injury, is uncommon as a cause of battle injury. When blunt trauma occurs, it is usually in the context of a tactical vehicle having detonated an antitank mine or improvised explosive device. A unique complex of injuries may be seen in such circumstances:

- Closed fractures of the axial skeleton and extremities
- Blunt head trauma
- Blast overpressure involving the ears
- If the vehicle's hull is penetrated, flash burns and inhalation injury from fumes produced by the explosion.

Bullets from small arms and fragments from explosive munitions are the two sources of penetrating wounds on the modern battlefield. In the wars of the past century, wounds made by explosive devices have been responsible for more than two thirds of all casualties. The United States experience in the Vietnam War was similar: about 65% of all casualties had penetrating missile wounds caused by fragments from explosive munitions.[9] In the most recent Iraq and Afghan conflicts, the majority of military casualties sustained a penetrating injury from one of six mechanisms: gunshot wound, improvised explosive device, landmine, mortar, bomb, or grenade.

MEASURING SURVIVAL OUTCOMES OF COMBAT INJURIES

The medical outcome of combat trauma is usually quantified in terms of morbidity and mortality rates. One group that is excluded from traditional statistical reporting includes those who are wounded in action (WIA). The WIA rate is determined by those injured, admitted to a military treatment facility, and returned to duty within 72 hours.

Such patients represent 50% of those injured in a combat. However, this statistic is included in the denominator of the mortality statistics.

Traditional combat mortality rates are measured by two statistics: killed in action (KIA) rates and died of wounds (DOW) rate. They differ not only in terms of time of death, but, more importantly, where death occurred. Approximately 80% of fatally wounded service members in World War II and Vietnam died on the battlefield; only 20% died after entering the medical system. Death before entering the medical system equates to dying before reaching the first echelon of care (battalion-aid station):

$$\%\text{KIA} = \frac{\text{Deaths before MTF}}{\text{KIA} + (\text{WIA} - \text{RTD})}$$

$$\%\text{DOW} = \frac{\text{Died after reaching MTF}}{\text{WIA} - \text{RTD}} \times 100.$$

(KIA: Killed in action; MTF: Military treatment facility; WIA: Wounded in action; RTD: Return to duty).

Mortality outcome data are presented not only as the gross number of casualties who are classified as KIA or DOW, but also as normalized statistics (i.e. as the percentage of the total casualty population, or the percentage of the admitted or hospitalized population, respectively). Modern epidemiological statistics refer to this value as a case fatality rate (CFR):

$$\text{CFR} = \frac{\text{KIA} + \text{DOW}}{\text{KIA} + \text{WIA}} \times 100.$$

Based on historical data, it is customary to assume that about 20% of the battle casualty population will be KIA, although data vary. The magnitude of the percentage KIA depends upon at least three medical factors:

- The lethality of the weapons
- The feasibility and effectiveness of first aid
- The length of time required for evacuation from the battlefield to a medical treatment facility.

The magnitude of the percentage of the population who die of wounds depends upon at least two medical factors:

- Adequacy of surgical care (e.g. if no neurosurgical care can be given, the number of casualties who have head wounds who die will increase)
- Casualty load and triage considerations (e.g. during a mass casualty situation, it may be necessary to place certain casualties in the expectant category, resulting in a greater number of casualties who will die of wounds).

Given a highly functioning medical system, about 3–5% of hospitalized casualties can be expected to die. In most wars, about half of the casualties who die of wounds can be expected to succumb within the first 24 hours. Recently, the percentage rate of KIA has been cut almost in half during the Iraq/Afghan war (from 20% to 13%) and the percentage rate of DOW have remained essentially unchanged (from 3.5 to 4.8%). The standardized CFR has also been cut in half over the past 50 years (15–19 vs. 9.4%).[10]

APPROACH TO MILITARY COMBAT CASUALTY CARE

Damage Control Resuscitation

Resuscitation strategies have undergone significant transition over the past several decades. A significant literature has been built around the concept of damage control surgery.[11,12] As a natural extension to such an approach of abbreviated laparotomy, a hemostatic resuscitation strategy has been advocated with associated improved outcomes.[13-15]

Following Advanced Trauma Life Support guidelines, resuscitation has traditionally involved large amounts of crystalloid fluids for resuscitation. This has been associated with higher risks of abdominal compartment syndrome and mutliorgan failure.[16,17] Strong evidence now exists that a balanced resuscitation with component blood products that approach reconstituted whole blood (e.g. 1 unit packed red blood cells, 1 unit plasma, 1 unit platelets, ± 1 unit cryoprecipitate) is independently associated with an improved survival (Fig. 33.8).[18] The primary goal of damage control resuscitation is to prevent the development of an acutely coagulopathic trauma patient. In order to stem the loss of clotting factors through dilutional coagulopathy with crystalloid fluids, permissive hypotension may be permitted with the exception of those patients with obvious brain injury. During the early period of resuscitation, a blood pressure targeting 90 mm Hg may be maintained until surgical care can be provided.

Patients who meet criteria for massive hemorrhage requiring high-volume transfusion should be identified early and the blood bank alerted. Due to a storage lesion associated with older banked blood, the concept of "Last In, First Out" has become military doctrine in combat resuscitation. That is, the "freshest" units of blood products are utilized in patients requiring massive transfusion.

Adjunctive measures include active core rewarming, the use of recombinant factor VIIa (rFVIIa) and tranexamic acid. Although a survival benefit has not been demonstrated with the use of rFVIIa, studies have demonstrated a decreased use of blood products after its administration.

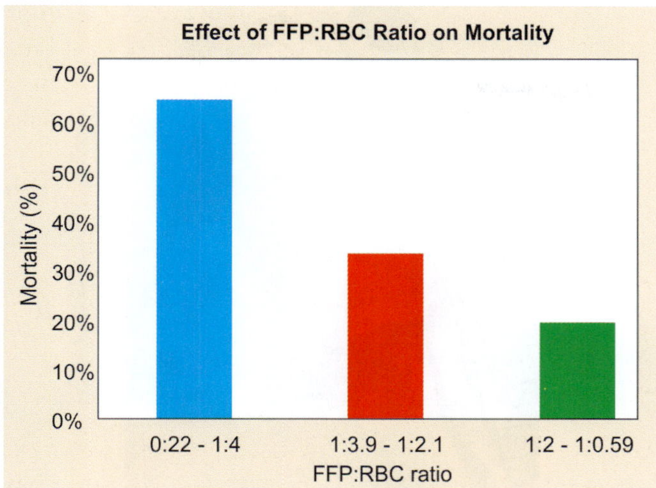

Fig. 33.8: Balanced fresh frozen plasma to red blood cell hemostatic resuscitation. Strong evidence supports balanced resuscitation that approaches whole blood, resulting in improved survival. (FFP: Fresh frozen plasma; RBC: Red blood cell).
Source: Borgman MA, Spinella PC, Perkins JG, et al. The ratio of blood products transfused affects mortality in patients receiving massive transfusions at a combat support hospital. J Trauma. 2007;63(4):805-13.

This becomes critically important when patients are at risk of massive hemorrhage, and replacement products may be unavailable at lower echelons of care. Limited studies support the use of tranexamic acid, an antifibrinolytic agent, in combat casualty care, although the side effect profile of tranexamic acid is favorable in coagulopathic patients.[19] Military damage control resuscitation has had a profound effect on combat mortality and the mitigation of trauma-related complications. Such an approach has been translated back to the civilian community with promising results (*see* Chapter 32, "Initial Surgical Care of the Trauma Patient," for further details).[20-23]

APPROACH TO COMBAT WOUND CARE

Wound debridement and irrigation is the most commonly performed procedure in the combat zone. Rapid evacuation of hematoma, removal of dirt, and surgical debridement of devitalized tissue are associated with decreased systemic complications.[24] Such debridement should be performed under the most sterile conditions as permitted in the austere environment. While one must aggressively debride all nonviable tissue, extension of debridement should be placed in the context of ultimate soft tissue coverage. Wound length should be preserved for possible reconstruction at higher echelons of care.

High-energy war wounds have a zone of injury that evolves over time. Wounds that appear viable during initial evaluation may progress to frank tissue necrosis within days. As opposed to traditional elective general surgery, serial wound evaluation in the operating room is key to ultimate tissue preservation. The war surgeon should understand the mechanism of injury and the likelihood for wound progression over time. Debrided wounds should undergo a relook procedure within 24 hours. Initial serial debridement may be required every 24–48 hours until the wound appears stable.

Irrigation with a *p*H-balanced solution should be used as an adjunct to sharp debridement but does not substitute for a scalpel. Bacterial loads within wounds will logarithmically diminish with increasing volumes of fluid. Wounds may require 3–10 L of irrigation based on size.

Temporary wound coverage should be utilized with moistened gauze. Once a wound appears stable for >48–72 hours, negative pressure wound therapy may be considered. Utilization of such a device requires a hemostatic wound bed. Once the wound enters this subacute phase of care, negative pressure wound therapy assists with the development of granulations and contracture of the overall size of the wound. High-energy war wounds should never be primarily closed due to natural zonal progression and risk of wound sepsis. Secondary closure may be performed once a wound enters the subacute phase. It may be loosely closed, with or without closed suction drainage. In cases of large wound defects without dermal coverage, split-thickness skin grafts may be required.

Antimicrobials should be initially utilized but discontinued as quickly as possible. The use of long-term antibiotics in patients with superficial war wounds should not substitute for surgical judgment as to when sharp debridement is required. Deep tissue antimicrobial-impregnated polymethylmethacrylate beads may be considered for grossly infected wounds or wounds with a tenuous blood supply.

Traumatic war wounds are at high risk of containing retained foreign bodies. Case-by-case decisions should be judiciously made with experienced surgeons as to whether removal is warranted. Serial debridement allows adequate time for dirt and debris to be removed. However, in some cases large retained foreign bodies deeply embedded are not easily accessible. Indications for removal include proximity to joint spaces and blood vessels. As patients move through various echelons of care, the risk of retaining surgical foreign bodies also increases. At the time of definitive wound closure, X-rays should be obtained to exclude the presence of gossypibomas (retained surgical sponges) or other retained surgical items.

ABDOMINAL TRAUMA AND DAMAGE CONTROL SURGERY

Staged surgery for combat injury is the result of damage control principles.[11] However, the decision to operate on patients who sustain blunt abdominal injury secondary to high kinetic energy transfer in combat is less straightforward. Protective body armor may protect the patient from penetrating missiles after an explosion, but cannot exclude abdominal injuries. Echelon III facilities may have computed tomogram imaging capability, but this is certainly not the case at the forward surgical hospital. When available, focused abdominal sonography should be used in addition to clinical examination. Patients with obvious signs of peritonitis will undergo a laparotomy. Endovascular or interventional approaches are not feasible at most levels of care in the combat zone. Laparoscopy for trauma, especially in the combat zone, is highly unreliable to rule out intra-abdominal injury and is not recommended. Nonoperative management should only be offered when the facility has holding capacity to closely monitor a patient.[25]

If a patient moves by air evacuation, it must be ensured that the risk of hemorrhage is minimal. High-grade injuries (Grade III or IV) that may be conservatively managed in a civilian environment are often considered too high risk for potential failure in a combat zone. Therefore, high-grade spleen or renal injuries are more likely to undergo resection versus organ preservation.

VASCULAR INJURY

Hemorrhage remains the number one cause of preventable mortality on the battlefield. Rates of vascular injury during World War II and the Vietnam War were on the order of 1–3%. The rates of vascular injury in Iraq and Afghanistan approached 12%. It is proposed that a fivefold increase may be related to the mechanism of improvised explosive. Extremity vessel injury accounts for 70–80% of cases, with 5–10% in the torso.

Prehospital care, to include self-aid buddy care, involves direct pressure to exsanguinating wounds and the placement of a compressive tourniquet. The tourniquet has had a storied history where it has fallen in and out of favor. Over the past 10 years of combat casualty care, the tourniquet has been responsible for both improved limb salvage and reduced mortality (Fig. 33.9).[26]

Hard signs of vascular injury such as hemorrhage or ischemia mandate immediate exploration of wounds.

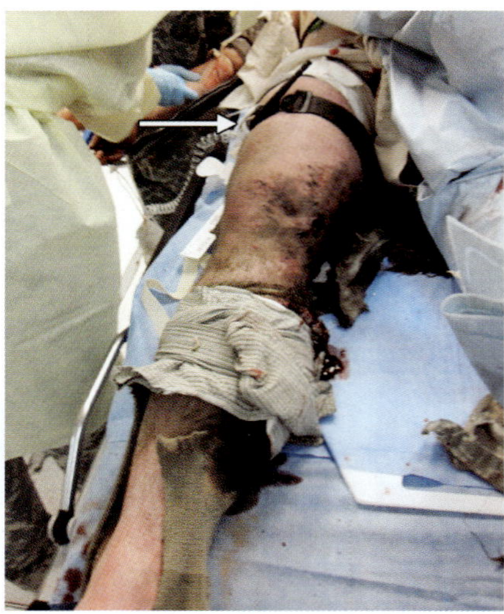

Fig. 33.9: Tourniquet placement (arrow). Tourniquet use in the absence of physiological shock is strongly associated with improved survival. Early use (prehospital) has been associated with an improved limb salvage and survival advantage.

Soft signs (e.g. proximity, fracture pattern) may be used in the context of the overall patient condition to determine the need for surgical exploration (Flowchart 33.1) (*see* Chapter 42, "Vascular Trauma," for further details). The ankle–brachial index remains a standard evaluation tool at every echelon of care.

Blood products, including the need for possible whole blood transfusion, should be made available prior to the release of a tourniquet. Between two and four units of packed red cells per extremity should be expected for transfusion of combat-related vascular injury. This is in addition to a balanced hemostatic resuscitation (i.e. plasma and platelet transfusion). Angiography has limited value in the diagnosis of extremity vascular injury at this level of care because of the limited expertise with advanced technology in the Echelon II combat environment. It is acceptable to ligate veins and some peripheral arteries with the paramount doctrine of "life over limb."

Lower and upper extremities are the most common sites of operative vascular injury. Proximal and distal controls remain a key principle in both civilian and military vascular trauma management. At the forward surgical hospital, resources or time may not allow definitive repair such as an interposition graft of reversed saphenous vein. In such cases, a temporary intravascular shunt is appropriate (Fig. 33.10) (*see* Chapter 35, "Case Study: Vascular Injury in Combat and Austere Settings," for an illustrative case). This is especially the case when segmental loss of a vessel is present with a viable distal extremity. Typical

Flowchart 33.1: Approach to vascular trauma: Suggested algorithm by the Joint Theater Trauma System (Central Command).

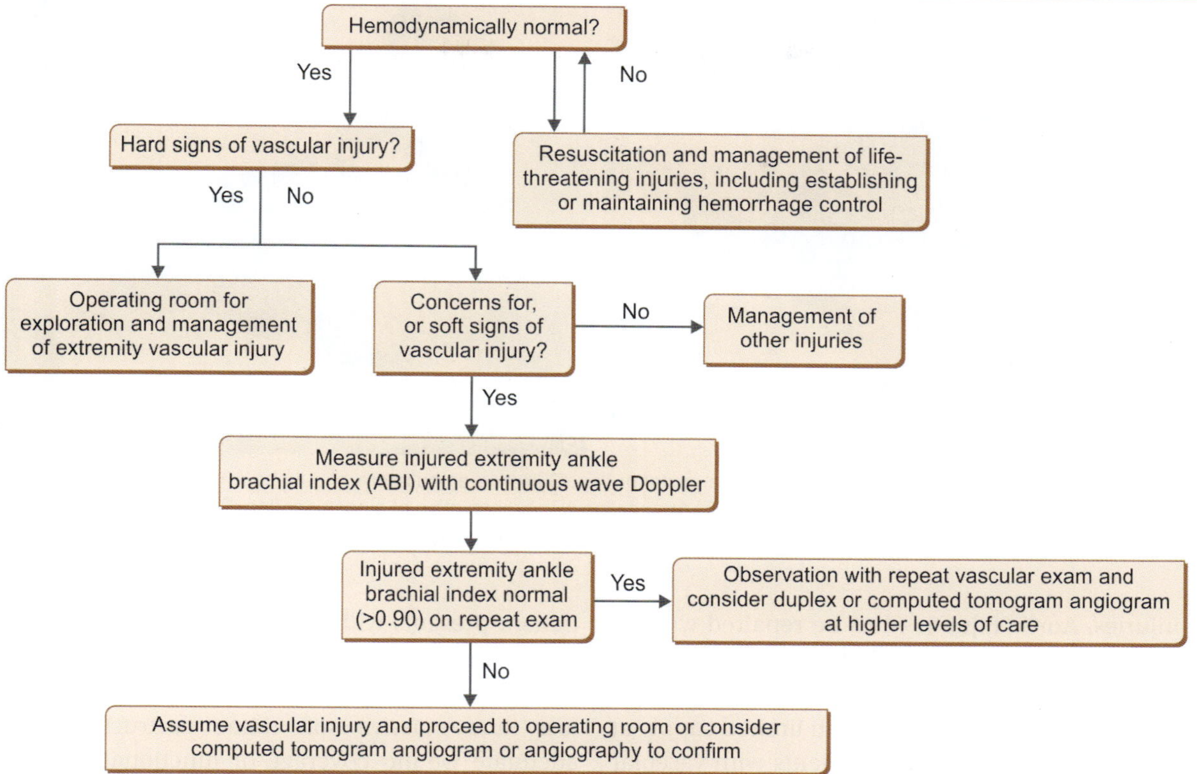

Source: US Department of Army. (2013). JTTS Clinical Practice Guidelines.[online] Available from http://www.usaisr.amedd.army.mil/clinical_practice_ guidelines.html. [Accessed June 1, 2013].

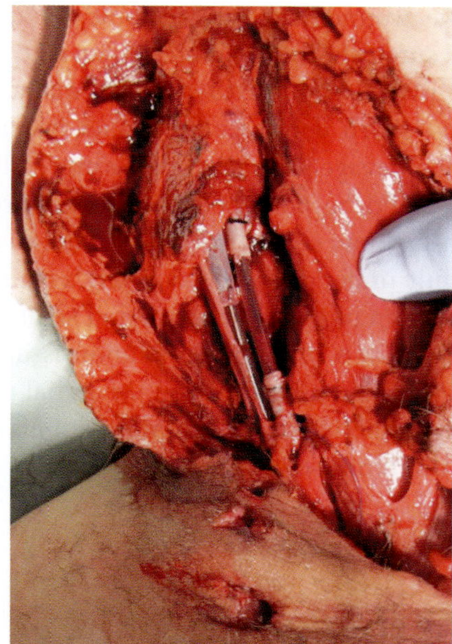

Fig. 33.10: Temporary vascular shunt (artery and vein). Temporary vascular shunts have resulted in increased limb salvage. If time permits, it is recommended to shunt the venous injury as well to decrease future morbidity and promote collateral development (e.g. edema and vasculitis).

shunts vary from 8 to 14 Fr and may remain patent at lengths up to 15–30 cm. Shunts are secured with a ligature at both the proximal and distal ends, with a typical "in-situ" use from 6 to 12 hours. Regional anticoagulation is typically used on the basis of the patient's clinical status, but systemic anticoagulation is rarely necessary. Many patients with major vascular injuries requiring a temporary vascular shunt are coincidentally coagulopathic with contraindication to anticoagulation.

Thrombectomy catheters should be used as a key tool to both slow blood loss during reconstruction and remove distal thrombus prior to definitive vessel repair. Once the repair is complete, viable tissue should be mobilized to cover the graft. Failure to do so incurs a risk of rupture within the subsequent week. Finally, prophylactic fasciotomies should be performed in both upper and lower extremities when the ischemic time exceeds 3–4 hours. The risk of developing a clinically significant extremity compartment syndrome is high among combat casualties, even in light of a hemostatic resuscitation.

Torso injuries are less common due to body armor. Injuries to the abdominal vascular structures represent

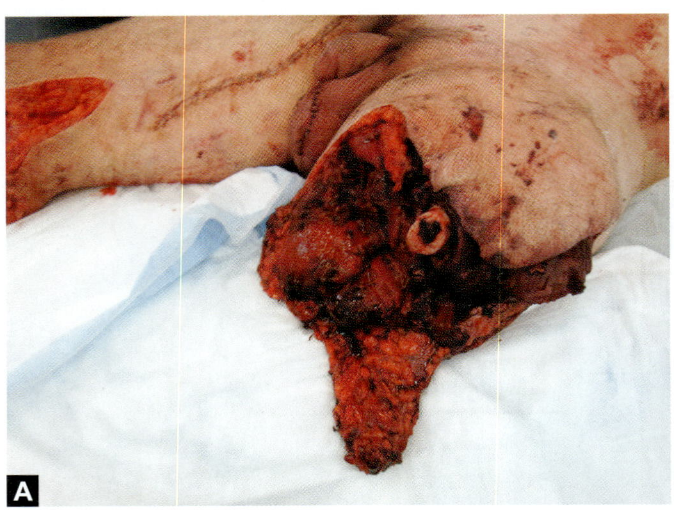

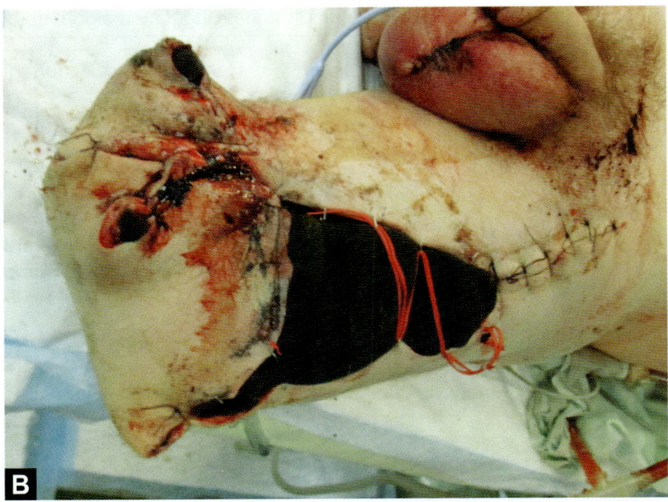

Figs. 33.11A and B: (A) Amputation with preservation of a posterior flap. Guillotine amputations should be avoided. Soft tissue, even if questionably viable, should be preserved for wound coverage. (B) Amputation with preservation of a posterior flap. Preservation of a posterior flap is maintained during this staged procedure. A temporary negative pressure sponge is being placed for planned re-exploration.

<3% of injuries. Aortic injuries must be repaired with an interposition prosthetic graft. Similarly, mesenteric, renal, and iliac arteries should be repaired with interposition or prosthetic grafts. Prosthetic grafts are in limited supply at the forward surgical hospital, and patients with vascular injuries often require urgent evacuation to the Echelon III hospital where a vascular/trauma surgeon is present. Vena cava injuries may be repaired if the lumen remains uncompromised and a tangential injury is present; temporary vascular shunts are of limited value. Of note, most abdominal venous structures can be ligated for patients in extremis. However, venous congestion in the gastrointestinal tract or lower extremities is to be expected with commensurate morbidity. Additional information on vascular trauma is contained in Chapter 42, "Vascular Trauma".

PRINCIPLES OF EXTREMITY AMPUTATION

As previously mentioned, the zone of injury surrounding a wound is highly dependent on the mechanism of injury. Crush injury, massive hemorrhage requiring supranormal resuscitation, and comorbid conditions [e.g. sepsis, renal failure, acute respiratory distress syndrome (ARDS)] all contribute to the decision-making process of extremity amputation.

Traumatic amputation occurs at the time of injury in the field. Surgical management may include debridement and vascular control of the remaining distal portion of the limb. A primary amputation will occur when the patient presents with a mangled extremity and the decision is made not to pursue limb salvage. Indications to forego limb salvage include segmental nerve loss, bone loss, and massive soft tissue destruction precluding adequate wound coverage or functional limb recovery. Current doctrine holds that extremity amputation after a combat injury should be limited to preserve limb length and eventual soft tissue coverage (Figs. 33.11A and B).

Extensive wound inspection should be undertaken with liberal surgical extension to evaluate all tissue levels and fascial planes. As described in the management of war wounds, sharp debridement should be undertaken and dilutional lavage should be performed. All vascular structures should be identified and ligated proximal to the most distal bony structure. The decision to amputate is never lightly undertaken. It is typically a team decision with consultation of the orthopedist and senior surgeons when available. If a primary amputation is undertaken, the wound should not be closed at the initial procedure. Additionally, guillotine or circular amputations should be avoided as this limits soft tissue coverage.

MOVEMENT ALONG A CONTINUUM OF CARE

As emphasized throughout this chapter, combat surgery is not just the application of surgical techniques, but a system in which first aid, evacuation, and operation are tightly integrated over time and distance. This concept of combat surgery should be viewed in terms of the echelons

Flowchart 33.2: Medical treatment facilities and the echelons of care as prescribed by Military Doctrine. Operations are performed at the forward surgical team (FST), and the third and fourth echelon hospitals. The FST performs emergency life-saving surgery, whereas the higher echelon hospitals perform the initial operations on the remaining casualties. This is the full deployment for a major war; a lesser conflict would see fewer medical treatment facilities and the fourth echelon might be absent.

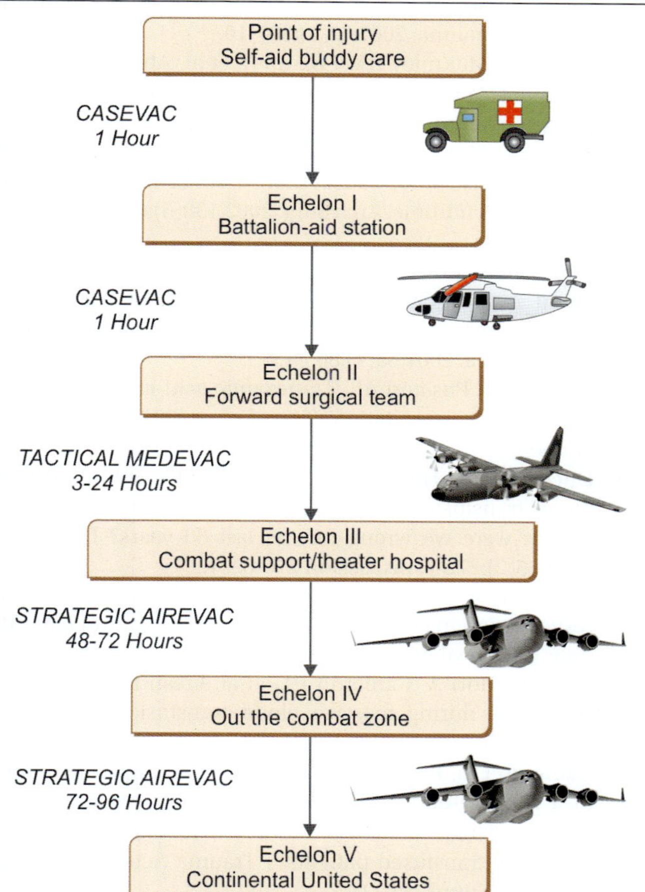

(CASEVAC: Casualty evacuation; MEDEVAC: Medical evacuation; AIREVAC: Air evacuation).

of care, as shown in Flowchart 33.2. Communication between echelons of care is critical, and a deployable electronic medical record system has been established for the transmittal of critical patient information and operative procedures. En-route critical care deserves special attention as this may be one of the most important advances in modern combat casualty trauma care. During the Korean and Vietnam conflicts, the average length of stay before patient movement to the continental United States was 45 days. With advances in en-route care, current military doctrine stipulates that patients must continue to progress along the continuum of care as early as physiologically possible. This is, in part, due to a smaller footprint during combat operations and fewer large fixed facilities in the area of combat operations. As a result of enhanced capability, rapid aeromedical transport of patients from the point of injury to their final destination outside the theater of operations may occur in 4–5 days.

A major advancement in the past decade of combat surgery has been the co-development of long-range transport of critically ill trauma patients by a mobile intensive care unit. With a smaller footprint in the war zone, critical care transport teams were required to minimize a bottleneck of intensive care beds at the Echelon III facility. With advances in critical care and the miniaturization of equipment (ventilators, transport monitors, and suction devices), the types of patients qualifying for urgent transport transitioned from stable casualties to some of the most critically ill polytrauma patients only hours or days postinjury.

As a natural evolution of these teams, several augmentation specialty teams developed for the critical care management of select patients. This includes a burn team to manage large burn surface casualties and a lung failure team for patients with severe ARDS. The lung failure team also provides extracorporeal membrane oxygenation as a rescue treatment for combat casualties. Such advanced technology and expertize has never previously been observed in a combat zone.

PAST, PRESENT, AND FUTURE

It has often been said that the only benefactor of war has been the advancement of medical knowledge. Many of the advances in postwar surgery and the increased interest in treating trauma have developed from the vast experience of war surgeons. The experiences of many former war surgeons who served in Vietnam largely fueled the explosive increase in civilian trauma services that occurred during the late 1960s and 1970s. Until the end of the 1970s, the war surgery experience of the 20th century played a dominant role in shaping the evolution of civilian trauma surgery. A new generation of war surgeons who experienced the longest sustained conflict in American history will continue to contribute to the trauma community.

Much of what was important in war surgery (such as the emphasis on staged operations as exemplified by delayed primary closure of soft tissue wounds) has been incorporated into civilian trauma surgery. Many advancements in military surgery have translated into civilian practice. Likewise, many of the resource-intensive capabilities, once thought impossible at a combat-support hospital, are now routinely present. This includes angiography, renal replacement therapy, and magnetic resonance imaging.[27]

Such a system will work only if evacuation is looked upon as an integral part of the surgical care. Medical command and control would have the crucial duty of integrating triage, treatment, and evacuation throughout the echelons, and there is little doubt that evolving techniques of telemedicine will have a role. Viewed as such, the distinguishing feature of war surgery is less an exercise in the application of arcane techniques and more a system in, which resuscitation, operation, stabilization, and evacuation are tightly integrated, not over the dimensions of a city as in civilian trauma, but over continents.

REFERENCES

1. Debakey M. Emergency War Surgery, 3rd edition. Washington, DC: Walter Reed Army Medical Center, Borden Institute; 2004.
2. Burris DG, FitzHarris JB, Holcomb JB (Eds). Emergency War Surgery, 3rd edition. Washington, DC: Borden Institute; 2004.
3. American College of Surgeons Committee on Trauma. Resources for Optimal Care of the Injured Patient. Chicago, IL: American College of Surgeons; 2006.
4. US Department of the Army. (2013). JTTS Clinical Practice Guidelines. [online] Available from http://www.usaisr.amedd.army.mil/clinical_practice_guidelines.html. [Accessed June 1, 2013].
5. Eastridge BJ, Costanzo G, Jenkins D, et al. Impact of joint theater trauma system initiatives on battlefield injury outcomes. Am J Surg. 2009;198(6):852-7.
6. US Department of the Army (Ed). Planning for Health Services Support. Washington, DC: US Department of the Army; 1994. pp. 8-55.
7. Wolf SJ, Bebarta VS, Bonnett CJ, et al. Blast injuries. Lancet. 2009;374(9687):405-15.
8. Proud WG. The physical basis of explosion and blast injury processes. J R Army Med Corps. 2013;159(Suppl 1):i4-9.
9. Owens BD, Kragh JF Jr, Wenke JC, et al. Combat wounds in operation Iraqi freedom and operation enduring freedom. J Trauma. 2008;64(2):295-9.
10. Holcomb JB, Stansbury LG, Champion HR, et al. Understanding combat casualty care statistics. J Trauma. 2006; 60(2):397-401;20.
11. Rotondo MF, Schwab CW, McGonigal MD, et al. "Damage control": an approach for improved survival in exsanguinating penetrating abdominal injury. J Trauma. 1993;35(3): 375-82; discussion 382-3.
12. Rotondo MF, Bard MR. Damage control surgery for thoracic injuries. Injury. 2004;35(7):649-54.
13. Holcomb JB. Fluid resuscitation in modern combat casualty care: lessons learned from Somalia. J Trauma. 2003;54 (5 Suppl):S46-51.
14. Holcomb JB. Damage control resuscitation. J Trauma. 2007;62(6 Suppl):S36-7.
15. Holcomb JB, Jenkins D, Rhee P, et al. Damage control resuscitation: directly addressing the early coagulopathy of trauma. J Trauma. 2007;62(2):307-10.
16. Balogh Z, McKinley BA, Cox CS Jr, et al. Abdominal compartment syndrome: the cause or effect of postinjury multiple organ failure. Shock. 2003;20(6):483-92.
17. Balogh Z, McKinley BA, Cocanour CS, et al. Supranormal trauma resuscitation causes more cases of abdominal compartment syndrome. Arch Surg. 2003;138(6):637-42; discussion 642-3.
18. Borgman MA, Spinella PC, Perkins JG, et al. The ratio of blood products transfused affects mortality in patients receiving massive transfusions at a combat support hospital. J Trauma. 2007;63(4):805-13.
19. Rappold JF, Pusateri AE. Tranexamic acid in remote damage control resuscitation. Transfusion. 2013;53(Suppl 1): 96S-9S.
20. Duchesne JC, Hunt JP, Wahl G, et al. Review of current blood transfusions strategies in a mature level I trauma center: were we wrong for the last 60 years? J Trauma. 2008;65(2):272-6; discussion 276-8; 21.
21. Duchesne JC, Kimonis K, Marr AB, et al. Damage control resuscitation in combination with damage control laparotomy: a survival advantage. J Trauma. 2010;69(1):46-52.
22. Mitra B, Mori A, Cameron PA, et al. Fresh frozen plasma (FFP) use during massive blood transfusion in trauma resuscitation. Injury. 2010;41(1):35-9.
23. Campion EM, Pritts TA, Dorlac WC, et al. Implementation of a military-derived damage-control resuscitation strategy in a civilian trauma center decreases acute hypoxia in massively transfused patients. J Trauma Acute Care Surg. 2013;75(2 Suppl 2):S221-7.
24. Haury B, Rodeheaver G, Vensko J, et al. Debridement: an essential component of traumatic wound care. Am J Surg. 1978;135(2):238-42.
25. Zonies D, Eastridge B. Combat management of splenic injury: trends during a decade of conflict. J Trauma Acute Care Surg. 2012;73(2 Suppl 1):S71-4.
26. Kragh JF Jr, Walters TJ, Baer DG, et al. Survival with emergency tourniquet use to stop bleeding in major limb trauma. Ann Surg. 2009;249(1):1-7.
27. Zonies D, DuBose J, Elterman J, et al. Early implementation of continuous renal replacement therapy optimizes casualty evacuation for combat-related acute kidney injury. J Trauma Acute Care Surg. 2013;75(2 Suppl 2):S210-4.

34

Trauma in the Elderly, in Pregnancy, and in Children

Graeme J Pitcher, Gerald P Kealey

Key Points

- Trauma care for patients in the three special interest groups, the old, the young, and the fetomaternal unit, needs to be tailored to each group's special needs.
- The reduced physiological reserves of the elderly patient mandate proactive monitoring and prompt yet prudent therapeutic strategies.
- Communication about end-of-life care should be opened early and candidly with high-risk elderly trauma patients and their families, but such discussions should not supersede the normal goals of care.
- Injured pregnant women pose the challenge of caring for two separate individuals, one of whom is inaccessible and extremely vulnerable.
- Favorable fetal outcome after maternal injury depends entirely on the adequacy of the care of the injured mother. Good maternal resuscitation and recognition of injuries to the fetoplacental unit that jeopardize both parties are essential.
- Injured children have an age-specific array of different injuries as well as unique physiological and social dynamics that need to be addressed in order to provide good quality, comprehensive care.

TRAUMA IN THE ELDERLY

Epidemiology

Although the threshold for consideration as elderly is obviously a matter of some controversy, most literature addressing the special medical needs of this patient group use the age of 65 years or greater. United States census data from 2010 demonstrate the progressive aging of the population. There is a 57% female gender preponderance.[1] The percentage of the US population over 65 years of age is 13% (up from 12.5% in 2000) and represents a total of 40 million people, an increase of 14% since the 2000 census. By the year 2050 that number is expected to rise to 88 million.[2] Elderly trauma victims have a higher and disproportionate mortality when compared with younger age cohorts. Data from 2008 to 2012 at the University of Iowa, a level one trauma center that serves a predominantly rural population, revealed that patients > 65 years of age comprised 23% of trauma admissions and contributed to 50% of all trauma mortalities. The overall mortality for trauma patients < 65 years of age is 4.3%, whereas that for the older group was 8.5%. These poorer outcomes in elderly patients have been a consistent finding over the period of study.[3,4]

Physiologic Changes in the Elderly

Cardiovascular

The aging heart shows age-dependent degenerative changes, even in good health. These include progressive diastolic and end-diastolic dysfunction, decreased cardiac output, and frequent age-related hypertension. Cardiac output and stroke volume decrease by 0.5–1.0% per year starting in middle age in individuals without overt cardiac disease. The aging healthy heart has lesser ventricular reserves and therefore may not be able to mount an adequate response if and when disease or traumatic injury results in a hypermetabolic state. Every degree centigrade rise in core temperature necessitates an 8–12% rise in oxygen consumption, carbon dioxide production, minute ventilation, and cardiac output. When compounded by a low hemoglobin level, demand ischemia may develop, resulting in failure of substrate delivery and peripheral end-organ hypoxia and anaerobic metabolism. This predisposes to the development of end-organ failure, multisystem organ failure, and death.[5] In addition to this normal aging of the heart, coronary artery and valve diseases are common issues in the aging human and these contribute significantly to trauma morbidity.[6] Many senior citizens develop rhythm and rate abnormalities, hypertension and congestive heart failure prior to any traumatic event. A recent review of the University of Iowa trauma registry revealed that 58% of all elderly trauma patients were taking some form of anticoagulation or antiplatelet medications prior to injury. The concomitant use of β-blockers, calcium channel blockers, and antihypertensive medications further complicated the management of this patient group. A thorough and complete review of any and all cardiac medications and history of interventions is crucial in order to provide optimal management.

Pulmonary

The architecture and functional characteristics of the lungs show age-related degenerative changes that are predictable and quantifiable. The vital capacity decreases with age, resulting in a loss of total lung capacity. There are emphysematous changes in the parenchyma of the lungs resulting in an increase of dead space and reduced elasticity and compliance of the lung tissue. Mid-maximal expiratory flow rate decreases with age. The functional residual capacity (FRC) decreases with age, and when the FRC is less than the closing volume of the lungs, atelectasis occurs. The elderly patient is intrinsically predisposed to atelectasis, ventilation/perfusion mismatch, and inflammatory disease of the lungs. The addition of an acute traumatic injury poses a very high risk of acute respiratory failure. This situation is life threatening and requires prompt diagnosis and the expeditious provision of supportive care. These steps may include oxygen supplementation, continuous SaO_2 monitoring, noninvasive ventilation, intubation, and ventilation in an orderly and pre-emptive approach. Hypoxia and hypercarbia are dangerous and deadly to any group of patients and must be avoided or remedied emergently.[7] Pneumonia and ventilator dependence are a constant risk in the elderly trauma patient. Careful application of preventative protocols reduces the risk of ventilator-associated pneumonia and the aspiration and contamination of the pulmonary tree by oral secretions. Assessment of the aspiration risk for the individual patient can be done at the bedside by trained nursing personnel. Intensive care protocols should include daily ventilator weaning assessment and careful review of cardiopulmonary status with a constant effort directed toward timely and appropriate withdrawal of ventilatory support and prevention of pulmonary infections.

Renal

Renal insufficiency has been documented to substantially increase mortality in any patient group regardless of the primary diagnosis. The aging kidney loses 1% of the creatinine clearance rate per year after age 30. Timely and adequate restoration of circulating blood volume and maintenance of cardiac output are the most effective measures to forestall renal dysfunction. Low cardiac output states, nephrotoxic drugs, and hypovolemia must be avoided or promptly remedied. If acute kidney injury (AKI) develops, then renal replacement therapy is indicated for a duration necessitated by the course of the illness. Even though the mortality rate of AKI in the elderly is high and the prognosis for recovery of renal function poorer than in young patients, advanced age alone should not be a contraindication to the use of such treatment.[9]

Management and Assessment of the Elderly Trauma Patient

The advanced trauma life support (ATLS) protocol should be used (for more details *see* Chapter 31, "Initial Trauma Evaluation and Resuscitation"). Life-threatening injuries are identified and assigned the highest priority. Elderly patients should be triaged to higher level trauma centers or academic hospitals.[10] Resuscitation should be focused on the provision of adequate ventilation and oxygenation, ensuring adequate tissue perfusion. The base deficit, lactate levels, arterial blood gases, urine output, and all routine end points of resuscitation must be monitored, and trends toward normalization established. Adequate oxygen carrying capacity and red cell mass must be maintained. Although there are no strong data to mandate the use of more aggressive invasive monitoring, there is a trend to the use of pulmonary artery catheters in this group to refine the endpoints of resuscitation.[11]

Head Injury

The most frequent cause of death in the elderly trauma victim is neurological trauma. Starting at about 45 years of age, increasing age is linearly associated with higher mortality rates and poorer neurological outcomes.[12,13] Patients with a Glasgow coma scale (GCS) score of <8 who are >65 years of age have a predicted mortality of 74%, compared to 18% in the age group 18–40 years.[14] Careful and repeated evaluation and assessment of neurological function is essential, and a computed tomographic (CT) scan of the head and cervical spine is a crucial diagnostic study. Confusion and delirium is common in elderly head-injured patients, rendering neurological evaluation difficult. Repeated CT imaging and a high index of suspicion may be the only way to detect expanding intracranial mass lesions in a timely manner. Preexisting anticoagulation and antiplatelet use in the elderly head-injured patient poses an especially common and dangerous problem. Such patients should be carefully examined, imaging obtained, and their coagulation profile restored to normal in an expeditious manner. This might necessitate the use of fresh frozen plasma, activated factor VIIA, tranexamic acid, vitamin K, cryoprecipitate, or prothrombin concentrate as appropriate.[6] Consultation with a hematologist is often essential in determining the best therapeutic option.

Thoracic Injury

The thoracic spine frequently develops a kyphotic curvature with aging, resulting in a loss of total lung capacity. The bony skeleton of the thorax becomes less mobile and more brittle with stiffening of the rib joints and osteoporosis. This results in more frequent rib fractures, pulmonary contusions, and hemopneumothoraces. These problems should be identified in the initial assessment, and tube thoracostomy should be placed where needed. When respiratory insufficiency is identified, steps must be taken to provide timely and adequate ventilation and oxygenation to the patient. Careful assessment of the thoracic and lumbar vertebrae must be done to evaluate for vertebral body fractures and potential spinal cord injury.[14]

Abdominal Injury

Elderly trauma patients with multiple injuries have a high incidence of intra-abdominal injuries. Diminished physiologic reserves make them intolerant of prolonged periods of hemodynamic instability. These factors lead the trauma surgeon to be faced with earlier decisions about operative and nonoperative management of abdominal injuries. This should also prompt an earlier consideration of damage control procedures in such patients. The damage control procedure is focused on control of the life-threatening injuries, truncating the operative procedures to achieve only the immediate lifesaving goals. Hemostasis is achieved, blood flow to vital organs is restored, and intestinal contamination is controlled as expeditiously as possible. The abdomen is packed with sponges where necessary, and left open to minimize the risk of abdominal compartment syndrome. The patient is then transferred to an intensive care setting, where normothermia, repletion of coagulation factors, and hemodynamic stability are achieved. Once stable, the patient is then returned for definitive management of all injuries in a timely manner. Decisions must be based on the individual patient's overall physiological status and pre-existing health status. There is evidence that nonoperative management of splenic injuries fails more frequently in the older patient group than in their younger counterparts.[15] Operative repair of solid visceral injuries in the monitored safety of the operating room seems to be safer than poorly conceived nonoperative management.

Orthopedic Injury

Osteoporosis and low bone density predispose to fractures of all kinds in the elderly trauma patient. Blunt chest injury and rib fractures are very common. These injuries contribute to the increased mortality of blunt chest injury in this group. Pelvic fractures result in mortality rates that are three to five times higher in the elderly. The elderly patient with a pelvic fracture is more likely to require interventions to achieve hemostasis and has a peculiar propensity to suffer lateral compression fractures.[16] Cervical spine injuries more frequently involve multiple levels, occur commonly in the higher spine at the C1 or C2 level, and are often unstable. Hip and femur fractures are classic geriatric injuries that necessitate operative management in an early and expeditious manner to preserve life and function.[14]

End-of-Life and Palliative Care Issues

Everything that has a beginning has an end. The injured elderly patient has an uncertain prognosis due to the constellation of challenges described in the preceding sections. The patient, their families, or caregivers must be fully informed of the gravity of the situation and probable outcomes as candidly as the available information permits. The patient, if lucid, retains the right to self-determination. If there is a living will or a durable power of attorney concerning health care decisions, goals of care are more easily determined. If none of these standards pertain, then decisions must be made that are based on the patient's best interest. When the patient has no advance directive and cannot communicate, then usually the next of kin and/or the entire family are included in all discussions to establish goals and limits of care. The legitimate spokesperson or persons must be acknowledged and identified in this process in order to protect the legal status of the physician and hospital. These discussions may take place over days and can be extremely trying for all parties involved. The involvement of a palliative care specialist and the advice of an ethics consultant may be invaluable in difficult cases.[17]

TRAUMA IN PREGNANCY

Epidemiology

Trauma is said to complicate 6–8% of pregnancies in the United States. In developing countries with population pyramids skewed toward younger age and greater birth rates, the problem is, if anything, more common. Mechanisms of injury include motor vehicle accidents (MVAs), falls, burns, and assaults. At our institution, 2% of injured women of childbearing age were found to be pregnant at the time of injury. Most injuries were caused by MVAs. There was a significant fetal morbidity and mortality. Fetal loss occurred in 7% of mothers admitted for injury and an additional 2% reported considering seeking a voluntary abortion as a result of the trauma.[3]

In reported series, assaults (most commonly due to domestic violence) predominate as the cause of fetal and maternal death.[18,19] The burden of serious trauma in pregnancy seems to be disproportionately shouldered by women of lower socioeconomic class, lower maternal age, unmarried status and those who abuse alcohol or drugs, or who were exposed to domestic violence as children.[20,21] This information has important implications for preventative strategies.

Physiologic Changes of Pregnancy

The physiologic changes of pregnancy[22] are well known and are summarized in Table 34.1. Blood volume expansion seen in late gestation is protective to the mother, as she can tolerate significant blood volume loss before a change in heart rate or blood pressure. This may be protective for the mother but in states of compensated maternal shock may be associated with splanchnic vasoconstriction with an attendant compromise in uterine and hence fetal blood flow. Crystalloid resuscitation and prompt administration of type specific blood are the cornerstones of fluid resuscitation. Inotropic agents should be avoided if possible, because they may aggravate uterine vasoconstriction. Frank maternal shock is very dangerous to the fetus, and fetal death occurs in approximately 80% of women presenting in this state.[23] Although pregnancy is widely deemed to be a hypercoaguable state, few guidelines exist for the use of prophylactic anticoagulation. Clinical judgment should be exercised, and when necessary, either unfractionated heparin or low molecular weight heparin (LMWH) can be used. If LMWH is selected, the standard dose should be increased by 20% to compensate for the greater volume of distribution as well as a higher glomerular filtration rate.[24] Warfarin is contraindicated as it crosses the placental barrier, is teratogenic in early pregnancy, and can cause fetal bleeding complications in later gestation.

Table 34.1 Physiologic and anatomic changes associated with pregnancy.

Cardiovascular	Cardiac output increases second and third trimester
	Heart rate increases
	Systolic blood pressure decreases (nadir 30 weeks)
	Electrocardiographic axis left shift
	Oxygen consumption increases 30–60%
Blood volume and fluid	Plasma volume increases 40%
	White blood count elevated
	Fibrinogen and other clotting factors elevated
	Decreased albumin and serum oncotic pressure
Respiratory	Increased minute ventilation with hypocapnia
	Decreased functional residual capacity
	Lower esophageal sphincter pressures—prone to aspiration
Renal	Increased glomerular filtration rate and low creatinine
	Proteinuria common
	Ureteric dilatation
Gastrointestinal	Decreased gastric motility
Musculoskeletal	Laxity of all ligaments
	Widening of symphysis pubis and sacroiliac joints

Source: Hill CC, Pickinpaugh J. Physiologic changes in pregnancy. Surg Clin North Am. 2008;88:391-401, vii.

Management

The cornerstones of management of the complex feto-maternal unit represented by the injured pregnant woman are rapidly instituted and comprise high-quality maternal resuscitation and accurate fetal monitoring. Women of childbearing age may not be obviously pregnant and even a second- or third- trimester gravid uterus can be missed on abdominal examination in the obese. All pregnant trauma patients > 20 weeks' gestation should be transferred to a center that is capable of managing both complex injuries as well as providing multidisciplinary obstetric care.[25]

Resuscitation should proceed along the normal lines recommended by ATLS, with the mother immobilized in the supine position, rotated slightly to the left to relieve vena caval compression caused by the gravid uterus. If the mother's condition is critical, all necessary treatment should be given with no delays caused by the need to evaluate the fetus. Monitoring of fetal heart tones is recommended as early as feasible as part of the primary survey. Tocodynamometry should be commenced as soon as feasible. The ideal duration of monitoring should be determined by the circumstances of the case as well as the severity of trauma, but should be continued for 2–6 hours at least. [26,27] Evaluation of the mother should include a specific pregnancy oriented physical examination (Table 34.2). The early involvement of an obstetrician to guide these aspects of care is mandatory.

All X-rays needed to diagnose injury in the mother should be performed. A missed injury due to reluctance to expose the fetus to radiation is a potential disaster for both mother and child. The effects of radiation at different stages of gestation are represented in Table 34.3. Intravenous (IV) contrast appears to be safe for use in pregnancy, but gadolinium is teratogenic and should always be avoided. Ultrasonography is a useful screening test for hemoperitoneum and solid visceral injury and needs to be augmented with CT scanning when indicated as in the nonpregnant patient. The dose estimated to accrue to the fetus in a typical abdominal CT scan is 30–43 mGy (3–4.3 rad),[28] well within safety limits if used prudently.

Table 34.2 Specific examination of the pregnant woman.

Abdominal	Pelvic skeletal stability
	Height of fundus
	Presence of uterine contractions, tenderness, or irritability
	Assessment of fetal position
Vaginal	Perineal inspection
	Bleeding
	Amniotic fluid
	State of cervix and dilatation

Fetomaternal hemorrhage refers to the passage of fetal blood into the maternal circulation and is known to occur in 9% to 30% of women who sustain an injury during pregnancy.[29] Important consequences are isoimmunization of Rh-mothers by Rh+ fetuses and fetal compromise by hypovolemia. The latter is rare but all Rh-mothers should undergo a Kleihauer Betke assay. If fetomaternal hemorrhage is detected, then 300 µg Rh immune globulin should be given. This dose will suffice for most cases, but if the volume of hemorrhage exceeds 30 mL, then more may be required.

Special Considerations

Abruptio Placentae

Abruptio placenta refers to a separation in the plane between the uterus and the placenta. It is seen after trauma with an increasing frequency depending on the severity of the injury, and can be present in patients with no apparent injury.[30] Ultrasonography may not detect the condition with sufficient accuracy, and it is suggested by a history of significant trauma with uterine tenderness and vaginal bleeding. In patients beyond 23–24 weeks, tocodynamometry is the most sensitive predictor of abruption after trauma.[29] Consequences range from none to fetal demise, and therefore fetal monitoring and intervention based on clinical course and the state of viability of the fetus is recommended.

Table 34.3 Summary of American College of Radiology practice guideline for imaging pregnant or potentially pregnant adolescents and women with ionizing radiation.

Age of conception	*<5 rad (50 mGy)*	*5–10 rad (50–100 mGy)*	*>10 rad (100 mGy)*
1–14 days	None	Probably none	None
15–56 days	None	Potential effects uncertain, or of questionable significance	Possible malformations increasing in incidence with increasing dose
9th–15th weeks	None	Potential effects uncertain, or of questionable significance	Intelligence quotient (IQ) deficit and mental retardation with increasing incidence and severity with increasing doses
16th–25th weeks	None	None	IQ deficits not detectable at diagnostic doses
> 27th weeks	None	None	Not applicable to diagnostic medicine

Uterine Rupture

This is a rare dramatic event, occurring in < 0.6% of injured pregnant women. It is suggested by maternal shock with hemoperitoneum and an abnormal fetal position with an indistinctly palpable fundic height. Fetal mortality rates are high and heart sounds are usually not detectable during resuscitation. Oftentimes pregnancy is not suspected, but discovered at surgery. Management is by laparotomy and evacuation of the fetus. Hemostasis is achieved by uterine repair or hysterectomy, as dictated by the circumstances.

Perimortem Cesarean Section

When a pregnant woman with a viable fetus is deteriorating despite normal resuscitative attempts or has an obviously lethal injury, then cesarean section should be considered.[31] Fetal and maternal outcomes are improved if this is undertaken within 5 minutes of maternal cardiac arrest—the so-called "5 minute rule". In a surprisingly large number of cases, there is a dramatic improvement in maternal status allowing survival. This is attributed to relief of the aortocaval compression by the gravid uterus[32] and more effective cardiopulmonary resuscitation after emptying of the uterus.[33]

Penetrating Abdominal Trauma

Gunshot wounds and stab injuries occur in about 10% of women who sustain abdominal injury during pregnancy. Maternal mortality is significant, and fetal mortality from 40% to 73% has been reported.[34] Upper abdominal injuries are associated with maternal bowel injury, whereas lower abdominal injury tends to cause uterine and fetal injury. Management is usually by surgical exploration, although conservative management may be warranted for stable mothers with stable fetuses where injury is in the lower abdomen.[35]

TRAUMA IN CHILDREN

Epidemiology

In the United States and worldwide, trauma is the commonest cause of death in children after the first year of life. When considering the mechanism of injury, falls predominate in the age group 0–9 years while MVAs predominate in the age group 10–18 years. Penetrating injury seems to be increasing in frequency, particularly in the adolescent group, and in those from urban and less affluent communities.[36] Patterns of injury differ between different countries and regions, depending on the state of urbanization and other geopolitical circumstances. Children living in areas affected by war and other forms of social upheaval are particularly at risk and are all too commonly injured or killed.[37] "Nonaccidental" injury caused by child abuse or neglect continues to affect scores of children and is most likely to cause severe or life-threatening injuries in the younger child. At the University of Iowa, abuse or neglect was suspected in 11% of admissions to hospital in children < 18 years of age and represents the commonest cause of severe head injury in the infant.[3] Targeted injury prevention programs have made some impact in developed countries but are woefully absent in many parts of the world.

Management of Pediatric Trauma Patients

Resuscitation in the Field

It is universally agreed that all pediatric trauma patients should be resuscitated according to the management priorities suggested by ATLS and then appropriately immobilized for transport when needed. This should include in-line spinal immobilization and stabilization of fractures. The child's airway should be secured and vascular access obtained. There has been considerable debate over whether prolonged attempts at stabilization—"stay and play"—at the scene are preferable or whether rapid transfer to a center for definitive care—"scoop and run"—results in better outcomes. No simple generalizations are possible and the answer will certainly depend upon factors such as the quality of prehospital care and the experience of such providers and the distances involved in transfer.[38] The fortunately rare patient with evidence of life-threatening internal bleeding should be transported without delay, as prompt surgical intervention may be their only hope of survival. The need for prolonged cardiopulmonary resuscitation in the field carries a grave prognosis for survival and neurological outcome, particularly if this needs to be continued during transfer to the treating hospital.[39]

Airway and Ventilation

The airway remains the most frequently mismanaged component of pediatric resuscitation. This is probably a result of anatomic unfamiliarity and the poor application of size- and age-specific interventions. Tube misplacement—either too deep or in an esophageal position—and the use of inappropriate-sized tubes remain distressingly common. The infant larynx is situated in a more anterior position than the adult and a large tongue and floppy epiglottis need to be negotiated in order to intubate. A straight Miller-type blade is generally preferred in children under 2 years of age and is used by picking up the epiglottis directly with the tip. The subglottic area is the narrowest portion of the child's airway and the most vulnerable to injury by pressure or direct trauma. For this reason, uncuffed endotracheal tubes are traditionally recommended, but cuffed tubes with carefully monitored cuff pressures are increasingly being used by more experienced providers for the benefits of improved airway protection. Tube size is generally determined by the diameter of the external nares or the diameter of the child's fifth finger. The tube size for an uncuffed tube can be estimated using the equation:

$$\text{Size} = [\text{age (years)}/4] + 4$$

In the event that intubation is unsuccessful and an airway needs to be urgently established, needle cricothyroidotomy is indicated. Ventilator-induced lung injury should be avoided by the use of tidal volumes of 7–10 mL/kg.

Fluid Resuscitation

A common error is the failure of recognition of pediatric hypovolemia. Tachycardia, pallor, poor perfusion, and mental status changes are the hallmarks of pediatric shock. Hypotension can be absent until the late stages of shock when decompensation occurs and is often an ominous sign. It can be safely assumed that a tachycardic, injured child is hypovolemic until proven otherwise.

Vascular access should be achieved by placement of a peripheral IV line of suitable bore, usually in named large peripheral veins, such as the saphenous, cephalic, or antecubital veins. If this strategy fails after two attempts in a severely shocked patient, then insertion of an intraosseous catheter or the performance of a cutdown to access the great saphenous vein should be employed. Central lines have a greater complication rate, especially in small children and should generally be avoided.

The initial fluid of choice to restore intravascular volume remains lactated Ringers or normal saline. An initial bolus of 20 mL/kg should be given and can be repeated. In children with traumatic brain injury, resuscitation with hypertonic saline, usually in a concentration of 3%, is becoming more widespread.[40]

Special Considerations

Head Injuries

Traumatic brain injury continues to be the commonest cause of traumatic death in all age groups of children. The burden of morbidity carried by these patients and their families and the expense to the medical systems that care for these children are enormous.[41] It has been long accepted that children (with the possible exception of infants) have more favorable outcomes from head injury than their adult counterparts.[42] Patterns of injury depend on age. Infants are vulnerable to nonaccidental injury, falls, and vehicular trauma; toddlers to falls; and older children and adolescents are often injured by bicycle accidents and vehicle trauma and assaults, respectively.

The child's large brain relative to their body mass is also poorly protected by a thin skull, rendering it very vulnerable to direct injury and the effects of acceleration and deceleration forces. This produces the primary injury to the brain parenchyma—typically lacerations, small hematomas, and axonal injury from shearing forces. Children have a higher incidence of diffuse injury without surface hemorrhages or collections requiring surgical drainage, more typically seen in adult trauma patients. This primary injury cannot be treated or ameliorated.

There are then two discrete types of secondary injury:

1. Hypoxemia, hypotension, hypercarbia, brain compression as a result of expanding hematomas, metabolic abnormalities such as hypoglycemia and electrolyte abnormalities, seizures, and cerebral edema may result in secondary injury. The avoidance and treatment of these physiologic and metabolic derangements and their sequelae remains the backbone of head injury care.
2. A dangerous syndrome of malignant or accelerated severe cerebral edema (more commonly in young children after high-speed vehicular trauma and thought to be due to disturbed autoregulation) can occur in a delayed fashion up to days after the initial traumatic event. If this is not recognized and rapidly treated, death and poor outcomes are the norm.

Intracranial pressure monitoring is recommended for children with a GCS score of 8 or less. Cerebral perfusion pressure (CPP; the pressure gradient providing for cerebral blood flow) is defined as:

$$\text{Mean arterial pressure} - \text{intracranial pressure}$$

Mortality and poor neurological outcomes have been consistently observed with CPP < 40 mm Hg in children, and the objective of care should be to maintain CPP in the range of 50–55 mm Hg. Established cerebral edema is now treated with a two-tiered approach.[43]

First-tier management consists broadly of sedation and analgesia, neuromuscular blockade and mild hyperventilation with CSF drainage via a ventriculostomy and hyperosmolar therapy using either hypertonic saline or

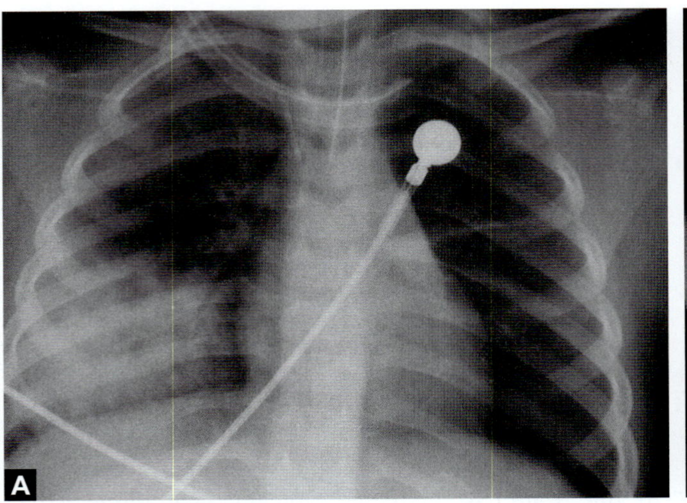

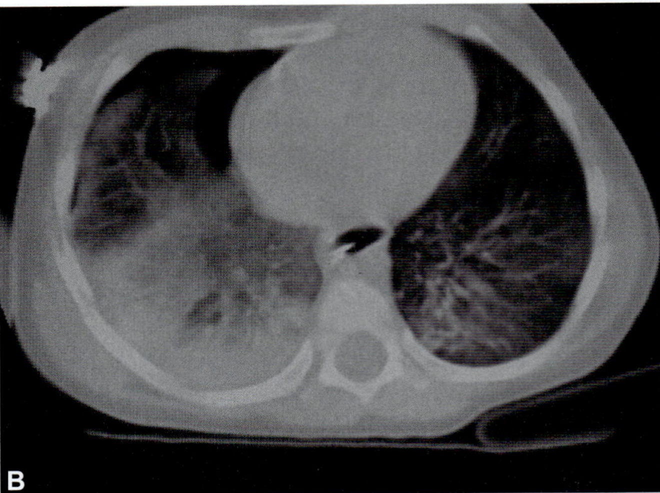

Figs. 34.1A and B: An 11-year-old boy with blunt thoracic trauma. (A) X-ray suggests contusion of right lower lobe. (B) Computed tomography identifies small pneumothorax and accurately delineates extent of pulmonary contusion.

mannitol. Second-tier management in patients with ongoing intracranial hypertension includes consideration of the need for high-dose barbiturate therapy, hypothermia, lumbar drainage, or decompressive craniectomy. The latter is a treatment option for children with severe diffuse injury who show evidence of progression of intracranial hypertension despite medical management.[44] Favorable outcomes can be achieved with timely intervention in well-selected patients before ischemic brain damage has occurred, but its role remains controversial. Early neurosurgical consultation in such patients is mandatory.

Thoracic Injury

Blunt injury to the chest causes a similar spectrum of injuries in the child as in the adult. The cartilaginous and supple chest wall of the child results in fewer fractures and affords less protection to the internal organs, resulting in a propensity for children to suffer pulmonary contusion without rib fractures. Contusion may not be evident on early plain chest films and the development of respiratory distress mandates repeated films when the injury may become evident. Contusions are much more readily diagnosed with a chest CT scan (Figs. 34.1A and B). Supportive management is usually effective. Fluid restriction is no longer advocated. Blunt aortic injury occurs much less frequently, with the exception of teenagers who appear to be at a similar risk to young adults for this injury.

Abdominal Injury

Abdominal injury occurs relatively frequently in childhood. Blunt injury accounts for most cases but penetrating injury from stabs, gunshots, and other accidental penetrations appear to be increasing, especially in inner city communities and in regions affected by conflict. The standard of care of penetrating injury in childhood remains exploratory laparotomy, with selective conservatism and laparoscopy being applied in selected cases by some. Children who are unstable should be explored with a generous midline vertical incision to afford rapid, good quality access to the pelvis and diaphragmatic hiatus for vascular control.[45]

In blunt injury, the liver and spleen are the most commonly injured organs. Traumatic pancreatitis is common, especially after blunt handlebar type injuries or lap belt injuries with hyperflexion. Serum amylase estimation should be performed on all children with suspected blunt abdominal injury to detect this injury. Hollow organ injury occurs less commonly but may be difficult to detect in a timely manner in patients undergoing conservative treatment.

The cornerstones of clinical care are as follows:

- Clinical evaluation and the recognition of need for early operative intervention.
  - Signs of peritonitis.
  - Clear signs of abdominal injury with hemodynamic instability unresponsive to resuscitation.
- Obtaining imaging studies in patients selected for nonoperative management. Contrast-enhanced CT scanning is the most helpful in this regard. Focused abdominal sonography in trauma (FAST) is not widely used or thoroughly validated for use in children,[46] partially as a result of the high incidence of significant abdominal injury without free fluid in this group.[47] Diagnostic peritoneal lavage is no longer used except

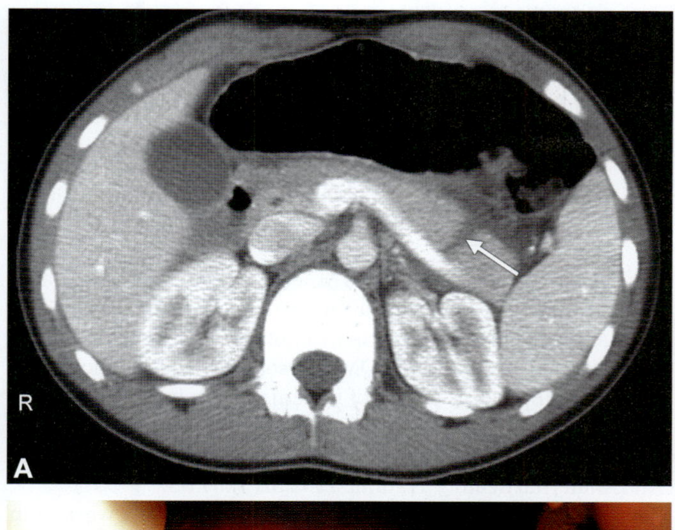

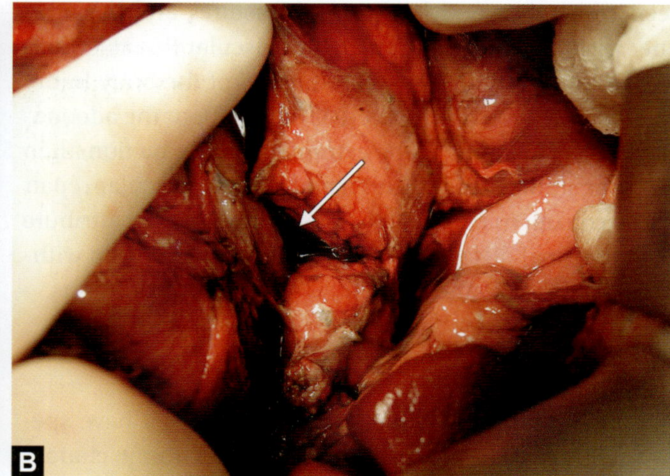

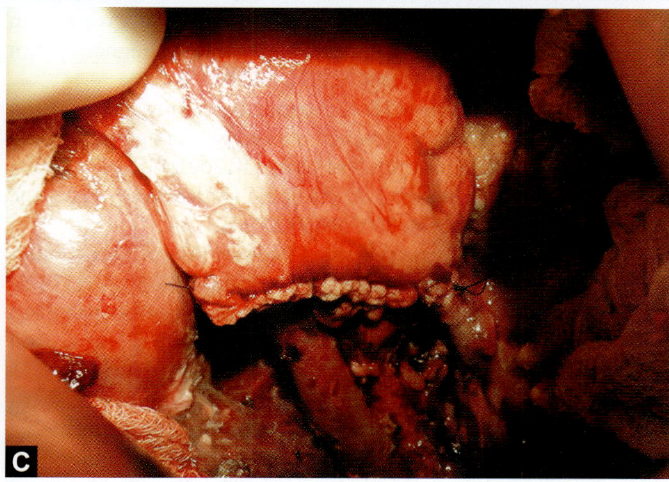

Figs. 34.2A to C: (A) Computed tomographic scan showing clear pancreatic transection in the tail of the pancreas, (B) operative findings, and (C) end result of operative distal pancreatectomy.

when CT is not available or in the hemodynamically unstable trauma patient with a negative or equivocal FAST examination.

- Institution of nonoperative management including hemodynamic monitoring, fluid therapy, blood transfusion as needed, bowel rest, and serial examinations.
- Prompt interventions for identified failure of nonoperative management or the development of complications.

The vast majority (>95%) of splenic injuries of all radiological grades can be managed successfully nonoperatively. In the unusual case where an operation is needed for hemostasis, splenic salvage should be attempted, especially in the young child < 10 years of age. Liver injury success rates are almost as good but are occasionally complicated by the development of complications such as bile leak, hemobilia, and symptomatic abdominal fluid collections, many of which can be managed by interventional radiological techniques.[48] If emergency operative intervention is necessary for unstable patients with severe liver lacerations, packing and embolization are generally safer than heroic attempts at hepatic resection. Traumatic pancreatitis is usually managed conservatively, but in the context of complete pancreatic transection, operative management by distal pancreatectomy will lead to a more rapid recovery (Figs. 34.2A to C).[49]

A legitimate concern is whether children are adversely affected by a delay in diagnosis of bowel injury, recognized by clinical criteria such as increasing pain, tenderness, fever or ileus while undergoing nonoperative management. It is the authors' contention that such an injury detected diligently and treated promptly does not add unduly to the burden of morbidity and does not compromise the safety of nonoperative management.[50]

Orthopedic and Limb Injury

Children with multiple long bone fractures can suffer disproportionate blood loss and should be managed with aggressive immobilization and resuscitation. In contrast, pelvic fractures are rarely life threatening in children.[8] Vascular compromise as a result of arterial injury is typically seen with supracondylar humeral fractures and posterior knee dislocations. Recognizing the vascular threat is vitally important. In most cases, reduction of the bony injury will restore blood flow. If there is doubt about the adequacy of vascular supply to the extremity after reduction, then vascular studies are indicated and prompt vascular repair is undertaken to restore flow to the extremity. To attribute any abnormal distal pulse findings to arterial spasm without excluding an arterial injury is potentially hazardous.

SUMMARY

The elderly, pregnant women, and children all have specific patterns of injury, physiologic and anatomic characteristics and present unique therapeutic and rehabilitative challenges. A focused approach, tailored to their special requirements, is essential for good outcomes after injury. All three of these patient groups are best treated in higher level trauma services, academic centers, or specialized units by teams of caregivers with experience in their care.

REFERENCES

1. 2010 Census Summary File. (2010). Available from http://www.census.gov/population/www/cen2010/glance/index.html. [Accessed July 31, 2013].
2. Department of health and human services. Administration on aging. 2013. Available from http://www.aoa.acl.gov/Aging_Statistics/future_growth/future_growth.aspx#age.
3. University of Iowa Hospitals and Clinics Trauma Database, 2008- 2010. (2010).
4. The 2011 Iowa Health Facts. (2011). Available from http://www.public-health.uiowa.edu/factbook/. [Accessed July 31, 2013].
5. Scalea TM, Simon HM, Duncan AO, et al. Geriatric blunt multiple trauma: improved survival with early invasive monitoring. J Trauma. 1990;30(2):129-34; discussion 34-6.
6. Ferraris VA, Ferraris SP, Saha SP. The relationship between mortality and preexisting cardiac disease in 5,971 trauma patients. J Trauma. 2010;69(3):645-52.
7. Lumb A. Nunn's Applied Repiratory Phsysiology, 7th edition. Edinburgh: Churchill Livingstone; 2010.
8. Ismail N, Bellemare JF, Mollitt DL, et al. Death from pelvic fracture: children are different. J Pediatr Surg. 1996;31(1):82-5.
9. Pascual J, Liaño F, Ortuño J. The elderly patient with acute renal failure. J Am Soc Nephrol. 1995;6(2):144-53.
10. Mangram AJ, Mitchell CD, Shifflette VK, et al. Geriatric trauma service: a one-year experience. J Trauma Acute Care Surg. 2012;72(1):119-22.
11. Brown CV, Shoemaker WC, Wo CC, et al. Is noninvasive hemodynamic monitoring appropriate for the elderly critically injured patient? J Trauma. 2005;58(1):102-7.
12. Mosenthal AC, Lavery RF, Addis M, et al. Isolated traumatic brain injury: age is an independent predictor of mortality and early outcome. J Trauma. 2002;52(5):907-11.
13. Hukkelhoven CW, Steyerberg EW, Rampen AJ, et al. Patient age and outcome following severe traumatic brain injury: an analysis of 5600 patients. J Neurosurg. 2003;99(4):666-73.
14. Jacobs DG. Special considerations in geriatric injury. Current opinion in critical care. 2003;9(6):535-9.
15. Peitzman AB, Heil B, Rivera L, et al. Blunt splenic injury in adults: multi-institutional Study of the Eastern Association for the Surgery of Trauma. J Trauma. 2000;49(2):177-87; discussion 87-9.
16. Henry SM, Pollak AN, Jones AL, et al. Pelvic fracture in geriatric patients: a distinct clinical entity. J Trauma. 2002;53(1):15-20.
17. Annas GJ. Judging Medicine. Clifton, NJ: Humana Press; 1988.
18. Dannenberg AL, Carter DM, Lawson HW, et al. Homicide and other injuries as causes of maternal death in New York City, 1987 through 1991. Am J Obstet Gynecol. 1995;172(5):1557-64.
19. Fildes J, Reed L, Jones N, et al . Trauma: the leading cause of maternal death. J Trauma. 1992;32(5):643-5.
20. Castro R, Peek-Asa C, Ruiz A. Violence against women in Mexico: a study of abuse before and during pregnancy. Am J Public Health. 2003;93(7):1110-16.
21. Quinlivan JA, Evans SF. A prospective cohort study of the impact of domestic violence on young teenage pregnancy outcomes. J Pediatr Adolesc Gynecol. 2001;14(1):17-23.
22. Hill CC, Pickinpaugh J. Physiologic changes in pregnancy. Surg Clin North Am. 2008;88(2):391-401, vii.
23. Rothenberger D, Quattlebaum FW, Perry JF, et al. Blunt maternal trauma: a review of 103 cases. J Trauma. 1978;18(3):173-9.
24. Jacobsen AF, Sandset PM. Venous thromboembolism associated with pregnancy and hormonal therapy. Best Pract Res Clin Haematol. 2012;25(3):319-32.
25. Sasser SM, Hunt RC, Faul M, et al. Guidelines for field triage of injured patients: recommendations of the National Expert Panel on Field Triage, 2011. MMWR Recommendations and reports: Morbidity and mortality weekly report Recommendations and reports/Centers for Disease Control. 2012;61(RR-1):1-20.
26. Pearlman MD, Tintinallli JE, Lorenz RP. A prospective controlled study of outcome after trauma during pregnancy. Am J Obstet Gynecol. 1990;162(6):1502-7; discussion 7-10.
27. Barraco RD, Chiu WC, Clancy TV, et al. Practice management guidelines for the diagnosis and management of injury in the pregnant patient: the EAST Practice Management Guidelines Work Group. J Trauma. 2010;69(1):211-4.
28. Damilakis J, Perisinakis K, Voloudaki A, et al . Estimation of fetal radiation dose from computed tomography scanning in late pregnancy: depth-dose data from routine examinations. Investigative radiology. 2000;35(9):527-33.
29. Chames MC, Pearlman MD. Trauma during pregnancy: outcomes and clinical management. Clin Obstet Gynecol. 2008;51(2):398-408.
30. Schiff MA, Holt VL. Pregnancy outcomes following hospitalization for motor vehicle crashes in Washington State from 1989 to 2001. Am J Epidemiol. 2005;161(6):503-10.
31. Vanden Hoek TL, Morrison LJ, Shuster M, et al. Part 12: cardiac arrest in special situations: 2010 American Heart Association Guidelines for Cardiopulmonary Resuscitation and Emergency Cardiovascular Care. Circulation. 2010;122 (18 Suppl 3):S829-61.

32. Katz V, Balderston K, DeFreest M. Perimortem cesarean delivery: were our assumptions correct? Am J Obstet Gynecol. 2005;192(6):1916-20; discussion 20-1.
33. Katz VL. Perimortem cesarean delivery: its role in maternal mortality. Semin Perinatol. 2012;36(1):68-72.
34. Petrone P, Talving P, Browder T, et al. Abdominal injuries in pregnancy: a 155-month study at two level 1 trauma centers. Injury. 2011;42(1):47-9.
35. Awwad JT, Azar GB, Seoud MA, et al. High-velocity penetrating wounds of the gravid uterus: review of 16 years of civil war. Obstet Gynecol. 1994;83(2):259-64.
36. Tracy ET, Englum BR, Barbas AS, et al. Pediatric injury patterns by year of age. J Pediatr Surg. 2013;48(6):1384-8.
37. Creamer KM, Edwards MJ, Shields CH, et al. Pediatric wartime admissions to US military combat support hospitals in Afghanistan and Iraq: learning from the first 2,000 admissions. J Trauma. 2009;67(4):762-8.
38. Smith RM, Conn AK. Prehospital care—scoop and run or stay and play? Injury. 2009;40 (Suppl 4):S23-6.
39. Murphy JT, Jaiswal K, Sabella J, et al. Prehospital cardiopulmonary resuscitation in the pediatric trauma patient. J Pediatr Surg. 2010;45(7):1413-9.
40. Bell MJ, Kochanek PM. Pediatric traumatic brain injury in 2012: the year with new guidelines and common data elements. Crit Care Clin. 2013;29(2):223-38.
41. Schneier AJ, Shields BJ, Hostetler SG, et al. Incidence of pediatric traumatic brain injury and associated hospital resource utilization in the United States. Pediatrics. 2006; 118(2):483-92.
42. Luerssen TG, Klauber MR, Marshall LF. Outcome from head injury related to patient's age: a longitudinal prospective study of adult and pediatric head injury. J Neurosurg. 1988;68(3):409-16.
43. Adelson PD, Bratton SL, Carney NA, et al. Guidelines for the acute medical management of severe traumatic brain injury in infants, children, and adolescents. Chapter 17. Critical pathway for the treatment of established intracranial hypertension in pediatric traumatic brain injury. Pediatr Crit Care Med. 2003;4(3 Suppl):S65-7.
44. Rutigliano D, Egnor MR, Priebe CJ, et al. Decompressive craniectomy in pediatric patients with traumatic brain injury with intractable elevated intracranial pressure. J Pediatr Surg. 2006;41(1):83-7; discussion 83-7.
45. Pitcher GJ. Ballistic trauma in children. In: Brooks AJ (Ed). Ryan's Ballistic Trauma, 3rd edition. London: Springer-Verlag; 2011. pp. 529-48.
46. Scaife ER, Rollins MD, Barnhart DC, et al. The role of focused abdominal sonography for trauma (FAST) in pediatric trauma evaluation. J Pediatr Surg. 2013;48(6):1377-83.
47. Emery KH, McAneney CM, Racadio JM, et al. Absent peritoneal fluid on screening trauma ultrasonography in children: a prospective comparison with computed tomography. J Pediatr Surg. 2001;36(4):565-9.
48. De Magnee C, Forgues D, Mercier G, et al. Complications after conservative treatment of blunt liver trauma in children. Acta chirurgica Belgica. 2012;112(4):261-7.
49. Jobst MA, Canty TG, Sr, Lynch FP. Management of pancreatic injury in pediatric blunt abdominal trauma. J Pediatr Surg. 1999;34(5):818-23; discussion 23-4.
50. Bensard DD, Beaver BL, Besner GE, et al. Small bowel injury in children after blunt abdominal trauma: is diagnostic delay important? J Trauma. 1996;41(3):476-83.

Case Study: 35 Vascular Injury in Combat and Austere Settings

Jamison S Nielsen, David H Zonies

THE PROBLEM

Vascular injuries are frequently encountered in modern combat environments, representing 12% of all nonreturn to duty wounds.[1] Whether in war or civilian practice, two principles of vascular trauma remain constant: immediate hemorrhage control and prevention of distal ischemia. Hemorrhage control takes immediate priority in order to prevent exsanguination. Next, the operative surgeon must balance the various options to restore distal perfusion in a highly variable patient. During a damage control approach,[2] formal vascular repair would be time consuming, requiring dedicated attention from the surgeon, specialized supplies, availability of blood products, and (ideally) a stable patient.

Combat surgery, austere environments, natural disasters, and other resource-limited situations may preclude formal vascular repair for several reasons:

- *Personnel:* Mass casualty situations demand prioritization of "life over limb." This is accentuated when there may only be a single surgeon available. A time-consuming formal vascular repair may not be possible if another patient is in extremis. Additionally, complex vascular repairs may be at the limits of the surgeon's expertise or experience.
- *Patient factors:* The development of acute coagulopathy of trauma exacerbated by hypothermia and acidosis increases operative times and increases mortality risk.[3,4]
- *Supplies:* Ideal performance of a vascular repair requires radiographic capability for angiography, a continuous wave Doppler, a vascular instrument set, embolectomy catheters, graft materials, and blood products.

An alternative to formal vascular repair is the use of a temporary shunt. Vascular shunts can decrease the operative time during damage control surgery, liberate the surgeon to address other life-threatening injuries, and allow time to transport the patient to another facility with more robust resources.

THE TYPICAL CASE

A young male was severely injured while on patrol when his vehicle made contact with an improvised explosive device and rolled down an embankment. He was evacuated to a Forward Surgical Team staffed by two general surgeons, an anesthetist, and a complement of seven nursing and technician staff members. Seven additional patients from the incident were also transported for care, each with varying degrees of injury. At least two of these patients required urgent surgical intervention.

Primary Survey

- *Airway:* Intact airway with cervical spine protection
- *Breathing:* Bilateral breath sounds present
- *Circulation:* Hypotension (blood pressure 86/48 mm Hg), tachycardia of 120 beats/minute
- *Disability:* Glasgow coma scale score of 15, equal and reactive pupils
- *Exposure:* Diffuse fragmentation/peppering wounds, open left thigh wound.

The focused secondary survey revealed abdominal distention with ecchymosis and peritoneal signs. His left thigh had a tourniquet in place and release resulted in rapid hemorrhage. The patient's hemoglobin was 6.5 g/dL with a pH 7.25. A central venous catheter was placed for rapid delivery of crystalloid and blood products. He was immediately transported to the surgical tent.

Limited staff mandated triage and early transport in the setting of a mass casualty event. The patient was taken to the operative suite first based on severity of symptoms, though at least two other patients required operative intervention. The patient underwent an exploratory laparotomy with hematoma evacuation, hepatic laceration packing and hemostasis, and splenectomy. The fascia was left open with a negative pressure dressing applied. Left thigh exploration revealed a rapidly hemorrhaging arterial injury. Proximal and distal vascular control was obtained.

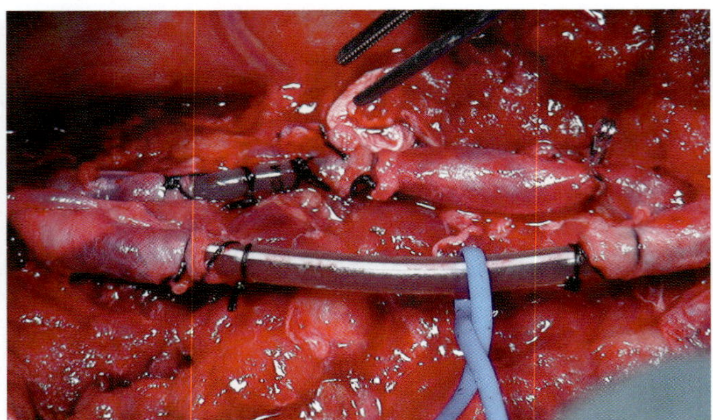

Fig. 35.1: Placement of temporary vascular shunts to the superficial femoral artery (identified with vessel loop) and femoral vein with shorter shunt in place.

A 4-cm defect was noted in the superficial femoral artery and a shorter venous defect. At this point, the patient's acidosis had worsened; he was diffusely coagulopathic, with a temperature of 35.8°C. Due to the patient's worsening condition and other patients awaiting operative repair, temporary vascular shunts were utilized. Commercially available shunts were inserted into the open proximal and distal portions of the exposed artery and vein and secured with silk sutures (Fig. 35.1). No anticoagulation was employed. A four-compartment left leg fasciotomy was then performed.

Within hours, the patient was evacuated to the next higher echelon of care, a Role III Combat Support Hospital. For transport a tourniquet was placed but left loose in the event that a shunt became dislodged.[5] At the higher level facility, the shunts were removed, the superficial femoral artery edges were sharply debrided, and a reversed saphenous vein bypass graft was performed with vein harvested from the opposite limb. The injured femoral vein was mobilized, debrided, and a primary repair was accomplished. His abdomen was closed. The patient was evacuated from the combat zone to the next level of care with distal triphasic pulse waveforms. One week later, he was discharged to rehabilitation with a functional left lower extremity.

MANAGEMENT OPTIONS

Acute hemorrhage in trauma demands immediate vascular control. Proximal and distal maneuvers using vascular clamps, Rummel tourniquets, or encircling (Potts) vessel loops are employed. Prior to vessel exposure, measures such as compression, the use of tourniquets, or missile tract balloon tamponade may be employed. After hemorrhage has ceased, or at least slowed, three options remain: ligation, temporary shunting, or formal repair. Not all options can be applied to every situation. For example, ligation would not be an ideal choice for the portal vein, but may be an excellent solution for an isolated arterial injury distal to the trifurcation of the leg.

Ligation may be an appealing option for vessel injuries with large defects or during damage control surgery. Almost any vein ligation in the body can be tolerated.[6] Caveats to this rule include the inferior vena cava and the portal vein. Attempts should be made to repair the vena cava, but if ligation is required to save the patient, bilateral lower extremity fasciotomies should be performed due to subsequent diffuse lower body edema. Ligation of the portal vein is poorly tolerated with likely resultant bowel infarction, portal hypertension, varices development, upper gastrointestinal bleeding, splanchnic fluid sequestration, and high mortality.[7] Few arteries can routinely be ligated, although those with collateral flow, duplicated systems, or distal branches have better tolerance. Examples of arteries that usually tolerate ligation include the radial, ulnar, distal profunda femoris, individual tibial branches, distal mesenteric branches, celiac, and internal iliac arteries.

For major vessels requiring repair, options include primary closure or anastomosis, prosthetic or autologous bypass grafting, or patching. In the setting of damage control surgery, a shunt may be employed as a bridge to definitive repair. Temporary vascular shunting during recent combat operations was associated with improved outcomes when used as a damage control adjunct.[8] There are several commercially available shunts, but many forms of sterile tubing can serve the purpose if necessary. The following lists represent vessel eligibility for shunting.[1]

Consider for Shunting

- Subclavian artery (difficult)
- Axillary artery
- Brachial artery
- Common femoral artery
- Superficial femoral artery
- Popliteal artery
- Large extremity veins
- Aorta
- Iliac arteries
- Carotid artery

Poor Candidates for Shunting

- Radial and ulnar arteries
- Profunda femoris artery

- Tibial arteries
- Vertebral arteries
- Portal vein
- Mesenteric vessels
- Jugular vein

If transport of the patient is anticipated, the shunt should be protected and labeled. Additionally, a tourniquet should be loosely placed in the event that the shunt becomes dislodged. Attempts should be made for definitive repair at the earliest opportunity to mitigate the risks of shunt thrombosis or dislodgement.

REFERENCES

1. Cubano MA. Emergency War Surgery, 4th edition. Washington, DC: Borden Institute; 2014.
2. Rotondo MF, Zonies DH. The damage control sequence and underlying logic. Surg Clin North Am. 1997;77(4):761-77.
3. Parr MJA, Alabdi T. Damage control surgery and intensive care. Injury. 2014;35:713-22.
4. Hess JR, Brohi K, Dutton RP, et al. The coagulopathy of trauma: a review of mechanisms. J Trauma. 2008;65(4): 748-54.
5. Blackbourne LH. First to cut: trauma lessons learned in the combat zone. San Antonio: US Army Institute of Surgical Research; 2012.
6. Hirschberg A, Mattox KL. Top Knife: The Art & Craft of Trauma Surgery. Castle Hill Barnes: TFM Publishing; 2005.
7. Pearl J, Chao A, Kennedy S, et al. Traumatic injuries to the portal vein: case study. J Trauma. 2004;56:779-82.
8. Gifford SM, Aidinian G, Clouse WD, et al. Effect of temporary shunting on extremity vascular injury: and outcome analysis from the Global War on Terror vascular injury initiative. J Vasc Surg. 2009;50(3):549-55.

Case Study: Operative Repair of Traumatic Diaphragmatic Liver Herniation with Subsequent Reperfusion Injury 36

James ML Williamson, Christopher P Armstrong

THE PROBLEM

Acute diaphragmatic rupture following blunt trauma is frequently overlooked, but is thought to have an incidence of 7% and a mortality rate of up to 28%. It typically affects the left hemidiaphragm (two-thirds of patients) and is bilateral in 2% of cases. Herniation of the abdominal viscera is due to a higher intra-abdominal pressure compared to the lower intrathoracic pressure. Herniation can either be acute or chronic and may be associated with respiratory or circulatory embarrassment. Computed tomogram (CT) scanning can delineate the extent of injuries sustained in the stable trauma patient and help to plan management. Diaphragmatic repair can be performed through a thoracic or abdominal incision, with the latter allowing full assessment of the peritoneal cavity.

THE TYPICAL CASE

A 47-year-old woman cyclist skidded off her bicycle on ice and was subsequently hit by a car that pushed her into a ditch and trapped her. The emergency services extracted her after an hour and transported her to the emergency department.

The primary survey revealed a patent airway, tachypnea (respiratory rate of 28 and saturations in the low 90s with poor air entry to the right lower chest), tachycardia (heart rate 107/min), and blood pressure of 120/68 mm Hg. Abdominal examination showed a tense, peritonitic abdomen with generalized guarding. Completion of the primary and subsequent secondary survey detected pelvic tenderness (a subsequent binder was placed) and hypothermia (temperature 33.5°C). Chest radiography showed a white-out in the right lower chest. Urgent CT scanning showed that most of the liver, hepatic flexure of the colon, gastric antrum, and some small bowel loops had herniated into the thoracic cavity (Figs. 36.1A and B), consistent with a right diaphragmatic rupture. There were imaging findings of bilateral pulmonary contusions, multiple rib fractures, right lower lobe collapse, and a leftward mediastinal shift. Free intra-abdominal gas and fluid were also noted, with thickened small bowel loops consistent with vascular

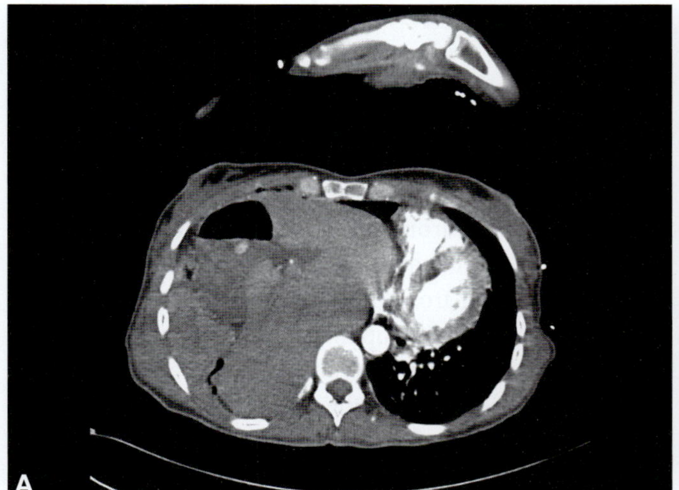

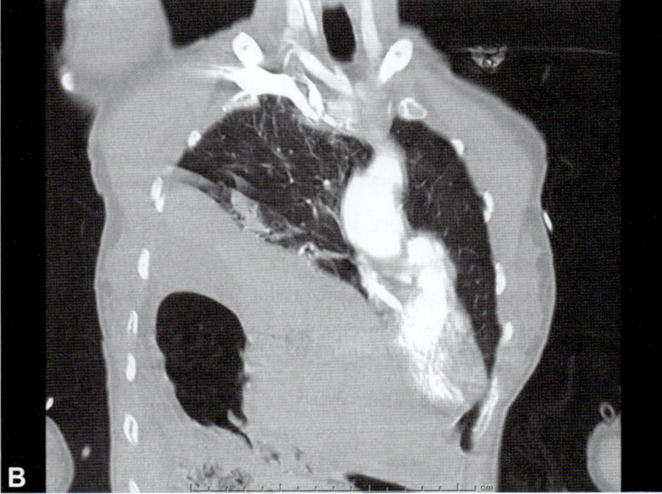

Figs. 36.1A and B: Coronal (A) and axial (B) CT images showing liver herniation into the thoracic cavity, with resultant compression of the right lung. The gas-filled colon can also be seen herniating into the chest.

compromise. Extensive pelvic fractures were also noted—bilateral superior and inferior pubic rami fractures, bilateral sacral ala fractures, and fractures of both iliac bones adjacent to the sacroiliac joints—plus fractures of the transverse processes of L2 and L3. Given the radiological findings, the patient underwent resuscitative laparotomy and pelvic fixation.

Operative findings confirmed that the liver had rotated and herniated into the chest through a ruptured right hemidiaphragm, and there were traumatic perforations of the mid small bowel and descending colon. The liver was derotated and reduced, prior to oversewing of the diaphragmatic defect. A chest drain was placed. The small bowel perforation was oversewn, the colonic perforation was resected, and continuity was restored with a stapled anastomosis. The pelvic fractures were stabilized with an external fixator. Postoperatively the patient was transferred to the intensive care unit (ICU).

After a period of stability, she deteriorated acutely some 12 hours later with abdominal distension and cardiac arrest, and cardiopulmonary resuscitation was commenced; she regained cardiac output transiently, but fresh blood was seen in her chest drain and she went into asystole. It was thought that she had bleeding intra-abdominally, so she underwent immediate relaparotomy.

At operation very high intra-abdominal pressure was noted: the liver was grossly enlarged and tense, suggesting a dramatic reperfusion injury with subsequent swelling and resultant abdominal compartment syndrome. Cardiac output was regained following decompression, but the patient was unstable suggesting active hemorrhage. Therefore, the right diaphragm was opened (which did not reveal any bleeding), and the pericardium was opened: a small tear at the base of the right atrium was identified (from presumed chest compressions) and was sutured to staunch the hemorrhage. The abdomen was left open and covered with a Bogota bag before further resuscitation in the ICU.

No other injuries were identified at relook laparotomy 24 hours later, although the liver was still engorged; a vacuum-assisted closure (VAC) dressing was applied.

In ICU, she received a tracheostomy and total parental nutrition and was slowly weaned off inotropic support. After five subsequent laparotomies and VAC changes, the abdomen was eventually closed some 3 weeks later. After a protracted period in the ICU of 63 days, she returned to the ward and was eventually discharged some 3 months after her accident.

DIAGNOSTIC DILEMMAS

This case illustrates some of the challenges in dealing with polytrauma and presents a series of dilemmas to the clinician. After the extraction of the patient and assessment within the emergency department, the first dilemma is whether the patient is stable enough to undergo urgent CT scanning. Computed tomogram scanning was performed in this case as the patient was not cardiovascularly compromised (apart from tachycardia), and this allowed full assessment of the extent of injury. If patients are not stable, they should undergo resuscitative laparotomy (or thoracotomy). Given the injuries shown on CT scanning, the next dilemma revolved about how and when to proceed to operative intervention. The presence of free gas combined with tachycardia mandated laparotomy to visualize and repair the injuries. The diaphragmatic repair was performed intra-abdominally after the liver had been reduced; inspection of the thoracic cavity could be obtained through the diaphragmatic defect, and a chest drain allowed the lung to re-expand and the pneumothorax to resolve. The third dilemma concerned the management of the two bowel perforations. In this instance, a decision to repair both of these perforation sites was made (rather than create stomas), and they healed satisfactorily. Many surgeons would advocate simple resection of the sites of perforation and a relook laparotomy at 24–48 hours (with definitive repair), which may have limited the subsequent abdominal compartment syndrome.

The cardiac arrest presented a series of important dilemmas: first, how best to manage the patient once cardiac output had been regained and then subsequently lost. The presence of blood within the chest drain implied that the arrest was secondary to hypovolemia. Thus, it appeared that the only chance of a successful resuscitation was to staunch the hemorrhage and replace circulating volume. However, upon reopening the abdomen, the patient regained cardiac output, suggesting abdominal compartment syndrome. The liver had swollen to twice its normal size, in keeping with a reperfusion injury. The ongoing bleeding from the chest demanded assessment of the thoracic cavity; reopening the diaphragmatic repair gave convenient access. As no active bleeding from the chest could be identified, the pericardium was opened to reveal a cardiac perforation secondary to rib fractures from cardiopulmonary resuscitation. The atrial laceration was safely repaired. There was no real dilemma regarding management of the abdomen; it could not be closed, so a series of staged laparotomies and abdominal VAC dressings was required to decompress the abdomen as the liver returned to normal size.

MANAGEMENT OPTIONS

The management options in this case reflect the surgical problems that evolved during the admission. As discussed, perhaps damage control surgery could have been performed during the initial laparotomy, which would have left the abdomen alone for a planned relook. This plan may have prevented the abdominal compartment syndrome (and subsequent cardiac arrest) at the expense of ongoing contamination from the intestinal perforations. Most centers would advocate the use of a wound management system—the abdominal VAC—although this could have been managed differently with simple wound care. Given the length of time until the wound was closed (even with the VAC system), it is unlikely that a staged wound closure or even use of deep tension sutures could have been appropriate.

Patients with isolated diaphragmatic injury, without abdominal injury, may be best served by thoracotomy and repair as this allows better visualization. However, patients must be stable enough to withstand single lung ventilation. Video-assisted thoracoscopic surgery can also be used to visualize the diaphragm and enable repair. Most centers would advocate the use of nonabsorbable sutures to repair diaphragmatic injuries (either in a continuous or interrupted fashion), with the judicious use of a nonabsorbable patch to close large defects. The use of a thoracotomy tube to provide drainage is advocated. The management of pulmonary contusions is usually supportive and may require mechanical ventilation, as in this case; CT scanning is highly specific at predicting the requirement for invasive ventilation.

FURTHER READING

1. Carvillo C, Fogler RJ, Shafton GW. Delayed gastrointestinal reconstruction following massive abdominal trauma. J Trauma 1993;34:233-5.
2. Cohn SM, Dubose JJ. Pulmonary contusion: an update on recent advances in clinical management. World J Surg. 2010;34:1959-70.
3. Haciibrahimoglu G, Solak O, Olcmen A, et al. Management of traumatic diaphragmatic rupture. Surg Today. 2004;34:111-4.
4. Hanna WC, Ferri LE, Fata P, et al. The current state of traumatic diaphragmatic injury: lessons learned from 105 patients over 13 years. Ann Thorac Surg. 2008;85:1044-8.
5. Mihos P, Potaris K, Gakidis J, et al. Traumatic rupture of the diaphragm: experience with 65 patients. Injury. 2003;32:169-72.
6. Schein M, Wittman DH, Aprahamian CC, et al. The abdominal compartment syndrome—the physiological and clinical consequences of raised intra-abdominal pressure. J Am Coll Surg. 1995;180:745-53.
7. Williamson JML, Rees JRE, Streets CG, et al. Management of liver trauma. Br J Hosp Med. 2013;74:432-8.

37

Neck Injury

Philip Barker

Key Points

- The neck represents a crossroad for vital structures entering or leaving the head, thorax, and upper limbs. A thorough knowledge of the related anatomy is vital.
- Blunt and penetrating traumas require distinct avenues of approach to avoid missed injuries.
- Surgical access for zone 1 injuries demands a familiarity with sternotomy and the upper mediastinum.
- Zone 3 injuries often require endovascular interventions.
- Multislice helical computed tomography (CT) with contrast and three-dimensional (3D) reconstruction is the investigation of choice for the majority of neck injuries.
- Selected neck injuries may, in some cases, be managed conservatively.

INTRODUCTION

The neck and its contained structures represent the anatomical crossroads for survival of the brain and upper limbs, the visceral organs of the thoracic cavity, and the integrity of neurological continuity of the spinal cord. It is also of vital anatomical importance for the maintenance of a patent airway for breathing and phonation, as well as providing the structure and function of the upper digestive tract. Interruption in one or more of these critical pathways can lead to major life-threatening events which, if not properly managed in a timely fashion, may lead to massive, long-term morbidity, or prove rapidly fatal. It is not within the scope of this chapter to cover injuries to the spine and spinal cord, which are covered in Chapter 38B, "Cervical Spine and Spinal Cord Trauma".

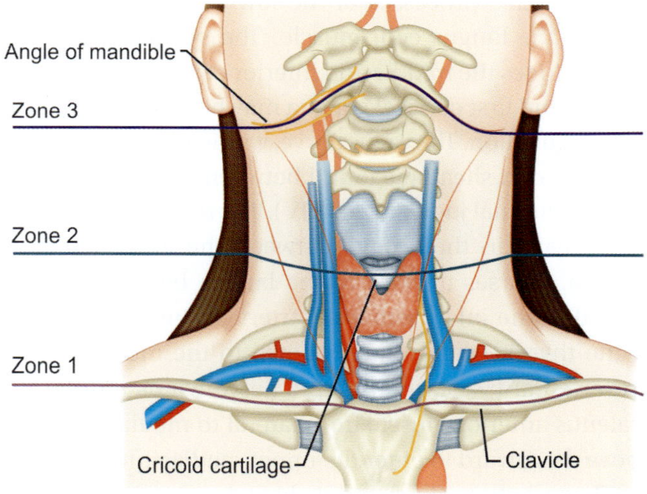

SURGICAL ANATOMY

The neck is usually divided into three zones for ease of description and because injuries in each zone are frequently treated differently. Zone 1 begins at the sternal notch and extends upward to the cricoid cartilage; zone 2 extends from the cricoid cartilage to the angle of the mandible; zone 3 reaches from the angle of the mandible to the base of the skull (Fig. 37.1). It is important to remember that in penetrating injuries while the visible wound may be in one zone, the compelling injury may be in quite another zone, or even within the thoracic cavity. To illustrate this point, the author treated a case of a stab wound on the right side of the neck in zone 1, but the compelling injury was deep within the mediastinum where the point of the weapon had transected the innominate artery and trachea. Thus, the surgical approaches to a wound in any of these zones of the neck may differ radically.

Fig. 37.1: Three zones of the neck. Zone 1 begins at the sternal notch and extends upward to the cricoid cartilage; zone 2 extends from the cricoid cartilage to the angle of the mandible; zone 3 reaches from the angle of the mandible to the base of the skull.

Zone 1 is a junctional zone both to the arm via the axilla, and to the chest cavity via the thoracic outlet. It contains the common carotid artery (CCA), and the first (and only easily accessible) part of the vertebral artery, arising from the first part of the subclavian artery. The sympathetic trunk lies just medial and posterior to the first part of the vertebral artery. The second and third parts of the subclavian artery lie behind and lateral to the scalenus anterior muscle, which separates the artery from the subclavian vein and its tributaries, which lie anterior to that muscle. The innominate vein may traverse zone 1 horizontally just above the sternal notch in infants and small children. The thoracic duct, which is prone to many variations,[10,11] usually enters the left subclavian vein. The roots, trunks, and divisions of the brachial plexus are also found in this zone, along with the dome of the pleura (covered by Sibson's fascia), the remaining scalene muscles, the inferior belly of the omohyoid muscle, and several named nerves. These nerves, detailed from posterior to anterior, begin with the sympathetic trunk, behind and outside the carotid sheath and separated from the transverse processes of the lower cervical vertebrae only by the longus colli muscle. The sympathetic trunk here includes the middle and inferior cervical ganglia. The inferior and first cervical ganglia may be fused to form the stellate ganglion. The vagus nerve, within the posterior part of the carotid sheath, is found between the carotid artery and the internal jugular vein (IJV). The recurrent laryngeal nerve, lying in the groove between the esophagus and trachea, courses upward to the larynx, being intimately related to the inferior thyroid artery at the lateral aspect of the thyroid gland. Bound down to the muscle by the prevertebral fascia, the phrenic nerve winds around the scalenus anterior muscle from lateral to medial and from above downward to enter the upper mediastinum.

The ansa hypoglossi and its branches loop around and (usually) in front of the carotid sheath. Division rarely results in significant clinical consequences. Similarly, the three cutaneous nerves that cross the clavicle just deep to the platysma muscle supply sensation to the skin of the upper chest and have considerable territorial overlap, and hence section of one or two is not noticed.

In addition to these structures, zone 1 is home to the cervical esophagus below the inferior constrictor muscle, and the trachea below the cricoid cartilage, wrapped around by the lateral lobes of the thyroid, with its isthmus, lying across the first-to-third tracheal rings. The inferior parathyroids may be found deep to the lower lateral poles of the thyroid.

Zone 2 defines the most accessible surgical field. It contains the CCA and its division into internal and external branches; the confluence of the common facial vein with the IJV, the fascial sling marking the junction of the superior and inferior bellies of the omohyoid muscle overlying the carotid sheath, the larynx, and lower pharynx. The vagus and recurrent laryngeal nerves remain at risk in zone 2, as does the sympathetic chain, immediately posterior to the carotid sheath and lying on the longus colli muscle covering the transverse processes of the cervical vertebrae, through which courses the second (intraosseous) part of the vertebral artery. The upper poles of the thyroid and the superior parathyroids embrace the lateral aspects of the thyroid cartilage beneath the insertion of the sternothyroid muscle. This zone is full of lymph nodes, and in the upper reaches of the zone the submandibular ganglion and the lateral part of the submandibular gland may be found just beneath the body of the mandible. The lower pole of the parotid gland may encroach on the junction between zones 2 and 3.

Zone 3 is the least accessible to the surgeon. It contains the lower pole of the parotid gland, the branches of the external carotid artery (ECA), and the upper reaches of the cervical internal carotid artery (ICA). The vertebral artery remains in its bony canal in this zone up to the level of the axis where it leaves the lateral foramen and courses initially horizontally (3rd part) and then vertically (4th part) to join with its opposite partner to form the basilar artery. The IJV remains lateral to the carotid arteries throughout zone 3.

The hypoglossal nerve is found usually just deep and inferior to the posterior belly of the digastric muscle, where it loops around and anterior to both the internal and external carotid arteries to pass into the floor of the mouth lateral to the hyoglossus muscle.

The spinal accessory nerve, after leaving the jugular foramen of the skull, traverses downward to pierce the anterior aspect of the sternomastoid muscle around its junction of upper and middle thirds, supplying motor fibers to that muscle, and leaving its posterior border around the junction of the middle and lower thirds to enter and provide motor fibers to the trapezius muscle. This nerve is at particular risk if the mastoid insertion of the sternomastoid muscle is detached from the skull to gain access to the upper reaches of the ICA.

Cervical Fascia

The deep fascia of the neck is of surgical importance. It consists essentially of three layers: (1) The general investing layer of fascia; (2) The pretracheal fascia; and (3) The prevertebral fascia.

The general investing layer is remarkable for the frequency with which it splits into two. It splits to enclose two muscles: the trapezius and sternomastoid. It splits to enclose two salivary glands: the submandibular and parotid. It splits to form two spaces: the lower part of the roof of the posterior triangle, and the suprasternal space (of Burns). Superficial to the general investing layer lies the platysma muscle, and in between the fascia and this muscle are the superficial veins of the neck, including the anterior and external jugular. If the platysma muscle is divided and these superficial veins are injured, they will not be able to retract and will continue to bleed unless the deep fascia is also divided, as they are attached to the latter. Once the deep fascia is also divided, the veins retract and usually stop bleeding.

On the deep surface of the sternomastoid muscle, the general investing layer gives off two sheets of fascia, the pretracheal and prevertebral fasciae. Between these two layers are found the CCA, the IJV, and the vagus nerve. The fascia immediately surrounding these structures is known as the carotid sheath[46] (Fig. 37.2). The pretracheal fascia passes in front of the carotid system and splits to enclose the thyroid gland. Superiorly, it attaches to the hyoid bone, and inferiorly it dives down in front of the trachea into the superior mediastinum to blend with the pericardium.

The prevertebral fascia passes posterior to the carotid system, the pharynx, larynx, esophagus, and trachea, but in front of the vertebrae and the prevertebral muscles. As it passes backward over the scalene muscles, it forms the floor of the posterior triangle, covering the brachial plexus and the subclavian artery. Here the prevertebral fascia sends with those structures a prolongation as a tubular sheath—the axillary sheath—which extends down to the elbow. Superiorly, the fascia is attached to the base of the skull. Inferiorly, it extends into the superior mediastinum, fading away on its posterior wall.

The extension of both the pretracheal and prevertebral fasciae into the superior mediastinum explains why, in undiagnosed injuries or anastomotic repairs that leak, particularly aerodigestive contents, contaminants may track down along these fascial planes into the chest and give rise to potentially lethal mediastinitis.

INJURY PATTERNS

Neck soft tissue injuries, as opposed to orthopedic injuries, are divided by mechanism into blunt and penetrating. The reason for this is because the management of each differs significantly. In the latter surgical intervention is frequently required, and the zones of the neck have greater therapeutic implications.

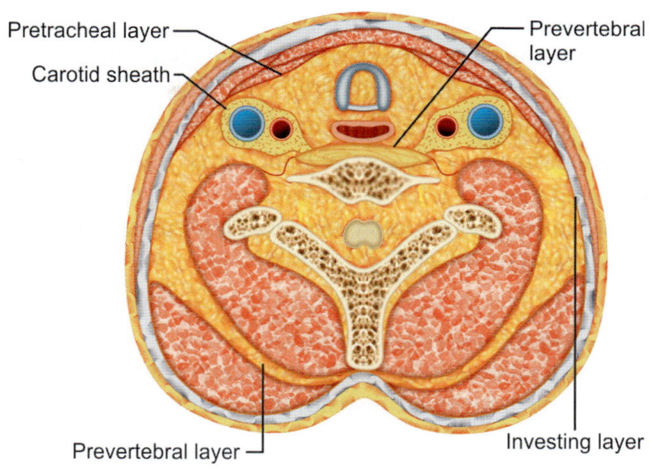

Fig. 37.2: The deep cervical fascia and its divisions.

Blunt Neck Trauma

Blunt neck injury is challenging for two main reasons; first, it may not be obvious initially and frequently presents late with complications, and second, because of the high density of vital structures in the region. For the first reason, a true incidence is hard to establish from published data, but it is probably a missed diagnosis in many initial assessments.

Some mechanisms of blunt injury are obvious, such as attempted hanging or strangulation, accidental injuries from clotheslines, or the shoulder strap of seat-belts, or a direct blow to the neck. Others are more subtle and involve deceleration injuries, often with head and facial trauma, or hyperextension forces with rotation, which may disrupt the brachial plexus, but may also produce an intimal tear of the carotid or vertebral arteries, leading to later thrombosis and neurological sequelae. Blunt laryngotracheal injuries account for $<1\%$ of injuries seen at trauma centers and esophageal ruptures are very rare and often discovered late after complications such as mediastinitis have set in.

Signs and Symptoms of Blunt Neck Trauma

These will depend on the structures involved. Stridor, hoarseness, dyspnea, subcutaneous emphysema, hemoptysis, and supraclavicular retraction indicate an airway injury. Pain or difficulty on swallowing, occasionally associated with hypersalivation and drooling may point to an esophageal injury. Hematoma, bruit, thrill, absent or diminished pulses in either the neck or upper limbs, particularly with neurological signs, suggest vascular compromise. A deviated trachea alone should arouse suspicion of possible vascular injury with a displacing hematoma, if an intrathoracic cause for a shifted mediastinum can be excluded.

Subtle neurological signs such as a Horner's syndrome may alert the clinician to a sympathetic chain injury, possibly associated with spinal injury.

The patient's use of intercostal and accessory muscles for breathing may suggest phrenic nerve damage, and a fractured clavicle with an underlying fracture of the first rib should raise suspicion of probable vascular injury to the subclavian vessels.

Approximately 50% of patients with blunt carotid artery injury will not manifest external evidence of neck injury, and most patients will present with delayed focal, cerebral, or ischemic neurological symptoms, up to several days or even weeks post-injury.[47]

The incidence of blunt carotid artery injury reported in the literature varies from 5% to 10% of all carotid artery injuries, but Biffl's work has suggested that higher figures may be obtained if screening is performed on patients with high-risk mechanisms of injury. His seminal study in 1998 showed an increase in incidence of blunt carotid artery injury from 0.1% (of all blunt trauma admissions) in his prescreening period to 0.86% in the postscreening period, most of whom were asymptomatic. In one year alone (1997), his unit managed 20 cases detected by screening, which was more than in the seven previous years combined.[1]

Management of Blunt Neck Trauma

Cervical spine and spinal cord injuries can lead to major neurological complications and may be missed if not suspected and examined for. Full advanced trauma life support (ATLS) protocols with cervical spine protection are crucial to prevent iatrogenic spinal cord injury.

Penetrating Neck Trauma

Penetrating neck trauma represents approximately 5–10% of all trauma cases that present to emergency departments in the USA.[2] About 30% of these cases are accompanied by injury outside of the neck zones. Penetrating neck trauma has been a significant cause of injury and death for centuries. The advent of gunpowder and the subsequent widespread use of firearms have increased the incidence of penetrating neck injuries and the mortality rate associated with them.

Historically, military conflict has provided significant opportunities for the advancement of trauma surgery, including the management of penetrating cervical injuries The current mortality rate in civilians with penetrating neck injuries ranges from 3% to 6%. During World War II, the mortality rate was 7%, and, in World War I, it was 11%. Higher mortality rates occur with injuries to large vessels, such as the carotid or subclavian arteries and veins.[2]

Recent experience with casualties from the Iraq war treated at Walter Reed Army Medical Center reported the CCA as the most frequently injured cervical vessel.[2]

Mechanisms of penetrating neck injury are usually obvious. Stabs, impalement, bullets, or fragments from explosive devices are generally self-evident, but more unusual items may cause penetrating injury and may confuse or mislead the clinician. Bone fragments from adjacent injured persons in an explosion may become missiles and cause injury, and glass fragments may not be easily seen if appropriate oblique X-rays are not taken so that foreign material is not hidden by underlying bone. Some plastics are radiolucent to standard X-rays, hence helical multislice CT is the gold-standard investigation, with or without computed tomography angiography (CTA).

Signs and Symptoms of Penetrating Neck Trauma

The presentation of penetrating neck trauma will depend on the anatomical structures involved. Clearly, where major vascular injury has occurred, there may be massive external hemorrhage or a rapidly expanding hematoma within the neck, sometimes associated with airway compression. Aerodigestive damage may produce bubbling or mucus discharge from the wound. Neurological injury will manifest according to which nerve is involved. The sympathetic trunk may present as a Horner's syndrome; a phrenic nerve injury as respiratory distress; and brachial plexus involvement will produce signs appropriate to the distribution of the injured nerves. Vagal injury is unlikely to be diagnosed preoperatively.

The key to diagnosis remains in the history as well as the physical signs, as bleeding from a venous injury may have ceased by the time the patient reaches the ER. Careful questioning of the patient or paramedics who brought the patient may elicit a history of massive blood loss at the scene, even if the wound is now no longer bleeding. Suspicion of injury and meticulous investigation is imperative if injuries are not to be missed.

Management of Penetrating Neck Trauma

Before World War II, nonoperative management was the standard for all penetrating neck injuries, but this had a mortality of around 15%.[4] Subsequent policy mandated obligatory exploration of all wounds that penetrated the platysma muscle. This created an enormous operative burden and more recent studies have shown up to 60%

nontherapeutic rates of exploration, more commonly with stab wounds than wounds caused by projectiles.[5,6] It has been suggested that even up to 80% of transcervical gunshot wounds may be managed conservatively with appropriate investigation.[7]

The trend to selective conservative management has been driven not only by high rates of negative explorations, but also by significantly improved imaging modalities and endovascular techniques that allow for stenting or embolization of vascular injuries in some instances (for more details *see* Chapter 15, "Diagnostic and Interventional Radiology"). Conservative management is, however, only an option in centers where repeated, high-quality clinical observation is available by both nurses and physicians, along with immediate access to emergency surgery.[3]

Because of the relative surgical inaccessibility of zones 1 and 3 compared to zone 2, management may differ according to the anatomical site of the injury. Nevertheless, as with all injuries, patient management proceeds along ATLS principles, treating first the immediate threat to life. In recent years, however, due to the number of significant military injuries with massive hemorrhage seen in global conflicts, there has been a paradigm shift to accommodate a change from the classic ATLS dictum of, "Airway, Breathing, Circulation", (ABC) priorities for treatment, to a "Circulation–Airway, Breathing, Circulation," (C-ABC), where catastrophic external bleeding is the compelling management issue (for more details *see* Chapter 31, "Initial Trauma Evaluation and Resuscitation").[8] If a patient is rapidly losing his or her blood volume onto the floor in front of the clinician, then arrest of that hemorrhage is the first priority.

Exsanguinating hemorrhage from a penetrating neck wound should not be approached blindly with hemostats plunged into the wound in a desperate fashion to staunch the flow of blood. This course of action is very likely to cause more damage and accelerate the process of exsanguination. If direct pressure with a rolled gauze swab is not sufficient, then it is possible to apply a tight bandage to the neck with a pressure dressing beneath it, so long as the opposite arm of the patient is elevated vertically alongside the ear on the side opposite the injury, and incorporated into the bandage. This maneuver will allow the contralateral carotid artery to remain uncompressed beneath the raised arm at the same time as allowing for an effective pressure bandage to be applied to the rapidly bleeding wound on the other side of the neck. This technique only works for injuries in zone 2. Torrential hemorrhage from zones 1 or 3 may be slowed or even stopped by inserting a Foley catheter into the wound and inflating the balloon. More than one catheter may be required as in the case shown in Figure 37.3 where three Foley catheters were inserted into a stab wound in zone 3 and the edges of the wound rapidly approximated to produce an effective tamponade that stopped the hemorrhage.

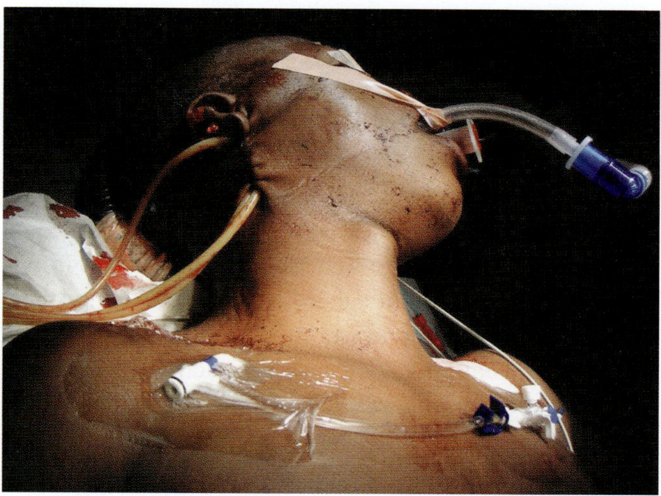

Fig. 37.3: Use of three Foley catheters and approximating sutures to arrest hemorrhage from zone 3 injury.

At no stage, however, should transfer to the operating room (OR) be delayed in favor of investigation when the patient's clinical condition mandates emergency surgery. Although a CTA would be highly desirable in suspected vascular injury in either zone 1 or 3, a hypotensive, rapidly bleeding patient will only succumb in the CT scanner, further enhancing its reputation as a place to die. Such a patient needs emergency surgery, which, in itself, constitutes both a diagnostic and therapeutic intervention.

Airway Injury

With the caveat (vide supra) to attend to obvious, external, torrential, life-threatening bleeding when present, the airway remains the first priority in both blunt and penetrating trauma.

Signs of airway injury have already been discussed, and the clinician needs to be prepared for both difficult intubation and the possible need for a surgical airway. Equipment and expertise for both are necessary. Cricothyroidotomy, using a scalpel and a tracheostomy tube, is still a quick and efficient way of gaining rapid access to secure a definitive airway. However, the advent of modern percutaneous tracheostomy sets, using the Seldinger technique, has made the older technique less commonplace.

Particular caution needs to be exercised where a penetrating wound in zone 1 results in an injury within the upper mediastinum, with the likelihood of an intrathoracic hematoma compressing the trachea, or even an intrathoracic tracheobronchial laceration.

Where a tracheal injury is present in zone 1, it may be turned into a definitive airway by placing an endotracheal or tracheostomy tube through the wound itself and inflating the cuff. This is not ideal, however, as the wound may be dirty and such a maneuver may introduce contamination to the distal airway. Simply advancing the endotracheal tube beyond the injury may be all that is necessary. Airway compromise inferior to the sternal notch may require bronchoscopic placement of a tube beyond the site of injury, even if this means temporary one-lung ventilation, advancing the tube into the right mainstem bronchus. If the patient has survived to get to the emergency room with an intrathoracic airway injury, it is likely that they will get to the OR for repair. However, it is prudent to be prepared to perform a rapid sternotomy should the patient's condition deteriorate.

Zone 1 Injuries

Zone 1 wounds with a high likelihood of vascular injury should not be explored through the root of the neck. This approach courts disaster. Proximal control of the subclavian vessels cannot be adequately achieved without access to the upper mediastinum. This is best obtained by a full, median sternotomy. All the major arch vessels are accessible by this route, including the proximal left subclavian artery. Although it is a posterior arch structure, it is not difficult to reach. The poorly-healing and painful "trap-door" combination of a supraclavicular approach and a partial sternotomy with left anterior thoracotomy incision, is time-consuming, obsolete, and unnecessary. While dissecting the origin of the left subclavian artery, care must be taken to avoid the recurrent laryngeal nerve as it winds around behind the ligamentum arteriosum beneath the arch at this point. The right recurrent laryngeal nerve winds around behind the first part of the right subclavian artery where it lies posterior to the right sternoclavicular joint.

A supraclavicular extension to the median sternotomy can be performed a finger's breadth above and parallel to the medial two thirds of the clavicle, to control the distal subclavian and proximal vertebral artery when injuries to either of these vessels in the root of the neck need repair. The subclavian artery becomes the axillary artery at the outer border of the first rib and control of the latter for injuries immediately behind the clavicle is readily obtained by an infraclavicular incision a thumb's breadth beneath the clavicle and parallel to its lateral two thirds. It is helpful to have the arm out at a right angle so that the fibers of the pectoralis major muscle can be separated and not divided for this infraclavicular exposure. It is greatly facilitated also by division of the pectoralis minor muscle high up at its insertion to the coracoid process of the scapula. It has never been necessary in the author's experience to divide or resect the clavicle, which takes longer to perform, longer to repair, and longer to heal. It is a straightforward matter to tunnel a bypass graft, if required, beneath the clavicle between the two parallel incisions.

Where the injury is to the brachiocephalic trunk or its branches, it is important to identify the origin of the left CCA as this may, on occasion, arise from the lateral aspect of the brachiocephalic trunk, and not from its usual position on the aortic arch. Thus, clamping the root of the trunk for proximal control would occlude both common carotids in such a case, with disastrous and fatal results.

Safe dissection of the proximal vertebral artery involves a thorough knowledge of the anatomy of the root of the neck. The key muscle is the scalenus anterior, which separates the subclavian vein anteriorly from the artery immediately posteriorly. To find the scalenus anterior muscle, the clavicular head of the sternomastoid muscle must be divided and the scalene fat pad beneath it removed. This is always present, even in the leanest of individuals, and contains numerous small lymph nodes and blood vessels, which need to be ligated. Occasionally, the thoracic duct traverses this fat pad. Care must be taken before dividing the cylindrical anterior scalene muscle as the phrenic nerve, bound down upon it by the prevertebral fascia, winds around the muscle from lateral to medial to enter the upper mediastinum. The origin of the vertebral artery is usually found just on the posteromedial border of the scalenus anterior muscle. It is embryologically derived from the fusion of seven intersegmental arteries and, as such, is subject to considerable developmental variation. It may be thin and tortuous, it may be duplicated or it may be absent. It is seldom responsible for neurological sequelae following ligation or embolization. However, it may be the source of continued, brisk, troublesome bleeding, even when proximal control has been achieved, as a result of retrograde flow from above through the Circle of Willis. This fact needs to be remembered when faced with otherwise unexplained, rapid, ongoing hemorrhage where proximal control was expected to halt the flow.

Repair of arch vessels is preferable to ligation where possible. This may be done by direct suture, by using a vein patch if narrowing the vessel seems inevitable, or by interposition grafting, which may be performed by using either vein or polytetrafluoroethylene (PTFE). If the patient's hemodynamic status does not allow for repair, an intraluminal shunt may be placed. Ligation is possible in some circumstances.

The CCA is easily accessible in zone 2 and in zone 1 (after division of the sternum). Repair is the procedure of choice, but ligation may be performed, usually without neurological sequelae, particularly in a young, fit patient, as cross-filling via the ECA and the circle of Willis is sufficient to maintain cerebral perfusion. Clinical dilemmas concerning the management of carotid artery injuries will be discussed later in this chapter.

The vertebral artery is only accessible to the surgeon in Zone 1 for its first few centimeters, before it enters the foramina of the transverse processes of the proximal six cervical vertebrae. Repair is therefore unusual. Ligation of the vertebral artery very rarely results in any neurological fallout. If endovascular intervention is readily available, embolization may be performed as an alternative to surgical exploration. Intraluminal balloon tamponade at surgical exploration using a Fogarty catheter may also arrest hemorrhage. The catheter is inserted up the vertebral artery, the balloon inflated, and the catheter left in place for 48 hours, after which the balloon may be gently deflated in the OR, and the catheter carefully withdrawn if there is no further bleeding. Should that occur, the balloon may be reinflated for a further 48 hours and the procedure repeated.

Zone 1 injuries to the trachea should be repaired with interrupted absorbable sutures in one layer, without narrowing the lumen. Inspection of the posterior aspect of the trachea is important to identify a through-and-through laceration or other injury requiring repair. If the esophagus is also injured, then an interposed muscle patch from one of the adjacent strap muscles is placed between the suture lines of the trachea and esophagus. Massive injuries to the esophagus with tissue loss may require a temporary cutaneous esophagostomy or placement of a polyethylene glycol tube for feeding, and a pharyngostomy for diversionary drainage. The key to effective immediate esophageal repair is good apposition of the mucosal layer with interrupted sutures. A two-layered closure is preferred, but the longitudinal muscle of the esophagus does not hold suture material well. The repair may be facilitated by the passage of a nasogastric tube, which acts as a stent. Both these tracheal and esophageal injuries should be drained externally using a sump-type drain. Oral feeding is withheld following repair of esophageal injuries until a barium swallow at 7–10 days demonstrates no leakage at the repair site.

The thoracic duct is a structure particularly prone to anatomical variation.[9] As such, its presence in an unusual site may be unexpected. Major variations include doubling, right-sided, or bilateral termination, and rarely, azygous vein termination. The duct may also pass posterior to the vertebral and subclavian arteries en route to its venous termination. Multiple studies of the duct termination indicate that variation is the rule, with < 40% joining the left venous confluence.[10-12] Ligation of any divided major lymph channels is required to prevent a troublesome chylous fistula.

The thyroid gland on occasion may be the source of significant bleeding. Resection or oversewing of damaged glandular tissue is appropriate after identifying and preserving the recurrent laryngeal nerve as it courses upward in the groove between the esophagus and trachea to pass under the inferior constrictor muscle before entering the larynx.

Zone 2 Injuries

This zone can be readily accessed by an incision along the full length of the anterior border of the sternomastoid muscle, with good exposure of the carotid sheath obtained by division of the central tendon of the omohyoid muscle, the only strap muscle of the neck to cross the sheath obliquely. Within the sheath lie the CCA medially, the IJV lateral to it, and the vagus nerve, lying posteriorly between the two. Behind and outside the carotid sheath lies the sympathetic chain, running vertically on the longus colli muscle, that separates it from the transverse processes of the cervical vertebrae. Dissection to expose the CCA and IJV within the sheath needs care as the common facial vein crosses in front of the CCA to enter the IJV just below the angle of the jaw. Inadvertent division or avulsion of the common facial vein before ligation will produce brisk and tiresome hemorrhage. Dissection of the contents of the carotid sheath is not possible until this critical landmark vein is divided.

Injuries to the carotid bulb or proximal ICA can be reconstructed using an interposition graft if simple lateral suture is not possible. Alternatively, the proximal ECA may be divided a few centimeters from its origin, and the distal end ligated. The distal ICA is then transposed to the proximal stump of the divided ECA. Shunts may be used if there is poor backflow from the divided distal end of the ICA, but they need not be used routinely. Their use, however, obviates the need for undue haste in repair, particularly if an interposition graft is used. In these cases, the shunt is passed through the lumen of the graft before anastomosis to the native artery. Wherever grafts are used, the distal anastomosis should be completed first.

If there is massive hemorrhage from the CCA and the patient's hemodynamic status is precarious, then the vessel should be ligated. Backflow from the ECA to the ICA is usually brisk enough to protect from neurological sequelae. Most injuries to the CCA, if proximal to the bulb and not readily reparable, should be ligated without hesitation. Similarly, if there is no backflow or thrombus in the ICA, and the patient is already deeply comatose, efforts at futile surgery should be abandoned and the ICA simply ligated. This issue will be further discussed at the end of this chapter.

The ECA may be repaired if injuries to that vessel are simple and readily accessible. In all other cases, the ECA may be ligated without consequence. Similarly, undue time is not spent repairing the IJV. Ligation of one IJV is not attended by morbidity. However, if both IJVs are injured, repair of one should be attempted in the hemodynamically normal patient to avoid cerebral hypertension and edema.

Venous injuries are prone to thrombosis and tamponade, and many are found incidentally at arterial exploration. Many more probably go unrecognized. The true incidence is therefore not established. If a major venous injury is encountered during surgical exploration, the patient should be placed in the Trendelenburg position to avoid air embolism. If simple lateral suturing is insufficient to effect repair, ligation of the vein should be performed.[13] Whatever method of repair is used, there is a high incidence of thrombosis, and the long-term outcome is not known.[14] Ligation of the subclavian vein may be performed, but there will be swelling of the associated arm and shoulder for about a week following, which may be quite alarming if not anticipated.

With CCA injuries, a coincidence of 18% with esophageal injury has been reported[15] and if a vascular repair is performed in the same procedure as a repair to the aerodigestive tract, then interposition of a partially divided strap muscle between the two is made. The operative approach to the esophagus may be from behind or in front of the carotid sheath. The posterior approach is safer but limits exposure, whereas the anterior approach, which gives wider access, requires identification and division of the middle thyroid vein and the inferior thyroid artery. The recurrent laryngeal nerve is at risk in this exposure. The landmark omohyoid muscle should have already been divided at the same time as division of the common facial vein, on the initial approach to the carotid sheath.

Vascular repairs in these combined injuries should ideally be made with autogenous tissue if time and the patient's condition permit, but in reality it is more common to use prosthetic material such as PTFE. All suture lines should, in any case, be wrapped with viable muscle flaps. In these situations, tracheostomy should be avoided if at all possible to prevent contamination of the vascular anastomosis.

In a major subclavian artery injury, following proximal and distal control, an interposition graft can be easily tunneled beneath the clavicle. Alternatively, a carotid-subclavian bypass may be performed. Although autologous vein is the preferred conduit, prosthetic material is quicker and easier to use. Animal experimental work has shown that this does not lead inevitably to graft infection, even in the presence of contamination (DERA, Porton Down, UK, Dr P Watkins; personal communication, 2003).

Not all subclavian vascular injuries are associated with absent distal pulses. A lowered blood pressure by 10% in the arm of the injured side compared with the unaffected side is enough to warrant a CTA study if time allows, or immediate exploration if the patient is in shock.

Zone 3 Injuries

The major concern with zone 3 injuries is injury to the upper reaches of the ICA and vertebral artery.

The second part of the vertebral artery runs through the bony canal of the upper six cervical vertebrae, and is surgically inaccessible without special expertise through zone 3. Hence, hemorrhage from this vessel is best approached by identifying it in its first part in zone 1, and ligating it there. If this does not result in cessation of bleeding due to backflow, then a Fogarty catheter is passed up the artery and the balloon inflated as previously mentioned. Usually this can be removed in the or after 48–72 hours. If the bleeding site can be visualized directly in the bony canal, it may be plugged with bone wax. Alternatively, endovascular embolization instead of surgical exploration may be performed if the patient's condition allows. One such vertebral artery injury, associated with a high-IJV injury was treated successfully by the author using a Fogarty catheter within the vertebral artery, and a Foley catheter passed alongside it to tamponade the vein.

The key to improve exposure of the upper ICA is the division of the posterior belly of the digastric muscle. Care must be exercised in division of this muscle as the hypoglossal nerve runs in close association with it. Usually visible just inferior to the muscle belly, the nerve crosses in front of both the ICA and the ECA, the occipital branch of the ECA hooking over it to course backward at this point, and acting as a landmark for the surgeon. The nerve then runs forward, below, and parallel to the lingual nerve, on the lateral surface of the hyoglossus muscle to enter the mouth.

Once the digastric muscle has been divided, considerable extra exposure of the ICA is obtained. Even higher exposure may be needed and osteotomy techniques are described to divide the neck of the mandible or sublux or even dislocate the temporomandibular joint anteriorly. These procedures take time and are not without complications. Another method of accessing the upper portion of the ICA is to divide the mastoid attachment of the sternomastoid muscle, (leaving a short tendinous stump for later reattachment) and reflecting it backward and downward, taking care to identify and preserve the spinal accessory nerve as it enters the junction of the upper and middle thirds of that muscle. If repair cannot be affected by this additional exposure, ligation or intraluminal balloon tamponade may be required to arrest life-threatening hemorrhage.

Wherever possible, a CTA should be obtained for zone 3 injuries, and endovascular techniques employed preferentially over operative approaches. But in the face of catastrophic, on-going bleeding, surgical ligation may be the only option.

Transcervical Neck Injuries

When stabs or projectiles cross the midline of the neck, or a severe blunt force raises the suspicion of damage to the visceral component of the neck, it may be difficult to establish the extent of injuries from unilateral exploration alone. No hesitation should be made in performing bilateral incisions along the anterior border of the sternomastoid muscles. These can be extended further, if necessary, by joining the two incisions at their lower extent in a "U"-shape. The superiorly-based flap can now be lifted deep to the platysma muscle in the same way as for thyroid surgery. The resultant exposure is excellent for both sides, as well as for the midline structures of the neck.

Nerve Injuries

Nerve injuries to the spinal cord, brachial plexus, or other critical nerves, such as the phrenic, must be suspected on initial examination of the patient, or noted at the time of surgery. Spinal cord injuries are not discussed here, but should be looked for in the emergency room, and not discovered later with embarrassment in the intensive care unit (*see* Chapter 38B, "Cervical Spine and Spinal Cord Trauma," for details on spinal cord injuries). Neural repairs are time-consuming and not appropriate in the acute trauma setting in most instances. However if time, technology, (excellent lighting and magnification of the operative field), and expertise are available, then they may be considered for repair at the initial presentation. The default option is to identify and mark divided or damaged nerves, either with metal clips or easily seen, nonabsorbable sutures, for delayed repair in an otherwise fully recovered patient.

Clinical Dilemmas in the Management of Carotid Artery Injuries

Ambroise Paré treated a carotid injury in a duelist by ligation in 1552 with an outcome of aphasia and left hemiplegia.[16] In 1798, Abernethy ligated a carotid artery for hemorrhage in a patient gored by a bull, but the patient died 30 hours later. The first successful carotid ligation is credited to David Fleming, a captain on the HMS Tonnant, who in 1803 "cut down upon and tie(d) the carotid artery below the wound" in a sailor attempting suicide.[17] Ligation remained the principal form of therapy for the remainder of the nineteenth century and the first half of this century. Cerebral complication rates of 30–33% and mortality rates of 45–50% continued through World Wars I and II.[18,19] With the development of modern vascular techniques and rapid triage in the Korean War, operative repair became acceptable and appeared to lower the mortality rate to 10%.[18] The Vietnam War brought improved outcomes mainly because of further refinements in triage, rapid transportation, and resuscitation. However, another swing of the pendulum occurred in 1970 when Cohen et al., reporting on their experience in Vietnam, suggested that restoration of vascular continuity was directly responsible for the deaths of some of their patients who had presented with neurological deficits.[20]

Based on Wylie's work with patients undergoing revascularization for acute thrombotic strokes,[21] Cohen's group postulated (without autopsy evidence) that revascularization of neurological deficits was converting ischemic infarcts into hemorrhagic ones. They concluded that ligation should be the treatment of choice for "many" patients with neurological impairment. Bradley's 1973 report of two patients who presented with preoperative neurological deficits, and who were found to have hemorrhagic cerebral infarctions on autopsy after repair of their carotid injuries, further strengthened the argument for ligation of the carotid arteries in patients with neurological impairment.[22]

In recent decades, however, numerous studies[15,23-27] have revisited the issue and strongly argue for the benefits of revascularization, when feasible, in all patients with carotid artery injuries. The recognition by a number of authors[4,28] that neurological deterioration after repair is probably the result of cerebral edema, and not hemorrhagic infarction, has further bolstered their argument. However, it has become clear that extrapolation from observations made in elderly patients who have undergone revascularization after atherosclerotic strokes[21], to those made in the young trauma population is hardly valid.[4,14]

Modern data suggest that repair should be attempted in all patients, even those in coma. First, the severity of the neurological deficit is not always possible to ascertain. The depressed mental status may be due to shock, intoxication, sedation, paralysis for airway control, or a combination of these. Second, strong evidence exists in the literature that the ischemic insult, rather than reperfusion hemorrhage, is the major cause of untoward outcome in these patients.[4,14] The concept of limiting ischemic damage by reperfusing the "ischemic penumbra" around an area of irreversible infarction may account for the clinical observations of improvement seen after restoration of flow in certain patients with preoperative neurological deficits.[14] In a review of 722 cases, Unger et al.[29] found no evidence to support coma as a contraindication to the repair of carotid injuries. Although clearly a poor prognostic sign, they felt that the presence of coma should not contraindicate repair.

In both blunt and penetrating injuries, part of the problem has lain with making the diagnosis, limited by the resolution of radiological imaging. Subtle, minimal intimal flaps were not easy to detect. Initially, direct, four-vessel angiography via the aortic arch was regarded as the gold standard for diagnosis. Certainly, this produced excellent pictures, but at a price of a 1–2% stroke rate, and a significantly invasive procedure, often requiring general anesthesia. The early four and eight-slice CT scanners allowed for the much less invasive CTA, but trials concluded that the images produced were not adequate.[30] However, the 16-slice, 3D, helical CTAs available since 2001 were deemed at least as good as, if not better than direct four-vessel angiography, and this has become the new gold standard.[31,32] In the last decade, technology has advanced rapidly, with 64-slice (and even 4D, 256-slice) helical CT scanners now commonplace, but no further trials have been published comparing the more advanced instruments with the old, historical "gold standard" of direct four-vessel angiography.[33]

Nevertheless, the debate over conservative management versus aggressive surgery in blunt vascular carotid artery injury continues, though no randomized controlled trials have been published to provide level 1 evidence. Though the Eastern Association for the Surgery of Trauma remains undecided,[34] the Western Trauma Association feels more confident of recommending conservative anticoagulation for most blunt vascular injuries, unless they are easily accessible to the surgeon (e.g. zone 2), or, for grade 5 injuries (on the Abbreviated Injury Score (AIS), of the extracranial internal carotid artery involving >50% of the vessel circumference[4]) endovascular interventions. They do not advocate aggressive surgical management in those with completed stroke.[35]

In addition to direct injury from penetrating objects, high-energy missiles, passing in proximity to vascular structures, but without actual contact, may produce a shock wave that induces a "percussion injury" to vessels. Here, the shock wave causes a sudden stretching and distortion of the vessel such that the intima of an artery is ruptured without any external laceration to the adventitia. The intima then rolls up like a blind, forced up by antegrade blood flow, and thrombus forms behind it, occluding the lumen. Neurological sequelae may follow if the cerebral perfusion pressure within the Circle of Willis is compromised. These injuries may be suspected on surgical exploration by the appearance of the artery. It may appear "bruised" at the point of intimal rupture, or have a sudden, unexpected narrowing in transverse diameter, with diminished or absent pulsation beyond the narrowing.

Diagnosis of significant penetrating neck arterial injury is based on the presence or absence of hard or soft physical signs (for details *see* Chapter 42, "Vascular Trauma"). Significant penetrating injury is defined as one that extends deeper than the platysma muscle. However, no attempt to probe or insert a finger into the wound should be made as it may dislodge a clot and start torrential bleeding. Exploration of the wound using good lighting by an experienced surgeon may be performed under local anesthesia,

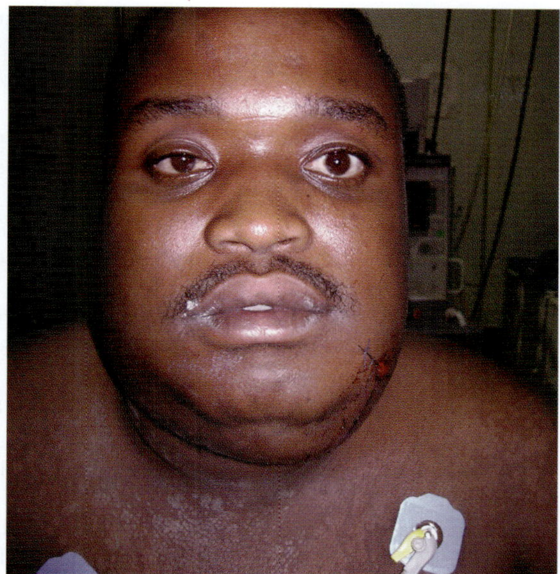

Fig. 37.4: Sutured wound on the left neck in a patient with a right Horner's syndrome.

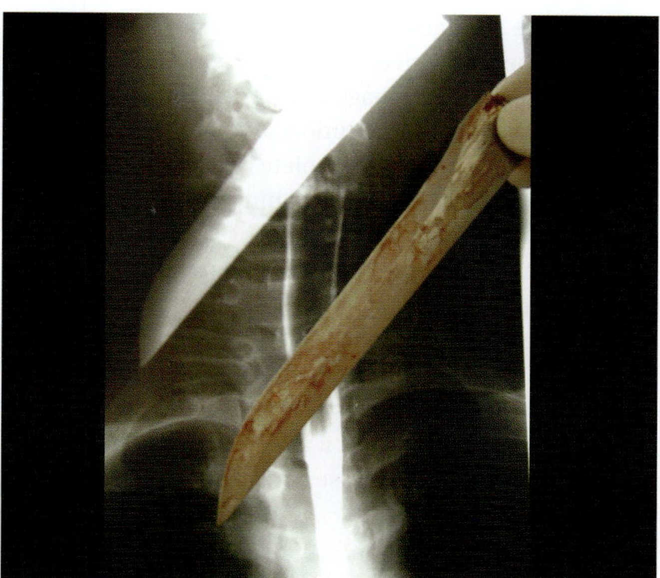

Fig. 37.5: Knife blade removed from patient's neck shown in Figure 37.4.

but if doubt exists whether the platysma muscle has been breached, it is better to err on the side of caution rather than assume an entirely superficial wound. Oblique injuries, by definition, will not divide anatomical structures in the same vertical plane as the entry wound, making even local exploration potentially hazardous and prone to misinterpretation.

Hard signs of vascular injury will include obvious pulsatile hemorrhage from the wound, an expanding hematoma, a cervical bruit or thrill, and an absent or diminished carotid pulse. Soft signs will include a nonexpanding cervical hematoma, a pulse deficit in the superficial temporal artery, signs of air embolism, active bleeding from an oropharyngeal or neck wound, widened mediastinum, ipsilateral Horner's syndrome, or dysfunction of cranial nerves IX–XII.

Signs of significant damage to other organs may be similar to those found in blunt injury such as dyspnea, stridor, hoarseness, surgical emphysema, dysphonia, dysphagia, hemoptysis, hematemesis, neurological deficit, and shock. In penetrating injuries, additional clues may be present, such as bubbling through a neck wound, saliva or mucus in the wound, or a foreign body present in the wound. It is important to look carefully for the latter. In a case a patient presented 2 days after a stab wound to the neck, which was regarded as inconsequential and sutured, developed a Horner's syndrome on the contralateral side to the sutured wound and a 15 cm knife-blade was removed from the neck on subsequent exploration. The blade had snapped off the knife-handle in the attack, crossed the midline behind the esophagus, and became embedded in the sympathetic chain on the opposite side from the entry wound[36] (Figs. 37.4 and 37.5).

ADJUNCTS TO DIAGNOSIS OF NECK INJURIES

Multidetector, helical CT scanning with CTA is now the first choice of investigation in the majority of these injuries and has the added advantage of 3D reconstruction.[37-40] If aerodigestive injury is suspected, then a combination of direct visualization via laryngoscopy and flexible bronchoscopy may aid in excluding injury to the upper airway. Flexible esophagoscopy can be used to detect an esophageal injury with less risk of procedure-related complications than rigid esophagoscopy (i.e. rupture and complications from general anesthesia). However, concerns exist regarding the introduction of oropharyngeal flora into the tissue planes of the neck when performing upper endoscopy in the presence of a perforation because visualization of the central lumen is aided by continuous gas insufflation through the endoscope. These concerns are probably more theoretical than real as any oropharyngeal perforation found will be explored, repaired, and drained, reducing the chances of local wound sepsis.

Esophageal endoscopy or a contrast swallow will each only detect around 60% of perforations, but if combined, can achieve a diagnostic accuracy approaching 90%. However, these invasive adjuncts of aerodigestive endoscopy and contrast esophagoscopy are being used less and less as the diagnostic resolution of modern CT scanners increasingly renders them obsolete (vide infra).

Duplex ultrasonography is noninvasive and of value in experienced hands for evaluation of vascular pathology in zone 2 injuries. Some have even suggested that it supplants angiography in zone 2.[41] It is of considerably less use in zones 1 and 3 because of underlying bony structures. It has no use where there is significant subcutaneous emphysema. Its appeal lies in the rapidity and repeatability of the procedure, but if not performed by the same skilled operator, may give rise to significant interoperator errors of interpretation.

FUTURE MANAGEMENT OF NECK TRAUMA

Notwithstanding the classical three-zone approach to neck trauma described originally by Monson in 1969 and adopted in this chapter,[42] it would be wrong to think that it is not changing. Several recent articles have challenged this traditional concept, suggesting that a return to careful physical examination and the liberal use of modern multidetector (multislice) CT scanners with CTA render the invasive investigations of endoscopy of the aerodigestive tract and contrast esophagography obsolete. [39,40,43,44,45] Instead of being rigidly bound by anatomical landmarks in decision-making, Shiroff's group propose a "no zone" approach, with critical decisions being made on the clinical signs supported by high-resolution CTA.[40] Whether this move away from the practice of the last 45 years will be readily adopted by the trauma community remains to be seen.

REFERENCES

1. Biffl WL, Moore EE, Ryu RK, et al. The unrecognized epidemic of blunt carotid arterial injuries: early diagnosis improves neurologic outcome. Ann Surg. 1998;228(4):462-70.
2. Alterman DM. Penetrating neck trauma. [Online] Available from http://emedicine.medscape.com/article/433306-overview#a0104 [Accessed June 2013].
3. Woo K, Magner DP, Wilson MT, et al. CT angiography in penetrating neck trauma reduces the need for operative neck exploration. Am Surg. 2005;71(9):754-8.
4. Johnson ML. Penetrating neck trauma. In: Pietzman AB, Rhodes M, Schwab CW, Yealy DM, (Eds). The Trauma Manual. Philadelphia, PA: Lippincott-Raven; 1998. Pp. 187.
5. Millar RH, Duplechain JK. Penetrating wounds of the neck. Otolaryngol Clin North Am. 1991;24(1):15-29.
6. Tisherman SA, Bokhara F, Collier B, et al. Penetrating zone II neck trauma. J Trauma. 2008;64(5):1392-405.
7. Demetriades D, Theodorou D, Cornwell E, et al. Transcervical gunshot injuries: mandatory operation is not necessary. J Trauma. 1996;40(5):758-60.
8. Hodgetts TJ, Mahoney PF, Russell MQ, et al. ABC to <C>ABC: redefining the military trauma paradigm. Emerg Med J. 2006;23(10):745-6.
9. Schieber W. The demonstration of thoracic duct abnormalities by lymphangiography. ANGIOLOGY. 1974;25:73-87.
10. Thompson A. Variations of the thoracic duct associated with abnormal arterial distribution. J Anat Physiol. 1884; 18(4): 416-25.
11. Butler CS. On an abnormal thoracic duct. J Med Res. 1903; 10(1):153-6.
12. Johnstone DW. Anatomy of the thoracic duct and chylothorax. In: Shields TW, LoCicero J, Reed CE, Feins RH (Eds). General Thoracic Surgery. Philadelphia, PA: Lippincott Williams and Wilkins; 2011. Pp. 827.
13. Nair R, Robbs JV, Muckart DJ. Management of penetrating cervicomediastinal venous trauma. Eur J Endovasc Surg. 2000;19:65-9.
14. Kumar SR, Weaver FA, Yellin AE. Cervical vascular injuries: carotid and jugular venous injuries. Surg Clin North Am. 2001;81(6):1331-44.
15. Ramadan F, Rutledge R, Oller D, et al. Carotid artery trauma: A review of contemporary trauma center experiences. J Vasc Surg. 1995;21(1):46-56.
16. Paré A. The Apologie and Treatise of Ambroise Paré Containing the Voyages Made in the Divers Places with Many Writings Upon Surgery. In: Key G (Ed). London: Falcon Education Books; 1957.
17. Fleming D. Case of rupture of the carotid artery and wounds of several of its branches, successfully treated by tying the common trunk of the carotid itself. Med Chir J Rev. 1817;3:2-4.
18. Rich N, Spencer FC. Carotid and vertebral injuries. In: Rich N, Spencer FC, (Eds). Vascular Trauma. Philadelphia: WB Saunders; 1978.
19. Makins GH. Gunshot Injuries to the Blood Vessels. Bristol: John Wright & Sons; 1919.
20. Cohen CA, Brief D, Mathewson CJ. Carotid artery injuries: an analysis of eighty-five cases. Am J Surg. 1970;120:210-4.
21. Wylie EJ, Hein MF, Adams JE. Intracranial hemorrhage following surgical revascularization for treatment of acute strokes. J Neurosurg. 1964;21:212-5.
22. Bradley EL. Management of penetrating carotid injuries: an alternative approach. J Trauma. 1973;13:248-55.
23. Liekweg WG, Greenfield LJ. Management of penetrating carotid arterial injury. Ann Surg. 1978;188:587-92.
24. Brown MF, Graham JM, Feliciano DV, et al. Carotid artery injuries. Am J Surg. 1982;144:748-53.
25. Karlin RM, Marks C. Extracranial carotid artery injury: current surgical management. Am J Surg. 1983;146:225-7.

26. Weaver FA, Yellin AE, Wagner WH, et al. The role of arterial reconstruction in penetrating carotid injuries. Arch Surg. 1988;123:1106-11.
27. Ledgerwood AM, Mullins RJ, Lucas CE. Primary repair vs ligation for carotid artery injuries. Arch Surg. 1980;115:488-93.
28. Meyer FB, Piepgras DG, Sandok BA, et al. Emergency carotid endarterectomy for patients with acute carotid occlusion and profound neurological deficits. Ann Surg. 1986;203: 82-9.
29. Unger SW, Tucker WS, Mrdeza MA, et al. Carotid arterial trauma. Surgery. 1980;87:477-87.
30. Berne JD, Reuland KS, Villarreal DH, et al. Sixteen-slice multi-detector computed tomographic angiography improves the accuracy of screening for blunt cerebrovascular injury. J Trauma. 2006;60:1204-10.
31. Miller PR, Fabian TC, Croce MA, et al. Prospective screening for blunt cerebrovascular injuries: analysis of diagnostic modalities and outcomes. Ann Surg. 2002;236:386-93; discussion 393-5.
32. Biffl WL, Egglin T, Benedetto B, et al. Sixteen-slice computed tomographic angiography is a reliable noninvasive screening test for clinically significant blunt cerebrovascular injuries. J Trauma. 2006;60:745-51; discussion 751-2.
33. Mori S, Endo M, Nishizawa K, et al. Comparison of patient doses in 256-slice CT and 16-slice CT scanners; Br J Radiol. 2006;79:56-61.
34. Bromberg WJ, Collier BC, Diesel LN, et al. Eastern Association for the Surgery of Trauma. Blunt cerebrovascular injury. J Trauma. 2010;68(2):471-7.
35. Biffl WL, Cothren CC, Moore EE, et al. Western Trauma Association Critical Decisions in Trauma: screening for and treatment of blunt cerebrovascular injuries. J Trauma. 2009;67:1150-53.
36. Dubois-Marshall S, De Kock S. Two days with a broken knife blade in the neck—an interesting case of Horner's syndrome. Emerg Med J. 2011;28(7):629-31.
37. Schneidereit NP, Simons R, Nicolaou S, et al. Utility of screening for blunt vascular neck injuries with computed tomographic angiography. J Trauma. 2006;60:209-15; discussion 215-16.
38. Berne JD, Norwood SH, McAuley CE, et al. Helical computed tomographic angiography: an excellent screening test for blunt cerebrovascular injury. J Trauma. 2004;57:11-7; discussion 17-9.
39. Inaba K, Branco BC, Menaker J, et al. Evaluation of multidetector computed tomography for penetrating neck injury: a prospective multicenter study. J Trauma Acute Care Surg. 2012;72(3):576-83; discussion 583-4.
40. Shiroff AM, Gale SC, Martin ND, et al. Penetrating neck trauma: a review of management strategies and discussion of the 'No Zone' approach. Am Surg. 2013;79(1):23-9.
41. Fry WR, Dort JA, Smith RA, et al. Duplex scanning replaces arteriography and operative exploration in the diagnosis of potential cervical vascular injury. Am J Surg. 1994;168(6): 693-5; discussion 695-6.
42. Monson DO, Saletta JD, Freeark RJ. Carotid vertebral trauma. J Trauma. 1969;9:987-97.
43. Bell RB, Osborn T, Dierks EJ, et al. Management of penetrating neck injuries: a new paradigm for civilian trauma. J Oral Maxillofac Surg. 2007;65(4):691-705.
44. Osborn TM, Bell RB, Qaisi W, et al. Computed tomographic angiography as an aid to clinical decision making in the selective management of penetrating injuries to the neck: a reduction in the need for operative exploration. J Trauma. 2008;64(6):1466-71.
45. Offiah C, Hall E. Imaging assessment of penetrating injury of the neck and face. Insights Imaging. 2012;3(5):419-31.
46. Du Plessis DJ. Synopsis of surgical anatomy. In: Fasciae, 11th edition. Bristol, England: John Wright & Sons Ltd; 1975. P. 207.
47. Cipolle MD. Blunt neck injury. In: Pietzman AB, Rhodes M, Schwab CW, Yealy DM (Eds). The Trauma Manual. Philadelphia, PA: Lippincott-Raven;1998. P. 195.

38A

Brain Injury

Alex B Valadka

Key Points

- Traumatic brain injury (TBI) is the leading cause of death and disability from trauma.
- Hematomas and other well-defined mass lesions may coexist with diffuse injuries like ischemia and axonal injury.
- A cornerstone of management is prevention, prompt detection, and treatment of such secondary cerebral insults as hypotension and hypoxia. The injured brain is especially vulnerable to the deleterious effects of such deviations from normal homeostasis.
- Initial assessment of patients makes use of the Glasgow Coma Scale and other key components of the neurologic examination, along with prompt computed tomogram scanning.
- Management of elevated intracranial pressure moves along a stepwise progression of interventions that become more aggressive and potentially more prone to be associated with complications.
- Outcome from severe TBI has changed little over recent decades, perhaps because our limited understanding results in our managing a variety of underlying pathophysiologic processes with the same generic treatment algorithm.

INTRODUCTION

Lessons learned from many completed clinical trials and from several ongoing large multinational studies may permit us to stratify our classification of traumatic brain injury (TBI) into specific subtypes based on pathophysiology and clinical relevance. In turn, such a categorization scheme may result in treatments that are tailored more specifically to individual patients.

EPIDEMIOLOGY

Traumatic brain injury is arguably the most important type of single organ system injury encountered by the trauma surgeon. Brain injury affects outcome in half of all deaths from trauma,[1] and it has been estimated that one third of the huge cost of trauma can be attributed to TBI.

Traumatic brain injury is present in roughly one third of trauma center patients. The mortality rate in those with TBI is higher than that for trauma patients without TBI (60% vs. 40%). Gunshot wounds to the head (GSWH) result in some of the highest mortality rates (almost 90%). The GSWH patients comprise <2% of the admissions to trauma centers in the United States, but account for 10% of the deaths in trauma centers. Generally, the mortality rate of TBI patients is little influenced by the presence of extracranial injury except when this injury overwhelms a relatively minor brain injury.

Traumatic brain injury is the most important cause of traumatic death and remains a major challenge in trauma care.[2,3] As with trauma, in general, TBI most commonly affects young males. Historically, motor vehicle accidents have predominated as the single most common cause of TBI.[4] Falls are the most common mechanism of injury for both younger and older patients. In some parts of the United States, GSWHs are the most common form of TBI.[5]

KINEMATICS

A good knowledge of the mechanics of TBI is helpful in anticipating and understanding the accompanying pathophysiology.

Blunt Injury

Blunt tissue damage is caused by loading, deceleration, viscous response, and blast. Loading mechanisms are responsible for most bony fractures, whereas deceleration is the mechanism traditionally deemed responsible for intracranial injury. Direct contact between the head and an

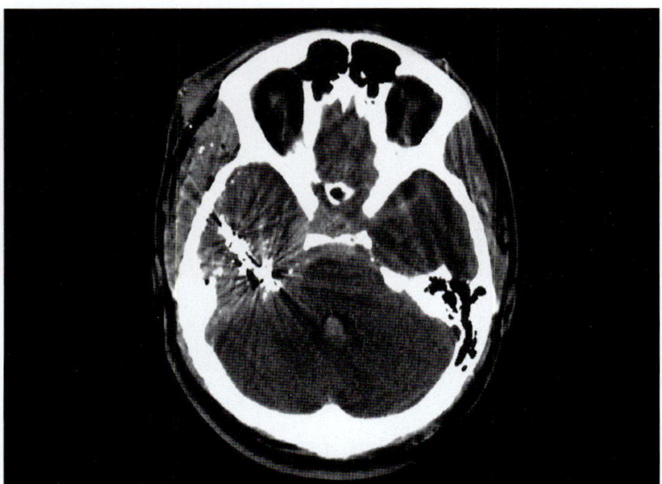

Fig. 38A.1: Gunshot wound to the head. Bullet track in right temporal lobe contains undriven bone fragments.

external surface is the most common type of deceleration, but rapid rotation or sudden noncontact acceleration/deceleration may also be causative. The brain and the skull are of different masses, so the brain has a delayed response to deceleration and may collide with the rough surfaces on the inside of the skull while also distracting from the contralateral surface. Brain deformation and axonal stretching may occur. This is believed to result in diffuse axonal injury (DAI). Subdural hematomas (SDHs) arise from tearing of veins in the potential subdural space or from separation of the inner from the outer layers of the dura.

The most common cause of TBI is vehicular trauma. As the vehicle suddenly decelerates, the head may rapidly flex forward and impact a rigid surface. This type of flexion, deceleration, or hyperextension mechanism explains not only the pathology of the brain injury, but also the frequently accompanying cervical spine and spinal cord injury discussed in Chapter 38B, "Cervical Spine and Spinal Cord Trauma".

Penetrating Injury

Bullets and other projectiles destroy tissue that is directly in their path (Fig. 38A.1). The volume of tissue destroyed in this fashion is increased by a projectile's tendency to tumble and roll in three dimensions. In addition, the cavitation produced by a bullet generates a region of low pressure, which destroys more brain tissue by sucking it into this space. Finally, bullets may cause pressure waves that are transmitted throughout the brain parenchyma. Such pressure waves can cause a temporary cessation of respiratory drive which, if for a sufficient duration, can lead to death if respiration is not supported.[6,7]

Besides damage caused by transmission of energy from the bullet to the brain, other histologic sequelae of penetrating brain injury can include any of the various types of intracranial hematoma described below, as well as the creation of a large tract of necrotic tissue that in many ways mimics a large contusion. The undriven bone, blood, skin, and other debris can act as a nidus for infection. Even tangential gunshot wounds can produce serious intracranial pathology.[7]

Penetrating injury results in a higher mortality rate than blunt injury because of the highly focused kinetic energy imparted by the bullet and secondary fragments. The resulting combination can cause massive brain damage. On the other hand, a low-velocity, low-caliber bullet passing through the frontal lobe may cause relatively minor injury because the kinetic energy available for transfer of vulnerable tissue is less.

When clinical circumstances permit, time invested in elucidating a detailed history is often rewarding, as is a careful examination of the skin to identify external evidence of injury.[8,9]

PATHOPHYSIOLOGY

Traditionally, closed TBI has been divided into two main categories: diffuse injury and mass lesions. These two types often coexist.

Diffuse Injury

Although the appearance of diffuse injuries on head CT scans may be less dramatic than that of large-mass lesions, they often have a much greater impact on a patient's long-term outcome.

Diffuse brain injuries may be considered in two broad categories: DAI and ischemia.

Diffuse Axonal Injury

Diffuse axonal injury describes the physical disruption or "breakage" of long axon cylinders throughout the brain after traumatic injury. If enough neurons sustain such physical disconnection of the nerve cell body from its axon, severe neurologic dysfunction may result from the overwhelming loss of normal neuronal connections. Although Strich[10] assumed that this loss of axonal continuity occurs immediately upon impact, subsequent work has suggested that frank axonal disruption may not occur for several hours after injury.[11] The shearing and rotational forces operant during the physical impact of the head injury appear to set into motion a series of changes that require a certain amount of time to produce axonal discontinuity. The existence of this time interval suggests that there may be a window of opportunity for therapeutic intervention to arrest and possibly reverse axonal disruption. Moreover, it has been demonstrated that the mammalian central nervous system is able to replace some axonal terminations that have been lost after experimental TBI. These findings have raised hope that one day it may be possible to prevent and treat DAI. At present, there is no specific treatment.

Ischemia

The ischemia, which frequently occurs after TBI, differs from that caused by stroke. The term "ischemic stroke" most commonly refers to interruption of blood flow in a specific vascular distribution due to thrombosis or embolism. Although this type of impairment of blood flow can occur after TBI, it is not seen nearly as frequently as global ischemia or regional hypoperfusion from disturbances of autoregulation, especially during the first few hours after injury. Global ischemia can also result from a decrease in systemic blood pressure or an increase in intracranial pressure (ICP), both of which can decrease the cerebral perfusion pressure (CPP).

A decrease in global or regional cerebral blood flow (CBF) below the ischemic threshold of 18 mL/100 g/min has been demonstrated in almost one third of severe TBI patients in whom CBF was measured 3.1 ± 2.1 hours after injury.[12] Such patients fare much worse than those whose blood flow does not fall into the ischemic range. Patients whose jugular venous oxygen saturation ($S_{jv}O_2$) drops below the critical threshold of 50% (indicating increased cerebral extraction of oxygen from the blood because delivery of blood is inadequate to meet the brain's metabolic requirements) during the first 5 days after severe TBI have been shown to have a worse outcome.[13] These physiologic observations about the importance of ischemia after TBI are supported by autopsy studies reporting that >90% of brains from patients who died from TBI exhibited ischemic damage.[14]

Mass Lesions

Four common types of mass lesion are subdural hematoma, epidural hematoma (EDH), intracerebral hematoma (ICH), and cerebral contusion.

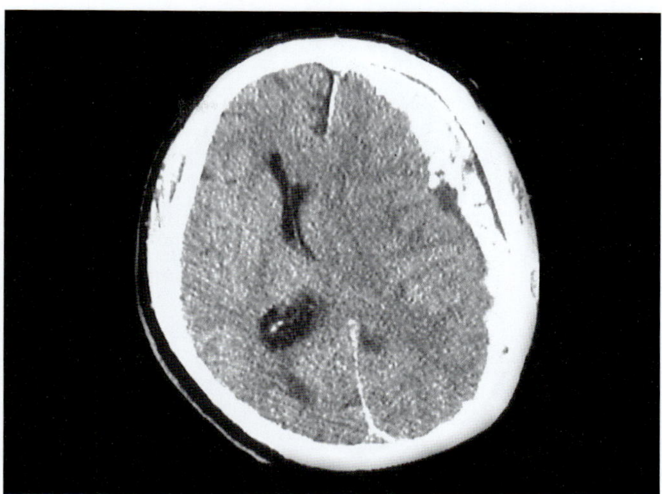

Fig. 38A.2: Subdural hematoma.

Subdural Hematoma

An SDH (Fig. 38A.2) is the most common type of traumatic intracranial hematoma. It has traditionally been said to originate from tearing of small veins that bridge the potential space between the cortex and the overlying dura, but others suggest that it may originate more commonly from splitting of the inner portion of the dura from the outer layers.

Historically, SDHs have been associated with a poor outcome. This may be due, in part, to their frequent coexistence with cerebral contusions and to their common occurrence in the elderly. Also, the same mechanical forces that cause sufficient tissue disruption to create an SDH may cause DAI, further contributing to poor outcomes. A statistically significant decrease in mortality rate has been reported if an SDH is evacuated within 4 hours of injury, but this result has been difficult to reproduce.[15] However, physiologic evidence supports the common sense notion that patients fare better if a large hematoma is evacuated promptly.[16]

Epidural Hematoma

An EDH (Fig. 38A.3) occurs between the outer layer of the dura and the inner layer of the skull. Traditional teaching ascribes it to a fracture of the squamous portion of the temporal bone, which lacerates the middle meningeal artery. Classically, an EDH is associated with a so-called lucid interval: the patient may be knocked unconscious for a few minutes after a blow to the head and then regains consciousness, but eventually, the enlarging blood clot produced by ongoing hemorrhage from the lacerated

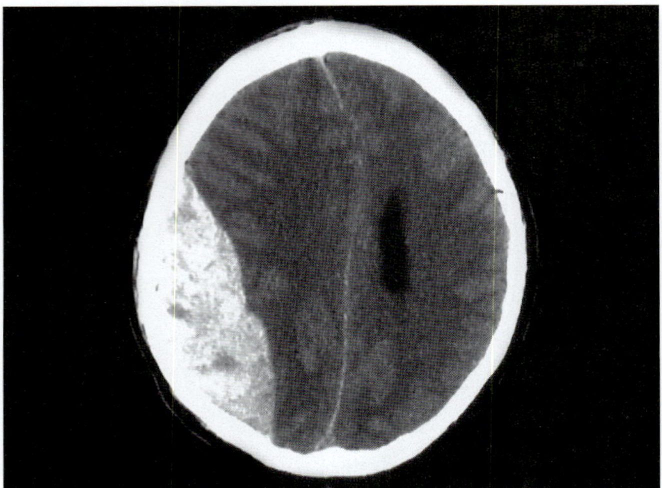

Fig. 38A.3: Epidural hematoma.

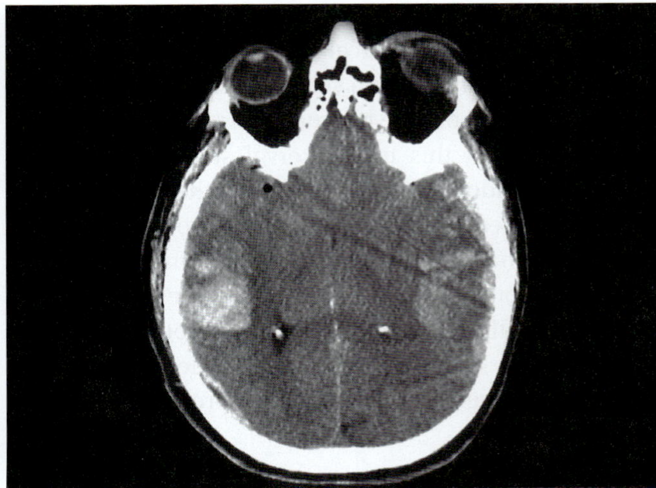

Fig. 38A.4: Large bilateral temporal contusions.

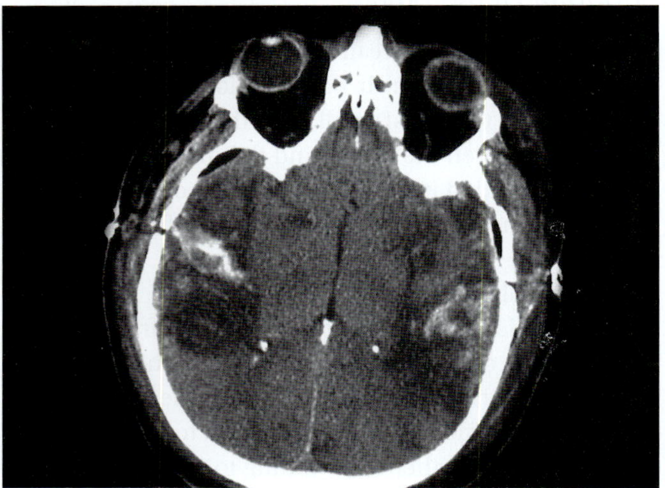

Fig. 38A.5: Follow-up computed tomogram (CT) scan from patient whose initial CT scan is shown in Figure 38A.4. Three days have elapsed since admission. Large dark areas represent edema around the contusions.

middle meningeal artery exerts such a pronounced mass effect that cerebral herniation occurs and the patient dies. Laceration of the middle meningeal artery is, however, not as common a cause of EDH as classical teaching suggests. More commonly, EDHs are caused by oozing of blood from the edges of skull fractures.

Perhaps the most important point to remember about EDHs, especially those caused by ongoing brisk arterial hemorrhage, is that an excellent outcome can often be achieved if they are evacuated promptly, before a patient begins to exhibit neurologic deterioration from a mass effect.

Intracerebral Hematoma and Cerebral Contusion

A traumatic ICH is a solid collection of blood within the brain parenchyma. It originates from disruption of a blood vessel and can occur anywhere in the brain.

A contusion may best be thought of as an area of focal breakdown of the blood–brain barrier in which extravasated red blood cells mix freely with brain parenchyma (Figs. 38A.4 and 38A.5). An alternative way to view a contusion is as a "bruise" of the brain. Although contusions, like traumatic ICHs, can occur anywhere in the brain, they have a predilection for the inferior parts of the frontal lobes and for the anterior and inferior parts of the temporal lobes bilaterally. In these regions, the brain may suddenly impact the rough surface of the skull base after the head abruptly stops moving during trauma.

Shear injuries appear as small hyperdense lesions frequently seen on CT scans of TBI patients. They are thought to occur as the mechanical forces of the trauma cause parts of the brain to move at different speeds and directions. This results in physical disruption of, and hemorrhage into, the brain tissue that lies between areas that are moving with different velocities.

Clinically, traumatic ICHs and contusions behave similarly. Smaller lesions can be managed nonoperatively. Larger lesions may require prompt surgical evacuation.

Other Hemorrhagic Lesions

Subarachnoid Hemorrhage

Trauma is the most common cause of SAH. Significant SAH after trauma may produce vasospasm or narrowing of a focal region or regions of the cerebral vasculature that may be severe enough to cause an ischemic stroke. However, for reasons that are not completely clear, vasospasm after traumatic SAH does not seem to occur nearly as often as after SAH resulting from a ruptured cerebral aneurysm. An exception may occur in blast-induced injuries.

Intraventricular Hemorrhage

Isolated intraventricular hemorrhage is rarely produced by trauma. If large enough, an intraventricular blood clot could interfere with flow of cerebrospinal fluid (CSF) and cause obstructive hydrocephalus. Otherwise, the prognosis is determined by the extent of coexistent injury to the brain parenchyma.

Skull Fractures

An isolated linear skull fracture rarely requires any special treatment. However, surgical intervention may be necessary if a fracture is depressed. One commonly used indication for surgery is that one edge of the fracture projects inward to such an extent that it lies inside the plane of the inner table of the skull at the other edge of the fracture. The likelihood of dural and cortical lacerations is higher with such fractures. The presence of an open depressed skull fracture (i.e. one in which a scalp laceration overlies the fracture) should lower one's threshold for surgical debridement and elevation of the fracture.

Extreme caution should be exercised when contemplating elevation of a depressed fracture that overlies a major dural venous sinus. Uncontrolled release of the tamponade that such a fracture may be exerting on the venous sinus may produce disastrous, and even fatal, hemorrhage.

RESUSCITATION AND EVALUATION

The initial resuscitation of a TBI patient is the same as for all trauma patients. Even before the patient reaches the hospital, resuscitation should be initiated by prehospital personnel. Emphasis is placed on airway, breathing, and circulation.[17] Evaluation and resuscitation proceed simultaneously. More thorough assessment includes the standard emergency department (ED) radiologic and laboratory studies, in addition to a careful secondary survey. These fundamental principles are often forgotten by physicians who are inexperienced in resuscitating TBI patients. It is all too easy to blame a "central process" for abnormalities in blood pressure, cardiac rhythm, respiratory pattern, temperature, urine output, and a host of other physiologic parameters. However, it is essential to remember that TBI patients are not an exception to basic principles of resuscitation; *see* Chapter 31, "Initial Trauma Evaluation and Resuscitation," for more details.

Table 38A.1 Glasgow Coma Scale

Score	*Component of examination*
	Motor
6	Obeys commands
5	Localizes stimulus
4	Withdraws from stimulus
3	Flexes arm
2	Extends arm
1	No response
	Verbal
5	Oriented
4	Confused
3	Recognizable words/phrases
2	Makes sounds
1	No response
	Eye opening
4	Spontaneously
3	To voice
2	To pain
1	Remain closed

Severe TBI patients are best cared for in an intensive care unit (ICU). Every attempt should be made to move them from the ED to the ICU as quickly as possible. Before this can be carried out safely, however, the ED evaluation should be completed and the patient stabilized. From this perspective, any emergency operations, including trauma craniotomies and laparotomies, are viewed as temporary stops in the operating room en route to the final destination (i.e. the ICU).

NEUROLOGIC ASSESSMENT

A detailed neurologic examination is often not possible during the initial assessment in the ED. However, the most essential information can be obtained quickly by determination of the Glasgow Coma Scale (GCS)[18] score (Table 38A.1) and an assessment of pupillary reactivity.

The GCS evaluates function in three areas: motor, verbal, and eye opening. The specific responses are scored according to a numbered scale. The advantage of the GCS is that it eliminates the use of such ambiguous terms as obtunded, lethargic, stuporous, semicomatose, etc. Although other coma grading schemes have been proposed, none enjoys both the widespread use and the simplicity of the GCS.

Patients who have a GCS score of 13–15 are often classified as having mild TBI. Patients who have a GCS score of 9–12 are considered to have moderate TBI, and those with a GCS score of ≤ 8 are usually described as having severe TBI. It is has commonly been stated that approximately 80% of all TBIs are mild, 10% are moderate, and 10% severe, but recent increased awareness of mild TBI and an apparent decrease in the incidence of severe TBI seem to have skewed this distribution away from the severe end of the spectrum toward the mild side.

Most patients with severe TBI will not obey commands (i.e. have a motor score ≤ 5). Such inability to follow simple one-step commands, such as to hold up two fingers, is a simple but useful definition of coma.

Problems with the use of the GCS may arise when some of its components cannot be assessed. For example, accurate determination of the verbal score is not possible if a patient has been endotracheally intubated in the field or has undergone a tracheostomy before neurologic examination. Periorbital swelling may make assessment of eye opening impossible. To avoid potential confusion, it is best to document the score for each of the three components of the GCS in addition to the summed GCS score.

The GCS does not assess pupil reactivity. The importance of this finding is that a dilated pupil that does not decrease in size in response to bright light may indicate the presence of cerebral herniation. Compression of the third cranial nerve by herniating brain tissue may cause inactivation of the pupilloconstrictor fibers on the periphery of the nerve. Their inactivation causes the pupil to dilate and become unresponsive to light. Although this physical finding may be caused by ocular trauma, the presence of a dilated or "blown" pupil mandates immediate evaluation for a large-mass lesion that requires emergency surgical evacuation.

Because of the overwhelming importance of the neurologic examination in TBI patients, any sedating, anesthetic, or paralyzing drugs should be withheld until after a reliable neurologic assessment has been carried out.

DIAGNOSTIC EVALUATION

Imaging

The radiologic test of choice for evaluating TBI is CT scanning.[19] Patients with severe TBI should undergo CT scanning as soon as they are stable enough to leave the ED. Patients with moderate TBI should also be scanned promptly, although the urgency of obtaining a CT scan in these patients may be less than that for severe TBI patients.

Deciding when to obtain a CT scan for patients with mild TBI is more problematic. Several studies have put forth clinical criteria that may be used to help decide when a CT scan is appropriate after an apparently minor TBI. Concerns about exposing patients, and especially children, to radiation have weakened enthusiasm for the practice of aggressively scanning all such patients. Similarly, follow-up scanning is probably not needed in most mild TBI patients whose neurological examinations remain stable. Using plain radiographs as a screening device to detect signs of injury to justify a CT scan adds little to the evaluation of the vast majority of cases.[20] Consideration should be given to scanning patients who have a prolonged loss of consciousness, severe headaches, or prolonged amnesia after an apparently minor blow to the head. If CT scanning is expected to be delayed, an alternative is to admit such patients to the hospital for a brief period of time in order to observe them carefully for any signs of neurologic deterioration.

Magnetic resonance imaging (MRI) is sometimes used to search for evidence of subtle or diffuse injury that might not be evident on CT scanning, especially in patients who are not neurologically improving after injury. At the present time, however, the value of this practice is debated because patient management is rarely affected by the additional information that MRI provides over CT scanning. Ongoing investigations in this area may help to clarify the role of MRI in acute TBI.

Serum Markers

Serum markers of TBI are currently of intense interest. A diagnostic test based on rapid detection of specific proteins in a drop of blood could facilitate diagnosis of TBI on the battlefield or the athletic field. Serial measurements could help clinicians track the evolution of all severities of TBI. Numerous candidate proteins have been identified and are undergoing rigorous testing.

CONFLICTING TREATMENT PRIORITIES

The coexistence of severe TBI with another immediately life-threatening injury often requires difficult treatment decisions to be made without delay. Providing the best possible care for such patients requires that physicians from the different specialties involved communicate openly and honestly to avoid potential conflicts about treatment priorities. A common situation in which this potential conflict occurs is the coexistence of severe TBI and hemodynamic instability. If such patients are taken for an immediate laparotomy, the neurosurgeon has several options, including any of the following:

- Placing an ICP monitor
- Performing an air ventriculogram in the operating room (and then if this demonstrates major midline shift, performing a craniotomy while the laparotomy is proceeding)
- Carrying out empiric surgical exploration and decompression on the side of a dilated pupil
- Waiting until the laparotomy is completed before obtaining a CT scan.

If a patient is hemodynamically stable despite the demonstration of free fluid on abdominal sonography, it is often possible to obtain a head CT scan while preparations are being made for a laparotomy. This option became more feasible with the advent of spiral CT scanning, which can complete a head CT scan in seconds. Another change in practice is the widespread adoption of leaving the abdomen open in anticipation of a planned return to the operating room for definitive hemostasis or for the expected development of abdominal compartment syndrome. This practice shortens the duration of an emergency laparotomy and makes it more reasonable simply to wait until the laparotomy is completed, and then obtain a head CT scan.

Another potential conflict arises when thoracic aortic injury is suspected. Like hypotension from abdominal trauma, severe aortic trauma is one of the few injuries that may be more immediately life threatening than severe TBI. If a TBI patient suspected of having such a lesion can be taken for aortic imaging immediately, the brain injury should take second priority. Practically speaking, however, a TBI patient can usually be taken to the CT scanner while the angiography suite is being prepared. In current practice, the widespread use of CT angiography to evaluate these injuries means that a head CT scan can be performed before the chest is scanned. If a patient is found to have both a large intracranial mass lesion and another injury requiring surgical intervention, clear communication between the neurosurgeon and the trauma surgeon is required to optimize patient outcome.

The advent of endovascular techniques to treat these injuries has shifted the debate to the question of how soon after injury anticoagulation may be used in a TBI patient. Fortunately, it is now recognized that many of these injuries may be safely treated by observation for several days before endovascular intervention. This may allow sufficient time to pass so that the intracranial risks of anticoagulation are minimized when the endovascular procedure is performed.

Although not immediately life threatening, long bone fractures are common in TBI patients. Any immediate intervention needed for the brain injury takes priority. However, the question is the timing of treatment of long bone fractures. The answer depends upon the status of the patient's cerebral metabolism, including ICP readings. In some cases, when a trauma craniotomy has not been complicated by brain swelling and a patient has remained hemodynamically stable during anesthesia, the orthopedic surgeons can proceed with fracture fixation immediately upon closure of the craniotomy while the patient is still under the same anesthesia. On the other hand, we do not endorse fixation of long bone fractures in the presence of malignant intracranial hypertension, hemodynamic instability, severe adult respiratory distress syndrome, or other problems until the patient's condition has improved considerably.

DEFINITIVE CARE

Secondary Insults

The most important principle underlying the ICU management of TBI patients is to prevent secondary insults.[21] Unlike the primary injury, which occurs at the time of impact and is beyond the control of the physician, secondary injury refers to any subsequent deviation from normal physiologic status that can have an adverse effect on neurologic function. This concept may sound overly simplistic. However, its importance arises from the fact that the acutely injured brain is exquisitely sensitive to even minor metabolic disturbances that it might normally tolerate. In the laboratory, this heightened vulnerability of the brain was elegantly demonstrated by Jenkins et al.,[22] who caused a relatively minor experimental TBI in rodents and then followed it with a relatively minor ischemic insult. Although either one of these insults administered by itself was well tolerated, their sequential occurrence produced extensive neuronal necrosis in the hippocampus.

Many secondary insults may occur in the clinical arena. They include hypotension, hypoxia, ischemia, elevated ICP, hyperthermia, hyperglycemia, seizures, delayed or recurrent intracranial hematomas, hypo- or hyperosmolality, and infections. Constant vigilance is required to prevent these abnormalities and, when they occur, to detect and treat them promptly.

Table 38A.2	Specific management goals.
MAP	>80 mm Hg
ICP	<20 mm Hg
PaO_2	>10.7 kPa (80 mm Hg)
SaO_2	>90%
$PaCO_2$	~ 5.3 kPa (40 mm Hg)
Serum Na	135–145 mmol/L (135–145 mEq/L)
Serum glucose	4.4–10 mmol/L (80–180 mg/dL)
Hemoglobin	>5 mmol/L (8.0 gm/dL)
Temperature	<38°C (100.4°F)
Nutritional support	Begin within 2–3 days

(MAP: Mean arterial pressure; ICP: Intracranial pressure).

Our management protocol centers on the following:

- Prompt evacuation of intracranial mass lesions
- Aggressive monitoring in the ICU
- Vigilance in preventing and treating secondary insults.

Some specific target values for physiologic parameters are listed in Table 38A.2.

Flowchart 38A.1: Progression of treatments used for refractory intracranial hypertension.

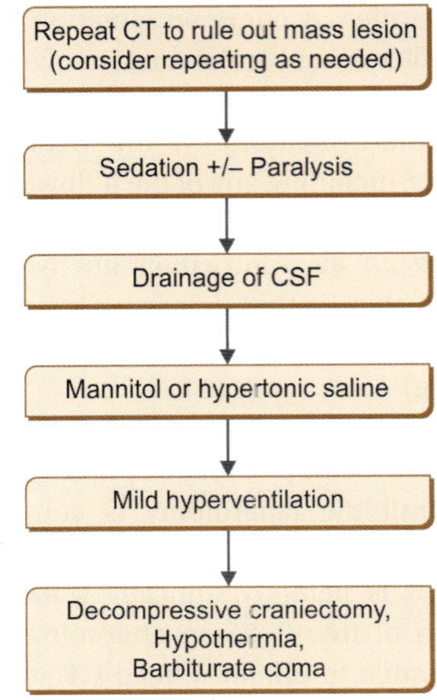

(CSF: Cerebrospinal fluid).

Management of Elevated ICP

Because elevated ICP is the most common secondary insult of cerebral origin, protection of the injured brain from refractory intracranial hypertension is one of the major thrusts of neurosurgical critical care. Narayan et al. recommended that the ICP be monitored in patients with severe TBI and abnormal CT scans and in those with normal scans if two of the following three features are present: age >40 years, posturing on motor examination, or systolic blood pressure <90 mm Hg.[23] We have adopted a more aggressive approach, inserting ventriculostomies or other ICP monitors in patients who are not obeying commands or who deteriorate to this level, as well as in selecting other patients in whom ICP control may become difficult.

The long established practice of aggressive ICP monitoring in severe TBI patients has been challenged by a South American study in which patients treated with ICP monitors and protocolized treatment of elevated ICP were compared to a group in which clinical and CT findings were used to decide whether to initiate a standardized series of interventions to lower ICP.[24] The use of ICP monitoring failed to improve outcome. This study should not be interpreted as justification for ignoring ICP in TBI patients. It must be remembered that both groups underwent treatment for an elevated ICP; in one group, elevated ICP was diagnosed with an ICP monitor, and in the other, it was diagnosed by more qualitative techniques. In the future, an improved ability to classify TBI may lead to more precise targeting of which patients truly benefit from invasive ICP monitoring.

Most centers use 20 mm Hg as the cutoff in adults above which ICP should be treated (normal adult ICP range 10-15 mm Hg). Such treatment proceeds in a stepwise fashion, similar to that described in the Guidelines for the Management of Severe Traumatic Brain Injury.[25] One algorithm for controlling elevated ICP is shown in Flowchart 38A.1.

If a recent CT scan has not been obtained, one is repeated promptly in case the ICP begins to rise. Any delayed or recurrent mass lesions are evacuated.

Control of elevated ICP may be achieved through sedation with opiates or benzodiazepines, together with pharmacological paralysis with neuromuscular blocking drugs. These agents are used to decrease and control patient agitation because bucking and straining can increase the ICP. However, the use of neuromuscular blocking drugs without specific indications has been questioned.[26]

If the ICP remains elevated, drainage of CSF through an external ventricular drain (EVD) may be tried. Because EVDs permit drainage of CSF, they may be considered as therapeutic devices (not just monitoring devices). For this reason, we prefer EVDs over other types of ICP monitors.

If the ICP continues to rise despite these maneuvers, mannitol or hypertonic saline may be administered. Part of the effectiveness of mannitol is said to arise from its osmotic effect, drawing water from the brain's extracellular fluid. Muizelaar et al. have demonstrated that mannitol also has a rheological effect, decreasing the viscosity of blood. As a result, the arteries can decrease in diameter because the reduced viscosity allows the amount of blood flowing through the narrowed arteries to remain unchanged.[27] The decrease in vascular diameter decreases cerebral blood volume (CBV), which has a beneficial effect on the ICP.

Mannitol can be administered frequently as necessary provided that the resultant free water losses are carefully measured and, when necessary, replaced. When serum osmolality exceeds 320 mmol/kg (320 mOsm/L), it is probably wise to avoid mannitol to prevent renal damage. In recent years, many clinicians have begun using hypertonic saline instead of mannitol, but solid data to recommend one treatment over the other are lacking. Similarly, the now-common practice of prophylactically raising serum osmolality in hopes of preventing an increase in ICP lacks a firm evidentiary basis.

Mild hyperventilation may be necessary if intracranial hypertension persists. Decreasing the $PaCO_2$ reduces cerebral arteriolar diameter and therefore CBV, which may help to lower the ICP. However, CBF also decreases as the vessels become narrow. Hyperventilation is not a first-line treatment for elevated ICP because of its demonstrated deleterious effect on outcome in TBI patients,[28] but in cases of refractory intracranial hypertension, we may decrease the $PaCO_2$ from our usual value of 40 mm Hg down to as low as 30 mm Hg, or perhaps slightly lower. We monitor $S_{jv}O_2$ or brain tissue PO_2 while we decrease the $PaCO_2$ in order to detect a potential decrease in CBF that is significant enough to trigger cerebral ischemia. If this happens, we increase the $PaCO_2$ back up to safe levels.

It should be noted that hyperventilation may be a useful temporizing measure in patients suspected of harboring a large-mass lesion. The slight decrease in CBV afforded by hyperventilation may temporarily lower the ICP and buy enough time to transport a patient to the operating room. This practice is reasonable when a mass lesion is likely, as in patients who exhibit a progressive decline in mental status with unilateral pupillary enlargement and progressive contralateral hemiparesis. In the absence of a mass lesion, however, or when a mass lesion has already been ruled out, the risks of hyperventilation may outweigh its benefits.[28]

Persistence of intracranial hypertension despite all these measures is an ominous sign. Potential interventions for such cases include barbiturate coma, induced hypothermia, or decompressive craniectomy (DC). The initiation of a barbiturate coma is a major undertaking, comparable to placing a patient under general anesthesia for a prolonged period of time. We may employ pulmonary artery pressure monitoring in such cases and have a very low threshold for initiating the use of pressors to support the arterial blood pressure. Hypothermia and DC are discussed in the following section.

Recent Trends in the Management of Severe TBI

Hypothermia

Hypothermia has been shown to be effective in mitigating the deleterious effects of experimental TBI in laboratory animals. Preliminary reports also suggested a benefit in the clinical setting. These studies, however, were based on small series of patients, and long-lasting benefit was difficult to demonstrate.[29] Several prospective multicenter trials of hypothermia failed to demonstrate a benefit in TBI patients.[30,31] One possible reason is that TBI is a very heterogeneous disease entity that includes many different types of pathophysiology. Beneficial effects of hypothermia in certain subgroups may have been masked by the lack of efficacy in other groups. This speculation is supported by a retrospective analysis of data from two North American hypothermia trials that found a strong protective effect if hypothermia was initiated within 90 minutes of the start of surgery to evacuate a traumatic intracranial mass lesion.[32] No such benefit was seen in patients with diffuse brain injury.

Decompressive Craniectomy

This procedure has witnessed a resurgence of popularity in recent years. Proponents of this practice argue that if the ICP cannot be controlled, then outcome can be improved by removing large portions of the skull and widely opening the dura to permit the injured brain to swell. After the cerebral edema has subsided, the removed bone can be replaced and the dura can be closed properly. Routine use of this practice was reported to be of little benefit in the 1970s.[33] Subsequent claims of its effectiveness were based on case series, historical controls, case reports, or similar types of data. An Australian prospective study of early DC in patients with diffuse brain injury concluded that this intervention not only failed to help patients, but was actually associated with worse outcomes.[34] This study was controversial for several reasons, including an imbalance between intervention and control groups in the proportion of patients with unreactive pupils. Posthoc adjustment for this variable changed the outcome of the intervention group from being worse than that of controls to not being significantly different, yet it should be noted that DC still failed to improve the outcome. An additional complicating factor associated with DC is that several variations exist in the technique used for performing this procedure, as well as in timing and indications. A just-concluded trial examined the benefits of DC as a last-stage intervention in potentially salvageable patients after a standardized protocol of progressively more aggressive nonsurgical interventions failed to control elevated ICP in TBI patients.[35] Results are pending at the time of writing this chapter.

Brain Tissue Oxygen Monitoring ($PbtO_2$)

Some clinicians use brain tissue $PbtO_2$ monitoring to guide their assessment of cerebral metabolism. Debate continues on the optimal placement of these devices. If placed in tissue that appears normal on CT scanning, the $PbtO_2$ monitors may reflect the status of global cerebral metabolism. But if placed near contused or otherwise injured tissue, the probes may be measuring oxygen metabolism in the focal area of injury. Those who advocate the latter approach point out that it is the injured tissue that is most in need of careful monitoring and of efforts to do everything possible to preserve its viability. A larger debate is whether the use of such monitors actually improves patient outcomes. This is similar to the discussion that has arisen recently regarding the use of ICP monitoring in severe TBI patients, with the difference being that the questions about the utility of $PbtO_2$ monitoring are being asked before this practice becomes disseminated throughout the clinical community. A midphase multicenter American study funded by the National Institutes of Health will hopefully shed at least some light on the answer to this question.[36]

Cerebral Perfusion Pressure Augmentation

To counteract the deleterious effects of hypotension, some authors in the past had advocated that CPP be maintained over 70 mm Hg (9.3 kPa) in patients with severe TBI.[37] However, initial reports describing the effectiveness of this practice were based on uncontrolled case series. A randomized, prospective trial investigated a similar management strategy.[38] Although CBF-targeted therapy was successful in reducing the frequency of cerebral ischemia as measured by jugular venous desaturation, it did not translate into greater success in controlling ICP or, more importantly, in improving clinical outcome. Moreover, the CBF-targeted patients had a significantly ($p < 0.05$) higher likelihood of developing adult respiratory distress syndrome. Therefore, although it seems well established that there is a "floor" below which the CPP should not fall, there may also be a "ceiling" above which additional augmentation of CPP may not provide extra benefit and may, in fact, cause harm.

COMPLICATIONS AND SEQUELAE

Refractory Intracranial Hypertension

Perhaps the most dreaded complication of severe TBI is the development of refractory intracranial hypertension. Depending upon the definition used, an elevated ICP can be expected in approximately 25–50% of severe TBI patients, and refractory intracranial hypertension develops in approximately 12–15%. Mortality rates exceeding 80% have been reported if intracranial hypertension cannot be controlled.

Complications of ICP Monitoring

The use of ICP monitors has slight but definite risks. The incidence of hemorrhage related to the insertion is 1–6% or even higher if more liberal definitions are used. Most such hemorrhagic complications are minor. The incidence of ventriculostomy placement causing an intracranial hematoma to require surgical evacuation is probably around 1.4%.[23] A more common complication of EVDs is infection. Depending upon how infection is defined and how aggressively it is sought, rates of 2–10% or more have been reported. Ventriculostomies have a higher infection rate than intraparenchymal monitors. Although widespread practice for many years has been the routine replacement of ventriculostomy catheters every 5–7 days in order to prevent infection, other data suggest that the same catheter may be left in place for a much longer period, with replacement required only if infection develops.[39]

CSF Fistulas

Another frequent source of infection is CSF fistulas, most commonly from fractures through the aerated sinuses at the base of the skull. Most of these fistulas close with simple elevation of the head of the bed. If CSF is not already being diverted through a ventriculostomy catheter and there is no concern about an elevated ICP causing cerebral herniation through the foramen magnum, diversion of CSF via a lumbar drain may be necessary. Persistent leakage may require surgical reconstruction of the skull base to obliterate the fistula.

Disorders of Coagulation

Disorders of coagulation have been well described after TBI. Coagulopathies are associated with a worse prognosis, at least partly because of the increased likelihood of delayed traumatic intracerebral hematomas (DTICHs). Most neurosurgeons are aware of the high incidence of coagulopathy after TBI and treat it aggressively. Although the benefit of administering plasma, platelets, or specific clotting factors after TBI awaits rigorous proof, the rationale for such treatments is intuitive, and a few neurosurgeons are willing to let obvious coagulopathy go untreated. Aggressive use of ICP monitoring and frequent CT scanning may be useful for early detection and prompt treatment of DTICHs.

Focal Ischemia

Focal ischemia can also develop after TBI. Sometimes the cause is obvious (e.g. prolonged compression of the posterior cerebral artery from cerebral herniation through the tentorial hiatus), but in other cases the cause is less clear. Possibilities include vasospasm, regional disruption of cerebral hemodynamics from the existence of isolated islands of altered autoregulation, or damage to an arterial wall from distortion of vasculature by mechanical forces during the traumatic impact.

Post-traumatic Seizures

Post-traumatic seizures are commonly classified as "early" or "late" according to the time of their occurrence, within or beyond 7 days of injury. Evidence suggests that anticonvulsant prophylaxis with phenytoin or carbamazepine prevents seizures for the first week after injury, while lower-quality evidence suggests a role for levetiracetam as well. After the first week, it does not appear to have much benefit in maintaining patients on this prophylaxis if they have never had a seizure. Some authorities have pointed out that the decrease in early seizure rates has not been shown to translate into improved long-term functional outcome in patients.

Hydrocephalus

Hydrocephalus can result from the primary brain injury itself or from a subsequent complication, such as ventriculitis. It may require treatment with a ventriculo peritoneal shunt or other CSF diversionary procedure.

Other Complications

TBI patients are susceptible to the full spectrum of systemic injuries and complications that occur in trauma patients who do not have TBI. For the most part, these are managed as if the patient does not have a brain injury. One common exception to this arises with injuries to the aorta or other major vessels. A trauma surgeon may include deliberate lowering of blood pressure as part of the management of these injuries, but as discussed above, hypotension is one of the most devastating secondary insults that can befall a TBI patient. Consequently, close co-operation between the neurosurgical and the trauma teams is recommended in such cases to maximize the patient's likelihood of achieving the best possible outcome from all of his or her injuries.

OUTCOME

The Glasgow Outcome Scale (GOS)[40] (Table 38A.3) is one of the most widely used schemes for classifying outcome after TBI. At major trauma centers with experience in treating these patients, the lowest mortality rate that can realistically be expected after severe TBI is probably 30–36%. Fewer than 5% of patients remain vegetative and approximately 15% remain severely disabled. Moderate disability can be expected in roughly 15–20% of patients, and >25% will achieve a good recovery.[41] At first glance, these outcomes are not as good as those described in some

Table 38A.3 Glasgow Outcome Scale.

Score	*Category*	*Description*
5	Good recovery	Able to live and work independently despite minor disabilities.
4	Moderate disability	Able to live independently despite disabilities. Can use public transportation, work with assistance/supervision, etc.
3	Severe disability	Conscious but dependent upon others for self-care. Often institutionalized
2	Persistent vegetative state	Not conscious, but may appear "awake"
1	Death	Self-explanatory

recent reports. However, many of those reports are based on series of patients who were not randomized or who were selected for various protocols by specific criteria. In addition, clinical trials of various drugs often exclude the most severely injured patients, those who are brought to the hospital after a specific time from injury, those with no known next of kin, those outside a certain age range; or those who fail to meet various other study requirements. This failure to enroll patients least likely to do well may explain the exceptionally good outcomes in many of these reports. As TBI rates increase among the elderly, whose outcomes are worse because they have more comorbidities, less CNS plasticity, and a greater likelihood of taking anticoagulant or platelet aggregation-inhibiting medications, TBI outcomes for the overall population will worsen.

For moderate TBI, the likelihood of good recovery or moderate disability is 60% and 25%, respectively. The probability of severe disability is approximately 7%, and the likelihood of death or a persistent vegetative state is also 7%.[42]

Patients with mild TBI have an extremely low mortality rate. Outcome in this group of patients is usually discussed in terms of cognitive, emotional, and behavioral disturbances, but the likelihood of developing such symptoms after mild TBI has been quite difficult to define because similar complaints are prevalent in the general population. The existence of such problems in people with an apparently high level of function emphasizes that even patients with good GOS scores can have severe functional deficits. Detailed neuropsychological testing is often helpful to quantify deficits in such patients. Post-traumatic stress disorder and other emotional sequelae often complicate the assessment of outcome in this population.

Concussion is a subtype of mild TBI characterized by transient neurologic deficits and normal brain imaging studies. Recovery is usually prompt, but perhaps 10–15% of such patients may develop longer-lasting symptoms. Many purported treatments have been proposed, but their effectiveness has not been demonstrated in rigorous studies. In the special case of sports-related concussion, most authorities agree that return to contact sports while an athlete is still suffering from the effects of a prior concussion is not recommended because a second concussion can worsen and prolong existing symptoms, and because of the potential development of the rare but catastrophic second-impact syndrome, categorized by rapid, severe, and often fatal cerebral edema.

Repeated concussions or even "subconcussive" blows to the head have been speculated to lead in some cases to chronic traumatic encephalopathy, characterized by abnormal accumulations of τ protein in the brain and the onset of any of a wide variety of neurological or psychiatric symptoms. This entity is controversial, and much still needs to be learned.

Blast injury is frequently encountered by military personnel (*see* Chapter 33, "Military Surgery," for more details). Many features mimic those seen after the more common mechanisms of TBI, but in severe cases, patients with blast injury to the brain may be predisposed to suffer from marked cerebral edema, cerebral vasospasm, and development of traumatic intracranial aneurysms.

Gunshot wounds to the heads have a different outcome curve. In a civilian setting, almost 90% of these injuries are fatal. Among patients who are alive upon arrival at a hospital, mortality rates approximate or even exceed 60%. On the other hand, moderate disability or good recovery will be achieved by 30–40% of patients, with <10% remaining persistently vegetative or severely disabled.[43] These data suggest that if bullets do not cause overwhelmingly devastating injuries from massive tissue destruction, direct passage through vital brainstem centers, or lethal pressure waves, they will probably produce relatively minor neurologic deficits.

Many TBI patients benefit from aggressive rehabilitation. The degree to which this intervention actually improves neurologic function is unclear. However, even if neurologic function does not improve, rehabilitation is enormously valuable for teaching both the patient and family and friends how to maximize the patient's level of function within the limits imposed by temporary or permanent disabilities.

CLINICAL TRIALS

Essentially, all potential therapies for TBI have failed to show benefit when subjected to well-conducted clinical trials.[44] Among some practitioners, this string of "failures" has produced a certain amount of cynicism about the effectiveness of any intervention for TBI.

Fortunately, the reality is not nearly so bleak. For a condition as heterogeneous and mysterious as TBI, a great deal has been learned about the proper design and execution of clinical trials. In retrospect, many trials have been conducted in very unsophisticated ways, even though they were considered to be the state-of-the-art at the time.

For example, it is being increasingly recognized that TBI is a heterogeneous condition. Not all patients who are comatose after a blow to the head are going through the same pathophysiologic processes. Those with large-mass lesions may require immediate craniotomy; those with DAI may require little TBI-specific care; and those with diffuse cerebral edema may be difficult to treat by any method. It is unrealistic to expect these different disease processes to all respond to the same treatment. By analogy, using abdominal pain as an entry criterion for a therapeutic trial is unacceptable because of the tremendous variety of underlying causes of abdominal pain, such as appendicitis, peptic ulcer disease, pancreatic cancer, diverticulitis, and ischemic bowel. No single treatment can be effective for all these diseases, and thus the trial would fail.

Statistical analysis of TBI trials has become much more sophisticated over the years. The GOS[40] is a five-item outcome measure (eight items in the GOS-Extended), yet TBI trials have historically dichotomized outcomes into "favorable" or "unfavorable." Much of the ability to discriminate between outcomes is lost when outcome scales are dichotomized. By analogy, a pass–fail system to grade students in school is not as informative as the traditional five-item scale based on letter grades (such as A, B, C, D, F). Other statistical techniques may tailor the definition of an acceptable outcome according to a patient's injury severity. For example, severe disability may be a poor outcome for a patient who initially had a GCS score of eight, but some might consider that to be a good outcome for a patient who arrived with a GCS score of three and fixed, dilated pupils.

Even something as basic as preclinical evaluation of potential treatments has sometimes been conducted in ways that are now recognized to be less than ideal. Rigorous criteria have now been published.[45,46]

In recognition of the heterogeneity of TBI and of the impossibility of conducting enough clinical trials in a timely manner to address the large number of unanswered important clinical questions, many TBI investigators have revived interest in the use of high-quality clinical databases. The best known of these is the Traumatic Coma Data Bank (TCDB), which collected data over three decades ago but still influences patient management today. Current ongoing efforts include the Transforming Research and Clinical Knowledge in Traumatic Brain Injury study,[47] which includes serum biomarkers, MRI studies, and detailed neuropsychological assessments in its evaluations. The Collaborative European NeuroTrauma Effectiveness Research in Traumatic Brain Injury is a comparable study based in Europe.[48] It is hoped that such large high-quality multinational databases may be as influential as the TCDB has been in improving care of TBI patients worldwide.

SUMMARY

Prevention and treatment of secondary cerebral insults begin before a TBI patient arrives in the ED. Assessment and stabilization proceed thoroughly but rapidly so that a head CT scan can be obtained as soon as possible. Intracranial mass lesions or life-threatening systemic injuries require immediate treatment in the operating room. In the ICU, every attempt is made to avoid secondary cerebral injury and to support the intrinsic efforts of the CNS to recover. Meticulous attention to numerous details is required if patients are to achieve their best possible recovery.

REFERENCES

1. Kraus JF. Epidemiology of head injury. In: Cooper PR (Ed). Head Injury, 2nd edition. Baltimore, MD: Williams & Wilkins; 1987.
2. Gennarelli T, Champion HR, Sacco WJ, et al. Mortality of patients who have a head injury and extracranial injury treated in trauma centers. J Trauma. 1989;29: 1193-202.
3. McMahon CG, Yates DW, Campbell FM, et al. Unexpected contribution of moderate traumatic brain injury to death after major trauma. J Trauma. 1999;47:891-7.
4. Frankowski RF, Annegers JF, Whitman S. Epidemiological and descriptive studies, Part I: The descriptive epidemiology of head trauma in the United States. In: Becker DP, Povlishock JT (Eds). Central Nervous System Trauma Status Report. Richmond, VA: William Byrd Press; 1985.
5. Levy ML, Masri LS, Levy KM, et al. Penetrating craniocerebral injury resultant from gunshot wounds: gang-related injury in children and adolescents. Neurosurgery. 1993;33: 1018-25.
6. Carey ME, Sarna GS, Farrell JB, et al. Experimental missile wound to the brain. J Neurosurg. 1989;71:754-64.
7. Stone JL, Lichtor T, Fitzgerald LF, et al. Civilian cases of tangential gunshot wounds to the head. J Trauma. 1996;40:57-60.
8. McSwain N. Kinematics of injury. In: Mattox K, Feliciano D, Moore EE (Eds). Trauma, 4th edition. New York, NY: McGraw Hill; 1999.
9. Mayberry JC. Blunt injury mechanism. In: Trunkey DD, Lewis FR (Eds). Current Therapy of Trauma. 4th ed. St. Louis, MO: Mosby; 1999.
10. Strich SJ. Shearing of nerve fibers as a cause of brain damage due to head injury. Lancet. 1961;2:443-8.
11. Povlishock JT. Traumatically induced axonal injury: pathogenesis and pathobiological implications. Brain Pathol. 1992;2:1-12.
12. Bouma GJ, Muizelaar JP, Stringer WA, et al. Ultra-early evaluation of regional cerebral blood flow in severely head-injured patients using xenon-enhanced computerized tomography. J Neurosurg. 1992;77:360-8.
13. Gopinath SP, Robertson CS, Contant CF, et al. Jugular venous desaturation and outcome after head injury. J Neurol Neurosurg Psychiatr. 1994;57:717-23.

14. Graham DI, Adams JH, Doyle D. Ischaemic brain damage in fatal non-missile head injuries. J Neurol Sci. 1978;39:213-34.
15. Wilberger JE, Harris M, Diamond DL. Acute subdural hematoma: morbidity and mortality related to timing of operative intervention. J Trauma. 1990;30:733-6.
16. Gopinath SP, Cormio M, Ziegler J, et al. Intraoperative jugular desaturation during surgery for traumatic intracranial hematomas. Anesth Analg. 1996;83:1014-21.
17. Committee on Trauma of the American College of Surgeons. Advanced Trauma Life Support Instructor Manual. Chicago, IL: American College of Surgeons; 1993.
18. Teasdale G, Jennett B. Assessment of coma and impaired consciousness. Lancet. 1974;2:81-4.
19. Valadka AB, Ward JD, Smoker WRK. Brain imaging in neurologic emergencies. In: Prough DS, Traystman RJ (Eds). Critical Care: State of the Art, volume 14. Anaheim, CA: Society of Critical Care Medicine; 1993.
20. Masters SJ, McClean PM, Arcarese JS, et al. Skull X-ray examinations after head trauma. Recommendations by a multidisciplinary panel and validation study. N Engl J Med. 1987;316:84-91.
21. Becker DP, Miller JD, Ward JD, et al. The outcome from severe head injury with early diagnosis and intensive treatment. J Neurosurg. 1977;47:491-502.
22. Jenkins LW, Moszynski K, Lyeth BG, et al. Increased vulnerability of the mildly traumatized rat brain to cerebral ischemia: the use of controlled secondary ischemia as a research tool to identify common or different mechanisms contributing to mechanical and ischemic brain injury. Brain Res. 1989;477:211-24.
23. Narayan RK, Kishore PR, Becker DP, et al. Intracranial pressure: to monitor or not to monitor? A review of our experience with severe head injury. J Neurosurg. 1982;56:650-9.
24. Chesnut RM, Temkin N, Carney N, et al. A trial of intracranial-pressure monitoring in traumatic brain injury. N Engl J Med. 2012;367:2471-81.
25. Brain Trauma Foundation. (2007). Guidelines for the management of severe traumatic brain injury. 3rd edition. New York, NY: Brain Trauma Foundation. [online] Available from https://www.braintrauma.org/pdf/protected/Guidelines_Management_2007w_bookmarks.pdf [Accessed December 24, 2014]
26. Hsiang JK, Chesnut RM, Crisp CB, et al. Early, routine paralysis for intracranial pressure control in severe head injury: is it necessary? Crit Care Med. 1994;22:1471-6.
27. Muizelaar JP, Wei EP, Kontos HA, et al. Mannitol causes compensatory cerebral vasoconstriction and vasodilation in response to blood viscosity changes. J Neurosurg. 1983;59:822-8.
28. Muizelaar JP, Marmarou A, Ward JD, et al. Adverse effects of prolonged hyperventilation in patients with severe head injury: a randomized clinical trial. J Neurosurg. 1991; 75:731-9.
29. Marion DW, Penrod LE, Kelsey SF, et al. Treatment of traumatic brain injury with moderate hypothermia. N Engl J Med. 1997;336:540-6.
30. Clifton GL, Miller ER, Choi SC, et al. Lack of effect of induction of hypothermia after acute brain injury. N Engl J Med. 2001;344:556-63.
31. Clifton GL, Valadka A, Zygun D, et al. Very early hypothermia induction in patients with severe brain injury (the National Acute Brain Injury Study: Hypothermia II): a randomised trial. Lancet Neurol. 2011;10:131-9.
32. Clifton GL, Coffey CS, Fourwinds S, et al. Early induction of hypothermia for evacuated intracranial hematomas: a post hoc analysis of two clinical trials. J Neurosurg. 2012;117: 714-20.
33. Cooper PR, Rovit RL, Ransohoff J. Hemicraniectomy in the treatment of acute subdural hematoma: a reappraisal. Surg Neurol. 1976;5:25-8.
34. Cooper DJ, Rosenfeld JV, Murray L, et al. Decompressive craniectomy in diffuse traumatic brain injury. N Engl J Med. 2011;364:1493-502.
35. Hutchinson PJ, Corteen E, Czosnyka M, et al. Decompressive craniectomy in traumatic brain injury: the randomized multicenter RESCUEicp study. Acta Neurochir Suppl. 2006; 96:17-20.
36. ClinicalTrials.gov. (2014). Brain Tissue Oxygen Monitoring in Traumatic Brain Injury (TBI) (BOOST 2).[online] Available from https://clinicaltrials.gov/ct2/show/NCT00974259 [Accessed December 24, 2014.]
37. Rosner MJ, Rosner SD, Johnson AH. Cerebral perfusion pressure: management protocol and clinical results. J Neurosurg. 1995;83:949-62.
38. Robertson CS, Valadka AB, Hannay HJ, et al. Prevention of secondary ischemic insults after severe head injury. Crit Care Med. 1999;27:2086-95.
39. Holloway KL, Bames T, Choi S, et al. Ventriculostomy infections: the effect of monitoring duration and catheter exchange in 584 patients. J Neurosurg. 1996;85:419-24.
40. Jennett B, Bond M. Assessment of outcome after severe brain damage. Lancet. 1975;1:480-4.
41. Marshall LF, Gautille T, Klauber MR, et al. The outcome of severe closed head injury. J Neurosurg. 1991;75:S28-36.
42. Stein SC. Outcome from moderate head injury. In: Narayan RK, Wilberger JE, Povlishock JT (Eds). Neurotrauma. New York, NY: McGraw-Hill; 1995.
43. Valadka AB. Penetrating cranial trauma. In: Batjer HH, Loftus CM (Eds). Textbook of Neurological Surgery. Philadelphia, PA: Lippincott Williams & Wilkins; 2003.
44. Maas AI, Roozenbeek B, Manley GT. Clinical trials in traumatic brain injury: past experience and current developments. Neurotherapeutics. 2010;7:115-26.
45. Landis SC, Amara SG, Asadullah K, et al. A call for transparent reporting to optimize the predictive value of preclinical research. Nature. 2012;490(7419):187-91.
46. Narayan RK, Michel ME, Ansell B, et al. Clinical trials in head injury. J Neurotrauma. 2002;19:503-57.
47. Yue JK, Vassar MJ, Lingsma HF, et al. Transforming research and clinical knowledge in traumatic brain injury pilot: multicenter implementation of the common data elements for traumatic brain injury. J Neurotrauma. 2013;30:1831-44.
48. Maas AI, Menon DK, Steyerberg EW, et al. Collaborative European NeuroTrauma Effectiveness Research in Traumatic Brain Injury (CENTER-TBI): A prospective longitudinal observational study. Neurosurgery. 2015;76:67-80.

38B

Cervical Spine and Spinal Cord Trauma

Sumeet Ahuja, Manish K Kasliwal, Vincent C Traynelis

Key Points

- Understanding the pathophysiology and early management of various cervical spine and spinal cord injuries is very important as these injuries are frequently encountered in any emergency department or outpatient clinic receiving trauma victims.
- Morbidity resulting from a missed diagnosis of cervical spine trauma or inappropriate treatment can have devastating neurological consequences for the patient as well as a significant medicolegal impact on the involved healthcare providers.
- When upper or lower cervical spine injuries are suspected, immediate immobilization, a thorough physical, including a careful and neurologic examination, and appropriate radiographic evaluation are imperative.
- Various traumatic injuries like occipitocervical dislocations that once were rare due to high mortality at the scene of injury are now seen more often in emergency departments but have a high potential to go unnoticed if not carefully sought.
- Though controversy remains surrounding cervical spinal clearance and the management of specific injuries, there has been an emerging consensus on management recommendations based on the best available evidence.

INTRODUCTION

Spinal cord injury (SCI) is one of the most devastating injuries for patients, their families, and all involved health professionals. Despite several basic science and clinical advances, there is still no cure for SCI. A high index of suspicion for spinal injury and SCI must be maintained, particularly when caring for the patient who has sustained multiple trauma. Injuries to the spine below the cervical region are discussed in Chapter 41, "Pelvic, Lumbar and Thoracic Spine and Spinal Cord Injuries". The importance of evaluation and protection of the cervical spine is underscored by continued reports of neurologic deterioration that occurs after patients are admitted to hospitals. Prompt diagnosis and appropriate management of traumatic spine and SCIs can reduce morbidity and mortality rates. While assuring appropriate resuscitation of the patient, the early management of such injuries includes maintaining adequate perfusion and oxygenation of the spinal cord, alleviating neural compression, the use of adjunctive medical measures and maintenance or restoration of proper spinal alignment. Even though the timing of surgery has been controversial, early decompression within 24 hours after SCI has been found to be safe and beneficial in recent studies making prompt diagnosis of these injuries of paramount importance.[1]

EPIDEMIOLOGY

Acute injuries of the spine and spinal cord are among the most common causes of death and disability resulting from trauma. Cervical spine injuries occur in 3–4% of all trauma patients.[2] Spinal cord injury is much rarer occurring in only about 12,000 people per year in the United States. Because of the association with traumatic brain injury, the risk of spinal injury can be stratified by level of consciousness, occurring in only 2.8% of alert compared with 7.7% of nonevaluable patients.[3] Estimates of the number of patients living with SCI in the United States range from 185,000 to 400,000. Approximately 2000 US hospital beds are required each year for the care of these patients.[4] According to Kraus and colleagues, of the individuals who sustain SCIs each year, 4,200 die before reaching the hospital and an additional 1,500 patients die during the initial hospitalization.[5] Neurologic deficit is associated with about half of spinal injuries. SCIs, like most traumatic injuries, tend to occur in a young, predominantly male population, although a second peak is observed in the elderly.[6,7] The most common etiologies for spinal injury are motor vehicle accidents (50%), followed by falls (20%) and sports or recreational mishaps (15%).[6,7] The cervical region is the segment of the spine most frequently injured in vehicular crashes, especially when shoulder and lap belt restraints are not worn.

Spinal column injury is a general term that encompasses insult to either or both the spinal cord and vertebral column with its supporting ligaments. Approximately half of spinal column injuries are bone fractures, one-third are fracture-subluxations and <10% consist of subluxation alone. Traumatic disc herniation may also occur. Although cervical spine fractures account for 20–30% of all spine fractures, cervical spinal cord injuries make up more than half of all SCIs. Of patients who have cervical fractures, 10% harbor a second spinal fracture at a noncontiguous level. The thoracolumbar junction is the next most common site of fracture (20%) and these injuries are discussed in detail in Chapter 41, "Pelvic, Lumbar and Thoracic Spine and Spinal Cord Injuries".

INITIAL MANAGEMENT AND NEUROLOGIC ASSESSMENT

Organized trauma systems, improvements in prehospital care, advances in surgical stabilization techniques, and the development of specialized centers for rehabilitation have all contributed to improving outcomes after cervical SCI. Despite these advances, prevention of injuries altogether, or, at a minimum, prevention of additional secondary injury will have the greatest impact on overall outcomes. For this reason, evaluation and treatment of trauma to the spine, spinal cord, and nerve roots requires a systematic approach integrated into the overall management of the trauma patient. Early diagnosis of injury, preservation of spinal cord and nerve root function, and restoration of spinal alignment and stability are the keys to successful management. Because motor vehicle accidents, falls, and sports-related injuries all have the potential for cervical spine injury, all accident victims must be assumed to have an unstable cervical spine until proven otherwise. Key factors such as airway, breathing, and hemodynamic function are essential when managing any trauma patient.[8] It is important to recognize the need to optimize these parameters and resuscitate the entire patient. Once these issues are appropriately addressed, proper attention can then be directed to clinical and radiographic examinations of the spine.[9]

Assessment of the circulation can be difficult in the setting of acute trauma. Loss of peripheral muscle tone through paralysis combined with interruption of the sympathetic nervous system can result in systemic hypotension or neurogenic shock.[8] Neurogenic shock may or may not accompany the flaccid paralysis and areflexia below the level of injury in the acute period after SCI. Loss of sympathetic innervation contributes to this phenomenon via multiple effects. Decreased peripheral resistance reduces preload to the heart and pathways for reflex tachycardia may be disrupted. Neurogenic shock can result in venous pooling and decreased cardiac preload, which is exacerbated by the lack of reflex, sympathetically-mediated, tachycardia. Unlike patients with hypotension as a result of acute blood loss, patients with spinal shock often appear to be well-perfused peripherally with pink and warm extremities. It is critical to distinguish between hypovolemic and neurogenic shock. Attributing hypotension to neurogenic shock is a diagnosis of exclusion, even in the setting of a dense neurologic deficit that is obviously caused by SCI. Hypovolemia must be the leading presumed cause of hemodynamic compromise in a trauma patient. Current treatment guidelines call for correcting the systolic blood pressure if <90 mm Hg and maintaining a mean arterial pressure of 85–90 mm Hg for about 7 days postinjury.[8]

Neurologic dysfunction resulting from SCI can complicate the assessment of other body systems. Loss of sensation may mask other symptoms, such as those associated with an acute abdomen or a compartment syndrome. High cervical injuries can alter respiratory dynamics through effects on the phrenic nerve (C3, 4, and 5). Damage attributable to the lower cervical and upper thoracic cord can lead to paralysis of the accessory respiratory muscles, such as the intercostal muscles, and altered respiratory function as the patient breathes by the use of the diaphragm alone, which may result in hypoventilation. Reduced expected vital capacity and inspiratory capacity can further contribute to global hypoxemia. Respiratory complications are common after cervical spinal cord injuries, and the incidence increases markedly in the presence of other bodily injuries. Furthermore, all cervical spinal cord lesions have the potential for the development of ascending levels of dysfunction because of increasing spinal cord hemorrhage or edema. Therefore, respiratory decompensation can occur at any time during the early stages of resuscitation. Because relative hypoxia can further damage an injured cord, all patients, regardless of the level of their injury, should receive supplemental oxygen. Respiratory function should be reassessed frequently and intubation performed as necessary. Respiratory insufficiency should be suspected in all patients with cervical cord injuries. High cervical cord injury, as in a patient with no arm function (i.e. above the outflow to the phrenic nerves at C3–5), may be associated with paralysis of one or both diaphragms, as well as the intercostals. Inadequate ventilation in a quadriplegic or quadriparetic patient is another indication for early intubation.[8]

Management of the patient with a suspected spinal injury begins at the scene of the trauma. The potential for an unstable spine must be considered at the accident scene even if the initial priorities of airway, breathing, and circulation are addressed. Attention to spinal immobilization during extrication and transport serves to prevent new deficits or worsen the neurologic injury that may have occurred.[10,11] Three to twenty five percent of SCI occurs after the initial insult, during transit or management before hospital arrival. This is not surprising as approximately 40% of cervical spine injuries are clinically unstable with potential to result in SCI, if not recognized.[12]

Key principles of extrication include the effective use of a stiff cervical collar and spine board as well as logrolling the patient. Soft collars allow complete neck movement in all planes and should not be used. Often supportive blocks (head pads) can be used. Sand bags and tape are insufficient.[12] Nasotracheal or orotracheal intubation, if needed, should not be delayed. If possible, airway management should be carried out in a manner that minimizes cephalic and cervical motion. During such maneuvers, most vertebral motion will occur in the upper cervical spine.[13] Appropriate spinal precautions must be maintained in the hospital setting because at least 5% of patients exhibit the onset or worsening of neurologic deficit after arriving in an emergency department. Spinal cord ischemia or progressive edema is the cause in some of these cases, but clearly some patients are injured by complacent or inadequate spinal precautions after they reach professional care.

A thorough neurologic examination is mandatory for all trauma patients. If a deficit is detected, it must be discerned whether the patient has a "complete" or "incomplete" SCI.

Complete Versus Incomplete Injury

The importance of a thorough neurological examination cannot be overemphasized as it has a significant influence on the long-term prognosis for recovery and management. Often its sensitivity is reduced by the patient's inability to report symptoms due to conditions such as distracting pain, mild head injuries, or intoxication. A complete injury implies absolutely no neurologic function below the level of SCI. An injury is termed incomplete if any neurologic function is present caudal to the level of cord damage. Functions that may be preserved include perianal sensation or rectal sphincter contraction (sacral sparing), sensation (including deep touch, pain and temperature, or proprioception), and any voluntary movement. Preservation of the deep tendon reflexes and/or sacral reflexes, such as the bulbocavernosus reflex, does not support an incomplete injury. If there is a deficit, the spinal "level" of injury must be determined from the most rostral functional dermatome or myotome with at least antigravity strength. Patients may have asymmetric levels of injury.

Though various classical syndromes have been described for classification of incomplete SCI as will be mentioned later, the American Spinal Injury Association (ASIA) international standards for neurologic and functional classification of SCI are recommended as the preferred neurologic examination tool for clinicians involved in the assessment and care of acute SCI patients.[3,14] The neurologic examination is performed using standards established by the ASIA and should be recorded in a timely manner (Fig. 38B.1). This neurologic examination involves detailed testing of motor and sensory function and perineal function. Motor function of key muscle groups in the arms and legs is assessed from grades 0 to 5. Several sensory functions including pinprick, light touch, and proprioception or vibratory function are tested in both the upper and lower extremities. Sensory function is graded 0, 1, or 2 (absent, hypoesthesia, and normal, respectively). Deep tendon and pathologic reflexes are determined. Hyper-reflexia and findings of clonus, Babinski signs, or Hoffmann signs are indications of spinal cord compression, although in cases of acute SCI, areflexia is common. The level of SCI is defined as the lowest-functioning root level with at least grade 3 motor function. Examination of the perineum is an important component of the clinical examination. The perianal skin is tested for pinprick sensation. Digital rectal examination is performed assessing tone and the presence of voluntary contraction. Finally, sacral reflexes are assessed. The anal wink is obtained by gently scratching the perianal skin and observing a contracture. The bulbocavernosus reflex is tested during digital rectal examination by compression of the glans penis or clitoris or alternatively by pulling on a Foley catheter. During this maneuver, an anal contracture should occur.

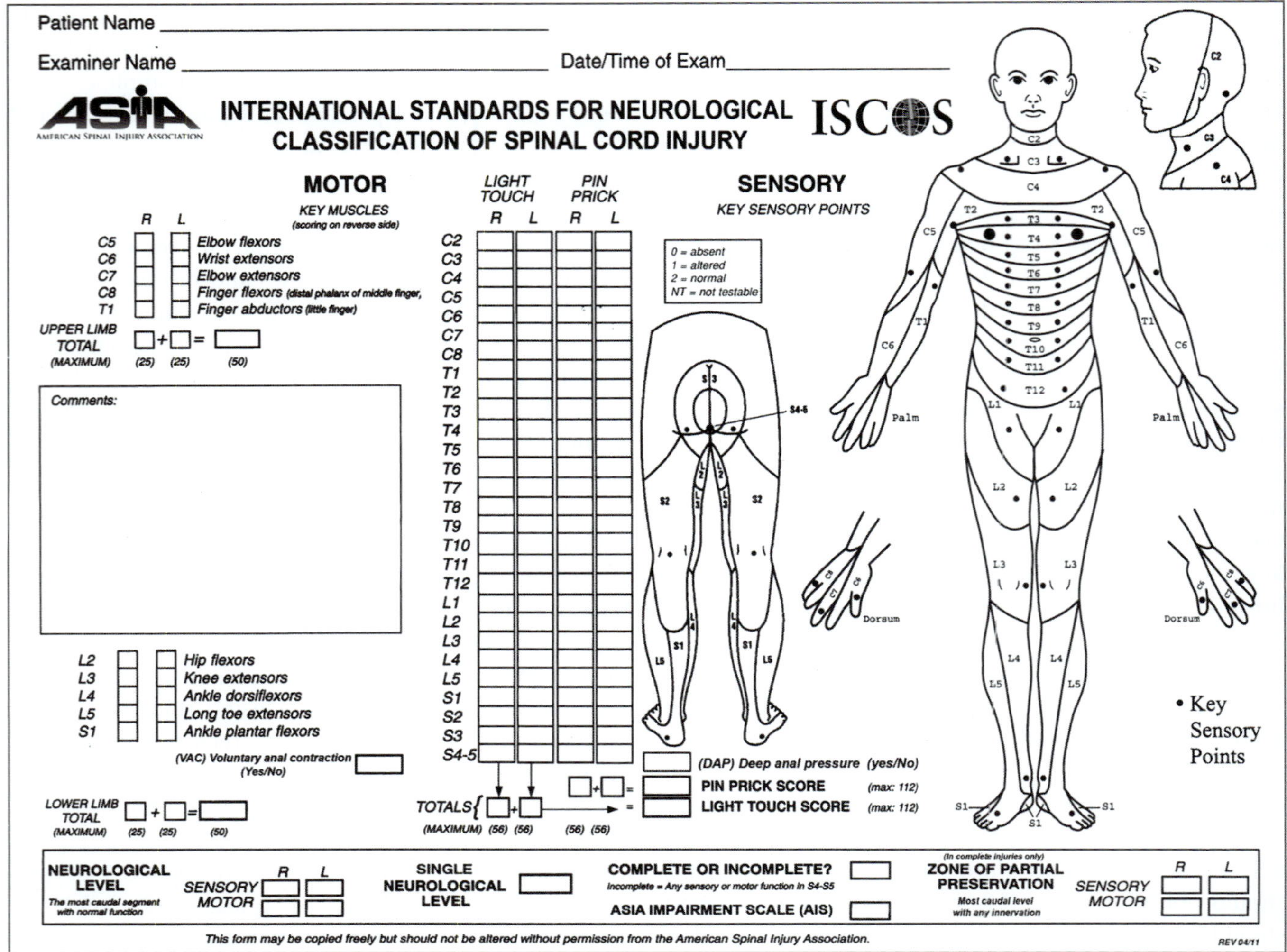

Patient Name ____________________

Examiner Name ____________________ Date/Time of Exam ____________________

ASIA — American Spinal Injury Association

INTERNATIONAL STANDARDS FOR NEUROLOGICAL CLASSIFICATION OF SPINAL CORD INJURY — ISCOS

MOTOR — KEY MUSCLES (scoring on reverse side)

	R	L	
C5			Elbow flexors
C6			Wrist extensors
C7			Elbow extensors
C8			Finger flexors (distal phalanx of middle finger)
T1			Finger abductors (little finger)

UPPER LIMB TOTAL (MAXIMUM) ☐+☐= ☐ (25) (25) (50)

Comments:

	R	L	
L2			Hip flexors
L3			Knee extensors
L4			Ankle dorsiflexors
L5			Long toe extensors
S1			Ankle plantar flexors

(VAC) Voluntary anal contraction (Yes/No) ☐

LOWER LIMB TOTAL (MAXIMUM) ☐+☐=☐ (25) (25) (50)

	LIGHT TOUCH R	LIGHT TOUCH L	PIN PRICK R	PIN PRICK L
C2				
C3				
C4				
C5				
C6				
C7				
C8				
T1				
T2				
T3				
T4				
T5				
T6				
T7				
T8				
T9				
T10				
T11				
T12				
L1				
L2				
L3				
L4				
L5				
S1				
S2				
S3				
S4-5				
TOTALS (MAXIMUM)	(56)	(56)	(56)	(56)

SENSORY — KEY SENSORY POINTS

0 = absent
1 = altered
2 = normal
NT = not testable

(DAP) Deep anal pressure (yes/No) ☐

PIN PRICK SCORE (max: 112) ☐

LIGHT TOUCH SCORE (max: 112) ☐

• Key Sensory Points

NEUROLOGICAL LEVEL (The most caudal segment with normal function) — R / L — SENSORY ☐☐ MOTOR ☐☐

SINGLE NEUROLOGICAL LEVEL ☐

COMPLETE OR INCOMPLETE? ☐ Incomplete = Any sensory or motor function in S4-S5

ASIA IMPAIRMENT SCALE (AIS) ☐

ZONE OF PARTIAL PRESERVATION (In complete injuries only) Most caudal level with any innervation — R / L — SENSORY ☐☐ MOTOR ☐☐

This form may be copied freely but should not be altered without permission from the American Spinal Injury Association.

REV 04/11

Fig. 38B.1: Chart illustrating ASIA grading of spinal cord injury severity.

Interpretation of the perineal examination depends on the level of injury and time from injury. In cervical cord injuries, the perineal function may be initially absent, but the bulbocavernosus reflex may return in several days, indicating resolution of spinal shock, which is an initial depolarization of axonal tissue after injury. If the patient has not made any distal recovery at this time, the prognosis is grave. In some cases, only sacral function is spared, changing the patient from complete to incomplete with a dramatic change in prognosis. Injuries at the conus or cauda equina that have retained perineal function or bulbocavernosus reflex have an improved prognosis for recovery of bladder and bowel function.

Various incomplete injury patterns seen after cervical spine trauma can be described as mentioned below:[15]

- *Central cord syndrome* is a cervical cord injury manifested by weakness that is greater in the upper than lower extremities and sensory loss can be patchy and variable. The typical injury pattern is hyperextension in the setting of pre-existing canal stenosis as it might occur from degenerative disease and evidence of damage to the bony spine may be absent.[16] This is due to somatotopic organization in which proximal motor function is represented at the more central portions, while the distal musculature is represented in the more peripheral portions of the spinal cord. Sixty-percent of these injuries may also be associated with fracture subluxations and acute disc herniations.
- *Anterior cord syndrome* is caused by infarction in the distribution of the anterior spinal artery, which supplies the anterior two-thirds of the cord. The syndrome presents with preservation of posterior column function (proprioception and vibration), but loss of the function of corticospinal tract (motor) and spinothalamic tract (pain and temperature). Typical mechanism is flexion-compression injury.

- *Brown-Séquard syndrome* is caused by hemisection of the cord resulting in loss of ipsilateral motor and proprioception function and contralateral pain and temperature sensation 1–2 levels below the injury level. Also ipsilateral hyper-reflexia, clonus, loss of superficial reflexes, and a positive Babinski sign can be seen.
- *The posterior cord syndrome* is rare. Injury is isolated to the posterior columns of the spinal cord, sparing the anterior two-thirds. Deep pressure, vibration, and joint sensation are affected.

Immediate Medical Therapy

Appropriate medical therapy should be instituted if there is any evidence of SCI. Although many avenues of research are being explored, use of methylprednisolone remained the standard of care for a number of years based on the result of National Acute Spinal Cord Injury Studies (NASCIS) trials.[17-20] Historically methylprednisolone was used in acute SCI based on tenuous data that was available.[17-20] More thorough and recent data have shown that methylprednisolone does not have any true benefit in SCI in the short- and long-term, and in fact evidence points to increased morbidity and mortality.[21] Therefore, the use of methylprednisolone in acute cervical SCI is not recommended. Recent research in the use of GM1 ganglioside has shown no statistically significant difference in its use for acute SCI and is also not currently recommended in acute cervical SCI.[21]

RADIOGRAPHIC EVALUATION OF THE SPINAL COLUMN

After the primary survey, neurological examination, and external assessment of the spine, the next step in identifying specific spinal injuries is an imaging evaluation. The diagnostic studies performed should be chosen so that they provide maximal information in a relatively short time. Imaging modalities include plain radiographs, fluoroscopy, computed tomogram (CT) scanning with multiplanar reconstruction, magnetic resonance imaging (MRI), and myelography. Specific choices for imaging of trauma patients may vary depending on the specific logistics involved at each center. Though the need of imaging and the best imaging modality remained nebulous in the past, there has been an emerging consensus on this aspect except in certain cases. It has long been recommended that all trauma patients undergo radiographic evaluation of the cervical spine. Hoffman et al. proposed five criteria commonly known as NEXUS (National Emergency X-Radiography Utilization Study) criteria that classified patients as having a low probability of injury.[22] When applied to 34,069 patients undergoing cervical spine radiography (CSR), these criteria identified all but 8 of the 818 patients who had cervical spine injuries (sensitivity of 99%). Of these 8 patients, falsely identified as being unlikely to have an injury, only 2 had what was previously defined by the authors as a "clinically significant" injury. According to the authors, use of the criteria would have avoided imaging in 12.6% of the overall 34,069 patients studied. In another similar effort, the Canadian C-Spine Rule (CCR) investigators developed an algorithm based on three determinations: a high-risk factor necessitating radiography; low-risk factors, one or more of which allow assessment of range of motion; and active assessment of range of motion. In a subsequent study of 8,924 patients in which the incidence of cervical spine injury was 1.7%, the CCR was found to be 100% sensitive and 42.5% specific for "significant" injuries.[23] Based on the NEXUS and CCR studies, imaging is not indicated in an awake asymptomatic patient without neck pain or tenderness who is neurologically intact without a distracting injury (e.g. upper extremity limb fracture), and able to complete full range of motion. With more powerful data available, recent guidelines have bolstered this historic generally accepted recommendation.[9]

Even though radiographic evaluation of the spinal column began with plain films of the cervical spine traditionally,[24] inadequate evaluation of the complete cervical spine and various other shortcomings along with wider availability of multidetector computed tomogram (MDCT) imaging have challenged this concept. In fact, MDCT is the imaging modality of choice in an awake symptomatic patient, as it has been proven to be more sensitive and specific than CSRs in detecting spinal column injury.[9] If CT is not available, then three-view CSR is the alternative imaging of choice. If CT is not available and CSR is used, a lateral cervical radiograph is adequate only when visualization includes the base of the occiput through the C7–T1 articulation. Commonly, a swimmer's view is required for adequate assessment of lower cervical structures. However, oblique swimmer's views only slightly improve the sensitivity and, therefore, have been deemed cost-inefficient.[25] The sensitivity of lateral radiographs alone to detect a fracture is 85%.[26] The addition of an open-mouth odontoid and an anteroposterior view increases the sensitivity to 92% and provides a negative predictive value of 99%.

In patients with an unremarkable CT and continued neck pain, management, including adjunct imaging, is based on lesser medical evidence and is partly determined by subjective clinician decision-making. Various options typically include (1) continued cervical immobilization until asymptomatic, (2) discontinue immobilization based on physician's discretion, and (3) discontinuation of immobilization after normal flexion/extension radiographs or a normal MRI. Magnetic resonance imaging is recommended to be done within 48 hours due to a decrease in sensitivity after this time window. There is some evidence to suggest the superiority of MRI as compared to flexion/extension lateral cervical radiographs.[9] This is important as dynamic radiographs are appropriate only for the alert patient and lateral flexion/extension views in the acute setting may be inadequate in almost one-third of cases.[27]

In the obtunded patient who cannot be reliably evaluated, initial recommendations are the same as for awake symptomatic patients and consist of an MDCT scan. Adjuvant modalities such as dynamic fluoroscopy and MRI have been used to further assess ligamentous injuries and cervical stability. The efficacy of dynamic fluoroscopy is limited because of a high rate of inadequate visualization of the entire cervical spine, especially at the cervicothoracic junction.[28] Magnetic resonance imaging is highly sensitive in detecting soft tissue and ligamentous injuries, but it is much more time intensive and is not as readily available as CT imaging. With recent technological advances, the imaging quality and resolution of CT scans have dramatically improved. It has been proposed that with modern MDCT scanners, a negative CT scan alone is sufficient for cervical spine clearance in obtunded patients.[29,30] However, there are other studies that have shown that CT scan can miss clinically important cervical injuries.[31,32] A meta-analysis by Panczykowski et al.[16] reported that following a protocol of clearing the cervical spine based on CT imaging alone in obtunded patients, the incidence of unstable cervical spine injury among the studies of negative CT scans approximates to 1 in every 4,776 patients.[30] The most recent guidelines from the American Association of Neurological Surgeons (AANS)/Congress of Neurological Surgeons (CNS) Joint Guidelines Committee, recommend CT imaging as the initial imaging modality of choice in the obtunded patient (Level I recommendation).[9] Subsequent to a negative CT scan, the recommendations become weak (Level II) and in patients in whom there is a high clinical suspicion of injury yet have a normal high-quality CT imaging study, the decision for further patient management is left to physicians trained in the diagnosis and management of spinal injuries. A Level III recommendation following a negative CT scan was either to continue cervical immobilization until asymptomatic, discontinue cervical immobilization following a normal MRI study obtained within 48 hours of injury, or discontinue cervical immobilization at the discretion of the treating physician.

Radiographs of the thoracic and lumbar spines are appropriate in the setting of a cervical injury, a neurologic deficit attributable to the thoracolumbar level or when the patient is unable to reliably deny spinal pain or tenderness. High-energy mechanisms of injury, such as ejection from a motor vehicle, are also indications for radiographic interrogation. Appropriate plain radiographic imaging of these spinal segments includes lateral and anteroposterior views. All painful regions should be evaluated radiographically.[15]

CERVICAL SPINE INJURIES

The cervical spine is the most commonly injured segment of the spinal column, and cervical spine injuries account for just over half of all spinal injuries. The cervical region is highly mobile, allowing a wide range of physiologic motion in multiple planes. For practical purposes, the cervical spine can be subcategorized into upper and lower segments based on the anatomy, biomechanics, and the differences in the patterns of injury between these two regions. The upper cervical spine consists of the occiput, atlas, and axis. These three structures along with their strong ligamentous attachments are often referred to as the craniocervical junction (CCJ). This osseoligamentous complex surrounds and protects the upper cervical spinal cord, the brain stem, and lower cranial nerves and is anatomically and functionally distinct from the motion segments in the subaxial cervical spine (C3 to C7) that explains the distinct patterns of injury that occur at the CCJ. The articulations at the craniovertebral junction (O–C2), which can be thought of as a single physiologic segment that is highly dependent upon ligamentous support for stability, are complex. The transverse ligament is of particular importance here because it maintains the relationship between the atlas and the odontoid process of the axis. Overall, the axis (C2) is the most commonly involved level of injury. In the subaxial cervical spine, C5 is the most commonly fractured vertebra and C5–6 is the most common site of subluxation.

Occipital Condyle Fractures

Most injuries to the occipital condyles are caused by high-energy trauma to the head and neck. The incidence of occipital condyle fractures (OCFs) is reported to range from 3 to 16%.[33] The clinical presentation of these injuries can range

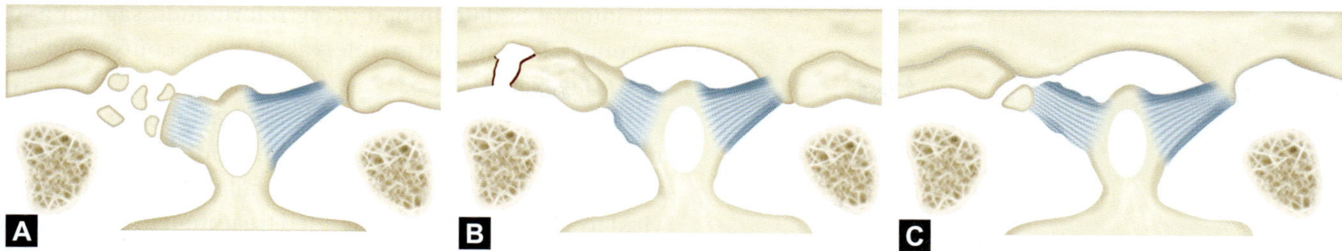

Figs. 38B.2A to C: Schematic diagrams illustrating classification for fractures involving the occipital condyles. (A) Type I, (B) type II, and (C) type III.

from minimal deficits to frank quadriparesis. Patients may complain of high cervical pain, torticollis, headaches, and impaired mobility. The most severe neurologic deficits are often seen with concurrent head injury. Up to 31% of these patients may exhibit acute lower cranial nerve deficits.

Although radiographs may show some abnormal soft tissue swelling in the presence of an OCF, these injuries are often extremely difficult to detect with conventional radiography. A computed tomogram scan with reconstruction is the imaging modality of choice in the diagnosis and classification of these fractures[33,34] with MRI being useful to assess the integrity of the craniocervical ligaments.[35]

Occipital condyle fractures can be classified into three types as per the classification by Anderson and Montesano: type I (comminuted), type II (extension of a linear basilar skull fracture), and type III (avulsion of a fragment) (Figs. 38B.2A to C).[36] Type I injuries are impaction fractures of the condyle from axial loading. These fractures tend to be comminuted. The tectorial membrane and the alar ligaments are usually intact. Unilateral type I fractures are stable, but bilateral fractures may be unstable. Type II injuries are part of a more extensive basioccipital fracture that involves one or both occipital condyles. The common mechanism of injury is a direct blow to the skull. The tectorial and alar ligaments are intact, and the fracture is usually stable. Type III injuries are avulsion fractures near the alar ligament insertion that result in medial displacement of the condylar fracture fragment from the inferomedial aspect of the occipital condyle into the foramen magnum. The mechanism of injury is a forced rotation of the head combined with lateral bending. Type III fractures are potentially unstable injuries owing to avulsion of the alar ligaments. Type I and type II fractures can be treated with a rigid cervical orthosis. Type III injuries can be treated initially with an orthosis or halo vest. However, posterior occipitocervical fusion may be necessary for chronic pain, neurologic deficit, or associated atlanto-occipital ligamentous injury or evidence of instability.[35,37]

Occipitoatlantal Dislocation

Occipitoatlantal dislocation (OAD) is associated with a high mortality rate at the scene of injury that accounts for its rarity in the clinical setting being seen in only about 1% of patients presenting to a hospital with cervical trauma.[38] Nearly all patients with this injury die at the scene of injury as a result of anoxia induced by respiratory arrest. Of patients autopsied after fatal cervical spine injury, 19% had an OAD.[39] However, with better safety mechanisms, patients with unstable injuries to the occipitocervical junction are more frequently surviving the site of injury. Ligamentous disruption is required to separate the skull from the spine. Because of distracting injuries and subtle radiographic findings, the chance of missing this injury is fairly substantial. The dislocation can be classified into three types according to the direction of dislocation of the occiput with respect to the atlas as described by Traynelis, et al.[40]: Type I OAD consists of anterior displacement of the occiput with respect to C1; type II OAD is primarily a longitudinal distraction with separation of the occiput from the atlas; and type III OAD exists when the occiput is posteriorly dislocated from C1 (Fig. 38B.3A to C). More recent grading schemes have focused on the presence or absence of instability and its severity, without emphasis on the direction of the dislocation; however, all of these injuries should be considered highly unstable until proven otherwise.[41]

While about 20% of patients presenting to trauma centers with acute traumatic atlanto-occipital dislocation (AOD) may have a normal neurologic examination, most of the patients will suffer deficits of the cranial nerves, brain stem, and upper cervical spinal cord and likely vertebral artery injury. The most common mechanism is from an extension-rotation force. Patients with vertebral artery insufficiency at this level may exhibit the Wallenberg syndrome, consisting of ipsilateral defects of cranial nerves V, IX, X, and XI; an ipsilateral Horner syndrome; dysphagia; and cerebellar dysfunction.

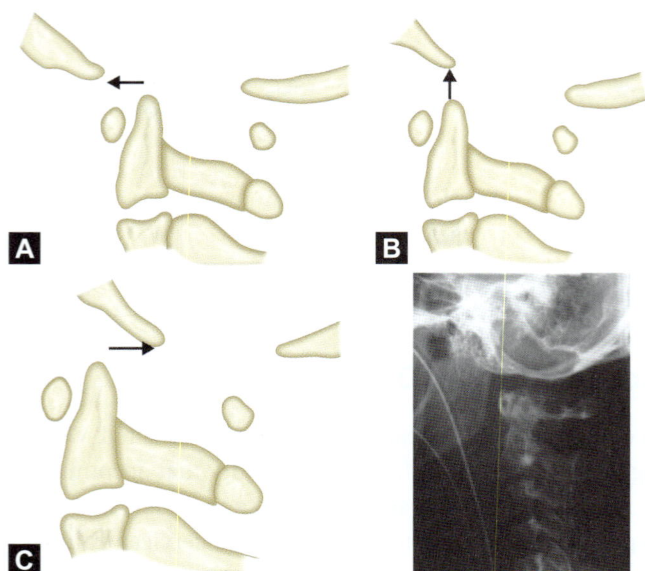

Figs. 38B.3A to C: Schematic drawings demonstrating the classification of occipitoatlantal dislocation (OAD). (A) Type I: anterior displacement of the occiput with respect to the atlas; (B) Type II: vertical displacement; (C) Type III: posterior displacement and a lateral radiograph showing OAD (lower right).

Axial traction should be avoided in cases of OAD because it reproduces the distractive mechanism of injury and is associated with a risk of damaging the spinal cord, medulla, or vertebral arteries and causing neurologic deterioration. Initial workup includes lateral cervical X-rays to determine traditional measures of instability such as Powers' ratio, X-line method, condylar gap method, basion-dens interval (BDI), and basion-axial interval (BAI) (Fig. 38B.4). Basion-axial interval when combined with the BDI is known as the Harris method.[42] The anatomic landmarks required for application of these methods make diagnosing OAD using plain lateral cervical X-rays challenging. Hence even though, the use of Harris lines on plain X-rays is often recommended for diagnosis of OAD, in the event of a nondiagnostic film in the presence of clinical suspicion of swelling of vertebral soft tissue, CT scanning, or MRI is recommended. Therefore CT scanning or MRI is recommended with OAD suspicion even in the setting of normal or indeterminate lateral X-rays. Findings of a prevertebral soft tissue shadow and subarachnoid hemorrhage on a brain CT scan are also prompting factors for CT scanning or MRI of the cervical spine. Dedicated studies using CT scanning to diagnose OAD have supported the use of the BDI[43] (with 10 mm as the cutoff) and the condyle to C1 interval (CCI) as a particularly sensitive imaging parameter for the diagnosis of AOD. Condyle to C1 interval is determined using reformatted sagittal and coronal CT scans and an interval >4 mm is concerning for AOD (Fig. 38B.4).[44]

Treatment depends upon prompt restoration of alignment and internal fixation. Traction is not recommended. External immobilization has a high failure rate. Craniocervical fixation is the recommended treatment in most cases of traumatic AOD. All occipitocervical dislocations should be treated initially by immediate application of a halo vest. Because the majority of these injuries are unstable, posterior occipitocervical fusion is the procedure of choice that can be done using a variety of techniques including posterior wiring and structural grafting, Ransford loop fixation with wiring or plate/rod, and screw fixation with structural grafting.[45]

Atlas Fractures

The first cervical vertebra is a thin ring of bone that has broad horizontally oriented articular surfaces. Atlas fractures account for 4–15% of all cervical injuries and occur as isolated fractures in only 56% of cases.[46,47] Approximately 40% of atlantal injuries are associated with a fracture of the axis, so emphasizing the importance of evaluating the CCJ as a single unit.[46]

Atlantal fractures can be classified from types I–V. Type I fractures involve the posterior arch alone. Type II fractures involve the anterior arch alone. Type III fractures are bilateral posterior arch fractures associated with a unilateral or bilateral anterior arch fracture. Type IV fractures involve the lateral mass. Type V fractures are transverse fractures of the anterior arch.[47] The most common atlantal fracture is Jefferson's fracture—the result of axial loading that produces bilateral spreading of the lateral masses with bilateral fractures of both the anterior and posterior atlantal ring. It is best visualized on the open-mouth odontoid radiograph as lateral migration of the lateral masses of C1 relative to the axis.

The transverse ligament plays a crucial role in determining atlantoaxial stability. Atlas fractures have often been defined as stable or unstable based on the inferred integrity of the transverse ligament. According to the rule of Spence, if the sum total of overhang of the lateral masses of C1 relative to C2 is at least 7 mm, then the transverse ligament is likely disrupted (Fig. 38B.5).[48] A combined lateral mass displacement on the open-mouth anteroposterior view exceeding 6.9 mm is indicative of transverse ligament insufficiency, but this measurement may not be sensitive enough to detect all unstable injuries.[49] Magnetic

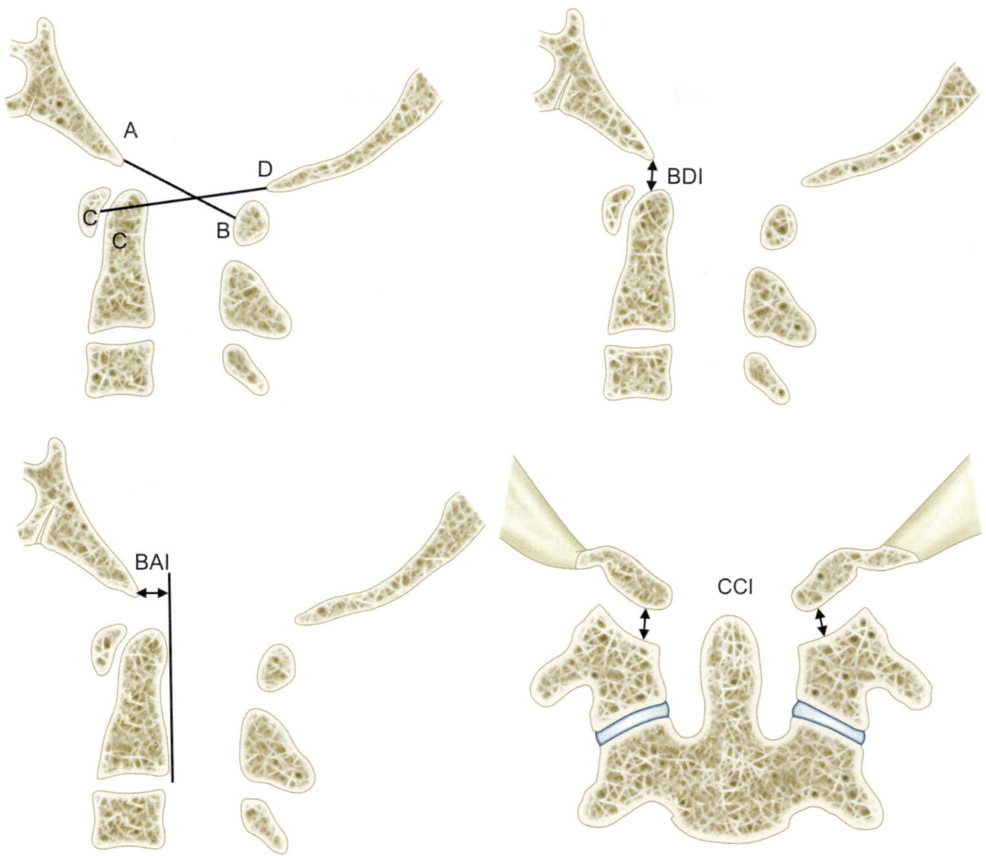

Fig. 38B.4: Schematic drawings of the midsagittal section through the craniocervical junction demonstrating various radiological parameters for diagnosis of occipitoatlantal dislocation: Powers ratio (Upper left) is the ratio of the basion-posterior atlas arch to the opisthion-anterior arch (AB/CD) and is abnormal at values >1. The basion-dens interval or BDI (upper right) is abnormal in the presence of a displacement between the basion and the dens of >10 mm in adults or >12 mm in pediatric patients. Basion-axial interval or BAI (lower left) is considered abnormal when there is anterior displacement of ≥12 mm or posterior displacement of ≥4 mm between the basion and posterior C2 line. This when combined with the BDI, is known as the Harris method. Condyle to C1 interval or CCI (lower right) is the distance between the occipital condyle and the superior articular facet of the atlas and is considered abnormal when it is >2 mm in adults or more than 5 mm in pediatric patients.

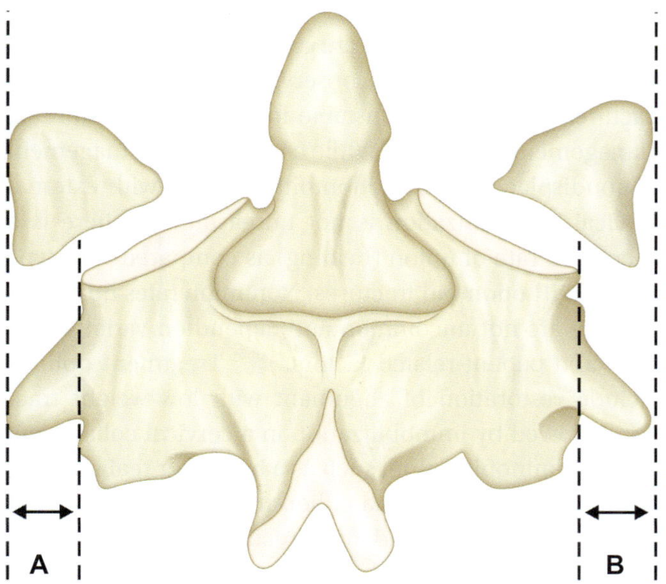

Fig. 38B.5: Coronal schematic illustration demonstrating lateral mass overhang in the setting of transverse alar ligament rupture where total lateral mass displacement (A + B) of ≥7 mm indicates transverse alar ligament rupture.

resonance imaging can be used to help assess the continuity of the transverse ligament in those cases in which the ligament status is unclear. Dickman et al. found that MRI was highly sensitive for diagnosing ruptures of the transverse ligament and classified transverse atlantal ligament (TAL) injuries into two types.[49] Type I injuries involve the mid-portion of the transverse ligament or the insertion point of the tubercle. These injuries are incapable of healing with external immobilization. Type II injuries, which involve fractures and avulsion of the tubercle for insertion of the transverse ligament, are capable of healing with external immobilization alone.

Most of these patients are neurologically intact. Patients will often complain of severe suboccipital discomfort and a sense of instability. Neurologic injury is uncommon in the case of isolated fractures of the atlas. The majority of atlantal fractures are commonly treated with external immobilization. Operative intervention is reserved for highly unstable injuries and is often dictated due to the presence of an associated C2 fracture. Treatment of isolated fractures of the atlas based on the specific atlas fracture type and the integrity of the TAL is recommended. For an isolated fracture of the atlas with an intact TAL, cervical immobilization is recommended. For isolated fractures of the atlas with disruption of the TAL, either cervical immobilization alone or surgical fixation and fusion is recommended.[50] In the presence of atlas fractures, instability can be seen with unacceptable bilateral overhang of the C1 over the C2 lateral masses or with a unilateral sagittal split that allows asymmetric subluxation of the C1 lateral mass, thus permitting the occipital condyle to settle onto the C2 lateral mass and create a cock-robin-type deformity.[51]

Axis Fractures

The axis (C2) is the largest cervical vertebra and has the most irregular shape, making it susceptible to a variety of fracture types. Axis fractures account for almost 20% of all acute cervical spinal fractures, with accompanying neurologic compromise relatively rare, of the order of 10%.[52] Axis fractures may be subdivided into odontoid fractures, hangman's fractures, and miscellaneous fractures. This last category includes fractures of the body, pedicle, lateral mass, laminae, and/or spinous process.

Fractures involving the odontoid process are the most common C2 injury. Odontoid fractures may be classified into three types according to Anderson and D' Alonzo (Fig. 38B.6).[53] Type I fractures are uncommon and involve the tip of the dens; a type II fracture is the most common odontoid fracture and occurs at the junction of the odontoid process with the body of the second cervical vertebra (Fig. 38B.6); and a type III fracture is a fracture that extends downward into the cancellous portion of the body and is really a fracture through the body of the axis. There are various other modifications of this classification; Hadley et al. in 1988 described the type IIA odontoid fracture as a comminuted fracture of the base of the odontoid with associated free fracture fragments.[54] This fracture subtype is markedly unstable and uniformly leads to nonunion, irrespective of the direction or degree of initial dens placement.

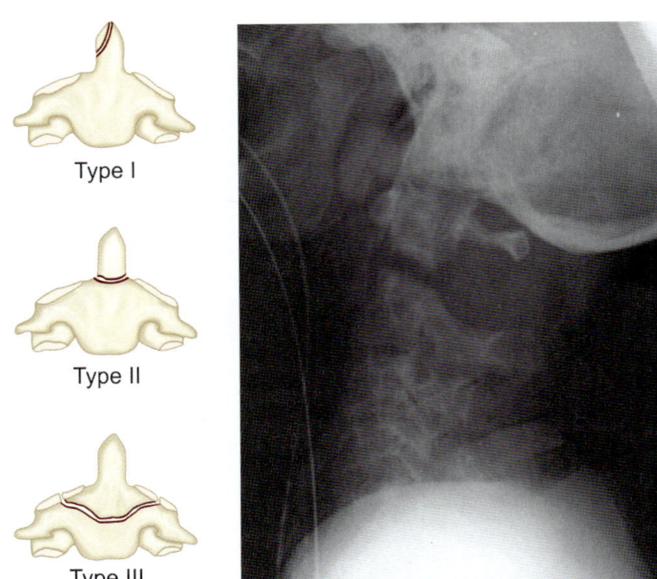

Fig. 38B.6: Schematic drawings demonstrating the three types of odontoid fractures along with a lateral radiograph showing a type II odontoid fracture.

Types I and III fractures are generally stable injuries and are successfully managed conservatively. Type II odontoid fractures are generally unstable injuries and the optimal management is variable. While conservative management of nondisplaced type II odontoid fractures with external cervical immobilization is not unreasonable, there is a decreased rate of union (healing) as compared with type I or type III odontoid fractures. Nonunion rates up to 30% or more are not uncommon and depend on various fracture- and patient-related factors.[52,55,56] Treatment options include restoration of alignment with low-weight traction followed by immobilization in a cervical collar, rigid external immobilization, such as a halo after realignment, or internal arthrodesis via either an anterior or posterior approach.[57] Current guidelines recommend serious consideration of surgical stabilization and fusion in patients

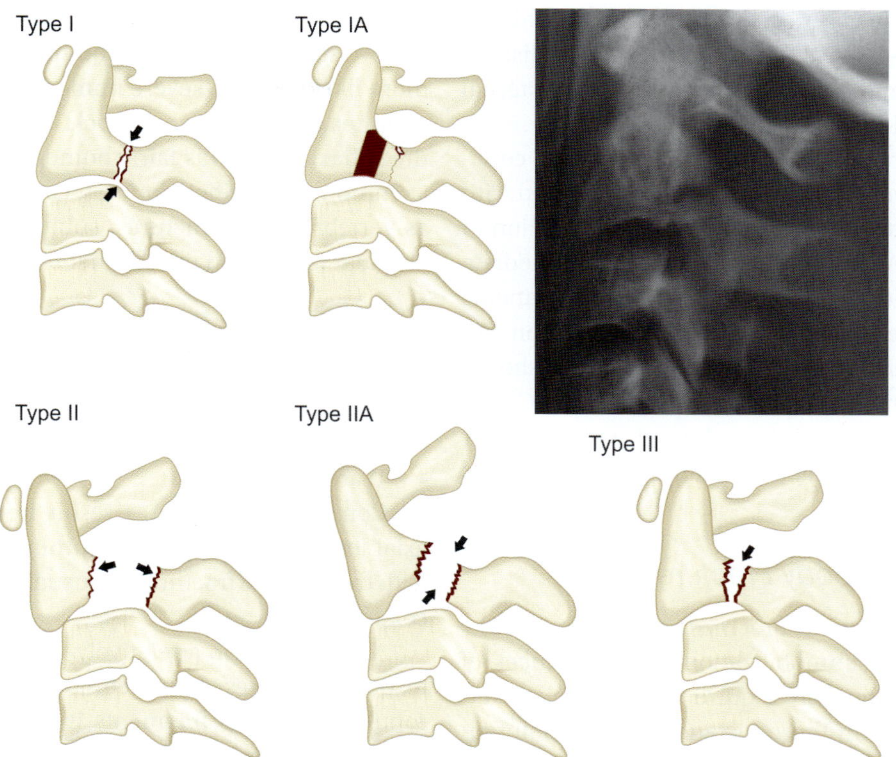

Fig. 38B.7: Diagram illustrating five injury patterns seen in traumatic spondylolisthesis along with a lateral radiograph showing a hangman's fracture.

>50 years of age with type II fractures. Most clinicians argue that odontoid type IIA fractures should be considered for early surgical stabilization and fusion considering the uniformly higher rate of nonunion irrespective of the direction or degree of initial dens placement.[46] Odontoid displacement of >5 mm is highly predictive of nonunion in type II and III fractures, and is commonly treated with early internal arthrodesis. Surgical stabilization and fusion of type II and type III odontoid fractures with dens displacement of 5 mm, comminution of the odontoid fracture, and/or inability to achieve or maintain fracture alignment with external immobilization are recommended.[52,55,56] All type II and III fractures treated with collar or halo immobilization should have close radiographic and clinical follow-up due to the possibility of nonunion and need for delayed surgical fixation. Evidence shows nearly 100% fusion rates in type I fractures treated with cervical immobilization.[55] Angulation of the fracture line is also critical in the decision-making process regarding surgical approaches. Surgical treatment may be performed by either anterior odontoid screw fixation or posterior C1–C2 arthrodesis with instrumentation.[55]

The hangman's fracture (traumatic spondylolisthesis of the axis) is defined by bilateral fractures of the pars interarticularis and is the second most common fracture of the axis (38%). It can be caused by a variety of mechanisms including combinations of extension, flexion, distraction, and axial loading of the cervical spine.[57] The fracture line passes through the neural arch of the axis. These fractures are best classified using the classification system given by Effendi, modified by Levine and Starr that describes five injury patterns (Fig. 38B.7).[57-59] Type I fractures are not displaced or have <3 mm displacement and have no angulation and are caused due to hyperextension and axial loading. Subtype IA are atypical, unstable fractures from side bending forces, typically creating an oblique fracture through one pars interarticularis and anterior to the pars within the body of the contralateral side. Type II injuries involve >3 mm translation, and a subtype, type IIA, involves significant angulation but minimal translation with the mechanism being hyperextension and secondary flexion–distraction. The type IIA subgroup, which results from flexion and distraction, has a more horizontal fracture pattern, kyphosis relatively greater than translation, and associated C2–C3 disk and posterior longitudinal ligament injuries. Type III injuries are caused by flexion–compression and involve severe angulation and translation and may involve unilateral or bilateral facet dislocation. Although surgery is indicated in cases of severe angulation, which is associated with C2–C3 disc or posterior articular disruption, types I and II may be treated effectively with external fixation (halo or rigid cervical collar).[55,57-59]

Isolated type I fractures can be treated in a rigid cervical collar for 8–12 weeks. Type II fractures are treated with initial traction in extension followed by immobilization in a halo vest. Type IIA fractures are treated with immediate application of a halo vest. Traction is avoided in patients with type IIa injuries because even minimal traction can cause severe over distraction. All type III fractures should be treated with surgical reduction and posterior C2–C3 fusion. Internal fixation can be achieved with posterior pedicle screws at C2 into the C2 vertebral body and lateral mass screws at C3.[55]

Miscellaneous C2 Body Fractures

Isolated C2 body fractures are most often successfully treated with external immobilization. Rare instances of ligamentous disruption may require urgent surgical stabilization and fusion. In these instances, high-resolution CT scanning with multiplane reconstructions and MRI are highly recommended, if available. In instances of comminuted body fractures, evaluation of the vertebral artery is highly recommended with computed tomography angiography, magnetic resonance angiography, or the most accurate alternate study available.[55]

Combination Fractures of the Atlas and Axis

Combination fractures are more likely associated with neurological injury compared to isolated fractures. Most combination patterns are successfully treated with external immobilization. However, current guidelines recommend consideration of surgical stabilization and fusion in C1-type II dens fracture combinations, and a C1-hangman's fracture combination with >11° angulation of C2–C3. This is because of a higher incidence of instability and higher nonunion rates (compared to other combination types) when treated with cervical immobilization alone.[60]

Subaxial Cervical Spine Injuries

Approximately 70% of traumatic cervical spine pathology occurs in the subaxial segment (C3–C7) and includes a broad range of fracture and dislocation injuries.[6] The incidence of neurologic morbidity associated with subaxial cervical spine injuries is increased as compared to the injuries of the craniovertebral junction, most likely because of greater spinal canal volumes at the upper cervical levels. Further, an SCI at the craniovertebral segment is more likely to have severe immediate ramifications, such as apnea and neurogenic shock. The vertebral anatomy of the subaxial region is fairly homogeneous from C3 to C6. Commonly identified injuries can be broadly classified as vertebral body fractures, subluxations and dislocated articular facets, and miscellaneous other fractures.

Vertebral Body Fractures

Common fractures of the vertebral body include:
- Compression fractures
- Burst fractures
- Teardrop fractures.

Compression fractures result from mild flexion and axial loading and do not compromise the canal. Patients with these stable fractures are usually treated with cervical collars.

Axial loading in a relatively neutral position may lead to burst fractures. Canal compromise secondary to retropulsion of bone fragments is common. Cervical burst fractures are unstable injuries. Although they may heal in many patients with rigid external immobilization, anterior decompression and stabilization is frequently preferable, particularly for patients with incomplete injuries. Anterior plate stabilization usually provides adequate stabilization in those patients requiring an operation.[61]

Teardrop fractures are primarily hyperflexion injuries, but they may also occur when extreme axial loading occurs with the spine in a flexed position (Fig. 38B.8). These injuries are identified by a small fracture across

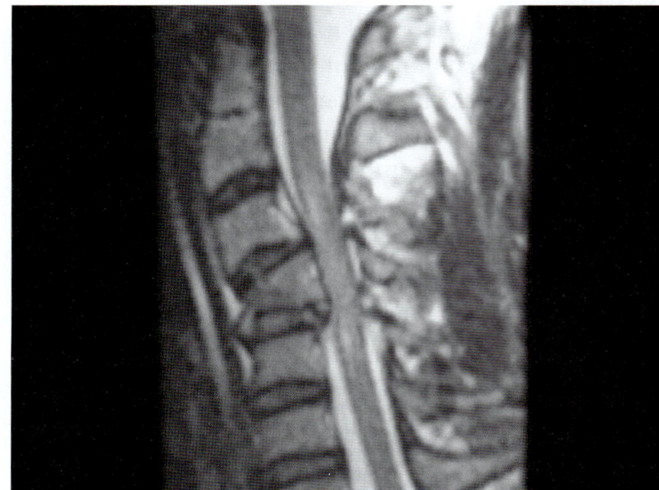

Fig. 38B.8: Lateral T2-weighted magnetic resonance imaging of C4 teardrop fracture.

the anteroinferior aspect of the vertebral body and posterior ligamentous incompetence. Flexion/axial loading injuries are devastating injuries due to the propensity for neurologic injury and often are the result of diving or other sports-related activities. Patients commonly present with a neurologic injury. Options for treatment include rigid external immobilization or surgical intervention. As with severe burst fractures, if there is a partial neurological deficit decompression with reconstruction of the anterior, load-bearing column is strongly recommended.

Subluxations and Dislocated Articular Facets

Anteroposterior subluxations are a commonly encountered problem in the subaxial cervical spine. Cadaveric studies of the cervical spine have shown that listhesis or horizontal subluxation of ≥3.5 mm or angulation of one vertebral body relative to another >11 degrees indicates ligamentous instability.[62] Such subluxations are seen in the subaxial cervical spine and may be associated with facet injuries or pure dislocations. Treatment is aimed at early realignment, most commonly with traction, followed by fusion.

Facet dislocation is a pathologic entity in that the inferior articular process of the upper vertebra lies anterior to the superior process of the lower vertebra (Fig. 38B.9). The articular processes may or may not have an associated bone fracture. Neurologic injury is common and there is significant potential for neurologic deterioration in patients with these injuries with relatively high rates of neurologic morbidity. Approximately 80% of unilateral locked facets are associated with some neurologic deficit, and this figure approaches 100% for bilateral locked facets.[63]

Head rotation or rotation associated with flexion causes forward and upward translation of the opposite facet, which when severe causes unilateral facet dislocation and in many cases facet fracture as well. On lateral views, unilateral facet dislocations result in 10–25% vertebral body rotation with CT imaging demonstrating that the inferior facet of the rostral vertebra is anterior to the superior facet of the caudal vertebra. Malalignment of the spinous process is evident on anteroposterior views. Use of cervical traction is generally required for realignment. Proper spinal alignment is then maintained either with a rigid external orthosis (halo) or with internal fixation. Open reduction with internal fixation is recommended for irreducible injuries or those that fail to stay reduced.

Bilateral facet dislocation results from hyperflexion with or without rotation. There will always be associated

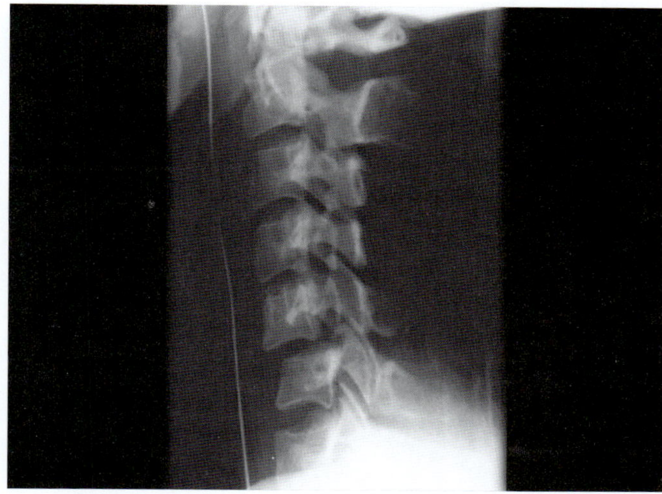

Fig. 38B.9: Lateral radiograph showing a cervical facet dislocation.

disruption of the posterior ligamentous complex, making these injuries highly unstable as a result of the ligamentous destruction required for such a deformity to occur. Lateral radiographs usually reveal 50% or greater anterolisthesis of the superiorly involved vertebral body with variable amounts of angulation. Fractures of the facets, lamina, and spinous processes are common. Posterior interspinous widening is usually present. Traction should be used to restore alignment. Treatment with an external orthosis commonly fails because the instability is so severe, and internal arthrodesis is usually recommended.

In patients with a cervical dislocation, early closed reduction with traction is an important part of treatment. Reduction can simplify surgical treatment as well as provide prompt decompression of the neural tissues in neurologically impaired patients. While the current evidence supports obtaining closed reduction in an awake patient before obtaining an MRI, it is generally recommended that in an unexaminable patient who cannot cooperate with the examination, a prereduction MRI is prudent to get an understanding of the status of the spinal cord and any potentially offending soft tissue or bony structures placing the spinal cord at risk. Surgical treatment for facet dislocations can involve anterior, posterior, or a combined approach, depending on the presence or absence of disc herniation, facet fracture, and status of the posterior ligamentous complex.

Though various subaxial cervical spine injuries have been classified into different types, there has been a trend towards development of classification systems to simplify the overall management of these groups of patients. Two new systems have been developed on the basis of modern

Table 38B.1 Subaxial Cervical Spine Injury Classification and Severity Scale (SLICS).

Morphology	
No abnormality	0
Compression	1
Burst fracture	+1 = 2
Distraction	3
Rotation/translation	4
Discoligamentous complex	
Intact	0
Indeterminate	1
Disrupted	2
Neurological status	
Intact	0
Root injury	1
Complete cord injury	2
Incomplete cord injury	3
Continuous cord compression (in setting of neurodeficit)	+1
Treatment	
SLICS ≤ 3: nonoperative	
SLICS = 4: consider for operative or nonoperative intervention	
SLICS ≥ 5: operative	

imaging that allows quantification of stability over a range to assess severity of injuries (CSISS and SLIC) and neurologic examination (SLIC), and can aid in identifying patients who clearly require nonoperative or operative treatment.[63,64] The Cervical Spine Injury Severity Score (CSISS) is based on an independent analysis of four columns (anterior, posterior, right, and left lateral columns).[63] The anterior column includes the body, disc including the annulus, anterior and posterior longitudinal ligaments, and transverse processes. Each lateral column is scored separately and includes the facet projections, lateral mass, pedicles, and facet joint capsules. The posterior column includes the lamina, spinous process, ligamentum flavum, and nuchal ligaments. The Subaxial Cervical Spine Injury Classification (SLIC) system evaluates fracture morphology, the discoligamentous complex, and neurologic function, creating a comprehensive system to aid treatment decision-making.[64] The overall injury score is obtained by summing the scores from each category (Table 38B.1). The SLIC score is the sum of the individual components. A patient with a SLIC score of 3 is treated nonoperatively, whereas surgery is recommended in a patient with a score of 5. A patient with a score of 4 can be treated either operatively or nonoperatively. Current guidelines strongly advocate the SLIC classification system. Robust evidence suggests that it is a powerful tool in choice of treatment with reliability and decreased variability. Most of the fracture patterns can be assigned a final score after analyzing the morphology, the discoligamentous complex, and neurologic function that can help with clinical decision-making to a certain extent. [65]

Miscellaneous Other Fractures

Miscellaneous other fractures include fractures of the lamina, spinous processes, and lateral masses. Most of these injuries are not associated with major instability or neurologic dysfunction and are successfully treated with a rigid cervical collar. Thorough evaluation of these injuries that includes CT imaging is prudent because identification of one of these fractures on plain films may be associated with an occult fracture of the vertebral body. Magnetic resonance imaging is an excellent means to detect ligamentous injury.

In the United States, penetrating spinal injuries generally comprise about 12% of all spinal injuries, although this rate may be triple in certain metropolitan areas.[66] Gunshot wounds cause more neurologic morbidity than stab injuries because 50% of individuals injured by a gunshot have a functional cord transection.[67] Spinal stability is not always a clinical issue. Treatment is directed toward removal of foreign bodies, dural closure, and antibiotic coverage.[67] The primary goal of spinal surgery is usually to minimize the risk of infection.

Patients may injure the cervical spine without evidence of fracture or dislocation. A tear of the annulus fibrosis may result in a traumatic herniated intervertebral disc. The clinical presentation can be variable. Patients with intractable pain or a neurologic deficit attributable to the herniated disc may benefit from surgical decompression and fusion. Patients who have cervical pain and tenderness, full neurologic function and no radiographic pathology after appropriate evaluation may have a "whiplash" or ligamentous strain injury. Patients with cervical strain are best treated with analgesics, muscle relaxants and passive stretching exercises.

SPINAL CORD INJURY WITHOUT RADIOGRAPHIC ABNORMALITY

Spinal cord injury without a radiographic abnormality (SCIWORA) is an entity with clinical evidence of spinal cord dysfunction after trauma, but nondiagnostic radiographic analysis including plain radiographs, CT scanning, and MRI. The SCI may be either complete or incomplete—the latter is more likely to recover function. Spinal cord injury without radiographic abnormality is most common in children because their immature spines predispose them to SCI.[68,69] The neurologic deficits associated with SCIWORA are usually more severe in children than adults and the prognosis for full recovery poorer.[68,69] Treatment includes medical optimization and external immobilization.

CONCLUSION

Cervical spine injuries occur in about 2–6% of blunt trauma victims. Due to the potential to result in adverse neurologic sequelae, the importance of prehospital care, spine precautions, appropriate radiological assessment, clearance, and appropriate management of the cervical spine cannot be overemphasized. There has been tremendous progress in the understanding of the pathophysiology and radiological evaluation of patients with cervical spine and SCI. Recent data have started to demonstrate the potential benefit of early surgery in patients with cervical cord injury. Though not without limitations, the development of a newer Subaxial Cervical Spine Injury Classification and Severity Scale classification system represents an improvement in the classification of injured patients providing certain objective measures to decide the need for surgical intervention. The role of MRI in acute cervical spine trauma and the value of stem cell treatment in acute cervical SCI remain key areas of future research.

REFERENCES

1. Fehlings MG, Vaccaro A, Wilson JR, et al. Early versus delayed decompression for traumatic cervical spinal cord injury: results of the Surgical Timing in Acute Spinal Cord Injury Study (STASCIS). PloS One. 2012;7:e32037.
2. Muchow RD, Resnick DK, Abdel MP, et al. Magnetic resonance imaging (MRI) in the clearance of the cervical spine in blunt trauma: a meta-analysis. J Trauma. 2008;64:179-89.
3. Hadley MN, Walters BC, Aarabi B, et al. Clinical assessment following acute cervical spinal cord injury. Neurosurgery. 2013;(72 Suppl 2):40-53.
4. DeVivo MJ, Fine PR, Maetz HM, et al. Prevalence of spinal cord injury: a reestimation employing life table techniques. Arch Neurol. 1980;37:707-8.
5. Kraus JF, Franti CE, Riggins RS, et al. Incidence of traumatic spinal cord lesions. J Chronic dis. 1975;28:471-92.
6. Bohlman HH. Acute fractures and dislocations of the cervical spine. An analysis of three hundred hospitalized patients and review of the literature. J Bone Joint Surg Am. 1979;61:1119-42.
7. Davis D, Bohlman H, Walker AE, et al. The pathological findings in fatal craniospinal injuries. J Neurosurg. 1971;34:603-13.
8. Ryken TC, Hurlbert RJ, Hadley MN, et al. The acute cardiopulmonary management of patients with cervical spinal cord injuries. Neurosurgery. 2013;(72 Suppl 2):84-92.
9. Ryken TC, Hadley MN, Walters BC, et al. Radiographic assessment. Neurosurgery. 2013;(72 Suppl 2):54-72.
10. Gillingham J. The problem of head and spinal injuries: prevention of the second accident. Med Sci Law. 1970;10:104-9.
11. Gunby I. New focus on spinal cord injury. JAMA. 1981;245:1201-6.
12. Theodore N, Aarabi B, Dhall SS, et al. Transportation of patients with acute traumatic cervical spine injuries. Neurosurgery. 2013;(72 Suppl 2):35-9.
13. Sawin PD, Todd MM, Traynelis VC, et al. Cervical spine motion with direct laryngoscopy and orotracheal intubation. An in vivo cinefluoroscopic study of subjects without cervical abnormality. Anesthesiology. 1996;85:26-36.
14. ASIA/IMSOP. International Standards for Neurological and Functional Classification of Spinal Cord Injury–Revised 1996. Chicago, IL: ASIA; 1996.
15. Radcliff KE, Kepler CK, Delasotta LA, et al. Current management review of thoracolumbar cord syndromes. Spine J. 2011;11:884-92.
16. Aarabi B, Hadley MN, Dhall SS, et al. Management of acute traumatic central cord syndrome (ATCCS). Neurosurgery. 2013;72 Suppl 2:195-204.
17. Bracken MB, Shepard MJ, Holford TR, et al. Methylprednisolone or tirilazad mesylate administration after acute spinal cord injury: 1-year follow up. Results of the third National Acute Spinal Cord Injury randomized controlled trial. J Neurosurg. 1998;89:699-706.
18. Bracken MB, Shepard MJ, Holford TR, et al. Administration of methylprednisolone for 24 or 48 hours or tirilazad mesylate for 48 hours in the treatment of acute spinal cord injury. Results of the Third National Acute Spinal Cord Injury Randomized Controlled Trial. National Acute Spinal Cord Injury Study. JAMA. 1997;277:1597-604.
19. Bracken MB, Shepard MJ, Collins WF, et al. A randomized, controlled trial of methylprednisolone or naloxone in the treatment of acute spinal-cord injury. Results of the Second National Acute Spinal Cord Injury Study. N Engl J Med. 1990;322:1405-11.
20. Bracken MB, Shepard MJ, Collins WF Jr, et al. Methylprednisolone or naloxone treatment after acute spinal cord injury: 1-year follow-up data. Results of the second National Acute Spinal Cord Injury Study. J Neurosurg. 1992;76:23-31.
21. Hurlbert RJ, Hadley MN, Walters BC, et al. Pharmacological therapy for acute spinal cord injury. Neurosurgery. 2013;(72 Suppl 2):93-105.
22. Hoffman JR, Wolfson AB, Todd K, et al. Selective cervical spine radiography in blunt trauma: methodology of the National Emergency X-Radiography Utilization Study (NEXUS). Ann Emerg Med. 1998;32:461-9.
23. Stiell IG, Wells GA, Vandemheen KL, et al. The Canadian C-spine rule for radiography in alert and stable trauma patients. JAMA. 2001;286:1841-8.
24. Harris JH, Jr. The Radiology Of Acute Cervical Spine Trauma, 2nd edition. Baltimore: Williams & Wilkins; 1987:10-109.
25. Rethnam U, Yesupalan RS, Bastawrous SS. The Swimmer's view: does it really show what it is supposed to show? A retrospective study. BMC Med Imaging. 2008;8:2.

26. Ross SE, Schwab CW, David ET, et al. Clearing the cervical spine: initial radiologic evaluation. J Trauma. 1987;27: 1055-60.
27. Insko EK, Gracias VH, Gupta R, et al. Utility of flexion and extension radiographs of the cervical spine in the acute evaluation of blunt trauma. J Trauma. 2002;53:426-9.
28. Traynelis VC, Kasliwal MK. Cervical clearance. J Neurosurg. 2011;115:536-9; discussion 9-40.
29. Chew BG, Swartz C, Quigley MR, et al. Cervical spine clearance in the traumatically injured patient: is multidetector CT scanning sufficient alone? Clinical article. J Neurosurg Spine. 2013;19:576-81.
30. Panczykowski DM, Tomycz ND, Okonkwo DO. Comparative effectiveness of using computed tomography alone to exclude cervical spine injuries in obtunded or intubated patients: meta-analysis of 14,327 patients with blunt trauma. J Neurosurg. 2011;115:541-9.
31. Menaker J, Philp A, Boswell S, et al. Computed tomography alone for cervical spine clearance in the unreliable patient—are we there yet? J Trauma. 2008;64:898-903; discussion-4.
32. Stassen NA, Williams VA, Gestring ML, et al. Magnetic resonance imaging in combination with helical computed tomography provides a safe and efficient method of cervical spine clearance in the obtunded trauma patient. J Trauma. 2006;60:171-7.
33. Bloom AI, Neeman Z, Slasky BS, et al. Fracture of the occipital condyles and associated craniocervical ligament injury: incidence, CT imaging and implications. Clinical radiology. 1997;52:198-202.
34. Leone A, Cerase A, Colosimo C, et al. Occipital condylar fractures: a review. Radiology. 2000;216:635-44.
35. Theodore N, Aarabi B, Dhall SS, et al. Occipital condyle fractures. Neurosurgery. 2013;72 Suppl 2:106-13.
36. Anderson PA, Montesano PX. Morphology and treatment of occipital condyle fractures. Spine. 1988;13:731-6.
37. Capuano C, Costagliola C, Shamsaldin M, et al. Occipital condyle fractures: a hidden nosologic entity. An experience with 10 cases. Acta Neurochir. 2004;146:779-84.
38. Powers B, Miller MD, Kramer RS, et al. Traumatic anterior atlanto-occipital dislocation. Neurosurgery. 1979;4:12-7.
39. Alker GJ, Jr, Oh YS, Leslie EV. High cervical spine and craniocervical junction injuries in fatal traffic accidents: a radiological study. Orthop Clin North Am. 1978;9:1003-10.
40. Traynelis VC, Marano GD, Dunker RO, et al. Traumatic atlanto-occipital dislocation. Case report. J Neurosurg. 1986; 65:863-70.
41. Bellabarba C, Mirza SK, West GA, et al. Diagnosis and treatment of craniocervical dislocation in a series of 17 consecutive survivors during an 8-year period. J Neurosurg Spine. 2006;4:429-40.
42. Harris JH, Jr, Carson GC, Wagner LK, et al. Radiologic diagnosis of traumatic occipitovertebral dissociation: 2. Comparison of three methods of detecting occipitovertebral relationships on lateral radiographs of supine subjects. AJR. 1994;162:887-92.
43. Dziurzynski K, Anderson PA, Bean DB, et al. A blinded assessment of radiographic criteria for atlanto-occipital dislocation. Spine. 2005;30:1427-32.
44. Pang D, Nemzek WR, Zovickian J. Atlanto-occipital dislocation–part 2: The clinical use of (occipital) condyle-C1 interval, comparison with other diagnostic methods, and the manifestation, management, and outcome of atlanto-occipital dislocation in children. Neurosurgery. 2007;61:995-1015; discussion
45. Theodore N, Aarabi B, Dhall SS, et al. The diagnosis and management of traumatic atlanto-occipital dislocation injuries. Neurosurgery. 2013;(72 Suppl 2):114-26.
46. Hadley MN, Dickman CA, Browner CM, et al. Acute traumatic atlas fractures: management and long term outcome. Neurosurgery. 1988;23:31-5.
47. Kakarla UK, Chang SW, Theodore N, et al. Atlas fractures. Neurosurgery. 2010;66:60-7.
48. Spence KF, Jr, Decker S, Sell KW. Bursting atlantal fracture associated with rupture of the transverse ligament. The J Bone Joint Surg Am. 1970;52:543-9.
49. Dickman CA, Greene KA, Sonntag VK. Injuries involving the transverse atlantal ligament: classification and treatment guidelines based upon experience with 39 injuries. Neurosurgery. 1996;38:44-50.
50. Ryken TC, Aarabi B, Dhall SS, et al. Management of isolated fractures of the atlas in adults. Neurosurgery. 2013;72 Suppl 2:127-31.

Additional references appear in the online version of this book.

39

Thoracic Trauma

Elias Zigiriadis, Martin D Smith, Tugba H Yilmaz, Elias Degiannis

Key Points

- Approximately 85% of patients with thoracic trauma do not need surgery but can be dealt with by basic invasive procedures immediately on admission to hospital.
- It is of paramount importance to identify immediate life-threatening injuries during the primary survey and potential life-threatening injuries during the secondary survey. Advanced life support principles should be adhered to.
- The clinician should always be alert to the possibility of breaching two cavities in the presence of penetrating trauma—the abdominal and thoracic cavities.
- A significant number of patients with thoracic trauma will need critical-care unit bed availability for physiological support.

INTRODUCTION

Thoracic trauma is a significant cause of mortality. Many trauma patients die on scene and a significant number after reaching hospital. Many of these latter deaths could be prevented with prompt diagnosis and treatment. Only 15% of patients with chest trauma will require surgical intervention. The rest can be initially managed with basic procedures, which should be performed by the emergency department/trauma surgeons. Cooperation between emergency physicians and trauma doctors based on ATLS principles drastically decreases the number of avoidable deaths in patients with chest trauma.

INITIAL MANAGEMENT

The primary survey begins with the airway, and major problems related to that should be immediately corrected. Airway patency and air exchange should be assessed by listening for air movement at the patient's nose and mouth and by auscultating the lungs; by inspecting the oropharynx for foreign body obstruction; and by observing for associated intercostal and supraclavicular retraction. Laryngeal injury with major thoracic trauma can present acutely or subacutely, causing dramatic airway obstruction. Posterior dislocation or fracture dislocation of the sternoclavicular joint can cause obstruction of the airway by producing external compression to the trachea. This injury can be recognized by the presence of stridor, a change in voice and obvious trauma to the base of the neck with a palpable defect in the region of the sternoclavicular joint. Evidence of a threatened airway should lead to the establishment of a definitive airway, preferably by endotracheal intubation. Assessment of breathing should be performed next or simultaneously with the assessment of the airway. Respiratory expansion of the chest wall should be observed together with simultaneous percussion and auscultation of the chest. It is important to be alert to the possibility of subtle signs of chest injury or hypoxia presenting as increased respiratory rate and progressive shallow breathing. It is of paramount importance to understand that cyanosis is a late sign of hypoxia in trauma patients and also that its absence does not necessarily indicate adequate tissue oxygenation or airway. It is important during the primary survey to be able to identify and initiate treatment of airway obstruction, tension pneumothorax, open pneumothorax, flail chest and pulmonary contusion and cardiac tamponade. These are life-threatening conditions, and they can be tackled by establishment of a definitive airway, insertion of an intercostal drain, ventilation or even emergency department thoracotomy/emergency thoracotomy depending on the type of injury.

The secondary survey must identify the potential life-threatening injuries: simple pneumothorax, hemothorax, pulmonary contusion, tracheobronchial tree injury, blunt cardiac injury, traumatic aortic disruption, traumatic diaphragmatic injury and blunt esophageal rupture. After excluding the immediate life-threatening and potentially life-threatening chest injuries, further investigations will probably be required to identify and treat more "exotic" thoracic injuries.

SPECIFIC INJURIES

Thoracic Wall Injuries

Fractured Ribs

Fractures of the ribs constitute one of the most common injuries encountered with chest trauma. Although rib fractures occur in all ages, the thoracic cage is easier to fracture in older people than in children as the ribs have lost their elasticity. Contusion of the lung in children can occur without the presence of rib fractures due to the elasticity of the thoracic cage.

Usually rib fractures do not significantly impair pulmonary function. They are, however, a marker of severe energy transfer. Fractures of the first and second ribs are associated with injuries of the thoracic aorta, subclavian artery, and brachial plexus. Third to seventh rib fractures are common causes of hemopneumothorax and pulmonary contusions. Fractures of the lower ribs (eight to twelve) can result in diaphragmatic injury or injury of the upper abdominal viscera (liver, colon, and spleen).[1, 2] In both scenarios of the patient with fracture of the first or second rib or fractures of ribs 10 through 12, a physiologically stable patient should undergo a computed tomogram (CT) scan of the chest and/or abdomen, given the high association of aortic and abdominal injuries respectively. On examination, in most cases, the patients present with focal pleuritic chest pain and point tenderness. When there are only one or two rib fractures present, the patient can be discharged home provided that there is no underlying pulmonary pathology (chronic obstructive pulmonary disease), the chest X-ray (CXR) does not show any parenchymal injury, there is no evidence of hemopneumothorax, and with analgesia the patient is able to cough adequately. The patient must be able to cough comfortably so that atelectasis and subsequent respiratory tract infections are avoided.[3] In the presence of three or more fractures, the patient should be admitted for pain control. In patients with multiple rib fractures, a high thoracic epidural anesthesia will result in lower morbidity rates than when parenteral narcotics are used.[4] An epidural is performed if the patient can be monitored in an intensive care environment and is extremely effective for pain relief and hence respiratory failure requiring ventilation may be avoided. An intrapleural block may be used if the patient has a chest tube in situ, and the patient is carefully monitored in a critical care environment. This technique is not appropriate if the chest drain is bubbling, as a tension pneumothorax can occur in the presence of an active air leak while the intercostal drain is clamped for 15 minutes after the intrapleural instillation of local anesthetic. Bilateral intrapleural blocks should not be used. An intrapleural block is achieved by instilling local anesthetic within the pleural cavity through a chest tube, but unfortunately it does not always provide effective pain relief for rib fractures. It can provide effective temporary analgesia for pain caused by the tip of the drain, which can otherwise be very difficult to treat. Twenty milliliters of ropivacaine with adrenalin is injected as proximal as possible into the intercostal drain via a 23G butterfly needle through a three way tap. The insertion of the butterfly needle is as close to the skin as possible to minimize dead space. After injection, the chest tube is clamped for 15 minutes to prevent the local anesthetic from running out. This block can be repeated every 4 hours, the maximum safe dose of ropivacaine is 3.5 mg/kg every 4 hours.[1]

An intercostal nerve block can provide analgesia for patients with isolated fractured ribs. The intercostal nerve can be blocked at the costal angle, one finger breadth lateral from the spinous process. The block can also be done in the midclavicular line because the local anesthetic spreads anteriorly and posteriorly over several centimeters affecting all the branches of the nerve. The local anesthetic is rapidly absorbed from the very vascular area with a low risk of toxicity. The effect of an intercostal block usually lasts 4–8 hours after which it can be repeated. For severely displaced rib fractures, it is better to call an anesthesiologist to insert an epidural or paravertebral indwelling catheter for a continuous block in order to maintain analgesia for several days.[1]

Certain patients with displaced and movable rib fractures who do not require assisted ventilation, but rather are experiencing persistent, unrelenting pain with breathing, coughing, or mobilization from the prone position, could have their fractures stabilized surgically to alleviate their pain. This reduces their risk of long-term pain and disability.[5,6]

A small percentage of rib fractures do not heal and manifest a nonunion months-to-years after their injury. A fibrous capsule envelopes the fracture as bony union has not occurred. The chronic nonunion may cause intermittent discomfort associated with movement of the fracture and can be quite disabling. For treatment, the fibrous callous enveloping the nonunion is resected and a plate is placed to fixate the rib ends.[7]

Flail Chest

A flail chest is defined as a fracture of two or more ribs in two or more places on each rib resulting in paradoxical movement of a segment of the chest wall. This paradoxical movement (recession of the chest wall on inspiration) may sometimes become apparent after 24 hours. On plain radiographs, multiple rib fractures in a flail pattern may be seen. This may be difficult to detect if the fractures run through the costochondral joints. Most flail chests, however, may be clearly visible on a CT scan.[8] Its diagnosis is a marker of the severity of the force causing the trauma. The blunt force required to disrupt the integrity of the thoracic cage and result in a flail chest typically produces an underlying pulmonary contusion. This abnormal movement in turn causes a decrease in vital capacity and ineffective ventilation, resulting in pulmonary insufficiency. Compliance of the ribs is an equally important factor as is the force of impact. In the elderly, low-energy trauma can cause a flail chest whereas in children only 1% of major impact injuries result in a flail chest.[9]

Traditional treatment uses positive pressure ventilation to internally splint the chest until fibrous union of the fractured ribs occurs. However, intubation and ventilation are still often required, especially in patients with severe injuries. Continuous positive airway pressure via a tight-fitting face mask is effective management of a flail chest in a cooperative patient (without facial fractures) and may avoid intubation and ventilation, and reduce the incidence of complications associated with these type of injuries including hospital acquired pneumonias.[9] Hospital stay may also be reduced. Close monitoring of the patient's respiratory rate and $PaCO_2$ levels is required. As with all pulmonary injuries, the cornerstones of treatment include analgesia and aggressive physiotherapy. Recently the concept of mechanical rib cage stabilization for flail chests has evolved. It is still quite controversial as definitive outcomes data are not available. The potential indications for operative fixation of the ribs include inability to wean the patient off the ventilator, persistent pain due to malunion not controlled by noninvasive analgesia, deformity of the chest wall that affects ventilation, and prior to closure of the chest wall after thoracotomy for other reasons. Small randomized trials of patients with a flail chest showed that patients with fixation of the thoracic cage had shorter ICU stay and an earlier return to work when compared with patients requiring ventilation. There is a suggestion that mechanical stabilization of a flail chest could be beneficial in a selected group of patients.[10-12]

Sternal Fractures

Sternal fractures are uncommon and affect about 4% of patients involved in motor vehicle accidents (MVAs). They occur more frequently in older patients and are usually caused by the impact of the steering wheel on the sternum. They are usually transverse and affect the upper half of the sternum. The definitive diagnosis in most cases is by a lateral CXR as the anterior–posterior view does not show the fracture in most cases. Sternal fractures are associated with cardiac contusions. In most instances, analgesia and physiotherapy are sufficient treatment, but in the presence of a severely displaced fracture with disruption of the sternocostal junctions, operative reduction and fixation may be required. Posterior dislocation or fracture dislocation of the sternoclavicular joints can also result in both tracheal and superior vena cava (SVC) compromise due to extrinsic compression in which case surgical reduction of the fracture will be necessary.[13]

Chest Wall Deformity/Defect

Chest wall deformities are characterized by a variety of traumatic circumstances and are the result of severely displaced rib fractures that visibly deform the chest wall, with or without soft tissue loss. Minimal-to-moderate size defects ($< 10 \times 10$ cm) can be caused by penetrating missiles or impalement with surrounding objects during MVAs. Repair of both rib fractures and soft tissue may be indicated to restore an incompetent segment of chest wall even if the patient does not require mechanical ventilation. Unrepaired segments may lead to chest wall herniation. Operations that deal with chest wall defects (extensive tissue loss) can be lengthy as they are associated with tissue transfer procedures and should only be considered as part of the initial management of patients who do not have severe trauma. Under normal circumstances in polytrauma patients, temporary closure should be achieved by creating skin flaps or using prosthetic materials until the patient is physiologically stable to undergo the more extensive and definitive repair.

Lung Injuries

Pulmonary Contusion and Laceration

Pulmonary contusion is a result of bleeding into the pulmonary parenchyma and usually occurs beneath fractured ribs or a flail segment in adults. It may be present in children in the absence of fractured ribs (due to the elasticity of the rib cage). It is the most commonly diagnosed intrathoracic injury in victims of blunt trauma and is an independent risk factor for pneumonia and adult respiratory distress syndrome. Significant contusions are often not diagnosed until 24 hours after admission as the CXR findings are typically delayed and often underestimate the degree of the pulmonary injury. A CT scan provides excellent information about the anatomical distribution of the pathology and the diagnosis of other associated injuries.

Respiratory dysfunction arises due to a combination of lack of pulmonary function in the contused segment and remote lung injury mediated by cytokines released by trauma to the lung parenchyma. In case of bleeding into the bronchial tree, normal parts of the lung can be flooded with blood, including the contralateral lung. In cases with extensive alveolar and vascular disruption, the patient may suffer air embolism. Arterial blood gases should be performed in all patients with significant lung contusions in order to assess the need for mechanical ventilation.

Treatment relies on recognition of pulmonary contusion, and consists of adequate analgesia, good physiotherapy, and supplemental oxygen (this may vary from observation and oxygen administration to mechanical ventilation).[14] In patients with pulmonary contusion, avoidance of over transfusion with intravenous fluids is sensible, but restriction of fluid as a treatment is not advised. The majority of patients with penetrating thoracic trauma can be managed nonoperatively.

Pneumothorax

Pneumothorax related to thoracic trauma typically occurs when air escapes from a lacerated or punctured lung into the pleural space. Much less frequently, pneumothorax can be related to disruption of the tracheobronchial tree or a hollow viscus (esophagus). The air is trapped in the pleural cavity and may or may not be under pressure. A simple pneumothorax leads to partial collapse of the lung and is treated by insertion of a chest tube. If the air is under pressure, the pneumothorax is called a tension pneumothorax; otherwise it is called a simple pneumothorax. Pneumothoraces can be classified as closed or open. Open pneumothorax is related to a traumatic injury to the chest wall, and air enters the pleural cavity through the chest wall defect. If the patient with an open pneumothorax attempts to breathe spontaneously, air will enter and exit the wound with each respiration, giving rise to the term "sucking chest wound". If the opening in the chest wall is approximately 2/3 the diameter of the trachea, air passes preferentially through the chest wall defect with each respiratory effort, because air tend to follow the path of least resistance. Effective ventilation is thereby impaired, leading to hypoxia and hypercarbia. In the presence of an open pneumothorax, the defect should be closed by a sterile occlusive dressing taped securely on three sides in order to provide a flutter valve effect. A chest tube will then be inserted as soon as possible at a place away from the wound. Definitive closure of the thoracic defect is required.

A tension pneumothorax may complicate a simple pneumothorax and quite frequently is caused when mechanical ventilation with positive pressure ventilation is applied to patients with visceral pleural injury. The air is forced into the thoracic cavity without escape, leading to complete collapse of the affected lung, displacement of mediastinum to the opposite side, decreased venous return and compression of the opposite lung, and the diaphragm being pushed inferiorly (Fig. 39.1). The intercostal spaces on the affected side are increased. The diagnosis should be a clinical one and should not be delayed for radiological confirmation. The patient presents with chest pain, respiratory distress, tachycardia, tracheal deviation, neck vein distension, hyper-resonant chest on the affected side, and lack of breath sounds. Immediate decompression of a tension

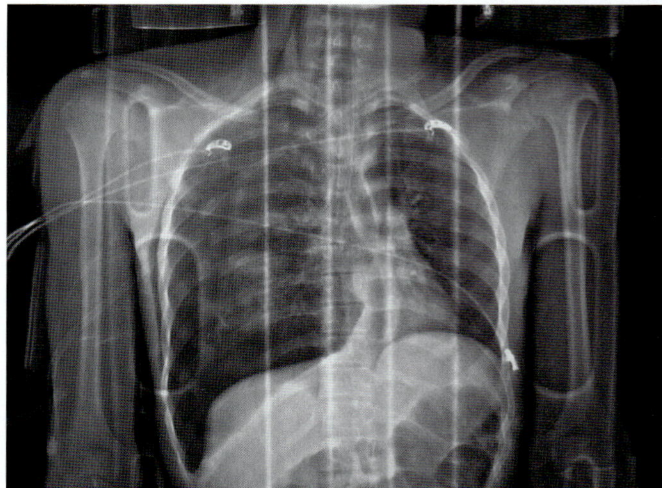

Fig. 39.1: Right-sided tension pneumothorax.

pneumothorax should be performed by inserting a large-caliber needle into the second intercostal space in the mid-clavicular line of the affected hemithorax. This should be followed by insertion of a chest tube through the fifth intercostal space just anterior to the mid-axillary line.

Hemothorax

The thoracic cavity can hold up to 3 L of blood. A hemothorax can result from injury of the thoracic wall or thoracic viscera following blunt or penetrating trauma. It is also possible to develop a hemothorax from blood originating from the base of the neck or abdomen if there is a communication via a tract between the base of the neck and the thoracic cavity or the peritoneal and pleural cavity through a diaphragmatic defect. A hemothorax is referred to as massive when there is >1500 mL blood in the pleural space. Usually a massive hemothorax is caused by laceration of the intercostal arteries, internal thoracic vessels, central lung injuries, heart, or great vessel injuries. Bleeding from the lung parenchyma is rarely massive due to the low systolic pulmonary artery pressure and the high thromboplastin levels in the lungs. A minimal hemothorax presenting as blunting of the costophrenic angle on CXR can be managed conservatively.

Hemothoraces that are bigger than the amount required to obscure the costophrenic angle on an erect CXR should be drained. If there is still a hemothorax despite a functioning chest tube (preferably a curved one), an additional tube is inserted. A post insertion CXR is routinely done. One has to be alert for malfunctioning chest tubes (i.e. an occluded tube or tube holes outside the chest cavity in the subcutaneous tissues) when an initially high volume loss suddenly ceases. If there is a retained hemothorax present after a few days, thoracoscopic drainage should be considered at an early stage, usually within the first 5 days before the clot is organized, making drainage difficult. However, if the initial drainage after placement of a chest tube is >1500 mL blood or the blood loss continues at a rate of 300 mL/h for 3–4 hours post insertion, this is an indication for thoracotomy. Furthermore a patient who is unstable despite aggressive volume resuscitation may also need a thoracotomy. The CXR should be repeated to make sure that there is no retained clot in the pleural cavity giving you the false impression that bleeding has stopped. There are no data supporting decreased hemorrhage or mortality by clamping the chest tube while preparing the patient for surgery. Consider autotransfusion of blood from the chest cavity to reduce the need for donor blood. If specific autotransfusion containers are not available, the normally available collection containers with 500 mL normal saline and 1000 U heparin added can be used.

Without doubt, access to most viscera of the pleural cavity is best achieved by a posterolateral thoracotomy, although in the common scenario when the patient is undergoing a thoracotomy for bleeding, an anterolateral thoracotomy is indicated as it is quicker and allows the surgeon to deal easily with cardiac injuries and injuries to most other thoracic cavity viscera. Both thoracotomies are usually via the 5th or 6th intercostal space. On the right, the posterolateral incision permits access to the distal thoracic trachea, right bronchus, carina, proximal 3 cm of the left bronchus, right lung, chest wall, and the whole of the esophagus. A left posterolateral thoracotomy provides access to the aorta, proximal left subclavian artery, (only for initial control in exceptional circumstances), the distal left bronchus, the left lung, and the distal esophagus. For a posterolateral thoracotomy, the patient should be placed in a full lateral position. The lower leg is flexed and the upper leg is kept straight with a pillow separating the legs. For better stability and spreading of the ribs, a pillow is placed beneath the chest wall perpendicular to the patient. The upper part of the chest is then strapped at the shoulders with either an Elastoplast or strapping belts. The same is done at the hips to hold the lower body in position. The surgeon should stand behind the patient and make a curvilinear incision extending from anterior to the tip of scapula—one fingers breadth below it—and curving posteriorly toward the vertebral column, but stopping approximately 5 cm short of it. The chest wall muscles are divided individually. The scapula is elevated with a scapular retractor. The plane between the scapula and the chest wall is avascular. The counting of the ribs is accomplished by sliding your hand under the scapula to the apex of the chest. The first rib can be difficult to feel and usually the highest palpable rib is the second one (while identifying the first or the second rib it must be remembered that there is usually a step between these two ribs that is not present between the second and the third). By counting the ribs this way, the fifth and sixth ribs are identified and the pleural cavity is entered through this intercostal space, along the superior border of the rib. At this point, if the patient has been intubated with a double lumen endotracheal tube, the surgeon can notify the anesthesiologist to isolate the respective lung. The surgeon should be vigilant not to injure the underlying lung, something that can easily take place if the lung is not isolated or is adherent to the pleura due to a previous inflammatory process. The ribs are spread using a Finochietto retractor and is done gradually to avoid iatrogenic rib fractures. However, in situations where torrential bleeding occurs, fracturing of the ribs is unavoidable. Both the surgeon and assistant should take care to avoid injury from rib fracture spikes. At the conclusion of the operation, two chest tubes are inserted, one is placed anteriorly at the apex and the other, a curved one, is placed posteriorly at the base of the pleural cavity. The tubes are attached to underwater sealed bottles and connected to a Gomco or gentle wall suction once in the critical care unit for better drainage of the pleural space. The thoracotomy is approximated by using a few figure-of-eight sutures, passing above and below the fifth and sixth ribs. The muscles are approximated by continuous suturing in layers.

EMERGENCY DEPARTMENT THORACOTOMY

The aims of emergency department thoracotomy (EDT) are the resuscitation of patients with penetrating cardiothoracic injuries by evacuating the hemopericardium and repairing the cardiac injury, controlling thoracic hemorrhage, and reducing subdiaphragmatic blood loss and preventing and treating air embolism. Sometimes open cardiac massage is required in combination with any of the above. Preserving and redistributing the remaining blood volume improves coronary/carotid arterial flow, increasing the left ventricular stroke work index and myocardial contractility. All critically injured patients who present in extremis to the emergency department with penetrating trauma and signs of life [pupillary response to light, respiratory effort, response to pain, or cardiac activity on electrocardiogram (EKG)] should undergo EDT.

Even in the absence of the above signs of life, two subgroups of patients with penetrating trauma should undergo EDT.

- Nonintubated patients who underwent cardiopulmonary resuscitation (CPR) for < 5 minutes before arrival in the emergency department[15,16]
- Intubated patients who underwent CPR for < 10 minutes before arrival in the emergency department.

In both these categories, EDT should be done even in the absence of cardiac electrical activity.

In penetrating chest trauma, witnessed cardiac arrest in the emergency department is considered a clear indication for EDT. Persistent postinjury hypotension (i.e. systolic blood pressure of < 60 mm Hg) not responding to copious fluid resuscitation also constitutes a clear indication for EDT, particularly if cardiac tamponade, intrathoracic hemorrhage, or air embolism cannot be excluded. Refractory moderate post injury hypotension (i.e. systolic blood pressure of < 80 mm Hg) suspected to be due to intrathoracic hemorrhage or intra-abdominal hemorrhage is a relative indication for EDT. The patient's age and comorbidities as well as logistic issues have to be taken into consideration.[17,18]

Table 39.1 Emergency department thoracotomy should be terminated if:

• Irreparable cardiac damage has occurred
• The patient is identified as having massive head injuries
• Pulseless electrical activity is established
• Systolic blood pressure is < 70 mm Hg after 20 minutes
• Asystolic arrest has occurred[20]

Emergency department thoracotomy in blunt trauma should be performed rarely, if ever, in patients with cardiopulmonary arrest because of a very low survival rate and poor neurological outcome. Trauma surgeons caution against this indication as results have been dismal. However, some authorities perform EDT for blunt trauma, but they limit this strictly to those patients who arrive with vital signs present or a witnessed cardiopulmonary arrest.[19]

Emergency department thoracotomy is a "team event". It should not be prolonged unduly, but should have specific end points (Table 39.1). If an injury is repaired and the patient responds, he or she should then be moved to the operating room for the definitive repair or closure.

The doctor undertaking EDT must be able to perform a thoracotomy fast, be able to open the pericardium and to suture the heart, to clamp the hilum of the lung, and clamp the descending aorta. The instruments available in the emergency department are often limited making surgical expertise of vital importance. The patient undergoes immediate endotracheal intubation coupled with reliable venous access and aggressive fluid replacement. A left anterolateral thoracotomy with the patient in the supine position is performed. Although elevation of the left arm increases the extent of the operative field, abduction of the arm is sufficient for satisfactory intraoperative exposure in most cases.

The skin incision extends from the lateral border of the left sternocostal junction inferior to the nipple, to the mid-axillary line laterally, usually in the fifth intercostal space. In females, a submammary incision is performed. The muscles are divided in the same line as the skin

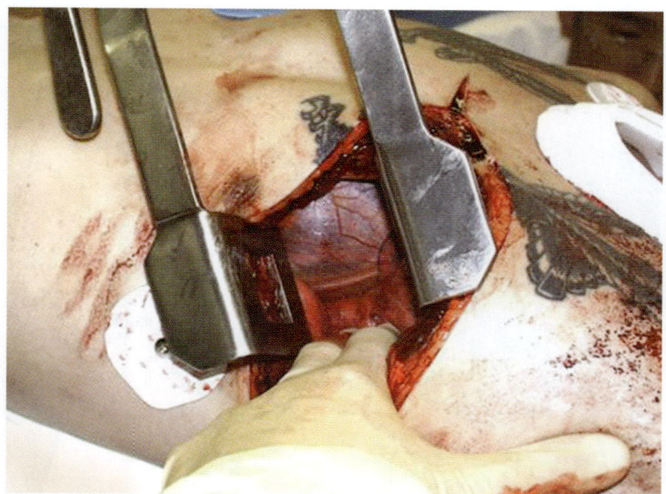

Fig. 39.2: Hemopericardium.

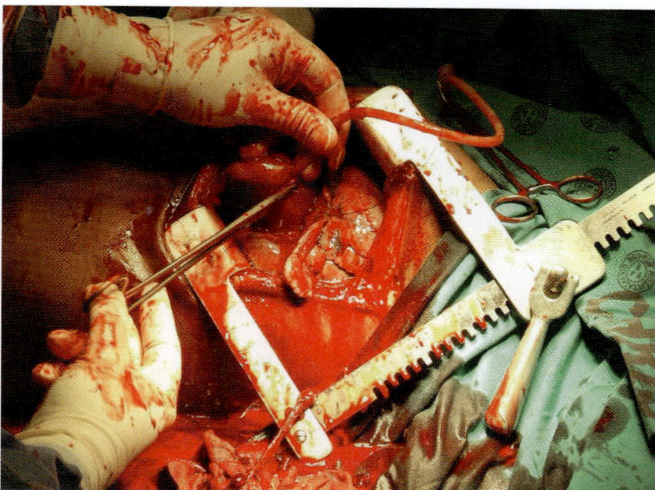

Fig. 39.3: A Foley catheter inserted through the cardiac wound facilitates suturing of the defect.

incision, usually with coagulation electrocautery, but rapid incision with a scalpel is acceptable. Care is taken not to injure the lungs on opening the pleura. A rib spreader is introduced and opened up rapidly. This almost invariably leads to fracture of ribs and caution must be taken by the surgeon and the assistants not to injure themselves on the rib fracture fragments while inserting their hands in the thoracic cavity. To avoid injury, it is advisable to cover the edges of the incision with abdominal swabs. If better access to the thoracic cavity is required, the costal cartilages of the corresponding ribs can be divided. At the end of the operation, it is important to look for the intercostal arteries corresponding to the divided cartilages and ligate them if severed.

The surgeon should initially look at the pericardium to exclude cardiac tamponade. Besides seeing a hole in the pericardium, a hemopericardium is evident by the white-bluish color of the pericardium produced by the underlying intrapericardial clot (Fig. 39.2). As the pericardium is very tense, it is difficult to open it by using mosquitoes; therefore the pericardium is carefully nicked with the scalpel blade at an area anterior to the phrenic nerve and the incision is extended vertically superiorly and inferiorly with scissors, always paying attention to the location of the phrenic nerve. If the heart is beating, repair is delayed until initial resuscitation measures have been completed. If it is not beating, suturing precedes resuscitation.

The injury to the heart is repaired with 3-0/4-0 non-absorbable sutures, interrupted figure-of-eight, or pledgeted mattress sutures, depending on the preference of the individual surgeon. Care is taken to avoid injury to the coronary vessels. In certain cases, if hemorrhage from the cardiac injury makes suturing difficult, insertion of a Foley catheter and inflation of the balloon with water can control the bleeding to allow for accurate suturing of the defect (Fig. 39.3). If the laceration is too long for a Foley catheter insertion, the assistant´s finger can be placed horizontally on the whole length of the laceration to control the bleeding. This is followed by careful insertion of stitches under the assistant´s finger while there is simultaneous retraction of the finger distally to the initial stitches. In situations in which the bleeding is torrential, compression of the right atrium or occlusion of the inferior vena cava and probably also the SVC can allow vital time for the surgeon to occlude the gap in the myocardium. It is always important to look for and identify the through and through injury to the heart that results in a simultaneous posterior wound. This necessitates elevation of the heart en bloc so that kinking and inflow occlusion are avoided (Fig. 39.4). This can cause bradycardia and cardiac arrest. Bathing of the heart in warm saline usually helps reversion back to a normal rhythm. Closure of the pericardium leaving only a 2 cm defect distally is desirable.

Cardiac massage where required in EDT should be done with both hands, one anteriorly and one posteriorly to the heart after opening the pericardium (Fig. 39.5). Cardiac massage with one hand compressing the heart against the vertebral column is less efficient and can cause severe injury to the left ventricle. Defibrillation with internal paddles may be needed, delivering between 10 and 50 joules. Intra-cardiac epinephrine can also be administered either in to the left or the right ventricle or systemically.[17]

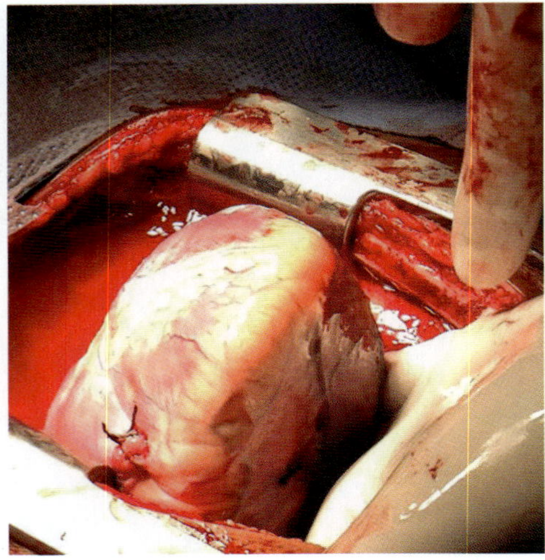

Fig. 39.4: Heart raised off its bed. There are an anterior and small posterior defect, which have been sutured.

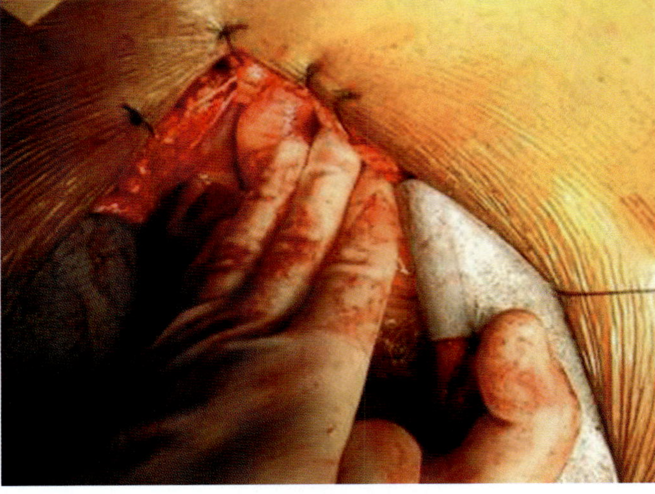

Fig. 39.5: Open cardiac massage using both hands.

The rationale for clamping the descending thoracic aorta in EDT is preservation and redistribution of the remaining blood volume, improvement of coronary/carotid arterial flow, reduction of subdiaphragmatic blood loss, increase of the left ventricular stroke work index and myocardial contractility. There are also adverse effects from thoracic aortic cross clamping; these are decreased blood flow to the abdominal viscera to approximately 10%, decreased renal perfusion to approximately 10%, and decreased blood flow to the spinal cord again to approximately 10%. This also induces anaerobic metabolism, hypoxia/lactic acidosis and imposes a tremendous afterload onto the left ventricle. We do not know the safe duration of cross clamping nor the incidence of reperfusion injury. Although thoracic aortic occlusion has been tolerated for as long as 75 minutes without spinal cord sequelae, clinical experience with elective thoracic aortic procedures indicates that 30 minutes is generally the threshold for reversible normothermic ischemia. The resulting hypoxia induces the elaboration, expression and activation of inflammatory cell adhesion mechanisms and mediators that have been linked to organ dysfunction and multiple organ failure.[17]

Although the suggested routine use of thoracic aortic clamping in patients with massive intra-abdominal hemorrhage makes physiological sense, its association with a significant improvement in the overall survival of these patients has yet to be clearly established. For clamping the descending aorta the left lung is elevated medially, the pleura is bridged at either side of the aorta, allowing for a long vascular clamp to be placed. In desperate situations, compression of the descending aorta with the fist against the vertebral column can be helpful when followed by clamping. Application of the vascular clamp without opening of the periaortic pleura is not advisable as it easily slips. The surgeon must be careful not to include the esophagus when clamping the aorta.

In penetrating injuries of the lungs that are bleeding profusely: if they are at the periphery, placement of a large Satinsky clamp including copious parenchyma of the lung will control the bleeding. Tractotomy has no place in the EDT scenario. Bleeding from a large vessel near the hilum or uncontrollable bleeding from the parenchyma can be best dealt by clamping of the hilum. This is achieved by initially retracting the lung anteriorly and inserting the left hand round the lower pole of the lung (sometimes tearing the inferior pulmonary ligament), and controlling the hilum between the index and the third finger of the left hand. A large Satinsky clamp is then taken with the right hand and the hilum is clamped from the opposite direction (the clamp is inserted from right to the left and the hilum is clamped just medially to the fingers of the surgeon). The same can be achieved by placing the Satinsky clamp to the hilum directly from above, in this case avoiding the maneuver of releasing the inferior pulmonary ligament. If a Satinsky clamp is not available in desperate situations, control of the hemorrhage can be achieved by a 180° twist of the lung at its hilum.

In the presence of bleeding from the right side of the heart or if the right side of the chest has to be accessed, the sternum is split transversely ("clamshell" incision) at the line of the skin incision (Fig. 39.6). When crossing the

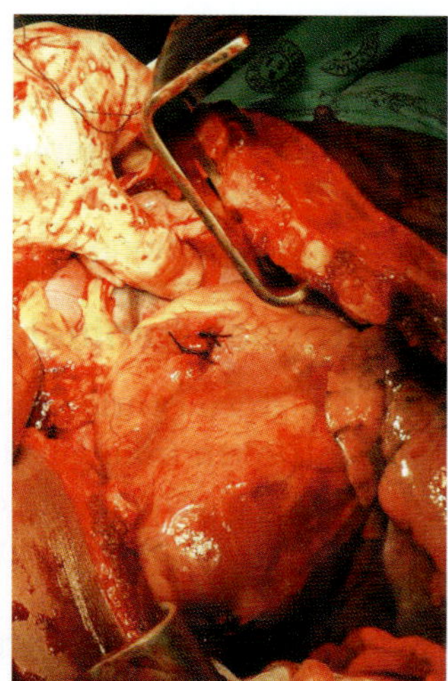

Fig. 39.6: Clamshell incision giving access to both thoracic cavities.

sternum from left-to-right, the incision should be carried upward to the 4th intercostal space to stay above the right nipple, thus facilitating exposure of the upper mediastinal structures (e.g. innominate artery bifurcation). The sternum is divided by a Gigli saw, a power saw, or if these are not available, the Lebsche knife is ideal, always making sure that upward traction is applied when the latter is hit with the hammer. A bone cutter is another alternative, albeit time consuming. The internal thoracic arteries must be ligated even if there is no obvious bleeding from them at the time of transection. In the hypovolemic patient, they can retract and not bleed when first divided. It is important to look for them within the areolar tissue posteriorly and immediately lateral to the sternum and ligate them before closing the incision.

Major air embolism can be a subtle clinical entity following thoracic trauma and is probably more common than recognized. The typical scenario involves a patient sustaining a penetrating chest wound who develops precipitous shock after endotracheal intubation and positive end expiratory pressure ventilation (PEEP). The shock results from global myocardial ischemia produced by coronary air emboli arising from traumatic alveolar-venous communications. A similar process may occur in patients with blunt lacerations of the lung parenchyma. Pulmonary hilum cross clamping is of paramount importance to prevent further pulmonary venous air embolism. Air should be aspirated from the left ventricle with the patient in the Trendelenburg position. In addition, vigorous cardiac massage may assist movement of air out of the coronary arteries. Venting of air from the root of the aorta prevents further egress into the coronary and other major arteries.

If the resuscitative thoracotomy is successful, attention should turn rapidly to the control of chest wall bleeding. These patients have systemic acidosis, are frequently hypothermic and often receive massive transfusions, resulting in significant coagulopathy. Divided muscles and tissues of the chest wall can bleed significantly when systemic perfusion is restored. Early attention to the hemostasis of these tissues will prevent continued blood loss while other injuries are treated. If the patient is successfully resuscitated, immediate transport to the operating room is mandatory. Results of EDT are based on the site of injury. In penetrating thoracic injuries, the presence of cardiac tamponade appears to be a favorable condition for improved survival.[21,22]

BLUNT CARDIAC TRAUMA

The reported incidence of blunt cardiac injury (BCI) varies widely from 15 to 52%.This is mainly due to the fact that the injury ranges to a wide spectrum of pathology from a mild contusion to rupture of the heart, usually due to a sudden increase in intracardiac pressure secondary to severe abdominal compression.[23] Blunt trauma to the heart can also cause blunt coronary artery injuries; usually the left anterior descending artery as it lies anteriorly in the chest and beneath the sternum. This injury can lead to myocardial infarction, arrhythmias, and ventricular failure. Valvular injuries are rare and are due to compressive forces of blood during contraction that leads to valve, chordae tendinae, and papillary muscle rupture. The aortic valve is most commonly involved followed by the mitral. Blunt cardiac injury is usually part of a multisystem trauma and should be suspected in chest trauma patients.[24]

The patient can present with angina-like chest pain or progressive dyspnea. The presence of a pericardial friction rub, S3 heart sound, or crepitations on auscultation should alert the physician to the diagnosis of cardiac contusion. The presence of raised central venous pressure or hypotension nonresponsive to fluid resuscitation in the absence of a source of major hemorrhage can also suggest cardiac contusion. Unfortunately no single test or combination of tests has proven consistently reliable in detecting BCI.[25.]

Patients with suspicion of BCI should undergo a CXR, EKG, and cardiac enzymes testing. A negative EKG does not exclude cardiac contusion. Common EKG changes range from nonspecific ST and T-wave changes, minor arrhythmias or complex arrhythmias. There can also be EKG ischemic changes such as ST elevation or T-wave inversion. Troponin T and troponin I are the recommended enzymes to be tested on admission and 8 hours later. Patients with abnormal values are further evaluated by color flow echocardiography, which is the gold standard for diagnosis. Echocardiography can reveal regional wall motion abnormalities, pericardial effusion, and valvular dysfunction. Patients diagnosed with BCI should be treated expectantly or symptomatically depending on the symptoms and EKG findings.[24] If pericardial fluid on the echocardiogram suggests tamponade, the patient should be treated by a subxiphoid pericardial window proceeding to a sternotomy if required or to anterolateral thoracotomy if moribund. The natural history of cardiac contusion in the majority of cases is benign, with arrhythmias or heart failure resolving within a few days after administration of appropriate medical management.

PENETRATING CARDIAC TRAUMA

In the last three decades, there have been numerous publications on the subject of penetrating cardiac injuries including a number of large series. Controversial issues remain; they relate to the diagnostic procedures that may be indicated and the therapeutic strategy best suited to each patient. These controversies are partly a reflection of differences in personal surgical preferences and logistical organization of trauma care. To a large extent, however, they stem from a lack of consistent stratification of patients. An elaborate scoring system for the purpose of predicting outcome has been devised, but attempts as classifying patients to inform rational management decisions have been rare and incomplete. In clinical practice, one can classify patients into five categories:[26]

Category 1: Lifeless

In this category are patients presenting with a thoracic wound who are unconscious with no sign of life (no respiratory effort, palpable pulse, or recordable blood pressure) and who have not been intubated and started on CPR after a witnessed cardiac arrest 5 minutes before arrival to the emergency department.

Category 2: Critically Unstable

These are patients with a penetrating thoracic injury, presenting with profound hypotension and impending cardiac arrest. The clinical picture is accounted for by either massive hemorrhage from the heart or severe cardiac tamponade.

Category 3: Cardiac Tamponade

These patients present with a thoracic wound and a clinical picture typical of cardiac tamponade (slight-to-severe hypotension and raised central venous pressure in the absence of tension pneumothorax).

Category 4: Thoracoabdominal Injury

These patients have a high epigastric wound or multiple lacerations of the trunk, often from gunshot or shotgun injury. The diagnosis of cardiac tamponade is clouded by the presence of an obvious abdominal injury.

Category 5: Benign Presentation

These patients present with a penetrating thoracic wound but are hemodynamically stable and without symptoms or signs of either hemorrhage or cardiac tamponade.

Management

The Lifeless Patient

Treatment consists of immediate intubation followed by thoracotomy and cardiorrhaphy in the resuscitation area. No procedure short of this heroic intervention would be adequate. However, reserve EDT for the lifeless patient whose vital signs have been preserved, at least for some time in the prehospital period.

The Critically Unstable Patient

This patient presents with signs of life but the clinical picture is dominated by profound hypotension and impending cardiac arrest. As in the previous category, diagnostic procedures would be detrimental, apart from e-FAST if available in the emergency department. Immediate endotracheal intubation and fluid replenishment are required. Some of these patients may regain sufficient hemodynamic stability and proceed to urgent thoracotomy in the operating room while others may remain unresponsive to resuscitation and require thoracotomy in the resuscitation area. It is clear from the literature that emergency room thoracotomy is more successful in this category of patients than in those who are "lifeless".

The Patient with Cardiac Tamponade

A high degree of suspicion based on the location of the thoracic wound in relation with this entity is usually sufficient to suggest the diagnosis of penetrating cardiac injury.

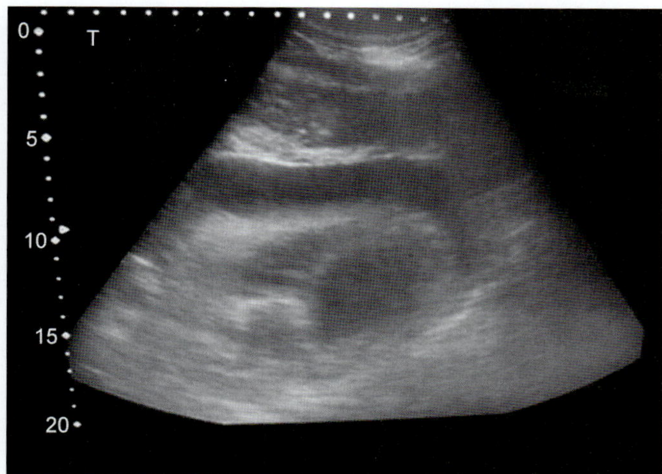

Fig. 39.7: e-FAST exam showing large amount of pericardial fluid in patient with cardiac injury.

The presence of both tracheal deviation and hyper-resonance of the chest will rule out a tension pneumothorax. A number of diagnostic methods have been recommended to increase clinical accuracy, of which e-FAST is the diagnostic "gold standard" (Fig. 39.7). The globular heart on the CXR is present in < 40% of cases. There is no place for needle pericardiocentesis as a therapeutic measure. Even a young patient with mild cardiac tamponade may deteriorate rapidly and have a cardiac arrest. In experienced hands, clinical judgment combined with a low threshold for intervention results in an extremely low rate of negative thoracotomy in patients with a clinical picture of cardiac tamponade. Nowadays, in most instances patients with hemopericardium are diagnosed before the development of the cardiac tamponade clinical picture as early diagnosis is achieved with the routine application of e-FAST in the emergency department.[27]

The Patient with Thoracoabdominal Injury

The diagnosis of cardiac tamponade may be masked by the presence of obvious abdominal signs due to peritonitis or more often by hemorrhage. An accurate preoperative diagnosis is often difficult, but is sometimes made; the clinician must then exercise clinical judgment in deciding which lesion is addressed first or whether a two team approach is indicated. In some cases, the cardiac tamponade is suspected only on completion of the laparotomy, either because the surgeon is worried about the presence of a precordial wound or because control of the intra-abdominal bleeding does not result in the expected improvement of the patient's condition. In this situation, a diagnostic pericardial window before closure of the abdomen has been shown to be safe and reliable. Needless to say that in certain cases a positive preoperative or intraoperative e-FAST exam can facilitate diagnosis and decision making, probably avoiding a diagnostic pericardial window.

The Patient with Benign Presentation

A number of patients with a penetrating precordial injury present with no symptoms or clinical signs of either cardiac tamponade or intrathoracic hemorrhage: nevertheless, the alert clinician should be concerned about the presence of a thoracic wound, especially in the precordium. The CXR may be normal. All these patients should be investigated by e-FAST, cardiac echo or even a CT angiogram of the mediastinum. Two arguments may support an aggressive management plan for all patients with penetrating cardiac injury, however minor. The first is the uncertainty about the long-term outcome of patients with an undrained hemopericardium. The entity of post-traumatic chronic constrictive pericarditis has been described in both the experimental and the clinical setting. The second is the danger of sudden and irremediable deterioration (even under hospital observation) that may occur several days after the initial injury. Clinical observation alone is insufficient for this type of patient therefore the above-mentioned investigations are performed. In cases of doubt, assessment is made via a subxiphoid pericardial window.

Always be very alert with a patient who has sustained penetrating trauma to the cardiac box who lies very quietly looking unwell or becomes aggressive trying to lift himself off the bed. This is a clinical picture that could be related to cardiac injury.

The ideal incision for access to the heart with penetrating trauma is a median sternotomy. On the other hand if the patient is moribund, a left anterolateral thoracotomy should be performed either in the emergency department or operating room as it gives quicker access to the heart.

All patients with repaired penetrating cardiac injuries should be auscultated daily for cardiac murmurs as there may be intracardiac defects secondary to the injury, and all patients with penetrating cardiac trauma should have an echocardiogram prior to discharge and 1 month later.

Pericardial Window

A subxiphoid pericardial window is required in cases where a pericardial blood collection cannot be excluded clinically or via investigations. A subxiphoid pericardial window is also particularly useful in patients with atrial injuries. These patients can present late and be hemodynamically stable irrespective of the presence of a significant defect of the atrial wall. This is a result of pressure equilibrium between the endopericardial and atrial pressures. This equilibrium is quite fragile and it is possible that under certain circumstances, the atrial pressure will be greater than that of a limited hemopericardium and result in a pericardial tamponade. On performing a pericardial window, start with a 5 cm incision from the xiphisternum inferiorly and open the linea alba. Do not open the peritoneum. The plane to work in is that of the preperitoneal fat. Insert a pair of scissors, tip facing in the preperitoneal fat space under the xiphisternum in a horizontal plane and open the limbs of the scissors. The pericardium is visualized right in front of you. Raise the pericardium with two hemostats and divide it in between. If there is any blood, aspirate it. If there is no further bleeding after aspiration, insert a drain and close the pericardial incision around it. The drain should be removed within 48 hours if no recurrence of bleeding occurs. If on opening the pericardium and aspirating, there is still blood collecting in the pericardial sack, convert to a median sternotomy, and deal with the problem. We do not recommend a transdiaphragmatic pericardial window. It is surprising how easy it is to fail to locate the pericardium on opening the diaphragm through the abdomen, but the best bet is to go through the central tendon of the diaphragm.[28]

BLUNT TRAUMATIC AORTIC INJURIES

In 93% of patients with rupture of the aorta after blunt trauma, it occurs just distal to the left subclavian artery. This is secondary to bending, torsion, sternal bone compression, and a "water hammer" contraction of the aorta. The isthmus of the aorta is the area that usually gives way as its tensile strength is only 63% of the rest of aorta.[29,30] The intra-aortic pressure rises considerably due to the above-mentioned mechanism of trauma, sometimes to 1500 mm Hg. This high pressure rise in conjunction with rotational forces results in aortic rupture at the weakest point, the isthmus. The patient can present with retrosternal or interscapular pain, dyspnea, pseudocoarctation syndrome, systolic murmur, and hemothorax. Hoarseness and cough can coexist in certain cases. Typical radiological features of traumatic injury include a widened mediastinum (>8 cm at T4 level) in the erect CXR that is taken at the standard distance from the patient's chest (in the trauma patients, take into consideration that in most instances the CXR is taken in the supine position and therefore a normal mediastinum can sometimes appear widened particularly in the overweight patient), opacification of the aortopulmonary window, depression of the left main bronchus, deviation of the trachea to the right, obliteration of the aortic contour, deviation of the nasogastric tube to the right, and presence of a left apical cap.[31] The presence of certain skeletal injuries can be associated with aortic injury including sternal, scapular, first or second rib, bilateral clavicles, thoracic vertebral body fractures, or thoracic vertebral dislocation. It is worth mentioning that in 10% of cases with rupture of the thoracic aorta, the mediastinum is not enlarged in the erect CXR and many times there is absence of the radiological signs that indirectly suggest the injury. It is therefore advised to consider aortic rupture in all patients with a high-energy deceleration injury. Mediastinal widening has a 90% sensitivity and a 100% specificity. [32,33]

Computed tomographic scanning has replaced conventional angiography as the gold standard for diagnosis with a sensitivity and specificity approaching 100% (96.2% vs. 99.8%), and can differentiate between hematomas secondary to aortic rupture or to hematomas that are related to SVC, brachiocephalic vein, thoracic spine, and sternal injuries that rarely require any intervention. It also provides the surgeon with useful information related to the aortic dimensions proximal and distal to the aortic injury, distance from the left subclavian artery, length of vascular injury, and any anatomical variants present.[34]

Transesophageal echocardiography is operator-dependent and has a high risk in the presence of a patient with an unstable cervical spine. In the past, it was an important tool but does not compare favorably to CT investigation. It is useful as a CT alternative if the patient cannot be moved to the CT suite due to physiological instability or if there are absolute contraindication to the administration of contrast. The above have been confirmed by the American Association for the Surgery of Trauma (AAST1 and AAST2) studies, which showed that CT angiography has surpassed transesophageal echography and standard angiography in diagnostic accuracy.[34a]

The use of intravascular ultrasound is mainly for problem solving in situations where differences in opinion exist.

The initial management varies. A patient with active extravasation of contrast requires immediate surgery or endovascular stent placement. The risk of rupture is highest during the first four hours following injury. With aggressive blood pressure management, the risk of rupture is 1.5% and without 12%. The use of β-blockers reduces wall stress and force of ejection. Fluids are restricted and further blood pressure control may require the addition of Nitrocine (glyceryl trinitrate). The systolic blood pressure is best maintained between 90 mm Hg and 110 mm Hg.[35,36]

Polytrauma patients are not ideal surgical candidates and the best timing and modality of treatment will vary. Sudden hypotension at any stage on medical treatment should alert the team to the possibility of free rupture necessitating early intervention. Demetriades et al. reported that the mortality in the early intervention group (<24 hours) was 16.5% vs. the late intervention group (>24 hours) 5.8%.[37] Estrera et al. in a series of 145 patients concluded that the reasons for a better outcome with delayed repair are due to better fluid resuscitation, attending to other life-threatening injuries, and an optimal operating environment.[38,39]

Rupture of the ascending thoracic aorta necessitates primary repair or use of an interposition graft in the presence of cardiopulmonary bypass. Smaller injuries in a suitable position can be directly repaired.

Injuries of the aortic arch require more complex repair, i.e. coupled with cardiopulmonary bypass and deep hypothermia, and circulatory arrest in difficult injuries.

Rupture of the descending thoracic aorta is the commonest site of injury and can be treated by either endovascular aortic repair (EVAR) or open surgical repair. The advantages of placing an endovascular stent are that it can be done with the use of local anesthesia, there is less blood loss, with good acceptability in high-risk polytrauma patients, and less incidence of paraplegia. This was shown in the $AATS_2$ study that included 193 patients, 65% of patients underwent EVAR (the majority were <55 years old with no associated major injuries). The patients in the EVAR group were older and had more extrathoracic injuries (abdominal trauma index >3) than the 35% of patients who were treated by open surgery. The injury severity score in the two groups was comparable. A comparison of mortality between the two groups favored EVAR by 7.2% versus 23.5% in the open surgery group. The incidence of device-related complications was high at 20%, and the study did show that high volume centers had lower complication rates.[39-42]

The long-term patency rates of the EVAR stent grafts are not fully known and reports of collapse and fracture of the devices have been reported in addition to thrombosis with subsequent paraplegia. Subclavian artery occlusion during stent deployment is generally well tolerated; however, some patients do develop left upper extremity ischemia and require a carotid to subclavian artery bypass or subclavian carotid transposition. Problems with current stent grafts are sizing, poor conformation to the arch, the risk of cumulative radiation at follow-up (avoided by doing MRI), and the need for anticoagulation in the polytrauma patient. Also a problem may develop in young patients due to the natural growth history of the aorta leading to unfolding and subsequent graft dislodgement, and changes in the wall consistency as the aorta increases by 1.5 mm in diameter per decade.[43]

The longest follow-up of blunt traumatic aortic injury patients is 8.7 years and showed no significant survival advantage noted at 4 years between the two procedures (open 16% vs. 11% EVAR).[44] The device sizing remains a problem and oversizing results in endoleak, infolding, collapse, acute occlusion, and death. Newer devices include curved and fenestrated grafts for the aortic arch. Follow-up CT angiography intervals are recommended during the first year at 6 and 12 months, followed by every 6 months for the second year and then yearly thereafter. Clinical practice guidelines for grading of aortic injury were published by Azizzadeh et al.:[45] grade I-intimal tear, grade II-intramural hematoma, grade III-pseudoaneurysm, and Grade IV-rupture. However, there are no prospective randomized controlled trials comparing open repair to EVAR. The Society of Vascular surgeons guidelines suggests endovascular repair be performed preferentially that in itself is a level IIC evidence and therefore weak. Murad et al.[46] compared the two groups in 7,768 patients and found the intervention rate is higher in the EVAR patients. There was no difference in mortality; however, the incidence of spinal ischemia, renal failure, and graft infections was higher in the open surgical group.

The management of grade I aortic injuries (intimal tear) should be conservative as Azizzadeh et al.[45] showed that most will heal spontaneously. The decision to intervene should be guided by the progression of the defect and symptoms. Most that will progress do so within 4 weeks. Good radiological investigative tools are required along with patient's compliance for follow-up in order to safely manage this grade of aortic injury.

DIAPHRAGMATIC INJURIES

The diaphragm can sustain both penetrating and blunt trauma. Stab wounds typically penetrate the anterolateral or posterior peripheral muscle fibers but gunshot wounds can cause perforations anywhere. Penetrating trauma between the nipple and umbilicus should be considered for diaphragmatic injury.[47] Diaphragmatic rupture from blunt trauma usually affects the posterior and lateral portions of the central tendon. In blunt trauma, the inherited weakness of the left hemidiaphragm and the protective effect of the liver to the right hemidiaphragm account for the higher incidence of left hemidiaphragm herniation. The symptomatology appears when viscera herniate into the thoracic cavity through the diaphragmatic defect as is frequently the case with blunt trauma acutely. Delayed presentation can occur after previous blunt or penetrating trauma. In those cases, the patient can develop respiratory distress and hypotension as the abdominal viscera herniate into the pleural cavity and exert pressure onto the lungs and mediastinum. In such a clinical presentation, it is important to differentiate between pneumothorax and cardiac tamponade. The thoracic pressure increases due to the mass effect of the abdominal viscera in the thoracic cavity leading to decreased venous return and decrease of diastolic filling pressures, which leads to decreased stroke volume and cardiac output. Positive pressure ventilation by increasing the pulmonary pressure can prevent herniation of the abdominal viscera into the chest (Fig. 39.8). This is exactly opposite to Ambu bag ventilation, which by distending the intrathoracic stomach and intestines, can compromise the patient's ventilation.[47] The patient can present with dyspnea, orthopnea, chest pain, Kehr's sign (acute pain in the tip of the shoulder due to the presence of blood or other irritants in the peritoneal cavity when a person is lying down and the legs are elevated), and on clinical examination with diminished anterior chest wall excursion. In penetrating trauma, usually the diaphragmatic defect is small and at least initially there is no herniation inside the chest cavity. On the other hand in blunt trauma, CXR may show obliteration of the left cardiophrenic angle, elevation of left hemidiaphragm, or herniation of stomach or colon through a large defect of the posterolateral diaphragm. Insertion of a nasogastric tube can facilitate the diagnosis by showing on a CXR curling of the tube inside the chest cavity in the herniated stomach. On the right, the protective effect of the liver to herniation of hollow viscera into the right chest makes the radiological diagnosis more difficult. In rare cases of very extensive rupture of the diaphragm on the right, the liver herniates into the chest. A CT scan has difficulties in diagnosing injury of the diaphragm without herniation as the diaphragm is often tangential to the scanning plane and there is no fat or air to help distinguish the diaphragmatic tissue from other soft tissue structures. Magnetic resonance imaging (MRI) has been promising for this type of plain diaphragmatic rupture but further studies are required to come to a solid conclusion on its sensitivity. Thoracoscopy and laparoscopy are the two methods with which a definitive diagnosis of diaphragmatic injury without herniation can be established.[47,48]

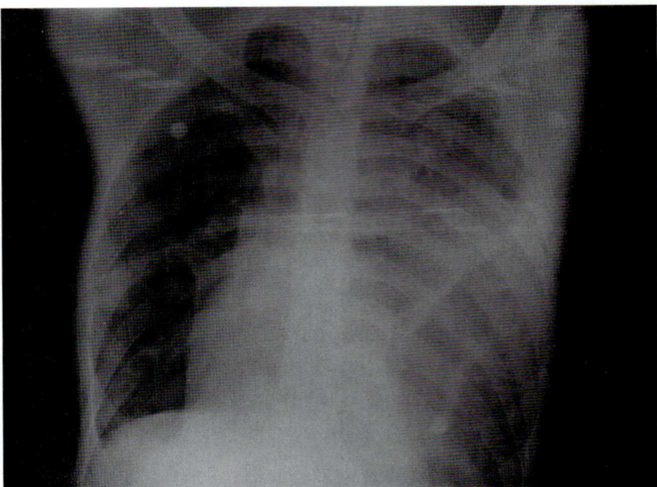

Fig. 39.8: Chest X-ray of a patient with a left-sided diaphragmatic injury with abdominal contents migrating to the thoracic cavity.

A type I diaphragmatic injury is a contusion. A type II diaphragmatic injury (laceration ≤2 cm) can be easily repaired with simple full thickness interrupted sutures using nonabsorbable material. Type III injuries (a laceration up to 10 cm in length) can also be repaired primarily (Fig. 39.9). Type IV injuries (a laceration exceeding 10 cm in length with tissue loss <25 cm^2) can, most of the time, also be repaired primarily, which will result in a decreased diaphragmatic surface area that does not result in significant reduction in ventilation. Type V injuries (laceration with tissue loss >25 cm^2) are commonly associated with major chest wall injury caused by crushing or a close range shot gun injury. Primary repair of the diaphragm in this case will create a lot of tension leading to the possibility of tearing of the repair. To avoid this complication, the anterolateral and posterior attachments of the diaphragm to the ribs are divided and elevated and attached two or three interspaces higher after the more central tear has been repaired. This decreases the tension of the repair and will not jeopardize its integrity. In rare cases of type V injury, the tissue loss is such that it necessitates the use of mesh to breach the defect. Acute presentation of

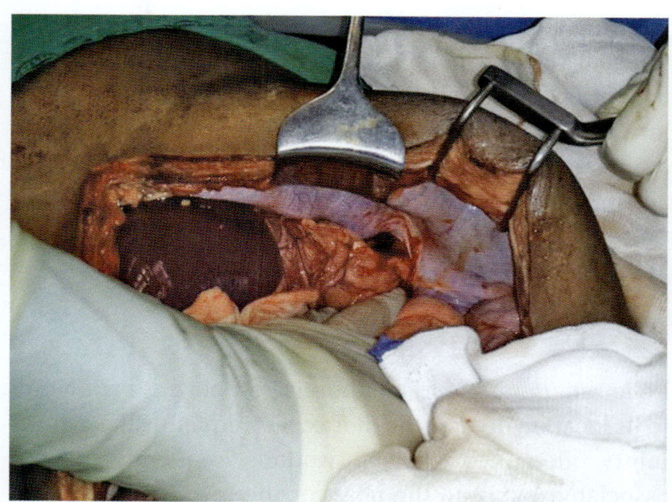

Fig. 39.9: Diaphragmatic injury with abdominal contents migrating to the left thoracic cavity.

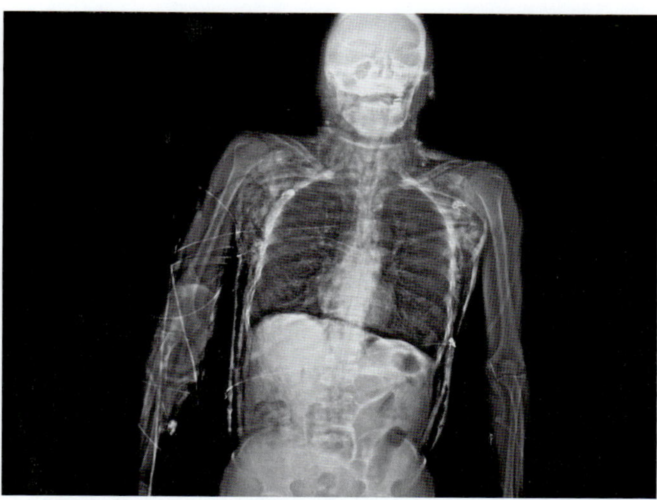

Fig. 39.10: Extensive subcutaneous emphysema after tracheal injury.

diaphragmatic herniation after a previous injury of the diaphragm is related to a high incidence of strangulation that may lead to death in up to 25% of patients.

This high mortality led certain centers to adapt an aggressive policy for the diagnosis of diaphragmatic injury (laparoscopy/thoracoscopy) in every patient in a stable condition presenting with penetrating trauma below the nipples.[49]

TRACHEOBRONCHIAL INJURIES

These can be due to blunt or penetrating trauma and can also be associated with concomitant esophageal or spinal trauma. The majority of penetrating injuries are due to stab and gunshot wounds. In the civilian setting, these injuries are limited to trauma caused by the direct path of the bullet or knife. In the military setting, where high-energy gunshot wounds are inflicted, there can also be injury to the tracheobronchial tree secondary to the shock wave that radiated laterally from the tract of the high-energy missile. Penetrating trauma to the intrathoracic part of the trachea and bronchi is almost exclusively due to missiles and is commonly found in association with a transmediastinal gunshot wound that can also be associated with injuries to the heart and great vessels.[50]

Blunt tracheobronchial injuries are commonly secondary to deceleration forces as happens with motor vehicle accidents and the level of the injury is usually at the level of the proximal bronchi. Acute compression of the chest wall especially if the glottis is closed can increase the pressure within the airway to such an extent to cause rupture at the junction of the membranous and cartilaginous portions of the airway. The cervical trachea can also be involved in blunt trauma through a direct blow when the neck is hyperextended, therefore crushing the trachea against the vertebral bodies. In rare cases, sudden hyperextension of the neck as in an unsupported posterior impact injury can cause complete transection of the trachea; luckily with the peritracheal fascia remaining intact in certain cases, this maintains patency of the airway while definitive treatment is accomplished.[51]

The clinical presentation is variable and extends from asymptomatic to those patients with stridor, dyspnea, hemoptysis, hypoxia, and subcutaneous emphysema (Fig. 39.10). Often the patient may present with a massive air leak via the chest tube and a second chest tube may be required to overcome it. In such instances, a tracheobronchial injury should be suspected, particularly when the lung does not expand with chest tube drainage and there is concomitant subcutaneous emphysema and a pneumomediastinum.

The CXR may show a pneumomediastinum or pneumothorax that can be related to a pleural effusion. Occasionally air surrounding a bronchus and the "fallen lung sign" can be seen. This latter sign is pathognomonic of a complete disruption of a mainstem bronchus. The bronchus is transected and the affected lung drops down onto the diaphragm with the lung completely collapsed and sitting at the medial aspect of the corresponding hemidiaphragm. A CT scan may assist with the diagnosis of tracheal and bronchial injuries, particularly with three-dimensional CT reconstruction of the trachea-bronchial tree in difficult diagnostic cases. Still most recommend a bronchoscopy for definitive diagnosis. A flexible bronchoscope may miss the injury if passed through an endotracheal tube that is traversing the injury. A rigid bronchoscopy has the benefits that it allows ventilation through the instrument and it is easier to evacuate blood and debris through it. Three-dimensional reconstruction of the tracheobronchial tree, visualizing the lumen from inside, could replace bronchoscopy in the future as a diagnostic tool.

If tracheobronchial injuries are suspected, the surgeon should be alert to the possibility of sudden ventilatory deterioration. The patient should not be sedated or converted to positive pressure ventilation if he is maintaining an airway and is breathing spontaneously with adequate oxygenation. It is preferable to perform invasive diagnostic procedures near or inside the operating room due to the possibility of airway deterioration. The presence of a surgeon comfortable with operating on the injury site is of paramount importance.[50]

Small injuries can be treated conservatively. A cervical tracheal defect can sometimes be converted into a tracheostomy. A tracheostomy can be used to bypass a proximal injury that can be repaired at a later stage, if required. Primary repair of a tracheal laceration can be done in certain cases. Resection of the trachea is uncommon but necessary in the presence of extensive loss of tissue.

For restructuring the upper thoracic trachea after extensive injury, the site of the injury can be approached with a collar incision or an upper-half median sternotomy. The patient is intubated via the oropharyngeal route with the tip of the tube distal to the tracheal injury. The affected tracheal segment is encircled, and the anesthesiologist is notified to ensure that the endotracheal tube bulb is not penetrated accidently during the repair maneuvers. The involved segment is resected having placed stay sutures at the 3 and 9 o'clock positions distal to the resection margin. The oropharyngeal endotracheal tube is pulled back gently after deflating the cuff and the distal trachea is reintubated with a sterile cuffed tube of a slightly smaller size. The insertion of this cuffed tube makes it easier to work with when placing sutures posteriorly. Posterior interrupted absorbable sutures are placed starting at the 12 o'clock position and proceeding to 3 and 9 o'clock. These include sutures taking 2–3 mm bites of the membranous portion of the trachea. On completion of the anastomosis of the posterior half of the trachea, the anesthesiologist removes the "distal" endotracheal tube and advances the proximal one distally to bridge the anterior gap of the tracheal resection site. The anterior half of the trachea is repaired by using absorbable interrupted sutures that encircle the tracheal rings. If possible it is always better to extubate the patient at completion of the operation. The very distal intrathoracic trachea, carina, and bronchi are repaired in a similar fashion. The access to the right bronchus, carina, and proximal 2 cm of the left bronchus is achieved by a right posterolateral thoracotomy. The rest of the left bronchus is approached by a left posterolateral thoracotomy.[52]

ESOPHAGEAL INJURIES

Penetrating trauma to the thoracic esophagus is rare due to its location deep in the thorax. Subsequently this type of injury, often due to gunshot wounds, frequently involves associated injury to the heart or the mediastinal vessels with fatal outcome. The patient's survival with this type of injury is dependent on a high index of suspicion leading to early diagnosis. A plain CXR frequently may show a pleural effusion, subcutaneous emphysema, a pneumomediastinum, a pneumothorax, and mediastinal air-fluid levels. Initially a chest tube is inserted until a diagnosis of esophageal injury is confirmed. Transmediastinal injuries are initially investigated with a contrast CT scan if the patient is physiologically stable. An attempt to identify the bullet tract is made and one proceeds to further investigations if it is in close proximity to the esophagus. Ideally a contrast study to exclude esophageal injury follows; however, this can miss injuries if not carefully performed. A barium swallow is relatively inert and is better than a Gastrografin swallow in showing hollow viscous leaks. Water-soluble contrast agents like gastrografin, which have historically been the initial agent of choice of radiological detection of esophageal injury, can cause severe pneumonitis if aspirated and can miss small leaks. For patients with a level of consciousness that is low but with a good gag reflex, one can still administer contrast via a Foley catheter that is positioned high in the esophagus with the balloon inflated to prevent aspiration of the contrast material. In intubated patients, administration of contrast can be given via a nasogastric tube positioned near the area of interest. Esophageal leak can also be confirmed by asking the patient to swallow methylene blue and observe for a leak from a previously inserted chest tube (for pleural effusion on CXR). Although this is pathognomonic of the presence of an esophageal defect, it cannot localize its site. Esophagoscopy is performed in cases where an esophageal injury is still suspected in the presence of a normal swallow. When a flexible esophagoscopy is performed to avoid missing esophageal injuries, the esophagus should be vigorously inflated so that one can observe the lumen of the esophagus without the presence of any mucosal folds. Bubbling in a chest tube bottle every time the esophagus is insufflated during the esophagoscopy is also a sign of an esophageal leak but does not localize its site accurately.

It is of paramount importance to diagnose and repair the esophagus within 24 hours from the time of the injury, as delay beyond this time is related to increased morbidity and mortality.[53-55]

Injuries of the proximal and mid-third of the esophagus are best approached via a right posterolateral thoracotomy. The distal third of the esophagus can also be approached via the same incision, although a left posterolateral thoracotomy can also be applied depending on the circumstances.

There are certain principles guiding the management of a perforated endothoracic esophagus. First, mediastinal contamination must be controlled, usually by debridement, copious washouts, and placement of several chest tubes in the area of the contaminated tissues and spaces. Second, primary repair with interrupted full-thickness sutures including approximately 4 mm of the esophageal mucosa even in cases where the presentation is delayed. Third, an attempt to buttress the repair with healthy surrounding tissue should be practiced (e.g. intercostal muscle and diaphragmatic flap). Following the esophageal repair, it is common to provide total parenteral nutrition or insert a feeding jejunostomy tube for enteral nutrition. A contrast esophagogram is usually performed on the seventh postoperative day. Some surgeons place the tip of the nasogastric tube immediately above the repair to act as a sump tube to aspirate the saliva. In cases where primary repair is not successful, insertion of an esophageal T tube through the esophageal injury has been recommended in an attempt to create a controlled esophageal pleurocutaneous fistula. Exclusion of the injured esophageal segment by creating a diverting esophagostomy and stapling the gastroesophageal junction, until the perforation heals has also been suggested. In rare occasions in the presence of a severe esophageal injury in a physiologically stable patient, resection of the esophagus can be performed with either immediate or delayed reconstruction depending on the degree of local sepsis.[50]

REFERENCES

1. Morse CR, Allan JS. Chest wall pleural space and lung parenchyma. In: Sheridan RL (Ed). The Trauma Handbook of Massachusetts General Hospital. Philadelphia: Lippincott Williams & Wilkins; 2004.
2. Richardson DJ, et al. Complex thoracic injuries. Surg Clin North Am. 1996;76(4):725-48.
3. Shields TW, et al. General Thoracic Surgery. Philadelphia: Lippincott Williams &Wilkins; 2000.
4. Moon MR, Luchette FA, Gibson SW, et al. Prospective randomized comparison of epidural versus parenteral opioid analgesia in thoracic trauma. Ann Surg. 1999;229(5):684-91.
5. Lee RB, Bass SM, Morris JA Jr, et al. Three or more rib fractures as an indicator for transfer to a level one trauma centre: a population based study. J Trauma. 1990;30:689.
6. Stawicki SP, Grossman MD, Hoey BA, et al. Rib fractures in the elderly: a marker of injury severity. J Am Geriatr Soc. 2004;52:805.
7. Todd SR, McNally MM, Holcomb JB, et al. A multidisciplinary clinical pathway decreases rib fractures—associated infections morbidity and mortality in high risk trauma patients. Am J Surg. 2006;192(6):806-11.
8. Gavelli G, Canini R, Bertaccini P, et al. Traumatic injuries: Imaging of thoracic injuries. Eur Radiol. 2002;12:1273.
9. Tanaka H, Yukioka T, Yamaguti Y, et al. Surgical stabilization or internal pneumatic stabilization? A prospective randomized study of management of severe flail chest patients. J Trauma. 2002;52(4):727-32.
10. Granetzny A, et al. Surgical versus conservative treatment of flail chest. Evaluation of pulmonary status. Interact Cardiovasc Thorac Surg. 2005;4:583-7.
11. Gunduz M, Unlugenc H, Ozalevli M, et al. A comparative study of continuous positive airway pressure (CPAP) and intermittent positive pressure ventilation (IPPV) in patients with flail chest. Emerg Med J. 2005;22(5):325-9.
12. Velmahos GC, Vassiliu P, Chan LS, et al. Influence of flail chest on outcome among patients with severe thoracic cage trauma. Int Surg. 2002;87(4):240-44.
13. Chiu W, D'Amelio L, Hammond J. Sternal fractures in blunt chest trauma: a practical algorithm for management. Am J Emerg Med. 1997;15:252.
14. Sutyak JP, Wohltmann CD, Larson J. Pulmonary contusions and critical care management in thoracic trauma. Thoracic Surg Clin. 17(1):11-23.
15. Copass MK, Oreskovich MR, Bladergroen MR. Prehospital CPR of the critically injured patient. Am J Surg. 1984; 148:20.
16. Mattox KL. Prehospital care of the patient with injured chest. Surg Clin North Am. 1989;69:21.
17. Biffl WL, Moore EE, Harken AH. Emergency department thoracotomy. In: Mattox KL, Feliciano DV, Moore EE (Eds) Trauma, 4th edition. New York: McGraw-Hill; 2000. pp. 245-60.
18. Velmahos GC, Degiannis E, Souter I, et al. Outcome of a strict policy on emergency department thoracotomies. Arch Surg. 1995;130:774.
19. Asensio JA, Tsai KJ. Emergency department thoracotomy. In: Definitive Surgical Trauma Care, Course Manual, Melbourne and Sydney 2003.
20. Boffard KD (Ed). Manual of the Definitive Surgical Trauma Care. London: Arnold; 2003.
21. Velmahos GC, Degiannis E, Souter I, et al. Penetrating trauma to the heart: a relatively innocent injury. Surgery. 1994;115:694.

22. Ivatury RR. Emergency Department Thoracotomy. In: Definitive Surgical Trauma Care, Course Manual, Melbourne and Sydney 2003.
23. Doll D, Glapa M, Bonanno F, Smith MD, et al. Traumatic rupture of the cardiac auricle after forceful blunt abdominal trauma. Unfallchirurg. 2007;110(7):637-9. German.
24. Cooke DT, MacGillivary TM. Blunt and penetrating injuries of the heart and central vessels. In: Sheridan RL (Ed). The Trauma Handbook of Massachusetts General Hospital. Philadelphia: Lippincott Williams & Wilkins; 2004:328-41.
25. Clancy K, Velopulos C, Bilaniuk JW, et al. Screening for blunt cardiac injury: An Eastern Association for the Surgery of Trauma practice management guideline J Trauma Acute Care Surg. 2012;73(5 Suppl 4):S301-6.
26. Saadia R, Levy RD, Degiannis E, et al. Penetrating cardiac injuries: clinical classification and management strategy. Br J Surg. 1994;81(11):1572-5. Review.
27. Degiannis E, Loogna P, Doll D, et al. Penetrating cardiac injuries: recent experience in South Africa. World J Surg. 2006 Jul;30(7):1258-64.
28. Degiannis E, Yilmaz TH, Doll D. Penetrating cardiac trauma. In: Velmahos GC, Degiannis E, Doll D (Eds). Penetrating Trauma: Practical Guide on Operative Technique and Perioperative Management. Berlin: Springer-Verlag; 2012.
29. Siegel JH, Smith JA, Siddiqi SQ. Change in velocity and energy dissipation on impact in motor vehicle crashes as a function of the direction of crash: key factors in the production of thoracic aortic injuries, their pattern of associated injuries and patient survival. A crash injury research engineering network (CIREN) study. J Trauma. 2004;57:760-77.
30. Siegel JH, Belwadi A, Smith JA, et al. Analysis of the mechanism of lateral impact aortic isthmus disruption in real-life motor vehicle crashes using a computer-based finite element numeric model: with simulation of prevention strategies. J Trauma. 2010; 68:1375-95.
31. Dehmeri S. ACR appropriateness criteria-blunt chest trauma-suspected aortic injury. Emerg Radiol. 2012;19:287-92.
32. Plurad D, Green D, Demetriades D, et al. The increasing use of computed tomography for trauma. J Trauma. 2007;62: 631-5.
33. Demetriades D, Gomez H, Velmahos GC, et al. Routine helical computed tomographic evaluation of the mediastinum in high-risk blunt trauma patients. Arch Surg. 1998;133:1084-8.
34. Degiannis E, Boffard K. Critical decisions in trauma of the thoracic aorta. Injury. 2002;33:317-22.
34a. Demetriades D, Velmahos GC, Scalea TM, et al. Diagnosis and treatment of blunt thoracic aortic injuries: changing perspectives. J Trauma. 2008;64:1415-19.
35. Fabian T. Prospective study of blunt aortic injury helical CT is diagnostic and antihypertensive therapy reduces rupture. Ann Surg. 1998;227:666-77.
36. Degiannis E, Bowley D, Smith MD. New concepts in blunt injury of the thoracic aorta. S Afr J Surg. 2003;41;60-1.
37. Demetriades D, Velmahos G, Scalea T, et al. Blunt thoracic aortic injuries: early or delayed repair. Results of an American Association for the Surgery of Trauma prospective study. J Trauma. 2009;66:967-73.
38. Estrera AL, Gochnour DC, Azizzadeh A, et al. Progress in the treatment of blunt thoracic aortic injury: 12-year single institution experience. Ann Thorac Surg. 2010;90:64-71.
39. Maggisano R, Nathens A, Alexandrova NA, et al. Traumatic rupture of the thoracic aorta: should one always operate immediately? Ann Vasc Surg. 1995;9:44-52.
40. Pate JW, Gavant ML, Weiman DS, et al. Traumatic rupture of the aortic isthmus: program of selective management. World J Surg. 1999;23:59-63.
41. Wahl WL, Michaels AJ, Wang SC, et al. Blunt thoracic aortic injury: delayed or early repair? J Trauma. 1999;47:254-9.
42. Hemmila MR, Arbabi S, Rowe SA, et al. Delayed repair for blunt thoracic aortic injury: is it really equivalent to early repair? J Trauma. 2004;56:13-23.
43. Fernandez V, Mestres G, Maeso J, et al. Endovascular treatment of traumatic thoracic aortic injuries: short- and medium-term follow-up. Ann Vasc Surg. 2010;24:160-6.
44. Patel HJ, Hemmila MR, Williams DM. Late outcomes following open and endovascular repair of blunt thoracic aortic injury. J Vasc Surg. 2011;53(3):615-21.
45. Azizzadeh A, Keyhani K, Miller CC III, et al. Blunt traumatic aortic injury: initial experience with endovascular repair. J Vasc Surg. 2009;49:1403-8.
46. Murad MH, Rizvi A, Milgor R, et al. Comparative effectiveness of the treatment of the treatment for thoracic aortic transection. J Vasc Surg. 2011;53:193-9.
47. Stein S, SchultzIII JT. Abdominal trauma 2: diaphragm and abdominal wall. In: Sheridan RL (Ed). The Trauma Handbook of Massachusetts General Hospital. Philadelphia: Lippincott Williams & Wilkins; 2004. pp. 402-12.
48. Steyn E. Penetrating injuries to the diaphragm. In: Velmahos GC, Degiannis E, Doll D (Eds). Penetrating Trauma: A Practical Guide on Operative Technique and Perioperative Management. Berlin: Springer-Verlag; 2012. pp. 287-90.
49. Lucas CE, Ledgerwood AM. Diaphragmatic injury. In: Cameron JL (Ed). Current Surgical Therapy. St Louis Missouri: Mosby; 1998. pp. 944-47.
50. Fynn-Thompson F, Allan JS. Chest Trauma 2: tracheobronchial and oesophageal injuries. In: Sheridan RL (Ed). The Trauma Handbook of Massachusetts General Hospital. Philadelphia: Lippincott Williams & Wilkins; 2004:315-27.

Additional references appear in the online version of this book.

40

Abdominal, Urologic and Perineal Injuries

Selman Uranüs, Sascha Flohé

Key Points

- Splenic injuries can successfully be managed nonoperatively in the adult patient provided that there is no ongoing hemorrhage. Surgical exploration and total splenectomy are required when there is bleeding and the patient is unstable, and partial splenectomy or splenorrhaphy is not possible.
- Hepatic injuries can be managed nonoperatively in the majority of cases if the patient is hemodynamically stable and there is no indication for emergent laparotomy.
- The incidence of "missed" gastric injuries can be reduced if a thorough examination of the stomach is made at laparoscopy or laparotomy. If there is an anterior gastric wall injury, the posterior wall of the stomach and pancreas should be evaluated carefully to exclude a through and through injury.
- The major complication following repair of a duodenal injury is a duodenal fistula or an obstruction. Other serious complications include an intra-abdominal abscess, pancreatitis, sepsis, and a bile duct fistula or stenosis.
- Grade I and II pancreatic injuries are considered minor and are managed conservatively or by external drainage, if needed. Grade III–V pancreatic injuries are complex and require resection and internal and external drainage.
- The diagnosis of a small bowel injury requires a high index of clinical suspicion. Abdominal tenderness is an important finding. A computed tomogram (CT) scan and an adjunctive peritoneal lavage are usually diagnostic. Laparoscopy can both increase diagnostic accuracy and contribute to definitive treatment.
- Nondestructive colon wounds in the absence of peritonitis can be repaired primarily, and selected patients with destructive, penetrating intraperitoneal colon wounds can undergo resection and primary anastomosis. Patients in shock, with underlying disease, appreciable associated injuries, or peritonitis should be managed by damage control surgery with temporary closure of the abdominal wall using negative-pressure wound therapy. In these cases resection and colostomy are the therapeutic aims.
- A renal injury should be suspected if there is gross or microscopic hematuria. A CT scan with intravenous contrast is the diagnostic study of choice to detect a renal injury in a hemodynamically stable patient with multiple intra-abdominal injuries due to blunt trauma.
- Perineal injuries are serious surgical problems as there are usually extensive associated injuries. Fifty percent have an associated pelvic fracture. Exsanguination is the cause of immediate death and later deaths are due to sepsis. In most cases, a diverting colostomy is needed to repair the pelvic floor and the anogenital region.

INTRODUCTION

Injury to the various abdominal structures is caused by either blunt or penetrating mechanisms of injury. The relative proportion of each of these injury patterns is widely variable and depends upon geographic location and demographics. The socioeconomic environment has a pronounced influence on the prevalence of blunt and penetrating trauma as well as on the ratio of blunt to penetrating trauma. Populations characterized by high levels of aggression potential and low levels of education comprise individuals with high rates of risk-taking behavior[1,2] associated with excess alcohol consumption and drug abuse, motor vehicle accidents (MVAs), and violent crime.[3] In more economically advantaged regions and countries, the incidence of penetrating injury is lower. The incidence of penetrating trauma is higher in metropolitan areas throughout the world than in areas of lower population density.

An important trend associated with the escalation in violence is a marked increase in the use of higher-velocity guns. Although handguns that fire low-velocity cartridges continue to be the most commonly used weapons, there has been a marked increase in the availability and use of medium- and high-velocity weapons.

These factors are important considerations in patient management. Low-velocity wounds produce damage as a result of direct injury to vital structures. High-velocity weapons produce wounds with large haloes of destruction to surrounding structures. Wide debridement is necessary for the more destructive wounds, and organ injury repair generally requires more complex techniques.

Although shotgun wounds are seen in rural areas as a result of accidents, these weapons are also commonly used by criminals because of their devastating effect at close range and because they do not require accurate aim. The distance to the target is important because small pellets lose energy quickly and dissipate rapidly unless the gun has a tight choke. If there are a few small pellets in the abdominal cavity, the holes in the hollow viscera usually seal and those in solid viscera rarely cause problems. It is a common practice in this situation to observe the patient and perform laparotomy only, if evidence of peritonitis or blood loss develops.[4]

Besides gunshot wounds, stabbings are also on the rise. These injuries are caused by pointed and cutting objects such as knives, screwdrivers, broken glass, and pointed sticks. Depending on size, form, and direction of the wound, stabbing can cause life-threatening injuries that must be diagnosed and treated promptly. A stab directed at a slant to the side can penetrate both thorax and abdomen and also injure the diaphragm. Even stable patients should have a careful exploration, possibly even laparoscopy.

There is a wide array of injury mechanisms for blunt trauma. Currently, MVAs cause 60–90% of blunt injuries, the proportion depending upon geographic factors (i.e. associated industrial, agricultural, and outdoor activity). Injuries that result from blunt trauma can be caused by direct impact, compression between fixed objects (e.g. automobile dashboard and spinal column) and shearing forces associated with rapid deceleration. Crushing injuries are commonly produced in industrial and agricultural environments. The impact of seatbelts, passive restraints, and airbags on the type and severity of injury is substantial. Although each of these safety features can produce specific injury types, especially if improperly used, they usually dissipate the energy associated with impact and clearly reduce the degree of injury (especially neurologic injury).

Laparoscopy is a good option for patients with unclear abdominal symptoms that cannot be clarified noninvasively. It also has therapeutic potential as mesenteric lacerations, stab injuries to the diaphragm, and minor intestinal lesions can be sutured. The prerequisite for laparoscopy is, however, hemodynamic stability.

With increasing experience and better technology, laparoscopy is playing an increasing role in trauma care, especially in diagnostics. The evaluation of blunt and penetrating thoracoabdominal trauma for the presence of intestinal and diaphragmatic injury presents a diagnostic challenge to the trauma surgeon. Diagnostic laparoscopy is an essential and safe modality.

SURGICAL ANATOMY

Anatomic considerations are important to understand the patterns of injury produced by both blunt and penetrating trauma. The abdomen can be defined by two planes:

- Cephalocaudal
- Dorsal/ventral.

The abdominal contents are contained superiorly by the diaphragm and inferiorly by the musculature of the pelvic floor. Diaphragmatic contraction and relaxation produce substantial changes in the size of the abdominal cavity. At end-inspiration, the diaphragmatic excursion is at approximately the level of the ninth or tenth thoracic vertebra, whereas at end expiration the diaphragm ascends to around the level of the fifth thoracic vertebra. Nearly all penetrating wounds to the torso have the potential to produce intra-abdominal injury depending upon the trajectory, but those associated with greatest risk occur between the nipple line and the gluteal crease.

Cephalocaudal Divisions of the Abdomen

Cephalocaudally, the abdomen can be divided into the upper, mid, and lower abdomen.

The upper abdomen is contained within the space between the diaphragm and the lower costal margin. The liver and spleen are contained within this region and receive some protection from both direct impact and crushing injury by the rib cage. The medial component of the upper abdomen, the epigastrium, is relatively unprotected; many severe injuries are produced in this region, which is occupied by the stomach, pancreas, and great vessels and also most of the major arterial branches to the abdominal viscera.

The mid-abdomen lies between the lower costal margins and the anterior superior iliac spines. Penetrating injuries in this area usually result in intestinal and renal wounds. Occasionally, the transverse colon and pancreatic neck can also be affected, depending on the direction of the force. All midline wounds have the potential to injure the aorta and vena cava. Seatbelt injuries and direct impact in this area can result in injuries of the mid-to-distal small bowel and, occasionally, degloving-type injuries to the abdominal wall. As the magnitude of these latter injuries often is underappreciated initially, subsequent morbidity is high. The skin is avulsed from the underlying fascia and variable amounts of necrosis of skin and abdominal wall muscle result.

The lower abdomen is divided into the false and true pelvis. The false pelvis is the upper portion contained within the iliac bones and extending to the area of the sacral promontory (first sacral vertebra). The true pelvis extends below the sacral promontory. Penetrating wounds in this region can injure the small bowel, rectosigmoid colon, rectum, genitourinary system, and iliac vessels. Blunt trauma results in pelvic fracture, occasionally bladder and bowel rupture, and urethral transection.

Dorsal/Ventral Plane Divisions of the Abdomen

The dorsal/ventral plane divides the abdominal cavity into three regions:

- The anterior abdominal wall is located ventral to the anterior axillary lines
- The flanks are located between the anterior and posterior axillary lines
- The back lies dorsal to the posterior axillary lines.

There are two important clinical considerations for penetrating injuries in these areas. As wounds to the flanks are more frequently tangential to the peritoneal cavity than anterior wounds, they are often selected for nonoperative management. Diagnostic techniques for wounds according to these various anatomic locations are discussed in Chapter 31, "Initial Trauma Evaluation and Resuscitation". The second important consideration is the fact that back wounds less commonly penetrate into the abdomen because of the extremely thick paraspinal musculature in the area. The distance from skin to retroperitoneum is 10–20 cm in most individuals. Stab wounds do not usually penetrate this barrier. Low-velocity missiles are more likely to penetrate than stab wounds, but less likely if they enter the anterior abdomen or flanks. Blunt impact to the flanks or back should arouse suspicion of kidney or renal arterial injury.

SPLENIC INJURY

Introduction

The treatment of splenic injury has changed over the past decade from prompt splenectomy in all cases to splenic salvage when possible. The most important factor influencing this change is the recognition of the risk of infection after splenectomy.

Pathophysiology

The spleen is the most important peripheral immune organ and contains more lymphatic tissue than all the lymph nodes in the human body taken together.[5] As the spleen is connected to the circulatory system and for its size and weight is very well-perfused, it plays a central role in the immune system. In contrast to lymph nodes and mucosal-associated lymphoid tissue, there are no afferent lymphatic vessels in the spleen, and it mainly reacts to disseminated blood-borne antigens such as circulating bacteria in septicemia. In order to provide the immunological functions, about 25% of the original weight of a normal-sized spleen should be available, along with an adequate arterial blood supply.[6,7] The branches of the splenic artery supply the individual segments of the spleen and are end arteries. The upper polar artery sometimes originates directly from the celiac trunk, but it can also branch off the splenic artery earlier and so continue to the upper pole. Blood flow is toward the stomach in the short gastric arteries, which go from the gastrolienal and gastrophrenic ligaments to the gastric fundus. These arteries normally do not anastomose with the left gastroepiploic artery and thus are end arteries.[8] The segmental arteries and their branches have no connections except for a few intersegmental anastomoses with each other and so are end arteries as well. With ligature of the main artery, pressure in the spleen can drop so that blood flow is reversed; going from the stomach to the spleen, the spleen atrophies but does not become totally necrotic.[5]

The deficiency in the clearance of intravascular antigens in asplenic patients is the basis for infectious complications, including overwhelming postsplenectomy infection (OPSI), increased early and late septic morbidity, and increased septic mortality. Overwhelming postsplenectomy infection is a life-threatening event that usually develops suddenly in a healthy person. Symptoms begin with a sore throat, fever, or malaise and progress quickly to headache, vomiting, and hyperexia; hypotension, septic shock, and death can follow within 24–48 hours. Disseminated intravascular coagulation has also been associated with OPSI. The incidence of OPSI is given as 1–5%.[9] The overall mortality is 50–80%.[10,11] The risk of developing OPSI is greatest in the first year after splenectomy.[12] The best and most effective measure for preventing OPSI is orthotopic conservation of the spleen.

An orthotopically preserved spleen with its natural vascular supply and an adequate residual parenchymal mass of at least 25% are prerequisites for normal hematologic and immunologic function.

The two major aims when dealing with splenic injuries are as follows:

- Controlling active hemorrhage
- Achieving surgical repair while preserving as much of the damaged organ as possible.

If there is no ongoing hemorrhage from the splenic injury, direct treatment is not required. In recent years, there has been an appreciable shift away from operative management toward nonoperative management.[13]

Operative Management

The need for operative treatment concerns essentially blunt trauma. The diagnosis of splenic injury is made based on one of three general criteria:

1. Physical examination suggests splenic injury due to evidence of ongoing hemorrhage and peritoneal signs.
2. The patient is hemodynamically unstable, physical examination is equivocal, and abdominal focused assessment with sonography study demonstrates gross intraperitoneal blood [in exceptional cases, diagnostic peritoneal lavage (DPL) can be done to confirm the diagnosis].
3. The patient is hemodynamically stable and a CT scan or ultrasonography demonstrates splenic injury.

The first two situations require emergency laparotomy, whereas the third is currently the typical scenario that prompts nonoperative management.[13,14] It should be emphasized, however, that death from splenic hemorrhage is common and is one of the more frequent causes of preventable death.[5,14]

Splenectomy

When operative management is selected, the surgical options are total or partial splenectomy or splenorrhaphy. Splenectomy is indicated for the shattered spleen if there is ongoing hemorrhage and is usually required for hilar injuries where hemostasis is hard to achieve. Splenectomy may also be indicated for the polytraumatized patient with moderate splenic hemorrhage, so as to expedite laparotomy and minimize the risk of postoperative bleeding.

If there is slight-to-moderate bleeding, a spleen-preserving partial resection can be considered in a polytraumatized patient if adequate hemostasis can be achieved temporarily by tamponading the spleen with moist and warm pads.

A midline abdominal incision is the best approach for both splenectomy and a spleen-preserving procedure. A left subcostal incision may provide excellent exposure to the spleen but this approach cannot be recommended for trauma patients because of its very limited access to other parts of the abdominal cavity. Additionally, the subcostal incision seriously damages muscles and fascia and also has a higher long-term scar hernia rate and poorer cosmetic results. Hence, it is not preferred to the midline incision.

Anatomic and technical considerations are important components of management. The spleen can be considered to have two separate blood supplies:

- The supplemental blood circulation through the vessels in the ligaments
- The main blood supply from the splenic artery and vein and their branches.

There are two possible approaches to the hilar vessels:

- The anterior approach via the omental bursa on the edge of the tail of the pancreas; suitable for elective surgery
- The posterior approach dorsolateral from the spleen; suitable for trauma.

Control of bleeding and ligation of the hilar vessels are very important for a fast and safe splenectomy. The approach in a trauma patient should be posterior, with fast mobilization of the entire spleen and the tail of the pancreas (Table 40.1). First, the caudal ligamentous connection to the left colonic flexure is severed between ligatures or by coagulation. To do this step and to sever the peritoneal reflection dorsolateral to the spleen

Table 40.1 Suggested steps for splenectomy in trauma

1.	Exert traction and countertraction by pulling the stomach and omentum medially and exposing the short gastric vessels
2.	Divide lower pole attachments with omentum and colonic flexure
3.	Dissect the dorsolateral peritoneal fold from caudal to cranial up to the gastroesophageal junction
4.	Elevate the spleen together with the pancreatic tail
5.	Place laparotomy pads in the splenic fossa
6.	Divide the short gastric vessels
7.	Deliver the spleen into the wound by elevating the pancreas, leaving the left adrenal in place*
8.	Divide the splenic artery and vein

*During splenic mobilization, pressure is exerted broadly over the spleen in a ventral and medial direction to avoid further splenic injury and decapsulation.

as safely as possible, the surgeon uses the nondominant hand and a laparotomy pad to compress the spleen medially and carefully pull it forward, taking greatest care to avoid further tears to the capsule by intact ligamentous connections. This maneuver reduces bleeding from the spleen and makes it easier to get to the organ; the view of the spleen and especially its dorsal surface is nonetheless hindered by blood and coagulate, in spite of careful suctioning. For this reason, the dorsolateral peritoneum is incised without direct view, with the finger of the hand holding the spleen guiding the tip of the scissors. Adequate traction enhances the view of the appropriate plane. Any tendency to pull the spleen too forcefully toward anteromedial during dissection may cause additional capsular avulsion and bleeding.

Two other technical points merit mention. First, the lienophrenic ligament should be divided 1–2 cm from the posterior splenic capsule. Closer division causes further splenic injury and capsular avulsion, whereas division further away means dissection behind the kidney and into the diaphragm muscle. Maintaining the proper distance from the spleen allows visualization and mobilization of the posterior pancreas along with the spleen, as well as visualization of the anterior portion of Gerota's fascia and the anterior surface of the left adrenal gland, which are left in place. The second technical point is to divide the lienophrenic ligament adequately supermedially to the area of the gastroesophageal junction. When this division is complete, the spleen and tail of the pancreas can be delivered to the level of the subcutaneous fat. Care must be taken medially to avoid injuring the stomach. If a final short gastric vessel is encountered, division allows complete separation and medial rotation of the stomach and visualization of the entire lesser sac.

When the spleen has been mobilized into the wound, laparotomy pads are placed in the splenic fossa to stop oozing bleeding and their placement makes it easier to hold the spleen on the abdominal wall. The main splenic artery and vein can be seen on the superior and posterior aspects of the pancreas. These vessels are then divided and ligated, and the spleen is delivered from the field. Table 40.1 outlines the steps for this technique of splenectomy, as described by Zollinger.[15]

After splenectomy, active immunization with pneumococcal vaccine should be administered as soon as possible when the patient is afebrile and in good general condition. Splenectomized patients should be informed of their immune deficiency, and they should be prescribed antibiotics generously when an infection sets in.

Splenorrhaphy

For splenic preservation, the choice of procedure depends not only on the clinical findings but also on the surgeon's experience in splenic surgery and the equipment available at the particular hospital. In elderly patients, the indication for splenic salvage should be chosen carefully.

Splenorrhaphy became an important issue in the latter 1970s. Interest was spurred by the recognition of postsplenectomy sepsis as a complication. At the peak of its application, splenorrhaphy accounted for approximately 50% of operations carried out for splenic injuries.[16] In recent years, a high proportion of these patients has been managed nonoperatively and splenorrhaphy is used much less frequently. Nonetheless, there remain occasional circumstances in which splenorrhaphy is appropriate. Patients with a severe splenic injury generally have other organ injuries, have lost a lot of blood, and are usually in shock, so the reconstruction and conservation of the spleen should not take significantly more time and require more blood than a splenectomy. In both splenic salvage and splenectomy, the first step is the same: complete mobilization of the spleen and rotation onto the abdominal wall. Only in this position is it possible to make the right decision as to saving or removing the spleen. Several laparotomy pads placed in the splenic fossa and left upper quadrant maintain exposure during repair.

There are three basic techniques for splenorrhaphy:

- Superficial hemostatic agents (argon beam coagulation, FloSeal, fibrin glue, Hemopatch, absorbable gelatin sponge)
- Partial splenectomy
- Mesh wrap.

The hemostatic techniques are indicated for superficial lacerations and are often combined with more extensive repairs of other organs. These are patients for whom the indication for laparotomy is not the spleen and whose splenic injury is treated in the context of other surgical procedures. Electrocautery and argon beam coagulation accomplish essentially the same goal. In general, electrocautery is only suitable for stopping minor superficial bleeds and is only seldom used in trauma. It tends to work most effectively at higher power settings (60–80 W) at which the current arc produces coagulation. At lower power, the metal tip of the cautery must be placed directly on the tissue, which then adheres with continued bleeding when the tip and eschar are removed. Purported advantages of argon beam coagulation include superior hemostasis and less damage to deeper tissue. However,

Table 40.2 Splenic Injury Grading System according to the American Association for the Surgery of Trauma.

*Grade**	*Type*	*Description of injury*
I	Hematoma	Subcapsular, <10% surface area
	Laceration	Capsular tear, <1 cm parenchymal depth
II	Hematoma	Subcapsular, 10–50% surface area, intraparenchymal, <5 cm in diameter
	Laceration	Capsular tear, 1–3 cm parenchymal depth that does not involve a trabecular vessel
III	Hematoma	Subcapsular, >50% surface area or expanding, ruptured subcapsular or parenchymal hematoma, intraparenchymal hematoma >5 cm or expanding
	Laceration	>3 cm parenchymal depth or involving trabecular vessels
IV	Laceration	Laceration involving segmental or hilar vessels producing major devascularization (>25% of spleen)
V	Laceration	Completely shattered spleen
	Vascular	Hilar vascular injury that devascularizes spleen

*Advance one grade for multiple injuries up to grade III.

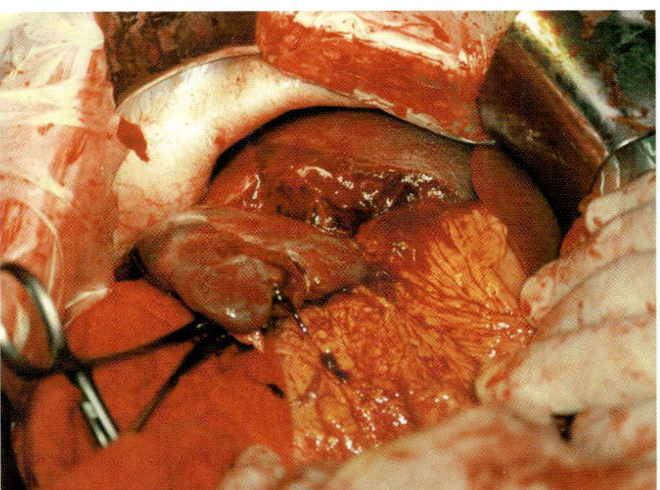

Fig. 40.1: Traumatic transection of the lower third of the spleen.

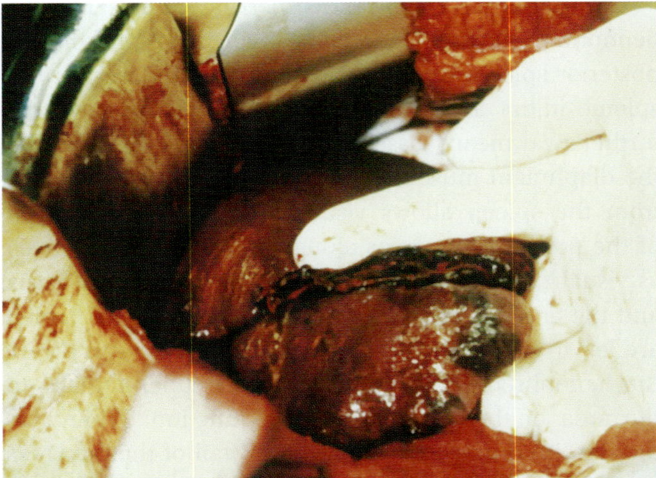

Fig. 40.2: Digital compression of the splenic tissue adjacent to the laceration.

no clear clinical advantage has been shown, and the argon beam device is more expensive. Fibrin sealing and collagen fleece are effective for less severe injuries as either the primary agent or as an adjuvant for achieving hemostasis. Localized active bleeding can be controlled effectively with a hemostatic matrix (FloSeal). This is an adjunct to hemostasis when control of bleeding by simple compression or suturing is ineffective or impracticable. Larger decapsulations with or without tissue loss can be covered and active nonpulsating bleeding can be stopped by using Hemopatch and similar substances.

Currently, most investigators rely on the organ injury scale classification developed by the American Association for the Surgery of Trauma to describe and stratify injury to the various intra-abdominal organs, including the spleen (Table 40.2).[17] The various suture repairs are not generally advisable for trauma because they are time consuming and involve more blood loss.

Stapling is simple and helps reduce operating time and blood transfusions. Injuries involving only one pole or half of the spleen can be treated with partial resection (Fig. 40.1). Stapler resection often makes organ conservation possible, and it represents a valuable alternative to the sutured partial splenectomy. The most suitable strategy for both quick and effective hemostasis and parenchymal preservation is resection with a TA stapler. Before the stapler is applied, the vessels supplying the segment to be resected should be selectively ligated or clipped to create an immediate demarcation. Then the splenic parenchyma should be compressed digitally adjacent to the injured area (Fig. 40.2). The compression presses the splenic parenchyma in the direction of the injury so that a thin layer of

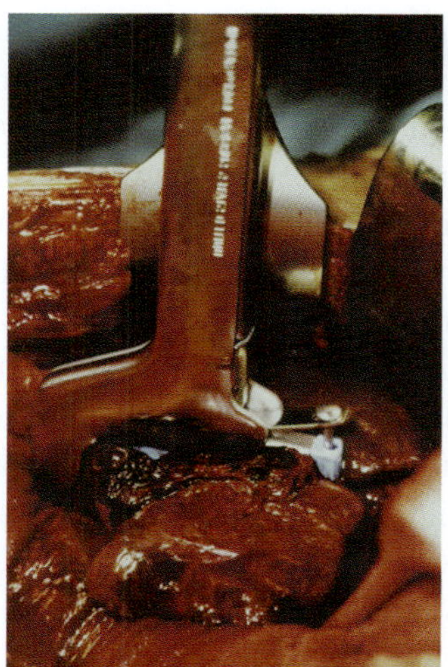

Fig. 40.3: Stapler resection of the lower third of the spleen.

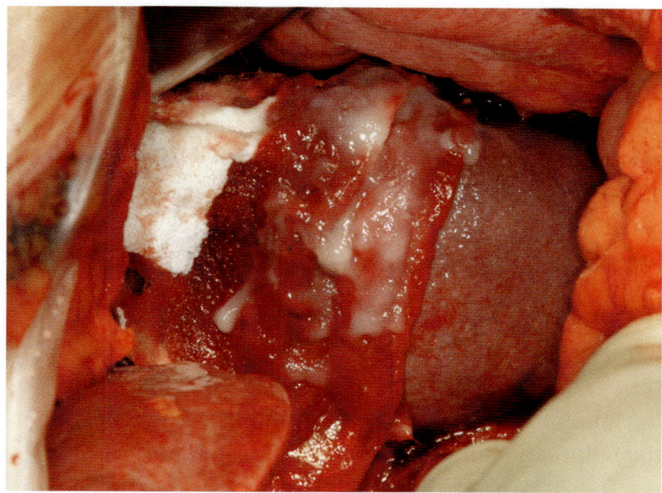

Fig. 40.4: Application of fibrin and collagen fleece after partial splenectomy to prevent after bleeding.

parenchyma and vessels with an intact capsule remain between the surgeon's fingers. The stapler can be applied and the resection performed without tearing the capsule (Fig. 40.3). The cut edge can be sealed with fibrin glue and collagen fleece (Fig. 40.4). The advantages of this technique are its simplicity and the reduction in time and blood loss.

The best course with severe injuries is splenorrhaphy with an absorbable mesh, which quickly and effectively stops the bleeding. When deep, extensive tears involve both hilar and diaphragmatic surfaces, this is the best approach. An appropriately sized piece of absorbable mesh with an absorbable thread is wrapped around the spleen, and the thread is pulled together on the hilar face to produce hemostasis without compromising intraparenchymal circulation. It is extremely important that the pouch be slightly smaller than the spleen itself, so that the thread lies on the margin when it has been pulled taut (Fig. 40.5). Because of the tension of the mesh on the hilar aspect, the splenic tissue forms a cone over the hilus. The mesh does not cover the tissue on the visceral surface and so there is a sufficiently large space around the hilus for vessels to enter and emerge. The conization itself compresses the splenic parenchyma on the concave surface, facilitating the desired hemostasis even in deep ruptures of this surface. On the convex diaphragmatic surface, the mesh lies taut over the surface and compresses the ruptured parenchyma. Any slight oozing of blood through the holes in the mesh can be arrested with fibrin glue and collagen fleece.

There are occasional reports in the literature of therapeutic laparoscopy in spleen trauma,[18-20] but it is not yet clear whether this is in fact a good option. Laparoscopy in stable patients with a spleen injury will not be needed since nonoperative management is the treatment of choice for stable patients. Unstable patients do not fulfill the basic criterion for laparoscopy, i.e. hemodynamic stability, and so should immediately undergo laparotomy. A stable trauma patient with a spleen injury will undergo laparoscopy not to treat the spleen trauma but, for example, to clarify an intestinal injury. Only in such cases does laparoscopy make sense. Spleen-preserving steps can of course be taken in the course of a diagnostic laparoscopy, but these measures are not to be interpreted as being applied primarily for the sake of preserving the spleen.

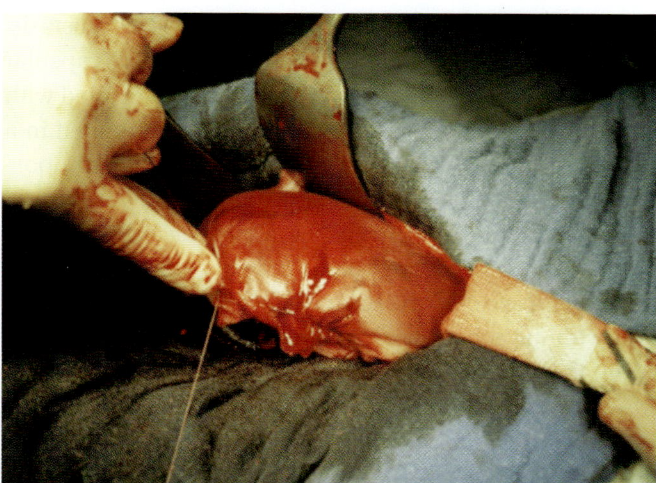

Fig. 40.5: Mesh splenorrhaphy: conization of the spleen when the thread is tautened.

Complications after orthotopic splenic salvage are minor and are usually avoidable when the procedure is correctly chosen and performed. The incidence and the effects of these complications are not greater or more severe, respectively, than for splenectomy (*see* Chapter 57, "Spleen," for details).

Nonoperative Management

Nonoperative management is limited to patients who are hemodynamically stable upon admission or after initial resuscitation. Glasgow coma scale/score, age, and hypotension upon admission do not have a significant effect on the failure rate for nonoperative management.[21]

The history of the surgical concepts applied to the spleen provides an understanding of how nonoperative management has evolved. In the past, it was thought that even minimal injuries to the spleen would continue to bleed and not respond to attempts at local hemostasis. As a consequence, small injuries produced by capsular avulsions from retraction of the omentum associated with an operation in the upper abdomen usually resulted in a splenectomy. It was also thought that blood was an important peritoneal irritant and that if the spleen was injured from blunt trauma, it would be apparent from physical examination. Following blunt trauma, the hematocrit might decrease over the first couple of days of hospitalization without apparent cause and on continued re-evaluation, the abdomen would seem more tender. Celiotomy was then performed but at operation only blood and clot were found around the spleen, and active hemorrhage was not usually observed. A splenectomy was performed and the diagnosis was "delayed" rupture of the spleen. Most of these cases were delayed diagnoses and in fact were instances of initial nonoperative management. Before the advent of DPL, many patients undoubtedly had splenic injuries that went unrecognized and caused no problems.

The use of DPL was reported by Root and colleagues in 1965.[22] It was extensively evaluated and reported over the ensuing 25 years, and its development coincided with the organization of trauma care. Its wide application resulted in a marked increase in laparotomies for splenic injury. Over time, many surgeons began to note that although there was no active bleeding at the time of celiotomy in a high proportion of cases, a splenectomy was usually performed. As noted above, splenic repair was developed following the recognition of postsplenectomy sepsis. Not surprisingly, the results with repair were quite good, yielding a high percentage rate of splenic salvage.

The introduction of CT scanning radically changed splenic injury management over the ensuing years. Wide application of CT scanning for trauma began in the early 1980s. It was initially used to study previously identified injuries from routine radiographic examinations, which included pulmonary, renal, and axial skeletal injuries. Computed tomography helped to recognize that several such patients had unrecognized injuries to the spleen and remained stable. These observations ushered in the formal concept of nonoperative management. It has always been emphasized that only hemodynamically stable patients are appropriate candidates and that they should be monitored closely so that they can undergo an urgent operation in case of continued or renewed bleeding. This policy implies that an operating room and personnel are available on short notice. All of these caveats continue to be applicable. An important change in management in many trauma centers over the years has been in the use of splenic organ injury scaling from CT scan findings as criteria for operative intervention. Initially, most centers observed stable patients with injury grades I–III and operated for grades IV–V. As a result, approximately one-third of patients were managed nonoperatively. It was believed that there would be a high rate of failure of nonoperative management due to continued bleeding from the injured spleen and consequent morbidity if nonoperative management was used for higher grade injuries. However, it was also noted that many of the higher grade injuries were either not actively bleeding or were not as extensive as suggested by CT scan findings. Consequently, several centers proceeded to use nonoperative management for higher grades of injury in stable patients. With this approach, approximately half of all splenic injuries could be managed nonoperatively.[23]

Failure of nonoperative management is an extremely important issue (*see* Chapter 44, "Case Study: Delayed Splenectomy Following Expectant Management of Splenic Trauma," for a description of such a case). If the rate is excessive and the hemorrhagic complications are substantial, the appropriateness of nonoperative management should be questioned. Reported rates of failure range from 3% to 48%.[23-26] There have been recent attempts to focus on the failures in order to select patients more accurately for operation. Patients whose injury on a CT scan is graded as IV–V have a higher incidence of failure than patients whose injury is lower grade (5% vs. 18%), but 82% of higher grade injuries (IV–V) have been managed successfully nonoperatively.[11] The extent of hemoperitoneum can also be used as a better predictor of failure of nonoperative therapy

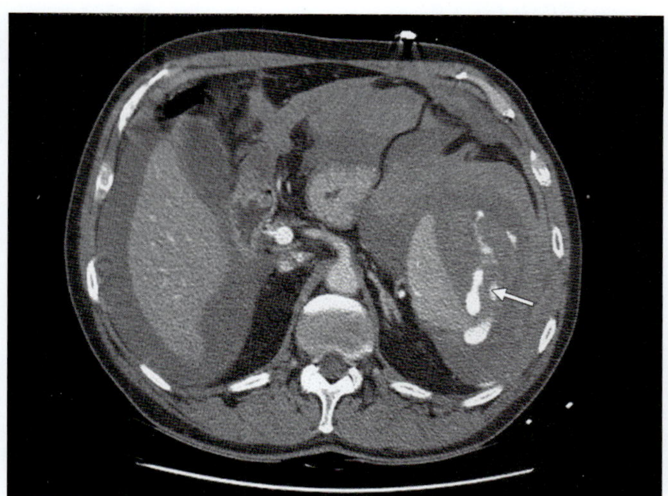

Fig. 40.6: Computed tomogram scan demonstrating "contrast blush" (arrow) from an injured spleen.

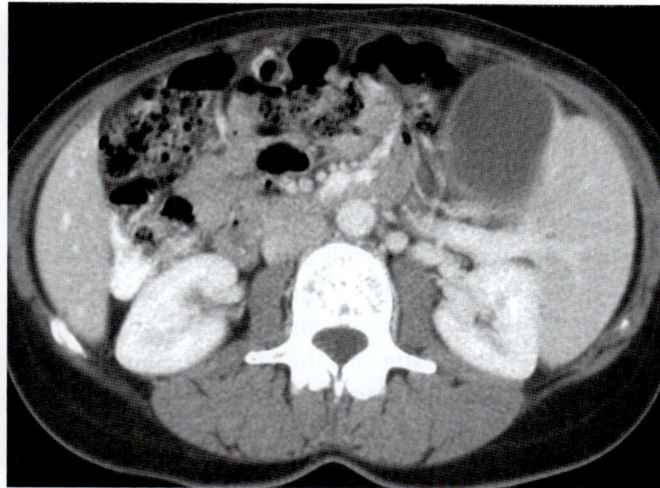

Fig. 40.7: Computed tomogram scan demonstrating a large post-traumatic splenic cyst.

than the grade of injury, but it is difficult to quantitate hemoperitoneum using current CT scanning technology. Most investigators use a scheme similar to the following to classify it:

- Minimal—blood around the spleen (1 unit)
- Moderate—blood around the spleen and down the left gutter (1-2 units)
- Major—blood around the spleen, in the gutter, and in the pelvis (>2 units).

If there is blood in more locations than these, the patient is usually unstable and is not a candidate for nonoperative management. The higher failure rates associated with major hemoperitoneum should generally indicate operative treatment, especially in those with multiple injuries.

Additionally, the presence of a contrast blush is another risk factor for nonoperative management.[27] Approximately 15% of patients undergoing planned nonoperative management were found to have a contrast blush on a CT scan (Fig. 40.6). Approximately 62% of the patients with a contrast blush failed to recover with nonoperative management and developed a true delayed rupture of the spleen. The contrast blushes proved to be false aneurysms of segmental branches of the splenic artery and gradual expansion of the false aneurysm resulted in splenic rupture when the aneurysm reached a critical size. Rupture occurred on an average of 3.5 days (range 1–9 days) after injury. Splenic rupture caused sudden acute pain and was associated with appreciable hemorrhage. One-third of patients with pseudoaneurysms that did not proceed to rupture apparently underwent thrombosis of the pseudoaneurysm.

There are insufficient data to objectively address when to obtain follow-up CT scan evaluations and when the patient should resume strenuous activity if splenic injuries are managed nonoperatively. For minor injuries (grades I–II), ultrasonography instead of CT scanning is a worthwhile option for follow-up. Healing usually occurs within a few weeks of injury. For higher grades, repeat examinations at 2-4-week intervals are carried out until substantial (but not complete) healing is apparent. In these cases as well, ultrasonography can replace CT scanning follow-up. Most grade IV–V injuries are essentially completely healed at 6–8 weeks, when normal activity can be resumed. If the patient is involved in strenuous physical activity, such as sports, it is advisable to obtain an ultrasound or CT scan after that interval to evaluate healing, and if healing is satisfactory, most surgeons believe that the patient can safely resume the activity. It has been suggested that after injury, the fibrosis associated with healing produces more resistance to subsequent injury than the normal spleen has. Rarely, splenic cysts have developed remote from such injury, which again are considered for surgery if their size exceeds 5 cm in diameter (Fig. 40.7).

Complications of splenic trauma other than immediate exsanguinating hemorrhage and delayed rupture are associated with splenectomy. These include postsplenectomy sepsis and left upper quadrant abscess. Subphrenic abscess most frequently occurs following penetrating trauma with associated hollow viscus injury and bacterial contamination of the empty splenic fossa. The risk is greatly increased if there is associated pancreatic injury. Efforts to repair the spleen are justified in this circumstance if the patient is stable. Drainage of the splenic fossa has not been shown to be advantageous unless pancreatic injury requires drainage.

LIVER INJURY

Hepatic trauma poses one of the greatest operative challenges of all injuries. The liver is the largest abdominal organ and, together with the spleen, the most frequently injured. Difficulties in operative management arise from the friable consistency of the tissue and the organ's extensive blood supply. Nutrient supply comes from the hepatic artery and portal vein and the large hepatic veins drain the liver directly into the inferior vena cava. In the last decade, death rates from hepatic injury declined from 12% to 5%. Four reasons appear to be responsible for the decrease in death rates as a result of hepatic bleeding:

- Decrease in the number of venous injuries requiring operation
- Improved management of major venous injuries
- Improved results with the concept of packing and reoperation
- Increasing availability of angiography and embolization.

As with splenic trauma, however, there is a marked trend toward nonoperative management, which presents fewer challenges and improves outcomes.

Operative Management

Considerations of hepatic vascular anatomy and injury patterns are a logical approach for selecting operative techniques and understanding the efficacy of nonoperative management. The branches of the hepatic artery and portal vein traverse the hepatic segments alongside the bile duct branches in the portal triads. Within the triads, the vessels are encased in fibrous tissue, which serves as a protective sheath. They form the architectural support for the liver and their main branches divide it into the eight hepatic segments (*see* Chapter 53, "Liver"). The right, middle, and left hepatic veins traverse the hepatic segments and have no protective wrapping (Fig. 40.8).

Blunt hepatic injuries usually produce shattering defects with crevices along anatomic divisions. Linear and stellate lacerations typically occur in the right lobe along:

- The line between segments VI–VII and V–VIII and the line between segments V–VI and VII–VIII
- The line between segments V–VIII and IV, which separate the right and left lobes (commonest area of important laceration)

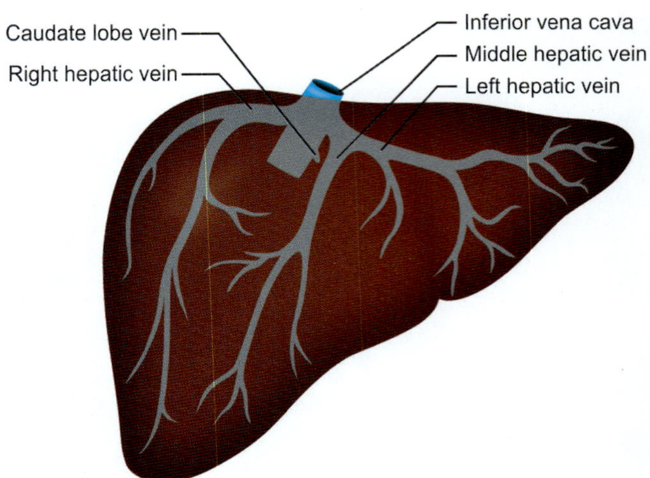

Fig. 40.8: Venous anatomy of the liver.

- In the left lobe along the falciform ligament separating segment IV from II–III.

As these lacerations occur along the planes of the main portal triads, the large hepatic arterial and portal vein branches are generally not injured. However, the major hepatic veins traverse these cleavage planes, so they are often torn. As the hepatic venous system is low pressure [2–5 cm H_2O (2–5 kPa)], the injuries are amenable to tamponade. These anatomic considerations become relatively unimportant for penetrating trauma, though, because the wounding agents can traverse any plane. Large caliber and high-velocity missile wounds usually produce very difficult operative problems and are highly lethal.

Although midline incisions are usually preferred for trauma celiotomy, subcostal incisions, which can be extended bilaterally, provide better exposure for major liver trauma. In the event of retrohepatic cava or main hepatic vein injury, extension via a right thoracoabdominal approach provides excellent exposure. Extension of the abdominal incision with a median sternotomy to gain proximal control of the vena cava is also an approach many surgeons favor. From experiences associated with liver transplantation, it has been learned that the median sternotomy can be carried out quickly and provides at least as good exposure as a right thoracoabdominal incision. The morbidity associated with the median sternal extension appears to be lower than with a right thoracoabdominal incision.

Upon entering the abdomen, rapid evacuation of blood and clot (by hand rather than with suction) is necessary to assess the organ injuries so that time is not wasted on less severe injuries while permitting ongoing hemorrhage

Table 40.3 Steps for hepatic mobilization.

Right lobe
• Complete division of the falciform ligament
• Division of the triangular ligaments anteriorly and posteriorly
• Division of accessory hepatic veins as necessary
• Delivery of the right lobe into the wound
Left lobe
• Complete division of the falciform ligament
• Division of the coronary ligament anteriorly and posteriorly

Sternotomy should be performed when proximal vena cava (intrapericardial) control is necessary.

Table 40.4 Initial steps for managing major liver injury.

• Rapidly evacuate intraperitoneal blood using laparotomy pads or towels to determine major source of hemorrhage.
• Mobilize the appropriate hepatic lobe.
• Assess the quality of liver hemorrhage.
• First assistant compresses the liver.
• Pringle maneuver (only helpful for arterial or portal venous injury, not hepatic vein injury).
• Individually ligate major bleeding vessels.

from more serious lesions. Once it becomes apparent that the liver is the major problem, it is important to assess the quality of hemorrhage. If the blood is dark, hepatic venous injury is the main problem. Red blood (oxygen saturated) indicates arterial or portal venous bleeding, and pulsatile bleeding differentiates the two because portal vein pressures are low. Other, less heavily bleeding organ injuries should be temporarily tamponaded with laparotomy pads so that attention can be focused on the liver. Severe splenic bleeding can also be controlled by splenic hilar clamping without losing too much time.

The injured hepatic lobe should be completely mobilized to allow adequate evaluation and treatment unless the injury can be well-defined with less dissection (Table 40.3). For lesions of the right lobe, the falciform ligament should be completely divided from inferior to superior and the triangular ligament divided anteriorly and posteriorly so that the right lobe is delivered into the wound, suspended from the vena cava by the hepatic vein. Complete mobilization usually requires division and ligation of 2–6 small veins that empty directly into the vena cava. When the left lobe is involved, the falciform and coronary ligaments should be divided. One instance in which division of the triangular or coronary ligaments should be avoided is when there is clot within them. This finding signifies probable retrohepatic injury to the vena cava and division may lead to rapid exsanguination or air embolization.

Following hepatic mobilization, discrete large vessel injuries should be sought and ligated. As mentioned above, noting the quality of hemorrhage can be most helpful. In approximately 90% of blunt injuries, the major bleeding arises from hepatic veins and is apparent by continuous welling up of dark blood within the liver crevice. Following hepatic mobilization, hemorrhage decreases if the first assistant compresses the liver while the treatment plan is made. When marked arterial or portal vein bleeding is encountered, compression of vessels in the porta hepatis (free edge of the lesser omentum), the Pringle maneuver, can be helpful. However, because hepatic vein bleeding is associated with retrograde bleeding from the vena cava, this maneuver is usually not effective for blunt trauma. A useful adjunctive approach is to use the finger fracture technique to expose a large bleeding vessel in a narrow crevice. Judgment is required to avoid exacerbating the situation. From a practical point of view, hepatic injuries can be divided in three groups. Type I superficial injuries with less intense bleeding do not require a Pringle maneuver. Such bleeds usually stop of their own accord and do not require surgical intervention. If laparotomy is needed due to any reason these liver lacerations can be treated with simple sutures, coagulation and hemostatic agents. Type II injuries require a Pringle maneuver. These are deeper parenchymal lesions losing both arterial and venous blood. They show a contrast blush on CT scanning and are almost always handled surgically. Type III injuries that do not respond to a Pringle maneuver involve damage to the hepatic vein and retrohepatic vena cava.

The initial steps for managing major liver injuries are outlined in Table 40.4. The goals in the operating room for major hepatic injury are as follows:

- Control hemorrhage
- Control bile leakage
- Debride dead liver tissue
- Drainage.

Seven procedures have been described specifically for treating liver injuries: resectional debridement and tissue sealing, mass liver suture, selective hepatic artery ligation (HAL), atriocaval shunting, total hepatic isolation, omental packing, and gauze packing. Individual vessel ligation should precede all of these.

Resectional Debridement and Tissue Sealing

Formal hepatic resection was abandoned in the 1970s because of unacceptable results. In unstable situations with ongoing hemorrhage, hypothermia and coagulopathy ensue quickly and formal resection is not appropriate. It can happen that lacerations nearly completely divide and devascularize one or more segments; resectional debridement is then appropriate for hemostasis and removal of nonviable liver to prevent coagulopathy and sepsis due to retention of necrotic hepatic tissue. Following ligation of exposed vessels, omental aprons and local hemostatic agents (fibrin glue in combination with collagen fleece) can help stop oozing from the raw surface. However, active bleeding from difficult accessible and surgically otherwise nonsuturable lesions can eventually be treated by using a flowable viscous hemostatic gel (Floseal).

Mass Liver Suture

For this technique, large atraumatic liver needles with absorbable sutures are placed from the surface of the liver to the depth of the laceration to exit through the surface on the opposite side of the liver laceration. The sutures are tied to close the laceration and provide tamponade. This traditional technique has been commonly used, but with two concerns about its application:

- The risk of injury to large vessels and bile ducts
- Lack of efficacy of producing hemostasis.

Omental and gauze packing techniques have largely supplanted mass suturing in recent years.

Hepatic Artery Ligation

Hepatic artery ligation occupies an interesting spot in surgical history. For many years, it was believed that right or left HAL would result in death as a result of hepatic necrosis and sepsis because of a paucity of collateral blood supply. Some of this rationale was based upon the fact that HAL generally does lead to sepsis and death. However, an important difference between dogs and humans is that canine portal blood commonly carries bacteria whereas in humans it is sterile. Hepatic artery ligation does not work well for blunt trauma because most of those injuries involve hepatic venous hemorrhage, but HAL can be helpful in managing deep penetrating wounds when there is arterial bleeding. Finger fracture type techniques can be used for such injuries, but these injuries may lead to extensive fracture for exposure and result in liver necrosis if the wound is such that the fracturing is nonanatomic and deep. If interventional radiology is available, a fast tamponade with laparotomy pads will stop the venous bleeding. The arterial bleeding can then be controlled with selective angioembolization.

Atriocaval Shunt

Atriocaval shunting was developed primarily to manage major hepatic vein and especially retrohepatic vena caval injuries. The technique was reported by Schrock and Blaisdell in 1968.[28] It is based upon the concept of hepatic isolation. Following hepatic mobilization, a tape is passed around the suprarenal inferior vena cava and a median sternotomy is performed followed by pericardiotomy and isolation of the right atrial appendage. A purse string is placed around the appendage and a chest tube with side holes cut in at the atrial end is passed through the right atrium into the vena cava. A tape is passed around the intrapericardial vena cava and then both caval tapes are secured around the tube. A Pringle maneuver is then performed; this sequence of occlusion effectively isolates the liver and permits venous return from the lower body, minimizing the hypotension that typically occurs in hypovolemic patients when the vena cava is occluded. Although anatomically appealing, it is a complex procedure and is even more difficult in the unstable patient. It is therefore rarely used today.

Total Hepatic Isolation

Total hepatic isolation is probably the best approach for managing retrohepatic venous injuries. It is relatively simple and not excessively time-consuming. The inferior vena cava is isolated at a convenient location and the suprahepatic vena cava is isolated after intrapericardial exposure via median sternotomy. Supraceliac clamping of the aorta is carried out to ameliorate the profound hypotension resulting from caval occlusion. This exposure is fairly straightforward following sternotomy. In all situations in which caval occlusion may be required, it is imperative that there be large-bore upper extremity venous access so that the anesthesia team can deliver appropriate fluid volumes. Following caval occlusion and aortic clamping, the venous injury can be identified and rapidly ligated or laterally repaired. Regardless of surgical expediency, these injuries are associated with a high mortality rate from hemorrhage or air embolization.

Omental Packing

Omental packing, reported by Stone and Lamb in 1975,[29] is an excellent technique for managing intrahepatic venous injuries, which account for most blunt hepatic trauma. The technique is simple, rapid, and can be performed effectively by surgeons who do not manage a large trauma volume or who have limited assistance. The technique works through tamponade by viable omental tissue. When a major liver laceration is encountered, the area is packed with laparotomy pads instead of extensively exploring the injury site and initiating more bleeding. The omentum is then dissected from its lateral attachments to the abdominal wall and along its avascular attachment to the transverse colon. The blood supply via the gastroepiploic vessels is preserved. Following this mobilization, either one large omental apron can be used or it can be divided in two in the middle with the corresponding gastroepiploic supply left intact on each side. In thin individuals, the entire omentum is required, and if they are extremely thin, this approach may not be practical because of insufficient omental tissue. In obese patients, it is often best to divide the omentum. The hepatic laceration is now explored and large vessels ligated and then the omental pack is tightly placed within the depth of the injury. It is secured firmly in place with a large running absorbable suture. Large sutures have less tendency to tear through the parenchyma. It can be helpful to buttress the liver edge with the divided falciform ligament or collagen fleece pledgets. The running suture should enter 1–2 cm from the edge of the laceration and travel 1–2 cm deep (this shallow technique minimizes damage to larger intrahepatic structures). As it exits the laceration, the suture is draped over the omentum and then passed through the laceration exiting the liver surface on the side opposite the initial needle entry at the same depth. A running suture is quick and provides firm and even distribution of pressure on the pack to maximize the tamponade effect. Figure 40.9 shows this technique. Tissue thromboplastin associated with an omental pack promotes coagulation in addition to the tamponade effect. To be maximally effective, the omentum should be packed quickly after major vessel ligation. There is always marked venous oozing from a number of small veins and these present a temptation to continue attempts at ligation and cauterization. Persisting with ligation of small veins leads to marked blood loss, hypothermia, and coagulopathy. The omental pack quickly stops such hemorrhage.

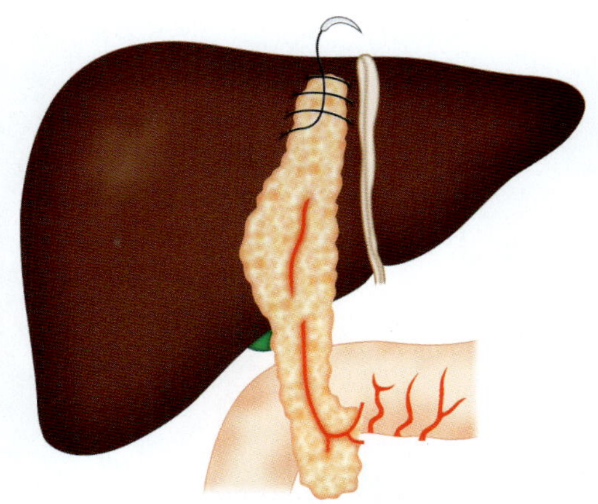

Fig. 40.9: Use of a viable omental pack to manage a fractured liver (crevice between segments IV and V–VIII). A pedicle of omentum is mobilized and sewn into the defect on the liver surface.

Gauze Packing

At the time of World War II, gauze packing was the procedure of choice for major hepatic wounds; the high rate of perihepatic sepsis led, however, to a trend to avoid the technique, and wide drainage was endorsed.[30] Gauze packing has been resurrected over the past 15 years and has been increasingly used since the onset of the era of nonoperative management. Mortality rates of 10–57% have been reported in recent years.[31-33] These results are acceptable considering that the technique is used for the most catastrophic injuries. Following attempts at ligating all large vessels, packs are placed above and below the liver to sandwich it in tightly and tamponade bleeding. It will not work satisfactorily if the arterial injuries have not been ligated. As in World War II, perihepatic sepsis remained high, reported at 30–83%.[32-34] After laparotomy, hypothermia and coagulopathy are corrected in the intensive care unit (ICU) and the patient is returned to the operating room within 1–2 days for pack removal. Evidence of marked ongoing liver bleeding requires early re-exploration to rule out mechanical bleeding. Early pack removal (at 24 hours) seems to reduce septic morbidity. Approximately 25–50% of patients require repacking because of the oozing with pack removal and a few require packing on the subsequent return to the operating room.

Drains

Drains should be used for major liver injuries in the absence of coagulopathy. Bile duct branches are routinely injured with these deep lacerations. Closed suction drainage in patients undergoing laparotomy for hepatic trauma may reduce bilomas and perihepatic infections.[22]

Nonoperative Management

Currently, >80% of liver injuries are treated nonoperatively. As with splenic trauma, it was similarly noted on CT scans

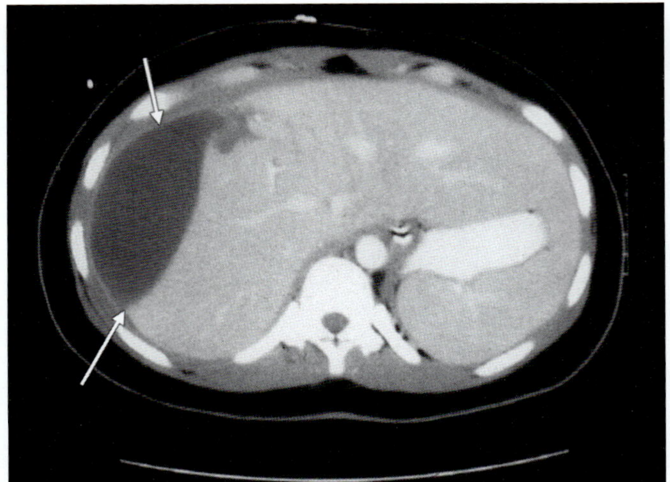

Fig. 40.10: Computed tomogram scan 2 weeks after liver injury demonstrating biloma (arrows).

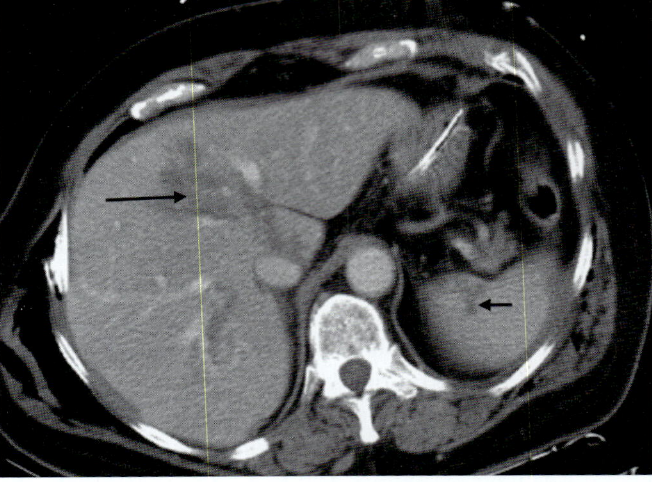

Fig. 40.11: Central liver injury with discrete blush (arrow) and splenic injury (arrow right).

obtained for other purposes that patients with previously unrecognized liver injuries often had no problems. One of the reasons for the reluctance to accept nonoperative management for liver injuries was a concern about bile leaks. Bile leaks and bilomas are found on occasion with nonoperative management (Fig. 40.10); they are not common and when they do develop they are usually easily managed by percutaneous drainage.

Early experiences were retrospective, and nonoperative management was generally undertaken only for highly selected patients with mild injuries; as a result 10–20% of cases were treated this way. With increasing experience, higher percentages of patients with liver injury are now managed nonoperatively. The failure rate of nonoperative management is lower than for splenic trauma. This finding is not surprising because of the anatomy of liver injury and because most bleeding is venous; the segmental vascular anatomy of the spleen is such that most splenic injuries involve an arterial branch. Liver injuries are usually tamponaded by the clot that forms in the area of injury. If, however, a significant contrast blush is noted on a CT scan and the patient is stable, angioembolization is a good option. Patients who are unstable or borderline stable should generally undergo laparotomy. A discrete blush or frank contrast extravasation does not unnecessarily predict the need of a trauma laparotomy (Fig. 40.11). Depending upon individual circumstances and absence of other organ injuries, these patients can also be managed nonoperatively.

Nonoperative management has been shown to have significantly lower blood transfusion requirements than operative management.[35] It appears that operative management sometimes precipitates bleeding that might not have been a problem if the injury had been left undisturbed.

The general rules for successful nonoperative management in liver injury are as follows:

- Unstable patients are not candidates for nonoperative management and require emergency laparotomy.
- Stable patients with all but the most trivial injuries should be initially monitored in an ICU with emergency operating room access in case the patient develops signs of ongoing hemorrhage.
- The length of observation should be based solely on clinical criteria. Patients with liver injuries may be safely discharged home in the presence of a normal abdominal examination and stable hemoglobin, regardless of the grade of injury.[36]

Complications

The major complications of liver trauma are perihepatic infection, biloma, and hemobilia. Perihepatic infection is mostly associated with penetrating trauma and hollow viscus injury. The infecting organisms develop from the gastrointestinal contamination. A synergistic effect of liver and hollow viscus injuries has been noted for intra-abdominal sepsis;[37] the combination yielded an intra-abdominal sepsis rate of 39%, whereas multivariate analysis found liver injuries to be an independent predictor of infection when associated with hollow viscus injury. Closed suction drains reduce the incidence of sepsis when compared with sump drains.[34] Bile leaks with biloma occur after both operative and nonoperative management. In operative cases,

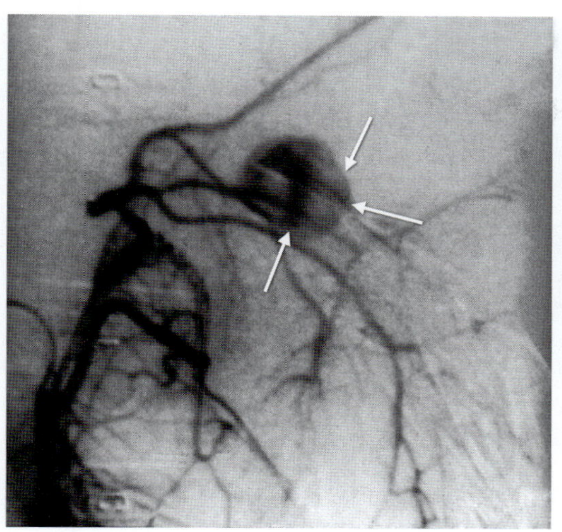

Fig. 40.12: Angiogram demonstrating hepatic artery pseudoaneurysm (arrows).

biloma increases the risk of perihepatic infection. Sterile bilomas are usually manifested by pressure symptoms and hyperbilirubinemia. Percutaneous drainage is usually successful, and leaks seal spontaneously within a couple of weeks.

Hemobilia can occur after either blunt or penetrating injury. It is thought that iatrogenic bile duct injury during mass hepatic suture can be responsible. Patients present several days to a few months after injury (most within 2 weeks). The classic presentation is upper gastrointestinal bleeding with fever, hyperbilirubinemia, and an elevated serum alkaline phosphatase. Hemobilia has been reported in 1.2% of operatively managed liver trauma cases.[38] Many cases are associated with false aneurysms of hepatic artery branches. Angioembolization is the treatment of choice if the false aneurysm is detected when small. Adjunctive percutaneous drainage of surrounding infection may be required. If the pseudoaneurysm is detected after it has grown to a large size, it begins to compress surrounding liver tissue and this may result in a progressive halo of hepatic necrosis, which becomes infected (Fig. 40.12).[38] This situation is life threatening; angioembolization and/or formal hepatic resection may be required.

EXTRAHEPATIC BILIARY INJURY

Blunt injuries to the extrahepatic bile ducts and gallbladder are rare. These are frequently insidious and difficult to diagnose due to the absence of irritation to the peritoneal cavity, a fact that is not always appreciated. Occasionally early diagnoses are made because of the presence of free peritoneal fluid without associated solid visceral injury on a CT scan or as an incidental finding at laparoscopy or laparotomy. In the case of a ruptured gallbladder, 2–3 L of bile can be present in the peritoneal cavity, yet the only symptoms are fullness and jaundice. At the time of surgery, there may be a shaggy, bile-stained inflammatory exudate on the peritoneal surfaces, but patients can make a good recovery after cholecystectomy and drainage.

Bile duct injuries present a more difficult problem. They generally occur in one of the two locations:

- The left hepatic duct where it exits from the liver
- The distal common bile duct.

They are occasional incidental findings at laparotomy. Any bile staining in the area of the porta hepatis requires exploration for bile duct or duodenal injury. More frequently, bile duct injuries are diagnosed when the patient develops jaundice. If the injury is diagnosed before there is marked inflammation, repair with a Roux-en-Y jejunostomy is appropriate. If there is a distal duct injury and appreciable inflammation or the patient is unstable, cholecystojejunostomy is an acceptable approach. However, these anastomoses often stricture after a few years, and secondary choledochojejunostomy may be required. Management of hepatic duct injuries is difficult. Hepaticojejunostomy should usually be performed, but the anatomy may mean that the proximal duct retracts into the liver, and the additional fact that this duct is small makes exposure and anastomosis difficult. It is important to avoid injury to the other uninvolved duct. The area where the injured duct is avulsed should be carefully oversewn to avoid compromising the other duct. In the absence of infection, if the anastomosis of the injured duct fails, that lobe should atrophy without clinical consequences if the other lobe drains normally.

GASTRIC INJURY

Perhaps the most famous gastric injury is that reported by William Beaumont. It is the case of the French Canadian Alexis St Martin who sustained a close-range gunshot wound to the left upper quadrant. Beaumont managed this nonoperatively, and St Martin survived for 58 years afterward with a gastrocutaneous fistula and died at the age of 78 years.

In 1901, American President William McKinley was shot in the abdomen and had several gastric wounds repaired at laparotomy.[39] He died 8 days later. Although this approach was initially controversial, it became standard therapy as improvements in surgical technique, anesthesia, asepsis, and instrumentation resulted in a decrease in morbidity and mortality rates.

Anatomy

Although the stomach may be protected by the lower rib cage at times, it is easily distended and fairly mobile. As it is fixed at the gastroesophageal junction and the pylorus, it is vulnerable to injury even though it is fairly mobile. It has an excellent blood supply from the left and right gastric, the left and right gastroepiploic, and the short gastric arteries. There is a rich network of collaterals between these vessels, which may contribute to extensive gastric bleeding. The fact that the gastric wall is thick and has a strong submucosal layer may explain why blunt gastric rupture is so uncommon.[40]

Most cases of gastric trauma result from MVAs. Other series have reported injuries secondary to falls, cardiopulmonary resuscitation, and direct violence. Isolated gastric injury is rare, but is associated with a low morbidity and mortality. The mechanism of injury, location of injury, and type of repair used all affect patient outcomes with gastric injury. Current series have reported mortality rates that range from 0% in isolated blunt injury to 52% for those combined with arterial and colonic injuries.[41,42]

Gastric injury after penetrating trauma is quite common. A review of gastric trauma noted the incidence of abdominal penetrating injury to be 7–20%.[40] Two large series of penetrating gastric injuries reported associated injuries in 74% and 84% of patients; the liver, diaphragm, and colon were most commonly injured.[42,43] The mortality rates in these series were 11% and 13.1%, respectively.

Diagnosis

Patients with a blunt gastric rupture often have a history of consuming a large meal before the traumatic event. They may present with hypotension and have appreciable abdominal pain and tenderness as a result of the chemical peritonitis caused by the spilled gastric acid.

An upright chest radiograph or lateral decubitus abdominal film is sometimes used to search for free air. However, these films are difficult to obtain in many trauma patients because of the associated injuries or hypotension. In one series, no patients had free air, but there was a 16–66% incidence of free air reported in four other series.[44]

As all gunshot wounds to the anterior abdomen come to laparotomy, gastric injuries are usually diagnosed at the time of laparotomy. For those who have penetrating injuries to the left upper quadrant, the presence of hematemesis or a grossly bloody nasogastric aspirate is highly suggestive of a gastric injury, and this should be thoroughly sought for at operation. In the instance of a stab wound, either of these findings should prompt laparotomy or laparoscopy without further delay.[42] It must be remembered that the stomach is fairly mobile and can be injured even after a stab wound to the lower abdomen (Fig. 40.13).[45]

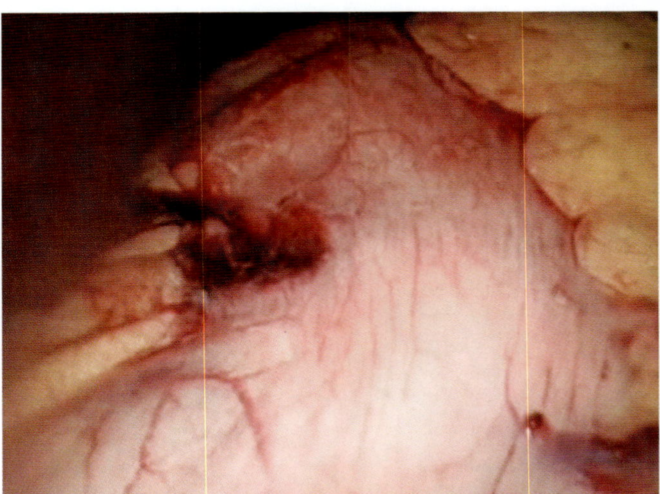

Fig. 40.13: Stab wound to the lesser curvature of the gastric corpus detected during diagnostic laparoscopy.

Operative Management

An injury on the anterior surface of the stomach should be easily identified. One must be thorough on intraoperative examination to ensure that an injury is not obscured by the gastrohepatic or gastrocolic ligament. If there is any doubt, these ligaments should be divided to search for an injury. Most gastric injuries can easily be treated by simple suturing (Fig. 40.14).

If there is an injury to the anterior surface, particularly a penetrating injury, one should also assume that there is an injury to the posterior stomach. Missed gastric injuries are among the most common of "missed" injuries. The gastrocolic ligament should be divided and the lesser sac entered to examine the posterior stomach. The pancreas must also be examined.

Careful attention must be paid to the gastroesophageal junction. Care must also be taken when exploring the distal anterior stomach or the first portion of the duodenum that a posterior injury is not missed; a Kocher maneuver facilitates exposure. Division of the gastrohepatic ligament

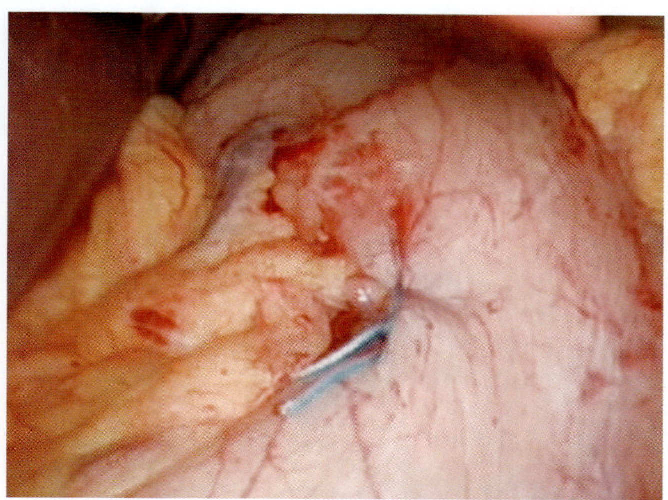

Fig. 40.14: Laparoscopic suture closure of the stab injury shown in Figure 40.13.

facilitates exposure of the lesser curve of the distal stomach as well. Once an injury is identified, the wound should be debrided and closed.

Diaphragmatic injury should also be sought. Appreciable pleural contamination can result in empyema. Empyema is the most frequent complication in those who have a combined penetrating gastric and diaphragmatic injury.[42] An association has been demonstrated between the development of an empyema and the presence of an intra-abdominal injury.[46]

Complications

Most complications of gastric trauma are infectious in nature. An intra-abdominal abscess is most likely to occur, complicating 50–75% of cases of blunt rupture. This sequence likely occurs because many of these patients have full stomachs at the time of their injury and the peritoneal cavity becomes contaminated with the food particles and the numerous oral floras that are present in the full stomach.

DUODENAL INJURY

An isolated injury to the duodenum is relatively uncommon and occurs in 3–5% of patients who sustain intra-abdominal injury.[47-49] Penetrating trauma accounts for approximately 80% of these injuries. The infrequency of duodenal injury is explained by the retroperitoneal location of the duodenum. This fact also makes the diagnosis of a duodenal injury difficult. The morbidity and mortality rates associated with duodenal injury are high.

Anatomy

The duodenum is the first portion of the small intestine and extends from the pylorus to the ligament of Treitz. Its four component portions and its relationships are described in Chapter 69, "Small Bowel". The first portion is the most mobile. It is covered by peritoneum on at least the anterior surface, and it lies at approximately the L1 vertebral body. The second, third, and fourth portions typically do not have a peritoneal covering.

The blood supply of the duodenum is shared with the pancreas and originates from both the celiac axis and the superior mesenteric artery.

Associated Injuries

Although isolated duodenal injuries have been reported,[56,57] they are the exception. Of 1,095 patients with duodenal injury, 87% had associated injuries (98% of these with penetrating trauma and 84% of those with blunt injuries).[52,54] There is an average of 2.9 associated injuries following penetrating trauma and 1.6 after blunt injury;[52] the liver is the most commonly injured organ.[58]

Diagnosis

Diagnosing duodenal injury remains a challenge. A key to making the diagnosis is a high index of suspicion, which is facilitated by a history covering the mechanism of injury (e.g. a marked blow to the midepigastrium or a head-on collision with bending of the steering wheel). A duodenal injury should also be considered in people who have had a fall from a height.[56]

Although signs of peritoneal irritation should be evaluated, physical examination may reveal no findings of a duodenal injury because of its retroperitoneal location. External signs of abdominal trauma should be sought, such as a seatbelt mark or some other type of bruising or abrasion to the midepigastrium, which suggest the possibility of a duodenal injury.

Laboratory studies offer little help. Leukocytosis is neither sensitive nor specific. Hyperamylasemia has been suggested as a diagnostic marker for duodenal injury; although an elevated amylase level may suggest the diagnosis, normal levels do not rule it out.

Radiologic studies are useful. Plain films may reveal the presence of air outlining the right kidney, in the retroperitoneum along the psoas, or in the retrocecal region.[57,59] Other less specific findings on a radiograph include obliteration of the psoas margin and segmental ileus in or

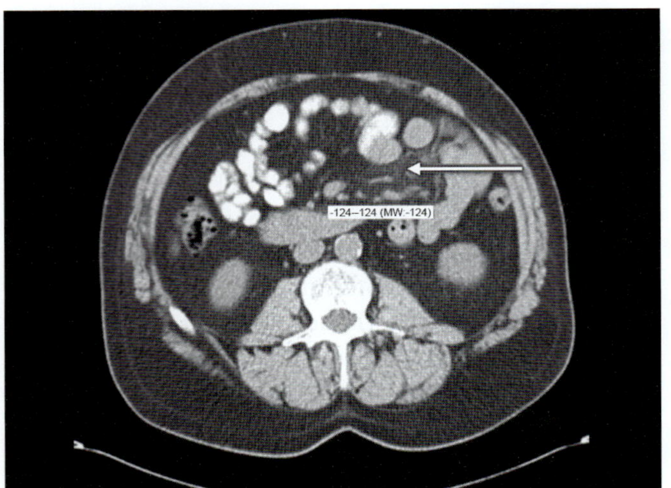

Fig 40.15: Duodenal injury (arrow). Marked inflammation of paraduodenal fatty tissue.

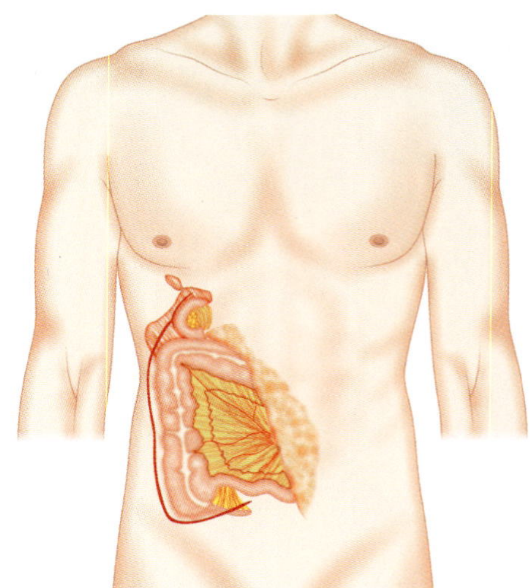

Fig. 40.16: Cattell-Braasch maneuver (right medial visceral rotation) allowing access to the right retroperitoneal space, including the duodenum and retropancreatic area.

near the duodenum. Abnormalities can be noted on plain films in approximately 50% of cases. If these findings are encountered, a contrast study of the upper gastrointestinal tract with water-soluble contrast medium with the patient lying on the right side should be considered.[55] If there is no extravasation, the patient may be given thin barium. This examination may show the "coiled-spring sign"[60] or the "stacked coin sign",[61] both of which are diagnostic of a duodenal hematoma.

A CT scan, particularly with the spiral technique, is a fairly reliable method for diagnosing duodenal injury. Patients should receive both oral and intravenous contrast. Extraluminal gas or extravasated oral contrast in the right anterior pararenal space is diagnostic of a duodenal perforation.[62] Thickening of the duodenal wall and fluid in the right anterior pararenal space can also be seen in patients who have either a duodenal hematoma or perforation (Fig. 40.15). The sensitivity of a CT scan for the diagnosis of blunt duodenal injuries is 70%.[59]

Operative Management

All four portions of the duodenum need to be explored. A generous Kocher maneuver is performed until the left renal vein and superior mesenteric vessels are visualized. This procedure allows visualization of the anterior and posterior aspects of the second and third portions of the duodenum.

The Cattell-Braasch maneuver (right medial visceral rotation) allows visualization of the third portion (Fig. 40.16).[63,64] It involves incising along the white line of Toldt and mobilizing the right colon medially. The retroperitoneal attachments of the small bowel can then be incised from the right lower quadrant up to the ligament of Treitz so that the small bowel can be reflected up and out of the abdomen. The fourth portion of the duodenum can be well-visualized by incising the ligament of Treitz.

Factors that determine the technique of repair include the severity of injury, the presence of associated injuries (specifically pancreatic or common bile duct injury), the time from injury to treatment, and the overall condition of the patient. Most duodenal wounds can be closed primarily by single or two layer sutures. Devitalized tissue should be debrided. Longitudinal defects may be closed in a transverse manner to prevent narrowing of the lumen.

Because of the unique anatomy of incomplete peritoneal covering and the physiology of the duodenum, possible breakdown of the suture line with resultant duodenal fistula formation or intra-abdominal sepsis is a cause of great concern. As approximately 10 L of fluid traverse the duodenum daily, including bile and pancreatic enzymes, several procedures have been developed to protect the repair. Although older publications on severe duodenal injuries all favor diverticulization and pyloric exclusion (PEX), newer work shows that when primary suture repair and PEX were compared, there were no differences in morbidity (including complications specific to the duodenal repair), mortality, and length of stay in intensive care and hospital between the two groups.[54,60] Due to the complexity of the anatomy and depending on the injury pattern under some circumstances, PEX and the triple tube technique can be

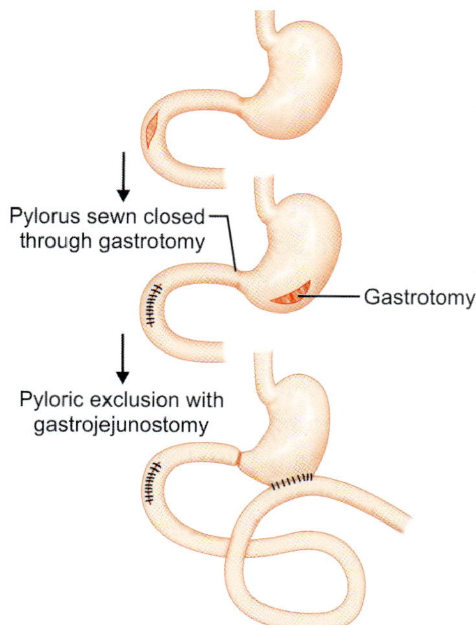

Fig. 40.17: Pyloric exclusion for duodenal injury. The exclusion of the pylorus allows healing of the duodenal injury.

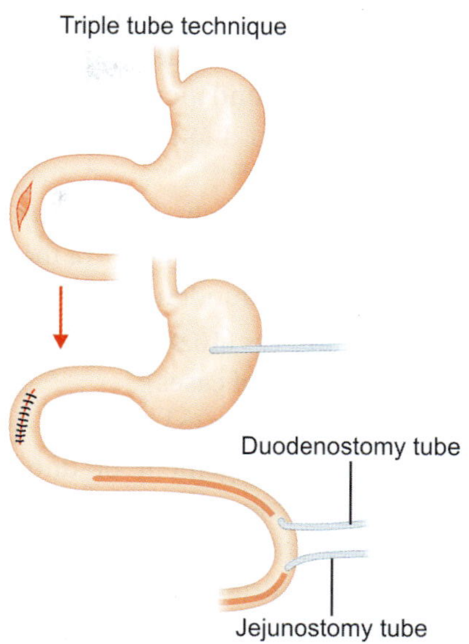

Fig. 40.18: "Triple tube" technique to manage duodenal injury. The area proximal and distal to the area of the injury is drained; feeding is through the distal jejunostomy tube.

advantageous. The concept of duodenal diverticulization consists of the repair of the duodenal injury followed by antrectomy, gastrojejunostomy, and tube duodenostomy.[65] This procedure is occasionally performed, but has been largely supplanted by the simpler technique of PEX suggested by Vaughn and colleagues.[66] This consists of primary repair followed by side-to-side gastrojejunostomy along the greater curvature (Fig. 40.17). Following gastrotomy, the pylorus is closed from inside the stomach using absorbable sutures. There was a 5% incidence of fistula among 75 patients who underwent PEX. Of the patients who had radiographic evaluation within a period ranging from 2 months to 3 years, all had a patent pylorus. Because of a low incidence of marginal ulceration, vagotomy is not required.

The "triple tube" technique in conjunction with duodenorrhaphy has also been advocated (Fig. 40.18).[64] Repair of the duodenal wound is followed by placement of a gastrostomy and two jejunostomies. The first jejunostomy tube (afferent) is placed in a retrograde fashion to drain the duodenal contents. The second (efferent) tube is placed in an antegrade fashion and used for feeding and installation of proximal tube effluent when there are large drainage volumes. When this technique was used on 237 patients, the incidence of duodenal fistula was 0.5%,[64] which is the lowest incidence reported to date. Of 44 patients in the series who did not have tube decompression, eight developed fistulas and there were three consequent deaths. A 9% incidence of duodenal fistula has been reported with a resultant 4% mortality rate following duodenorrhaphy and tube decompression.[67,68]

Large duodenal wall defects pose a serious challenge. Closure of such defects causes luminal narrowing, and the patient is usually too unstable for resection of the defect by pancreatoduodenectomy. Highly specialized repair techniques have been proposed for these unique situations. These include repair of the remnant antrum with a patch, delayed repair with a small intestinal submucosa patch, and the use of a serosal patch from the jejunum.[65,66]

Intramural duodenal hematoma may develop from blunt injury, usually as a result of shearing of blood vessels. It can be diagnosed with an upper gastrointestinal series from the characteristic signs described above. A CT scan may reveal thickening of the duodenal wall and fluid in the right anterior pararenal space. This injury can usually be managed conservatively with nasogastric suction and parenteral nutrition.[56,57] The hematoma should resolve within 7–14 days. If it does not resolve within this time, the liquified hematoma should be evacuated surgically.

Morbidity and Mortality Rates

The two major complications of duodenal injuries are as follows:

1. Fistula
2. Duodenal obstruction.

Duodenal fistula occurs as a result of suture line breakdown, usually around the fifth postoperative day. The clinical picture consists of acute deterioration with tachycardia, fever, hypotension, and increasing abdominal pain and tenderness. The rate of duodenal fistula ranges from 0% to 16.2% (average 6.6%).[47,48]

Duodenal obstruction results from narrowing of the lumen during repair and occurs in <2% of the cases.[47,48]

Other complications of duodenal injury include:

- Intra-abdominal abscess (10.9–18.4% of cases)
- Pancreatitis (2.5–14.9% of cases)
- Bile duct fistula (1.3% of cases).

The principles of management of duodenal fistula are the same as for any enterocutaneous fistula. There needs to be extensive drainage of the fistula followed by either total parenteral nutrition or enteral feeds through a jejunostomy. Meticulous skin care at the fistula site is essential because the duodenal drainage damages the skin. Any associated intra-abdominal abscesses require drainage. Duodenal fistulas that occur after PEX are end fistulas, which usually close spontaneously.[49-52] Those that occur after simple repair are lateral fistulas, which have a high output and may not close spontaneously. In the face of an uncontrolled fistula or clinical deterioration, the patient may undergo early re-exploration with duodenal exclusion (duodenal diverticulization or PEX).[49,52,53] The influence of PEX on the outcome is controversial. A recent multivariable analysis using propensity score did not show any statistically significant differences in mortality or occurrence of septic abdominal complications between those patients undergoing primary repair only or PEX. Some suggest that the use of PEX in patients with severe duodenal injuries may contribute to longer hospital stays and confers no survival or outcome benefit.[54]

Mortality rates following duodenal trauma range from 5.3% to 30% (average 17%).[34,35] Early death is usually from exsanguination due to an associated vascular injury. Late deaths following duodenal injury (6.5–12.5%) are usually related to sepsis and multiorgan dysfunction.

Death is related to several factors. Perhaps the most important is the timing of the diagnosis after the injury. Blunt injuries or a missed injury following exploration for penetrating trauma can lead to a delay in diagnosis. Lucas and Ledgerwood demonstrated a 40% mortality rate in patients undergoing surgery >24 hours after injury compared with a 14% mortality rate for those operated on within 24 hours.[55] Other factors that contribute to the mortality rate include the presence of associated injuries to the pancreas or the common bile duct, and blunt trauma as the cause of the injury.

PANCREATIC INJURY

Pancreatic injury occurs in 3–12% of patients with severe abdominal trauma.[69] Its retroperitoneal location affords the pancreas some protection from injury, but at the same time makes the diagnosis of injury difficult.

Diagnosis

It is often more difficult to make a diagnosis of blunt pancreatic injury than of penetrating pancreatic injury. Physical examination may raise the suspicion of a retroperitoneal injury if there is epigastric pain out of proportion to the examination.[69] Any soft tissue ecchymosis in the epigastrium should be noted. However, these findings are nonspecific, and physical examination is often limited by distracting injuries, intoxication, or marked central nervous system injuries.

Because a delay in diagnosis can result in appreciable morbidity and mortality rates, surgeons have tried to identify other ways to assist in making the diagnosis of pancreatic injury. As the pancreas is one of the main sources of amylase, an elevation in serum amylase following injury would seem to be a good diagnostic test, but it has been reported that only 8% of patients with an elevated serum amylase level had blunt pancreatic injury.[70,71] Current means of determining levels of pancreatic amylase have not improved the ability to diagnose pancreatic injuries,[72,73] though serum amylase may be valuable as an indicator of pancreatic injury when patients with elevated levels are identified.

The modality of choice for evaluating possible pancreatic injury in hemodynamically stable patients with blunt abdominal trauma is CT scanning,[74] particularly spiral CT technology. Subtle findings can be identified, including the presence of intra-abdominal or extra-abdominal fluid, fluid in the lesser sac, pancreatic hematoma or laceration, focal edema at the injury site, thickening of the left anterior renal fascia, fluid in the pararenal space, and fluid between the splenic vein and pancreatic parenchyma.[69,70] However, early scanning following injury may not reveal these findings, which are caused by hemorrhage and edema. Follow-up CT scans can be valuable to diagnose pancreatic injuries.[75]

Although CT scanning can be unreliable in the early diagnosis of pancreatic trauma, magnetic resonance cholangiopancreatography is very useful in trauma patients to show peripancreatic fluid collections and the ductal

Table 40.5 Pancreatic injury grading scale according to the American Association for the Surgery of Trauma.

Grade*	Type	Description of Injury
I	Hematoma	Minor contusion without duct injury
	Laceration	Superficial laceration without duct injury
II	Hematoma	Major contusion without duct injury or tissue loss
	Laceration	Major laceration without duct injury or tissue loss
III	Laceration	Distal transection or parenchymal injury with duct injury
IV	Laceration	Proximal transection or parenchymal injury involving ampulla†
V	Laceration	Massive disruption of pancreatic head

*Advance one grade for multiple injuries to the same organ.
†Proximal pancreas is to the patient's right of the superior mesenteric vein.

anatomy. Magnetic resonance cholangiopancreatography is a safe, noninvasive test that shows active leakage from the pancreatic duct and thus pancreatic disruption; it can be used in conjunction with clinical data to select patients for either interventional or conservative treatment.[75]

Emergency endoscopic retrograde cholangiopancreatography (ERCP) is safe and accurate in both children and adults, and may allow definitive treatment of ductal injury with stenting in selected patients.[76] Several authors have reported the value of emergency ERCP for diagnosing pancreatic ductal injury.[71,72,77] It has been proposed that laparotomy is not indicated if ERCP demonstrates no evidence of ductal injury. However, ERCP requires highly skilled personnel who are not normally available 24 hours a day.

Anatomy

The pancreas is situated deep in the retroperitoneum and traverses the posterior abdomen in an oblique fashion. The head is wrapped by the duodenum and the tail is intimately associated with the hilum of the spleen. The superior mesenteric vessels mark the neck of the gland. Injuries to the patient's right of these vessels are considered proximal, whereas injuries to the left are distal. The blood supply of the pancreas is shared with the duodenum and is derived from the celiac axis and superior mesenteric artery.

Associated Injuries

Associated injuries are the rule. The aorta, portal vein, or vena cava is injured in over 75% of cases of penetrating pancreatic trauma.[67] These associated injuries account for many of the deaths. Hemorrhage is the cause of death in most patients who do not survive the first 48 hours. Overall mortality rates range from 10% to 30%.

Grading of Injuries

The American Association for the Surgery of Trauma grading scale has replaced previous scales (Table 40.5). Grade I and II injuries are considered to be minor, whereas grades III, IV and V injuries are more complex.

Operative Management

Pancreatic injury should be sought after hemorrhage and contamination have been controlled. All central abdominal hematomas must be explored. The gastrocolic ligament is incised to enter the lesser sac. The stomach is retracted superiorly and the transverse colon inferiorly to allow visualization of the body and tail of the gland. Mobilization of the hepatic flexure and a Kocher maneuver are required to visualize the head and uncinate process completely. The tail and posterior aspect of the gland can be well-visualized by medial rotation of the colon, spleen, and tail of the pancreas.

All missile and knife tracts in the area of the gland require exposure and inspection. If parenchymal injury is noted, it is necessary to evaluate the duct for injury as well. Signs of parenchymal injury include:

- The presence of a central retroperitoneal hematoma
- Edema around the gland and in the lesser sac.

Signs of ductal injury include:

- Direct visualization of a ductal injury
- Complete transection of the gland
- Bile staining of the retroperitoneum.

Suspicious signs of ductal injury are:

- Laceration of more than one-half of the gland
- Central perforation
- Severe maceration.

Pancreatography is rarely indicated for the assessment of the duct. Intraoperative ERCP should be carried out rather than duodenotomy or distal pancreatic transection.

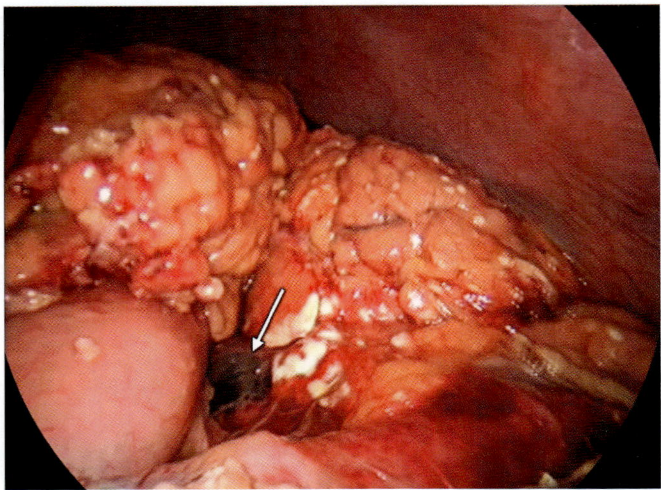

Fig. 40.19: Grade II pancreatic injury with superficial laceration and pseudocyst (arrow).

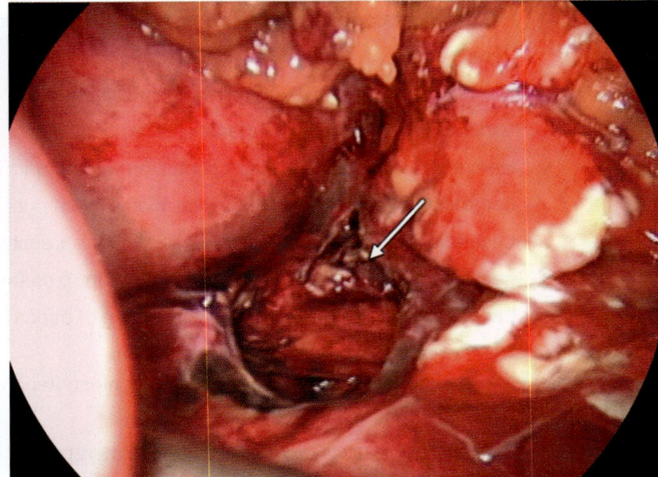

Fig. 40.20: Laparoscopic removal of necrosis (arrow) and lavage in the grade II pancreatic injury shown in Figure 40.19.

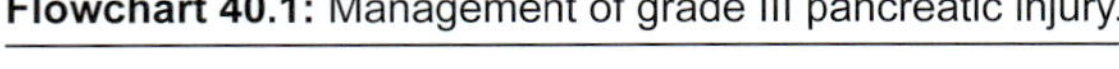

Flowchart 40.1: Management of grade III pancreatic injury.

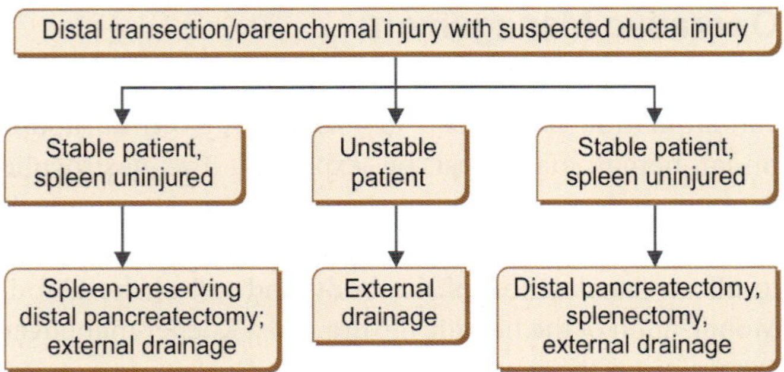

Minor Injuries (Grades I and II)

When there is no associated ductal injury, treatment of these injuries can be deferred. They are appropriately managed laparoscopically or by using an open technique with external drainage alone.[67,74-79] A hematoma or pseudocyst (Fig. 40.19) is evacuated and the area is lavaged (Fig. 40.20). The type of drainage catheter to be used seems to be the only question in the management of these minor injuries. In a prospective randomized study, closed suction drainage systems were superior to sump drainage systems because the patients treated with sump drainage systems showed an increased incidence of intra-abdominal infections.[80]

Distal Transection or Parenchymal Injury with Suspected Ductal Injury (Grade III)

The procedure of choice for grade III injuries (Flowchart 40.1) is distal pancreatectomy (Figs. 40.21 and 40.22). Complex procedures, such as distal pancreaticojejunostomy, are no longer widely practiced. They pose an unnecessary risk to the patient because a distal pancreatectomy is well-tolerated. Resection of up to 80% of the gland is well tolerated with no ill effects on carbohydrate metabolism in otherwise healthy patients.

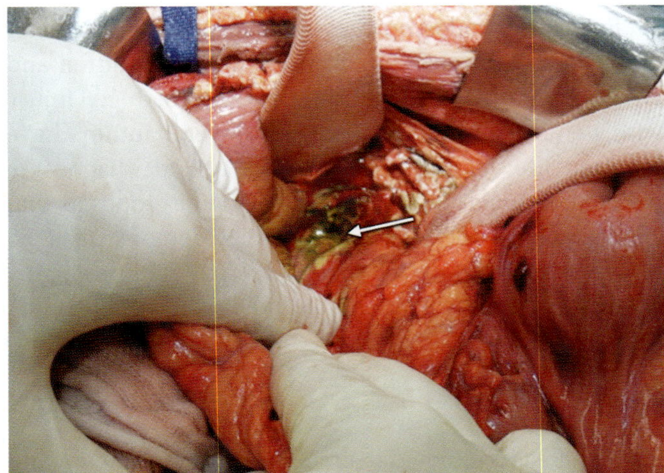

Fig. 40.21: Grade III injury with bile staining through the necrotic pancreatic tissue (arrow).

It is possible to preserve the spleen and perform a distal pancreatectomy in 50% of cases, and this operation is indicated in hemodynamically stable patients. It prevents overwhelming postsplenectomy sepsis and lowers the incidence of left subphrenic abscess.

There are several options for managing the transected pancreas. Stapling is quick and easy (Fig. 40.22). If the stump is not stapled, it should be closed with overlapping

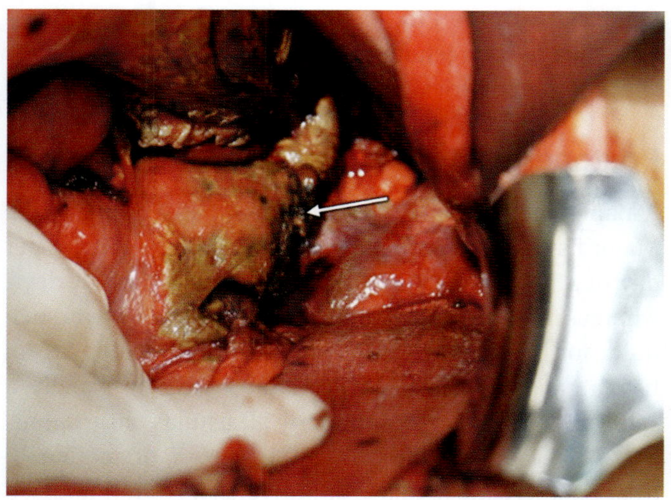

Fig. 40.22: Left pancreatectomy in the grade III injury shown in Figure 40.21. The arrow points to the stapling line adjacent to the portal vein.

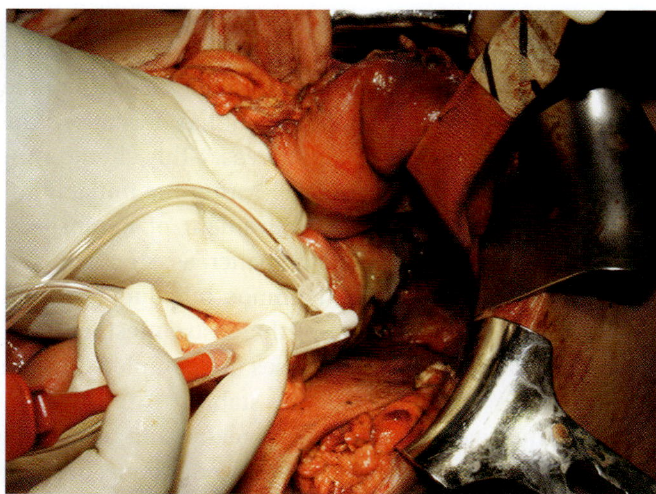

Fig. 40.23: Fibrin sealing and collagen tamponade of the stapling line to prevent pancreatic fistula.

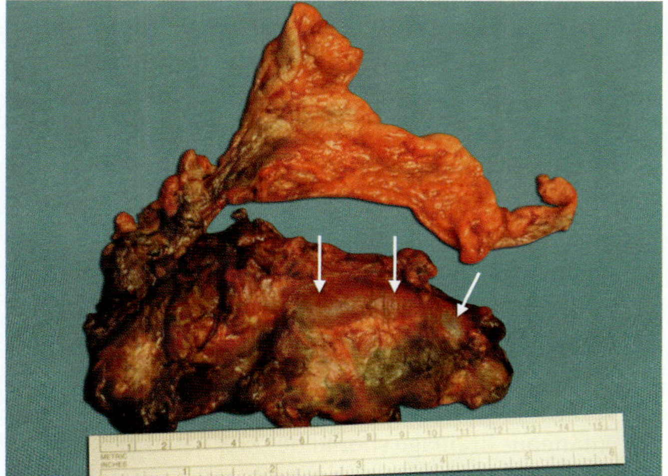

Fig. 40.24: Total necrosis of the pancreatic tail in grade III injury with ductal involvement (view from dorsal). Bile has stained the tissue green. The arrows point out the splenic vein.

interrupted U-type polypropylene stitches. Precise ligation of the duct and application of fibrin glue, preferably with a collagen fleece, may decrease fistula development (Fig. 40.23). The pancreatic bed should be drained with a closed suction drainage catheter (Fig. 40.24).

Proximal Transection or Contusion with Ductal Injury (Grade IV)

As most injuries to this area of the pancreas result in death because of the involvement of the neighboring major vascular structures, experience is limited. Management options include distal resection (up to 95%), internal drainage via pancreaticoenteric anastomosis, wide external drainage alone, and duodenal diversion procedures (Flowchart 40.2). There has been a definite movement toward conservative management of these injuries. Wide external drainage rather than resectional therapy has become the accepted method of management (Fig. 40.25).[69,81]

Flowchart 40.2: Management of grade IV pancreatic injury.

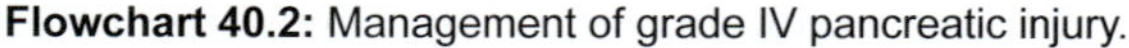

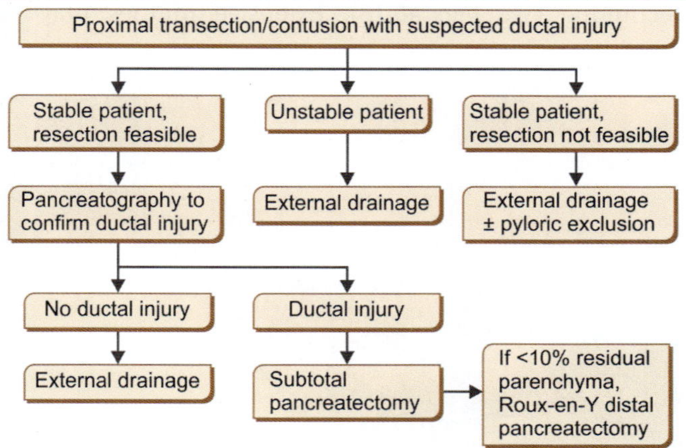

Massive Disruption of the Pancreatic Head (Grade V) and Combined Pancreaticoduodenal Injury

Associated injuries are common because of the proximity of major vascular structures and the relationship of the duodenum to the pancreas. These associated injuries are the usual cause of death. If the injuries are sufficiently extensive, pancreatoduodenectomy may be required, but this is a major undertaking in a critically injured patient. Reported mortality rates range from 46% to 60%.[82,83] It has been recommended that pancreatoduodenectomy be carried out only if the traumatic event has devitalized the duodenum and head of the pancreas.[84] This should preferably be a two-stage procedure. [85] After the initial damage control operation and achievement of hemostasis, all resected organs including the pancreas, stomach, and jejunum are stapled off. The common bile duct is ligated and drained. The continuity of the gastrointestinal tract and the biliodigestive anastomoses are completed in the following days, when the patient is stable. [86]

For extensive combined pancreatic and duodenal injuries that do not require pancreatoduodenectomy, it is preferable to decompress the duodenal and proximal pancreatic secretions (Flowchart 40.3). This maneuver may diminish activation of the pancreatic enzymes and subsequent autodigestion of the peripancreatic tissue. Diversion can be accomplished through the "triple tube" technique (*see* Fig. 40.18). Extensive injuries may be managed with the PEX technique (*see* Fig. 40.17). Placement of a feeding jejunostomy is indicated for all patients with complex injuries.

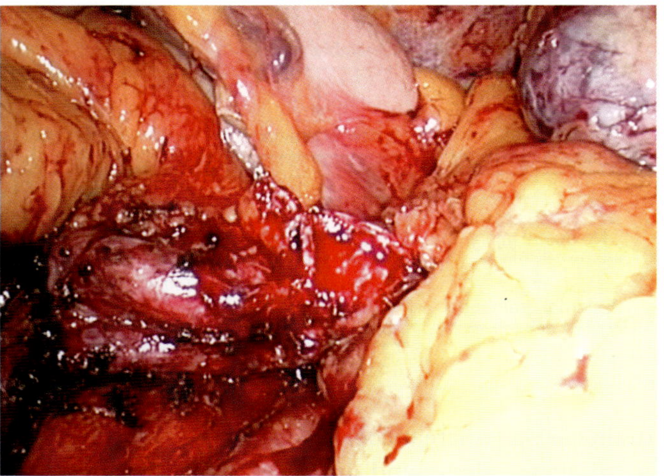

Fig. 40.25: Grade IV pancreatic injury treated by external drainage after primary hemostasis.

Postoperative Management

A pancreatic fistula is the most common complication. Major fistulas are defined as those draining >100 mL per day of a fluid with a high amylase content for >31 days, whereas minor fistulas drain <100 mL per day of such fluid for 13–31 days. Recent reported incidences of fistula range from 5% to 40%.[65,70,78,79] This is usually a self-limiting problem, and nearly all fistulas close spontaneously within 3 months.[87] The use of octreotide to treat a pancreatic fistula is controversial. No randomized prospective studies have proven a beneficial effect in trauma patients and retrospective reviews have reported conflicting results. Amirata and colleagues were largely successful in preventing pancreatic complications while using octreotide prophylactically.[88] However, Nwariaku and colleagues showed no benefit for it in their retrospective review.[89] Further prospective studies are needed before octreotide can be recommended for treatment of fistulas after pancreatic trauma.

Other complications of pancreatic trauma include a pancreatic abscess, a pseudocyst, and pancreatitis:

- A pancreatic abscess usually requires operative intervention; this can sometimes be drained by entering the retroperitoneum and abscess through the twelfth rib. Predictors of abscess formation include the presence of ductal and colon injury; if technically possible, percutaneous drainage should be considered.
- Pseudocyst formation is relatively uncommon and can usually be handled by percutaneous drainage, which may convert it to a fistula that should heal spontaneously. Rarely, a cystojejunostomy can be required to treat a recurrent pseudocyst.

Flowchart 40.3: Management of grade V pancreatic injury.

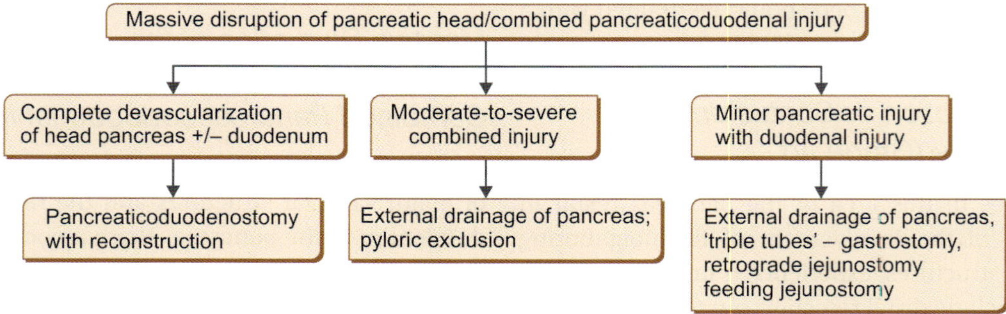

- Pancreatitis is manifested as abdominal pain, nausea, and hyperamylasemia. It usually runs a benign course and should be managed in the same way as nontraumatic cases.

SMALL BOWEL AND MESENTERIC INJURY

Most small bowel injuries are the result of penetrating trauma, but blunt small bowel injuries are increasingly seen following high-speed MVAs often due to the seatbelt. Mesenteric tears or hematomas also have this same blunt mechanism, with devascularization and subsequent full-thickness necrosis of the segment of small bowel or life-threatening hemorrhage from the mesentery (Fig. 40.26).

Anatomy and Physiology

The mesenteric small bowel (jejunum and ileum) begins at the ligament of Treitz and runs to the ileocecal valve. Its blood supply is from the superior mesenteric artery, which gives off multiple jejunal and ileal branches that form the arcades within the mesentery. It must be remembered that important digestive functions can be lost after resection of small bowel. Resection of the terminal ileum will compromise the ability to absorb vitamin B12 and bile salts. Short-bowel syndrome can develop if approximately <90 cm of the small bowel is left intact.

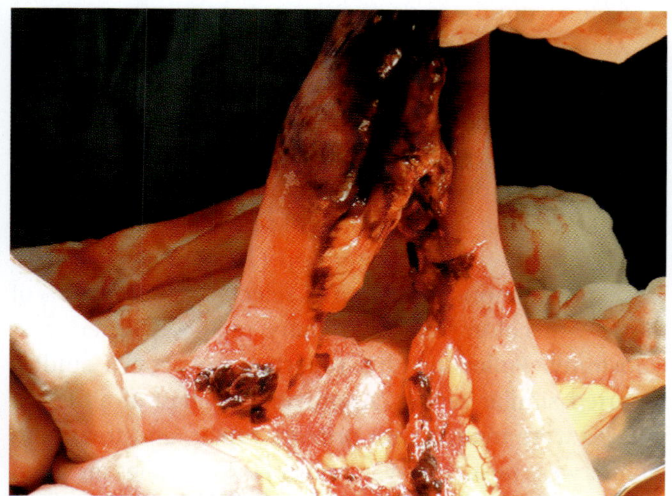

Fig. 40.26: Severe mesenteric laceration including laceration of the small bowel.

The bacterial load increases appreciably from the ligament of Treitz to the ileocecal valve. In the proximal jejunum, the bacterial load is usually < 10^4 organisms/mL, and the predominant organisms are gram positive. Moving distally, the bacterial load increases; typically there are as many as 10^8 organisms/mL. These observations have an impact on antibiotic selection for prophylaxis and therapy.

Diagnosis

The diagnosis of blunt small bowel or mesenteric injury may be difficult to make. Physical examination is often hard to evaluate because of distracting injuries or the patient's use of intoxicating substances; however, abdominal tenderness has been reported in 75% of patients with a blunt intestinal injury.[90]

Diagnostic peritoneal lavage can be a useful adjunct for making a diagnosis of blunt small bowel injury. Peritoneal contamination with intestinal contents produces peritoneal inflammation, which is manifested as an elevated white blood cell count in the lavage fluid. Several studies have, however, shown that this response may take 3 hours to appear,[91-93] and if DPL is performed >7 hours after injury, the lavage white blood cell count may be falsely elevated and result in an unnecessary laparotomy.[94]

The high resolution of scans with spiral CT technology has improved the means of detecting injury to the small bowel and mesentery. Sherck and colleagues described a constellation of CT findings (Table 40.6) that suggest small bowel injury,[95] but these findings do not necessitate laparotomy. In a more recent paper, CT had a sensitivity

Table 40.6 Computed tomography findings suggestive of small bowel perforation.[82]

	Sensitivity (%)	*Specificity (%)*	*Positive accuracy (%)*
Gastrointestinal contrast extravasation	19	100	100
Extraluminal gas*	46	99	85
Bowel wall thickening (>3 mm)	35	99	50
Bowel dilatation	15	98	22
Mesenteric thickening	4	99	3
Unexplained free fluid†	73	96	34

*Without extra-abdominal source (pneumothorax or pneumomediastinum) or previous diagnostic peritoneal lavage

†Without associated solid organ injury, bladder rupture or previous peritoneal lavage

of 64%, an accuracy of 82%, and a specificity of 97%.[96] In unclear cases, adjunctive laparoscopy or laparotomy can be helpful (Fig. 40.27).

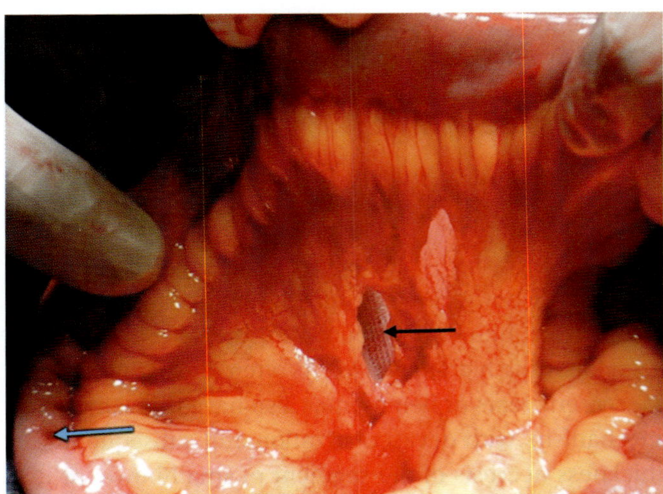

Fig. 40.27: Demarcation line of small bowel ischemia (blue arrow) due to mesenteric damage with only a small nonbleeding injury (black arrow), not visible on contrast CT scan.

Management

Damage control surgery may be required in the unstable patient, as described in Chapter 32, "Surgical Care of the Trauma Patient". Otherwise, general surgical principles are followed to control bleeding, resect severely traumatized non-viable small bowel and restore gastrointestinal continuity. Minor injuries can be sutured, taking care to avoid narrowing the bowel lumen. The peritoneal cavity is then irrigated copiously to remove any spilled bowel contents.

COLON INJURY

The main issue with injuries to the intraperitoneal colon is when to perform primary repair rather than colostomy. If the complication rate is either the same or less with primary repair, this approach is superior because of the higher costs associated with colostomy and its subsequent takedown. Penetrating injuries are primarily discussed because blunt injuries are rare.

Management

Colostomy is the usual treatment for a blunt injury, but in selected cases with minimal associated injury, primary repair may be acceptable.

Approximately 20% of abdominal gunshot wounds produce colonic injury. In the case of penetrating injury, there are sufficient data to provide some definitive conclusions. In World War II, the poor results following primary repair led to the dogma of obligatory colostomy for colon injury.[97] This approach was also applied to civilian trauma and became the standard of care until the late 1970s when surgeons began questioning whether colostomy and exteriorization were required for all wounds. The first prospective study addressing the controversy included 278 patients and was reported in 1978.[98] If the injury was severe, the patient was treated with a colostomy (the standard of care), but patients whose injuries were not severe were randomized to either primary repair or colostomy. The criteria for severity were strictly defined as follows:

- Shock—preoperative blood pressure <80/60 mm Hg
- Hemorrhage—intraperitoneal blood loss of >1 L
- Associated organ injury—injury of more than two intra-abdominal organ systems
- Contamination—major peritoneal soilage by feces
- Time after injury—operation commenced >8 hours after injury
- Colon wound—so destructive as to require resection
- Abdominal wall—major loss of substance or requiring mesh replacement.

Of the 278 patients, 139 required colostomy by the severity criteria and the remaining patients were randomized. Of those receiving primary repair, there were no leaks and the intra-abdominal sepsis rate was roughly half that of the colostomy group (15 vs. 29%, $P < 0.05$). This study demonstrated that in selected patients (50% of those with colon injury), primary repair is superior to colostomy. Following this report, retrospective studies reported similar results. Approximately half of all colon injuries were treated with primary repair, and treatment failures were rare. However, none of these studies included the more seriously injured patients, and these studies included few destructive wounds requiring resection and anastomosis.

A second prospective study was subsequently reported in which all patients with colon wounds not requiring resection received primary repair regardless of the degree of shock and associated injury.[99] There were no instances of suture line failure in the 102 cases studied. Subsequently, three prospective, randomized trials were conducted in nonselected patients.[100-102] There were a total of 99 primary repairs in these three studies with only one instance of suture line failure and no deaths. It appears that primary repair is appropriate for all nondestructive wounds regardless of the associated injury.

The most analytic evaluation of colon injury management was performed by the Eastern Association for the Surgery of Trauma (EAST), which was published as part of the organization's trauma management guidelines project.[103] The guidelines project is available on the EAST website (www.east.org). A standardized evidence-based process has been established for the guideline project. Articles are classified as class I (prospective randomized), class II (prospective or controlled retrospective), or class III (retrospective) in a similar fashion to methodologies established by the Canadian and the US Health Preventive Task Forces. Confidence levels for management recommendations are level I (well supported by class I and class II data), level II (supported by class II and strongly by class III data) and level III (management options not supported by controlled studies). For the colon injury guideline recommendations, 113 articles published over 18 years were evaluated:

- Five class I articles involving 399 patients with nondestructive colon wounds randomized to primary repair versus colostomy
- Four class II articles involving 490 patients
- Eighteen class III articles involving 1,272 patients.

There were five leaks among the class I and class II primary repairs and 15 leaks among the class III repairs, yielding an overall leak rate of 1% for the 1,861 cases of primary repair.

Less experience has been reported for primary anastomosis of destructive colon wounds. There were 40 anastomoses in four class I studies, 12 in one class II study, and 303 in 14 class III studies. There were 18 anastomotic leaks among these 355 cases, yielding a failure rate of 5%.

The EAST evaluation produced the following recommendations:

Level I

There are sufficient class I and class II data to support a standard of primary repair for nondestructive colon wounds in the absence of peritonitis.

Level II

Patients with penetrating intraperitoneal colon wounds that are destructive can undergo resection and primary anastomosis, if they:

- Are hemodynamically stable without evidence of shock
- Have no severe underlying disease
- Have minimal associated injuries
- Do not have peritonitis.

A Cochrane database with a total of 705 patients who sustained significant colonic injuries shows that primary closure is at least as safe as fecal diversion. The numbers of deaths are similar in both the primary repair (1.94%) and the diverted groups (1.74%). Total complications, total infectious complications, abdominal infections, and wound complications all favored primary repair.[104]

A very recent study identified that outcomes after colonic injury in the setting of damage control laparotomy were similar regardless of the surgical management strategy. Based on these findings, a strategy of diversion over anastomosis cannot be strongly recommended.[105]

Colostomies performed after colon and rectal trauma can be closed within 2 weeks if a colonoscopy or contrast enema is performed to confirm distal colon healing. This recommendation does not pertain to patients with nonhealing bowel injury or unresolved wound sepsis and those who are not stable.

Colonoscopic exploration is advised to rule out colon cancer or polyps before colostomy closure in trauma patients who otherwise have no indications of being at risk for these conditions.

RECTAL INJURY

Management

The three main issues in the management of rectal injuries are:

- Primary repair
- Distal rectal washout
- Retrorectal drainage.

There is much less experience with rectal wounds than with intraperitoneal colon wounds, and so definitive evaluation is impossible at present and prospective multicenter trials are required. Another problem with data analysis is that rectal wounds are lumped together in most analyses rather than stratified according to anatomic location, although anatomic considerations are quite important. The main reason that rectal wounds have received different treatment from injuries of the more proximal large bowel is the lack of serosa, which is important for secure suture repair. This, however, is not true for the entire rectum. The rectum is 15–20 cm long and runs from the sacral promontory to the anal verge. In the upper two-thirds, the anterior and lateral surfaces are covered with serosa; there is no serosa on the posterior aspect. If injury involves only the portion that has a serosa, should the wound be handled differently from more proximal colon wounds? The lower one-third is completely extraperitoneal and does not have a serosal covering.

The largest reported series of rectal trauma included 100 injuries over 10 years.[106] The authors recommended retrorectal drainage and distal washout, but the recommendations were not strongly supported by the data. In a prospective study, 48 patients were randomized over 45 months to retrorectal drainage with closed suction drains versus no drains. There were no retrorectal infections, and the authors concluded that drainage was not necessary.[107] However, the data were not analyzed in relation to the location of the rectal injury, and it is questionable whether there were enough injuries in the lower rectum in this small series to avoid a type II statistical error.

Retrospective experience with 58 rectal wounds managed over 5 years was recently reported from our institution.[108] Ten wounds were managed by primary repair without a suture line failure; 72% of the 58 cases had extraperitoneal involvement, while the remaining patients underwent colostomy. There were three presacral infections, all of which occurred in wounds to the extraperitoneal lower third of the rectum. Washout had no measurable impact. Analysis of the drainage technique used demonstrated that two of eight undrained patients developed rectal wound-related infections compared with one of 30 drained patients ($P = 0.11$). The infection in the drained patient produced purulent drainage through the exit wound, which went through the sacrum, and the patient was not systemically ill. The two infections in undrained patients were large presacral abscesses and produced septic shock (Fig. 40.28). They occurred in patients with undrained extraperitoneal rectal wounds.

If the lower rectal wound is explored and repaired, it effectively becomes intraperitonealized and drainage is likely to be of no benefit. However, if the wound is not explored, there is a threat of marked retroperitoneal sepsis, which can probably be prevented by retrorectal drainage. Wounds of the upper rectum do not benefit from drainage, but the extraperitoneal surface should be explored if there is a possibility of injury.

According to the recommendations of the American Society of Colon and Rectal Surgeons, intraperitoneal rectal injuries generally can be treated as equivalent colon trauma with primary repair without fecal diversion. However, diversion should be considered for most extraperitoneal rectal trauma. Whether primary repair of the injury is mandatory in the setting of proximal diversion is at the discretion of the surgeon. Selective application of presacral drains may be appropriate in inaccessible rectal wounds or when there are wide areas of tissue destruction.

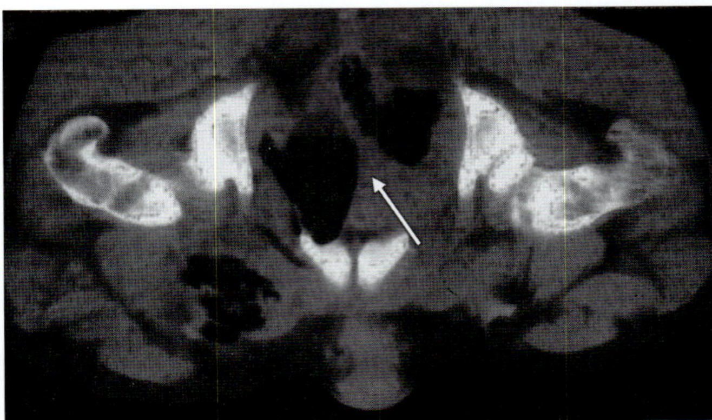

Fig. 40.28: Large presacral abscess (arrow) 1 week following a gunshot wound to the retroperitoneal rectum.

RENAL INJURY

Blunt trauma accounts for 70–90% of renal injuries. At least 90% of the blunt injuries are minor contusions that require no surgical intervention. Penetrating injuries are generally of greater impact and there is a greater chance of kidney loss. Renal injury should be suspected if the patient has gross or microscopic hematuria. Many authors, however, have reported that the degree of hematuria does not correspond to the severity of injury, so it is necessary to define which trauma patients with hematuria have a high-risk of major renal injury.

Diagnostic Imaging

Intravenous urography (IVU) was once the starting point in the evaluation of hematuria, but there has been appreciable controversy about which patients require this test. As many authors have shown that IVU is neither indicated nor cost-effective when it is ordered for every suspected renal trauma,[109-111] a more selective approach is warranted. Klein and colleagues considered that any patient with >30 red blood cells/high power field on admission, urinalysis warranted further imaging.[111] Mee and McAninch have since proposed the following criteria for determining which patients with suspected renal trauma require further diagnostic imaging:

- Any hematuria following penetrating trauma to the flank or abdomen
- Gross hematuria following blunt trauma
- Microscopic hematuria in a patient in shock following blunt trauma.[112]

There are both retrospective and prospective data to support the use of an IVU to evaluate microscopic hematuria in patients in shock following blunt trauma.[109,110,113,114]

Improved resolution with spiral CT scanning as well as the additional information gained from a CT scan provides distinct advantages over IVU studies. When intravenous contrast is given for the CT scan, the extent of renal lacerations, perfusion of the kidney, extravasation of urine, devascularization of renal segments, and the presence of perinephric hematomas can all be determined accurately. In view of these distinct advantages, a CT scan should be the initial diagnostic study in hemodynamically stable patients who may have multiple intra-abdominal injuries following blunt trauma.[115]

According to the guidelines of the European Association of Urology, CT scanning is the gold standard method for the radiographic assessment of stable patients with renal trauma. A CT scan is more sensitive and specific than IVU, ultrasonography, or angiography. In a retrospective study, the positive rate during evaluation of 298 patients was 96% by CT scanning, 91% by double-dose intravenous IVP, and 79% by ultrasonography.[116,117]

The "one-shot" IVU is often advocated before transporting an unstable patient with potential renal trauma to the operating room. The rationale behind this policy is to demonstrate the presence of two kidneys, although this should not be difficult to see at laparotomy. Stevenson and Battistella have demonstrated that this study was unwarranted.[118] In their study, 8% of patients with a normal IVU had renal injuries identified at operation and 26% of patients with an abnormal IVU had no renal injury identified at operation. Interestingly, no patient in their series of 239 patients over 4.5 years had a solitary kidney identified by a one-shot IVU. Patel and Walker reported similar results in their review of "one-shot" IVUs before laparotomy for penetrating trauma in proximity to the kidneys.[119] They reported a sensitivity, specificity, and a positive predictive value of 25%, 76%, and 20%, respectively. The "one-shot" IVU did not alter the surgical management of any patient.

Staging

Renal trauma can be classified in several different ways. The simplest is based upon the mechanism of injury. Injuries can then be divided into minor or major injuries:

- Minor injuries are contusions and superficial lacerations.
- Major injuries are deep lacerations that involve the corticomedullary junction, the collecting system, or major renal vessels.

A more precise anatomic classification has been put forward by the American Association for the Surgery of Trauma (Table 40.7).[120] It grades injuries on a scale of I–V (I is the least severe and V is the most severe). These grading scales can be used to help determine patient management, but clinical judgment must also be used and consideration given to underlying renal function, the amount of bleeding from the injury, and the presence of associated injuries.

Table 40.7 Renal injury grading scale according to the American Association for the Surgery of Trauma.

*Grade**	*Type*	*Description of injury*
I	Hematoma	Contusion or hematoma without devascularization
	Laceration	Partial thickness laceration
II	Laceration	Laceration <50% of circumference
III	Laceration	Laceration >50% of circumference
IV	Laceration	Full-thickness laceration with extension into the perineum
V	Vascular	Devascularized segment

*Advance one grade for multiple injuries up to grade III

Management

Blunt Injuries

Approximately 85–90% of blunt injuries can be classified as minor injuries, i.e. contusions, superficial lacerations of the cortex, and rupture of a renal fornix. As injuries of these types heal spontaneously, management is nonoperative.

The management of major renal injuries is unclear. Major injuries include deep lacerations that involve the corticomedullary junction, injury to the collecting system, and renal vascular injuries. Such injuries may cause urinary extravasation or they may be associated with devitalized fragments. The controversy surrounding these injuries arises from whether they require immediate surgical intervention or can be managed nonoperatively.[121]

Hussman and colleagues identified major renal lacerations with associated devitalized fragments as a predictor of failed nonoperative management (83% of those patients who required delayed surgical intervention).[122] Patients with a renal laceration and a devitalized fragment had a 38% incidence of complications if there was no other associated injury. However, if there was another intra-abdominal injury that required laparotomy, but the kidney injury was still managed expectantly, the incidence of complications jumped to 85%. By contrast, opponents of early surgical intervention point out that the chance of renal loss following early surgical intervention is greatly increased. No randomized prospective studies compare early intervention with expectant management, so the controversy persists.

The management of major renal lacerations associated with extravasation of urine is also unclear. Historically, these injuries were treated surgically to prevent persistent extravasation, delayed hemorrhage, or hypertension, but there has been a movement toward a more conservative approach, since most appear to heal spontaneously. Matthews and colleagues noted that 87% of renal lacerations associated with extravasation healed spontaneously.[123] For those associated with persistent complications, such as a urinoma, endourologic, or percutaneous drainage techniques can be used to assist in management.

Penetrating Injuries

Penetrating injuries to the kidney typically warrant surgical exploration. Minor injuries can be managed with minor debridement, oversewing of vessels, and packing with omentum or perinephric fat, but the best management for penetrating injuries is unclear. Selective management of gunshot wounds and stab wounds may be possible. Carroll and McAninch used a CT scan to distinguish between minor and major injury[124] and so avoided an operation in 8 patients. Similarly, Eastham and colleagues used both IVU and a renal angiogram to evaluate stab wounds in proximity to the kidney;[125] 63% of the patients could be managed nonsurgically or with angiographic embolization.

General Principles of Operative Management

An attempt at renal salvage is possible for stable patients but those who are unstable and have life-threatening renal injuries should undergo a nephrectomy rather than prolonged attempts at salvage. All devitalized segments should be debrided. Large bleeding vessels should be controlled with suture ligatures. Horizontal mattress sutures can be used to obtain hemostasis along the cut edge of the kidney following partial nephrectomy. A free piece of omentum or peritoneum can be used to buttress the cut surface as well. The kidney can also be wrapped with a piece of absorbable mesh to repair major lacerations,[126] and injuries to the collecting system can be repaired with fine absorbable sutures.

RENOVASCULAR INJURIES

Renovascular injuries typically result from blunt trauma, except in large urban trauma centers where penetrating trauma is the more common etiology.[127] In general, patients with penetrating injuries are severely injured and have a substantial chance of renal loss and complications. Hematuria may be a feature. Injury causes either thrombosis of the main renal artery or partial or complete laceration of the main renal artery, a segmental branch or the renal vein. Nonfunction of one kidney on IVU or lack of enhancement on a CT scan is indicative of renal artery thrombosis. A renal angiogram is the gold standard for diagnosis, but by the time the diagnosis is made, it is usually too late to salvage the kidney. Cass recommended that repair should be undertaken within 12 hours to have any chance of salvage.[128] Guerriero, however, considered that repair is needed to be done within 3 hours of injury to salvage the kidney.[129] An attempt should be made to revascularize the kidney for patients with only a single kidney or bilateral renovascular injuries. Revascularization can be performed by resecting the damaged portion of the artery followed by an end-to-end anastomosis provided that there is no tension on the anastomosis, in which case an interposition graft or some other type of bypass is required.

Lacerations to the renal artery, segmental arterial branches, or renal vein usually present as large central hematomas. These injuries can be either primarily repaired or ligated. Primary repair is undertaken with fine monofilament sutures, such as a 6-0 polypropylene. If the patient is unstable or has other life-threatening injuries, nephrectomy is indicated. Overall, the results of attempted repair of renovascular injuries are discouraging. Carroll and colleagues were able to preserve complete kidney function in only 14% of patients with renovascular injuries.[127]

PERINEAL INJURY

Although perineal injuries are uncommon, they are of great importance because they often present complex management problems. The high energy transfer is indicated by the extensive associated injuries as well as the high mortality rate. Over 50% of these patients have a pelvic fracture, which may in turn result in injury to the genitourinary tract, rectum, anus, or vagina. The mortality rate ranges from 32% to 60%,[130-133] and exsanguination is a cause of early death. Spleen and liver injuries are seen in 15–20% of patients.[134] For those who survive the initial injury, the cause of death is usually sepsis.

Evaluation

After adequate resuscitation, the patient should be given broad-spectrum antibiotics and in stable patients a CT scan is completed, which can give important information about the depth of injury and the organs involved. There can also be further injuries to other intra-abdominal organs that require prompt attention. A preoperative

CT scan can prevent an unnecessary laparotomy. Unstable patients with a perineal injury should be transferred to the operating room for evaluation. Initially any source of appreciable bleeding from the perineum should be controlled. Evaluation of the wound requires placement into the lithotomy position for the examination of the perineum as well as rigid sigmoidoscopy and vaginal speculum examination. Care must be taken when placing patients with unstable pelvic fractures into the lithotomy position.

Management

Exploration, Diversion, and Feeding Jejunostomy

Laparotomy, rather than a CT scan or DPL, is indicated to evaluate associated intra-abdominal injury as well as to create a diverting colostomy. Diversion of the fecal stream can be accomplished via a loop sigmoid colostomy, end colostomy with mucus fistula, or loop colostomy with the distal limb stapled off to provide complete diversion. This diversion of the fecal stream is necessary to prevent further contamination of these complex wounds and the development of sepsis. Washout of the distal rectum is also important. A feeding jejunostomy tube should be placed as the final step. This tube feeding helps maintain nutrition for a patient who is in a highly catabolic state and requires operations for debridement. Placement of a feeding jejunostomy tube means that enteral feeds can be administered right up to the time of operation with little risk of aspiration, whereas oral feeding has to be stopped 6–8 hours before surgery.

Perineal Wound Care

Perineal injuries are typically of a degloving type, so there is often extensive skin and soft tissue destruction. They require extensive debridement and washout with a pulsatile irrigation setup. The pulsatile irrigation system helps to significantly reduce bacteria counts in the wound.[135] In wounds in which major undermining of the perineal skin creates large skin flaps that look healthy, it is tempting to tack the flaps down loosely to obtain early closure, but this maneuver predisposes the patient to life-threatening sepsis. Although the skin may appear viable, the blood supply has usually been destroyed. The wound requires daily debridement and washout with a pulsatile irrigation system and gauze packing to prevent pelvic sepsis caused by the presence of devitalized tissue in the perineum.[131] Wound closure can be accomplished with split-thickness skin grafts or, sometimes, rotational or free flaps. During this time, fractures should be stabilized to allow mobilization of the patient and help prevent complications such as pneumonia, deep venous thrombosis, and fat emboli syndrome.

BLADDER INJURY

Most bladder injuries are the result of blunt trauma, most commonly MVAs. They indicate that a large amount of energy has been transferred to the victim. Associated injuries occur in approximately 85–90% of patients, who have an average of 2.9 injuries per patient.[136,137] Pelvic fractures are the most commonly associated injury, occurring in 70–93% of patients with bladder injury;[136-138] however, bladder injury occurs in only 5–10% of patients with pelvic fractures.[136-138] Mortality rates following bladder injury range from 12% to 44%.[17,138,139]

Diagnosis

Hallmarks of bladder injury include lower abdominal pain and tenderness in a conscious patient, microscopic or gross hematuria, inability to void, or incomplete recovery of fluids used to irrigate the Foley catheter. As urine may be absorbed by the peritoneum, there may be an elevation in blood urea nitrogen following intraperitoneal bladder rupture. There may also be an associated urethral injury, so one should check for blood at the external urethral meatus or the presence of a high-riding prostate before insertion of a Foley catheter. Either of these findings demands a retrograde urethrogram (*see* Chapter 41, "Pelvic, Lumbar and Thoracic Spine and Spinal Cord Injuries," for further discussion of urethral injuries).

A retrograde cystogram is the standard technique for evaluating bladder injuries and should be performed when there is any indication of bladder injury. It is performed by administering 300–400 mL of water-soluble contrast under gravity fill via a urethral catheter. Anteroposterior films are taken following instillation of contrast and again after drainage and irrigation of the bladder with saline. This drainage film is essential. Multiple studies have shown this technique to be 100% accurate at detecting injuries.[140] False negatives usually occur from improperly performed studies with <250 mL of contrast instillation or omission of a postdrainage film. Only a properly performed cystography should be used to exclude bladder injury.

A CT scan has also been shown to be useful for diagnosing bladder injuries. A CT cystogram can be performed by instilling 150 mL of water-soluble contrast into the bladder and then clamping the Foley catheter.

Findings to look for include:

- Free intraperitoneal contrast
- Focal extraperitoneal contrast
- A low-attenuation paravesical fluid collection.[141]

Bladder injury secondary to penetrating injury is usually identified at laparotomy, when the pelvis and bladder should be thoroughly explored. The bladder is explored by a cystotomy on the dome of the bladder; all bladder walls, the bladder neck, and the orifice of each ureter are thoroughly inspected.

Management

Numerous reports indicate that extraperitoneal bladder rupture can be managed by Foley catheter drainage alone.[142] Even in the presence of extensive retroperitoneal or scrotal extravasation, nonoperative management results in spontaneous healing in 10–14 days in 74–87% of cases.[142,143] Obstruction of the catheter by clots or tissue debris must be prevented for proper healing.

Healing can occur despite complex rupture and retroperitoneal extravasation of contrast as high as the kidneys, into the thigh via the obturator foramen, into the scrotum via the inguinal canal, up the anterior abdominal wall, or into the penis.[116,142,144] It is important to maintain adequate drainage of the bladder to prevent complications. Kotkin and Kock[143] recommend a catheter size of 22F or greater to establish adequate drainage. Surgical repair and drainage may be required if adequate drainage cannot be established.

Once a diagnosis of intraperitoneal rupture of the bladder has been made, surgical exploration and repair are indicated. The rupture should be repaired in three layers using absorbable sutures to establish a watertight closure. A suprapubic catheter should be placed through a separate stab incision. This should be a large tube (20 or 22F) to help establish adequate drainage postoperatively. A suprapubic catheter is well-tolerated by patients, and decreases the incidence of urethritis and catheter-associated epididymo-orchitis in males.

Complications

Despite good success overall with nonoperative management of extraperitoneal bladder rupture, several complications may arise, including delayed healing, vesicocutaneous fistula, sepsis, bladder calculus formation, poor drainage as a result of retained clots, and even death. Complications have been noted in 26% of patients,[143] but it was not possible to predict who was at risk for them. Death is usually a result of associated injury rather than the bladder injury itself.

Postoperative Management

A cystogram should be obtained at two days if extraperitoneal rupture has been managed with catheter drainage. If the films show no extravasation, the Foley catheter can be removed, but if leakage persists, the Foley should remain in place. If leakage persists for several weeks, a percutaneous suprapubic catheter may be placed and the Foley removed. A cystogram can be repeated weekly until there is no further evidence of leakage. At this point, the suprapubic catheter can be clamped and removed if there is no evidence of voiding dysfunction. The puncture site closes spontaneously in about 24 hours.

For patients with an intraperitoneal rupture, the cystogram should be performed at 2 weeks. If there is no evidence of leakage, the suprapubic catheter can be clamped for a voiding trial. If there is no evidence of dysfunction, the catheter can be removed.

URETERAL INJURIES

Unlike kidney injuries and extraperitoneal bladder ruptures, injuries to the ureter usually require either endoscopic or open surgical repair.

A distinction is made between incomplete and complete injuries. For the former, the continuity of the ureter wall is preserved and the treatment of choice is endoscopic catheter splinting. Depending on the extent of injury, the catheter can usually be removed after 2 to 6 weeks but after 3 months at the latest. Reconstruction is mandatory with complete transection. During the reconstruction, neither devascularizing extensive dissection nor tension should be applied to the ureter. To prevent stenosis at the anastomosis, both ends of the ureter should be widened with a lengthwise incision (Figs. 40.29A and B). Care should be taken that the ureter is not twisted and that the anastomosis is not under tension.

The surgical method to be preferred depends on the level and the extent of the injury:

- Injuries to the pyeloureteral transition or the proximal section: The ureter is mobilized as necessary and implanted directly in the kidney pelvis; a double-J stent through the anastomosis diverts drainage percutaneously from the kidney pelvis.
- Injuries to the middle third: After mobilization of both ends and limited resection of the injured area,

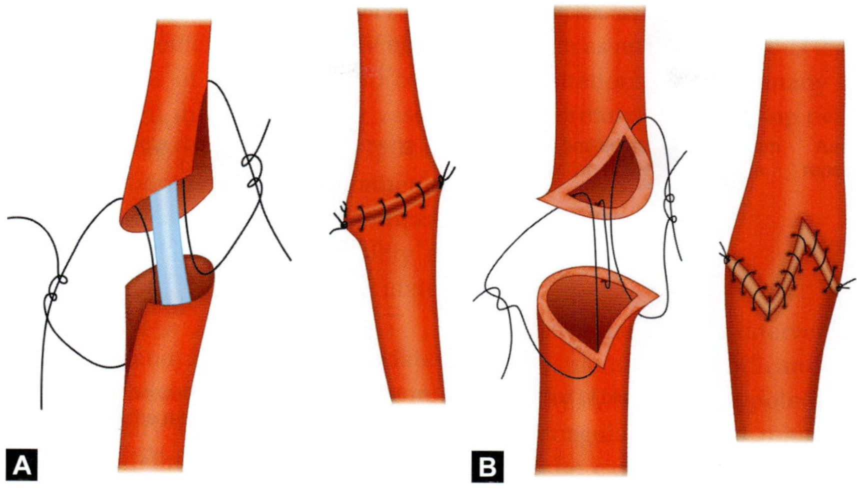

Figs. 40.29A and B: Uretero-ureteral anastomosis after lengthwise incision of both ends stented with a double-J stent (in blue) to prevent stenosis.

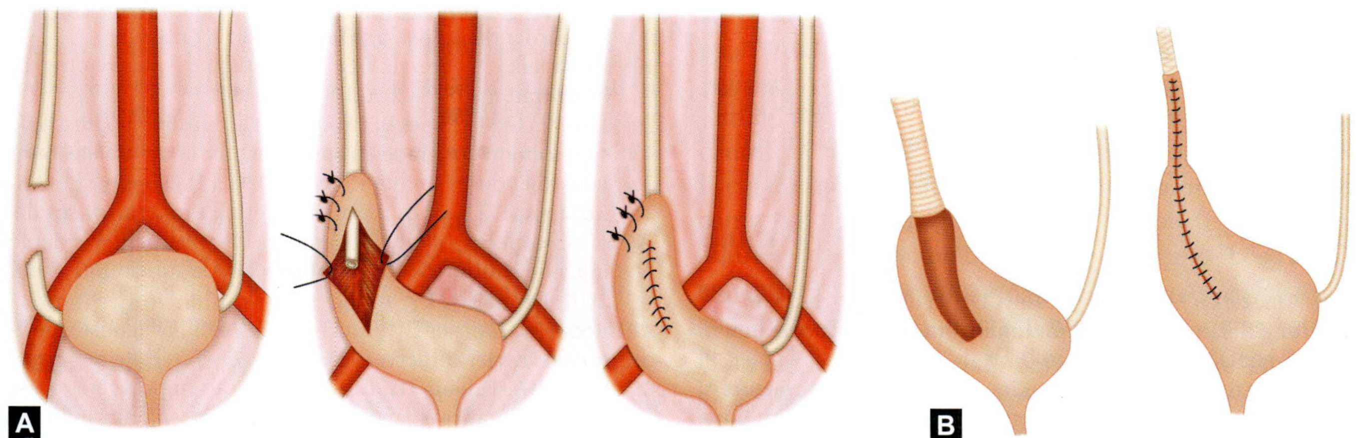

Figs. 40.30A and B: The most commonly used ureterocystoneostomy techniques: (A) psoas-hitch; (B) Boari tubulization.

both ends are widened with a lengthwise incision and anastomosed over a double-J stent with 4/0 atraumatic monofilament single button sutures.

- Injuries to the pelvic section: The best approach is implantation of the proximal end in the bladder, i.e. ureterocystoneostomy. The most commonly used technique is the psoas-hitch method (Figs. 40.30A and B); to mobilize the urinary bladder, it is partially dissected from the peritoneum and the bladder pillars and urachus are partially severed, so that a lappet of the bladder wall can be grasped and drawn up over the iliacal vessels. Then the anterior wall of the bladder is opened transversely; the spatulated ureter is drawn into the bladder lumen through a perforation in the posterior wall and fixed there with single button sutures. The lappet of the bladder is fixed to the psoas minor tendon with multiple sutures to assure that the ureter anastomosis is tension free. The bladder is closed with a lengthwise running suture and decompressed for 1 week with an indwelling catheter.
- Lengthy defects: If the distance between the proximal ureter and the bladder cannot be bridged, a trans-ureteroureterostomy is an option (Fig. 40.31). The ureter in question is drawn in the contralateral direction behind the root of the mesentery and ventral from the aorta and vena cava and implanted end-to-side in the healthy ureter.

In the postoperative course suture insufficiency can result in urinomas and subsequent abscesses, which are rare but possible complications. A ureter stenosis can be a

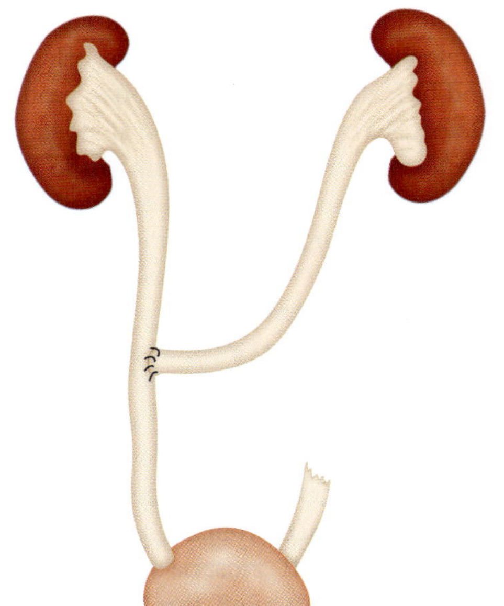

Fig. 40.31: Transureteroureterostomy.

late complication with kidney damage from urinary retention. For this reason, regular renal sonograms should be scheduled after reconstructive ureter surgery.

REFERENCES

1. Mackersie RC, Davis JW, Hoyt DB, et al. High-risk behavior and the public burden for funding the costs of acute injury. Arch Surg. 1995;130:8840-9.
2. Redeker NS, Smeltzer SC, Kirkpatrick J, et al. Risk factors of adolescent and young adult trauma victims. Am J Crit Care. 1995;4:370-8.
3. Spain DA, Boaz PW, Davidson, DJ, et al. Risk-taking behaviors among adolescent trauma patients. J Trauma. 1997; 43:423-6.
4. Glezer JA, Minard G, Croce MA, et al. Shotgun wounds to the abdomen. Am Surg. 1993;59:129-32.
5. Uranüs S. Physiology of splenic function. In: S.Uranüs (Ed). Current Spleen Surgery. Munich: Zuckschwerdt Verlag; 1995. pp. 11-4.
6. Van Wyck DB, Witte MH, Witte CL, et al. Critical splenic mass for survival from experimental pneumococcecemia. J Surg Res. 1980;28:14-21.
7. Witte MH, Witte CL, Van Wyck DB, et al. Preservation of the spleen. Lymphology. 1983;16:128-33.
8. Roth H, Zachariou Z, Daum R. Die arterielle Blutversorgung des oberen Milzpoles bei Stammarterienverschluß. Chirurg. 1987;58:828.
9. Francke EL, Neu HC. Postsplenectomy infection. Surg Clin North Am. 1981;61:135-41.
10. Green JB, Shackford SR, Sise MJ, et al. Late septic complications in adults following splenectomy for trauma: a prospective analysis in 144 patients. J Trauma. 1986;26:999-1007.
11. Malangoni MA, Dillon CD, Klamer TW. Factors influencing the risk of early and late serious infection in adults after splenectomy for trauma. Surgery. 1984;96:775-80.
12. Linet MS, Nyren Olof, Adami HO, et al. Causes of death among patients surviving at least one year following splenectomy. Am J Surg. 1996;172:320-3.
13. Uranüs S, Pfeifer J, et al. Nonoperative treatment of blunt splenic injury. World J Surg. 2001;25(11):1405-07.
14. Uranues S, Kilic YA. Injuries to the spleen. Eur J Trauma Emerg Surg. 2008;34(4): 355-61.
15. Zollinger Jr RM, Zollinger RM. (Eds). Splenectomy. Atlas of Surgical Operations, 6th edn. New York: Macmillan; 1988; 266-9.
16. Pachter HL, Hofstetter SR, Spencer FC. Evolving concepts in splenic surgery: splenorrhaphy versus splenectomy and postsplenectomy drainage: experience in 105 patients. Ann Surg. 1981;194:262-9.
17. Moore EE, Cogbill TH, Jurkovich GJ, et al. Organ injury scaling: spleen and liver (1994 revision). J Trauma. 1995;38:323-4.
18. Basso N, Silecchia G, Raparelli L, et al. Laparoscopic splenectomy for ruptured spleen: lessons learned from a case. J Laparoendosc Adv Surg Tech. 2003;13(2):109-12.
19. Dissanaike S, Frezza EE. Laparoscopic splenectomy in blunt trauma. JSLS. 2006;10(4):499-503.
20. Mostafa G, Matthews BD, Sing RF, et al. Elective laparoscopic splenectomy for grade III splenic injury in an athlete. Surg Laparo Endosc Percutan Tech. 2002;12(4):283-6.
21. Kornprat P, Uranues S, Salehi B, et al. Preliminary results of a prospective study of nonoperative treatment of splenic injuries caused by blunt abdominal trauma. Eur Surg. 2007;39(1):33-8.
22. Root HD, Hamser CW, Mckinley CR, et al. Diagnostic peritoneal lavage. Surgery. 1965;59:633-7.
23. Davis KA, Fabian TC, Croce MA, et al. Improved success in nonoperative management of blunt splenic injuries: embolization of splenic artery pseudoaneurysms. J Trauma. 1998;44:1008-15.
24. Godley CD, Warren RL, Sheridan RL, et al. Nonoperative management of blunt splenic injury in adults: age over 55 years as a powerful indicator for failure. J Am Coli Surg. 1996;183:133-9.
25. Shackford SR, Molin M. Management of splenic injuries. Surg Clin North Am. 1990;70:595-620.
26. Smith JS, Cooney RN, Mucha P. Nonoperative management of the ruptured spleen: a revalidation of criteria. Surgery. 1996;120:745-51.
27. Schurr MJ, Fabian TC, Gavant M, et al. Management of blunt splenic trauma: computed tomographic contrast blush predicts failure of nonoperative management. J Trauma 1995;39:507-13.
28. Shrock T, Blaisdell FW, Mathewson C Jr. Management of blunt trauma to the liver and hepatic veins. Arch Surg. 1968;96:698-704.
29. Stone HH, Lamb JM. Use of pedicled omentum as an autogenous pack for control of hemorrhage in major injuries of the liver. Surg Gynecol Obstet. 1975;141:92-4.
30. Madding GF. Injuries of the liver. Arch Surg. 1955;70:748-56.

31. Ivatury RR, Nallathambi M, Gunduz Y, et al. Liver packing for uncontrolled hemorrhage: a reappraisal. J Trauma. 1986;26:744-53.
32. Svoboda JA, Peter ET, Dang CV, et al. Severe liver trauma in the face of coagulopathy: a case for temporary packing and early re-exploration. Am J Surg. 1982;144:717-21.
33. Feliciano DV, Mattox KL, Jordan GL Jr. Intra-abdominal packing for control of hepatic hemorrhage: a reappraisal. J Trauma. 1981;21:285-90.
34. Fabian TC, Croce MA, Stanford GG, et al. Factors affecting morbidity following hepatic trauma: a prospective analysis of 482 injuries. Ann Surg. 1991;213:540-8.
35. Croce MA, Fabian TC, Menke PG, et al. Nonoperative management of blunt hepatic trauma is the treatment of choice for hemodynamically stable patients: results of a prospective trial. Ann Surg. 1995;221:744-55.
36. Parks NA, Davis JW, Forman D, et al. Observation for nonoperative management of blunt liver injuries: how long is long enough? J Trauma. 2011;70(3):626-9.
37. Fabian TC, Croce MA, Payne LW, et al. Duration of antibiotic therapy for penetrating abdominal trauma: a prospective trial. Surgery. 1992;112:788-95.
38. Croce MA, Fabian TC, Spiers JP, et al. Traumatic hepatic artery pseudoaneurysm with hemobilia. Am J Surg. 1994; 168:235-8.
39. Lorie FL. Historical aspects of penetrating wounds of the abdomen. Int Abstr Surg. 1948;87:521.
40. Durham R. Management of gastric injuries. Surg Clin North Am. 1990;70:517-27.
41. Siemens RA, Fulton RL. Gastric rupture as a result of blunt trauma. Am Surg. 1977;43: 229-33.
42. Edelman DA, White MT, Tyburski JG, et al. Factors affecting prognosis in patients with gastric trauma. Am Surg. 2007;73(1):48-53.
43. Coimbra R, Pinto MCC, Aguiar JR, et al. Factors related to the occurrence of postoperative complications following penetrating gastric injuries. Injury. 1995;76:463-6.
44. Brunsting LA, Morton JH. Gastric rupture from blunt abdominal trauma. J Trauma. 1987;27:887-91.
45. Murr P, Moore EE, Dunn El, et al. Stabbed stuffed stomach syndrome. N Engl J Med. 1979;300:615.
46. Coselli JS, Mattox KL, Beall AC. Re-evaluation of early evacuation of clotted hemothorax. Am J Surg. 1984;148: 786-90.
47. Asensio JA, Feliciano DV, Britt LD, et al. Management of duodenal injuries. Curr Probl Surg. 1993;30:1021-100.
48. Asensio JA, Stewart BM, Demetriades D. Duodenum. In: Ivatury RR, Cayten CG (Eds). The Textbook of Penetrating Trauma. Philadelphia: Williams and Wilkins; 1996. pp. 610-30.
49. Levinson MA, Peterson SR, Sheldon GF, et al. Duodenal trauma: experience of a trauma center. J Trauma. 1982;24:475-80.
50. Gray's Anatomy. New York: Gramercy Books; 1977.

Additional references appear in the online version of this book.

41

Pelvic, Lumbar and Thoracic Spine and Spinal Cord Injuries

Sascha Flohé, Selman Uranüs

Key Points

- ❒ An understanding of the mechanism of injury and pathoanatomy is essential to prescribe treatment in pelvic and spinal column injuries.
- ❒ Pelvic ring disruption can result in severe hemorrhage and pelvic organ injury. It is frequently associated with other distant organ injuries and carries a mortality of >40%.
- ❒ Rapid pelvic stabilization and bleeding control in patients with pelvic fractures may be life-saving.
- ❒ Pelvic ring injuries can be classified by the direction of force, namely anteroposterior (AP) compression, lateral compression, vertical shear, or combinations thereof.
- ❒ Likewise, spine injuries are classified as wedge compression fractures, stable burst fractures, unstable burst fractures, flexion-distraction injuries, or shear injuries.
- ❒ Spine injuries may be associated with complete or incomplete spinal cord injury with distal paralysis.
- ❒ Treatment of all pelvic and spine fractures, both operative and nonoperative, aims to create anatomic restoration, stability, long-term fracture healing, and restoration of function.
- ❒ In acetabular fractures, the anatomical reduction in the weight-bearing portion of the joint is the primary goal of surgery.
- ❒ The treatment of unstable pelvic fractures demands stabilization of the posterior portion and eventually also the anterior portion of the pelvic ring.

PELVIC INJURIES

Epidemiology and Mechanism

Fractures of the pelvis and acetabulum have been associated with a variety of injury mechanisms. In healthy adults, high-energy injuries, such as those caused by motor vehicle accidents (MVAs), falls from a height, or collisions as a pedestrian in which a large change in velocity occurs, are associated with dislocated fractures of the pelvis with disruption of both the anterior and posterior portions of the pelvic ring. These fractures are frequently combined with injuries to the pelvic viscera as well as with remote organ injury. In older individuals with osteoporosis, as well as in those with other pathologic conditions that result in increased bony fragility, low-energy trauma (such as falls from a standing position) can cause pelvic fractures. These low-energy injuries usually result in stable fractures and are only rarely associated with substantial pelvic visceral injury but can result in severely displaced multifragmentary fractures. The incidence of pelvic fractures is from 19-36 per 100,000 of the population per year.

Principally pelvic ring injuries can be divided into several groups based on the mechanism of injury as follows:

- Force in an AP direction through the pelvis
- Lateral compression mechanism of injury to the pelvis
- Vertical (posteriorly and superiorly directed) shear force
- A combination of these mechanisms.

Understanding the mechanism of injury and the vectors of force transmission to the pelvis can help the treating physician predict the potential patterns of injury that may be associated with a given type of pelvic fracture.

Pathophysiology and Classification

Because of the rigidity of the pelvis, generally speaking a break at one point of the ring must be accompanied by a disruption at a second point. Exceptions are direct blows, which include acetabular fractures and pediatric fractures as children have an increased flexibility of the ring. In many cases, the second break is not directly evident. Nevertheless the degree of disruption of the pelvic ring is the basis for most classifications of pelvic injuries. In the middle of the 19th century, the first classification of pelvic fractures was introduced by Joseph-François Malgaigne, who first realized that fractures occur in the anterior and/or posterior pelvic ring. Meanwhile pelvic ring injuries are most commonly classified according to the Tile classification[1] or the Arbeitsgemeinschaft für Osteosynthesfragen (AO) classification, and the Young and Burgess classification, which all follow more or less the same principles defining the injury pattern based on the predominant force leading to the fracture dislocation. In the AO classification, the pelvic ring belongs to the region 6/1, the further subdistribution follows the components of the Tile-classification described below.

Lateral compression injuries

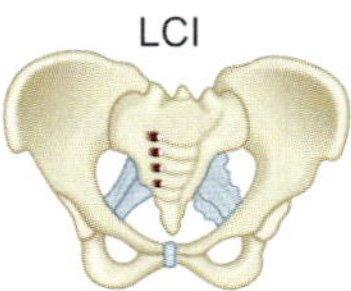
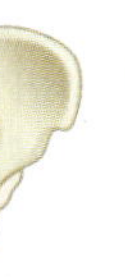

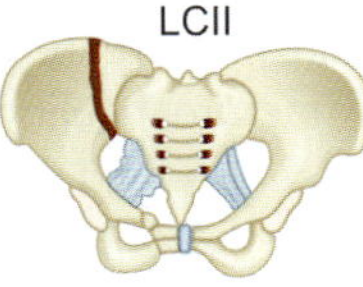

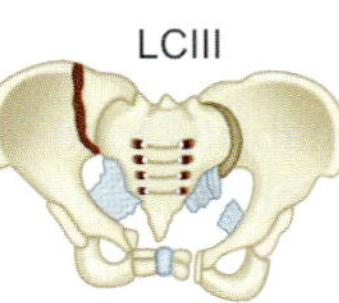

Anteroposterior compression injuries

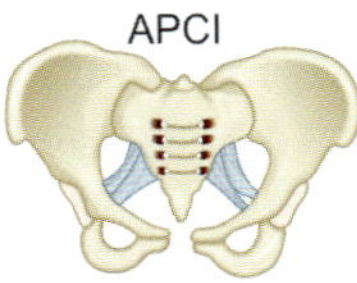
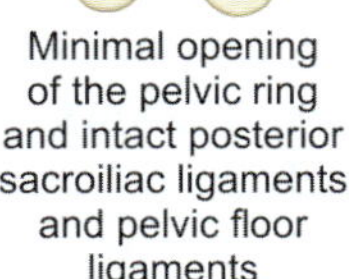

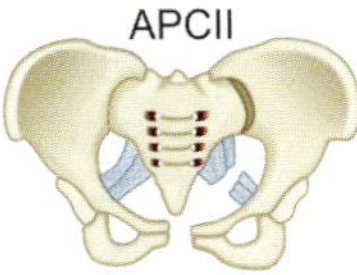

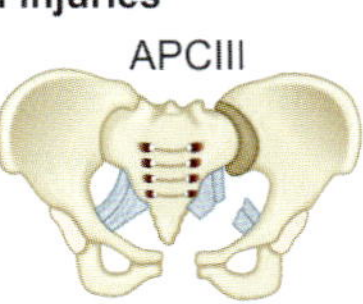

Vertical shear injury

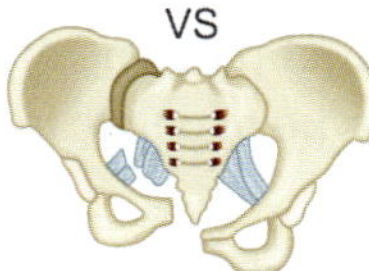

Combined mechanical injury

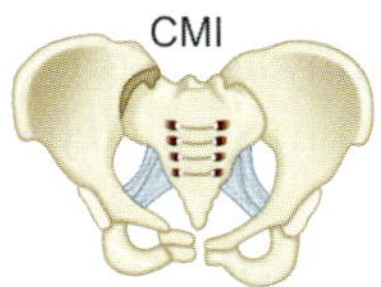

Fig. 41.1: The Young and colleagues[2-4] classification of pelvic ring injuries. *Source:* Adapted with permission from Burgess AR. Fractures of the pelvis. Part I. The pelvic ring. In: Rockwood CA Jr, Green DP, Bucholz RW (eds). Fractures in Adults, 3rd edition. Philadelphia: JB Lippincott; 1991. pp. 1399-442.

No classification system obviates the need for a thorough understanding of the relevant pathoanatomy of a particular injury; however, classification systems can be useful if they allow the treating physician to organize information about an injury in a way that helps with treatment decisions. Many classification systems for pelvic ring injuries have been developed, but two are particularly useful. The classification system of Young and colleagues describes pelvic ring disruptions in terms of the mechanism of injury, with a goal of predicting patterns of associated organ system injury and potential for instability (Fig. 41.1).[2-4] The Tile classification system segregates injuries by the type and direction of instability they produce, with a goal of determining definitive treatment needs (Table 41.1).[1]

Table 41.1 Tile classification of pelvic ring injuries.

Type description
A Stable pelvic ring injury
A1 Fractures not involving ring; avulsion injuries
A1.1 Anterior superior spine
A1.2 Anterior inferior spine
A1.3 Ischial tuberosity
A2 Stable, minimal displacement
A2.1 Iliac wing fractures
A2.2 Isolated anterior ring injuries
A2.3 Stable, undisplaced, or minimally displaced fractures of pelvic ring
A3 Transverse fractures of the sacrum or coccyx
A3.1 Undisplaced transverse sacral fractures
A3.2 Displaced transverse sacral fractures
A3.3 Coccygeal fracture
B Rotationally unstable; vertically stable pelvic ring injury
B1 External rotation instability; open book injury
B1.1 Unilateral injury
B1.2 <2.5 cm displacement
B1.3 >2.5 cm displacement
B2 Internal rotation instability; lateral compression injury
B2.1 Ipsilateral anterior and posterior injury
B2.2 Contralateral anterior and posterior injury (bucket-handle) fracture
B3 Bilateral posterior rotational unstable injury
C Rotationally and vertically unstable pelvic ring injury
C1 Unilateral injury
C1.1 Fracture through ilium
C1.2 Sacroiliac dislocation and/or fracture dislocation
C1.3 Sacral fracture
C2 Bilateral injury, one side rotationally unstable, one side rotationally and vertically unstable
C3 Bilateral injury, both sides rotationally and vertically unstable

Source: Modified with permission from Kellam JF, Browner BD. Fractures of the pelvic ring. In: Browner BD, Jupiter JB, Levine AM, Trafton PG (Eds). Skeletal Trauma. Fractures, Dislocations, Ligamentous Injuries. Philadelphia: WB Saunders; 1992. pp. 849-97.

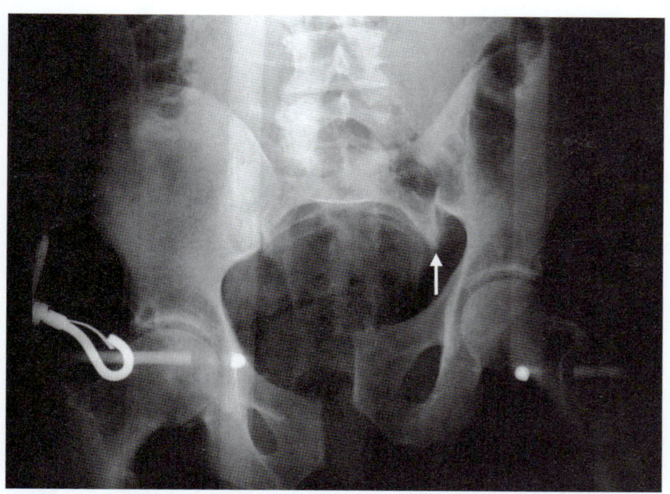

Fig. 41.2: Pelvic disruption (arrow) associated with a posteriorly and superiorly (vertically) directed force. The injury resulted in both rotational and vertical instability. This is a vertical shear injury in the Young et al. classification and a type C1.2 injury in the Tile classification.

The Young and Burgess classification[2-4] defines four basic injury patterns: lateral compression, AP compression, vertical shear, and combined mechanism. The lateral compression and AP compression injuries are each further subdivided into three groups of ascending injury severity. The value of this classification lies in its ability to correlate the pelvic fracture with associated body system injuries and the potential for hemodynamic instability secondary to intrapelvic blood loss.[5] Brain injury compounded by shock is the likely cause of death in patients who have lateral compression injuries, whereas severe AP compression injuries are associated with the largest retroperitoneal hemorrhages.

Although the Tile classification system does not address the likelihood of associated body organ system injury, it does help predict which injuries require stabilization before the onset of unprotected weight bearing.[6] Tile A injuries are stable and early mobilization is possible. Tile B injuries have some degree of horizontal plane or rotational instability. Tile C injuries (Fig. 41.2) have both rotational instability and the potential for posterior and/or superior (vertical) displacement with stress. Tile A injuries are most common and account for >50% of all pelvic ring fractures, while B and C fractures occur less often and each make up about 20% of all pelvic fractures.

Beside the bony structures, viscus organs and various anatomical structures can be associated with pelvic ring injuries. Especially dislocated C-fractures with a complete interruption of both the anterior and posterior portions of the pelvic ring have a high incidence of accompanying injures. First, pelvic fractures are a potential bleeding source with possible blood loss of ≥5 L making disrupted pelvic fractures a cause of life-threatening bleeding. The origin of the blood loss is mostly venous and is caused by an injury of the presacral venous plexus. Arterial bleeding from branches of the internal iliac artery (e.g. obturator artery or pudendal artery) occurs in about 10% of cases. Especially in transforaminal sacral fractures, injury of the lumbosacral nerve plexus occurs frequently with neurological deficits. Sacral nerve roots can be affected by displaced sacral fractures with sensation failure in the perianal region and rectal, and bladder dysfunction. This diagnosis might be missed initially in a multiple injured patient.

Injuries of the bladder and urethra are present in about 15–20 % of complex cases. It is important to clarify the exact location of the bladder injury. While an intraperitoneal injury always needs surgical repair, a retroperitoneal bladder injury can regularly heal conservatively after placement of a transurethral urinary catheter. Eventually an additional suprapubic bladder catheter is necessary. A typical sign of an intraperitoneal bladder injury is a large amount of free fluid on the Focused Assessment with Sonography in Trauma (FAST) exam without any evidence of liver or spleen injury. Injuries of the bladder can be caused by a fragment from the rami ossis pubis or indirectly by disruption of the pubic symphysis. Urethral injuries are found frequently in combination with symphysis disruption. These injuries have a high rate of secondary strictures. Delayed repair has been reported to result in a lower stricture rate than primary repair in the emergency situation. Important for male patients is the fact that in dislocated pelvic fractures, erectile dysfunction is also a frequent sequel. Finally, vagina and rectosigmoidal injuries and also vaginal lacerations can occur in patients with dislocated pelvic ring fractures. These injuries often are associated with perianal lacerations and hence are considered as open pelvic fractures with a high-risk of severe infectious complications. Pelvic ring fractures with soft tissue injuries or accompanying lacerations of vessels, injuries to urinary tract structures, or other visceral organs in the small pelvis (the cavity of the pelvis below the brim or below the superior aperture) are defined as "complex pelvic fractures". Mortality of complex pelvic fractures is >20%, while it is <5 % in "simple" type A fractures.

Initial Care

Although pelvic injury is common in multiple injured patients, an analysis of treatment error in multiple trauma patients revealed delayed diagnosis or treatment of pelvic fractures as one of the reasons for potentially preventable deaths.[7] Therefore, just as in any other trauma patient, the evaluation of an individual with a possible pelvic injury is performed according to the advanced trauma life support standards. In the trauma workup under the priority C for circulation, the clinical and radiological exam of the pelvis is demanded. Attention must be paid to the establishment of adequate venous access, particularly after high-energy injuries, because pelvic ring injuries can be associated with massive hemorrhage that is often underestimated due to its retroperitoneal location and hence the diagnosis and treatment of the hemorrhage is delayed.

During the secondary survey, attention should be paid to the resting alignment of the legs. Pelvic ring injuries associated with lateral displacement of one of the hemipelves may cause an external rotation deformity of the associated leg. If there is marked vertical displacement of one of the hemipelves, a leg length discrepancy may result. Both vascular and neurologic injuries can occur in association with pelvic trauma, so attention should be paid to the neurologic and vascular assessments of the legs. Injuries of the lumbosacral nerve plexus can occur as a result of dislocated sacral fractures. Therefore, the neurological examination should also include the perianal region and assessment of sphincter function.

Careful attention should also be paid to the examination of the soft tissues surrounding the pelvis. Areas of ecchymosis, abrasions, or open wounds should arouse suspicion of an underlying pelvic ring injury. Bleeding from pelvic fractures can cause edema in the labia or scrotum. Associated gonad or genitalia injury can occur and should be suspected in the presence of contusions or ecchymoses. Open wounds reflective of an open fracture are found in the perianal or genital region and can be missed due to a cursory examination that may have later detrimental consequences.

Pelvic stability can be ascertained by applying pressure to the iliac wings. Stress should be applied in both AP and lateral manners. Any gross motion is abnormal and should preclude any further clinical evaluation of pelvic stability as excessive motion may exacerbate retroperitoneal bleeding. Every patient with abnormal pelvic instability has to be treated by stabilization of the pelvis as soon as possible in order to prevent further blood loss. In the field or in the emergency department, pelvic sheeting or stabilization with other external devices is the treatment of choice (Fig. 41.3). Traction and internal rotation of the legs helps to reduce the pelvic ring and supports the external stabilization. More rigid external stabilization by an external fixator of pelvic C-clamp is performed in case of persisting hemodynamic instability as an emergency procedure (*see* "Emergency Management" below).

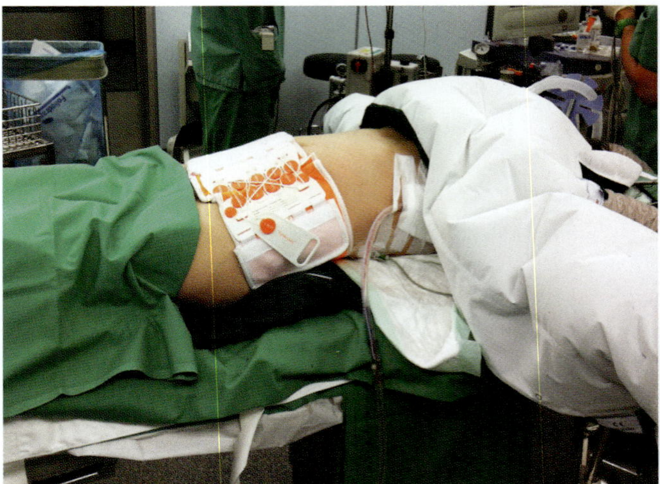

Fig. 41.3: Pelvic binder (T-POD) as initial external stabilization for C-type pelvic fracture before external fixation in the operation room.

All patients with suspected pelvic ring injuries require a digital rectal examination. Blood in the rectum may be a sign of an open fracture that has violated the rectal mucosa. Sigmoidoscopy should be carried out if a rectal injury is suspected. A high-riding prostate is a sign of disruption of the prostatic urethra. Another common sign of urethral disruption associated with pelvic ring injury is blood at the penile meatus. If any evidence suggests urethral disruption, a retrograde urethrogram should be performed before insertion of a Foley catheter.

Women with pelvic fractures require a pelvic examination that includes a careful speculum inspection of the vaginal wall for evidence of intravaginal lacerations.

Diagnosis

Among the radiographs routinely obtained during the evaluation process for trauma patients is the AP view or an urgent computed tomogram (CT) scan of the pelvis. The purpose is to seek evidence of pelvic trauma that could be associated with life-threatening hemorrhage. This view can also be used to look for sacral fractures, displaced sacroiliac (SI) joint disruptions, symphysis pubis disruptions, iliac wing fractures, and acetabulum fractures. Although some minimally displaced fractures may not be easily visualized on this single view, most fractures or dislocations that result in a markedly increased intrapelvic volume are

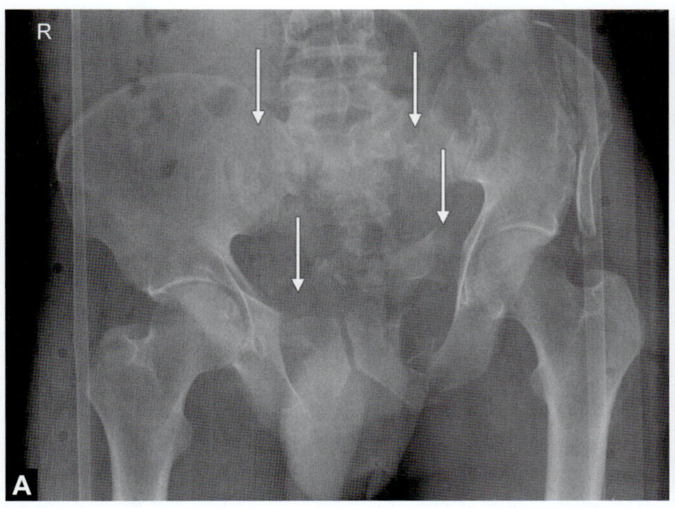

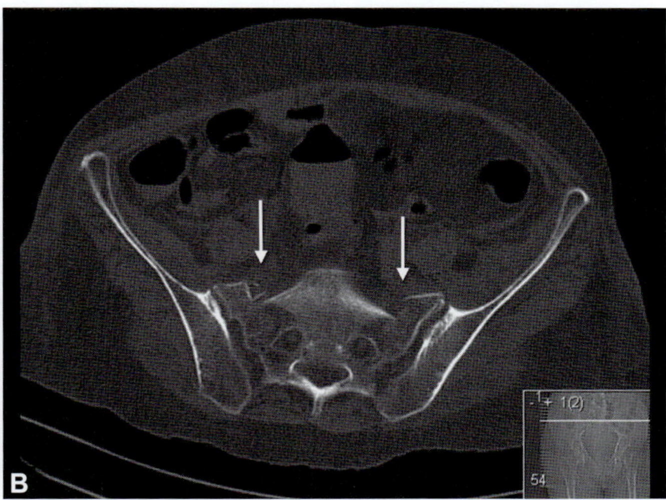

Figs. 41.4A and B: (A) Pelvic ring injury (arrows). Pelvic ring injuries that markedly increase intrapelvic volume can be readily identified with a single screening anteroposterior radiograph of the pelvis obtained during the initial evaluation process of patients who have been subjected to high-energy trauma. (B) Computed tomogram scan of the pelvis: posterior pelvic ring disruption with a fracture dislocation involving the right and the left side of the sacrum with transforaminal fractures on both sides (arrows).

readily apparent and therefore can confirm or rule out the pelvis as a source of major blood loss in the emergency setting (Figs. 41.4A and B). Inlet and outlet radiographs are useful to delineate fracture lines not readily visualized on the AP pelvic radiograph and also to determine the direction of displacement. The inlet (or caudad) view is taken with the patient supine and the X-ray beam directed 40° caudad. The outlet (or cephalad) view is also taken with the patient supine; however, in this case the X-ray beam is directed 40° cephalad.

A CT scan is the best method available for visualizing posterior pelvic ring disruptions. Displacement in all planes is readily visualized when cross-sectional scans are reformatted to produce sagittal and coronal plane reconstructions. Three-dimensional CT reformation of the pelvic image gives the best understanding of the injury and is very helpful for the surgical strategy. In all patients with signs for relevant blood loss, CT-scanning should be performed with intravenous contrast and examination of an arterial phase to rule out major arterial bleeders. The presence of intravenous contrast extravasations (ICE) is a strong indicator for the need for angiographic bleeding control. Any patient with macrohematuria or displaced fractures of the anterior pelvic ring should get an additional scan with intravesical contrast to rule out or to confirm and specify the presence of a bladder injury. Foley catheters should be inserted cautiously. If blood is on the meatus or a high riding prostate is found on rectal examination, urethrography is indicated. Blind attempts at transurethral catheterization cause further harm in the face of undiagnosed pre-existing injuries of the urethra.

Magnetic resonance imaging (MRI) can usefully delineate soft tissue injuries associated with pelvic ring disruptions; however, MRI plays no role in emergency diagnostics. Magnetic resonance imaging may be of particular value in stable patients to specify suspected vascular, nerve, or genitourinary injuries. In addition, MRI has proved useful for delineating occult fractures in elderly patients after low-velocity falls when plain films are initially normal.

Emergency Management

High-energy fractures or ring disruptions are frequently associated with substantial bleeding. Fluid resuscitation including blood and coagulation factors should begin during the primary survey. It is important to recognize that high-energy pelvic fractures or ring disruptions may be associated with exsanguinating retroperitoneal hemorrhage.[8] When the screening AP radiograph and/or clinical examination demonstrates evidence of a pelvic fracture with substantial displacement or evidence of increased intrapelvic volume, multiple large-bore upper extremity peripheral intravenous catheters or high-flow central lines should be inserted even in the absence of hemodynamic instability. For the patient who presents in extremis, early administration of uncross-matched blood is necessary. As these patients often lose massive amounts of blood, correction of coagulopathy is also necessary. The principles of a balanced resuscitation with correction of acidosis,

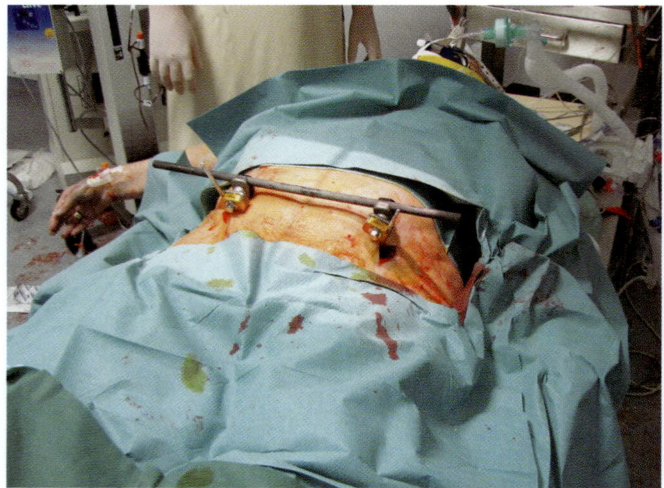

Fig. 41.5: Pelvic ring stabilized with a supra-acetabular external fixator as an urgent procedure in the emergency room in a patient with hemodynamic instability: the reduction in the pelvic volume limits retroperitoneal hemorrhage.

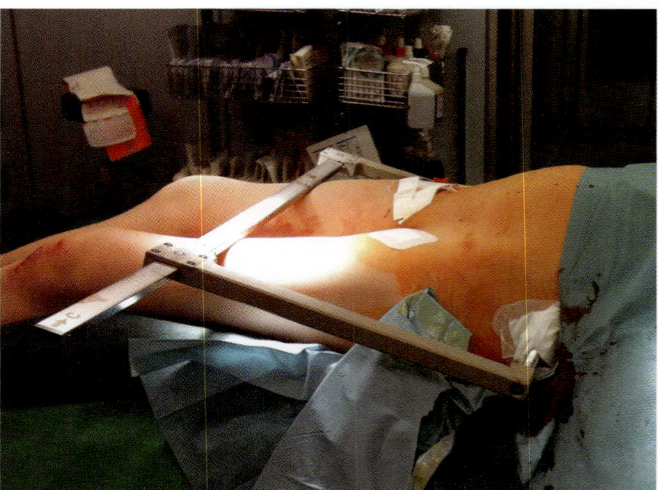

Fig. 41.6: Pelvic ring stabilized with C-clamp: the C-clamp applies maximal compression to the sacroiliac-joint and the sacrum and allows stabilization in C-type fractures of the pelvis.

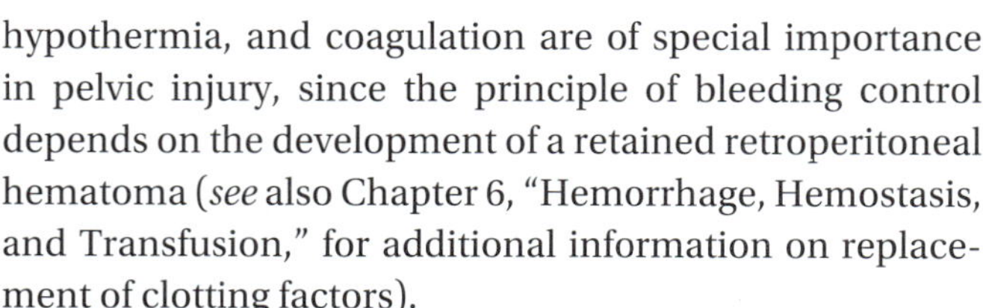

hypothermia, and coagulation are of special importance in pelvic injury, since the principle of bleeding control depends on the development of a retained retroperitoneal hematoma (*see* also Chapter 6, "Hemorrhage, Hemostasis, and Transfusion," for additional information on replacement of clotting factors).

The primary goal of all emergency surgical procedures for displaced pelvic ring fractures in patients with hemodynamic instability is the reduction in the pelvic volume by external stabilization devices. Pelvic sheeting or similar devices are the nonoperative procedures of choice; however, prolonged external compression with such devices may cause serious soft tissue injuries and complicate care in the critical care unit. For this reason, external stabilization by an external fixator (Fig. 41.5) or a pelvic C-clamp (Fig. 41.6) should be applied as an emergency surgical procedure in the operation room or in rare cases in extremis in the emergency department. The external fixator should be preferably applied in the supra-acetabular region since with this location in combination with long pins in the os ileum a certain rigidity of the posterior pelvic ring can be achieved. However, all ventral applied external fixation constructs only achieve a limited stability to the SI-joint region posteriorly. The external fixator in the iliac crest reveals less stability of the pelvic ring; however, it is an effective method of rapidly stabilizing the pelvic ring as a prerequisite for tamponading retroperitoneal hemorrhage. Anterior frames can be applied quickly for this purpose in the trauma resuscitation area even without an image intensifier. Although long-term stabilization for vertically unstable injuries is not possible using this technique, temporary stability sufficient to allow adequate resuscitation to occur can be reliably achieved in most cases. Pelvic clamps have been designed to provide maximal posterior pelvic compression in cases of wide posterior displacement. From a biomechanical point of view, a pelvic C-clamp assures maximal stability of the posterior pelvic ring. However, their use can be associated with severe complications related to the need for blind insertion of pins.

When hemodynamic stability cannot be achieved despite aggressive fluid resuscitation and external fixation (if appropriate), pelvic angiography or retroperitoneal packing may be indicated. Most commonly, in approximately 90% of cases, retroperitoneal hemorrhage secondary to pelvic ring injuries occurs as a result of venous bleeding. The major venous bleeding locus is the presacral venous plexus. In the rare instances of substantial arterial or arteriolar bleeding, angiographic embolization may control the hemorrhage. Branches of the internal iliac artery such as the obturator artery or internal pudendal artery may be possible bleeding sources. Extremely displaced pubic arch fractures should raise awareness for such dangerous situations. Retroperitoneal pelvic packing is a rather simple method that allows for rapid control of retroperitoneal bleeding. Via a vertical or horizontal suprapubic incision, blunt retroperitoneal dissection is used (most of the time this is already accomplished by the retroperitoneal hematoma) to advance to the location of the (SI) joint. Tamponade of the bleeding is achieved by the placement

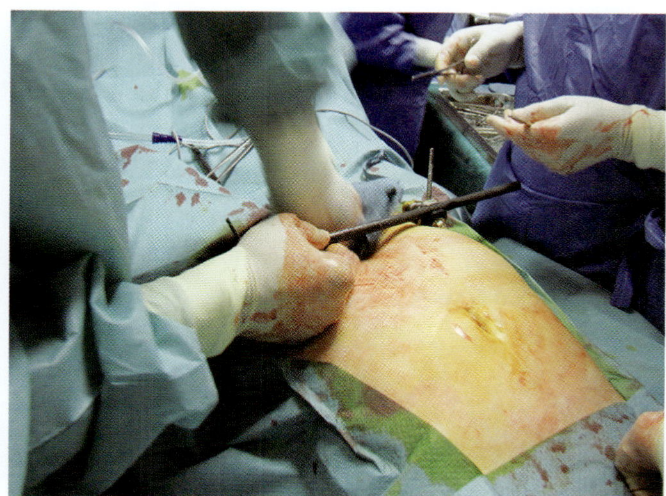

Fig. 41.7: Pelvic packing in a patient with persisting hemodynamic instability: If the patient stays in severe shock even after external stabilization of the pelvis, either pelvic packing or angioembolization is the next step to control the bleeding.

of surgical towels just ventral to the sacral bone (Fig. 41.7). This emergency procedure quickly controls retroperitoneal hemorrhage, but does need an external fixation (C-clamp or external fixator) as counterpart. There exists an ongoing debate whether angioembolization or pelvic packing is the first choice of treatment in case of persisting hemodynamic instability after external mechanical stabilization. While American guidelines give a strong recommendation for angioembolization as first treatment for persisting bleeding after stabilization, European guidelines suggest to pack the retroperitoneum or to embolize as first steps after mechanical stabilization. Good quality trials comparing both strategies do not exist.[9-11] However, these two techniques of bleeding control do not exclude each other but can easily be combined in whatever sequence.

Aggressive fluid and especially blood substitution is the baseline treatment for all patients with bleeding pelvic injuries. The correction of the trauma-induced coagulopathy is the prerequisite for the retroperitoneal tamponade and all procedures mentioned above have only a very limited rate of success in a patient with uncorrected coagulation disorders.

A large retroperitoneal hematoma after pelvic fracture affects gut motility eventually leading to a paralytic ileus. Another rare but dangerous early sequel of large retroperitoneal hematomas especially in multiple injured patients is the development of an abdominal compartment syndrome. Therefore, monitoring of intra-abdominal pressures is mandatory in these patients (*see* Chapters 40, "Abdominal, Urologic and Perineal Injuries," and 80, "Case Study: Abdominal Compartment Syndrome Following Repair of a Ruptured Aortic Aneurysm," for more information).

Open unstable pelvic ring injuries have been associated with a 50% mortality rate.[12] Early deaths are usually associated with hemorrhage or injuries to other body organ systems. Large open perineal wounds may limit the potential for intrapelvic tamponade of retroperitoneal hemorrhage, increasing the likelihood of exsanguination.[13] Late deaths usually occur secondary to sepsis and multiple organ failure. Early colostomy and rectal washout to divert the fecal stream away from the site of open injury is a hallmark of treatment. Although small anterior abdominal wounds or intravaginal wounds that communicate with the pelvic fracture can be successfully managed without a diverting colostomy, open pelvic fractures with perineal wounds mandate diversion of the fecal stream to prevent late sepsis (*see* Chapter 40, "Abdominal, Urologic and Perineal Injuries," for additional information).

Definitive Treatment

Evaluating the posterior pelvic ring stability is of important value for a definitive treatment decision. In type A fractures, the posterior portion of the pelvic ring and the SI-joint are stable, so that these fractures are principally treated nonoperatively. To permit early mobilization in the context of nonoperative management for a pelvic ring injury, the treating physician must diagnose the injury as being both rotationally and vertically stable for these injuries. Crutch walking with protected pain by limited weight bearing on the injured side can begin as soon as the patient's pain is sufficiently controlled. Type C fractures are by definition unstable and are normally not suitable for nonoperative treatment. The evaluation of the stability of the posterior portion of the pelvic ring can be insecure in laterally compressed type B fractures. In these cases, early radiological controls are recommended to notice secondary dislocations.[14]

Nonoperative management for unstable pelvic ring injuries is possible, especially in undisplaced fractures. Injuries with pure rotational instability have historically been treated with pelvic slings. Problems with this management technique include poor control of pelvic rotational alignment and the need for a prolonged period of recumbence. As external fixation is minimally invasive and readily provides for the restoration of rotational stability after pelvic trauma, there are now few indications to use pelvic slings for the management of fractures with rotational instability.

For vertically unstable injuries, skeletal traction can be used to prevent cephalad migration of injured hemipelves or to restore vertical alignment after injury. Traction can be applied through a distal femoral or proximal tibial pin. Approximately 1/10th of the patient's body weight of traction is generally necessary to prevent vertical displacement.

The use of skeletal traction for managing vertically unstable pelvic ring injuries presents problems associated with prolonged recumbence, including inadequate pulmonary toilet and sacral decubitus pressure ulcer formation. Improvement in surgical techniques for open reduction and internal fixation as well as the establishment of percutaneous techniques to treat displaced pelvic fractures has decreased the need to manage many vertically unstable pelvic ring injuries by bed rest with skeletal traction. Therefore, traction for the treatment of vertically unstable injuries is nowadays rather uncommon.

Principles of Operative Management

Operative treatment is typically chosen for the management of unstable pelvic ring injuries.[14] The goals of operative treatment are to:

- Provide sufficient stability to allow early mobilization with protected or ideally full weight bearing
- Correct any misalignments that, if uncorrected, may lead to marked leg length discrepancy
- Provide pain relief during the rehabilitation phase of treatment.

As a rule of thumb, the following principles can be applied for the surgical strategies for unstable pelvic ring fractures:

- Open book injuries of the symphysis or similar type B1 fractures are treated by isolated procedures of the anterior pelvic ring
- Rotational and vertically unstable fractures are stabilized both at the posterior and anterior pelvic ring.

Surgical Stabilization of the Anterior Portion of the Pelvic Ring

For rotationally unstable injuries, procedures are used to reduce and stabilize the anterior portion. Open reduction and internal fixation of displaced anterior pelvic ring injuries with associated rotational instability have been used successfully for certain injury patterns.

Pure pubic symphysis disruptions with a distance >2.5 cm can be approached through a Pfannenstiel incision or through an extension of a midline laparotomy incision and are ideally suited for open treatment. Open reduction is best achieved with large reduction forceps with points placed in the obturator foramina (Fig. 41.8). Symphyseal plates should be placed posterior to the insertion of the rectus muscle and screws should be drilled in the plane of the pubic arch in order to assure good stability. When the sites of instability include fractures through the pubic arch substantially lateral to the symphysis pubis, more extensive exposures are necessary to allow open reduction and internal fixation. External fixation with an iliac crest external fixator or with a supra-acetabular anterior frame (more stable) represents an alternative technique to address more complicated fractures of the anterior portion of the pelvis. Pin tract infection after external fixation may develop, especially in obese patients.

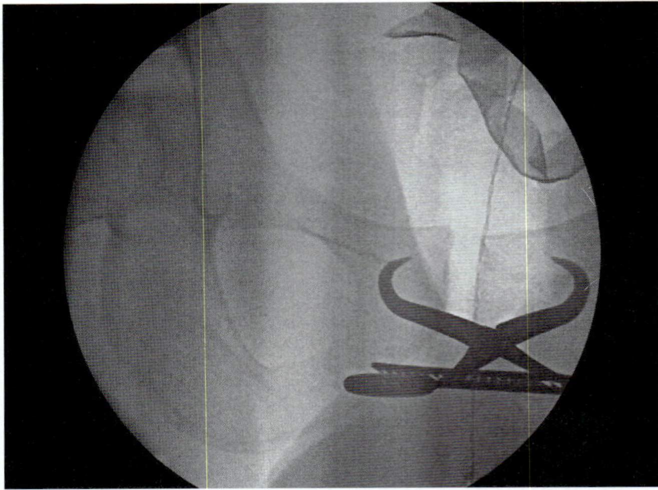

Fig. 41.8: Open reduction and temporary fixation with reduction forceps: in open book injuries with pubic symphysis disruption, a very quick reduction can be achieved by positioning large reduction forceps with points into the obturator foramen on both sides.

Surgical Stabilization of the Posterior Portion of the Pelvic Ring

The SI-joint and the posterior pelvic ring are of crucial importance for pelvic stability. For type C injuries with associated vertical instability, selection of appropriate treatment is contingent on a complete understanding of the relevant pathoanatomy of the injury. In these injuries, stabilization of both the posterior and the anterior portion of the pelvic ring is desirable.[14]

Percutaneous cannulated screws are the treatment of choice to stabilize SI-joint dislocations or lateral sacral fractures. Their placement requires a thorough understanding of the radiographic anatomy of the posterior pelvis and technical proficiency with fluoroscopic visualization of the posterior portion of the pelvic ring. The proximity

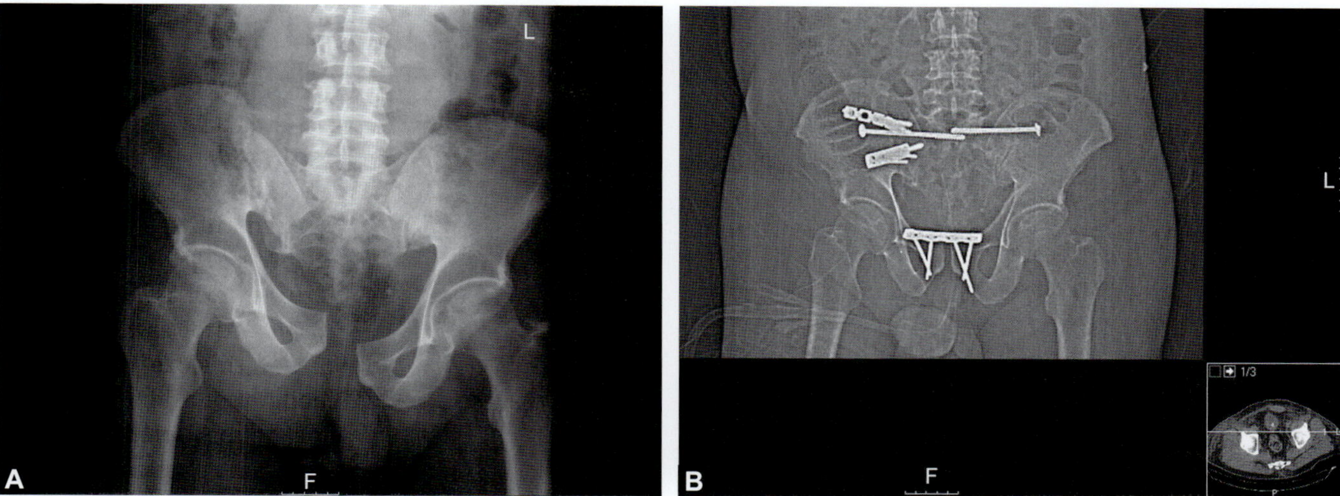

Figs. 41.9A and B: Open reduction and internal fixation of a pelvic C3 fracture by combined techniques. This example shows a combination of typical osteosynthesis of the anterior and posterior part of the pelvic ring. The right-sided posterior fracture was a transiliacal instability that was stabilized by open reduction and plating from a ventral approach. The symphysis disruption was fixed with open reduction and plating; the left-sided posterior instability was treated with percutaneous iliosacral screw fixation.

of the iliac vessels and lumbosacral nerve roots to the sacral ala requires extreme care during their insertion to ensure that the guidewires, drills, and screws remain completely within the bone at all times. Modern navigation techniques have been described to work safely in experimental and clinical settings; however, this technique is not yet generally available. Although percutaneous screws can also be used to stabilize some extremely lateral sacral fractures in much the same manner as they are used for SI-joint disruptions, treatment of fracture lines that are more medial and involve the sacral foramina or sacral spinal canal require more careful thought. Screws that create compression across medial fracture lines may impinge on nerve roots with resultant palsy. Fully threaded screws that avoid interfragmentary compression may not provide sufficient stability. It remains a matter of debate whether to place one or two screws passing the SI-joint. Placing two screws in the S1 sacral corpus or placing one screw in the S1 and one in the S2 vertebrae are options; however, the latter is technically demanding due to the small size of the pedicle and the corpus of S2. The number of screws and their position depend on bone quality, the anatomy of the sacrum as well as type of fracture. Open reduction with internal fixation using sacral bars or plates that span both iliac wings has been used successfully for some injuries, but great care must be taken to avoid iatrogenic neurologic injury. The use of dorsal iliac plates has been associated with high reported rates of soft tissue complications. In case of bony fragments in the sacral foramina and the need for open reduction, a laminectomy and open exploration of the nerve roots has to be taken into consideration. For all open posterior approaches, it is essential to wait until all posterior ecchymosis has resolved and any areas of abrasion have re-epithelialized before embarking on any posterior pelvic operative procedure. Even if operative treatment can be accomplished without neurologic or soft tissue complication, rigid fixation may be difficult to achieve and postoperative traction may be necessary to prevent late displacement. Transiliacal instabilities of the dorsal portion of the pelvic ring have to be reduced and treated by an anterior approach along the iliac crest. The first 2 cm of the lateral part of the sacrum can be considered a safe zone. A more central screw placement will affect the lumbosacral plexus. Two plates in an angle of at least 30° should be placed to assure a stable osteosynthesis. Depending on the type of fracture, all stabilization principles may have to be combined in order to achieve a stable condition in disrupted pelvic rings (Figs. 41.9A and B).[14]

A special type of injury is bilateral sacrum fractures that can occur even without a disruption of the anterior portion of the pelvic ring. In this case, there exists a complete separation of the spine from the pelvic ring. Sacroiliac screws alone give only limited stability. Additional fixation of the spine with the pelvis by screw rod systems is the only method that allows mobilization with full weight bearing. Pedicle screws placed in one or two lumbar vertebra and in the ilium are combined with SI-screws in a triangular type of construction, which results in a stable osteosynthesis allowing mobilization with full weight bearing (Figs. 41.10A and B).[15]

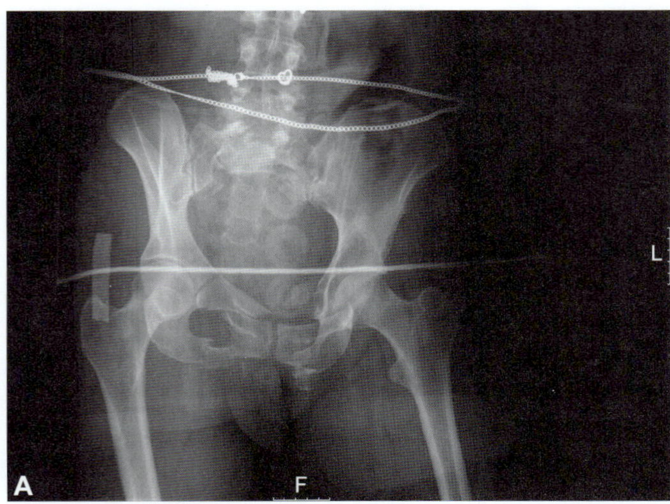

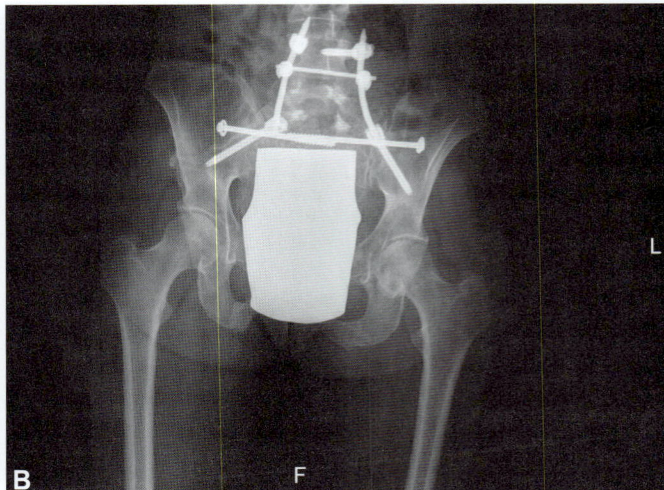

Figs. 41.10A and B: Spinopelvic fixation in a bilateral sacral fracture: this example shows a severe bilateral sacral fracture that results in a complete separation of the spine from the pelvic ring. Due to the fracture zone, iliosacral screw fixation alone gives only limited stability. For this reason, iliosacral screws were combined with a spinopelvic fixation from L4 to the ileum. The anterior portion of the pelvic ring was not addressed in this patient.

Principally in patients with type C pelvic fractures that have a complete disruption of the posterior and anterior portions of the pelvis, the fixation of the posterior part is absolutely mandatory. If the patient could benefit from early mobilization, additional fixation of the anterior portion gives maximal stability for this purpose and should be taken into consideration. The anterior external fixator is a minimal invasive technique for this aim. Normally bony consolidation begins after 3–4 weeks in this region, so that only short treatment periods with an external fixator are necessary. In multiple trauma patients, accompanying pulmonary or brain injuries often delay the mobilization process, so that in these patients the osteosynthesis of the posterior portion alone is assumed to be sufficient.

Outcome

The goal of any surgical procedure for pelvic ring injuries is to achieve and maintain adequate alignment until healing or fusion occurs. As with any operative procedure for a fracture or dislocation, there will be a failure of fixation with late deformity if adequate healing is not present before the onset of weight bearing. Therefore, early unprotected weight bearing after operative treatment of unstable pelvic ring injuries is generally not possible.

Sacral fractures and other pelvic bony injuries heal in 6–10 weeks. Soft tissue injuries, such as pure SI-joint dislocations or pubic symphysis disruptions, require 8–12 weeks before sufficient stability is present to allow weight bearing. Only fractures of the pubic arch begin to consolidate after 3–4 weeks. When nonoperative modalities (such as traction or protected weight bearing) are used, times to union are similar. Determination of the exact time when sufficient healing has occurred to allow onset of weight bearing depends upon a combination of clinical and radiographic findings as follows:

- Clinical findings include the absence of pain and tenderness at the site of injury
- Radiographic findings include evidence of bony callus formation across the fracture site.

Acetabular Fractures

Fractures of the acetabulum occur by forcing the femoral head into the pelvis, which is caused either by a blow on the side as, e.g. by a fall from a height or by a dashboard injury with a blow on the front of the knee, which typically destroys the dorsal part of the acetabulum. Acetabular fractures combine the complexity of pelvic fractures with those of joint destruction. Due to the limitations in surgical exposure, the operative reconstruction of the hip joint may be challenging.

Evaluation of the patient with a fracture involving the acetabulum begins with a physical examination, just as with any other pelvic injury. Special attention should be paid to the distal neurologic examination because many injuries of the acetabulum especially those of the posterior wall or posterior column are associated with disrupted sciatic nerve function.

Radiographic evaluation of the acetabulum should include Judet views.[16] Letournel described a series of radiographs that help to determine the exact pathoanatomy of a particular acetabulum fracture.[16] These views include the standard AP view pelvis, an AP centered on the involved hip joint, and 45° iliac and obturator oblique views of the hemipelvis. The iliac oblique view usefully shows the anterior lip and the posterior column of the acetabulum. Conversely, the obturator oblique view demonstrates the posterior wall and the anterior column. Although nowadays a pelvic CT scan with two- or three-dimensional reconstruction is the standard preoperative diagnostic study, the knowledge of the standard radiographic views is crucial for the interpretation of intra-operative fluoroscopic imaging.

Classification

Several classifications of acetabular fractures are currently popular. Letournel classified acetabular fractures in a system based on the anatomy of particular injuries.[17] This classification has been modified and further specified; however, the principles described by Letournel remain the basis for most classifications. Acetabular fractures are divided into five "simple" and five "complex" fracture types. Simple fracture patterns include anterior wall, posterior wall, anterior column, posterior column, and transverse fractures. Complex or associated fracture patterns include T-type, posterior wall plus posterior column, transverse plus posterior wall column, and anterior column plus posterior hemitransverse fractures. This classification system is useful for planning an operative treatment strategy for fractures associated with substantial intra-articular displacement or instability. The predominant dislocation and the classification of the fracture type help to select the suitable approach for the surgical repair.

Management

Early protected ambulation is possible without initial operative treatment for:

- Stable fractures
- Fractures without substantial intra-articular displacement and without an intra-articular fragment
- Fractures that involve mainly nonweight-bearing portions of the joint.

Undisplaced or minimally displaced fractures that extend into the weight-bearing portion of the articular surface may also be treated nonoperatively with early mobilization. Early radiological follow-up is recommended to detect secondary dislocation.

The weight-bearing portion of the acetabulum, also referred as the acetabular dome can be determined by the area of 45° medial from the vertical axis of the joint (so called "Matta-angle") in a plain radiograph in AP, ala, and obturator views. Open treatment is necessary to restore articular congruity for displaced fractures. Matta has demonstrated that the incidence of post-traumatic arthritis is lower and functional outcomes are improved for cases in which operative restoration of articular congruity is achieved.[18]

The operative approach chosen varies depending upon the site of greatest displacement and the complexity of the fracture. The anterior ilioinguinal approach is selected for dislocated fractures of the anterior column. The Kocher–Langenbeck approach gives a good exposition of the posterior wall and posterior column. In general, when the anterior and posterior portions of a displaced fracture segment move as a single unit, a single anterior or posterior approach will suffice.[19] If, as is common with associated fracture patterns, anterior and posterior displacements are both present and manipulation of independent fracture fragments is necessary to achieve reduction, a combination of anterior and posterior approaches are necessary. Alternatively, an extensive approach, such as the extended iliofemoral approach that exposes both the anterior and posterior columns can be used, but is associated with a higher rate of complications. Special pelvic reposition tongues are helpful in acetabular surgery. A combination of lag screws and plating allows stabilization of the joint, however, only for protective weight bearing (Figs. 41.11A and B). Minimal invasive limited approaches and computer-navigated osteosynthesis are performed in specialized centers and do not represent standard care yet. Principally weight bearing is limited for 6–10 weeks after acetabular osteosynthesis. In elderly patients, primary hip arthroplasty with special hip revision implants such as the Burch–Schneider cage represents a good alternative to joint reconstruction and also allows full weight bearing immediately after surgery. Management of acetabular fractures requires a thorough familiarity with the relevant clinical anatomy. There is great potential for severe disability after these injuries, yet with appropriate treatment excellent long-term results, even after some severe complex injuries, can be achieved. Complications the surgeon has to be aware of are a high risk for deep vein thrombosis and pulmonary embolism, iatrogenic nerve injuries and

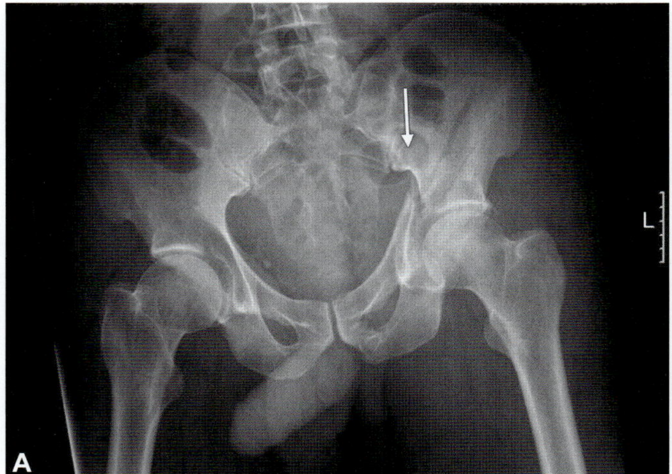

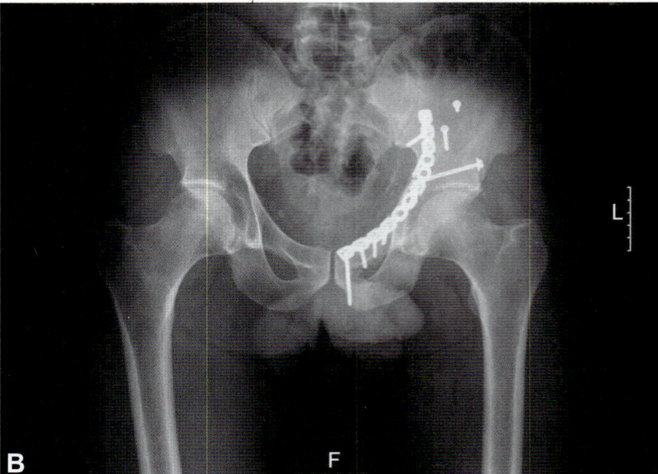

Figs. 41.11A and B: Fracture involving the left acetabulum (arrow). There is extension of the fracture line into the iliac wings superiorly and medial subluxation of the femoral head. It is a complex two column fracture, with the major dislocation of the anterior column. Open reduction and osteosynthesis with hip joint reconstruction was done in this example from a ventral over an ilioinguinal approach. Surgical treatment for these injuries is aimed at restoration of articular congruity to decrease the risk of post-traumatic arthritis associated with these injuries.

especially after dorsal surgical approaches the development of periarticular ossifications is rather common. The use of appropriate deep venous thrombosis prophylaxis is mandatory (*see* Chapter 88, "Venous Diseases").

THORACIC AND LUMBAR SPINE AND SPINAL CORD INJURIES

Epidemiology and Mechanism

Injuries to the spine and spinal cord occur as a result of a variety of mechanisms. The potentially devastating consequences of such injuries require early recognition of abnormalities and a high index of suspicion for injury after blunt trauma. For every multiple injured patient, a spinal injury has to be ruled out by clinical examination and/or radiologic examinations. Falls from a height and MVAs are the most common cause of spinal cord injuries. Men are four times more likely than women to sustain traumatic spinal cord or column injury. Cervical spine injuries are covered separately in Chapter 38B, "Cervical Spine and Spinal Cord Trauma".

Pathophysiology

Injuries of the spinal cord and column have been described with numerous classification systems. The most thorough appreciation of a particular injury comes from a complete understanding of the pathoanatomy specific to that injury.

Spinal cord injuries may be complete or incomplete; the distinction is important:

- A complete spinal cord injury is one in which there is no motor or sensory function distal to the level of injury
- An incomplete lesion is one in which neurologic function exists distal to the level of injury and that has the potential for functional recovery.

A state of complete spinal areflexia, known as spinal shock, after spinal cord injuries may make determination of the presence of a complete spinal cord injury difficult. No injury can be defined as complete until spinal shock has resolved, as defined by the return of function in sacral reflex arcs (such as the bulbocavernosus reflex). If there has been no recovery 24–48 hours after the injury, the injury is determined to be a complete lesion and no later recovery can be expected.

The neurologic deficit after spine injury may be at the level of the spinal cord, conus medullaris, cauda equina, or nerve roots, depending upon the level and type of injury to the spinal column. Normally, the spinal cord ends at L1 or L2 and the L1/L2 disk level marks the end of the spinal cord and the beginning of the cauda equina. In the thoracolumbar part of the spine, the spinal canal is wide; in the middle part of the thoracic spine, the channel is very narrow. For this reason, complete transections of the spinal cord in the thoracolumbar region are very rare.

The initial injury to the neural elements is usually from blunt trauma secondary to compression by displaced bony or soft tissue elements. Secondary injury can be caused by continued compression, epidural hematoma, and ischemia.

Classification of Spine Injuries

Five major categories of injury to the thoracic and lumbar spine have been described. Injuries vary, depending upon:

- The specific anatomic structures or spinal columns involved
- The deforming forces applied to the spine at the time of injury.[20]

An understanding of both is essential to determine which injuries are inherently stable and which are at risk for progression of deformity or late neurologic injury.

Wedge Compression Fracture

A wedge compression fracture typically occurs as a result of compression force applied to the anterior column of the spine secondary to a flexion or axial loading force. There is no posterior ligamentous injury and no major failure of the middle osteoligamentous column. The pure wedge compression fracture is, typically, a stable injury. Wedge compression fractures occurring at two or more vertebral levels in the upper thoracic spine can cause progressive kyphosis and therefore secondary spinal cord compression. Multiple adjacent wedge compression fractures should be observed carefully, because currently no adequate orthotic device corrects upper thoracic kyphosis once it starts to develop. Normal kyphosis ranges from 30° to 45°. Kyphosis of >60° may require operative intervention.

Stable Burst Fracture

A stable burst fracture involves failure of the anterior and middle spinal columns secondary to an axial loading and/or flexion mechanism. Because, by definition, there is no disruption of the posterior elements, these are stable injuries and can often be treated nonoperatively eventually with bracing and early mobilization. Characteristics of a stable burst fracture include mainly the missing posterior column involvement and reduction in the vertebra body height below 1/3rd. Most stable burst fractures heal without progression of deformity, do not cause progressive pain, and are not associated with a progressive neurologic deficit. Nonoperative management is usually sufficient.

Unstable Burst Fracture

An unstable burst fracture is an injury with compressive axial failure of the anterior and middle spinal columns that also involves complete disruption of the posterior elements. These unstable injuries can lead to increasing deformity, pain, and late neurologic deficits if not appropriately managed (Fig. 41.12).

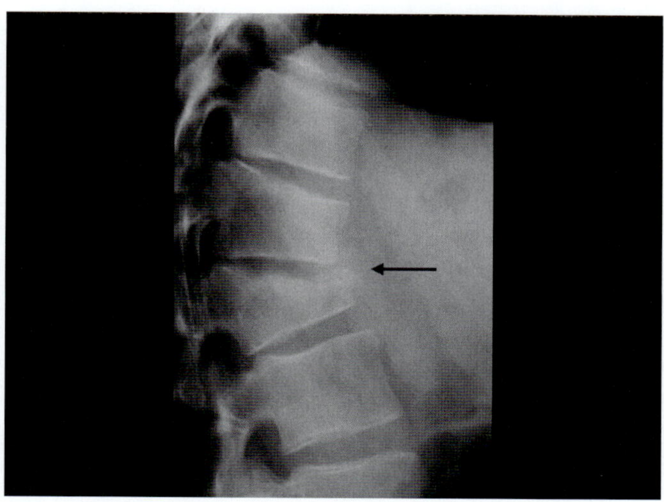

Fig. 41.12: Unstable burst fracture of L1 (arrow) sustained as a result of a motor vehicle accident. There is disruption of the anterior, middle, and posterior osteoligamentous columns, >50% loss of anterior vertebral body height, and >20°–30° of kyphosis relative to normal sagittal plane alignment at the injured segment.

Flexion–Distraction Injury

Flexion-distraction is a potentially serious injury that involves ligamentous disruption of the middle spinal column and posterior elements (Fig. 41.13). A flexion force applied to the thoracic spine usually results in a facet subluxation or dislocation. The anterior aspect of the vertebral bodies is crushed, whereas the posterior elements are distracted. These types of fractures develop after a considerable energy input to the trunk. Therefore associated injuries, especially of retroperitoneal organ (pancreas, kidneys), can be found and complicate the patients' recovery (*see* Chapter 40, "Abdominal, Urologic and Perineal Injuries," for details).

Shear Fracture

Shear fracture is defined as an injury of the spine that results from a shearing failure of all three osteoligamentous columns. These are among the most unstable of all thoracolumbar spinal injuries and are associated with the highest incidence of paraplegia and complete neurologic deficit. Treatment of these injuries is directed toward reduction, stabilization, rapid mobilization, and early rehabilitation.

AO Classification

The AO classification of thoracolumbar spine injuries according to Magerl follows similar principles. The AO classification describes three different main types of

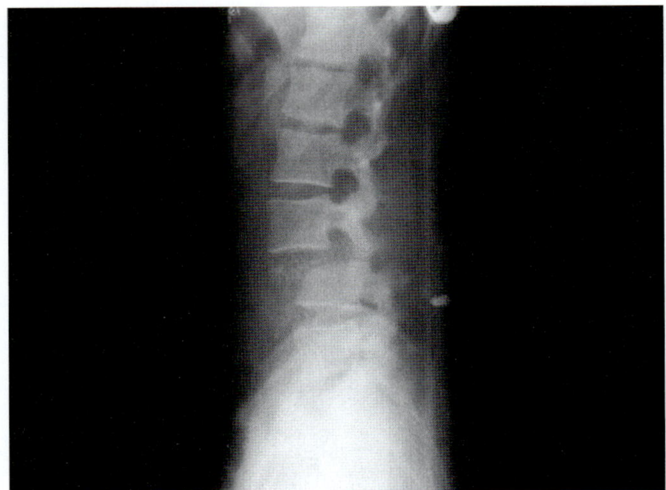

Fig. 41.13: Flexion–distraction injury involving all three osteoligamentous columns of the spine. This injury at L3–L4 involved the bony endplate anteriorly and soft tissue structures posteriorly and was associated with a complete neurologic deficit. This type of injury is often associated with the use of a lap belt without supplemental shoulder restraints.

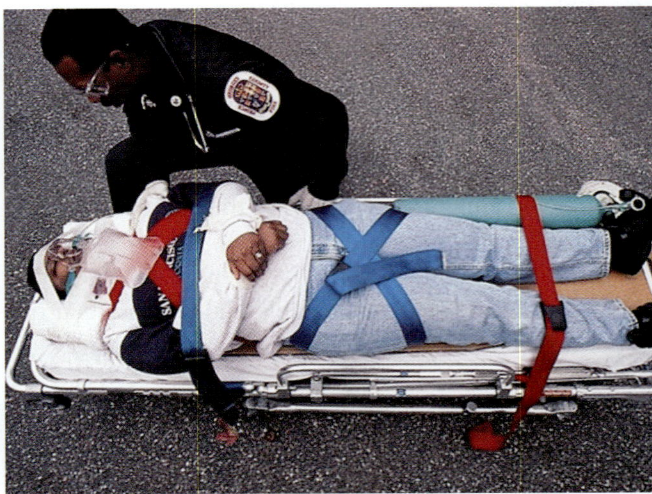

Fig. 41.14: Initial care of patients with potential spinal injuries begins in the field. The patient is completely immobilized on a long backboard. A rigid cervical collar and paracervical rolls are placed to protect the cervical spine.

fractures. Type A fractures include all types of compression fractures caused by axial loading. Stable and unstable burst fractures and wedge fractures represent the different subgroups of the type A injuries. Flexion-distraction injuries are classified as type B fractures where there is a complete disruption of the anterior and posterior parts of the vertebral column. In many cases, the posterior disruption is only present as a ligamentous injury, so that the bony deformation of the vertebral body may occur just like an incomplete cranial burst fracture. Clinical and radiological exams (MRI) may help to differentiate these two types, which is of importance since type B fractures are unstable and may need surgical stabilization. Finally type C fractures are caused by axial loading and rotational forces on the spine and affect parts of the spinal column. Spinal cord injuries are most frequent in this fracture type.

Initial Management

Initial care of patients with potential spinal injuries begins in the field. The spine must be immobilized and protected until the presence of a spinal injury has been excluded. Strict adherence to placement of a rigid cervical collar and to paracervical rolls is essential. The thoracic and lumbar spine is protected by using a long backboard (Fig. 41.14). During the secondary survey, the patient should only be moved when needed by log rolling to prevent iatrogenic neural injury. During the evaluation, the cardiopulmonary status is continuously monitored. After high thoracic or cervical spine injuries, a patient may develop neurogenic shock with clinically significant hypotension and bradycardia.

Intravenous administration of methylprednisolone for spinal cord injuries with neurological disorders is not anymore recommended for routine use. Adverse effects in terms of infectious complications overcome the very moderate and questionable benefits of a potential improvement in the neurologic status after spinal cord injury.

Diagnosis

Patients who have sustained injuries associated with high-energy trauma should be assumed to have spinal injuries until proven otherwise through physical examination and a complete radiographic evaluation. In the alert patient, physical examination includes palpation of the entire spine. Areas of localized tenderness suggest injury. Visual inspection for abrasions is important. Abrasions or contusions along the abdomen may suggest seatbelt injuries to the spine or flexion-distraction injury. Neurologic examination should be detailed and findings from manual muscle testing, sensory evaluation, and assessment of anal sphincter tone, bulbocavernosus reflex, deep tendon reflexes, and the Babinski response should all be documented.

Imaging of the thoracic and lumbar spine, when indicated, should include AP and lateral plain radiographic images. Noncontiguous spinal injuries occur in 5–20%

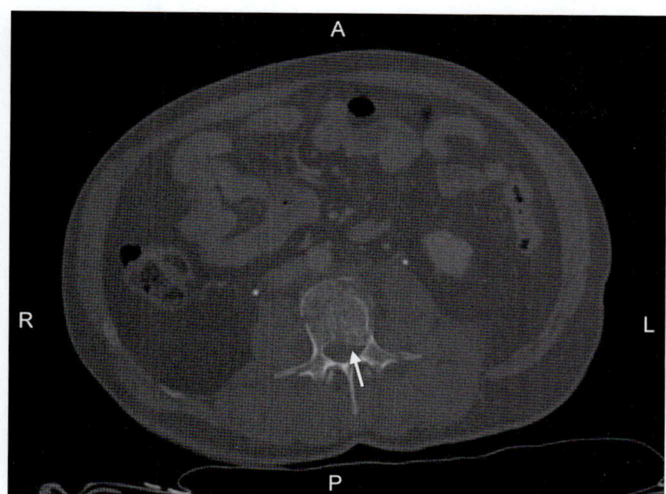

Fig. 41.15: Burst fracture at the thoracolumbar junction revealed by computed tomogram scan. There is involvement of all three osteoligamentous columns and marked retropulsion of bone from the vertebral body into the spinal canal, particularly on the left side (arrow). This injury was associated with an incomplete neurologic deficit.

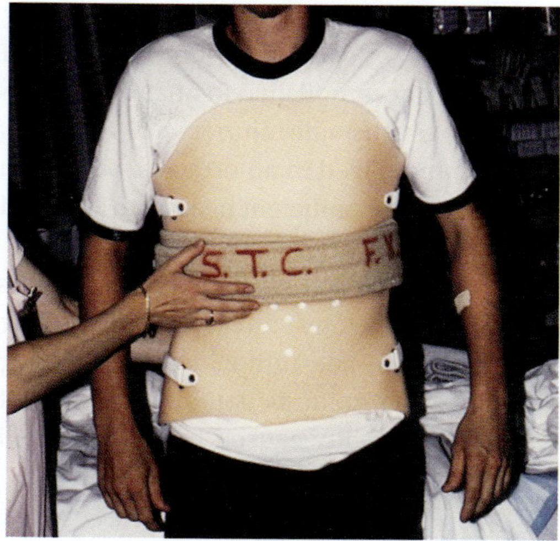

Fig. 41.16: Total contact orthosis. This may be applied to treat inherently stable thoracic or lumbar spine injuries or to provide some additional stability for otherwise relatively stable spinal injuries that are managed nonoperatively with early mobilization. This patient sustained a stable burst fracture at T12 that was treated nonoperatively. Before mobilization, this molded orthosis was applied.

of patients with spinal fractures; therefore, a patient with one spinal injury should routinely undergo radiographic evaluation of the entire spinal column.

After recognizing a spinal fracture on plain radiographs, CT evaluation should be considered. The true extent of canal compromise may be under-represented on plain images and is more accurately visualized with CT imaging (Fig. 41.15). Due to a considerable amount of missed injuries in plain radiographs, a liberal use of CT evaluation, if available, is recommended also as a primary screening method. For cervical spine injuries, CT evaluation is nowadays the first diagnostic tool; in lumbar spine injuries, it is increasingly used.

Magnetic resonance imaging can be very helpful in supplementing CT scans for patients with spinal cord injury. Although CT scanning better delineates bony fracture patterns, MRI better demonstrates neural pathology and soft tissue injuries. Bone scans can help delineate occult pathology and especially osteoporotic fractures. In addition MRI is helpful to detect osteoligamentous or disk injuries in flexion-distraction mechanisms.

Definitive Management

The goals of treatment for thoracolumbar spinal injuries are as follows:

- Anatomic restoration of coronal and sagittal plane alignment
- Maintenance of that alignment
- Neural decompression when necessary
- Long-term fracture and fusion mass healing.[21]

For each patient, the goals must be clearly defined and the appropriate treatment methods used. Therefore, the trauma patient with a marked sagittal or coronal plane deformity of the spine (i.e. traumatic kyphosis, axial compression, and/or translation), but no neurologic deficits, only needs to undergo correction of alignment and rigid fixation; canal decompression is unnecessary.

However, the patient with kyphosis, bone fragments that impinge on neural tissues and an incomplete neurologic deficit requires realignment, canal decompression, stabilization, and fusion.

Nonoperative Management

Braces can be used to treat inherently stable fractures (Fig. 41.16).[22] The type of brace depends upon fracture pattern, level of injury, and degree of stability. A total contact orthosis can be applied for fractures between T6 and L4. Patients can be rapidly mobilized out of bed in braces that are used for 4–6 months after injury. Stable injuries at the thoracolumbar junction can be managed with commercially available hyperextension braces. In spite of a broad application of different braces for the nonoperative treatment of thoracolumbar spine fracture, the effectiveness of bracing is controversial. Although high-quality trials are missing, evidence for the effectiveness of braces for thoracolumbar fractures is missing.[23]

Unstable injuries of the thoracic and lumbar spine require restoration of stability before mobilization. This can be principally accomplished in one of the two ways:

- With time, most unstable injuries will heal and patients can then be mobilized in an orthosis, but 3–6 months' time is required for sufficient healing to allow this to be achieved safely
- If operative management for unstable injuries is absolutely necessary, bed rest must be maintained with the patient positioned flat until clinical and radiographic evidence of bony union is obtained. Such treatments have a high morbidity caused by the immobilization and are nowadays rarely done.

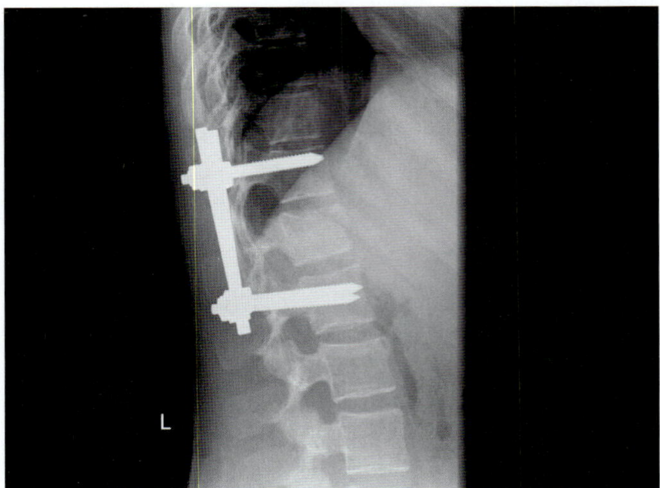

Fig. 41.17: Unstable burst fracture of L1 treated by posterior spinal instrumentation and fusion from T12 to L2. Healing of the fusion and consolidation of the fusion mass must ultimately occur or the instrumentation will fail.

Operative Management

Operative treatment can restore stability sufficiently to allow early mobilization of patients with unstable thoracic or lumbar spine injuries.[24] Spinal instrumentation can be used to correct sagittal or coronal plane deformity and to restore sufficient stability to allow for early mobilization. The purpose of spinal instrumentation is to maintain alignment until bony union occurs.[25] Dorsal instrumentation with pedicle screws and an internal fixator overspanning the fractured vertebra is a standardized established technique (Fig. 41.17). Recently, minimal invasive dorsal instrumentation techniques are available that allow similar stabilization without dorsal exposure of the spine.

Spinal instrumentation is carried out in conjunction with spinal fusion when used in the treatment of thoracic or lumbar spinal trauma. Healing of the arthrodesis and consolidation of the fusion mass are the ultimate goal of the operative procedure. Dorsal fusion techniques as well as transpedicular bone grafting do not regularly lead to complete vertebral fusion. Spinal instrumentation eventually fails if the fusion mass does not adequately heal.[26] For this reason, dorsal spinal instrumentation should be removed after 6–9 months to prevent breakage.

Operative treatment is also indicated for decompression of the spinal canal in cases of incomplete neurologic injury. Decompression of the spinal canal may result in an improvement in neurologic function distal to the zone of injury for injuries with an incomplete neurologic deficit.[27] Spinal decompression can be achieved anteriorly and posteriorly.[28,29] Direct posterior decompression for injuries above the level of L2 must rely on indirect reduction in the middle spinal column because direct exposure by retraction of the cauda equina or spinal cord is dangerous.[30,31] When operative treatment is indicated to decompress the spinal canal, concurrent stabilization should be performed. The choice of anterior or posterior stabilization is often based on the choice of approach for the treatment of the neurologic component of the injury.[32] In some complex cases with fracture dislocation (type C fractures), both anterior and posterior approaches may be necessary to accomplish both adequate decompression and stabilization (Fig. 41.18). In patients with fracture dislocation and a partial neurologic deficit, urgent spinal cord decompression and surgical stabilization are generally recommended. However, surgeons should be aware of the fact that there is no evidence that even in these cases surgical management has a better outcome than nonoperative treatment. In patients with complete paraplegia, spine stabilization is thought to shorten hospital stay and ease nursing and therefore is also the conventional surgical practice. However, also for this indication there does not exist any good evidence from the surgical literature. In an unstable fracture without neurological deterioration, surgical stabilization will allow early mobilization and enhance rehabilitation. A recent Cochrane review based on two randomized trials did not reveal any difference in outcome between patients with thoracolumbar spine fracture treated with or without surgery.[33]

A special entity of spinal column fractures with increasing incidence represents osteoporotic compression fractures, which may cause severe deformity of the spine as well as immobilizing pain with its adverse side effects in elderly patient. Beside the therapy of the underlying disease osteoporosis, the treatment of the fracture itself may

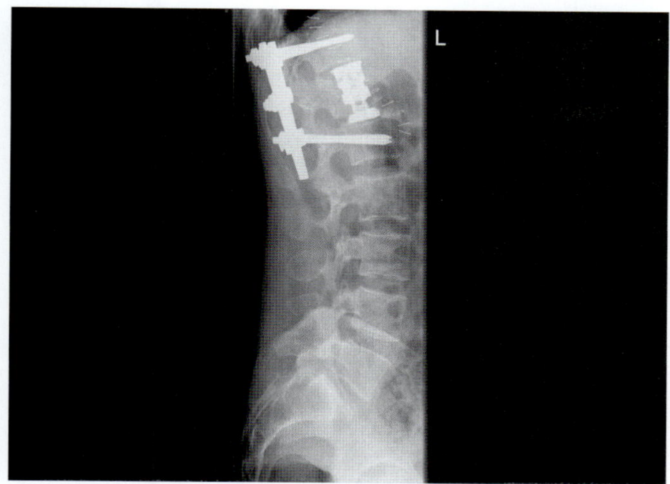

Fig. 41.18: Lumbar unstable burst fracture treated by posterior spinal instrumentation and a ventral fusion with cage. 360° fusion and consolidation is normally achieved, and implant removal is not necessary. Cages can be combined with plates for additional stability.

be challenging for spine surgeons. Cement augmentation for vertebral compression fractures as vertebroplasty and after balloon reposition as kyphoplasty are very popular procedures due to their minimal invasive character. Both procedures are considered safe and often lead to rapid pain relief. Cement extravasation is a complication that is more frequent after a vertebroplasty. For this reason, many surgeons prefer to do a kyphoplasty, since with this technique at least theoretically the compressed vertebra can be reduced. Adjacent fractures of the next vertebral body are a common problem after all cement augmentation procedures.

Complications

Complications of the treatment of thoracic and lumbar spinal injuries are common. Late deformity can occur if there is inadequate stability before mobilization. Consequences of deformity include chronic back pain and abnormal posture. Severe deformity can lead to late neurologic deficits due to secondary spinal canal stenosis.

Late deterioration of neurologic function after spine injury is rare. Exceptions to this general rule are patients with severe inflammatory and degenerative conditions that can result in abnormal spinal mechanics. Patients with ankylosing spondylitis and diffuse idiopathic skeletal hyperostosis have a predisposition to late neurologic deterioration after seemingly minimal injuries. The reasons for this are twofold:

- First, because of the extent of fusion of the spinal column above and below the level of injury in these patients, the amount of leverage at the site of injury is markedly increased, which results in major forces imparted to the injury site with only minor movements of the patient.
- Second, there is an increased risk of epidural hematoma at the injury site in these patients.

Therefore, patients with ankylosing spondylitis or diffuse idiopathic skeletal hyperostosis who present with even minor spinal trauma should be carefully evaluated and immobilized at all times until a thorough understanding of the injury has been obtained. The indication for surgical stabilization should be liberal if no general medical contraindication exists.

The incidence of deep venous thrombosis is higher after spinal cord injury than perhaps after any other medical disease or injury. Some studies estimate that >70% of patients with complete spinal cord injuries develop clinically significant proximal deep venous thrombosis, and the incidence of fatal pulmonary embolism in this patient population approaches 5% in the absence of prophylaxis. Prophylaxis against pulmonary embolism must be used in this patient population. No single treatment modality has been clearly shown to be the most effective (*see* Chapter 88, "Venous Diseases," for more details).

REFERENCES

1. Pennal GF, Tile M, Waddell JP, et al. Pelvic disruption: assessment and classification. Clin Orthop. 1980;151:12-21.
2. Young JWR, Burgess AR, Brumback RJ, et al. Lateral compression fractures of the pelvis: the importance of plain radiographs in the diagnosis and surgical management. Skeletal Radiol. 1986;15:103-9.
3. Burgess AR, Eastridge BJ, Young JWR, et al. Pelvic ring disruptions: effective classification system and treatment protocols. J Trauma. 1990;30:848-56.
4. Dalal SA, Burgess AR, Siegel JH, et al. Pelvic fracture in multiple trauma: classification by mechanism is key to pattern of organ injury, resuscitative requirements, and outcome. J Trauma. 1989;29:981-1002.
5. Burgess AR. Fractures of the Pelvis. Part I. The Pelvic Ring. In: Rockwood CA Jr, Green DP, Bucholz RW (Eds). Fractures in Adults, 3rd edition. Philadelphia: JB Lippincott; 1991. pp. 1399-442.
6. Tile M. Fractures of the Pelvis and Acetabulum, 2nd edition. Baltimore: Williams & Wilkins; 1995.
7. Tien HC, Spencer F, Tremblay LN, et al. Preventable deaths from hemorrhage at a level I Canadian trauma center. J Trauma. 2007;62:142-6.
8. Kellam JF, Browner BD. Fractures of the pelvic ring. In: Browner BD, Jupiter JB, Levine AM, Trafton PG (Eds). Skeletal Trauma. Fractures, Dislocations, Ligamentous Injuries. Philadelphia: WB Saunders; 1992. pp. 849-97.

9. Cullinane DC, Schiller HJ, Zielinski MD, et al. Eastern Association for the Surgery of Trauma practice management guidelines for hemorrhage in pelvic fracture—update and systematic review. J Trauma. 2011;1:1850-68.
10. Published online -www.awmf.org/leitlinien/detail/ll/012-019.html
11. Ben-Menachem Y, Handel SF, Ray RD, et al. Embolization procedures in trauma: the pelvis. Semin Intervent Radiol. 1985;2:158.81.
12. Rothenberger DA, Velasco R, Strate R, et al. Open pelvic fracture: a lethal injury. J Trauma. 1978;18:184-7.
13. Maull KI, Sachatello CR, Ernst CB. The deep perineal laceration—an injury frequently associated with open pelvic fractures: a need for aggressive surgical management. J Trauma. 1977;17:685-96.
14. Pohlemann T, Culemann U. Pelvic ring. In: Rüedi T, Buckley RE, Moran CG (Eds). AO Manual of Fracture Management, 2nd edition. Stuttgart: Thieme/AO Publishing; 2008.
15. Sagi HC, Militano U, Caron T, et al. A comprehensive analysis with minimum 1-year follow-up of vertically unstable transforaminal sacral fractures treated with triangular osteosynthesis. J Orthopad Trauma. 2009;23:313-9.
16. Letournel E, Judet R (Eds). Fractures of the Acetabulum, 2nd edition (translated by RA Elson). New York: Springer-Verlag; 1993.
17. Letournel E. Acetabulum fractures: classification and management. Clin Orthop. 1980;151:81-106.
18. Matta JM. Fractures of the acetabulum: accuracy of reduction and clinical results in patients managed operatively within 3 weeks after the injury. J Bone Joint Surg. 1996;78A: 1632-45.
19. Matta JM, Letournel E, Browner BD. Surgical management of acetabular fractures. Instr Course Lect. 1986;35:382-97.
20. Denis F. Spinal instability as defined by the three-column spine concept in acute spinal trauma. Clin Orthop. 1984;189: 65-76.
21. Levine AM. Lumbar and sacral spine trauma. In: Browner BD, Jupiter JB, Levine AM, Trafton PG (Eds). Skeletal Trauma. Philadelphia: WB Saunders Co; 1992. pp. 805-48.
22. Mumford J, Weinstein JN, Spratt KF, et al. Thoracolumbar burst fractures: the clinical efficacy and outcome of non-operative management. Spine. 1993;18:955-70.
23. Giele BM, Wiertsema SH, Beelen A. et al. No evidence for the effectiveness of bracing in patients with thoracolumbar fractures. Acta Orthop. 2009;80:226-32.
24. Dickson JH, Harrington PR, Erwin WD. Results of reduction and stabilization of the severely fractured thoracic and lumbar spine. J Bone Joint Surg. 1978;60A:799-805.
25. Rosenthal RE, Lowery ER. Unstable fracture-dislocations of the thoracolumbar spine: results of surgical treatment. J Trauma. 1980;20:485-90.
26. Riebel GD, Yoo JU, Fredericksin BE, et al. Review of Harrington rod treatment of spinal trauma. Spine. 1993;18:479-91.
27. McAfee PC, Bohlman HH, Yuan HA. Anterior decompression of traumatic thora-columbar fractures with incomplete neurological deficit using a retroperitoneal approach. J Bone Joint Surg. 1985;67A:89-104.
28. Hardaker WT Jr, Cook WA Jr, Friedman AH, et al. Bilateral transpedicular decompression and Harrington rod stabilization in the management of severe thoracolumbar burst fractures. Spine. 1992;17:162-71.
29. Harrington RM, Budorick T, Hoyt J, et al. Biomechanics of indirect reduction of bone retropulsed into the spinal canal in vertebral fracture. Spine. 1993;18:692-9.
30. Doerr TE, Montesano PX, Burkus JK, et al. Spinal canal decompression in traumatic thoracolumbar burst fractures: posterior distraction rods versus transpedicular screw fixation. Orthop Trauma. 1991;5:403-11.
31. Edwards CC, Levine AM. Early rod-sleeve stabilization of the injured thoracic and lumbar spine. Orthop Clin North Am. 1986;17:121-45.
32. Kaneda K, Abumi K, Fujiya M. Burst fractures with neurologic deficits of the thoracolumbar-lumbar spine. Results of anterior decompression and stabilization with anterior instrumentation. Spine. 1984;9:788-95.
33. Abudou M, Chen X, Kong X, et al. Surgical versus non-surgical treatment for thoracolumbar burst fractures without neurological deficit. Cochrane Database Syst Rev. 2013;5:CD005079.

42

Vascular Trauma

Martin Veller, John D Corson

Key Points

- Vascular trauma is associated with high mortality and morbidity rates, usually due to hemorrhagic shock, ischemia, and/or reperfusion injury.
- Following trauma, there should be a high index of suspicion for the presence of a vascular injury.
- The presence of normal limb pulses does not exclude an arterial injury.
- A patient with hard signs of vascular trauma requires immediate surgical or endovascular intervention.
- Early imaging of a patient with a suspected vascular injury can prevent devastating complications.
- Arterial injuries usually require a procedure to maintain flow whereas most venous injuries can safely be ligated.
- Endovascular therapies are being increasingly used in the management of vascular trauma.

INTRODUCTION

Injuries to major arteries or veins can be very challenging to treat. A systematic approach to their management ensures optimal outcomes. Particular emphasis on recognizing vascular injuries early, minimizing the associated hemodynamic instability by controlling hemorrhage, and avoiding the consequences of prolonged ischemic cell damage have made the greatest impact on outcomes.[1]

HISTORICAL PERSPECTIVE

Many of the innovations in the treatment of vascular trauma occurred as a consequence of war and other violent conflicts. Ambroise Paré, a French barber surgeon with extensive experience of managing war injuries in the 16th century, is credited with establishing the value of arterial ligatures to control bleeding vessels in preference to the traditional use of stypics or hot cautery, such as boiling oil.[2] This simple innovation reduced mortality from hemorrhage and minimized the pain and trauma associated with the use of the traditional methods.

Early amputation was the primary treatment for severe limb injuries during the American 19th century military conflicts.[3] The high mortality rates, up to 80% for high thigh wounds, were predominantly caused by sepsis. Lister's epoch-making work on antisepsis, published in 1867, was too late to benefit the victims of these fierce campaigns.[4,5] Although the principles of antisepsis were slow to be adopted, they changed the practice of surgery, in particular when the excellent results that German surgeons obtained in applying these techniques in the surgical treatment of limb injuries during the Franco-Prussian war of 1877 became known.[6]

During World War I (1914–18), arterial ligation, which was the standard treatment for a major arterial injury, frequently resulted in a major amputation following a limb arterial injury.[7] Following carotid artery ligation, the mortality rate was reported to be 44%.[8] World War II (1939–45) brought no significant improvements, with 40% amputation rates reported after major arterial ligation for extremity vascular injury and specifically a 73% amputation rate for popliteal artery ligation.[9] At that time, wounds were radically debrided and left open if they were >8 hours old because of the threat of infection—above all, the organisms causing gas gangrene. It was not until the availability of antibiotics such as penicillin in the 1940s that the repair of battlefield arterial injuries became a realistic option.[10] During the Korean conflict (1950–53), the major shift in the management of vascular injuries occurred as a result of the application of innovations that were also being introduced into civilian surgical practice, especially the use

Table 42.1 Pathophysiology of vascular trauma.

Hemorrhage
Hemorrhagic shock occurs more commonly following penetrating injuries
Blood loss may not be obvious in chest, abdominal, or retroperitoneal injuries
Thrombosis, ischemia, and reperfusion injury
Thrombosis typically follows blunt trauma due to intimal injury
As blood flow may be maintained initially despite injury, it is important to frequently reassess for deterioration of the distal circulation
The degree of ischemia following occlusive injury depends upon the adequacy of collateral flow and is variable
Oxygen-free radicals play a major role in reperfusion injury
False aneurysm
Develops more frequently after a penetrating injury
May initially go undiagnosed or be confused with a simple hematoma
Arteriovenous fistula
Direct continuity between an artery and vein, or a short fistula tract joining the two, may be present
Diagnose by Branham's sign: slowing of the pulse rate following temporary obliteration of the fistula
Arterial spasm
Muscular arteries develop spasm when traumatized
Usually self-limiting provided no other arterial injury is present
Only make this diagnosis if other etiologies of arterial injury have been excluded

of autogenous vein bypass grafts.[11] Early repair of arterial injuries resulted in a lowering of the amputation rate to 12.7% with further refinements being introduced during the Vietnam War (1964–72).[12,13]

The improvements in outcomes of battlefield vascular trauma in Korea and Vietnam would not, however, have been possible without other important parallel developments in the management of severely traumatized patients: improved, rapid evacuation of battlefield casualties, sophisticated surgical facilities within the sphere of conflict, military surgeons with specialized vascular training, and the availability of heparin and antibiotics among many other factors. Subsequent additional lessons have also been learnt, during the wars in Iraq (2003–2011) and Afghanistan (2001–2014), and in regions exposed to high civilian trauma volumes and civil unrest.[14-21] Among these are the refinements in the diagnosis of vascular injuries, the recognition of the importance of repairing certain venous injuries, and an understanding of the pathophysiology of reperfusion injury. These advances have led to ongoing improvements in outcomes, with amputation rates of 1–5% currently being reported for civilian vascular trauma despite increased levels in the severity and extent of injuries that are currently being managed in most major trauma centers (*see* Chapter 33, "Military Surgery," and Chapter 35, "Case Study: Vascular Injury in Combat and Austere Settings," for more information).

ETIOLOGY OF VASCULAR TRAUMA

The type of injury, be it penetrating or blunt, and the associated force by which it is applied to any tissue, including blood vessels, determine the immediate and late consequences and therefore also guides management (Table 42.1). Other determinants of outcome include the location of such injuries, the manner in which the vessel is affected (pathophysiology of the injury), and the hemodynamic consequences (Fig. 42.1).

In civilian trauma practice, the most frequent causes of vascular injuries are motor vehicle accidents (MVAs), bullet wounds—mostly from handguns but also rifles and shotguns, wounds caused by sharp instruments and objects, falls, and rarely burns (flame and chemical). As is the case in all trauma, the severity and extent of injury is largely determined by the amount of kinetic force transferred to the tissues, which is the reason that in high-energy transfer trauma (such as high velocity MVAs and high velocity gunshot injuries), vascular injuries can be found at sites remote from the point of impact.

The heightened awareness of injury prevention has nearly eliminated acute work-related vascular injuries in most parts of the industrialized world, with most emphasis now being directed at addressing chronic vascular injuries. However, iatrogenic vascular injuries are increasing, particularly as a consequence of the use of minimal

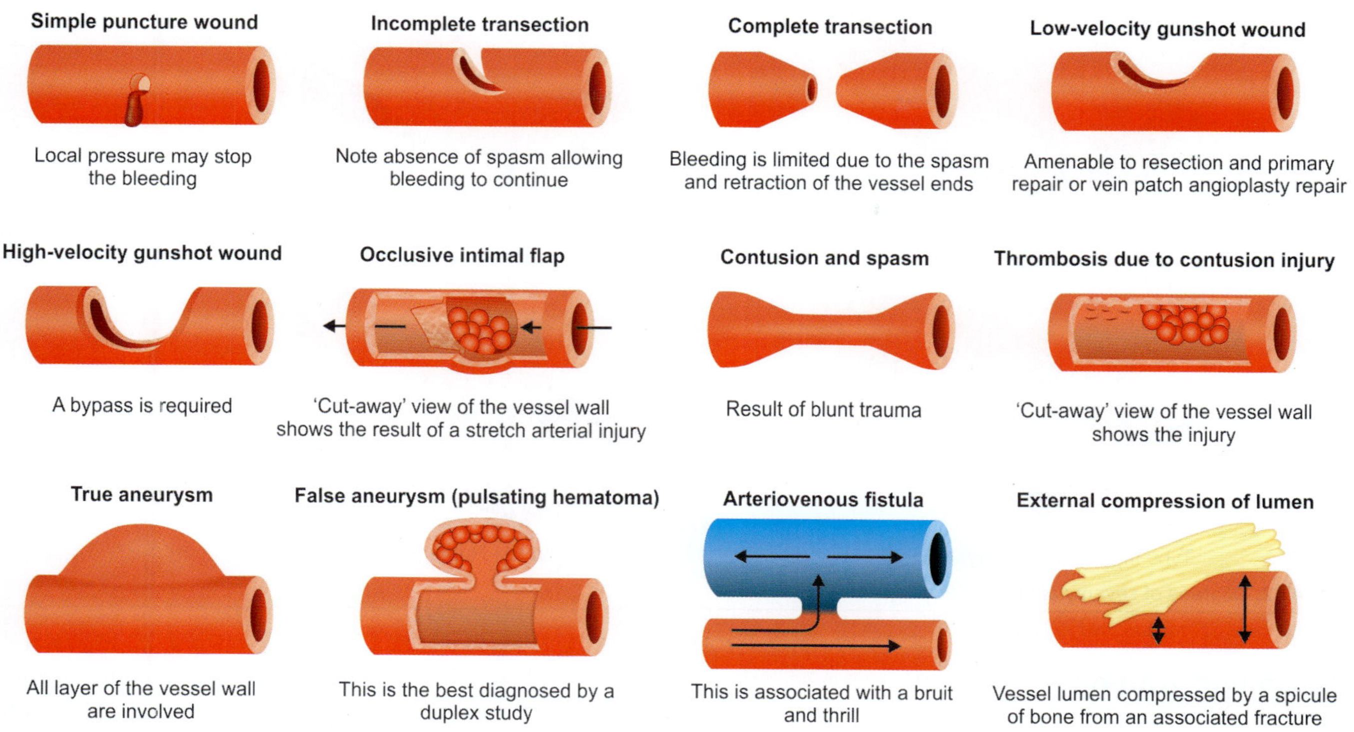

Simple puncture wound
Local pressure may stop the bleeding

Incomplete transection
Note absence of spasm allowing bleeding to continue

Complete transection
Bleeding is limited due to the spasm and retraction of the vessel ends

Low-velocity gunshot wound
Amenable to resection and primary repair or vein patch angioplasty repair

High-velocity gunshot wound
A bypass is required

Occlusive intimal flap
'Cut-away' view of the vessel wall shows the result of a stretch arterial injury

Contusion and spasm
Result of blunt trauma

Thrombosis due to contusion injury
'Cut-away' view of the vessel wall shows the injury

True aneurysm
All layer of the vessel wall are involved

False aneurysm (pulsating hematoma)
This is the best diagnosed by a duplex study

Arteriovenous fistula
This is associated with a bruit and thrill

External compression of lumen
Vessel lumen compressed by a spicule of bone from an associated fracture

Fig. 42.1: Pathophysiology of common types of arterial trauma.

access interventions[22] (*see* Chapter 14, "Vascular Access," and Chapter 15, "Diagnostic and Interventional Radiology," for more information on iatrogenic vascular injury).

Penetrating Trauma

In low-energy vascular trauma such as that caused by knives, small caliber handguns and other sharp objects including teeth from bites, the blood vessel injury is caused by direct contact with the injuring object and may vary from a simple small puncture to complete vessel transection. Occasionally, after blunt trauma, a sharp spicule of bone from a fracture may perforate an artery simulating a penetrating injury.

When increasing levels of kinetic energy are transmitted to the tissues, such as in high-velocity gunshot and explosive shrapnel injuries, blood vessels may also be contused and even disrupted at sites remote from the immediate injury tract; mostly because of the damaging effects of cavitation. These high-energy injuries are often recognized by the smaller entry and larger exit wounds. Shotgun injuries, while not usually being high-velocity, cause the most severe penetrating vascular injuries because of the many tracts caused by the multiple missiles, especially when these are concentrated as a result of being fired at close range.

Blunt Trauma

The diffuse application of major force to the body results in mostly crushing injuries within the soft tissues and is often associated with long bone fractures and joint dislocations. Blunt trauma vascular injuries generally have a worse prognosis than penetrating trauma vascular injuries. The mechanism causing injury to blood vessels can be one of, or a combination of, crushing, stretching (traction), shearing, and torsion. The degree of arterial injury, which is dependent on the force applied, varies from a mild external contusion to major intimal disruption with thrombosis, and even complete arterial transection (Fig. 42.2). Many blunt arterial injuries, particularly those associated with intimal damage with an intact media-adventitia complex, and usually caused by extensive stretching of the artery, can be difficult to recognize and may present with late complications such as stroke (following blunt trauma to the carotid arteries)[23] or acute limb ischemia (often associated with dislocations).[24,25] For the same reason, a false aneurysm or arteriovenous fistula may occur after blunt arterial trauma, but less frequently than after a penetrating arterial injury.[26] Associated or isolated venous injuries are also commonly found following blunt trauma.

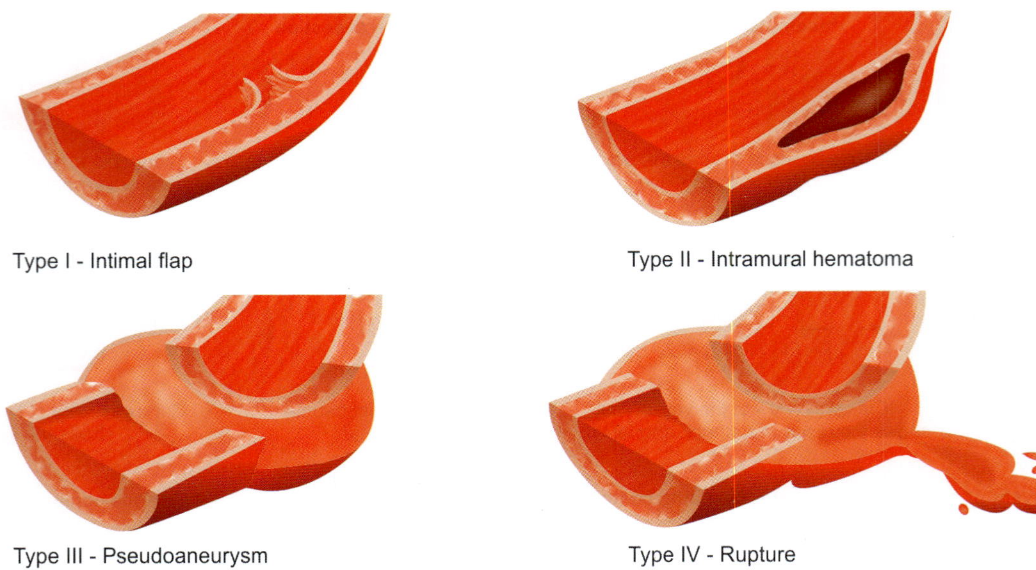

Fig. 42.2: Degrees of severity of blunt arterial injuries.

Iatrogenic Trauma

Vascular injuries occurring in the course of therapeutic or diagnostic procedures fall broadly into the following groups: those that occur as a result of diagnostic or intentional endovascular interventions on blood vessels, those in which a vascular injury occurs in the course of a procedure unrelated to a blood vessel, and those that occur as a consequence of inadvertent intra-arterial injections.[27-34] Many, if not all, iatrogenic vascular injuries are preventable.

The incidence of iatrogenic vascular injuries after vascular diagnostic and therapeutic procedures, even with the introduction of the Seldinger technique, used to be around 10%. With the advent of ultrasound-guided needle puncture and use of micropuncture techniques, these complications are now less frequent but still are a source of substantial morbidity and even occasional mortality. The most frequent mechanisms by which such injuries are induced are dissection with potential malperfusion, rupture, and false aneurysm formation. The underlying common reasons that lead to such injuries are as follows:

- Faulty technique or routine
- An error in judgment or management
- Failure to correctly identify the anatomy
- Failure to correctly interpret angiograms and other forms of vascular imaging or the results of laboratory studies.

Iatrogenic injuries to blood vessels after nonvascular surgical procedures may occur after an operation on any part of the body. The highest incidence of such iatrogenic injuries occurs after orthopedic procedures, but even relatively straightforward general surgical procedures, such as a groin hernia repair, may be associated with iatrogenic vascular complications such as bleeding, arterial thrombosis, or a false aneurysm, mostly as a result of the failure to appreciate local anatomy or poor surgical technique.[28,30,35] Not all iatrogenic injury is caused by an invasive intervention, e.g. cervical spine manipulation may result in serious iatrogenic trauma to the carotid or vertebral arteries,[36] and the inappropriate use of limb restraints or tourniquets may result in limb ischemia.[37]

EPIDEMIOLOGY OF VASCULAR TRAUMA

Injuries to major arteries or veins are found in approximately 3% of civilian cases of major trauma and are estimated to affect >450,000 individuals annually in the United States of America (USA). Most of these injuries are found in men aged between 15 years and 49 years. The crude mortality in patients with vascular trauma is approximately 10%.[20,21]

The most frequent cause for vascular trauma varies widely across the world. In regions where MVA rates are high, much of the vascular trauma is blunt in nature. The incidence of penetrating injuries in a country is dependent mostly on the frequency with which firearms are found in that society. As a consequence, in Europe and Scandinavia, stabbing is the most common mechanism for penetrating vascular trauma, whereas in the USA gunshot wounds are more frequently the cause of penetrating injuries.[20] In many parts of the world, there is an increasing incidence of penetrating vascular trauma as a result of urban violence due to gang warfare related to the illegal distribution of narcotic drugs.

PATHOPHYSIOLOGY OF VASCULAR TRAUMA

Hemorrhage

Hemorrhagic shock occurs more commonly after penetrating as opposed to blunt vascular trauma. The extent of bleeding depends upon whether an injured artery is completely or partially transected. After complete transection, the divided arterial ends retract and then constrict, which usually results in thrombosis and cessation of bleeding. More frequently, however, the artery is only partially transected and will continue to bleed because the injury site is held open as the vessel attempts to retract.

A dangerous situation develops when blood loss is not clinically obvious. Such occult blood loss is frequently encountered with penetrating trauma to the thoracic and retroperitoneal vessels, and with blunt pelvic trauma causing severe fractures. It may also occur after an angiographic or endovascular procedure where the access is in the groin and the entry point into the artery, or rarely in the vein, is mistakenly made above the inguinal ligament that may then result after catheter withdrawal in occult bleeding into the retroperitoneum.[38] A high index of suspicion is needed to diagnose these potentially extremely dangerous conditions expediently. A marked reduction in blood volume usually occurs before the correct diagnosis is made.

Thrombosis

Both penetrating and blunt arterial injuries may present with partial or complete thrombosis as a result of intimal injury when an intimal flap limits flow or a platelet plug forms at the injury site. These changes may lead to an occluding or nonoccluding arterial thrombosis. When blood flow is maintained, this may result in embolization of thrombus. It is important to frequently reassess the circulation in a patient with suspected vascular trauma to look for changes in perfusion and ischemic symptoms as a result of distal embolization or progression of the initial arterial injury to thrombosis. The trauma team should also be alert to the development of other complications following vascular trauma.

Ischemia

In acute ischemia of aerobic tissues, hypoxia associated with a decreased supply of nutrients causes irreversible tissue destruction and cell death when the ischemia lasts longer than the availability of inherent energy reserves within the affected tissues. A process known as the ischemic cascade causes the resultant damage as a result of a buildup of metabolic waste products, inability to maintain the cell membranes, mitochondrial damage, and eventual leakage of autolyzing proteolytic enzymes into the cell and surrounding tissues.

The degree of ischemia that develops after an occlusive arterial injury depends upon the adequacy of the collateral blood flow and varies in different regions of the body. Occlusion of an end artery is associated with the most severe ischemia. When a major artery is injured, but there is preservation of the main collateral supply to the limb (e.g. via the profunda brachial artery in the arm or profunda femoral artery in the leg), adequate distal blood flow is usually maintained and limb-threatening ischemia does not occur. Also, an isolated occlusive injury to the profunda femoris artery is well-tolerated if the superficial femoral artery is widely patent; indeed, the injury may not be clinically obvious. In contrast, however, an elderly atherosclerotic patient with a chronic superficial femoral artery occlusion who develops a traumatic profunda femoral artery thrombosis will have evidence of marked acute distal ischemia because of the loss of major collaterals. A single crural artery thrombosis is relatively innocuous because there is an adequate compensating supply of blood to the lower extremity through the remaining infrapopliteal vessels. Indeed, a single patent crural artery is usually adequate to maintain limb viability, provided there is adequate runoff into the foot.

Reperfusion Injury

If blood flow is restored to the ischemic aerobic tissues before the cellular energy reserves are fully depleted, complete recovery can be anticipated. The abrupt return of arterialized blood—reperfusion—to already injured tissues can, however, also inflict additional local tissue and remote organ damage—as a result of inflammatory, thrombotic, and metabolic consequences, which may be significantly more dangerous when compared to the initial ischemic episode.

Several mechanisms have been implicated in reperfusion injury, including alterations in cellular oxygen levels and pH, and the release of arachidonate metabolites, cytokines, proteases, complement, and oxidants. Reactive oxygen metabolites and polymorphonuclear leukocytes have been implicated in the pathobiology of reperfusion injury.[39] During ischemia adenosine triphosphate is catabolized to yield hypoxanthine. Hypoxic stress triggers the conversion of nicotinamide adenine dinucleotide reducing xanthine dehydrogenase to the oxygen radical producing xanthine oxidase. Oxygen-free radicals and other similar molecules created by the highly oxidative state interact with most cellular structures. For example, they form lipid-free radicals by removing hydrogen from polyunsaturated fatty acids, which initiates a chain reaction in the phospholipid bilayer of organelle membranes causing extensive additional cell injury. Another mechanism causing damage is the inactivation of nitric oxide by oxygen-free radicals. Nitric oxide prevents leukocyte and platelet adhesion and its inactivation results in leukocyte adherence to the vascular endothelium with resultant induction of inflammation and endothelial injury often at sites remote from the site of ischemia. Such remote organs particularly susceptible to reperfusion injury include the lungs, kidneys, heart, and brain. The extent of the reperfusion injury is dependent on the extent of ischemic injury, the longer the period of ischemia, the more severe the reperfusion injury and the worse the associated tissue damage.

Arterial Spasm

Muscular arteries spasm when traumatized. This is usually self-limiting, provided there is no other injury to the artery. When "arterial spasm" is thought to be a likely diagnosis, an important question to resolve is whether there is any associated arterial injury. In view of the negative consequences of missing a major arterial injury, a basic vascular trauma principle requires that a specific arterial injury is excluded before a diagnosis of "arterial spasm" is confirmed.[40]

In younger individuals, the major arteries are especially prone to spasm and thrombose when directly traumatized or handled surgically. This may partly explain the high incidence of iatrogenic thrombotic complications in the smaller arteries of infants and children that are often only discovered when a chronic arterial occlusion is noted many years after an invasive arterial diagnostic study. In view of the high-risk of thrombosis, invasive diagnostic arterial studies in children should be carried out only when there is no appropriate less invasive diagnostic option.

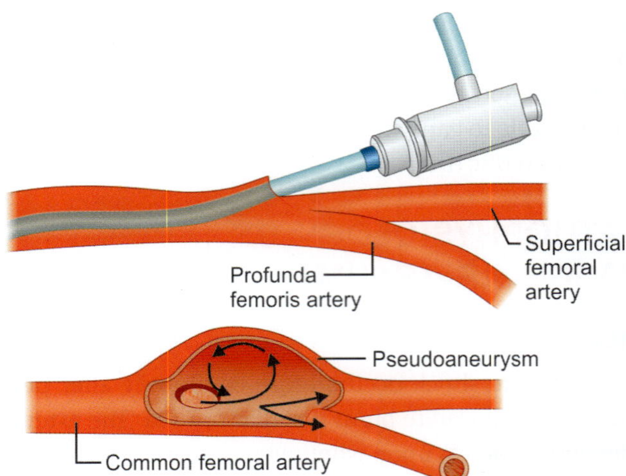

Fig. 42.3: Mechanism for the development of an iatrogenic femoral artery false aneurysm following cardiac catheterization. After the introducer sheath is removed, the arterial defect is usually sealed by a hemostatic plug that forms when pressure is applied to the site. If a hemostatic plug does not seal the arterial defect, a false aneurysm may form. The wall of the false aneurysm is formed by the surrounding tissues.

False Aneurysm

Occasionally, a blunt traumatic injury causes a false aneurysm as a result of disruption of a portion of the weakened and injured arterial wall. A false aneurysm (pulsating hematoma) more often develops after a penetrating injury rather than after a blunt arterial injury.[26] A false aneurysm may develop as an iatrogenic complication of an angiogram (Fig. 42.3).

If the arterial puncture site does not develop an occluding thrombotic platelet plug, blood then flows out from the arterial lumen through the site of arterial wall penetration into the surrounding tissues, which form a pseudoaneurysmal sac. An acute false aneurysm is usually associated with evidence of local bruising and an obvious arterial pulsation. False aneurysms may expand and cause local pain and may later rupture; some thrombose spontaneously (< 4 cm diameter).[33] A small false aneurysm may initially be undiagnosed or be confused with a simple hematoma. An expanding hematoma, in which there is continued bleeding through the arterial puncture site, must not be confused with a false aneurysm.

Arteriovenous Fistula

An injury that simultaneously penetrates an artery and its neighboring vein may result in an arteriovenous fistula—there may be direct continuity between the artery and vein,

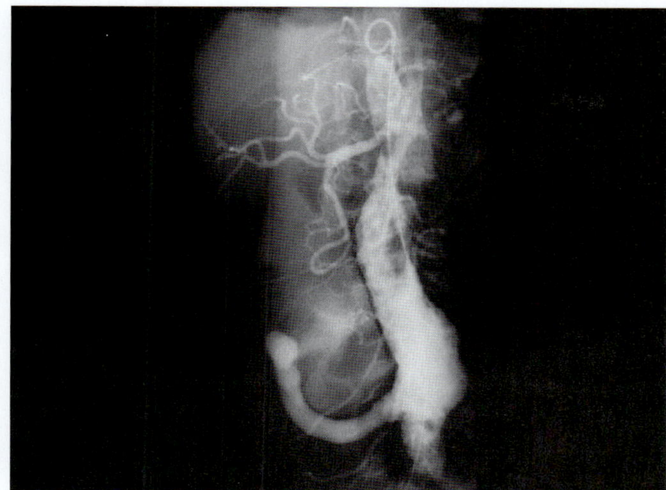

Fig. 42.4: Aortocaval fistula. This was discovered in a patient who had initially presented with heart failure. Note the aneurysmal dilatation of the aorta. The only notable history was a previous nephrectomy many years ago.

or a short fistula tract may join the two structures.[41] For example, inadvertent puncture of the profunda femoris artery and vein may result in an arteriovenous fistula because of the close proximity of the vessels.

A large fistula may cause hemodynamic compromise and result in a hyperdynamic state with increased cardiac output. The classic diagnostic sign is a slowing of the pulse rate during temporary obliteration of an arteriovenous fistula (Branham's sign). Cardiac failure may result if a large arteriovenous fistula is neglected (Fig. 42.4). A large central arteriovenous fistula may be associated with diminished peripheral pulses and in some patients symptoms of claudication. Small peripheral arteriovenous fistulae are usually hemodynamically unimportant. It is unusual for an arteriovenous fistula to close spontaneously.

SIGNS AND SYMPTOMS OF VASCULAR TRAUMA

In the polytraumatized patient, the clinical signs and symptoms of vascular injury may be obscured by the presence of other injuries. Therefore, evidence of a vascular injury should usually be looked for using objective modalities, especially if the patient has a substantial injury in the vicinity of a major vessel.

Evidence of an arterial injury is classified as definite in the presence of "hard" clinical signs or equivocal if the signs are "soft" (Table 42.2).[42] Hard signs confirm the presence of an arterial injury that usually requires some form of immediate surgical or endovascular intervention. Imaging

Table 42.2 Signs of extremity arterial trauma.

"Hard" signs	*"Soft" signs*
External arterial bleeding	Proximity of injury to major blood vessel
Pulse deficit	Injury to adjacent nerve
Expanding or pulsatile hematoma	Small/moderate stable hematoma
Bruit or thrill	Unexplained shock in a patient with a truncal injury
Signs of ischemia or compartment syndrome	Dislocation of a major joint
Major abnormality on noninvasive vascular testing	Excessive swelling or detection of minor abnormality on noninvasive vascular testing

studies are not usually required when hard signs of an arterial injury are present. An exception would be when there are hard signs in a stable patient with a shotgun injury because of the possibility of multiple puncture wounds to the vessels. Patients with soft signs usually require further diagnostic studies to exclude the presence of a significant arterial injury. Proximity alone, however, does not mandate an additional diagnostic evaluation unless this soft sign is associated with an injury that was caused by a high-kinetic force, or if it is associated with other evidence of vascular injury such as an ankle brachial index (ABI) < 0.9 (*see* below). Using these signs to categorize patients into those who need intervention or additional diagnostic evaluation has been shown to be safe with a diagnostic accuracy approaching 100% and a missed arterial injury rate of < 1%.

Acute ischemia is usually recognized by the presence of the "six Ps"—a painful, pallid, pulseless, paresthetic, paralytic, and poikilothermic limb. However, in a severely injured patient, these classic findings may not be as obvious and diagnostically useful. Confounding factors include the presence of painful fractures, hemodynamic instability, hypothermia, and head or other injuries. In such circumstances, a comparison between an injured and uninjured extremity is valuable and diagnostic as there may be marked differences in pulses, coolness, capillary return, appreciation of light touch, and degree of intrinsic muscle function.

Although the absence of a palpable distal pulse always suggests the possibility of an arterial injury, the presence of a palpable pulse does not reliably exclude it. Up to 20% of patients with an extremity arterial injury have a palpable distal pulse because the injury is either nonocclusive or because of the presence of rich collaterals around a short arterial segmental occlusion. The latter occurs in up to 10%

of trauma patients and is particularly frequent in vascular injuries around the shoulder. For this reason, if distal pulses are present, the onus is on the treating clinician to consider the presence of a significant arterial injury, particularly if the trauma is in proximity of a major vessel. This is usually done using appropriate diagnostic studies, especially if the patient requires operative treatment for associated injuries, but serial observations by a skilled examiner may occasionally be an alternative.[43]

The presence of leg swelling, hematomas, wounds, splints, and dressings may limit and prevent an accurate physical examination. A limb with a fracture or dislocation should initially be splinted and the status of the distal circulation evaluated. Occasionally the pulse status worsens after reduction of a fracture or dislocation due to arterial thrombosis or entrapment.

An arterial injury may be difficult to diagnose in an individual with known pulse deficits as a result of chronic atherosclerotic peripheral vascular disease. Various diagnostic studies may be needed to make the diagnosis as described below.

DIAGNOSIS OF VASCULAR TRAUMA

It is important to make a prompt diagnosis of a vascular injury in order to limit the ischemic sequelae and improve the functional outcome. Neglected or undiagnosed arterial injuries are often associated with appreciable complications.

Plain Radiography

Plain radiography with biplanar views identifies the presence of foreign bodies, the proximity of penetrating objects to major vessels, and the presence of other associated injuries. Radiopaque markers should be placed on the entry and exit wounds, when present, to identify the specific details of injury more precisely and determine the potential track of a penetrating injury. Specific orthopedic injuries, especially those associated with elbow or knee dislocations or fractures, are frequently associated with vascular injuries and therefore extremity radiographs should be carefully evaluated to identify such orthopedic injuries.[25]

Noninvasive Vascular Studies

Noninvasive vascular studies are useful when evaluating a patient with a suspected vascular injury, not only to identify the presence of a vascular injury but also to quantify, when present, the degree of ischemia (Fig. 42.5).[44-46] In contrast to angiographic diagnostic procedures, noninvasive studies are objective, quick to perform, repeatable, and relatively inexpensive.

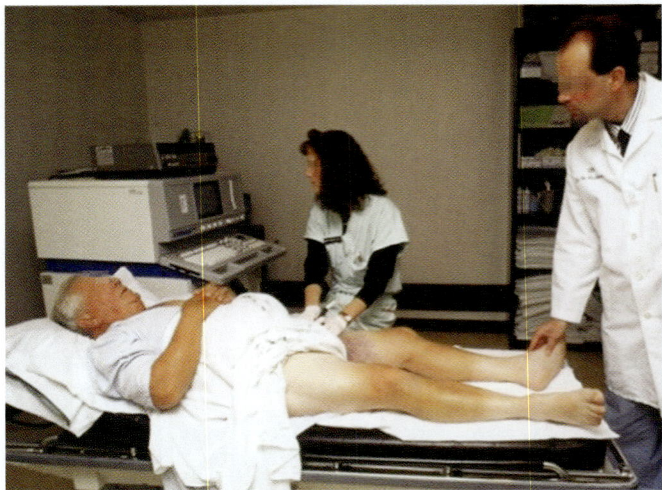

Fig 42.5: A large femoral false aneurysm was found on an ultrasound exam in this patient who had recently had undergone cardiac catheterization.

Segmental limb pressure studies or pulse volume recordings can be difficult to obtain in an injured extremity, because of pain and swelling from associated soft tissue or bone injuries. However, the distal arterial systolic blood pressure can be measured in most patients with extremity trauma. In the lower extremities, a blood pressure cuff is placed just above the ankle and a handheld Doppler device is used to detect pulsatile arterial flow in the posterior tibial, dorsal pedis, or peroneal arteries at the ankle level beyond the cuff as it is slowly deflated. The highest systolic pressure in any of the major vessels at the ankle is recorded and an ABI is calculated by dividing the highest recorded ankle systolic blood pressure by the highest brachial artery systolic pressure reading. A reduction in the distal arterial systolic pressure by 10 mm Hg or more and in the ABI of 0.1 or more suggests an arterial injury. In both blunt and penetrating trauma, the finding of an ABI of <0.9 has a sensitivity of 87% and a specificity of 97% in making the diagnosis of an arterial injury. An ABI of ≥ 0.9 has a negative predictive value of 96%. As a consequence when the ABI is ≤ 0.9, further evaluation is mandated, while if it is above this level, these patients are observed. Similar studies can be utilized in the upper extremities to diagnose an arterial injury and the degree of ischemia.

A color duplex ultrasound scan, focusing on the region of the suspected injury site, can provide valuable diagnostic information.[47] Duplex ultrasound studies are useful for

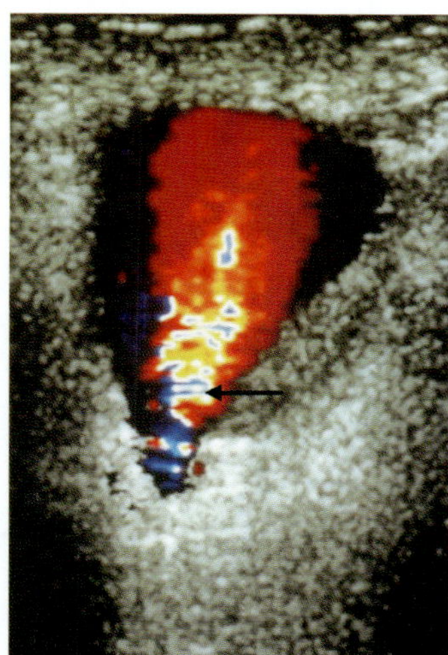

Fig. 42.6: Color duplex ultrasonography shows a jet flow of blood during systole into a femoral false aneurysm (arrow).

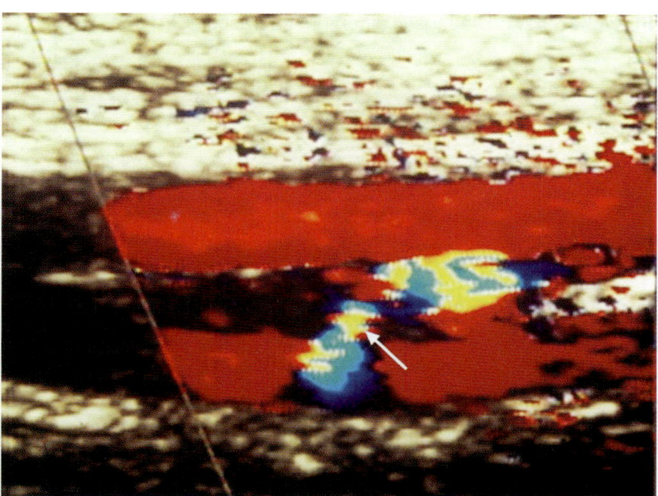

Fig. 42.7: Arteriovenous communication between the profunda femoris artery and the superficial femoral vein following cardiac catheterization (arrow).

screening for arterial injury, especially when proximity of injury to the artery is the only indication for evaluation.[48,49] These studies, if normal, limit the need for angiography in many individuals. Duplex ultrasound studies are especially useful to identify a complication, such as a false aneurysm or an arteriovenous fistula, and may also identify an intimal arterial injury (Figs. 42.6 and 42.7). Duplex studies are, however, highly "technician-dependent" and may be of limited value in the acute phase of trauma. In addition, the area of suspected injury may be difficult to study if there are open wounds or marked swelling, or if an external fixator device or cast is in place. In addition, access may be difficult because of the lack of patient cooperation or anatomic limitations (e.g. a bony structure, such as the clavicle). A combination of a careful physical evaluation and duplex examination may limit the need for many angiographic studies. Some have suggested that duplex ultrasonography should be instituted as the primary diagnostic procedure of choice for penetrating neck trauma[50] (*see* Chapter 37, "Neck Injury," for more discussion).

Angiography

Conventional angiography has been for many years the standard by which to diagnose arterial injury (Fig. 42.8). However, it is invasive, costly, and time consuming, and there is a high incidence of negative studies and a small but important incidence of complications. In addition, an angiogram may be oversensitive in detecting minor degrees of arterial trauma. Conventional angiography has therefore been abandoned in favor of newer imaging angiography techniques such as computed tomogram angiography (CTA)[51] and more recently magnetic resonance angiography (MRA).[52] The value of these two imaging modalities lies in the substantial additional three-dimensional anatomic evidence obtained. Each has its own limitations (CTA—requires contrast, MRA—long examination times and use of gadolinium). Both studies are costly and usually can only be performed in hemodynamically stable patients, and additionally not every facility worldwide that receives trauma patients has access to these imaging modalities. Both modalities, when compared to conventional angiography, are accurate.

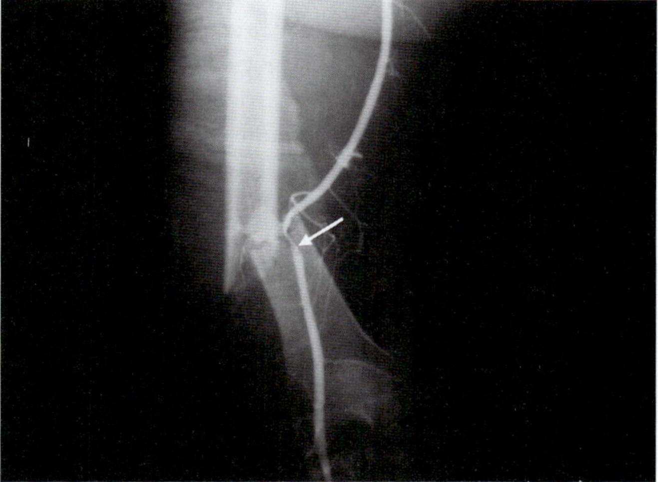

Fig. 42.8: Distal superficial femoral artery traumatized at the site of a fracture of the distal third of the femur (arrow).

Flowchart 42.1: Diagnostic algorithm for vascular trauma.

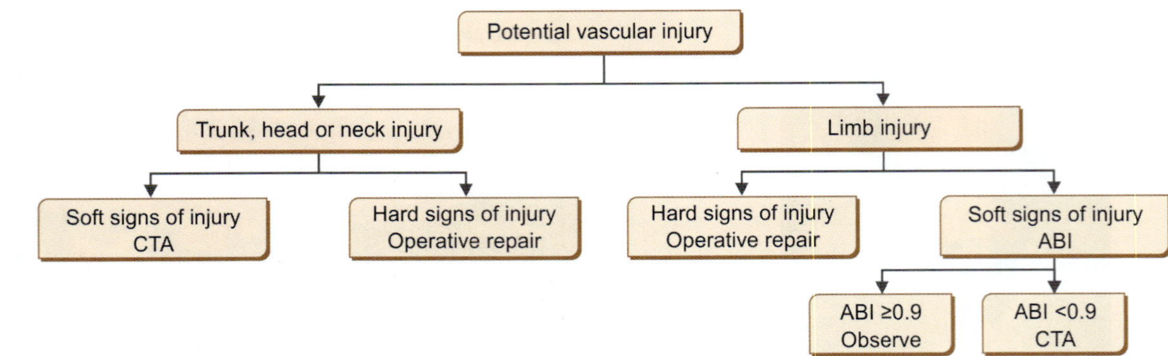

(CTA: Computed tomogram angiography; ABI: Ankle brachial index).

In most patients, the suspected site of the arterial injury is reasonably obvious. If there, however, is a question of arterial trauma at an inaccessible site or at more than one level, or if there is a possibility of widespread arterial injury as a result of a shotgun wound or concern about the track of a missile injury that has no exit wound, an expedient radiologic investigation can be very useful. In practice, a form of angiography is usually carried out to either confirm the specifics of an arterial injury in a stable patient with one or more "hard" signs following blunt trauma or to exclude an arterial injury in a patient with "soft" signs. Conventional angiography will be required if endovascular therapy is the chosen treatment option.

Importantly, in many trauma centers, angiography is done in a radiologic suite remote from the emergency room and for that reason usually can only be done when patients are hemodynamically stable. In hemodynamically unstable trauma patients, limited "single-shot" angiograms (for extremity injuries) can be performed in the emergency department if it is essential to make the diagnosis of a vascular injury prior to urgent transfer into the operating room.[53] Most such patients should be operated on without delay, particularly when there is uncontrollable hemorrhage. If required, additional diagnostic procedures can be performed in the operating room usually after life-saving "damage control" surgery has been completed.

A recent trend in high-volume trauma centers has been to equip emergency department resuscitation rooms with high-quality radiographic equipment usually in the form of ultrafast CT. Thus, all the diagnostic information needed to allow appropriate planning of all surgical procedures is acquired in the emergency department and delays resulting from transportation to and from the radiology department are avoided.

When carrying out any form of angiography in a trauma patient, it is important to visualize the normal arteries both proximal and distal to the site of injury. Findings may include extravasation of contrast from a transected vessel, a complete arterial cutoff as a result of occlusion, luminal irregularities caused by an intimal injury or thrombus, filling of a false aneurysm, or rapid venous filling caused by the presence of an arteriovenous fistula. As a result of the acuteness of a thrombosis at the site of an arterial injury and therefore poor collateralization, angiography may not always define the distal runoff beyond the injury site adequately, especially for an injury that involves the distal popliteal artery or the trifurcation.

INITIAL ASSESSMENT OF TRAUMA PATIENTS

The advanced trauma life support protocol should always be followed in all trauma patients (Flowchart 42.1) (*see* Chapter 31, "Initial Trauma Evaluation and Resuscitation," for further details). In regard to vascular injuries, hemorrhage control is a priority. Any obvious bleeding is controlled with immediate local pressure usually using a gauze pad and applying digital pressure over this. Some caution should be exercised when initially applying digital pressure as a result of sharp objects that may be hidden in the wound. An adjunct to local pressure is the placement of one or more Foley catheters into a wound tract.[54] The bulbs of the catheters are then inflated to the point that they stop the bleeding. This technique of hemorrhage control is particularly suitable for penetrating wounds in zones 1 and 3 of the neck (*see* Fig. 37.3 in Chapter 37, "Neck Injury"). Tourniquets have a limited role in the management of extremity arterial injuries as their misuse can cause significant harm. An attempt to place hemostats on bleeding vessels in the emergency room is discouraged because of the risk of additional iatrogenic injuries, particularly to adjacent nerves and because of the crushing force of the hemostats that may worsen the extent of the vascular injury. Adequate intravenous access must be quickly established with two large-bore intravenous catheters at sites away from the injured area. Ongoing significant bleeding, as evidenced by hemodynamic instability or because local control cannot be achieved mandates immediate surgical exploration.

After the primary survey and appropriate associated interventions to maintain life are completed, a more complete comprehensive secondary survey is performed. At this point, priorities must be defined depending upon the presence and extent of other major life-threatening injuries, such as burns, head, chest, or abdominal trauma.

Removal of hemostatic pressure bandages or other devices should only occur once the patient is hemodynamically stable and when sufficient information has been obtained to manage the potential recurrent life-threatening hemorrhage expeditiously. It is usually necessary to do so in an operating room using appropriate anesthesia or local analgesia.

The optimal time to manage a major arterial injury is shortly after its occurrence because this allows for the simplest repair and minimizes the development of early or late complications. Therefore, all significant arterial injuries should ideally be treated expeditiously after diagnosis. Late repair of complications of vascular trauma, such as secondary hemorrhage, sepsis, a false aneurysm, or an arteriovenous fistula, is usually much more complex.

MANAGEMENT OF VASCULAR TRAUMA

Nonoperative

With the increasing use of CTA and MRA, many vascular injuries are now found that do not require additional therapy.[55] Such minor arterial injuries, usually defined angiographically, include:

- Evidence of minimal arterial wall disruption
- An intimal defect of < 5 mm in length
- A small false aneurysm or
- An adherent or downstream protruding intimal flap. Minor arterial injuries progress or cause distal embolization in <10% of cases. Patients with such minor degrees of arterial injury are observed. This usually consists of serial observations of the distal circulation to identify any progression of the injury.[56] Follow-up should be long enough to identify late complications such as an arteriovenous fistula. This approach has its limitations because many trauma patients often do not return for follow-up evaluation after hospital discharge.

Operative

Damage Control

Extensive therapeutic interventions in a severely traumatized patient often significantly worsen their physiological stability by inducing hypotension, hypothermia, acidosis, hypocoagulability, and many other factors. In order to limit the extent of this "second-hit" phenomenon, early interventions are ideally limited to those that are both life-saving and life and limb sustaining. In addition, if possible, such procedures are truncated, to allow rapid reversal of the above physiological derangements. It is rarely appropriate for the first set of operations in a severely injured patient to last > 60 minutes. In the vascular trauma setting, this is also applicable. This is achieved by rapid control of bleeding from arteries and large veins, effective packing of confined spaces with laparotomy pads for control of hemorrhage from small vessels (e.g. in pelvic injuries), early ligation of bleeding veins and those arteries supplying tissues that are unlikely to develop ischemia, and the use of temporary shunts in limb arteries where there is a threat of ischemia (*see* Chapter 35, "Case Study: Vascular Injury in Combat and Austere Settings," for a case example of the use of a temporary arterial and venous shunt).

Repair of vascular injuries is only justified in the severely traumatized patient if it can be achieved rapidly—usually by direct repair of the vessel—and is highly likely to be effective.

General Principles of Surgical Management

Adequate surgical exposure is essential to ensure visualization and safe control of the injured blood vessel proximal and distal to the site of the injury. When other specialty teams are to be involved in the operating room, it is important to discuss the optimal placement of incisions preoperatively. This situation arises most frequently with the orthopedic team. Intraoperatively the extent of injury to major veins, nerves, bones, joints, and soft tissue must be carefully assessed and decisions made concerning the surgical priorities and sequence of repair of the identified injuries. The injured vessels and all wounds must be

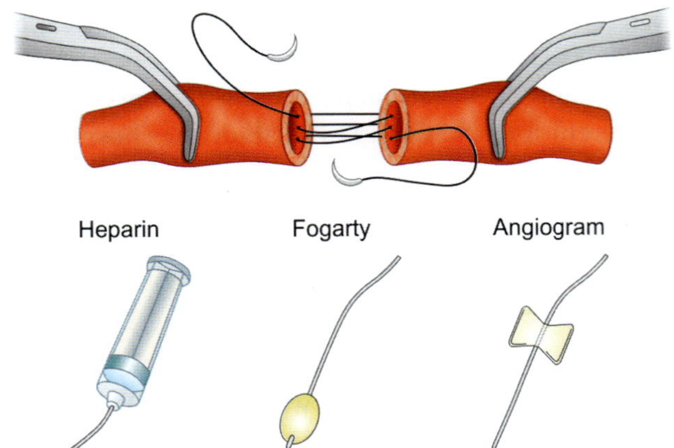

Fig. 42.9: General principles of arterial repair. Injured vessels are first controlled with vascular clamps. Regional heparin is utilized. A Fogarty catheter is used to remove thrombus both distally and proximally. An angiogram will confirm the patency of the distal circulation. A tension-free anastomosis is performed.
Source: Redrawn with permission from Baylor College of Medicine.

adequately debrided and irrigated. In low-velocity injuries, the extent of debridement can be determined by the naked eye. Arterial debridement at least 1 cm beyond any visible abnormality is required when treating high-velocity and blast injuries.

The general principles of arterial repair are shown in Figure 42.9.

In a patient with an arterial injury that cannot be primarily repaired, a bypass is required for revascularization. Ideally this is done with autogenous vein—an autogenous artery is infrequently used. Therefore, if possible, an uninjured lower limb should be prepped and draped to allow harvesting of a segment of great saphenous vein in case an interposition vein bypass graft is required. If there is no available autogenous vein, a prosthetic conduit is used but prosthetic bypass grafts are usually reserved to replace injured segments of large vessels with a diameter >6 mm.[16,57,58]

Intraoperatively, arterial spasm can be ameliorated by topical application of warm papaverine or nitroglycerine-soaked sponges or by controlled sequential hydrostatic distension.[59] Hydrostatic dilatation is also very useful to reverse spasm of a vein bypass conduit. The pressure should ideally be kept below 300 mm Hg (40.0 kPa) to minimize endothelial injury to the vein conduit.[60]

When the arterial repair has been completed and just before restoration of blood flow, a Fogarty catheter is passed distally to remove any thrombus that may have formed distal to the site of the injury. Occasionally, proximal passage of a Fogarty catheter is also required if there is concern about the arterial inflow. After passage of the Fogarty catheters, the arterial tree is flushed then filled with heparinized saline, the final suture is placed and flow is restored by first releasing the distal then the proximal arterial clamp.

The adequacy of the reconstruction should be confirmed by a continuous wave Doppler, duplex ultrasound study, or an angiogram intraoperatively. Before awakening the patient, the status of the distal pulses should be critically assessed. A revisional procedure may be required if a technical problem is identified.

Postoperatively the distal pulses should be assessed by serial physical examinations to confirm the continued patency of the reconstruction. In the severely traumatized patient with other major injuries, hypothermia or evidence of hemodynamic instability, the early clinical assessment of the distal circulation may be unreliable. Therefore, noninvasive vascular studies, such as measurements of the ABI, can be used to quantify serially the adequacy of the distal circulation. Postoperative color duplex ultrasound studies can also be useful both to confirm a satisfactory reconstructive result or define a technical problem threatening long-term patency. Re-exploration is carried out if there is evidence of continued ischemia, early failure of the arterial reconstruction or evidence of a technical problem that might compromise the patency of the reconstruction.

Endovascular

Catheter-directed therapies reduce the morbidity associated with the treatment of some vascular injuries.[52] The endovascular techniques used include stent graft placement, coil and microsphere embolization, and occasionally temporary balloon occlusion (Fig. 42.10).[60-63] Frequently, the diagnosis of the vascular injury and the subsequent treatment can be carried out expediently in a well-equipped angiography suite. These techniques are mostly used in patients in whom the acute vascular injury site is surgically inaccessible. Such patients must be sufficiently hemodynamically stable to allow treatment to be undertaken in a suitable radiologic or surgical angiographic suite. Randomized studies supporting endovascular treatment in the trauma setting are limited due to the difficulty in performing such studies and because of the significant gains noted in observational studies. The general lack of long-term follow-up data in such studies is also of concern—particularly because stents and other items left in the vessels are designed for other pathologies

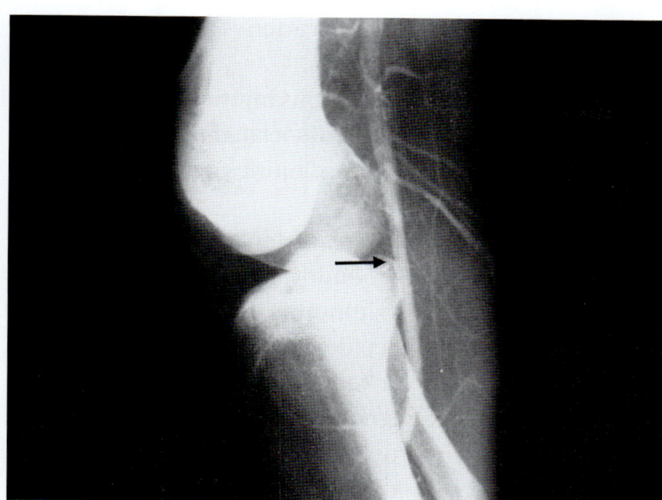

Fig. 42.10: Posterior knee dislocation demonstrating the mechanism of damage to the popliteal artery. Site of blunt trauma (arrow).

and are also now being used in patients expected to survive for ≥ 60 years. Occasional late infections of the endovascular materials have been reported.[64]

The currently used common application of endovascular therapies are for injuries of central or relatively inaccessible vital arteries that are treated by placement of an endovascular stent graft. Other situations where endovascular therapy has been shown to be useful include:

- Embolization as an adjuvant therapy in "damage control" of severe solid viscus and pelvic trauma.
- Treatment of arterial complications in critically ill patients with coexisting injuries or medical comorbidities.
- Treatment of false aneurysms and arteriovenous fistulas of nonessential arteries, such as branches of the hypogastric or profunda femoris artery, can be satisfactorily treated by catheter techniques to occlude the vessels.
- The late treatment of complications of arterial trauma.

MANAGEMENT OF SPECIFIC INJURIES

Penetrating Trauma

In cases of penetrating vascular trauma, the injury tract should usually only be explored after proximal and distal control of the injured vessels is obtained. An impaled device should not be removed or manipulated until potential bleeding can be adequately controlled in an operative setting. Once the injury tract has been explored in the operating room and all foreign bodies, debris, and hematomas have been removed, the arterial injury can be fully assessed.

Arterial reconstruction should be attempted unless the patient is markedly unstable. Small nonessential injured arteries can be ligated. After a simple stab wound, an artery can often be primarily repaired without luminal narrowing by closing the defect with carefully placed 6-0 Prolene sutures. It is important to remember that an entry site on the anterior aspect of an artery may be associated with a similar defect on the posterior aspect of the artery. Lateral suturing of an arterial wall defect should in most cases be avoided as it may restrict the diameter of the lumen, especially in small arteries. Vein patch angioplasty closure is a safe technique to repair an arterial wall defect and preserve an adequate lumen. If, however, the defect is circumferential or very large, a segment of the injured artery may need to be excised. In this case, a primary end-to-end anastomosis can be achieved in most cases by mobilizing the artery for a few centimeters both proximally and distally. It is essential that such a repair is tension-free. Small collateral arterial branches may need to be sacrificed to allow satisfactory mobilization. If a tension-free nonstenotic suture line cannot be achieved, a short interposition reversed vein bypass graft should be placed. Adequate soft tissue coverage of the reconstruction is essential to avoid desiccation of the arterial tissues and vein bypass graft that usually results in disruption and secondary hemorrhage.

Blunt Trauma

After blunt trauma, the extent of the intimal injury is usually much greater than the external appearance of the artery might suggest. An intraoperative duplex ultrasound study or some form of angiogram can be useful to identify the site and extent of intimal injury. Accurately localizing the site of the injury may limit the extent of revascularization procedure required. In practice, most arteries with blunt injury need to be explored as appreciable intimal injuries are usually found.

Most arterial injuries associated with compound fractures should be directly explored. An exception is when there is a thrombotic arterial injury associated with a closed fracture and no other complications of the arterial injury. A bypass as opposed to direct repair is usually required in such circumstances if revascularization is necessary.

It is important that the orthopedic and vascular teams define a plan preoperatively for managing the patient that allows for the least amount of limb ischemia. At the time of

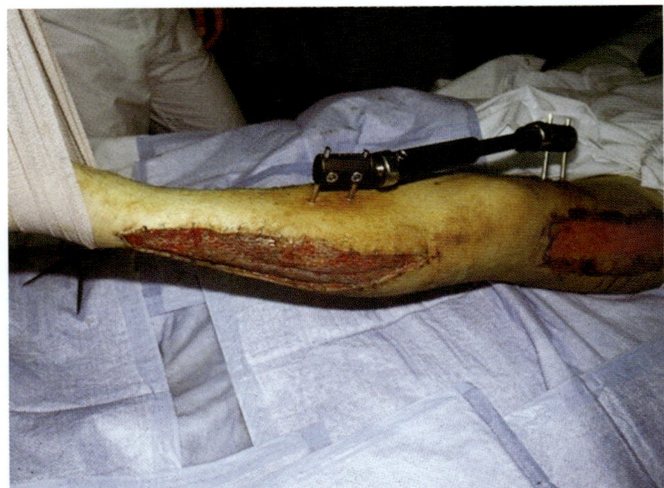

Fig. 42.11: External fixator. The use of external fixators has revolutionized the treatment of complex orthopedic fractures. This patient required an immediate fasciotomy following arterial repair and was returned to the operating room for a split-thickness skin graft several days later.

the exploration of the arterial injury, any associated orthopedic injury must be stabilized. A variety of external and internal fixation devices are available for this purpose. External fixators are especially useful when dealing with contaminated compound fractures (Fig. 42.11). If application of these devices results in a marked delay in revascularization, one option is to use a temporary arterial and/or very occasionally a venous shunt. In such circumstances, it is important to monitor the function of the shunt to avoid further ischemic compromise. Most vascular surgeons, however, prefer to perform the revascularization procedure before any definitive orthopedic stabilization procedure to limit the duration of ischemia. When revascularization is carried out before bone stabilization, allowance must be made for the correct (i.e. final) length of the limb after reduction of the fracture. It is also important to "guard" the vascular reconstructive procedure to ensure that it is not damaged during the orthopedic procedure. Before the patient leaves the operating room, it is critical to ensure that the vascular reconstructive procedure is functioning appropriately and that close monitoring of its function continues postoperatively.

Venous Injuries

Large vein injuries often bleed more than an equivalent arterial injury mainly because venoconstriction does not control bleeding from a transected vein. External pressure, when it can be applied, nearly invariably arrests venous hemorrhage. However, surgical control of venous bleeding is often more difficult than with arteries and can be associated with substantial blood loss.

The diagnosis of occult venous injuries is usually made on imaging performed for associated arterial injuries. Combined arterial and venous injuries occur in up to 50% of cases of vascular trauma.

If venous injury requires intervention, the options are ligation or surgical or endovascular repair.[65-70] Minor veins can be ligated with impunity. For major vein injury, it is not always easy to decide whether repair is appropriate and the necessity for repair is not clear. In some circumstances, the maintenance of early venous patency is important as it improves the chances of limb salvage, especially if there is an associated arterial injury and marked ischemia. Ligation of a major vein markedly increases the swelling in the injured extremity as a result of the compromised venous outflow. The decision to repair a major venous injury is therefore determined by factors, such as the extent of the venous injury and the state of other veins in the area, as well as the presence and extent of other injuries, and the overall status of the patient. In the lower extremity, a single (unpaired) popliteal vein and the common femoral vein should be repaired. Often a lateral repair can be carried out rather than an interposition graft. If a major proximal vein is ligated, fasciotomies should be carried out. Anticoagulation may be valuable to maintain venous patency if there is no contraindication to its use. However, the majority of complex venous repairs, which include interposition grafts and extensive local repairs, occlude over time. Postphlebitic syndrome may result when major veins are ligated or occlude.

Specific injuries of the vena cava, renal and hepatic veins and the portal vein are discussed respectively in Chapter 39, "Thoracic Trauma," and Chapter 40, "Abdominal, Urologic and Perineal Injuries".

False Aneurysm

Iatrogenic false aneurysms can be amenable to different treatment options, which include observation with serial follow-up ultrasound studies, thrombin injection, direct arterial repair, or rarely endovascular intervention.[33,81] Occlusion by ultrasound-guided compression, while well-described in the literature and associated with a high success rate, is associated with significant patient discomfort and for this reason has now been eclipsed by the use of direct thrombin injection that can be utilized in most circumstances.[72]

The natural history of iatrogenic femoral artery false aneurysms has been extensively studied. Most iatrogenic femoral false aneurysms, with a diameter <4 cm and with a small neck, thrombose spontaneously. As a consequence, it is safe to observe with serial ultrasound studies most small asymptomatic iatrogenic false aneurysms of the common femoral artery, when these arise after arterial catheterization.

Iatrogenic femoral artery false aneurysms that are symptomatic, or >4 cm in diameter or have a neck with a diameter >10 mm require treatment to avert local complications or rupture. If thrombin injection is unsuccessful, a surgical approach is required. In our experience, the wall of an iatrogenic false aneurysm can be opened directly and, with direct pressure proximally and distally, the small arterial defect can simply be closed with a single 6-0 Prolene suture.

The surgical principles followed when surgically treating a traumatic false aneurysm are to gain proximal and distal arterial control in order to repair the arterial defect and evacuate the laminated thrombus in the aneurysmal sac.[26]

False aneurysms of nonessential arteries such as branches of the hypogastric or profunda femoris artery can be treated satisfactorily by catheter techniques to occlude the artery. A covered stent may be utilized to treat a surgically inaccessible false aneurysm of a major artery.[73-76]

Arteriovenous Fistula

A small asymptomatic iatrogenic arteriovenous fistula discovered initially after arterial catheterization may be followed up conservatively by serial observations, especially if the patient has appreciable or unstable coronary artery disease.[33] Occasional successes have been reported with ultrasound-guided compression to treat an iatrogenic arteriovenous fistula, particularly in the presence of a long fistula tract.[72]

Most traumatic arteriovenous fistulae are amenable to surgical treatment where the underlying surgical principle is to maintain arterial continuity. Covering the arterial entry site of an arteriovenous fistula with a stent graft is also an option, especially to treat an inaccessible arteriovenous fistula but it is essential to ensure that insertion of the stent graft does not dislodge a thrombus often found in the artery distal to the fistula.[77,78]

REPERFUSION INJURY

Currently, the only known method to minimize this injury is to ensure a good level of hydration of the patient and to minimize the extent of the antecedent ischemia. Few if any additional modalities are available to attenuate reperfusion injury.[79] Free radical scavengers, such as mannitol, and agents that modify xanthine oxidase activity, such as allopurinol, have been extensively studied but are only generally beneficial if given before the onset of acute ischemia. This is, however, not compatible with the trauma setting. The role of remote ischemic preconditioning that describes a phenomenon of brief ischemia reperfusion being applied to tissues distant to the point of ischemia is currently under study. This maneuver has been demonstrated to reduce infarct size in myocardial ischemia and elsewhere and may have potential in the trauma setting.[80,81] The mechanism and how the stimulus is transmitted to the ischemic tissues are currently unknown.

In addition to the detrimental cardiovascular systemic effects that occur after reperfusion, the release of lactic acid, potassium, metabolites, and toxins into the circulation have further detrimental systemic and cardiovascular effects. In the presence of muscle ischemia, there are high blood levels of myoglobin, which block the renal tubules causing acute kidney injury.[82] It is important to attempt to avert this problem by maintaining hemodynamic stability, adequate hydration, and by the use of forced alkaline diuresis (usually >300 mL/h with a urine pH between 6 and 7), and to maintain a normal acid-base status. A common formula is to use an infusion of 0.45% saline solution at 166 mL/h containing 75 mL 8.5% sodium bicarbonate and 250 mL of mannitol. The development of multisystem organ failure (MSOF) after an attempt at salvage of an acutely ischemic limb may be an indication for an urgent amputation, which can be life-saving when carried out expediently. The major error is to ignore the early signs of MSOF and attribute them to previous rather than ongoing muscle ischemia.

EXTREMITY COMPARTMENT SYNDROME

After fractures, crush injuries, revascularization, bleeding, burns, or even just severe shock there is a build-up of tissue pressure in the fascial compartments. When fascial compartment pressures are high, this can cause tissue ischemia and eventually necrosis as a result of a reduction of the arterial perfusion pressures in the confined spaces. This will result in ischemic muscle contractures and permanent nerve damage if the elevated compartmental pressure is not reduced.[83] A diagnosis of compartment

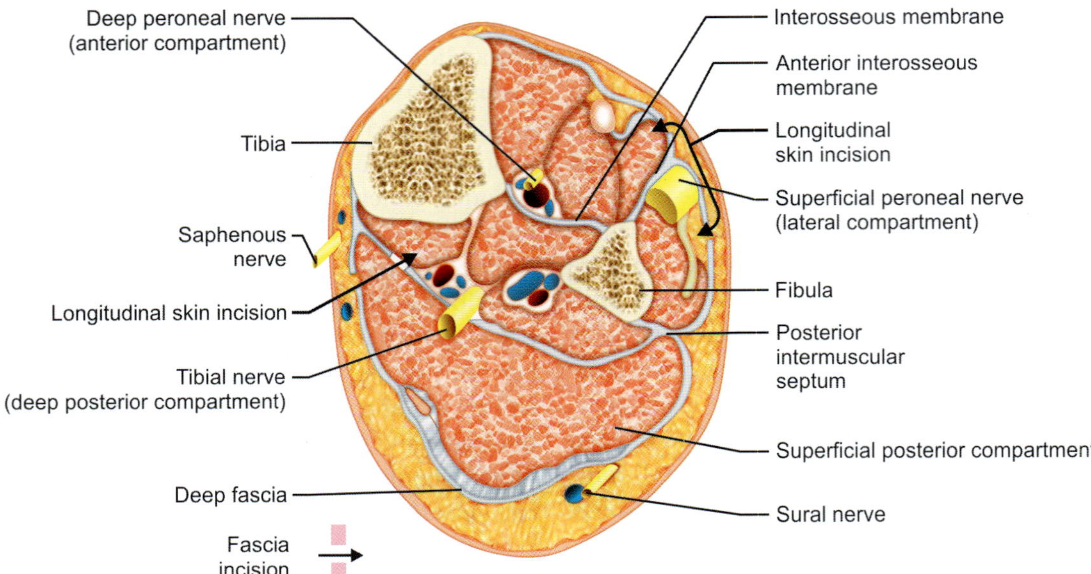

Fig. 42.12: Fasciotomy. Cross-sectional view of the left leg from below. The anterior and lateral compartments are decompressed through an anterolateral lateral incision. The skin incision is placed just anterior to the fibula and the skin is undermined anteriorly and posteriorly to expose these two separate compartments. The incision on the medial side of the leg opens the superficial posterior compartment. At a deeper plane, the deep compartment is then released.

syndrome should be considered if there is a disproportionate amount of pain in an injured upper or lower limb. The pain is accentuated by passive stretching. Physical findings include swelling and tenderness of the compartments. Paresthesia, hypoesthesia, and anesthesia may be found initially, followed shortly thereafter by paralysis. It is important to realize that a compartment syndrome may be present even if distal pulses are present. The various muscle compartments in the lower leg are shown in Figure 42.12. An urgent fasciotomy should be carried out if symptoms and signs of a compartment syndrome develop.

When there is a delay in the revascularization of an acutely ischemic extremity, a prophylactic fasciotomy should be considered because of the anticipated swelling from reperfusion injury. It is probably safest to err on the side of over rather than under use of fasciotomies in patients at risk of a compartmental syndrome.[84] Other indications for a fasciotomy include the presence of a marked soft tissue crush injury or a major vascular or venous injury. The rapidity with which a compartment syndrome develops is extremely variable. For this reason, this potential complication should always be considered postoperatively. Monitoring of the compartmental pressures may be useful when attempting to assess the need for a fasciotomy postoperatively.

Various techniques for releasing the tension in the compartments in the lower leg have been described. A fibulectomy relieves tension in all compartments, but is considered to be too extensive a procedure. The two incision four-compartment fasciotomy, shown in Figure 42.12, provides the greatest guarantee of release of pressure in all compartments with minimal surgical morbidity.[85] A four-compartment fasciotomy through one lateral incision can be carried out (incision 3–4 cm posterior to the fibula), but is not as effective as the two-incision approach. Closed subcutaneous fasciotomies should be avoided because they are not as effective as a four-compartment fasciotomy and may lull the surgical team into a false sense of security. Options for closing fasciotomy wounds include delayed primary closure, split-thickness skin grafting, or gradual mechanical dermal apposition. The latter option appears to be very satisfactory and cost-effective.

SPECIFIC VESSEL INJURIES

Cervical, Mediastinal, and Upper Extremity Vessels

Innominate Artery

Blunt trauma involving the innominate artery generally results in disruption of the proximal component of this artery, which in survivors of such trauma is usually held together by the adventitia. Penetrating trauma usually affects the more distal parts of the artery. In the past, repair of innominate artery injuries was only possible through a median sternotomy but with developments in endovascular technologies this surgery can now often be avoided. Endovascular repair is only feasible, however, if individuals with appropriate skills and equipment are available and if the injury to the vessel allows for placement of an endovascular device into safe landing zones. For this latter reason, injuries in close proximity of the aorta and of the right common carotid artery are usually treated by open repair.

If an open repair is required, the proximal part of the innominate artery usually needs to be replaced especially after blunt trauma with a prosthetic bypass graft that originates from the aorta and not the proximal stump of the innominate artery, as this is usually friable and does not hold sutures well. The proximal end-to-side anastomosis onto the ascending aortic arch is performed using a side biting aortic clamp that can usually only be safely placed with the aid of moderate hypotension. After the proximal anastomosis is completed, the graft is then sutured end-to-end to the distal innominate artery, or its branches. This approach allows for the shortest duration of cerebral ischemia. For occasional penetrating wounds, a lateral sutured arteriorrhaphy, a prosthetic patch arteriorrhaphy, or short interposition graft may be all that is required after debridement of the injury.

Subclavian Artery

The subclavian artery is more frequently injured as a result of penetrating trauma. Although the subclavian artery is sheltered by the clavicle and the sternum, blunt injuries do still occur secondary to posteriorly displaced first rib fractures or fragmented clavicular fractures. As a result of the proximity of the brachial plexus, associated nerve injuries are often encountered. Marked ischemia after injury to this vessel is rarely encountered because of a rich upper extremity arterial collateral circulation.

Injuries to the extrathoracic subclavian artery are often tamponaded by the surrounding soft tissues. Surgical control and repair of such injuries may be aided by division of the clavicle, which should be stabilized with wires or screws after the vascular repair in order to optimize early mobility. Endovascular repair of these injuries, if available, has now generally replaced the need for open repair, particularly in injuries requiring delayed repair. In our experience, such endovascular repair is durable despite the substantial movement of the affected artery and the young age of the average patient.

Injuries to the intrathoracic subclavian artery can result in substantial hemorrhage into the pleural cavity. Operative control of such bleeding usually requires a median sternotomy for a right subclavian artery injury and a left third intercostal space anterior thoracotomy for a left subclavian artery injury. Endovascular approaches, usually through the ipsilateral brachial artery, are gaining favor for the management of selected intrathoracic arterial injuries in hemodynamically stable patients.

Axillary Artery

Most injuries to the axillary artery are penetrating. Such injuries often involve the accompanying vein and nerve plexus. Blunt trauma to the axillary artery may occur after an acute shoulder fracture or dislocation or result from chronic repetitive injuries. These latter injuries are seen in baseball pitchers, swimmers, rowers, and weightlifters. Less vigorous activities can also result in an axillary artery injury, as in patients with thoracic outlet syndrome, especially in the presence of a congenital anomaly, such as a cervical rib. Improper use of crutches can also result in an extrinsic compressive injury to the axillary artery. Blunt axillary artery trauma can result in aneurysm formation with distal embolization and digital ischemia.

Injuries to the distal part of the axillary artery are exposed through an infraclavicular incision that can be extended into the deltopectoral groove for further distal control. Patients with an injury to the proximal axillary artery may require exposure of the distal subclavian artery through a supraclavicular incision to achieve safe proximal arterial control. As a result, endovascular options, when available, are often favored.

Brachial, Radial, and Ulnar Arteries

Blunt brachial artery injuries as opposed to penetrating injuries are rare but do occur in association with elbow dislocations. These are mostly posterior (>80%) and are often associated with median or ulnar nerve injuries. In children, blunt brachial artery injuries are frequently associated with supracondylar humeral fractures. Brachial artery injuries may also be iatrogenic as a result of catheterization. The brachial artery and the radial and ulnar arteries are relatively easy to expose when traumatized so either direct repair of a short segment injury or an interposition bypass for a longer segment injury are the best management options. Thrombectomy of the distal vessels must be done prior to completing the revascularization procedure. In cases of prolonged ischemia or venous injury, a fasciotomy may be necessary.

Thoracic aortic and other vascular chest injuries are discussed in Chapter 39, "Thoracic Trauma". Carotid and vertebral artery injuries are discussed in Chapter 37, "Neck Injury".

Abdominal and Pelvic Vessels

In civilian trauma centers, roughly one in six individuals presenting with abdominal trauma have a significant vascular injury. The risk of a vascular injury is highest with penetrating abdominal trauma. Indeed, abdominal vascular injuries account for a substantial proportion of all vascular injuries seen, approximately one-quarter of the arterial injuries and nearly one-half of the venous injuries in many of the published trauma unit audits. Central abdominal vascular trauma, particularly due to penetrating injuries, is associated with a high mortality because of the potential for a large-volume hemorrhage before and during treatment, as well as the frequent presence of other major injuries and further bleeding complications caused by the coagulopathy associated with the subsequent shock, hypothermia, and other pathophysiological consequences of major trauma.

Vascular injuries after abdominal trauma present with hemorrhage and hemodynamic instability, an intra-abdominal hematoma (mostly in the retroperitoneum) or with thrombosis. For patients with hemodynamic instability, which includes not only hemodynamic parameters but also metabolic evidence of hypoperfusion such as a raised base deficit and lactic acidosis, rapid transfer to the operating room is mandated. Very rarely, intra-abdominal hemorrhage can be partially controlled by use of an emergency room thoracotomy and cross-clamping of the descending thoracic aorta. This maneuver has only been demonstrated to have benefit in penetrating injuries of the abdomen and pelvis.[86] An alternative method for temporary aortic occlusion is to use resuscitative balloon occlusion of the aorta (discussed in detail in Chapter 32, "Initial Surgical Care of the Trauma Patient").

During an emergency laparotomy, obvious hemorrhage from an arterial source is immediately controlled with digital pressure and subsequently with vascular clamps. Bleeding from a venous source, particularly if it appears to be from a midline retroperitoneal vein or veins, is controlled in the first instance with laparotomy pads packed in a systematic manner into all quadrants of the abdominal cavity. Urgent control of the intra-abdominal aorta can be achieved by placement of an aortic occlusion clamp at the level of the diaphragmatic hiatus (*see* also Chapter 40, "Abdominal, Urologic and Perineal Injuries").[87] The aorta is easily identified as it passes through the left crus of the diaphragm. The presence of a nasogastric tube helps to identify the esophagus, which needs to be retracted to the left. The left lobe of the liver is mobilized and retracted to the right, and the peritoneum over the left diaphragmatic crus is incised transversely over the pulsating abdominal aorta. Careful finger dissection through the left crus of the diaphragm on either side of the aorta then frees up adequate space to allow safe placement of an atraumatic aortic occluding clamp. Once the arterial injury is controlled, the aortic clamp can be released to restore flow to the visceral organs.

Exposure of the infrarenal aorta is achieved by incising through the retroperitoneum directly over the aorta. The transverse colon is retracted upwards and the small bowel to the right. Exposure of the suprarenal aorta is usually accomplished by left medial visceral rotation. Any further maneuvers to manage the vascular injury, be it by ligation, local suture, patch repair, or bypass grafting, should only be performed once hemodynamic and physiological stabilities have been achieved. For most abdominal arterial injuries, some form of repair that restores vascular continuity is required. In our view, most abdominal and pelvic venous injuries should be ligated, particularly in severely traumatized patients or if other coexisting major injuries are present. Vascular shunts are generally not a suitable alternative in abdominal vascular trauma, even in circumstances where damage control maneuvers are being considered.

The subset of hemodynamically unstable patients with thoracoabdominal trauma present a particular challenge because of the inability to determine which cavity most of the bleeding is arising from. In recent years, the use of a Focused Assessment with Sonography for Trauma examination performed rapidly by traumatologists in the emergency room has been useful to identify whether to explore the chest or abdomen initially.[88]

The presence of a large central retroperitoneal hematoma should alert the surgeon to the possibility of an injury to the one or more of the visceral arteries or veins. Hence medial visceral rotation is required to inspect all potential vessels for evidence of injury including the aorta, celiac trunk, superior mesenteric artery, both renal arteries, left renal vein, portal vein, and inferior vena cava. Injuries to these vessels should ideally be repaired but ligation of venous structures and on occasion an artery should be considered when the patient is hemodynamically unstable or if significant other injuries are present.

All expanding abdominal retroperitoneal hematomas should be explored. Pelvic hematomas associated with pelvic fractures should not be opened; these are mostly due to venous injury and usually tamponade once the pelvic fracture is stabilized. On occasion extraperitoneal packing of a pelvic hematoma is required. A stable lateral retroperitoneal hematoma can be left undisturbed but is best further evaluated later by a CT scan.

A postoperative CTA or MRA should always be considered to assess the result of the vascular repair and to exclude the presence of missed vascular injuries, especially when a damage control surgical approach is used during the initial procedure. Revascularization of a thrombosed visceral artery may be required in a very small number of patients within a few hours after the initial procedure when the patient is stabilized.

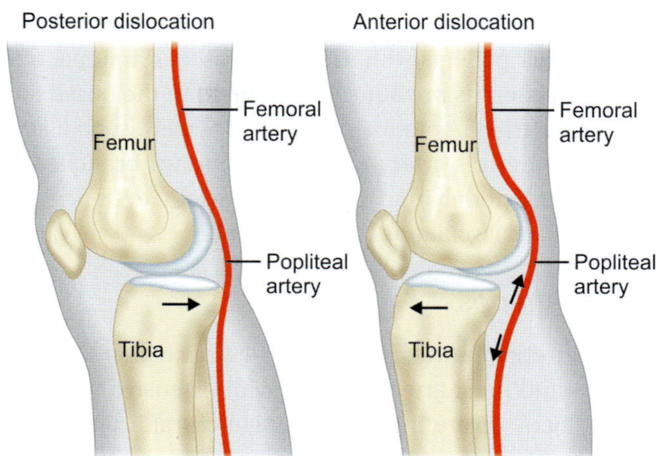

Fig. 42.13: Knee dislocation and arterial trauma. In a posterior dislocation of the knee, the popliteal artery impinges on the posterior aspect of the tibial plateau to cause a localized arterial injury. In an anterior dislocation of the knee, the popliteal artery undergoes a stretch injury.

Lower Limb Vessels

Femoral, Popliteal, and Crural Arteries

The femoral artery as already mentioned is a frequent site for iatrogenic injury and treatment of such complications has already been discussed. The superficial femoral artery may be injured bluntly usually in association with a fracture of the femoral shaft. However, penetrating trauma is the most common mechanism of injury to this artery. Although lower limb ischemia is usually less obvious with injuries of the superficial femoral artery than when the popliteal artery is injured, due to the adequacy of flow provided by an intact profunda femoris artery, it is best to perform a direct repair or place an interposition bypass graft in order to relieve future possible claudication symptoms and avoid the development of late local complications of the vascular injury.

Popliteal artery injuries comprise up to 10% of civilian arterial injuries. After penetrating injuries to the popliteal artery, the amputation rate is still substantial, being reported in most series to be above 10%.[89] Blunt trauma to the popliteal artery is associated with a higher risk for amputation, especially if the ischemia time is >6 hours.[90]

The popliteal artery is classically injured in association with a perigeniculate fracture or a dislocation of the knee (Fig. 42.13). Appreciable force is usually associated with these injuries, which are usually caused by automobile dashboard injuries, motorcycle accidents, or falls. The reported incidence of arterial injury after a knee dislocation is 30%. Approximately half of these individuals have hard signs of arterial injury and require immediate surgical exploration. In those without hard signs of arterial injury approximately 25% will have evidence of arterial injury other than arterial spasm if some form of angiography is performed. A knee dislocation is categorized by displacement of the tibia in relation to the femur. In an anterior knee dislocation, the artery is stretched and the intima disrupts, whereas in a posterior knee dislocation the artery is directly damaged by impingement on the posterior aspect of the tibial plateau. Less commonly, medial, lateral, or rotational dislocations occur. The association between an unstable knee caused by a distal femur fracture, tibial plateau fracture, or knee dislocation and a major arterial injury is sufficiently frequent that it was traditionally taught that all patients with these types of injuries needed to be investigated by an angiographic study to visualize the distal superficial femoral, popliteal, and proximal crural arteries to exclude a vascular injury. Currently, however, if no hard signs of arterial injury exist, which may include a negative high-quality duplex ultrasound evaluation, an angiographic study is not performed. Serial clinical evaluation of the arterial circulation by an experienced clinician is the current standard practice for the management of such patients.[21] The presence of a normal ABI >0.9 and normal peripheral perfusion implies either minimal or no arterial injury. Minor degrees of popliteal arterial injury do not require operative intervention but these patients should be monitored closely in case there is any deterioration in the status of the distal circulation.

When applying these principles based on pulse palpation to other patients with suspected vascular trauma, one should be alert as previously mentioned to the possibility of missing an injury to major nonaxial vessels, such as the profunda femoris artery or other important branches. A significant arterial injury may be present even though normal distal circulation is maintained.

Crural Arteries

Crural arterial injuries account for 8% of civilian vascular injuries and most are associated with extensive fractures to the leg. A severe injury to a single crural artery is followed by limb loss in approximately 10% of cases, whereas such injury to two crural vessels results in limb loss in over 50% of cases.[9,11] The absence of the posterior tibial or dorsalis pedis pulses during the secondary survey is in the first instance managed with splinting of the tibial fractures. In most instances, this maneuver returns adequate blood supply to the foot to maintain viability. If the distal pulses are not restored, this indicates a significant injury that requires surgical intervention. Angiography may be useful to identify the site and extent of injury. Usually an interposition vein bypass is required to restore the distal circulation. It is preferable that two crural arteries are preserved, but it is possible to salvage a foot with revascularization of a single crural artery provided there is good runoff to the foot.

PRIMARY AMPUTATION

The policy of life over limb must always be adhered to. A severely mangled extremity with major crush injury, major nerve injury, segmental bone loss, and appreciable soft tissue loss may be best treated with a primary amputation (Fig. 42.14).[91] This is always a difficult decision to make, but a careful analysis of the overall clinical situation should determine the optimal plan. The option of primary amputation should be discussed preoperatively by a multidisciplinary team but temporary arterial and venous shunts may be placed, while a decision is made between an attempt at limb salvage and primary amputation. Parameters to determine the need for a later amputation after a salvage attempt should also be discussed. These include the presence of sepsis, myoglobinuria, organ failure, continued tissue loss, and if the injury to the limb is so severe that a satisfactory functional outcome cannot be anticipated particularly as a result of injury to major nerves. Even if limb salvage is achieved but the patient has a late nonunion of a long bone in that limb, ischemic contractures, or an insensate foot, a later delayed amputation may be the best alternative. A number of injury severity scoring systems have been used to determine the need for immediate amputation.[92] These scoring systems, though complex and subjective, are of value in decision making because they define injuries that carry a high risk of amputation. They do not, however, predict success or failure and they are in no way a substitute for good clinical judgment. Currently available injury severity scores are not predictive of the functional recovery of patients who undergo successful limb reconstruction.[93]

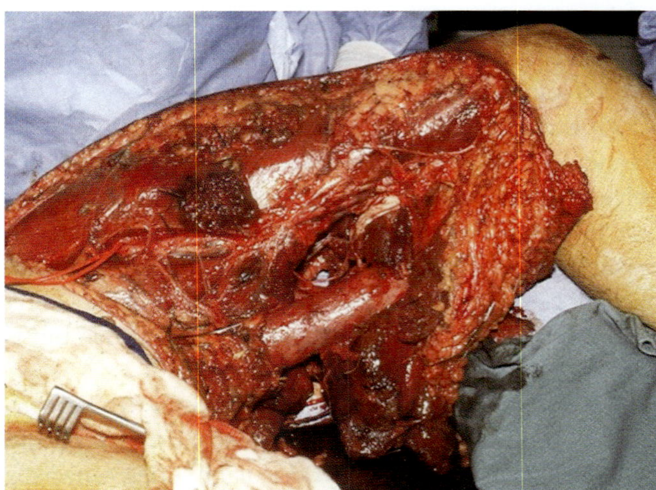

Fig. 42.14: Extensive left thigh injury requiring a high-thigh amputation.

Limb replantation may be an option for selected patients with traumatic extremity amputations of the upper extremity.[94]

PEDIATRIC VASCULAR TRAUMA

In children, the same principles for management of vascular trauma mostly apply as in adults. However, there are some differences as pediatric patient's vessels are much smaller and more easily develop spasm when traumatized or handled. Also there are future growth issues to be considered and the durability of a reconstruction may need to last over nine or even ten decades. Hence, revisional procedures may be required over time if there are hemodynamic size issues or reconstructive failures. Chapter 122, "Preoperative Management of the Pediatric Patient," and Chapter 19, "Surgical Management of Children and Neonates," detail further differences between surgical pediatric and adult populations.

Certain pediatric iatrogenic injuries can pose difficult management decisions.

When complications of limb ischemia occur in an infant with an umbilical artery catheter, the catheter is immediately removed and the infant is heparinized with a bolus of heparin 100 units/kg and then an infusion of 25 units/kg/h. The infant is also volume resuscitated and warmed, if needed.[95] Because a surgical approach is fraught with difficulties due to vessel size and spasm, it is usually not advised unless there is an aortic thrombosis with severe bilateral limb ischemia and/or evidence of visceral artery ischemia. The presence and extent of an aortic thrombosis can be documented by a duplex ultrasound scan. If aortic thrombosis is documented, a transperitoneal approach to the aorta is used and through an aortotomy the thrombus is removed and embolectomy catheters are introduced into occluded outflow or visceral vessels to remove thrombus from their lumens.

Experience with thrombolytic agents in young children is limited.[96] In neonates, there is the potential for increased bleeding complications because of the immaturity of the coagulation system. Higher doses of thrombolytic agents may be required in neonates because of their lower levels of plasminogen compared with adults. More information on their use in neonates is needed and surgery remains the best option when there is severe extremity ischemia secondary to an aortic thrombosis after an umbilical artery catheter has been removed.

A late complication of an umbilical artery catheter is an infected false aneurysm.[97] These are treated in a similar fashion as those that develop in adults (*see* Chapter 82, "Aneurysmal Disease," for more details).

The prevalence of thrombosis is 20–40% after placement of a femoral artery catheter.[98] If there is evidence of ischemia, the catheter is removed immediately (Flowchart 42.2) and the infant heparinized. If the limb is viable but ischemic, a trial of heparin for several hours will result in improvement in most cases. If there is no return of either a palpable femoral pulse or a detectable distal Doppler signal, a surgical revascularization procedure is required.

Femoral artery thrombosis in a child is associated with potential growth retardation in the affected limb. Taylor et al.[99] reported an 8% incidence of clinically marked limb growth retardation after femoral artery catheterization in children under 5 years of age. These children should be monitored for arterial occlusion, and those detected should be monitored for leg growth retardation. Gait abnormalities do not occur unless the limb length disparity is >2 cm. Annual bone length radiographs should be carried out if there is a discrepancy of 1 cm. Future leg-lengthening procedures may be required for marked length discrepancies, and arterial repair may be required in the future for symptomatic patients.

Flowchart 42.2: Management of acute ischemia of the lower extremity after femoral artery catheterization.

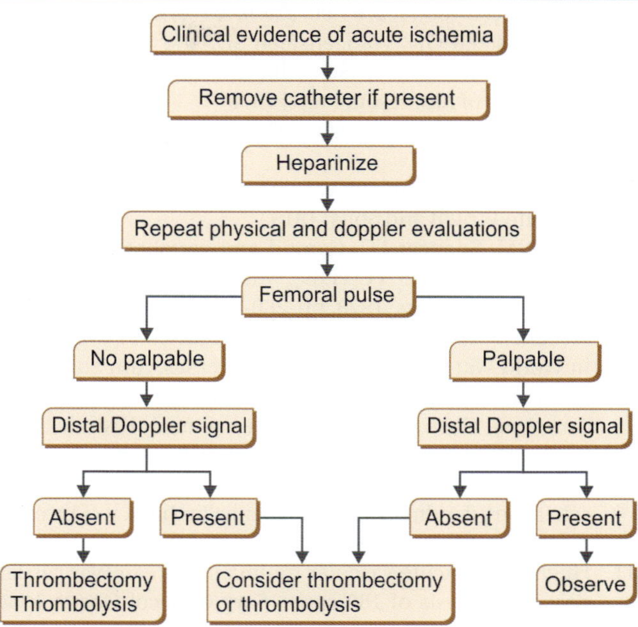

Occasionally, a transfemoral catheter may tear or rupture an external iliac artery during a therapeutic procedure. Vascular reconstruction is required to control the bleeding and the internal iliac artery from the contralateral extremity can be used as a free graft or the ipsilateral internal iliac artery can be rotated to replace the injured external iliac artery.[100]

One should be especially alert for arterial injury with fractures or dislocations of the humerus that can be associated with a brachial artery injury. Volkmann's ischemic contracture should rarely occur if the appropriate principles of trauma management are followed in the pediatric population.[101]

REFERENCES

1. Brohi K, Cole E, Hoffman K. Improving outcomes in the early phases after major trauma. Curr Opin Crit Care. 2011;17:515-9.
2. Keynes G. The Apologie and Treatise of Ambroise Pare'. London: Falcon Educational Books; 1951.
3. Aldea PA, Aldea GS, Shaw WW. A historical perspective on the changing methods of management for major trauma of the lower extremity. Surg Gynecol Obstet. 1987;165: 549-62.

4. Lister J. On a new method of treating compound fracture, abscess, etc. with observations on the conditions of suppuration. Lancet. 1867:1, 2, 95-96, 326-9, 357-9, 387-39, 507-09.
5. Wangensteen OH, Wangensteen SD. The Rise of Surgery; From Empire Craft to Scientific Discipline. Minneapolis: University of Minnesota Press; 1978
6. Ellis H. A History of Surgery. Cambridge University Press. 2002. p. 137.
7. Makins GH. On Gunshot Wounds to the Blood Vessels. Bristol: John Wright and Sons; 1919.
8. Rich NM, Spencer FC. Carotid and vertebral injuries. In: Rich NM, Spencer FC (Eds). Vascular Trauma. Philadelphia: WB Saunders; 1978. pp. 260-86.
9. Debakey MD, Simeone FA. Battle injuries of the arteries in World War II: an analysis of 2471 cases. Ann Surg. 1946; 123:534-79.
10. American Chemical Society International Historic landmarks. Discovery and development of Penicillin. Available from http://www.acs.org/content/acs/en/education/whatischemistry/landmarks/flemingpenicillin.html. [Accessed April 23, 2015].
11. Hughes CN. Acute vascular trauma in Korean War casualties: An analysis of 180 cases. Surg Gynecol Obstet 1954; 99:91-100.
12. Rich NM, Baugh JH, Hughes CW. Acute arterial injuries in Vietnam: 1000 cases. J Trauma. 1970;10(5):359-69.
13. Rich NM, Rhee P. A historical tour of vascular injury management from its inception to the new millennium. Surg. Clin. North Am. 2001;81(6):1199-215.
14. White JM, Stannard A, Burkhardt GE, et al. The epidemiology of vascular injury in the wars in Iraq and Afghanistan. Ann Surg. 2011;253(6):1184-9.
15. Sherif AA. Vascular injuries: experience during the Afghanistan war. Int Surg. 1992;77(2):114-7.
16. Mattox KL, Feliciano DV, Burch J, et al. Five thousand seven hundred and sixty cardiovascular injuries in 4,459 patients. Epidemiologic evolution 1958–1987. Ann Surg. 1989;209(6):698-705.
17. Sugrie M, Caldwell BW, Damours SK, et al. Vascular injury in Australia. Surg Clin North Am. 2002;82(1):211-9.
18. Barros D'Sa AAB. Twenty years of vascular trauma in Northern Ireland. Br Med J. 1995;31:1-2.
19. Oegiannis E, Velmahos GC, Levy RD, et al. Penetrating injuries of the iliac arteries: a South African experience. Surgery. 1996;19:146-50.
20. Austin OMB, Redmond HP, Burke PE. Vascular trauma: a review. J Am Coll Surg. 1995;181:91-106.
21. Martin RR, Mattox KL, Burch JM. Advances with vascular injuries with blunt and penetrating limb trauma. World J Surg. 1992;16:938-9.
22. Giswold ME, Landry GJ, Taylor LM,et al. Iatrogenic arterial injury is an increasingly important cause of arterial trauma. Am J Surg. 2004;187(5):590-92.
23. Singh RR, Barry MC, Ireland A, et al. Current diagnosis and management of blunt internal carotid artery injury. Eur J Vasc Endovasc Surg. 2004;27(6):577-84.
24. Bunt TJ, Malone JM, Moody M, et al. Frequency of vascular injury with blunt trauma-induced extremity injury. Am J Surg. 1990;160(2):226-8.
25. Schlosser V, Spillner G, Breymann TH, et al. Vascular injuries in orthopedic surgery. J Cardiovasc Surg. 1982;23:323-7.
26. Rich NM, Hobson RW 2nd, Collins G Jr. Traumatic arteriovenous fistulas and false aneurysms: a review of 558 lesions. Surgery. 1975;78(6):817-28.
27. Orcutt MB, Levine BA, Gaskill HV 3rd, et al. Iatrogenic vascular injury: a reducible problem. Arch Surg. 1985;120:384-5.
28. Adar R, Bass A, Walden R. Iatrogenic complications in surgery; five years' experience in general and vascular surgery in a university hospital. Ann Surg. 1982;196:725-9.
29. Nehler MR, Lawrence WA, Whitehill TA, et al. Iatrogenic vascular injuries from percutaneous suturing devices. J Vasc Surg. 2001;33:943-7.
30. Nordesgaard AG, Badily KC, Osborne RW, et al. Major vascular injuries during laparoscopic procedures. Am J Surg. 1995;169:543-5.
31. Kinmonth JB, Sheperd RC. Accidental injection of thiopentone into arteries. Br Med J. 1959;2:914-8.
32. Woodburn KR, Murie JA. Vascular complications of injecting drug misuse. Br J Surg. 1996;83:1329-34.
33. Kresowik TF, Khoury MD, Miller BV, et al. A prospective study of the incidence and natural history of femoral vascular complications after percutaneous transluminal coronary angioplasty. J Vasc Surg. 1991;13:328-36.
34. Messina L, Brothers T, Wakefield T, et al. Clinical characteristics and surgical management of vascular complications in patients undergoing cardiac catheterization: interventional versus diagnostic procedures. J Vasc Surg. 1991;13:593-600.
35. Wilson JS, Miranda A, Johnson BL, et al. Vascular injuries associated with elective orthopedic procedures. Ann Vasc Surg. 2003;17(6): 641-4.
36. Rothwell DM, Bondy SJ, Williams JI. Chiropractic manipulation and stroke: a population-based case-control study. Stroke. 2001;32(5):1054-60.
37. Van der Spuy L. Complications of the arterial tourniquet. South Afr J Anaesth Analg. 2012;18(1):14-18.
38. Kent K, Moscucci M, Mansour K, et al. Retroperitoneal hematoma after cardiac catheterization: prevalence, risk factors, and optimal management. J Vasc Surg. 1991;13: 328-36.
39. Zimmerman BJ, Granger DN. Mechanisms of reperfusion injury. Am J Med Sci. 1994;307(4):284-92.
40. Samson R, Pasternak BM. Traumatic arterial spasm—rarity or nonentity. J Trauma. 1980;20:607-08.
41. Hegarty MM, Angorn IB, Gollogly J, et al. Traumatic arteriovenous fistulae. Injury. 1975;7(1):20-28.
42. Fox N, Rajani RR, Bokhari F, et al. Penetrating lower extremity arterial trauma: evaluation and management. J Trauma. 2012;73(5):S315-20.
43. Frykberg ER, Crump JM, Dennis JW, et al. Non-operative observation of clinically occult arterial injuries: a prospective evaluation. Surgery. 1991;109:85-96.

44. Johansen K, Lynch K, Paun M, et al. Non-invasive vascular tests reliably exclude occult arterial trauma in injured extremities. J Trauma. 1991;31:512-14.
45. Lynch K, Johansen K. Can Doppler pressure measurement replace "exclusion" arteriography in the diagnosis of suspected arterial injuries in penetrated extremities? Ann Surg. 1991;214:734-41.
46. Bergstein JF, Blair JF, Edwards J, et al. Pitfalls in the use of color-flow duplex ultrasound for screening of suspected arterial injuries in penetrated extremities. J Trauma. 1992; 33:395-402.
47. Helvie MA, Rubin JM, Silver TM, et al. The distinction between femoral artery pseudoaneurysms and other groin masses: the value of duplex scan. Am J Roentgenol. 1988; 150:1177-80.
48. Francis H III, Thai ER, Weigelt JA, et al. Vascular proximity: is it a valid indication for arteriography is asymptomatic patients? J Trauma. 1991;31:512-4.
49. Gillespie DL, Woodson J, Kaufman J, et al. Role of arteriography for blunt or penetrating injuries in proximity to major vascular structures: an evolution in management. Ann Vasc Surg. 1993;7:145-9.
50. Ginzburg E, Montalvo B, LeBlanc S, et al. The use of ultrasonography in penetrating neck trauma. Arch Surg. 1996; 131:691-3.

Additional references appear in the online version of this book.

43

Thermal Injury

Philip Barker

Key Points

- Burns represent a frequently unrecognized source of major pathology, particularly in low-income countries.
- Children and the elderly are especially at risk and carry the highest mortality.
- An understanding of the pathophysiology of the burn wound is crucial to proper management and resuscitation.
- Special types of burn (e.g. electrical, inhalational) demonstrate singular characteristics requiring early recognition and specific management.
- Modern biosynthetic materials have enhanced closure of the burn wound.
- Early surgical excision +/- grafting is key to successful outcome.
- Special areas (face, hands, feet, and perineum) require specialized expert management.
- The metabolic response and increased nutritional needs of patients with larger burns should not be underestimated.
- Cold injuries are best divided into local tissue damage and systemic hypothermia.
- The physiology of lowering core body temperature and effects of rewarming must be understood.
- Localized cold injuries must be managed appropriately if tissue loss is to be minimized.
- Prevention by protective clothing and avoidance of harsh conditions would reduce morbidity and mortality due to cold injury.

INTRODUCTION

Since people discovered fire and developed the skills to make it, they have sustained injuries from it. Similarly, as humans dispersed and moved from the accepted "cradle of humankind" in Africa to colder climes, or populations were overtaken by a glacial maximum, when ice sheets were at their maximum extension, covering most of North America, Europe, and Asia, their exposure to cold resulted in local cold injuries and systemic hypothermia. Burn injury is far more common than cold injury, not only because clothing has reduced the likelihood of the latter, but because for a large percentage of the world's population cooking and heating is still done on open fires, and, in addition, fire is still widely used as an effective and terrifying weapon. Burn injury is a ubiquitous threat in the military environment, and war burns have been described for >5,000 years of written history. Fire was probably utilized as a weapon long before that.

BURNS

Definition

A burn is an injury to the skin or other tissues primarily caused by heat, either flame or contact with hot materials including liquids. It may also be due to radiation, radioactivity, electricity, friction, or contact with chemicals. Respiratory damage resulting from steam and smoke inhalation, along with the toxic effects of the products of combustion, is also considered to be a burn.

Demographics

Globally, burns are a serious public health problem. At least 80% of the world's population lives on less than \$10 a day[1] and more than half the world's population—about 3 billion people—cook their meals with wood, dung, coal, and other solid fuels over open fires or on primitive stoves inside their homes. That simple act is killing 1.5 million people every year, according to a report by the World Health Organization.[2]

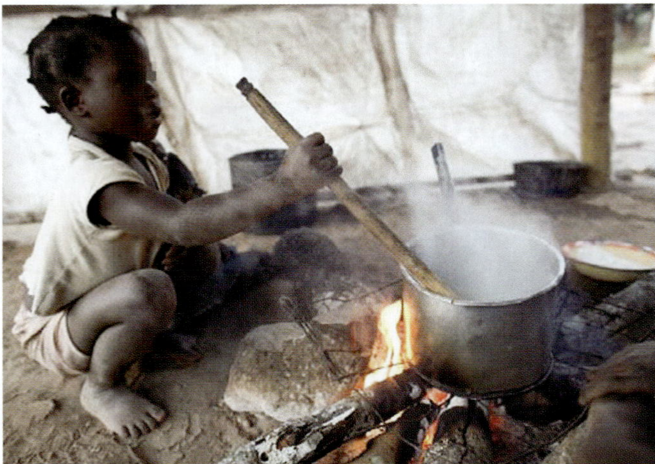

Fig. 43.1: Burn injuries to children in low- and middle-income countries can lead to lifelong disabilities and disfigurements.

Fire-related deaths rank among the 15 leading causes of death among children and young adults aged 5–29 years old (Fig. 43.1). Over 95% of fatal fire-related burns occur in low- and middle-income countries. South-East Asia alone accounts for just over one-half of the total number of fire-related deaths worldwide and females in this region have the highest fire-related burn mortality rates globally. Among age groups, children <5 years and the elderly >70 years have the highest fire-related burn mortality rates. In addition to those who die, millions more are left with lifelong disabilities and disfigurements, often with resulting stigma and social rejection. Furthermore, the societal knock-on has the effect of worsening the outcome for the family of a burn victim. Burns cause children to stop going to school because they cannot use their hands to write; mothers cannot pick up their babies because they can no longer bend their arms; and fathers lose their jobs because they can no longer work, plunging poor families deeper into poverty.

The suffering caused by burns is even more tragic as many burns are so eminently preventable. High-income countries have made considerable progress in lowering rates of burn deaths through a combination of proven prevention strategies and through improvements in the care of burn victims. Most of these advances in prevention and care have been incompletely applied in low- and middle-income countries. Increased efforts to do so would likely lead to significant reductions in rates of burn-related death and disability.[19]

The devastation caused by burns in the developing world is enormous, but the demographic statistics for burns in the United States seem to have shown no significant change in almost the last 20 years (Tables 43.1 and 43.2).

Table 43.1 Selected statistics on admissions to US burn centers, 1995–2005.
Burn injuries receiving medical treatment per year: 500,000
Fire and burn deaths per year: 4,000
Hospitalizations for burn injury per year: 40,000
Survival rate: 94.4%
Total body surface area (TBSA) burned: 38% of admitted patients exceeded 10% TBSA, and 10% exceeded 30% TBSA.
Most included severe burns of such vital body areas as the face, hands, and feet
Gender: 70% male, 30% female
Ethnicity: 62% Caucasian, 18% African–American, 12% Hispanic, 8% other
Burn cause: 46% fire/flame, 32% scald, 8% hot object contact, 4% electrical, 3% chemical, 6% other
Place of occurrence: 43% home, 17% street/highway, 8% occupational, 32% other

Source: Data from the American Burn Association.

Table 43.2 Selected statistics: 2002–2011 burn admissions to US burn centers.
Burn injuries receiving medical treatment: 450,000
Fire and burn deaths per year: 3,400
Hospitalizations related to burn injury: 40,000, including 30,000 at hospital burn centers
Survival rate: 96.1%
Gender: 69% male, 31% female
Ethnicity: 59% Caucasian, 19% African-American, 15% Hispanic, 7% other
Admission cause: 44% fire/flame, 33% scald, 9% contact, 4% electrical, 3% chemical, 7% other
Place of occurrence: 69% home, 9% occupational, 7% street/highway, 5% recreational/sport, 10% other

Source: Data from the American Burn Association.

However, when reading these statistics, it is important to appreciate that the population of the United States has increased by 30 million (from 281,421,906 in 2000 to 311,800,000 in mid-2011) during this time. So in relative terms, there has been a decrease in burn deaths.

First Aid and Emergency Room Treatment

Whatever "treatment" is used, the first principle of dealing with a burned casualty is to stop the burning process— without risk of the rescuer becoming another casualty. Rushing in to extract a person from a burning fuel truck where fuel has been spilled over the road may not be the most sensible course of action, nor attempting to pull an electrocution victim off a high tension cable if they are still in contact. Heroic rescues have been achieved on occasion, but many more attempts have resulted in increasing the casualty load.

Before the receiving team tackles the burn wound itself, it is imperative that as detailed a history as possible is taken from the patient, from witnesses, or the rescuing paramedic team. The casualty may have had to jump from a burning building, or have been extricated from a car crash, and there may be associated injuries that will be overlooked if the resuscitation team concentrates solely on the burn wound. If the patient is found to be clinically shocked in the early stages after a burn, it is wise not to attribute this to the burn, but look carefully for occult associated injuries. Advanced trauma life support (ATLS) principles should apply. The administration of supplemental oxygen, while routine in ATLS protocols, becomes critical where the suspicion of an inhalational burn exists.

Management of the wound upon arrival in the emergency room (ER) has changed significantly in the last two decades. It is no longer appropriate for the nursing staff to smother the patient in thick layers of silver sulfadiazine cream, followed by roll upon roll of crepe bandages. The procedure is painful for the patient, time-consuming, and messy for nursing staff, and quite unnecessary. Many studies have shown that using cling film (Glad Wrap) has distinct advantages; it is quick and easy to apply, sterile, and reduces pain, wound contamination, and fluid losses. Furthermore, it is inexpensive, widely available, nontoxic, and transparent, which allows for wound monitoring without dressing removal.[13-15] One caveat is that it should not be applied to limbs circumferentially, to avoid any possibility of a tourniquet effect; it should be unrolled lengthwise, along the limb. The cling film may be retained without adverse effects for up to 72 hours, by which time a first debridement should have been performed, and a definitive dressing applied.

The relatively modern concept of first aid is believed to have originated from the military battlefield,[8] where soldiers were taught how to bandage and splint their wounded comrades. The Prussian surgeon, General Friedrich Von Esmarch, is attributed with the earliest written description of first aid (his work was translated into English in 1882) and he recommended that burnt surfaces should be protected from air, and anointed well with oil (lamp oil, salad oil, castor oil, or carron oil from a chemist) or painted over with grease or butter, or powdered with flour, starch, or charcoal to alleviate the pain.[9]

Local Management

Throughout history, a variety of acute treatments have been used for burn injuries, although most of these agents have little or no scientific evidence to support their use.

From the earliest records (around 1500 BC), an exotic and eclectic mix of substances has been recommended including mud, excrement, plant extracts, frogs boiled in oil, fermenting goat dung, pig fat, resin, bitumen, honey, bran, cork, ashes, wine, and myrrh.[3-6] Galen (AD 129-199) was the first to be credited with application of cold water for burn treatment, but a direct reference to him is unknown.[6,7]

By 1901, the recommendations for first aid treatment of burns/scalds were clearly segregated according to wound depth.[10] The application of flour, whiting, or powdered chalk was recommended for burns where the skin was "merely reddened," but a covering with oils (carron, olive, salad, linseed, almond, or cod-liver), Vaseline, lanoline, or cold cream was recommended, where the skin was blistered or charred.

It was not until 1965 that the use of cold water treatment started to appear in St John Ambulance first aid manuals, also with recommendations to not apply any lotions to the burn and for the patient to go to a hospital.[11] The manuals stated that the immediate need after a burn injury was to "lessen the spread of heat in the tissues and alleviate pain by immersing the part in cold water if possible (or any other nonflammable fluid to hand), then keep the part dry and clean". By 1969, guidelines had progressed to irrigation with cold water, followed by cold compresses, and then covering the burn with a clean/sterile cloth. These are the recommendations still promoted by many organizations today[12], but much of the world's population has neither knowledge of them nor access to information about them. Consequently, traditional methods of first aid are still applied, if any at all. These can consist of applications of egg, butter, oil, toothpaste, chocolate, papaya, and banana leaves, among a host of other concoctions. Ice and iced water should not be used as this may deepen the burn wound by extending the zone of stasis such that it becomes part of the zone of coagulation (necrosis). Inadequate resuscitation will do the same thing (Fig. 43.2).

Escharotomies

Full thickness (FT) burns can produce a constricting eschar in any part of the body where the burn is circumferential. Relieving incisions through the insensate skin and

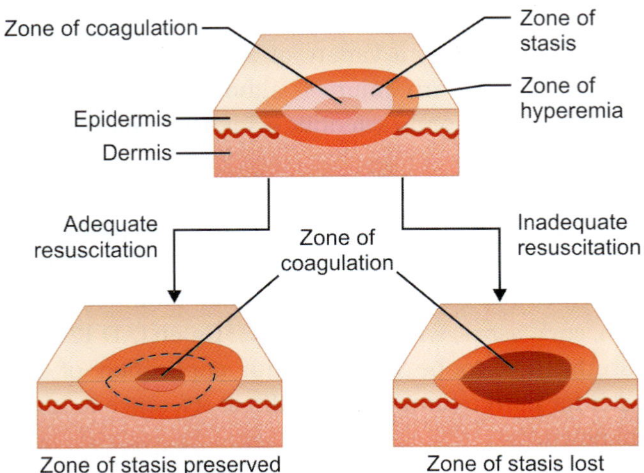

Fig. 43.2: These three zones of a burn are three dimensional, and loss of tissue in the zone of stasis will lead to the wound deepening as well as widening.

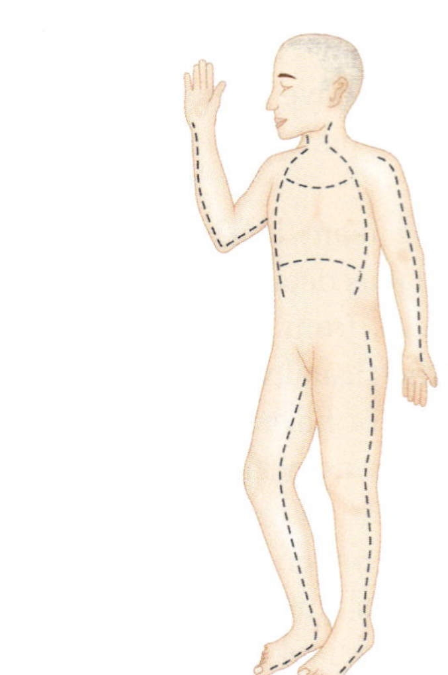

Fig. 43.3: Escharotomies.

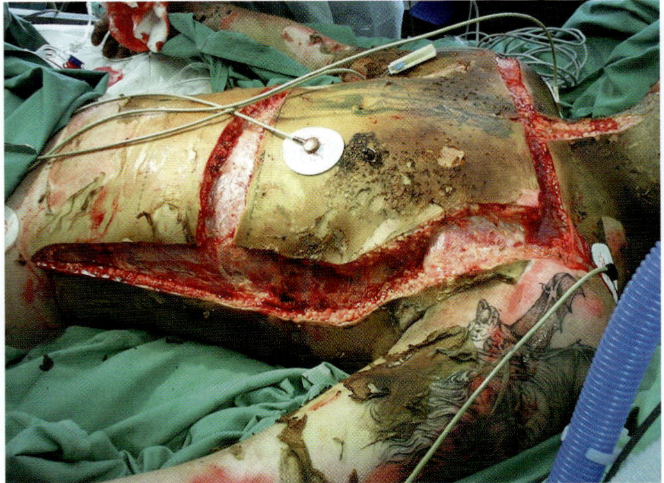

Fig. 43.4: Patient with escharotomies to prevent ischemia of limbs and compromised ventilation of the thorax.

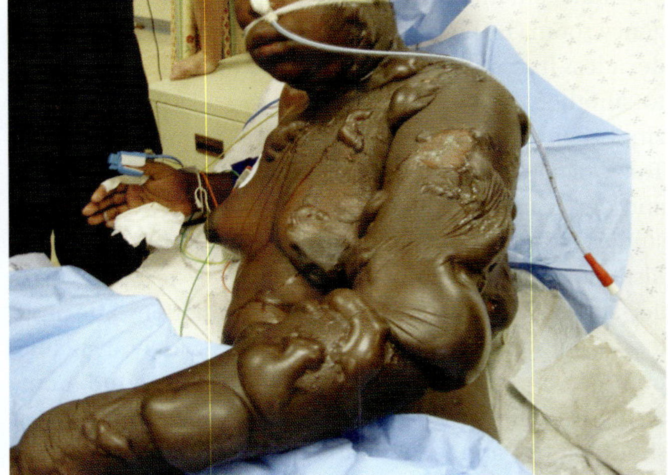

Fig. 43.5: Leaking blisters and soaked bedsheets on the skin of a burn patient.

superficial fat (escharotomies) may be required to prevent ischemia of limbs or, if the eschar constricts the thorax, compromised ventilation (Figs. 43.3 and 43.4).

Blisters

The management of blisters in burn wounds continues to fuel debate. Those in favor of leaving them intact argue that they constitute a sterile and comfortable "dressing" over an otherwise raw, painful, but superficial exposed wound, and that to burst or remove them will predispose the burn to subsequent infection (Fig. 43.5). The argument to remove blisters is based on a number of practical observations: first, that not all blistered burns are superficial[16,17,35,36], and if a deep partial thickness (DPT) burn is found, it may require split skin graft (SSG); second, that some blisters are tense and across joints, and need to be evacuated or removed to allow movement and rehabilitation of the joint; third, that even if blisters are left intact initially, they frequently then burst during the patient's hospitalization, leaking copious amounts of sticky, proteinaceous fluid, and take up unnecessary nursing time; last, that the application of cling wrap over any exposed burned surfaces significantly reduces pain and keeps the wound sterile until the first surgical debridement in the operating room (OR).

General Management

Analgesia

Burns are often intensely painful, and analgesia is frequently given too little and too late. Small, repeated, intravenous (IV) doses of opiates, titrated to patient comfort, are required and should be administered at the same time as exposing the burn and applying cling wrap. Exposed nerve endings are exquisitely sensitive to the slightest of air currents, and for this reason superficial partial thickness (SPT) burns, which retain these nerve endings in the dermis, are very much more painful than deeper or FT burns, where such dermal elements are lost.

Fluid Resuscitation

Not all burn patients need IV fluid resuscitation. Although figures vary between different burn centers across the world, a figure of 15% total body surface area (TBSA) burn would generally be accepted to indicate the need for IV fluid therapy. Some countries still feel there should be a difference between the threshold for IV therapy in children (usually taken as <12 years), where they prefer a 10% TBSA trigger to IV therapy, reserving 15% for adults.

If the patient is extensively burned, it is still possible and acceptable to place IV cannulae even through a FT eschar. When an IV line is set up for any burns patient, blood should be sent at the same time for biochemistry analysis including urea and creatinine, electrolytes, glucose, typing and cross matching, as well as routine hematology. Any suggestion of an inhalational component should prompt an arterial blood gas (ABG) sample to be drawn for standard ABGs along with a lactate level, and carbon monoxide (CO) estimation, if possible.

Types of Fluid and Rates of Administration

The amount of IV fluid required is calculated by a formula. Up until relatively recently the Parkland formula has been used extensively throughout the world. This formula is mathematically expressed as: Amount of fluid required in 24 hours (mL) = 4 × Patient's weight (kg) × Percent TBSA burned.

For example, a person weighing 75 kg with burns of 20% TBSA would require 4 × 75 × 20 = 6,000 mL of fluid replacement within 24 hours. The first half of this amount is delivered in the first 8 hours and the remaining fluid is delivered in the next 16 hours. The "first 24 hours" is taken from the time of burn, not the time of presentation to the ER.

Studies over the last decade have suggested that this formula may provide too much fluid if rigidly adhered to, and that not enough attention is given to the physiological response in terms of urine output. For adults, this should be no more than 0.5 mL/kg/h. Where this is exceeded, or the infused volume of fluid is allowed to gradually increase even beyond the prescribed 4 mL/%TBSA/kg/24 h, then the phenomenon of "fluid creep" may occur.[18] Fluid creep from overinfusion may manifest as the abdominal compartment syndrome with the inevitable leak of fluid into the interstitium and generalized edema.

To avoid this complication, various alternative formulae have been suggested, some using colloids, in an attempt to maintain the capillary oncotic pressure, while others have simply reduced the fluid volume infused. The Brooke formula suggests halving the volume of the Parkland formula to 2 mL/%TBSA/kg/24 h, but this has not found general acceptance. More recently, the compromise volume of 3 mL%TBSA/kg/24 h has been tried, but the most important factor in preventing the complication of fluid creep is to monitor the urine output, and, in adults, not let it increase beyond 0.5 mL/kg/h. Children <12 years should attain a urine output of 1 mL/kg/h, and infants up to 2 mL/kg/h. Urine volumes in excess of these figures should prompt a reduction in the volume of IV resuscitation fluids.

It should be noted that those patients who fall into the category of needing full IV resuscitation will need bladder catheterization. It is important that the urine is tested for blood and myoglobin—particularly in electrical burns, where myonecrosis is both common and a potential cause of renal failure and/or compartment syndrome, especially in the limbs. The residual volume of urine in the bladder on catheterization, once tested, should be discarded and not be included as part of the subsequent physiological response to infused fluid.

Although it is now generally agreed that the administration of colloids in the first 24 hours is not indicated, as the leaky capillaries will also lose the larger molecules, there is as yet no consensus over the use of colloids in the second 24 hours. Marginal benefits have been described, but have not translated into improved survival, and there is often a further capillary leak after the colloid infusion is stopped.[17] Generally, Ringer's lactate (RL) is the crystalloid solution of choice.

Several very important conceptual differences exist in pediatric burn resuscitation. Intravenous fluid resuscitations are usually required for patients with smaller burns. Some centers would argue for IV resuscitation from

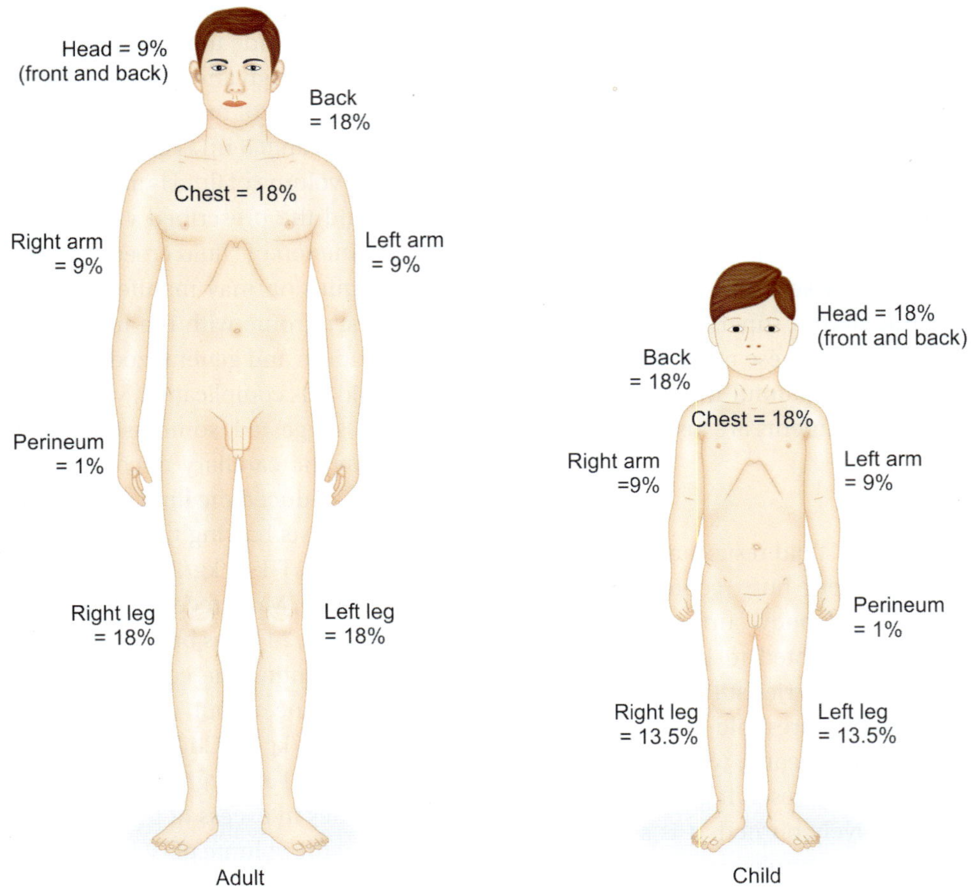

Fig. 43.6: Differences in total body surface area percentages between adults and children.

10% TBSA upwards in children. Venous access in small children may be a difficult issue, and an interosseous line is an acceptable alternative in the short term.

Most routinely used resuscitation formulae were developed using adult patients and are almost exclusively weight-based. Since the linear relationship between weight and surface area does not exist in children, use of these formulae results in under- or over-resuscitation. Children have proportionally larger body surface areas (BSAs) than adults and burn TBSA must be estimated using pediatric modifications to Lund–Browder tables, which demonstrate the relatively larger head and small thighs (Fig. 43.6).

Pediatric burned patients should therefore be resuscitated using formulae based on BSA, which can be calculated from height and weight using a standard nomogram or formulae.

Dubois formula: BSA (m^2) = ht (cm)$^{0.725}$ × wt (kg)$^{0.425}$ × 0.007184

Jacobson formula: BSA (m^2) = [ht (cm) + wt (kg) – 60]/100

The pediatric resuscitation protocol from Shriners Burns Hospital (Cincinnati) is based on the original Parkland formula:

4 mL/kg per %TBSA + 1500 mL/m^2 BSA

First 8 hours – RL solution + 50 mEq sodium bicarbonate per liter

Second 8 hours – RL solution

Third 8 hours – RL solution + 12.5 g of 25% albumin solution per liter

Many other formulae may be obtained from the literature, but the critical point is that children require more fluid for burn shock than adults with similar %TBSA. Due to their small body weight to BSA ratio, fluid losses are proportionally greater in children. Normal blood volume in children is approximately 80 mL/kg body weight, and neonates, 85–90 mL/kg, compared to the adult whose normal blood volume is 70 mL/kg. Evaporative water losses in a 20% TBSA burn in a 10 kg child are 475 mL or 60% of the circulating volume, while the same size burn in a 70 kg adult causes the loss of 1100 mL, or only 25% of the blood volume. For this reason, children may manifest a shock state very soon after the burn injury if resuscitation is delayed, even within 30 minutes.[115]

Recommended physiological end points are also higher in children, with urine output closer to 1 mL/kg/h being a more appropriate goal. Children approaching 50 kg are probably better served by adult resuscitation calculations (0.5 mL/kg/h urine output). Children under a year lose their renal medullary concentrating capacity secondary to washout of the medulla during resuscitation and the immature kidney's inherent inability to concentrate. As a result, hyponatremia is frequently seen in the first 48 hours after injury; so regular monitoring and replacement will be necessary.

Another concern with this population is the limited hepatic glycogen reserve, which can be exhausted quickly and sometimes requires a change from RL solution to dextrose 5% in RL solution to prevent life-threatening hypoglycemia. For this reason, blood sugar monitoring every 4–6 hours should be routine during the hypermetabolic state, especially for patients with larger burns.

Nasogastric Feeding

Those with 15% TBSA or more will also need a nasogastric tube (NGT) to be placed. Despite the theoretical complication of acute gastric dilatation, which is extremely rare, nasogastric (NG) intubation is required for feeding. As a general rule, burned patients lose their appetites, and the obligatory catabolism associated with the burn is worsened by lack of calorie input. A dietitian should, ideally, form part of the burns team, and aim to provide 100% of the total calorie requirement down the NGT, with any oral intake regarded as a bonus. Although there is evidence that absorption from the gut is delayed in the early hours after a major burn[20], the aim should be to start NG feeding within 18 hours if possible, and certainly within 24 hours. This should also help to prevent the acute duodenal ulcer (Curling's) that early endoscopic studies suggested may occur.[21] Additionally, sucralfate down the tube between feeds may also be beneficial in ulcer prevention. Curling's ulcer is now a rare finding.

Antibiotics

Prophylactic antibiotics are not indicated in the acute stages after a burn. Studies have shown that a burn remains sterile for up to 72 hours after injury[22,23], by which time some definitive debridement with grafting or dressing should have been performed. Nevertheless, tetanus prophylaxis should be given.

Special Types of Burn Injury

Electrical Injury

Electrical injuries, although relatively uncommon, are inevitably encountered by most emergency physicians. Adult electrical injuries usually occur in occupational settings, whereas children are primarily injured in the household setting. The spectrum of electrical injury is broad, ranging from minimal injury, to severe multiorgan involvement, to death. Electrical injuries are estimated to cause approximately 500–1,000 deaths per year in the United States (US).[24] They are responsible for 3–5% of all burn unit admissions and cause 2–3% of emergency department burn visits in the pediatric population.

An electrical current can produce an array of injuries as the current passes through the body. Most of the damage is beneath the skin surface and therefore the actual injury can easily be underestimated. Tissue damage results from heat generated by the passage of electric current through the body as well as direct thermal injury caused by the ignition of clothing.[25]

Electricity is generated by the flow of electrons, the current, across a potential gradient through a conductive material. The voltage (V) represents the magnitude of this potential difference and is usually determined by the electrical source. Ohm's law states that the current [(I) in amps] through a conductor between two points is directly proportional to the potential difference [(V) in volts] across the two points when the resistance [(R) in ohms] is constant.[26,27]

The type and extent of an electrical injury are determined by voltage, current strength, resistance to flow, the duration of contact with the source, the pathway of flow, and the type of current (i.e. direct or alternating).

Voltage: Electrical injuries are typically divided into high-voltage and low-voltage injuries, using 500 V or 1000 V as the cutoff. In the US and Canada, typical household electricity provides 110 V for general use and 240 V for high-powered appliances, while industrial electrical and high-tension power lines can have >100,000 V.[24]

Current: The current is a measure of the amount of energy that flows through a body. That energy is perceptible to the touch at a current as low as 1 mA. A narrow range exists between perceptible current and the "let go" current: the maximum current at which a person can grasp and then release the source of the current before muscle tetany makes it impossible to let go. The "let go" current for the average child is 3–5 mA; this is well below the

Table 43.3 Physiological effects of different electrical currents.

Effect	Current (milliamperes)
Tingling sensation/perception	1–4
Let-go current–children	3–4
Let-go current—women	6–8
Let-go current—men	7–9
Skeletal muscle tetany	16–20
Respiratory muscle paralysis	20–50
Ventricular fibrillation	50–120

15–30 mA threshold of common household circuit breakers. For adults, the "let go" current is 6–9 mA, slightly higher for men than for women. Skeletal muscle tetany occurs at 16–20 mA. Ventricular fibrillation can occur at currents of 50–100 mA (Table 43.3).[30]

Resistance: The resistance of body tissues varies with their electrolyte and water content. Blood vessels, muscles, and nerves have high electrolyte and water content, and thus low resistance, and are good conductors of electricity—better than bone, fat, and skin.[28.] Heavily calloused areas of skin are excellent resistors, whereas a moderate amount of water or sweat on the skin surface can decrease its resistance significantly.

Type of circuit: Electrical current can flow in one of two types of circuits: direct current (DC), in which the direction of flow of electrons is constant, or alternating current (AC), in which the direction changes in rhythmic fashion. Alternating current (AC) is the most common type of electricity in homes and offices, standardized to a frequency of 60 cycles/sec (Hz).

High-voltage DC often causes a large, single muscle contraction that throws the victim away from the source, resulting in a brief duration of contact with the current. In contrast, AC of the same voltage is considered to be approximately three times more dangerous than DC, because the cyclic change of flow of electrons causes muscle tetany that prolongs victims' exposure to the current. Muscle tetany occurs when fibers are stimulated at 40–110 Hz; the standard 60 Hz of household current is within that range. If the source contact point is the hand, when tetanic muscle contraction occurs, the extremity flexors contract, causing the victim to grasp the source, resulting in prolonged contact with the current.

Tissue damage from electrical injury may be obvious at the cutaneous contact site or sites, but often also involves underlying tissues and organs along the path of the current. The amount of heat generated in these is proportional to the tissue resistance. Current density (current per unit cross-sectional area) is the next main determinant of tissue damage, with severity of injury being inversely proportional to the cross-sectional area traversed by current. Therefore, severe injuries to the extremities are common, and marked injuries to the torso are rare. Superficial tissues in a limb may be normal, whereas muscles surrounding bone may be nonviable because of the longer duration of heating caused by the slower heat dissipation from bone.[29] This is critically important as it means that myonecrosis and a compartment syndrome may occur in limbs where the outward appearance is normal.

Types of Electrical Burns

Electrical burns can cause a variety of injuries through several different mechanisms.

Direct contact: Current passing directly through the body will heat the tissue causing electrothermal burns, both to the surface of the skin as well as deeper tissues, depending on their resistance. It will typically cause damage at the source contact point and the ground contact point.

Electrical arcs: Current sparks are formed between objects of different electric potential that are not in direct contact with each other, most often a highly charged source and the ground, as with lightning (*see* "Lightning Injuries" below). The temperature of an electrical arc can reach 2,500–5,000°C, resulting in deep thermal burns where it contacts the skin. These are high-voltage injuries that may cause both thermal and flame burns in addition to injury from DC along the arc pathway.

Flame: Ignition of clothing causes direct burns from flames. Both electrothermal burns and arcing currents can ignite clothing.

Flash: When heat from a nearby electrical arc causes thermal burns but current does not actually enter the body, the result is a flash burn. Flash burns may cover a large surface area of the body but are usually only partial thickness.

With all electrical burns, in order to avoid becoming another victim, would-be rescuers should ensure that any electric current is switched off before attempting to remove the casualty from the source.

Lightning Injuries

Because the effects of a lightning strike can be variable and diffusely spread over the body, most authors characterize lightning injuries as mild, moderate, or severe.

Mild lightning injury is rarely associated with burns, but persons struck often report loss of consciousness, amnesia, confusion, tingling, and numerous other nonspecific symptoms. Mild lightning burns are invariably superficial with little or no deep-tissue damage.

Moderate lightning injury may cause seizures, respiratory arrest, or cardiac standstill, which spontaneously resolves with resumption of normal cardiac activity. Much of the symptomatology mirrors that of mild lightning injury, but superficial burns are much more common, both initially and in a delayed fashion. These patients may have lifelong symptoms of irritability, sleep disorders, and paresthesias.

Patients with severe lightning injury usually present with extensive flash burns and cardiopulmonary arrest, which is often complicated by a prolonged period in which they do not receive cardiopulmonary resuscitation (CPR). This delay is attributable to the fact that these individuals are often in an isolated location when injured. Survival is rare in this group unless a bystander expeditiously begins CPR.[31]

Chemical Burns

Most acids produce a coagulation necrosis by denaturing proteins, forming a coagulum (e.g. eschar) that limits the penetration of the acid and can usually be adequately dealt with by simple dilution with copious amounts of water. Alkalis, or bases, typically produce a more severe injury known as liquefaction necrosis. This involves a saponification of fats as well as a denaturing of proteins, which may allow the burn to penetrate deeply into the tissues. Hydrofluoric acid is somewhat different from other acids in that it also produces a liquefaction necrosis.

The severity of a chemical burn is related to a number of factors, including the length of the contact time and the pH, concentration, volume, and the physical form of the agent. The ingestion of solid pellets of alkaline substances results in prolonged contact time in the stomach, thus, more severe burns. In addition, concentrated forms of some acids and bases generate significant heat when diluted or neutralized, resulting in a combination of thermal and caustic injury.

The mainstay of treating chemical burns is persistent and prolonged irrigation. Attempts to neutralize either acids or alkalis are futile and time-wasting, with the exception of hydrofluoric acid, which may cause significant systemic toxicity due to fluoride poisoning. Treatment of hydrofluoric acid burns includes applying 2.5% calcium gluconate gel to the affected area. If the proprietary gel is not available, it can be constituted by mixing 10% calcium gluconate solution with three times the volume of a water-soluble lubricant (e.g. KY gel). If pain persists for >30 minutes after an application of calcium gluconate gel, further treatment is required. Subcutaneous infiltration of calcium gluconate is recommended at a dose of 0.5 mL of a 5% solution per cm^2 of surface burn extending 0.5 cm beyond the margin of involved tissue. Further details can be obtained from other sources.[32]

Inhalational Injury

Inhalational burns continue to cause serious concerns because not only are they a potent source of mortality, but also the correct management remains undecided due to lack of controlled clinical trials.

There are *different types of inhalational burn damage*, categorized according to anatomy and pathology. *Anatomically*, they may be classified according to the level of airway affected; (i) the upper airway burn, i.e. the supraglottic compartment, down to and including the vocal cords of the larynx, and (ii) the lower airway or bronchioalveolar burn. *Pathologically*, inhalational injury can occur by (i) *cell injury* and pulmonary parenchymal damage by heat and irritants, (ii) *hypoxemia* by interruption of oxygen delivery by asphyxiants, (such as CO, carbon dioxide and hydrogen cyanide) and (iii) end-organ damage by *systemic absorption* of toxic gases (among others, hydrogen cyanide, chlorine, formaldehyde, ammonia, sulfur dioxide, and phosgene) through the respiratory tract.

Anatomic Classification

Upper airway burn: The heat generated during combustion can cause significant thermal injury to the upper airway, and particulate matter produced during combustion (soot, cokes, and chars) can mechanically clog and irritate the airways, causing reflex bronchoconstriction. Intense heat from flame, vapor, and steam can all produce significant edema that gives rise to the classic symptoms of a hoarse voice and barking cough, sometimes accompanied by carbonaceous sputum, although the latter is more commonly a feature of the lower, bronchioalveolar burn. Laryngeal edema is not always manifest in the early stages after an airway burn, and is usually maximal at around 12–36 hours, which can lull the unwary into a state of false security while the airway is not immediately compromised and the voice remains normal. Suspicion of an airway burn should be possible with a history of fire in a confined space, obvious steam burns and scalding of the face, or a raised CO level >5%. Patients at risk should not be discharged from hospital despite their protestations of feeling well, and careful observation and early intubation are essential if a disaster is to be averted. Frantic attempts to intubate an imminently closing larynx should not occur if staff have been vigilant in anticipation.

It will usually be possible to extubate the patient at 48 hours if there is no other damage to the lower airway.

Bronchioalveolar burn: Deep inhalational burns produce an intense reaction, but it takes time to evolve, so that what is initially seen is not the end-pathology. While this is true of all elements of a burn injury in the early stages, it is particularly so of the inhalational component. In the same way that it may take up to 24 hours post-burn for laryngeal edema to compromise the upper airway, so in deeper, alveolar burns, the pathology develops progressively over 3–5 days. Once pneumonia and adult respiratory distress syndrome have set in, ventilation can be difficult, so the decision to ventilate needs to be taken early if it is felt that the bronchioalveolar burn is still evolving. There are, however, few reliable clinical data on which to base this decision and no published randomized clinical trials to date.

Pathologic Classification

Cell damage: The clinical picture of respiratory compromise following inhalational burn injury is the result of thermal or chemical damage to the epithelial cells of the intrathoracic and extrathoracic airways. Secondary insult with bacterial pneumonia may occur days after inhalation, causing further cytotoxic damage. Ciliary function is impaired by the initial injury, leading to accumulation of airway debris. The inflammatory cascade initiates neutrophil infiltration. Vascular hyperpermeability leads to a large amount of fluid flux from the circulating plasma to the interstitial spaces. This lung edema formation is even more severe when the thermal injury is associated with smoke inhalation. Macrophages within the alveoli are destroyed, allowing bacteria to proliferate. Lack of an intact epithelial barrier further facilitates the development of pneumonia.[33]

Some units have attempted to ameliorate the alveolar clogging from casts and exudate by instilling heparin or acetylcysteine down the endotracheal tube, but again, no randomized controlled clinical trials are reported to demonstrate conclusively that these measures improve survival or reduce the incidence of post-burn pneumonia. Recent experimental work has suggested that the urinary trypsin inhibitor, ulinastatin, may reduce the inflammatory response in the lung parenchyma, and improve survival[42], but studies in burned humans have yet to be performed.

Hypoxemia results from a decrease in inspired oxygen concentration at the scene of injury, a mechanical inability to exchange gas because of airway obstruction or parenchymal pulmonary damage, and inhibition of oxygen delivery and tissue use by toxins. With the advent of sophisticated intensive care support, patients who survive the acute injury and are successfully transported to an intensive care unit now rarely die from isolated pulmonary injury.[74] However, the presence of multiorgan dysfunction, a common sequela of hypoxemia, substantially raises morbidity and mortality rates.

Carbon monoxide is produced from both smoldering and flaming combustion and is one of the commonest products of combustion. It does not directly injure the lung; its toxic effect results from a displacement of oxygen from hemoglobin-binding sites, thereby decreasing the oxygen-carrying capacity of the blood. Lethal concentrations of CO can be generated in the immediate vicinity of the ignition within 10 minutes.[34] It not only has a 250-fold greater affinity for hemoglobin than oxygen but also shifts the oxyhemoglobin dissociation curve to the left. This shift results in further tissue hypoxia because the hemoglobin is less able to unload oxygen. Carbon monoxide reacts with myoglobin to worsen impaired tissue oxygen uptake by decreasing facilitated diffusion of oxygen into muscle. Carbon monoxide also interacts with several heme-containing enzymes of the electron transport chain, reducing tissue oxygen availability even more.

Cyanide, produced by the combustion of many nitrogen containing compounds, causes tissue asphyxiation through the inhibition of intracellular cytochrome oxidase. It blocks the final step in oxidative phosphorylation and prevents mitochondrial oxygen use. Affected cells convert to anaerobic metabolism, and lactic acidosis results. The organs most sensitive to cellular hypoxia are the central nervous system (CNS) and the heart. The CNS reacts to low concentrations of cyanide by stimulating hyperventilation, thereby increasing inhalation of the agent.

There are some clues that a severe bronchioalveolar burn injury may be present; the initial ABGs may demonstrate a V:Q mismatch—a shunt—despite the administration of increased inspired oxygen (FiO_2). The degree of shunting may be expressed as a percentage (%), and readily available tables in anesthetic textbooks allow the % shunt to be read off the graph of a plot of inspired oxygen against the partial pressure of arterial oxygen

(FiO_2 vs. PaO_2). It is important not to use hemoglobin saturation (SaO_2) as this is colorimetrically derived, and, percutaneous saturation monitors are unreliable where CO poisoning is a likely factor.[37,38] Carbon monoxide is eliminated through the lungs and the half-life of CO in the body at room air temperature is 3–4 hours. Supplemental oxygen increases the dissociation of CO from carboxyhemoglobin, thus turning it back into hemoglobin. One hundred percent oxygen via a nonrebreather mask reduces the half-life to 30–90 minutes, and hyperbaric oxygen (HBO) at 2.5 atmospheres pressure with 100% oxygen reduces it to 15–23 minutes.[39-41] However, it is controversial whether HBO actually offers any extra benefits over normal high flow oxygen, in terms of increased survival or improved long-term outcomes.

The value of determining the degree of shunt may be in selecting those patients whose prognosis is dismal, whether ventilated or not. Personal observation by the author suggests that patients with a shunt >20% on presentation do badly; with no access to either HBO or extracorporeal membrane oxygenation, there was 100% mortality in this group, irrespective of TBSA burned. However, it may be important to lower the initial CO level before assessing the percent shunt and deciding whether or not to ventilate. These studies are yet to be performed.

Repeated flexible bronchoscopy for pulmonary toilet to improve ventilation has been tried, but there are no controlled trials data to support or refute its use.

Toxic effects of inhaled gases/vapors: All fires produce noxious asphyxiant gases, with CO and hydrogen cyanide being the most common products of combustion. Other by-products produced by combustion of furniture and fabric (aldehydes), or rubber and plastics (chlorine gas, ammonia, hydrocarbons, various acids, and ketones) produce injury when inhaled. Exposure to metal fumes and fluorocarbons, systemic toxins typically released during industrial fires, is rare in the pediatric population. Children are more likely to be affected by toxins from household products and products of smoke, including CO and cyanide poisoning.[62]

Tables of inhaled toxins and their effects can be found at appropriate websites.[51] The clinical manifestations will depend on the concentration of these gases in the inhaled air.

Closure of the Burn Wound

The burn wound is analogous to an intestinal evisceration. If this comparison seems excessively dramatic, consider that each demonstrates a loss of domain. For the intestine to be hanging on the outside of the abdominal wall, it is obvious that it needs to be inspected, cleaned, repaired where necessary, and then returned to its proper place, and the wound closed. Unless this is done swiftly, the exposed gut will lose heat and fluid, desiccate, and become infected.

Similarly, where skin and dermal elements are lost, the loss of domain pertains to the body's ability to thermoregulate, retain moisture, resist bacterial invasion, and remain waterproof, without pain. The sooner the burn wound is "closed," the less effect this loss of domain will have on the body as a whole. This wound closure is therefore the priority in burn management. Temporary cover using cling wrap has already been described above.[13,36] It should be noted that its use is as an initial dressing (up to 72 hours) in the first aid and ER scenarios, or after exposing wounds for assessment on ward rounds. It is not a form of skin closure.

Superficial Partial Thickness Burns

Superficial partial thickness burns will heal on their own within 10–14 days without scarring if they remain infection free. After initial debridement including removal of blisters and inspection of the burn base to ensure no deeper elements, the SPT burn may either be treated open with topical antibiotic ointments or covered with a silver containing compound and the dressing undisturbed for 4–5 days. Skin substitutes like biobrane are useful for areas like the face and hands.[49,50,63-68] The practice of daily, or even twice daily, dressings for uninfected burns is unnecessary, painful for the patient, and delays healing by removal of the new epithelium at each dressing change. If left alone, the wound will re-epithelialize faster.

Except for large %TBSA or suspicion of abuse, most SPT burns may be treated as outpatients.

Deep Partial Thickness and Full Thickness Burns

In many hospitals around the world, burned patients are neglected in a corner of the ward until time can be found to deal with them surgically. By this time, often weeks after the burn injury and hundreds of painful dressings, the patient is malnourished, emaciated, with contracted and infected wounds, and there is little hope of a full functional, cosmetic, or emotional recovery. Despite many seminal publications in the literature over the last 50 years demonstrating significant reductions in morbidity, mortality, and hospital stay, the exhortation to early wound closure by timely excision and grafting has been frequently ignored for the most part, outside of established burn centers.[43-48]

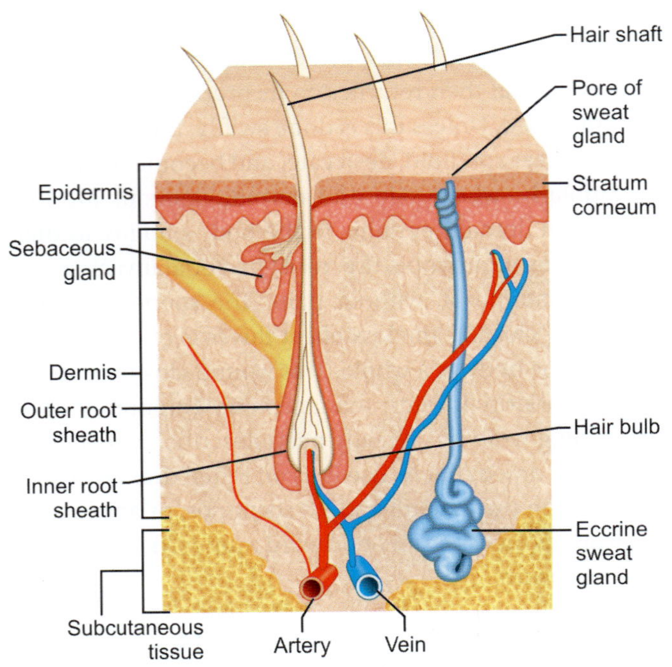

Fig. 43.7: Layers and structures of the skin.

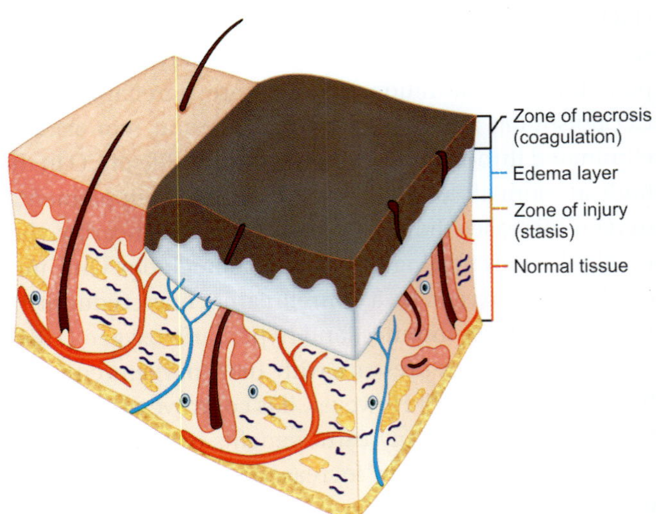

Fig. 43.8: Superficial partial thickness. It involves the entire epidermis to basement membrane and no more than the upper third of the dermis. Rapid re-epithelialization occurs in 1–2 weeks. Because of a large number of remaining epidermis cells and good blood supply, there is a very small zone of injury or stasis beneath the burn eschar. *Courtesy* of Smith & Nephew, Inc.

Definitive closure of the burn wound means providing what has been lost, i.e. skin. Ideally, this should be an autologous autograft to avoid the immunological rejection of cadaveric or porcine skin. However, sufficient autologous skin may not be available, and synthetic "skin substitutes" may be necessary to provide donor sites time to heal before reharvesting. The decision to graft or not is based on experience and the depth of the burn wound.

Management strategies are largely dependent on depth and percentage TBSA of the burn wound, but are also influenced by limitations of the particular treatment center.

Assessment of Burn Wound Depth

The nomenclature of 1st, 2nd, 3rd, and 4th degree burns is outdated and has been replaced by more accurate terminology based on a more pathological description (Fig. 43.7) of damaged epidermal and dermal elements.

Simple erythema (1st degree) in lighter-skinned races or sunburn is not included in the assessment of the percentage burn of TBSA. Though painful, it is treated entirely symptomatically and will not be discussed further.

Superficial Partial Thickness (2nd Degree)

Superficial partial thickness burns (Fig. 43.8) are characterized by being moist, often blistered, red, and intensely painful. The surface epithelium has been burned away leaving exposed nerve endings unprotected. Sweat glands and hair follicles are still intact, and a pulled hair will be retained. If pressed, the red, moist surface of the burn will blanche, and then capillary refill will restore its redness in a short time.

These burns are often caused by scalding liquids or steam, and should heal without grafting or scarring in around 10–14 days.

Deep Partial Thickness (Deeper 2nd Degree)

Deep partial thickness (DPT) burns (Fig. 43.9) can be hard to assess as they are often patchy and initially indeterminate in extent. They are often caused by flame or prolonged contact with sticky liquids, such as cooking oil, tar, or porridge that adhere to the skin. When the red area is pressed, there is no longer any blanching as the capillaries are ruptured and the red cells are now "tattooed" into the burned dermis. This is called "fixed skin staining" and is pathognomonic of a DPT burn. The DPT burn may be mixed with areas of FT or SPT burn. Deep partial thickness burns will take a long time to re-epithelialize as the majority of the skin dermal elements, such as sweat glands and hair follicles, where epithelial cells are generated, are largely destroyed. Residual hairs are easily removed by gentle traction or wiping with a swab.

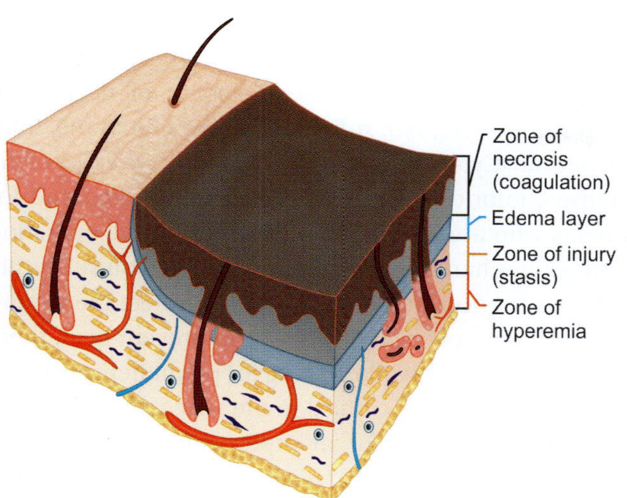

Fig. 43.9: Deep partial thickness. Destruction of the epidermis occurs to the basement membrane plus the middle third of the dermis. Re-epithelization is much slower (2–4 weeks) due to fewer remaining epidermal cells and less blood. More collagen deposition will occur, especially if not closed by 3 weeks. The depth of wound has a significant risk of conversion. The zone of stasis is much larger than in the superficial partial thickness injury because of less blood flow and more initial injury to the remaining epidermal cells.
Courtesy of Smith & Nephew, Inc.

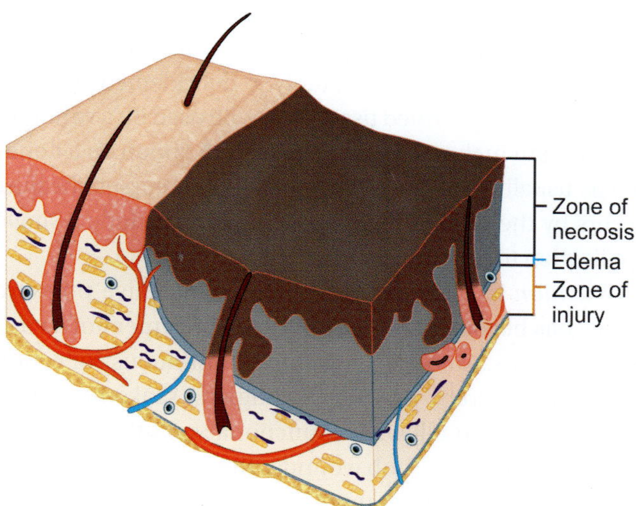

Fig. 43.10: Full thickness (FT). It involves the entire epidermis and at least two-thirds of the dermis, leaving very little dermis and epidermal cells to regenerate. Spontaneous healing is very slow, over 4 weeks. Sharp debridement is needed to remove eschar. Scarring is usually severe if not skin grafted and there is a high risk of infection. Inflammation-induced conversion to a FT burn is common. The function of a re-epithelialized deep partial thickness burn is poor due to fragility of the epidermis and the rigidity of the scar laden dermis.
Courtesy of Smith & Nephew, Inc.

Because of the patchy nature of DPT burns, it is often wise to wait for 5–7 days to see which areas become clearly either SPT or DPT, and then apply an SSG only to the latter. Although conservative management will eventually achieve healing in DPT burns, the incidence of infection, scarring, and contracture is high if this course of action is adopted.

Full Thickness (3rd Degree)

Full thickness burns (Fig. 43.10) are thick, leathery, often charred, and show marbling of the skin, which is pale yellow or white with obvious capillary thrombosis. The dermis has been completely destroyed down to subcutaneous fat, sometimes down to muscle or even deeper (4th degree). This distinction is not important clinically, as all FT burns will need a full, tangential excision of the burn wound and either SSG or, depending on the part of the body (e.g. face), FT (Wolfe) grafts, or plastic surgery pedicle flap-transfer techniques.

Modern Wound Dressings and Prevention of Infection

The immediate goal of managing the acute burn is to close the wound; however, infection is a constant threat to the burn patient. Immune suppression is a consequence of any major injury and this is compounded in the burn patient by loss of the barrier to infection as well as the presence of eschar (dead, burned tissue), which is a protein-rich, avascular medium ideal for bacterial growth. Typically the wound is first colonized by skin commensals and then endogenous respiratory and gut flora, and nosocomial microbes. The two mainstays of infection prevention are topical antimicrobials and maintenance of a moist environment with good management of exudate. There is no role for prophylactic systemic antibiotics[14-17,22,23,36] and IV antibiotics are reserved for systemic signs of infection.

The antimicrobial effects of silver have been known since the 19th century, and silver impregnated creams and dressings used on burns with good effect for many decades. More recent advances in nanocrystalline technology have allowed much greater bioavailability of silver, (e.g. Acticoat) with significant improvements in antibacterial and anti-inflammatory action.[49,50]

Hydrofiber is a soft, nonwoven dressing composed of sodium carboxymethylcellulose. It is a conformable material that can absorb a large amount of wound exudate, but prevents lateral spread of that fluid across the wound and locks in both the exudate and bacteria. The saturated hydrofiber is then transformed into a soft gel, which creates a moist environment. The gel aids the removal of nonviable tissue from the wound by autolytic debridement without damaging newly formed tissue. It can be used on a variety of wounds, but in the burn patient is a good option on a donor site as usually with only one application complete healing occurs by the time of removal. Other uses include a single application to SPT wounds.[63]

Vacuum-assisted closure or topical negative pressure (TNP) has become popular for the management of a variety of wounds. Among its benefits is continuous collection of exudate, thereby avoiding soiling and strikethrough of dressings. It also allows for functional splinting, particularly useful in upper limb wounds. The condition for application is that the wound must be a clean, debrided wound, as it remains sealed for a couple of days. Other benefits include reduced edema. It may also be used as a reliable form of graft fixation. In extensive wounds, to obtain a good seal can be challenging.[64]

Surgical Principles and Wound Coverage

Debridement

Debridement is the removal of all necrotic or nonviable tissue from the wound bed. Tangential excision is specific to burns and is the layered and serial excision of thin layers of the burn until punctate bleeding occurs in the deeper viable layers of the dermis. This is performed using either a Humby–Braithwaite knife (or a variant thereof) or an electric dermatome. Control of blood loss and the temperature of the patient are vital during the procedure. A dedicated burns OR is optimal for the surgical treatment of these patients. The temperature is set at 30°C. Timing of this process is also important. Early burn wound excision within 48–72 hours has now been shown to be the gold standard of care.[43-48] It reduces the inflammatory response, shortens hospital stay, and decreases scar hypertrophy, but at the cost of increased need for blood transfusions. Techniques for minimizing blood loss are described later.

A newer technique now available is the *hydrosurgery system*. This consists of a graded power console that propels saline through a handheld cutting and suction device. The stream of pressurized saline functions as a knife. Where traditional tangential excision lacks precision, the Versajet system offers the opportunity for preservation of the deeper dermal elements and is ideal for DPT wounds. It is also useful in difficult and contoured areas like the nose, eyelids, ears, and hands.

Permanent and Temporary Cover

Currently there is no product that performs as well as an autologous SSG for permanent closure of deep burn wounds. However, *skin substitutes* such as Biobrane, Integra, or TransCyte have a role for temporary coverage of the extensive injuries where donor sites are limited and for patients who are too sick for a more extensive operation that includes harvesting of donor sites. The skin substitute functions to provide good pain relief, protect the wound from infection, promote healing, and prevent heat, fluid, and electrolyte loss while waiting for permanent coverage with autologous skin. Critical to the success of these skin substitutes is the need for an impeccable wound bed free from any sign of infection or necrosis. In the same way that the presence of such tissue will cause any autologous skin graft to fail, skin substitutes will not adhere and similarly fail.

A *human cadaver allograft* is another option for temporary wound coverage. It may also be used as a biological overlay dressing over widely meshed autografts. Adherence to the wound bed makes the use of an allograft desirable due to the decreased microbial contamination. Although it is ultimately rejected, it allows time for donor sites to heal or the physiology of the patient to recover until autologous skin can offer permanent closure. Bacterial and viral contamination remains a risk as with any biological product, but the risk is low.

The cultured epithelial autograft (CEA) was promoted as an option for permanent wound closure, but results have not been overwhelmingly successful.[65-67] The culture of keratinocytes takes weeks to produce, and is extremely fragile when used on a wound bed with no underlying dermis, as in FT burns. However, it can be useful as an adjunct in hastening the healing of donor sites or partial thickness wounds. It may also be sprayed on to widely meshed grafts to fill the interstices and speed up epithelial coverage.

Management Strategies

The approach to SPT wounds that will heal spontaneously and deeper wounds that will not is different. Appropriate management becomes vital in the large surface area burns, as the management of the wound plays a large role in the systemic response to the burn and subsequent complications.

Superficial Partial Thickness Burns

As long as the wound stays infection-free and does not progress in depth, healing will occur in SPT burns. The option for dressing chosen depends often on the site of the wound, and it is rarely necessary—and never desirable—to "mummify" any part of the patient in swathes of bandages. Such practice is wasteful of nursing time and resources, means painful dressing changes for the patient, does not reduce costs, and delays recovery as it is impossible for an occupational therapist to work under such constraints. Furthermore, it may be socially isolating if the head and face is bandaged so that the patient can no longer interact with either staff or other patients. The torso is best covered and the dressings held in place by a combination of adherent (e.g. Op-site) or elasticated (e.g. Netelast) products. The "special areas" of the hands, feet, face, and perineum are dealt with separately.

Biobrane is one of the several skin substitutes that can be applied by either skin clips or sutures to burns. It must be compressed by bandaging for 48 hours to adhere, so that when the bandages are removed the membrane is transparent. It is ideal for SPT burns as it reduces analgesic requirements, protects from contamination, and is retained in place until re-epithelialization is completed beneath it, whereupon it separates naturally from the new underlying skin. If this dressing is not available, other skin substitutes may be tried.

Use of skin substitutes in large surface area SPT burns offers physiological closure of the wound and attenuates the systemic inflammatory and catabolic response. Ideally it should be done early in the first 48–72 hour window while the burn is still sterile, with a precise superficial debridement and coverage with a skin substitute as one procedure. Subsequently no further dressings should be required, which further decreases pain and nursing workload, but the more important benefit is the decreased incidence of burn wound infection. Synthetic skin substitutes have been shown to have good cosmetic outcomes in SPT burns of the face and are considered by many the standard of care.[43,68] Hydrofiber dressings or TNP are other options in the management of partial thickness wounds that may be more cost-effective than skin substitutes.

Deep Partial Thickness and Full Thickness Burns

Excision Techniques: The FT wound must be excised early and covered. In wounds <30 %TBSA this can be done in one procedure, with immediate autologous meshed split-thickness skin grafting. The split-thickness skin graft is taken from donor sites using either a freehand technique using a Watson, Humby, or Braithwaite knife (the Goulian adaptation is excellent for small, difficult and delicate areas), or an air-driven or electric dermatome.

Debridement (as described above) is different from excision, so the "set" of the blade (depth of cut) of either the knife or dermatome is greater for tangential excision than for taking an SSG.

Blood loss can be significant in both procedures, but may be minimized by using tourniquets for the limbs, or the "tumescent technique" on the torso. The latter technique uses 2 mL of 1:1000 adrenaline (epinephrine) + 40 mL 0.5% plain bupivacaine added to 1 L of warm normal saline. A 19-gauge, 3.5-inch spinal needle is attached to the giving set of the bag, which is placed in a pressurized infusion device and the injection given subdermally. The raised skin should feel cold (and look white in Caucasian races). Once the skin has been harvested (for SSG) or the burn excised (by tangential excision), adrenaline-soaked abdominal packs (5 g in 1 L warm normal saline) can be applied to the wound bed, with a significant reduction in blood loss.

Split-thickness skin grafts are secured by skin clips, tissue glue, or sutures, depending on the site, and then covered with several layers of paraffin gauze to prevent movement, followed by dry gauze, and bandaging.

If infection has been a problem, activated nanocrystalline silver (Acticoat; Smith and Nephew, London, UK) may be applied and secured in place with water-soaked gauze and bandages. The dressing will remain bacterially active for up to 4 days, and has anti-inflammatory properties.

The choice of site for harvesting skin depends on the location of the burn, and what skin is available. For example, neck skin is good for the eyelids; inner arm skin is good for the face. For both of these sites, it is preferable not to mesh the graft (make expansion holes by means of a graded mesher), but use it as a complete "sheet". Sheet grafts only require a few tiny perforations to be made with a scalpel point to allow for the escape of any underlying trapped exudate. Meshing grafts can be a very useful way of expanding the area covered by a harvested piece of skin. Meshing plates and rollers are graded in ratios from 1.5:1 up to 9:1 depending on the degree of expansion required. The larger ratio meshed grafts potentially cover a much greater area for the amount of skin harvested, but at the cost of reduced cosmetic appearance.

Wherever possible, harvested skin should be matched for color, texture, and hair growth of the recipient bed. When skin substitutes are not an option, reharvesting of donor sites is usually possible within 10–14 days.

Local limitations, such as limited operating time or availability of blood, may mean a staged procedure for even moderate sized burns. In wounds >30% TBSA, sufficient donor areas are lacking and the magnitude of the surgical insult becomes greater, so staged procedures are inevitable. It is preferable not to spend >1 hour at a time on any one procedure. Prolonged OR sessions increase the metabolic stress on the patient and the potential for blood loss and hypothermia, even in especially heated ORs. It should be remembered that every operation to harvest skin for SSG is making a further open surgical wound. Excision of the burn wound is the most important priority. Coverage options depend on the availability of autologous skin for SSG or commercial skin substitutes that some institutions may not have. It may be necessary to resort to only topical antimicrobial dressing coverage between operations. In such situations, mortality and morbidity is high.

Additional options in very large %TBSA burn injuries include very widely meshed grafts (3:1 to 6:1) overlaid with a cadaveric allograft sandwich or CEA. Some surgeons test their excision bed with application of allograft initially, and only perform autologous grafts a few days later. Cultured epithelial autograft has also been used on donor sites to accelerate healing both for enabling donor site reharvesting and to decrease the %TBSA of wounds, so diminishing the systemic inflammatory and catabolic responses.

Special Areas: Hands, Feet, Face, and Perineum

Hands: The critical element of dealing with hand burns is preservation of function. Because the hand is (usually) dependent and the skin of the dorsum is lax, edema appears rapidly. This impairs flexion at the metacarpophalangeal joints. Simple elevation of the burned hand will reduce pain and the tendency to swell, and facilitate early movement and functional recovery.

If no other first aid is available, then placing a plastic bag over the injured hand will reduce pain and prevent further contamination, but layering on cling-film each side of the hand followed by copious applications of cold, running water is better. The practice of smothering the hand in silver sulfadiazine cream and leaving it contained in a plastic bag for days is to be avoided. Such practice results in a hand that is swollen, with all previously normal unburned skin now totally macerated, swilling in a pool of foul liquid. Wrapping in boxing glove-type dressings will rapidly result in stiff, contracted hands, so wherever possible leave the hands exposed or with minimal dressings.

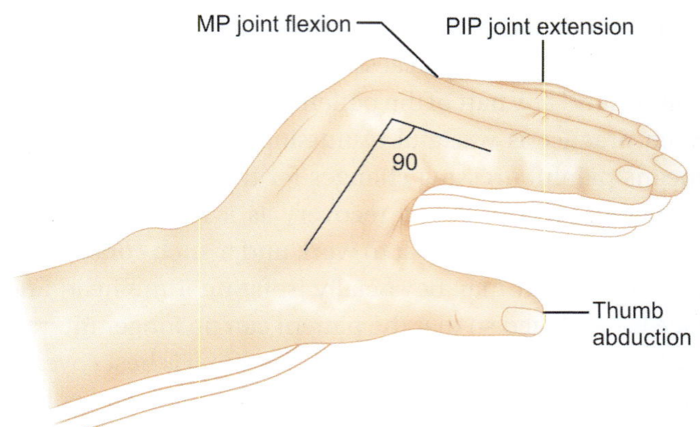

Fig. 43.11: "Intrinsic-plus" position of the hand.

Mupirocin ointment applied over the hands keeps the dermis supple, stops the burn desiccating and cracking, and allows for early mobilization. A night splint to maintain the "intrinsic-plus" position (Fig. 43.11) and prevent contracture of the collateral ligaments and interosseous muscles is recommended. The splint should be applied to the volar surface of the forearm and hand, with the wrist slightly dorsiflexed, the metacarpophalangeal joints at a right angle, the thumb abducted, and the fingers (separately bandaged) in full extension. If the fingers are affected, individual and interdigital Vaseline gauze wrapping will prevent syndactyly, which can occur at an alarmingly rapid speed and is both difficult and time-consuming to reverse.

Superficial partial thickness burns are best dealt with this way, but DPT burns may be covered by a biosynthetic skin substitute such as Biobrane that is available in gloves of different sizes. Skin grafting and splinting the fingers is not easy and an hour of operating time should be allocated for each full hand burn. Zeal for early postoperative mobilization must be tempered by the need to allow any SSG to "take" adequately, or hours of meticulous operative technique will be wasted by failed grafts. If SSGs are applied to the fingers, it is suggested that at least three full days are allowed before any attempt is made to remove the splint. A hand that is still splinted and immobile >5 days will take many months of rehabilitation to regain former function.

Where there are FT burns of the hand, then early, adequate escharotomies are needed within hours of the injury if digital necrosis is to be avoided. Escharotomy may not be sufficient for a circumferential FT burn of the forearm that may require decompression by fasciotomy. If this is done, it should include decompression of the carpal tunnel. Escharotomies of the hand include dorsal incisions along the interosseous web spaces, and digital escharotomies along the radial side of the thumb and the ulnar sides of the fingers to preserve an unaffected pinch-grip without scarring.[69]

Feet: As in the hand, the risk of syndactyly exists for adjacent burned toes, and individual dressings also apply here.

Although the function of the foot is less dextrous than the hand, the aim is to provide a sensate, plantigrade foot that can take weight, with sufficient skin cover that is durable enough for this task. Split skin is not robust enough cover for the sole where rotation or free flaps may be needed, though it is adequate for the dorsum of the foot. Contractures of the toes are common but usually easily corrected by minor orthopedic procedures and 10–14 days of K-wire fixation.

Of much greater concern are the tendinous contractures of the sole and the ankle joint that occur. These are harder to correct and pose a much greater challenge to patient and surgeon alike. The basic technique of incisional release and skin grafting is useful, but rotational flaps to cover the sole of the foot that has sustained an FT burn are not easy or universally successful.[70] Although it is not usually referred to in most modern textbooks on burns, consideration should be given to primary below-knee amputation as a way to swifter and more successful recovery with today's modern prosthetics. The alternative may involve many months in hospital with multiple operations and, in the end, a poorly functional, insensate foot with residual ankle contracture and an antalgic gait.

Face: The face is not only the window from which we look out on the world, but it is also the window the world uses (for the most part) to look in on us. Injury to the face, especially by disfiguring burns, is therefore perhaps the most emotive and psychologically challenging of all the areas of burn care. This short chapter is clearly not the place to address the many issues surrounding such a topic, so the subject will be curtailed to emphasizing a few brief principles. The reader is encouraged to seek greater depth in more extensive and specialized volumes.

On the positive side, many burned faces are those of children who have sustained scalds from either boiling water or steam. Most of these are SPT and heal well within 10–14 days with no requirement for surgery and no residual scarring.

Infection is always a problem in the face area as *Staphylococcus* and *Streptococcus* bacterial organisms are commensals in the mouth and nose of most people, and *Pseudomonas aeruginosa* is a commensal organism present in the external auditory meatus. For this reason, mupirocin ointment is used liberally around the mouth and nose, and chloramphenicol ointment in the ears and eyes. These ointments may also be applied to grafts. Biobrane may be used to cover a graft and hold it in place, or used directly onto a SPT facial burn.[68]

Where deeper burns occur, they are usually the result of flames or a deliberate attack with a caustic substance. Because the face is so contoured and heterogeneous in depth of skin from area-to-area, it is often burned to different depths in different places; the eyelid will burn faster than the cheek, the ear will burn faster than the chin. However, when it is clear how much of the face will require grafting, it is best managed expeditiously with early tangential excision and grafting. The Goulian knife and Versajet are of particular use here. Individual burn surgeons frequently have their own "favorite" donor sites for facial skin, and plastic surgical and burn textbooks will give advice based on these experiences. A personal preferred donor site for SSG is the skin of the upper, inner arm for the face and eyelids, and FT (Wolfe) grafts taken either from behind the ear or a fold of neck skin for eyelids. These Wolfe grafts are used for eyelids as inlay grafts after the initial SSG has contracted and pulled back the lid, exposing the cornea. The SSG is used for temporary cover of the burned eyelid and allows the surgeon to close the eye by tarsorrhaphy. Around 10 days later, the tarsorrhaphy will have opened and the SSG contracted. This is now split transversely, and a small Wolfe graft inlaid in the gap that opens up when the lid is once again pulled down (or up) by tarsorrhaphy. Full thickness grafts do not usually contract, and the eyelid should now function normally.

Skin substitutes may again be useful here, and Biobrane may allow the patient to be pain-free while allowing time for burns of indeterminate depth to declare themselves. It should be clear by 5 days which areas of burn need grafting. If grafting is required, then unmeshed, complete sheet grafts are preferred and are attached along embryological and anatomical lines. These give the best cosmetic results. Although some bandaging is necessary to obtain adhesion of both the Biobrane and SSG, this should be retained for only 48 hours—or as short a time as necessary—to avoid the "mummification syndrome" of totally wrapping the patient's head in bandages, which results in significant psychological discomfort and sensory isolation.

Perineum: The perineum is a notoriously difficult place to bandage; the application of diapers coated with silver sulfadiazine cream seems to be both effective and comfortable for most patients. In infants and toddlers, it is appropriate to leave them exposed to run around, placing the diapers only at night. Most patients (of all ages) will have urinary catheters from the outset. If constant soiling of the burn is a problem, then consideration should be given to a temporary colostomy to divert the fecal stream. Despite best efforts, there will be some almost inevitable soiling, but most patients are remarkably tolerant of their own fecal organisms. Larger texts should be consulted for detailed treatments.[52]

Hypermetabolic Response in Burns

The hypermetabolic response in burn patients is characterized by a hyperdynamic circulatory response with massive protein and lipid catabolism, total body protein loss, muscle wasting, peripheral insulin resistance, increased energy expenditure, increased body temperature, increased infection risk, and stimulated synthesis of acute phase proteins located in the liver and intestinal mucosa. Early recognition and treatment of these profound metabolic changes improves clinical outcome.[52]

These responses occur in all trauma, surgical, or critically ill patients, but the severity, duration, and magnitude are uniquely severe for burn patients. Marked and sustained increases in catecholamine, glucocorticoid, glucagons, and dopamine secretion initiate the cascade of events leading to the acute hypermetabolic response with its ensuing catabolic state. This complex response is not well understood. Interleukins 1 and 6, platelet-activating factor, TNF, endotoxin, neutrophil-adherence complexes, reactive oxygen species, nitric oxide, and coagulation and complement cascades have been implicated in regulating this response to burn injury. Once these cascades are initiated, their mediators and by-products appear to stimulate the persistent and increased metabolic rate associated with altered glucose metabolism seen after severe burn injury.[55,56]

The metabolic rate increases proportionally to the increase in burn size.[60] A 15–25% TBSA burn injury initiates a catabolic response, including impaired immunity and fluid shifts.[75] Adults with a 25% TBSA burn injury develop a metabolic rate between 118% and 210% of that predicted by Harris-Benedict equations for basal metabolic rate.[76] Those with burns >40% TBSA always experience hypermetabolism.[56] A further increase in hypermetabolism occurs in patients with burns of 50–60% TBSA, after which there is minimal further increase in catabolic rate.[68]

The hypermetabolic state begins within 5 days of a major burn injury and may persist for as long as 1 year.[56,60] A prospective, longitudinal study found that children with burn injuries >40% TBSA develop a metabolic rate of 180% of the basal metabolic rate during the acute admission, persist with an elevated rate of 150% following complete wound closure, and maintain a 110% rate at 1 year.[54,61]

The persistent and profound catabolism in major burns hampers rehabilitative efforts and delays the meaningful return of individuals to society. The simplest, effective anabolic strategies for severe burn injuries are: early excision and grafting of the wound; prompt treatment of sepsis; maintenance of environmental temperature at 86–89.6°F (30–32°C) continuous feeding of a high carbohydrate, high protein diet, preferably by the enteral route; and early institution of vigorous and aerobic resistive exercise programs. To further keep erosion of lean body mass to a minimum, administration of anabolic agents—recombinant human growth hormone, insulin, oxandrolone or anticatabolic drugs, such as propranolol, are alternative approaches. Exogenous continuous low-dose insulin infusion, β-blockade with propranolol, and use of the synthetic testosterone analog, oxandrolone, are the most cost-effective and least toxic pharmacological treatments to date.[61]

Nutritional Support

Patients with burns >40% TBSA can lose up to 25% of their body weight in the first 3 weeks following injury if maintained on an oral diet alone. For this reason, a dietician is an essential member of the burns team. All patients with a major burn (>15% TBSA) should have a NGT or fine-bore feeding tube for early enteral nutrition. This should ideally be started within 18 hours of the burn.[36,57] Not only does this help in the early replacement of calories, but it also protects against gut bacterial translocation and systemic sepsis. It may in addition protect against the development of the rare Curling's ulcer.[21,117]

The aim should be, in pediatric patients at least, to provide 100% of their calorie requirements down the tube, and any further food they can take orally is a bonus. Meeting the nutritional needs of burn patients is essential to the healing process. At least a dozen formulae have been developed to calculate the requirements of each patient based on the size of the burn, the total surface area of the patient, the presence or not of sepsis and body weight. Probably the best known for adults is the modified Harris-Benedict equation (based on their original work on basal energy expenditure), and one of the three age-adjusted Galveston formulae for children. The two Curreri formulae (for adult and junior) address the needs of both. However, as Dickerson et al., have pointed out, there are inaccuracies in all of them.[76]

This nutrition should be provided enterally for the reasons given earlier and parenteral feeding held in reserve for those with prolonged ileus or intolerance of enteral feeding. There are no clear guidelines on the duration of supplemental feeding, but sense dictates at least until all burn wounds are closed. There is a bewildering array of commercially available nutritional products, some of which are very costly and have little advantage over a simple diet of milk and eggs.[71]

Outcomes

The chances of survival after major burn injury have increased markedly during the past 50 years. In the 1940s when organized burn care was in its infancy, only 50% of patients with burns involving 40% TBSA survived. Today, over 50% of all patients with burns involving 80% TBSA can survive such injury. In select groups of patients such as children <15 years of age the lethal area (LA) 50 (LA 50 = the percentage of the TBSA burned corresponding to a 50% survival rate) approaches 90% TBSA. This marked improvement in survival may be attributed to a number of therapeutic developments as:

- Development of successful resuscitation formulae and the prevention of early acute renal failure
- Early excision of burn wounds and prompt wound closure with autograft and skin substitutes
- Advances in critical care
- Provision of appropriate nutritional requirements
- Prevention of burn wound infection with effective topical antimicrobial agents
- Routine care of severely burned patients in specialized multidisciplinary burn centers.[29]

The strongest predictors of death in burn patients include advanced age, extent of burn injury, and the presence of smoke inhalation injury.[58,59] In 1998, a retrospective analysis was made of the records of all 1,665 patients with acute burn injuries admitted to the Shriners Burns Institute, Boston, and Massachusetts General Hospital from 1990 to 1994. Three risk factors for death were identified: age >60 years, >40% of BSA burned, and inhalation injury. The mortality formula developed in the study predicted 0.3%, 3%, 33%, or approximately 90% mortality, depending on whether none, one, two, or three of these risk factors were present. A large increase in the proportion of patients who chose not to be resusitated complicated comparisons of mortality over time.[73]

The relationship between age and survival is biphasic, with the highest mortality rates in infants and elderly patients and the lowest mortality rates in children and young adults with similar injuries. The presence of smoke inhalation injury may increase the mortality rate by as much as 20% over that predicted from the age of the patient and the extent of injury. When pneumonia complicates smoke inhalation, the mortality rate may rise to 60% above the predicted level. Developments in ventilator management and critical care, however, may be associated with improved outcomes, even for patients who have smoke inhalation injury complicating burn trauma.[74]

Other comorbid factors such as mechanical trauma and pre-existing medical conditions might be expected to influence outcome from burn injury. However, CNS injury is an independent predictor of poor outcome, probably because of the inability to protect the injured brain during large volume resuscitation. The presence of long bone skeletal fractures has not been associated with a worse outcome. Diabetes mellitus, hypertension, and heart disease are also not associated with worse outcomes.

More people are surviving more extensive injuries, which means that burns centers must place a greater focus on rehabilitation and quality of life for those survivors.

COLD INJURY

Exposure to cold can produce various injuries that occur as a result of the human inability to adapt to cold.[77] These injuries can be divided into localized injury to a body part or parts (peripheral cold injuries), generalized cooling of the entire body (systemic hypothermia), or a combination of both. Among the civilian population, especially in densely populated cities, cold injuries are quite frequent, although sporadic. However, unlike civilians, who spend only 5–10% of each day outdoors, soldiers in tactical situations can be exposed to an extreme environment for ≥30% of each day, which may precipitate epidemics of cold injuries.[78]

Much knowledge about the incidence and circumstances surrounding cold injury has been gleaned from the extensive military experiences of the past.[79] Hannibal lost nearly half his army of 46,000 due to frostbite during a 2 week crossing of the Pyrenean Alps. During the revolutionary war, it is recorded that in 1778 Washington lost 10% of his army to cold-related casualties during a single winter.[80]

Baron Dominique Larrey, Surgeon General to Napoleon's forces during his Russian campaign of 1812–1813, produced the first classic descriptions of frostbite and trench foot, and noted the disastrous effects of refreezing that occurred after bonfire thawing and subsequent marching in still freezing conditions. He also noted that the number of cold-induced injuries was much greater during periods of wet, near-freezing conditions as opposed to similar periods when conditions were dry, but below freezing. He described the loss of all but 360 troops in a division of 12,000 men due to cold.[81]

Military expeditions since that time have also fared badly from cold injuries. Both world wars and the Korean conflict included one million frostbite injuries. German troops underwent 15,000 amputations due to cold injury in the winter of 1942. Even in the Vietnam war, there were substantial numbers of nonfreezing cold injuries due to wet environments and a temperature range of 34.9–39.9°F (1.6–4.4°C).

Physiology

Body temperature may fall as a result of heat loss by radiation, evaporation, conduction, and convection. Radiation causes 55–65% of the body's heat loss. Evaporation occurs via the skin and airway and accounts for 30% of the heat loss. Normally, in a dry environment, only 15% of the body's heat loss results from conduction. However, the thermal conductivity of water is approximately 30 times that of air, so the body loses heat rapidly when immersed in water or covered in wet clothing, leading to a rapid decline in body temperature. Convection accounts for a minor amount of heat loss, but it becomes more significant in a windy environment—the wind-chill factor. The amount of heat dissipated by any of these mechanisms is proportional to the temperature difference between the body and the environment.

Normal thermoregulation involves a dynamic balance between heat production and control of heat loss, with the aim of providing a constant core temperature. This is achieved in part by adjustment of central thermogenesis, and in part by maintaining a differential temperature gradient between the body core and the peripheries directly exposed to the environment; the amount of heat gained from or lost to the environment is closely and rapidly regulated in response to changing circumstances. Two types of cutaneous receptors are involved: cold and warm. Exposure to cold increases activity in the afferent fibers from the cold receptors, which stimulate the preoptic nucleus of the anterior hypothalamus; direct reflex vasoconstriction reduces blood flow to the cooling skin. Colder blood also reaches temperature-sensitive neurons in the hypothalamus. The hypothalamus then initiates various responses that either increase heat production or reduce heat loss: immediate responses via the autonomic nervous system, more delayed responses through the endocrine system, adaptive behavioral responses, extrapyramidal skeletal muscle stimulation, and shivering. The resulting enhancement of muscle metabolism can increase heat production by as much as 500%.[85,86]

Systemic Hypothermia

Hypothermia is defined as any body temperature below 95°F (35°C). It is subdivided into four different grades: mild, 89.6–95°F (32–35°C); moderate, 82.4–89.6°F (28–32°C); severe, 68–82.4°F (20–28°C); and profound at less than 68°F (20°C).[112]

Predisposing Factors

Older people are particularly susceptible to accidental hypothermia because thermoregulatory ability is progressively impaired with age. They may also have a reduced ability to generate heat because of reduced lean body mass, impaired mobility, inadequate diet, and reduced shivering in response to cold. Sympathetically activated thermogenesis in brown adipose tissue is attenuated from the end of infancy. In addition, older people are susceptible to increased heat loss through a reduced ability to vasoconstrict appropriately, are less able to discern changes in temperature, may have abnormal adaptive behavioral responses, and may be prone to exposure to cold through falls or illness. Predisposing socioeconomic factors may be particularly relevant to the elderly. Indeed, some elderly people suffer recurrent episodes of hypothermia, suggesting that they may have a particular predisposition to thermoregulatory failure that can be precipitated by a relatively minor insult.

In addition to this age-related impairment of adaptability to a fall in temperature, various pathological conditions may be implicated in the development of hypothermia. For example, central thermoregulatory ability can be impaired as a result of a stroke, CNS trauma or infection, tumors, hemorrhage, and uremia, Parkinson's disease, multiple sclerosis, and Wernicke's syndrome.[87] Overt or covert psychiatric disease as well as smoking, diabetes mellitus, homelessness, fatigue, improper clothing, previous cold injury, high altitude, extremes of age, and male gender have all been implicated in both local and systemic cold injury.[84]

Poor control of the peripheral vasculature through autonomic dysfunction can also contribute to hypothermia in those with diabetes, infection, and cardiac failure. Reduced heat production occurs in endocrinopathies such as hypothyroidism, hypoadrenalism, and hypopituitarism. Hypoglycemia alone can predispose to hypothermia, particularly in the context of alcohol ingestion.[88,110] Pancreatitis and diabetic ketoacidosis also need to be considered as precipitating causes of hypothermic episodes, even if they are not clinically apparent. Pancreatitis has been suggested as either a sequela or precipitant of hypothermia, though the association has been questioned in recent years.[111]

Perhaps the most frequent precipitating factor in older people is sepsis, which in several series has been found in about 80% of elderly patients with hypothermia.[89-91] In the 9–10% of patients in whom an infection results in hypothermia rather than fever, there is a significantly worse prognosis: mortality is approximately doubled, perhaps in part because of the higher rate of shock in these patients.[92] Sepsis may predispose to hypothermia either by causing a failure of vasoconstriction, or by inducing an abnormal hypothalamic response. The mechanism for this remains unclear, but there is evidence of an increased cytokine response, with raised levels of TNF-α and interleukin-6, and elevated prostacyclin and thromboxane B2 metabolites in hypothermic septic patients.[93]

Some pharmacological agents, e.g. barbiturates, opioids, tricyclic antidepressants, and benzodiazepines, can cause central thermoregulatory failure, and phenothiazines can both impair central thermoregulation and also inhibit peripheral vasoconstriction in response to cold by their α-blocking activity.[94] Other α-blockers such as prazosin have been reported to cause hypothermia, and the elderly seem particularly susceptible to this effect of α-blockade.[95,96] Lithium toxicity has been reported to lead to a reduction in core temperature.[97] Ethanol can lead to peripheral dilatation, impaired shivering, hypoglycemia, and environmental exposure to cold, as well as having a direct effect on the hypothalamus,[98] by which it lowers the thermoregulatory set point, resulting in a fall in core temperature.[99] Valproic acid has also been reported to cause hypothermia in a handful of cases, but the mechanism is unknown.[100]

The end point of accidental hypothermia can, therefore, be considered as a failure of thermoregulatory control, which may have both underlying predisposing causes, including age, various pathologies both acute and chronic, and pharmacological agents, and also more immediate precipitating factors. These precipitating factors may vary between acute exposure to severe cold in an otherwise previously fit individual, through a more prolonged period in a less cold environment (so-called chronic hypothermia),[101] to a relatively brief exposure to mild cold in the context of illness, often sepsis, or enforced immobility such as after a fall.

For a previously fit, younger victim of cold exposure, the outlook is generally good in the absence of apnea or circulatory arrest, and rewarming alone generally leads to full recovery. The more commonly encountered situation in clinical practice, however, is when an elderly person becomes hypothermic because of another condition, and the outcome is then generally determined by the nature of this underlying illness. Attention, therefore, needs to be directed to finding and treating this precipitating condition—often sepsis—in parallel with measures to deal with the hypothermia.

Signs and Symptoms

Hypothermia affects multiple organs. Initially, the metabolic rate increases, with tachycardia, tachypnea, increased muscle tone, and peripheral vascular resistance plus maximal shivering. With continued hypothermia, the metabolism progressively declines, with bradycardia and hypoventilation and subsequent carbon dioxide retention. The shivering mechanism of thermoregulation stops at 87.8°F (31°C). The heart rate drops to half its normal rate at 82.4°F (28°C), and ventricular contractility decreases. The risk of ventricular fibrillation increases at temperatures below 82.4°F (28°C). Cerebral metabolism is decreased 6–7% per 1.8°F (1°C) drop in temperature, which results in a declining level of consciousness. Autoregulation of cerebral blood flow is impaired at temperatures below 77°F (25°C). The symptoms of hypothermia vary depending on the severity of the cold injury. In mild hypothermia, clinical symptoms are often vague and include dizziness, fatigue, joint stiffness, nausea, and pruritus. The skin is pale and cool as a result of peripheral vasoconstriction. The patient may exhibit lethargy, flat affect, impaired judgment, and mild confusion progressing to motor incoordination, ataxia, and slurred speech. As hypothermia worsens, the victim's behavior may become increasingly bizarre, with paradoxical undressing,[102] and terminal burrowing being exhibited.[103] In severe hypothermia, mental status is further impaired, leading to hallucinations, stupor, and coma.

Atrial and ventricular arrhythmias are common with moderate hypothermia. The Osborn (J) point, an upward deflection at the junction of the QRS complex, and the ST segment, can usually be seen on the electrocardiogram (EKG). The patient may appear clinically dead, with non-palpable peripheral pulses, fixed and dilated pupils, loss of ocular reflexes, and stiff extensor posturing. Cardiac standstill usually occurs at 68°F (20°C).

Diagnosis

The diagnosis of hypothermia is easy if the patient is a mountaineer stranded in cold weather. However, it may be more difficult in an elderly patient who has been exposed to a cold external environment. In either case, the rectal temperature should be checked with a low-reading thermometer. The diagnosis of accidental hypothermia has proved elusive, largely because ordinary clinical thermometers do not record temperatures below 35°C. Rectal temperature measurements are also influenced by probe placement. An inaccurate reading may result if the rectal probe was inserted into cold feces or to a depth of <15 cm.

Other methods of determining core body temperature include infrared tympanic thermometers, esophageal probes in intubated patients, and bladder thermistors embedded in urinary catheters. The tympanic probe accurately measures hypothalamic temperature (provided the external auditory meatus is clear of wax) and responds swiftly to reflect variations in core body temperature.[85]

Management of Systemic Hypothermia

Field first aid and prehospital management: The general principles of prehospital management are to prevent further heat loss, rewarm the body core temperature in advance of the shell, and avoid precipitating ventricular fibrillation. The application of these principles depends on the patient's core temperature, the equipment available, and the presence of complicating illnesses or injuries.

Mild Hypothermia

For a person with mild hypothermia [≥ 91.4°F (33°C)], found in a cold environment, the first priority is to search for other injuries in that person and/or other affected individuals. The second priority is to increase the patient's core temperature towards normal, before and during transport to the hospital. The patient should be moved into a tent or other dry shelter for protection from the wind. Wet clothing should be removed by cutting along the seams. Insulation, such as a sleeping bag, should be placed under and over the patient, who should not be allowed to stand or sit and whose head should be covered. A fire should be built or a stove lit. No fluids should be given by mouth. The patient should be transported to the hospital in an ambulance heated to 30°C.

Severe Hypothermia

Severe hypothermia [82.4°F (28°C)] should be treated as a life-threatening emergency. Attention should be directed first to the cardiopulmonary system. If the patient is breathing, humidified oxygen (10 L/min) should be administered using a nonrebreathing reservoir mask. If the patient is not breathing, ventilation should be initiated with a bag-valve-mask ventilator or a pocket mask connected to a humidified, heated oxygen delivery system.

The patient should not be hyperventilated because this may induce ventricular fibrillation. If bradycardia and hypotension are evident, do not perform cardiac compressions because this, too, may precipitate ventricular fibrillation. To avoid inappropriate chest compressions, prehospital personnel must examine the patient for a full minute before diagnosing pulselessness. If the patient is pulseless, external cardiac compressions with ventilations should be initiated unless the exterior chest wall is frozen and not compressible. Cardiopulmonary resuscitation should continue until the patient is evaluated and treated in the hospital.

Always follow the dictum that patients with severe hypothermia are never dead until they are warm and dead. Even with prolonged cardiac arrest, resuscitation is possible. Many physicians who are specialists in hypothermia believe that patients with severe hypothermia should not be rewarmed in the field, but, rather, kept in a "metabolic icebox" until in a hospital setting in which physiologic monitoring and advanced life-support equipment are available.

Hospital treatment: Upon the patient's arrival in the emergency department, the physician must focus on cardiopulmonary function. If the patient is still not breathing, endotracheal intubation should be undertaken to maintain the airway. Cricothyroidotomy may be needed if the skin is frozen. Central venous pressure monitoring is useful to determine the results of volume expansion in patients with severe hypothermia and hypovolemic shock. Rapid ultrasound evaluation of the inferior vena cava in experienced hands can also determine the degree of vascular filling.

Baseline laboratory determinations should include a complete blood cell count; levels of blood glucose, electrolytes, phosphate, creatinine, amylase, lactic dehydrogenase, and creatine kinase; prothrombin time; activated partial thromboplastin time (aPTT); and ABG values. These laboratory studies should be repeated as indicated. Toxicology is recommended for any patient whose history is unknown or who may have ingested a drug or poison. An initial 12-lead EKG should be obtained, after which the patient should have continuous cardiac monitoring. Intensely cold skin may preclude adequate transmission of electrical impulses to the EKG electrodes. A Foley catheter is introduced into the bladder to monitor urine output and to provide specimens for urinalysis including myoglobin levels, and toxicology screening.

Treatment of hypothermic patients should include volume expansion, cardiopulmonary support, and rewarming. Blood volume should be expanded using crystalloid solutions such as dextrose saline, warmed to 104-113°F (40-45°C), to maintain blood pressure and coronary perfusion.

Although severe cardiac arrhythmias in hypothermic patients may represent an immediate threat to life, most rhythm disturbances (e.g. sinus bradycardia, atrial fibrillation, or flutter) require no therapy and revert spontaneously with rewarming. Ventricular fibrillation may be refractory to therapy until the patient is rewarmed to at least 93.2°F (34°C). At core body temperatures below 30°C, the heart is usually unresponsive to defibrillation, pacemaker stimulation, and cardioactive drugs.

Patients with ventricular fibrillation should receive 1-2 attempts at electrical defibrillation once the temperature is >82.4°F (28°C). One dose of 10 mg/kg of bretylium (Bretylol) may be given; it is the only antiarrhythmic drug effective at low temperatures. If this is unsuccessful, CPR should be started or continued together with active rewarming until the patient's core body temperature is >89.6°F (32°C). As the myocardium warms, the rhythm may revert spontaneously or in response to electrical defibrillation.

Coagulopathy is an underappreciated cause of morbidity in patients with moderate and profound hypothermia. Platelets are sequestered in frostbitten areas and in the lungs, causing thrombocytopenia and failure of platelets to develop a clot. The aPTT becomes prolonged as core temperatures decrease. The combination of a prolonged aPTT and thrombocytopenia produces clinical disseminated intravascular coagulation. The passage of an NGT through friable nasal passages may produce torrential bleeding.

Rewarming Techniques

Passive rewarming involves effective insulation of the patient, allowing the patient's spontaneous metabolic heat to rewarm the body. With this technique, the patient is covered with one or two blankets and rewarmed at a room temperature of 77-91.4°F (25-33°C). The increase in core temperature varies from 0.9-3.6°F (0.5-2°C)/h; 24 hours may be required to achieve a normal temperature. If the increase in temperature is <0.9°F (0.5°C)/h, the presence of a complicating disease, such as hypothyroidism, should be considered.

Active rewarming involves the internal or external addition of heat to the body. Active external rewarming works best for patients with mild or moderate hypothermia because it applies exogenous heat to the surface of the body in the form of warm packs, heating blankets, radiant heat, and warm water immersion.

Active external rewarming may precipitate hypovolemic rewarming shock by decreasing the circulating blood volume secondary to peripheral vasodilation in a patient already hypovolemic from another cause. This peripheral vasodilation paradoxically causes central cooling by shunting stagnant, cold blood to the core, thus further chilling the myocardium, depressing contractility, and increasing its vulnerability to ventricular fibrillation.

The safest method of active rewarming of patients with severe hypothermia is internal rewarming that increases the core temperature. Active core rewarming should be used in patients with core temperatures <32°C (90°F), who are hemodynamically unstable, or in whom more conservative rewarming methods have failed. Internal or core rewarming has the advantage of minimizing rewarming shock by warming the central core circulation first. Heat may be added internally by heated humidified inhalation, peritoneal dialysis, mediastinal irrigation, gastrointestinal tract irrigation, arteriovenous shunting including hemodialysis or extracorporeal bypass.[85]

More detailed system responses to hypothermia can be found in Mallett's excellent review.[86]

Localized Cold Injuries

It is important to realize that those with localized cold injuries may well have systemic hypothermia as well, and examination of the patient should take this into account. In a hypothermic patient, whole body warming should take priority over the localized injury. Once the patient's core temperature has reached 95°F (35°C), peripheral warming can begin.[104]

Freezing cold injury (which includes frostnip and frostbite), and nonfreezing cold injury (commonly called trench or immersion foot) will be covered here. Nonfreezing cold injuries (NCFIs) occur at 32-59°F (0-15°C), while freezing injuries occur below 32°F (0°C) in dry conditions, and this can be exacerbated by wet tissues, wind chill, and altitude. The diagnosis of freezing and nonfreezing injuries can generally be made on the basis of history and clinical manifestations.

Ill-defined conditions such as chilblains, and rarer disorders such as cold urticaria and erythrocyanosis, will not be covered.

Nonfreezing Cold Injury

Trench foot: This is a medical condition caused by prolonged exposure of the feet to damp, unsanitary, and cold conditions. It is one of many immersion foot syndromes. The use of the word "trench" in the name of this condition is a reference to trench warfare, mainly associated with World War I. The feet may become numb, affected with erythrosis or cyanosis as a result of poor vascular supply, and may begin to have a decaying odor due to the early stages of necrosis setting in. As the condition worsens, the feet may also begin to swell. Advanced trench foot often involves blisters and open sores, with subsequent gross fungal infections. A warm-water trench foot variant can occur in the tropics where it was troublesome in the Vietnam War, and was known as "paddy foot" (jungle rot).[105]

If left untreated, trench foot usually results in gangrene, which can necessitate amputation. If trench foot is treated properly, complete recovery is normal, though it is marked by severe short-term pain when feeling returns. As with other cold-related injuries, trench foot leaves sufferers more susceptible to it in the future.

Hyperemia appears to be an important part of the pathogenesis, probably in the generation of free radicals and vascular endothelial damage.[107] If the NFCI part is then rapidly rewarmed, as if it was a freezing injury, or inadvertently in a hot shower in routine post-exercise hygiene, this augments the hyperemia and worsens outcome.[108] Accordingly, joint treatment policy[109] strongly recommends that NFCI should be allowed to *rewarm slowly* and not rapidly, unlike freezing cold injury. It is possible that HBO may have value in early treatment too, although no trials appear to have assessed that use. Gross tissue damage following NFCI is relatively rare in peacetime experience, and after *initial slow* rewarming, management should follow the standard conservative protocol employed in freezing injury.

Freezing Cold Injury

Frostnip: The mildest form of peripheral cold injury is frostnip, which is reversible and resolves completely within 30 minutes of starting to rewarm. It tends to affect acral structures (nose, ears, hands, and feet), where blood flow is most variable because of richly innervated arteriovenous anastomoses. Frostnip most often occurs in skiers exposed to fast-moving, very cold air. Simple warming either by pressure from a warm hand or by placing the affected hand in the patient's opposite axilla is sufficient treatment but the subject remains at considerably greater risk for some months of sustaining a further freezing cold injury. The differentiation of frostnip from frostbite is largely on history of exposure and response to rewarming. Mild exposure plus a rapid response to rewarming is indicative of frostnip. In the early stages, the two conditions can look clinically very similar, with blanching and numbness of affected parts. If symptoms or signs persist beyond 30 minutes of rewarming, the subject has frostbite, not frostnip (Fig. 43.12).

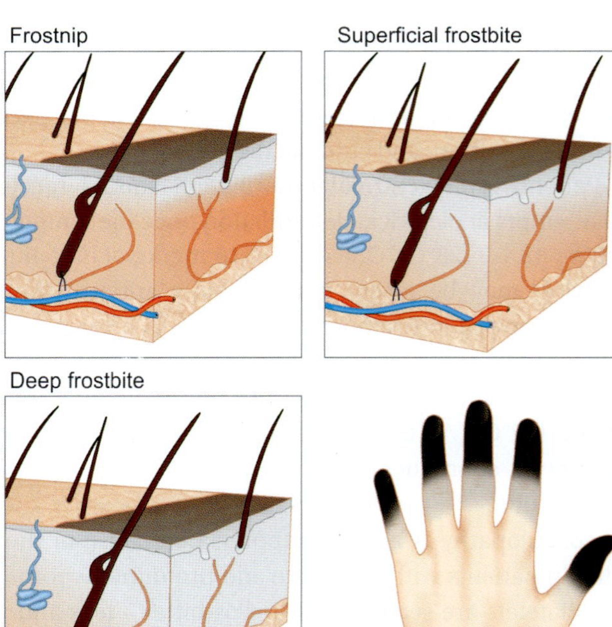

Fig. 43.12: The mildest form of peripheral cold injury is frostnip, which is reversible and resolves completely within 30 minutes of starting to rewarm.

Frostbite: The exact prevalence of frostbite is uncertain, and in the past the military accounted for the majority of cases. With increasing world travel, and more participants in skiing, mountaineering, and other winter leisure pursuits, there has been a steady rise in the prevalence among civilians.

Predisposing risk factors: A number of factors increase the risk of developing frostbite, including behavioral aspects such as the individual's clothing, consumption of alcohol, and other drugs, and access to (and use of) appropriate shelter. Physiological factors such as dehydration, hypoxia, and high altitude also appear to increase the risk of developing frostbite. Certain medical conditions such as diabetes, peripheral vascular disease, Raynaud's phenomenon, psychiatric illness, and previous frostbite predispose to the condition. Certain mechanical factors may affect the risk of developing frostbite such as tight, wet, or inadequate clothing, prolonged contact with a conducting material (e.g. bare metal), and exposure to high winds. In most situations where frostbite develops, more than one factor will be involved and each will have a synergistic effect with the others. While any area may be affected, certain areas are more susceptible because of site, pressure, poor insulation, or susceptibility to wetting. Examples include the face, tips of the nose and ears, fingers and hands, toes, feet, and male genitalia (Fig. 43.13).

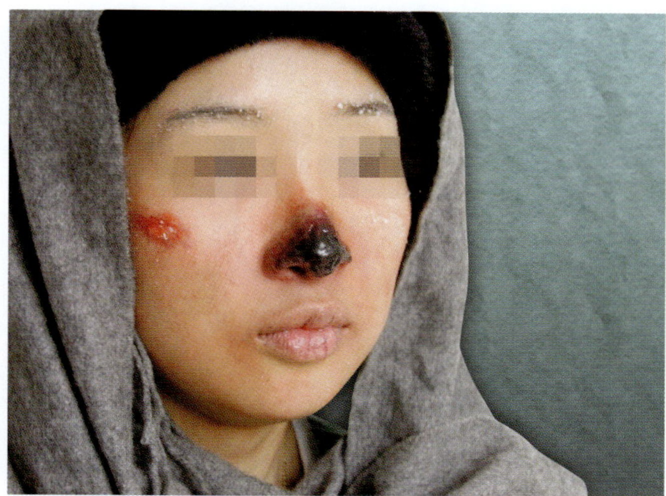

Fig. 43.13: Certain areas are more susceptible to frostbite because of site, pressure, poor insulation, or susceptibility to wetting.

Pathophysiology: The mechanisms of peripheral cold injuries can be divided into those phenomena that affect cells and extracellular fluids (direct effects) and those that disrupt the function of the organized tissue and the integrity of the circulation (indirect effects).[113] Generally, no serious damage is seen until tissue freezing occurs. During frostbite, initially extracellular ice crystals many times the size of individual cells form as fluid shifts from the cells to the extracellular space, producing intracellular dehydration. The cell content becomes hyperosmolar, and toxic concentrations of electrolytes may cause cell death.[114] A reversal of this process probably occurs during thawing of frozen tissues. Usually, no gross rupture of the cell membrane is evident until deeper freezing produces intracellular ice crystals and tissue necrosis then occurs. After tissue thawing, vasodilation and leakage from capillaries occur, causing tissue edema. Alternating freeze-thaw cycles potentiate the vascular injury and lead to ischemic infarction.

The indirect effects of frostbite, a fulminating vascular reaction and stasis, are associated with the release of prostaglandins that have been implicated in progressive dermal ischemia. Both prostaglandin F2 and thromboxane A2 cause platelet aggregation and vasoconstriction. Therapy with antiprostaglandin agents and thromboxane inhibitors has been shown in experimental and clinical studies to increase tissue survival.[85,104,106]

Clinical manifestations: Patients with frostbite may present with multisystem disorders (e.g. systemic hypothermia, blunt trauma, and substance abuse). The health professional must detect these multisystem injuries and appropriately triage care according to the most life-threatening injuries.

Diagnosis of frostbite is usually straightforward, but an awareness of the risk is important. Frostbite is usually painful initially but may not be. If a cold extremity becomes numb, frostbite is the likely cause. The skin may become white and blanched in appearance and tissues feel "woody" to the patient. If a large area becomes frostbitten, it may become purple due to sludging of blood.

Several days after the injury, frostbite can be classified into four degrees of severity. In first-degree frostbite, hyperemia and edema are evident. Second-degree frostbite is characterized by hyperemia and edema, with large, clear blisters that may extend the entire length of the limb, digit, or facial feature (Fig. 43.14). Third-degree frostbite manifests as hyperemia, edema, and vesicles filled with hemorrhagic fluid that are usually smaller than those of second-degree frostbite and do not extend to the tip of the involved digit. Fourth-degree frostbite, the most severe type, involves complete necrosis with gangrene and loss of the affected part.

The classification of frostbite into four degrees of severity is not universally favored by clinicians, who find

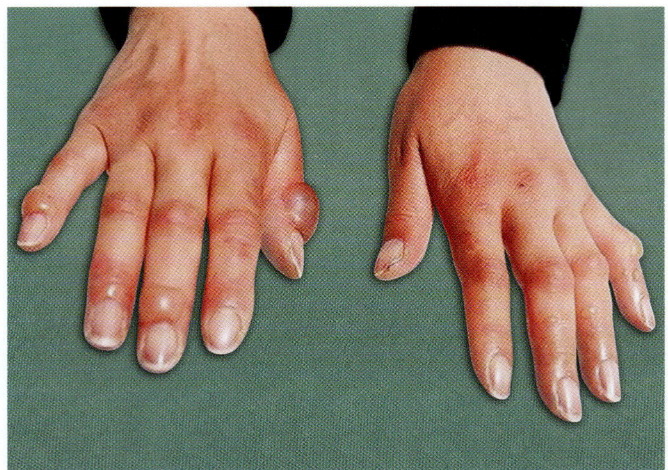

Fig. 43.14: Second-degree frostbite is characterized by hyperemia and edema, with large, clear blisters that may extend the entire length of the limb, digit, or facial feature.

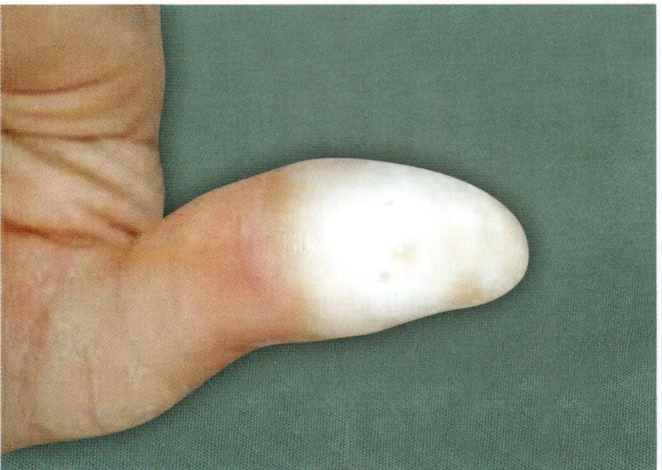

Fig. 43.15: Superficial frostbite (first- and second-degree frostbite) involves the skin and subcutaneous tissues. The skin is cold and waxy white.

assessing the full extent of tissue injury difficult in the acute setting. A simpler classification divides frostbite injury into two types: superficial or deep. Superficial frostbite (first- and second-degree frostbite) involves the skin and subcutaneous tissues. The skin is cold and waxy white (Fig. 43.15). The frozen part is anesthetic but becomes painful and flushed with thawing. Edema develops and clear bullae filled with serous fluid appear within the first 24 hours. Deep frostbite (third- and fourth-degree frostbite) involves the muscle, tendons, neurovascular structures, and bone, in addition to the skin and subcutaneous tissues. The frozen part is hard, wood-like, and anesthetic. It appears ashen-gray, cyanotic, or mottled and may remain unchanged even after rewarming. Edema develops, but bullae may be absent or delayed. Bullae, if present, are filled with hemorrhagic fluid.

Principles of management: First, the part(s) must be protected from further cold injury. Remove any jewelry, put on dry gloves/mitts/socks, if possible, and adjust boots to accommodate any swelling.

Do not, in the field, deliberately thaw the part until it can be rapidly rewarmed in a water bath in a situation from which evacuation can be arranged without further risk to damaged tissue. This will normally be base camp for mountain and military scenarios. If above 4,000 m and if available, give oxygen. When available, give aspirin 300 mg daily to facilitate the microcirculation, prevent platelet clumping, and inhibit potentially damaging toxins.

On arrival at a hospital or secure base, the patient should first be checked for *systemic hypothermia* and treated, if diagnosed, by *slow* rewarming with insulation in a warm environment. This will include hydrating the patient with warm drinks.

Once the core temperature is >95°F (35°C), the *frostbitten part* should be *rapidly* rewarmed by immersion in warm (not hot) water, at around 104-107.6°F (40-42°C) (baby bath temperature). The bath should contain a large enough volume of water to minimize cooling by the cold body part and to facilitate easy top-ups with warm water to maintain the temperature. The damaged part should not be in contact with the side of the bath. Additional hot water is added to the bath only after the extremity is removed from it. After hot water is added, the bath is stirred and the temperature retested before the extremity is reintroduced. An antiseptic can be added to the water, if available. Full thawing may take an hour or more. The thawing process may be very painful and strong analgesics may be needed by injection.

Once thawed, the *frostbitten part* must not be used. A patient with frostbitten toes or feet must not be allowed to walk on them. A patient with frostbitten fingers or hands will be unable to use a walking stick, ice axe, or crutch and will need help with dressing, eating, and going to the toilet. The damaged part should be loosely bandaged with dry, protective, nonadherent dressings, and well padded, especially between the digits.

Take daily digital photos and photos of all procedures for medical records and to facilitate e-mail transmission if advice is needed. Tetanus prophylaxis is required and systemic antibiotics if tissue destruction is apparent. Unlike burns that are sterile for around 72 hours after injury, cold injuries carry no such protection.

Adjunctive treatments: Various therapeutic adjuncts have been tried with mixed results. Few have been subjected to rigorous clinical trials. Sympathectomy, IV dextrans, vasodilators and, more recently, thrombolytic agents, and HBO have been tried with some anecdotal success, but no multicenter trials have been published to date.

Heggers et al. recommended a therapeutic approach devised to prevent the progressive dermal ischemia of frostbite. The combination of the systemic prostaglandin inhibitor ibuprofen and the topical antithromboxane agent aloe vera was used to inhibit localized thromboxane production, which had been implicated as the cause of dermal ischemia.[106]

As with burns blisters, so with frostbite blisters, opinion differs as to correct management. Some suggest that bursting blisters is undesirable, but if inevitable, to do so with a sterile needle or blade.[104] Others feel that clear blisters should be debrided immediately, and aloe vera applied directly to the debrided wound, whereas hemorrhagic blisters should be left intact, but still treated with aloe vera. The aloe vera is reapplied to the frostbitten wounds every 6 hours. When the hemorrhagic blisters rupture, the blisters are then debrided, facilitating application of the aloe vera to the wound.[85]

Iloprost is a prostacyclin analog with profound vasodilatory properties and has been used with some success. It is used in arterial surgery to mimic the effect of a sympathectomy. Intra-arterial reserpine has been used in frostbite to prevent vasospasm. The use of pentoxifylline, a methylxanthine derived phosphodiesterase inhibitor, has been shown to enhance tissue survival.[104]

In 2007, Bruen et al. reduced the incidence of amputation in frostbite injury with thrombolytic therapy. From 2001–2006, their patients with severe frostbite within 24 hours of injury underwent digital angiography and treatment with intra-arterial tissue plasminogen activator (tPA) if abnormal perfusion was documented. These patients were compared with those treated from 1995–2006 who did not receive tPA. In their study, 32 patients with digital involvement were identified. Seven patients received tPA (6 within 24 hours of injury). The incidence of digital amputation in patients who did not receive tPA was 41%. In those patients who received tPA within 24 hours of injury, the incidence of amputation was decreased to 10%. The authors concluded that the use of tPA represents the first clinically significant advancement in the treatment of frostbite in >25 years[116], but no multicenter studies have been published to date.

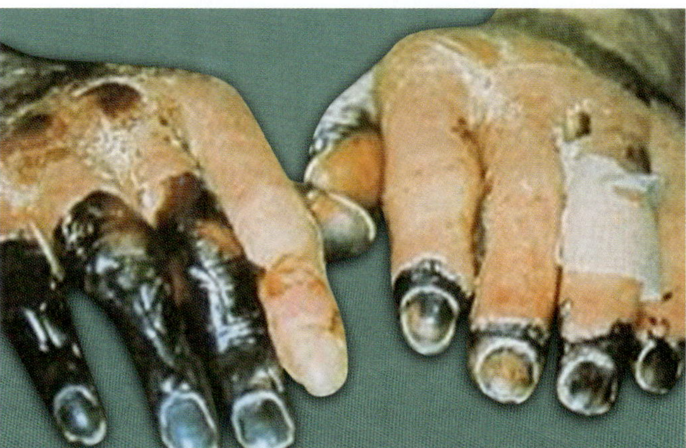

Fig. 43.16: Over time, clear demarcation of necrotic tissue occurs as shown here. Autoamputation is a late result.

Surgery may be required, but may need to be delayed. It can take several months to be certain which tissues are truly nonviable and require amputation. Clear demarcation of mummified tissue and autoamputation may make this easier (Fig. 43.16).

CONCLUSION

Thermal injuries constitute a surgical and physiological challenge. They require a thorough knowledge of the evolution of the pathology and timely intervention if complications are to be avoided. With greater survival in high %TBSA burns, emphasis must now focus on rehabilitation and psychological support. In cold injury, anticipation of risk and prevention are key.

REFERENCES

1. Shah A. Poverty Facts and Stats; Global Issues. [Online] Available from http://www.globalissues.org/article/26/poverty-facts-and-stats [Accessed December 2015]
2. West L. Indoor pollution from cooking fires kills 1.5 million people annually. [Online] Available from http://environment.about.com/od/pollution/a/stovepollution.htm [Accessed June 2013]
3. Nunn JF. Ancient Egyptian Medicine. London: British Museum Press; 1996.
4. Majno G. The Healing Hand—Man and Wound in the Ancient World. Cambridge: Harvard University Press; 1975.
5. Haeger K. The Illustrated History of Surgery. London: Harold Starke (Medical); 1998.
6. Artz CP. History of burns. In: Pruitt BA (Ed). Burns: A Team Approach. Philadelphia, PA: WB Saunders Company; 1979.
7. Cuttle L, Kimble RM. First aid treatment of burn injuries. Wound Pract Res. 2010;18:(1);6-13.
8. Pearn J. The earliest days of first aid. BMJ. 1994;309(6970):1718-20.

9. Esmarch F. First Aid to the Injured. Five Ambulance Lectures. (Translated by HRH Princess Christian). 1st ed. London: Smith, Elder and Co.; 1882.
10. Cantlie J. First Aid to the Injured. 5th edition. London: St John Ambulance Association; 1901.
11. St John Ambulance Association. First Aid. Manual of St John Ambulance Association, the St Andrew's Ambulance Association and the British Red Cross Society. 2nd edition; 1965.
12. http://www.mayoclinic.com/health/first-aid-burns/FA00022 [Accessed December 2015].
13. Wendling P. (2008). Think plastic wrap as wound dressing for thermal burns. Am Coll Emerg Phys. [Online]Available from http://www.acep.org/content.aspx?id=40462.
14. Hudspith J, Rayatt S. First aid and treatment of minor burns. BMJ. 2004;328(7454):1487-9
15. Burns; Clinical Practice Guidelines; The Royal Children's Hospital Melbourne, Australia; [Online] Available from http://www.rch.org.au/clinicalguide/guideline_index/Burns/[Accessed June 2013].
16. Hettiarachy S, Papini R. Initial management of a major burn: II—assessment and resuscitation. BMJ. 2004; 329(7457): 101-3.
17. Oliver R. Burn resuscitation and early management. [Online] Available from http://emedicine.medscape.com/article/1277360 [Accessed December 2015].
18. Pruitt BA Jr. Protection from excessive resuscitation: "pushing the pendulum back". J Trauma. 2000;49(3):567-8.
19. Scheven D, Barker P, Govindasamy J. Burns in rural KwaZulu Natal. Epidemiology and the need for community health education. Burns. 2012;38(8):1224-30.
20. Carter EA, Udall JN, Kirkham SE, et al. Thermal injury and gastrointestinal function. I. Small intestine nutrient absorption and DNA synthesis. J Burn Care Rehab. 1986;7:469-74.
21. Czaja A, McAlhany JC, Pruitt BA. Acute gastroduodenal disease after thermal injury: an endoscopic evaluation of incidence and natural history. N Engl J Med. 1976;29:925-9.
22. Erol S, Altoparlak U, Akcay MN, et al. Changes of microbial flora and wound colonization in burned patients. Burns. 2004;30:357-61.
23. Wysocki AB. Evaluating and managing open skin wounds: colonization versus infection. AACN Clin Issues. 2002;13: 382-97.
24. Spies C, Trohman RG. Narrative review: Electrocution and life-threatening electrical injuries. Ann Intern Med. Oct 2006;145(7):531-7.
25. Cushing TA, Wright RK, Electrical Injuries in Emergency Medicine. [Online] Available from http://emedicine.medscape.com/article/770179-overview#aw2aabb62b2
26. Millikan RA, Bishop ES. Elements of Electricity. American Technical Society. 1917:54.
27. Heaviside O. Electrical Papers; 1. Macmillan and Co. 1894; p 283.
28. Price T, Cooper MA. Electrical and Lighting Injuries. In: Marx J, Hockberger R, Walls R (Eds). Rosen's Emergency Medicine. Vol 3. 5th edition. Mosby; 2002. pp. 2010-2020.
29. Mozingo DW. Thermal injury. In: Corson JD, Williamson RCN (Eds). Surgery. London: Mosby, 2001.
30. Koumbourlis AC. Electrical injuries. Crit Care Med. 2002; 30(11 Suppl):S424-430
31. Cooper MA. Lightning injuries. [Online] Available from http://emedicine.medscape.com/article/770642-overview#a0101 [Accessed June 2013].
32. Wilkes G. Hydrofluoric acid burns treatment & management. [Online] Available from http://emedicine.medscape.com/article/773304-treatment#a1126. [Accessed June 2013].
33. Enkhbaatar P, Traber DL. Pathophysiology of acute lung injury in combined burn and smoke inhalation injury; Clin Sci. 2004;107:137-43.
34. Gann RG, Bryner NP. Combustion products and their effects on life safety. [Online] Available from fire.nist.gov/bfrlpubs/fire08/PDF/f08043.pdf [Accessed December 2015]
35. Pomahac B. http://www.brighamandwomens.org/Departments_and_Services/surgery/services/burntrauma/pdf/Burn_Injury_Manual 2010.pdf; p 24.
36. Barker P. Burns. In: Boffard KD (Ed.). Manual of Definitive Surgical Trauma Care, 3rd edition. London: Hodder Arnold; 2011. pp. 194-203.
37. Vegfors M, Lennmarken C. Carboxyhaemoglobinaemia and pulse oximetry. Br J Anesth. 1991; 66(5):625-6.
38. Barker SJ, Tremper KK. The effect of carbon monoxide inhalation on pulse oximetry and transcutaneous PO_2. Anesthesiology. 1987;66(5):677-9.
39. Weaver LK. Clinical practice. Carbon monoxide poisoning. N Engl J Med. 2009;360(12): 1217-25.
40. Shochat GN. (2012). Carbon monoxide toxicity in emergency medicine. [Online] Available from http://emedicine.medscape.com/article/819987-overview#a0104.
41. Raub JA, Mathieu-Nolf M, et al. Carbon monoxide poisoning-a public health perspective. Toxicology. 2000;145(1): 1-14.
42. Fang Y, Xu P, et al. Ulinastatin improves pulmonary function in severe burn-induced acute lung injury by attenuating inflammatory response. J Trauma. 2011;71(5):1297-304.
43. Heimbach DM. Early burn excision and grafting. Surg Clin North Am. 1987;67(1):93-107.
44. Hunt JL, Sato R, Baxter CR. Early tangential excision and immediate mesh autografting of deep dermal hand burns. Ann Surg. 1979;189(2):147-51.
45. Deitch EA. A policy of early excision and grafting in elderly burn patients shortens the hospital stay and improves survival. Burns. 1985;12(2):109-14.
46. Engrave LH, Heimbach DM, et al. Early excision and grafting vs. nonoperative treatment of burns of indeterminant depth: a randomized prospective study. J Trauma. 1983; 23(11):1001-4.
47. Jackson D, Topley E, et al. Primary excision and grafting of large burns. Ann Surg. 1960;152:167-89.
48. Barrow RE, Herdon DN. History of treatments of burns. In: Herndon DN (Ed). Total Burn Care, 3rd edition. Saunders Elsevier; 2007.
49. Strohal R, Schelling M, et al. Nanocrystalline silver dressings as an efficient anti-MRSA barrier: a new solution to an increasing problem. J Hosp Infect. 2005;60(3):226-30.
50. Fong J, Wood F. Nanocrystalline silver dressings in wound management: a review. Int J Nanomedicine. 2006;1(4):441-9.

Additional references appear in the online version of this book.

Case Study: 44
Delayed Splenectomy Following Expectant Management of Splenic Trauma

James ML Williamson, James C Hewes

THE PROBLEM

The spleen is involved in 0.17–1.30% of all traumatic injuries presenting to hospital. Injury frequently results from impact or crushing trauma, typically following road traffic collisions and falls onto protruding objects. Management is dependent upon the cardiovascular stability of the patient and the grade of injury; currently two thirds of all splenic injuries are managed expectantly, with an overall nonoperative management rate of 90%. Intervention is required in cases of hemodynamic instability or ongoing bleeding. Splenic artery embolization and spleen-preserving measures, including partial splenectomy, may be considered as alternatives to splenectomy, with a view to reducing the risk of postoperative sepsis.

THE TYPICAL CASE

A 48-year-old alcoholic man presented with abdominal pain following an unwitnessed collapse while intoxicated. Although further clinical details were uncertain, he was complaining of severe upper abdominal pain and nausea. His previous medical history included chronic pancreatitis and a duodenal ulcer, for which he was taking a proton pump inhibitor. Examination revealed that he was pale and in shock (pulse 120 bpm, blood pressure 90/46 mm Hg). Abdominal examination elicited generalized upper abdominal tenderness, but no signs of distension, peritonism, or bruising. Initial blood tests noted a low hemoglobin (8.5 g/dL [85 g/L]; normal 13-17 g/dL [130-170 g/L]), elevated C reactive protein (CRP) (0.01 g/dL [110 mg/L]; normal <0.0005 g/dL [<5 mg/L]) and a normal serum lipase. Urgent computed tomography revealed a large splenic hematoma with extracapsular extension containing a faint blush of contrast, which suggested active bleeding. The splenic artery was tortuous and the pancreas calcified and atrophic. He was cautiously fluid resuscitated and became hemodynamically stable, allowing him to be observed on the intensive care unit (ICU).

After a period of stability of a few hours, he became hemodynamically unstable and his hemoglobin fell to 5.9 g/dL (59 g/L). Management options were considered, and he proceeded to splenic angiography. The angiogram did not show a definitive point of bleeding, and it was therefore decided to perform empirical Gelfoam embolization of the main splenic artery with resultant stasis of flow in this vessel. Postangiography the patient was transferred back to the ICU for further resuscitation with fluid, blood products and inotropic support. He made a steady improvement over the next 5 days and was weaned off inotropes, but CRP was persistently elevated.

On day 7 his temperature became elevated, CRP increased to 45 g/dL (450 g/L) and he started showing signs of cardiovascular instability. Repeat CT showed an enlarged heterogeneous spleen consistent with the previous embolization, with both an increased size of the perisplenic hematoma (Fig. 44.1) and locules of gas within the collection. There was associated free intra-abdominal fluid.

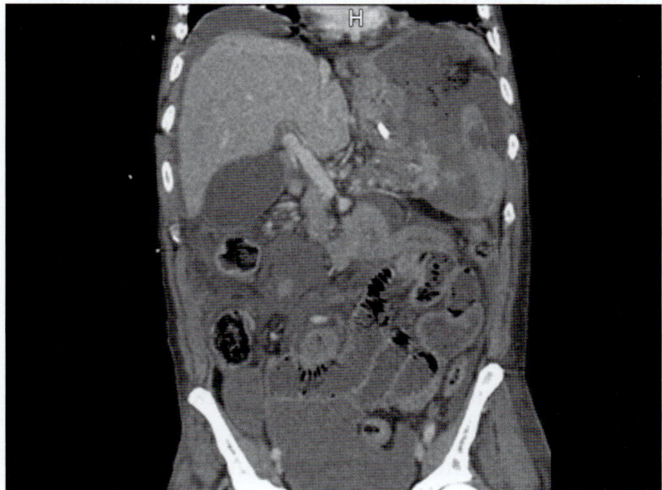

Fig. 44.1: Computed tomography showing a grade IV splenic laceration and a large perisplenic hematoma. Note locules of gas within the collection, denoting infection with a gas-forming organism.

Given the presence of sepsis secondary to the infected hematoma, a laparotomy was performed. At operation a large perisplenic hematoma was evacuated. There was ongoing oozing from the spleen that could not be adequately controlled; therefore, a splenectomy was performed after ligation of the splenic vessels close to the hilum. Copious peritoneal lavage was performed, and drainage tubes were placed in the splenic bed and pelvis. Postoperatively the sepsis resolved, but he had ongoing discharge of turbid fluid from the splenic bed drain: the fluid was analyzed biochemically and revealed an elevated amylase level of 25,000 units consistent with a pancreatic fistula. The patient made a protracted recovery, receiving his splenic vaccinations 2 weeks postoperatively (HiB and meningitis combined vaccine plus pneumococcal vaccine) and was discharged on lifelong penicillin V. The fistula was managed conservatively, and he was discharged on day 40 with a drain in place. The drain then became dislodged and he represented to hospital 12 days later with increasing abdominal pain and an elevated CRP (25.5 g/dL [255 g/L]). Further CT revealed a 4 cm collection in the splenic bed. He was commenced on intravenous antibiotics, and an urgent endoscopic retrograde cholangiopancreatogram (ERCP) was performed. At endoscopy a distal pancreatic ductal stone was seen; pancreatic sphincterotomy was performed, and a pancreatic drain was placed.

DIAGNOSTIC DILEMMAS

This case highlights some of the difficulties in managing patients with splenic hematomas and underlying lacerations. The key diagnostic dilemma relates to the initial management of the hematoma: he had a grade II laceration and was hemodynamically stable after fluid resuscitation. It is acknowledged that two thirds of all splenic lacerations can be managed expectantly, with success rates of 90%, and this is particularly recommended for minor injuries. Thus, the initial expectant management, with intensive care support and regular surgical review, seemed appropriate especially in view of the potential for portal hypertension, given his history of alcohol abuse and chronic pancreatitis. An alternative management plan would have been to proceed to immediate laparotomy after resuscitation; this intervention would have allowed early splenectomy plus full visualization of the abdominal cavity to exclude other injuries but at the expense of postsplenectomy complications.

The second dilemma relates to the management of ongoing bleeding: whether to perform arterial embolization or proceed to operation. Given the arterial contrast blush noted on the initial CT and the patient's preadmission status, it seemed prudent to attempt angiography to identify the source of bleeding and control it if possible. Partial splenic embolization can be highly successful in controlling ongoing hemorrhage. The subsequent ischemia can be limited to the wedge supplied by the vessel. Unfortunately the site of hemorrhage could not be identified, which led to the third dilemma: whether to embolize the whole splenic artery or proceed to laparotomy. Embolization is likely to cause some infarction of the spleen, although this may be mitigated by the collateral arterial supply via the short gastric vessels, while laparotomy is not without risk in an unstable patient. In this case embolization was performed, and it controlled the source of bleeding at the cost of an infected hematoma, which led to the fourth dilemma.

We now faced a fourth dilemma: although the infected splenic hematoma could theoretically have been managed conservatively with antibiotics and radiological drainage, its size in conjunction with the patient's overall instability indicated that it was time to abandon nonoperative measures. At this stage there was no option for splenic preservation, and thus total splenectomy could not be avoided. A pancreatic fistula occurred as a result of the operation despite a careful dissection, and the final dilemma relates to how to manage this complication. Most cases of pancreatic fistula can be managed conservatively. Octreotide may decrease pancreatic secretions, while ERCP with sphincterotomy or pancreatic duct stenting will decompress the pancreatic system. Reoperation and over-sewing of a pancreatic leak is seldom advocated. In this case, the leak was managed conservatively, but the dislodgment of the abdominal drain indicated an endoscopic maneuver to decrease the fistula output.

MANAGEMENT OPTIONS

The main question with any splenic injury is whether or not to operate, and over the last two decades conservative management has been increasingly adopted. This expectant plan does require the support of intensivists, surgeons and interventional radiologists, as well as an understanding that patients may require later intervention. Patients with minor splenic injuries can almost always be safely managed in this manner, but patients with more serious injuries (grade 3–4 or above) or with multiple comorbidities may require transfer to a specialist trauma or hepatopancreatobiliary center. Recognition of ongoing bleeding or failure of an expectant management plan is also vital and should prompt the need for further intervention.

Splenic embolization can be very successful in staunching hemorrhage but at the potential risk of splenic infarction. The degree of necrosis can be limited by selective embolization and collateral flow via the short gastric vessels. Embolization does not deal with a pre-existing hematoma, which can become secondarily infected, as in this case. Operative intervention is also successful in managing splenic injury; some injuries can be managed with spleen-preserving techniques (splenorrhaphy, suture repair, partial splenectomy), but the overall stability of the patient is paramount and often a quick and definitive total splenectomy is best. No definitive recommendations exist for the placement of drains; most surgeons place them to drain any blood, prevent infection and detect any pancreatic fistulae. Pancreatic injury is a well-recognized complication of splenectomy and is generally managed conservatively.

There is a 1–2% lifelong risk of developing overwhelming postsplenic infection following traumatic splenectomy, with children being at greatest risk and adults with trauma probably at lowest risk. Most cases present within 2 years. Infection with *Streptococcus pneumoniae* (50–90%) is the most common, with *Neisseria meningitidis* and *Haemophilus influenzae* type b also being implicated. Patients typically present with severe sepsis (pyrexia, malaise, vomiting, and ultimately circulatory collapse) following an insidious infection. Overwhelming postsplenic infection is associated with a mortality rate of 50–70% within 48 hours.

FURTHER READING

1. Brady RRW, Bandari M, Kerssens JJ, et al. Splenic trauma in Scotland: demographics and outcomes. World J Surg. 2007;31:2111-6.
2. Davies JM, Lewis MPN, Wimperis J, et al. Review of guidelines for the prevention and treatment of infection in patients with an absent or dysfunctional spleen: prepared on behalf of the British Committee for Standards in Haematology by a Working Party of the Haemato-Oncology Task Force. Br J Haematol. 2011;155:308-17.
3. Renzulli PR, Schnüriger B, Schoepfer AM, et al. Management of blunt injuries to the spleen. Br J Surg. 2010:97:1696-703.
4. Rose AT, Newman MI, Debelak J, et al. The incidence of splenectomy is decreasing: lessons learned from trauma experience. Am Surg. 2000:66:481-6.
5. Sclafani SJA, Shaftan GW, Scalea TM, et al. Non-operative salvage of computed tomography-diagnosed splenic injuries: utilization of angiography for triage and embolization for hemostasis. J Trauma. 1995;39:818.
6. Williamson JML. Splenic injury: diagnosis and management. Br J Hosp Med. 2015;2:204-29.

Case Study: 45

Management of a Patient with Multiple Stab Injuries to the Chest

James ML Williamson, Christopher P Armstrong

THE PROBLEM

Blunt injury to the chest is the most common type of trauma sustained in the civilian population; when penetrating injuries are seen, they are predominantly from low-velocity bladed weapons rather than missiles. Stab injuries to the chest are usually minor and can be managed conservatively unless they involve one of the vital thoracic structures. Most patients (80%) who do require intervention only need insertion of a chest tube for drainage of a pneumothorax and/or hemothorax. Traumatic pseudoaneurysms may rupture and should usually be treated. Treatment options include endoluminal intervention in the form of a stent, embolization, or open surgical repair. A persistent pneumothorax (lasting longer than 7 days) raises the possibility of a bronchopleural fistula and may require operative intervention.

THE TYPICAL CASE

A 65-year-old man was rushed to the emergency department after being stabbed multiple times by his schizophrenic neighbor. He was assessed in accordance with advanced trauma life support protocols; his airway was patent and he was oxygenating well on 100% oxygen. There was tachypnea (respiratory rate of 30/min), poor air entry to the right lung base, and associated hyperresonance to percussion. He was tachycardic (110 beats/min) and normotensive (blood pressure 130/80 mm Hg). Jugular venous pressure was not elevated, and heart sounds were normal. Inspection of the chest revealed five stab wounds measuring 3–4 cm in length, one to the right hemithorax and four to the left, including a stab injury close to the mediastinum. These wounds were inspected and irrigated under local anesthesia and did not appear to be deep. Abdominal examination and secondary survey were unremarkable apart from superficial cuts to both forearms and hands. A thoracotomy tube was inserted in the right midaxillary line in the 5th rib space: this was connected to an underwater seal and drained 400 mL of blood immediately, thereby decreasing his tachypnea and oxygen requirement.

Hematological investigation was unremarkable, with a hemoglobin of 13.7 g/dL (137 g/L). An urgent contrast-enhanced computed tomography (CT) scan of the chest and abdomen confirmed a moderate right hemopneumothorax, with no extravasation of arterial contrast. The chest tube was in a satisfactory position and there was a small left-sided pneumothorax and a small amount of mediastinal air. There was no evidence of great vessel or cardiac injury. To the left of the sternum in the first rib interspace, there was a 2 × 3-cm hematoma with an associated pseudoaneurysm arising from the left internal mammary artery (LIMA). No intra-abdominal injuries were identified. Despite the patient's condition stabilizing following fluid resuscitation and chest drainage (tachypnea and oxygen requirement decreased), he continued to bleed into his chest drain (at 100 mL/h). Urgent angiography confirmed a small pseudoaneurysm at the origin of the LIMA, which was not actively bleeding but was thought to be the most likely source of hemorrhage; thus the whole LIMA was embolized successfully with multiple microcoils (Figs. 45.1A and B). Thereafter, he was transferred to the surgical intensive care unit (SICU) for observation.

The patient stabilized with simple supportive measures. His chest tube remained patent, and the bleeding stopped within 24 hours; hemoglobin dropped to a nadir of 10 g/dL (100 g/L), but he remained cardiovascularly stable. Repeat chest X-rays on days 1–3 following admission revealed that the small left-sided pneumothorax had resolved, but the right-sided pneumothorax remained. The chest tube was attached to suction for 48 hours and the lung re-expanded. However, after the suction was discontinued the pneumothorax reaccumulated and persisted, necessitating supplemental oxygenation. A second chest CT scan was arranged to look for evidence of a bronchopleural fistula, but no obvious cause of pneumothorax was identified (Fig. 45.2).

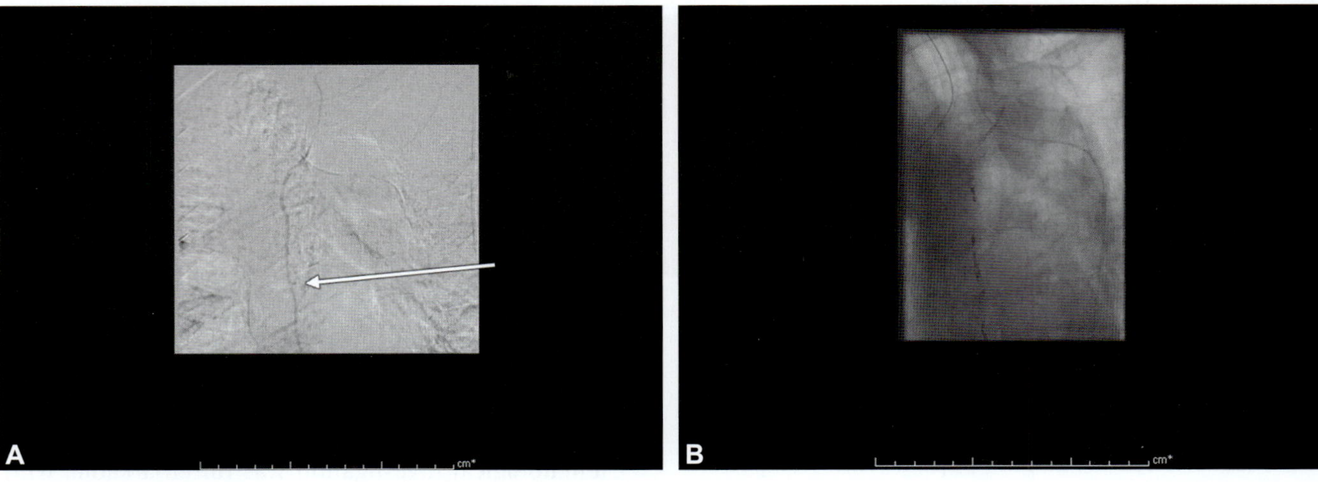

Figs. 45.1A and B: Pulmonary angiogram highlighting left internal mammary artery. (A) No active extravasation of contrast can be seen, but small pseudoaneurysm is identified (arrow). (B) Successful coil embolization—no contrast seen within the left internal mammary artery.

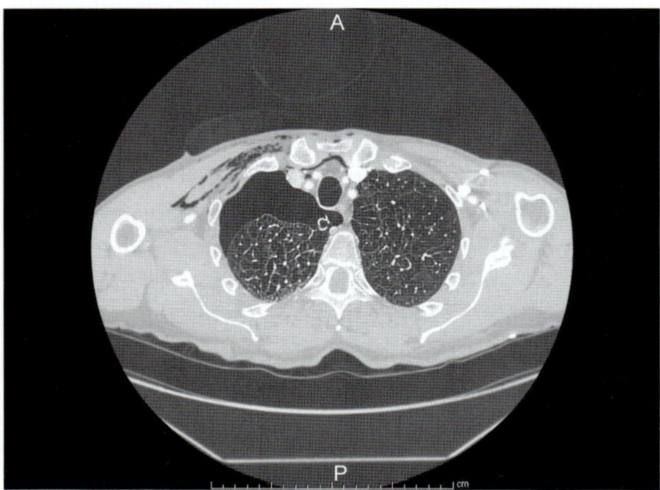

Fig. 45.2: Chest computed tomography scan showing persistent pneumothorax and associated lung collapse with thoracotomy tube lying anteriomedially. Surgical emphysema identified over the anterior right chest wall and small residual pneumomediastinum.

Surgical intervention was considered, but a second period of suction proved successful in completely resolving the pneumothorax and the chest tube was removed. The patient continued to improve and was discharged 17 days following admission after declining follow-up psychological support for his trauma.

DIAGNOSTIC DILEMMAS

This case illustrates some of the common themes regarding low-velocity thoracic penetrating trauma. Most cases of injury are superficial and do not cause major injury, but they do need accurate assessment. There are three main dilemmas relating to this case: first, with regard to his initial management within the emergency department; second, regarding the management of the LIMA pseudoaneurysm; and last, regarding the management of persistent pneumothorax. No other major intrathoracic structures were injured from any of the stab sites, despite the proximity of the mediastinal wound to the heart. A symptomatic hemopneumothorax should always be drained; in addition to allowing the lung to re-expand, drainage of the blood will improve both hypoxia and hypercarbia by increasing the amount of lung parenchyma available for gas exchange. In this patient, ventilation improved following insertion of the chest tube, and neither the initial nor the ongoing blood loss necessitated thoracotomy. An urgent CT scan revealed the extent of injuries. The presence of the LIMA pseudoaneurysm presented the first diagnostic dilemmas to the clinicians, whether to manage the pseudoaneurysm expectantly or perform endoluminal or operative intervention. Angiography allowed further assessment of the aneurysmal site; the lack of extravasation of contrast did not alter the risk of ongoing bleeding, so a decision was made to intervene. The size of the vessel meant that deployment of an arterial stent (to exclude the aneurysmal sac from the circulation) was not possible and thus the LIMA was embolized with coils. Open thoracotomy could have also achieved a similar outcome in addition to excluding other injuries, but adequate visualization of a bleeding vessel in the presence of a hematoma can be difficult and the endoluminal approach seemed a safer approach. As the LIMA runs within the chest wall, it is unlikely that thoracoscopy would have identified the source of hemorrhage, but it would have allowed assessment of the thoracic cavity.

The reaccumulation of this patient's pneumothorax after the first period of suction to the thoracic tube presented an opportunity to review management. Persistent pneumothorax is generally associated with a bronchopleural fistula, which usually requires operative intervention. The cardiovascular stability of this patient and the clinical impression that his injuries seemed insufficient enough to cause a fistula meant that operative intervention was avoided. Bronchoscopy was considered, but as no major injury was seen on a chest CT scan, a second period of suction was employed, which proved to be successful.

MANAGEMENT OPTIONS

Any penetrating chest trauma can injure the heart, great vessels, and hilar structures, in addition to the lung parenchyma. Occasionally a cardiac injury requires an immediate thoracotomy in the emergency room. Clinical examination should seek signs of (1) cardiac tamponade: Beck's triad of elevated venous pressure (distended neck veins), falling arterial pressure and muffled heart sounds; (2) hemothorax; (3) pneumothorax (either tension or simple); or (4) a sucking chest wound. A chest tube (with prior decompression of a tension pneumothorax) is usually the definitive management for drainage of the pleural cavity, but pericardiocentesis is at best a temporizing maneuver for drainage of the pericardial sac. An immediate thoracotomy can relieve cardiac tamponade and allow the surgeon to stanch hemorrhage from the heart, lungs, and great vessels, but it should only be used in extremis as a life-saving measure. Thoracotomy is indicated in massive blood loss: immediate drainage of 1500 mL blood after chest tube insertion or ongoing hemorrhage of > 200 mL/h for 4 hours.

The injuries sustained in this case did not mandate a thoracotomy as either an initial or subsequent intervention. Theoretically, angiography and coil embolization of the LIMA could have been delayed as there was no active bleeding, but further bleeding seemed a distinct possibility. The size of vessel precluded stent deployment, hence the decision to embolize. Embolization of the LIMA is unlikely to have an adverse effect as the blood supply to the anterior chest (including the breast and sternum) and abdominal wall involves multiple collateral branches. Most cases of pneumomediastinum resulting from trauma do not require drainage and resolve spontaneously, as in this case. Mediastinal sepsis may be solely managed with antibiotic therapy but often does mandate radiological or operative drainage.

FURTHER READING

1. American College of Surgeons Committee on Trauma. Advanced Trauma Life Support for Doctors, 8th edition. Chicago: American College of Surgeons, 2012.
2. Carrillo EH, Schmacht DC, Gable DR, et al. Thoracoscopy in the management of posttraumatic persistent pneumothorax. J Am Coll Surg. 1998;186:636-9.
3. Martin M, Schall CT, Anderson C, et al. Results of a clinical practice algorithm for the management of thoracostomy tubes placed for traumatic mechanism. Springer Plus. 2013;12:642.
4. Pineda AM, Valdez GD, Mihos CG, et al. Coil embolization for spontaneous rupture of the left internal mammary artery secondary to lupus vasculitis. J Am Coll Cardiol. 2014;63:290.
5. Van Waes OJF, Van Riet PA, Van Lieshout EMM, et al. Immediate thoracotomy for penetrating injuries: ten years' experience at a Dutch level I trauma center. Eur J Trauma Emerg Surg. 2012;38:543-51.
6. Wise D, Davies G, Coats T, et al. Emergency thoractomy: "how to do it." Emerg Med J. 2005;22:22-4.

46 Case Study: Secondary and Tertiary Blast-Related Injuries

Mark W Bowyer

THE PROBLEM

Injuries as a result of explosions have been traditionally associated with war but are becoming more prevalent civilian terrorist actions, as seen in recent attacks in Madrid, Paris, London, Oslo, and Boston as well as being a near-daily occurrence in the Middle East. These incidents usually result in multiple casualties with severe injuries, requiring surgical teams to make rapid diagnostic and treatment decisions based on minimal information in chaotic circumstances. Most surgeons have little or no experience with the management of blast-related injuries, but would be well advised to gain a basic understanding of the pathophysiology and implications for management of these often complex and devastating injuries.

THE TYPICAL CASE

A 14-year-old Iraqi male was brought by helicopter to the emergency room of a military role three (civilian level one trauma center equivalent) combat support hospital in Iraq, 30 minutes after being injured in a homicide bombing in a local cell-phone shop. He was one of 21 casualties received within the subsequent 30 minutes from the same incident.

The patient was rapidly assessed and was awake and talking with normal vital signs, complaining only of an inability to move his legs and loss of sensation below his nipples. He had no visible signs of injury other than a 3-mm puncture wound in the mid-back and several superficial scratches and abrasions. The patient had a negative portable chest X-ray and focused abdominal sonogram for trauma and was triaged initially into the delayed category. A contrast-enhanced computed tomogram (CT) scan was ultimately obtained and was remarkable for an obvious transection of the thoracic spine and a retained foreign body in the back (Fig. 46.1). Further review of the CT scan documented the presence of an intact nail that had entered through the small puncture wound on the back, whose tip appeared to be in close proximity to the abdominal aorta.

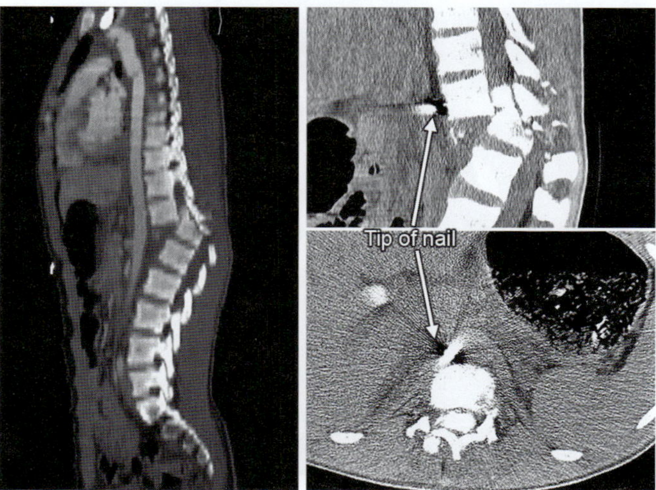

Fig. 46.1: Contrast-enhanced computed tomogram scan showing transection of the lower thoracic spine and a retained foreign body (nail) whose tip (arrow) appears to be in close proximity to the abdominal aorta.

Given the concern for a potential injury to the abdominal aorta, the patient was taken to the operating room for exploration through a generous midline incision. A left-to-right visceromedial rotation was undertaken to expose the abdominal aorta, and the nail tip was found to be adjacent to but not violating the aorta and was removed. There were no other intra-abdominal injuries noted.

Once all of the patients involved in this mass casualty event had received initial care and the chaos resolved, a systematic re-evaluation of every patient was undertaken to include re-review of all films and tertiary physical examination. When this patient's CT scan was re-reviewed it was obvious that there was an injury to the thoracic aorta (Fig. 46.2) that was clearly visible on the initial CT scan (Fig. 46.1) but was missed, likely due to focusing on the obvious dramatic spinal injury.

The patient was taken back to the operating room and underwent thoracic aortic resection and repair with Dacron interposition grafting via a left posteriolateral thoracotomy, as full interventional radiology capability was not available in this deployed military hospital. The patient tolerated this procedure well and was subsequently returned to the operating room for spinal fixation by the orthopedic team.

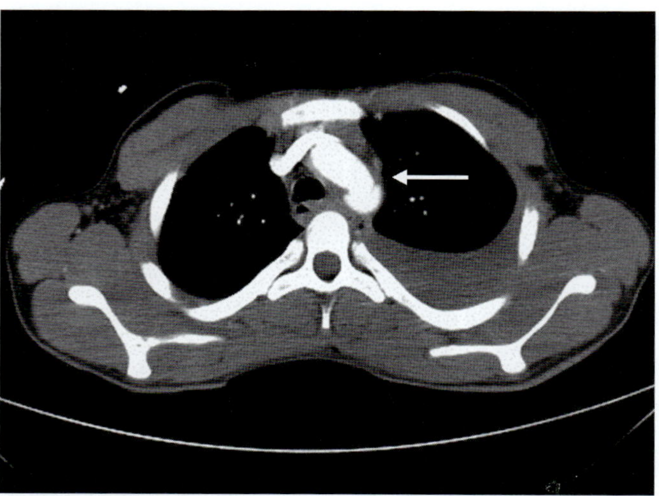

Fig. 46.2: Contrast-enhanced computed tomogram scan showing traumatic transection of the thoracic aorta (arrow) and blood in the left chest.

DIAGNOSTIC DILEMMAS

Blast injuries have the propensity to create a multitude of devastating injuries based upon proximity to the blast and the circumstances associated with it. Classically, the injuries caused by an explosion are divided into primary, secondary, and tertiary (Fig. 46.3). The surgeon caring for blast injuries should have an understanding of the potential injuries and must maintain a high index of suspicion so as not to miss potentially life-threatening injuries. Primary injuries are caused by the blast pressure wave and include injuries to the tympanic membranes, lungs, bowel, and brain. These injuries are most pronounced in individuals closest to the blast and the manifestation of these injuries in initial survivors are rarely (but can be) life-threatening, as those who are likely to die from these injuries usually do so at the scene. Of much more importance is secondary injury, which is caused by rapidly moving fragments of the explosive as well as objects in the environment propelled by the initial blast. These flying projectiles can cause both penetrating and blunt injury, and the treatment considerations are similar to nonblast penetrating and blunt injury. The major difference with blast injury is the potential number of projectiles and the ability to determine which of these has caused major injury. Victims of blast are often "peppered" with multiple small penetrating wounds that may seem innocuous

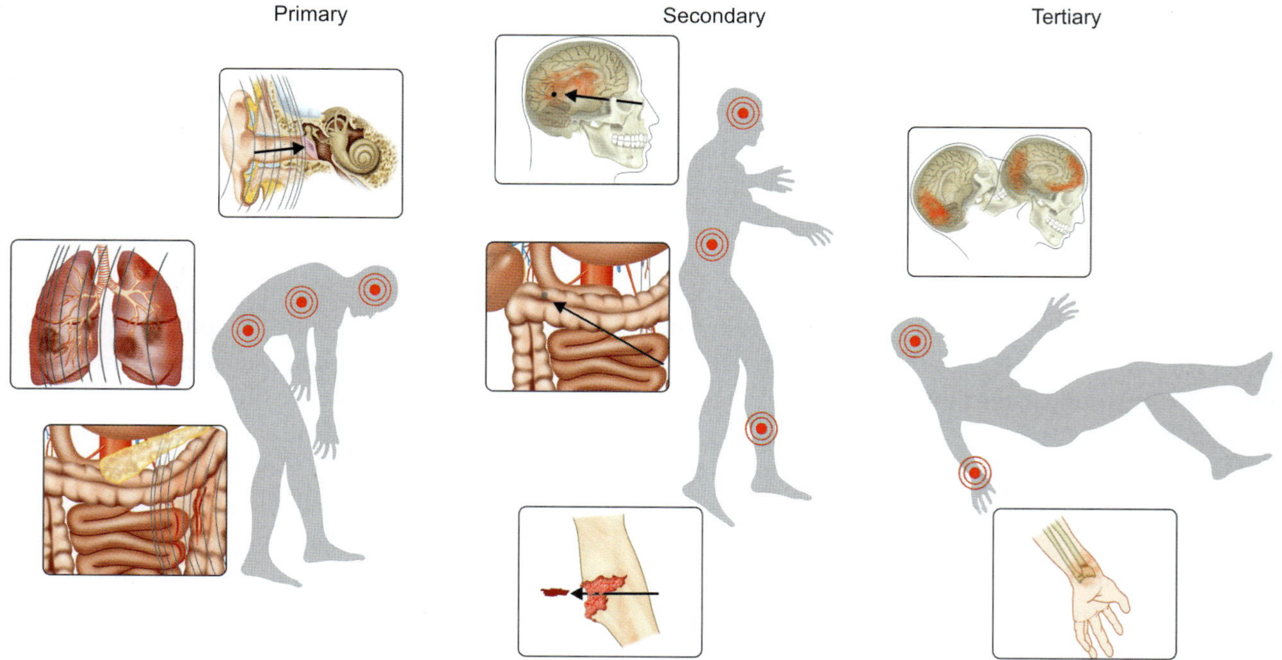

Fig. 46.3: A graphic representation of the potential injuries sustained from a blast injury.

at first glance but may be a harbinger of significant internal injury, as seen in this case. Tertiary injuries from blast are caused by the individual being propelled by the blast into another structure such as a wall or the ground with resultant potential for significant blunt trauma. These patients should be evaluated and treated like nonblast victims of falls with similar concerns for potential injuries.

The patient presented here had a significant spinal injury that was likely a result of a tertiary mechanism in which he was forcefully propelled into another object, which also explains the thoracic aortic injury that is associated with deceleration. The finding of a spinal injury in this patient suggests a large blunt force mechanism and should be a marker for concern for associated injures that are found in up to 80% of blast-related spine fractures.

The practitioner caring for victims of blast injury must keep in mind the multitude of potential associated injuries and perform an exhaustive and comprehensive search to exclude them.

MANAGEMENT OPTIONS

As victims of blast are fortunately rare in most of the world, surgeons who do not deal with such injuries routinely should make themselves aware of the pathophysiology of blast injury and the associated potential injuries. Such events are unpredictable, chaotic, and usually involve multiple or mass casualties stressing even the most prepared surgeon or system. The optimal management of blast victims is to stick to the basic principles of Advanced Trauma Life Support and rapidly address any life-threatening injuries discovered in the primary survey. Patients should also be rapidly triaged by the most experienced individual with consideration of resources available. A high index of suspicion for possible injuries should be maintained and aggressively ruled out. Penetrating and blunt injuries resulting from blast require management similar to nonblast injuries. Potential blast injury to the lung and bowel must be kept in mind as the presentation can be subtle and presentation delayed. Seemingly innocuous wounds should not be overlooked and may be harbingers of serious internal injury. Pan CT scanning, if available, should be routinely performed in victims of blast. If a CT scanner is not available, careful and repeated physical examination with a low threshold for surgical exploration should be the norm.

FURTHER READING

1. Eastridge BJ. Things that go boom: injuries from explosives. J Trauma. 2007;62(6 Suppl):S38.
2. Patzkowski JC, Blair JA, Schoenfeld AJ, et al. Skeletal Trauma Research Consortium. Multiple associated injuries are common with spine fractures during war. Spine J. 2012;12:791-7.
3. Proud WJ. The physical basis of explosion and blast injury processes. J R Army Med Corps. 2013;34:159 (Suppl 1):i4-9.
4. Wolf SJ, Bebarta VS, Bonnett CJ, et al. Blast injuries. Lancet. 2009;374(9687):405-15.

Section 3

Gastrointestinal Surgery

Section Editors: *James W Maher, Robin CN Williamson, MRB Keighley, Andrew de Beaux*

Parts

47

Benign Diseases of the Esophagus

James G Bittner IV, James W Maher

Key Points

- Gastroesophageal reflux (GER) is a common condition that is accompanied by hiatal hernia in 80% of patients. Reflux esophagitis is associated with reduced pressure of the lower esophageal sphincter (LES) or inappropriate relaxation of the sphincter.
- The initial treatment of reflux esophagitis is through changes in lifestyle and diet, plus medications that reduce gastric acid output. When the diagnosis of reflux is objectively confirmed, surgical therapy should be considered in individuals who: (1) have failed medical management, (2) opt for operation despite successful medical management due to quality-of-life considerations, (3) have complications of reflux, or (4) have extraesophageal manifestations of acid reflux.
- Benign strictures are the end result of acid-peptic reflux. Annular strictures can generally be managed by endoscopic dilatation with acid suppression or operation; however, longitudinal (transmural) strictures may require operative treatment.
- Barrett's esophagus is diagnosed by the demonstration of intestinal metaplasia of the lower esophagus in response to chronic reflux. It is a premalignant condition in a small percentage of patients, so regular biopsy surveillance is needed. The presence of Barrett's esophagus is considered by many to be a clear indication for an anti-reflux operation, although there is little evidence to suggest that correction of reflux prevents cancer.
- All symptomatic paraesophageal hiatal hernias should be repaired if the patient is medically fit, particularly those with acute obstructive symptoms or gastric volvulus.
- Achalasia and symptomatic epiphrenic esophageal diverticula are most effectively managed with laparoscopic myotomy, which can be performed safely and with minimal morbidity in appropriately selected patients.

SURGICAL ANATOMY

The esophagus, unlike the rest of the digestive tract, is conceptually a simple organ. Its sole function is to convey food from the mouth to the stomach, where the digestive process begun in the mouth continues. The esophagus, which is essentially a hollow muscular tube lined with stratified squamous epithelium, is collapsed at rest and extends from the cricoid cartilage in the neck to the upper end of the stomach within the peritoneal cavity. It is the narrowest part of the gastrointestinal tract. Muscular sphincters are present at both the proximal and distal ends.

Anatomic Relationships

The elongated course of the esophagus within three major body regions (neck, thorax, and abdomen) is associated with a variety of unique relationships to other organs. The anatomic aspects of the esophagus that are of primary clinical interest are its relationships to the pharynx, cervical and intrathoracic structures above, and to the diaphragm and stomach below.

The esophagus in the neck is a midline structure located immediately behind the trachea. In the chest it continues in the midline directly posterior to the trachea and anterior to the vertebrae, but deviates slightly toward the left as it passes behind the left main bronchus (Fig. 47.1). The aortic arch indents the esophagus proximally, as does the left atrium distally. Distal to the carina, the esophagus deviates slightly to the right and is covered on the right by the parietal pleura and the azygos vein as the vein enters the vena cava. Just above the diaphragm, the esophagus again deviates toward the left just posterior to the pericardium and passes anterior to the aorta into the abdomen.

The association of the esophagus with the diaphragm is of considerable importance. The esophageal hiatus is composed of loops of diaphragmatic muscle, which

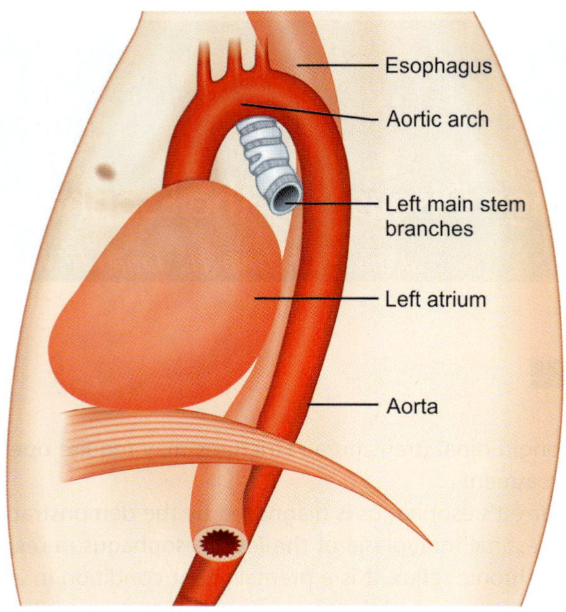

Fig. 47.1: Lateral view of esophagus. This shows esophageal indentations in its relationship to aortic arch, left mainstem bronchus and left atrium.

originate on the vertebral bodies of L2–L4 and are known as crura. Their anatomy is quite variable, but, the loops pass superiorly to form the margins of the hiatus and insert on the tendinous portion of the diaphragm. The right crus most commonly forms the margin of the hiatus, with variable contributions from the left crus.

The phrenoesophageal ligament anchors the esophagus to the hiatus. This tough collagenous membrane is an extension of the abdominal transversalis fascia. It lies between the parietal peritoneum and the diaphragmatic muscle and inserts in a fan-like fashion over a wide zone around the circumference of the esophagus (Fig. 47.2). The attachment of the phrenoesophageal ligament explains the fact that, even in the presence of hiatus hernia, the lower esophagus may still be exposed to the positive pressure environment of the abdomen.

The esophagus differs from most of the rest of the digestive tract in having no mesentery and no serosal layer. The loose envelope of the mediastinum that surrounds it allows the esophagus extraordinary mobility. Deglutition may result in vertical movements of the esophagus of approximately 2.5 cm.[1] This lack of fixation explains the feasibility of the surgical practice of stripping the esophagus bluntly from its mediastinal bed to accomplish esophagectomy.

Compression of the esophagus by muscular sphincters and adjacent organs produces narrowings that are of clinical importance and can be recognized on both fluoroscopy and endoscopy. The cricopharyngeal sphincter is

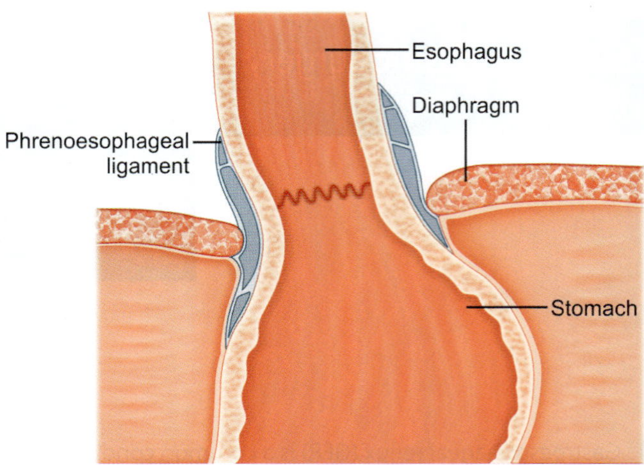

Fig. 47.2: Relationship of the phrenoesophageal ligament to the diaphragm and esophagus. Note the fan-like insertion over several centimeters on the esophagus.

seen approximately 15 cm from the incisors endoscopically, whereas the pulsation of the aortic arch is at approximately 22–23 cm. The narrowing of the lower esophageal sphincter (LES) is typically encountered at 38–44 cm from the incisors.

Microscopic Anatomy

The esophagus is well suited to transport food. It consists of a thick muscular coat with both an external longitudinal layer of muscle and an internal circular layer. Both layers are striated in the upper third with a gradual transition to smooth muscle in the distal two thirds of the organ. This arrangement makes good teleological sense because initiation of deglutition should be voluntary, whereas emptying of the esophagus should be automatic. The longitudinal layer inserts on the dorsal side of the cricoid cartilage with some fibers continuing into the inferior pharyngeal constrictor muscle, whereas others travel directly down toward the stomach. The inner circular layer of muscle also originates from the cricoid cartilage.

The fibers of the circular muscle layer form incomplete circles with overlapping ends (Fig. 47.3). The density of circular muscle fibers increases and produces a gradual thickening of this layer 3 cm above the junction with the stomach. On the lesser curvature side of the esophagus, these circular muscle fibers maintain their orientation and form "clasp fibers" producing a high-pressure zone that can be measured with esophageal manometry and is commonly referred to as the LES. On the greater curvature side, the circular muscle changes its orientation to form the gastric sling, which extends as a loop that both originates and inserts on the lesser curvature.[1] The sling fibers are thought to prevent gastric distention from effacing the esophagogastric junction producing reflux.

At the upper border of the esophagus, the cricopharyngeus muscle loops around the hypopharynx and forms another high-pressure zone. It is tonically contracted at

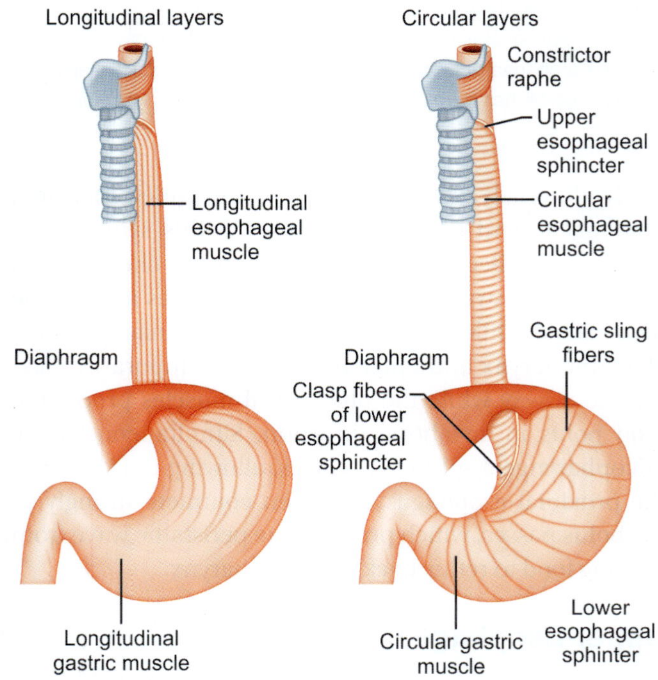

Fig. 47.3: Muscular layers of the esophagus. Longitudinal layers are shown on the left. Circular layers demonstrating gastric sling fibers and clasp fibers, which constitute the lower esophageal sphincter, are shown on the right.

rest and closes the esophageal opening against the edge of the cricoid cartilage.

The esophagus is lined by durable stratified squamous epithelium that can tolerate the physical and chemical trauma associated with the wildly diverse substances that humans choose to consume as food. Submucosal mucous glands lubricate the esophageal lining and may be important in neutralizing irritants. The esophageal mucosa is reddish proximally and becomes paler distally. It can be easily distinguished from the salmon-colored gastric mucosa at the squamocolumnar junction. This junction is also referred to as the ora serrata or Z line.

Blood Supply

Arterial

The arterial blood supply of the cervical esophagus is from the inferior thyroid arteries (Fig. 47.4). The thoracic segment derives its arterial supply from direct esophageal branches from the aorta and bronchial arteries. Distally there are esophageal branches from the inferior phrenic and left gastric vessels.

Venous

Venous drainage partially imitates the arterial supply, but there is an extensive collateral system in the submucosa. These submucosal collaterals drain into larger submucosal channels that run longitudinally throughout the esophagus and drain via perforating veins into the azygos and hemiazygos systems and ultimately into the superior vena cava. In the abdomen, these veins connect via the

Arterial blood supply
Inferior thyroid artery
Superior left bronchial artery
Right bronchial artery
Inferior left bronchial artery
Aortic esophageal artery
Left gastric artery
Inferior Phrenic artery

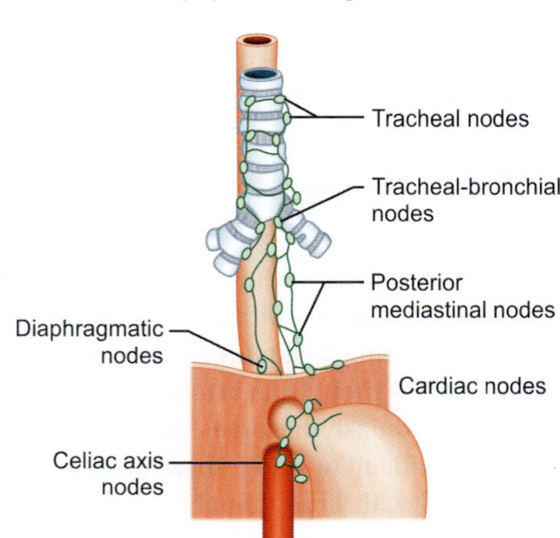

Fig. 47.4: Arterial blood supply and lymphatic drainage of the esophagus.
Source: Adapted with permission from Ellis.[2]

coronary (left gastric) vein with the portal venous systems. This collateral connection between the portal and systemic veins becomes clinically important when elevated portal pressures causes the longitudinal veins to form esophageal varices.

Lymphatic Drainage

The lymphatic drainage of the esophagus is not well understood. Most studies come from the distribution of lymphatic metastases noted in patients with esophageal cancer.[3] Lymphatic spaces run vertically in the submucosa before penetrating the esophageal wall to drain into regional nodes. These nodes extend along the esophagus and communicate liberally with each other and with the tracheal, subcarinal, mediastinal, gastric, celiac, aortic, and even cervical nodes (*see* Fig. 47.4). The thoracic duct also provides considerable drainage.

Innervation

Parasympathetic innervation of the esophagus is provided by the vagus nerves and branches of the recurrent laryngeal nerves. The vagal nerves form a plexus around the esophagus. As this plexus approaches the esophageal hiatus, it coalesces into two major trunks, with the left vagus emerging anteriorly and the right vagus posteriorly on the surface of the esophagus. Sympathetic innervation derives from the splanchnic nerves and direct branches from the celiac plexus. There are also multiple ganglia between the longitudinal and circular muscle layers (Auerbach's plexus) and in the submucosa. These ganglia seem to play important roles in local regulation of blood flow and muscle contraction. The full physiologic effects of the vagus nerve are largely unknown since over 80% of vagal fibers are afferent to the brain.

PHYSIOLOGY

Swallowing

The initiation of swallowing in the oral cavity and hypopharynx is voluntary. It begins with insertion of food into the mouth where chewing facilitates an admixture of the food with saliva, but the propulsion of food from the mouth to the hypopharynx quickly becomes an automatic and rapid event that is difficult to study. These events are normally accomplished with little thought unless there are neuromuscular or anatomic disorders that interfere with them. Under such circumstances swallowing may be both difficult and, if aspiration occurs, hazardous.[7]

Table 47.1 Sequence of events in swallowing.

Sequence of events in swallowing
Tongue pushes bolus into hypopharynx
Tongue rises to close oral cavity
Palate rises to close nasopharynx
Larynx elevates and moves forward to close supraglottis and open hypopharynx
Pharynx contracts to propel bolus to esophagus
Cricopharyngeal sphincter relaxes to receive bolus
Esophageal peristaltic wave propels bolus toward stomach
Lower esophageal sphincter relaxes at the onset of deglutition and then re-establishes its resting pressure as bolus passes into stomach

Traditionally, swallowing has been divided into oral, pharyngeal, and esophageal phases.[4,5] This sequence of events is detailed in Table 47.1. When the chewed food is ready to be swallowed, the tongue opposes itself to the hard palate while the soft palate seals the nasopharynx. Next, the larynx and epiglottis elevate, temporarily closing the airway while the pharyngeal muscles propel the food bolus in an aboral direction. Simultaneously, the cricopharyngeal sphincter relaxes, allowing food to enter the proximal esophagus, and then contracts strongly as the bolus passes, which prevents the peristaltic wave from causing food to reflux back into the pharynx.

Upper Esophageal Sphincter

The upper esophageal sphincter (UES) pressure is primarily created by the cricopharyngeus muscle with a contribution from the inferior pharyngeal constrictor muscles.[6] The tonic contraction of the UES is maintained by direct vagal innervation and continuous vagal discharge at rest. These discharges cease at the time of sphincter relaxation, and relaxation is aided by upward displacement of the larynx, which elevates the sphincter by approximately 2 cm. The sphincter closes with a contraction that has an amplitude approximately twice as high as resting pressure.

Esophageal Body

The striated muscle of the upper esophagus derives its excitatory innervation directly from vagal fibers. The smooth muscle portion is differently innervated. In the longitudinal muscle, there are only stimulatory fibers that act from cholinergic stimulation of excitatory neurons in the myenteric plexus. The circular muscle, however, contains both excitatory and inhibitory neurons in the myenteric plexus.

Coordination of the movements of the entire esophagus is centrally controlled, but the mechanism is obscure. Three types of pressure waves are seen in the esophagus (Fig. 47.5):

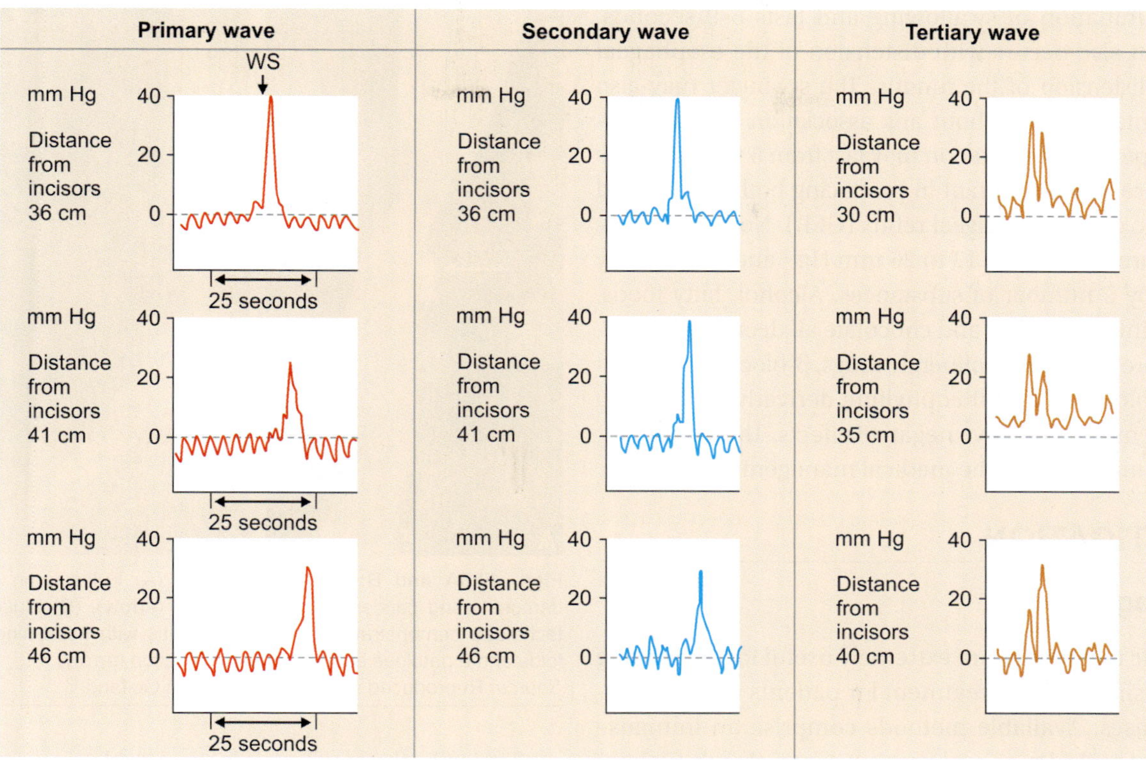

Fig. 47.5: Manometric representation of primary, secondary, and tertiary waves. (WS: Wet swallow).

1. Primary peristalsis is a voluntary propulsive contraction that sweeps down the esophagus in association with swallowing.
2. Secondary peristaltic waves are not associated with a swallow, but are initiated by either retained esophageal content or esophageal distension.
3. Tertiary contractions are not propulsive, but may occur either after swallowing or spontaneously.

Primary peristalsis varies in response between wet and dry swallows. Over 96% of wet swallows result in complete peristalsis, whereas only about two thirds of dry swallows produce complete peristaltic contractions.[8] The peristaltic wave travels at 2–5 cm/s, with slower velocity in the proximal esophagus and more rapid response distally. Contraction amplitudes approach 50 mm Hg in the proximal esophagus and 70 mm Hg in the distal esophagus.[9] Individuals over 80 years of age show a marked decline in amplitude of peristaltic contractions without necessarily exhibiting disordered motor activity. Many normal individuals also exhibit longer double-peaked contractions in the distal esophagus. Peristaltic waves with triple peaks are abnormal.

Secondary peristalsis is a peristaltic sequence that occurs without deglutition and is usually seen in response to irritation, typically by acid. An acid bolus in the esophagus generally produces a secondary peristaltic sequence within 5–15 seconds. This response reduces the remaining acid to a minuscule amount.

Tertiary contractions (simultaneous) occur with approximately 4% of swallows. Spontaneous tertiary contractions occur slightly less than once per minute. Tertiary contractions produce no symptoms. Radiologically they may produce "curling" of the esophagus.

Lower Esophageal Sphincter

For many years, investigators maintained that no LES could be identified anatomically, but microdissection studies of Liebermann-Meffert have shown that there is indeed an anatomic sphincter at the junction of the esophagus and stomach.[1] Like all sphincters it maintains a basal tone, relaxes with swallowing, and then contracts following passage of the peristaltic wave.[10]

The resting tone of the sphincter seems to be intrinsic. Small strips of muscle cut from the region of the "clasp" fibers demonstrate a tonic contraction. The exact mechanisms controlling relaxation and contraction are unclear but may be mediated by the swallowing center in the vagal nuclei.[1] Relaxation of the LES commences simultaneously with the initiation of swallowing and lasts 6–9 seconds. Relaxation also occurs with distension of the esophageal body or distension of the fundus. The sphincter may also relax spontaneously without any association with deglutition. The periods of relaxation may last from 5 to 30 seconds and are probably important in producing both normal and pathologic gastroesophageal reflux (GER). Normal sphincter pressure varies from 13 to 26 mm Hg[11] and is adversely affected by a number of substances. Alcohol, fatty foods, peppermint, coffee, tea, and chocolate all decrease sphincter pressure as do anticholinergic drugs, β-blockers, calcium channel blockers, and theophylline derivatives. Smoking and large meals also have negative effects. These relationships are important in the medical management of reflux.

INVESTIGATION

Radiology

Radiologic techniques are extremely useful for diagnosing and choosing the best treatment for patients with esophageal diseases. Available methods comprise an immense number of techniques and maneuvers to search for specific abnormalities. It is incumbent upon the surgeon to provide the radiologist with sufficient clinical data to allow selection of the techniques most likely to yield the desired information. There is also no substitute for the surgeon personally examining the radiographs with the radiologist who performed the study to extract maximum diagnostic information.

If perforation is suspected, water-soluble contrast material should be used, because it is readily absorbed from the abdominal and thoracic cavities unlike barium, which may potentiate abdominal and pleural sepsis. Nevertheless, these water-soluble contrast media have important drawbacks since they do not coat the mucosal surface as well as barium and may thus give less mucosal detail and can miss small perforations. Therefore, if perforation is suspected but not confirmed by water-soluble media, the study should be repeated with barium suspension. Additionally, water-soluble media is hyperosmotic and if aspirated may produce a severe pneumonia, pulmonary edema, and laryngospasm. Barium should be used in all patients at risk of aspiration. As many patients at risk of perforation are also at risk of aspiration, the risk-versus-benefit ratio must always be considered when choosing the most appropriate contrast agent. It is appropriate for the surgeon to discuss the choice of contrast and technique with a knowledgeable radiologist in this situation.

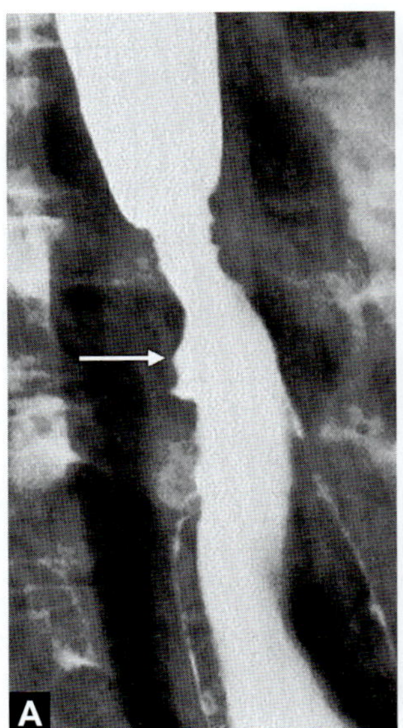

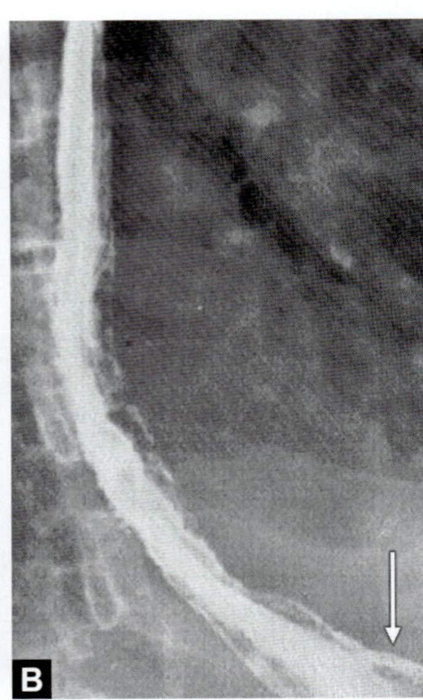

Figs. 47.6A and B: Barium swallows. (A) Full-column technique demonstrating cancer of the esophagus (arrow). (B) Mucosal relief technique demonstrating reflux esophagitis with thickening of distal folds and a patulous esophagogastric junction (arrow).
Source: Reproduced with permission from Gelfand.[12]

Typically, the esophagus is examined using single contrast to delineate the organ in both a distended and flaccid state. The full-column techniques (Fig. 47.6A) are well suited for demonstrating esophageal strictures, cancer, rings, and postoperative changes, whereas mucosal-relief techniques (Fig. 47.6B) are better suited for demonstrating subtle mucosal abnormalities such as small cancers, varices, and reflux esophagitis.

Double-contrast techniques involve the patient ingesting carbon dioxide producing granules along with a small amount of water and then drinking barium. The carbon dioxide distends the esophagus, while the barium shows the fine mucosal detail. This technique requires more cooperation from the patient and is more difficult to perform.

If the patient is thought to have a swallowing disorder, the fluoroscopic examination should be videotaped for examination by the ordering physician. These recordings graphically illustrate the complicated events of swallowing, and slow motion allows a precise analysis of abnormalities encountered. Videofluoroscopy is extremely helpful in patients who have motility disorders, aspiration, or cricopharyngeal diverticula.

Another helpful technique involves ingestion of a marshmallow followed by dilute barium suspension. This semisolid bolus may help to localize areas of poor esophageal transport by lodging proximal to subtle obstructions, whether mechanical or functional.

Table 47.2 Diseases with impaired oropharyngeal motility.	
Cerebrovascular accidents	Cricopharyngeal dysphagia
Bulbar palsy	Myasthenia gravis
Amyotrophic lateral sclerosis	Muscular dystrophy
Multiple sclerosis	Systemic lupus erythematosus
Parkinson's disease	

Poor Oropharyngeal Motility

Many conditions are associated with poor oropharyngeal motility, dysphagia and in severe cases, aspiration (Table 47.2). These conditions are associated with inadequate transport of the food bolus through the oropharyngeal cavity. Most commonly the examiner is already aware of the precipitating condition. The questions to be answered include:

- Is the tongue able to form the bolus and pass it into the pharynx?
- Is the pharyngeal swallow effective?
- Is there laryngeal penetration or aspiration and, if so, with which substances?

The answers are obtained by administering barium-food mixtures of varying density (e.g. cookie, pudding, milkshakes, and liquids); this technique is known as the barium cookie examination. It is usually performed in tandem with a speech pathologist, who is experienced in disorders of swallowing and who can use the information gleaned to plan an effective feeding regimen that minimizes or eliminates aspiration. The study may also indicate that swallowing is inadequate with all consistencies of food and that tube feeding is necessary.

On radiologic examination, the cervical esophagus seen begins at approximately the C5–C6 level and has no normal indentations. The thoracic esophagus normally exhibits indentations at the aortic arch, the left main bronchus and the left atrium. The esophagus narrows as it passes through the esophageal hiatus. There is also a transiently widened area of the esophagus just proximal to its entry into the stomach, termed the esophageal vestibule.

Endoscopy

The indications, technique and subtleties of upper gastrointestinal endoscopy are discussed elsewhere. The lumen of the esophagus is readily and safely examined with the flexible fiberoptic endoscope. The endoscope can be easily passed in most cases under direct visualization through the cricopharyngeus into the proximal esophagus. Exceptions to this rule include patients who have cricopharyngeal diverticula and cervical vertebral osteophytes, in whom passage of the endoscope may be both difficult and potentially hazardous. Endoscopy is indicated for all patients who have any degree of dysphagia. Dysphagia is never a trivial symptom. All strictures must be biopsied regardless of their duration because it is well known that long-standing strictures may harbor an occult carcinoma.

Endoscopic Ultrasound

In the 1980s, ultrasound probes attached to endoscopes were introduced. This marriage of technologies is of immense use in the staging of esophageal cancer. Newer scopes also allow for fine-needle aspiration biopsy of nodes. This type of examination identifies the five layers of the esophageal wall and allows tumors to be staged by the depth of their invasion. The patient can also be examined for lymph node metastases by noting abnormalities in normal lymph node architecture such as:

- Heterogeneous echoes within the node
- A distinct border
- Spherical shape.

Endoscopic ultrasound is approximately 85% accurate in staging the local tumor and 90% correct in assessing lymph nodes.[13,14]

High-Resolution Esophageal Manometry

The modern use of manometry to study esophageal motility began in the 1950s.[15-17] The technique utilized multilumen catheters connected to pressure transducers at 10 cm intervals in the esophagus to determine the amplitude, velocity, and coordination of swallowing events. High-resolution manometry (HRM) of the esophagus is a newer technique that provides a more precise assessment of esophageal motility than the older techniques. The catheter used has apertures spaced approximately 1 cm apart to produce a pressure over time picture in which the pressure is color coded for ease of visualization. The advantages of HRM over conventional manometry include the fact that HRM is technically easy to perform (catheter does not need to be repositioned during study), allows for real-time simultaneous monitoring of the LES, esophageal body, and upper esophageal sphincter (UES), permits visualization of small and/or isolated segments of dysfunctional esophagus, and compensates for esophageal shortening and movement of the LES during swallows.

The technique of conventional manometry is accomplished by the passage of an array that consists of a multichannel catheter with from three to six lumens. These

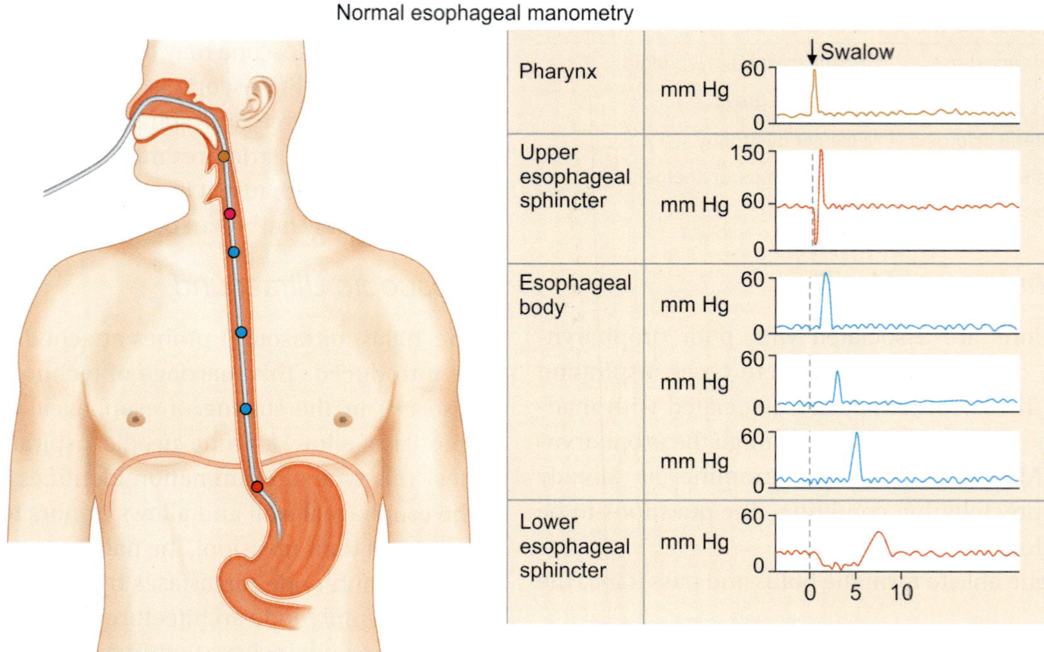

Fig. 47.7: Esophageal manometry catheter tracings at corresponding levels during a single primary peristaltic wave.

catheters are perfused continuously with water and are connected to external pressure transducers. The catheters have side-holes that are spaced 5 cm apart such that the whole assembly measures pressures at 5 cm intervals along the entire length of the esophagus. The catheter is also marked at 1 cm intervals allowing the operator to determine the length from the incisors to the pressure monitoring aperture. As the catheter assembly is withdrawn through the esophagus and LES, it provides a pressure profile as seen in Figures 47.7 and 47.8. Traditionally, the catheter is slowly withdrawn at 1 cm intervals until the LES is seen. The patient is then given 5 mL sips of water and asked to swallow. A belt transducer placed around the chest allows monitoring of respiration and correlation of respiratory variations. In the abdomen, inspiration is associated with an increase in pressure, whereas in the chest inspiration is associated with negative variations in pressure. Identification of the point at which these associations change allows the diaphragmatic hiatus to be distinguished.

Techniques and protocols learnt from conventional manometry continue to be applied to HRM, but a major difference is that the stationary pull through maneuver is no longer required with HRM. The standard HRM clinical protocol uses 10 wet swallows in the supine position in the fasting patient. The addition of multiple rapid swallows may be of value, and needs to be added to the standard protocol. Use of bolus consistencies other than liquid need to be further studied, and diagnostic value may be augmented with the use of high-resolution impedance manometry. When evaluating patterns of activity, several discrete manometric profiles can be appreciated by HRM. HRM has particularly high sensitivity and positive predictive value for the diagnosis of LES relaxation errors, with very low false positive rates. The gain in sensitivity in the diagnosis of achalasia is significant.

Table 47.3 identifies the characteristics that should be reported in any manometric study. Individual manometric findings are addressed under individual disease entities. Esophageal manometry is indicated whenever the physician suspects a motor abnormality in a patient who has symptoms of dysphagia, odynophagia, or atypical chest pain.

Ambulatory 24-Hour pH Monitoring

This test is used to detect increased esophageal exposure to gastric juice. Foregut symptoms are not sufficiently specific to allow differentiation of disease entities by symptoms alone. In the absence of endoscopic or biopsy evidence of esophagitis, it is necessary to demonstrate pathologic esophageal acid exposure objectively before considering surgical therapy. This technique involves transnasal placement of an indwelling pH probe 5 cm above the LES.

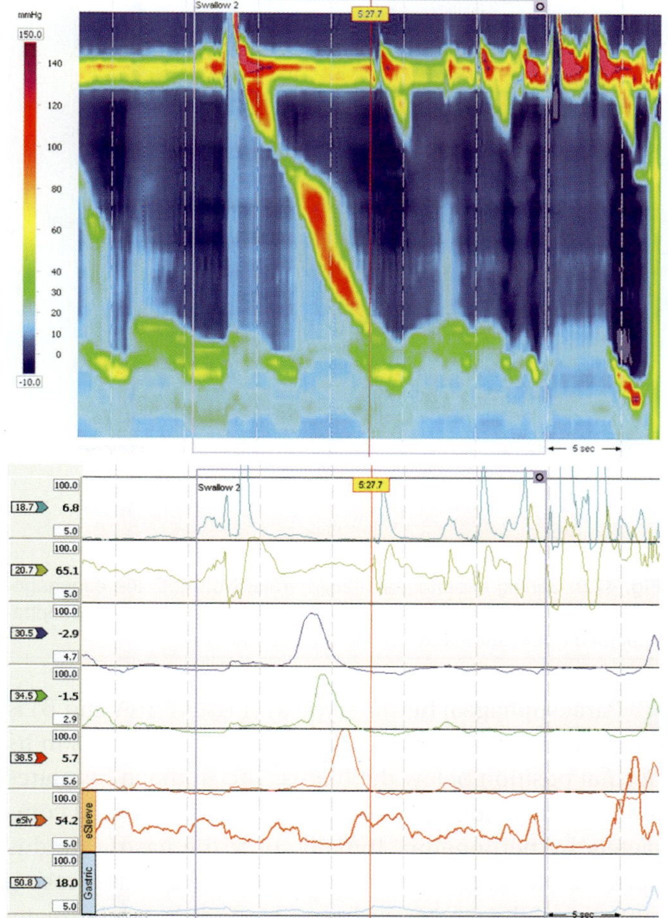

Figs. 47.8: High-resolution manometry with the corresponding standard manometry below. Pressures are color-coded and the actual propagation velocities, percentage of propagated swallows and pressure amplitudes are reported.

This probe is connected to a recorder and is worn by the patient over a 24-hour period. Formerly the probe was passed transnasally and required the indwelling catheter to be worn for the duration of the test. Patients uniformly detested this test, and it has been largely supplanted by the Bravo probe where the probe is endoscopically pinned to the esophageal mucosa and wirelessly transmits its signal to an external receiver (the probe typically passes in the stool within a few days). The results are analyzed by computer to determine acid exposure. Measurements include:

- The cumulative time at which the esophageal pH is below 4.0 during the total, upright, and supine periods
- Number of reflux episodes below pH 4.0 per 24 hours-Duration of these episodes expressed as the number of episodes lasting longer than 5 minutes per 24 hours, the time in minutes of the longest recorded episode and the percentage of time the pH is below 4.0.

Table 47.3 Characteristics reported at esophageal manometry.

Lower esophageal sphincter
Pressure (normal > 10 mm Hg)
Sphincter length (normal > 2 cm)
Relaxation (complete or partial)
Point of respiratory reversal (marks the hiatus)
Double pressure peaking (associated with hiatus hernia)
Double respiratory reversal (associated with hiatus hernia)
Peristalsis
Velocity of contraction (2–5 cm/s)
Amplitude of contraction (normal >50 mm Hg)
Presence of double peaks (normal)
Presence of triple peaks (abnormal)
Upper esophageal sphincter
Pressure
Relaxation
Coordination of relaxation with pharyngeal contraction

Table 47.4 Normal values for esophageal exposure to pH <4 (24-hour pH study). 95% confidence limits are DeMeester score less than 14.72.

Component	*Mean*	*Standard deviation*	*95th Percentile*
% of total time	1.51	1.36	4.45
Upright time (%)	2.34	2.34	8.42
Supine time (%)	0.63	1.0	3.45
Number of episodes	19.00	12.76	46.90
Number >5 min	0.84	1.18	3.45
Longest episode (min)	6.74	7.85	19.80

With permission from DeMeester and Stein, 1989.[18]

Table 47.4 quantifies the normal values for these variables. The upper limits of normal are defined at the 95th percentile. Twenty-four hour monitoring is the ideal way of determining pathologic reflux. Nevertheless, there are a few situations in which the test may be misleading. It does not adequately measure exposure to duodenal reflux. Further, bacterial or fungal overgrowth may occur in patients who have achalasia producing fermentation within the esophagus and resultant abnormal acidic pH values, without GER. This finding is characterized by a gradual drop in pH to acidic values rather than the abrupt drops characteristic of GER; pH then rises abruptly as the patient swallows saliva neutralizing the fermented content. Nevertheless, the computer program will interpret this as reflux. Since the proton pump inhibitors suppress acid secretion leading to false negative studies, they should be stopped for at least 2 weeks before the study.

GASTROESOPHAGEAL REFLUX AND HIATAL HERNIA

The symptom complex that, for most of the last century, was attributed to the presence of a sliding hiatal hernia is actually caused by reflux of the stomach contents into the distal esophagus. This seemingly obvious association, which underpins all current therapy, was unknown to surgeons and physiologists before the 1950s. Phillip Allison was the first to postulate this explanation.[19] He believed that gastroesophageal competence was related to a pinchcock valve formed by the diaphragmatic hiatus and that reflux was related to a failure of this mechanism. Allison believed that if the hiatus could be restored to a normal anatomic configuration, reflux would be eliminated. He designed an operation that reduced the hiatal hernia and narrowed the hiatus posteriorly. The high failure rate associated with Allison's operation does not in any way minimize the importance of his conceptual contribution. Furthermore, this concept has led to all of our current therapies for GER including a number of extremely effective operative antireflux procedures.

Association of Reflux with Hiatal Hernia

What is the importance of the hiatal hernia in the genesis of GER? There is probably some relationship since 80% of patients who have reflux have a sliding hiatal hernia, yet 80% of patients with hiatus hernia are asymptomatic.[20] Further, hiatal hernia is ubiquitous. When provocative maneuvers are used by the radiologist, hiatal hernia can be demonstrated in over 50% of the population.[21] The importance of hiatal hernia and its contribution to reflux remains an enigma for the present, but a sliding hiatal hernia is clearly not the cause of pathologic GER. Therefore, the so-called incidental antireflux procedure in an asymptomatic patient who has hiatal hernia is never indicated. Such an operation invariably leads to a patient who suffers all the side effects of the operation without reaping any benefit. This statement refers only to "sliding hiatal hernia." There are two general types of hiatal hernias:

1. Sliding (type 1)
2. Paraesophageal (type 2).

The sliding hiatal hernia (Fig. 47.9) is defined by a cephalad (upward) displacement of the esophagogastric junction and proximal stomach through the hiatus into the posterior mediastinum. The stomach is covered anteriorly by a sac of peritoneum, whereas the posterior stomach is bare. In most patients, the esophagus is normal in length and the hernia reduces easily in the upright position.

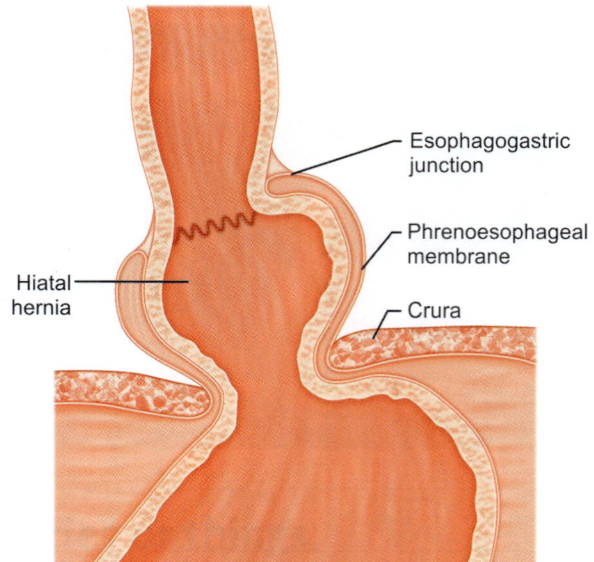

Fig. 47.9: Sliding esophageal hiatal hernia. Note that the esophagogastric junction is above the diaphragm and that the phrenoesophageal membrane still inserts on the esophagus itself.

Paraesophageal hernia (type 2) (Figs. 47.10A and B) is one in which the esophagogastric junction remains in its normal position below the hiatus. The stomach herniates into the chest next to the esophagus and is covered completely by peritoneum. Initially, only the gastric fundus herniates through the hiatus, but eventually increasing amounts of the greater curvature of the stomach herniate, until finally the entire stomach enters the chest giving the appearance of the "upside-down stomach" or "gastric volvulus." A paraesophageal hernia where the esophagogastric junction is displaced above the diaphragm is referred to as a type 3 hernia while a paraesophageal hernia with herniation of colon, spleen or pancreas is termed type 4. Even asymptomatic paraesophageal hernias are of clinical importance and are discussed separately later in this chapter.

Pathophysiology

Twenty-four hour pH monitoring of normal subjects has amply demonstrated that postprandial reflux occurs in everyone.[18] What then distinguishes normal individuals from patients who develop GER disease? It has become apparent that at least four factors are important in the etiology of this disease:

1. Efficacy of the antireflux mechanism
2. Content of the refluxed material (e.g. acid, pepsin, pancreatic enzymes, bile, and pancreatic juice)
3. Tissue resistance of the esophageal mucosa
4. Esophageal clearance of refluxed material.

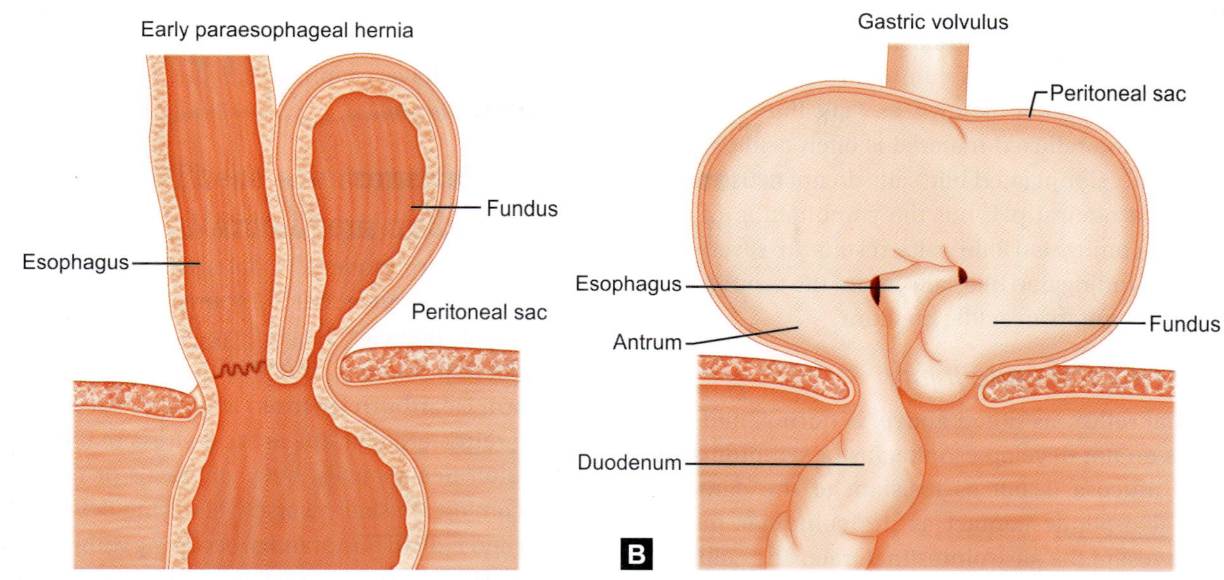

Figs. 47.10A and B: Paraesophageal hernia. (A) Herniated fundus (note the esophagogastric junction is in the normal position). (B) Gastric volvulus with entire stomach in the chest.

Reflux esophagitis can be defined as inflammation of the esophageal lining caused by GER, but the symptom complex associated with GER is not solely limited to patients with histologic evidence of reflux esophagitis. The symptomatic response of patients to reflux varies widely, and there is a poor correlation between symptoms and the severity of microscopic or macroscopic findings of esophagitis. Patients who have a normal histologic appearance, typical reflux symptoms and abnormal 24-hour pH findings are said to have pathologic GER.

Antireflux Mechanism

The LES is the major barrier to GER. The LES pressure must approach zero to allow an episode of reflux.[22] Many authors have attributed GER to a low LES pressure,[23-25] but more recently investigators have shown that many patients who have reflux esophagitis have normal sphincter pressures.[26,27] Much of the disparity in these studies can probably be explained by patient selection. Patients who have severe reflux esophagitis and those in surgical series tend to have LES pressure lower than the general population of patients with symptomatic reflux. Overall, at least 50% of patients with reflux have LES pressures below 10 mm Hg. What is not clear is whether the defect in sphincter pressure produces the esophagitis or whether the esophagitis damages the sphincter resulting in low sphincter pressures. There is evidence to support both hypotheses. It is possible that both are correct: hypotension may be either primary or secondary, and it is seldom possible to determine which is operative in an individual patient.

In patients who have reflux with normal resting LES pressure, the mechanism of reflux appears to be prolonged inappropriate relaxations of the LES. Simultaneous recordings of LES pressure and intraesophageal pH demonstrate that these relaxation episodes may occur:

- Spontaneously, following normal peristaltic contractions
- Spontaneously (not in association with a peristaltic event)
- In association with failed peristaltic events
- When subjects are aroused from sleep.[28]

Therefore, reflux appears to be principally related to a low-LES pressure, although not necessarily a low resting LES pressure.

Content of Refluxed Material

The composition of the refluxed material is another important element in the development of esophagitis. Altering the composition of the refluxate is the principal mechanism underpinning medical therapy. Both acid and pepsin play important roles. Pepsin is activated at pH values below 3.2, and even small amounts of activated pepsin can produce protein digestion and severe esophageal injury.[29] Patients who have gastric hypersecretion secondary to duodenal ulcer disease or Zollinger-Ellison syndrome may also develop severe esophagitis secondary to the high concentration of acid and a high volume of secretion.[30,31]

Esophageal injury may also be caused by reflux of duodenal content through the stomach and into the esophagus. This reflux is seen most commonly after a previous gastric operation and is known as "alkaline esophagitis," although the refluxed material is often acidic or only weakly alkaline. Conjugated bile salts do not cause mucosal injury at a neutral pH, but the combination of acid, pepsin, and conjugated bile salts results in severe esophagitis.[32] Unconjugated bile salts injure the esophagus in an alkaline but not in an acidic medium.

Mucosal Resistance to Injury

Postprandial reflux, as noted above, is normal and most individuals do not develop esophagitis or symptoms. The squamous mucosa is not as resistant to the damaging effects of acid-peptic contact as the columnar mucosa seen in the rest of the gastrointestinal tract. The columnar epithelium of Barrett's esophagus is much more resistant to the acid injury of reflux, and esophagitis is generally confined to the squamous mucosa that lies above.

Squamous mucosa is normally impermeable to acid, but prolonged exposure produces back-diffusion of acid across the mucosa. If acid exposure is not overwhelming, the mucosa responds with increased cell turnover that may compensate for the cellular injury. This process accounts for the increased thickness of the basal cell layer and prominent papillae in patients who have pathologic reflux without macroscopic or microscopic esophagitis. These changes may also be seen in experimental models and are associated with an increased turnover in the basal layer.[33]

Acid Clearance

As postprandial reflux is ubiquitous, there must be a mechanism that clears acid from the esophagus and restores the normal intraluminal esophageal pH. This mechanism has two components:

1. The primary peristaltic wave clears most of the refluxed acid from the esophagus
2. Swallowed saliva neutralizes the remaining acid, causing the intraluminal pH to return to normal values.

Some patients with reflux exhibit normal acid clearance times, whereas others show delayed acid clearance. Approximately 30–40% of patients with severe esophagitis display a high rate of failure of primary peristalsis to travel all the way from the proximal to the distal esophagus. The pathogenesis of peristaltic abnormalities is not known, but it does not appear to normalize when the esophagitis heals. This failure of peristalsis is particularly important in patients with scleroderma, who exhibit both a low LES pressure and aperistalsis and thus have particularly severe esophagitis. Salivary flow appears to be normal in most patients who have esophagitis,[34] but not in those with Sjögren's syndrome.

Clinical Features

The symptoms of reflux are secondary to the irritating effects of gastroduodenal contents that have flowed cephalad across an either temporarily or permanently incompetent sphincter. This refluxed material can produce protean manifestations, but the classic manifestation is heartburn. Heartburn (pyrosis) is typically described as a burning retrosternal or epigastric distress that commonly occurs after heavy meals, between meals or nocturnally. The discomfort is usually worse when lying down or bending over and is often postprandial occurring within 1–2 hours of eating. Heartburn is almost ubiquitous. Among normal subjects 36% complain of heartburn at least once per month, and 7% note daily heartburn.[35] The incidence of heartburn is increased in pregnancy, with 25% of pregnant women complaining of daily symptoms. There may also be excessive belching and regurgitation of small amounts of sour or bitter gastric contents into the throat. This symptom is dissimilar from vomiting because it is effortless and is not accompanied by nausea. No retching is involved. This form of regurgitation may occur at night, resulting in sudden awakening with a choking feeling.

Some patients may also have a squeezing type of substernal pain that can be difficult to distinguish from angina because it may radiate into the neck, jaw, shoulders, or back. DeMeester noted that there was pathologic reflux in nearly 50% of patients who had chest pain and negative investigations for coronary artery disease.[36] At one time it was speculated that this type of pain was secondary to esophageal spasm, but recent studies have failed to confirm this association.

Pulmonary symptoms may be important because they can reflect regurgitation with nocturnal aspiration. This process may lead to aspiration pneumonia, bronchitis, or asthma. Radionuclide scans have documented episodes of pulmonary aspiration with bronchospasm in asthmatic patients.[37] Other airway manifestations include cough, laryngitis, vocal cord granulomas, subglottic stenosis, laryngospasm, hoarseness, and loss of dental enamel. The best way to demonstrate the association of reflux with pulmonary symptoms is a Bravo probe with both the distal esophageal probe and a more proximal probe which allows correlation of pulmonary symptoms with episodes of proximal reflux.

Dysphagia may indicate the development of an esophageal stricture, or it may be secondary to esophagitis without stricture. Dysphagia should never be treated as a trivial symptom. The development of dysphagia mandates esophagoscopy to rule out the possibility of cancer.

Investigation and Diagnosis

Clinical symptoms are not adequate for confirming a diagnosis of GER. Regurgitation in the supine position is a relatively reliable symptom, but the pain of pyrosis may be very similar to the pain of biliary tract disease, peptic ulcer disease or gastritis. Many clinicians advocate a trial of acid suppression to make the diagnosis, but if this does not result in prompt relief, or if symptoms recur when therapy is stopped, a diagnostic evaluation should be carried out.

Radiology

Radiologic assessment of the esophagus is not a particularly sensitive way to detect reflux, but barium examinations can be used to demonstrate hiatal hernia and to document reflux. Radiologic assessment is very useful in detecting esophageal shortening secondary to esophagitis or stricture. Ulcerations of the esophagus that occur in squamous mucosa tend to be linear. Punched-out ulcers occur in columnar mucosa. A punched-out esophageal ulcer implies the presence of Barrett's esophagus. Similarly, strictures tend to occur at the squamocolumnar junction. A midesophageal stricture suggests the presence of Barrett's esophagus.

Endoscopy

Endoscopy is less sensitive than pH assessment in detecting reflux, but it is extremely useful in eliminating other possible diagnoses. It allows the endoscopist to evaluate the configuration of the LES and whether gastric contents are refluxing into the esophagus. The presence or absence of a hiatal hernia and the position of the squamocolumnar junction can also be evaluated. Endoscopic esophagitis is classified according to objective criteria, as shown in Table 47.5.

Table 47.5 Endoscopic classification of esophagitis.

Grade	*Features*
1	(Minimal) erythema and dilation of capillaries or friability
2	Linear erosions and ulceration
3	Confluent erosions with a pale bed of granulation tissue
4	Stricture with or without changes of grade 3

The endoscopic diagnosis of grade 1 esophagitis is not reproducible from observer to observer. The diagnosis of grade 2 esophagitis (linear erosions; Fig. 47.11) is clear-cut and is sufficient to confirm the diagnosis without pH studies.

Confirmation of the diagnosis of esophagitis requires biopsy-proven esophagitis or obvious ulcerations, preferably documented by endoscopic photographs. Strictures should always be biopsied and brushed for cytology regardless of the duration of time for which they have been present. There is a well-known propensity for chronic strictures to harbor an occult carcinoma.

24-Hour pH Monitoring

24-hour pH studies are the gold standard for determining whether a patient has pathologic GER. They should be used to document reflux in patients who have symptoms of reflux and normal mucosal biopsies before any consideration of surgical therapy. Other indications for this test are noted in Table 47.6.

High-Resolution Esophageal Manometry

HRM or conventional manometry is not necessary in every patient who presents with symptoms of GERD. Despite

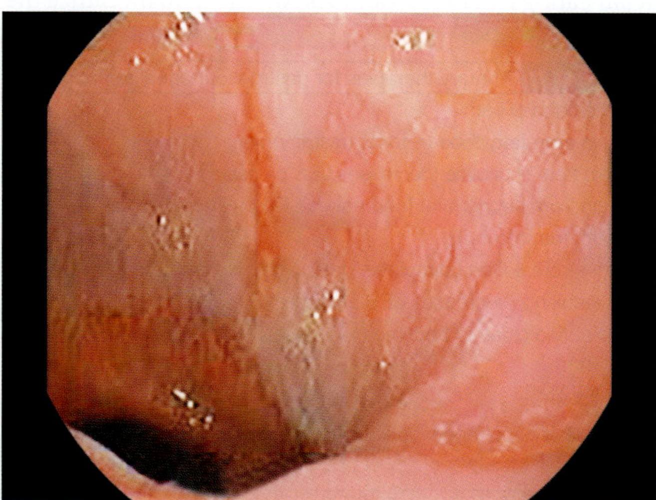

Fig. 47.11: Linear erosions are visible on endoscopy.

Table 47.6 Indications for 24-hour ambulatory pH monitoring.

Normal endoscopic biopsy in a patient who has reflux symptoms
Poor response to acid suppressive therapy and normal biopsy
Pulmonary symptoms with suspected reflux
Noncardiac chest pain

the importance of the LES, a low sphincter pressure is not synonymous with the diagnosis of GER. Manometry may be indicated in patients who fail to respond to medical therapy, especially if they have suspected scleroderma or other collagen vascular disease. The presence of aperistalsis and an extremely low LES pressure confirms the diagnosis of scleroderma.

Manometry should always be performed in any patient being considered for an antireflux operation to rule out scleroderma, unsuspected achalasia, diffuse esophageal spasm (DES), or weak peristalsis. Many believe that antireflux surgery is to be avoided in these situations.

Medical Management

Medical therapy should include a phased approach. Alterations in lifestyle, avoidance of certain medications and changes in diet may result in substantial relief of symptoms (Table 47.7). Gravity should be used to aid the patient in clearing refluxed acid from the esophagus either by elevating the head of the bed on 15 cm (6 in.) blocks or the use of a foam wedge to elevate the upper body. These maneuvers do not decrease the number of reflux episodes, but do appear to improve acid clearance.[38] Foods that decrease acid clearance should be avoided. Patients should be instructed to eat smaller meals and to avoid eating for several hours before sleep to minimize the amount of gastric content available for reflux. Weight loss also improves reflux symptoms, possibly by decreasing intra-abdominal pressure.

Table 47.7 Primary therapies for gastroesophageal reflux.
Elevate head of bed
Abstain from fatty food (retards gastric emptying)
Abstain from chocolate (decreases LES pressure)
Abstain from peppermint (decreases LES pressure)
Abstain from alcohol
Abstain from coffee (stimulates gastric acid production)
Stop smoking (decreases LES pressure)
Avoid eating close to bedtime (reduces volume of material available to reflux)
Lose weight

(LES: Lower esophageal sphincter).

The second line of therapy works by decreasing the damaging nature of the refluxed material. Antacids are widely available and function by neutralizing stomach acid, raising pH and preventing the activation of pepsin. They have the advantage of working promptly to relieve symptoms. Antacids should be administered approximately 1 and 3 hours after eating to neutralize meal-induced secretions and whenever symptomatic relief is needed.

H_2-Receptor Antagonists

When lifestyle measures and antacids are not successful, the next line of therapy includes H_2-receptor blockade to decrease the quantity of acid available for reflux. Cimetidine and its competitors ranitidine and famotidine work by competitively inhibiting H_2 receptors. They have no effect on LES pressure. H_2-receptor blockade decreases the symptoms of heartburn and improves the endoscopic appearance of the mucosa. Side effects include headache, constipation, fatigue, dizziness, and thrombocytopenia. Cimetidine also interferes with the metabolism of drugs such as warfarin. All of these drugs are now available in reduced dosage as over-the-counter medications in the United States and other developed countries.

Prokinetic Agents

These agents work by increasing LES pressure and improving gastric emptying. Their doses, mechanisms of action and side effects are shown in Table 47.8. Metoclopramide is a weak prokinetic with many side effects, while cisapride, a potent prokinetic, is no longer available in the United States.

Cytoprotective Agents

The only cytoprotective agent that has demonstrated activity against GER is sucralfate. Sucralfate binds to

Table 47.8 Prokinetic agents.

Agent	Dose	Mechanism of action	Side effects
Metoclopramide	10 mg 30 min before meals and at bedtime	Increases LES pressure, improves gastric emptying	Sedation, agitation, extrapyramidal syndromes
Bethanechol	10–25 mg before meals and at bedtime	Increases LES pressure, improves acid clearance, improves gastric emptying	Cholinergic: diarrhea, cramps, salivation, urinary frequency
Cisapride	10 mg 30 min before meals and at bedtime	Increases LES pressure, increases amplitude of peristalsis, improves gastric emptying	Dizziness, faintness, cramping, cardiac arrest

(LES: Lower esophageal sphincter).

inflamed and ulcerated areas in the esophagus. It prevents back-diffusion of hydrogen ions, absorbs bile salts, and prevents pepsin-induced damage to the esophagus. Sucralfate in a dose of 1 g q6h produces marked improvement in symptoms and endoscopic appearance. There may be advantages to dissolving it in water and administering it as a slurry.

Proton Pump Inhibitors

The mainstay of medical therapy is the use of a proton pump inhibitor. Oral omeprazole and lansoprazole both result in endoscopic healing of esophagitis in over 90% of patients. The usual dose of omeprazole is 20 mg orally daily, whereas lansoprazole is given as 15–30 mg orally daily. The once daily dosage helps to improve compliance.

Acid-reducing drugs only reduce the caustic nature of the refluxate; they do not combat regurgitation. Therefore, although heartburn may virtually disappear, regurgitation may remain bothersome. Early concerns about the development of gastric carcinoids in patients on prolonged omeprazole therapy have not materialized, although some patients develop enterochromaffin-like cell hyperplasia of uncertain importance. A more worrying consideration is that proton pump inhibitors seem to hasten the onset of atrophic gastritis in patients who are infected with *Helicobacter pylori*,[39] and atrophic gastritis is a premalignant condition. It has been recommended that *H. pylori* status be tested in all patients treated with long-term proton pump inhibitors and that positive patients be treated to eradicate the bacteria. It remains to be determined whether eradication of *H. pylori* in these patients will prevent atrophic gastritis.

Operative Management

Although medical therapy achieves excellent results in many patients with GER disease, some fail to achieve satisfactory relief or develop complications of their reflux that do not respond to medical therapy or choose surgical therapy for other reasons. The indications for operation are listed in Table 47.9. The need for documentation of pathologic reflux esophagitis, either by biopsy or by 24-hour pH monitoring, cannot be overemphasized. When the diagnosis of reflux is objectively confirmed, surgical therapy should be considered in individuals who (1) have failed medical management, (2) opt for operation despite successful medical management due to quality of life considerations, (3) have complications of reflux, or (4) have extraesophageal manifestations of acid reflux.

Table 47.9 Indications for operation for reflux.

Intractable symptoms secondary to:
Esophagitis documented by biopsy
Pathologic gastroesophageal reflux documented by 24-hour pH monitoring (in the absence of esophagitis)
Complications of reflux that are not amenable to medical therapy
Stricture
Bleeding
Asthma
Laryngeal irritation related to reflux
Cough

Goals of Operation

Three goals should be pursued in any operation to treat GER. First, the barrier to GER must be re-established either by increasing LES pressure, restoring the esophagus to its normal intra-abdominal position, or both. All the currently available operations meet this goal. All of the current antireflux procedures increase LES pressure by wrapping the esophagogastric junction with fundus. In general, the magnitude of the increase in LES pressure is proportional to the completeness of the wrap (Fig. 47.12).[40] Second, the surgically created barrier to reflux must relax in response to deglutition like the normal LES. The fundus of the stomach, which is generally used to construct the wrap, participates in the receptive relaxation of the normal sphincter, although relaxation is not always complete. Third, most procedures restore the barrier to reflux, which

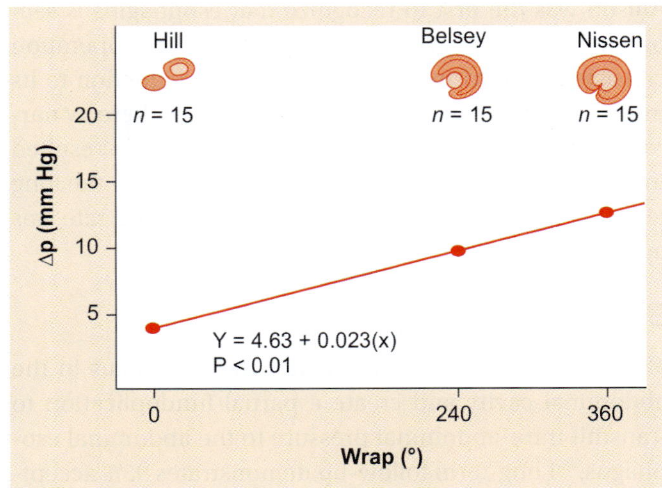

Fig. 47.12: Changes in sphincter pressure. Δp is change in lower esophageal pressure (mm Hg) associated with the wrap with various antireflux procedures.
Source: Adapted from DeMeester et al.[40]

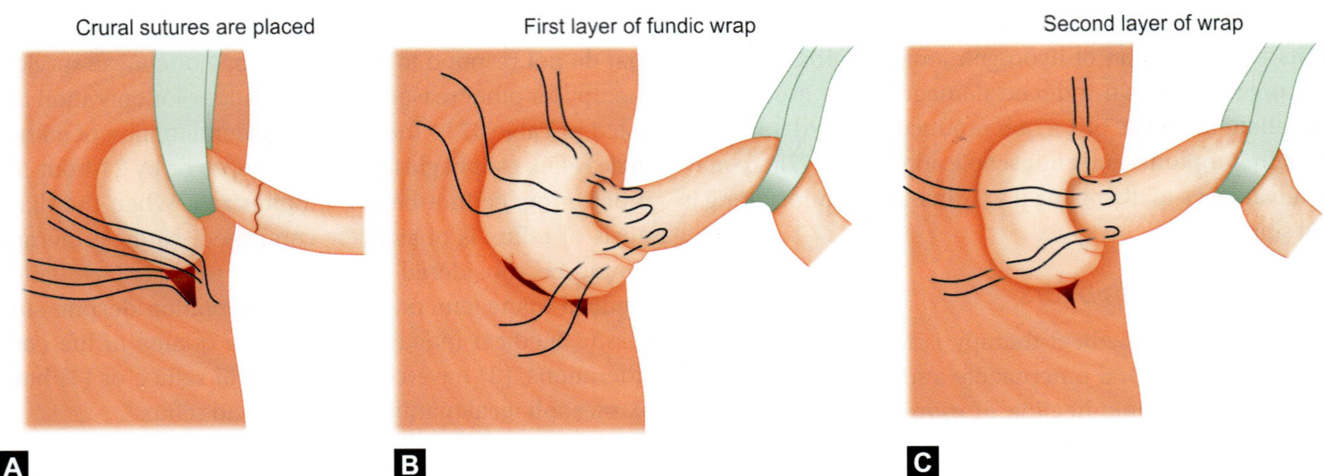

Figs. 47.13A to C: Belsey's Mark IV operation. (A) Following esophageal mobilization, crural sutures are being placed to be tied later. (B) The first layer of the fundic wrap is created using mattress sutures. (C) The second layer of the wrap is created using mattress sutures that also help to reduce the wrap below the hiatus.

by augmenting sphincter pressure also forms a potential antegrade barrier to deglutition. Unless the patient has adequate amplitude of peristalsis to overcome this potential barrier, dysphagia may be a problem. This possibility is the primary reason for obtaining manometry in patients before surgical therapy. Partial fundoplication may be considered in patients with indications for operation but with underlying low amplitude peristalsis or a high (80%) proportion of failed swallows; however, these operations may have a higher failure rate.

Allison's Technique of Crural Closure

Allison was the first to recognize that esophagitis is secondary to reflux of acid from the stomach.[19] His operation consisted of restoring the esophagogastric junction to its intra-abdominal position and maintaining it there by narrowing the hiatus with sutures. This restoration resulted in an short-term increase in LES pressure, but in the long term (as reported by Allison himself) the failure rate was approximately 50%.[41,42]

Belsey's Mark IV Operation

The procedure attempts to anchor the esophagus in the abdominal cavity and create a partial fundoplication to transmit intra-abdominal pressure to the abdominal esophagus.[43] Long-term follow-up demonstrates 95% acceptable results at 5 years,[44] falling to approximately 30% at 15 years.[45]

This transthoracic operation relies on maintaining the length of intra-abdominal esophagus, so preoperative evaluation must ensure that there is no esophageal shortening. The operation is performed through the left sixth interspace. The esophagus is mobilized to the level of the aortic arch to aid in reduction of the stomach and esophagus into the abdominal cavity. A 270° fundoplication increases LES pressure, and sutures maintain the reduction of the esophagogastric junction below the diaphragm by suturing the wrap to the hiatus (Figs. 47.13A to C).

Most patients can be managed adequately without a nasogastric tube, but an overnight tube will prevent nausea and retching with the possibility of gastric dilatation and disruption of the sutures. Belsey recommended a barium swallow on the seventh postoperative day as a baseline study.[46] The most feared complication is leakage from the esophagus or stomach at the site of the fundoplication. It should be suspected in patients who have tachycardia and/or fever, who should receive a contrast study.

This procedure is still in use by many thoracic surgeons, but the need for thoracotomy, with its attendant morbidity, has markedly diminished its use since the advent of laparoscopy. Further, although the 5-year rates of reflux control are good, the 10-year results are less satisfactory.

Nissen's Fundoplication

Nissen is reported to have discovered the principle of fundoplication serendipitously in a patient whose cardia he had excised for an esophageal ulcer. He wrapped the fundus around the anastomosis to decrease the possibility of anastomotic leakage, and 16 years later he noted that

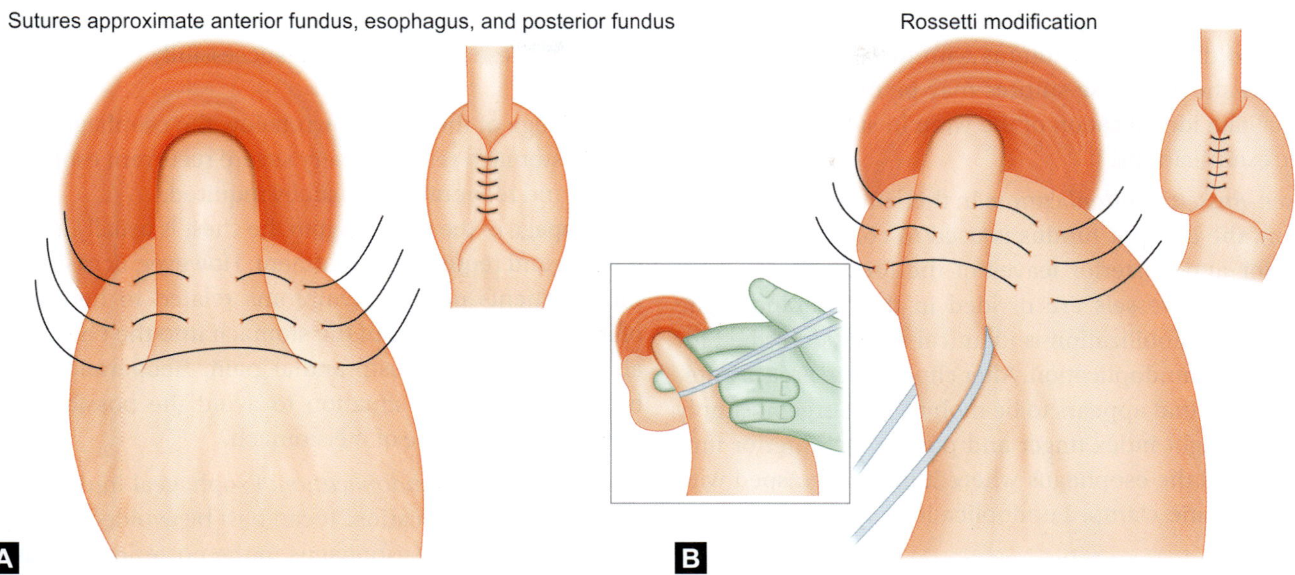

Figs. 47.14A and B: Classic Nissen's fundoplication. (A) The mobilized posterior fundus is brought posterior to the esophagus. Nonabsorbable sutures approximate anterior fundus, esophagus, and posterior fundus to create the wrap. (B) The Rossetti modification of Nissen's fundoplication (lower inset): the mobile anterior fundus is pushed posterior to the esophagus by the surgeon's hand and then sewn to more anterior fundus to create the fundoplication (upper inset).

the patient had not developed esophagitis.[47] His original technique for esophagitis involved mobilization of the fundus to allow it to be brought behind the esophagus and sutured to the anterior fundus, including esophageal bites (Fig. 47.14A).[48] Later, he introduced a modification that used the anterior fundus without fundic mobilization or division of the vasa brevia. The anterior fundus was brought posterior to the esophagus and was then sutured to itself (Fig. 47.14B). This procedure is widely referred to as Rossetti's modification or the Nissen-Rossetti.[49] Both techniques may be performed laparoscopically.

Original Nissen's fundoplication: Many surgeons dissect the esophagus in the abdomen, but this requires dissecting through the phrenoesophageal ligament, which may be stout in patients without a sliding hiatal hernia. It is safer to dissect the esophagus in the posterior mediastinum above the hiatus where there are only areolar attachments. The initial dissection and encirclement of the esophagus are shown in Figures 47.15A and B. Mobilization of the fundus may be carried out from the angle of His downward in thin patients, but in obese patients, it is more easily begun by opening the lesser sac on the greater curvature several inches below the hiatus. Vasa brevia may be ligated using ultrasonic shears or bipolar vessel sealing device.

Crural repair is advocated to prevent herniation of the completed repair into the chest,[50] with potential risks of ulceration and healing.[51] However, it has been shown both experimentally and clinically that a fundoplication functions quite well in the chest should the crural repair dehisce.[52,53] The fundoplication described originally by Nissen was 3–6 cm long. Over the years many modifications have been suggested to reduce the incidence of complications. Most surgeons now follow the recommendations of Donahue who advocated the "floppy" fundoplication. This is a 1.0–2.5 cm wrap constructed over a large (54–60 F) intraesophageal bougie.[54] A loose wrap minimizes the risk of

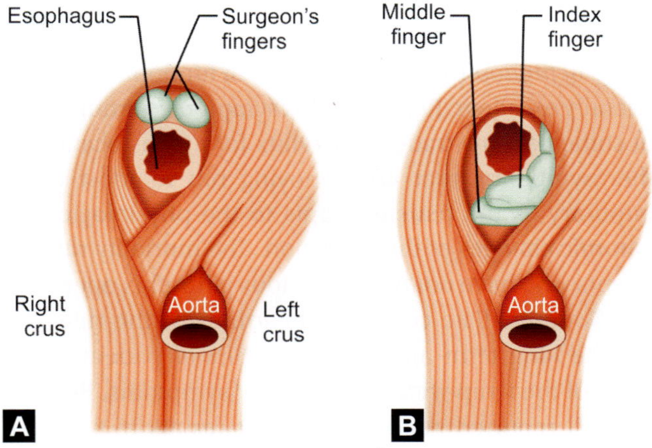

Figs. 47.15A and B: Nissen's fundoplication. (A) Cross-section demonstrating the surgeon's fingers dissecting anterior to the esophagus. (B) The surgeon's fingers encircle the esophagus superior to the diaphragm including all tissue anterior to the aorta until the esophagus is completely encircled.

postoperative dysphagia. The anterior fundus is approximated to the posterior fundus with three permanent sutures as shown. These sutures may be marked with clips to facilitate identification of the wrap in subsequent radiologic examinations.

Nissen-Rossetti fundoplication: In this simplified fundoplication, the anterior fundus is used to construct both the anterior and posterior leaves of the fundoplication. No short gastric vessels are divided in this operation. The esophageal mobilization is identical to that described for the original fundoplication. After choosing an area of anterior fundus that appears to be mobile, the surgeon simply takes the right index finger and pushes the anterior fundus behind the esophagus where it may be grasped with an atraumatic clamp. Fundoplication is then performed as before.

There is no convincing evidence that the classic fundoplication gives a looser wrap with less postoperative dysphagia. To the contrary, the lack of fundic mobilization may make the fundus less likely to migrate through the hiatus into the chest, while the use of the anterior fundus makes the wrap less likely to migrate distally on the stomach.

Results of fundoplication: The results of fundoplication are generally excellent. Relief of reflux symptoms is immediate, but some patients trade their reflux for a constellation of other symptoms that are annoying but in most cases temporary as the patient adapts to the physiologic and anatomic changes of the operation. The mortality rate for patients who have not had a previous antireflux operation is <1 %. Immediate control of heartburn is the rule, but over the long term approximately 10% of patients have failure of the wrap with recurrence of symptoms. Rossetti and Hell reported good or excellent results in 87.5% of patients followed up to 20 years.[55] Of patients who develop recurrent reflux symptoms, 63% do so within 3 years of their operation. Another 30% have reappearance of symptoms within 3–10 years of their operation and the remaining 7% of recurrences take place after >10 years.[46] Therefore, a reasonable estimate of the recurrence rate of any operation requires a 10-year follow-up.

Failure of the wrap to control reflux is usually related to one of two mechanisms:

1. Disruption may occur secondary to prolonged retching, but in most cases there is no precipitating event that can be identified. Disruption is best identified by a barium swallow. If there is partial dehiscence of the wrap, its residual ability to prevent reflux may be judged by 24-hour pH studies and endoscopic biopsy. Often these patients can be successfully treated medically.
2. Slippage of the wrap down below the esophagus onto the stomach results in very severe recurrent esophagitis, and reoperation is usually required.

Slippage of the wrap-up into the chest is usually asymptomatic and requires no treatment. However, occasionally these patients develop symptoms related to herniation of increasing amounts of the stomach into the chest, notably bloating and postprandial pain. Reoperation may be required in this situation to avoid the possibility of intrathoracic rupture of the stomach.

Complications of fundoplication: Esophageal injury is the most feared complication. It can best be avoided by careful dissection of the esophagus in the posterior mediastinum. If the perforation is not recognized promptly, the mortality rate is higher. Unexplained fever, tachycardia, or leukocytosis in the postoperative period merits an immediate upper gastrointestinal study with water-soluble contrast to evaluate for perforation. The fundus may also leak secondary to intraoperative injury or fundoplication sutures pulling through the gastric wall. Reoperation has been the standard therapy for leak; however, some authors have reported acceptable results with endoscopic stenting of leaks. Splenic injury occurs in approximately 1% of cases. It can usually be treated with splenic salvage techniques, rarely splenectomy is necessary.

From 12% to 15% of patients have temporary dysphagia. If it is troublesome, simple dilatation with a 50 F Maloney bougie usually solves the problem. Few patients have permanent dysphagia, provided preoperative manometry demonstrates adequate amplitude of peristalsis and the wrap is performed in a "floppy fashion." If the wrap is performed too tightly or peristalsis was poor, the patient may develop severe dysphagia. A barium swallow may reveal an aperistaltic esophagus with a "bird's beak" deformity. Results of manometry in this situation are indistinguishable from those of achalasia; however, the previous history of GER makes the diagnosis clear. Correction of this problem ordinarily requires takedown of the Nissen's fundoplication and performance of a partial fundoplication. Avoiding this serious complication is the most compelling reason for performing preoperative manometry.

Woodward described the postfundoplication or "gas-bloat" syndrome[56] characterized by excessive flatus, early satiety and left subcostal postprandial discomfort. These symptoms have several origins. At least 20–30% of patients are unable to belch effectively following fundoplication. Therefore, all swallowed gas must be passed per rectum. Many of these patients are air swallowers, and this aggravates the problem. Furthermore, the fundus used for the wrap is no longer available to be involved in gastric accommodation of larger volumes of food. These symptoms are helped by administration of metoclopramide, bethanechol chloride, or erythromycin to hasten gastric emptying. They are self-limiting and are seldom a problem beyond 6 months. Most patients consider them a good trade for their previous disabling reflux symptoms.

Approximately, 20% of patients are unable to vomit after fundoplication. If they develop a flu-like syndrome, they will retch (dry heaves), and this can cause disruption of the wrap requiring reoperation. The ability of the fundoplication to function as a competent one-way valve may also create problems if the patient develops a bowel obstruction. A distal obstruction in this situation may cause a closed-loop obstruction with possible rupture of the stomach; this process can be avoided by prompt insertion of a nasogastric tube.

Gastric ulcer is another potential complication after fundoplication, whether or not the wrap has slipped into the chest. In those patients without intrathoracic herniation of the wrap, the ulcer occurs in the usual site for ulceration at the junction of antrum and corpus and should be treated like any other gastric ulcer. H. pylori status should be determined, and the patient should be treated if positive. The patient should also be carefully questioned about ingestion of nonsteroidal anti-inflammatory drugs (NSAIDs). Treatment with proton pump inhibitors is indicated.

Patients in whom the wrap has assumed an intrathoracic position present a slightly different problem. Although *H. pylori* and NSAIDs play a role, the intrathoracic position of the wrap may also add a mechanical component to the picture and these patients may develop ulcers within the intrathoracic wrap. These patients should be treated medically, but rarely they fail to respond or present with severe hemorrhage or perforation that may require a lifesaving operative procedure.

Reoperations for Failure of Fundoplication

Reoperations are more challenging because the previous operation can result in severe adhesions in the left upper quadrant. Laparoscopic redo fundoplication is possible assuming the surgeon has sufficient experience with these difficult operations. Redo procedures are probably best undertaken by surgeons who have extensive experience at carrying out esophageal operations because they are:

- Difficult
- Associated with a higher mortality rate
- Associated with a lower success rate.

Patients with multiple previous procedures may be optionally approached through a transthoracic route that allows the surgeon to avoid the severe adhesions commonly associated with the previous abdominal approaches.

Postoperative care: Postoperative care is similar to that described for the Belsey's Mark IV procedure. Metoclopramide is started along with resumption of oral intake. This drug helps to decrease the incidence of gas-bloat symptoms in the early postoperative period. It is continued for 6 weeks. Patients may be discharged when they are tolerating a regular diet.

Laparoscopic Nissen's Fundoplication

Many surgeons thought that the superior results obtained with proton pump inhibitor therapy of reflux esophagitis would eventually eliminate the need for antireflux operations. However, these agents are expensive and may be required lifelong. Further, many patients develop tolerance to these inhibitors with escalating dose requirements, and symptoms of regurgitation may still be troublesome. In this context, the ability to perform antireflux procedures with laparoscopic techniques makes these procedures much more attractive to patients. Morbidity due to pain and disability are reduced, and most patients can return to work within 1–2 weeks. Laparoscopic fundoplication can be performed using the same techniques that have been developed and refined over the last 30 years.[57-59]

Technique: Pneumoperitoneum is achieved in the usual fashion. Some surgeons find it helpful to insert an endoscope into the stomach to facilitate identification of the esophagus. The esophageal hiatus is usually easily identified in patients who have a hiatal hernia. In patients who do not have a hiatal hernia it is marked by the presence of the esophagogastric fat pad (Belsey's fat pad). Details of this operation are beyond the scope of this text, but as in the open procedure, the esophagus is mobilized and encircled (Figs. 47.16A and B). The crura are cleared of their attachments to the stomach. The esophagus is retracted, and the crura are sutured with interrupted permanent sutures. The crural aperture should not be narrowed too tightly against the esophagus because this may produce dysphagia.

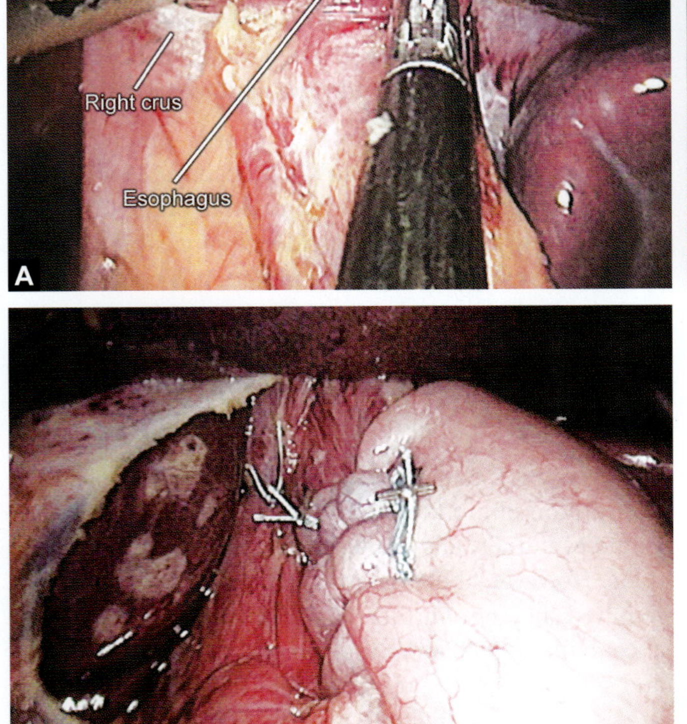

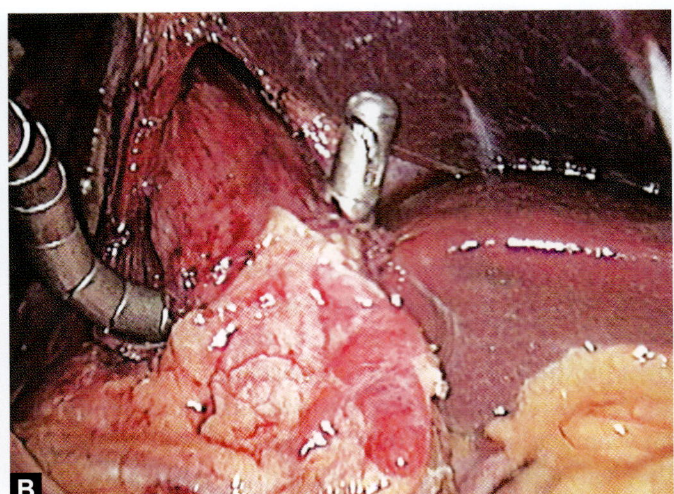

Figs. 47.16A to C: Laparoscopic Nissen's fundoplication. (A) Dissection anterior to the esophagus using two blunt graspers. (B) The esophagus is encircled by a retractor to facilitate dissection of the crura. (C) Completed laparoscopic fundoplication.

The next step is the fundoplication. The debate between the classic Nissen and the Nissen-Rossetti modification was addressed by Watson and colleagues, who performed a prospective double-blind randomized trial of fundoplication with and without division of the short gastric vessels.[60] The perioperative outcome, complications, dysphagia scores, relief of heartburn, and overall satisfaction did not differ between the two groups. Measured physiologic parameters including LES pressure, esophageal acid exposure, and radiologic evaluation were also comparable. The wrap is performed with permanent sutures including bites of anterior fundus, esophagus, and posterior fundus (Fig. 47.16C). Three sutures suffice to construct a 2.0 cm wrap. The bougie is removed. Some surgeons advocate leaving a nasogastric tube overnight to avoid gastric distention and potential retching on the first postoperative night; however, many feel this is unnecessary.

These patients are usually discharged on the first postoperative day. Some surgeons find it helpful to obtain a barium swallow on patients early in the morning after operation to rule out an occult perforation. If the barium swallow is normal, the patient is started on a diet. Metoclopramide is then given orally 10 mg 30 minutes before meals and at bedtime. When the patient is comfortable and tolerating food, he or she may be discharged.

Complications: Complications of laparoscopic fundoplication are similar to those following open fundoplication. However, the usual early discharge from the hospital places more responsibility on patients to let the surgeon know if they have unusual pain or fever, so patients must be advised accordingly.

Complications specific to the pneumoperitoneum include subcutaneous emphysema and pneumothorax. Both of these can usually be treated expectantly because of

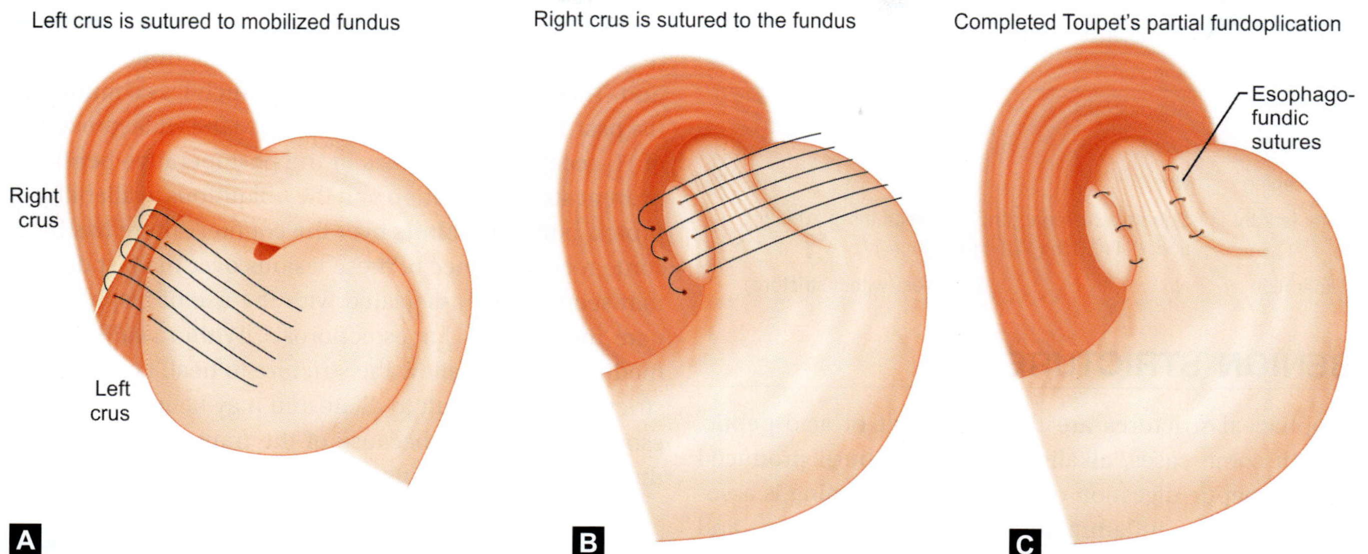

Figs. 47.17A to C: Toupet's partial fundoplication. (A) The left crus is sutured to mobilized fundus with three interrupted nonabsorbable sutures. (B) The right crus is sutured to the fundus in a similar fashion. (C) Completed Toupet demonstrating completed partial wrap.

the high solubility of carbon dioxide. Symptomatic pneumothorax can usually be treated nonoperatively, since CO_2 usually reabsorbs quickly.

Other Antireflux Procedures

Toupet's partial fundoplication: A posterior partial fundoplication was described by Toupet in 1963.[65] It was thought to produce less morbidity than a Nissen's fundoplication because the procedure left patients able to belch, and it was associated with less dysphagia because the wrap was not circumferential. Two randomized trials of this procedure versus open Nissen's fundoplication have suggested that the control of reflux is similar for the two procedures.[66,67] The technique is illustrated in Figures 47.17A to C. McKernan adapted laparoscopic technology to this procedure.[68]

Although the results of open Toupet's procedures seem to be largely comparable with those of an open Nissen's fundoplication, both in terms of control of reflux and durability, there is disagreement about how the results of the laparoscopic adaptation of Toupet's procedure compare with those for laparoscopic Nissen's fundoplication. Hunter and colleagues reported a nonrandomized laparoscopic series of 184 patients comparing the classic Nissen's fundoplication with the Nissen-Rossetti and Toupet's procedure. Dysphagia occurred in 54% of the Nissen-Rossetti patients compared with 17% and 16% of patients undergoing the classic Nissen's and Toupet's procedures, respectively.[69] An increased incidence of dysphagia has been reported in small series that compared the Nissen-Rossetti with the Toupet.[67,70] Conversely Laws and colleagues[70] randomized 40 patients to receive either a laparoscopic classic Nissen (with division of the short gastric vessels) or a laparoscopic Toupet's procedure. There was no difference between the groups postoperatively in terms of Visick score or incidence of dysphagia requiring dilatation. All these studies suffer from lack of objective measurements of efficacy. Jobe and colleagues[71] reported a series of 100 patients undergoing laparoscopic Toupet's fundoplication: 20% (15/74) complained of recurrent heartburn at a mean of 22 months postoperatively. Twenty-four hour pH studies were abnormal in 90% of these patients (9/10). Twenty-four hour pH studies were also performed in 31 asymptomatic patients at follow-up, and 39% of these patients (12/31) had pathologic acid reflux. Jobe therefore suggested that this procedure should not be used in patients who have GER disease and normal esophageal peristalsis. It is probably best reserved for those who have diminished peristalsis (<50 mm Hg), in whom a 360° fundoplication might be associated with a high degree of dysphagia.

Dor's fundoplication: The Dor fundoplication is an anterior partial fundoplication that is roughly equivalent in intent and results to the Toupet. Some surgeons use this procedure to cover the extended cardiomyotomy in achalasia patients.

Table 47.10 Characteristics of esophageal strictures.

Type	*Annular*	*Longitudinal*
Scarring	Submucosal	Transmural
Dilatation	Easy	Difficult
Shortening	No	Yes
Site; length	Squamocolumnar junction; 0.4–0.8 in (1–2 cm)	Distal third; >0.8 in (2 cm)
Ulceration	No	Yes (within stricture)

BENIGN STRICTURE

Esophageal strictures are the end result of acid-peptic, and in some cases, alkaline reflux. The burn produced by acid-peptic digestion of the esophageal lining is associated with an inflammatory infiltrate, ulceration, and submucosal edema. The normal healing process results in accumulation of collagen, which ultimately cross-links and then contracts. The collagen may be laid down primarily in the submucosal layer or, in more severe cases, may be transmural involving the esophageal muscularis and periesophageal tissues. The degree of fibrosis is probably related to the repetitive nature of the injury. Contraction of the collagen, when inflammation is limited to the submucosal layer, produces a stricture that is primarily annular. If the fibrosis is transmural, the contraction takes place in both the circumferential and longitudinal dimensions. It therefore produces a lesion characterized by both cross-sectional narrow of the lumen and some degree of longitudinal esophageal shortening.

These distinctions between fibrosis limited to the submucosa and transmural fibrosis have important implications in judging the response of a stricture to dilatation. Strictures may be conveniently divided into two types: annular and longitudinal (transmural) (Table 47.10).

Annular strictures are 1–2 cm long and nearly always occur at the squamocolumnar junction. Once they start to cause dysphagia, symptoms of heartburn may actually disappear because the stricture tends to reduce reflux and allow the ulcerations to heal. The presence of an esophageal stricture above the anatomic gastroesophageal junction (i.e. in the upper or middle third) should always alert the clinician to the probability that the patient has Barrett's esophagus. These strictures are ordinarily easy to dilate because of their submucosal nature (even if they appear tight).

Longitudinal strictures are longer than 2 cm and typically show severe ulceration within the stricture itself. They are typically seen in patients who have a history of prolonged nasogastric intubation, prolonged vomiting (e.g. hyperemesis gravidarum), or gastric outlet obstruction. These strictures have become much less common in the past 15–20 years, possibly owing to the widespread use of H_2-receptor antagonists in the postoperative period to prevent stress ulceration and the ubiquitous availability of proton pump inhibitors over the counter. There has been some recrudescence of these lesions over the last decade that seems to be associated with the use of bisphosphonate medications for osteoporosis. Withdrawal of these medications may allow the stricture to heal. Longitudinal strictures are difficult to dilate and may be more prone to esophageal rupture because of the transmural nature of the scarring. They are also prone to recurrence.

Dysphagia should never be treated as a trivial symptom. All cases of dysphagia should be investigated with endoscopy and in most cases barium swallow, which helps to identify longitudinal strictures. All strictures require both endoscopic brushings for cytology and endoscopic biopsy to rule out dysplasia or cancer. The addition of brushings to biopsy increases the diagnostic accuracy in patients with cancer from about 60% to over 90%. Even longstanding strictures should be investigated because they have a well-known propensity to harbor an occult carcinoma.

Strictures that appear to be annular may be dilated at the time of the original endoscopy. Dilatation is most easily performed using either Savary dilators inserted over a guidewire or a "through the scope" balloon dilator. The Savary system is preferred by the senior author because it gives the endoscopist tactile feedback about the severity of the stricture and the ease of dilatation. If the stricture dilates easily, it may be safely dilated to the 45–50 F range at the first session. If the stricture is tight and dilates with difficulty, it may be safer to limit the dilatation to two or three consecutively sized dilators at a single session. Dilatation may then be repeated at 1- to 2-week intervals until a final size of 45–50 F is reached. Once the stricture has been satisfactorily dilated, a decision should be made about whether medical or surgical therapy should be pursued. In the interim, aggressive therapy with proton pump inhibitors should be instituted to aid in preventing recurrent ulceration and stenosis. Esophageal stents may be very helpful in malignant strictures but should be avoided in peptic strictures since they promote reflux.

Medical Management

As an esophageal stricture represents the end stage of severe esophagitis, it is tempting to conclude that all patients who have an esophageal stricture merit surgical therapy. Nevertheless, as noted above, the degree of esophagitis correlates poorly with symptoms. Many of these patients have been virtually asymptomatic until they develop dysphagia.

Endoscopic Dilatation

If the stricture can be dilated, these patients are usually quite willing to undergo dilatation once or twice a year if an operation can be avoided. Treatment of annular strictures with dilatation plus H_2-receptor antagonists or proton pump inhibitors gives satisfactory results in 75% or more of patients treated,[72] although the definition of success is loose in most medical series. The choice between decision for medical and surgical therapy should be based on:

- The patient's general condition
- The response to dilatation
- Whether dilatation results in severe recurrent reflux symptoms
- Whether there is ulceration within the stricture itself, which indicates the possibility of a transmural stricture.

The traditional method of dilatation employs Jackson dilators through a rigid esophagoscope. It requires a general anesthetic and the considerable skills associated with rigid esophagoscopy. Following the initial dilatation with the rigid scope, the stricture is dilated on a chronic basis using graduated Maloney dilators passed blindly under topical anesthetic. This venerable technique has now been largely supplanted by flexible endoscopy with the use of the Savary wire-guided dilators.

Technique using Savary dilators: Use of Savary dilators requires preliminary endoscopy. If the flexible endoscope, which is usually sized at 29–32 F, is able to pass the stenosis, it is passed into the stomach. The Savary wire with its spring-tip is then passed into the stomach. An assistant should be assigned to control the end of the wire outside the patient because this may injure the endoscopist, the assistant or the patient. The patient's eyes should be covered with a towel. If the stricture cannot be passed with the endoscope, the wire should be passed through the stricture under direct vision until resistance is met. Following passage of the wire, the endoscope should be withdrawn over the wire without moving the wire. The caliber of the stricture should also be estimated from its appearance at endoscopy. A dilator of the corresponding diameter should then be chosen. The wire is passed through the channel of the dilator until it emerges from the blunt end of the dilator. The dilator is advanced over the wire without allowing the wire to move. The next larger size is then chosen and the procedure is repeated until the stricture is either completely dilated (at least 45 F) or undue resistance to passage of the dilator is encountered. The endoscope should now be passed again to examine the result. If the stricture has been completely dilated, the lumen may be maintained with periodic dilatation. If the stricture cannot be satisfactorily dilated at one sitting, the procedure should be repeated at weekly intervals until satisfactory swallowing is restored. The patient should then be counseled to return at yearly intervals or sooner if dysphagia begins to recur.

Complications: The main complication of esophageal dilatation is esophageal perforation. Early detection of this complication requires a low threshold of suspicion on the part of the endoscopist to obtain a water-soluble contrast swallow for any patient experiencing pain or fever following dilatation. The possibility of perforation is not remote. Skinner and Belsey noted a mortality rate of 22% for patients treated with dilatation and medical therapy, but their report predated H_2-receptor antagonists, proton pump inhibitors and the Savary wire-guided dilator system.[43]

Operative Management

Dilatation and Antireflux Procedure

Annular strictures can be treated quite satisfactorily by dilatation combined with an antireflux procedure. In this situation, the fibrosis is limited to the submucosa. If the stricture is dilated and reflux is prevented, there is a high likelihood of a good result. Some authors have reported satisfactory results with dilatation and Hill's gastropexy in 85% of patients with a stricture,[64] whereas Bushkin described satisfactory results in 100% of patients who had a Nissen's fundoplication.[56,61-63] Both Hill and Payne have reported that dilatation combined with either a Hill's or Nissen's fundoplication produces satisfactory results in 90% of cases.[73,74]

Longitudinal strictures are more difficult to dilate. In such strictures, dilatation results in hemorrhage, formation of granulation tissue, fibroblast proliferation, deposition of collagen, and finally cross-linking and contraction of collagen in all three dimensions. Contraction in the circumferential dimension produces recurrent stenosis, whereas contraction in the longitudinal direction produces esophageal shortening. These are biologic realities that cannot be altered by either medical therapy or an

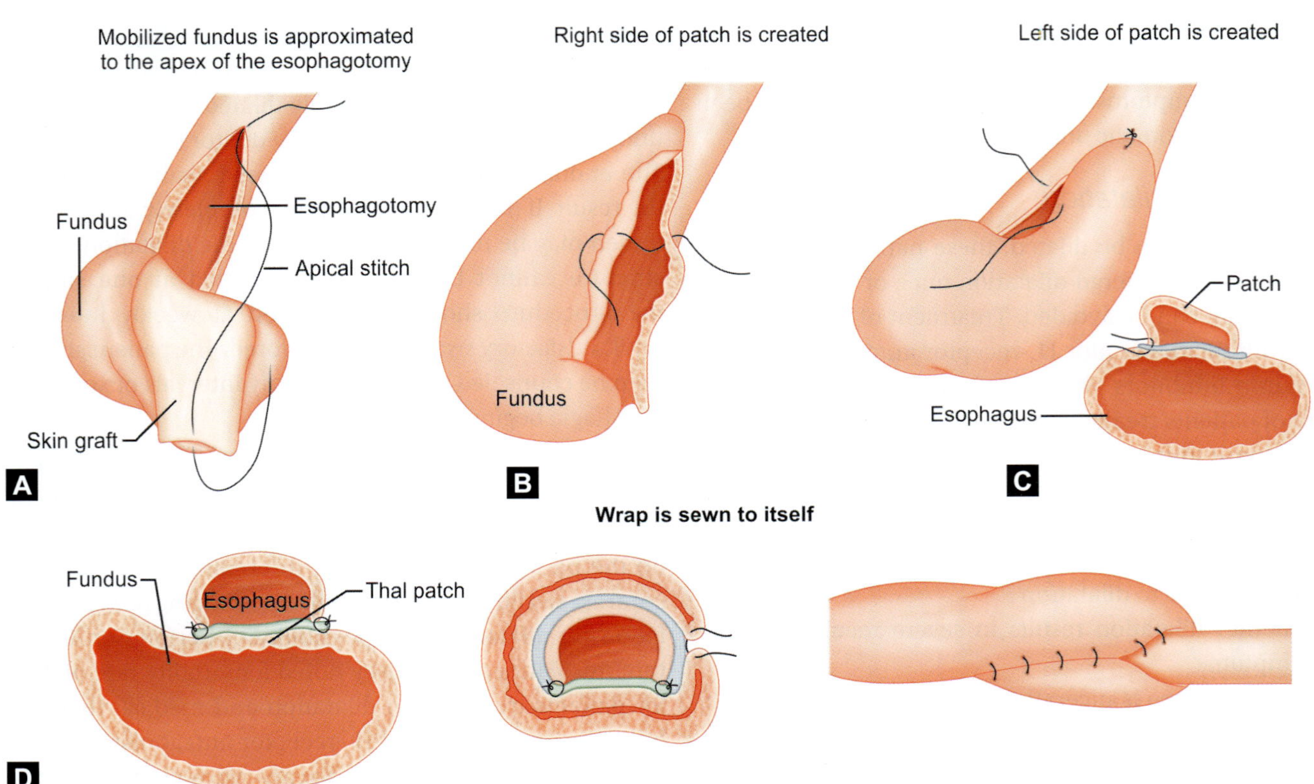

Figs. 47.18A to D: Combined Thal fundic patch–Nissen fundoplication. (A) The mobilized fundus and skin graft is approximated to the apex of the esophagotomy with a single stitch. (B) The right side of the patch is created with interrupted nonabsorbable sutures. (C) The left border of the patch is created in a similar fashion. (D) The wrap is then brought circumferentially around the esophagus and sewn to itself.

antireflux procedure. Orringer[75] has advocated intraoperative dilatation combined with a Collis gastroplasty and Nissen's fundoplication, but the need for long-term intermittent dilatation was seen in nearly 20% of these patients. The surgeon has only two choices for the patient with a transmural longitudinal stricture:

1. A Thal fundic patch combined with Nissen's fundoplication
2. Esophageal resection with jejunal or colonic interposition.

Combined Thal Fundic Patch–Nissen Fundoplication

The Thal fundic patch was originally used alone in patients who had acid-peptic esophageal strictures.[76] It soon became apparent that although this procedure was quite effective in opening the stricture, there was inevitable production of severe reflux esophagitis since reflux was not being prevented. Woodward added fundoplication to the Thal patch and demonstrated its effectiveness. Hollenbeck and Woodward reported that the Thal-Nissen procedure produced satisfactory results for transmural strictures in 87% of 45 patients and no deaths.[77]

Technique: The Thal fundic patch uses well-established plastic surgical principles to replace part of the strictured esophageal wall with the pliable fundus lined by a skin graft. The skin graft prevents resurfacing of the fundic wall by granulation tissue, which heals by contraction. The skin graft therefore minimizes contraction of the fundic patch.

The esophagus is encircled through a left thoracotomy with a Penrose drain. The hiatus is opened radially, and the fundus is mobilized. A large dilator is then advanced per os to the upper border of the stricture. The esophagus is opened longitudinally over the tip of the dilator, and the esophagotomy is extended distally from the upper border of the stricture to the esophagogastric junction (Figs. 47.18A to D). The Thal fundic patch is fashioned and sewn to the margins of the esophagotomy (Figs. 47.18A to D). The fundus is wrapped around the esophagus and sutured to itself to create a 360° fundoplication. The wrap is then sutured to the diaphragm circumferentially to prevent herniation of the stomach into the chest after reducing as much fundus below the diaphragm as possible.

A nasogastric tube is inserted before completion of the procedure. The patient is not fed orally for 10 days. On the

10th day, a water-soluble contrast radiographic examination of the esophagus is performed. If there is no leak the nasogastric tube is discontinued and the patient is started on a diet. The chest tube draining the patch is not removed until the patient is tolerating a diet.

Complications: The key factor in the postoperative care of patients following a Thal–Nissen procedure is the early recognition of an esophageal leak. Fever or tachycardia necessitates immediate radiographic examination with water-soluble contrast to exclude the possibility of a leak. If the X-ray is negative, greater accuracy can be achieved by repeating the examination with thin barium. The chest tube output should be watched daily, and if there is any question of leakage the drained fluid should be sent for amylase determination. Elevated amylase levels indicate the presence of an esophagocutaneous fistula. If a fistula is present and is well drained by the chest tube, the patient should be started on broad-spectrum antibiotics and maintained on parenteral nutrition. If the fistula is poorly drained, the patient will remain toxic with fever and tachycardia. A CT scan of the chest and upper abdomen will show any undrained fluid collections. These may be drained percutaneously or with surgical resection of a rib over the underlying empyema cavity. It is counterproductive to try closing the fistula because the sutures will simply pull through the edematous, infected tissue. If the fistula is well drained, the patient will survive and the fistula will heal. The need for this operation is rare since longitudinal strictures have become rare, but when other treatments fail to resolve a longitudinal stricture it is quite valuable. The Collis–Nissen, popularized by Orringer, is not useful with a longitudinal stricture since the stricture cannot be successfully dilated.

Resection and Visceral Interposition

The only real alternative to the Thal–Nissen procedure for patients who have a transmural stricture is resection. Reconstruction is accomplished with:

- Esophagogastrostomy[78]
- Colonic interposition[79]
- Jejunal interposition.[80]

Esophagogastrostomy, even using an antireflux technique, is a poor choice for the patient who has a benign stricture because resection of the LES produces recurrent reflux even when combined with an antireflux procedure. Long-term follow-up of such patients in one series with esophagogastrostomy revealed recurrence of stricture in 25% and recurrent esophagitis in 87%.[78] It has been reported that transhiatal esophagectomy with cervical esophagogastrostomy results in nocturnal regurgitation in only approximately 10% of patients.[81] These results have undoubtedly been helped by the availability of proton pump inhibitors.

Belsey[80] reported good results in patients with transmural strictures treated by colonic interposition. The mortality rate was 5%, and there were no late strictures or esophagitis. Other investigators have reported mortality rates ranging from 7% to 20%, with recurrent stricture occurring in up to 27% of cases.[82,83] Merendino[81] had satisfactory results with jejunal interposition in a small group of patients with an 8% mortality rate, but Ferrer and Bruck reported a 15% mortality rate and 15% of the jejunal loops had to be discarded because of an inadequate blood supply. Polk[85] more recently has reported excellent results with jejunal interposition, with a 3% mortality rate and a need for reoperation in approximately 9%. The author uses visceral interposition only in:

- Patients who have transmural strictures in whom there is insufficient stomach for a Thal–Nissen procedure because of a previous gastric operation
- Patients who have caustic strictures

These patients are becoming rare.

Technique: The appropriate jejunal segment is isolated through a midline laparotomy or by laparoscopy, while the esophageal resection and actual interposition of jejunum between esophageal stump and gastric fundus can generally be carried out through a left thoracotomy.

Colonic interposition is performed in a similar fashion to jejunal interposition. Some authors advocate reconstruction with left colon, although many prefer the right colon because the distal ileum provides a better fit through the thoracic outlet.

Complications: Early complications and care of patients with jejunal or colonic interpositions is identical to that of patients receiving the Thal–Nissen procedure. However, there are two extra anastomoses with these operations, and each has the additional disadvantage of possible vascular compromise of the interposed visceral segment.

Ischemia may be quite subtle and indolent, and diagnosis may require early diagnostic endoscopy. Arterial insufficiency is usually evident at the time of operation, but venous infarction is insidious and may take days to become clinically evident. This is an especially important consideration with the colon. Ischemia is the real disadvantage of resection of the stricture and colonic or jejunal interposition. There is no ready fallback position; a bridge has been burned. If the interposed segment dies, the patient is left with the possibility of a permanent esophageal fistula. A patient's own esophagus, no matter how diseased, is almost always a better means to transport food from the mouth to the stomach than anything the surgeon can construct.

CAUSTIC STRICTURE

Caustic burns of the gastrointestinal tract are most commonly seen in children, in whom the ingestion is accidental, or in adults trying to commit suicide. The most severe injuries are caused by ingestion of lye-containing drain cleaners, which produces liquefactive necrosis. Acid ingestion produces coagulative necrosis, which commonly involves the gastric antrum. Other less common fluids that may injure the gastrointestinal tract include bleach and ammonia solutions. The early stages of the injury include acute necrosis and inflammation, but if the esophageal muscularis is involved, scarring and contraction may eventually produce strictures that are both transmural and extensive. Occasionally, the burn may penetrate the full thickness of the esophageal or stomach wall producing mediastinitis or peritonitis.

Initial Treatment

Initial therapy requires a precise determination of what was swallowed, how much, when the injury occurred and whether the ingestion was intentional or accidental. Immediate flexible endoscopy is indicated to determine the extent and grade of the injury. The grade of the injury is depicted in Table 47.11.

Patients with necrosis should be fed parenterally initially, whereas those with lesser degrees of injury may be fed orally. Grades 0–2 usually heal without sequelae. Third-degree injuries heal within about 3 months, and no definitive therapy should be undertaken before that period unless there is evidence of acute perforation.

Pain is not generally helpful in judging the need for operation because the nerve endings are destroyed. Extensive grade 3 injuries of the stomach and esophagus or bloody emesis are strong evidence of full-thickness injury. Other findings may include leukocytosis, progressive acidosis, and disseminated intravascular coagulation. If there is extensive gastric necrosis at an emergency operation, the patient should undergo a total gastrectomy and/or transhiatal esophagectomy with cervical esophagostomy and feeding jejunostomy. If the injury is less severe and resection seems to be unnecessary, the patient may be treated with a feeding jejunostomy. If resection is undertaken, re-establishment of intestinal continuity may be performed later using the techniques described previously for esophageal resection.

Table 47.11 Caustic injuries.

Grade of injury	*Description*
0	Normal
1	Edema
2	Mucosal erosion
3	Mucosal necrosis

Later Management

Strictures develop in approximately 50% of patients with grade 3 injuries. They may be treated by dilatation in less severe cases, but it must be remembered that these are transmural strictures and dilatation is therefore going to be less successful. Furthermore, patients who have lye strictures have an increased incidence of developing esophageal cancer. If dilatation is unsuccessful, the patient may require visceral interposition. Bypass of the strictured lesion is an option because evidence suggests that cancer usually occurs only in a functioning esophagus, but many surgeons prefer resection to eliminate the possibility of cancer in the bypassed segment. Continuity should be re-established using colonic or jejunal interposition. The author prefers not to use the stomach in this situation because of the possibility of injury to the intragastric collateral blood supply from the caustic ingestion.

Long-Term Management

Patients treated without resection or bypass should have periodic endoscopy to rule out cancer in the esophagus or antrum. Suicidal patients need expert long-term psychiatric care of the precipitating condition.

BARRETT'S ESOPHAGUS

In 1950, Norman Barrett described a columnar epithelium lining of the lower esophagus as a distinct condition[86] that differed from the usual patient with a short esophagus in whom an attenuated segment of stomach is drawn into the chest. In the condition described by Barrett, there was oral displacement of the squamocolumnar junction into the esophagus above the junction of the tubular esophagus and the stomach. It was not until manometry became available that it was possible to confirm that this was

Table 47.12 Types of mucosa in Barrett's esophagus.

Type	*Characteristics*
Fundic and body	Clusters of glands containing parietal cells and chief cells identical to gastric body; least common variety
Junctional	Gastric cardiac mucosa with deep clusters of mucous glands; identical to gastric cardiac mucosa
Specialized or intestinal	Villous surface; intestinal goblet cells; most commonly is in apposition to squamous mucosa. Associated with adenocarcinoma

indeed esophagus lined by columnar epithelium. It exhibited both characteristic esophageal peristalsis and a lower esophageal high-pressure zone.

It was initially thought that the condition was congenital, but it is now generally accepted that it is related to loss of the squamous lining secondary to reflux with replacement by columnar mucosa. This process has been documented both by the development of Barrett's lining in patients with reflux who did not originally have this condition and by the development of Barrett' mucosa in experimental animals in which reflux has been produced and the distal esophageal mucosa excised.[87] Presumably loss of the squamous lining leads to replacement from the gastric cardia mucosa, which regenerates approximately five times faster than esophageal squamous mucosa. As the reflux progresses, more and more of the esophagus becomes lined by the columnar lining. Patients also develop strictures at the squamocolumnar junction and punched-out ulcers within the columnar epithelium. As noted earlier, the presence of a punched-out ulcer within the esophagus or a stricture above the esophagogastric junction is considered to be synonymous with Barrett's esophagus. Some patients have small patches of ectopic mucosa, usually within the cervical esophagus, which are of congenital origin and are not related to reflux.

Three varieties of metaplastic mucosa are seen in patients who have Barrett's esophagus (Table 47.12).

Endoscopic Appearance

The endoscopic appearance of Barrett's esophagus is quite characteristic. The junction of the squamous and columnar mucosa is shown in Figure 47.19. A firm diagnosis of Barrett's esophagus requires an endoscopic biopsy. This biopsy must be taken from the tubular esophagus, and the lining must extend >2 cm into the tubular esophagus. Often, this is an area of some diagnostic ambiguity, especially if fundic or junctional-type epithelium is present. Most experts require intestinal-type metaplasia to make the diagnosis, although others feel there is some risk of malignancy in the other variations. The diagnosis is also made easier if esophageal-type submucosal glands are seen or there is penetration of the columnar epithelium by submucosal gland ducts, but the tiny biopsy specimens typical of the usual endoscopic biopsy are seldom deep enough to include these features.

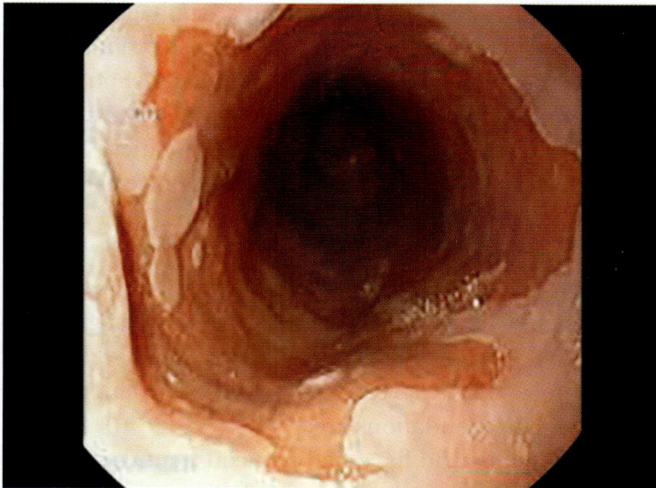

Fig. 47.19: Endoscopic appearance of Barrett's mucosa. Note the salmon colored tongues of mucosa extending cephalad.

Barrett's mucosa is clearly associated with the development of adenocarcinoma of the esophagus, but the magnitude of this predisposition is not clear. Cameron reported an incidence of approximately 376/100,000.[88] The prevalence of cancer in patients diagnosed with Barrett's esophagus is close to 10%, but this figure is misleading because many patients who have Barrett's esophagus are relatively asymptomatic and so remain undiagnosed. Among patients who have Barrett's esophagus and who do not have esophageal adenocarcinoma at the time of diagnosis, the incidence of development of cancer varies between 1/81 and 1/441 cases/person years.[89-91] Despite these relatively reassuring figures, the incidence of adenocarcinoma of the esophagus has shown a marked increase in both the United States and Europe, and the reason for this increase is not known.

Management

The treatment of Barrett's esophagus is controversial. Many surgeons have advocated that all patients who have Barrett's esophagus, regardless of their symptomatic status, should undergo an antireflux operation in the belief that preventing further reflux damage prevents the development of cancer in these patients. Some have suggested that prevention of reflux causes regression of Barrett's esophagus. There is no good evidence to support either of these premises.

Patients who have Barrett's esophagus should have an antireflux operation to provide symptomatic relief if they do not receive adequate relief with medical therapy. Patients who have strictures may likewise be treated with either:

- Dilatation and medical therapy
- Dilatation with an antireflux procedure

Presently, patients who have Barrett's esophagus need periodic endoscopic surveillance to detect severe dysplasia, which precedes the development of adenocarcinoma. The current recommendations are:

- For patients who have had two consecutive endoscopies that show no dysplasia, surveillance endoscopy is recommended at an interval of every 3 years.
- If dysplasia is noted, another endoscopy should be performed with extensive biopsy sampling (especially from areas with mucosal irregularity) to look for invasive cancer, and the histology slides should be interpreted by an expert pathologist.
- For patients with verified low-grade dysplasia after extensive biopsy sampling, yearly surveillance endoscopy is recommended.
- For patients with verified high-grade dysplasia, treatment should be individualized. If there is accompanying mucosal irregularity, the area should be evaluated by endoscopic mucosal resection, primarily to determine if there is submucosal invasion.

The formerly accepted standard of care for patients who developed severe dysplasia was esophagectomy since 43% of patients who had severe dysplasia were found to have an invasive cancer in the resected specimen.[92] However, new techniques such as the HALO360 system (BÂRRX Medical, Sunnyvale, CA, USA), which uses a balloon-based array of closely spaced electrodes to deliver radiofrequency energy to ablate the esophageal mucosa, inflict a uniform, circumferential thermal injury whose depth is controlled to vary the power, density, and duration of the energy applied. Reports utilizing this technique demonstrates the feasibility of eradicating dysplastic Barrett's epithelium with endoscopic ablation, but has not established the long-term benefit of the techniques for cancer prevention. Further, the procedures often leave behind residual foci of metaplastic epithelium, and partially ablated Barrett's epithelium can heal with an overlying layer of squamous epithelium that "buries" metaplastic tissue (with its neoplastic potential) and hides it from the endoscopist.

Endoscopic mucosal resection commonly is performed using a "suck and cut" technique. The endoscopist elevates the dysplastic area by injecting fluid into the submucosa, the elevated mucosa is suctioned into a cap and a polypectomy snare is then deployed around the suctioned mucosa to remove it. A similar variation utilizes elastic bands around the suctioned mucosal segment without the submucosal fluid injection. The banded segment is removed with a polypectomy snare. Early reports comparing this therapy with esophagectomy suggest that survival is similar, although metachronous cancers occur in 5–21%.

The question is whether this sort of treatment prevents the development of cancer.[95] Current studies involve a few highly specialized centers. Proof would require large-scale cooperative studies with suitable controls and extended follow-up over many years.

PARAESOPHAGEAL HERNIA

Presentation

Paraesophageal hernia (type 2) occurs when there is herniation of the gastric body into the chest, while the gastroesophageal junction remains anchored below the diaphragm. Patients are classified as having a type 3 hernia if they have components of both the paraesophageal and sliding hernia. As the hernia enlarges, increasing amounts of the mobile greater curvature of the stomach herniate into the chest anterior to the gastroesophageal junction until the entire stomach is upside down within the chest with the pylorus being located at the diaphragm. This configuration is referred to as a gastric volvulus or "upside-down stomach." These hernias account for <5% of hiatal hernias, the rest being type 1 or "sliding." Many physicians are not familiar with this type of hernia because it is less common. They associate hiatal hernias with symptoms of reflux and, if these symptoms are absent, ignore the condition.

Paraesophageal hernias symptoms are nonspecific and may include:

- Postprandial breathlessness (due to lung compression)
- Early satiety
- Dysphagia.

A careful history may reveal a previous history of reflux that has gradually disappeared over time. These hernias may first present acutely with respiratory distress, bleeding from a gastric ulcer or gastritis, incarceration, rupture, or gangrene of the intrathoracic stomach.

Skinner and Belsey[44] described a group of 21 asymptomatic patients managed with medical therapy. There was a 30% incidence of life-threatening complications within 3 years of diagnosis that included perforation, bleeding, and infarction.

Diagnosis is usually apparent from a simple lateral chest radiograph, which demonstrates an air-fluid level in the posterior mediastinum. A barium swallow will confirm the diagnosis. Endoscopy should be performed to rule out esophagitis.

Controversy exists as to whether these hernias should be managed by simple reduction of the hernia, excision of the sac and narrowing of the hiatus, or whether all patients should have an antireflux procedure in addition. Advocates of the antireflux procedure point out that many of these patients have reflux documented by either biopsy proven esophagitis or an abnormal 24-hour pH study. Furthermore, some patients who do not have documented reflux preoperatively demonstrate symptomatic reflux postoperatively that requires therapy. Reflux is less of a problem than it was in the past now that effective medical therapy is available. Many prefer to add an antireflux procedure at the time of repair for the reasons cited above, but this is not mandatory if the patient does not have reflux. All symptomatic paraesophageal hiatal hernias should be repaired, particularly those with acute obstructive symptoms or those that have undergone gastric volvulus.

Operative Management

Most paraesophageal hernia repairs are undertaken laparoscopically via a transabdominal approach. The stomach is manually reduced into the abdomen, and the esophagus is encircled as for any other esophageal procedure. The sac should be completely excised to reduce the possibility of hernia recurrence, using either electrosurgery or harmonic shears. These patients seem to have excess fat in the posterior mediastinum, which makes the laparoscopic excision of the sac much more tedious. Once the sac has been excised, the esophagus can be mobilized longitudinally and the hiatus should be narrowed with permanent synthetic sutures.

If an antireflux procedure is to be performed, it is then carried out. In patients who have documented reflux, a Nissen's fundoplication is preferred for its greater efficacy in eliminating reflux. Many surgeons also add an anterior gastropexy with or without gastrostomy to fix the greater curvature to the anterior abdominal wall, so minimizing its mobility if the closure of the muscular crura fails. Some may regard this as a redundant approach to the problem, but it may reduce the risk of recurrence. Successful results are obtained in over 90% of patients.

For a number of years there was a great deal of sentiment supporting placement of mesh to reinforce the hiatus at the time of paraesophageal hernia repair. Initially, synthetic mesh was used but was abandoned when it became apparent that it was prone to erosion into the stomach or esophagus. This often necessitated esophageal resection to salvage the situation. This was supplanted by biologic mesh which does appear to be better tolerated but, in randomized trials, does not reduce the recurrence rate.[93]

Patients who have evidence of strangulation of the intrathoracic stomach may be approached from above the diaphragm through the chest. This route allows a more complete assessment of the problem with the possibility of a proximal gastrectomy and esophagogastrostomy if appropriate.

MOTOR DISORDERS AND DIVERTICULA

Successful completion of a swallow requires an enormously complex series of events that must be perfectly timed. The oropharyngeal aspects of the swallow must be integrated seamlessly with normal esophageal function. Sphincters must relax and then contract in the appropriate sequence, and there must be a normal peristaltic contraction in the body of the esophagus. When there is an abnormality in the above process, the most common symptom is dysphagia. However, dysphagia is not usually very helpful in defining the site of the dysfunction. Likewise, cough may signal aspiration, but is not helpful in determining whether this is caused by oropharyngeal dysfunction or reflux. Chest pain may also result from esophageal causes or from reflux.

The capabilities and limitations of manometry and fluoroscopy in the evaluation of oropharyngeal causes of dysphagia have been described earlier in this chapter. The neurologic and muscular diseases that produce dysphagia are described in Figure 47.7. An operation is not indicated in these patients and may make the dysphagia worse. However, these patients can be helped by careful fluoroscopic evaluation of swallowing of foods with different consistencies to determine which causes the fewest problems. This study allows modification of the diet.

The upper esophageal sphincter is difficult to evaluate because of its short length and movement with swallowing. Certain findings in symptomatic individuals occasionally warrant surgical therapy.

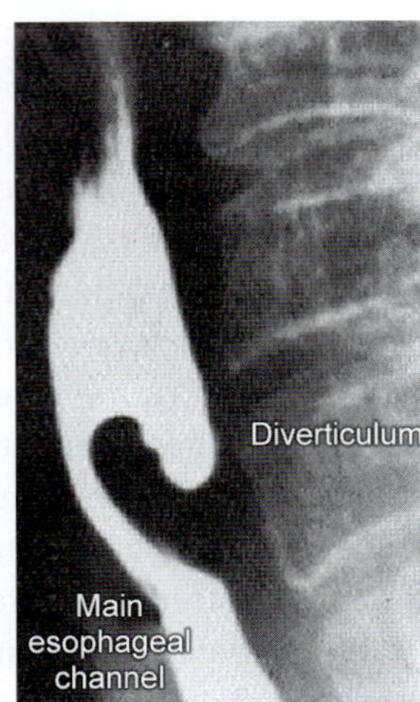

Fig. 47.20: Zenker's diverticulum.

A cricopharyngeal bar may be seen on fluoroscopy in some patients with dysphagia. Most individuals with this finding are asymptomatic. These patients should be carefully evaluated to exclude neurologic or muscular causes. Selective use of cricopharyngeal myotomy may improve swallowing and carries minimal risk.[95]

ZENKER'S DIVERTICULUM (PHARYNGEAL POUCH)

Zenker's diverticulum is a false diverticulum (containing only mucosa and submucosa) characterized by outpouching of the mucosa and submucosa in the posterior midline of the esophagus between the cricopharyngeus muscle and the inferior constrictor muscle. Its radiologic appearance is seen in Figure 47.20. Typically patients have dysphagia localized to the cervical esophagus and may, especially in advanced cases, suffer from aspiration of the contents of the diverticulum or bad breath caused by fermentation within a large diverticular sac.

Pathophysiology

The cause of Zenker's diverticulum can be demonstrated manometrically in approximately 50% of patients. These patients commonly have discoordination of the relaxation–contraction response of the upper esophageal sphincter, which relaxes and contracts prematurely. The sphincter is therefore contracting at the precise time that the pharyngeal contraction reaches the area, thereby producing a high pressure at the weak area between the inferior constrictor and the cricopharyngeus (Killian's dehiscence), which results in the diverticulum. Once this process begins, it tends to increase in an inexorable fashion.

Medical Management

There is no effective medical therapy for this disease.

Operative Management

Cricopharyngeal Myotomy with or without Excision or Diverticulopexy

The operation is performed through an incision that parallels the sternocleidomastoid and is deepened medial to the carotid sheath (*see* Fig. 47.21). Once the diverticulum is exposed, its neck is dissected down to its exit site from the cricopharyngeal-inferior constrictor intersection. The cricopharyngeus muscle is then elevated over a right-angle clamp and is divided using electrosurgery. Smaller diverticula essentially disappear once the myotomy is finished, and no further treatment is necessary. Larger diverticula may be excised with a stapler or treated by diverticulopexy, tacking the diverticulum in a position where it will not be dependent. Most surgeons drain the neck if the diverticulum has been excised.

Complications include leakage from the esophagus, which can usually be managed by simple drainage, and is relatively rare, especially if the sac is not excised. Other complications include temporary recurrent laryngeal nerve injury, wound infection, and incomplete relief of dysphagia. Postoperative stricture formation may occur if the suture line encroaches on the lumen. This can easily be treated with dilatation. The incidence of all these complications is approximately 1%. Approximately 90% of patients become completely asymptomatic.[96]

Dohlman's Endoscopic Technique

Dohlman[97] has described an endoscopic technique that divides the wall between the esophagus and diverticulum. This procedure is performed under a general anesthetic and uses a special endoscope, which has a split that forms anterior and posterior lips. The posterior lip is inserted into the diverticulum while the anterior intubates the esophageal lumen. The wall between the esophagus and diverticulum appears as a horizontal ridge. An operating microscope facilitates division of this wall with electrocautery or a carbon dioxide laser. Recurrence rates have averaged 7%, as has the incidence of mediastinitis. This procedure lacks any advantage except the absence of a visible scar. Many have now substituted a GIA type stapler advanced through the laryngoscope to divide the cricopharyngeus (Fig. 47.22).

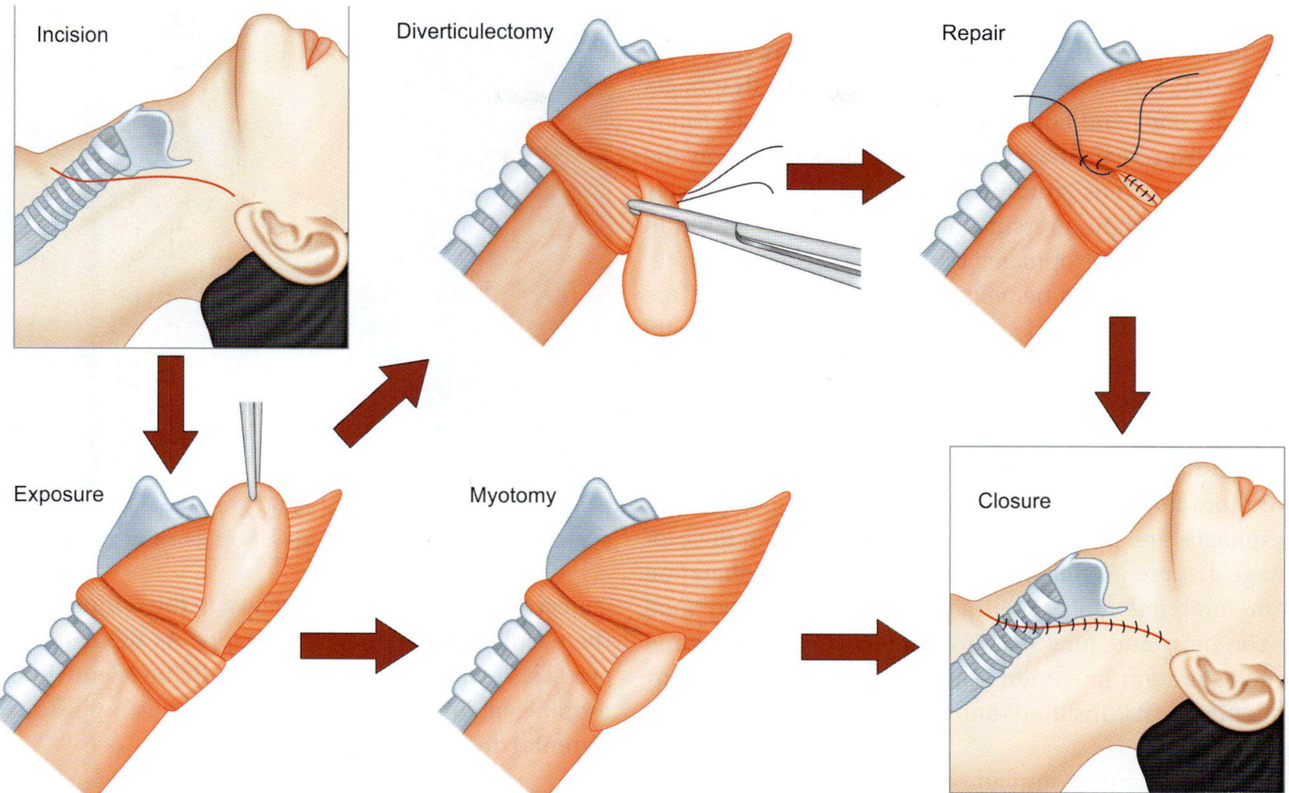

Fig. 47.21: Repair of Zenker's diverticulum. Technique of repair demonstrating both cricopharyngeal myotomy and diverticulectomy. The myotomy is represented by a diamond-shaped incision towards the back of the cricopharyngeus.

ACHALASIA

Pathophysiology

The term achalasia is of Greek origin and translates as "failure to relax." The allusion refers to the LES, which exhibits a lack of receptive relaxation in achalasia. This term ignores the fact that there is also a generalized failure of peristaltic function in the esophagus. There are therefore two components of achalasia:

1. A hypertensive, nonrelaxing LES
2. An aperistaltic esophagus.

Examination of the dorsal motor nucleus and the vagus nerve may reveal mild degenerative changes, and many studies have shown reduced numbers of ganglion cells in the myenteric plexus. Nevertheless, the etiology of this disease is not clear.

Achalasia gives a picture similar to that of Chagas' disease, which shows a loss of ganglion cells within the myenteric plexus secondary to infestation with the protozoan *Trypanosoma cruzi:* Affected patients have cardiomegaly, megaesophagus, and megacolon. There is no satisfactory experimental model for achalasia, although a bilateral high cervical vagotomy will produce an achalasia-like picture in dogs.

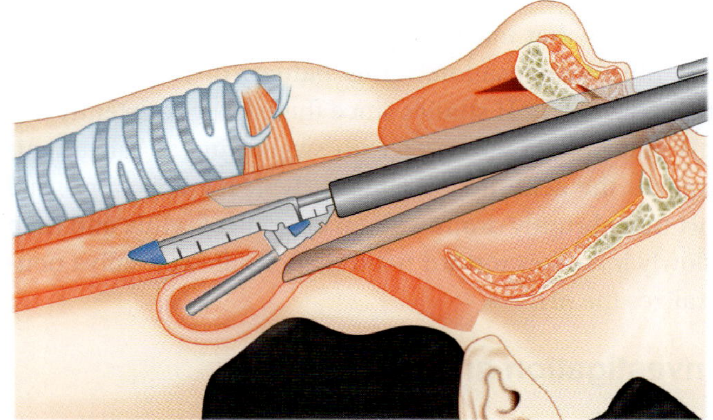

Fig. 47.22: Modified Dohlman division of septum of diverticulum with Endo-GIA stapler.

Clinical Features

Achalasia has no predilection for gender and may occur at any time in life. The onset of dysphagia may be subtle, and patients commonly have symptoms for years before seeking medical care. The degree of dysphagia may vary from day to day, but these patients frequently have dysphagia for both solids and liquids from a very early stage. Many patients learn maneuvers that can help them to empty the esophagus such as grunting or straining. They rely solely on the hydrostatic pressure of the column of food and liquid within the esophagus to aid in esophageal emptying. This process can be helped by the contraction of the striated muscular portion of the esophagus, which still functions. Increasing intrathoracic pressure with the Valsalva maneuver may also aid in achieving emptying of the esophagus.

Chest pain due to esophageal spasm is a frequent symptom and may actually precede the development of dysphagia. The increased hydrostatic pressure in the esophageal lumen leads to gradual esophageal dilatation with food retention. Regurgitation of undigested food is common and may lead to nocturnal aspiration and even aspiration pneumonia. Weight loss occurs in many patients, but it is insidious and must be carefully sought or it will be missed.

Some patients complain of burning epigastric pain that may be mistaken for heartburn. This fact is paradoxical because these patients have a high-pressure sphincter that does not relax. Recent studies have shown that there may be fermentation of rotting food within the esophagus that may produce an acid pH and the resultant burning sensation.[98] This pattern of reflux is easily recognized on pH studies since there is a consistently low pH that rapidly increases with swallowing as saliva neutralizes the acid. Reflux patients typically have a normal pH that abruptly drops with an episode of reflux and then slowly increases toward neutral, as swallowed saliva neutralizes the pH.

Investigation and Diagnosis

Physical examination is unhelpful. Diagnosis relies on manometric and radiographic criteria.

Radiology

Barium swallow can be quite helpful in achalasia. It should be carried out in the supine position so that the esophagus does not empty by gravity. The esophagus typically shows varying degrees of dilatation, although this sign may be absent early in the disease. The typical finding is a smooth symmetrical "bird's beak" distally (Fig. 47.23) in contrast to the "apple core"-type of narrowing seen in esophageal cancer. When the patient is placed in the upright position, the esophagus may begin to empty. As the disease progresses, retained food will frequently be seen within the esophageal lumen. Occasionally, there is a pulsion (epiphrenic) diverticulum.

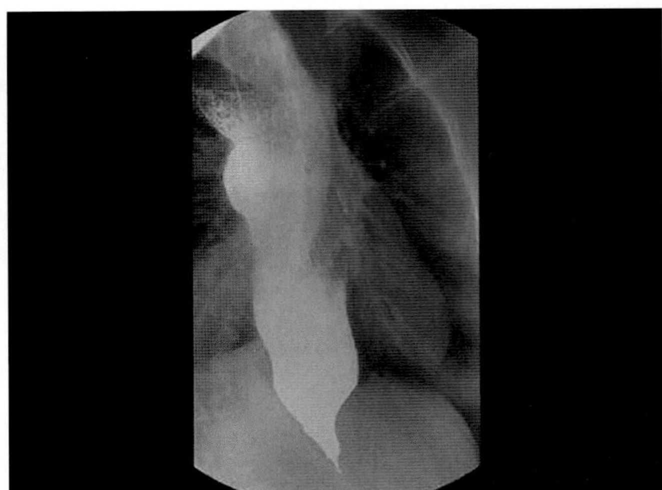

Fig. 47.23: Achalasia—barium swallow. This barium swallow demonstrates the bird's beak of achalasia and esophageal dilation.

High-Resolution Esophageal Manometry

A diagnosis of achalasia is best made by manometry. Typically, these patients demonstrate an increased LES pressure that does not relax in response to deglutition, although some patients may demonstrate incomplete relaxation (Fig. 47.24). Occasionally, the sphincter may appear to relax. This finding usually represents movement of the measuring aperture away from the sphincter during the longitudinal shortening of the esophagus that may occur during swallowing. It is important to differentiate this finding from true receptive relaxation of the sphincter because the latter is incompatible with achalasia. The two can be more easily distinguished by utilizing HRM compared to conventional manometry.

The other characteristic finding is aperistalsis. Some patients demonstrate rises in pressure with swallowing, but these increases in pressure are simultaneous rather than peristaltic. They indicate the presence of esophageal dilatation and are referred to as a "common-cavity" phenomenon.

Some patients demonstrate high-pressure simultaneous contractions in addition to the usual findings of achalasia. These high-pressure waves are usually associated with chest pain and the condition is termed "vigorous achalasia."

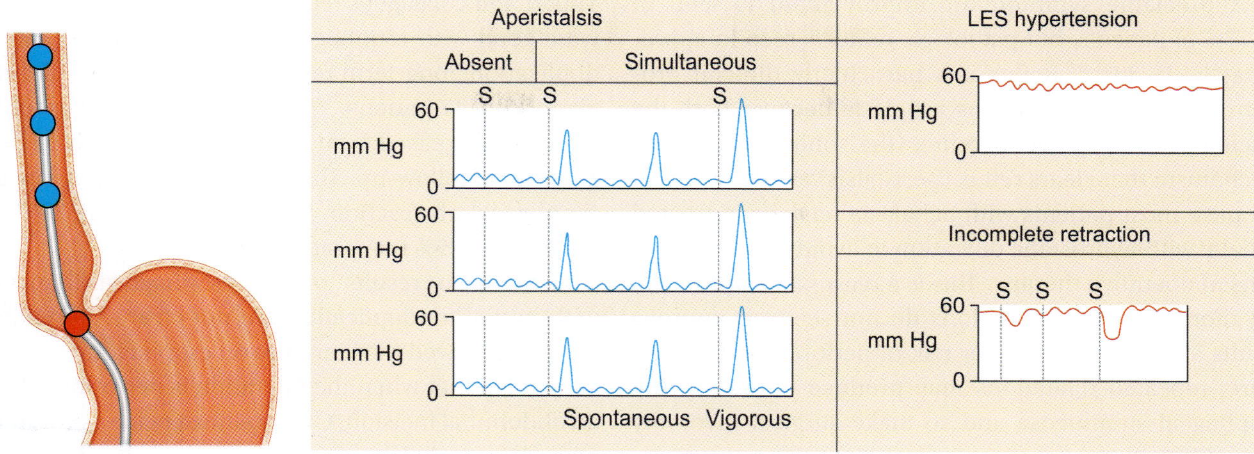

Fig. 47.24: Achalasia—esophageal manometry. Manometry demonstrates aperistalsis, incomplete or absent relaxation of the LES and common cavity pressure waves characteristic of esophageal dilation. (LES: Lower esophageal sphincter; S: Swallow).

24-Hour pH Monitoring

Some patients with achalasia exhibit a pattern on 24-hour pH monitoring that is thought to represent fermentation of retained food (above). Following pneumatic dilatation or surgical myotomy, patients may have symptoms that represent pathologic reflux caused by disruption of the sphincter. The pattern of fermentation is interpreted by the 24-hour pH study as pathologic reflux. It is therefore extremely helpful to have a baseline pH study before therapy so that post-treatment symptoms can be properly interpreted.

Endoscopy

Endoscopic examination should be carried out in all patients for two major reasons. The first is to establish the diagnosis. An infiltrating carcinoma of the cardia may produce a picture that is indistinguishable from achalasia except by endoscopy with biopsy; this condition is known as pseudoachalasia. Strictures must also be ruled out. The typical endoscopic examination demonstrates a dilated esophagus with retained food. The distal esophagus may be tortuous and difficult to navigate. The gastroesophageal junction is closed, but the endoscope will pass through with gentle pressure and produces a "pop" sensation that is typical of achalasia.

Endoscopic evaluation is also helpful immediately preoperatively to document that the esophagus is clean and empty of food before the operation, thus preventing aspiration at the time of induction of anesthesia. If it is not empty, it should be emptied with a lavage tube.

Medical Management

Commonly used medical therapies include smooth muscle relaxants such as long-acting nitrates and calcium channel blockers. These medications tend to reduce LES pressure, but the amount of symptomatic relief obtained is inconsistent and generally not long-lasting. Use of a standard rigid dilator may produce relief for 2–3 days, but because the standard 45–50 F circumference dilators do not disrupt esophageal muscle, no long-term relief should be expected.

Hydrostatic or Pneumatic Balloon Dilatation

Dilatation of the distal esophagus to a diameter above normal is effective in eliminating dysphagia because it tends to rupture the LES. These dilators used to be fluid-filled bags, and the inflation diameter was limited by a layer of cloth. Currently, they are flexible nonstretch balloons inserted over a guidewire placed during endoscopy. These balloons are 30–40 mm in diameter. Inflation of the balloon typically produces severe chest pain. Many endoscopists believe that if the patient does not experience this pain, the procedure has not been successful. Despite the fact that blood is often seen on the balloon, the esophageal perforation rate is only 5%. Patients should either be observed overnight to rule out perforation of the esophagus, which is usually signaled by continuing chest pain and tachycardia, or undergo postdilatation contrast studies if they are to be discharged. Most perforations are quite localized, and many can be managed by placement of a nasoesophageal tube for suction, parenteral antibiotics, and parenteral nutrition.

Appreciable symptomatic improvement is seen in 60–77% of patients, but pathologic reflux is seen in approximately 25–30%.[97] Reflux is a particularly difficult problem in the patient who has achalasia because both the mechanism that prevents reflux (the sphincter) and the mechanism that clears reflux (peristalsis) are deficient. In the past, most patients with achalasia have been treated initially with hydrostatic dilatation to avoid the complications of operative therapy. This is a reasonable approach, but more than two dilatations do not seem to improve results and there is a higher risk of perforation. Furthermore, repeated dilatations may produce fibrosis in the esophageal submucosa and so make surgical myotomy more difficult.

Botulinum Toxin Injection

Botulinum toxin injection into the LES does lower its pressure and give some symptomatic relief in patients who have achalasia, but the result is transient. Furthermore, the fibrosis induced by the injections may render myotomy difficult if it is required later.

Operative Management

The best method for achieving surgical relief of the dysphagia associated with achalasia is controversial. Most investigators believe that a complete myotomy cannot be assured unless the incision is extended well down onto the stomach. This maneuver invariably produces reflux, which they manage with either a Toupet or Dor partial fundoplication.[99-102] Other surgeons believe that an esophagomyotomy that extends <1 cm past the squamocolumnar junction will relieve dysphagia without producing significant pathologic reflux. Ellis demonstrated that at 10–20 years following transthoracic esophagomyotomy as described above, 88% of patients remain improved over their preoperative status and only 5% develop symptomatic reflux.[98] The lack of clinically important reflux with this approach is probably related to the fact that the limited myotomy does not traverse the gastric sling fibers. Furthermore, a limited transthoracic or transabdominal esophagomyotomy does not disturb the phrenoesophageal membrane. These surgeons believe that relieving one physiologic obstruction with myotomy and then adding another potential obstruction in the form of an antireflux procedure is counterintuitive.

Early results with either type of approach are very good. However, the surgeon cannot restore the patient's peristalsis, and the esophagus must empty passively. Topart and colleagues reported that although early results were good with esophagocardiomyotomy plus 360° fundoplication, long-term results included return of dysphagia in 14 of 17 patients.[103] Furthermore, distal esophageal diameter increased from 3.9 cm preoperatively to 6 cm at 10 years of follow-up. This result suggests that low grade esophageal obstruction was produced by the 360° wrap. There was a 29% reoperation rate.

Long-term results of the esophagocardiomyotomy with partial fundoplication are not clear. Andreollo and Earlam reviewed the literature on esophagomyotomy and concluded that when the operation is performed through an abdominal incision, GER is almost twice as common as when it is carried out through a thoracic incision, regardless of whether an antireflux procedure is performed.[104]

Thoracoscopic and laparoscopic techniques have now been adapted for esophagomyotomy. The controversies about the extent of myotomy and the addition of an antireflux procedure are the same.[105-109] Early results with these procedures mimic the results of the open procedures, but the morbidity is much less. The endoscopic approaches have now become standard therapy.

Thoracoscopic Esophagomyotomy

Preparation: The esophagus must be empty before the operation. Endoscopy on the day before operation allows retained food to be emptied from the stomach. After the esophagus is clean, the patient should remain on clear liquids until the operation. If weight loss is severe, the patient should have preoperative measurement of nutritional parameters preoperatively, with appropriate nutritional supplements if these indicate malnutrition.

Technique: A double-lumen endotracheal tube is useful to improve exposure. Insertion of a flexible endoscope into the esophagus before turning the patient helps the surgeon to determine the proper extent of myotomy. The procedure is performed through a standard 4 or five trocar approach. A third rib trocar is used to retract the collapsed left lung. The esophagus is dissected free from the mediastinum and encircled with a drain that is secured outside the chest with clamps. The traction exerted aids in exposure of the distal portion of the myotomy, which is begun approximately 10 cm above the hiatus. It is extended through the longitudinal and circular layers. The submucosa is easily recognized as it protrudes out through the myotomy. The myotomy is carried out with the hook cautery, harmonic scalpel or both, taking care not to cauterize the submucosa (Fig. 47.25). Bleeding should be

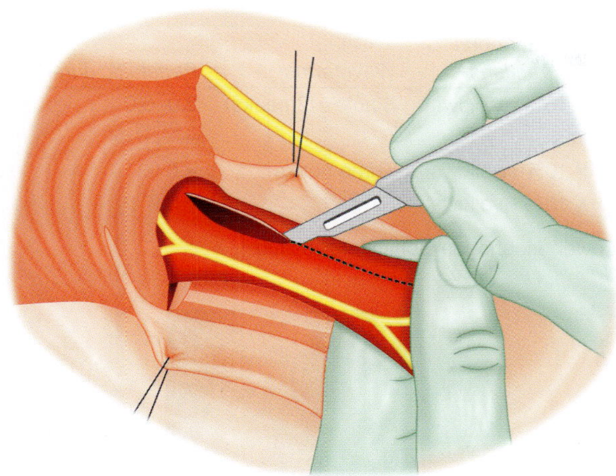

Fig. 47.25: Transthoracic esophagomyotomy. Technique of esophagomyotomy with electrocautery.

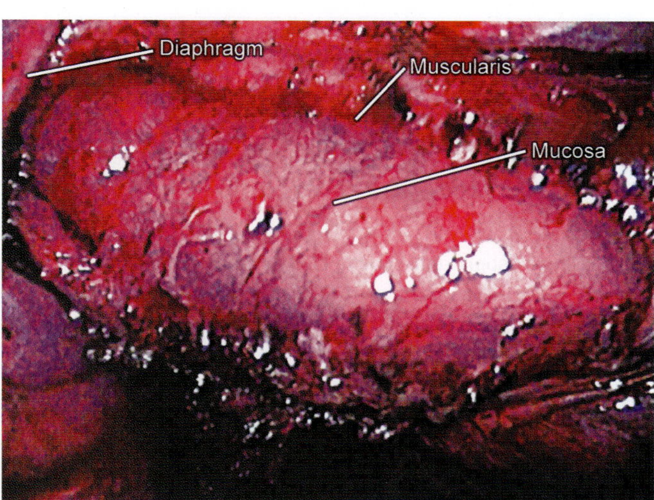

Fig. 47.26: Thoracoscopic view of completed esophagomyotomy.

controlled with thrombin-soaked collagen sponge. The myotomy is extended <1 cm past the squamocolumnar junction. Extending the myotomy far enough onto the stomach to relieve obstruction is the biggest challenge of the thoracoscopic approach. A standard vein retractor, inserted through one of the trocar openings may be used to retract the crura to facilitate this maneuver. The completed myotomy is shown in Figure 47.26. The transition to stomach can be recognized in several ways. There is a slight darkening of the columnar mucosa and the surgeon will notice the presence of submucosal transverse veins on the cardiac submucosa along with the fat from Belsey's fat pad. Nevertheless, the squamocolumnar junction is most easily recognized internally with the flexible endoscope; the esophagogastric junction (which was previously closed) will open with only gentle insufflation after the obstruction is relieved. A single chest tube is used to drain the chest, and it may be removed in the recovery area if the chest radiograph shows complete lung expansion.

These patients may resume a regular diet the next morning. They are instructed to chew their food well and to drink plenty of liquids with meals, since they still have an aperistaltic esophagus. Solid food empties primarily by peristalsis, whereas liquids empty primarily by gravity. Adding liquids to food therefore aids passive esophageal emptying. Patients are discharged when they are comfortable on oral analgesics.

Complications: Most investigators have reported no deaths following esophagomyotomy. Mucosal perforations occur, and are usually obvious when the esophagus is insufflated under irrigation, but they should be rare and may be repaired with fine sutures when they occur. If a perforation occurs near the distal end of the myotomy, some prefer to close the myotomy, rotate the esophagus and perform the myotomy on the opposite side. This maneuver is problematic from the thoracoscopic approach.

Residual dysphagia occurs in <5% of patients. Patients who still have dysphagia and a manometric high-pressure zone may benefit from another myotomy. If the previous operation was performed through the chest, the reoperation should be performed through the abdomen and vice versa.

Reflux is found in <5% of patients. In most cases, it can be treated with standard medical therapy. If reflux is severe, an antireflux procedure with a partial fundoplication or even resection is occasionally appropriate.

Transabdominal Esophagomyotomy with Antireflux Procedure

Laparoscopic transabdominal esophagomyotomy requires that the phrenoesophageal ligament must be opened anteriorly. The myotomy is started on the esophagus itself above the gastroesophageal junction and extended proximally 4–5 cm. Distally, it may be extended onto the stomach for 2–3 cm as an extended myotomy or <1 cm as in the traditional approach. If extended myotomy is performed, a Dor or Toupet fundoplication may be performed as previously described in this chapter to prevent reflux.

These patients are commonly discharged the next day. A contrast radiograph may be obtained to document the

Table 47.13 Classification of motility disorders.

Condition	*LESP (mm Hg)*	*LES relaxation*	*Peristaltic amplitude (mm Hg)*	*Simultaneous contractions*	*Waveforms*	*Peristaltic duration (s)*
Normal	10–45	Yes	30–190	< 10% swallows	Single (<2 peaks)	2.0–6.0
Achalasia	>45	No or incomplete	Aperistalsis	Yes	–	–
DES	Normal	Yes	Normal or increased	> 10% swallows	Three peaks	> 6.0
Nutcracker	Normal	Yes	>180	< 10% swallows	Single	> 6.0

(DES: Diffuse esophageal spasm; LES: Lower esophageal sphincter; LESP: Lower esophageal sphincter pressure).

lack of leak and relief of obstruction on the morning following operation if indicated. The patient is then begun on a regular diet.

Resection for End-Stage Disease

The results of myotomy when esophageal dilatation has progressed to the stage of megaesophagus or sigmoid (tortuous) esophagus are not as good as the results for lesser degrees of dilatation. Some patients still have severe dysphagia because the sigmoid curling of the esophagus leaves the esophagogastric junction in a position in which the esophagus will not empty dependently. In some of these patients and in those who have severe postmyotomy reflux, esophageal resection may relieve obstruction. Resection may be performed through a transhiatal approach with cervical esophagogastrostomy. Transhiatal resection of megaesophagus is associated with an increased incidence of intraoperative hemorrhage during the esophagectomy.

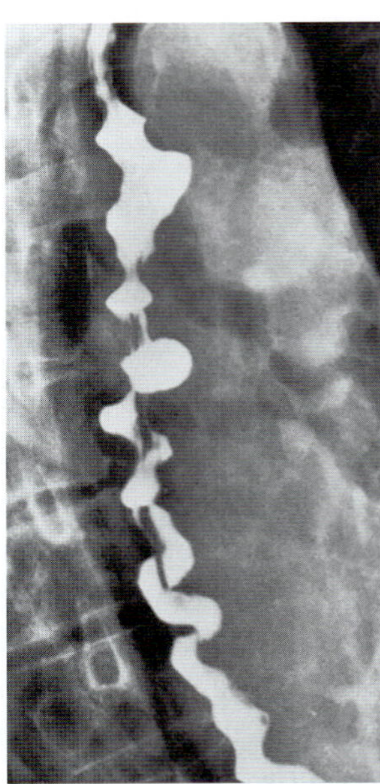

Fig. 47.27: Corkscrew appearance of the esophagus in diffuse esophageal spasm.

DIFFUSE ESOPHAGEAL SPASM

Diffuse esophageal spasm is a primary motor disorder characterized by chest pain and dysphagia. Its pathophysiology is unknown. On manometry, these patients exhibit simultaneous contractions that occur in at least 10% of all wet swallows. The contractions may be repetitive (at least three peaks) and of increased duration (>6 seconds). The patient must also demonstrate normal peristaltic sequences. The contractions are usually of normal amplitude, but there may also be some high-pressure contractions. Diffuse esophageal spasm must be distinguished from "nutcracker esophagus" (also known as high-amplitude peristaltic contractions), which is also associated with chest pain. The manometric criteria are defined in Table 47.13.

Clinical Features

All patients have chest pain, which may be crushing in nature and difficult to distinguish from angina. Dysphagia may occur, but is usually less prominent than the chest pain.

Investigation and Diagnosis

The diagnosis is made by manometry, but it may be suggested by barium swallow, which demonstrates a corkscrew appearance in approximately one third of patients (Fig. 47.27). In some patients, the described manometric abnormality is induced by reflux, but these patients complain primarily of reflux symptoms. Patients in whom the disorder is primary complain mainly of chest pain. Some cases may eventually progress to vigorous achalasia.

Medical Management

Smooth muscle relaxants such as nitrates and calcium channel blocking agents produce a decrease in the amplitude and duration of peristalsis, but most have been studied only in uncontrolled trials. The duration of relief from symptoms is often short. The likelihood of long-term medical control of symptoms is about 60%. Medical therapy is also effective for nutcracker esophagus.

Operative Management

Surgical Total Esophageal Myotomy (Open or Thoracoscopic)

Surgical intervention for DES consists of a long esophageal myotomy. This procedure is quite effective in relieving dysphagia, but less predictable in eliminating chest pain. The myotomy should be extended throughout the hypertrophied esophageal muscularis. The operation is best accomplished through the right chest and may be performed with thoracoscopic techniques. Good results are obtained in approximately 85% of patients.[110] The procedure has also been used in a few patients who have a nutcracker esophagus, with some reduction in chest pain.[111,112] Patients who have pathologic reflux should undergo treatment of their reflux. Only patients who have recalcitrant DES should undergo surgical therapy.

ESOPHAGEAL DIVERTICULA

Types

Esophageal diverticula can be classified by either location or etiology. Zenker's diverticula are the most common diverticula. Parabronchial diverticula are found near the bifurcation of the trachea, and epiphrenic diverticula arise in the lower third of the esophagus, a short distance above the diaphragm. Diverticula may be either:

- True diverticula containing all layers of the esophageal wall
- False diverticula containing only mucosa and submucosa

Traction diverticula occur when the esophageal wall is pulled out by external traction and are usually true diverticula. Pulsion diverticula occur when intraluminal forces push the lumen outward and are usually false. These categories emphasize pathophysiology and are therefore useful in planning treatment.

Diagnosis is made by videofluoroscopy, which allows the radiologist to detect associated abnormal motor activity of the body or GER.

Traction Diverticula

Pathophysiology

Traction (parabronchial) diverticula are most commonly seen in the middle third of the esophagus. These lesions occur on the right side if they are below the trachea and on the left side if they are above the trachea. Anatomically, this is where the esophagus lies in closest approximation to parabronchial lymph nodes. Most of these diverticula occur secondary to granulomatous infections (e.g. tuberculosis and histoplasmosis) of the parabronchial nodes, which become adherent to the esophagus and produce traction on the esophageal wall as the scarred nodes contract. In some cases, this retraction may produce a diverticulum. Occasionally, the necrosis may be severe enough to produce a perforation of the esophagus with subsequent epithelialization of the abscess cavity or formation of a nonmalignant tracheoesophageal fistula causing recurrent pneumonia.

Most parabronchial diverticula have a wide mouth that lies inferior to the apex of the cavity. As this position produces easy dependent drainage, there are seldom associated symptoms. Sporadic patients present with substernal pain, dysphagia or rarely bleeding. Only symptomatic patients should be considered for surgical excision.

Management

Traction diverticula may be approached through an ipsilateral thoracotomy. A nasogastric tube should be used. The diverticula usually originate on the anterior esophageal wall. Dissection on the anterior wall leads the surgeon to the lesion. The diverticula are densely adherent to surrounding tissues. Closure may be achieved with staples or sutures. In some cases, the adherent diverticulum should be left in situ and the esophagus closed without attempting complete excision. It is advisable to reinforce the closure with a pleural flap because of the dense scarring. Adequate drainage is assured by leaving a chest tube near the closure. The tube is not removed until the patient is consuming a general diet.

It is sensible to obtain a radiographic examination with contrast before pulling out the nasogastric tube and resuming oral intake.

Pulsion Diverticula

Pathophysiology

Pulsion (epiphrenic) diverticula are typically located just above the diaphragm and are therefore referred to as epiphrenic. They are typically pseudodiverticula composed of mucosa and submucosa. Epiphrenic diverticula are often associated with abnormal motor activity, which may present either as a clearly defined syndrome such as achalasia or DES or as less well-defined manometric phenomena. Debas and colleagues[113] reviewed 65 patients

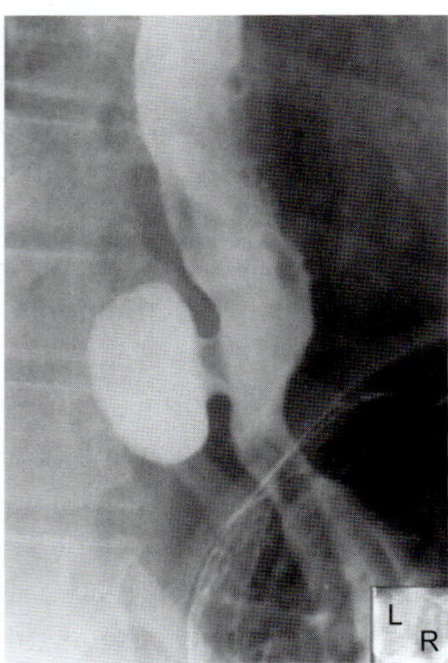

Fig. 47.28: Epiphrenic diverticula of the seen on barium swallow.

for associated motility disorders: 50 patients (77%) had abnormal studies. Of these 21 patients had diffuse spasm, 13 had achalasia, and 16 had poorly defined motility disorders (some included discoordination between the peristaltic wave and relaxation of the LES). Of the patients exhibiting normal motility, 13 had a hiatal hernia. The early symptoms are those associated with the associated motility disorder (dysphagia, chest pain, heartburn). When the lesions become large, they no longer drain dependently. These patients may experience aspiration, regurgitation of food eaten several days previously, halitosis, bleeding, or dysphagia.[114]

Investigation and Diagnosis

Diagnosis is made by cinefluoroscopic barium swallow (Fig. 47.28). Manometry is mandatory to define any associated motility disorder. Twenty-four hour pH studies should be used to identify pathologic reflux. These studies allow the surgeon to tailor the procedure to the patient's pathophysiology, so increasing the probability of achieving a satisfactory result. Many of these patients have other associated disorders such as colonic and small intestinal motility disorders that only become evident postoperatively but are preferably identified before operation. Esophagoscopy should be performed just before operation to clean out any retained food and to avoid missing the occasional esophageal cancer within the diverticulum.

Management

Between 12% and 25% of patients with epiphrenic diverticula have symptoms that are severe enough to warrant excision. In general, these lesions are best approached through the left chest because of the high incidence of associated pathology. Even lesions in the right chest may be easily rotated for excision from the left side. Some laparoscopists advocate approaching these lesions through a laparoscopic abdominal approach, opening the mediastinum. The esophagus is dissected free from the posterior mediastinum and encircled with a Penrose drain. The sac is easy to identify and is dissected back to the neck, where it is excised with a stapled or sutured technique. The muscular defect should also be closed for reinforcement.

The diverticulectomy is then supplemented by the appropriate concomitant procedure. Modified Heller myotomy should be performed for achalasia using Ellis' technique of limiting the myotomy to an extension of only 0.5–1.0 cm past the squamocolumnar junction. The myotomy is oriented to avoid the suture line from the excision. If the patient has diffuse spasm, long esophagomyotomy is the procedure of choice. If there is discoordination between the sphincteric relaxation and the peristaltic contraction, the modified Heller myotomy technique should be used. Patients with concomitant GER should undergo an antireflux procedure, preferably with a fundoplication that is <360° in circumference to avoid obstruction. Postoperative care is identical to that described for the patient with a parabronchial diverticulum.

The Mayo Clinic has reported on 33 patients who underwent excision combined with appropriate complementary procedures (e.g. esophagomyotomy).[115] There were three postoperative deaths (9%). Long-term results were excellent, good, fair, and poor in 48%, 27%, 17%, and 8% of cases, respectively. This operation has appreciable risks and should only be undertaken for those who have severe symptoms. The procedure may also be performed using laparoscopic or thoracoscopic techniques. It should be emphasized, however, that no compromise should be made in the procedure to accommodate the less invasive approach.[116-119] The surgeon should perform the same procedure that he or she would perform through the open approach, the only difference being the size of the incisions.

ESOPHAGEAL PERFORATION (BOERHAAVE'S SYNDROME)

Presentation

Perforation of the esophagus constitutes a true emergency. It most commonly occurs following diagnostic or therapeutic procedures. Spontaneous perforation is referred to as Boerhaave's syndrome, for the Dutch physician who first described it. It accounts for only 15% of cases of esophageal perforation, foreign bodies for 14%, and trauma for 10%. Pain is a striking and consistent symptom and strongly suggests esophageal rupture has occurred, particularly if located substernally in a patient with a history of vomiting or in the cervical area following instrumentation of the esophagus. If subcutaneous emphysema is present, the diagnosis is almost certain; only the site remains to be determined.

Spontaneous rupture of the esophagus is associated with a high mortality rate because of delays in recognition and treatment. A history of vomiting defines the diagnosis; however, in a small number of patients, the injury occurs without any history of emesis. When the chest radiogram of a patient with an esophageal perforation shows free air or an effusion in the pleural space, the condition is often misdiagnosed as a pneumothorax or pancreatitis. If the chest radiogram is normal, a mistaken diagnosis of myocardial infarction or dissecting aneurysm might be made.

Spontaneous rupture usually occurs into the left pleural cavity just above the gastroesophageal junction (GEJ). During vomiting, high peaks of intragastric pressure can be recorded, frequently exceeding 200 mm Hg, but because extragastric pressure remains almost equal to intragastric pressure, stretching of the gastric wall is minimal. Since the GEJ usually is in the abdomen and exposed to intra-abdominal pressure, the pressure transmitted to the esophagus is much less than if the GEJ is in the negative thoracic pressure environment. If the glottis remains closed, the pressure in the lower esophagus may equal intragastric pressure producing rupture. Some patients may tear only the cardiac mucosa cardia following emesis producing hemorrhage; this is termed Mallory-Weiss tear.

Diagnosis

The clinical manifestations of esophageal perforations include tachycardia, fever, subcutaneous emphysema, pain, dysphagia, and shortness of breath. Cervical esophageal perforations typically present with neck pain and crepitus involving the neck or upper thorax. Abdominal and thoracic esophageal perforations complain of subxiphoid, epigastric, or retrosternal pain.

The need for diagnostic studies depends on the circumstances. Iatrogenic endoscopic injury may need no further diagnostic studies if the injury is seen directly. When the presence or nature of esophageal injury is not known, various diagnostic studies can be helpful. Chest X-ray findings are not reliable but may suggest the diagnosis (Table 47.14).

Table 47.14 Chest film findings in esophageal perforation.

Etiology	*Cervical perforation post instrumentation*	*Thoracic perforation emetogenic*
Cervical crepitus	Common	Uncommon
Mediastinal emphysema	Uncommon	Common
Pneumothorax	Uncommon	Common
Widened mediastinum	Uncommon	Common
Pleural effusion	Uncommon	Common

Chest X-ray findings are often nonspecific, and an upper gastrointestinal series or chest CT scan with oral contrast material may confirm the diagnosis. Water-soluble contrast material is recommended to avoid barium mediastinitis. Chest CT scanning is reported to be 95% sensitive for the diagnosis of esophageal perforation. The use of flexible endoscopy is limited to the operating room, where can help delineate the area of injury for definitive surgical repair.

The management of esophageal perforation depends on etiology, location, and time since injury. Delay in diagnosis produces continued contamination, release of inflammatory mediators, and resulting sepsis. The diagnosis of iatrogenic perforation is usually suspected shortly after the incident and thus usually has an improved prognosis. Spontaneous perforations are more likely to be missed and carry a worse prognosis.

Prognosis is also affected by site. Cervical perforations typically are most often localized and have a mortality of <10%. Thoracic and abdominal perforations are typically not well contained and are associated with mortality rates of up to 25% or higher if the diagnosis is missed.

Management

Initial management of esophageal perforation involves fluid resuscitation of the patient, H_2-blockers or proton pump inhibitors to reduce gastric acid secretion, broad-spectrum antibiotics, and NPO status. Nasogastric tube placement should only be done under fluoroscopic guidance to prevent inadvertent passage of tube through the injury.

Surgical treatment for esophageal perforation is the traditional foundation of therapy; however, nonoperative treatment can sometimes be useful. Nonoperative therapy traditionally had a 20–40% mortality rate. However, if the perforation is well-contained or internally drained (meaning most of the extravasated contrast drains back into the esophagus) and the patient is not septic, nonoperative management may be attempted. This is especially true in those who are poor operative candidates or have a much delayed diagnosis. Nevertheless, most thoracic and abdominal leaks require operation.

The goals of surgery are (1) to prevent further contamination when possible by closing the leak and to (2) drain the leak. The latter is the most important since the leak will heal if systemic sepsis can be avoided. The key to avoiding sepsis is prompt evacuation of extravasated esophageal contents into the drain. There are four possible treatments: (1) primary repair and drainage, (2) diversion and esophageal exclusion, (3) esophagectomy with immediate or delayed reconstruction, and (4) internal diversion by placement of a covered esophageal stent.

Primary repair of the leak is possible when the tissue quality of the esophagus is of sufficient integrity to allow accurate and secure placement of sutures to close the injury. Most patients suitable for primary repair present within 24–48 hours of injury. Cervical perforations lend themselves to primary closure because the contamination tends to be minimal and the repair can be well drained. Thoracic and abdominal perforations with minimal mediastinal and intra-abdominal contamination and no systemic sepsis may also be closed primarily. Repairs should be buttressed with diaphragmatic, pleural, or pericardial patches. Intercostal muscles flaps may also be used but should not be wrapped circumferentially around the esophagus because of the risk of subsequent bone formation. All injuries should be widely drained. The authors have found that a penrose drain sutured to a chest tube allows placement of the soft drain directly adjacent to the leak diminishing the risk of erosion of the stiff chest tube.

If there is extensive contamination and devitalized esophageal tissue, the surgeon may consider: exclusion and diversion, and/or esophagectomy. Exclusion and diversion utilizes a cervical esophageal fistula to divert saliva and a gastrostomy to minimize reflux of gastric contents into the esophagus. The esophagus is stapled without division distal to the perforation to prevent gastric reflux. The distal esophagus will usually eventually recanalize and the esophagostomy can be closed in the neck after recovery. The mediastinum is debrided and the perforation is repaired as well as is practicable. Wide mediastinal drainage is mandatory. If the perforation is associated with esophageal cancer, severe stricture, or megaesophagus, the surgeon should give strong consideration to esophagectomy with either primary or delayed reconstruction.

Recently, there has been a wave of enthusiasm for internal exclusion of the perforation by placing an endoscopic covered stent placed across the perforation combined with drainage[120]. This technique has been surprisingly successful even with delayed presentation of the leak, possibly because it achieves the effects of esophageal exclusion without thoracotomy. Its ultimate utility will require further study. Problems with displacement or migration of the stent may require more than one procedure and the need for concomitant drainage must be emphasized.

REFERENCES

1. Liebermann-Meffert D, Duranceau A. Anatomy and embryology. In: Orringer MB (coed). Esophagus, Vol. 1. In: Zuidema G (Ed). Shackelford's Surgery of the Alimentary Tract, 4th edition. Philadelphia: WB Saunders; 1997.
2. Ellis FH Jr. The esophagus. In: L Davis (Ed). Christopher's Textbook of Surgery, 8th edition. Philadelphia: WB Saunders; 1964. p. 593.
3. Akiyama H. Surgery for carcinoma of the esophagus. Curr Probl Surg. 1980;17:53-120.
4. McEwan-Alvarado G. Physiology of deglutition. Tex Med. 1969;65:82-6.
5. Payne WS, Olsen AM. The origin, form and function of the esophagus. In: The Esophagus. Philadelphia: Lea & Febiger; 1974. pp. 1-25.
6. Sokol EM, Hellmann P, Wolf BS, et al. Simultaneous cineradiographic and manometric study of the pharynx, hypopharynx and cervical esophagus. Gastroenterology. 1966;51:960-74.
7. Castell DO. The Esophagus. Boston: Little Brown; 1992. p. 19.
8. Duranceau AC, Devroede G, Lafontaine E, et al. Esophageal motility in asymptomatic volunteers. Surg Clin North Am. 1983;63:777-86.
9. Humphries IJ, Castell DO. Pressure profile of esophageal peristalsis in normal humans as measured by direct intraesophageal transducers. Dig Dis. 1977;22:641-5.
10. Fyke FE, Code CF, Schlegel FJ. The gastroesophageal sphincter in healthy human beings. Gastroenterologia. 1956;86:135-50.
11. Hellemans J, Vantrappen G. Manometric measurements of the resting pressure in the lower esophageal sphincter. In: Hellemans J, Vantrappen G (Eds). Diseases of the Esophagus. New York: Springer Verlag; 1974. pp. 48-60.
12. Gelfand DW. Gastrointestinal Radiology. New York: Churchill Livingstone; 1984. pp. 51-3.
13. Heyder N. Endoscopic ultrasonography of tumours of the oesophagus and the stomach. Surg Endosc. 1987;1:17-23.

14. Kouzu T, Ogino Y, Jocson R, et al. Evaluation of preoperative stage of esophageal cancer by endoscopic ultrasonography. In: Siewert JR, Holscher AH (Eds). Diseases of the Esophagus. Berlin: Springer Verlag: 1988. pp. 164-9.
15. Kramer P, Ingelfinger FJ. Motility of the human esophagus in control subjects and in patients with esophageal disorders. Am J Med. 1949;7:168-73.
16. Kramer P, Ingelfinger FJ. Cardiospasm, a generalized disorder of esophageal motility. Am J Med. 1949;7:174-9.
17. Butin JW, Olsen AM, Moersch HJ, et al. A study of esophageal pressures in normal persons and patients with cardiospasm. Gastroenterology. 1953;23:278-91.
18. DeMeester TR, Stein HJ. Gastroesophageal reflux disease. In: Moody FG, Jones RS, Kelly KA, et al. (Eds). Surgical Treatment of Digestive Disease, 2nd edition. Chicago: Year Book Medical Publishers; 1989. p. 65.
19. Allison PR. Reflux esophagitis, sliding hiatus hernia and the anatomy of repair. Surg Gynecol Obstet. 1951;92:419-31.
20. Skinner DB. Esophageal hiatus hernia. In: Sabiston DC, Spencer FC (Eds). Gibbons Surgery of the Chest, Vol 2, 4th edition. Philadelphia: WB Saunders; 1983. pp. 773-92.
21. Stilson WL, Sanders I, Gardiner GA, et al. Hiatual hernia and gastroesophageal reflux. A clinicoradiological analysis of more than 1,000 cases. Radiology. 1969;93:1323-7.
22. Dodds WJ, Dent J, Hogan WJ. Mechanisms of gastroesophageal reflux in patients with reflux esophagitis. N Engl J Med. 1982;307:1547-52.
23. Cohen S, Harris LD. The lower esophageal sphincter. Gastroenterology. 1972;63:1066-73.
24. Pope CE. A dynamic test of sphincter strength: its application to the lower esophageal sphincter. Gastroenterology. 1967;52:779-86.
25. Winans CS, Harris LD. Quantitation of lower esophageal sphincter competence. Gastroenterology. 1967;52:773-8.
26. Bombeck CT, Battle WS, Nyhus LM. Preoperative manometry in the choice of operations for gastroesophageal reflux. Am J Surg. 1973;125:99-107.
27. DeMeester TR, Johnson LF, Joseph GJ. Patterns of gastroesophageal reflux in health and disease. Ann Surg. 1976; 184:459-70.
28. Dent J, Dodds WJ, Friedman RH, et al. Mechanism of gastroesophageal reflux in recumbent asymptomatic human subjects. J Clin Invest. 1980;65:256-67.
29. Goldberg HI, Dodds WJ, Gee S, et al. Role of acid and pepsin in acute experimental esophagitis. Gastroenterology. 1969;56:223-30.
30. Casten DF. Peptic esophagitis, hiatal hernia and duodenal ulcer. Am J Surg. 1967;113:638-41.
31. Dodds WJ, Dehn TG, Hogan WJ, et al. Severe peptic esophagitis in a patient with Zollinger-Ellison syndrome. Am J Roentgenol. 1971;113:237-40.
32. Henderson RD, Mugaske FL, Jeejeebhoy KN, et al. Synergism of acid and bile salts in the production of experimental esophagitis. Can J Surg. 1973;16:12-7.
33. Livstone E, Sheahan D, Behar J. Studies of esophageal epithelial cell proliferation in patients with reflux esophagitis. Gastroenterology. 1977;73:1315-9.
34. Sonnenberg A, Steinkamp U, Weise A, et al. Salivary secretion in reflux esophagitis. Gastroenterology. 1982;83: 889-95.
35. Nebel OT, Fornes MF, Castell DO. Symptomatic gastroesophageal reflux: incidence and precipitating factors. Am J Dig Dis. 1976;21:953-6.
36. DeMeester TR, O'Sullivan GC, Bermaduz G. Esophageal function in patients with angina type chest pain and normal coronary angiograms. Ann Surg. 1982;196:488-98.
37. Reich SB, Early WC, Ravin TH. Evaluation of gastropulmonary aspiration by a radioactive technique. J Nucl Med. 1977;18:1079-81.
38. Johnson LF, DeMeester TR. Evaluation of elevation of the head of the bed, bethanechol and antacid foam tablets on gastroesophageal reflux. Dig Dis Sci. 1981;26:673-80.
39. Kuipers EJ, Lundell L, Klinkenberg-Knol EC, et al. Atrophic gastritis and Helicobacter pylori infection in patients with reflux esophagitis treated with omeprazole or fundoplication. N Engl J Med. 1996;335:750-51.
40. DeMeester TR, Johnson LF, Kent AH. Evaluation of current operations for the prevention of gastroesophageal reflux. Ann Surg. 1974;180:511-25.
41. Brennan TG, Tnndade LM, Rozycki ZJ, et al. The influence of the lower esophageal sphincter pressure on the outcome of hiatus hernia repair. Br J Surg. 1974;61:201-5.
42. Allison PR. Hiatus hernia; a 20 year retrospective survey. Ann Surg. 1973;178:273-6.
43. Baue AE, Belsey RHR. The treatment of sliding hiatus hernia and reflux esophagitis by the Mark IV technique. Surgery. 1967;62:396-406.
44. Skinner DB, Belsey RHR. Surgical management of esophageal reflux and hiatus hernia. Long term results with 1030 patients. J Thorac Cardiovasc Surg. 1967;53:33-54.
45. Hiebert CA, O'Mara CS. The Belsey operation for hiatus hernia; a 20-year experience. Am J Surg. 1979;137:532-5.
46. Belsey RHR. Transthoracic partial fundoplication (Belsey repair). In: Jamieson GG (Ed). Surgery of the Oesophagus. London: Churchill Livingstone; 1988. pp. 255-9.
47. Jamieson GG, Duranceau AC. The development of surgery for gastroesophageal reflux disease. In: Jamieson GG (Ed). Surgery of the Oesophagus. London: Churchill Livingstone; 1988. pp. 233-43.
48. Nissen R, Eine E, Einfat HE. Operation zur Beeinflussung der Refluxochitis. Schweiz Med Wochenschr. 1956;86: 590-92.
49. Rossetti M. Zur Technik der Fundoplicatio. Acta Chir. 1978;3: 235-40.
50. Polk HC Jr. An approach to reflux esophagitis complicating sliding hiatal hernia. In: Schwartz SI (Ed). Modern Techniques in Surgery. New York: Futura Publishing; 1980. pp. 1-23.

Additional references appear in the online version of this book.

48

Peptic Ulcer Disease

John M Kellum

Key Points

- Duodenal ulcer disease has decreased in prevalence for unknown reasons.
- At least 90% of duodenal ulcers can be healed by drugs such as H -receptor antagonists, proton-pump inhibitors, and antibiotics active against *Helicobacter pylori* (either alone or in combination).
- Apart from the rare recalcitrant duodenal ulcer, operation is reserved for the complications of perforation, bleeding, and obstruction. Proximal gastric vagotomy, which can be accomplished laparoscopically, has the lowest incidence of side effects and death but the highest rate of recurrent ulcer, whereas the situation is reversed for vagotomy and antrectomy.
- Acute erosive gastritis or stress ulceration can arise in vulnerable patients because of decreased splanchnic perfusion and disruption of the normal mucosal barrier. Prophylactic measures include antacid administration via a nasogastric tube, oral sucralfate, or intravenous infusion of an H-receptor antagonist.
- Gastric ulcer complications are often seen in older individuals who are taking nonsteroidal anti-inflammatory drugs (NSAIDs).
- In chronic gastric ulcer, the main indication for operation is to exclude a carcinoma. Distal gastrectomy with Billroth I or II anastomosis should have mortality and recurrence rates $< 5\%$.
- Postgastrectomy syndromes include dumping (early and late), diarrhea, reflux alkaline gastritis, atony of the stomach following Roux-en-Y reconstruction for bile gastritis, afferent limb syndrome, bezoar, and bone disease. Both drug therapy and remedial operations may be required for those with persistent symptoms.

ANATOMY AND FUNCTION OF THE STOMACH AND DUODENUM

The stomach is a reservoir of the digestive tract in which ingested food is stored, saturated in hydrochloric acid and activated pepsin, ground into a semiliquid (chyme) by the antrum, and then propelled into the duodenum by gastric peristalsis. The pylorus relaxes intermittently to deliver the chyme to the duodenum.

The stomach has two borders—the concave lesser curvature and the convex greater curvature (Fig. 48.1). The two join cephalad at the cardia, where the esophagus enters. On the right, the esophagus continues smoothly into the lesser curvature; on the left, there is a definite indentation, the angle of HIS, which becomes more obvious when the uppermost portion of the stomach, the fundus, is full. The major portion of the stomach, the corpus (or body), blends into the pyloric portion, except along the lesser curvature, where a notch, the incisura angularis, marks the boundary between them. The pyloric portion is divided into the antrum, which narrows down, and the pylorus into which it enters. The antrum actually extends higher on the lesser than on the greater curvature and extends cephalad to the incisura.[1] External landmarks of the pylorus are a circular ridge of sphincter muscle and the subserosal pyloric vein. The duodenum has a total length of about 25–30 cm. As a result of its intraperitoneal position, the first portion of the duodenum is freely movable whereas the remaining portions are retroperitoneal. The radiologic designation "duodenal bulb" refers to the most proximal end of the first portion of the duodenum, which is slightly dilated when the organ is filled and then more sharply separated from the stomach because of the pyloric contraction.

Blood Supply

Stomach

Although there are many variations in the arrangement of blood vessels, six vessels provide the main blood supply:

- The left and right gastric arteries supply the lesser curvature

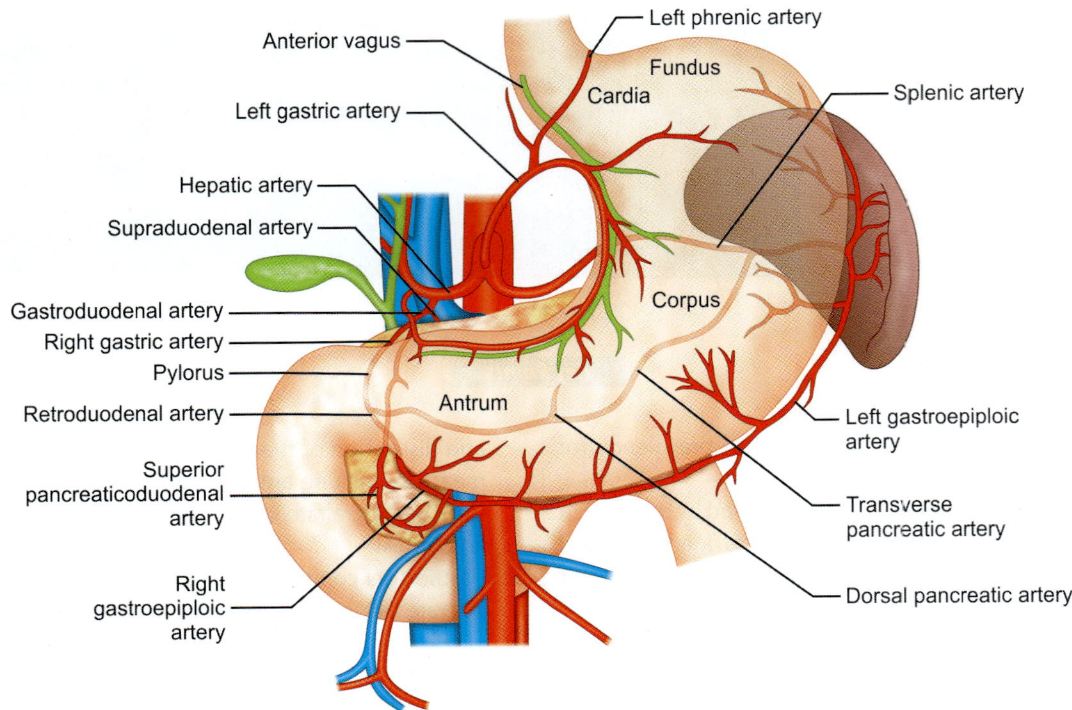

Fig. 48.1: Anatomy and blood supply of the stomach and duodenum. The stomach is divided into the fundus, body (corpus), and antrum. The blood supply to the stomach is carried by six major vessels: the left and right gastric arteries, the right gastric and left gastroepiploic arteries, the splenic artery via the short gastric arteries, and the gastroduodenal artery. The remaining vessels supplying the stomach are the superior pancreaticoduodenal artery, the supraduodenal artery, the retroduodenal artery, the transverse pancreatic artery, the dorsal pancreatic artery, and the left inferior phrenic artery. The anterior (left) vagus is shown dividing into a gastric and a hepatic branch. Just behind it is also shown the posterior (right) vagus dividing into a gastric and celiac branch.

- The right and left gastroepiploic arteries supply the greater curvature
- The splenic artery supplies the area of the fundus by way of the short gastric arteries
- The gastroduodenal artery sends branches to the area of the pylorus.
- In general, venous effluent from the stomach parallels the arterial supply. The venous equivalent of the left gastric artery is the coronary vein.

Duodenum

The blood supply of the duodenum is carried by
- The supraduodenal and retroduodenal arteries
- The superior pancreaticoduodenal artery, which arises from the gastroduodenal artery
- The inferior pancreaticoduodenal artery, which arises from the superior mesenteric artery.

Innervation

The parasympathetic nerve supply to the stomach is from the vagus nerves, which control tonic and phasic contractions and the secretion of acid and pepsin. The left and right vagal trunks give off numerous branches and are somewhat inconstant in their relations at the diaphragm. They parallel the lesser curvature anteriorly (left vagus) and posteriorly (right vagus) and distribute branches to the cardia, fundus, and corpus (body). Opposite the body of the stomach, they are called the "nerves of Latarjet." Distally they distribute branches to the antrum known as the "crow's foot." The left or anterior vagus nerve gives off a hepatic branch, which also sends fibers to the area of the pylorus, as well as to the gallbladder. The posterior vagus nerve gives off a large branch to the celiac plexus, and the remaining nerve goes to the posterior wall of the stomach. The ability of the stomach to accommodate large portions of food and liquids without increasing its pressure is a vagally mediated function termed "receptive relaxation." Very little is known of the role of vagal innervation outside the stomach, pancreas, and gallbladder, and >80% of vagal fibers are afferent to the brain.

The gastric sympathetic innervation is derived from spinal segments T5–T10. Pain of gastroduodenal origin is sensed through afferent fibers of sympathetic origin.

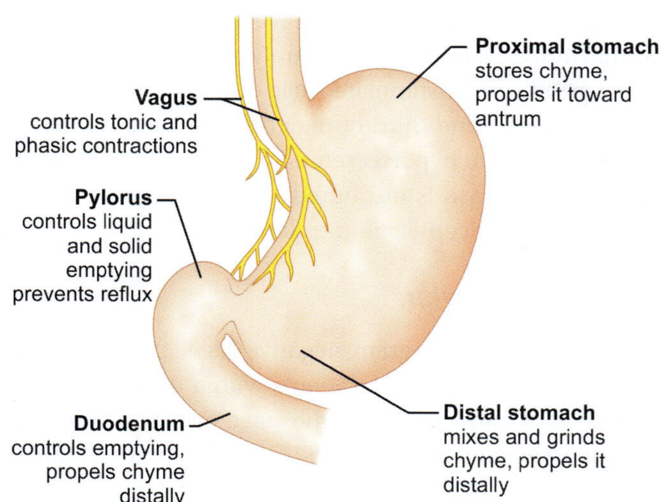

Fig. 48.2: Anatomic components of gastric motility and their roles in gastric emptying.

Gastric Secretion

Gastric secretion is divided into three phases:

1. The first or cephalic phase represents the response to sight, smell, and taste of food and is mediated through vagal activity, which directly stimulates the parietal cells and releases gastrin from the antrum. This cephalic phase and the gastric phase are synergistic, so that elimination of either reduces maximal acid output (MAO) by 70%.
2. The second or gastric phase results from the mechanical stimulation of distension acting through vagal reflex arcs and directly releasing gastrin from the antrum by contact with food.
3. Finally, food entering the duodenum initiates the third or intestinal phase of acid secretion, which appears to be mediated through several pathways, including absorbed peptides in the portal circulation stimulating parietal cell secretion and gastrin release from endocrine cells of the proximal duodenum. This phase accounts for only 5% of MAO.

The stomach accomplishes its functions of trituration (mechanical breakdown of food) and emptying by the interaction of two distinct motor regions:

1. A proximal region, consisting of the fundus and proximal one-third of the gastric corpus
2. A distal region, consisting of the distal two-thirds of the corpus, the antrum, and the pylorus.[1]

Confirmation of the division between the two gastric regions has been established by myoelectric and motility criteria. Pacesetter potentials—the cyclic potential changes in gastric smooth muscle that determine the frequency, direction, and velocity of propagation of peristaltic contractions—are present in the distal stomach. By contrast, pacesetter potentials and the peristaltic contractions they trigger do not occur in the proximal stomach, which instead is characterized by slow sustained tonic contractions. The distinct motor patterns of the two regions of the stomach are in keeping with their unique physiologic roles in digestion. The proximal stomach functions primarily to receive and store food and to transfer ingested liquids from the stomach to the duodenum. This process is known as accommodation and is mediated by vagal innervation. The distal stomach functions mainly to retain, grind, and empty solids and to prevent duodenogastric reflux; it is also vagally mediated (Fig. 48.2).

Histology of Gastric Mucosa

The histology of gastric mucosa varies with the area of the stomach, and the different types of cells have specific functions:

- In the fundus and body of the stomach, parietal cells manufacture and secrete hydrochloric acid and gastric intrinsic factor whereas chief cells make and secrete pepsinogen—acid and pepsin work synergistically to digest food.
- In the antrum, most of the cells are mucus secreting or gastrin cells, which synthesize, store, and secrete gastrin.

DUODENAL ULCER

The incidence of duodenal ulceration has declined over the past 40 years. This decline is only partially explained by the introduction of potent antisecretory agents because it predated these agents. The decline could be partly explained by a decrease in smoking, but it is just as likely that the reasons may be related to wider use of broad-spectrum antibiotics or other unknown factors.

Etiology

Peptic ulcers have multiple etiologies, and no single pathophysiologic defect applies to every case. The gastric and duodenal mucosa is protected from the damaging effects of gastric acid and pepsin[3] by the following factors:

- Surface epithelial cells secrete mucus, which provides an unstirred layer immediately adjacent to the epithelial surface and is an effective barrier to pepsin

Table 48.1 Factors that affect gastroduodenal mucosal integrity.

Protective factors	*Damaging factors*
HCO_3^-	H^+
Mucus	Pepsins
Blood flow	Smoking
Growth factors	Ethanol
Cell renewal	Bile acids
Prostaglandins	Ischemia
	Nonsteroidal anti-inflammatory drugs
	Hypoxia
	Helicobacter pylori

- Continuous bicarbonate secretion by the gastric and duodenal surface epithelial cells into the overlying mucus layer results in a pH gradient in which the pH varies from approximately 7 at the epithelial surface to <2 in the gastric or duodenal lumen
- Gastric mucosal cells also have apical membranes and tight junctions that are impermeable to the back-diffusion of acid into the cell.[4]

Other factors that are important in the maintenance of mucosal integrity include blood flow and the ability of epithelial cells to renew themselves rapidly and to migrate along the basal membrane to areas of minor injury, a process referred to as reconstitution.[5] Cytokines and growth factors also play a role in mucosal defense, and so do prostaglandins by stimulating mucus and bicarbonate secretion and blood flow (Table 48.1).

A number of interacting factors serve as defensive mechanisms for the maintenance of the gastroduodenal mucosa. Ulcers arise when there is an imbalance between the mucosal defense mechanisms and injurious factors such as acid and pepsin. The major factors that disrupt mucosal resistance resulting in ulcer development include NSAIDs, *Helicobacter pylori* infection, mucosal bicarbonate secretion, cigarette smoking, and gastric secretion.[6] Additional factors that appear to be important in the development of ulcers include genetic predisposition, bile reflux, and underlying medical illnesses, including cirrhosis and chronic obstructive pulmonary disease.

Pathophysiology

Acid Secretory Status

Gastric acid and pepsin are essential factors in the process of ulcer formation. Although patients who have duodenal ulcers as a group have higher mean basal or pentagastrin-stimulated acid outputs than normal subjects, acid secretion in most patients who have an ulcer is within the normal range. Duodenal ulcers rarely occur in patients who have a pentagastrin-stimulated acid output of <12 mmol/h, and only about one-third of patients who have a duodenal ulcer are true hypersecretors of gastric acid. In many cases, the increase is attributed to an enlarged mass of acid and pepsinogen-secreting glands.

Helicobacter pylori

Helicobacter pylori is a gram-negative flagellated rod found in the antrum of >95% of patients with a duodenal ulcer as well as in most patients who have gastric ulcers that are not associated with NSAIDs. In 1994, the US National Institutes of Health issued its consensus statement that *H. pylori* is an insidious bacterium and a major etiologic factor in peptic ulcer disease.[7] Available evidence strongly suggests that >50% of the world population is infected with *H. pylori.*[8] Most individuals acquire *H. pylori* early in life, and most studies have demonstrated an inverse relationship between socioeconomic status and prevalence of infection. Humans appear to be the only reservoir for *H. pylori* infection. A variety of host factors are considered as contributory to the pathogenesis of peptic ulcer disease resulting from *H. pylori* infection. Factors such as gender, smoking, diet, genetics, acid secretory profile, and Lewis blood group antigens may modulate the clinical response to *H. pylori* infection.[9] It should be noted that there is no state of colonization with *H. pylori*. The presence of the bacterium is synonymous with infection and there are always pathologic changes.

The gastritis caused by *H. pylori* is characterized by an inflammatory response with gastric epithelial injury.[10] Adherence of *H. pylori* to gastric epithelial cells seems to be required for bacterial infection of the gastric mucosa. There are a number of mechanisms by which *H. pylori* leads to gastric mucosal injury[11]:

- The first toxin identified from *H. pylori* strains, known as vacuolating cytotoxin, induces vacuole formation in cells
- Ammonia produced through urease activity may be toxic to gastric epithelial cells
- *H. pylori* protease and lipase degrade gastric mucus and disrupt the phospholipid-rich layer at the apical epithelial cell surface, allowing cell injury from back-diffusion of gastric acid
- *H. pylori* infection increases gastric acid secretion in patients who have duodenal ulcer, and eradication of *H. pylori* returns acid secretion to normal

- Infection of the gastric antrum increases gastrin release[12]: certain cytokines released during *H. pylori* gastritis, such as tumor necrosis factor-a and specific products of *H. pylori* such as ammonia, release gastrin from G cells
- Finally, there is evidence that the immune and inflammatory responses during infection with *H. pylori* induce autoimmune-mediated damage to gastric epithelium.[13]

Nonsteroidal Anti-inflammatory Drugs

Nonsteroidal anti-inflammatory drugs may cause gastric or duodenal ulcers de novo or exacerbate an underlying ulcer diathesis.[14] Chronic NSAID use is associated with the development of mucosal ulceration in 20% of patients. There is an estimated 40-fold increase in gastric ulcers and an eightfold increase in duodenal ulcers among daily NSAID users. Long-term users of NSAIDs are seven times more likely to have a serious gastrointestinal hemorrhage or perforation than the normal population. Further NSAID use may produce ulceration anywhere in the GI tract.

The NSAIDs apparently produce gastric damage by two independent mechanisms:

- An irritative topical effect
- A systemic effect (e.g., indomethacin suppositories can produce gastric ulcers).

Chronic NSAID injury is thought to arise from the inhibition of cyclo-oxygenase, resulting in decreased mucosal prostaglandin synthesis and impaired mucosal defense.

Clinical Features

Pain is the most common complaint of patients who have a duodenal ulcer. Pain is often exacerbated by certain foods and alcohol. Patients may inadvertently intensify their pain by taking antacids that contain aspirin, for example, Alka Seltzer, BC Powders, and Goody Powders. The pain is often periodic and occurs in the upper epigastrium. Usually patients do not have the pain during meals, but they are often awakened by pain in the early morning, which is then relieved by antacids. About 20% of patients who require treatment for perforated or bleeding duodenal ulcer do not have an antecedent history of ulcer pain. The symptoms are generally nonspecific; other pathology such as reflux esophagitis, gastritis, and pancreatobiliary disease must be considered and excluded.

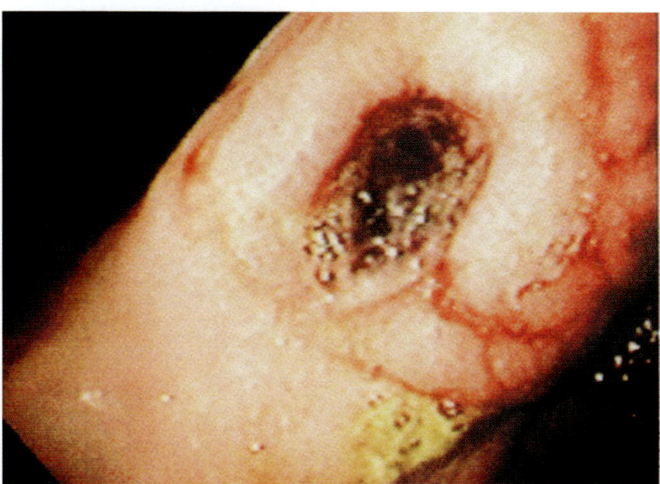

Fig. 48.3: Duodenal ulcer on endoscopy.

Diagnosis

Endoscopy

The diagnostic accuracy of endoscopy is >95%, and it is superior to radiography for defining the presence of lesions of the stomach and duodenum (Fig. 48.3). In addition to demonstrating the actual presence of the lesions, endoscopy allows biopsy and can show whether there is active bleeding. Also, endoscopy can demonstrate other pathologies such as Mallory-Weiss tears of the gastroesophageal junction, acute mucosal erosions, gastritis, duodenitis, and marginal ulcers, which are not well demonstrated by upper gastrointestinal radiographs. Biopsies should be sent to test for *Helicobacter* infection. (For additional information *see* Chapter 13, "Principles of Endoscopy.")

Upper Gastrointestinal Radiographs

The radiologic diagnosis of duodenal ulceration is 75% accurate. Barium studies may show an actual crater deformity indicative of active disease (Fig. 48.4) or merely demonstrate scarring of the duodenal bulb caused by previous ulceration. About 95% of duodenal ulcers occur in the duodenal bulb, and 5% are postbulbar. If a postbulbar ulcer is present, the diagnosis of Zollinger–Ellison syndrome must be considered and excluded by testing (*see* later). Some ulcers occur in the pyloric canal, and these are often called "channel" ulcers. Secondary radiologic signs indicative of an active duodenal ulcer are mucosal edema and spasm. Although postbulbar ulcers may occur anywhere in the duodenum distal to the bulb, 75% occur proximal to the duodenal papilla. They are often small and buried in folds. With healing, the duodenal ulcer becomes

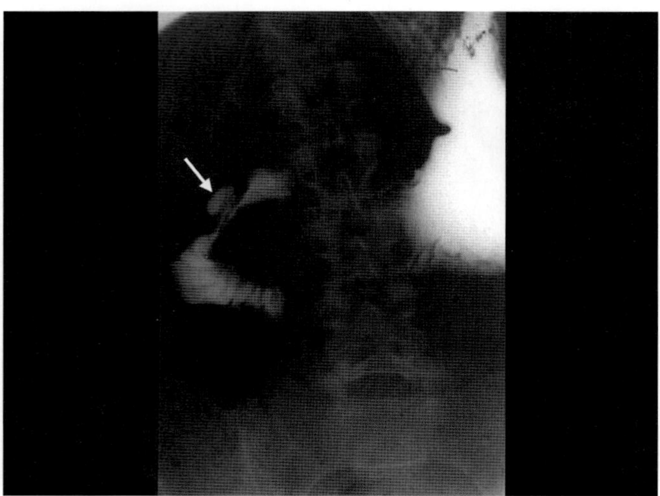

Fig. 48.4: Large postbulbar ulcer of the duodenum. Ulcer is arrowed on this upper gastrointestinal barium study. Its presence indicates active duodenal ulcer disease.

smaller and may disappear altogether. A "cloverleaf" deformity of the duodenal bulb seen in healed ulcer disease is the consequence of fibrosis in the wake of inflammation.

Gastric Analysis

Gastric analysis refers to the measurement of acid output both in the fasting state (basal acid output) and in response to pentagastrin stimulation (MAO). It is not possible to diagnose duodenal ulcer by means of gastric analysis alone. Gastric analysis has fallen into disfavor because it lacks precise correlation with disease and the test is uncomfortable for the patient. The last two indications for gastric analysis were:

- Patients with suspected Zollinger-Ellison syndrome (where secretin stimulation can confirm or exclude the diagnosis)
- Patients with recurrent ulceration following a previous operation, in whom a measurable acid response to sham feeding confirms the presence of residual vagal innervation. Considering the potent antisecretory drugs available, this finding is probably no longer important.

Gastrin

Increased levels of circulating gastrin, secreted by gastrinomas of the pancreas or duodenum, are a feature of Zollinger-Ellison syndrome.

Increased gastrin levels are seen with all antisecretory agents and are directly related to the associated degree of acid suppression.[15] Gastrin concentrations revert to normal within 2–4 weeks of discontinuing the antisecretory agent.

Hypergastrinemia is also seen in patients with pernicious anemia (from loss of acid inhibition of antral gastrin release) and in the rare patient who might have had antral exclusion, which results in permanent sequestration of antral mucosa in the alkaline environment of the duodenum. Hypergastrinemia can also be observed in chronic renal failure and occasionally in patients with pyloric obstruction.

Hypergastrinemia associated with the conditions mentioned earlier can be distinguished from Zollinger–Ellison syndrome by the serum gastrin response to a "secretin stimulation test." Secretin infusion in normal individuals typically suppresses gastrin levels. However, in gastrinoma patients, secretin infusion increases serum gastrin levels.

Helicobacter pylori

Various noninvasive tests are available that are both rapid and reliable, including *H. pylori* antibody and the urea breath test. Although the serology and blood tests are widely available and inexpensive, the urea breath test is not only more sensitive and more specific but also more expensive. When endoscopy is not clinically indicated, the primary diagnosis of *H. pylori* infection can be made serologically or with the urea breath test. When endoscopy is clinically indicated, the primary diagnosis should be established by biopsy, urease testing, and/or histology.

Testing for confirmation of eradication after treatment should be delayed for at least 4 weeks after completion of therapy. The urea breath test is the noninvasive test of choice for confirmation of eradication. Antibody testing is not generally useful to confirm *H. pylori* eradication because specific antibody levels may remain elevated after successful treatment. If endoscopy is clinically indicated after treatment, obtaining multiple biopsy specimens from the gastric body and antrum for both histology and urease testing is recommended to exclude persistent infection. Recently, a stool test for *Helicobacter* antigen has become available, which detects active infection without the need for endoscopy or stopping PPI (proton pump inhibitor) therapy. This test may end up eventually replacing the others.

Medical Management

Medical therapy includes avoidance of agents that damage gastroduodenal mucosal integrity and administration of medications that provide protection (Table 48.2).

Table 48.2 Medical therapy for duodenal ulcer disease.

Avoid ulcerogenic agents
Nonsteroidal anti-inflammatory drugs
Cigarette smoking
Promote mucosal defense
Sulfated disaccharides (e.g., sucralfate)—protective coating
Prostaglandins (e.g., misoprostol)—cytoprotection
H_2-receptor antagonist (e.g., cimetidine)—secretory inhibition
Proton pump inhibitors (e.g., omeprazole)—H^+, K^+-ATPase inhibition
Eradicate Helicobacter pylori
Colloidal bismuth (e.g., bismuth subsalicylate)—protective coating, eradicates *H. pylori* Proton pump inhibitors
Antibiotics (e.g., clarithromycin and metronidazole)—eradicates *H. pylori*

The PPI omeprazole (40 mg/day) is highly efficacious in the treatment of NSAID-associated gastric ulcers and may be more effective than H_2-receptor antagonists. Although the mechanism of NSAID-associated ulceration is an alteration in mucosal defense, the marked acid inhibition provided by omeprazole permits healing of these ulcers since conversion of pepsinogen to activated pepsin is prevented by a pH level >3.5. Prostaglandin analogs such as misoprostol have also been shown to enhance gastric ulcer healing during continued NSAID use. Once NSAID-associated ulcers have healed, prophylactic therapy with H_2-receptor antagonists may be considered to prevent recurrent ulcers.

Abstinence from Ulcerogenic Agents

For patients who have NSAID-associated gastric or duodenal ulcers, the offending agent should be discontinued whenever possible. The history may be difficult to elicit.[16] Many patients do not consider these substances as medications. Patients must be asked what they take for pain or headaches. If NSAIDs are discontinued, both gastric and duodenal ulcers respond rapidly to conventional antiulcer treatment.[17] For some patients who have inflammatory conditions or arthritis, it may not be feasible to discontinue NSAIDs despite active ulceration. Duodenal ulcers and small (<5 mm in diameter) gastric ulcers will heal within 8 weeks of starting H_2-receptor antagonists despite continuation of NSAIDs. The healing rate of larger (>5 mm) gastric ulcers, however, appears to be markedly slower on H_2-receptor antagonist therapy.

Antacids

Antacids have been used for centuries to treat patients with acid-peptic disease and to exert their therapeutic effects by neutralizing gastric acidity. In addition, they appear to promote gastric mucosal defensive mechanisms by stimulating mucus and bicarbonate secretion, prostaglandin release, mucosal regeneration, and mucosal blood flow. Only the aluminum oxide-hydroxide-based formulations have undergone sufficient clinical investigation in ulcer treatment. Many of these formulations also contain magnesium oxide-hydroxide, which contributes to the acid-neutralizing capacity and counteracts the constipating effects of aluminum. Excellent duodenal ulcer healing rates may be achieved with daily doses of antacids with as little as 120–200 mmol of buffering capacity. Healing rates of approximately 70% can be achieved with 4 weeks of therapy.[18]

H_2-Blockers

These agents produce reversible competitive inhibition of the histamine H_2 receptor of the parietal cell, thereby reducing intracellular cAMP and acetylcholine, both of which stimulate acid secretion by increasing intracellular calcium. The H_2-receptor antagonists inhibit not only histamine-stimulated acid secretion but also basal secretion and secretion in response to sham feeding, pentagastrin, and meals in a dose-dependent fashion.[19] All available H_2-receptor antagonists are efficacious in the treatment of duodenal ulcer disease, yielding overall ulcer healing rates of 75% after 4 weeks and 85–90% after 8 weeks of therapy.[19]

A number of randomized trials have compared once-daily bedtime doses with the equivalent dosage administered in twice-daily regimens. Healing rates are equivalent, with the nightly schedules completely suppressing nocturnal acid secretion and having little effect on daytime intragastric acidity.[19] Therefore, for those with uncomplicated duodenal ulcers, once-daily evening or nocturnal regimens offer ease of administration, improved patient compliance, lower cost, and less risk of drug interactions.

Proton Pump Inhibitors

The enzyme hydrogen/potassium ATPase is the final common step in the acid secretory process of the parietal cell referred to as the proton pump. Restoration of acid secretion after proton pump inhibitor administration requires synthesis of new hydrogen/potassium ATPase by the parietal cell. Omeprazole in doses of 20–40 mg/day has proved efficacious in the treatment of acute duodenal ulcers.[20] It produces healing rates of 69% at 2 weeks and 93% at 4 weeks. Proton pump inhibitors also appear to provide more rapid pain relief than H_2-receptor antagonists, with most studies demonstrating earlier pain relief at 1–2 weeks.[20]

Protective Barrier Drugs

Sucralfate: This is a complex salt of sucrose in which hydroxyl groups are replaced by sulfate and aluminum hydroxide. Within an acidic milieu, there is dissociation of aluminum hydroxide into solution, leaving negatively charged sulfate groups, which bind electrostatically to positively charged proteins, mucins, and cells. A protective barrier is therefore formed that limits diffusion of injurious bile salts, pepsin, and acid, so retarding further proteolytic digestion. Sucralfate also has trophic effects on gastric mucosa that may be important in ulcer reepithelialization and stimulating growth of the mucosa. Sucralfate appears to stimulate prostaglandin synthesis, bicarbonate secretion, mucus production, mucosal blood flow, and mucosal regeneration.

Sucralfate is efficacious as both an acute cytoprotective topical agent and a chronic therapeutic agent in peptic ulcer disease.[21] At a dose of 1 g qds (q6h), sucralfate is as effective as H_2-receptor antagonists in the acute therapy of duodenal ulcers. Overall cumulative healing rates with sucralfate are 70% at 4 weeks and 85% at 8 weeks.[19]

Bismuth compounds: Bismuth compounds have been used extensively in the treatment of dyspepsia, peptic ulcer disease, and diarrheal illnesses in the past. More recently, colloidal bismuth sulfate and bismuth subsalicylate have been used in combination with antibiotics in an effort to eradicate *H. pylori.*[22] Bismuth compounds are complex bismuth salts that precipitate in an acidic milieu to form insoluble crystals of bismuth oxychloride and bismuth citrate.

The mechanism of action of the bismuth compounds in peptic ulcer disease seems to be enhancement of mucosal defense mechanisms[22]:

- Bismuth crystals bind preferentially to ulcer craters, creating a protective barrier against acid-peptic digestion
- Bismuth enhances mucosal production of prostaglandin E_2 and bicarbonate secretion
- Finally, bismuth compounds have direct antibacterial action against *H. pylori,* eradicating this organism in one-third of ulcer patients.

Ulcer healing rates with colloidal bismuth sulfate approach 85% at 4 weeks and 95% at 6 weeks. Most importantly, bismuth compounds may have a marked impact on reducing subsequent ulcer recurrence. Twelve-month ulcer relapse rates were reported to be lower with colloidal bismuth sulfate therapy (59%) than with H_2-receptor antagonists (85%).[23]

Prostaglandin Analogs

The mechanisms by which prostaglandin analogs heal ulcers include:

- Stimulation of mucus and bicarbonate secretion
- Enhancement of mucosal blood flow
- Inhibition of acid secretion.

One agent, misoprostol, is approved for the prevention of ulceration in patients on chronic NSAIDs. At antisecretory doses, prostaglandin analogs appear to be more effective than placebo in the acute treatment of gastric and duodenal ulcers but are probably less effective than H_2-receptor antagonists. As a result of their marked side effects (especially diarrhea) and their limited efficacy, they play little role in the acute treatment of duodenal ulcer disease. They should never be used in pregnant women.

Anti-Helicobacter pylori Regimens

A variety of combination regimens, including one, two, or three antimicrobial agents with an H_2-receptor antagonist or a proton pump inhibitor, are being used to treat *H. pylori* infection with eradication rates ranging from 70% to 90%. The US Food and Drug Administration has approved three combination regimens for the treatment of *H. pylori* infection in patients with active duodenal ulcer disease (Table 48.3).

Selection of therapy should be based on efficacy, safety, drug interaction potential, antibiotic resistance, tolerability, convenience, and cost. The likelihood of compliance with the treatment regimen is an important consideration. Poor compliance with treatment can lead to unsuccessful bacterial eradication and the development of antibiotic resistance.

Table 48.3 Treatment regimens for *Helicobacter pylori* infection.

Omeprazole 40 mg/day + clarithromycin 500 mg tds (q8h) for 2 weeks, then omeprazole 20 mg/day for 2 weeks
Ranitidine bismuth citrate (RBC) 400 mg bd (q12h) + clarithromycin 500 mg tds (q8h) for 2 weeks, then RBC 400 mg bd (q12h) for 2 weeks
Bismuth subsalicylate 525 mg qds (q6h) + metronidazole 250 mg (q6h) + tetracycline 500 mg qds (q6h) for 2 weeks + H_2-receptor antagonist for 4 weeks
Lansoprazole 30 mg + amoxicillin 1 g + clarithromycin 500 mg bd (q12h) for 2 weeks

INDICATIONS FOR OPERATIVE MANAGEMENT OF DUODENAL ULCER

The indications for operative treatment of duodenal ulcers have changed considerably in the past 10–20 years. Traditionally, they included intractability, perforation, obstruction, and bleeding. With the decrease in the incidence of peptic ulcer disease, the development of potent H_2-receptor antagonists and proton pump inhibitors, increasing evidence regarding the role of *H. pylori*,[24] and the increased availability and use of NSAIDs, intractability should be eliminated as an indication for operation in duodenal ulcer disease. Furthermore, the early and late complications and side effects of operations for duodenal ulcer can be debilitating in many patients (Table 48.4; *See* "Postgastrectomy Syndromes" later in this chapter). Operations to treat complicated ulcer disease, including cases of perforation, obstruction, and hemorrhage, should be approached with current knowledge of the etiology and medical treatments for peptic ulceration.

Perforation

Erosion of an anterior duodenal ulcer through the full thickness of the duodenal wall results in free perforation into the peritoneal cavity. This complication occurs in 5–10% of patients who have a duodenal ulcer and may be the initial presentation of the disease. The pain is usually sudden and intense and results in patients seeking immediate medical attention. However, debilitated patients and those on corticosteroids may have minimal symptoms of peritonitis and present late in the disease when septic or in shock. Chest radiographs demonstrate pneumoperitoneum in up to 75% of cases (Fig. 48.5). In a minority of patients, the omentum or liver seals the perforation before severe peritoneal soilage occurs. The clinical presentation in these patients may be atypical and lead to the misdiagnosis of pancreatitis, cholecystitis, or appendicitis. An upper gastrointestinal series with water-soluble contrast may demonstrate a sealed perforation. If pneumoperitoneum is absent, a computed tomogram (CT) scan may demonstrate subhepatic or lesser sac fluid collections (Fig. 48.6).

Duodenal ulcer perforation is an indication for operation in most patients. Some authors have advocated a nonoperative approach for selected patients:

- Without generalized peritonitis
- Without continuing duodenal leakage as confirmed by water-soluble contrast study
- For those who have absolute contraindications for laparotomy.[25]

Table 48.4 Side effects of operations for duodenal ulcer.

Early postoperative complications	*Long-term side effects*
Afferent loop obstruction	Alkaline reflux gastritis
Anastomotic leak	Anemia
Duodenal stump leak	Dumping syndrome
Efferent loop obstruction	Gallstones
Gastric atony	Gastric remnant cancer
Gastric outlet obstruction	Malnutrition
Hemorrhage	Postprandial hypoglycemia
Acute pancreatitis	Postvagotomy diarrhea
	Weight loss
	Reflux esophagitis
	Small bowel obstruction

Fig. 48.5: Massive pneumoperitoneum caused by a perforated duodenal ulcer.

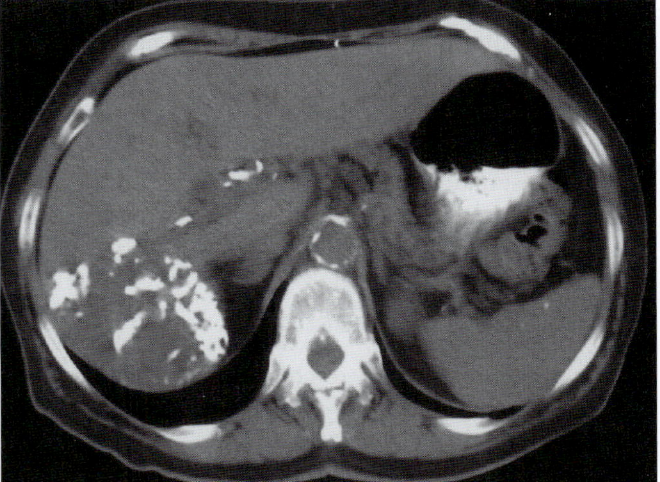

Fig. 48.6: Extravasation of contrast into the peritoneal cavity from a perforated duodenal ulcer.

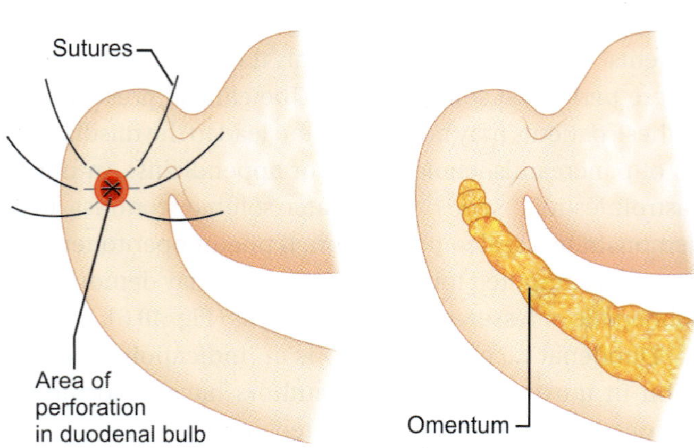

Fig. 48.7: Omental onlay patch for a perforated duodenal ulcer.

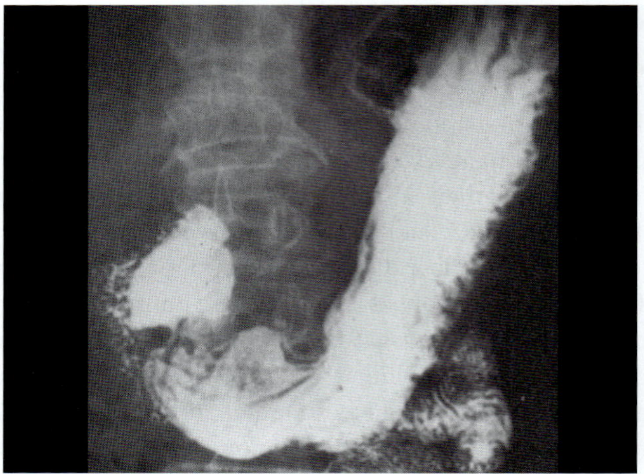

Fig. 48.8: Gastric outlet obstruction due to chronic peptic ulceration. Upper gastrointestinal barium radiograph. Note the elongated configuration of the stomach, which is displaced inferiorly.

Treatment in these cases consists of intravenous fluids, nasogastric suction, broad-spectrum antibiotics, and H_2-receptor antagonists. Implementation of this approach should be extremely selective.

In a large prospective study evaluating perforated duodenal ulcers, three factors predicted death:

- Preoperative shock
- Perforation for longer than 24 hours
- Concomitant medical illness.[26]

Therefore, nearly all patients who have a perforated duodenal ulcer should undergo expeditious resuscitation and operation.

Simple closure of the perforation can be achieved by suture plication of the ulcer if possible and then application of an omental patch (Fig. 48.7). This maneuver can be performed by either formal laparotomy or laparoscopy. In the past, there was enthusiasm for an acid-reducing procedure in certain cases of perforated duodenal ulcer because of the high recurrence rates (affecting nearly two-thirds of patients).[27] However, this practice is changing with the present understanding of the etiology of ulcer disease and the fears of suture-line dehiscence, mediastinitis, and long-term side effects of these surgical procedures.[28]

Gastric Outlet Obstruction

Gastric outlet obstruction remains an important indication for operation in peptic ulcer disease. Most patients requiring admission to the hospital with emesis from gastric outlet obstruction secondary to ulcer disease do not have a fixed obstruction, but rather ulcer-induced inflammatory edema or impaired antral motility. Upper gastrointestinal radiographs will demonstrate an elongated, dilated, hypotonic stomach, with delays in transit of contrast into the duodenum (Fig. 48.8).

Patients who have gastric outlet obstruction caused by inflammatory edema can be successfully treated with nasogastric tube decompression, intravenous rehydration, and an H_2-receptor antagonist. Total parenteral nutrition should be instituted early for those with severe malnutrition. Endoscopy, which can be both diagnostic and therapeutic, should be performed to confirm the mechanical nature of the obstruction and rule out the presence of a neoplasm. Endoscopic dilatation of these strictures has shown promise.[29] After the acute ulcer has healed, balloon dilatation of short gastroduodenal strictures can be accomplished by endoscopy.

If dilatation of peptic strictures combined with aggressive medical management is unsuccessful, a number of operative options remain. Before any operation, a thorough history should be taken directed toward delineating the use of NSAIDs, and appropriate diagnostic tests should be performed to check for the presence of *H. pylori.* The operation selected for obstructing duodenal ulcer should relieve the mechanical emptying problem, and there should be plans for subsequent aggressive medical management of the ulcer diathesis.

A variety of operations have been conducted, ranging from vagotomy and antrectomy to stricturoplasty alone. If there is active inflammation or dense scarring to the pancreas, duodenal mobilization for antrectomy can be hazardous. This maneuver can be avoided by mobilizing the duodenum completely before dividing the stomach. If there is dense scarring, antrectomy is best avoided.

Various methods have been proposed for handling a scarred and inflamed duodenum after antrectomy. If a posterior ulcer has eroded into the pancreas, the scarred duodenum can be sutured to the ulcerated area of the pancreas (Fig. 48.9). Decompression of the duodenum with a temporary duodenostomy tube is useful to control pancreatobiliary secretions following antrectomy and Billroth II anastomosis (Figs. 48.10A and B). The duodenostomy tube can then be pulled out at a later date.

Stricturoplasty can relieve the gastric outlet obstruction caused by a peptic ulcer without adding the irreversible effects of a vagotomy. A horizontal incision through the narrowed segment, followed by vertical closure, is performed in a fashion analogous to a Heineke-Mikulicz pyloroplasty (Figs. 48.11A and B). Other investigators advocate a concomitant proximal gastric vagotomy at the time of stricturoplasty to treat the ulcer disease.[29]

Hemorrhage

Most patients who have acute hemorrhage from duodenal ulcers stop bleeding spontaneously.[30] However, hemorrhage remains the principal cause of death from peptic ulcer disease. Bleeding duodenal ulcers are usually situated on the posterior wall of the duodenal bulb. Penetration of the ulcer through the duodenum with erosion into the gastroduodenal artery or one of its branches can result in rapid hemorrhage. Patients may present with hematemesis when hemorrhage is severe, but only with melena if the bleeding is slow or there is no duodenogastric reflux. The diagnosis is made by early endoscopy to localize the bleeding source and achieve hemostasis.

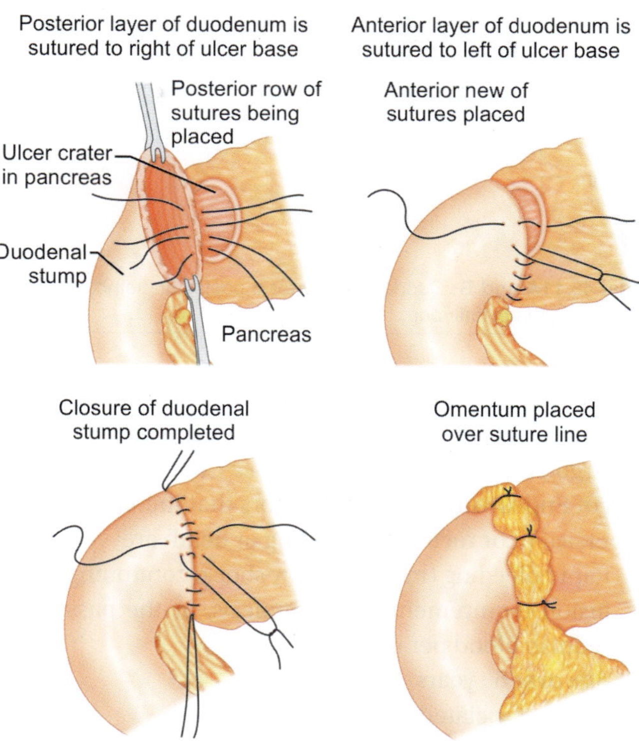

Fig. 48.9: Treatment of the duodenal stump following antrectomy when a posterior duodenal ulcer has penetrated into the pancreas. The posterior layer of the duodenum is first sutured to the right of the ulcer base. The anterior layer of the duodenum is then also sutured to the pancreas, to the left of the ulcer crater. Omentum is placed over the duodenal closure to prevent leakage.

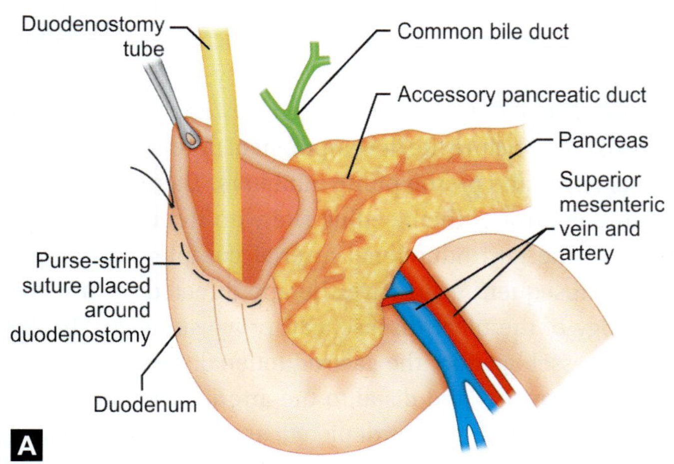

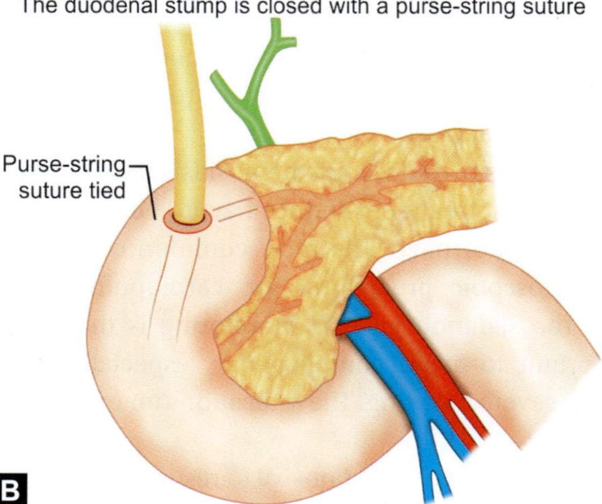

Figs. 48.10A and B: Treatment of the "difficult" duodenal stump following antrectomy. The accessory pancreatic duct is in close approximation to the area of closure of the duodenum. A duodenostomy tube is placed in the duodenal stump and closed with a purse-string suture. The tube is then brought out through the abdominal wall to drain pancreatobiliary secretions. Some surgeons prefer to close the duodenum primarily and bring the tube out through a small lateral duodenotomy.

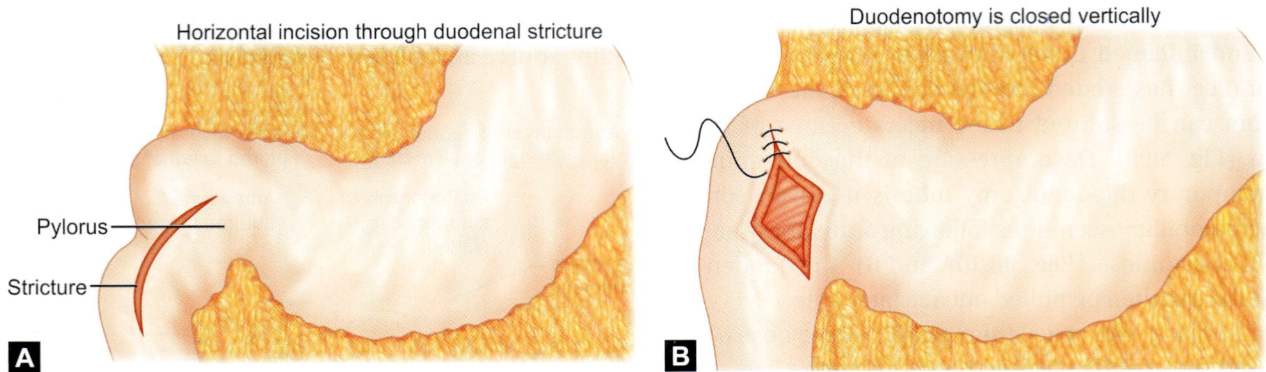

Figs. 48.11A and B: Duodenoplasty for a postpyloric stricture. The longitudinal incision is converted to a transverse suture line and does not transgress the pyloric ring.

Endoscopy plays an important role in treating bleeding duodenal ulcers. Selected high-risk patients should undergo endoscopic hemostasis (*see* Chapter 13, "Principles of Endoscopy"). Clinical factors that increase the risk of persistent or recurrent bleeding or death are:

- Rapid bleeding (manifested by shock, continuing transfusion requirements, hematemesis, or the passage of reddish blood per rectum)
- Age over 60 years
- Major associated diseases
- In-hospital bleeding
- Rebleeding episodes after admission.[31]

Endoscopic findings of pulsatile bleeding or oozing from the ulcer or the finding of a visible vessel or sentinel clot in the ulcer are also indications for endoscopic hemostatic treatment.[32] Interventions commonly used include electrocoagulation devices, heater probes, endoscopic clips, and injection methods. Heater probes and bipolar electrocoagulation are the preferred methods, but injection therapy with vasoconstrictors or sclerosing agents is also safe and efficacious.

Complications of endoscopic hemostasis include perforation, necrosis, treatment-induced acute hemorrhage, and delayed hemorrhage. The most common complications of endoscopic procedures are cardiopulmonary, related to the sedation given.[33] Monitoring is therefore very important to avoid complications, especially in a patient with severe bleeding. The indications for operation include:

- Severe hemorrhage unresponsive to resuscitation
- Prolonged bleeding with cumulative loss of 50% or more of the estimated blood volume
- Recurrence of hemorrhage after initial control with medical or endoscopic measures
- A second hospitalization for ulcer hemorrhage
- A coexisting additional indication for operation.[30]

Endoscopic findings of a visible vessel, pulsatile bleeding, or active oozing not only are indications for endoscopic hemostatic treatment (*see* earlier) but also correlate with ongoing or recurrent bleeding that requires operative intervention.[34] An aggressive operative approach should be considered when one or more of the indications for operation are present and endoscopy demonstrates one of the aforementioned findings.

The operation selected for the patient who has a bleeding duodenal ulcer should arrest the hemorrhage, and there should be subsequent plans for aggressive medical management of the ulcer diathesis. Previous surgical dictum stated that the choice of operation depended upon the age and condition of the patient and the size, location, and bleeding rate of the ulcer. Historically, vagotomy and pyloroplasty with suture ligation of the bleeding ulcer or vagotomy and antrectomy were advocated for bleeding duodenal ulcer.[35] However, this policy arose before the knowledge of the etiologic role of *H. pylori* and the role of NSAIDs and before the development of potent H_2-receptor antagonists and proton pump inhibitors. Therefore, simple suture control of the bleeding site with three-vessel ligation of the gastroduodenal arterial complex, combined with subsequent aggressive therapy directed toward the etiology of the ulcer disease, can prove sufficient. In the three vessel ligation, the gastroduodenal artery is suture-ligated proximal and distal to the arterial opening with a simple suture ligature as depicted; a third suture is placed around the site of the hole in the vessel as a horizontal mattress to control the transverse pancreatic branch, which usually enters posteriorly and accounts for many rebleeding episodes (Fig. 48.12).

OPERATIONS FOR DUODENAL ULCER

Operations used historically for the operative treatment of duodenal ulcer include vagotomies, gastric resections, drainage procedures, or combinations thereof. Each operation has specific effects on gastric secretion and motility and has variable results regarding postoperative recurrence and the subsequent development of postgastrectomy symptoms (Table 48.5).

Vagotomy

Three alternative types of vagotomy are proximal gastric, total gastric, and truncal. The purpose of vagotomy is to denervate the acid-producing fundal and body mucosa, so eliminating the cephalic phase of gastric secretion. An unavoidable side effect of any vagotomy is altered gastric motility and gastric emptying although the degree of disrupted motility varies with the completeness of vagotomy (Fig. 48.13).

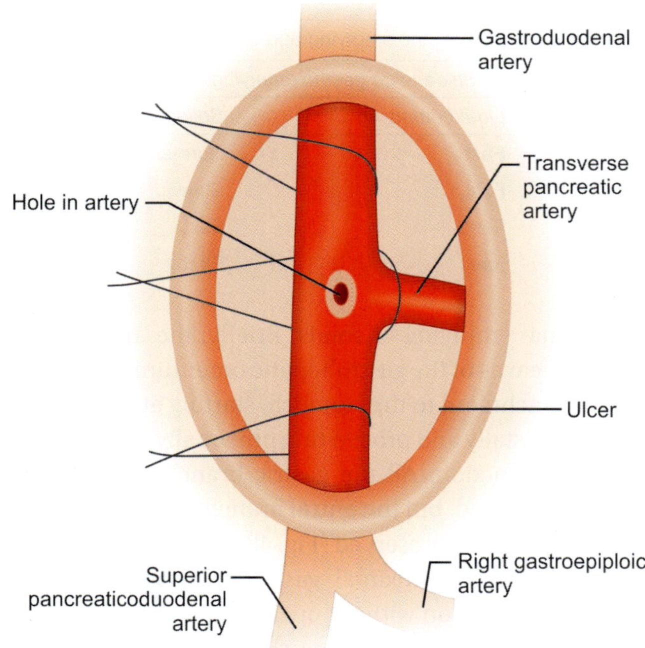

Fig. 48.12: Principles of three-point ligation of the bleeding site of a duodenal ulcer penetrating the gastroduodenal arterial complex. The gastroduodenal artery is suture-ligated proximal and distal to the arterial perforation. The third suture is a horizontal mattress suture placed around the site of the vascular perforation to control the transverse pancreatic branch. Failure to do this may be an important cause of recurrent hemorrhage in the immediate postoperative period.

In proximal gastric (highly selective) vagotomy, the vagal branches to the fundus and corpus are divided, leaving intact the branches to the antrum, pylorus, and remainder of the gastrointestinal tract. Proximal gastric vagotomy does not require an additional operative procedure to drain the stomach. It abolishes gastric receptive relaxation and impairs accommodation and storage in the proximal stomach.

After proximal gastric vagotomy, intragastric pressure increases and gastric distention leads to more rapid gastric emptying of liquids. The quickening of gastric emptying is usually not sufficient to result in dumping or diarrhea. Most importantly, the strength of antral peristaltic contractions, gastric trituration, and gastric emptying of digestible and indigestible solids are not altered. Also, the antropyloric mechanism that retains solids and prevents duodenogastric reflux is maintained.[36]

Truncal Vagotomy

In truncal vagotomy, the vagal nerves to the stomach and the rest of the gastrointestinal tract receiving vagal innervation are divided. Truncal vagotomy is usually combined with pyloroplasty or gastroenterostomy to facilitate gastric emptying. It has effects on proximal gastric motor physiology that are similar to those of proximal gastric vagotomy. However, unlike proximal gastric vagotomy, truncal vagotomy has marked effects on distal gastric motor function. It weakens distal gastric peristalsis, impairs trituration, and delays gastric emptying of both digestible and indigestible solids.[37] Therefore, another operative procedure is necessary to improve the delayed emptying. Distal gastric resection, pyloroplasty, and gastroenterostomy all decrease

Table 48.5 Incidence of recurrent ulcer and postgastrectomy syndromes after operation for duodenal ulcer.

Original operation	*Incidence of recurrence (%)*	*Incidence of postgastrectomy syndromes (%)*	*Mortality rate (%)*
Proximal gastric vagotomy	10	5	0.1
Truncal vagotomy and drainage	7	20–30	<1
Truncal vagotomy and antrectomy/Billroth I or Billroth II	1	30–50	0–5
Truncal vagotomy and antrectomy/Roux-en-Y	5–10	50–60	0–5

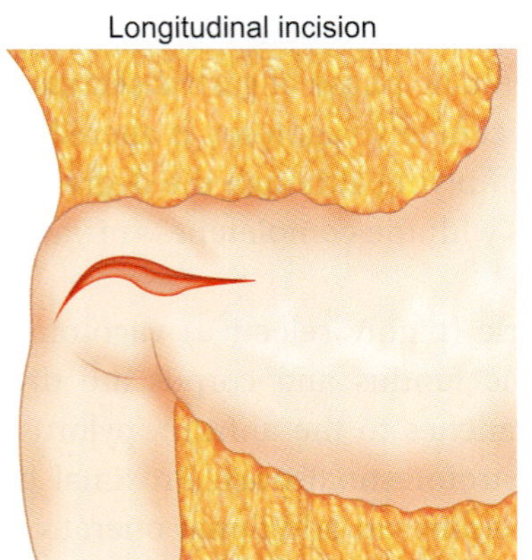

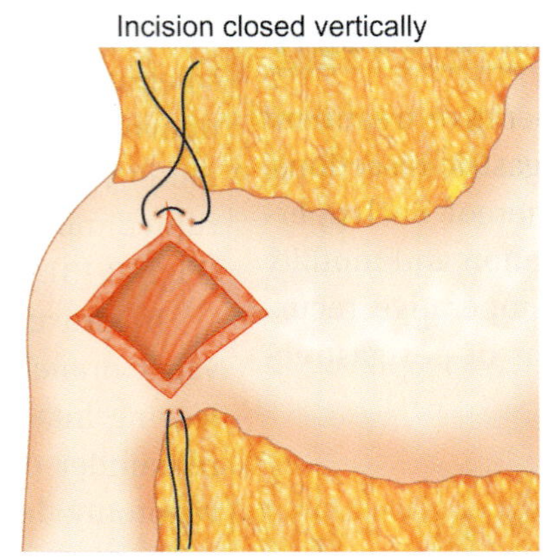

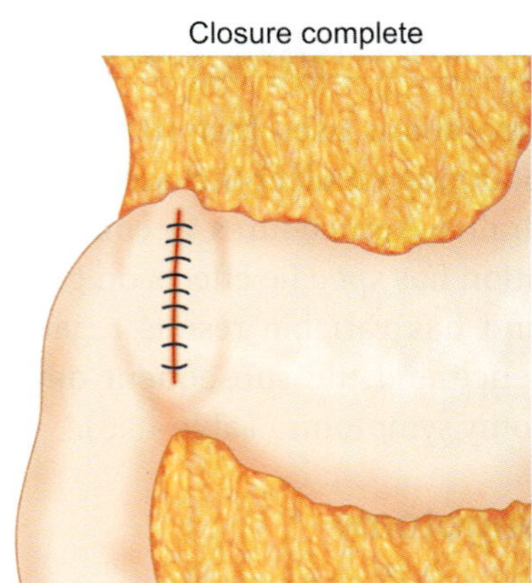

Fig. 48.13: Heineke-Mikulicz pyloroplasty. A longitudinal incision is made through the distal stomach, pylorus, and proximal duodenum. This incision is then closed in a vertical fashion, which destroys the sphincter.

Table 48.6 Operations historically performed for peptic ulcer disease and their effects on gastric emptying and gastric mobility.

	Effects of operations for peptic ulcer disease on gastric emptying and gastric mobility		
Operation	*Antral innervation*	*Liquid emptying*	*Solid emptying*
Proximal gastric vagotomy	Preserved	Fast	Normal
Truncal vagotomy	Divided	Fast	Slow
Truncal vagotomy and drainage	Divided	Fast	Fast
Truncal vagotomy and antrectomy	Divided	Fast	Fast

the resistance to outflow from the stomach and thus enhance the gastric emptying of solids after total gastric or truncal vagotomy (Table 48.6).

Vagotomy and Pyloroplasty

Combining vagotomy with pyloroplasty produces alterations in gastric motility that are the net result of the two procedures. Both proximal and distal gastric motility are impaired after vagotomy, as is vagally induced acid secretion. Pyloroplasty has little effect on the functions of the proximal stomach, but the disruption of the pylorus results in impaired trituration, rapid gastric emptying of solids, and increased duodenogastric reflux. There are multiple techniques for pyloroplasty; of these, the Heineke-Mikulicz (Fig. 48.13), the Jaboulay (Fig. 48.14), and the Finney (Fig. 48.15) are the most commonly used.

After vagotomy and pyloroplasty, the incidence of ulcer recurrence is approximately 7% and the risk of postgastrectomy symptoms approximately 20–30% (*see* Table 48.5).

Proximal Gastric Vagotomy

Proximal gastric vagotomy impairs receptive relaxation and accommodation in the proximal stomach, resulting in rapid emptying of liquids, but normal antral contractions and normal emptying of solids. Briefly, the anterior and posterior leaves of the gastrohepatic omentum are divided at their attachment to the stomach, starting at the incisura angularis distally and proceeding proximally to the esophagogastric junction. All the gastric branches of the vagi should be divided, but the antral branches of the nerves of Latarjet should be preserved (Fig. 48.16).

The appeal of proximal gastric vagotomy is that it offers acid reduction without opening the gastrointestinal tract and without denervating the rest of the gastrointestinal tract. Most importantly, it has the lowest mortality rate. Of all operations for the treatment of duodenal ulcer, proximal gastric vagotomy has the highest incidence of ulcer recurrence (~10%) and the lowest risk of postgastrectomy symptoms (~5%) (*see* Table 48.5). It should not be done for pyloric channel ulcers because of a high recurrence rate. This procedure is also readily adaptable to laparoscopic techniques, but since the introduction of antibiotic therapy for H. pylori, it has seldom been required.

Recently, some enthusiasm has been directed toward posterior truncal vagotomy and anterior seromyotomy performed laparoscopically.[38] The technique is efficacious in terms of reducing acid secretion, thus sustaining ulcer healing as well as truncal vagotomy and drainage, and it

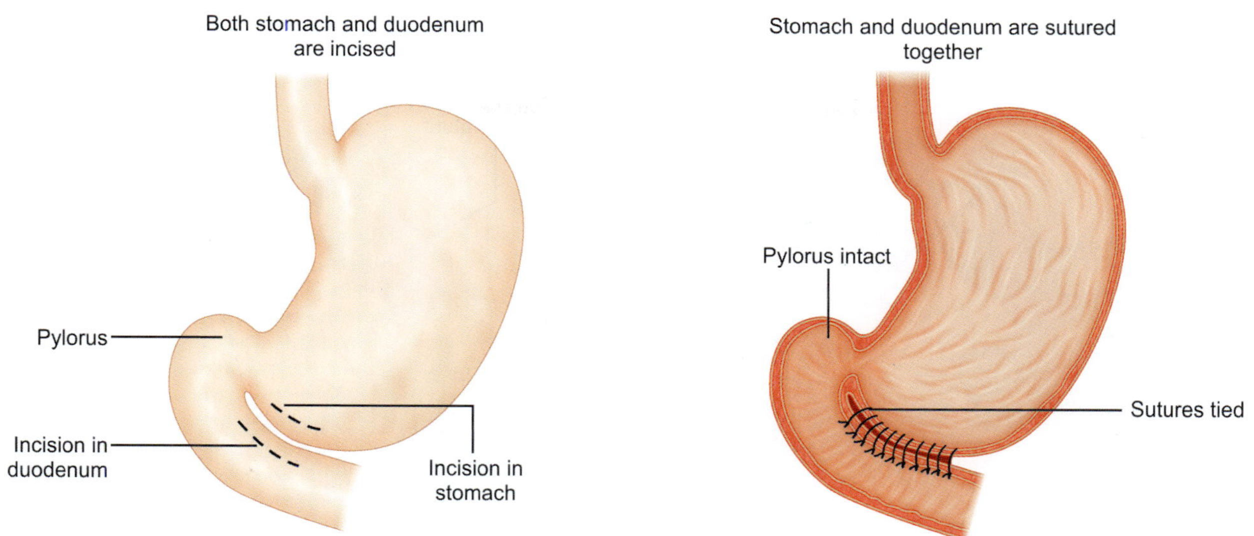

Fig. 48.14: Jaboulay pyloroplasty. A two-layer anastomosis is made between the stomach and duodenum. In this drainage procedure, the incision is not carried through the pylorus.

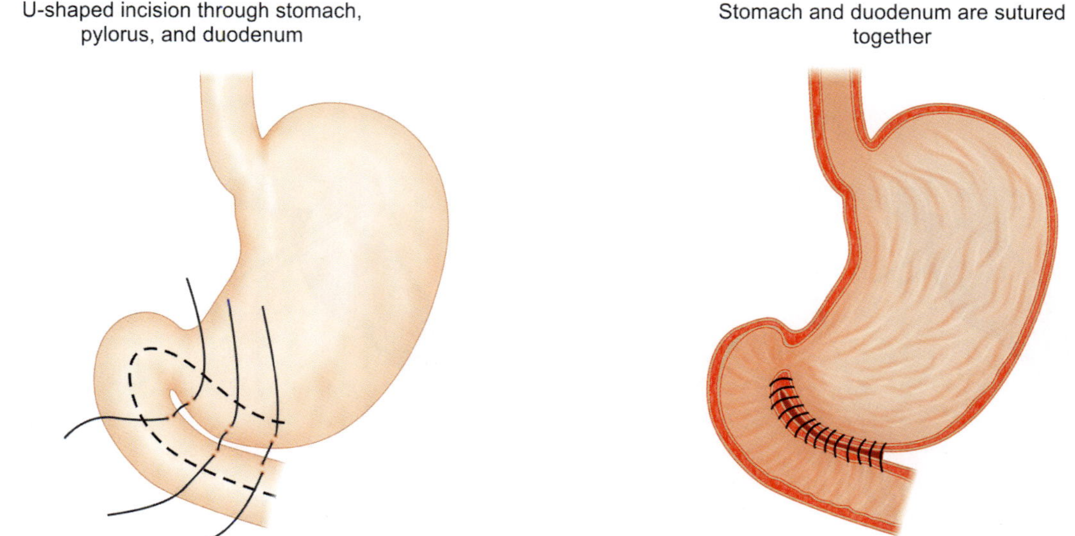

Fig. 48.15: Finney pyloroplasty. A two-layer anastomosis is made between the stomach and duodenum using a U-shaped incision through the distal stomach, pylorus, and proximal duodenum.

is associated with few postprandial symptoms. However, long-term follow-up will be needed to assess adequately this "minimally invasive" procedure.

Vagotomy and Antrectomy

The most common gastric resection used for the treatment of duodenal ulcer disease is removal of the distal stomach and pylorus with either a gastroduodenal anastomosis or a gastrojejunal anastomosis. Vagotomy and antrectomy eliminate both the cephalic and gastric phases of gastric secretion. As mentioned previously, vagotomy results in impaired receptive relaxation and accommodation and rapid gastric emptying of liquids. As resection of the distal stomach becomes more extensive, accommodation and storage are more likely to be impaired, resulting in more rapid gastric emptying of liquids. Antrectomy abolishes antral trituration and results in rapid gastric emptying of solids. Loss of the pylorus destroys the distal gastric mechanism that prevents duodenogastric reflux.

In performing an antrectomy, the external landmark for the antral-fundal junction on the lesser curvature of the stomach is the incisura angularis. A line drawn

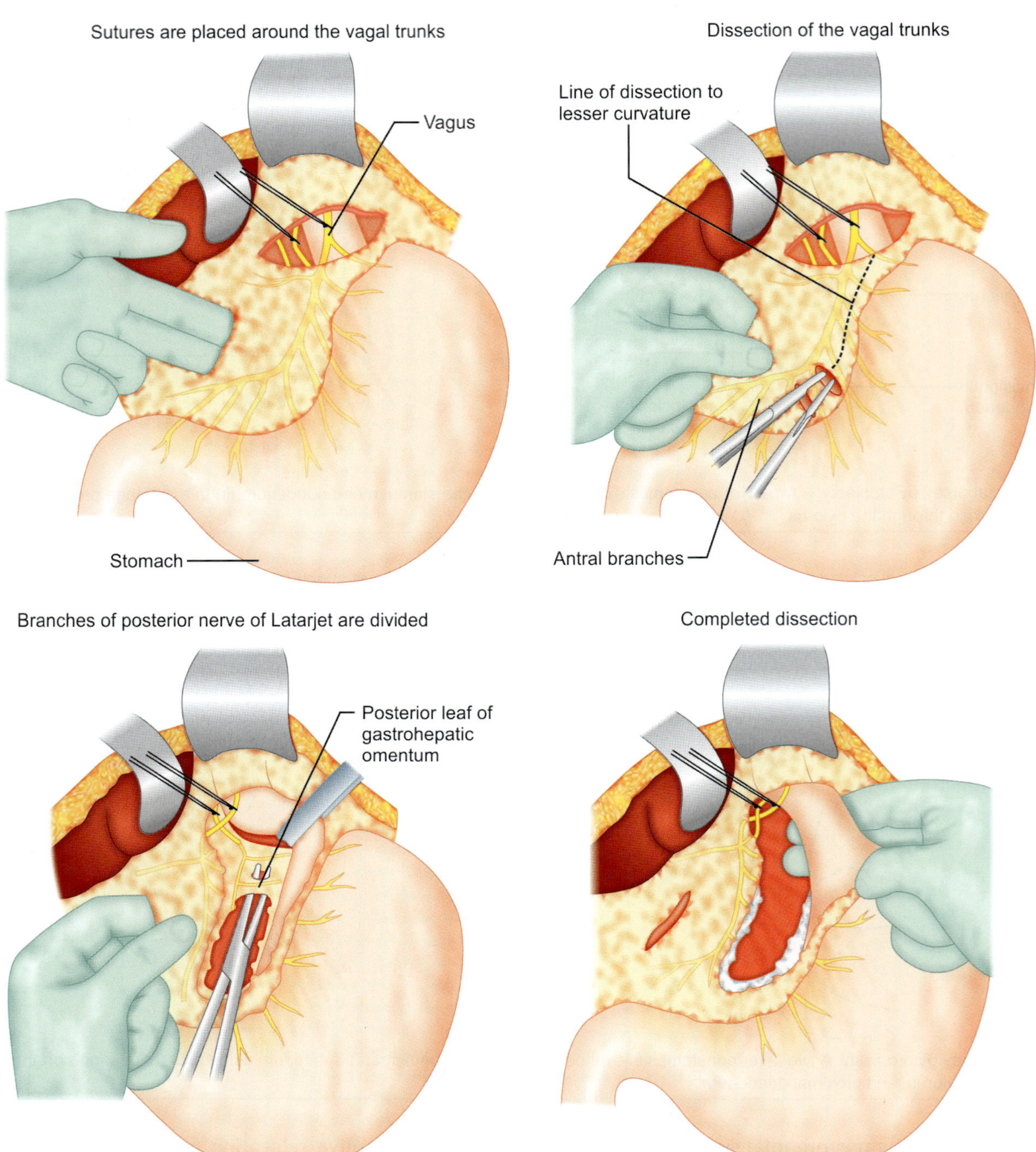

Fig. 48.16: Proximal gastric vagotomy. The esophagus is mobilized and sutures are placed around the vagal trunks. Subsequent dissection is carried adjacent to the lesser curvature. The perpendicular branches of the anterior nerve of Latarjet along with the accompanying vessels are divided between hemostats beginning proximal to the so-called crow's foot. The branches of the posterior nerve of Latarjet are isolated and divided. The lesser curve is devascularized and denervated, beginning 7 cm proximal to the pylorus. The esophagus is dissected for a distance of 5–7 cm to the level of the muscularis to divide any additional vagal branches.

inferiorly and 45° to the left down to the greater curvature approximates the junction of the antrum and fundus. Gastroduodenostomy appears to be preferable to gastrojejunostomy.

Patients who have a vagotomy and antrectomy have the lowest incidence of ulcer recurrence (1%), but a 30–50% incidence of postgastrectomy symptoms and a 0–5% mortality rate (*see* Table 48.5).

Postoperative Complications

Early postoperative complications include hemorrhage and leakage from the gastrointestinal tract. Hemorrhage in the immediate postoperative period usually results from bleeding at a suture line or failure to control bleeding from the ulcer.

The scarred inflamed duodenum can present difficulty during gastric resection for duodenal ulcer. The most serious common complication following resection is leakage from the duodenal stump in a Billroth II anastomosis or leakage at the gastroduodenostomy in a Billroth I procedure. Both result in peritonitis and are associated with ileus, sepsis, and a mortality rate of up to 15%. Resection is associated with a higher incidence of breakdown of the suture line than with drainage procedures because dissection is carried out in areas of ulcer scarring and the blood supply to the remaining structures may be compromised. The best way to handle a difficult duodenal stump is to avoid making one.

Another factor that contributes to leakage of a duodenal stump is obstruction of the afferent limb after construction of a gastrojejunostomy. This obstruction results in distention of the afferent loop with bile and pancreatic secretion, leading to increased pressure, which may cause breakdown of the suture line.

Patients who have leakage of a duodenal stump have an acute exacerbation of abdominal pain, typically on the 5th–7th postoperative day. The severity of the patient's symptoms is related to the degree of leakage. When the leak is sizable, there are activated pancreatic enzymes and duodenal content throughout the peritoneal cavity, resulting in symptoms of an acute abdomen. If the leak is small, the patient may have a low-grade fever or mild discomfort associated with a small upper abdominal abscess. A CT scan can provide evidence of the leak, but surgical exploration is diagnostic. Since duodenal stump blowout carries a 50% mortality rate, relaparotomy is justified for diagnosis and placement of adequate drains.

Recurrent Duodenal Ulcer

Etiology

The incidence of ulcer recurrence after a gastric operation depends upon several factors.[39] Recurrent ulcers are more common after an operation for an "intractable" duodenal ulcer than after an operation for a gastric ulcer. In addition, with the steady decline in operations for peptic ulcers, an increasing percentage of patients now seen with postoperative recurrent ulcers received the original operation for reasons unrelated to peptic ulcer. Before the increased use of NSAIDs in the population, the recurrence rate varied with the type of operation performed (*see* Table 48.5). Low ulcer recurrence rates were gained at the cost of more postgastrectomy complications and deaths. The occasional recurrent duodenal ulcer is due to Zollinger-Ellison syndrome (*see* later). Finally, and probably most importantly, behavioral risk factors play an important role for recurrent ulcers. Numerous studies suggest a causal relationship between chronic gastric ulceration and ingestion of NSAIDs.[40] In addition, cigarette smoking appears to play a pathogenic role in both duodenal and gastric ulceration. Postoperative ulceration has not been shown to be caused by *H. pylori* because most recurrent ulcers occur in *H. pylori*-negative stomachs. In addition, 50–90% of postgastrectomy patients are free of *H. pylori*.

Clinical Features

More than 90% of unoperated patients with primary peptic ulcer have pain, whereas the incidence of pain in patients who have postoperative recurrent ulcers is only about 40%. The pain in postoperative patients is typically vague and is difficult to distinguish from other postgastrectomy syndromes such as gastritis or delayed gastric emptying. Upper gastrointestinal bleeding is frequently the first symptom of postoperative recurrent ulcer, occurring in 40–60% of patients. A recurrent ulcer in the pyloric channel or duodenum or at a gastrojejunal anastomosis may lead to gastric outlet obstruction. Symptoms include nausea, early satiety, vomiting, and weight loss. However, these symptoms are identical to those produced by gastric atony. Perforation is a very uncommon presentation for a recurrent ulcer.

Diagnosis

The first diagnostic test in patients who have unexplained symptoms after a gastric operation is endoscopy. Upper gastrointestinal radiographs may play a role in determining the postoperative anatomy but frequently mistake postoperative changes for peptic ulcers. Recurrent ulcers nearly always occur within 1–2 cm of the gastrointestinal anastomosis, and biopsies should be obtained to exclude cancer. The most common causes or possible contributing factors for postoperative recurrent ulcers and the complementary diagnostic tests are shown in Table 48.7.

Table 48.7 Causes, investigation, and management of postoperative recurrent ulcer.

	Postoperative recurrent ulcer	
Causes and contributing factors	*Investigation*	*Management*
Ulcerogenic drugs and smoking	History, serum salicylate levels	Discontinue drug use or smoking
Helicobacter pylori infection	Endoscopy, serum antibodies	Treatment to eradicate *H. pylori* (*see* Table 48.2)
Nonabsorbable suture	Endoscopy	Remove suture
Zollinger-Ellison syndrome	Endoscopy, serum gastrin, secretin stimulation	Operation to excise tumor (gastrinoma)
Gastric cancer	Endoscopy	Operation—gastric resection
Gastric outlet obstruction	Endoscopy	Dilatation or operation
Bezoar and atony	Endoscopy	Remove bezoar
Bile reflux	Endoscopy	Cholestyramine, ursodeoxycholic acid, operation to divert bile
Retained antrum	Serum gastrin	Operation, resect retained antrum
Antral G-cell hyperplasia hyperplasia	Serum gastrin	Operation—antrectomy
Primary hyperparathyroidism	Serum calcium	Operation—parathyroidectomy
Incomplete vagotomy	Sham feeding test	Operation—completion vagotomy

Three diagnostic procedures should be performed for virtually all patients who present with recurrent ulcer:

- Initial endoscopy may help diagnose and even treat many causes of recurrent ulcer
- Serum gastrin levels should be determined in all patients—patients who have hypergastrinemia should undergo studies to determine the cause, which may be pancreatic islet cell tumor, retained antrum, G-cell hyperplasia, or administration of H_2-receptor antagonists or proton pump inhibitors
- Serum calcium concentrations should be determined in all patients and appropriate treatment instituted. Any patient with duodenal ulcer and hypercalcemia should be suspected of having the multiple endocrine neoplasia (MEN) type 1 syndrome with a parathyroid adenoma and a gastrinoma.

When acid is not the cause of postoperative ulcer recurrence, two other factors require evaluation:

- Presence of *H. pylori*
- Use of NSAIDs.

Although *H. pylori* has been implicated in recurrent ulceration in the intact stomach, its role in the recurrence of postoperative ulcer is unclear. Determining the presence of *H. pylori* by biopsy and serum antibodies may help in diagnosis. Urea breath tests can be unreliable after a gastric operation. Most importantly, a history of NSAID use should be elicited, and salicylate levels should be determined on more than one occasion to exclude surreptitious aspirin use.

Medical Management

Several studies have shown that H_2-receptor antagonists effectively treat postoperative recurrent ulcers,[41] but endoscopic evaluation of ulcer healing is required for all such patients. After healing, maintenance therapy with antisecretory medication is necessary. Discontinuation of maintenance treatment results in ulcer recurrence in nearly all patients. Cigarette smoking should be stopped if possible.

If *H. pylori* is found, it should be eliminated (*see* Table 48.3), even though its role in recurrent postoperative ulcers is unclear. Abuse of NSAIDs and aspirin should be rigorously excluded before recommending elective operation for intractable, recurrent, or complicated peptic ulcer. If NSAIDs or aspirin is being used, their intake should be stopped if at all possible. There is a substantial underreporting of NSAID use by patients. If these drugs are not discontinued, the patient will continue to have intractable and complicated ulcer disease. Proton pump inhibitors are sometimes effective, but outcome should be closely monitored. If stenosis is causing obstruction of the gastric outlet, endoscopic dilatation combined with potent acid suppression is of benefit only when ulcerogenic agents (aspirin and NSAIDs) are stopped. An operation may be unavoidable, but a relapse is a certainty with continued abuse of NSAIDs.

Operative Management

In the past, a number of authors proposed that all reoperations should include re-resection and revagotomy.[39] However, long-term morbidity is common with this approach, with as many as 45% of patients having unsatisfactory long-term outcomes. Ulcer recurrence, gastric emptying problems, bile reflux gastritis, and chronic pain combine to give poor clinical results. In most patients, antisecretory regimens and abstention from ulcerogenic medications are adequate. Therefore, only the minimal necessary operation should be performed, on the basis of the preoperative assessment. Scintigraphic determination of gastric emptying is required to demonstrate whether slowed gastric emptying may be contributing to recurrent ulceration in patients with a previous partial gastrectomy.

If serum gastrin levels and acid secretory studies implicate a gastrinoma as the cause of recurrent ulcer, exploration should be performed with the intent of identifying and removing the tumor. In the rare patient in whom no tumor is found, the medical management of Zollinger-Ellison syndrome may be successful in up to 90% of patients.

Revision or resection of obstructed gastroenterostomies with impaired motility should include a resection that leaves a small gastric remnant. Roux-en-Y gastrojejunostomy for the management of bile reflux gastritis is successful in eliminating alkaline reflux and bilious vomiting. However, 40% of patients develop nausea, vomiting, and abdominal pain—the Roux stasis syndrome (*see* "Postgastrectomy Syndromes" later this chapter).

STRESS ULCER

Etiology

Acute superficial ulcerative lesions of the gastroduodenal area have been called acute mucosal erosions, stress ulcers, acute peptic ulcers, erosive gastritis, hemorrhagic gastritis, and Curling's or Cushing's ulcers.

In stress ulceration, the stomach appears to be the target organ for metabolic alterations caused by a variety of diseases that result in multiple system organ failure. The high concentration of acid and digestive enzymes in the stomach and duodenum renders this area vulnerable during periods of sepsis, hypotension, or pulmonary insufficiency. An episode of shock often precedes acute mucosal bleeding.

The mechanism by which stress causes mucosal ulceration is multifactorial and includes:

- Decreased splanchnic perfusion
- Disruption of the mucosal barrier with back-diffusion of acid
- Decreased availability of energy substrates.

In both experimental and clinical studies, patchy areas of ischemia are detectable within 12 hours of the insult. Ischemia may initiate a series of cellular changes culminating in superficial infarction. If there is back-diffusion of acid, frank superficial ulcerations are more likely to develop. Some degree of acidity in the stomach is necessary to produce the erosive changes. Although a small amount of acid diffuses into the gastric mucosa normally, this quantity is likely to be greatly increased in conditions of stress. Finally, changes in energy substrates in the mucosa have been postulated to play an important role in the preservation of mucosal integrity. A number of experimental and clinical studies have observed that inadequate nutrition during severe stress increases the incidence of gastric erosions.

Diagnosis

Stress ulceration not only occurs most commonly in patients who have undergone episodes of shock or sepsis, but also appears to be a nonspecific end-result of a wide variety of insults such as drugs, head injuries, burns, cardiac operations, uremia, and malnutrition. Although bleeding usually begins about 7–10 days after the initial insult, it may appear within the first few days. Often it is heralded by 1–2 days of ileus and bilious nasogastric drainage. Small amounts of blood first appear in the nasogastric aspirate, followed by steady bleeding. Occasionally, hemorrhage is massive from the start. When bleeding first appears per rectum, a nasogastric tube should always be inserted for diagnosis of an upper gastrointestinal source.

Endoscopy is the most important diagnostic tool and is also a valuable therapeutic instrument (Fig. 48.17). Sequential endoscopy has shown that the lesions characteristically appear first in the fundus and progress to the junction of the body and antrum. The acute erosions of stress ulceration are superficial rather than deep, multiple rather than single, gastric rather than duodenal, and fundal rather than antral, and usually bleed rather than perforate. Upper gastrointestinal radiograph series obtained during bleeding episodes are rarely helpful because the

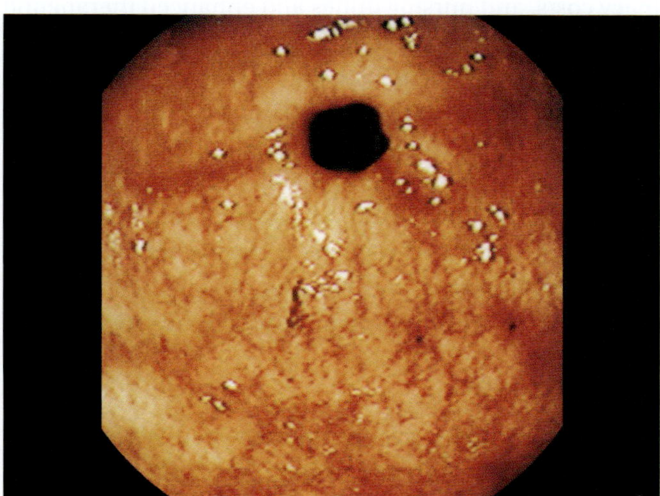

Fig. 48.17: Gastritis in a septic postoperative patient.

erosions are quite superficial. Selective celiac angiography will often demonstrate the point of bleeding and can then be used for subsequent arterial infusions of vasopressin.

At least 90% of patients stop bleeding in response to active nonoperative treatment, with <10% requiring operative intervention. For those who require an operation, the mortality rate can reach 30–50%. The mortality rate is higher for patients older than 60 years and in those who have sepsis.

Prophylaxis

All high-risk patients should be treated prophylactically. Regardless of the initial mechanism of mucosal damage, acid is required for mucosal destruction and bleeding. The mainstays of prophylaxis include antacids, H_2-receptor antagonists, PPI, and sucralfate.

The hourly administration of antacid by nasogastric tube to maintain the gastric pH >3.5 has proved to be effective prophylaxis.[42] If intragastric pH can be maintained >5, nearly 100% of acid is neutralized and pepsin is inactivated.

Cimetidine is considered to be as effective as antacids in preventing stress ulcerations. Although studies demonstrate that H_2-receptor antagonists can prevent stress ulceration, most studies demonstrate that it is easier to titrate gastric pH with antacids than with the standard intermittent dose regimens of H_2-receptor antagonists. In addition, continuous infusions of H_2-receptor antagonists provide more consistent maintenance of a gastric pH > 3.5 than the standard intermittent infusion doses. Theoretic advantages of continuous infusion of H_2-receptor antagonists include reduction in toxicity, decreased pharmacy costs, and nursing duties and enhanced therapeutic benefit.

Sucralfate has been evaluated for prophylaxis against stress ulceration. Controlled trials suggest that sucralfate, 1 g q6h, can be as effective as antacids or cimetidine. This form of protection is not antisecretory; it avoids bacterial overgrowth by allowing the intragastric pH to remain low. Critically ill ventilated patients receiving sucralfate have been shown to have a lower incidence of pneumonia than patients receiving prophylactic antisecretory agents.[43]

Management

Ideally, prophylaxis, prompt attention to sepsis, treatment of pulmonary insufficiency, restoring intravascular volume, reversing nutritional deficiencies, and decreasing gastric acidity will prevent stress ulceration. At the first sign of bleeding, gastric lavage with iced saline through a nasogastric tube should be initiated. About 90% of patients who present with upper gastrointestinal hemorrhage stop bleeding with this approach. Once acute bleeding has stopped, the gastric pH should be maintained at a pH >5 (or 7) with the agents listed previously. Definitive treatment of ongoing acute active gastrointestinal bleeding with any of these agents is usually unsuccessful. Further treatment to arrest hemorrhage must then be instituted. Treatment of the hemorrhage itself must not overshadow treatment of its cause. Stress bleeding should be regarded as evidence of untreated sepsis, and a diligent search for the cause is necessary. The stomach lining is exquisitely sensitive to sepsis. This has led stress hemorrhage to be referred to as the "canary in the coal mine."

Endoscopy has become the diagnostic tool of choice. With electrocautery and laser photocoagulation capabilities, the endoscope can function as therapy, although its effectiveness in stress gastritis has not yet been established. Selective angiographic catheterization of the splanchnic arterial circulation offers an additional means for controlling bleeding. Gastric bleeding can be effectively controlled by selective infusion of vasopressin into the splanchnic circulation through the left gastric artery. Vasopressin should be used with caution in patients who have ischemic cardiac disease or liver disease. Although effective in controlling blood loss, the use of selective intra-arterial infusion of vasopressin is not associated with an improved survival rate. An additional angiographic technique used to control acute bleeding is transcatheter embolization with a variety of hemostatic substances, including metal coils and oxidized cellulose.

Approximately 10% of patients who have acute bleeding from stress ulceration require operation despite medical, endoscopic, or angiographic interventions. Goals of operative therapy in stress ulceration include control of bleeding and reducing the mortality and recurrent bleeding rates. The ideal operation that fulfills these requirements is unknown. Vagotomy and drainage, vagotomy and antrectomy, vagotomy and subtotal gastrectomy, total gastrectomy, and gastric devascularization have all been used to treat hemorrhage from stress ulceration. Mortality rates for bleeding from stress ulceration range from 30% to 100%, regardless of the surgical procedure. As the outcome in these high-risk patients is grave, the most expeditious operation (simply oversewing isolated actively bleeding erosions alone) should be performed. An additional gastric resection or drainage procedure, vagotomy, or gastric devascularization is not recommended unless bleeding continues. Following operative therapy, care should be directed toward essential supportive measures including nutritional support, treatment of sepsis, and maintaining hemodynamic parameters.

GASTRIC ULCER

Etiology

Impaired mucosal defense is probably the principal mechanism in the development of gastric ulcers. Normally, the tight junctions of the epithelial cells maintain a barrier against the back-diffusion of acid into the mucosa. In the presence of "barrier breakers"—agents that disrupt the tight junctions—the acid back-diffuses into the mucosa, resulting in erosions and ulcers. Once the barrier is broken, histamine is released; this stimulates the secretion of more acid as well as vasodilatation and increased capillary permeability. Common gastric irritants implicated as "barrier breakers" include aspirin, NSAIDs, alcohol, and bile. *Helicobacter pylori* also causes gastric ulcers.

Pathology

Gastric ulcers are sharp, well-defined breaks in the mucosa. They usually occur at the junction of the fundal and antral mucosa, typically on the lesser curvature near the incisura angularis. However, the antrum varies in shape and size. The antrum-corpus junction may be found anywhere from the angularis to the cardioesophageal junction. In addition, the antrum increases in size with aging, and its junction with the fundal mucosa is more proximally located in the elderly. When a gastric ulcer is found in an unexpected area, gastric irritants, carcinoma, or the Zollinger–Ellison syndrome should be suspected.

In contrast to those who have duodenal ulcers, patients who have gastric ulcers tend to have normal or decreased gastric acid secretion, depending upon the degree of associated gastritis. In general, an ulcer near the pylorus or associated with a duodenal ulcer is generally accompanied by acid hypersecretion, whereas ulcers elsewhere in the stomach are usually characterized by hyposecretion.

Chronic gastritis is common in patients with duodenal or gastric ulcers.[44] Those with severe active gastritis have a greater likelihood of recurrent gastric ulcer. A gastric ulcer may be regarded not simply as a localized lesion, but as part of a generalized abnormality of the gastric mucosa. Therefore, the gastritis itself may be looked upon as contributing not only to the hyposecretion that accompanies gastric ulcer, but also to the susceptibility of the mucosa to discrete ulceration.

Clinical Features

Gastric ulcer is commonly associated with heartburn and dyspepsia. The pain is usually indistinguishable from duodenal ulcer pain, but a large meal may exacerbate the pain, which is relieved by antacids. Vomiting, fullness, and distension are other features. A gastric ulcer may also be silent if the etiologic agent is aspirin or NSAID. When the ulcer is large, penetrating, and on the posterior wall, the pain may penetrate to the back. Bleeding is often associated with aspirin, NSAID use, or alcohol abuse. Patients with a gastric ulcer may lose weight as a result of early postprandial pain, but marked weight loss suggests a neoplasm.

Diagnosis

Endoscopy is the diagnostic procedure of choice for gastric ulcers. The gastric ulcer can be directly examined, photographed, and biopsied for later histologic examination. The experienced endoscopist can often recognize malignant ulcers. Multiple biopsies provide the most direct means of identifying a possible malignancy.

The differentiation between benign and malignant ulcers by radiographs is approximately 95% accurate but can be difficult. About 95% of gastric ulcers are located on or near the lesser curvature, and the majority have been reported in the region of the incisura angularis (Fig. 48.18).[45] There seems to be no tendency for malignant ulcers to occur more frequently on the greater curvature of the stomach than elsewhere.

Medical Management

The management of gastric ulcers is similar to that of duodenal ulcers except that the elimination of barrier breakers is even more important and the question of whether a gastric ulcer represents a gastric cancer must be addressed. Patients who have gastric ulcers should stop smoking and avoid aspirin, corticosteroids, NSAIDs, and alcohol. Those patients who need aspirin or corticosteroids for other disorders can continue to take them as long as H_2-receptor antagonists or misoprostol therapy is instituted.

Results

Misoprostol (100–200 μg q6h) has been demonstrated to be efficacious in the prevention of NSAID-associated gastric ulceration. Sucralfate appears to be ineffective in the prevention of NSAID-associated gastric ulceration.

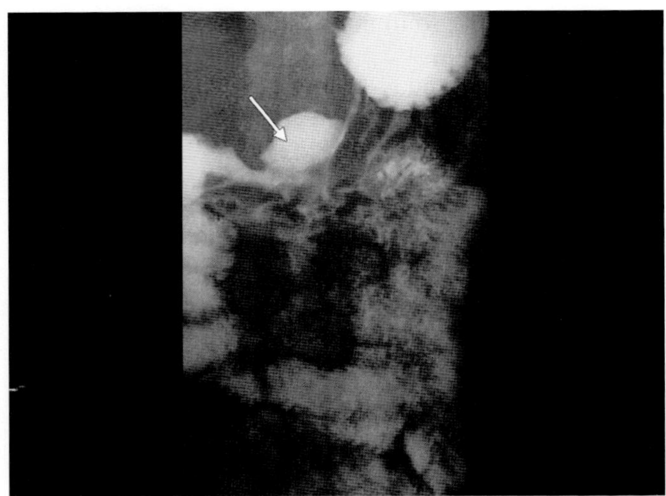

Fig. 48.18: Large benign ulcer on lesser curvature of the stomach (arrow). Upper gastrointestinal barium study.

The role of antacids in the treatment of gastric ulcers is less clear than it is for duodenal ulcers. Moderate to large doses (>500 mmol/day) are effective in expediting gastric ulcer healing. In comparative trials, antacids appear comparable to H_2-receptor antagonists for overall gastric ulcer healing, although the time to healing may be longer with the use of antacids.

The H_2-receptor antagonists are well established as effective agents for acute gastric ulcer therapy. Although most patients have normal or even reduced acid secretion, reducing gastric acidity with H_2-receptor antagonists promotes ulcer healing. As with duodenal ulcers, healing rates for gastric ulcers increase with increasing duration of treatment. The average time for complete ulcer healing is approximately 2–4 weeks longer for gastric ulcers than for duodenal ulcers, which may be attributable to their greater size. As with duodenal ulcers, nocturnal dosing of H_2-receptor antagonists is equal in efficacy to the more frequent dosing regimens for healing uncomplicated gastric ulcer. Omeprazole 20–40 mg/day appears to be slightly superior to H_2-receptor antagonists for acute gastric ulcer therapy.[15]

Sucralfate is efficacious for the acute treatment of a gastric ulcer with healing rates of 60% at 4 weeks and 80% at 8 weeks of therapy.[21] Bismuth compounds also appear to be effective in the therapy of acute gastric ulcers, having comparable efficacy to that of H_2-receptor antagonists.

Elective Operative Management

The main indication for elective operative treatment of a gastric ulcer is to exclude a malignancy. Failure of a newly diagnosed gastric ulcer to heal completely within 12 weeks of medical therapy or failure of a recurrent ulcer to respond to medical therapy should increase the suspicion of a gastric cancer. Most studies of operative treatment of gastric ulcer are from the 1970s to early 1980s, before medical therapy changed the environment.[46] Numerous surgical procedures have been described for each type of gastric ulcer and reflect the operative treatment of duodenal ulcer. However, with the knowledge that gastric ulcer results from a generalized abnormality of the gastric mucosa, total excision of the ulcer alone for histologic evaluation to rule out malignancy, followed by aggressive medical therapy, may be sufficient. If malignancy is found, further resection is warranted.

Many authors advocate a distal gastrectomy with either a Billroth I or Billroth II anastomosis for patients who have a gastric ulcer in the body of the stomach. The ulcer should be included in the resected specimen. The operative mortality rate for this procedure is <5%, with a recurrence rate of <5%.[46] An alternative procedure is a proximal gastric vagotomy and excision of the ulcer. The ulcer recurrence rates are similar for both gastrectomy with a Billroth I anastomosis and a proximal gastric vagotomy with ulcer excision.[47] When patients have a concomitant duodenal ulcer, some investigators advocate adding a vagotomy; however, this increases the incidence of postgastrectomy syndromes.

Peri- and Postoperative Complications

The acute complications of the operative treatment of gastric ulcers, like those for the operative treatment of duodenal ulcers, are:

- Hemorrhage
- Leak (*see* previously).

Long-term complications or postgastrectomy syndromes following operative treatment of gastric ulcers are discussed elsewhere.

Emergency Operative Management

Bleeding

As for hemorrhage caused by duodenal ulceration, the patient should be adequately resuscitated and prompt endoscopy should be performed to determine the source of bleeding. If operative treatment of a bleeding gastric ulcer is necessary, suture ligation of the ulcer alone with subsequent aggressive medical therapy, excision of the ulcer, or antrectomy are all acceptable procedures. More complicated procedures should be avoided. If ulcer excision is not possible, multiple biopsies should be taken to exclude the presence of gastric cancer.

Perforation

Nearly all patients with a perforated gastric ulcer should undergo operation, either by the traditional open method or laparoscopically. They should be resuscitated with intravenous fluids and be given broad-spectrum antibiotics and H_2-receptor antagonists. Acceptable procedures for treating perforated gastric ulcers include excision of the ulcer, biopsy, and simple closure of the perforation with an omental patch or an antrectomy. If the ulcer is excised, care must be taken to avoid gastric outlet obstruction at the excision site. Aggressive medical therapy with either proton pump inhibitors or H_2-receptor antagonists should be instituted on a long-term basis to decrease recurrence rates.

ALTERNATIVE CAUSES OF UPPER GASTROINTESTINAL HEMORRHAGE

This matter is considered in greater detail in the chapter on gastrointestinal bleeding (Chapter 73, "Upper and Lower Gastrointestinal Hemorrhage"), but some conditions merit a brief mention here.

Mallory-Weiss Syndrome

Mallory and Weiss were the first to describe clinical and autopsy findings in alcoholic patients who had bled from longitudinal tears of the cardia extending into the esophagogastric mucosa. The etiology of these tears was thought to be forceful vomiting. A large review of patients with the Mallory-Weiss syndrome demonstrated an association with alcohol in 60% and vomiting in 90% of patients.[48] In addition to vomiting, other etiologic conditions were blunt chest trauma, bouts of severe coughing, and marked increases in intra-abdominal pressure.

A Mallory-Weiss tear should be considered whenever a patient is bleeding vigorously from the upper gastrointestinal tract and there is no obvious diagnosis. Most patients who have Mallory-Weiss syndrome stop bleeding spontaneously. Hemostasis may be achieved using a Sengstaken-Blakemore tube or cautery techniques via endoscopy. If bleeding persists, an operation may be necessary. A long gastrostomy incision in the upper stomach is required for visualization of the tear, which can then be oversewn (narrow malleable retractors placed through the gastrostomy are helpful to achieve exposure of the gastroesophageal junction).

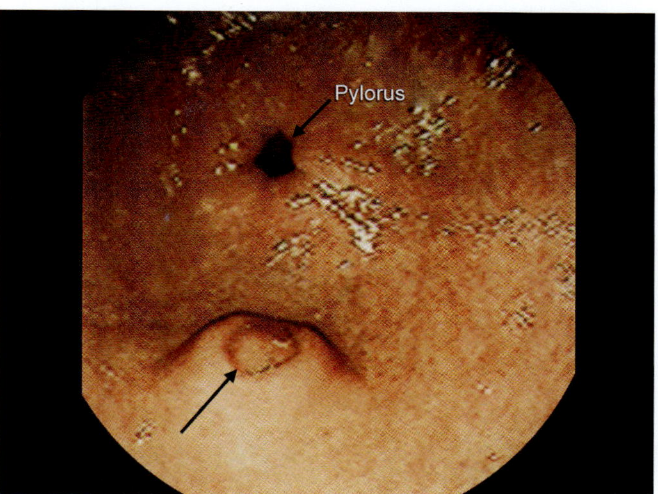

Fig. 48.19: Ectopic pancreatic rest (arrow). This was found in the gastric antrum during routine upper gastrointestinal endoscopy.

Benign Tumors

Leiomyomas, also referred to as gastrointestinal stromal tumors, and gastric polyps are discussed in Chapter 69, "Small Bowel".

Ectopic Pancreas

A mass of pancreatic tissue may be present within the wall of the stomach, usually occurring in the antrum or the prepyloric area (Fig. 48.19). Usually <3 cm in diameter, the tumor may project into the lumen of the stomach and can potentially cause pyloric obstruction. The mass of ectopic pancreas is composed of glands and intervening connective tissue. Islets of Langerhans may be decreased or absent. There may be ductal dilatation and cyst formation. The heterotopic pancreas characteristically has a large central duct, which can be filled with contrast media and detected by radiographs.

GASTROSTOMY

The indications for all types of gastrostomy are:

- To provide enteral access in patients who have either temporarily or permanently lost the ability to eat
- For gastric decompression.

Contraindications are similar for all types of gastrostomy and include uncontrollable ascites, coagulopathy, or a diseased gastric wall.

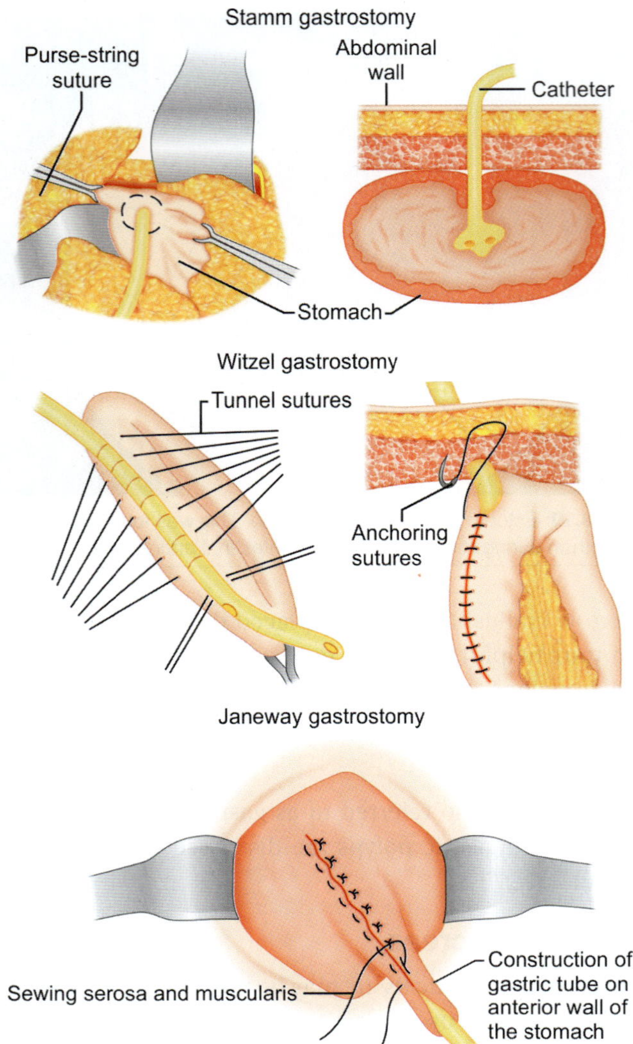

Fig. 48.20: Operative gastrostomies. In the Stamm gastrostomy, the stomach is opened inside a purse-string suture and a feeding tube is introduced into the stomach. The purse-string is secured, the feeding tube is brought out through the abdominal wall, and the serosa of the anterior gastric wall is secured to the posterior abdominal wall. In the Witzel modification, a serosa-lined passage is created through which the tube passes. The Janeway gastrostomy requires construction of a tube from a portion of the gastric wall. After the tube has been fashioned, it is passed through the abdominal wall via a separate incision.

Gastrostomies can be grouped into two types:

- Operative (open and laparoscopic)
- Percutaneous (endoscopic and nonendoscopic).

Operative gastrostomy is performed in the operating room under local or general anesthesia. Endoscopic gastrostomy can be performed at the patient's bedside or in the endoscopy suite. Nonendoscopic percutaneous gastrostomy requires fluoroscopy and is performed in a radiology suite.

Operative Gastrostomies

Operative gastrostomies include the Stamm, Witzel, and Janeway gastrostomies (Fig. 48.20); the Stamm gastrostomy is the most common in general use.

Placement of a gastrostomy tube can be performed laparoscopically, which also requires general anesthesia. The laparoscope is inserted through a supraumbilical trocar, and the stomach is insufflated. The anterior stomach is anchored under direct laparoscopic view using specially designed fasteners.

The pneumoperitoneum is decreased to allow the anterior stomach to be drawn up to the abdominal wall. The gastrostomy is made by inserting a needle through the skin in the center of the previously placed fasteners and into the stomach. A guidewire is passed through the needle into the gastric lumen, and the needle is removed. The tract is dilated, and the gastrostomy tube is passed into the stomach through a peel-away introducer catheter. A balloon on the end of the gastrostomy tube is then inflated, pulling the gastrostomy tube and gastric wall against the abdominal wall.

Percutaneous Gastrostomies

Percutaneous endoscopic gastrostomies have gained popularity since being introduced in 1981.[49] The patient's mouth is mechanically prepared with a topical anesthetic spray, while the abdomen is scrubbed with an antibacterial solution. An endoscope is passed into the stomach, and the esophagus, duodenum, and stomach are examined. The position of the endoscope is ascertained by observing:

- The position of the light transilluminating the abdominal wall
- The movement of the anterior gastric wall with indentation of the abdominal wall overlying the stomach.

A site for the feeding tube is selected, and the skin is infiltrated with local anesthetic. A stab incision is made through the skin. A plastic cannula over a needle is then placed through the abdominal wall and into the stomach (Fig. 48.21). The needle is removed, and a guidewire is placed through the cannula into the stomach. The intragastric portion of the guidewire is grasped with a snare, pulled through the mouth, and tied to the feeding tube. The guidewire protruding through the abdominal wall is then pulled with passage of the feeding tube through the mouth, esophagus, and stomach until resistance is felt. The endoscope is reintroduced to check the tube position

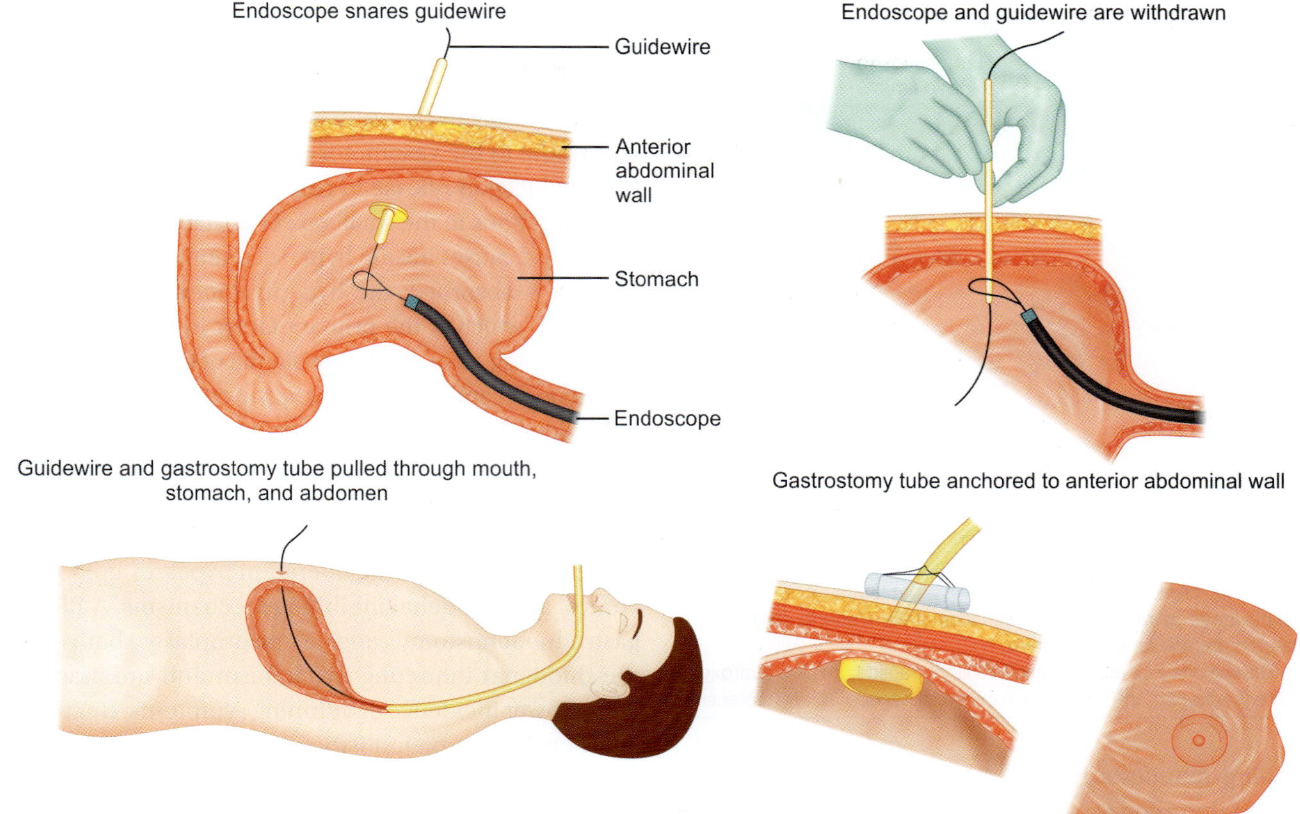

Fig. 48.21: Placement of percutaneous endoscopic gastrostomy tube. The endoscope is placed into the stomach and snares a guidewire that was placed through a stylet percutaneously. The scope is withdrawn along with the guidewire and the gastrostomy tube is then attached to the guidewire. The guidewire (along with the gastrostomy tube) is then pulled through the mouth, stomach, and abdomen, and the gastrostomy tube is anchored to the anterior abdominal wall.

and to rule out bleeding. The feeding tube is secured, and the gastrostomy tube is managed in a way similar to that for operatively placed tubes.

A percutaneous nonendoscopic gastrostomy procedure has been described that requires insertion of a nasogastric tube and distention of the stomach.[50] The abdomen is scrubbed with an antibacterial solution and the skin is infiltrated with local anesthetic. A catheter is inserted over a trocar through the abdominal wall and into the stomach. Its position is checked by instilling contrast into the stomach. The trocar is removed and replaced by a catheter, preferably with one inflatable balloon end.

Complications

Major complications of all gastrostomy tubes include hemorrhage, separation of the stomach from the abdominal wall, leakage and peritonitis, injury to the posterior stomach wall or adjacent organs, and early dislodgment. Minor complications include superficial wound infection and leakage of gastric contents into the abdominal wall, resulting in severe dermatitis. Deaths are only rarely associated with the procedure. Patients who die usually succumb to complications of their underlying disease. The only prospective study reported demonstrated no difference between the mortality rates for a Stamm gastrostomy performed under local anesthesia and a percutaneous endoscopic gastrostomy.[51] Aspiration has been noted in all types of gastrostomy. Patients known to have a history of aspiration may be better served by a jejunostomy feeding tube.

POSTGASTRECTOMY SYNDROMES

Dumping

Dumping syndrome can be separated into an early and a late form based on the time between ingestion of the meal and the occurrence of symptoms. However, both forms occur in response to the ingestion of a hyperosmolar carbohydrate-rich meal. Early dumping begins within 10–30 minutes after ingestion of the meal, whereas late

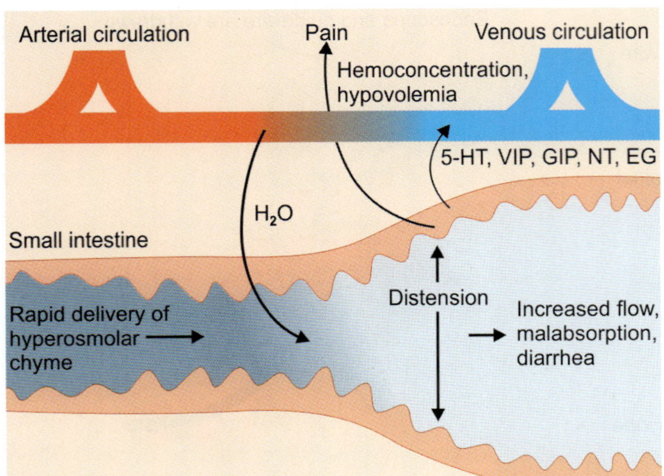

Fig. 48.22: Putative mechanisms for dumping syndrome. The density of shading represents the relative osmolarity of the various fluid compartments. With rapid delivery of hyperosmolar chyme, fluid shifts occur, leading the hemoconcentration and hypovolemia. The distended intestine leads to release of intestinal peptide. Patients then experience pain, faintness, and diarrhea.
(EG: Enteroglucagon; GIP: Gastric inhibitory peptide; 5-HT: 5-hydroxytryptamine (serotonin); VIP: Vasoactive intestinal peptide; NT: Neurotensin).

dumping manifests itself 2–4 hours after a meal. Both forms of dumping produce vasomotor symptoms such as diaphoresis, weakness, dizziness, flushing, and palpitations. Early dumping is also associated with gastrointestinal symptoms, which may include fullness, crampy abdominal pain, nausea, vomiting, and explosive diarrhea.

Mechanisms

The mechanisms that lead to the dumping syndrome include:

- Loss of gastric reservoir function
- Rapid emptying of hyperosmolar carbohydrates into the small intestine.

Both vagotomy and gastric resection decrease reservoir function. Vagotomy results in loss of receptive relaxation and accommodation,[52] whereas gastric resection decreases gastric capacity.[53]

Gastric emptying is speeded by both pyloroplasty and gastrojejunostomy.[54] Pyloroplasty results in loss of the control of gastric emptying, whereas gastrojejunostomy results in the loss of duodenal feedback inhibition of gastric emptying. Loss of reservoir function and rapid gastric emptying result in the rapid appearance of large amounts of carbohydrate-rich chyme in the small intestine (Fig. 48.22). This process leads to fluid shifts from the intravascular space into the bowel lumen,[55] producing the vasomotor and gastrointestinal symptoms of early dumping. The loss of intravascular volume and the release of enteric hormones, including serotonin,[56] gastric inhibitory peptide, vasoactive intestinal peptide,[57] and neurotensin,[58] contribute to the vasomotor symptoms of early dumping. Enteroglucagon release in response to high carbohydrate concentrations in the small bowel sensitizes the pancreatic B cells and causes insulin hypersecretion.[59] After the carbohydrate is absorbed, the hyperinsulinemia causes hypoglycemia, which is the primary factor in the symptoms of late dumping. Also, the hypovolemia of early dumping and the hypoglycemia of late dumping result in epinephrine (adrenaline) release, which contributes to the symptoms.

Operative procedures that cause rapid gastric emptying are associated with an increased incidence of dumping.[60] After a Billroth II resection, the incidence of dumping may exceed 50%, because the operation bypasses both pyloric control and duodenal inhibiting mechanisms. A Billroth I gastroduodenostomy and a pyloroplasty both retain the duodenal inhibiting mechanism and are associated with a lower incidence of dumping symptoms. By contrast, Roux-en-Y gastrojejunostomy rarely results in gastric emptying rapid enough to cause dumping and has been used to treat severe dumping symptoms if medical therapy fails. Proximal gastric vagotomy can also speed gastric emptying by impairing receptive relaxation and accommodation through vagal denervation. However, the effect is minimal, dumping occurring in only 1–6% of patients.[61]

Management

Dietary modification is the first line of therapy for the medical treatment of dumping. Most patients modify their diet appropriately to minimize their dumping symptoms. The most effective means is a diet low in simple carbohydrates and high in protein. The patient should be instructed to avoid all liquids during a meal, consuming them 30–45 minutes following the meal. For severe vasomotor symptoms, lying supine for 30 minutes postprandially may minimize the likelihood of syncope. Other medical therapies have included dietary additives that result in delayed glucose absorption and prolonged bowel transit time.[62] These dietary supplements are worth trying but may not be effective for patients who have severe symptoms, while their side effects, such as malabsorption and diarrhea, can be marked.

Octreotide acetate, a long-acting somatostatin analog, has been used with some success in treating severe dumping symptoms. Octreotide alleviates dumping by slowing gastric emptying, inhibiting insulin release, and decreasing enteric peptide secretion. Four controlled randomized trials have documented the short-term efficacy of octreotide treatment in patients who have severe dumping symptoms.[63] The initial octreotide dose is 50 μg subcutaneously, 2–3 times daily. In general, octreotide improves the symptoms in 90% of patients who have dumping unresponsive to other medical therapies.

Diarrhea

Diarrhea is common after vagotomy or gastric resection. Truncal vagotomy is responsible for the highest incidence (20%), followed by selective vagotomy (5%) and proximal gastric vagotomy (4%).[64] The diarrhea is usually episodic, lessens over the first year after operation, and rarely remains a severe problem. It is said that really intractable diarrhea occurs in only 1% of truncal vagotomy patients.

The mechanisms responsible for postvagotomy diarrhea are unknown, but the cause may be multifactorial. As the vagotomy performed becomes more selective, the incidence of postvagotomy diarrhea decreases, suggesting vagal denervation of the small bowel or biliary tree as a causal mechanism. Changes in the rate of gastric emptying may be a cause. Decreased receptive relaxation and rapid gastric emptying of liquid have been correlated with the presence of postvagotomy diarrhea.[65] In the past, surgeons have treated this with interposition of reversed ileal loops to slow transit but the need for these procedures has nearly vanished with the demise of surgical treatment of ulcers.

Reflux Gastritis

Up to 15% of patients undergoing a gastric operation develop the symptom complex of alkaline reflux gastritis. The symptoms include:

- Burning epigastric pain
- Nausea
- Bilious vomiting.

They can result in decreased food intake, weight loss, and anemia. More than 60% of gastrectomy patients exhibit histologic gastritis but are relatively asymptomatic. Reflux gastritis is a clinical syndrome and requires operative treatment more often than any other postgastrectomy syndrome.[66] It results when the pylorus is resected, bypassed, or destroyed, allowing intestinal contents to reflux into the stomach; the gastroenteric anastomosis must allow bile to contact the gastric mucosa. The highest incidence of alkaline gastritis occurs after Billroth II gastrojejunostomy,

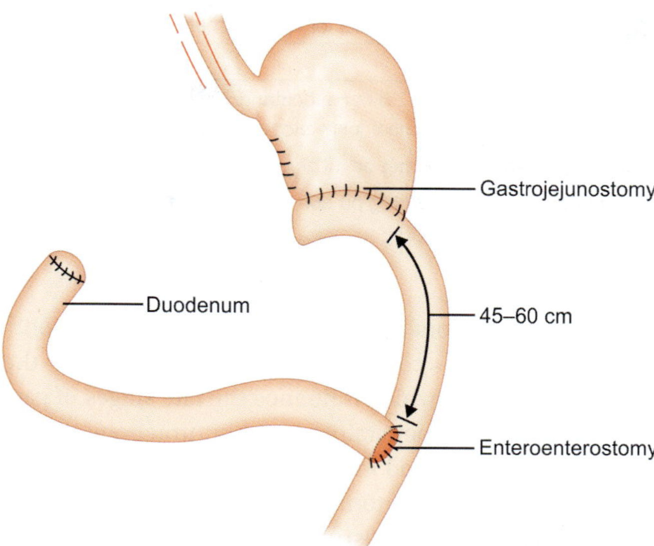

Fig. 48.23: Roux-en-Y gastrojejunostomy. Anatomic arrangement after truncal vagotomy and gastrojejunostomy. The length of the jejunum from gastrojejunostomy to enteroenterostomy (the Roux limb) is generally 45–75 cm.

followed by loop gastrojejunostomy, Billroth I gastroduodenostomy, and pyloroplasty.[67] Bile salts are thought to be the most injurious factor, but delayed clearance of bile may play an important role.[68]

A recent study has advocated feeding the bile acid ursodeoxycholic acid to symptomatic patients.[69] Ursodeoxycholic acid almost completely abolished nausea and vomiting and decreased both the intensity and frequency of epigastric pain. However, neither the macroscopic nor microscopic appearance of the gastric mucosa was altered by treatment.

The aim of operative treatment historically has been to divert upper intestinal contents completely away from the residual gastric pouch using a 40–60-cm Roux-en-Y gastrojejunostomy (Fig. 48.23). However, this maneuver may result in the Roux stasis syndrome.

Chronic Gastric Atony

Mechanisms

Patients complain of epigastric fullness and pain, nausea, and vomiting. They cannot tolerate solids but can usually tolerate liquids. In the chronic form, the symptoms become so severe that malnutrition and weight loss develop.

Gastric atony can result from a gastric operation, postoperative ileus, or medical conditions such as diabetes. It can also be seen after pylorus-preserving proximal pancreatoduodenectomy. Gastric atony secondary to a gastric

Table 48.8 Prokinetic agents for the treatment of chronic gastric atony.

Agent	Dose	Side effects
Bethanechol	Initial 2.5 mg subcutaneously; adjusted according to response; long-term use 10–30 mg po q6-8h	Parasympathetic side effects; long-term use associated with increased incidence of peptic ulcer
Metoclopramide	5–10 mg po or IV q6h	Dystonic reactions, dyskinesia
Cisapride	10–20 mg po q6h	Fewer antidopaminergic side effects than metoclopramide
Erythromycin	100–500 mg po or IV q6h	Nausea, vomiting

operation results from the loss of gastric vagal innervation.[70] The vagal branches control the tonic contractions of the proximal stomach, which influence the late stages of gastric emptying. The peristaltic antral contractions during the postprandial period are likewise under the control of the vagus nerves. Vagotomy results in the loss of these contractions, leading to disrupted antral trituration. Medical disorders that increase the risk of gastric atony include:

- Preoperative gastric outlet obstruction
- Diabetes mellitus
- Hypothyroidism
- Autonomic neurologic disorders
- Long-term narcotic use

Acute postoperative gastric atony results from the activation of neural reflexes that lead to the release of norepinephrine (noradrenaline) or other inhibitory substances from the gastric wall.[72] Norepinephrine acts directly on the gastrointestinal smooth muscle, blocks the release of acetylcholine from the parasympathetic neurons supplying the cells, and inhibits gastric action potentials and therefore contractions. The actions of norepinephrine result in gastric atony, slow emptying of liquids and solids, and an absence of interdigestive contractions.[73] Unlike the gastric atony seen after gastric operations, the postoperative form of gastric atony lasts only 3–5 days. By contrast, atony following gastric operations may last up to 6 weeks or even longer.

Management

The medical treatment of gastric atony following surgery involves the use of prokinetic drugs. Supportive care, including adequate nutritional support and intermittent or chronic gastric decompression, is also necessary. Disrupted motility because of long-term narcotic use should be addressed. Prokinetic drugs used for treating this group of patients include bethanechol, metoclopramide, cisapride, and erythromycin (Table 48.8). Operative intervention should be used only as a last resort and is seldom indicated.

There have been some suggestions that gastric electrical stimulation may be helpful for patients in whom gastric atony is present without previous surgery and even in some with previous gastric surgery. This device is approved by the Food and Drug Administration only for compassionate release but may be helpful for some individuals requiring long-term parenteral nutrition.

Roux-Stasis Syndrome

Mechanisms

The combination of vagotomy, antrectomy, and Roux-en-Y gastrojejunostomy causes delayed gastric emptying of both solids and liquids. From 10% to 50% of patients develop postoperative symptoms that include epigastric fullness, abdominal pain, nausea, and vomiting.[74,75] Gastric bezoars may form, and a number of patients develop malnutrition and weight loss.

Investigations into the Roux stasis syndrome have revealed that both the postvagotomy proximal gastric remnant and the Roux limb contribute to delayed gastric emptying. Vagotomy diminishes the tone of the remaining stomach. The Roux limb also adds to the pathophysiology of this syndrome. Scintigraphic studies of the Roux limb have demonstrated delayed transit, which may be attributable to its myoelectric patterns.[76] As in the stomach, action potentials (contractions) of the small intestine in health are controlled by pacesetter potentials that propagate from the duodenum distally down the jejunum. Construction of the Roux limb requires transection of the jejunum, which disturbs this pattern by interrupting the propagation of the pacesetter potentials and decreasing their frequency in the Roux limb.[77] Ectopic pacemakers then develop in the Roux limb. They generate pacesetter potentials that propagate toward the stomach. The orally propagating pacesetter potentials, with their associated orally propagating contractions, result in slower transit through the Roux limb.[78] Also, motility studies during fasting have demonstrated a higher frequency of phase III potentials in the Roux limb during fasting that are irregular and do not propagate as well as they do in health.[79]

Management

To treat the Roux stasis syndrome, chronic gastric atony should first be diagnosed by ruling out mechanical obstruction with either an upper gastrointestinal series or endoscopy. The medical treatment of Roux stasis syndrome includes:

- Nutritional support
- Stopping any narcotics
- Prokinetic drugs.

Common prokinetic medications used are the same as those for gastric atony. Treatment of chronic gastroparesis with bethanechol has a 30–40% success rate, whereas metoclopramide and cisapride are less effective in treating this condition.[80] Erythromycin, a macrolide antibiotic, has shown some benefit in experimental studies,[81] although only 40% of patients respond to the drug on a long-term basis.[80]

Operative treatment of the Roux stasis syndrome includes near-total gastrectomy. Removal of the atonic gastric remnant usually improves symptoms in 60–85% of patients.[82-84]

The best treatment for this syndrome is prevention. An alternative method of gastric drainage that does not involve the creation of a Roux-en-Y anastomosis has been recommended to avoid alkaline reflux gastritis. This operation has been designed to divert bile away from the stomach, like the standard Roux-en-Y gastrojejunostomy construction, but without the inherent motility disturbances. The "uncut Roux" gastroenterostomy is fashioned from a loop gastrojejunostomy with the afferent limb occluded by staples (Fig. 48.24). The staples prevent the flow of biliopancreatic secretions across the gastrojejunostomy (so preventing alkaline reflux gastritis), but allow normal aboral propagation of pacesetter potentials. Proximal to the staple line, the afferent and efferent loops of the gastrojejunostomy are anastomosed. In a canine study, the uncut Roux operation abolished ectopic pacemakers in the Roux limb and speeded the delayed gastric emptying found with the conventional Roux gastrojejunostomy.[85] Early reports suggest that the operation improves postoperative symptomatology in up to 60% of patients, but an unsatisfactory high rate of staple line dehiscence developed during follow-up.[86]

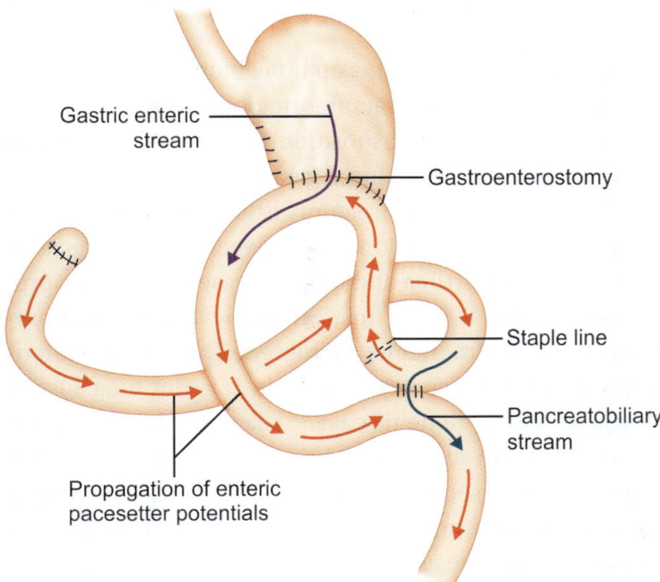

Fig. 48.24: "Uncut Roux" gastroenterostomy or Braun procedure.

Afferent Limb Syndrome

Blockage of the afferent limb is an important consideration in the differential diagnosis of postoperative vomiting. The typical complaint of patients who have this problem is crescendo epigastric pain occurring within 30–45 minutes of a meal that is relieved by projectile vomiting of bilious material that does not contain any recently eaten food. Pain is immediately relieved by the vomiting. The immediate cause of the vomiting is the explosive release of postprandial pancreatic and biliary secretions that exceed the volume of a near-completely obstructed afferent limb. As pressure builds in this loop, the patient experiences nausea and a dull ache in the upper abdomen, with a definite crescendo-decrescendo pattern. Vomiting occurs as the obstruction is relieved and the fluid in the duodenal loop passes into the gastric remnant. The patients are usually cachectic because they soon discover that they have no symptoms if they do not eat.

Afferent loop syndrome may be caused by several mechanisms. Kinking or herniation of a redundant afferent limb may result in partial obstruction, but anastomotic stricture, adhesions, stomal ulceration, jejunogastric intussusception, and carcinoma may also be responsible. If the obstruction of the afferent limb is chronic, the patient may develop hyperbilirubinemia as well as pancreatitis because of the chronic effects of increased luminal pressure in the duodenum.

Endoscopy frequently reveals the diagnosis by direct examination of the anastomotic site; any lesions can be identified and biopsied. The dilated afferent limb may also be visualized with an abdominal CT scan. Once the diagnosis is made, operative correction is indicated. The Billroth II anastomosis may be revised to a Billroth I or a Roux-en-Y gastrojejunostomy or to a simple enteroenterostomy between the afferent and efferent loops of bowel. The Roux-en-Y reconstruction is probably best avoided to prevent the Roux stasis syndrome.

Efferent Limb Obstruction

This syndrome complex results from partial or incomplete mechanical obstruction of the distal loops of intestine draining the stomach at or near the gastrojejunostomy. Symptoms consist of diffuse abdominal pain, nausea, and bilious vomiting. The main difference between the symptoms produced by this condition and those described for afferent limb syndrome is the presence of food in the vomited material.

Efferent limb syndrome may occur because of adhesions, recurrent cancer, carcinomatosis, or any condition that results in a near-total or total obstruction of the upper gut. Rarely, the jejunal segment is shown to intussuscept into the gastric lumen. Jejunogastric intussusception is usually recognized as the valvulae conniventes of the jejunum, as seen during endoscopy or on an upper gastrointestinal series. Although endoscopic reduction of an intussusceptum is theoretically possible, edema in the jejunal segment may prevent this approach being successful. The operative procedure may consist simply of lysis of adhesions. However, other operative findings may dictate the need for revision of the anastomosis or conversion to a Billroth I or Roux-en-Y gastrojejunostomy.

Bezoar

Collections of food and mucus or phytobezoars composed of vegetable matter sometimes form in the gastric remnant after partial gastrectomy, especially if a vagotomy has been performed. Autonomic neuropathy associated with diabetes mellitus is another predisposing condition. Patients complain of anorexia, epigastric fullness, nausea, or vomiting. The diagnosis is often apparent from upper gastrointestinal barium studies, but endoscopy may be needed to distinguish the bezoar from a neoplasm.

The bezoar can often be removed by vigorous and repeated gastric lavage through a large-bore orogastric tube. Fragmenting the lesion during endoscopy may facilitate removal by lavage. Some phytobezoars can be partially digested with cellulase and then broken up successfully by lavage. Rarely, operative removal is necessary. Medications that enhance gastric emptying may be tried to prevent recurrence. Nondigestible foods that predispose to the formation of bezoars should be avoided (i.e., orange pith, persimmons).

Bone Disease

Postgastrectomy bone loss has important consequences. Loss of bone mineral content is accelerated by gastric resection and becomes more pronounced with time after the gastric operation.[87,88] Abnormal bone loss has been estimated to affect 3–25% of patients who have had a gastric resection.[89] The process of bone demineralization appears to be more rapid after total than subtotal gastrectomy, but there is no clear difference between Billroth I and Billroth II resections.[90] An apparently slower rate of bone loss occurs after vagotomies without gastric resections.[91]

Bone biopsies in postoperative patients often reveal features of both osteoporosis and osteomalacia, but osteomalacia is the prevalent finding after gastric operations. Studies on patients who have subtotal gastrectomies have consistently revealed one or all of the features of osteomalacia, including:

- Bone pain
- Elevated serum alkaline phosphatase
- Depressed total serum calcium
- Decreased 25-hydroxyvitamin D;
- Elevated serum concentrations of parathyroid hormone
- Increased renal retention of absorbed enterally administered radiocalcium
- Widened osteoid seams on bone biopsies
- Occasional pseudofractures on bone films.[92]

There is also a predisposition to vertebral collapse in 2–36% of patients after partial gastrectomy.[93]

The cause of postgastrectomy osteomalacia is obscure. There is no clear relationship between the presence or absence of steatorrhea and bone disease, and the absorption of vitamin D is normal.[94] Blood levels of dihydroxyvitamin D are frequently increased. These observations suggest that a deficiency in vitamin D is not the cause of postgastrectomy bone disease.[95] Likewise, the absorption of radiocalcium appears to be normal in most patients after gastric resection.[95] Finally, an inadequate intake of calcium may not be a relevant factor. A number of reports[93,96] indicate adequate calcium intakes in postoperative patients in general and specifically in some patients who exhibit abnormal bone loss.[96]

Most reports indicate little bone loss among large numbers of patients studied many years after nonresective vagotomy operations.[91] A lower prevalence of bone disease after nonresective operations parallels the somewhat lower prevalence of iron deficiency after these operations. Both phenomena could be explained by the need of gastric acidification for efficient absorption and the less marked decrease in acid output after vagotomy without resection. Absorption of iron salts from food is demonstrably lowered by the hypochlorhydria induced by H_2-blocking agents in normal subjects,[97] but H_2-blockers and even sustained achlorhydria do not affect absorption of calcium from dairy products or calcium carbonate.[98] The pathogenesis of bone loss after gastric resections therefore remains a mystery.

Carcinoma

A relationship between a gastric operation for gastric and duodenal ulcer disease and the subsequent development of gastric cancer has been noted in a number of reports.[99] About 1% of the total number of gastric carcinomas develop in patients who have had a gastrectomy. In a large Danish study,[100] the risk of developing gastric cancer in patients undergoing a Billroth II subtotal gastrectomy was 3.2 times higher than normal after 25 years.

CONCLUSION

The above litany of complications that can follow a gastric operation leads to a simple conclusion: these syndromes are best avoided by focusing treatment on the known etiologies of ulcer disease that are amenable to medical therapy. Complications are best treated by the simplest procedure possible. Lester Dragstedt, who defined gastric hypersecretion as the cause of ulcers and introduced vagotomy to treat it, stated that "the stomach is a mighty handy organ to take to the dinner table." Although his operation has fallen out of common use, the truth of his statement remains and should be remembered by the modern-day surgeon.

REFERENCES

1. Oi M. Peptic ulcer and gastric acidity: a new look at an old aphorism, "the higher the ulcer, the lower the acidity." J Gastroenterol. 1995;30:122-7.
2. Peura DA. The report of the Digestive Health Initiative International Update Conference on Helicobacter pylori. Gastroenterology. 1997;113:S4-8.
3. Gisbert JP, Calvet X. Review article: Helicobacter pylori-negative duodenal ulcer disease. Aliment Pharmacol Ther. 2009;30:791-815.
4. Mitchell HM, Lee A, Carrick J. Increased incidence of Campylobacter pylori infection in gastroenterologists: further evidence to support person to person transmission. Scand J Gastroenterol. 1989;24:396-400.
5. Eagon JC, Kelly KA. Postgastrectomy syndromes. Surg Clin North Am. 1992;72:445-65.
6. Christensen A, Bousfield R, Christiansen J. Incidence of perforated and bleeding ulcers before and after the introduction of H_2-receptor antagonists. Ann Surg. 1988;207:4-6.
7. Scratcherd T. Gastroduodenal mucosal defense mechanisms. Curr Opin Gastroenterol. 1988;4:926-30.
8. Wallace JL. Gastric resistance to acid: is the "mucus-bicarbonate barrier" functionally redundant? Am J Physiol. 1989; 256:G31-8.
9. Silen W. Experimental models of gastric ulceration and injury. Am J Physiol. 1988;255:G395-402.
10. Soli A. Pathogenesis of peptic ulcer and implications for therapy. N Engl J Med. 1990;322(13):909-16.
11. Wyatt JI. Histopathology of gastroduodenal inflammation: the impact of Helicobacter pylori. Histopathology. 1995;26:1-15.
12. Dixon MF. Pathophysiology of Helicobacter pylori infection. Scand J Gastroenterol. 1994;201(suppl 201):7-10.
13. Beardshall K, Moss S, Gill J, et al. Suppression of Helicobacter pylori reduces gastrin releasing peptide stimulated gastrin release in duodenal ulcer patients. Gut. 1992;33:601-3.
14. Ernst PB, Crowe SE, Reyes VE. How does Helicobacter pylori cause mucosal damage? The inflammatory response. Gastroenterology. 1997;113:S35-42.
15. Soll AH, Weinstein WM, Kurata J, et al. Nonsteroidal anti-inflammatory drugs and peptic ulcer disease. Ann Intern Med. 1991;114:307-19.
16. Holt S, Howden CW. Omeprazole: overview and opinion. Dig Dis Sci. 1991;36:385-93.
17. Lanas A, Serrano P, Bajador E, et al. Evidence of aspirin use in both upper and lower gastrointestinal perforation. Gastroenterology. 1997;112:683-9.
18. Graham DY. Prevention of gastroduodenal injury induced by chronic nonsteroidal anti-inflammatory drug therapy. Gastroenterology. 1989;96:675-81.
19. Berstad A, Weberg R. Antacids in the treatment of gastroduodenal ulcer. Scand J Gastroenterol. 1986;21:385-91.
20. Isenberg JI, McQuaid KM, Laine LA, et al. Acid-peptic disorders. In: Yamada T, Alpers DH, Owyang C, et al. (Eds). Textbook of Gastroenterology. Philadelphia: JB Lippincott; 1991. pp. 1241-352.
21. Maton P. Omeprazole. N Engl J Med. 1991;324:965-75.
22. Lam S. Implications of sucralfate-induced ulcer healing and relapse. Am J Med. 1989;86(suppl 6A):122-6.
23. Gorbach S. Bismuth therapy in gastrointestinal diseases. Gastroenterology. 1990;99: 863-75.
24. Chiverton S, Hunt R. Initial therapy and relapse of duodenal ulcer: possible acid secretory mechanisms. Gastroenterology. 1989;96:632-9.

25. Sloan R, Cohen H. Common sense management of Helicobacter pylori—associated gastroduodenal disease. Gastroenterol Clin North Am. 1993;22:199-206.
26. Donovan AJ, Vinson TL, Maulsby GO, et al. Selective treatment of duodenal ulcer with perforation. Ann Surg. 1979; 189:627-36.
27. Boey J, Wong J. Perforated duodenal ulcers. World J Surg. 1987;11:319-24.
28. Boey J, Lee NW, Koo J, et al. Immediate definitive surgery for perforated duodenal ulcers: a prospective controlled trial. Ann Surg. 1982;196:338-44.
29. Feliciano DV. Do perforated duodenal ulcers need an acid decreasing surgical procedure now that omeprazole IS available? Surg Clin North Am. 1992;72:369-80.
30. Hooks VH III, Bowden TA Jr, Mansberger AR Jr, et al. Highly selective vagotomy with dilatation or duodenoplasty: a surgical alternative for obstructing duodenal ulcer. Ann Surg. 1986;203:545-50.
31. Stabile BE, Passaro E Jr. Duodenal ulcer: a disease in evolution. Curr Probl Surg. 1984;21:1-79.
32. Consensus Conference. Therapeutic endoscopy and bleeding ulcers. JAMA. 1989;262:1369-72.
33. Griffiths WJ, Neumann DA, Welsh JD. The visible vessel as an indicator of uncontrolled or recurrent gastrointestinal hemorrhage. N Engl J Med. 1979;300:1411-3.
34. Hart R, Classen M. Complications of diagnostic gastrointestinal endoscopy. Endoscopy. 1990;22:229-33.
35. Branicki FJ, Boey J, Fok PJ, et al. Bleeding duodenal ulcer: a prospective evaluation of risk factors for rebleeding and death. Ann Surg. 1990;211:411-8.
36. Hunt PS. Bleeding gastroduodenal ulcers: selection of patients for surgery. World J Surg. 1987;11:289-94.
37. Wilkinson AR, Johnston D. Effect of truncal vagotomy, selective vagotomy and highly selective vagotomy in man on gastric emptying and transit of a food-barium meal in man. Ann Surg. 1973;178:190-3.
38. Dozois RR, Kelly KA. Gastric secretion and motility in duodenal ulcer: effect of current vagotomies. Surg Clin North Am. 1976;56:1267-76.
39. Cuschieri A. Laparoscopic vagotomy: gimmick or reality. Surg Clin North Am. 1992;72:357-67.
40. Thirlby RC. Postoperative recurrent ulcer. Surg Clin North Am. 1994;23:295-311.
41. Hirschowitz BI, Lanas A. Intractable upper gastrointestinal ulceration due to aspirin in patients who have undergone surgery for peptic ulcer. Gastroenterology. 1998;114: 883-92.
42. Gugler R, Lindstaedt H, Miederer S, et al. Cimetidine for anastomotic ulcers after partial gastrectomy: a randomized control led trial. N Engl J Med. 1979;301:1077-80.
43. Zinner MJ, Zuidema GD, Smith PL, et al. The prevention of upper gastrointestinal tract bleeding in patients in an intensive care unit. Surg Gynecol Obstet. 1981;153: 214-20.
44. Ephgrave KS, Kleiman-Wexler R, Pfaller M, et al. Effects of sucralfate vs antacids on gastric pathogens: results of a double-blind clinical trial. Arch Surg. 1998;133:251-7.
45. Sipponen P, Seppala K, Aarynen, et al. Chronic gastritis and gastroduodenal ulcer: a case control study on risk of coexisting duodenal or gastric ulcer in patients with gastritis. Gut. 1989;30:922-9.
46. Oi M, Ito Y, Kumagai F, et al. A possible dual control mechanism in the origin of peptic ulcer. A study on ulcer location as affected by mucosa and musculature. Gastroenterology. 1969;57:280-93.
47. Thomas WEG, Thompson MH, Williamson RCN. The long-term outcome of Billroth I partial gastrectomy for benign gastric ulcers. Ann Surg. 1982;195:189-95.
48. Emas S, Grupcev G, Eriksson B. Ten-year follow-up of a prospective, randomized trial of selective proximal vagotomy with ulcer excision and partial gastrectomy with gastroduodenostomy for treating corporal gastric ulcer. Am J Surg. 1994;167:596-600.
49. Weaver DH, Maxwell JG, Castleton KB. Mallory-Weiss syndrome. Am J Surg. 1969;118:887-92.
50. Gauderer MW, Ponsky JL. A simplified technique for constructing a tube feeding gastrostomy. Surg Gynecol Obstet. 1981;152:83-5.

Additional references appear in the online version of this book.

49A

Esophageal Neoplasms

Jon Shenfine, Glyn Jamieson

Key Points

- Squamous carcinoma varies widely in incidence from one country to another. Possible reasons include dietary and viral factors as well as patterns of alcohol and cigarette consumption.
- In developed countries, an increasing incidence of adenocarcinoma of the lower esophagus is linked to gastroesophageal reflux and Barrett's esophagus.
- Esophageal cancer should be highly suspected in every patient beyond middle age who presents with dysphagia. The diagnosis is confirmed by endoscopy with biopsy.
- Surgery remains the mainstay of potential cure, but definitive radiotherapy or chemoradiotherapy may be used in carefully selected patients.
- Selection for operation requires an assessment of patient fitness (age, cardiorespiratory status) as well as the stage of the cancer as determined by computed tomography (CT) scan, positron emission tomography (PET) scan, bronchoscopy, and endoscopic ultrasound.
- Resection for cure may involve a left thoracoabdominal approach, a two-stage abdominal plus right thoracic approach, a three-stage approach incorporating a cervical incision or a transhiatal approach. Esophageal conduit reconstruction generally utilizes the stomach, but the jejunum and colon are alternatives. Minimal access techniques may widen the scope of operation, but their role remains in contention.
- Multidisciplinary postoperative care has contributed to a decline in the mortality rate of esophagectomy toward 5%. Pulmonary complications and anastomotic leakage are the most common causes of death.
- Neoadjuvant treatment with chemotherapy or chemoradiotherapy is now the standard of care for advanced but still operable disease. Chemotherapy, radiotherapy, dilatation, stenting, and thermal ablation can be used as palliation to relieve dysphagia.

INTRODUCTION

Esophageal cancer is a devastating diagnosis. By far the majority of patients at the time of presentation have advanced disease and a grim outlook. Untreated, the obstructive effect of the tumor in the esophageal lumen rapidly leads to increasing dysphagia, first for solids and terminally even for saliva, resulting in a miserable death. Although primarily a disease of the elderly, better healthcare has led to an aging population and thus an increasing incidence, but coupled to this there has been an independent and dramatic increase in the incidence of adenocarcinoma of the esophagus in developed nations over the last 30 years. We are also in an era of major changes in how to manage this disease—through minimally invasive surgical techniques, endoscopic treatments, and adjuvant/neoadjuvant multimodal therapies. Despite these advances, esophageal cancer remains of low public and media profile, perhaps as it remains of lower prevalence than cancers such as colorectal and lung and is less emotive than breast or prostate cancers.

EPIDEMIOLOGY AND ETIOLOGY

Adenocarcinoma of the Esophagus

In the 1940s, any consideration of esophageal cancer would have dealt almost exclusively with squamous cell carcinoma because adenocarcinoma of the esophagus then accounted for <5% of cases. In much of the Eastern world, this situation remains largely unchanged. However, in the Western world, over the last three decades, the incidence of adenocarcinoma of the lower esophagus and cardia has risen dramatically; at one point the rate of increase in incidence was 10% per year in the United States, but it has slowed to 1.5% more recently.[1,2] As a result, the incidence of adenocarcinoma of the esophagus was 0.1/100,000 in the first half of the 20th century in the United States, but it has now overtaken that of squamous cell cancer and probably accounts for two thirds of all esophageal cancer cases in the West, with an incidence of 4.8/100,000 in the white, male, US Caucasian population.[3]

This almost epidemic rise in incidence in esophageal adenocarcinoma is difficult to blame on one predisposing factor. A strong birth cohort effect (i.e. an increasing risk for successive generations) suggests that there are lifestyle and/or environmental factors with significant ongoing influence on the risk of developing esophageal adenocarcinoma. The main risk factors are generally acknowledged to be gastroesophageal reflux, obesity, and smoking, which may all act synergistically.[4] Although smoking rates are on the decline, it is without question that the prevalence of obesity has increased in the West, with successive generations in the United States becoming heavier at younger ages.[5] This situation has occurred hand in hand with an increase in the prevalence of reflux.[6] This is not the situation in the Eastern world, which may be responsible for the differences in incidence.

Adenocarcinoma of the esophagus probably develops in a series of steps: damage to the normal squamous mucosal lining of the esophagus leads to metaplastic replacement with columnar epithelium, termed Barrett's esophagus. Over time this mucosal change becomes increasingly dysplastic and eventually develops into frank adenocarcinoma. The damage probably stems from inflammation associated with gastroesophageal reflux, be this acid, bile, pepsin, or a mixture of these gastric and duodenal juices. The origin of the columnar cells remains unclear. The severity and chronicity of the mucosal damage are likely to be important, as demonstrated by a large cohort population-based Danish study.[7] The authors showed that patients with erosive esophageal reflux have a fivefold risk of developing Barrett's esophagus and an eightfold increased incidence of esophageal adenocarcinoma over patients with nonerosive reflux. Regardless, once Barrett's esophagus has developed, the relative risk of developing an esophageal adenocarcinoma increases to 40–125 times than that of the general population, although an individual's risk remains low at 0–3% per year.[8] Varying degrees of dysplasia can be distinguished prior to malignant transformation with highly dysplastic Barrett's esophagus, demonstrating a risk of at least 25% of developing adenocarcinoma, and patients who undergo resection of high-grade dysplasia uncover a hitherto unknown underlying adenocarcinoma of the esophagus in 40–57%.[9] Interestingly, Barrett's esophagus is not always visible beside an adenocarcinoma of the esophagus, with reported rates of 20–58% of cases, and the behavior of tumors with or without an associated columnar change is reported to be different.[10,11] However, this fact may be due to obliteration of the Barrett's epithelium by tumor and earlier diagnosis in patients with Barrett's changes.[12] It also remains possible that an as yet unidentified factor is responsible for the development of esophageal cancer—without the need for pre-existing columnar mucosa.

Squamous Cell Carcinoma of the Esophagus

The incidence of squamous cell carcinoma varies enormously, from 3–5/100,000 in Western populations to >100/100,000 population in Linxian county in Northern China, but in all areas the incidence is currently stable. High ethanol intake, cigarette consumption, and low socioeconomic status are the most important general risk factors, and there is some evidence for the role of human papillomavirus as a potential etiologic factor, akin to its role in squamous cancer of the cervix.[13] However, in areas in which there is a very high incidence of squamous cell carcinoma, dietary factors may be of primary etiological importance, e.g.:

- In Linxian county in China, it is thought that the method of preserving food is related to the high incidence, and this hypothesis is apparently confirmed by the fact that chickens in the area fed similar preserved foods develop an identical type of cancer.[14]
- In Golestan province in northern Iran, which has a similar incidence to that of Linxian county, the most likely main factor is the habit of drinking exceptionally hot black tea, although other factors such as vitamin deficiency and opium use may also be relevant.[15]

In a small number of cases, the development of squamous cancer is specifically linked to other disorders. Patients with achalasia have a sevenfold increased incidence regardless of treatment status.[16] Tylosis, a rare disease of hyperkeratosis of interphalangeal epithelium and soles of the feet, is also associated with squamous cell cancer (at an earlier age than sporadic cases). Finally, there is an association with caustic injuries, although the latent period for the development of a squamous cancer is probably 15–40 years.[17]

NATURAL HISTORY AND PRESENTATION

The most common presentation of esophageal cancer is difficulty in swallowing. Of 209 patients who had carcinoma of the esophagus seen at the Royal Adelaide

Hospital between 1979 and 1983, dysphagia was the presenting symptom in 89% and about 50% had retrosternal or epigastric pain or discomfort. Almost 80% noticed that they had lost weight. Only about two thirds of patients who had an adenocarcinoma arising in association with columnar-lined esophagus had complained of pre-existing heartburn.

Although they arise from different cells, the clinical course of adenocarcinoma and squamous cell cancer affecting the esophagus are probably similar as they:

- Are both mucosal in origin
- May be polypoid, ulcerative or infiltrative in type
- Tend to spread to lymphatics and then predominantly to liver and/or lungs.

The extensive submucosal lymphatic network of the esophagus ensures that upper esophageal lesions can spread caudally to abdominal lymph nodes and lower esophageal lesions can spread cranially to cervical lymph nodes (*see* section "Radical Lymph Node Resection").

Once a cancer has spread beyond the mucosa, the survival rate is poor regardless of treatment and if lymph nodes are involved, the survival rates are even worse (*see* section "Survival"). The only consistently good results following esophagectomy are when the cancer remains mucosal, with a cancer-specific survival of 94% for tumors confined to the mucosa and a cancer-specific survival of 88% for tumors that had invaded the submucosa but that remained confined by the muscularis propria.[18]

Without treatment, esophageal cancer progresses with catastrophic consequences: increasing esophageal obstruction leads to aspiration pneumonia and pneumonitis; friability of tumor tissue may cause anemia or frank hemorrhage; and penetration into surrounding structures can occur, such as into the airways to cause an aerodigestive fistula or into the aorta to cause an aortoesophageal fistula.

DIAGNOSIS

As a general rule of thumb, whenever an older patient develops difficulty in swallowing, even if only a single episode, cancer of the esophagus should be the provisional diagnosis until proven otherwise and prompt diagnostic studies should be undertaken. The diagnosis of esophageal cancer is almost always made by upper gastrointestinal endoscopy, but occasionally through contrast swallow radiography or even CT. Most clinicians favor direct inspection of the esophagus by endoscopy, which has the advantage of picking up subtle mucosal abnormalities that would be missed by other investigative modalities, e.g. Barrett's esophagus. In addition, the endoscopist can biopsy any lesion seen. Contrast radiology remains a useful tool, especially for patients who would tolerate endoscopy poorly (Figs. 49A.1 and 49A.2).

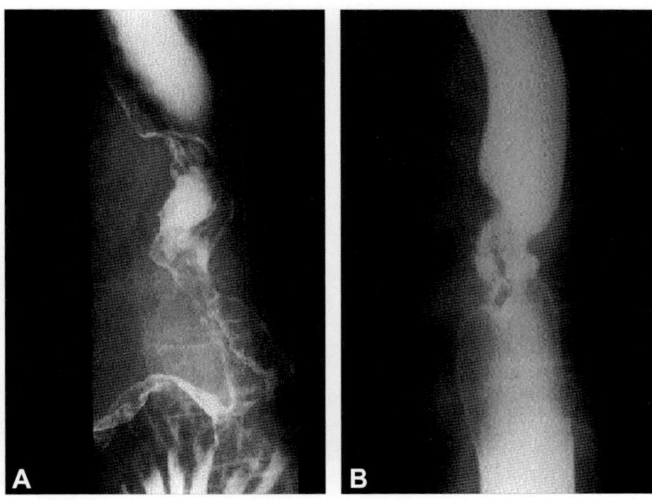

Figs. 49A.1A and B: Esophageal cancer—barium swallows. (A) A large polypoid cancer in the esophagus. (B) An "apple core" type infiltrative carcinoma of the esophagus.

Biopsy verifies the diagnosis and also determines the cell of origin. The overwhelming majority of cancers are squamous cell cancers, adenocarcinomas or undifferentiated variants of these two. Occasionally, other lesions are uncovered such as lymphoma of the esophagus, gastrointestinal stromal tumor (GIST), secondary melanoma, or small cell carcinoma.

Once a diagnosis of esophageal cancer is established, a battery of tests is required to determine the best options for management, whether these be potentially curative or purely palliative. This process is termed "staging." There are two main aspects to staging: first, staging of the disease, i.e. how advanced the disease; second, staging of the patient's fitness, i.e. whether they will tolerate certain aggressive therapies.

ESOPHAGEAL CANCER STAGING

CT, Endoscopic Ultrasound, and Positron Emission Tomography–CT

Staging esophageal cancer now utilizes a combination of investigations to determine the depth of infiltration of the cancer into the esophageal wall (T stage), the involvement of locoregional lymph nodes (N stage), and the presence of distant metastases (M stage). The first investigation is

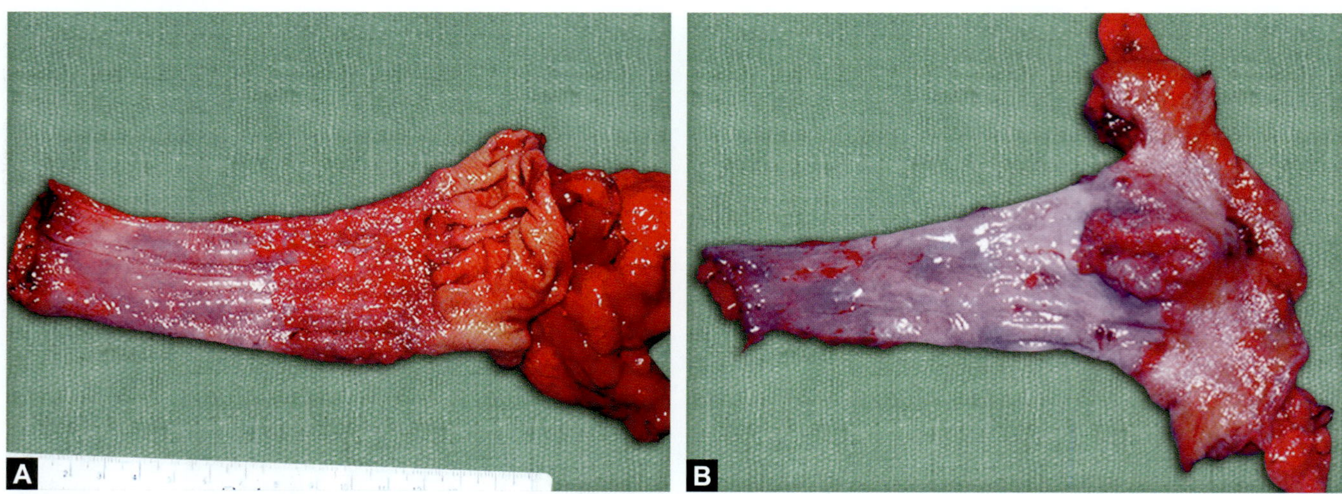

Figs. 49A.2A and B: Esophageal cancer—operative specimens. (A) Columnar-lined lower esophagus containing dysplastic cells. (B) Adenocarcinoma of the lower esophagus—protuberant type.

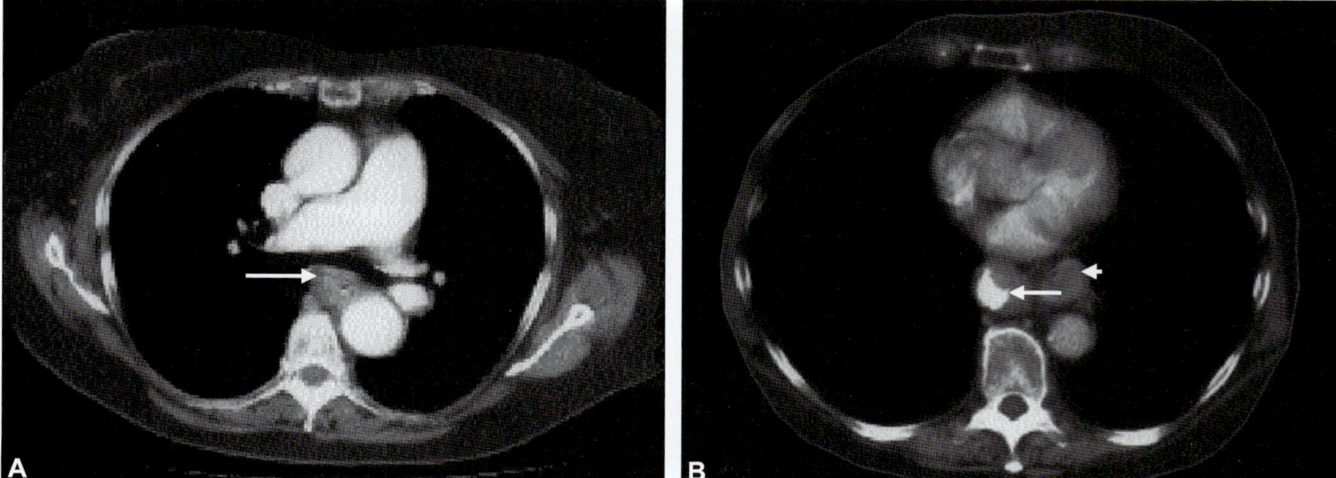

Figs. 49A.3A and B: Esophageal cancer—CT scans. (A) Thickened esophageal wall (arrow) caused by an esophageal cancer results in the lumen being eccentrically placed. (B) Dilated esophageal lumen with eccentric thickening of the esophageal wall (arrow) and a large nodal mass (arrowhead) lying anterior to the aorta.

a contrast helical CT scan (Figs. 49A.3A and B), which gives an accurate idea of the locoregional disease, i.e. the bulk of the tumor and local deposits/invasion as well as whether there is any distant spread (which for esophageal cancer is most commonly found in the lungs, liver, and adrenal glands). Computed tomography alone may be enough on which to base treatment. However, although CT can pick up any abnormally enlarged masses above 1 cm in diameter, it is not able to prove that these contain cancer, nor can it determine actual invasion of local adjacent structures rather than just abutment. As such, the sensitivity for CT alone for regional disease is around 60% and the specificity 83%.[19]

Endoscopic ultrasonography (EUS) helps in determining locoregional invasion, and certain features of local nodes can suggest metastatic cancer. However, like CT it is not completely reliable, with sensitivity of 80% and specificity of 70% for regional lymph node disease, and it is highly operator dependent.[19] Occasionally a fine needle aspiration (FNA) can be performed on a suspicious lymph node on CT or biopsied using EUS localization, with a corresponding increase in accuracy, as enlargement can be due to benign reactive inflammation rather than cancer.

Detection of cancer metastases by PET scanning is based on the abnormal glucose metabolism that cancers tend to utilize, so unlike CT and EUS that give anatomical detail, PET renders images of active biochemical metabolism, i.e. it can distinguish between benign and malignant lesions. The commonest tracer used is ^{18}F-fluoro-2-deoxy-D-glucose or FDG for short. Increasingly FDG–PET is combined with a CT scan so that direct overlay of images is possible between the metabolic PET scan and the anatomical CT. This is termed PET–CT. Positron emission tomography has the highest accuracy for the detection of distant metastases of these investigations, but false positives are still possible.

In summary, individually all three of these investigations are reasonably accurate, but they all have disadvantages and using and reviewing their images in combination minimize these and maximize the overall accuracy. Regardless, other specific investigations are still occasionally required.

Staging Laparoscopy

For tumors that cross the esophagogastric junction there is always a risk of peritoneal spread of disease, which is easily missed by conventional staging modalities. Laparoscopy can detect these occult peritoneal metastases (as well as liver metastases and metastatic lymph nodes), but it does have a small potential for associated morbidity.

Table 49A.1 TNM definitions.

Primary tumor (T)	
TX	Primary tumor cannot be assessed
T0	No evidence of primary tumor
Tis	Carcinoma *in situ*
T1	Tumor invades lamina propria or submucosa
T2	Tumor invades muscularis propria
T3	Tumor invades adventitia
T4	Tumor invades adjacent structures
Lymph node (N)	
NX	Regional lymph nodes cannot be assessed
N0	No regional lymph node metastasis
N1	Regional lymph node metastasis
Distant metastasis (M)	
MX	Presence of distant metastasis cannot be assessed
M0	No distant metastasis
M1	Distant metastasis

Source: Reprinted with permission from AJCC: esophageal and esophagogastric junction. In: Edge SB, Byrd DR, Compton CC, et al. (Eds). AJCC Cancer Staging Manual. 7th edition. New York, NY: Springer; 2010.

Bronchoscopy

If a tumor is situated in the proximal half of the esophagus and shows any signs of extraesophageal spread, then tracheal or major bronchial involvement should be considered, and a bronchoscopy should be carried out to exclude such invasion.

Ultrasound Scan

Focused nonendoscopic ultrasound scanning with or without contrast (microbubbles) can be a useful adjunct to staging: for example, to look closer at an unusual liver lesion identified on CT or with the addition of FNA to sample a suspicious cervical lymph node. Magnetic resonance imaging (MRI) is similarly useful to examine suspicious liver lesions in more detail.

Panendoscopy

As there is a 15% incidence of synchronous or metachronous naso- and oropharyngeal cancers in patients with squamous cell cancer of the esophagus, these patients should undergo panendoscopic assessment.

Stage of Disease

The most popular system of esophageal cancer staging is that of the Union Internationale Contre Le Cancer (UICC): the TNM (primary tumor, lymph node, and distant metastases) system. This system has recently been updated to the 7th edition (TNM7). The previous staging system reflected only the anatomical extent of cancer and did not take into account prognostic factors such as histology and nodal burden. TNM is usually combined with the recommendations of the American Joint Committee on Cancer; it is shown in Tables 49A.1 and 49A.2 to delineate an easy to understand "stage" (Table 49A.3).[20]

Table 49A.2 Stage groupings.

Stage	*T*	*N*	*M*
0	Tis	N0	M0
I	T1	N0	M0
IIA	T2	N0	M0
	T3	N0	M0
IIB	T1	N1	M0
	T2	N1	M0
III	T3	N1	M0
	T4	Any N	M0
IV	Any T	Any N	M1

Table 49A.3 Cancer stages.

Stage	*Definition*
I	Cancer confined to the mucosa and submucosa without involvement of lymph nodes
IIA	Cancer that has spread into the muscle or esophageal adventitia, but again without involvement of lymph nodes
IIB	Cancer that has spread no deeper than the main muscle coat (i.e. not as deeply as the adventitia) with involved lymph nodes
III	Cancer that has spread to the adventitia with involved nodes or any patient in whom the cancer has spread to involve structures outside the adventitia, such as pleura, aorta, pericardium, regardless of nodal status
IV	Any cancer with distant metastases

The major changes between TNM6 and TNM7 were the development of separate staging systems based on histology and regional lymph node involvement. This change reflects the belief that esophageal squamous cell cancer and adenocarcinoma represent two different disease entities with very distinct pathogenesis, epidemiology, and outcomes. Specific changes were:

- Subclassification of nodal (N) status according to the number of regional nodes containing metastases (at least 15 lymph nodes must have been resected)
- Reclassification of tumors at the gastroesophageal junction (GEJ) and/or the proximal 5 cm of the stomach that extend into the GEJ or esophagus as "esophageal" cancer
- Redefining of Tis (carcinoma in situ) as high-grade dysplasia
- Subclassification of T4 disease based on potential resectability of adjacent involved organs or structures

Perhaps the most important change is the emphasis on number of lymph nodes harvested as opposed to location, as recent data demonstrate that there may be increased survival based on the number of lymph nodes resected, although the evidence for this remains somewhat conjectural.[21]

MANAGEMENT CONSIDERATIONS

Assessment of Fitness

A radical transthoracic esophagectomy is essentially two major operations in one: abdominal and thoracic. It causes great physical stress to the body, with patients not only having to withstand the operative trauma but also the physiological trauma of prolonged one-lung anesthesia. Patients who are young and relatively fit with normal cardiac and pulmonary function have a low risk of operative death regardless of whether they develop postoperative complications. There are now many reported series in the literature with operative mortality rates of 2% or less, and the incidence of complications and mortality increases with worsening cardiorespiratory function and increasing age. Surgeons often take the view that biologic age, i.e. physiological age, is more important than chronologic age. As such, every patient's fitness has to be determined individually, although few surgeons would undertake an esophagectomy in a patient over 90 years of age irrespective of fitness. Indeed many surgeons choose nonoperative therapies for patients over 80 years of age, believing that esophagectomy carries too high a mortality rate for such patients. In most centers, objective assessment of fitness is based around pulmonary function testing and a gated heart scan, stress echocardiogram or similar. Cardiopulmonary exercise testing (CPET) is a noninvasive tool that can quantify an individual's exercise response. It has long been hoped that this would provide clinicians with an objective fitness measure to aid decision making. Unfortunately, studies to date have not confirmed this expectation. The clinical utility of CPET therefore remains uncertain, and further research in its use is underway in a number of centers.

Therefore, a good history, physical examination, pulmonary function tests (PFT), and resting ECG remain the mainstay of most units' fitness assessment, with a formal anesthetic review for those in whom doubt exists over fitness. The importance of fitness is that in "high volume" units, i.e. those carrying out >20 esophagectomies each year, selection of patients is probably the most important factor in determining operative mortality (*see* below). It was hoped that the introduction of minimally invasive approaches to esophageal resection would lessen the impact and thus allow operative treatment for a greater spectrum of patients, but so far this has not been the case (*see* below).

Patient Preference

With increasing public awareness of health and healthcare and available information on the internet, patients may have predetermined preferences about their intended treatment modality. Informed patient choice is an individual's prerogative and has to be respected within the bounds of evidence-based practice, but it does not mean that the surgeon should abrogate the right to provide their professional opinion as to the best course of action for a patient.

Optimization and Enhanced Recovery

Operative treatment remains the mainstay of potential cure for esophageal cancer, but is a major physical and physiological insult. There has been a move to centralization and treatment in high-volume centers that has been associated with reduced morbidity and mortality, but there remains substantial risk associated with the procedure and a long hospital stay when complications occur. Surgeons have long believed that patient's respiratory, cardiac, and nutritional function can be optimized before operation with an associated impact on their ability to recover. This belief has partly led to the development of "Enhanced Recovery after Surgery" or ERAS pathways, protocols, and programs—sometimes termed "fast-track surgery." A written, evidence-based, multidisciplinary step-by-step, goal-directed approach to the preoperative, perioperative, and postoperative care seems logical in terms of improving not only efficiency but the quality of patient care. However, the impact of ERAS pathways has mostly been seen in decreased length of stay rather than lower complication rates, which is probably a result of the complexity of the surgery and the factors that lead to complications.[22–24]

Nutritional support remains a contentious issue. Patients are not infrequently immunocompromised through their malignancy or through neoadjuvant treatment and have pre-existing malnutrition from cancer catabolism or the obstructive effects of their esophageal cancer. They are then subjected to a major surgical procedure with corresponding associated catabolism and have restricted oral intake until their newly fashioned esophagogastric anastomosis has healed.

Because of the catastrophic consequences of an anastomotic leak after esophagectomy, three questions arise. First, should patients undergoing esophagectomy be nutritionally optimized preoperatively? Second, should patients undergoing esophagectomy be fed immediately postoperatively? And third, should patients undergoing esophagectomy receive "immunonutrition"?

One question answered is that enteral nutrition is superior to parenteral nutrition.[25] However, achieving this preoperatively is difficult in esophageal cancer patients not least because of the urgency of operation, issues around their neoadjuvant therapy and the obstructive nature of the disease: e.g. because of dysphagia, they may require surgical placement of an enteral feeding tube and this may delay neoadjuvant chemotherapy. To get around this problem, preoperative dilatation, placement of nasojejunal feeding tubes and even placement of removable or biodegradable self-expanding stents have all been suggested. However, small published studies on the use of such stents preoperatively have not deemed them very useful.[26,27] Anecdotally, from the authors' experience, operating on patients after stent placement is associated with a great deal of periesophageal fibrosis. It is not to be recommended currently.

Despite the logic of feeding patients, it does appear surprisingly difficult to prove benefit. Numerous randomized studies of postoperative enteral feeding have failed to demonstrate measurable benefits in terms of complication rates, and in fact most concluded that there is a not insubstantial morbidity associated with the placement of feeding jejunostomy at the time of operation.[28] However, the studies have been underpowered, multicentered and confounded by the heterogeneity of the patient groups studied. The lack of quality studies means that we have to rely instead on the results from studies of other gastrointestinal surgery. These suggest that enteral nutritional support improves outcomes and that formal surgical jejunostomy tubes may be superior to nasally placed tubes for achieving this.[25]

If the evidence for nutritional support is inconsistent, then the evidence for immunonutrition (improvement of immune function by the provision of specific nutrients) is a minefield. Meta-analyses have suggested benefit in patients undergoing major gastrointestinal surgery, but a relatively large randomized study in esophagectomy and gastrectomy patients did not find any benefit.[29] Further trials are ongoing. Despite the logic, the benefits of nutritional support remain to be demonstrated.

The Multidisciplinary Team

Once staging investigations are complete, a decision has to be made regarding the optimal management of the patient with esophageal cancer, whether this be potentially curative treatment or purely palliative therapy. A multidisciplinary team approach to reviewing staging investigations has been shown to improve overall staging accuracy in patients with esophageal cancer, thereby helping to ensure that the selection of the correct management is made for the highest number of patients.[30] This policy leads to improved outcomes for those selected for operation or other definitive therapies and may also improve uptake to clinical trials.[31-33]

Surgical Management

The terms "operable" and "resectable" are often incorrectly interchanged. Operability relates to whether or not a patient has the necessary fitness to withstand surgery and whether removing the tumor would offer a reasonable chance of cure. In contrast, resectability relates to whether or not the tumor can safely be removed from the patient. As such, patients may have locally resectable disease but be rendered inoperable through fitness issues or distant metastatic spread, or conversely have operable but unresectable disease because of local invasion when operation would either fatally incapacitate them or risk leaving cancer behind.

Operative resection remains the mainstay of potentially curative treatment. The principles of surgery have remained constant since the first successful esophagectomy for cancer in 1913: resection of all detectable cancer tissue and reconstruction of the alimentary conduit. However, there are numerous operative approaches.

OPERATIVE APPROACHES

Left Thoracotomy

The first successful thoracic resection for esophageal cancer was performed in 1913 by Franz Torek. He used a left thoracotomy (Fig. 49A.4) to resect the esophagus and brought out an esophagostomy and gastrostomy. The patient fed herself using an external rubber tube to bridge between the stomas and lived for 13 years before dying at the age of 80 years of an unrelated disease. A number of esophagectomies were carried out using this approach, and most were unsuccessful. In 1941, it was reported that of 58 such operations carried out to that time, only 17 patients survived the procedure. Richard Sweet described a left thoracotomy approach to resection with a proximal gastric pull-up in 1945, and this became popular thereafter as "the Sweet procedure."[34] Although the anastomosis (which is distal to the aortic arch) is technically straightforward, it requires an incision in the diaphragm with only limited access to the abdomen and the esophagus is relatively inaccessible behind the aortic arch. Therefore, there is limited ability to clear lower one-third cancers by an adequate margin, and debilitating postoperative reflux is common with this approach (*see* below). It has lost popularity in the West as a result of these disadvantages, especially in an era of adenocarcinoma of the cardia, but remains the most popular approach in China.

View into left chest

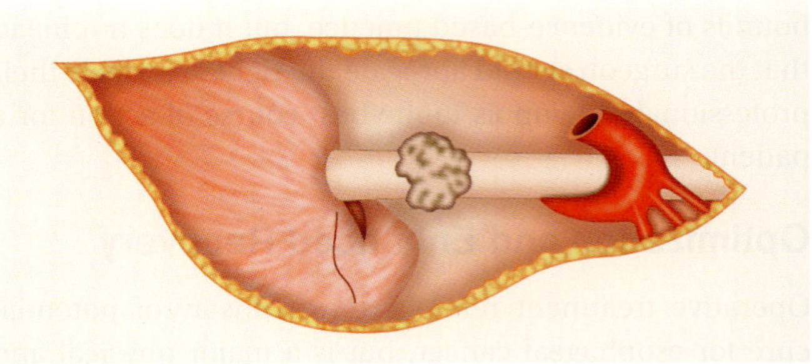

Diaphragm open with view into upper abdomen

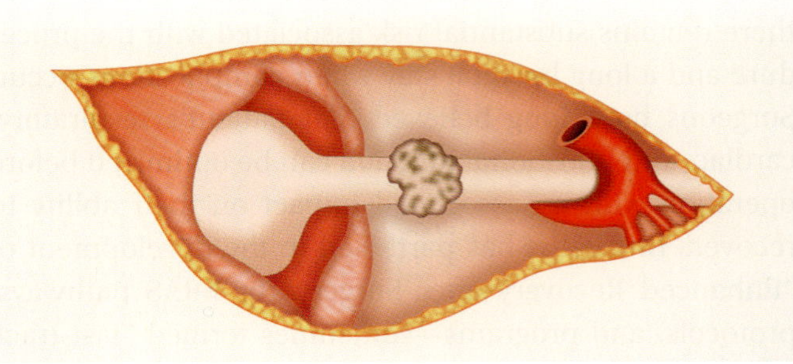

Stomach anastomosed to esophagus

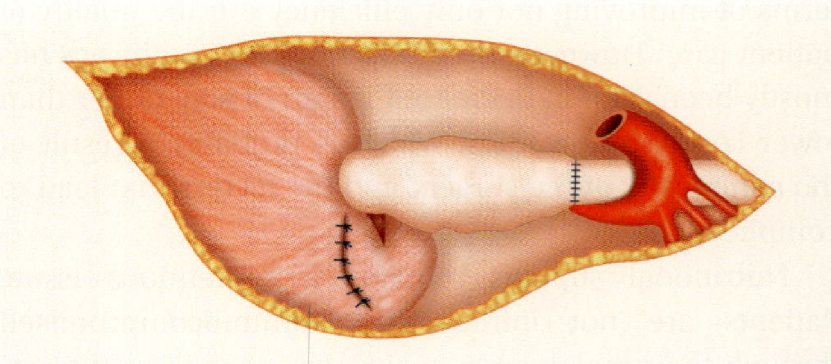

Fig. 49A.4: Left thoracotomy—On entering the chest a radial incision is made in the diaphragm (black line). The stomach is anastomosed to the esophagus distal to the aortic arch.

Left Thoracoabdominal Approach

Garlock and Klein stated that "one of the great technical advances in the last decade has been the development of the abdominothoracic approach" in 1954.[35] This approach (Fig. 49A.5) shares the same advantages and disadvantages

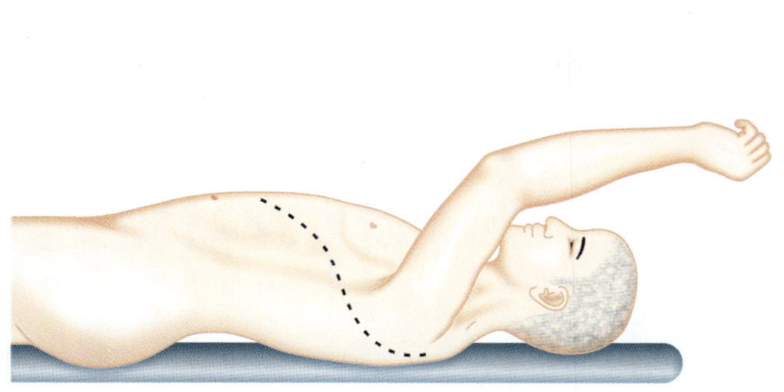

Fig. 49A.5: Left thoracoabdominal incision—Incision indicated by broken line extends across the costal margin, usually to the midline or beyond, in the abdomen.

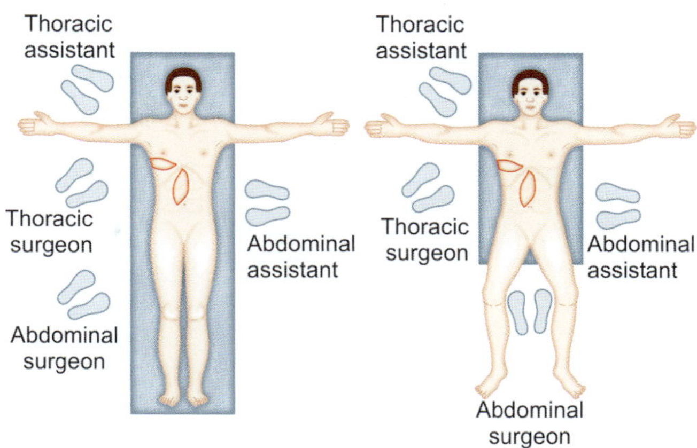

Fig. 49A.6: Ivor Lewis operation—Synchronous thoracic and abdominal approaches with the abdominal surgeon standing either to the patient's right or between the patient's legs.

as the "Sweet" approach, but provides better access to the abdomen. It remains in the armamentarium of general surgeons, although the incision across the costal margin is a painful one and in the West has been superseded by approaches that utilize the abdomen and right chest through separate incisions.

Abdominal and Right Thoracic Approach

Ivor Lewis first performed a two-stage approach in 1944 and reported this in 1946.[36] The stomach and lower esophagus are mobilized through a midline abdominal incision; this wound is then closed and the operation is completed through a posterolateral right thoracotomy. Lewis advocated the approach only for midesophageal cancers initially but later recommended this approach for lower esophageal cancers. Other surgeons independently undertook this approach, Norman Tanner in 1944 and Santy in 1947, so the procedure may be referred to as an Ivor Lewis, Lewis–Tanner and Lewis–Santy approach. It is the most popular method in the Western world for the surgical treatment of esophageal cancer, accounting for 67% of surgeon preferences in the mid-eighties, whereas a left-sided approach was preferred in only 21% of cases.[37] The approach has the advantages of:

- Ease of abdominal access for the abdominal procedure
- Excellence of access to the thoracic esophagus via a thoracotomy
- Excellent access to the thoracic esophagus without the hindrance of the aortic arch, as occurs from the left side (the azygos vein is usually divided), allowing an anastomosis to be made high in the apex of the chest in all cases

However, the patient needs to be repositioned during the operation. An alternative is the use of a right anterolateral thoracotomy as first described by Nanson (Fig. 49A.6).[38] This route allows the abdominal stage and the thoracic stage of the operation to be performed synchronously if two surgical teams are available. This approach is further facilitated by placing the patient in the lithotomy position, with the abdominal surgeon standing between the patient's legs (Fig. 49A.6).

Abdominal, Right Thoracic, and Cervical Approach

A variant of the two stage Ivor-Lewis approach was reported by McKeown in 1976. This introduces a third stage to the procedure with a cervical incision, dissection and placement of the esophagogastric anastomosis in the neck.[39] This procedure has the advantage that if anastomotic leakage occurs, it usually only produces a well-tolerated salivary fistula, whereas an intrathoracic leak can lead to life-threatening mediastinitis or empyema. The disadvantage to the approach is that the gastric tube does not always extend easily to the neck without compromising its blood supply, so that the leak and stricture rate is higher than with intrathoracic placed anastomoses (*see* below).

Transhiatal Esophagectomy

Resection of the esophagus without entering the pleural cavity was probably first undertaken successfully in 1933 by George Grey Turner (Fig. 49A.7). Orringer and his group in Michigan popularized this approach. The main theoretical advantage is the avoidance of opening the thoracic cavity, thereby causing less wound morbidity and a lower

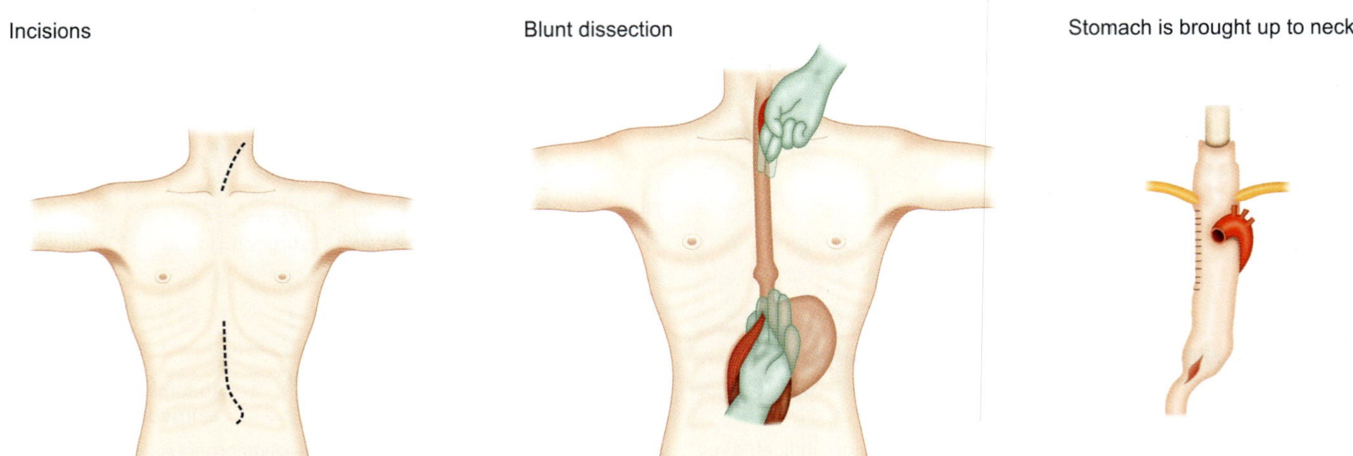

Fig. 49A.7: Transhiatal esophagectomy—The incisions are indicated with broken lines. Blunt dissection is carried out with hands in the mediastinum. The stomach is brought up to the neck for an esophagogastrostomy.

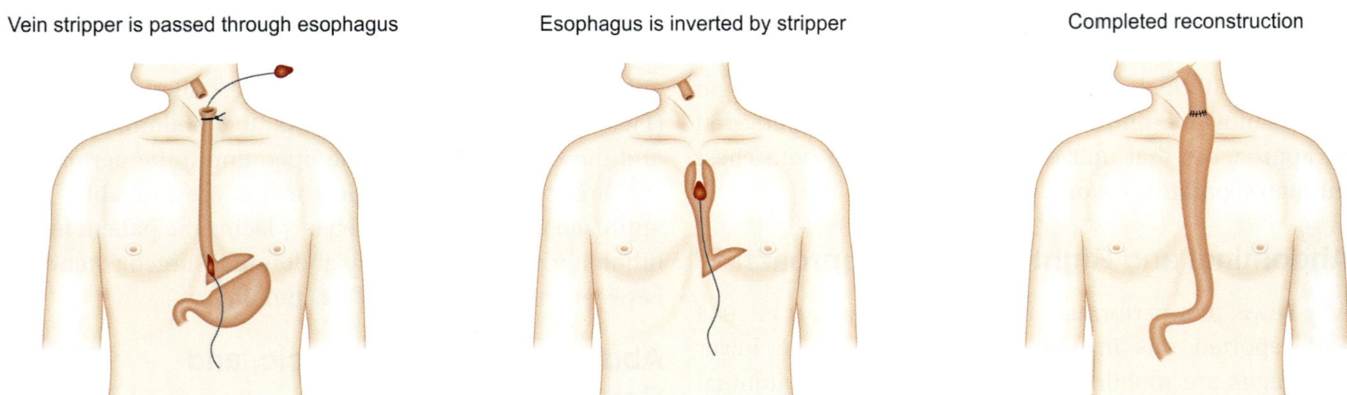

Fig. 49A.8: Eversion extraction transhiatal esophagectomy—The esophagus is inverted by a vein stripper and emerges everted.

rate of pulmonary complications. However, studies have produced conflicting results: there was a respiratory complication rate of 41% in a group of patients undergoing transhiatal esophagectomy versus 6% in a group undergoing transthoracic esophagectomy in one nonrandomized study.[40] In Giuli's overview, the respiratory complication rate was 24% in transhiatal patients versus 23% in transthoracic patients.[37] Other investigators found the respiratory complication rate to be 17% for patients having a transhiatal esophagectomy and 34% for patients having a transthoracic approach.[41] In a randomized study comparing the two operations, the incidence of pulmonary complications was about 20% in *both* groups.[42] The disadvantages of the technique are that of a cervical anastomosis and the lack of a radical nodal dissection in the chest. Regardless, this remains popular with acceptable results from several centers specializing in esophageal surgery. Variants of the transhiatal technique use esophageal "stripping" with a ring dissector or an eversion technique (as originally advocated by Akiyama et al. in 1975) (Fig. 49A.8).[43,44]

Minimally Invasive Esophagectomy

The dramatic expansion of laparoscopic and thoracoscopic surgery during the 1990s suggested a possible application for esophageal cancer.[45] Esophagectomy remains an extremely traumatic procedure, perhaps more than any other common surgical procedure. This fact is reflected in the morbidity and mortality rates associated with the procedure (*see* below) and in the poor overall survival (50% in the first 12 months after operation).[46] Some of the morbidity relates to the size of the incisions used for access to surgical cavities, so it was hoped that applying a minimally invasive approach to esophageal resection would be of great benefit to patients. Reports of abdominal and thoracic stages of esophagectomy being performed laparoscopically and thoracoscopically began to appear in the late 1990s, and it was hoped that this would reduce the surgical trauma and be reflected in reduced hospital stay, reduced postoperative pain, reduced operative complications, and improved quality of life.

The uptake of these approaches by surgeons has been rapid, but benefits have been slow to emerge and there is still no consensus that the outcomes are superior to conventional open surgery. In addition, questions have been raised over the safety and the oncological clearance possible with these approaches.[47] Various combinations of approaches may be utilized, including a totally minimally invasive esophagectomy with a laparoscopic abdominal approach and a thoracoscopic chest approach but also utilizing open approaches to either of these stages and the addition of a cervical incision and dissection and the use of an abdominal hand-port. These may be termed "hybrid" approaches. This variety inhibits our ability to compare approaches, together with the inherent, underlying clinical heterogeneity of patients which in most cases entails an individualized approach to surgical treatment.[48] Regardless, there have been numerous case series, at least six systematic reviews and one randomized study of minimally invasive techniques in esophageal resection. Biere and colleagues randomly assigned 115 patients to either an open or totally minimally invasive esophagectomy.[49] Short-term follow-up demonstrated improved outcomes for the minimally invasive group: they had a lower incidence of pulmonary complications, a reduced hospital stay, and better quality of life, with no compromise in the quality of the resected specimen. When reviewed together with other quality case series, a few points can be gathered in relation to minimally invasive esophagectomy:

1. Feasibility and safety:
    a. Minimally invasive techniques are feasible and safe.
    b. Similar morbidity and mortality rates occur.[50–52]
    c. There is a trend to reduced pulmonary complications and reduced intraoperative blood loss.[49,52]
    d. There is a marginally higher rate of postoperative gastric necrosis. Preconditioning of the conduit does not appear to improve this, but using a wide gastric conduit and placement of the anastomosis in the chest does.[50,53–55]
    e. A minimally invasive approach is no less traumatic option for patients deemed unfit for open operation. Patient selection and staging remain the same.[52]
2. Oncological effects:
    a. Resection rates and nodal yields appear to be comparable between open and minimally invasive approaches.[49]
    b. There is no increase in locoregional recurrence rates with a minimally invasive approach.[56]
    c. Overall and disease-free survival appear broadly comparable.[56,57]
3. Benefits:
    a. Minimally invasive approaches are associated with a reduced postoperative hospital stay.[49,50,58]
    b. There are short-term benefits in the recovery of postoperative health and related quality of life for a minimally invasive approach.[50,59]
    c. These effects diminish over time, and medium-term quality-of-life scores are comparable between open and minimally invasive approaches.[58]

In summary, there appear to be short-term benefits to a minimally invasive esophagectomy, but these approaches are probably best used on an individual basis and should not be viewed as a panacea to reduce complications or hospital stay. In fact, it can be argued that the impact of enhanced recovery programs has been greater with no associated concern over oncological clearance.[23]

Robotic Surgery

Conventional thoracoscopy has some limitations: port placement is hindered by the rib spaces, which in turn limits freedom of movement, and the standard two-dimensional view impedes hand–eye coordination. Robot-assisted surgery with improved optics (an enlarged three-dimensional field of view) and articulated instruments that allow fine control within a confined space should in theory complement the thoracoscopic approach. However, there have been reports of increased airway injuries, long operating times, and an extremely high cost.[60,61] The potential benefits of this new technology are being evaluated in a randomized study, but it is unlikely for the reasons elucidated earlier that substantial differences will be determined.[61]

RECONSTRUCTION

Gastric Conduit

The stomach is the most popular substitute for the esophagus when it is removed for cancer. In one review of 709 cases, stomach was used in 88%, colon in 8%, and small bowel in 4% of patients.[37] The reasons for the popularity of the stomach are obvious and well known:

- The stomach has an excellent and plastic blood supply
- It is relatively straightforward to mobilize
- Only one anastomosis is required—an esophagogastric anastomosis.

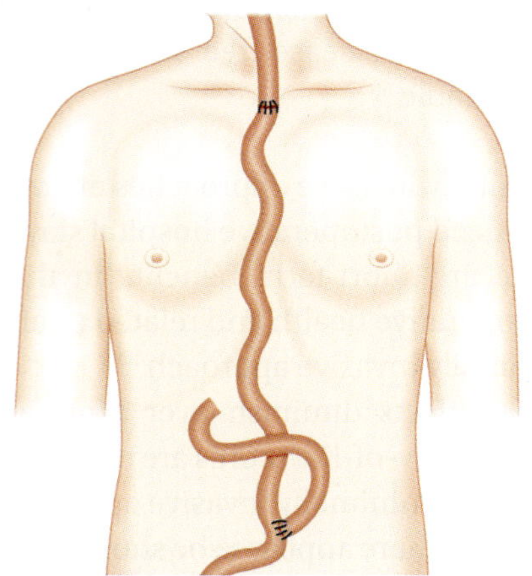

Fig. 49A.9: Esophageal resection with Roux-en-Y reconstruction using jejunum.

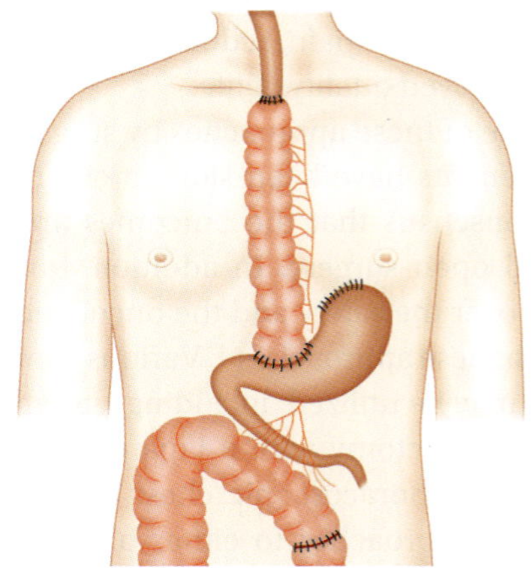

Fig. 49A.10: Esophageal resection with colonic interposition, retaining the stomach.

The vagal nerves are sectioned during cancer resection, so opinion is divided about whether some form of pyloric modification should accompany the transposition of the stomach into the chest or neck. Two randomized studies have suggested that pyloroplasty should be added: in both of these studies, delayed gastric emptying caused problems in some of those who did not have a pyloroplasty, while two and three patients, respectively, died as a result of aspiration almost certainly associated with delayed gastric emptying.[62,63] However, more recent studies have questioned this finding.[64] Additionally, the type of drainage procedure—whether formal pyloroplasty, pyloromyotomy or endoscopic balloon dilatation—is uncertain.[65,66] The height of the esophagogastric anastomosis in or above the chest is another technical factor worth emphasizing. A prospectively studied series of patients having esophagectomy showed that 5 of 17 patients who had apical thoracic anastomoses had endoscopic evidence of esophagitis compared to 19 of 20 patients who had a subhilar anastomosis in the chest.[67] A more recent report also supports the view that reflux symptoms are less likely the more proximal the anastomosis, with reflux esophagitis being found in 43% of 30 patients when the anastomosis was intrathoracic (with a 13% late-stricture rate) as opposed to 6% (with a 2% stricture rate) when the anastomosis was in the neck.[68] Finally, although the stomach has an excellent blood supply, this is sometimes suboptimal once the stomach reaches to the neck, hence the greater incidence of anastomotic leak and stricture formation in those who have a cervical anastomosis.[69]

Other Conduits

The jejunum can also be used as a neoesophageal conduit, but it is more difficult to make it reach the neck and its configuration often has a "gathered" look, which is not ideal for good ingestion. Furthermore, another anastomosis is required (i.e. a jejunojejunal anastomosis; Fig. 49A.9). Colon provides good length, but more extensive dissection is required than with the other two procedures, three anastomoses are required (i.e. esophagocolic, cologastric, and colocolic), and colon also has the reputation of being the most likely of the substitute organs to have an inadequate blood supply (Fig. 49A.10). In one report of 760 resections, the rate of ischemic necrosis was 1% for stomach, 11.3% for jejunum, and 13.3% for colon.[70] For this reason, the colon tends to be used only when the stomach is not available or if there is a wish to retain it as a functioning organ, which is often the case when esophagectomy is undertaken for benign disease.

RESULTS OF SURGICAL TREATMENT

The results of esophagectomy have varied dramatically over the 100 years since Torek's first successful resection. Perhaps the results are best considered under the headings of morbidity, mortality, and survival. A number of generalizations have to be made: results are often combined for resection of squamous cancer and adenocarcinoma; literature leak rates are usually quoted as those that are clinically relevant and almost certainly underestimate the actual leak rate; "30-day mortality" rates were reported in the past, however, intensive care support means that many critically ill patients can survive past 30 days, but eventually succumb to complications associated with their operation, so that the more accurate "in-hospital mortality" rate should be used.[71] Equally, 1-year survival after esophagectomy is almost never quoted and yet it can be argued that if a patient does not survive for 1 year after the operation it is scarcely worthwhile for the patient to undergo such a major procedure.

Morbidity

Esophagectomy is a daunting operation and one that should not be undertaken lightly, with overall complication rates hovering around 50%. The index complications in published series tend to be anastomotic leakage, chylothorax, and pulmonary complications, but wound infections, delayed gastric emptying, recurrent laryngeal nerve palsy, tracheoesophageal fistula, anastomotic strictures, and cardiac complications feature all too frequently.

Anastomotic Leak

Esophageal anastomoses have a reputation for higher leakage rates than other gastrointestinal anastomoses (Table 49A.4). Most case series report leak rates at somewhere between 5% and 10%.[23,24,32,52,72-77] However, it is likely that this is an underestimate, since a recent randomized trial for neoadjuvant treatment with excellent and comprehensive recording mechanisms put the overall leak rate at 23%.[71] Also, published leak rates do not usually break these down into true "anastomotic" leaks and "conduit failures."[78] In a large (n = 291) Western single center series from the modern surgical era, a leak rate of 6.5% (n = 19) was reported at a median of 8 (range 3–30) days postesophagectomy.[74] All "isolated" true anastomotic leaks (n = 13) were managed with targeted mediastinal drainage, intravenous antibiotics, and enteral nutrition; the mortality rate was 2 of 13 patients. In contrast, patients with gastric suture line dehiscence or gastric necrosis (n = 6) had a more severe clinical picture and required repeat thoracotomy with either revision of the conduit or resection and exclusion. Despite early intervention, the mortality rate was four of six patients. Any leak from an intrathoracic anastomosis carries a mortality risk through mediastinitis and sepsis; one benefit of a cervical anastomosis is that if a small leak occurs, a simple salivary fistula is usually the outcome with little systemic effect unless the leak tracks into the chest. However, regardless of the site of anastomosis, the study by Griffin and coworkers study clearly demonstrates a dichotomy: there appears to be one group of simple, isolated "true" anastomotic leaks and another more serious one associated with gastric necrosis. In the authors' experience, the former are usually small holes directly at the anastomotic line caused by a combination of a poor blood supply, a lack of serosal covering on the esophagus, tension on the anastomosis or a technical failure. These patients generally do well and can usually be managed nonoperatively if adequate drainage is possible and with intensive support. Computed tomography or ultrasound-guided percutaneous drainage to establish an external fistula avoids the need for repeat thoracotomy. The other groups are much more serious. These are caused by ischaemia of the conduit, most commonly seen at the "angle of sorrow," the area of the stomach between the gastric suture line and the anastomosis, leading to transmural necrosis or gastric suture line dehiscence. Rarely, complete or total gastric necrosis occurs—irreversible vascular failure of the conduit.[73] These cases require urgent repeat thoracotomy and either refashioning of the conduit and anastomosis if the ischemic area is small or resection of the conduit with temporary cervical esophagostomy and feeding jejunostomy.

Table 49A.4 Anastomotic leakage after esophagectomy.

Type of cancer	*Number of patients*	*Number of leaks (%)*
Adenocarcinoma	1191	145 (12.2)
Squamous cell cancer	1691	287 (17.0)
Adenocarcinoma and squamous cancer not considered separately	6463	662 (10.2)
Total	9345	1094 (11.7)

As a result of the potentially severe consequences of a leak, a variety of studies have scrutinized anastomotic techniques in an attempt to improve healing rates, while other studies have examined the causes of conduit failures. For example, there have been randomized studies of the superiority of the single-layer versus two-layer hand-sewn anastomosis, interrupted versus continuous suturing, stapled versus hand-sewn and circular versus linear stapling. Most of these have demonstrated no differences between groups in terms of leakage or stricture formation.[79] This conclusion suggests that it's not "how you do it" that matters. In fact, if one factor is more important than the others, it is the adequacy of the blood supply. This fact is underlined by the usually reported higher leakage rate of cervical anastomoses compared with thoracic anastomoses. In a series of 218 esophagectomies at the

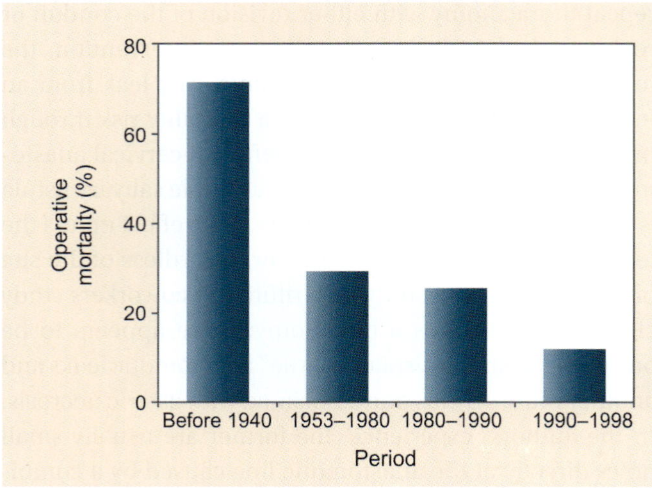

Fig. 49A.11: Mortality rate after surgery for esophageal cancer.

Royal Adelaide Hospital, the leak rate was 11% and 23%, respectively, for thoracic and cervical anastomoses and, as might be expected, the incidence of postoperative strictures was also higher following cervical anastomoses (14% vs 44%). In terms of gastric necrosis, as previously discussed in the section on minimally invasive surgery, the width of the conduit appears to be the most important factor, and preoperative conditioning appears to make little difference to avoid this disastrous consequence.[50,54]

Chylothorax

Resection of the thoracic duct is a slightly contentious issue among esophageal surgeons. Some surgeons always resect and ligate the duct both for oncological reasons and to reduce the risk of leakage.[80] Other surgeons feel this maneuver is unnecessary, yet the proximity of the thoracic duct and lymphatic channels to the esophagus render it vulnerable to inadvertent trauma when preserved. Persistent chyle leakage into the thoracic cavity or chylothorax rapidly leads to malnutrition, respiratory compromise, and immunosuppression through loss of lymphocytes and as a result increases the risk of major complications, length of stay in hospital, and mortality.[81] Unfortunately, there is no definition of what constitutes a chylothorax, although most surgeons would agree that high volume fluid loss (i.e. >500 mL/24 h) from a chest drain is suspicious and pleural fluid analysis for chylomicrons is diagnostic. Most series place the rate of chylothorax at 1–10%[48,71,74,81,82] Failure of the fluid loss to diminish in 24 hours after switching enteral feed to medium chain triglycerides would be an indication to reoperate and religate the duct. Early reoperation is associated with a high success rate.[83]

Table 49A.5 Operative mortality rate after esophagectomy.

Type of cancer	*Number of patients*	*Number of deaths (%)*
Adenocarcinoma	1232	139 (11.3)
Squamous cell cancer	2235	294 (13.2)
Adenocarcinoma and squamous cancer not considered separately	7931	817 (10.3)
Total	11,398	1250 (11.0)

Mortality

The mortality rate from esophagectomy for cancer has undoubtedly fallen during the past century (Fig. 49A.11 and Table 49A.5). In 1941, collected reports of 191 esophageal resections showed a 72% mortality rate. Earlam and Cunha-Melo collected a series from the world literature of all published cases up to 1980 (83,783 cases), and the operative mortality was 29%.[84] Muller and colleagues reviewed the published figures from 1980 to 1990 and found that among 43,070 patients who had a resection the mortality rate was 13%.[85] Although there are some discrepancies depending on the source of the data, large databases studies in the United States now show a mortality rate of at most 7.7%.[72,86]

A Danish series of 464 patients undergoing operations for esophageal cancer between 1985 and 1988 showed an overall hospital mortality rate of 16.6%. However, departments in this series performing >20 resections a year had a rate of 7%, implying that the mortality rate for departments performing <20 per year was considerably higher.[87] This volume effect has now been shown to be highly significant, with high-volume centers with specialist surgeons and multidisciplinary teams reporting lower mortality.[88-90] This finding has driven centralization of esophageal cancer services. However, once a certain level of expertise is reached, it seems likely that patient selection becomes more important for differing mortality rates.[91] If a patient is fit, relatively young and slim, there is little risk of operative death in experienced hands, but if the patient is unfit, old, and obese, there is a much higher risk of operative death. Although only anecdotal evidence, a small series of eight Chinese patients were operated on by one of the authors and it was found that operations took about half the time that similar operations take in Western patients. This was almost entirely due to the fat-free planes of the slim Chinese patients. This fact perhaps explains results such as those from a single center series in China of over 15,500 patients in which a very low mortality rate of 1.1% was recorded, a rate that most Western units can only aspire to.[75]

Table 49A.6 Survival rates after esophagectomy.

Type of cancer	Number of patients		Number of survivors (%)	
	1 year	5 years	1 year	5 years
Adenocarcinoma	286	1396	159 (55.6)	407 (29.0)
Squamous cell cancer	221	1146	119 (53.8)	241 (21.0)
Adenocarcinoma and squamous cancer not considered separately	975	4147	436 (44.7)	781 (18.8)
Total	1472	6689	714 (48.5)	1429 (21.4)

Survival

Blazeby et al. demonstrated the deleterious effects on the quality of life of patients undergoing esophagectomy.[92] Patients only regained their former quality of life if they survived at least 2 years following operation. In contrast, patients who died within 2 years of operation never regained their former quality of life. This is logical: there seems little point in putting patients through the rigors and risk of an esophagectomy if they are to die of their disease within 1–2 years of the procedure, and yet most potentially curative esophagectomies turn out to be essentially palliative procedures.

The 5-year survival figure after esophagectomy is gradually creeping upward (Table 49A.6). In the United States, around 1980 it was a dismal 5%; 20 years later it approached 15%.[93] However, recent publications are reporting 5-year survival rates following surgery of 40–50%.[21,71,94–96] This is a striking difference. Criticism of such figures is that the improvements in survival could simply reflect the more restrictive selection of better prognosis patients with no actual overall improvement in survival from the condition. Without a denominator, i.e. the numbers of the whole population, it is impossible to know if this is the case. A recent study from Germany looking carefully at surgical time cohorts has suggested that the differences are genuine.[96] It is likely that this improvement is multifactorial. The rising proportion of adenocarcinoma, with a differing biological behavior to squamous cancer, may account for some of the improvement, especially with the use of Barrett's surveillance programs and diagnosis at an earlier stage of disease. There have also been major changes in the use of multimodal neoadjuvant therapies, with randomized studies proving their impact on survival, and in addition we have reduced surgical mortality through the impact of multidisciplinary care, i.e. better anesthesia, intensive care and interventional radiology, centralization, and high-volume centers. However, some of the improvement must be attributed to more cautious selection criteria and the exhaustive battery of staging investigations that are now utilized.[71,95]

In addition, several points can be made in relation to long-term outcomes:

- Cancers involving the mucosa very rarely spread to draining lymph nodes and following esophagectomy are associated with 5-year survival rates >90%.
- As wall penetration of the cancer deepens, lymph node involvement increases and 5-year survival decreases; even penetration to the submucosa is associated with a leap in the risk of lymph node metastases to at least 20% and 5-year survival rates following esophagectomy of only 50–60%. Although cancers that have penetrated no deeper than the submucosa are designated "early" cancers, these figures suggest that only those confined to the mucosa should truly be called early esophageal cancer.[18]
- Once cancers extend into the main muscle coat of the esophagus, the rate of lymph node metastases is high and the 5-year survival falls to disappointingly low levels; in the Western world most esophageal cancers fall into this latter category.

Therefore to improve survival further, we either need to detect esophageal cancer at an earlier stage (perhaps through surveillance programs) or find better systemic therapies.

RADICAL LYMPH NODE RESECTION

The esophagus has a complicated, some say an erratic, distribution of draining lymph tissue. No discrete groups of lymph nodes are associated with the esophagus, so it is convenient to describe nodes according to the structures to which they lie in proximity, as if such discrete groups do exist. For example, paraesophageal nodes lie in proximity to the esophagus, paratracheal, subcarinal and bronchial nodal groups around the airways, paracardial nodes around the hiatus and left gastric, celiac, splenic, and hepatic nodes take their name from the local blood vessel with which they are associated.

Based on Halsted's principles, Andrew Logan from Edinburgh Royal Infirmary is credited with the concept of an en bloc radical lymphadenectomy for esophageal

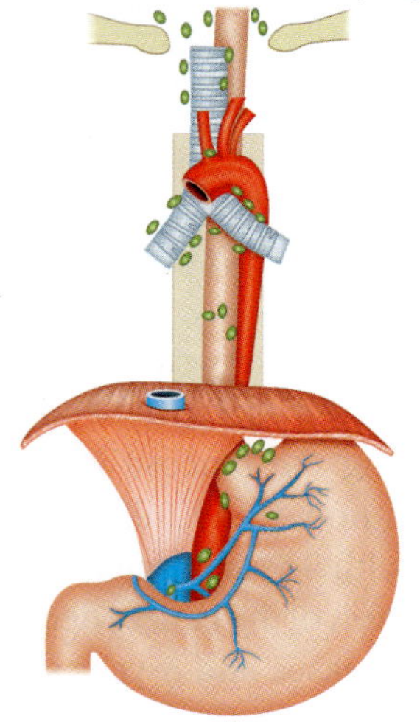

Fig. 49A.12: Type I two-field lymph node resection.

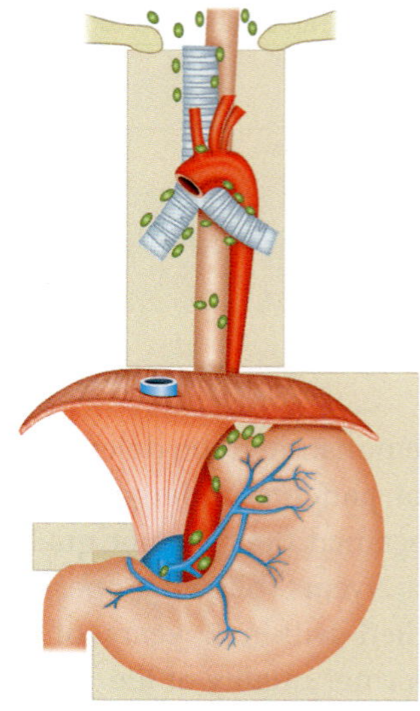

Fig. 49A.13: Type II two-field lymph node resection.

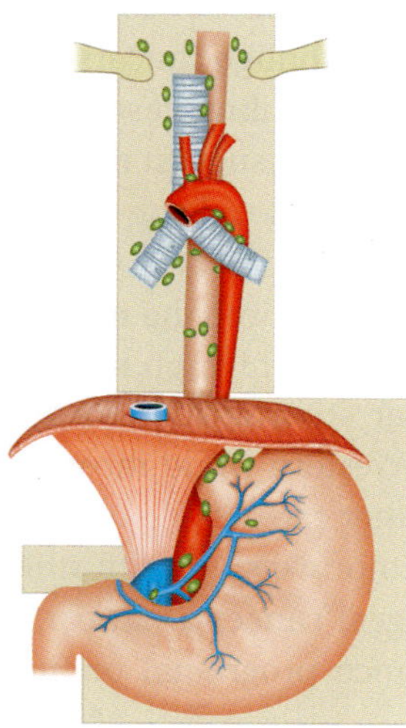

Fig. 49A.14: Three-field lymph node resection.

cancer, with a report in 1963 involving 251 patients.[97] This technique became popular in the East and in some US centers.[98,99] Various degrees of radicality have been proposed and followed. These are referred to depending on the fields of lymph nodes that are cleared. Thus, a "two-field lymphadenectomy" encompasses all lymph node and associated tissue in the chest phase, such as the thoracic duct distal to the aortic arch and carina en bloc with the esophagus together with the upper abdominal gastric first- and second-tier lymph nodes (Figs. 49A.12 and 49A.13). Equally a three-field lymphadenectomy, most commonly performed in Japan for squamous esophageal cancer, includes the previous two-field nodes as well as nodal stations above the carina and aortic arch in the chest and also neck nodes in a separate cervical surgical phase (Fig. 49A.14).

However, not all surgeons believe that these radical resections are necessary or beneficial. The esophagus has an anatomical position that makes resection challenging enough with high associated morbidity. It is unnecessary to increase the complexity and risk of the operation with a radical lymphadenectomy for early disease and, since the lymphatic drainage is unpredictable and occurs early in the clinical course of advanced disease, a radical dissection might offer little if any advantage.[100] "Radical" means different sets of nodes to different surgeons, and differing levels of radicality are possible within the confines of each surgical approach. It is interesting that Western surgeons who fiercely advocate radical subcarinal two-field lymphadenectomy have not embraced the Japanese three-field lymphadenectomy. However, the rationale for advocating the radicality of the two procedures is essentially the same, and cervical lymph node metastases can be detected in 25–37% of distal adenocarcinoma patients.[101,102]

So, is there a survival advantage that correlates with the radicality of the lymphadenectomy? Unfortunately, there are no controlled randomized studies directly comparing radicality using the same surgical approach. However, a number of studies have compared operations that we know have different radicality, i.e. transhiatal versus transthoracic approaches: Omloo and coauthors conducted this very study and found no difference in long-term survival but a "trend" to better survival in the more radical transthoracic group of patients.[103] Is this trend to better survival not enough to justify more radical surgery? Table 49A.7 reports the survival and nodal status of patients of well-known surgical groups advocating the procedures

Table 49A.7 Five-year survival rates reported with different techniques.

Technique	*Authors*	*Patients who had positive lymph nodes (%)*	*5-year survival (%)*		
			Overall	*Node negative*	*Node positive*
Transhiatal esophagectomy	Orringer et al.[104]	52	27	40	13
Ivor Lewis esophagectomy	King et al.[105]	68	23	47	8
Two-field resection	Altorki and Skinner[106]	79	18	40	10
Extended two-field resection	Isono et al.[107]	72	27	46	18
Three-field resection	Isono et al.[107]	61	34	57	23

listed.[104-107] Some interesting points emerge. In the Western series, as the radicality of the procedure increases so does the percentage of patients noted to have involved lymph nodes. Thus as more nodes are sampled, there is a greater chance of finding nodes that are involved, i.e. radical procedures stage patients more accurately. Therefore, if a patient has had a three-field lymphadenectomy and a painstaking examination of all the nodes removed is undertaken and no cancer is found, then the statement "node negative" can be made with some confidence. On the other hand, if the patient has a transhiatal resection and only three or four nodes are removed, and no cancer is found in the nodes, then clearly the term "node negative" is a relative statement at best. This fact could provide an explanation for the increased survival reported in Japanese series. That is, Japanese patients who are "node negative" are genuinely node "N0" patients, whereas many of the patients called "N0" in the Western series could actually be "N1" or "N2," and have a correspondingly worse prognosis. This is termed the stage migration phenomenon.

It is also of interest that in the collected series reported by Isono and colleagues, the incidence of positive lymph nodes recovered from their three-field resection patients was actually less than that recovered from their series of two-field resection patients.[107] As the lower third, middle third, and upper third esophageal cancers have incidences of cervical lymph node involvement of 19%, 27.5%, and 42.3% of cases, respectively, it seems inconceivable that the node positivity rate should fall for the three-field resections when compared with two-field resections, unless the three-field patients have earlier and therefore more favorable disease. This possibility seems quite likely because when surgeons and centers develop expertise in an area, unintended selection often occurs, as fitter patients and patients who have earlier disease are referred to the center. It is now well established that the use of historical controls is fallacious when treatment benefits for a new treatment are shown, a fact that highlights the need for randomized studies in this field. The other feature of this table is that the overall 5-year survival of Orringer's group performing the least radical of the operations (27%) is probably not statistically different from the 34% quoted by Isono and colleagues for three-field lymphadenectomy, given that greater selection is undertaken in patients chosen for radical lymphadenectomy.

There are, however, no doubts that metastatic involvement of draining lymph nodes is an important prognostic factor in esophageal cancer and the change in the TNM classification of esophageal cancer nodal involvement reflects this fact.[108,109] Extended lymphadenectomy improves staging accuracy, may enhance locoregional control, and may improve survival for those with limited numbers of involved nodes, but at a cost of increased morbidity; this is a balance that the surgeon has to weigh in every case.

OTHER TREATMENT MODALITIES

Salvage Esophagectomy

Recently, there has been an increasing use of chemoradiotherapy as definitive treatment in esophageal cancer. In squamous cell cancer of the esophagus, there are several studies showing that overall survival from this approach gives comparable results to surgical treatment.[110] The role of definitive chemoradiotherapy in adenocarcinoma of the esophagus is less certain.[111] The major problem with this approach is that when cure is not achieved, the cancer recurs or persists, leading to problematic dysphagia. Several small series suggest that, providing the patient is deemed fit enough, esophagectomy can still be undertaken with reasonable morbidity and mortality risk. This procedure is termed "salvage esophagectomy." Long-term comparable results to primary esophagectomy can be achieved thereafter.[112] This is an emerging role for esophagectomy and again demands the involvement of units specialized in the surgery of the esophagus.

Neoadjuvant Therapies

The role of adjuvant and neoadjuvant therapies has been debated and studied for many years, given the poor outcomes from surgery alone for advanced disease. The aims of any adjuvant therapy are to downstage local disease to enable an R0 resection and to sterilize micrometastatic disease, thereby improving long-term survival. Despite the logic of these statements, benefits have been surprisingly difficult to prove. Regardless, the last 10 years has seen a dramatic change in our management of patients with advanced disease, with two adjuvant modalities proving useful, both given preoperatively: chemotherapy and chemoradiotherapy.

Chemotherapy

Evidence for preoperative chemotherapy comes mostly from two studies performed by the United Kingdom (UK) Medical Research Council (MRC). The OE02 trial randomized 802 patients with potentially operable esophageal cancer (approximately 70% had adenocarcinoma) to preoperative chemotherapy (two cycles of cisplatin and 5-fluorouracil, 5-FU intravenously) followed by esophagectomy versus surgery alone.[113] Resection rates were higher in the neoadjuvant group, and survival at 5 years improved by 6%. A concurrent trial for gastric cancer (MRC ST02 or MAGIC trial) randomized 503 patients to three cycles of preoperative chemotherapy (epirubicin, cisplatin, and 5-FU) followed by surgery followed by a further three cycles of chemotherapy again versus surgery alone.[114] This trial demonstrated a significant survival benefit of 13% at 5 years. The importance of this study is that 26% of the patients had distal esophageal or GEJ cancers. This has prompted a third study, MRC OE05 in the United Kingdom, with longer and stronger preoperative chemotherapy, similar to the MAGIC regimen, being compared to the standard OE02 regimen. This study has now closed and we await the results. Preoperative neoadjuvant chemotherapy remains the standard of care in the United Kingdom for advanced disease and in many European centers as a result of these trials.

Chemoradiotherapy

The MRC studies proved the benefit of preoperative chemotherapy, but the local response to treatment was limited with low complete pathological response rates. The addition of preoperative radiotherapy seemed logical then to improve local response. Walsh and coauthors were the first to run a randomized study: 113 patients were allocated to surgery alone or the OE02 regimen plus 40 Gy of radiotherapy, with a significant survival advantage demonstrated in the chemoradiotherapy group at 3 years (32% vs 6%, $p = 0.01$).[115] There were limitations to the study, but several studies have followed. The most definitive has been the recently published CROSS trial from the Netherlands.[71] This study compared surgery alone to 41 Gy of radiotherapy plus carboplatin/paclitaxel chemotherapy. Survival was significantly improved from a median of 24 months for surgery alone to 49 months for the neoadjuvant group. The complete pathological response for the radiotherapy group was 29%.

There are still many unanswered questions. Does chemotherapy or chemoradiotherapy offer a survival advantage over the other? What is the best chemotherapeutic regimen? What is the optimal radiotherapy dose? How to we improve response rates? How do we select those that will respond? Unfortunately, there have been only limited studies in these areas and we await further information to guide our choices.

Palliative Treatments

Dysphagia

The principal symptom of esophageal cancer is dysphagia from esophageal obstruction, with 80–90% of all patients experiencing some degree of difficulty in swallowing in their clinical course. It is a particularly distressing symptom due to repeated aspiration, pulmonary infection, and the inability to swallow saliva. Although many patients who have advanced disease are not suitable for any treatment other than terminal nursing care, some patients with significant dysphagia have a life expectancy of many months if they are able to swallow satisfactorily. Relief of dysphagia, then, is a priority of any palliative care program. Relieving dysphagia not only improves quality of life but can lead to a serendipitous survival advantage through improved nutrition and the prevention of early death from aspiration.

There are several options for treatment of total or near-total obstruction. An ideal method of palliation would:

- Be suitable for all patients
- Restore normal swallowing
- Allow the resumption of a normal diet
- Have low associated morbidity and mortality rates

No single method achieves these goals. Dilatation can sometimes be helpful to achieve temporary dysphagia relief, but the perforation risk is high and the effect is short-lasting. As such, radiotherapy, chemotherapy, esophageal stenting, thermal ablation therapies, and surgical excision have been used and may all have a role. Whatever treatment is offered, quality of life must be balanced against potential morbidity and negative sequelae of the treatment as many of these patients are in the terminal phase of their illness.

Self-expanding metal stents were introduced to a fanfare in the 1990s as they were felt to offer prolonged and marked dysphagia relief with little associated morbidity. Randomized trials in palliative populations are hard to achieve due to ethical considerations and a high attrition rate, but there are two excellent studies of note. One of the authors ran a large multicenter study in the United Kingdom between a number of different endoscopic therapies and essentially concluded that there is no "palliative panacea" and that no single modality is more clinically effective than any other.[116] The choice of palliative therapy, then, should be determined by patient preference, tumor characteristics, and clinician experience. An interesting finding of this study was a small but significant survival "benefit" to nonstent therapies. Homs and coauthors in another well-planned multicenter study randomized patients to stenting versus a single dose of brachytherapy (intraluminal radiotherapy) for palliation of dysphagia and again favored the nonstent therapy.[117] As such, the first choice in palliation of dysphagia should probably be a nonstent option unless there is a specific contraindication. This policy leaves self-expanding metal stents for salvage therapy.

The REAL2 study established that in terms of palliative chemotherapy, a combination of epirubicin, oxaliplatin, and capecitabine is a reasonable first-line regimen for esophagogastric cancer patients, with a median response rate of 47.9% and a median overall survival of 11.2 months.[118] However, chemotherapy alone probably does not have a place in palliative therapy as dysphagia relief is poor, but combined with radiotherapy it may actually be the best palliative modality available; toxicities are generally well tolerated and dysphagia relief is high.[119]

Does Palliative Surgery Have a Role?

Palliative operations, either resection or bypass (usually taking the stomach substernally to join the esophagus in the neck), are superficially attractive as the form of treatment most likely to allow the patient to swallow relatively normally until death supervenes. However, the life expectancy of the patient who would benefit is usually only 3–6 months, and generally these forms of operation are too traumatic to justify their use, unless in exceptional circumstances.[120]

Tracheoesophageal Fistula

A malignant communication between the esophagus and the respiratory tree occurs only rarely in esophageal cancer but is a major therapeutic problem. Its occurrence is sometimes iatrogenic: treatment such as radiotherapy or chemoradiotherapy in a patient who has an esophageal cancer that has invaded the trachea or a major bronchus often induces necrosis of the tumor, followed by the establishment of a communication between the respiratory tree and the esophagus. Most patients who develop a tracheoesophageal fistula die of repeated aspiration, pneumonia, and lung sepsis.

A review of >600 tracheoesophageal fistulas of malignant origin showed that there is no ideal treatment for this incurable condition.[121] In planning treatment, it should be remembered that it is not the malignancy that kills the patient, but the recurrent respiratory infections. If chest infection can be controlled, these patients can live relatively symptom free for an extended period before dissemination of the disease finally overwhelms them. The simplest form of effective palliation is, if possible, occlusion of the fistula by an intraluminal stent either esophageal or endobronchial/endotracheal stent. If such an approach fails, the best option is diversion with a cervical esophagostomy and a feeding jejunostomy, with catheter insertion into the distal esophagus and a stapled closure of the GEJ.[121]

THE FUTURE

There are no doubts that large steps have been taken over the last 50 years in improving the outcomes of patients with esophageal cancer: centralization of services, high-volume multidisciplinary centers, and the use of neoadjuvant therapies. However, many questions remain unanswered. The areas that are likely to be of interest in the future are:

- The increasing use and role of definitive radiotherapy and chemoradiotherapy
- Tailoring of chemotherapeutic regimens through the use of biomarkers to assess sensitivity or response
- The development of minimally invasive approaches and defining of their role
- Increasing use of endoscopic ablation and resection
- Better neoadjuvant regimens and defining the role of chemotherapy versus chemoradiotherapy
- Awareness campaigns to increase the profile of the disease.

LEIOMYOMA OF THE ESOPHAGUS

In 1761, Morgagni described leiomyoma of the gastrointestinal tract. Sauerbruch performed the first surgical resection in 1932. Leiomyoma is the most common benign tumor of the esophagus, accounting for about 70% of such tumors. However, it is still 50 times less common than esophageal cancer.[122] A review of 838 cases of esophageal leiomyomas from the world literature revealed that 161 leiomyomas were found in 180,222 autopsies, an incidence of 1:1,120 autopsies.[122] There is a male preponderance of 2:1. Leiomyomas are found most frequently in the lower (56%) and middle thirds (33%) of the esophagus and less frequently in the upper third (11%).[122] This distribution is not surprising as the transition between striated and smooth muscle is not fixed and smooth muscle does occur in the upper one third in some patients.[123] Approximately 97% of leiomyomas are intramural; the remaining are polypoid intraluminal, or extraesophageal. Latter group may initially be subserosal. Most leiomyomas are solitary and 2–5 cm in diameter, although very large tumors weighing up to 5 kg do occur. Multiple lesions occur in <3% of cases and the condition of diffuse leiomyomatosis is even rarer.[122] Malignant transformation of leiomyoma is very rare and cannot be used as a justification for surgical removal of the esophagus.

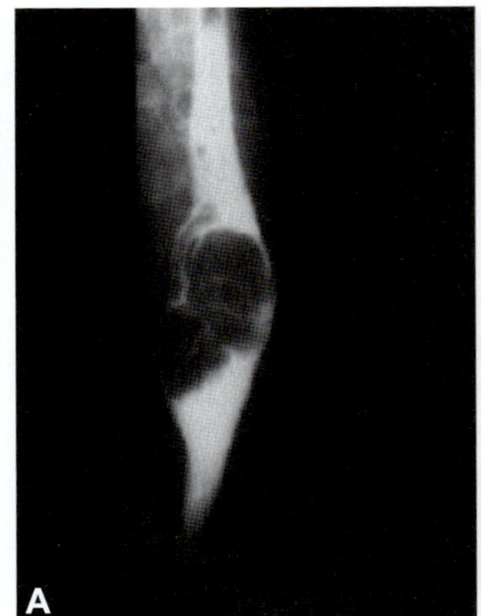

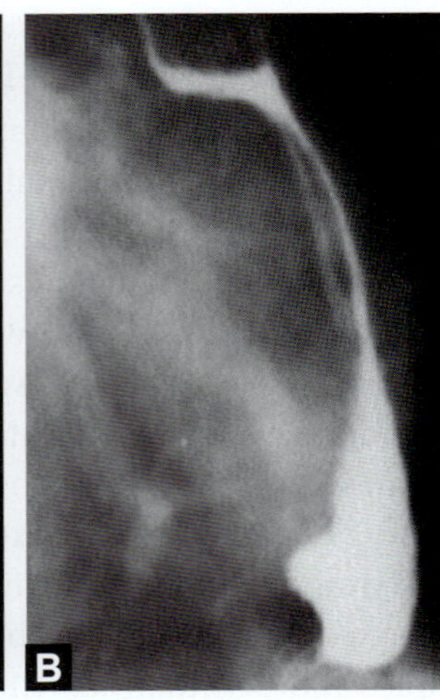

Figs. 49A.15A and B: Leiomyoma—(A) Polypoidal leiomyoma shown on barium radiograph. (B) Typical appearance of leiomyoma on barium radiograph.

Symptoms

Approximately 50% of leiomyomas are asymptomatic, with those larger than 5 cm in diameter being more likely to be symptomatic due to their mechanical effect. The most common symptoms are dysphagia, pain, and heartburn, which are usually long-standing, with 60% present for longer than 2 years.[122] The pain is usually described as a poorly localized ache or heavy pressure retrosternally or over the left chest. Hemorrhage has been reported, but is rare unless there is erosion of the overlying mucosa[123]; this is more likely to occur when the lesion lies at the esophagogastric junction. Other less common symptoms include weight loss, regurgitation, salivation, and asphyxia, or choking in the extremely rare case of pedunculated leiomyoma.

Investigation

A leiomyoma may be seen on chest radiography as a "bump" in the region of the right heart border or as a mediastinal mass; however, the barium swallow radiograph is diagnostic in most cases. Schatzki and Hawes described a characteristic smooth semilunar defect in the contour of the esophageal lumen, with intact mucosa, clear borders and a sharp angle between the tumor and normal esophageal wall (Figs. 49A.15A and B).[124] Mucosal folds may be obliterated over the tumor, but not the opposite esophageal wall (smear effect). In cases of very large tumors, the barium swallow image may be confused with that seen in achalasia because the esophagus dilates with the tumor growth and the tumor itself is mistaken for food residue. Endoscopy is useful for assessing the overlying mucosa, but if this is intact biopsy is unlikely to be helpful and in "typical" cases should be avoided as it causes a "perforation" of the mucosa that may complicate the eventual enucleation of the tumor. The main differential is a GIST. Small tumors may be missed by endoscopy as the mucosa is normal, the lesion is mobile, and the scope passes easily beyond it, but CT scans differentiate intramural leiomyomas from extrinsic lesions and vascular lesions. The most effective way of diagnosing the tumor as benign is EUS and contrast enhancement can aid the diagnosis.[125] Endoscopic ultrasonography shows a hypoechoic mass within the muscularis propria, with clearly delineated boundaries and an absence of nodal involvement. Endoscopic-ultrasonography-guided FNA may also be possible if the diagnosis remains in doubt.

Management

Treatment is necessary for those patients who are symptomatic or whose tumor is >5 cm in diameter and therefore likely to cause complications. Incidental tumors can be observed safely, with periodic follow-up as the risk of malignancy is slight.

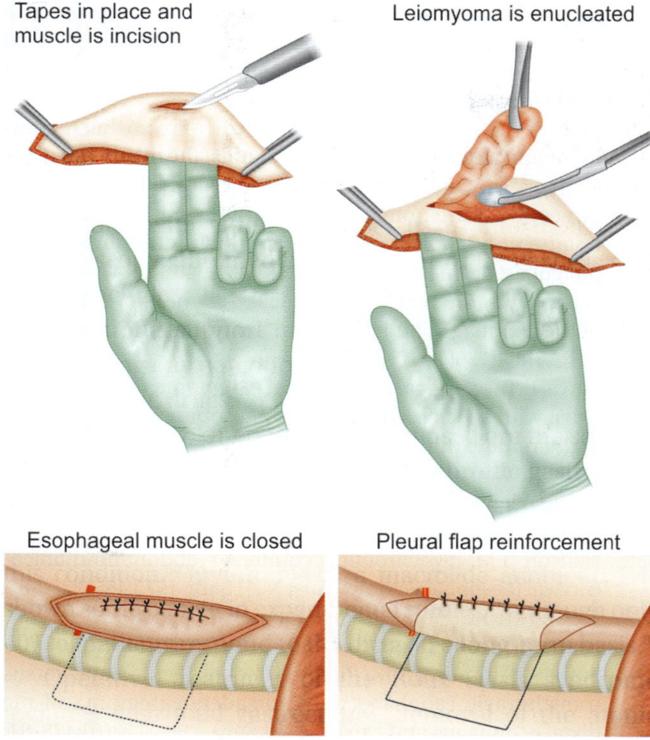

Fig. 49A.16: Excision and enucleation of leiomyoma of the esophagus. Tapes are placed above and below the bulging leiomyoma and the muscle over it is incision. The leiomyoma is enucleated by gentle blunt dissection and the muscle of the esophagus is then closed. The broken line indicates pleura to be raised for a flap which is sutured over the muscle to reinforce the repair.

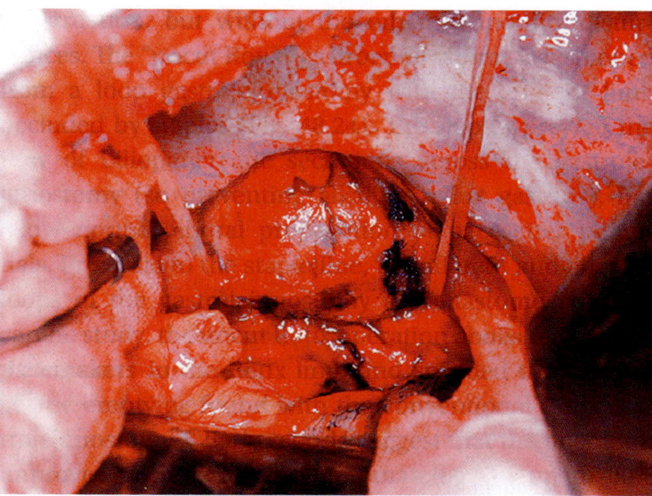

Fig. 49A.17: Tapes in place above and below a bulging leiomyoma.

The treatment of choice is enucleation of the tumor after splitting the overlying muscle layer (Figs. 49A.16 and 49A.17). A plane can be developed between the tumor and the mucous membrane unless there is inflammation or mucosal damage after biopsy. In terms of enucleation of the tumor, the operation is a minor one, and the advent of thoracoscopic surgery has changed the approach and removed the trauma of a thoracotomy.[126,127] The muscle layer of the esophagus should be reapproximated after removing the tumor to prevent the mucosa ballooning out through it as a pseudodiverticulum.[128]

REFERENCES

1. Hur C, Miller M, Kong CY, et al. Trends in esophageal adenocarcinoma incidence and mortality. Cancer. 2013; 119(6):1149-58.
2. Thrift AP, Whiteman DC. The incidence of esophageal adenocarcinoma continues to rise: analysis of period and birth cohort effects on recent trends. Ann Oncol. 2012;23(12): 3155-62.
3. Cook MB, Chow WH, Devesa SS. Oesophageal cancer incidence in the United States by race, sex, and histologic type, 1977-2005. Br J Cancer. 2009;101(5):855-9.
4. Lagergren J, Bergstrom R, Lindgren A, et al. Symptomatic gastroesophageal reflux as a risk factor for esophageal adenocarcinoma. N Engl J Med. 1999;340(11):825-31.
5. Ogden CL, Carroll MD, Curtin LR, et al. Prevalence of overweight and obesity in the United States, 1999-2004. JAMA. 2006;295(13):1549-55.
6. Ness-Jensen E, Lindam A, Lagergren J, et al. Changes in prevalence, incidence and spontaneous loss of gastro-oesophageal reflux symptoms: a prospective population-based cohort study, the HUNT study. Gut. 2012;61(10):1390-7.
7. Erichsen R, Robertson D, Farkas DK, et al. Erosive reflux disease increases risk for esophageal adenocarcinoma, compared with nonerosive reflux. Clin Gastroenterol Hepatol. 2012;10(5):475-80 e1.
8. Shaheen NJ, Sharma P, Overholt BF, et al. Radiofrequency ablation in Barrett's esophagus with dysplasia. N Engl J Med. 2009;360(22):2277-88.
9. Bennett C, Vakil N, Bergman J, et al. Consensus statements for management of Barrett's dysplasia and early-stage esophageal adenocarcinoma, based on a Delphi process. Gastroenterology. 2012;143(2):336-46.
10. Lerut T, Coosemans W, Van Raemdonck D, et al. Surgical treatment of Barrett's carcinoma. Correlations between morphologic findings and prognosis. J Thorac Cardiovasc Surg. 1994;107(4):1059-65; discussion 65-6.
11. Johansson J, Johnsson F, Walther B, et al. Adenocarcinoma in the distal esophagus with and without Barrett esophagus. Differences in symptoms and survival rates. Arch Surg. 1996;131(7):708-13.
12. Cameron AJ, Lomboy CT, Pera M, et al. Adenocarcinoma of the esophagogastric junction and Barrett's esophagus. Gastroenterology. 1995;109(5):1541-6.
13. Sur M, Cooper K. The role of the human papilloma virus in esophageal cancer. Pathology. 1998;30(4):348-54.
14. Clarke CA, Bodmer WF. Oesophageal cancer in China. Lancet. 1989;2(8678-8679):1525.
15. Islami F, Pourshams A, Nasrollahzadeh D, et al. Tea drinking habits and oesophageal cancer in a high risk area in northern Iran: population based case-control study. BMJ. 2009;338:b929.

16. Leeuwenburgh I, Scholten P, Calje TJ, et al. Barrett's esophagus and esophageal adenocarcinoma are common after treatment for achalasia. Dig Dis Sci. 2013;58(1):244-52.
17. Shenfine J. Chapter 19, Oesophageal emergencies. In: Griffin SM, Raimes SA (Eds). Oesophagogastric Surgery, 5th edition Edinburgh: Elsevier; 2009.
18. Griffin SM, Burt AD, Jennings NA. Lymph node metastasis in early esophageal adenocarcinoma. Ann Surg. 2011;254(5):731-6; discussion 6-7.
19. van Vliet EP, Heijenbrok-Kal MH, Hunink MG, et al. Staging investigations for oesophageal cancer: a meta-analysis. Br J Cancer. 2008;98(3):547-57.
20. Reid TD, Sanyaolu LN, Chan D, et al. Relative prognostic value of TNM7 vs TNM6 in staging oesophageal cancer. Br J Cancer. 2011;105(6):842-6.
21. Stein HJ, Siewert JR. Improved prognosis of resected esophageal cancer. World J Surg. 2004;28(6):520-5.
22. Li C, Ferri LE, Mulder DS, et al. An enhanced recovery pathway decreases duration of stay after esophagectomy. Surgery. 2012;152(4):606-14; discussion 14-6.
23. Preston SR, Markar SR, Baker CR, et al. Impact of a multidisciplinary standardized clinical pathway on perioperative outcomes in patients with oesophageal cancer. Br J Surg. 2013;100(1):105-12.
24. Low DE, Kunz S, Schembre D, et al. Esophagectomy—it's not just about mortality anymore: standardized perioperative clinical pathways improve outcomes in patients with esophageal cancer. J Gastrointest Surg. 2007;11(11):1395-402; discussion 402.
25. Markides GA, Alkhaffaf B, Vickers J. Nutritional access routes following oesophagectomy—a systematic review. Eur J Clin Nutr. 2011;65(5):565-73.
26. Lopes TL, Eloubeidi MA. A pilot study of fully covered self-expandable metal stents prior to neoadjuvant therapy for locally advanced esophageal cancer. Dis Esophagus. 2010;23(4):309-15.
27. Krokidis M, Burke C, Spiliopoulos S, et al. The use of biodegradable stents in malignant oesophageal strictures for the treatment of dysphagia before neoadjuvant treatment or radical radiotherapy: a feasibility study. Cardiovasc Intervent Radiol. 2013;36(4):1047-54.
28. Wheble GA, Benson RA, Khan OA. Is routine postoperative enteral feeding after oesophagectomy worthwhile? Interact Cardiovasc Thorac Surg. 2012;15(4):709-12.
29. Sultan J, Griffin SM, Di Franco F, et al. Randomized clinical trial of omega-3 fatty acid-supplemented enteral nutrition versus standard enteral nutrition in patients undergoing oesophagogastric cancer surgery. Br J Surg. 2012;99(3):346-55.
30. Davies AR, Deans DA, Penman I, et al. The multidisciplinary team meeting improves staging accuracy and treatment selection for gastro-esophageal cancer. Dis Esophagus. 2006;19(6):496-503.
31. Stephens MR, Lewis WG, Brewster AE, et al. Multidisciplinary team management is associated with improved outcomes after surgery for esophageal cancer. Dis Esophagus. 2006;19(3):164-71.
32. Adams R, Morgan M, Mukherjee S, et al. A prospective comparison of multidisciplinary treatment of oesophageal cancer with curative intent in a UK cancer network. Eur J Surg Oncol. 2007;33(3):307-13.
33. McNair AG, Choh CT, Metcalfe C, et al. Maximising recruitment into randomised controlled trials: the role of multidisciplinary cancer teams. Eur J Cancer. 2008;44(17):2623-6.
34. Sweet RH. Carcinoma of the midthoracic esophagus: its treatment by radical resection and high intrathoracic esophagogastric anastomosis. Ann Surg. 1946;124(4):653-65.
35. Garlock JH, Klein SH. The surgical treatment of carcinoma of the esophagus and cardia; an analysis of 457 cases. Ann Surg. 1954;139(1):19-34.
36. Lewis I. The surgical treatment of carcinoma of the oesophagus; with special reference to a new operation for growths of the middle third. Br J Surg. 1946;34:18-31.
37. Giuli R. Compte-rendu de la 8eme reunion de l'O.E.S.O. Depart de l'essai therapeutique mondial sur les cancers de l'oesophage. J Chir Paris. 1986;123:295-9.
38. Nanson EM. Synchronous combined abdomino-thoraco-cervical (oesophagectomy). Aust N Z J Surg. 1975;45(4):340-8.
39. McKeown KC. Total three-stage oesophagectomy for cancer of the oesophagus. Br J Surg. 1976;63(4):259-62.
40. Stark SP, Romberg MS, Pierce GE, et al. Transhiatal versus transthoracic esophagectomy for adenocarcinoma of the distal esophagus and cardia. Am J Surg. 1996;172(5):478-81; discussion 81-2.
41. Tilanus HW, Hop WC, Langenhorst BL, et al. Esophagectomy with or without thoracotomy. Is there any difference? J Thorac Cardiovasc Surg. 1993;105(5):898-903.
42. Goldminc M, Maddern G, Le Prise E, et al. Oesophagectomy by a transhiatal approach or thoracotomy: a prospective randomized trial. Br J Surg. 1993;80(3):367-70.
43. Akiyama H, Hiyama M, Miyazono H. Total esophageal reconstruction after extraction of the esophagus. Ann Surg. 1975;182(5):547-52.
44. Jamieson GG, Devitt PG, Game PA. Eversion extraction of the oesophagus. Aust N Z J Surg. 1989;59(7):567-70.
45. Cuschieri A, Shimi S, Banting S. Endoscopic oesophagectomy through a right thoracoscopic approach. J R Coll Surg Edinb. 1992;37(1):7-11.
46. Hirst J, Smithers BM, Gotley DC, et al. Defining cure for esophageal cancer: analysis of actual 5-year survivors following esophagectomy. Ann Surg Oncol. 2011;18(6):1766-74.
47. Mamidanna R, Bottle A, Aylin P, et al. Short-term outcomes following open versus minimally invasive esophagectomy for cancer in England: a population-based national study. Ann Surg. 2012;255(2):197-203.
48. Uttley L, Campbell F, Rhodes M, et al. Minimally invasive oesophagectomy versus open surgery: is there an advantage? Surg Endosc. 2013;27(3):724-31.
49. Biere SS, van Berge Henegouwen MI, Maas KW, et al. Minimally invasive versus open oesophagectomy for patients with oesophageal cancer: a multicentre, open-label, randomised controlled trial. Lancet. 2012;379(9829):1887-92.
50. Luketich JD, Alvelo-Rivera M, Buenaventura PO, et al. Minimally invasive esophagectomy: outcomes in 222 patients. Ann Surg. 2003;238(4):486-94; discussion 94-5.

Additional references appear in the online version of this book.

50

Obesity Surgery

Jacob A Greenberg, Guilherme M Campos

Key Points

- Obesity is defined as a body mass index (BMI) >30. Patients qualify for bariatric surgery with a BMI of 35 or greater with associated obesity-related comorbid conditions or with a BMI of 40 or greater.
- Obesity is associated with increasing rates of a large number of comorbid conditions including type-2 diabetes, obstructive sleep apnea, hypertension, as well as a variety of malignancies including breast, endometrial, and prostate cancer, among others.
- The surgical treatment of obesity includes (1) procedures designed to restrict gastric capacity (restrictive procedures) such as sleeve gastrectomy (SG) and adjustable gastric banding (AGB) and (2) procedures that combine reducing gastric capacity and different degrees of food bolus contact with the duodenum and the small bowel (malabsorptive component), such as Roux-en-Y gastric bypass (RYGB) and biliopancreatic diversion (BPD) with or without duodenal switch.
- The introduction of laparoscopic techniques has led to appreciable decreases in perioperative morbidity while maintaining excellent long-term outcomes.
- Bariatric surgery provides major and sustained weight loss in most patients, while it improves, cures, or markedly lowers incidence rates of obesity-associated diseases and reduces overall mortality.

INTRODUCTION

Over the past 40 years, there has been a dramatic increase in the rates of obesity in the United States and worldwide. According to the Center for Diseases Control and Prevention, approximately 35.7% of US adults and 17% of children and adolescents ages 2–19 years are obese (BMI >30).[1] In 2005, obesity was responsible for approximately 216,000 deaths in the United States, making it the third most common cause of preventable death behind smoking and hypertension.[2] Additionally, the World Health Organization estimates that the cost of obesity care accounts for 2–7% of total healthcare costs worldwide.[3] In the United States, the medical cost of obesity in 2008 was estimated at $147 billion dollars and is likely to be higher today.[4]

Obesity is a multifactorial disease with important societal and public health implications. Although the fundamental mechanism is an imbalance between caloric intake and energy expenditure, there is physiologic, biochemical, and genetic evidence that obesity and severe obesity are not simple disorders of willpower. In addition, several factors have contributed to the observed increasing rates of obesity over the last 40 years: major changes in the availability, composition, preservation methods and cost of available food products in the United States and worldwide, urbanization, and other changes in modern lifestyle. Important examples are the increase in consumption of sugar, high-fructose corn syrup, fats, and consumption of grain-fed over grass-fed livestock meats during recent decades.[5,6] High-fructose corn syrup and vegetable oils, products that did not even exist a couple of generations ago, are now ubiquitous in a variety of foods as added sugars and fats. Other factors that add to the complexity of the matter include the US government policy on farm subsidies, the marketplace involving food manufacturers, revenues from beverage and processed foods, among many others. The low cost of government-subsidized commodities like corn and soybeans make sugars and fats some of the cheapest food substances to produce. At the same time, prices for fruits and vegetables, grown with relatively little government support, have risen nearly 40% in the past 20 years.[7]

While societal changes and treatment strategies aimed at prevention of obesity are essential to stem the rising

Table 50.1 Categories of obesity.

Category	BMI
Underweight	<18.5 kg/m^2
Normal weight	18.5–24.9 kg/m^2
Overweight	25–29.9 kg/m^2
Obesity (class 1)	30–34.9 kg/m^2
Obesity (class 2)	35–39.9 kg/m^2
Extreme obesity (class 3)	≥40 kg/m^2

rates of obesity, treatment for the millions of individuals with established obesity and severe obesity are essential. For individuals with severe obesity, nonsurgical treatment modalities have high rates of failure and bariatric surgery should be offered as a therapeutic option.

Bariatric surgery has been shown to be cost-effective at approximately $18,000 per quality adjusted life year (QALY)[8] and when the operation is carried out in high-volume centers by expert surgeons, it is associated with the following: (1) a low risk of perioperative and long-term complications[9]; (2) major and sustained weight loss in most patients[10]; (3) improvements in or cure of obesity-associated diseases including type-2 diabetes; (4) a better quality of life[11]; and (5) increased life expectancy resulting from fewer cardiovascular and cancer-related deaths.[12,13]

ASPECTS OF OBESITY

Obesity Classification

The classification of obesity is based on body mass index (BMI). Body mass index is measured by dividing the patient's weight in kilograms by their height in meters squared. The categories of weight and obesity can be found in Table 50.1. Patients with BMI > 30 have increased death rates from cardiovascular disease and many specific cancers.[14] Additionally, BMI alone has been found to have a significant relationship with overall mortality in that overweight and obese patients, as well as underweight patients, have a higher risk of death from all causes than those with a BMI of 20.0–24.9.[15]

While BMI is currently the marker used to determine obesity, it does have limitations. In itself it is an inadequate measure to serve as the sole guide for individualized clinical decision making and to predict the future risk of disease because BMI reflects both fat and lean mass and does not identify the distribution of body fat and/or metabolic active adiposity.[16] In other words, BMI will overestimate obesity in people with a high percentage of lean body mass or muscle mass, such as bodybuilders or athletes. Similarly, BMI will underestimate obesity in patients with

Table 50.2 Obesity-related comorbidities.

Cardiovascular	Hypercholesterolemia
	Hypertension
	Cardiomyopathy
Pulmonary	Obstructive sleep apnea
	Obesity hypoventilation syndrome
	Pickwickian's syndrome
	Asthma
Gastrointestinal	Nonalcoholic steatohepatitis
	Cholelithiasis
	Gastroesophageal reflux disease
Endocrine	Type-2 diabetes mellitus
Orthopedic	Knee arthropathy
	Low back pain
	Weight-bearing joint pain
Psychologic	Depression
	Anxiety
Genitourinary	Stress incontinence
	Polycystic ovarian syndrome
	Infertility
	Gestational diabetes
	Poor maternal and fetal outcomes
Oncologic	Endometrial cancer
	Breast cancer
	Prostate cancer
	Colorectal cancer
	Esophageal cancer
	Hepatocellular carcinoma
	Ovarian cancer

a lower percentage of lean body mass such as the elderly and many individuals who have complications of their obesity at lower levels of BMI. Other measures of obesity that are more specific for intra-abdominal adiposity, such as the waist circumference, waist-hip ratio, or waist-height ratio, have been found to have stronger association with the risk of premature death and may play an increased role in the classification of obesity in the future.[17]

Obesity-Related Comorbid Conditions

While the association between obesity and type-2 diabetes, hypertension, hypercholesterolemia, and obstructive sleep apnea are well established, many other medical, psychiatric, and oncologic disorders are closely associated with obesity (Table 50.2). The comorbidities associated with obesity can have a massive impact on the overall health and psychological well-being of patients. Most of these comorbidities will correct to some degree with weight loss.[18,19]

Medical Treatment of Obesity

In order to achieve meaningful changes in obesity-related comorbidities, it is necessary to attain a minimum of 5–10% reduction in total weight.[20] In general, nonsurgical treatment options for weight loss, which include behavioral modification through diet and exercise as well as pharmacotherapy, fail to meet these goals in most subjects and have high weight regain rates.[20]

Two recent randomized controlled trials that were well designed and with appropriate follow-up support this notion. Appel and colleagues randomized 415 obese patients with a mean BMI of 36.6 to one of three behavioral interventions: (1) remote weight-loss support through the phone, internet, and e-mail; (2) in-person as well as remote support; and (3) a control group with self-directed treatment.[21] The percentage of patients who lost 5% or more of their initial weight was 18.8% in the control group, 38.2% in the remote support group, and 41.4% in the in-person support group.[21] Wadden and colleagues randomized obese patients to receive usual primary care physician counseling, monthly sessions with a lifestyle coach, or monthly sessions with a lifestyle coach plus either meal replacements or medication therapy.[22] After 2 years, initial weight loss of >5% was achieved by 21.5%, 26.0%, and 34.9% of study participants in each arm.[22]

Results with medical therapy are similar to those seen with behavioral modification. Until recently, the only medication approved for the treatment of obesity by the Food and Drug Administration (FDA) was Orlistat, whose mechanism of action is to prevent the absorption of ingested fat. As such, it has appreciable gastrointestinal side effects, such as steatorrhea, which make long-term compliance poor. In one long-term placebo-controlled study of Orlistat, 52.8% of patients lost >5% of their initial body weight, but only 26.2% lost >10%.[23]

Two additional medications have recently been approved for use by the FDA, lorcaserin and phentermine plus topiramate. Lorcaserin is a selective serotonin 2C receptor agonist that has not been found to cause serotonin-associated lesions of the heart valves. In a 2-year placebo-controlled trial, lorcaserin produced a >5% initial weight loss in 47.5% compared to 20.3% of patients in the control group.[24] Additionally, among the treated patients who were able to achieve a weight loss of >5% in the first year, 67.9% of patients who remained on lorcaserin for the second year of the trial were able to maintain this weight loss, compared to 50.3% who were placed on placebo for the second year.[24] In a 1-year randomized controlled trial of placebo versus high- and low-dose phentermine plus topiramate, the low- and high-dose medication groups lost an average of 8.1 kg and 10.2 kg, versus the 1.4 kg lost by the control group.[25]

While prevention, behavioral modification, and pharmacotherapy remain an integral part of the treatment regimen for obesity, it is clear that they are not as effective as bariatric surgery. The improvements seen in type-2 diabetes outcomes following bariatric surgery compared to medical therapy are even more profound. Two recent randomized controlled clinical trials have compared bariatric surgery to either regular or intensive medical therapy for the treatment of type-2 diabetes associated with obesity. In the STAMPEDE trial, patients who underwent laparoscopic SG or laparoscopic RYGB had statistically significant decreases in their hemoglobin A1C levels compared to patients placed on intensive medical therapy.[26] Additionally, they did so while decreasing the number of medications required to treat their type-2 diabetes, while control patients were placed on additional medications.[26] Mingrone and colleagues compared patients who underwent laparoscopic RYGB or laparoscopic BPD to patients on regular medical therapy.[27] At 2 years, type-2 diabetes underwent remission in 75% of patients in the RYGB group and 95% of patients in the BPD group compared to 0% in the medical-therapy group.[27]

Surgical Treatment of Obesity

Historically, there were a number of surgical procedures performed for the treatment of obesity. Many of these procedures, like jejunoileal bypass, were associated with high rates of long-term complications and treatment failure and are thus no longer performed. Others such as silicone ring gastroplasty, horizontal gastric bypass, and vertical banded gastroplasty (VBG) are seldom performed nowadays. They have fallen out of favor due to high rates of weight recidivism and/or the development of more standardized procedures that can be done using minimally invasive techniques.

In the early 1990s, roughly 20,000 bariatric procedures were performed annually in the United States.[28] This number increased to approximately 180,000 by 2006 and continues to climb slowly.[28] Many factors have led to this dramatic increase in the utilization of bariatric surgery in the United States, and include the introduction of laparoscopic minimally invasive techniques, the increasing rates of obesity, the recognition of obesity as a health hazard, the poor outcomes with behavioral and medical management of obesity and the reproducible good outcomes with bariatric surgery in high-volume centers.[29] Many individuals contributed to the introduction and standardization of laparoscopic minimally invasive techniques; noteworthy was the work of Dr Allan Wittgrove, with the publication of the first series of laparoscopic Roux-en-Y gastric bypass (RYGB) for morbid obesity in 1994.[30] Since then, most bariatric procedures have been performed utilizing minimally invasive techniques with similar weight loss and resolution of obesity associated disease outcomes,[11] but significant decreases in morbidity compared to open bariatric procedures.[9]

In the United States, four surgical procedures are now performed routinely for the treatment of obesity: RYGB, sleeve gastrectomy (SG), adjustable gastric banding (AGB), and biliopancreatic diversion with duodenal switch (BPD-DS). A review of the techniques and outcomes of these procedures will be presented later in this chapter.

Indications for Surgery and Choice of Operation

A decision favoring operative treatment must consider the potential benefits and risks of general anesthesia and an abdominal operation. Assessment of a patient's readiness for operation is a clinical judgment that should be made by a surgeon experienced in the operative management of obese patients in conjunction with other health allied professionals with expertise in the evaluation and management of obesity, such as a mental healthcare professional and a dietician.

In 1991, the National Institutes of Health (NIH) convened a panel of experts from a variety of specialties to review what were then the current data on the treatment of obesity in order to define a patient population that would most benefit from bariatric surgery. The NIH consensus criteria stated that in order to qualify for surgery, patients must have a BMI >40 or a BMI of 35–39.9 with specific obesity-associated comorbid conditions such as severe sleep apnea, type-2 diabetes, or hypertension.[31] They also recommended that patients must be well-informed, self-motivated, and of acceptable operative risk. Additionally, they must have failed previous nonsurgical treatment options, which include integrated diet, exercise, behavioral modification, and psychological support.[31] These criteria were adopted by the Centers for Medicare and Medicaid Services and eventually by most private insurance companies, and they remain to date the accepted indications for operative treatment.

While outcomes following bariatric surgery are superior to all other forms of obesity treatment, bariatric procedures may fail over the long term if there is no significant patient motivation to change lifestyle. In addition, it is recommended that bariatric surgical programs should include a multidisciplinary team for patient evaluation and a structured pathway for pre- and postoperative counseling and medical evaluation. Team members should include bariatric surgeons, health psychologists, nutritionists, and exercise physiologists. Patients should be advised and agree (1) to comply with lifestyle changes; (2) adhere to nutritional supplement prescriptions; (3) comply with eating behavior modifications; and (4) participate in long-term monitoring and follow-up evaluation.

Age alone is no longer a contraindication to operative treatment if a patient has comorbidities that would benefit from sustained weight reduction. Bariatric surgery in adolescents is still considered experimental, and should be done only in specialized medical centers under the supervision of an institutional review board.

When a surgeon specifically recommends an operation, there is an implied endorsement for the operation. Patients should be informed of the known expected benefits and risks of all available operative procedures. They should be given percentages of the incidence of negative effects with an adequate description of their type and severity.

Patients should know there is no accepted consensus regarding the optimal operation for every patient, and they should be given data from the better studies of comparative safety and efficacy of all procedures available, as well as the surgeon and center experience (*see* Section "Comparative Effectiveness of Current Bariatric Surgical Procedures").

The American Society for Metabolic and Bariatric Surgery and American College of Surgeons support the initiative for Centers of Excellence (COEs) in bariatric surgery. The requirements for these centers include the establishment of a multidisciplinary approach to the treatment of obesity as mentioned in the previous text. Additionally, COEs must perform a high volume of cases annually and commit to long-term follow-up of their patients. While there is some evidence that perioperative outcomes between COEs and non-COEs centers may not be significantly different,[32] there is clear evidence that higher volume hospitals have improved outcomes compared to lower volume hospitals[33,34] and that the support of a multidisciplinary team for successful and optimal management of these patients in the long term is of utmost importance.[35]

THE ORIGINAL PROCEDURES

A brief description of common bariatric surgical procedures used in the past is found below. It is still important that surgeons are aware of the particular anatomic changes and specific problems associated with these procedures.

Jejunoileal Bypass

Jejunoileal bypass was the prototype early operation used for the operative treatment of severe obesity. It achieved weight reduction by inducing rampant malabsorption associated with a surgically created short-gut syndrome. Jejunoileal bypass (Fig. 50.1) was first introduced clinically in 1954 and it was widely used in its many forms from 1964 to 1980. It was then abandoned because of frequent and severe complications, such as liver failure, fulminant diarrhea, electrolyte imbalances, nutritional deficiencies, recurring calcium oxalate stones, interstitial nephritis, and arthropathy,[36] as well as the publication of studies demonstrating the superiority of RYGB.[37]

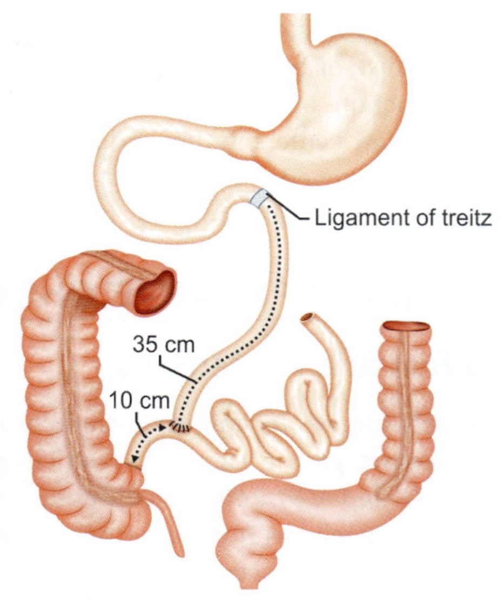

Fig. 50.1: Jejunoileal bypass.

Horizontal Loop Gastric Bypass Procedure

The pioneering design of the horizontal loop gastric bypass procedure (Fig. 50.2) was empiric and based on the observation that patients with subtotal gastrectomy frequently had sustained weight reduction. Horizontal loop gastric bypass consisted of division of the stomach into a small proximal pouch that was anastomosed to the upper jejunum just beyond the ligament of Treitz and the distal 90% of stomach, which was bypassed. Problems associated with bile-induced gastritis and esophagitis led to the procedure being abandoned in favor of the Roux-en-Y configuration.

Horizontal Gastroplasty

Horizontal gastroplasty (Fig. 50.3) was first performed in 1971 in an attempt to simplify the operative treatment of severe obesity by mechanically restricting excess caloric intake without inducing malabsorption. The original procedure consisted of a small proximal pouch connected to the distal stomach via an outlet on the greater curvature. This operation failed to sustain weight loss. It was abandoned because the unsupported outlet channel from the proximal pouch dilated and gastric restriction was no longer effective.

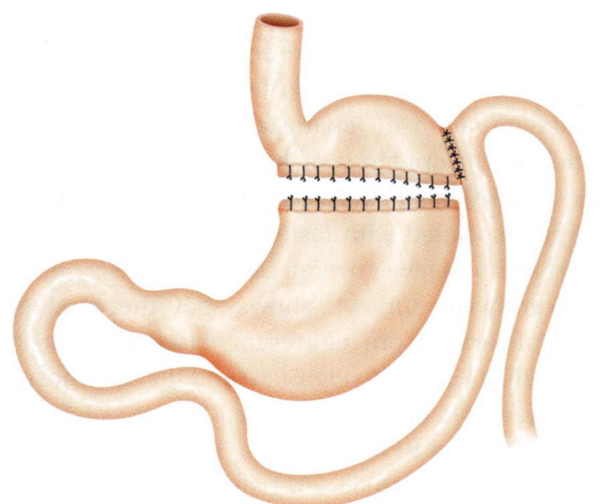

Fig. 50.2: Horizontal loop gastric bypass procedure.

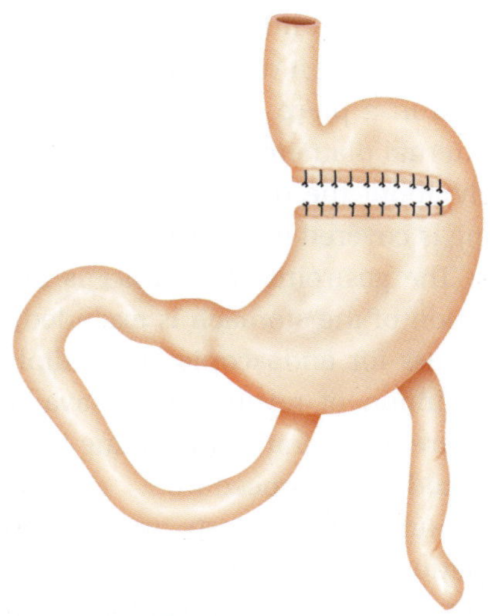

Fig. 50.3: Horizontal gastroplasty.

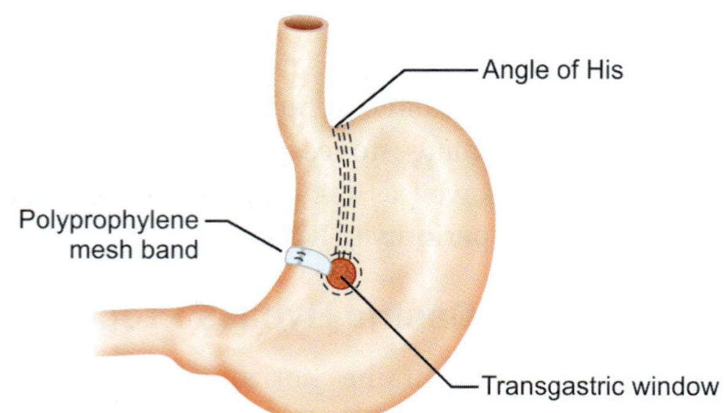

Fig. 50.4: Vertical banded gastroplasty (VBG) was introduced.

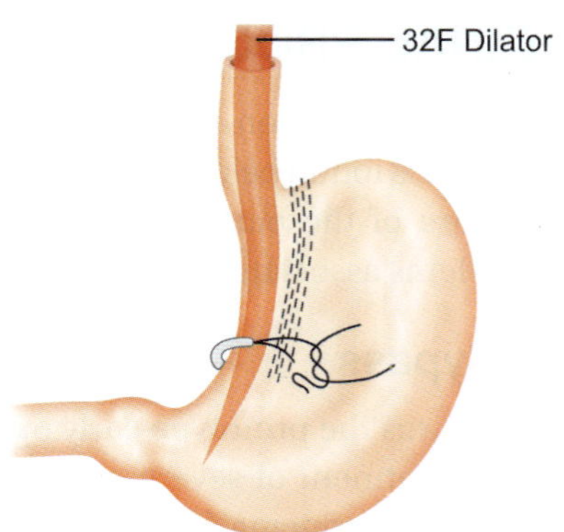

Fig. 50.5: Silastic ring vertical banded gastroplasty.

Many surgeons tried multiple variations of gastrogastrostomy or horizontal gastroplasty during the years 1975–1980. These operations were fraught with problems that included pouch enlargement, pouch outlet obstruction, reflux esophagitis, pouch outlet enlargement, staple line disruption, and failure to sustain weight loss.[38]

Vertical Banded Gastroplasty

In 1980, VBG was introduced (Fig. 50.4).[39] A transgastric window was created near the lesser curvature using a circular stapler. The window facilitated measurement of the pouch volume and provided easy access for the stapling device to construct the vertical partition. This operation provides a small food-receiving pouch. A collar of polypropylene mesh stabilizes the outlet channel of the pouch to a diameter of 1.1 cm. The mesh band is 1.5 cm wide and is sewn to itself to a circumference of 5 cm to prevent dilatation of the outlet channel. A technical alternative was Silastic ring VBG (Fig. 50.5), in which instead of using the mesh, the outlet channel from the pouch is supported by encircling it twice with a 3/0 polypropylene suture encased in a piece of radiopaque Silastic tubing 2.3 mm in external diameter and 4.2 cm long. The suture is tied snugly about the orifice over a 32-F dilator. The Silastic tubing is covered with a row of interrupted inverting sutures. The gastrointestinal tract is not bypassed. Since no portion of the stomach is excluded, VBG offers unfettered access for endoscopic and radiologic examinations. The option of reversibility is available for the patients who are intolerant of the eating behavior modifications induced by the procedure.

Vertical banded gastroplasty was a very common procedure performed during the 1980s and produced acceptable results in terms of weight loss and resolution of obesity-associated comorbidities. Large case series confirmed sustained weight loss at 5 years after operation in most severely obese patients.[40] However, revisional procedures were quite common and the technique fell out of favor because of better overall results with RYGB plus the introduction of AGB and minimally invasive techniques. Very few centers in the world still offer VBG, although it is still approved by many insurance companies and has better results than laparoscopic banding.[41]

THE CURRENT OPERATIVE CHOICES

Range of Bariatric Procedures

Current bariatric surgical techniques include procedures designed to restrict gastric capacity (restrictive procedures) such as SG and AGB, and procedures that combine reducing gastric capacity with malabsorption of different degrees. Malabsorption is accomplished by diversion of food away from the duodenum using different lengths of Roux-en-y small bowel reconstruction, such as RYGB and BPD or BPD-DS.

All of these procedures are routinely performed using laparoscopic techniques in most centers. The introduction and dissemination of laparoscopic techniques fostered the increased popularity of bariatric surgery.[29] Laparoscopic surgery has a steep learning curve, but in expert hands is associated with faster patient recovery, shorter hospital stay and fewer overall complications.[9,11]

A worldwide survey[41] shows that the total global number of bariatric procedures increased from 146,301 in 2008 to 340,768 in 2011 (Fig. 50.6) and that the most commonly performed procedures were RYGB (47%), SG (28%), AGB (17.8%), and BPD-DS (2.2%). In addition, the global trends from 2003 to 2008–2011 showed (1) a decrease in RYGB from 65% to 49% to 47%; (2) an increase, followed by a steep decline, in AGB from 24% to 42% to 18%; (3) a

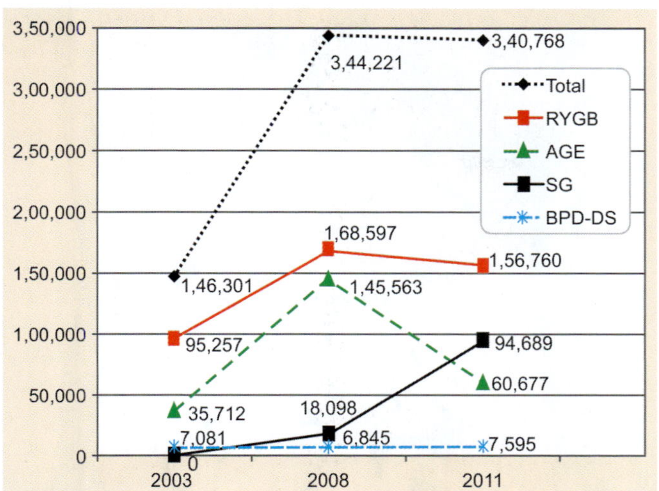

Fig. 50.6: Trends in numbers of procedures worldwide from 2003 to 2008 to 2011.

Source: Adapted from Buchwald H, Oien DM. Metabolic/bariatric surgery worldwide 2011. Obes Surg. 2013;23(4):427-36. (RYGB: Roux-Y gastric bypass; AGB: Adjustable gastric banding; SG: Sleeve gastrectomy; BPD-DS: Biliopancreatic bypass-duodenal switch).

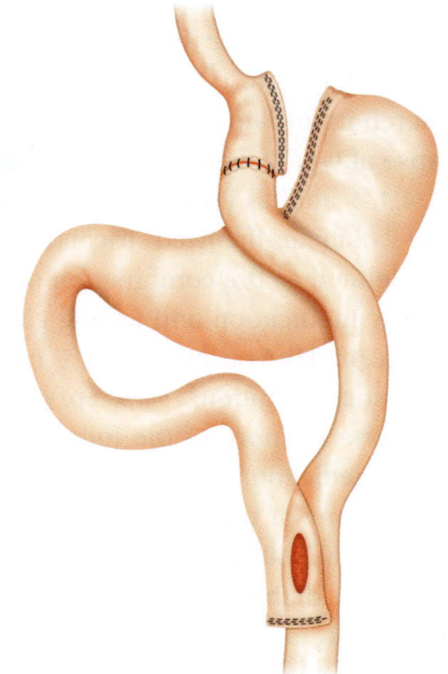

Fig. 50.7: The Roux-en-Y gastric bypass (RYGB).

marked increase in SG from 0% to 5% to 28%; and (4) a decline in the utilization of BPD-DS to 2%.These trends are illustrated in Figure 50.6.

These trends were similar in academic medical centers in the United States, where the utilization rates of these techniques from 2008 to 2012 showed that, though RYGB is still the most commonly used, it declined from 76% in 2008 to 60% in 2012.[42] The AGB decreased substantially (from 24% in 2008 to 4% in 2012) and was followed by a marked increase in SG from near zero in 2008 to 36% in 2012. It is estimated that BPD-DS represents about 2% of all procedures currently performed in the United States.[42]

Roux-en-Y Gastric Bypass

The RYGB (Fig. 50.7) is currently the most common procedure used to treat morbid obesity in the United States, Europe, and South America.[41] The concept of gastric restrictive surgery for the treatment of severe obesity was developed in 1965 by Mason and Ito.[43] The stomach is divided into a small, 30–50 mL proximal pouch based on the lesser curvature, and the jejunum is divided about 60 cm from the ligament of Treitz. An antecolic or retrocolic Roux-en-Y anastomosis is made between the proximal gastric pouch and the divided distal jejunum (alimentary limb). The bypassed stomach, duodenum and proximal jejunum are reconnected to the alimentary tract by a jejunojejunostomy, leaving a 100- to 150-cm alimentary loop. The Roux-en-Y configuration diverts the duodenal contents from the proximal pouch and prevents alkaline gastritis and esophagitis.

The safety profile of RYGB has been confirmed by multiple case series and large administrative database studies[33,44,45] and by the results of a prospective, multicenter, observational study of 4,340 consecutive patients at 10 clinical sites in the United States.[9] Severe complication and mortality rates were low overall (4.1% and 0.3%). The study also showed that complications and mortality were significantly lower in patients who had a laparoscopic as opposed to an open RYGB: complication and mortality rates laparoscopic, 4.8% and 0.2%; open, 7.8% and 2.1%, $p<0.01$. Similar data from a randomized controlled trial support the notion that laparoscopic RYGB is associated with fewer overall complications than open RYGB.[11]

A series of 608 patients with RYGB who were followed for 14 years was reported in 1995, with 98% of the patients included in the analysis.[46] The percentage of excess weight loss was 70%, 58%, 55%, and 49% at 2, 5, 10, and 14 years, respectively. The improvement in comorbidities with this sustained weight reduction included a reduction in the number of patients with hypertension from 58% to 14%, while type-2 diabetes remitted in 83%. The development of new cases (incidence rates) of type-2 diabetes was also reduced; only 1% of patients who had impaired glucose tolerance preoperatively progressed to type-2 diabetes in the postoperative period. It was estimated that 21–38% of these patients would have become diabetic without sustained weight reduction.

The largest report to-date to evaluate long-term remission and relapse of type-2 diabetes after RYGB is a multi-site study of 4,434 adults. Postoperative remission and relapse of type-2 diabetes followed strict criteria: *complete remission* was defined as the combination of discontinuing hypoglycemic medication and fasting glucose values <100 mg/dL and/or HbA1c levels <6.0% occurring >90 days after the last prescription; *relapse of type-2 diabetes* was defined as one or more of the following: restarting type-2 diabetes medication, one or more HbA1c measures ≥7%; and/or one or more fasting glucose measures ≥126 mg/dL.[47] Overall, 68.2% of all patients experienced an initial complete diabetes remission within 5 years after surgery and the median duration of remission was 8.3 years. Among those who initially remitted, 35.1% relapsed within 5 years. Significant predictors of complete remission and relapse were poor preoperative glycemic control, insulin use, and longer duration of diabetes.

Much interest and research is underway to define precisely and understand the mechanisms of diabetes remission and relapse, the optimal timing of operation in effecting a durable remission, and the relationship between remission duration and incident microvascular and macrovascular events. Nevertheless it is clear that bariatric surgery is currently the only available weapon that is capable of providing reliable and enduring rates of type-2 diabetes remission.

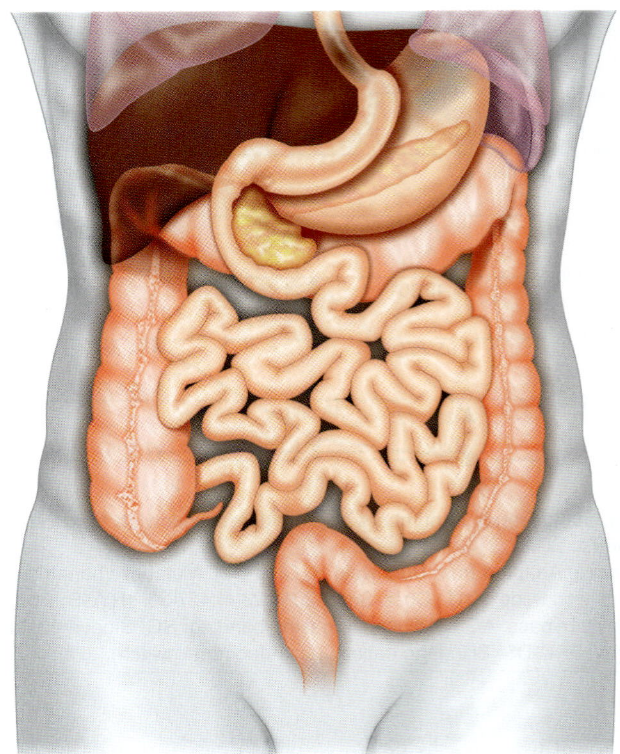

Fig. 50.8: Sleeve gastrectomy is performed by excising the left lateral portion of the proximal antrum starting about 3–5 cm from the pylorus, and the left lateral portion of the body and fundus over a bougie. The portion of stomach that has just been resected is shown more faintly behind the slimmed-down gastric sleeve in front.

Sleeve Gastrectomy

The SG was initially used as the gastric restrictive portion of the BPD-DS procedure. In late 1980, a few centers in the United States and in Europe[48-50] started using SG as the first of a two-step procedure so as to decrease operative time and perioperative morbidity and mortality with BPD-DS in the super-obese patient. However, it was noted that many patients did not need the second step (the BDP-DS part), as they would lose a substantial amount of weight with SG alone. Since then SG has been proposed and is currently accepted as a stand-alone bariatric procedure.[51,52]

Sleeve gastrectomy is performed by excising the left lateral portion of the proximal antrum starting about 3–5 cm from the pylorus, and the left lateral portion of the body and fundus over a bougie (Fig. 50.8). The best bougie size to provide optimal weight loss and reduce incidence of leaks at the top of the SG is still debated, but recent evidence suggests that a size of 40 F or greater may decrease leak rates without significant impact at weight loss at 3 years of follow-up.[53]

One of the series with longer-term follow-up of patients with SG comes from Belgium.[52] Himpens and colleagues reported a cohort of 31 patients in whom percentage weight loss was 73% at 3 years and 57% at 6 years.

Current relative contraindications for SG are patients with Barrett's esophagus, gastroesophageal reflux disease with esophageal mucosal injury such as erosive esophagitis, strictures, and ulcers, achalasia, large hiatal, or para-esophageal hernias, diabetic gastroparesis, and active Crohn's disease. Due to its relative simplicity compared to RYGB and much better results compared to AGB, the utilization of SG has increased markedly both in the US and worldwide.[41,42]

The results of SG are compared with those of other procedures in the section, "Comparative Effectiveness of Current Bariatric Surgical Procedures".

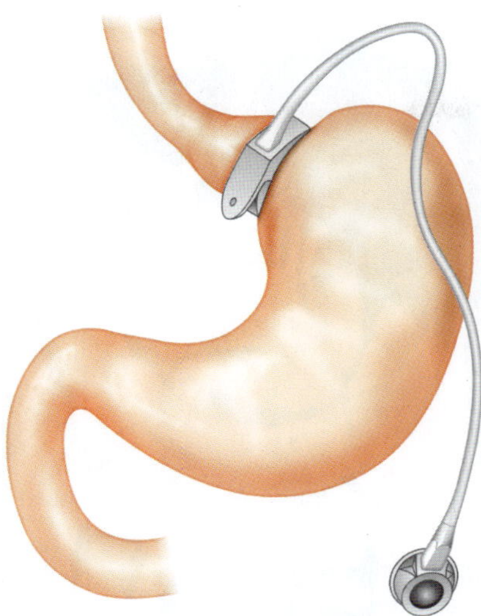

Fig. 50.9: The port is then secured to the anterior abdominal fascia in the subcutaneous tissue.

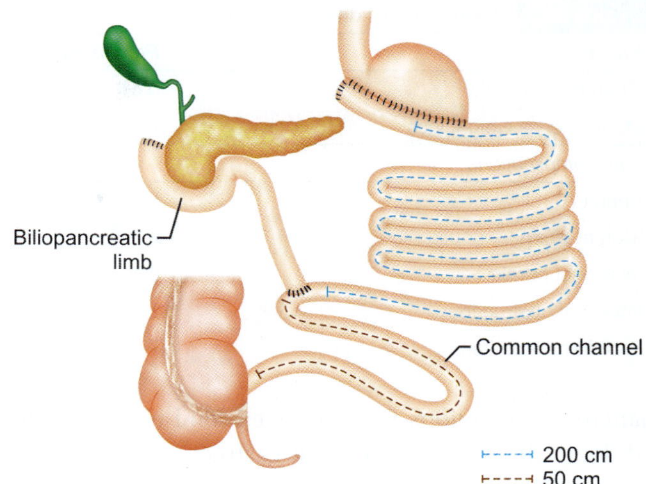

Fig. 50.10: Partial biliopancreatic diversion (BPD).

Adjustable Gastric Banding

AGB uses an inflatable belt-like silicone device that is placed around the superior portion of the stomach to create a small 30–50 mL gastric pouch above the band. The device is connected to tubing and to a port. The port is then secured to the anterior abdominal fascia in the subcutaneous tissue (Fig. 50.9). The port can later be accessed using a Huber needle in order to inflate or deflate the band, thus adjusting the inner diameter of the band.

The first report of the use of an AGB to treat morbid obesity was in 1986.[54] It is an attractive concept as it is adjustable, reversible, and potentially associated with less morbidity and cost, as no stomach stapling or transection is necessary. Since then, AGB designs have improved considerably. The technique was frequently used in Europe and in Australia in the 1990s with the publication of well-designed studies.[55,56]

Some of the best overall results with AGB come from a center in Australia, where long-term results were recently published.[57] O'Brien and colleagues reported results in 78% of 714 patients with at least 10 years of follow-up. There was no perioperative mortality during the index operation or for any revisional procedures. Percent excess weight loss (%EWL) was 47.1% at 15 years ($n = 54$) and 62% at 16 years ($n = 14$). The mean EWL for the 714 patients who were at or beyond 10 years follow-up was 47.0%. Revisional procedures were performed for proximal enlargement (26%), erosion (3.4%), port and tubing problems (21%) and band explant (5.6%), a total reoperation rate of over 50%.

In 2001, the FDA approved the first commercial AGB system to be used in the United States and its use increased until about 2008. However, the initial enthusiasm with the technique in the United States, Europe, and South America has faded with the publication of several case series showing a high failure rate, with a need for revisional surgery and device-related complications, along with better results from RYGB and SG in terms of weight loss and resolution of comorbidities.[58–62] While AGB is still considered an option in selected patients,[57] its use has declined considerably outside Australia.[41,42] The reasons for the differences in outcomes with AGB between continents and between centers within the same country are multifactorial: differences in patients' demographics, cultural, socioeconomic, racial, genetic, and behavioral background plus differences in the availability of medical resources, among other factors.

Currently, several brands of adjustable bands are available including the LAP-BAND System and Realize System (both approved by use in the United States). None have yet been shown clearly to be superior to the other.

Other results with AGB are presented in the section, "Comparative Effectiveness of Current Bariatric Surgical Procedures".

Biliopancreatic Diversion

In 1979, Dr Nicola Scopinaro described the operation known as a partial biliopancreatic diversion (BPD)[63] (Fig. 50.10). The operation has both gastric restrictive and malabsorptive components, with separation of bile and

Table 50.3 Biliopancreatic diversion results.

Result	*Percentage (%)*
Operative mortality	0.4
Mean excess weight loss	75.0
Late complications	
Anemia	5.0
Stomal ulcer	2.8
Incisional hernia	8.7
Intestinal obstruction	1.2
Protein malnutrition	7.0

pancreatic secretions from ingested food up to the distal ileum. It consists of a distal gastrectomy with a long Roux-en-Y reconstruction to anastomose the distal 250 cm of small intestine (the alimentary limb) to the stomach. The bypassed proximal small intestine (the biliopancreatic limb) is anastomosed to the ileum 50 cm proximal to the ileocecal valve to form the common channel. The stomach remnant volume has been adjusted to 200–500 mL, according to the patient's initial excess weight, gender, age, eating habits, and estimated compliance with postoperative eating behavior requirements. The residual stomach is referred to as the "ad hoc stomach".

The malabsorptive portion of the procedure is designed to delay the mixing of food with biliopancreatic secretions. This maneuver reduces digestion and intestinal absorption of fat, starch, and protein. Patients have two to four soft stools per day and may have excessive malodorous flatulence. The procedure is used in many centers in Europe and South America, but a modification to BPD-DS is preferred in the United States and some European Centers.[41]

In 1996, Scopinaro and colleagues reported a maximum follow-up of 115 months with a nearly 99% patient follow-up[64] (Table 50.3). At 10 years after initial operation, 90% of patients had excess weight loss > 50%, with a failure rate (i.e. loss of < 25% of excess weight) of 0.5%. A beneficial improvement in the comorbidities of patients who sustained weight reduction was observed. The proportion of patients with nutritional deficiencies is also presented in Table 50.3. As with other bariatric procedures, BPD is now routinely performed using laparoscopic surgical techniques.

Biliopancreatic Diversion with Duodenal Switch

The biliopancreatic diversion with duodenal switch (BPD-DS) is a modification of the original BPD. The difference between these two operations is that in the BPD-DS, an SG is performed by excising the left lateral portion of the proximal antrum starting (about 3–5 cm from the pylorus) plus the left lateral portion of the body and fundus over a 40–50 F bougie. The duodenum is transected between the first and second portion, and the divided distal 250 cm of jejunum (alimentary limb) is anastomosed to the postpyloric duodenum (Fig. 50.11). In both BPD and BPD-DS, the stomach pouch has a capacity of about 250 mL, and the same long Roux-en-Y reconstruction of the bowel is carried out with a common channel of 50–100 cm and an alimentary limb of 250 cm.[65]

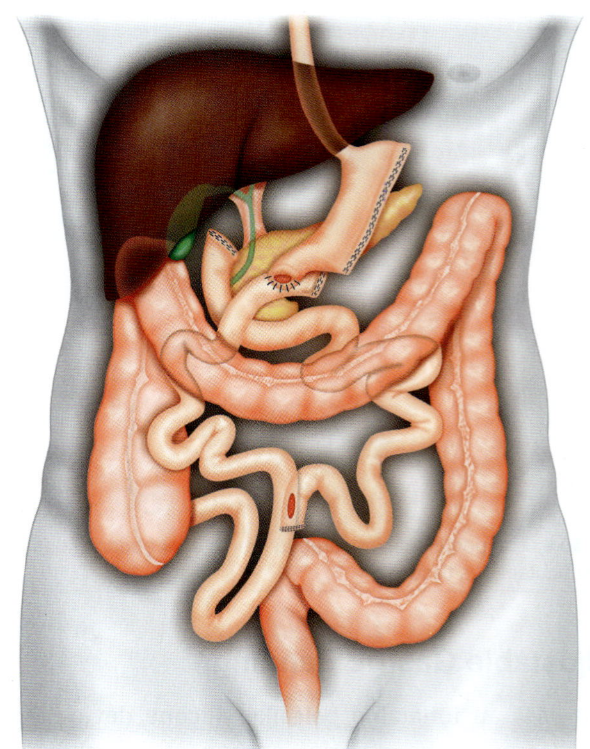

Fig. 50.11: Biliopancreatic diversion with duodenal switch (BPD-DS).

The BPD has excellent long-term weight loss as noted above, but unlike the BPD-DS, it seem to have a greater risk of postgastrectomy symptoms related to the distal gastrectomy and absent pylorus, including diarrhea, dumping, and marginal ulceration.[66] The rationale for using BPD-DS comes from studies on the prevention of postgastrectomy syndrome. In 1987, DeMeester demonstrated in dogs that preserving the pylorus prevented marginal ulceration.[67] Marceau and coworkers[68] were the first to describe a reduction in postgastrectomy symptoms associated with BPD by preserving the pylorus. In the United States, the procedure was popularized by the

Table 50.4 Weight loss, surgical procedure and remission of type-2 diabetes with current bariatric procedures.

	Total	AGB	RYGB	BPD-DS
No. of studies (*n* patients)		66 (8,599)	116 (15,560)	23 (3,127)
% EWL	55.9	46.2	59.7	63.6
% Resolved overall	78.1	56.7	80.3	95.1
% Resolved <2 years	80.3	55.0	81.6	94.0
% Resolved ≥2 years	74.6	58.3	70.9	95.9

Source: Adapted from Buchwald H, Estok R, Fahrbach K, et al. Weight and type-2 diabetes after bariatric surgery: systematic review and meta-analysis. Am J Med. 2009;122(3):248-56 e5.
(%EBWL: Percentage of excess body weight loss; AGB: Gastric band; RYGB: Gastric bypass; BPD-DS: Duodenal switch).

work of Hess.[69] Serious complications have been reported in 2.7–3.7% of cases, and the operative mortality in large series using an open approach is approximately 1%.[66] The operative mortality rate in large laparoscopic case series is currently lower.[70]

Marceau and colleagues[71] reported that BPD-DS patients continue to have 25% greater mean weight loss than those who underwent BPD with a distal gastrectomy.

In addition, serum calcium, iron, and hemoglobin levels were higher and parathyroid hormone levels were lower in patients with BPD-DS, and the need for revisions was also lowered from 18.5% with BPD plus distal gastrectomy to 2.7% with BPD-DS group. A beneficial improvement in the comorbidities of patients who sustained weight reduction was also observed.

COMPARATIVE EFFECTIVENESS OF CURRENT BARIATRIC OPERATIONS

AGB/RYGB/BPD-DS

A systematic review meta-analysis of 205 studies with 27,286 patients who received AGB, RYGB, or BPD-DS (Table 50.4) showed that BPD-DS patients had a greater percentage of excess weight loss than RYGB and AGB and also improved rates of type-2 diabetes remission.[60]

Valuable evidence was supplied by a randomized clinical trial comparing BPD-DS to RYGB in superobese patients (BMI, 50–60 kg/m^2).[72] This study demonstrated better weight loss at 1 year for BPD-DS, though at the expense of longer hospital length of stay and longer operating time. However, there was no significant increase in perioperative morbidity or mortality rate in the BPD-DS group. The mean reductions in BMI were 17.3 kg/m^2 (95% CI, 15.7–19.0 kg/m^2) after RYGB and 24.8 kg/m^2 (CI, 23.0–26.5 kg/m^2) after BPD-DS (mean between-group difference, 7.44 kg/m^2 [CI, 5.24–9.64 kg/m^2]; $P < 0.001$).

Although these results favor BPD-DS over RYGB and AGB in terms of weight loss and resolution of some comorbidities, the procedure is used in very few centers in the United States and is reserved for patients with a BMI > 60. Its limited popularity reflects some of the disadvantages and risks such as inconvenient diarrhea and malodorous flatulence, prevalent micronutrient and vitamin deficiencies and protein–calorie malnutrition, which have been documented in up to 25% of patients.[66]

AGB/SG/RYGB

Two large studies compared the results of these three operations.

One study, from the American College of Surgeons-Bariatric Surgery Center Network accreditation program,[73] reported outcomes in 28,616 patients. Weight loss, measured as reduction in BMI, and resolution or improvement in type-2 diabetes were significantly better for RYGB (reduction in BMI, 15/res. T2DM: 83%) than for SG (reduction in BMI, 12/res. T2DM: 55%) and AGB (reduction in BMI, 7/res. T2DM: 44%). AGB had the lowest rate of perioperative complication and SG had a lower reoperation/intervention rate compared to RYGB, though RYGB and SG procedures had similar risk-adjusted morbidity and readmission rates.

The other study came from the Michigan Bariatric Surgery Collaborative Group,[51] in which 2,949 SG patients were matched with equal numbers of RYGB and AGB patients on 23 baseline characteristics. Outcomes studied were perioperative 30-day complications, weight loss, quality of life, and comorbidity remission at 1, 2, and 3 years after operation.

Overall complication rates in SG patients (6.3%) were significantly lower than for RYGB (10.0%, $P < 0.0001$) but higher than for AGB (2.4%, $P < 0.0001$). An interesting finding was that serious complication rates were similar for

SG (2.4%) and RYGB (2.5%, $P=0.7$) but higher than for AGB (1.0%, $P<0.0001$). Excess body weight loss (EBWL) at 1 year was lower for SG compared to RYGB (EBWL: SG, 60% vs RYGB, 69%, $P<0.0001$), but was 77% higher for SG than for AGB (EBWL for AGB was only 34%, $P<0.0001$). Remission of obesity-associated diseases was similarly closer in between SG and RYGB and superior to AGB.

AGB/RYGB

Studies comparing RYGB to AGB are many. Most confirm superiority of RGYB over AGB in terms of weight loss and resolution of comorbidities that are similar to the results of the systematic review meta-analyses[60] and the two studies presented in the previous text.[51,73] Better studies were a randomized controlled trial[61] and two large two-cohort pair matched studies.[59,62]

An important concept confirmed by all the aforementioned studies is that though RYGB and SG have a higher 30-day perioperative complication rate when compared to AGB,[9,51,61,62,74] AGB has a steadily increasing rate of complications and reoperations over the subsequent months and years, and the overall rate of complications and reoperations may match or supersede those observed for RYGB.[58,59,61,74] Because RYGB has significantly better weight loss and resolution of comorbidities than AGB, AGB utilization has decreased considerably in the United States, Europe, and South America over recent years.[41,42]

SG/RYGB

Lastly, a prospective randomized trial compared SG to RYGB and best medical therapy.[26] It studied 150 patients with a BMI >30 and with type-2 diabetes. RYGB had better weight loss than SG at 1 year (BMI reduction, RYGB = 10 vs SG = 9, $P = 0.03$), but similar rates of type-2 diabetes remission (RYGB: 42% vs. SG: 39%, $P = 0.59$).

Due to the preservation of the pyloric sphincter, continuing duodenal contact with food bolus and absence of mesenteric defects, SG is not associated with rare complications seen long-term with RYGB, such as marginal ulcers and internal hernias. The SG is also an attractive alternative for patients who may be candidates for organ transplant, since it preserves normal alimentation pathway for absorption of oral medications.[75] The SG is an irreversible procedure, whereas RYGB and AGB can be reversed.

The decision-making process to choose the optimal procedure for a specific patient is complex and should take into account all individual characteristics such as age, obesity-associated diseases, performance status, and body habitus. Patients' preferences should also be taken into consideration, but a genuine effort should always be made to inform patients of the known expected benefits and risks of the available operative procedures, including the accepted literature as well as the individual surgeon and center experience.

IDENTIFICATION AND TREATMENT OF COMPLICATIONS AFTER BARIATRIC SURGERY

Fundamental to the practice of bariatric surgery is the need for early identification and treatment of perioperative and long-term complications associated with the operation. The spectrum, severity, timing, and type of complications vary with each procedure and with type of access used (open or laparoscopic).[9,34,44,45,53,59,61] All healthcare professionals involved in the care of bariatric surgical patients should be knowledgeable in identifying and directing appropriate treatment for these complications.

Specific complications seen with the three most commonly used procedures in the United States are briefly discussed in the following sections.

Roux-en-Y Gastric Bypass

- *Gastrojejunostomy (GJ) stricture*: These strictures following RYGB have been reported in 3–27% of patients. Patients usually present with symptoms of vomiting 3–6 weeks after the operation. Most patients can be successfully treated with outpatient endoscopic balloon dilatation. Some earlier series suggested that a higher stricture rate was associated with the use of a 21-mm circular stapler (18% stricture rate) compared to hand-sewn, linear stapler, and 25-mm circular techniques (2–5% stricture rate).[61,76] However, our recent personal experience and data from other large series[77] have shown that using a 21-mm circular stapler with a transoral anvil technique is associated with a similarly low stricture rate and possibly better long-term weight loss results due to the smaller diameter of the anastomosis. The anvil delivery technique (transoral through the gastric pouch staple line as opposed to transgastric above the gastric pouch staple line) may be more important than the anvil diameter in itself.
- *Postoperative bleeding*: Most episodes of bleeding occur in the perioperative period. In a systematic literature review of 3,464 cases, the frequency of postoperative bleeding in the gastrointestinal tract was higher after

laparoscopic RYGB than after open RYGB (1.93% vs 0.6%, respectively, $P = 0.008$).[45] However, the incidence of gastrointestinal bleeding after both laparoscopic and open RYGB in other series appears similarly low.[78,79] The main potential sources of bleeding are intraluminal (the gastric remnant, GJ, and jejunojejunostomy staple lines), intraperitoneal (mesenteric staple line and dissection planes), and the abdominal wall trocar sites.[78] Whereas bleeding from the GJ may manifest as hematemesis and permit endoscopic intervention, bleeding from the other sources may pose a diagnostic and treatment challenge. The decision to transfuse, use of therapeutic endoscopy, or reoperate is based on a combination of clinical factors and local experience. Bleeding may also occur months or years after RYGB.[78]

- *Small-bowel obstruction (SBO)*: This type of obstruction after laparoscopic RYGB has been reported in 1.5–5% of patients and can occur either early or late in the postoperative period. Causes of SBO early after the operation are usually adhesions, trocar site hernias, and obstruction at the jejunojejunostomy owing to narrowing or malpositioning (a "kink") of the biliopancreatic and alimentary limbs or postoperative hemorrhage producing an obstructive blood clot, whereas internal herniation through the mesenteric defects is the dominant cause of SBO months and years postoperatively.[44,80] SBO rates can be decreased by routinely closing all mesenteric defects during RYGB. The incidence of SBO is reportedly higher when a retrocolic Roux limb is used. The antecolic Roux limb eliminates a common site for obstruction, namely the transverse mesocolon.[81] Because radiologic examination with computed tomography, upper gastrointestinal series, or both may show false-negative results,[80] early surgical intervention should be considered in patients with sudden or severe symptoms to prevent the development of gangrenous bowel.
- *Leak from the GJ*: The GJ leak is one of the most feared complications after RYGB. The GJ leak and pulmonary embolism are the main causes of death. It is a rare complication nowadays in most series. Though earlier series reported rates as high as 3–5%,[45] rates not exceeding 1% are the norm in more recent years.[9] Many centers use routine postoperative radiological testing of the GJ via an upper gastrointestinal series. We have found this approach unreliable[82] and prefer selective use of CT with oral and intravenous contrast in the small subset of patients who have clinical manifestations of GJ leaks, such as tachycardia and/or a high white blood cell count. Early laparoscopy should be considered in any patient suspected of a GJ leak. The use of fully covered temporary endoscopic stenting currently plays a major role in treating GJ leaks.[83]
- *Gastrojejunal ulcers*: Gastrojejunal ulcers or marginal ulcers occur in 1–2% of patients following RYGB and are usually seen several months after operation. Risk factors for marginal ulcers are use of tobacco products and NSAIDs plus a large gastric pouch. Gastrojejunal ulcers manifest with new onset epigastric pain and/or bleeding or perforation.[84] Upper gastrointestinal endoscopy can be diagnostic and therapeutic in cases without perforation. Laparoscopic Graham patch maybe used in small perforations if advanced laparoscopic expertise is available, followed by modification of risk factors and acid suppression therapy.[85]

Adjustable Gastric Banding

- *Device-related malfunctions*: These types of malfunctions are seen after AGB in about 25% of patients. These include port malfunction, port erosion, tubing disconnection, band migration, and band leakage. Revisional surgery is usually required to reposition or replace the defective parts.[86]
- *Esophageal dilation and esophagitis*: Marked esophageal dilation, in some cases mimicking esophageal achalasia, is observed in as many as 50% of patients when routine barium esophagogram is obtained.[87] Esophageal dilation rates from 15% to 20% are reported in series in which routine esophagograms have not been obtained.[86] Band deflation followed by band removal is recommended. Esophagitis and new-onset reflux symptoms are reported in as many as 30% of patients.
- *Pouch dilation*: This is reported in 15–20% of patients. Treatment is band deflation,
- *Band erosion into the stomach*: Band erosion is a serious complication, reported in about 2–3% of patients in whom the pars flaccida technique has been used.[88] It is reported to occur at a median time of 33 months from initial operation (range: 11–170 months).[88] Common presentations include loss of satiety and recent infection of the port site. Higher rates (up to 7%) were reported using the perigastric technique.[55,57,86] Treatment is band removal, which can usually be done laparoscopically. A few centers have recommended staged band replacement,[88] while others offer staged conversion to another bariatric procedure.[58]

- *Gastric slippage*: This is reported to occur in 4–6% of patients.[57] It presents with acute onset of epigastric pain and needs immediate attention. Deflation of the band followed by serial examination may relieve symptoms, but emergent band removal maybe needed to salvage the patient from progressing to a perforated necrotic gastric slippage.[89]

Sleeve Gastrectomy

- *Leak*: This is the most feared complication after a SG. It is reported to occur in 0.6–2.6% of cases,[51,53,90] and it typically occurs at the most superior aspect of the staple line. It can present in the early postoperative period, up to few weeks after operation. The best evidence to-date suggests that, other than attention to the many technical detail of the procedure, the use of a bougie of 40 F or greater diameter to calibrate the SG may decrease leak rates without negative impact on long-term weight loss.[53,90] Treatment involves operative drainage and endoscopic stenting; however, these leaks take much longer to heal than leaks after RYGB and may ultimately require reoperation.[90]
- *Postoperative bleeding*: This problem occurs in about 1.1% of patients. The potential sources of bleeding are intraluminal, intraperitoneal (gastric staple line and dissection planes), and the abdominal wall trocar sites.[51] Intraluminal bleeding may manifest as hematemesis and permit endoscopic intervention. Similar to RYGB, the decision to transfuse, use of therapeutic endoscopy, or reoperate is based on a combination of clinical factors and local experience.
- *Sleeve stricture*: Strictures or stenosis may be related to operative technique but also to healed leaks and fistulas.[91] Treatment is difficult and involves endoscopic dilation, sleeve seromyotomy or wedge resection, or conversion to RYGB.

INNOVATIONS IN BARIATRIC SURGERY

Some of the recent innovations in bariatric surgery include the use of single-incision port techniques, endoscopic techniques, and robotic-assisted surgery. There are no current data to show that single-incision or robotic surgical techniques offer improved patient centered outcomes, other than improved cosmesis. Reported outcomes from single-incision transumbilical RYGB, AGB, and SG were generally similar to multiport laparoscopic surgery, with greater operative times and improved cosmetic outcomes for the single port.[92–94] Robotic-assisted RYGB, AGB, and SG have all been performed and found to have longer operative times, but similar leak rates to laparoscopic techniques.[95] The added cost of robotic and single-port technology, greater operative times, and the lack of evidence that provides improved patient-centered outcomes are the main barriers to a wider adoption of these techniques.

A variety of endoscopic devices are being created to treat obesity, failures of primary bariatric operations, and surgical complications. For treatment of obesity, space occupying devices such as the intragastric balloon, endoscopic suturing and stapling systems, and endoluminal liners to induce malabsorption have all been tested, and some are currently being used as primary treatment for obesity.[83,96] While the long-term impact of these innovations is unknown, it is clear that they will be incorporated as part of the available armamentarium to treat obesity, failures, and operative complications.

Another innovation in bariatric surgery is the idea of metabolic surgery, i.e. operative treatment for patients with active metabolic disease and comorbidities such as type-2 diabetes and a BMI < 35. Given the profound effects that certain bariatric surgical procedures have on diabetic outcomes, there has been great interest in modifications of standard bariatric techniques as a treatment for type-2 diabetes in patients who do not fit the traditional criteria for a bariatric operation. The International Diabetes Federation Taskforce on Epidemiology and Prevention of Diabetes convened a consensus working group, which felt that not only should bariatric surgery be an accepted option for patients with type-2 diabetes and BMI > 35, but should also be considered as an alternative treatment option in patients with BMI between 30 and 35 when diabetes cannot be adequately controlled by medical therapy.[97] While this is not currently accepted practice in the United States, as the literature regarding the effects of bariatric surgery on diabetes continues to mount there may be a shift toward offering bariatric surgery to patients with lower BMIs in the future.

CONCLUSION

Four bariatric surgical techniques are currently preferred: RYGB, SG, AGB, and BPD-DS. All these procedures can be performed using laparoscopic techniques, with an improved safety profile over the open techniques. The decision on which procedure should be used for a specific patient is complex. Patients should be informed of the known expected benefits and risks of all available operative procedures together with the experience of the surgeon and the center involved.

Bariatric surgery is cost-effective at approximately $18,000 per QALY.[8] When the operation is done in high-volume centers by expert surgeons, it is associated with a low risk of perioperative and long-term complication rates,[9] produces both substantial sustained weight loss in most patients,[10] improves, cures, or significantly lowers incidence rates of obesity-associated diseases, improves quality of life,[11] and reduces overall mortality.[12,13]

REFERENCES

1. CDC. Available from http://www.cdc.gov/obesity/data/facts.html. [Accessed September 23, 2014].
2. Danaei G, Ding EL, Mozaffarian D, et al. The preventable causes of death in the United States: comparative risk assessment of dietary, lifestyle, and metabolic risk factors. PLoS Med. 2009;6(4):e1000058.
3. WHO. Obesity: Preventing and Managing the Global Epidemic. Geneva: Switzerland; 2000.
4. Finkelstein EA, Trogdon JG, Cohen JW, et al. Annual medical spending attributable to obesity: payer-and service-specific estimates. Health Affairs. 2009;28(5):w822-31.
5. Sievenpiper JL, de Souza RJ, Jenkins DJ. Sugar: fruit fructose is still healthy. Nature. 2012;482(7386):470.
6. Block G. Foods contributing to energy intake in the US: data from NHANES III and NHANES 1999-2000. J Food Composition Anal. 2004;17(3-4):439-47.
7. Putnam J, Allshouse J, Kantor LS. U.S. per capita food supply trends: more calories, refined carbohydrates, and fats. Food Rev. 2002;25(3):2-14.
8. Picot J, Jones J, Colquitt JL, et al. The clinical effectiveness and cost-effectiveness of bariatric (weight loss) surgery for obesity: a systematic review and economic evaluation. Health Technol Assess. 2009;13(41):1-190, 215-357, iii-iv.
9. Longitudinal Assessment of Bariatric Surgery (LABS) Consortium. Perioperative safety in the longitudinal assessment of bariatric surgery. New Engl J Med. 2009;361(5):445-54.
10. Sjostrom L. Review of the key results from the Swedish Obese Subjects (SOS) trial—a prospective controlled intervention study of bariatric surgery. J Intern Med. 2013;273(3):219-34.
11. Nguyen NT, Goldman C, Rosenquist CJ, et al. Laparoscopic versus open gastric bypass: a randomized study of outcomes, quality of life, and costs. Ann Surg. 2001;234(3):279-89; discussion 89-91.
12. Sjostrom L, Narbro K, Sjostrom CD, et al. Effects of bariatric surgery on mortality in Swedish obese subjects. New Engl J Med. 2007;357(8):741-52.
13. Adams TD, Gress RE, Smith SC, et al. Long-term mortality after gastric bypass surgery. New Engl J Med. 2007; 357(8):753-61.
14. Prospective Studies Collaboration, Whitlock G, Lewington S, et al. Body-mass index and cause-specific mortality in 900 000 adults: collaborative analyses of 57 prospective studies. Lancet. 2009;373(9669):1083-96.
15. Berrington de Gonzalez A, Hartge P, Cerhan JR, et al. Body-mass index and mortality among 1.46 million white adults. New Engl J Med. 2010;363(23):2211-19.
16. Reis JP, Macera CA, Araneta MR, et al. Comparison of overall obesity and body fat distribution in predicting risk of mortality. Obesity. 2009;17(6):1232-9.
17. Pischon T, Boeing H, Hoffmann K, et al. General and abdominal adiposity and risk of death in Europe. New Engl J Med. 2008;359(20):2105-20.
18. National Institutes of Health. Clinical Guidelines on the Identification, Evaluation, and Treatment of Overweight and Obesity in Adults—the Evidence Report. Obesity Res. 1998;6(Suppl 2):51S-209S.
19. Rabl C, Campos GM. The impact of bariatric surgery on nonalcoholic steatohepatitis. Semin Liver Dis. 2012;32(1):80-91.
20. Franz MJ, VanWormer JJ, Crain AL, et al. Weight-loss outcomes: a systematic review and meta-analysis of weight-loss clinical trials with a minimum 1-year follow-up. J Am Dietetic Assoc. 2007;107(10):1755-67.
21. Appel LJ, Clark JM, Yeh HC, et al. Comparative effectiveness of weight-loss interventions in clinical practice. New Engl J Med. 2011;365(21):1959-68.
22. Wadden TA, Volger S, Sarwer DB, et al. A two-year randomized trial of obesity treatment in primary care practice. New Engl J Med. 2011;365(21):1969-79.
23. Torgerson JS, Hauptman J, Boldrin MN, et al. XENical in the prevention of diabetes in obese subjects (XENDOS) study: a randomized study of orlistat as an adjunct to lifestyle changes for the prevention of type 2 diabetes in obese patients. Diabetes Care. 2004;27(1):155-61.
24. Smith SR, Weissman NJ, Anderson CM, et al. Multicenter, placebo-controlled trial of lorcaserin for weight management. New Engl J Med. 2010;363(3):245-56.
25. Gadde KM, Allison DB, Ryan DH, et al. Effects of low-dose, controlled-release, phentermine plus topiramate combination on weight and associated comorbidities in overweight and obese adults (CONQUER): a randomised, placebo-controlled, phase 3 trial. Lancet. 2011;377(9774):1341-52.
26. Schauer PR, Kashyap SR, Wolski K, et al. Bariatric surgery versus intensive medical therapy in obese patients with diabetes. New Engl J Med. 2012;366(17):1567-76.
27. Mingrone G, Panunzi S, De Gaetano A, et al. Bariatric surgery versus conventional medical therapy for type 2 diabetes. New Engl J Med. 2012;366(17):1577-85.
28. Kohn GP, Galanko JA, Overby DW, et al. Recent trends in bariatric surgery case volume in the United States. Surgery. 2009;146(2):375-80.
29. Steinbrook R. Surgery for severe obesity. New Engl J Med. 2004;350(11):1075-9.
30. Wittgrove AC, Clark GW, Tremblay LJ. Laparoscopic gastric bypass, Roux-en-Y: preliminary report of five cases. Obes Surg. 1994;4(4):353-7.
31. NIH conference. Gastrointestinal surgery for severe obesity. Consensus Development Conference Panel. Ann Intern Med. 1991;115(12):956-61.

32. Dimick JB, Nicholas LH, Ryan AM, et al. Bariatric surgery complications before vs after implementation of a national policy restricting coverage to centers of excellence. J Am Med Assoc. 2013;309(8):792-9.
33. Gould JC, Kent KC, Wan Y, et al. Perioperative safety and volume: outcomes relationships in bariatric surgery: a study of 32,000 patients. J Am Coll Surg. 2011;213(6):771-7.
34. Nguyen NT, Paya M, Stevens CM, et al. The relationship between hospital volume and outcome in bariatric surgery at academic medical centers. Ann Surg. 2004;240(4):586-93; discussion 93-4.
35. Heber D, Greenway FL, Kaplan LM, et al. Endocrine and nutritional management of the post-bariatric surgery patient: an endocrine society clinical practice guideline. J Clin Endocrinol Metab. 2010;95(11):4823-43.
36. Halverson JD, Wise L, Wazna MF, et al. Jejunoileal bypass for morbid obesity. A critical appraisal. Am J Med. 1978; 64(3):461-75.
37. Griffen WO, Jr, Young VL, Stevenson CC. A prospective comparison of gastric and jejunoileal bypass procedures for morbid obesity. Ann Surg. 1977;186(4):500-9.
38. Linner JH. Comparative effectiveness of gastric bypass and gastroplasty: a clinical study. Arch Surg. 1982;117(5):695-700.
39. Mason EE. Vertical banded gastroplasty for obesity. Arch Surg. 1982;117(5):701-6.
40. Ridings P, Sugerman HJ. Vertical banded gastroplasty for the treatment of morbid obesity. Br J Surg. 1994;81(5):776.
41. Buchwald H, Oien DM. Metabolic/bariatric surgery worldwide 2011. Obes Surg. 2013;23(4):427-36.
42. Nguyen NT, Nguyen B, Gebhart A, et al. Changes in the makeup of bariatric surgery: a national increase in use of laparoscopic sleeve gastrectomy. J Am Coll Surg. 2013; 216(2):252-7.
43. Mason EE, Ito C. Gastric bypass in obesity. Surg Clin North Am. 1967;47(6):1345-51.
44. Campos GM, Ciovica R, Rogers SJ, et al. Spectrum and risk factors of complications after gastric bypass. Arch Surg. 2007;142(10):969-75; discussion 76.
45. Podnos YD, Jimenez JC, Wilson SE, et al. Complications after laparoscopic gastric bypass: a review of 3464 cases. Arch Surg. 2003;138(9):957-61.
46. Waters GS, Pories WJ, Swanson MS, et al. Long-term studies of mental health after the Greenville gastric bypass operation for morbid obesity. Am J Surg. 1991;161(1):154-7; discussion 7-8.
47. Arterburn DE, Bogart A, Sherwood NE, et al. A multisite study of long-term remission and relapse of type 2 diabetes mellitus following gastric bypass. Obes Surg. 2013;23(1): 93-102.
48. Almogy G, Crookes PF, Anthone GJ. Longitudinal gastrectomy as a treatment for the high-risk super-obese patient. Obes Surg. 2004;14(4):492-7.
49. Baltasar A, Serra C, Perez N, et al. Laparoscopic sleeve gastrectomy: a multi-purpose bariatric operation. Obes Surg. 2005;15(8):1124-8.
50. Gagner M, Gumbs AA, Milone L, et al. Laparoscopic sleeve gastrectomy for the super-super-obese (body mass index > 60 kg/m(2)). Surg Today. 2008;38(5):399-403.

Additional references can be found in the online version of this book.

Case Study: 51
Abdominal Pain after Roux-en-Y Gastric Bypass

Jacob A Greenberg, Guilherme M Campos

THE PROBLEM

Abdominal pain is a common chief complaint seen throughout emergency rooms across the globe. While the underlying cause of abdominal pain can be difficult to diagnose in all patients, it becomes more complex in patients who have previously undergone a Roux-en-Y gastric bypass (RYGB) for the treatment of morbid obesity. While post-RYGB patients can present with any of the causes of abdominal pain, such as appendicitis, diverticulitis, cholecystitis, pancreatitis, and others, there are specific causes that are directly related to the RYGB itself, such as marginal ulcer or internal hernia. The early detection and treatment of these causes of abdominal pain are crucial to avoid potentially devastating complications.

THE TYPICAL CASE

A 44-year-old woman presents to the emergency room of her local hospital with complaints of 6 hours of worsening, diffuse, crampy abdominal pain. Two years prior she underwent a laparoscopic RYGB for morbid obesity. At that time her BMI was 51 and she had a history of gastroesophageal reflux disease, obstructive sleep apnea, and hypertension. She has subsequently lost 150 pounds and her current BMI is 26. She has had close follow-up with her bariatric program and has had no postoperative issues until now. She states that the pain started earlier today, is not associated with vomiting, but she has not passed flatus since the pain began. The pain is diffuse throughout her abdomen and she has some mild tenderness to palpation. Her pain has not improved with a GI cocktail in the ER or after 2 mg of dilaudid IV.

DIAGNOSTIC DILEMMAS

Abdominal pain following RYGB is common. Like all other patients with abdominal pain, a detailed history and physical examination focusing on the quality, character, duration, and location of the pain is a mandatory first step. In this patient, the pain is crampy and colicky in nature, diffuse throughout her abdomen, and has grown progressively worse over the course of the day. For the last several weeks, she had mild abdominal cramps that did not appear to be associated with meals.

In terms of her initial operation, she underwent a standard laparoscopic RYGB with a 150-cm antecolic alimentary limb and a circular-stapled gastrojejunostomy. She has shown excellent postoperative behavioral modification, eating three small meals and two small snacks daily and exercising 45 minutes per day at least four times a week. She has been maintained on PPI therapy for acid suppression, does not smoke cigarettes, and does not take any NSAIDs. Additionally, she takes all of her recommended supplements including iron, calcium, and a multivitamin. Her nutritional laboratories were checked at her last visit to the bariatric clinic 3 months ago and were all within normal limits.

On physical examination, she is afebrile, has a heart rate of 95, a blood pressure of 135/70, and normal respirations and pulse oximetry. Her abdominal examination is mostly unremarkable save some mild diffuse tenderness to palpation without any obvious distention or tympany. She has no signs of peritonitis.

Her laboratories are all within normal limits with the exception of her white blood cell count, which is elevated to 13. A CT scan of the abdomen/pelvis is performed, which shows some fecalized and thickened loops of small bowel with no obvious transition point.

MANAGEMENT OPTIONS

This patient has a history and imaging study highly concerning for an internal hernia and a diagnostic laparoscopy is the most appropriate next step. At the time of laparoscopy, an internal hernia through the Petersen defect was identified with the small bowel herniating beneath the alimentary limb mesentery with venous and lymphatic congestion and bowel wall edema. The small bowel was reduced through the defect with rapid resolution of the congestion and edema. The mesenteric defect was closed with a running silk suture and the patient had an uncomplicated postoperative recovery.

Internal hernias may occur in about 2% of patients following laparoscopic RYGB. Depending on the orientation and route of passage (antecolic or retrocolic) of the alimentary limb, there are either two or three potential spaces where internal hernias may form. In a retrocolic alimentary limb, the small bowel can herniate cephalad through the defect in the colonic mesentery. In both retrocolic and antecolic alimentary limbs, the small bowel can herniate through the mesenteric defect at the jejunojejunostomy or where the mesentery of the alimentary limb travels over the mesentery of the transverse colon, commonly referred to as the Petersen defect. While the jejunojejunostomy and Petersen defects should be routinely closed at the initial operation, internal hernias may still develop in these spaces, especially in patients who have significant weight loss that leads to loss of fat in the mesentery. Without prompt recognition and treatment, internal hernias can lead to bowel ischemia and necrosis and are a potentially deadly long-term complication of RYGB.

All of the common causes of abdominal pain remain on the differential following RYGB, and these can frequently be diagnosed with a history and physical examination followed by appropriate laboratory and imaging studies. Common diagnoses, such as appendicitis and diverticulitis, appear with the same frequency after gastric bypass as they do in the general population.

Other causes of abdominal pain are more common after RYGB and need to be placed higher on the differential diagnosis. The timing between the surgery and the presentation of abdominal pain is also an important factor in diagnosing the cause of abdominal pain. Anastomotic leaks frequently occur within the first week following surgery and become increasingly rare beyond that. Strictures of the gastrojejunal anastomosis, which tend to present with persistent vomiting rather than frank abdominal pain, occur usually 3–8 weeks following surgery. Internal hernias, though reported early after an RYGB, are most commonly a late complication, occurring months to years following surgery. Cholelithiasis is common following RYGB, as rapid weight loss is associated with stone formation. Roughly 5–8% of patients will develop symptomatic cholelithiasis and laparoscopic cholecystectomy should be considered. Marginal ulcers at the gastrojejunostomy will occur also in about 1–2% of patients following RYGB. These can lead to significant upper gastrointestinal pain, bleeding or perforation. Marginal ulcers are usually associated with smoking, using tobacco products and NSAID use and patients should be counseled against use of these substances. Intussusception of the jejunojejunostomy and bezoars are other uncommon causes of abdominal pain following RYGB and can usually be identified on the CT scan. Abdominal pain post-RYGB can also be exacerbated by certain foods and by some nutritional deficiencies. Dumping symptoms occur in roughly 80% of patients following RYGB and are brought on by foods that are high in sugar and simple carbohydrate content. Vitamin B12 deficiency can also cause abdominal pain.

In summary, abdominal pain following RYGB is a common complaint and must be assessed rapidly to diagnose and treat the potentially life-threatening causes. Abdominal/pelvic CT scan assessed by a bariatric surgeon and a senior radiologist is an extremely helpful adjunct study. Early operative intervention is mandatory if there is a suspicion of internal hernia in order to prevent small bowel loss.

FURTHER READING

1. Aghajani E, Jacobsen HJ, Nergaard BJ, et al. Internal hernia after gastric bypass: a new and simplified technique for laparoscopic primary closure of the mesenteric defects. J Gastrointest Surg. 2012;16(3):641-5.
2. Al Harakeh AB. Complications of laparoscopic Roux-en-Y gastric bypass. Surg Clin North Am. 2011;91(6):1225-37.
3. El-Hayek K, Timratana P, Shimizu H, et al. Marginal ulcer after Roux-en-Y gastric bypass: what have we really learned? Surg Endosc. 2012;10:2789-96.
4. Greenstein AJ, O'Rourke RW. Abdominal Pain after gastric bypass: suspects and solutions. Am J Surg. 2011;201(6): 819-27.

Case Study: 52

Barrett's Esophagus with High-Grade Dysplasia—Is It Still Necessary to Perform Esophagectomy?

Jon Shenfine, Glyn Jamieson

THE PROBLEM

It has now been established that a columnar-lined lower esophagus (Barrett's esophagus) can progress to invasive adenocarcinoma. This process is thought to occur through a progression of cellular change, starting with metaplasia of the cells of the lower esophagus to columnar cells of intestinal type through various degrees of dysplasia to invasive adenocarcinoma. On an individual patient basis, it is not known whether dysplasia always progresses to invasive cancer. If such progression does always occur, its time course is almost certainly quite variable.

The problem in the management of such cases is compounded by three factors:

- Inflammatory changes associated with esophagitis make it difficult to distinguish between lower grades of dysplastic tissue and inflamed but nondysplastic tissue.
- If high-grade dysplasia is established, there is a strong likelihood of invasive carcinoma already being present.
- Perhaps most important, the usually recommended treatment for this condition is esophagectomy.

It is worth considering that a similar sort of dysplasia occurring in the female cervix is treated by a cone biopsy, a daycase procedure. High-grade esophageal dysplasia treated by esophagectomy, however, is an operation associated with a mortality rate of the order of 5–10%.

THE TYPICAL CASE

A 63-year-old journalist had a long history of symptomatic gastroesophageal reflux, which he had managed mainly by self-medication. Three years previously, he had undergone a successful coronary artery bypass operation and noted that his symptoms of reflux had improved considerably while he was in hospital for the procedure. Six months previously, he had noted some minor difficulty in swallowing and was therefore referred to a gastroenterologist who carried out an endoscopy, which showed 4 cm of columnar-lined lower esophagus; there was ulcerative esophagitis proximal to the columnar lining. No other abnormality was noted. Random biopsies were taken of the lower esophagus, and to the surprise of the endoscopist, one esophageal biopsy showed "low-grade dysplasia" in the columnar mucosa. The patient was treated with 40 mg omeprazole daily, and a further endoscopy was carried out 3 months later. The esophagitis had now healed, and the 4 cm of featureless columnar-lined lower esophagus was present, as before, without any evidence of other abnormality. Multiple biopsies were taken of the columnar-lined mucosa. On this occasion, the pathology report showed "high-grade dysplasia." The patient was referred for a surgical opinion.

DIAGNOSTIC DILEMMAS

The first dilemma is the difficulty that active inflammation can cause a pathologist in distinguishing between severely inflamed tissue and dysplasia. For this reason, it is wise to prescribe maximal antireflux therapy with a proton pump inhibitor, which usually cures any esophagitis present. The patient can then be re-examined and further biopsies taken so that the pathologist may be more confident if a diagnosis of dysplasia is made.

A second dilemma relates to the degree of dysplasia. Most clinicians believe that low-grade dysplasia is not of immediate concern, and it is possible that it is reversible with antireflux therapy or treatment with radio frequency ablation (RFA). However, equally, there is general consensus that high-grade dysplasia means that invasive carcinoma eventually develops in the not too distant future or has already developed at a site not biopsied in the lower esophagus. Therefore, it is very important for a pathologist to be confident of the degree of dysplasia, and this is a further reason why a second endoscopy with biopsy is performed and why a second specialist pathologist independently reviews the histology. Once high-grade dysplasia has been established, the dilemma becomes one of appropriate treatment.

MANAGEMENT OPTIONS

If one could be certain that high-grade dysplasia alone was present, then a number of avenues are possible. We could:

- Keep the area under frequent surveillance using a number of endoscopic aids such as chromoendoscopy or narrow band imaging
- Ablate the area using RFA
- Locally remove this area with endoscopic mucosal resection (EMR) or endoscopic submucous dissection
- Resect the esophagus as a formal esophagectomy

A CURATIVE RESECTION?

Our patient undergoes another endoscopy. There is an area of nodularity within the Barrett's segment and biopsies from this area are confirmed as high-grade dysplasia by two pathologists. He is counseled about his options of surveillance, ablation, EMR, or esophagectomy and he opts for the latter. He feels that he would cope better mentally with complete removal of his future risk and appreciates the short-term risks involved in a formal resection. He undergoes an Ivor Lewis esophagectomy shortly thereafter. On day 2 postoperatively, he develops atrial fibrillation that is managed medically. On day 7, there is enteric fluid in his chest drain; this is associated with signs of sepsis. A CT scan confirms an anastomotic leak that is fairly well controlled by his drain and he is managed conservatively. He initially improves, but on day 9, he has a cardiorespiratory arrest and dies. The postmortem notes that he had a myocardial infarction with thrombosis of his neocoronaries, secondary to septic shock, as a result of the anastomotic leak. His histopathology eventually comes through as a completely resected T1a intramucosal adenocarcinoma with no involved metastatic nodes.

CONCLUSION

The dilemma in a case such as this is that there is a 30–60% chance that underlying the area of high-grade dysplasia is an invasive adenocarcinoma; this rate is higher when there is an endoscopically visible abnormality. The benefits of EMR are that there is a tissue specimen for the pathologist to review (a big biopsy) to better inform decision making, and this may also be curative in itself. There has certainly been a swing to this approach in recent years, especially in older patients. The drawbacks are that this is not performed without some risk (perforation or bleeding) and that this does not deal with the remaining Barrett's, although this could subsequently be ablated with RFA. Esophagectomy remains an excellent treatment if a patient is deemed fit. This deals with all of the disease and is the preferred option in the presence of a "field change," i.e. multifocal high-grade dysplasia or when there is a confirmed underlying cancer. The cure rate for early esophageal cancer with surgery is high, with a 5-year survival rate of at least 90%. However, despite advances in surgery and postoperative support, esophagectomy comes with an appreciable short-term complication and mortality risk, and long-term morbidity is also significant. All this information should be considered and discussed with patients.

FURTHER READING

1. Bennett C, Vakil N, Bergman J, et al. Consensus statements for management of Barrett's dysplasia and early-stage esophageal adenocarcinoma, based on a Delphi process. Gastroenterology. 2012;143:336-46.
2. Hamilton SR, Smith RL. The relationship between columnar epithelial dysplasia and invasive adenocarcinoma arising in Barret's esophagus. Am J Clin Path. 1987;87:301-12.
3. Reid BJ, Weinstein WM, Lewin KJ, et al. Endoscopic biopsy can detect high grade dysplasia or early adenocarcinoma in Barrett's esophagus, without grossly recognisable neoplastic lesions. Gastroenterology. 1988;94:81-90.
4. Rice TW, Falk GW, Achkar E, et al. Surgical management of high grade dysplasia in Barrett's esophagus. Am J Gastroenterol. 1993;88:1832-6.
5. Sampliner RE, Hixson U, Fenneerty B, et al. Regression of Barrett's esophagus by laser ablation in an antacid environment. Dig Dis Sci. 1993;38:365-8.
6. Shaheen NJ, Sharma P, Overholt BF, et al. Radiofrequency ablation in Barrett's esophagus with dysplasia. N Eng J Med. 2009;360(22):2277-88.
7. Wright TA. High grade dysplasia in Barrett's oesophagus. Br J Surg. 1997;84:760-66.

53 Liver

Long R Jiao, Layton F Rikkers

Key Points

- Clarification of the anatomy of the liver and a better understanding of its pathophysiology provide a rational basis for major resectional procedures.
- Percutaneous and laparoscopic techniques have now replaced open operation for cysts and abscesses of the liver.
- Benign liver tumors include hemangioma, hepatic adenoma, focal nodular hyperplasia (FNH), and biliary adenoma. Diagnostic doubt and the potential for complications (including malignant change) govern the need for resection, which differs for each type.
- One of the commonest cancers worldwide, hepatocellular carcinoma (HCC) is seldom resectable and postoperative recurrence is common in any case. Partial hepatectomy remains the mainstay of treatment, although percutaneous ablative techniques are an alternative to resection for tumors < 3 cm; transplantation is usually thwarted by recurrence in the liver graft.
- The liver is the commonest site for metastatic carcinoma, and surgical excision with or without chemotherapy offers the chance of cure in selected cases.
- All patients should be considered for treatment in a specialist center.
- Some patients benefit from repeat resection for recurrent liver metastases.

INTRODUCTION

The liver simultaneously performs four broad functions, all essential for survival:

1. It extracts nutrients from the portal venous inflow.
2. It converts nutrients into substrates, which are then used by the rest of the body for energy and homeostasis.
3. It detoxifies noxious agents generated in the gastrointestinal tract (e.g. ammonia) or serum (e.g. drugs).
4. It aids in the digestion of nutrients by the secretion of bile into the bile canaliculi and ultimately into the bowel lumen.

The myriad of interrelated functions performed by the liver cannot be replaced by any means other than liver transplantation. Yet, the liver is able to perform most of these critical functions even when injured. Unlike many other human organs, the liver may recover from injury by regeneration.

The function of the liver was a puzzle to early scientists and philosophers. The human liver was known to occupy a large portion of the abdominal cavity and was therefore assumed to be important because of its relative size. Its abdominal location suggested a digestive function, but the need for such a large organ remained obscure. Attempts to explain the function of the liver before understanding hepatic anatomy were more philosophic than physiologic. The Babylonians postulated that the liver produced blood and was therefore the repository of the soul. The Greeks thought that the soul was elsewhere, but two of the four bodily humors (black bile and yellow bile) were excreted by the liver according to Hippocrates. The liver was therefore thought to be essential, but for no obvious reason. Its function was only understood when the gross and microscopic anatomies were more completely defined.

True understanding of hepatic anatomy became possible with the advent of microscopy. Using a magnifying glass, Kiernan made many critical and fundamental observations, which he reported in 1883.[1] He described a method for eliminating blood from the liver, so allowing examination of its parenchyma. He described the functional unit of the liver to be the lobule, with a central hepatic vein surrounded by the portal triads (Fig. 53.1). He correctly concluded that the liver is not a typical excretory gland because the lobules seemed more dependent upon

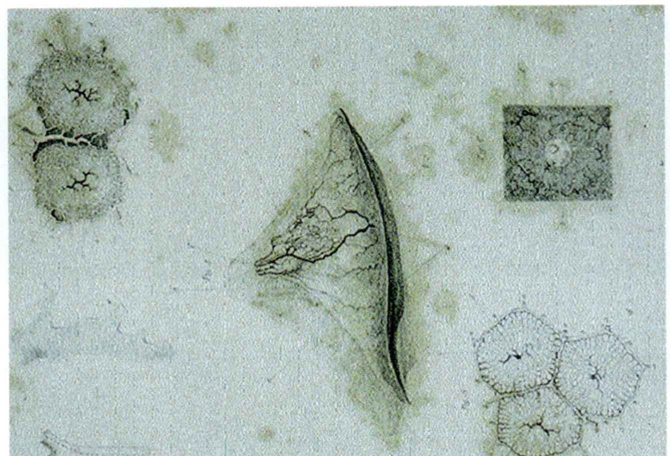

Fig. 53.1: Microscopic appearance of functional hepatic unit with central hepatic vein surrounded by portal triads.

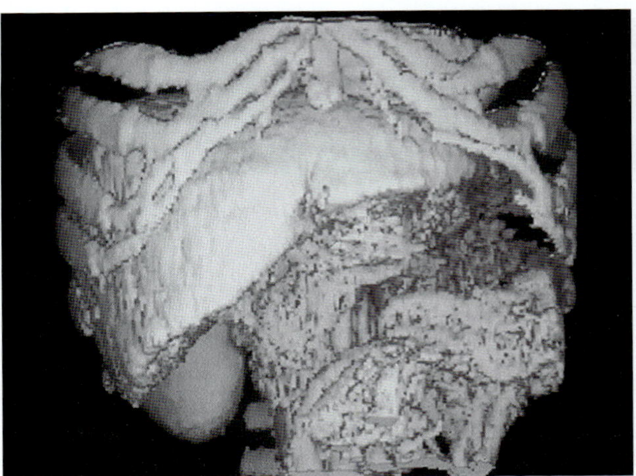

Fig. 53.2: Radiological reconstruction of upper abdominal and chest wall to show the relationship between liver and chest wall.

the portal and hepatic veins. He also concluded that the hepatic artery supplied only the structures of the portal triad, whereas the portal vein blood ultimately drained to the hepatic vein.

The sinusoidal pattern was appreciated with the advent of light microscopy. Delineation of the ultrastructural anatomy of the sinusoids was further refined by the use of transmission and scanning electron microscopy. The lobular structure, however, did not explain the mechanism of injury to the liver by toxins or by infectious agents. Hepatocytes were noted to respond differently to various injuries. Fibrosis and necrosis were most frequently noted in the region of the hepatic veins, whereas inflammation usually affected the portal triads. The physiology and anatomy of the lobular unit were unified by the classic contributions of Rappaport, who postulated and proved that the rationale for this differential susceptibility was related to blood flow. He showed that the acinus was based not on the hepatic vein (as proposed by Kiernan), but rather on the portal vein.

Operative treatment of the liver was first reported in penetrating battlefield wounds that exposed the injured organ. The first planned liver resections were undertaken only with the development of anesthesia and readily available banked blood. Refinements in the technique of hepatic resection have subsequently led to a decrease in the morbidity and mortality rates of this operative procedure since the 1940s. An understanding of the common causes of hepatic dysfunction and the scientific basis for the treatment of primary and secondary liver lesions is essential for effective operative therapy of liver diseases.[2]

SURGICAL ANATOMY

Embryology

During the third week of gestation, the liver arises from a duodenal bud and splits into hepatic and biliary components. The hepatic portion of this bud develops into hepatocytes, while the biliary component becomes the extrahepatic biliary system and gallbladder. The ultrastructure of the liver is ultimately formed by the ingrowth of umbilical veins, which form the sinusoids of the liver.

The fetal liver is responsible for production of blood, which ceases before birth. Two fetal structures are relevant to adult hepatic anatomy:

1. The ligamentum venosum is a remnant of the ductus venosum, which is a connection between the left portal vein and the left hepatic vein. The ligamentum venosum can be found deep to the bifurcation of the left portal vein between the left lateral segment and the caudate lobe.
2. The ligamentum teres (the residual umbilical vein) runs from the umbilicus to the left portal vein bifurcation and is found in the falciform ligament.

Lobar Structure

The bulk of the liver resides on the right side of the abdomen protected by the ribs (Fig. 53.2). At the right midclavicular line, the liver spans an area from the right nipple to the edge of the right costal margin. At the left midclavicular line, the superior margin is 1–2 cm below the nipple, and the most inferior extent is 3–4 cm above the costal margin. There is a large bare area (bounded by the triangular ligament on the right and the fissure for the ligamentum venosum on the left) above the liver, which attaches the liver to the diaphragm without intervening peritoneum. Posteriorly, the liver is fixed in place by the inferior vena cava (Fig. 53.3). The gallbladder rests on the posterior surface of the liver and a small portion of it is visible anteriorly with the liver in situ.

Blood Supply

The liver receives blood supply from both the hepatic artery and the portal vein (Figs. 53.4 and 53.5). The hepatic artery arises from the celiac trunk, runs to the right along the pancreas and joins the portal vein and the common bile duct in the free edge of the lesser omentum before entering the liver at the porta hepatis. The liver is drained by segmental hepatic veins, which enter the superior vena cava approximately 2 cm below the right atrium.

The portal blood supply and the hepatic venous drainage of the liver are relatively constant. The arterial blood supply, however, is anomalous in 20% of patients. This fact has implications for hepatic resection and for other upper gastrointestinal operative interventions such as gastrectomy, proximal pancreatectomy, and biliary procedures. The most common anomalies are aberrant origin of:

- Right hepatic artery from the superior mesenteric artery.
- Left hepatic artery from the gastric artery.

An aberrant right hepatic artery travels posterior and superior to the head of the pancreas to reach the porta

Anterior and posterior view of the liver

Anterior surface of the liver

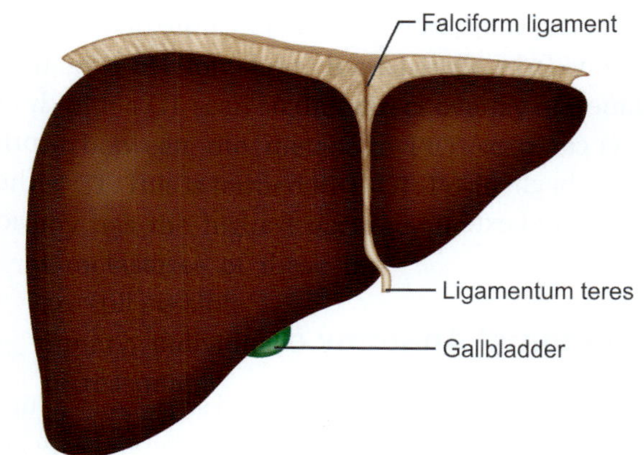

Posterior surface of the liver

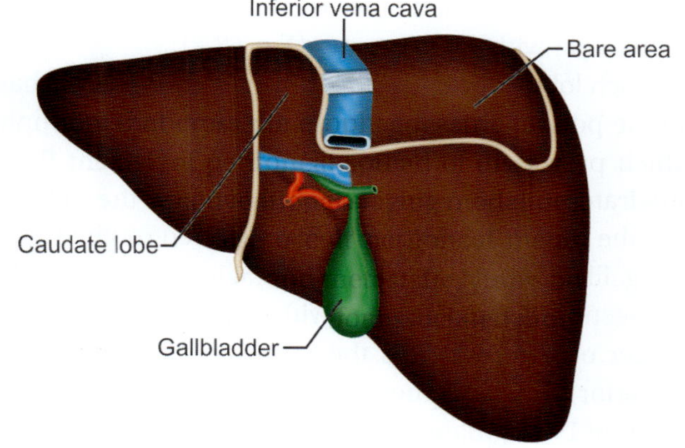

Fig. 53.3: Anterior and posterior surface of liver and its attachment.

Fig. 53.4: CT angiography showing the arterial supply to liver from hepatic artery arising from celiac axis.

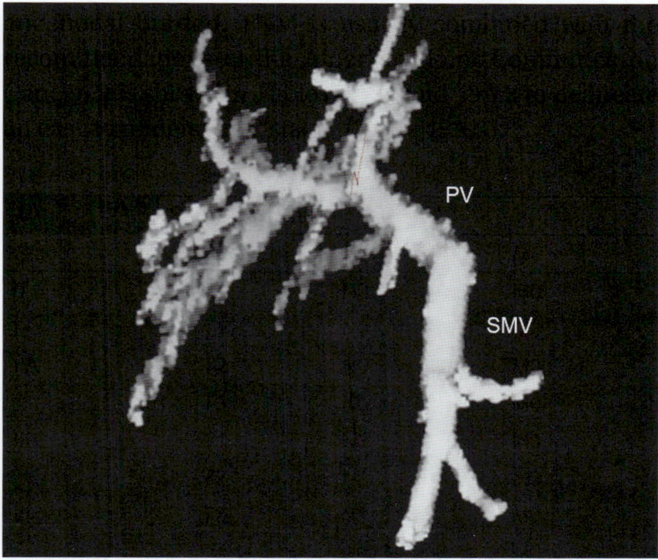

Fig. 53.5: CT angiography showing portal vein from superior mesenteric vein (SMV).

hepatis to the right of the pancreatic head (Fig. 53.6). This vessel can be identified in the porta hepatis below and behind the portal vein and common bile duct. An aberrant left hepatic artery may arise from either the right or left gastric artery and enters the liver at the falciform ligament via the gastrohepatic ligament.

Division into Lobes

The liver is anatomically divided into right and left lobes. Unlike in many other mammalian species, no external anatomic features of the human liver identify this division.

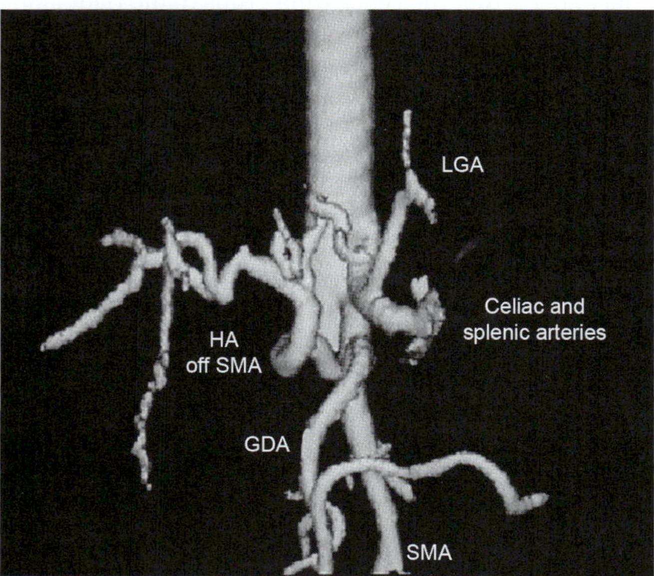

Fig. 53.6: CT angiography showing aberrant right hepatic artery arising from superior mesenteric artery (SMA).

The falciform ligament is present at the midline of the peritoneal cavity and appears to divide the liver into right and left lobes. Corrosion cast injections of the right and left portal veins, however, demonstrate that the two lobes are divided well to the right of the falciform ligament by a plane that runs between the gallbladder anteriorly and the vena cava posteriorly. With the liver *in situ* this principal plane begins approximately 1 cm to the left of the right nipple and extends obliquely to the vena cava adjacent to the spine.

Segmental Anatomy of the Liver

An understanding of the lobar and segmental structure of the liver is essential for the hepatic surgeon. The segmental anatomy of the liver has been most clearly outlined by Couinaud and Bismuth. Their classification divides the liver into right and left lobes via a plane that connects the gallbladder with the vena cava (Fig. 53.7).

Each lobe is divided into four anatomic segments based on the portal venous and hepatic arterial blood supplies, which parallel one another (Fig. 53.8). Segment IV (the quadrate lobe) of the left liver lies between the right liver and the left lateral segment. It is bounded on the right by the gallbladder fossa and the imaginary oblique plane connecting the gallbladder with the vena cava; the left border of segment IV is the falciform ligament and the posterior margin is the vena cava. The blood supply to segment IV originates from the left hepatic artery and left portal vein, which travel from the main portal vein inferior to the liver and into the falciform ligament. The portal

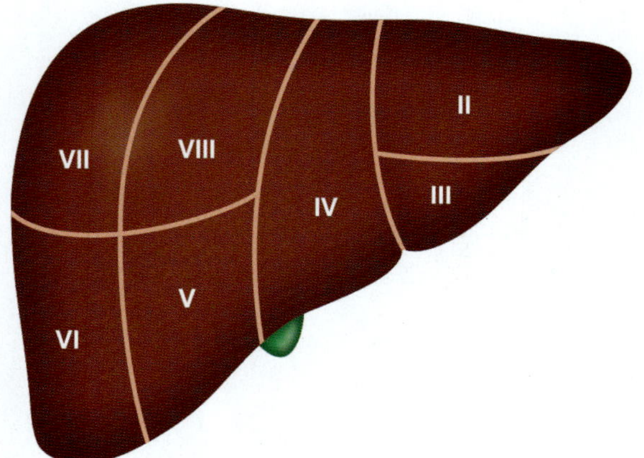

Fig. 53.7: Segmental anatomy of liver showing two lobes and Cantlie's line between gallbladder and super hepatic vena cava.

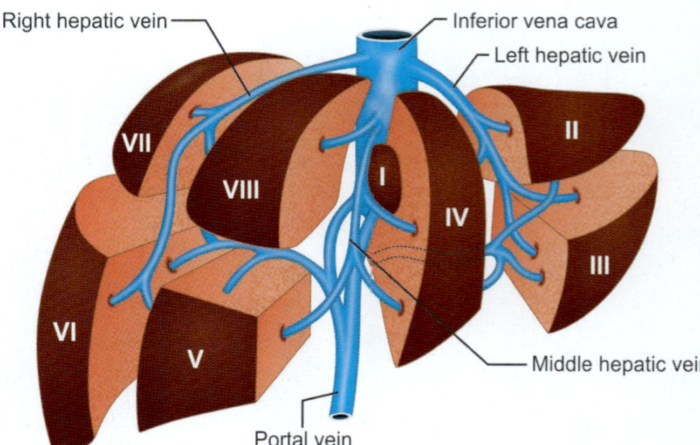

Fig. 53.8: Segmental anatomy of liver showing eight segments based on portal venous branches.

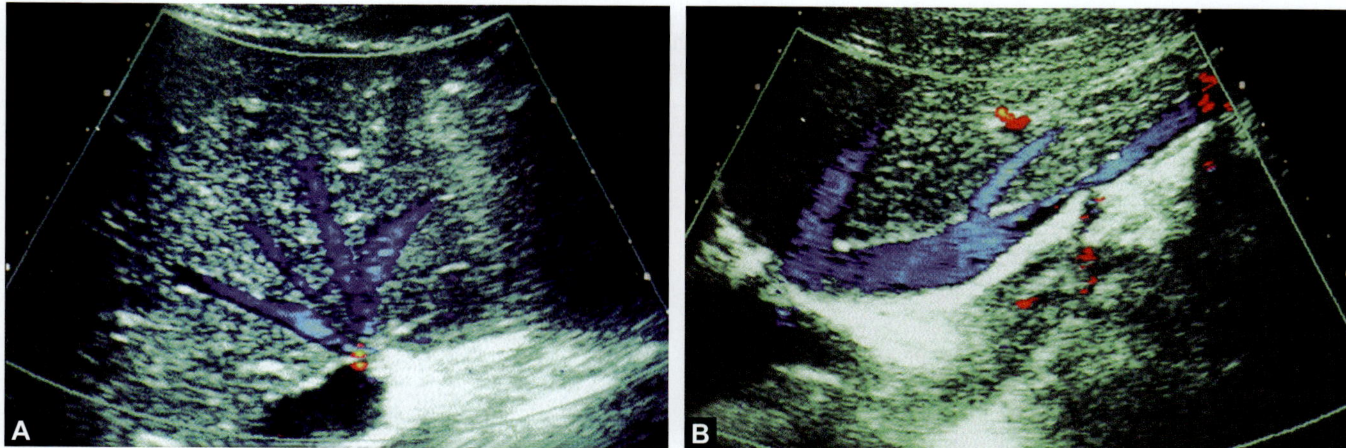

Figs. 53.9A and B: Duplex ultrasound showing three hepatic veins (A) and middle and left hepatic veins (B).

vein then divides into a branch to segment IV and other branches to segments II and III. The ligamentum venosum fixes the vessels in the falciform ligament posteriorly. The segmental blood supply therefore approaches segment IV from the left.

The numbering of hepatic segments when viewed inferiorly is similar to a counterclockwise revolution around the face of a clock (*see* Fig. 53.8):

- Segment I is the caudate lobe of the liver.
- Segments II and III are the superior and inferior portions of the lateral segment of the left liver.
- Segment IV is the quadrate lobe.
- Segments V–VIII comprise the right liver.

Segment V is most lateral, anterior, and inferior to the right portal vein bifurcation, segment VI is posterior to segment V, segment VII lies superior to segment VI above the right portal vein bifurcation, and segment VIII is superior to segment V.

The liver, with the exception of segment I, is drained by the right, middle, and left hepatic veins (Figs. 53.9A and B). The portal venous inflow can be visualized as a hand with four fingers (the portal veins after bifurcation in the falciform or the right lobe) approaching from below. The hepatic veins can be visualized as three fingers approaching from above and interdigitating with the four portal veins from below.

Histology

At the microscopic level, the portal triad (the hepatic artery, bile duct and portal vein) enters the liver perpendicular to the hepatic venous outflow (Fig. 53.10). The portal vein blood empties into the intralobular sinusoids and ultimately into the perpendicularly oriented central hepatic veins, which are lined by hepatocytes and surrounded by the perisinusoidal space of Disse. The liver parenchyma is organized into sheets of cells with the polygonal hepatocytes abutting adjacent hepatocytes as well as the sinusoids and space of Disse. The apical hepatocyte also abuts the bile canalicular radical (intralobular cholangiole).

The lobular structure of the liver is based on the acinar unit, which is centered on the portal triad (Fig. 53.11).

The lobular units of the liver have been divided into three portions based on the studies of Rappaport (Fig. 53.12):

- Zone 1 is adjacent to the portal venous inflow.
- Zone 2 lies between zones 1 and 3.
- Zone 3 is the area adjacent to the hepatic vein.

Zone 3 is the region of the liver acinus with the lowest oxygen tension and is therefore most susceptible to damage by toxins such as drugs and ethanol (Fig. 53.13). Liver regeneration begins in zone 1.

The sinusoidal space is also heavily populated by hepatic macrophages (Kupffer cells), which function similarly to peripheral macrophages and clear the sinusoids of debris, bacteria, and fungi. The Kupffer cells are also important for antigen presentation.

APPLIED PHYSIOLOGY

Normal Function

The organization of the hepatic acinus is intimately related to its function. The hepatocytes in Rappaport zone 3 have a different function to those in zone I. Synthetic enzymes such as those in the Krebs cycle are generally located in zone I, whereas enzymes involved in drug metabolism are found in zone 3 (Table 53.1).

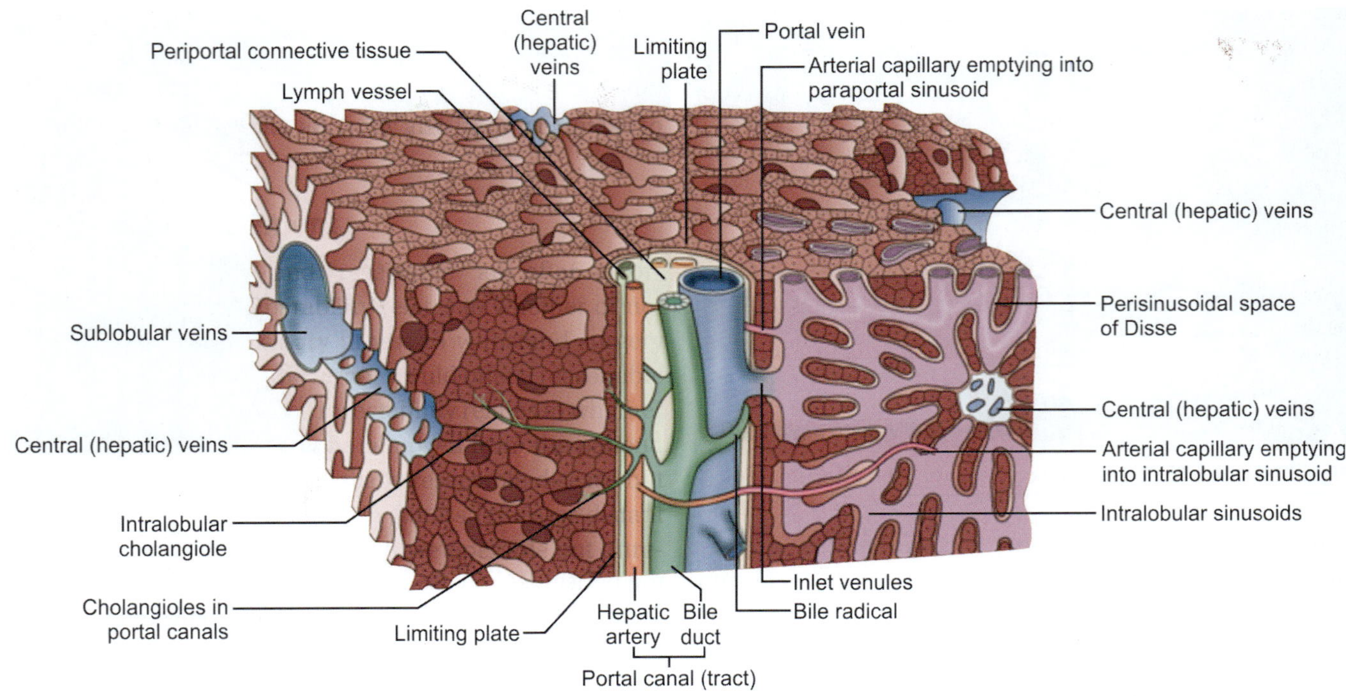

Fig. 53.10: Portal triads and plates of hepatocytes.

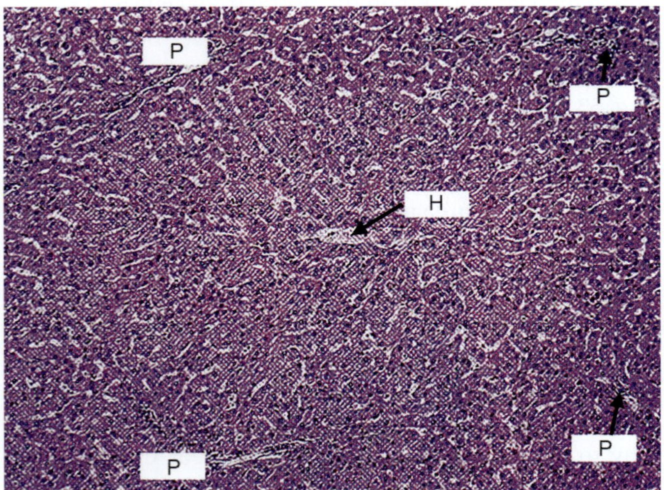

Fig. 53.11: Microscopic picture of liver acinar unit.

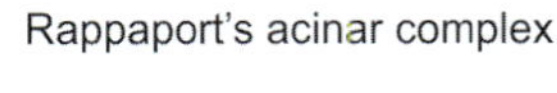

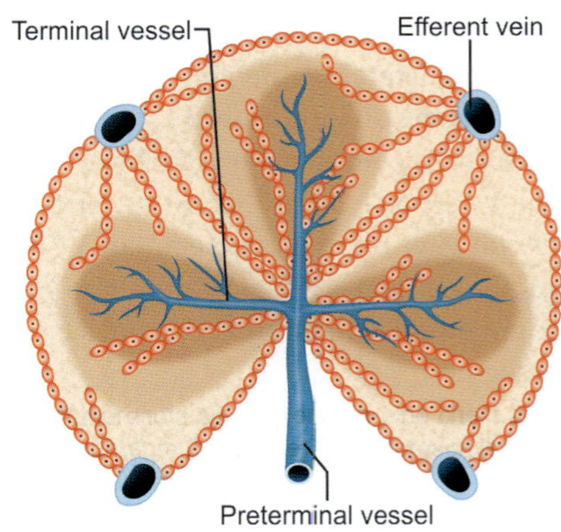

Fig. 53.12: Rappaport's acinar complex.

The histologic finding of bridging necrosis secondary to poisoning by ethanol and other toxins is localized to zone 3 and probably results from direct toxicity to hepatocytes that have the lowest oxygen tension. Why ethanol is toxic in some patients and not in others is poorly understood. Although bile formation occurs in both zones, bile salt-dependent formation tends to occur in zone I, whereas bile salt-independent formation is generally confined to zone 3.

Disordered Function

Abnormal liver function can be divided into deficient synthetic function, disorders of excretory function and obstruction of hepatic blood flow[3] (Table 53.2).

Loss of synthetic function results in the inability to metabolize precursor molecules into products such as albumin and proteins necessary for the coagulation cascade. The clinical manifestations of a decline in synthetic function include encephalopathy due to a lack of detoxification of noxious gastrointestinal tract chemicals, bleeding, and jaundice.

Disorders of excretory function may be congenital (Gilbert's disease, biliary atresia) or acquired (biliary obstruction secondary to choledocholithiasis or tumor). Patients with loss of excretory function are generally less ill than those who have hepatocellular failure, although patients who have superimposed biliary sepsis may be seriously ill at the time of presentation. Most patients who have bile stasis are therefore noted to be yellow by an acquaintance, have few if any systemic symptoms, and initially have normal synthetic hepatic function. Congenital surgical jaundice is typically caused by atresia of the extrahepatic biliary system. The operative management of infants with biliary atresia is more fully outlined in Chapter 125, "Gastrointestinal Surgery in Children".

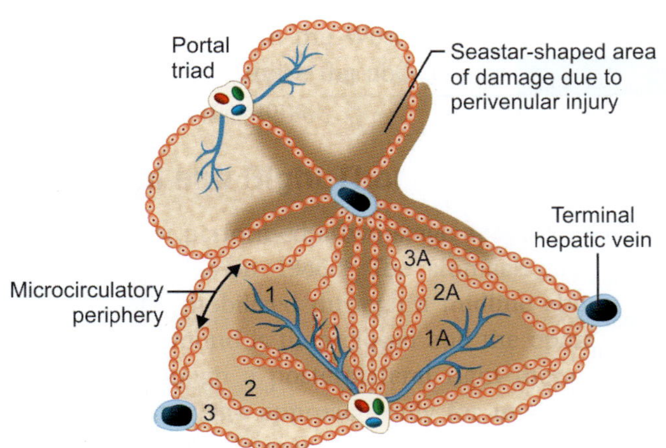

Fig. 53.13: Blood supply to liver acini showing areas susceptible to damage.

Obstruction to hepatic blood flow most commonly occurs in the cirrhotic liver secondary to increased resistance to blood flow caused by fibrosis of the acinar units. Less common causes are extrahepatic inflow occlusion from portal vein thrombosis or extrahepatic outflow resistance because of hepatic vein obstruction (Budd–Chiari syndrome; Fig. 53.14). The mechanism of obstruction to portal blood flow is important when designing treatment strategies for portal hypertension, but the clinical manifestations of portal hypertension are similar in all three patient groups. The pathophysiology and management of portal hypertension are discussed in detail in Chapter 54, "Portal Hypertension".

In the adult patient with jaundice, the clinical history generally leads to a presumptive diagnosis before obtaining laboratory tests. The history should concentrate on the chronicity of the patient's symptoms, any exposure to hepatotoxic drugs or skin puncture by needles contaminated with hepatitis viruses. Physical examination is focused on signs of chronic hepatocellular dysfunction such as ascites, spider angiomas, and a nodular liver. Examination of the stool for blood is an essential screening test for the presence of bleeding in cirrhosis or a bleeding ampullary tumor in obstructive jaundice. Laboratory tests should be specific and directed initially at common causes of jaundice:

- Serum bilirubin measurement is essential as an initial screening test.
- Serum transaminase levels (aspartate transaminase and alanine transaminase) provide a measure of hepatocellular damage.
- Serum albumin and coagulation studies (prothrombin time and partial thromboplastin time) measure the ability of the liver to synthesize essential proteins (Table 53.3).

Table 53.1 Metabolic function and pathologic damage to liver by zone.

Rappaport zone	*Metabolic functions*	*Oxygen tension*	*Pathologic damage*
1	Gluconeogenesis, bile salt-dependent bile formation	High	Ferrous sulfate, phosphorus
3	Glycolysis, bile salt-independent bile formation, P450 enzymes	Low	Necrosis in acute viral hepatitis, fibrosis in chronic hepatitis, most drug-induced necrosis (halothane, ethanol, acetaminophen, salicylates)

Table 53.2 Disorders of liver function.

Disorder	*Congenital causes*	*Acquired causes*
Loss of synthetic function	α I-antitrypsin deficiency	Acute or decompensated chronic hepatic failure
Loss of excretory function	Gilbert's disease	Sclerosing cholangitis, biliary obstruction (stone disease, biliary or pancreatic cancer), primary biliary cirrhosis
Obstruction to hepatic blood	Congenital hepatic fibrosis	Portal hypertension secondary to cirrhosis, hepatic vein obstruction (Budd-Chiari syndrome), extrahepatic portal vein obstruction

The patient who has jaundice secondary to hepatitis is initially managed supportively, and the etiology of the disease can generally be diagnosed by biochemical tests. By contrast, obstructive jaundice may be best managed by operative or interventional therapy. Unlike hepatitis serology, biochemical tests of hepatic function are not specific and do not differentiate the causes of biliary obstruction. The combination of a focused physical examination and radiographic evaluation of the biliary tract lead to a timely diagnosis and well-planned intervention.

A method for differentiating causes of obstructive jaundice is outlined in Table 53.4. High levels of serum bilirubin and alkaline phosphatase with normal transaminase levels and normal synthetic liver function are characteristic, but not diagnostic, of mechanical biliary obstruction. Patients with obstructive jaundice secondary to carcinoma of the pancreas tend to have painless and progressive jaundice. Patients with obstructive jaundice secondary to gallstone disease tend to have an acute onset of jaundice with abdominal pain, which may be complicated by superimposed sepsis secondary to ascending cholangitis.

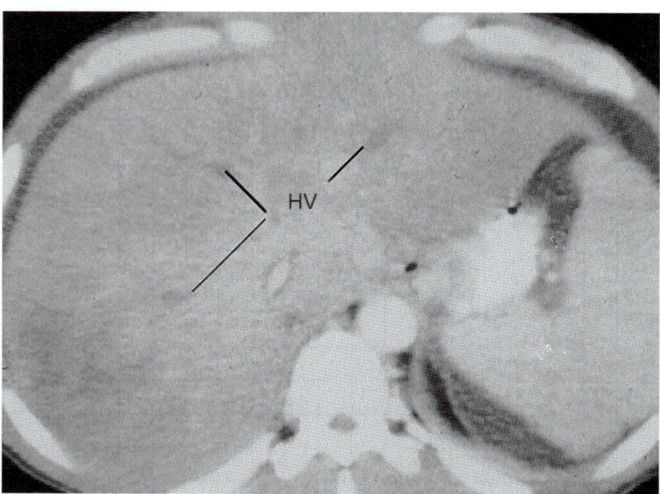

Fig. 53.14: Portal venous phase of CT scan of abdomen showing a total occlusion of three hepatic veins.

Regeneration

Unlike other solid organs, the liver can regenerate after maturity. In Greek tragedy, the Titan Prometheus saw the suffering of man, so he stole the fire of Zeus from his temple and brought it to man. When Zeus discovered this betrayal, he shackled Prometheus to a rock, opened his abdomen, and allowed an eagle each day to eat a portion of his liver. The liver regenerated every night and the eagle returned the next day for another meal. The Greeks therefore seemed to understand the regenerative power of the liver long before the biology of regeneration was known.

Table 53.3 Serum tests of liver function.

Diagnostic test	*Implications of abnormal value*
Bilirubin	
– Unconjugated	Prehepatic or hepatocellular dysfunction
– Conjugated	Biliary obstruction
Alkaline phosphatase	Biliary obstruction
Aspartate transaminase, γ-glutamyltransaminase	Hepatocellular damage (nonspecific)
Prothrombin time, partial thromboplastin time	Loss of hepatic synthetic function
Albumin	Loss of hepatic synthetic capacity
Ammonia	Hepatic encephalopathy

Table 53.4 Differential diagnosis of obstructive jaundice.

Feature	*Choledocholithiasis*	*Bile duct carcinoma*	*Pancreatic head carcinoma*	*Ampullary carcinoma*
Bilirubin level	Acute rise	Slowly increasing	Remorselessly increasing	Intermittent elevation (secondary to necrosis of tumor)
AST/GGT	Normal	Normal	Normal	Normal
Symptoms	Pain, fever	Generally none, weight loss	Generally none, weight loss, thoracic back pain	Generally none, weight loss
Stool guiac	–	–	–	+
Ultrasound	Dilated ducts, +/– stones	Dilated intrahepatic ducts	Dilated intra-and extrahepatic ducts	Dilated intra- and extrahepatic ducts
CT	+/– Stone at ampulla	No mass generally seen	Mass in head of pancreas	Negative or suggestion of duodenal mass
ERCP	Stone	Stricture at hepatic duct bifurcation	Stricture of distal common bile duct	Tumor of ampulla

[AST: Aspartate transaminase; ERCP: Endoscopic retrograde cholangiopancreatography; GGT: γ-glutamyltransaminase; Guiac (indicative of blood in stool)].

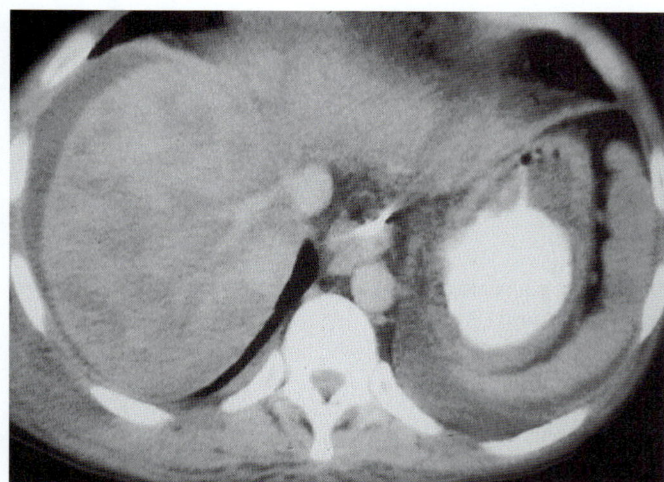

Fig. 53.15: CT scan of abdomen showing a patchy perfusion of liver on venous phase and a pleural effusion.

Table 53.5	King's College Hospital criteria for liver transplantation in fulminant hepatic failure.
Acetaminophen	
pH <7.30 (irrespective of grade of encephalopathy)	
or	
Prothrombin time >100 s and serum creatinine >300 μmol/l in patients who have grade III or IV encephalopathy	
Nonacetaminophen patients	
Prothrombin time >100 s (irrespective of grade of encephalopathy)	
or	
Any three of the following variables (irrespective of grade of encephalopathy)	
Age <10 or >40 years	
Etiology: nonA, nonB hepatitis, halothane hepatitis, idiosyncratic drug reaction	
Duration of jaundice before onset of encephalopathy >7 days	
Prothrombin time >50 s	
Serum bilirubin >300 μmol/l (17.5 mg/dl)	

An understanding of the mechanism of liver regeneration required the tools of molecular biology developed in the 20th century. Regeneration begins in Rappaport zone 1 of the acinus and results from a very orderly expression of cytokines and proteins. The most critical initiating factor in the complex cascade of regeneration is the synthesis of hepatocyte growth factor (HGF). In the first several hours after 70% hepatectomy in the rat, HGF is synthesized by the remaining hepatocytes. Hepatocyte growth factor is not only required for regeneration, but also loss of the *HGF* gene is a fatal mutation probably secondary to abnormal liver development. Hepatocyte growth factor expression is then followed by the rapid expression of transforming growth factor-α and a cascade of cytokines. This liver regeneration is ultimately stopped by the expression of transforming growth factor-β. This topic has been reviewed extensively.

Acute Liver Failure

Hepatic failure can occur either acutely or chronically. Fulminant hepatic failure is defined as the development of hepatic encephalopathy within 2 weeks of the onset of jaundice (Fig. 53.15). Subacute or subfulminant hepatic failure is generally defined by an interval of 2–8 weeks from jaundice to hepatic encephalopathy.

The management of acute hepatic failure is dependent upon:

- Early recognition
- Aggressive management of extrahepatic disease
- Availability of liver transplantation

The most frequent causes of acute hepatic failure are viral hepatitis and acetaminophen (paracetamol) poisoning. Less common causes include mushroom poisoning, idiosyncratic reaction to inhalational anesthetics such as halothane and Wilson's disease.

The survival of patients who have fulminant hepatic failure has improved, increasing from 15% to 50% in the past 30 years as a result of improved intensive care and the availability of liver transplantation. The differentiation of patients who are likely to die without transplantation from patients whose liver will regenerate is critical in the effective management of patients with acute hepatic failure. Criteria such as those developed by King's College Hospital (Table 53.5) serve as guides for decision making.

The lack of sufficient donor organs and the necessity for lifelong immunosuppression after transplantation have led to proposals for the conservative treatment of fulminant hepatic failure. These studies have focused on efforts to limit hepatic damage, accelerate regeneration, or support liver function temporarily with a bioartificial liver. The treatment of acute liver failure is outlined more fully in Chapter 118, "Liver Transplantation".

Cirrhosis and Chronic Liver Failure

Chronic liver failure has a slower and less dramatic onset than fulminant hepatic failure, but represents a much larger public health problem. Chronic liver disease is the ninth most frequent cause of death in the United States. Cirrhosis leads to a myriad of physiologic alterations, the most critical being:

- Failure to perform essential synthetic functions
- Failure to detoxify nutrients generated in the gastrointestinal tract

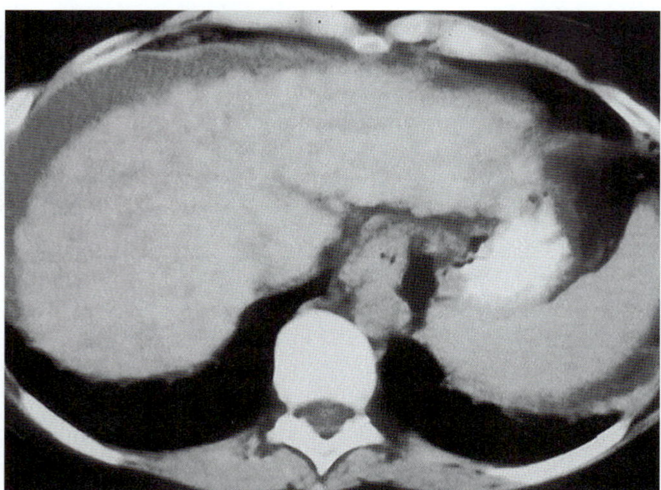

Fig. 53.16: CT scan of abdomen showing nodular appearance of cirrhotic liver and a pleural effusion.

The fibrosis of the liver, which is the histologic end point of cirrhosis, then leads to obstruction of intrahepatic blood flow and portal hypertension (Fig. 53.16). The chronic inflammation of cirrhosis is associated with the additional long-term risk of HCC. In a prospective surveillance study of 200 patients who had been newly diagnosed as having cirrhosis, HCC developed in 41% of the cohort with a yearly incidence of 5%.

Etiology

The most important etiologic agents for the development of cirrhosis are ethanol and chronic infection with the hepatitis C and B viruses, but their capacity to cause liver damage and cirrhosis varies (Table 53.6). Ethanol abuse is common, yet cirrhosis is only the ninth leading cause of death in the United States, so the majority of the ethanol-consuming population does not develop cirrhosis.

Many investigators have suggested that ethanol intake alone is not sufficient to cause cirrhosis and that dietary factors are also important. In one recent study, a group of alcoholics admitted to hospital for acute ethanol-related, but noncirrhotic, illnesses was compared with a group of alcoholics admitted for acute liver decompensation. Carbohydrate intake had a protective effect, whereas saturated fatty acid intake had a multiplicative (negative) effect. The quantity of ethanol consumed also influences the development of cirrhosis in retrospective case-control studies. The question as to why some chronic alcoholics develop cirrhosis and some do not may be explained in part by these models, but neither of these studies detected

Table 53.6 Relative probability of the etiology of cirrhosis.

Etiologic factor	*Proportion developing chronic infection after acute* episode (%)*	*Proportion developing cirrhosis (%)*
Ethanol	N/A	low
Hepatitis B	10	<2
Hepatitis C	60–80	20–40†

*Difficult to quantitate as most patients are asymptomatic at the time of acute disease

†Higher percentage in patients who have increased duration of disease.

a difference in total nutritional intake between the groups. Diet and the amount of hepatotoxin delivered to the liver are obviously important, but it is not clear how they interact. Another complicating factor in this complex model is the additive effect of chronic viral hepatitis to the development of cirrhosis in alcoholics. A group of patients who had newly diagnosed cirrhosis was compared with a cohort of nonalcoholic patients to assess the effect of nutrient intake and viral hepatitis infection on the development of cirrhosis in alcoholics. Both chronic viral hepatitis and a diet high in lipids, but low in carbohydrates and protein, were more prevalent in the patients who had cirrhosis. The addition of viral infection to ethanol intake, however, seems to have an additive rather than a synergistic effect, suggesting that the two agents act independently.

The most important prognostic factor in the development of cirrhosis is chronic infection with the hepatitis C virus. Hepatitis C infection (generally reported as the presence of antibody) was present in 72–80% of patients in a large multicenter cohort of patients with cirrhosis.[4] Other risk factors such as ethanol abuse (21%) or concomitant hepatitis B infection (3%) were also present, but 48% of cirrhotics in this series had hepatitis C as the only risk factor. Chronic infection with hepatitis C does not inevitably lead to cirrhosis. A large sample of patients who had a new diagnosis of chronic hepatitis C infection was identified, and the mode of acquisition of infection was determined. The presence of other factors associated with cirrhosis were identified, and the patients were followed over time. Of the entire cohort, 21% developed cirrhosis. The acquisition of infection by transfusion was more likely to result in cirrhosis than infection acquired as a result of intravenous drug use (23% vs. 7%). Longer duration of disease, excessive ethanol intake, and the presence of hepatitis B infection were risk factors for the development of cirrhosis.

Hepatocellular cancer developed in 18% of cirrhotic but in only 4% of the entire cohort of hepatitis C-positive patients.

Management

Treatment is aimed at preventing complications and death from HCV infection. As it takes decades for liver cirrhosis to develop following chronic HCV infection, efficacy of therapy is judged by the sustained virological response, a surrogate marker (rather than a clinical endpoint) defined as the absence of HCV RNA from serum by a sensitive PCR assay 24 weeks following discontinuation of treatment. Absence of detectable virus at the end of either a 24-week or 48-week course of therapy is referred to as an end-of-treatment response.

The most effective method for decreasing the number of patients with cirrhosis is to prevent a patient with hepatitis C infection from developing cirrhosis and ultimately hepatic fibrosis. The currently recommended therapy—the combination of a pegylated interferon-α and ribavirin—is based on the results of three pivotal, randomized, clinical trials that demonstrated the superiority of this combination treatment over standard interferon-α and ribavirin.[5-7] The drug (interferon α-2a or α-2b), which has received the most extensive evaluation, reduces the inflammatory process and may therefore prevent or modulate hepatic fibrosis. The clinical data to support the use of this relatively toxic drug are not completely convincing, however. Two groups of patients have been studied: cirrhotic patients and those with chronic hepatitis C infection without cirrhosis. A prolonged response and occasional clearing of infection is much more likely in patients who have chronic infection without cirrhosis. In cirrhotic patients interferon does not consistently reduce fibrosis, although a prolonged interferon response may be possible in 10–15% of patients. The rationale for interferon therapy in hepatitis B infection is even less clear. Most patients who have initial hepatitis B infection will not develop cirrhosis; therefore, the value of this drug depends upon identifying those at high risk for the development of cirrhosis.

Irrespective of the cause, the common end points of cirrhosis are portal hypertension and chronic liver failure. Portal hypertension may result in variceal bleeding, encephalopathy, ascites, and other manifestations of hepatic dysfunction and is discussed in depth in Chapter 54, "Portal Hypertension". An effective therapy for patients with complications of cirrhosis is hepatic transplantation. The indications for transplantation are discussed in Chapter 118, "Liver Transplantation".

INVESTIGATION

Liver Function Tests

The first diagnostic evaluation of a patient who has suspected hepatic disease should be aimed at assessment of the cause and severity of liver dysfunction. Some of the available diagnostic tests are outlined in Table 53.3. Abnormal liver function tests should lead to other tests that further define the pathology and generate a treatment plan. Abnormalities that suggest marked loss of liver function such as an elevated prothrombin time or hepatic encephalopathy should result in early transfer to a center specializing in the treatment of these very ill and complex patients.

In patients with evidence of acute viral hepatitis (elevated transaminases and bilirubin), the cause of the hepatitis can usually be determined by the assessment of viral serologies; little more in the way of diagnostic testing is necessary. Those with evidence of biliary tract obstruction or a more subtle mixture of vague symptoms, nonspecific physical findings and normal or mildly elevated serum tests should have an imaging study.

Imaging

Radiographic studies help delineate many hepatic diseases such as primary tumors or metastatic disease of the liver and disorders of the biliary system. The "best" imaging modality depends upon the disease process and the expertise of the institution.

Ultrasound Scanning

Ultrasound scanning has been the traditional first line of liver imaging. It is inexpensive and may be the only diagnostic radiologic procedure necessary for extrahepatic biliary tract disease, but its use is more limited as a tool for evaluating liver parenchymal pathology. As surgeons become more experienced at performing intraoperative ultrasonography, more reliable information may be obtained, such as the relationship of mass lesions to blood vessels.

The initial imaging procedure in patients who have obstructive jaundice is an ultrasound scan. Patients with biliary stone disease can be identified solely by ultrasound and can proceed to a definitive therapeutic procedure. When malignant biliary obstruction is suspected during an ultrasound examination, CT evaluation of the abdomen is mandatory further to delineate the pathology and identify extrabiliary disease. Intraoperative ultrasound scanning is critical for hepatic resection and is discussed later in this chapter.

Contrast-enhanced ultrasound (CEUS) or microbubble ultrasound scanning is now being used extensively in liver units for assessment of liver tumors.[8,9] Although operator dependent, it offers major advantages over CT or MRI in differentiating hepatic tumors from other lesions. It is a real-time dynamic imaging modality that depicts the enhancement pattern of tumors. The intravascular properties of microbubble contrast agents consistently demonstrate washout of malignancy and allows repeat observation of tumor vascularity after multiple injections of the agent, with an excellent safety profile and no nephrotoxicity. Contrast-enhanced ultrasound to determine the exact nature of an indeterminate lesion seen on CT or MRI and differentiate benign and malignant tumors: hemangiomas show delayed venous filling, FNH, and adenoma show early arterial filling; HCC shows arterial hypervascularity and often late partial washout, while metastatic liver disease shows arterial hypervascularity and complete rapid washouts.

Computed Tomography

This has the advantage of not only identifying lesions of the liver and pancreas, but also of defining the relationship of such lesions to the portal vein, hepatic artery and hepatic veins, and their relationship to adjacent structures such as the pancreatic head. Before resectional hepatic procedures, CT scanning is mandatory for operative planning as well as for the identification of extrahepatic pulmonary and peritoneal disease. In many cases, the resectability of a lesion can be determined solely from a contrast-enhanced CT[10] (Fig. 53.17).

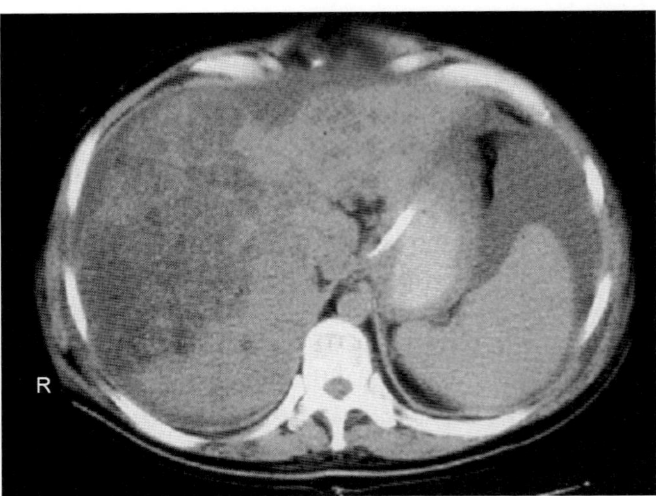

Fig. 53.17: CT scan of abdomen showing extensive metastases in liver and ascitic fluid.

Recent advances in CT technology, especially spiral CT and biphasic CT, have largely replaced arteriography and CT portography (CT after injection of contrast via the hepatic or superior mesenteric artery) in the preoperative assessment of patients who have liver tumors:

- Spiral CT with overlapping reconstruction of rapidly acquired images improves the images obtained by eliminating respiratory motion and by maintaining high levels of contrast for the duration of the scan.
- Biphasic CT incorporates the speed of spiral CT with a quickly administered intravenous contrast bolus and allows acquisition of images during the arterial phase of enhancement. This technique highlights arterially perfused lesions in the liver (primary or metastatic neoplasms) against the background of less enhanced liver parenchyma (Figs. 53.18A and B).

The resolution of contemporary biphasic CT is at least as good as that of CT portography in the detection of liver neoplasms. An arteriogram or a CT portogram is no longer required before undertaking hepatic resection. One pitfall of the increase in sensitivity of biphasic CT, however, has been a decrease in specificity due to the identification of false-positive liver lesions.

Magnetic Resonance Imaging

The role of MRI in the diagnosis of hepatic disease is less well defined. For patients who have diffuse liver disease such as cirrhosis, hemochromatosis, or fatty infiltration of the liver, MRI is quite effective in establishing a presumptive diagnosis and in serially evaluating patients who have known benign liver disease. Magnetic resonance imaging, particularly with the addition of gadolinium contrast enhancement, is superior to CT in the definitive diagnosis of hemangioma and will accurately detect hypervascular tumors such as hepatomas. Both the sensitivity and the specificity of MRI have been greatly improved by using a diffusing image and contrast (1) to detect and characterize small liver lesions, whether primary or metastatic (2) as a part of preoperative staging and (3) for post-treatment monitoring.[10,11]

Other Imaging Modalities

These are used when specific pathology is suspected. The liver-spleen scan using radiolabeled autologous blood is

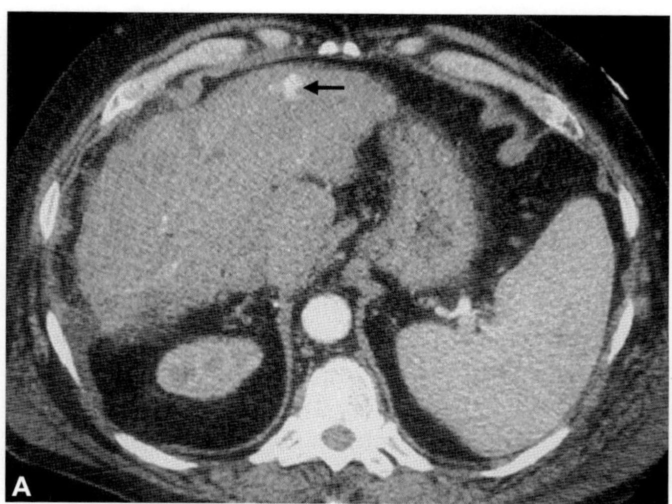

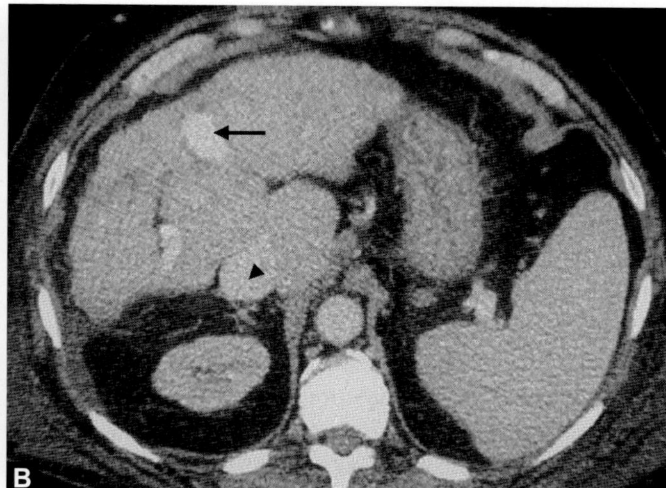

Figs. 53.18A and B: Biphasic CT scan of abdomen showing an arterial enhancing lesion suggestive of HCC (A) and a portal venous enhancing lesion suggestive of hemangioma (B).

less expensive than MRI and can also confirm that a mass lesion detected by CT is a hemangioma. Magnetic resonance spectroscopy with phosphorus-32 assesses hepatic functional reserve in patients who have cirrhosis and predicts the ability of a patient to withstand liver resection.[10,11]

Laparoscopy

Laparoscopic cholecystectomy has revolutionized biliary tract surgery. Laparoscopic treatment of benign and malignant liver lesions has now gained widespread acceptance in expert hands.[12,13]

Laparoscopy is a sensitive method for evaluating disease on the liver surface and peritoneum. Laparoscopic evaluation of the liver and peritoneal cavity before operative exploration in patients who have pancreatic carcinoma avoids a laparotomy in 10–15% of patients because of the detection of metastatic disease. By contrast, the incidence of peritoneal metastases and surface lesions in patients with CT criteria of resectability in primary HCC or metastatic colorectal carcinoma is quite low, so routine laparoscopy is probably not justified.

A subset of patients with lesions noted on CT, however, may benefit from the combined use of laparoscopy and laparoscopic ultrasound. Lesions as small as 2–3 mm can be detected by laparoscopic ultrasound scanning in the hands of an experienced practitioner (compared with the 1 cm resolution of spiral CT). The detection of multiple small lesions by laparoscopic ultrasound or by intraoperative ultrasound through a small subcostal incision precludes a large incision and therefore hastens recovery in the setting of unresectable disease.

Cholangiography

The biliary tract of patients who have intrahepatic or extrahepatic biliary disease may also be evaluated by means of more invasive imaging procedures: percutaneous transhepatic cholangiography (PTC) or endoscopic retrograde cholangiopancreatography (ERCP). In addition to the diagnostic imaging data, both tests offer access to the biliary tract for biopsy and the capacity for therapeutic intervention by placing stents or removing stones. The choice between ERCP and PTC is most effectively based on the suspected location of pathology:

- Endoscopic retrograde cholangiopancreatography is used for patients with jaundice and distal biliary obstruction.
- Percutaneous transhepatic cholangiography is preferable for patients with proximal obstruction of the extrahepatic biliary tract.

Endoscopic retrograde cholangiopancreatography may be inadequate for visualizing the intrahepatic bile ducts and for placing stents in many patients who have proximal biliary tract obstruction. Optimal imaging of the intrahepatic ducts in such patients requires PTC, which has the disadvantage of causing intra-abdominal hemorrhage in some patients, although the bleeding is generally not life-threatening. A percutaneous catheter may be left in position to decompress and to allow future access to the biliary tree.

Angiography

Angiographic investigation of the portal and hepatic blood supply to the liver may be useful in patients undergoing anatomic hepatic resections. Angiography allows the definition of aberrant anatomy such as a replaced right hepatic artery from the superior mesenteric artery or a replaced left hepatic artery from the right or left gastric artery. In general, however, this determination can be easily made during an exploratory operation by an experienced surgeon.

In patients with hilar cholangiocarcinoma angiography can identify encasement or obstruction of the portal vein or hepatic artery, which precludes curative resection. The use of biphasic CT and the routine use of intraoperative ultrasound mean that preoperative angiography is now rarely necessary. Biphasic CT defines the relationship of hepatic masses to vascular structures; it is as sensitive as CT portography and can detect encasement of the hepatic artery and portal vein. Angiography is more critical for the confirmation of suspected vascular invasion at the bifurcation of the portal structures, an area not well visualized by CT. The identification of vascular invasion by angiography precludes a laparotomy. Magnetic resonance angiography may be useful to evaluate the hepatic blood supply and avoid an invasive angiographic procedure.

Biopsy

Hepatic biopsy can be performed percutaneously, laparoscopically, or via laparotomy. Percutaneous biopsy remains the commonest method because of its low cost and because it can be carried out under local anesthesia. Laparoscopic liver biopsy has replaced open liver biopsy except for patients who have a contraindication to laparoscopy, such as previous upper abdominal operative procedures. The false-negative rate for percutaneous liver biopsy implies that a more direct method of biopsy may increase the yield among patients who have localized hepatic disease. When percutaneous biopsy is contraindicated by abnormal coagulation parameters or ascites, for example, laparoscopic liver biopsy can be performed with a low complication rate.[13] Laparoscopy has the additional advantage of providing direct visualization of the liver and peritoneum. The miniaturization of laparoscopic instrumentation may soon preclude the need for general anesthetic, and eventually the procedure may be used instead of percutaneous liver biopsy for most patients.

TRAUMA

The first successful hepatic resection for trauma was performed through a self-inflicted knife wound. Although 100 years have passed since then, the presence of a penetrating abdominal injury should still result in emergency laparotomy. The goals of exploration for penetrating hepatic injury are control of bleeding, removal of devitalized tissue, and assessment of concurrent injury.

The evaluation and management of blunt hepatic injury have evolved in recent years. The hemodynamically unstable patient who has suspected abdominal injury should be explored as an emergency. Liver injury in the stable patient does not necessarily require operative intervention, however.

The initial evaluation of a patient who has blunt abdominal trauma and the roles of CT and diagnostic peritoneal lavage are more completely discussed in Chapter 40, “Abdominal and Perineal Injuries”. Diagnostic peritoneal lavage is highly sensitive, but results in unnecessary laparotomy in many patients who have minimal self-limiting liver injury and has been supplanted by CT for the stable patient. A CT evaluation can identify the subset of patients with isolated liver injury and provide an assessment of the extent of hepatic damage, but does not clearly differentiate patients for whom an operation is necessary. When nonoperative management was prospectively evaluated in a series of patients with blunt trauma, fewer abdominal complications developed and less blood was transfused than for a cohort of patients who underwent operative management.[14] At the other extreme, transplantation has been reported in patients who have otherwise lethal liver injuries.

Postoperative complications of both penetrating and blunt hepatic injury (such as intrahepatic bile duct injury) can usually be treated by interventional techniques. Operative intervention for late complications is only necessary for patients who have failed to respond to nonoperative management.

LIVER CYSTS

Solitary Cyst

Cystic disease of the liver is a frequent finding on CT and MRI evaluation of the liver, but rarely requires operative intervention (Fig. 53.19). Occasionally, patients with solitary liver cysts present with severe abdominal pain, marked increase in abdominal girth or atypical findings (thick wall, necrotic debris in the lumen) on liver imaging.

Operative management of symptomatic patients is limited to unroofing of simple cysts. The operative fenestration of solitary cysts in symptomatic patients has a low complication rate and generally the patient’s symptoms

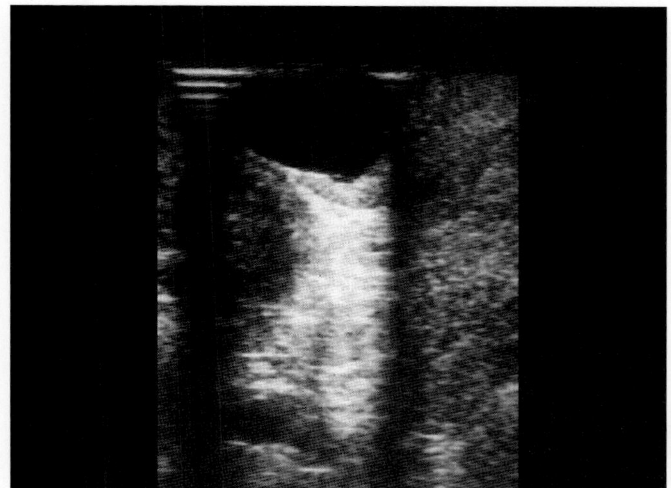

Fig. 53.19: Ultrasound appearance of a simple liver cyst.

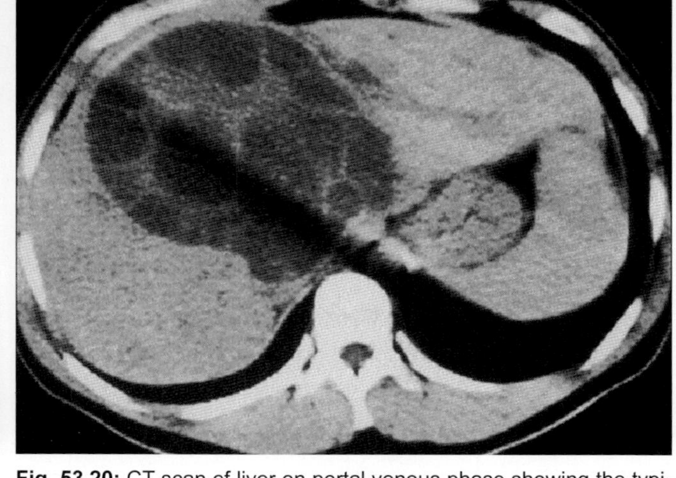

Fig. 53.20: CT scan of liver on portal venous phase showing the typical appearance of a hydatid cyst and daughter cysts.

resolve. Solitary cysts that about the liver capsule can be fenestrated laparoscopically with a low rate of operative complications and a short hospital confinement.

If at the time of exploration the cyst is filled with bile or has a thickened wall, or biliary cyst adenoma or cystadenocarcinoma is suspected (this can usually be confirmed by biopsy of cyst wall), then resection or cyst enucleation should be performed rather than fenestration.

Polycystic Disease

Polycystic liver disease often occurs in conjunction with polycystic renal disease. The patient's prognosis is determined not by the liver disease, but by the severity of renal insufficiency, which may complicate polycystic renal disease. Unlike solitary liver cysts, the cystic contents in polycystic disease may contain degenerated blood, probably from bleeding into the cysts. Most patients with polycystic liver disease are asymptomatic, although the occasional patient may present with severe abdominal pain or abdominal distension due to hepatomegaly. Less commonly polycystic disease may obstruct the biliary system or the hepatic venous outflow of the liver.[15]

Nonoperative methods such as percutaneous drainage will relieve symptoms, but the cysts tend to recur. The frequency of recurrence may be decreased by injection of sclerosing agents such as ethanol into the drained cyst.

Operative treatment of polycystic disease is accompanied by more potential complications and is less successful than the treatment of solitary liver cysts and should therefore be reserved for the occasional patient who has troublesome symptoms. Resection of the most severely involved areas of the liver has been studied in small groups of symptomatic patients and the results have been mixed. Resection achieved symptomatic relief in five of eight patients, with an operative complication rate of 38%. Similar results, including one death, were obtained in a second series.

Hydatid Cysts

Hydatid liver cysts caused by the parasites *Echinococcus granulosus* and *Echinococcus multilocularis* are endemic in countries bordering the Mediterranean and China,[16] but are uncommon in Western Europe and in the United States. *E. granulosus* is associated with cystic echinococcosis *and E. multilocularis* is associated with the more aggressive, but 50-fold less common, alveolar echinococcosis.

Patients who have cystic echinococcosis present with abdominal pain, fever, jaundice, urticaria, or an abdominal mass. Definitive diagnosis depends upon a positive serum immunoelectrophoresis or the detection of echinococcal antibodies in the serum plus cystic liver disease on CT or ultrasound scan (Fig. 53.20).

Screening evaluation for asymptomatic echinococcal disease consists of either serologic testing or screening ultrasound. Even in an endemic area echinococcal liver disease is rare; therefore, screening should be reserved for high-risk patient populations. In a serologic screening protocol, only eight cases of asymptomatic alveolar echinococcosis were detected in a population of 7,884 patients. The authors concluded that screening was cost-effective and reduced the risk of morbidity. Ultrasonographic screening for cystic hydatid disease has also been

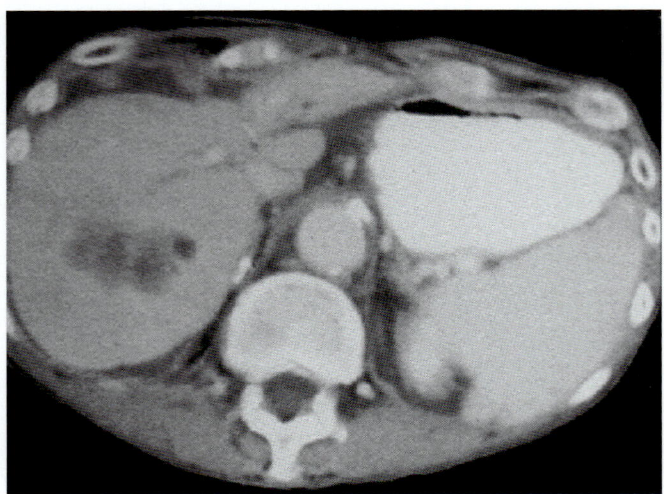

Fig. 53.21: CT scan of liver on portal venous phase showing a complex-looking cystic lesion suggestive of pyogenic liver abscess.

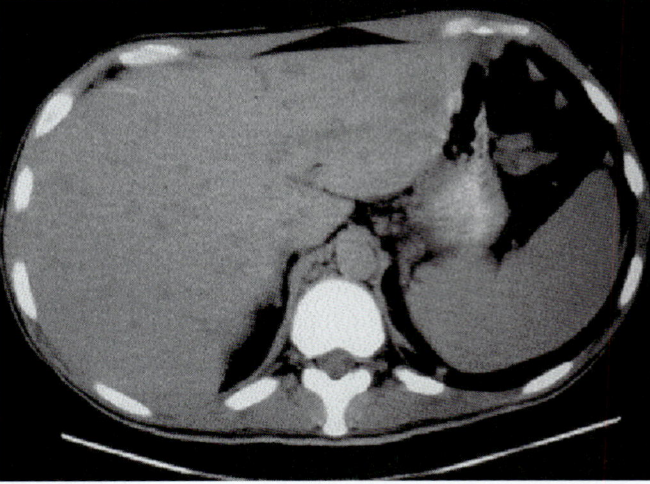

Fig. 53.22: Non-contrast CT scan of abdomen showing multiple low-attenuation areas suggestive of liver abscess.

studied in a population of 9,482 patients in an endemic area of Uruguay. Confirmation of positive cases was made in 48 of 51 patients explored surgically. The complications that these screening studies attempt to avoid include rupture into the biliary tree (17%) and infection of the cyst cavity (5%). The early cases discovered by screening may also be more amenable to nonoperative therapies.[16]

Alveolar echinococcal disease is associated with a mortality of 90% in untreated cases. Radical resection, if possible, followed by albendazole or mebendazole for at least 2 years is the treatment of choice. For those with unresectable disease, a longer duration of drug therapy is indicated, although the outlook is poor. Liver transplantation may be successful for patients who have deteriorating liver function.

The operative treatment of hydatid cyst based on resection of the cyst to include the pericyst either by cystectomy or partial hepatectomy is safe and effective. Attempts to avoid operative treatment by drug therapy with mebendazole or albendazole alone have not been effective. The sometimes successful combination of drug therapy with cyst aspiration rather than resection, however, does suggest that operative resection can be avoided in some cases. A prospective randomized trial that compared operative removal of the cyst with percutaneous drainage and concomitant albendazole demonstrated that percutaneous drainage combined with albendazole therapy was as effective as operative cystectomy.[17] In countries where there is a high incidence of cystic echinococcal disease, nonoperative therapy may be a more cost-effective treatment, although both operative therapy and drainage of the cyst combined with drug therapy are also effective. In the subset of patients who have intrahepatic biliary rupture, operative cystectomy, biliary lavage, and biliary drainage are mandatory.

LIVER ABSCESS

Pyogenic Abscess

The early diagnosis of pyogenic liver abscess depends upon a high index of suspicion in patients with who has fever, leukocytosis, right upper quadrant pain, and a history of biliary tract pathology. Pyogenic liver abscess is associated with ascending cholangitis, due either to benign or malignant biliary tract disease, in 30–40% of cases (Fig. 53.21).

Inflammatory diseases of the gastrointestinal tract with resultant hematogenous spread via the portal venous system are also common precipitating factors. Many patients, however, have no history of either biliary or gastrointestinal tract symptoms (Fig. 53.22).

In the subset of patients without an established infectious cause for their liver abscess, diabetes mellitus is a risk factor in 65% of cases. More than 50% of the abscesses in diabetic patients contain gas-forming organisms, which may explain the higher mortality rate in diabetics than nondiabetics (30 vs. 5%): however, in another study the presence of gas-forming organisms was not an independent negative prognostic variable.

With univariate analysis, the following factors were associated with death in 352 patients who had newly diagnosed liver abscesses:

- Patient age
- Gas-forming abscess
- Bilobar involvement
- Sepsis
- Bilirubin >2 mg/dL (35 μmol/L)
- Blood urea nitrogen (BUN) > 20 mg/dL (7.2 mmol/L)
- Serum creatinine > 2 mg/dL (176 μmol/L)
- Aspartate transaminase > 100 U/mL
- Albumin < 2.5 g/dL

When the positive variables were subjected to multivariate analysis, only age, BUN, creatinine, bilirubin, and albumin at the time of diagnosis remained predictors of death.

The most critical factor in the successful treatment of pyogenic liver abscess is early institution of broad-spectrum antibiotics, which can then be refined according to the sensitivity of the organisms cultured from the abscess cavity. The continuation of antibiotic therapy for 3–6 months generally cures the infection. For liver abscess secondary to cholangitis, the biliary obstruction must be relieved by either operative biliary bypass or biliary drainage and stenting via PTC or ERCP. After aspiration of the abscess for culture, pyogenic abscesses can be treated either by antibiotics alone or in combination with percutaneous aspiration, or percutaneous drainage with a catheter left in place or open operative drainage. Open operative drainage is reserved for patients who have failed to respond to percutaneous drainage or those who require another operative procedure (e.g. biliary bypass or appendectomy). Intravenous antibiotics alone are rarely successful without concomitant percutaneous drainage. The presence of multiple abscess cavities is not a contraindication to percutaneous drainage. When percutaneous drainage of single and multiple abscesses was compared retrospectively, no difference in abscess resolution was noted.[18] Two of 28 patients with solitary abscesses died of peritonitis after percutaneous drainage, compared with none of 10 patients with multiple lesions.

The success of nonoperative catheter drainage suggests that aspiration without prolonged drainage in combination with antibiotics may also eradicate infection. No comparative trial has been reported, although two studies have retrospectively reviewed this technique. Aspiration without drainage has the advantage of avoiding the discomfort and morbidity of an external tube. Ultrasound-guided needle aspiration without catheter placement was successful for 23 of 24 patients who had solitary liver abscesses: 18 were aspirated once and seven required subsequent aspiration, all within 10 days of diagnosis. A second series included 115 patients who had both solitary and multiple abscesses aspirated a mean of 2.2 times. No complications, deaths or recurrences were noted in any patient, and operative drainage was necessary for only two patients because of large abscess size.

Amebic Abscess

The pathogenic agent of amebic liver abscesses *(Entamoeba histolytica)* is environmentally acquired, survives in the gastrointestinal tract, and gains access to the portal venous system through the colon. The liver abscess forms after blockage of the portal venous radicals by the organism and subsequent hepatic necrosis, which results in a typical chocolate cyst. *E. histolytica* is endemic in the tropics and subtropics. Latency between colonic infection and hepatic infection may be as long as 6 months. Patients present with malaise, abdominal pain, fever, leukocytosis, and hepatomegaly. Almost all patients ultimately develop positive serology for *E. histolytica,* but stool examination for cysts is positive in only 30% of patients.[19]

Treatment with metronidazole alone is curative in most patients, although aspiration or percutaneous drainage of large amebic liver abscesses in addition to metronidazole may have a role in some cases. The presence of a cavity over 6 cm in diameter was associated with an accelerated resolution after percutaneous aspiration, but no difference in resolution was noted at 6 months in a retrospective study. A prospective randomized trial of metronidazole alone versus percutaneous aspiration plus metronidazole in patients who had lesions >5 cm in diameter revealed that clinical improvement was significantly faster and hospital stay shorter in the aspiration plus metronidazole group. Therefore, patients who have large amebic abscesses or those who are refractory to medical measures should be treated with metronidazole in combination with percutaneous drainage.

The presence of jaundice suggests a biliary communication with the cyst and is an indication for percutaneous drainage.

A perforated amebic liver abscess can be successfully treated with metronidazole plus percutaneous drainage complemented by operative drainage if necessary.

BENIGN LIVER TUMORS

Benign hepatic tumors can be categorized as:

- Tumors of the biliary system
- Tumors of the hepatic parenchyma
- Hemangiomas

All have malignant counterparts.

Hemangioma

This is the commonest benign tumor of the liver. The lesion is generally noted incidentally on CT or ultrasound scans performed for unrelated problems, and the diagnosis is definitively established by tagged red blood cell scan, MRI, or microbubble ultrasound. The periphery of a typical hemangioma is enhanced late in the arterial phase of a biphasic CT, with contrast diffusing to the center of the lesion during the portal phase. Most hemangiomas are asymptomatic, although if very large they occasionally cause pain because of pressure on the liver capsule or other organs. Symptomatic hemangiomas should be operatively removed by either enucleation or resection.

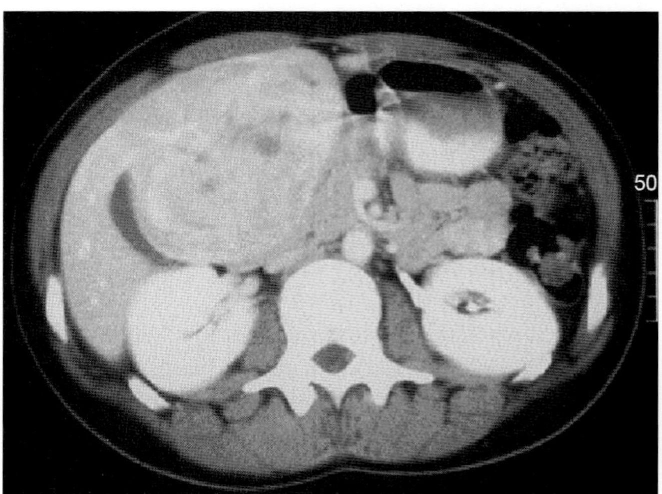

Fig. 53.23: CT scan of liver on portal venous phase showing a vascular lesion with displacement of surrounding structures.

Hepatic Adenoma

Hepatic adenoma and FNH (*see* below) are benign hepatic parenchymal tumors and are generally found incidentally at the time of radiographic evaluation for other diseases. The major diagnostic dilemma is differentiation of these two entities from HCC. Hepatic adenomas are associated with oral contraceptive use, and in contrast to FNH they often present as symptomatic lesions (Fig. 53.23). Regression of an adenoma, even with cessation of oral contraceptives, is uncommon. As up to one third of adenomas spontaneously rupture and bleed, most of these lesions should be resected. Radiographic evaluation with CT or MRI may be diagnostic, but resection is mandatory for the patient who has an atypical presentation (male, older, lack of oral contraceptive use) or an uncertain diagnosis. Peripheral or pedunculated adenomas are treated by resection of the lesion with a minimal clearance margin. In the patient who has large or centrally placed adenomas in whom major resection would be required for removal, enucleation may be preferable and is not associated with local recurrence. If the diagnosis of adenoma is not clear by imaging, the lesion should be treated as an HCC.

Focal Nodular Hyperplasia

In contrast to hepatic adenoma, FNH is usually not symptomatic at presentation. The incidence of FNH is increasing, probably as a result of the more frequent use of diagnostic imaging. Microbubble ultrasound, CT, and MRI detect FNH in most patients. On CT evaluation, FNH typically fills early with contrast, is not visible during the venous phase and may have a central scar. The fact that none these features rules out the diagnosis of HCC (Figs. 53.24 and 53.25) poses a therapeutic problem because at least 50% of these lesions will either resolve spontaneously or decrease in size during follow-up. Expectant treatment of patients who have suspected FNH, however, risks a delay in the operative treatment of a small HCC.

The perception that FNH is difficult to diagnose before resection has led to the biopsy and resection of many lesions for diagnostic reasons. Although many radiographic studies have reported the imaging characteristics of FNH, few studies have confirmed the radiographic diagnosis of FNH by operative resection. Focal nodular hyperplasia was diagnosed preoperatively by biphasic CT in 17 patients in one study and this diagnosis was confirmed for all patients at operation. In a second group of 33 patients who had adenoma or in whom adenoma and FNH could not be differentiated before resection, three were found to harbor HCC. Hepatocellular carcinoma did not convincingly arise in areas of FNH, but was associated with one adenoma. A clear radiologic or histologic diagnosis of FNH with long-term observation is therefore appropriate. Resection should be performed for patients who have equivocal radiographic findings.

Biliary Adenoma

This is typically cystic, and it is also less common than hepatic adenoma. Biliary adenomas are often discovered during the investigation of patients who have upper abdominal pain, fever, and jaundice. Differentiation from parasitic cysts may be a problem in endemic areas, although serologic evaluation generally excludes an infestation. These tumors are usually right-sided, solitary, multiloculated cysts that have an irregular cyst wall. Malignant

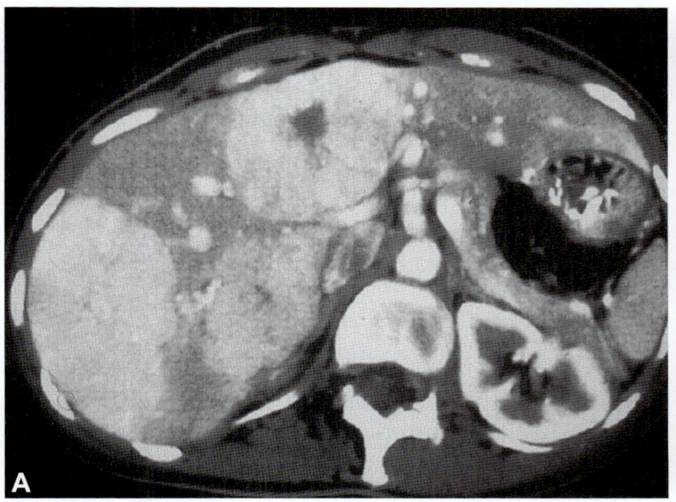

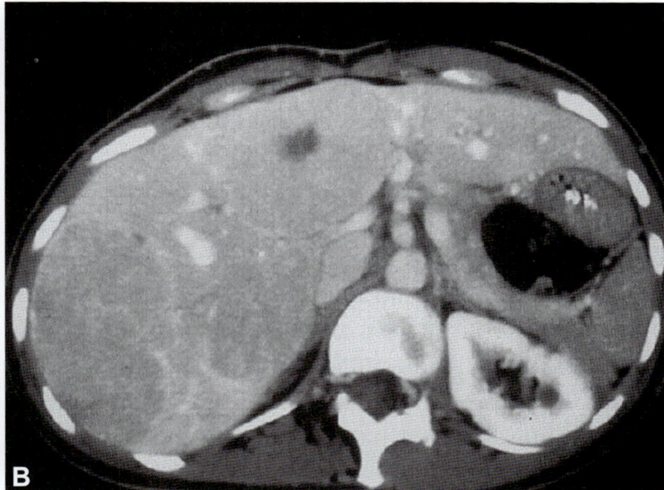

Figs. 53.24A and B: CT scan of liver showing enhancing lesions on arterial phase (A) and a near-total washout on portal venous phase (B) and central scarring suggestive of FNH.

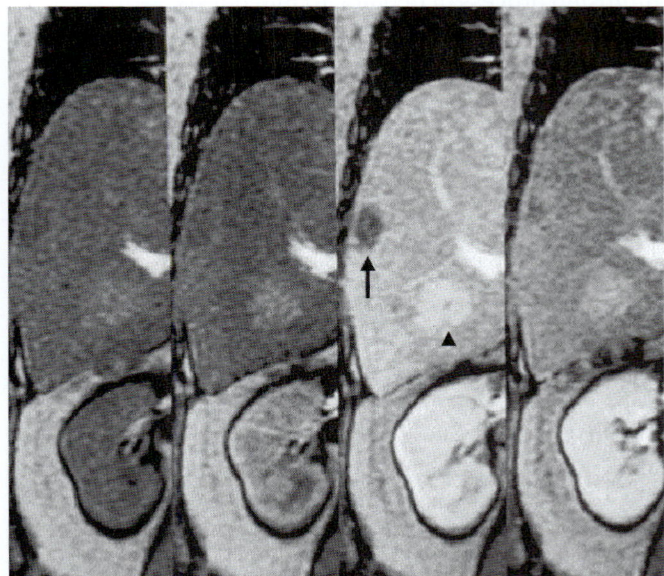

Fig. 53.25: MRI appearance of two liver lesions with totally different enhancing patterns.

transformation is common as is recurrence after incomplete excision. Biliary obstruction is also common, arising from either local obstruction or thick mucoid secretions. A complete resection is the treatment of choice for preventing recurrences.[20]

HEPATOCELLULAR CARCINOMA

More than one million deaths are caused each year worldwide by HCC. This tumor is most prevalent in Africa and East Asia, although the incidence in the United States is on the rise, probably because of an increase in the incidence of chronic viral hepatitis and cirrhosis.

Table 53.7 Etiology of HCC in patients who have cirrhosis.

Cause of cirrhosis	*Association with carcinoma*	*Mechanism*
Ethanol	+/–	Unknown
Hepatitis B	+ +	Integration into genome
Hepatitis C	+++	Unknown
Aflatoxins	+	Mutation of P53 codon 249

Epidemiologic studies have identified multiple risk factors associated with the development of HCC, including thorotrast (a radiologic contrast agent), ethanol, aflatoxins, chronic infection with hepatitis band C, hemochromatosis, Wilson's disease, and α_1-antitrypsin deficiency. The common end point of these disparate factors is the development of cirrhosis, which is a risk factor for HCC.

Molecular Biology

The long list of risk factors suggests that anything that causes chronic liver injury may result in HCC (Table 53.7). The mechanism for the transformation to carcinoma is almost certainly multifactorial. Chronic viral infection resulting in cirrhosis is the most important worldwide risk factor. Although the viral infection alone can occasionally result in HCC without cirrhosis, most patients who have viral hepatitis-induced HCC have cirrhosis.

Chronic infection with the hepatitis B virus results in cirrhosis and mutagenesis secondary to integration of the hepatitis B virus into the genome in a subset of patients infected acutely with hepatitis B. No universal proto-oncogene or suppressor gene mutation has been associated with hepatitis B infection. Hepatitis C infection is also associated with chronic hepatitis, cirrhosis, and subsequent HCC. Hepatitis C is less prevalent worldwide than hepatitis B, but appears to confer a higher risk for the development of HCC, probably because hepatitis C infection more often progresses to chronic infection and cirrhosis. Hepatitis B and hepatitis C infection may function independently in the pathogenesis of HCC. Most HCC patients have antibodies to either hepatitis B or C, but a few have antibodies to both hepatitis B and C. The number of chronically infected patients who do not have HCC confirms that infection alone is not sufficient for malignant transformation.

The mechanism of viral carcinogenesis is incompletely understood. Five different viral species cause hepatitis, but hepatitis A (single-stranded RNA) and hepatitis E (a labile RNA virus) do not cause chronic hepatitis. Hepatitis D (a defective RNA virus that encodes the delta antigen) can cause chronic hepatitis, but is not associated with HCC. The hepatitis B virus is a DNA virus that is associated with chronic infection, cirrhosis, and HCC. The hepatitis C virus is a single-stranded RNA virus that is also associated with chronic infection, cirrhosis, and HCC. The different types and differing end-results of infection with these viruses imply that chronic (but not acute) inflammation of hepatocytes together with some other as yet unknown stimuli result in a monoclonal proliferation of cells and subsequent development of HCC.

P53 Mutations

Although there is not a cause-and-effect relationship for a specific genetic event in all virally infected patients who develop HCC, several intriguing observations of mutations in the P53 tumor suppressor gene have been identified. Wild-type P53 (the usual situation in nontransformed cells) suppresses cell growth, whereas mutated P53 can result in unregulated cell growth. The most common genetic event associated with carcinogenesis is a G to T transversion at codon 249 of the P53 gene, which results in loss of the suppressor function of the gene and prolonged expression of the mutated product. This transversion is particularly common in HCCs in areas at high risk for both aflatoxin B1 and hepatitis B exposure, such as China and sub-Saharan Africa. The exposure of patients to aflatoxin has been difficult to quantitate and has relied on the surrogate mark of region and country of origin rather than aflatoxin exposure. Genetic testing of HCC has shown that patients from areas where there are high aflatoxin levels are more likely to have a codon 249 mutation than patients from low aflatoxin exposure areas. Genetic changes in P53 are also associated with hepatitis B infection alone, but the resultant P53 mutations in patients who have hepatitis B are present in other sites and not restricted to codon 249.

In patients from the United States who have chronic hepatitis B infection, the codon 249 transversion is uncommon. By contrast, four of seven patients who had HCC-positive P53 staining by immunohistochemistry did not have hepatitis B infection. The less specific mutation in P53 in patients who have not been exposed to aflatoxin suggests that noncodon 249 P53 mutations are unrelated to aflatoxin and this is not always a necessary step in the multistep process of hepatocarcinogenesis.

The overexpression of P53 by immunohistochemical staining was also present in hepatocytes within regenerating nodules adjacent to HCCs of eight of 12 patients who had chronic hepatitis B and cirrhosis. This finding indicates that either:

- P53 overexpression is a normal event in the regenerating liver and not a factor in carcinogenesis; or
- P53 expression and regeneration are early events, but not sufficient for malignant transformation in HCC.

Hepatocyte Growth Factor

The liver regeneration associated with cirrhosis, particularly cirrhosis associated with chronic hepatitis B and C infection, may also be a factor in the development of HCC. An important early response to various injuries such as hepatitis, trauma, or ischemia is the upregulation of mRNA for hepatocyte growth factor (HGF) and subsequent protein expression. HGF, which is produced in Kupffer cells and sinusoidal endothelial cells, but not hepatocytes, is a protein heterodimer with 38% homology to plasmin. Injury to the liver results in HGF production by lung, kidney, and spleen, indicating that the stimulus for HGF expression may be both paracrine and endocrine. Hepatocyte growth factor is the most potent mitogen for mature hepatocytes and may also act as a hepatotrophic factor. The HGP receptor, the product of the c-met proto-oncogene, is present on hepatocytes as well as various other epithelial cells. Hepatocyte growth factor may be important in cancer invasion, transformation, and metastasis, but the mechanism is not clearly understood.

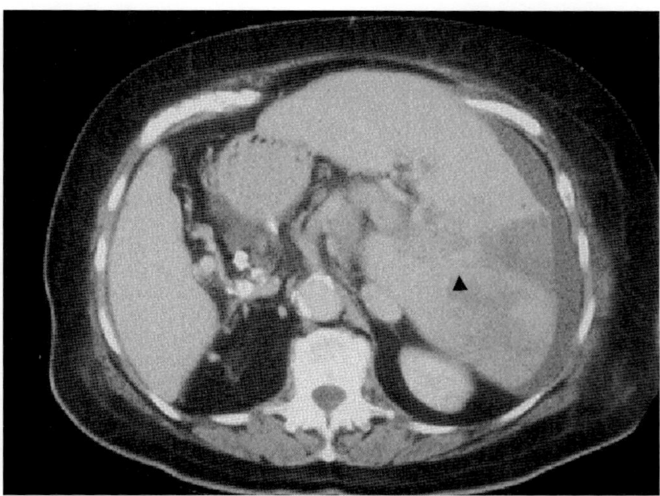

Fig. 53.26: CT scan of liver on arterial phase showing a normal-looking liver with a large exophytic HCC (arrowhead) arising from segment III of liver.

Diagnosis

Risk factors such as cirrhosis and chronic hepatitis B or C viral infection have a high-enough prevalence to justify routine screening for HCC in affected patients. In the absence of cirrhosis, HCC is generally detected after a diagnostic examination such as CT for vague upper abdominal symptoms (Fig. 53.26). Acute decompensation of liver function or new onset of hepatic failure is probably the commonest presentation in a patient who has stable cirrhosis.

Many HCCs express α-fetoprotein in the serum; therefore, this tumor-specific marker is an excellent tool for screening cirrhotic patients. An α-fetoprotein serum level >100 ng/mL (normal adult levels are <20 ng/mL) is suggestive of HCC. In patients with acute or chronic viral hepatitis alone α-fetoprotein may be elevated, but persistently elevated levels suggest HCC. Cholangiocarcinomas as well as poorly differentiated HCCs and some fibrolamellar variants of HCC may be associated with normal α-fetoprotein values.

The imaging procedure of choice in a patient with suspected HCC is a CT scan of the liver. An HCC lesion will appear hypodense when compared with the normal liver, and vascular invasion may be present. After the administration of intravenous contrast, the lesion will enhance during the arterial, but not the venous phase. MRI has a similar diagnostic accuracy to CT. Occasionally, regenerating nodules of the liver may be confused with HCC in a patient with a mildly elevated α-fetoprotein level. Borderline lesions may be followed with repeat CT scans and serial serum α-fetoprotein determinations.

Image-guided or laparoscopically guided liver biopsy should be reserved for patients who are thought to have a benign lesion, patients with technically unresectable disease or those with lesions that are unsuitable for operation. Image-guided liver biopsy is not necessary in a patient who has resectable disease and may in some cases result in seeding of the needle tract.

Nonoperative Treatment

Scope of Treatment

Many patients who have HCC confined to the liver are not candidates for hepatic resection because of underlying liver disease. Even in the subset of patients with resectable disease, postoperative recurrence is common. Many different nonoperative treatments have been tested both as primary therapy and in the adjuvant setting. They broadly consist of the following options in patients with HCC deemed unresectable:

- Systemic treatment with chemotherapy
- Local regional therapy
  - Transcatheter arterial chemoembolization or transarterial chemoembolization (TACE)
  - Radiofrequency ablation (RFA)
  - Ethanol injection
  - Other ablative therapies
    - Microwave
    - Cryotherapy
  - Selective internal radiation therapy (SIRT)
- Liver transplantation

A review of 37 randomized controlled trials for HCC found little benefit for chemotherapy.[21] Two recent studies have shown a marginal survival benefit in patients treated with biological agents.[22,23] In the first study, a multicenter controlled trial of 271 patients, median overall survival was 6.5 months (95% CI, 5.56–7.56) in patients treated with sorafenib, an oral multikinase inhibitor of the vascular endothelial growth factor receptor, compared with 4.2 months (3.75–5.46) in those who received placebo [hazard ratio (HR), 0.68; 95% CI, 0.50–0.93; p = 0.014]. The second study randomly assigned 602 patients with advanced HCC who had not received previous systemic treatment to receive either sorafenib (at a dose of 400 mg twice daily) or placebo. Median overall survival was 10.7 months in the sorafenib group and 7.9 months in the placebo group (HR in the sorafenib group, 0.69; 95% CI, 0.55–0.87; $p < 0.001$).

Transarterial Chemoembolization

This can be combined with extirpation (whether by resection or transplantation) to convert an unresectable lesion into a resectable lesion or to treat presumed micrometastatic disease and enhance survival. The finding that arterial embolization alone may result in tumor shrinkage in patients with unresectable disease suggests that embolization or embolization plus chemotherapy might be considered in some patients with resectable HCC. One series evaluated 185 patients with a new diagnosis of HCC for chemoembolization with lipiodol and doxorubicin. The embolization was possible in only 37% of patients. Patients who had small tumors were treated twice at 6-week intervals, whereas patients who had large tumors were treated three times. No patients who had unresectable disease before embolization were converted to a resectable status by therapy. Two of the 185 patients were alive and disease free after 2 years. Chemotherapy-related complications occurred in 22% of patients. The authors concluded that this treatment offered little benefit in advanced disease, but that results with small tumors were encouraging.[24]

Recent evidence suggests that TACE in combination with RFA offers much better 4-year survival in patients with HCC < 7 cm than RFA alone (61.8% vs. 45%).[25]

Other preoperative therapies such as chemoradiotherapy have converted some patients with unresectable disease to a resectable status. In the subset of patients converted to a resectable status by combined radiation and chemotherapy, no difference in survival or perioperative complications was noted in patients treated subsequently with resection as opposed to primary chemotherapy and radiotherapy. Similar nonrandomized series of pre-resection hepatic arterial chemoembolization demonstrated that tumor diameter was decreased by 31%, with normalization of α-fetoprotein serum levels in some patients, but very few patients ultimately underwent resection. The role of adjuvant therapy for liver transplant patients who have HCC has also not been validated in a prospective randomized trial. A variety of regimens of pre- or post-transplant adjuvant therapy resulted in 3-year survival rates of 30–50%.[26] These studies are flawed by the inclusion of patients with incidental HCC and by the use of historical controls. Chemotherapy, arterial embolization, or the combination of the two may therefore convert some patients who have unresectable tumors into operative candidates, but there is no coevidence that survival is improved.

Chemoprevention

Chemoprevention, in contrast to therapy, has the potential of greatly altering the natural history of patients with resected HCC and those risks of developing HCC. An acyclic retinoid (polyprenoic acid), which inhibits experimental hepatocarcinogenesis and induces differentiation and apoptosis in human hepatoma cell lines, has been evaluated for its ability to prevent recurrence and the development of second primary tumors in patients whose HCC was either resected or ablated by percutaneous ethanol injections. After a median follow-up of 38 months, 27% of the polyprenoic acid treated patients and 49% of the placebo group had recurrent hepatoma ($p = 0.04$).

Radiofrequency Ablation

Radiofrequency ablation (RFA) works by converting radiofrequency waves into heat. The alternating current passes from an electrode tip into the surrounding tissues and generates changes in the direction of ions and creates ionic agitation and frictional heating. The tissue heating drives extracellular and intracellular water out of the tissue, which results in tissue desiccation as a result of coagulative necrosis. Radiofrequency ablation has now been widely accepted as an effective modality for treating liver tumors that are unsuitable for resection,[27,28] and it can be delivered either percutaneously or at open operation.

Although there is no level 1 evidence on the best approach for RFA, whether delivered percutaneously, laparoscopically or by open operation, systemic review suggests that an operative approach offers a better outcome in terms of the completeness of RFA.[29] The size of lesions in the liver is also a major determining factor. For lesions over 5 cm, the results of RFA are extremely poor.

More and more patients with liver tumors are undergoing RFA even for resectable liver tumors. Data from a few randomized controlled trials suggest a similar overall survival result for small-sized tumors when comparing RFA with surgical resection. However, the disease-free survival was much better in patients who had surgical resection. A total of 180 patients were randomized to percutaneous RFA versus hepatectomy for < 5 cm hepatocellular carcinoma. Seventy one had ablation because 19 withdrew their consent. Ninety patients had surgical resection Only 1 patient died after surgical resection within the same hospital admission. Post-treatment complications were more frequent and severe after operation than ablation. The 1-, 2-, 3-, and 4-year overall survival rates after ablation were 96%, 82%, 71%, and 68%, while after operation they were 93%, 82%, 73%, and 64%. The corresponding disease-free survival rates fell from 86% to 46% over 4 years with ablation and from 87% to 52% with operation. Statistically, there was no difference between these two treatments. However, the authors concluded that ablation was as effective as surgical resection in the treatment of solitary and small HCC.[30]

Percutaneous Ethanol Ablation

Percutaneous ethanol ablation (PEI) requires multiple treatment sessions under ultrasound guidance until the entire lesion is treated. Ethanol ablation resulted in complete histologic tumor necrosis in 15 of 21 patients who had nonresectable disease in one series. Recurrence rates were high, but recurrence generally occurred in other areas of the liver. A second study noted local recurrence after 2 years in 14% of patients undergoing ethanol ablation and concluded that percutaneous tumor ablation was most successful for patients who have small (<3 cm) HCCs.

One systematic review and meta-analysis of published randomized controlled trials comparing radiofrequency with PEI including 396 patients treated by RFA and 391 treated by PEI reported that available evidence supported the superiority of RFA versus PEI, in terms of better survival and local control of the disease, for the treatment of patients with relatively preserved liver function and early-stage nonsurgical HCC but the higher rate of adverse events.[31]

Percutaneous Microwave Therapy

Another option for unresectable HCC is percutaneous microwave therapy. No serious complications have been reported, and the local tumor control appears to be similar to other ablative therapies (although follow-up remains short).

Cryosurgical Tumor Ablation

This is also an effective method of local control. The number of HCC patients treated by cryosurgical ablation is small compared with the large number of patients with metastatic colorectal carcinoma who have been treated with this modality. Acceptable local recurrence rates (0–24%) in several series suggest that tumor freezing effectively eradicates HCC.[32]

Selective Internal Radiation Therapy

During the last few years, selective internal radiation therapy using yttrium[90] radiolabeled microspheres (SIR-Spheres, SIRTEX Medical, Sydney, Australia) has become a treatment modality for patients with unresectable liver tumors. Results are encouraging.[33] A phase II study of 52 patients with intermediate (n = 17) and advanced (n = 35) HCC treated with SIRTEX showed a median overall survival of 15 months and 5 patients had a complete response (9.6%).[33,34]

Table 53.8 Methods of nonoperative management of unresectable HCC.

Therapy	*Randomized trial with positive results*	*Long-term survival*
	–	–
Chemoembolization	–	–
Interferon	–	–
Chemotherapy	+	+
Ethanol injection	–	+
Chemotherapy plus resection	–	+
Chemotherapy plus transplant	–	+

Summary

The treatment of unresectable HCC by ablative therapies has been effective in the hands of investigators skilled at these techniques. Local recurrence rates are low and certainly acceptable in these unresectable patients. The efficacy of any method other than hepatic resection should be tested in controlled clinical trials when dealing with potentially curable patients (Table 53.8).

OPERATIVE MANAGEMENT

Objectives and Key Steps

The objectives of hepatic resection for malignant disease are removal of all tumors leaving both a clear margin and an adequate, well-perfused liver remnant with intact biliary drainage. However, the decision to proceed to operation, which should be made by a multidisciplinary team, is often difficult as it involves many patient factors (Table 53.9).

The key intraoperative steps are as follows: (1) a full exploration of the peritoneal cavity, pelvis, retroperitoneum, and porta hepatis to exclude extrahepatic disease (usually a contraindication to resection); (2) examination of the liver with bimanual palpation and intraoperative ultrasonography to assess the extent of hepatic disease; (3) control of the vascular supply to and from the portion of the liver to be resected; (4) parenchymal transection. Open exploration may be preceded by diagnostic laparoscopy in selected cases.

The major technical challenge in liver resection is control of bleeding during transection of the parenchyma. Liver resection can be performed by different devices with

Table 53.9 Management of patients with liver tumor

Assessment of patients for liver surgery
• Healthy patients without comorbidity (requires routine blood tests)
• Patients with significant co-morbidity (requires formal cardiopulmonary exercise testing (CPEX) in addition to routine blood tests)
Surgical considerations
• To achieve a clear resection margin but leave adequate functioning liver remnant (>20% in healthy patients with a normal liver)
• To consider portal vein embolization to induce liver hypertrophy preoperatively in cases with insufficient future remnant liver volume
• To stage after systemic chemotherapy in patients with multiple liver metastases, and to consider 2-stage resection
Unresectable patients
• Systemic chemotherapy followed by re-assessment for operation
• Open, laparoscopic or percutaneous RFA to multiple liver metastases if disease remains unresectable
• Selective internal radiation therapy (SIRT) in combination with systemic chemotherapy
• Best supportive palliative care
Follow up
• Clinical examination
• Tumor markers
• Radiology
– CT/MRI
– Contrast ultrasound
– PET/CT

or without inflow occlusion (Pringle maneuver). Only limited data are available on the best transection technique. The most popular devices facilitating bloodless transection include the ultrasonic desiccator [e.g. Cavitron Ultrasonic Surgical Aspirator (CUSA), Tyco Healthcare, Mansfield, MA, USA], water jet dissector (e.g. Hydro-jet, Erbe, Tubingen, Germany), harmonic scalpel, monopolar and bipolar cautery devices, and the dissecting sealer (e.g. Tissuelink, Dover, NH). Parenchymal dissection has been performed under routine inflow occlusion with finger fracture technique (digitoclasy), in which liver parenchyma is crushed between finger and thumb, isolating vessels and bile ducts which can then be ligated and divided. This particular technique has subsequently been improved using surgical instruments such as small Kelly or Pean clamps (clamp crushing) for blunt transection. These devices have gained wide acceptance for hepatectomy, although only three randomized control trials comparing them exist to date. Other important advances in liver surgery that have contributed to improved perioperative outcomes include intraoperative ultrasound, use of vascular staplers, and reduction in bleeding by the development of low central venous pressure anesthesia.

Laparoscopic Liver Resection

Laparoscopy is useful for staging purposes, and laparoscopic resection is also gaining popularity over the last few years with around 30% of liver resections now performed by this technique. Compared with open operation, laparoscopic resection can result in reduced operative blood loss and earlier recovery without sacrificing oncologic clearance. When performed by experienced surgeons in selected patients it may be both feasible and safe.[12,13,35]

As with open resection, the most common perioperative complication is bleeding that usually arises from the liver parenchyma but has also been described as a result of portal vein injury and splenic laceration. The length of postoperative hospital stay following laparoscopic resection varies. Some series show no difference when compared to open operation, but on balance recovery time is shorter. The inpatient stay has been shown to be affected by the type of lesion and extent of resection. Those patients with more than two segments resected remained in hospital longer than those with one or fewer (8 vs. 6 days).

Selection of Patients

Extirpation of primary HCC results in long-term survival in some patients. The underlying disease process that predates the discovery of HCC increases the risk of hepatic resection and also increases the chance that another HCC will develop in the resected liver. Although the goal of operative therapy is to remove tumor for cure, the selection of appropriate candidates is critical. The prediction of whether patients have an adequate hepatic functional reserve, however, remains more an art than a science. The availability of liver transplantation and potential therapy for HCC makes even more critical the differentiation of patients who will tolerate resection from those who will not.

Patients who have Child's class C cirrhosis and a large HCC will not tolerate a major liver resection. By contrast, a noncirrhotic patient who has normal hepatic function and a resectable HCC should be treated operatively. The selection of operative candidates from among those with known cirrhosis and a tumor that necessitates a major resection is more difficult. Several diagnostic and functional tests may aid the surgeon in the decision-making process.

The retention of indocyanine green correlates with the degree of hepatic impairment and may differentiate operative from nonoperative candidates. A retrospective study compared patients who had a 15-minute indocyanine green retention rate of 20% or greater (indicative of impaired liver function) and those with a retention rate of 10% or less (indicative of normal liver function). The patients who had prolonged dye retention had lower serum albumin, higher bilirubin, worse Child's classification and higher prothrombin times than those who had normal dye retention. The patients who did not have impaired function tolerated significantly greater volume resection of the liver, which provided better resection margins. Despite the larger volume of resection, the operative mortality and morbidity rates were similar in the two groups.

A second report analyzed preoperative predictors of morbidity and mortality in a multivariate analysis. The most significant preoperative predictor of morbidity was the serum bilirubin level ($p > 0.005$). These retrospective studies are flawed, however, by evaluating only patients treated with resection and not the entire population of patients who have hepatocellular cancer. No measure of liver disease can accurately predict poor outcome (Table 53.10).

The recent trend away from anatomic lobectomies and toward smaller liver resections has extended resectional therapy to patients who have less hepatic reserve and more comorbid disease. The decreased hepatic reserve of many patients treated operatively has not translated into an increase in mortality rate, however. Several authors have reported a decline in mortality rate despite operating on patients who have more advanced liver disease. Among 229 patients undergoing curative resection (>50% of whom had comorbid disease such as diabetes mellitus), an operative mortality rate of 7% was reported. Child's class, sulfobromophthalein sodium retention (a test of hepatic reserve similar to indocyanine green, but with greater risk) and operative blood loss predicted the risk of death. In another series focusing on postoperative morbidity, 50% of patients developed a postoperative complication with a 2% overall mortality rate. Improvements in postoperative care, specifically nutritional support, do appear to reduce the mortality rate even in patients who have major complications. The incidence of postoperative complications was reduced from 55% to 34% by the addition of intravenous nutrition for 14 days in the perioperative period in one series, primarily because of a decrease in the number of septic complications.

Table 53.10 Negative prognostic variables in HCC patients revealed by various retrospective reviews.
Elevated serum bilirubin
Indocyanine green retention at 15 minutes of 20% or greater
Type of resection (lobectomy versus less extensive procedure)
Size of lesions
Number of lesions
Child's classification
Operative blood loss
Poor preoperative nutritional status
Presence of underlying cirrhosis
Portal vein invasion
High α-fetoprotein
Operative margin

Partial Hepatectomy

Hepatic resection is currently the most effective therapy for HCC. Numerous publications document that a subset of HCC patients will be cured of disease by hepatic resection alone. Several trends in the operative treatment of HCC have emerged over the past three decades. The overall 5-year survival of resected patients has increased from 5.4% (1958–1970) to 11.9% (1971–1982) to 46.2% (1983–1994) in one large series. The size of the tumors resected decreased over the same time period. In the first time period, only 2.6% of tumors were <3 cm in diameter compared with 33.4% in the 1983–1994 time period. The smaller tumor size allowed both more limited resections and re-resection for recurrence in some patients.

Clinical series must be interpreted in the context that patients who have less advanced tumors are now undergoing resection. The 5-year survival rate in multiple large retrospective series varies from 26% to 50%, with tumor size, histologic margin of resection, and liver reserve as the most significant prognostic factors. The decreased volume of the first resection allowed repeat resection for 37 of 48 patients in the series with the highest 5-year survival liver reserve and margin of resection were significant prognostic factors. Analysis of a large tumor registry confirmed

Table 53.11 Management options for patients with HCC.

Underlying liver disease	Extrahepatic disease	Technically resectable	Management
Any	Yes	Any	Palliative
Normal or mild impairment	None	Yes	Resection
Severe	None	Any	Transplant for <5 cm. less than three lesions or nonresective ablation (e.g. ethanol. cryosurgery)

the prognostic value of tumor size, operative margin, and underlying cirrhosis. In addition, serum α-fetoprotein, the number of tumors and portal vein involvement also had prognostic value.

The critical nontumor factor of underlying liver disease renders the traditional tumor node metastasis (TNM) staging system less useful for prognosis in patients who undergo operative resection, probably because underlying liver disease can limit the margin of clearance and is frequently the cause of perioperative death. The high intrahepatic recurrence rate for even small HCCs is related to serum albumin and alanine transaminase levels, which indicates that underlying hepatic reserve and ongoing hepatocellular inflammation have a more important influence on recurrence than tumor factors per se. Isolated recurrent tumors in the residual liver can be successfully treated. Patients who have recurrent tumors often present with slightly worse hepatic reserve, yet tolerate repeat hepatectomy well. Tumor recurrence does not result in a decreased survival in patients with re-resectable disease. In fact, when patients who have complete tumor resection during secondary excision were compared with those undergoing primary hepatic resection, no survival difference was noted.[36]

Some generalizations regarding prognostic factors for operative resection can be made. Many of these factors are beyond the control of the surgeon (α-fetoprotein, portal vein invasion, underlying hepatic reserve), but may influence the selection of patients for resection. If clear margins cannot be obtained at operation, resection should not be performed. Nor should resection be performed for patients with limited hepatic reserve, such as those with Child's class C cirrhosis. Underlying hepatic disease limits the role of anatomic right or left lobectomy, but adequate (1 cm) margins at operation are absolutely critical if a less extensive resection is to be attempted (Table 53.11).

Table 53.12 Retrospective reviews of survival after transplant or resection in single institution studies.

Series	Number of patients	Transplant survival	Resection survival
Bismuth	60	47 (3 years)	50
Lwatsuki and Starzl[37]	105	37 (5 years)	36
Mazzaferro et al.[43]	48	75 (4 years)	–

Aggressive resection of new or recurrent hepatocellular cancer is indicated for patients who have an isolated hepatic recurrence after previous curative resection.

Liver Transplantation

The excellent survival rate now achieved for patients who have benign liver disease treated with orthotopic liver transplantation has led to the application of this technique to patients who have HCC that is not amenable to resection. No prospective comparison of liver transplantation versus resection has been performed. Retrospective studies suggest that transplantation and resection are followed by similar short-term (<5 year) survival rates (Table 53.12).[37]

As expected based on resection data, the patients with small tumors had significantly better survival. Recurrence in the transplanted liver was less than in the liver remnant of a comparable group of patients treated with resection in all series that examined this variable. Transplant appears neither superior nor inferior to resection in these early nonrandomized trials. Patients who have small (<5 cm) HCCs with hepatic reserve that prevents resection should therefore be considered for transplantation (*see* Chapter 118, "Liver Transplantation").

Transplant patients generally had less hepatic reserve than resection patients, but otherwise groups tended to be comparable. No randomized series has been reported.

METASTATIC LIVER CANCER

Scope of Operative Management

Treatment of metastatic disease to the liver is the commonest indication for hepatic resection. Over the past 25 years, hepatic resection has evolved from a high-risk, resource-intensive procedure with limited application to a safe and commonly performed operation with broad indications. There has been a marked improvement in perioperative outcome, including reductions in mortality, blood loss, transfusion rates, and hospital stay. These

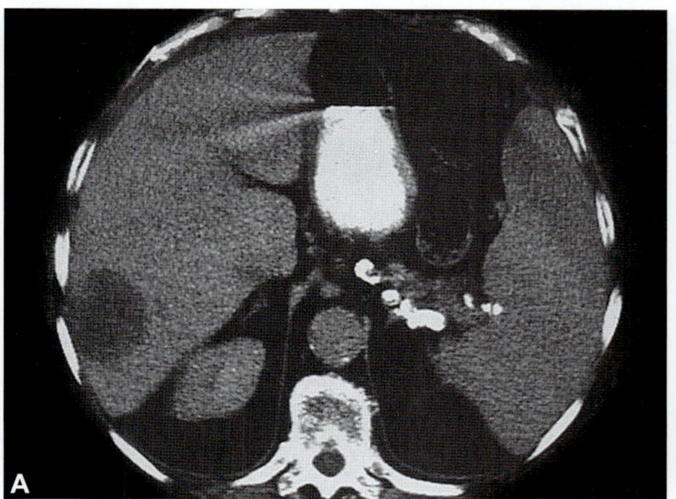

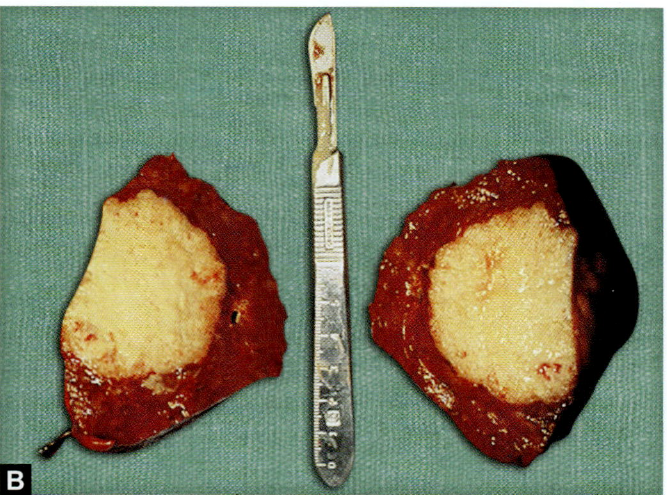

Figs. 53.27A and B: CT scan of liver showing a low-attenuation-mass lesion (A), and macroscopic appearance of the cut surface of resected colorectal liver metastasis (B).

improved perioperative results have allowed hepatic resection to become a more viable and effective treatment option for selected patients with primary liver tumors and metastases. The liver remains the most frequent site for hematogenous metastasis. Metastatic colorectal carcinoma is by far the commonest indication for hepatic resection in Western countries. Liver metastases from other primary tumors, such as neuroendocrine carcinoma and genitourinary tumors, are also treated effectively with liver resection and in selected cases from breast cancer. Various options are now available for management of metastatic disease if surgical resection is not possible such us systemic chemotherapy, selective internal irradiation therapy (SIRTEX) with or without combined chemotherapy and RFA.[33,34]

Primary Colorectal Cancer

Most metastatic tumors treated by liver resection arise from primary colorectal cancer. Metastatic colorectal cancer results in the death of most patients who have disease beyond the regional nodal basin. Approximately 10% of patients present with surgically resectable hepatic disease as a first recurrence, while systemic chemotherapy can now downstage metastatic disease from unresectable to resectable in another 10%. Two randomized controlled studies have shown an increased response rate as high as 78% by adding a biological agent to conventional chemotherapy, with a conversion rate of 30% from unresectable liver metastases to resectable disease.[38,39] A multicenter study of capecitabine, oxaliplatin plus bevacizumab as perioperative treatment of patients with poor-risk colorectal liver-only metastases not selected for upfront resection. In the CELIM study 34% of patients had a complete (R0) resection following systemic chemotherapy for initially unresectable hepatic metastases. The primary site for metastatic spread of colorectal carcinoma to solid organs is the liver, either in isolation or as a manifestation of other systemic or intraperitoneal disease (Fig. 53.27A and B). These metastases travel through the portal venous supply and become lodged in the liver. Metastatic liver disease is occasionally solitary, but more often multiple. All patients who have isolated liver metastases who are not treated operatively will die of disease within 5 years. The treatment of patients with or without resectable liver metastases will improve long-term survival. For resectable disease, up to 75% 5-year survival can be achieved with a combination of surgical resection and systemic chemotherapy, and 1 in 4 patients is alive at 10 years (www.livermetsurvey.org).[40] For initially unresectable disease, systemic chemotherapy can permit curative liver resection in up to 30% of patients, while those with metastases that are still unresectable after chemotherapy have a median survival of 12–18 months.

No consensus exists on the indications for surgical resection in metastatic colorectal cancer. In patients with multiple liver metastases, systemic chemotherapy is now the primary treatment with or without biological agents pending on K-ras status. Systemic chemotherapy can help patients with initially unresectable disease undergo potentially curative surgery (Figs. 53.28A and B). Portal vein embolization (PVE) is often used in conjunction with major right hepatectomy to induce a compensatory hypertrophy of the left lobe of the liver in patients whose future liver

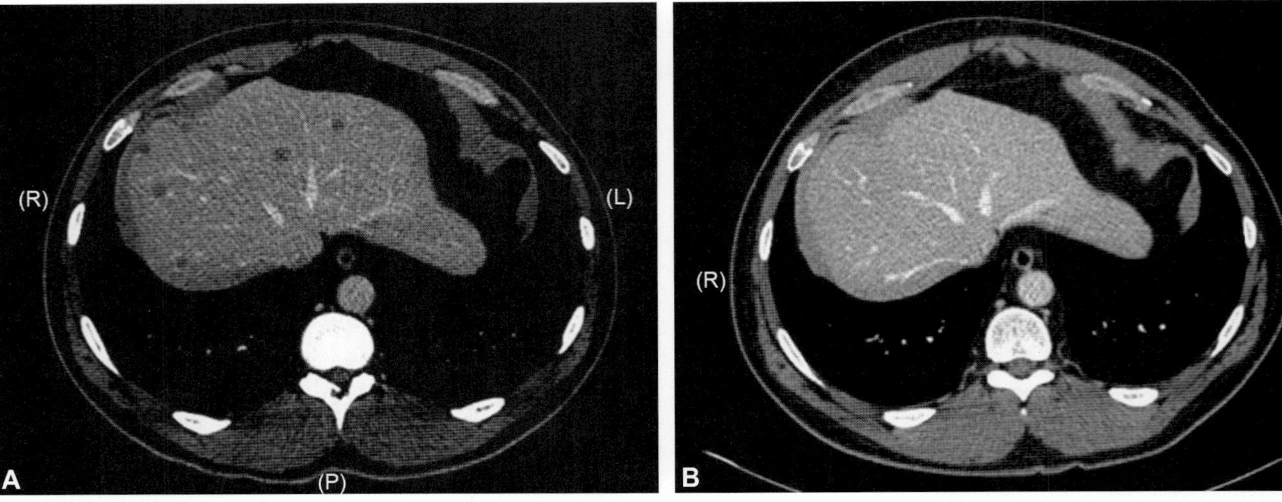

Figs. 53.28A and B: CT scan of liver on portal venous phase showing a complete response of multiple liver metastases to chemotherapy before (A) and after (B) treatment.

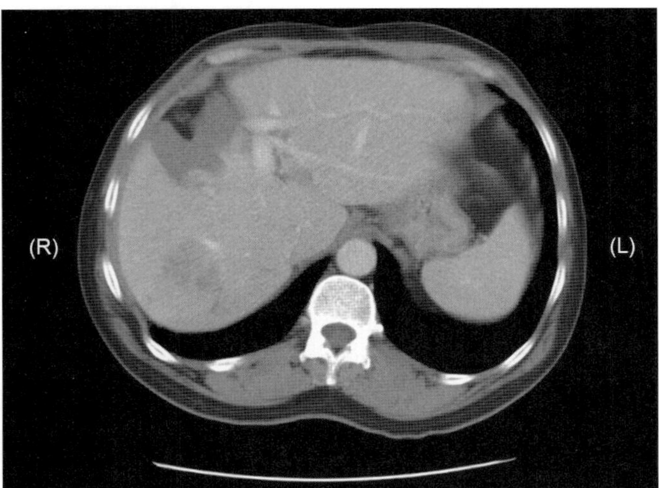

Fig. 53.29: CT scan of liver on portal venous phase showing post-chemotherapy and stage 1 liver resection prior to PVE and stage II liver resection: wedge resection of segment IV metastasis and a large liver metastasis in segment VI.

remnant (FLR) would otherwise preclude resection. For multiple bilobar disease, simultaneous right hepatectomy and left hemiliver wedge resections after PVE are performed, but it is now recognized that PVE can accelerate the relative growth of the metastases as opposed to the normal liver parenchyma. Metastases located in the FLR should be resected before PVE in a stage I resection (Fig. 53.29). After PVE is used to induce liver regeneration in an FLR, a second definitive stage II resection is performed within 6 weeks to achieve complete clearance of the liver metastases. Encouraging results from several series support this modified strategy of staged liver resection; the overall intention is cure, but the initial resection is used to clear the FLR of tumor.[41]

Neuroendocrine Tumors

The resection of metastatic neuroendocrine tumors has resulted in long-term survival and symptom relief in selected patients. These malignancies tend to grow in an indolent fashion, and the excellent survival statistics of patients treated with hepatic resection (70% at 5 years) may be a manifest of the natural history of the tumor. Orthotopic liver transplantation has also been used both for palliation and for cure in selected patients with neuroendocrine malignancies. In patients with either metastatic carcinoid tumors (15 cases) or metastatic islet cell carcinomas (16 cases), curative resection of the primary tumor and orthotopic liver transplantation was effective for carcinoid tumor (69% 5-year survival), but not for islet cell carcinoma (4% 5-year survival).

Repeat Hepatic Resection

Recurrence occurs in most patients who undergo a curative hepatic resection for colorectal cancer metastases. In 20–30% of patients only the liver is involved, and 10–25% of these patients have lesions amenable to repeat resection. Repeat hepatectomy is generally well tolerated and can result in long-term survival. The number of patients in any single series tends to be small, but 4-year survival rates can be as high as 43%. Although several authors state that no drop-off in survival occurs with repeat resection, the largest published series (144 patients) reported a 5-year survival rate of 16% compared with 25% for 1,626 patients after a first resection. The high recurrence rate suggests that patients who cannot be resected with a margin of at least 1 cm should not undergo operation. In selected patients, long-term survival is possible, however, after re-resection of metastases.

Regional Chemotherapy

Most patients who have metastatic liver disease are not operative candidates because the disease, although localized to the liver, is present throughout the organ. This factor has led to regional chemotherapy for patients with metastatic disease confined to the liver. Most clinical trials of regional therapy used a drug, such as 5-fluorodeoxyuridine, delivered continuously via an operatively placed hepatic arterial catheter and extracted during the first pass through the liver. Regional chemotherapy has been complicated by appreciable bile duct toxicity, however. A carefully planned placement of the catheter in the common hepatic artery with interruption of flow to the gastroduodenal artery and cholecystectomy may decrease the complication rate.

The efficacy of regional therapy has not been proved. Although many studies have demonstrated high response rates and promising early (<2 years) survival, improved long-term survival compared with systemic chemotherapy has not been achieved. For patients with unresectable disease, both the toxicity and the response rate are critical considerations; both regional and systemic chemotherapy have appreciable morbidity. Several well-designed randomized comparisons of systemic chemotherapy and regional chemotherapy are currently in progress. At this time, no active therapy is superior to the no-treatment option in unresectable metastatic colorectal carcinoma. Therefore, this large patient population should be encouraged to participate in clinical trials of systemic and regional chemotherapy.

Other Metastatic Liver Tumors

Resection of both primary HCC and secondary colorectal carcinoma in carefully selected patients is accepted practice. Many other cancer patients will develop liver metastases at some point in their disease, but in most of these, liver disease is only one of multiple sites of failure and should not be treated operatively (e.g. in those who have breast cancer, lung carcinoma, melanoma, sarcoma, and gynecologic cancer). Alternatively, the liver may be the primary site of metastatic disease, but the lesions are diffuse and thus unsuitable for resection (e.g. gas and pancreatic carcinoma). Carcinoid tumors often metastasize to the liver and cause symptoms because of their size or by producing hormones. Survival beyond 5 years has been reported following resection for isolated metastatic liver disease. As already stated, patients with other types of neuroendocrine tumors (such as nonfunctional islet cell tumors) generally derive no benefit from resection.

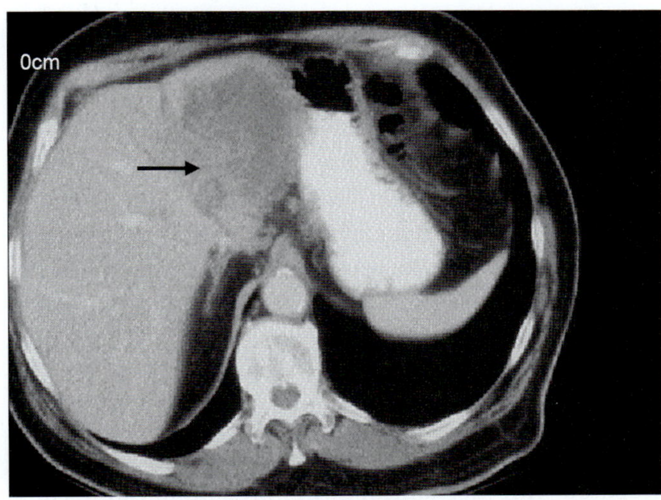

Fig. 53.30: CT scan of liver on portal venous phase showing intrahepatic cholangiocarcinoma.

Besides the hepatocyte, other cell types in the liver have malignant counterparts that can easily be confused with HCC. Intrahepatic cholangiocarcinoma arises from the bile duct epithelium and has many of the characteristics of extrahepatic biliary carcinoma, such as perineural invasion and early nodal metastasis (Fig. 53.30). The presentation is similar to that of HCC, but without elevation of α-fetoprotein. Radiotherapy and chemotherapy are not effective. In the rare patient who has localized, peripheral disease, resection is possible. The treatment of extrahepatic biliary malignancies is fully outlined in Chapter 55, "Gallbladder and Biliary Tree".

As in any organ, sarcomas may arise in the liver. The outcome of patients who have either differentiated (angiosarcoma) or undifferentiated sarcoma is uniformly poor. Operative resection or transplantation is seldom technically feasible.

PRINCIPLES OF LIVER SURGERY

Elective hepatic resection was once a rare and dangerous procedure, but is now routine and safe when carried out by experienced surgeons. Several aspects of hepatic surgery are responsible for the sharp decrease in morbidity rates observed over the past 20 years. Complications and deaths associated with hepatic resection are related to intraoperative blood loss and postoperative hepatic dysfunction. Any technical refinements that preserve hepatic function in a cirrhotic patient will contribute to a lower complication rate, while technical improvements that decrease blood loss reduce both morbidity and mortality rates. Furthermore, decreased blood loss may preclude the need for blood transfusion in patients undergoing operative procedures for malignancies.

Perioperative Precautions

All patients undergoing elective hepatic resection are prepared with mechanical bowel preparation to decompress the colon. A central venous line is placed before operation. At the time of liver transection, a central venous pressure below 10 mm Hg will decrease the amount of venous bleeding and, as a result, transfusion can often be avoided. Before complete exposure of the liver, the peritoneum is surveyed for evidence of extrahepatic disease which, if present, should terminate after a biopsy has been obtained. The preliminary liver examination can be performed either laparoscopically or via a small right subcostal incision. Laparoscopy is less invasive than open exploration and is better for evaluating the peritoneum, but exploration via a small incision has the added advantage of palpation of the celiac and portal nodal basins.

Operative Approach

When resection is feasible, either a bilateral subcostal incision with extension superiorly in the midline or a J-shaped incision into the right upper quadrant provides the best exposure of the liver. Almost all parts of the liver can then be approached following mobilization of the organ. A transthoracic incision is rarely required for access to tumors near the diaphragm.

Intraoperative Ultrasound

An essential component of hepatic surgery is intraoperative ultrasound scanning. The initial ultrasound survey of the liver can be performed either laparoscopically or at laparotomy. Ultrasonographic identification of unexpected lesions by affords the opportunity to treat other lesions and also identifies a subgroup of patients who have widespread disease that is not amenable to resection. Ultrasound scanning also delineates critical vascular structures in the vicinity of the tumor and assists in the design of a procedure to encompass the tumor with a 1 cm operative margin. The resolution of intraoperative ultrasound is superior to palpation and preoperative imaging with CT, ultrasound, and MRI and therefore often alters operative decision making. Previously undetected lesions were found by intraoperative ultrasound, but not seen by CT, in 10 of 19 prospectively studied patients. The resection procedure is also enhanced by intraoperative ultrasound imaging of the tumor margin before transection of the liver. In one study, the use of intraoperative ultrasound to determine the line of liver transection resulted in no positive operative margins in comparison with a 16% incidence before the routine use of ultrasound.

Mobilization and Vascular Control

All patients undergoing hepatic resection should have complete mobilization of the liver. This is accomplished by incising the peritoneum lateral to the liver and freeing the liver of its right diaphragmatic attachments. This dissection is continued until the liver is attached superiorly and inferiorly by the vena cava and the right lateral border of this vessel is completely exposed. The left lobe of the liver is similarly freed from its diaphragmatic attachments until the liver is attached only by the porta and the vena cava. This extensive dissection allows control of the vasculature if hepatic exclusion is used and provides good visualization of the entire liver surface. Standard hepatic lobectomy is accomplished by ligation of the right or left hepatic artery, portal vein, and bile duct in the hilum of the liver. The liver will then demarcate at the border of the right and left lobes. Glisson's capsule is incised with electrocautery, and the liver parenchyma is transected. Dissection through the surface of the liver is performed bluntly with ligation and division of all important vascular structures. The method of parenchymal transection varies widely. The principal technical consideration is the ligation of vessels after removal of surrounding liver and this can be accomplished by blunt dissection, an ultrasonic aspirator (CUSA), a water jet, laser radiofrequency, or other cauterization devices such as the harmonic scalpel, Ligasure, and staplers. No one method is superior in comparative studies of perioperative blood loss. However, radiofrequency-assisted liver resection would seem to offer the best hemostasis with minimal blood loss in experienced hands.[42]

For laparoscopic right hepatectomy, vascular isolation in the hilum and transection of the parenchyma without mobilization may offer an alternative to a difficult mobilization of the right lobe of liver. An anterior incision in the liver is carried to the vena cava using a dissector. The major hepatic vein is then ligated or stapled with a vascular stapler. The liver is mobilized laterally only when the resected area is completely devascularized.

Techniques to Limit Blood Loss

The morbidity and mortality rates as well as the survival rate following resectional liver surgery have decreased markedly in the past 20 years, and one reason is a decrease in operative blood loss as a result of improvements in operative technique. Although clearly not the only factor, the amount of perioperative blood loss predicts the risk of death after hepatic resection. When survivors were compared with patients dying of liver failure during the early postoperative interval, the patients who died had significantly greater blood loss (4,300 mL vs. 1900 mL). A clear understanding of the vascular anatomy of the liver limits blood loss and is one of the few variables amenable to control by the surgeon. Hepatic transection based on the segmental structure of the liver allows resection to be performed in a controlled and planned manner through relatively bloodless planes, as emphasized by Couinaud and Bismuth. These fundamental anatomic contributions have allowed the performance of major hepatic resection without blood transfusion even in a patient with cirrhosis. Over the last two decades, various cauterization devices have been developed for liver parenchymal transection. These devices have already had a major impact on liver surgery with a marked reduction in intraoperative blood loss and postoperative admission rates to intensive care.

Resection Techniques

The technical considerations relevant to hepatic anatomy vary according to the location of the lesion and the type of resection. An isolated segmental resection is best accomplished by parenchymal dissection without isolation of the segmental vessels in the hilum. Segmental resection has the potential to result in more blood loss than lobectomy and may be best carried out with vascular isolation of the liver (as discussed below).

Anatomic Left Hepatectomy

An anatomic left hepatectomy begins with control of the left hepatic artery, portal vein, and bile duct to the left of the portal vein bifurcation. This dissection is best performed 1–2 cm to the left of the hilum because the dissection is easier and the risk of injuring the right hilar structures is less. The left hepatic vein can be isolated either extrahepatically, intrahepatically, or near the end of the parenchymal resection.

Right Lobectomy

This is preceded by complete mobilization of the liver. The hilar structures are isolated, and the right hepatic artery and right portal vein are ligated. The distance from the bifurcation of the portal vein to the bifurcation of the right portal vein is <1 cm. Therefore, the right portal vein is usually divided near the bifurcation. The right hepatic artery, unlike the right portal vein, has a lengthy extrahepatic course and is easily isolated and divided.

Anomalies of the right hepatic artery are common, and the most frequent type (origin from the superior mesenteric artery) can be identified intraoperatively by the posterior location of the artery in the porta hepatis. A preoperative arteriogram defines the vascular anatomy well, but may be unnecessary if the surgeon is experienced. If there is uncertainty about the arterial anatomy, occlusion of the putative vessel before transection with observation of the liver for demarcation can avoid operative misadventures. The right hepatic vein is usually intrahepatic, but it can be ligated intrahepatically either before resection or as the final step after transection of the parenchyma.

Total Vascular Occlusion

Blood loss may be decreased by hepatic vascular isolation during parenchymal transection. This technique occludes inflow from the portal vein and hepatic artery. Back bleeding from the hepatic veins is prevented by occluding the inferior vena cava above and below the liver. One theoretic disadvantage of this technique is the possibility of hepatic dysfunction after transient liver ischemia. Several canine studies, however, suggest that the liver can sustain 60 minutes of normothermic ischemia without acute or long-term sequelae.

The cessation of inflow may also be accomplished by clamping the aorta above the celiac axis. Aortic clamping, however, is associated with a 33% increase in arterial pressure and a 40% decrease in cardiac index. By contrast, porta hepatis clamping is associated with a 14% decrease in arterial pressure and a 40% decrease in cardiac index. Although there are no acid-base abnormalities with either method and no difference in morbidity or mortality rate, the increase in arterial pressure associated with aortic clamping suggests that portal occlusion plus caval occlusion is preferable to aortic occlusion.

Blood loss has been compared retrospectively in cirrhotic patients submitted to resection by a standard technique, portal occlusion only, or portal plus caval occlusion. Blood loss was significantly less in those with vascular isolation, and it was lowest least in the portal plus caval occlusion group (2,900 vs. 1,200 vs. 765 mL, respectively). Thus, vascular isolation in the cirrhotic patient does limit blood loss in patients with cirrhosis.

Techniques Applicable in Cirrhosis

Postoperative complications in patients with cirrhosis correlate closely with preoperative hepatic function. Blood loss and transfusion have an adverse effect on postoperative hepatic function. Discussion of vascular exclusion of the liver is therefore particularly relevant for the cirrhotic liver. The cirrhotic liver has less reserve than the noncirrhotic organ and may be less tolerant of normothermic ischemia than the normal liver, but no data from animal experiments convincingly support this view. In a rat model, the cirrhotic liver was more resistant than the normal liver to ischemia, yet the animals had a slightly higher mortality rate after intermittent clamping than did noncirrhotic animals.

In humans, several retrospective studies have evaluated vascular isolation. In one study, the portal vessels were occluded for an average of 19 minutes in a group of 15 patients who had cirrhosis, with an operative mortality rate of zero and with less morbidity than a control group without inflow occlusion. Nor does the duration of occlusion appear to impact on morbidity or mortality rates. In a study comparing short (30–42 minutes) and long (50–75 minutes) occlusions, those with longer occlusion had higher transaminases at day 3 after resection, but both groups had a lower complication rate than when vascular occlusion was not used.

The advantage of decreased blood loss more than offsets any problem associated with vascular isolation in these retrospective series. Other groups have cooled the liver topically to prolong the ischemic interval safely. Although topical and portal venous cooling solutions did not seem detrimental, the role of hepatic hypothermia has not yet been established.

Another critical factor in limiting complications and death, especially in cirrhosis, is the amount of residual liver. Residual liver is most effectively preserved by limiting the extent of resection, but smaller resection volumes may result in either close or positive operative margins. In almost all series operative margin is an important prognostic factor: it must be free of tumor if long-term survival is to be achieved. The amount of negative margin that is required is unclear, but a 1 cm margin is generally considered adequate. When a 1 cm margin was compared with a margin that was < 1 cm but microscopically negative there was no difference in recurrence or disease-free survival in a retrospective review of patients who had HCC. Positive operative margins in colorectal carcinoma are associated with recurrence.

Patients with small liver tumors can be treated with either a major resection such as lobectomy or a less extensive procedure such as segmentectomy (with negative operative margins), with similar long-term survival. Segmental resection of small tumors may result in more blood loss than a lobectomy with preresection control of the hilar vessels, and it is probably best performed after complete vascular isolation, especially in patients who have cirrhosis. For those with large tumors who are capable of tolerating a major resection, lobectomy generally results in the highest likelihood of tumor-free margins and subsequent survival.

Radiofrequency Ablation

In patients with unresectable colorectal liver metastases (CLM) or recurrent disease, RFA is a useful adjunct to surgery and/or chemotherapy and can prolong survival. Radiofrequency ablation can be applied either percutaneously or operatively by the direct insertion of a radiofrequency probe into the cancer (whether primary or secondary) to achieve tumor necrosis within the cancer cells.[27,28] The use of RFA to ablate multiple deposits involving more than two lobes can downstage the disease and increase the resectability rate.[28] Intraoperative RFA has also been found to be a safe and effective option in our series of 57 patients with 297 inoperable liver metastases and no extrahepatic disease. The overall survival in this cohort was 72.5% at 1 year and 52.5% at 3 years following RFA. With regards to percutaneous RFA, a recent systematic review showed that RFA of unresectable CLM is a useful adjunct to surgery and/or chemotherapy and can prolong time without toxicity and survival.

REFERENCES

1. Kiernan F. Philos Trans. 1883;123:711-70.
2. Chen TS, Chen PS. Understanding the liver: a history. Westport: Greenwood Press; 1984.

3. Sherlock S, Dooley J. Diseases of the liver and biliary system. Oxford: Blackwell Science; 1997.
4. De Bac C, Stroffolini T, Gaeta GB, et al. Pathogenic factors in cirrhosis with and without hepatocellular carcinoma: a multicenter Italian study. Hepatology. 1994;20:1225-30.
5. Manns MP, McHutchison JG, Gordon SC, et al. Peginterferon alfa-2b plus ribavirin compared with interferon alfa-2b plus ribavirin for initial treatment of chronic hepatitis C. Lancet. 2001;1358:958-65.
6. Fried MW, Shiffman ML, Reddy KR, et al. Peginterferon alfa-2a plus ribavirin for chronic hepatitis C virus infection. N Eng J Med. 2002;347:975-82.
7. Hadziyannis SJ, Sette H Jr, Morgan TR, et al. Peginterferon-alpha2a and ribavirin combination therapy in chronic hepatitis C: a randomized study of treatment duration and ribavirin dose. Ann Intern Med. 2004;140:346-55.
8. Jang HJ, Yu H, Kim TK. Contrast-enhanced ultrasound in the detection and characterization of liver tumors. Cancer Imaging. 2009;19:96-103.
9. Cosgrove D, Lassau N. Imaging of perfusion using ultrasound. Eur J Nucl Med Mol Imaging. 2010;37:65-85.
10. Saini S. Imaging of the hepatobiliary tract. N Eng J Med. 1997;336:1889-94.
11. Niekel MC, Bipat S, Stoker J. Diagnostic imaging of colorectal liver metastases with CT, MR imaging, FDG PET, and/or FDG PET/CT: a meta-analysis of prospective studies including patients who have not previously undergone treatment. Radiology. 2010;257:674-84.
12. Rao A, Rao G, Ahmed A. Laparoscopic or open liver resection? Let systematic review decide it. Am J Surg. 2012;204:222-31.
13. Nguyen KT, Gamblin TC, Geller DA. World review of laparoscopic liver resection—2,804 patients. Ann Surg. 2009;250:831-41.
14. Rutledge R, Hunt JP, Lentz CW, et al. A statewide, population-based time-series analysis of the increasing frequency of nonoperative management of abdominal solid organ injury. Ann Surg. 1995;221:311-22.
15. Uddin W, Ramage JK, Portmann B, et al. Hepatic venous outflow obstruction in patients with polycystic liver disease: pathogenesis and treatment. Gut. 1995;36:142-5.
16. Xu M. Progress in surgical treatment of hydatid diseases in China. A clinical analysis of 22,005 surgical cases. Chin Med J. 1995;108:295-9.
17. Khuroo MS, Wani NA, Javid G, et al. Percutaneous drainage compared with surgery for hepatic hydatid cysts. N Eng J Med. 1997;337:881-7.
18. Hashimoto L, Hermann R, Grundfest-Broniatowski S. Pyogenic hepatic abscess: results of current management. Am Surg. 1995;61:407-11.
19. Wynants H, Van DEJ, Randria J, et al. Diagnosis of amoebic infection of the liver; report of 36 cases. Ann Soc Belg Med Trop. 1995;75:297-303.
20. Limongelli P, Pai M, Damrah O, et al. Cystic tumors of the biliary tract: a complete excision is crucial. Int Surg. 2009;194136-40.
21. Simonettt RG, Liberati A, Angiolini C, et al. Treatment of hepatocellular carcinoma:a systematic review of randomized controlled trials. Ann Oncol. 1997;8:117-36.
22. Cheng AL, Kang YK, Chen Z, et al. Efficacy and safety of sorafenib in patients in the Asia-Pacific region with advanced hepatocellular carcinoma: a phase III randomised, double-blind, placebo-controlled trial. Lancet Oncol. 2009;110:25-34.
23. Llovet JM, Ricci S, Mazzaferro V. Sorafenib in advanced hepatocellular carcinoma. N Eng J Med. 2008;359:378-90.
24. Ryder SD, Rizzi PM, Metivier E, et al. Chemoembolisation with lipiodol and doxorubicin: applicability in British patients with hepatocellular carcinoma. Gut. 1996;38:125-8.
25. Peng ZW, Zhang YJ, Chen MS, et al. Radiofrequency ablation with or without transcatheter arterial chemoembolization in the treatment of hepatocellular carcinoma: a prospective randomized trial. J Clin Oncol. 2013;131:426-32.
26. Cherqui D, Piedbois P, Pierga JY, et al. Multimodal adjuvant treatment and liver transplantation for advanced hepatocellular carcinoma. A pilot study. Cancer. 1994;73:2721-6.
27. Goldberg SN. Radiofrequency tumor ablation: Principles and techniques. Eur J Ultrasound. 2001;13:129-47.
28. Jiao LR, Hansen PD, Havlik R, et al. Clinical short-term results of radiofrequency ablation in primary and secondary liver tumors. Am J Surg. 2009;177:303-6.
29. Mulier Seal. Local recurrence after hepatic radiofrequency coagulation: multivariate meta-analysis and review of contributing factors. Ann Surg. 2005;2421158-7.
30. Chen MS, Li JQ, Zheng Y, et al. A prospective randomized trial comparing percutaneous local ablative therapy and partial hepatectomy for small hepatocellular carcinoma. Ann Surg. 2006;243:321-8.
31. Bouza C, López-Cuadrado T, Alcázar R, et al. Meta-analysis of percutaneous radiofrequency ablation versus ethanol injection in hepatocellular carcinoma. BMC Gastroenterol. 2009;11:9-31.
32. Adam R, Akpinar E, Johann M, et al. Place of cryosurgery in the treatment of malignant liver tumors. Ann Surg. 1997;225:39-48.
33. Jiao LR, Szyszko T, Al-Nahhas A, et al. Clinical and imaging experience with yttrium-90 microspheres in the management of unresectable liver tumours. Eur J Surg Oncol. 2007;33(5):597-602.
34. Mazzaferro V, Sposito C, Bhoori S, et al. Yttrium(90) radioembolization for intermediate-advanced hepatocarcinoma: a phase II study. Hepatology. 2012;22:123-5.
35. Bachellier P, Ayav A, Pai M, et al. Laparoscopic liver resection assisted with radiofrequency. Am J Surg. 2007;193:427-30.
36. Matsuda Y, Ito T, Oguchi Y, et al. Rational of surgical management for recurrent hepatocellular carcinoma. Ann Surg. 1993;217:28-34.
37. Iwatsuk S, Starzl TE. Role of liver transplantation in the treatment of hepatocellular carcinoma. Semin Surg Oncol. 1993;9:337-40.

38. Folprecht G, Gruenberger T, Bechstein WO, et al. Tumour response and secondary resectability of colorectal liver metastases following neoadjuvant chemotherapy with cetuximab: the CELIM randomised phase 2 trial. Lancet Oncol. 2010;11:38-47.
39. Wong R, Cunningham D, Barbachano Y, et al. A multicentre study of capecitabine, oxaliplatin plus bevacizumab as perioperative treatment of patients with poor-risk colorectal liver-only metastases not selected for upfront resection. Ann Oncol. 2011;22:2042-8.
40. Colon Cancer Collaborative Group. BMJ. 2000;321:521-2.
41. Tsim N, Healey AJ, Frampton AE, et al. Two-stage resection for bilobar colorectal liver metastases: R0 resection is the key. Ann Surg Oncol. 2011;18:1939-46.
42. Weber JC, Navarra G, Jiao LR, et al. New technique for liver resection using heat coagulative necrosis. Ann Surg. 2002;236:560-63.
43. Mazzaferro VI, Regalia E, Doci R, et al. Liver transplantation for the treatment of small hepatocellular carcinomas in patients with cirrhosis. N Engl J Med. 1996;334(11):693-9.

54

Portal Hypertension

J Michael Henderson

Key Points

- Defined as a portal venous pressure >10 mm Hg (1.3 kPa), portal hypertension usually results from the sinusoidal obstruction of liver cirrhosis.
- The prognosis depends upon the degree of hepatocellular dysfunction, which is assessed clinically by the Child–Pugh classification. Ascites and encephalopathy indicate decompensated liver failure.
- Presinusoidal obstruction [portal vein thrombosis (PVT)] and postsinusoidal obstruction (hepatic vein thrombosis or Budd–Chiari syndrome) should be distinguished from cirrhosis because liver function is generally preserved in these conditions.
- Splanchnic hyperemia contributes to the development of portosystemic collaterals.
- Emergency treatment of patients who present with bleeding esophagogastric varices includes drugs to reduce portal pressure, balloon tamponade, and endoscopic measures (injection, banding) aimed at thrombosing the varices.
- Long-term portal decompression can be achieved by radiologic or surgical means. Transjugular intrahepatic portosystemic stenting (TIPS) has encroached upon the role of operative shunts, whether partial or total. Liver transplantation is reserved for those with end-stage liver disease.

INTRODUCTION

Historic landmarks in the management of portal hypertension have largely focused around surgical events. In 1877, Eck declared that a portacaval shunt could safely be performed in humans based on his studies in eight dogs: seven of his animals died and the eighth ran away! The response was Pavlov's classic paper[1] in 1893 describing the effects of total portal diversion in dogs leading to liver failure and encephalopathy. Splenectomy, omentopexy, and various degrees of devascularization gained some acceptance in the early 1900s, but clearly they did not deal with the underlying portal hypertension. Endoscopic therapy for varices was initially introduced in the 1930s and resurfaced in the 1970s. It was initially provided by surgeons who used rigid endoscopes, then by gastroenterologists following the introduction of flexible endoscopy.

Surgical shunts in humans were first attempted in the early 1900s and came into the clinical arena in the 1940s.[2] Total shunts, partial shunts, and selective variceal decompression evolved over the next three decades and provided methods of surgical decompression. The 1990s saw a resurgence of interest in decompression of varices with the introduction of the radiologically placed intrahepatic shunt.[3] However, the greatest impact on portal hypertension has been the clinical coming of age of liver transplantation through the 1980s.[4] Transplantation deals not only with the consequences of portal hypertension but also with the underlying disease. Nowadays, all therapies must be judged against the need for, availability of and outcome of liver transplantation (*see* Chapter 118, "Liver Transplantation").

ETIOLOGY

Definition

Portal hypertension is present if portal venous pressure exceeds 10 mm Hg (1.3 kPa). Normal portal venous pressure is 5–10 mm Hg (0.7–1.3 kPa), which is sufficient to maintain a portal flow through the hepatic sinusoids of approximately 1 L/min.

Classification and Causes

Portal hypertension can be classified into presinusoidal, sinusoidal, and postsinusoidal causes (Fig. 54.1) that help to separate patients who have normal hepatocellular function from those who have hepatocellular damage. This separation has important implications in outcome.

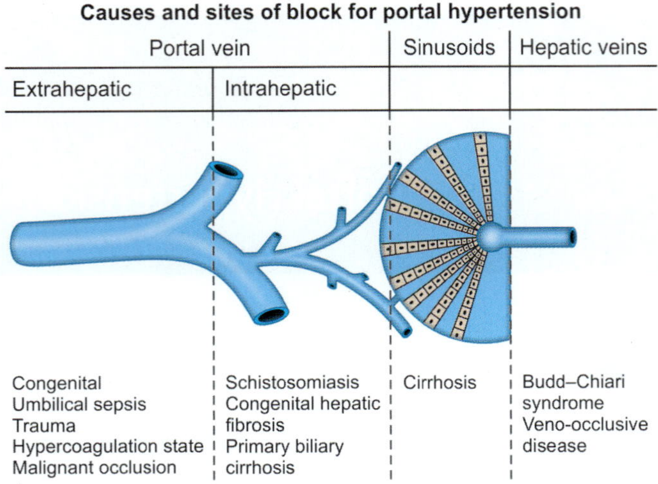

Fig. 54.1: Etiologies of portal hypertension. These are divided into those associated with normal liver function (presinusoidal) and those associated with liver damage (sinusoidal).

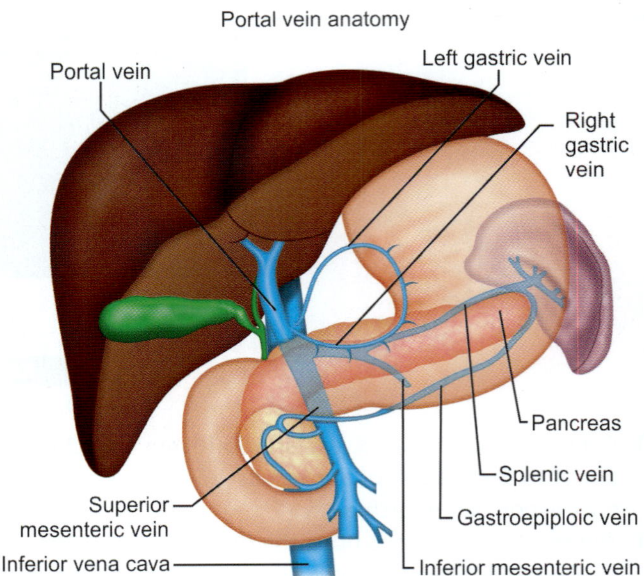

Fig. 54.2: Portal venous anatomy in portal hypertension. The superior mesenteric, splenic, and inferior mesenteric veins unite behind the neck of the pancreas to form the portal vein. The right and left gastric and gastroepiploic veins enter the portal and superior mesenteric veins, respectively.

Presinusoidal Portal Hypertension

This may be either extrahepatic or intrahepatic. Thrombosis of the extrahepatic portal vein or one of its major tributaries may lead to extrahepatic portal hypertension and occurs in early life associated with umbilical sepsis, or in older patients who have a hypercoagulable state. Other etiologies for portal or splenic vein thrombosis are tumors of the pancreas, pancreatitis, or metastatic nodes at the hepatic hilus. Isolated splenic vein thrombosis, e.g. in chronic pancreatitis or pancreatic cancer, produces left-sided portal hypertension involving the spleen and gastric fundus. It is important to identify this condition because it is cured by splenectomy.

Congenital hepatic fibrosis, schistosomiasis, and the early stages of primary biliary cirrhosis are pathologic processes that affect the presinusoidal terminal portal venules and result in intrahepatic presinusoidal portal hypertension.

All of the above etiologies have well preserved liver function, and the emphasis of management is on dealing with variceal bleeding.

Sinusoidal Obstruction

This is caused by cirrhosis, with viral hepatitis and ethanol abuse the most common etiologies. Less common causes of cirrhosis such as autoimmune liver disease, hemochromatosis, Wilson's disease, more advanced stages of primary biliary cirrhosis, sclerosing cholangitis, and α_1-antitrypsin deficiency should be considered if the etiology is less clear.

The importance of cirrhosis as the etiology for portal hypertension is that there is concurrent hepatocellular damage as well as the increased resistance to portal venous flow. Sinusoidal anatomy is destroyed, regenerative nodules form, fibrosis further obstructs portal venous flow and the normal metabolic processes are disrupted. The emphasis in this group of patients is on careful evaluation of liver function and an assessment of the activity of the underlying liver disease, its rate of progression and the hepatic reserve. The question to be answered is whether the cirrhosis is compensated or decompensated.

Postsinusoidal Portal Hypertension

This results from hepatic venous outflow obstruction, which falls under the broad category of Budd–Chiari syndrome. This is the least common cause of portal hypertension, but may be reversible if identified and treated early.

SURGICAL ANATOMY

The portal vein is formed behind the neck of the pancreas as the superior mesenteric joins the splenic vein (Fig. 54.2). The portal vein itself is approximately 6–8 cm long and 1–1.2 cm in diameter. It runs in the free edge of the lesser omentum from the pancreas to the right end of the porta hepatis. Two major tributaries of importance

Table 54.1 Zones of venous drainage at the gastroesophageal junction.

Zone	Site	Veins
1: Gastric	2–3 cm below the gastroesophageal junction (junctional zone)	Veins run longitudinally towards esophagus rather than via an irregular network as seen in the rest of the stomach
2: Palisade	2–3 cm above the gastric zone extending into lower esophagus	Evenly distributed longitudinal veins correspond to major mucosal folds of the esophagus; no perforating veins
3: Perforating	2 cm up the esophagus above the Ralisade zone	Large looping collaterals between internal and external venous plexuses of the esophagus
4: Truncal	8–10 cm up the esophagus above the perforating zone	4–5 longitudinal veins in the lamina propria and perforating veins from the submucosa to external venous plexus

in portal hypertension are the left gastric (coronary) and inferior mesenteric veins. These enter the portal system close to the splenic portal vein junction, the left gastric vein superiorly and the inferior mesenteric vein inferiorly.

The other important surgical anatomy in portal hypertension is the venous anatomy of the gastroesophageal junction, which has been extensively studied by several investigators.[5] Zones of venous drainage at the gastroesophageal junction are shown in Table 54.1.

PATHOPHYSIOLOGY

The major theories in the pathophysiology of portal hypertension have been the "backward" and the "forward" flow theories:

- Backward flow theory postulates that all consequences of portal hypertension result from obstruction to portal venous flow.
- Forward flow theory postulates that increased inflow to the portal venous system (usually because of splenomegaly) causes the changes that lead to the clinical findings of portal hypertension.

Evidence indicates that both theories contribute to the pathophysiology.[6] The stages in developing portal hypertension have been clarified to show that the primary event is an increased resistance to portal venous flow. The increased pressure on the splanchnic venous bed leads to the development of collaterals to bypass the blockage to flow. The compensatory increase in splanchnic inflow perpetuates and aggravates the portal hypertension. The major importance in clarifying this pathophysiology is that it has implications for clinical management, particularly in pharmacologic therapy.

Hemodynamic Pathophysiologic Changes

These can be broadly divided into splanchnic and systemic changes.[6] Portal venous pressure increases and is transmitted back into the whole splanchnic bed. The major sites for collateral pathway development are the natural watersheds for portosystemic collaterals:

- Gastroesophageal
- Perirectal
- Periumbilical
- Retroperitoneal.

Increased portal venous pressure, dilatation of the splanchnic venous bed and the development of collaterals all act as stimuli for splanchnic hyperemia. The marked increase in total splanchnic flow perpetuates the initial changes. Local release of nitric oxide through various mediators appears to be the relevant mechanism.

The systemic hemodynamic changes occur whatever the etiology of portal hypertension. In parallel with the splanchnic vascular changes of vasodilatation and hyperemia, there is an increase in plasma volume. Total systemic vascular resistance decreases, primarily in the splanchnic bed, but also to a lesser degree in the peripheral circulation. The clinical consequences are that a hyperdynamic systemic circulation develops with a high cardiac output and a low total systemic vascular resistance and a low normal blood pressure.

Natural History of Portal Hypertension

When cirrhosis is first diagnosed, approximately 30% of patients have compensated disease and 60% with decompensated disease have varices. About 8% of cirrhotic patients develop varices each year, and these can enlarge to cause bleeding. It follows that all patients diagnosed with cirrhosis should have a screening endoscopy to look for varices and determine the need to start therapy to reduce the risk of an initial bleed.[7]

The risk of the first variceal bleed may be predicted from:

- Variceal size
- Red color signs
- Portal pressure gradient > 12 mm Hg (1.6 kPa)
- Poor liver function.

An acute variceal bleed carries a mortality rate of approximately 30%, most deaths occurring among poorer risk patients with a Child score ≥ 8 points. Early rebleeding occurs in 20–50% of patients in the first 7–10 days after the first variceal bleed and is a poor prognostic sign. After the first 6 weeks, the rebleeding risk drops to approximately the same as before the initial bleed (i.e. about 30%). After an initial bleed, the risk of rebleeding is 75–80% within the first year.

CLINICAL PRESENTATION

The main clinical presentations of portal hypertension are variceal bleeding, ascites, hypersplenism, and encephalopathy. The major factor in determining the course and outcome is the status of the underlying liver disease. Approximately 90% of patients in the United States and Europe who present with portal hypertension have underlying cirrhosis, and the critical determinant is whether this is compensated or decompensated. Ascites and encephalopathy are the two clinical indications of decompensation. In contrast, variceal bleeding, splenomegaly, and hypersplenism or portal hypertension as an incidental finding are often with compensated disease and have a very different prognosis.

Classification of the severity of the underlying liver disease at the time of presentation of a patient who has portal hypertension is important. Child's classification has stood the test of time and has undergone several modifications. The modification most commonly used is that of Pugh[8] (Table 54.2). Child–Pugh A patients have a score of 5 or 6, Child–Pugh B patients have a score of 7–9, and Child–Pugh C patients have a score of 10–15.

Each of the clinical presentations referred above is discussed in more detail below.

INVESTIGATION

History and Physical Examination

The history should include exposure to hepatitis, excessive alcohol ingestion familial liver disease and relevant complications: upper or lower gastrointestinal bleeding, fluid accumulation, confusional episodes, and nonspecific symptoms of chronic liver disease such as fatigue and itching.

Table 54. 2 Child-Pugh classification.

Parameter	*1 point*	*2 points*	*3 points*
Bilirubin (mg/dl)	<2	2–3	>3
Albumin (g/dl)	>3.5	2.8–3.5	<2.8
Increase in prothrombin time (s)	1–3	4–6	>6
Ascites	None	Slight	Moderate
Encephalopathy	None	1–2	3–4

The grades are A for 5–6 points, B for 7–9 points and C for 10–15 points.

General physical examination includes a visual inspection for muscle wasting, jaundice, and spider angiomas, and in males for gynecomastia and testicular atrophy. Abdominal examination focuses on hepatosplenomegaly and ascites, but may also reveal prominent abdominal wall veins. Nonspecific findings suggestive of portal hypertension are mild persistent tachycardia and low blood pressure, which suggest systemic hemodynamic changes.

Hematology

Hematocrit may be reduced, either secondary to chronic bleeding or as a result of the expanded plasma volume. Platelet count may be < 100,000/mm^3 and white cell count < 4,000/mm^3 because of hypersplenism. Prothrombin time is used in calculating the Child–Pugh score (*see* above): prolongation of the international normalized ratio by > 1.5 indicates moderate liver impairment. A plasma fibrinogen level of < 100 mg/dL indicates advanced liver disease associated with poor synthetic function. The therapeutic implication is an increased risk of bleeding and the need to give fresh frozen plasma to patients who are bleeding or require any interventional procedure.

Biochemistry

In portal hypertension total body sodium is increased, but intravascular sodium is depleted, particularly following aggressive attempts at diuresis. A low blood urea nitrogen at presentation may indicate poor liver function, as the liver is the sole site of urea production in the body. An elevated blood urea nitrogen in a patient with cirrhosis suggests more severe renal insufficiency than suspected. The same principle holds true for serum creatinine: patients with advanced liver disease have a decreased lean body mass, so an elevated serum creatinine indicates more severe renal insufficiency than in a normal subject.

Other biochemical parameters of importance in investigating patients who have liver disease are elevated serum bilirubin and liver enzymes, aminotransferases, alkaline phosphatase, ↑γ-glutamyl transpeptidase, and reduced albumin.

Serology

Hepatitis A, B, and C serologies should be carried out routinely. For those who are positive for hepatitis B or C,

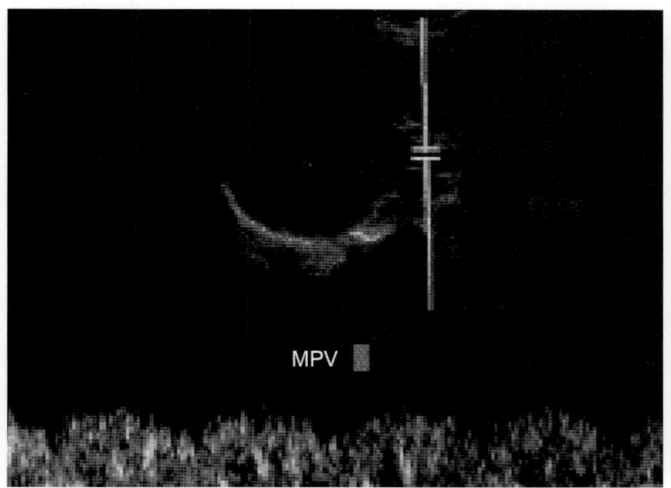

Fig. 54.3: Ultrasound scan with Doppler evaluation of the portal vein showing patency and prograde flow. (MPV: Main portal vein).

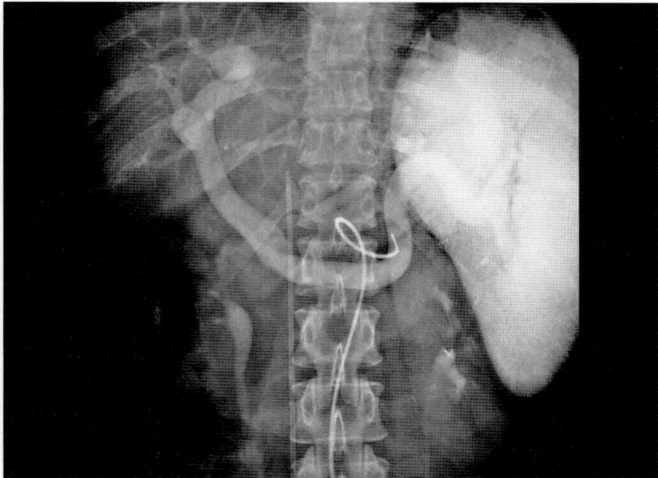

Fig. 54.4: Venous phase imaging of splenic artery injection demonstrating venous anatomy.

evidence of active viral replication should be sought by testing for hepatitis B DNA or hepatitis C RNA titers. Other serologic tests that help define the etiology of chronic liver disease are:

- Antimitochondrial antibody (primary biliary cirrhosis)
- Antinuclear antibody (for evidence of autoimmune hepatitis)
- Ceruloplasmin for Wilson's disease
- α_1-antitrypsin to reveal deficiency.

Endoscopy

All patients confirmed or suspected of having cirrhosis should have a screening upper gastrointestinal endoscopy. If varices are identified at screening, patients should be started on appropriate prophylactic pharmacologic therapy.

For a cirrhotic patient with upper gastrointestinal hemorrhage, endoscopy is the first step in evaluation of the bleeding site. Its major aims are to look for esophageal and/or gastric varices and portal hypertensive gastropathy. Other pathologies such as peptic ulcer disease, gastric antral vascular ectasia, or malignancies should be excluded.

The grading of severity of portal hypertensive changes has been extensively studied by Japanese and European workers. The classification of the severity of varices is based on size, extent, and the "color signs".[9]

Radiologic Imaging

For a patient who has established or suspected portal hypertension, abdominal vascular imaging is indicated. The initial imaging study is ultrasound with Doppler evaluation of the major vessels.[10] An ultrasound scan of the liver should inspect overall morphology; it is the initial screening procedure for focal intrahepatic lesions that may suggest hepatocellular carcinoma.

The vessel imaging focuses on the main portal vein, the splenic vein, the hepatic veins, and the infra- and intrahepatic inferior vena cava. The goal of this study in screening of patients who have portal hypertension is to evaluate portal vein patency and directional flow (Fig. 54.3). Portal vein size measurement and flow velocities have been extensively studied as measures of the severity of portal hypertension, but their value in clinical practice has not been established.

A CT scan or MRI of the abdomen may be indicated for some patients who have portal hypertension to evaluate the liver morphology in greater detail and to image the intra-abdominal venous system.

Not all patients need all of these studies, so centers must decide which modality provides the best clinically useful information in their experience.

Angiography

Angiography is sometimes indicated in patients with portal hypertension. Several techniques are used to visualize the portal venous system either through a transvenous or a transarterial approach.

The venous phase imaging can delineate the portal venous anatomy in patients being considered for decompressive shunt surgery. Splenic artery injection followed through the venous phase gives the best imaging of the splenic vein and its tributaries (Fig. 54.4). Superior mesenteric artery injection through the venous phase gives detail

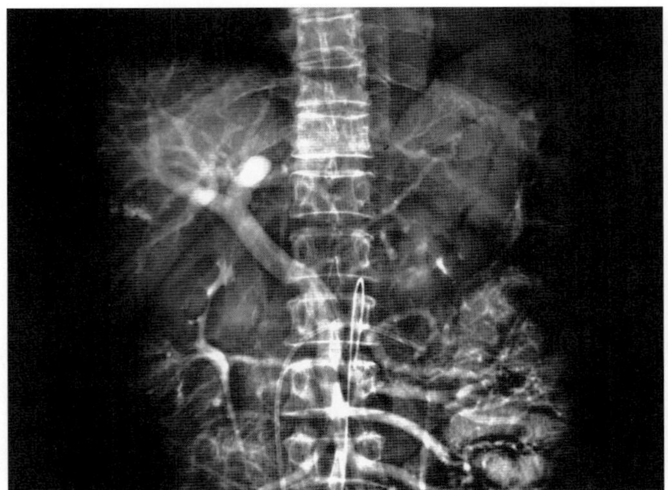

Fig. 54.5: Venous phase imaging of superior mesenteric artery injection demonstrating the superior mesenteric and portal veins.

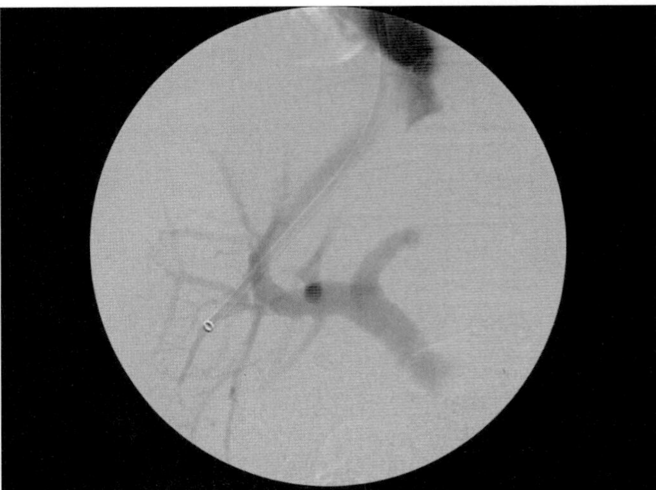

Fig. 54.6: Portal venous anatomy demonstrated by retrograde injection of carbon dioxide using a catheter wedged in the main right hepatic vein.

of the superior mesenteric and portal vein (Fig. 54.5). Identification of the site, size, and flow parameters of the major collaterals such as the left gastric and inferior mesenteric vein are best defined on arteriography. These studies provide data on the pathophysiology for specific patients that cannot be obtained by noninvasive methods.

Venography

This is used to assess the hepatic veins, the inferior vena cava, and the left renal vein and may be carried out by either a transfemoral or a transjugular approach. Hepatic venography combines both pressure measurements and imaging. Pressures are measured in the hepatic vein in both the occluded and free vein position, using the same principle as pulmonary pressure measurement with a Swan-Ganz catheter. The occluded pressure is an indirect measurement of hepatic sinusoidal pressure. The difference between the occluded and free pressure—the hepatic venous pressure gradient (HVPG)—is used as a clinical measurement of portal hypertension.

Wedged hepatic vein injection of contrast can reflux into the hepatic sinusoids and, in patients who have sluggish portal venous flow, into the main portal vein and/or its feeding tributaries (Fig. 54.6). Imaging of and pressure measurements within the inferior vena cava and left renal vein may be important in making decisions for surgical intervention. The vena cava may be compressed by an enlarged and cirrhotic liver, causing with distortion or a pressure gradient. The left renal vein has anomalies in 20% of the population, with a circumaortic vein present in 16% and a totally retroaortic left renal vein in 4%.

The transjugular route of venous access has become the preferred method because it allows easier intervention for liver biopsy and is the route when a TIPS is indicated.

Liver Biopsy

A histologic diagnosis will often help guide therapy, e.g. in hemochromatosis before phlebotomy or in Wilson's disease before copper chelation. For all types of cirrhosis, assessment of acute cellular injury and extent of fibrosis help judge the degree of underlying liver disease. Finally, image-guided biopsy may be required for focal lesions.

The different techniques for liver biopsy are: percutaneous, transjugular, or laparoscopic.

Quantitative Liver Function Testing

This field has received attention over the past 30 years, but has not achieved widespread clinical use. Quantitative tests can be broadly divided into those:

- Limited by hepatocyte function
- Dependent upon liver blood flow

Markers such as galactose, indocyanine green, antipyrine, or lidocaine (lignocaine) have been most widely used for quantitative testing. Other methods used to quantitate liver function include rates of urea synthesis and high first-pass clearance methods to estimate liver blood flow, such as sorbitol and galactose.

The major difficulty with quantitative liver function testing is the high inducibility of many of the pathways being studied, such as the P450 enzymes.

Table 54. 3 Treatment strategies for esophagogastric varices.
Pharmacologic therapy
Endoscopic therapy
Tamponade
Decompression—radiologic, surgical
Devascularization operation
Liver transplantation

Table 54.4 Time points in the treatment of esophagogastric varices.	
Prophylaxis to prevent the initial bleed	
Treatment of acute variceal bleeding	
Treatment to prevent recurrent variceal bleeding	– first-line treatment – second-line treatment
Treatment of end-stage liver disease	

MANAGEMENT OF ESOPHAGOGASTRIC VARICES

Esophagogastric varices can be treated with a variety of therapies (Table 54.3).[11] The time points of treatment become important in deciding upon the most appropriate therapy (Table 54.4). Each therapy is briefly reviewed and management schemes are presented for the different time points of presentation.

Pharmacologic Therapy

Patients with acute variceal bleeding may be treated initially with intravenous terlipressin or somatostatin or one of its analogs. In the elective situation, noncardioselective β-blockers and the long-acting nitrates are the main drugs used to lower portal pressure.

Acute pharmacologic therapy is most easily administered using octreotide infused at 50 μg/h. Such a regimen can help prevent early recurrent bleeding in patients who have presented with an acute variceal bleed. Glypressin has gained considerable popularity because of its longer duration of action (than vasopressin) and is an alternative to octreotide.

Oral pharmacologic therapy was introduced in 1980 when it was demonstrated that portal pressure could be lowered by about 20% with propranolol.[12] A similar effect can be obtained with the long-acting nitrates. The goal of oral pharmacologic therapy, which prevents variceal bleeding, is to:

- Reduce the HVPG to 12 mm Hg (1.6 kPa) or less
- Achieve a 20% pressure reduction from the baseline portal pressure measurement.

Other drugs such as α_2-agonists, calcium channel blockers, serotonin antagonists, and prokinetic agents have not shown clinical usefulness.[11]

Endoscopic Therapy

Endoscopic therapy for variceal bleeding was initially introduced in 1939 using the rigid esophagoscope, then revived in the 1970s and assured of its place in the treatment of variceal bleeding with the introduction of flexible endoscopy. It has a definite role in acute variceal bleeding and is a first-line therapy in preventing rebleeding. The two main techniques are sclerotherapy or variceal banding[13]:

- Sclerotherapy involves the use of one of several agents to thrombose a varix directly or to create fibrosis in the mucosa overlying a varix.
- In banding the varix is sucked into an applicator on the end of the flexible endoscope, and a rubber band is fired to strangulate the varix; the bands slough off in 7–10 days with minimal scarring and less ulceration than with sclerotherapy.

Endoscopic banding became the preferred approach with the introduction of multiple band ligators, when it was shown to be more effective with earlier obliteration of varices and fewer complications than endoscopic sclerotherapy.[13]

Tamponade

This is rarely indicated any more, except as a bridge to other treatment for the 10% of patients whose acute bleeding is not controlled endoscopically. The Sengstaken–Blakemore tube has both gastric and esophageal balloons. Attention to detail is essential in placing a tamponade tube. The tube must first be fully introduced into the stomach and confirmed with X-ray with a small amount of air placed in the gastric balloon. The gastric balloon should then be inflated to 300–350 mL and pulled up into the gastric fundus. This maneuver will control virtually all bleeding. Occasionally, persistent bleeding may occur above the gastric balloon in the esophagus, requiring inflation of the esophageal balloon to 40 mm Hg (5.3 kPa) as tested through a sphygmomanometer. Confirmation of the position of the tube should be obtained radiologically when both balloons are inflated. The tube should not be left in place for >12–24 hours and should only be used as a temporary measure while the patient is resuscitated and prepared for either repeat endoscopic therapy or decompression.

Table 54.5 Methods of decompression for portal hypertension and gastroesophageal varices.

TIPS	
Nonoperative, radiologic	
Portosystemic surgical shunts	
Total	Portacaval (using portal vein) Mesocaval, mesorenal, mesoatrial (using superior mesenteric vein)
Partial	Portacaval or mesocaval (interposition graft of restricted diameter to allow some prograde portal flow)
Selective variceal decompression	
Distal splenorenal shunt	

Decompression

This may be carried out by either radiologic or surgical methods, and the aim is to reduce intravariceal pressure below 12 mm Hg (1.6 kPa). This fall may be achieved by total, partial, or selective variceal decompression (Table 54.5).

Total decompression of portal hypertension is achieved when an anastomosis >12 mm in diameter is made between the portal vein or one of its major tributaries and the inferior vena cava or one of its major tributaries. This may be an end-to-side portacaval shunt or any type of side-to-side anastomosis.

A partial portosystemic shunt is achieved between these same vessels with any type of side-to-side anastomosis that is 8–10 mm in diameter. These shunts will reduce portal pressure to approximately 12 mm Hg (1.6 kPa) and control variceal bleeding. Pathophysiologically, the same outcome can be achieved radiologically by a TIPS.

Transjugular intrahepatic portosystemic stenting has become the most popular method for decompression since the 1990s because it avoids the risk of operations. It is a side-to-side portosystemic shunt and acts as a total or partial shunt depending upon its diameter, as outlined above.

Selective variceal decompression can be achieved by a distal splenorenal shunt, which selectively decompresses gastroesophageal varices through the spleen and splenic vein to the left renal vein; portal hypertension is maintained in the superior mesenteric and portal vein to maintain portal flow to the cirrhotic liver.

The difference in these types of variceal decompression lies in the degree of maintenance of portal venous perfusion. Loss of portal flow accelerates liver failure and increases the rate of encephalopathy.

Each method of decompression is discussed in more detail below.

Transjugular Intrahepatic Portal Systemic Shunts (TIPS)

Radiologic shunts have evolved over two decades. Initial animal studies demonstrated the feasibility of connecting the portal and hepatic veins. Angioplasty techniques developed in the 1970s and 1980s allowed a larger track to be made through the liver.[14] Finally, the development of expandable metal stents in the mid-1980s made it possible to keep the track open (Fig. 54.7), with improved patency when covered stents became available.[15]

It takes about 1–2 hours to place a TIPS, and it is best done under anesthesia. The right internal jugular vein is cannulated and either the right or middle hepatic vein is accessed. Coaxial catheter systems are used to maintain access to a major hepatic vein and other catheters are advanced:

- Initially to traverse the hepatic parenchyma
- Then to access the portal venous system
- Finally to allow the advancing balloon-dilating catheter into the track.

When the track has been dilated, a self-expanding stent is deployed and is dilated up to 10–12 mm. Attention to detail in placing the stent is important as it shortens during expansion. There must be sufficient but not excessive length at the portal and hepatic venous ends. The stent should not be advanced too far into the portal vein or protrude from the hepatic vein up into the suprahepatic vena cava.

Once the stent has been placed, the pressures in the portal vein, the stent, and the right atrium are measured. The goal is to reduce the portal-to-atrial pressure gradient to <12 mm Hg (1.6 kPa).

Contraindications to TIPS are hepatoma, polycystic liver, and right heart failure. The major complication is hemorrhage from either perforation of the liver capsule or the portal venous system outside the liver. Major complications occur in <2% of patients.

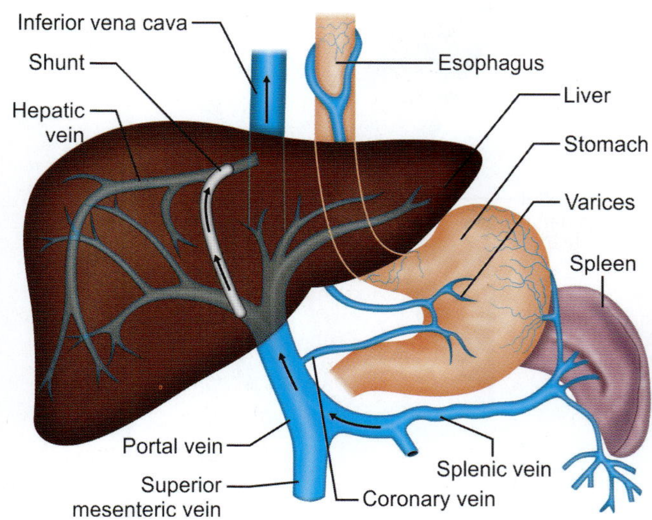

Fig. 54.7: Transjugular intrahepatic portosystemic shunting (TIPS). The metallic shunt maintains the transparenchymal track, which has been made through the liver between the portal and hepatic veins.

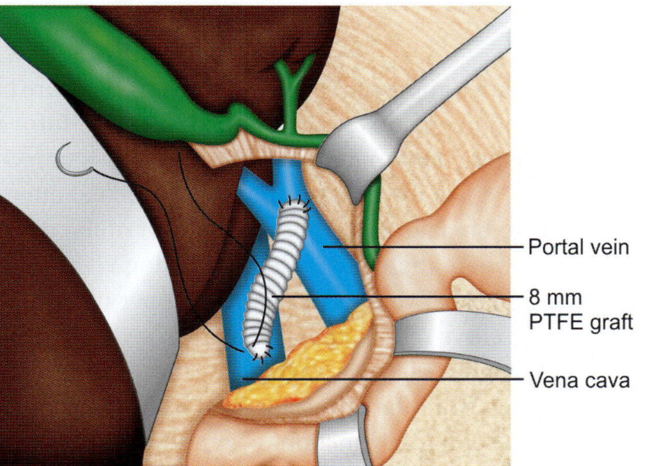

Fig. 54.9: Partial portosystemic shunt with an 8 mm graft between the portal vein and inferior vena cava. Exposure is the same as for the total portacaval shunt.

Total Portosystemic Surgical Shunts

The most common is a portacaval shunt (Fig. 54.8),[16] which requires dissection of the portal vein at the hepatic hilus and either direct anastomosis of the vein to the infrahepatic inferior vena cava or anastomosis using an interposition graft. Exposure is through a long right subcostal incision. The portal vein is approached by mobilization of the duodenum and retraction of the hepatic artery and bile duct to the left. The portal vein is isolated

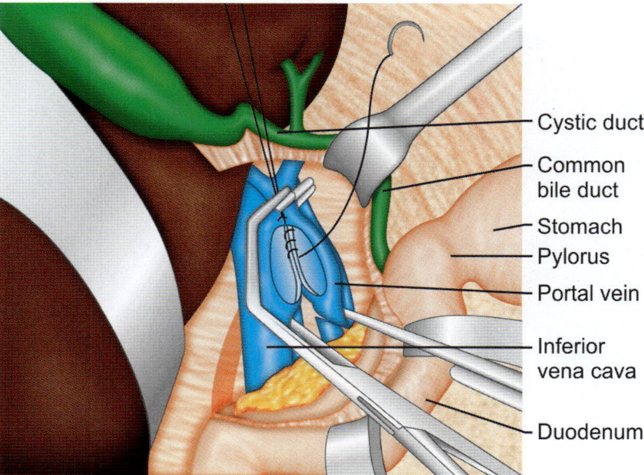

Fig. 54.8: Side-to-side portacaval shunt—with direct vein-to-vein anastomosis. The portal vein is dissected from the right side, posterior to the bile duct. The intrahepatic vena cava is fully mobilized. If there is a larger caudate lobe, an interposition graft may be used.

over an adequate distance to allow safe clamping for anastomosis. The inferior vena cava also needs to be mobilized sufficiently to complete the anastomosis safely. An interposition graft may be needed if the two vessels are separated by an enlarged caudate lobe.

Mesocaval, mesorenal, and mesoatrial shunts involve isolating the superior mesenteric vein just below the pancreas. The vein is identified by lifting up the transverse colon and dissecting at the base of the mesocolon. The middle colic vein is followed to the superior mesenteric vein, which is freed over sufficient distance for safe anastomosis. The decision about anastomosing it to the inferior vena cava or left renal vein is based on the surgeon's preference. To isolate the inferior vena cava, the third and fourth portions of the duodenum need to be mobilized and pushed cranially to expose an adequate length of vessel. An interposition graft is required using either 14–18 mm ringed polytetrafluoroethylene (PTFE) or an internal jugular vein graft. A mesoatrial shunt may be required if the intrahepatic inferior vena cava is obstructed (as with some patients with Budd-Chiari syndrome).

Partial Portosystemic Shunts

These may be placed in either the portacaval (Fig. 54.9) or mesocaval position. If the graft diameter is reduced to 8 mm with ringed PTFE graft, the portal venous system is only partially decompressed, allowing some maintenance of prograde portal flow.[17] At this size, the pressure is reduced to approximately 12 mm Hg (1.6 kPa), which is sufficient to control variceal bleeding.

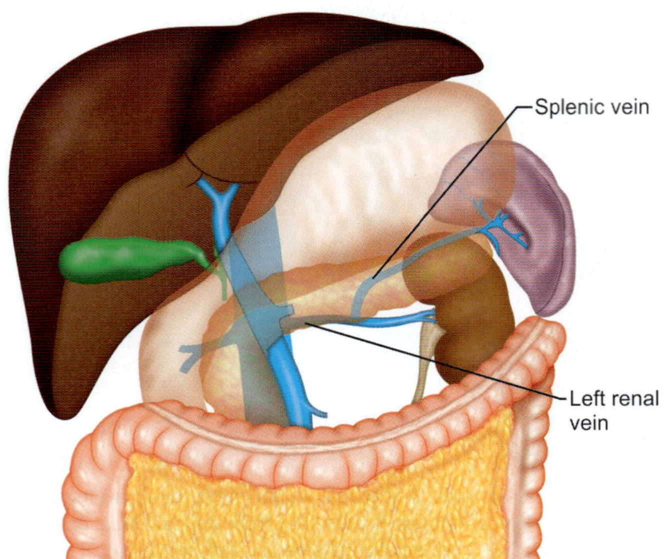

Fig. 54.10: Distal splenorenal shunt, with anastomosis of the splenic to the left renal vein. The gastric fundus, esophagus and spleen are decompressed. Portal hypertension and prograde portal flow are maintained.

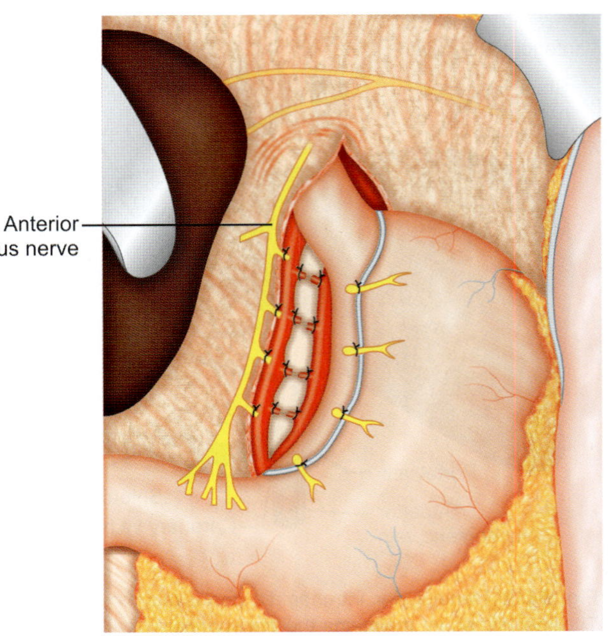

Fig. 54.11: Gastroesophageal devascularization interrupts all variceal inflow to most of the stomach and the distal 7 cm of the esophagus. Splenectomy and devascularization of the greater curve of the stomach complete the procedure.

Selective Variceal Decompression

This is most commonly achieved by a distal splenorenal shunt (DSRS) (Fig. 54.10).[18] Exposure is obtained through a bilateral subcostal incision, opening the gastrocolic omentum, and then mobilizing and elevating the inferior border of the pancreas. The splenic vein is identified and isolated from the back of the pancreas right up to its junction with the superior mesenteric and portal vein. The vein is divided at this point, and sufficient vein is freed from the back of the pancreas to allow it to be moved down to the left renal vein without kinking.

The second component to this operation is portal-azygos disconnection, which involves ligation of the left gastric vein at its entry into the portal or splenic vein and again just above the pancreas. More complete portal-azygos disconnection can be achieved by totally isolating the splenic vein from the pancreas and meticulously ligating the right gastric and gastroepiploic veins.

Devascularization Procedures

These have the components of splenectomy, gastric, and esophageal devascularization, and esophageal transection, with the goal of reducing inflow to bleeding varices (Fig. 54.11).[19] Their success depends upon the extent of the devascularization: the more extensive, the lower the subsequent rebleeding rate.

The operative approach requires sufficient exposure of the upper abdomen and left upper quadrant to perform a safe splenectomy and to mobilize fully both the stomach and at least 7 cm of the distal esophagus. Particular attention needs to be paid to the posterior aspect of the distal esophagus, where there are large penetrating veins from the paraesophageal venous plexus. The upper two thirds of the lesser curve of the stomach should be devascularized as for highly selective vagotomy. The whole of the greater curve should be devascularized from the pylorus to the gastroesophageal junction.

The role of esophageal transection is controversial because most patients have had extensive sclerotherapy and the thickened esophagus does not lend itself to stapled transection. Most surgeons therefore now omit this component.

Liver Transplantation

This is part of the surgical repertoire of managing patients who have portal hypertension and variceal bleeding. The indication for transplant remains end-stage liver disease, and for Child's class C patients, this treatment has altered the long-term outcome. Liver transplantation is dealt with in more detail in Chapter 118, so the technical aspects are not discussed here.

Flowchart 54.1: Management of variceal bleeding.

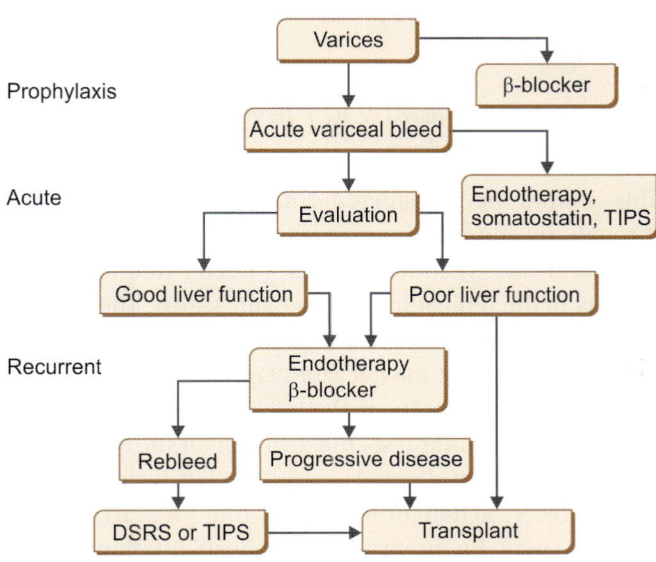

MANAGEMENT OF VARICEAL BLEEDING AT DEFINED TIME POINTS (FLOWCHART 54.1)

Prophylactic Therapy

Treatment should be initiated before the first variceal bleed because prophylactic therapy can reduce the risk of an initial bleed from 30% to 20%, and the mortality rate of that first bleed is approximately 30%. Most of the above treatments have been used for prophylaxis, but pharmacologic therapy is generally recommended nowadays.[11]

Total portosystemic shunts were tested with clinical trials in the 1960s; although the first bleed was prevented, there was an increased mortality rate in the surgical groups from encephalopathy and liver failure. No studies have looked at the role of TIPS in the prophylactic setting.

Sclerotherapy has been extensively studied in prevention of the initial bleed. Clinical trials have shown mixed results. Although a meta-analysis indicates that sclerotherapy is not recommended at present,[11] further randomized controlled trials of bleeding prophylaxis in high-risk patients may alter this recommendation.[20]

Pharmacologic therapy to prevent the first bleed has been most widely studied using β-blockers. The risk of bleeding was reduced in seven of nine randomized trials, while meta-analysis showed a significant decrease in the risk of bleeding for patients receiving β-blockers.[11] Side effects occur in approximately 20% of patients. An alternative pharmacologic option is isosorbide-5-mononitrate, which has a similar hemodynamic effect and clinical efficacy as that of β-blockers.

Acute Variceal Bleeding

This requires a team approach in management. General measures for these patients differ from those of the typical volume resuscitation for other bleeding patients. Volume resuscitation in the conventional manner with saline and/or Ringer's lactate will lead to ascites and/or edema. For those with cirrhosis, crystalloid administration should be limited. Resuscitation requires blood replacement and blood products. Other important measures in these patients include clearing the gastrointestinal tract of blood, protecting the airway and making an early diagnosis using endoscopy.

In patients with advanced liver disease, gastrointestinal bleeding can easily precipitate encephalopathy because blood in the gastrointestinal tract represents a heavy protein load.

Cirrhotics

Patients who have cirrhosis are susceptible to infection, so intravenous antibiotics should be given as a component of acute phase management.

Gastrointestinal tract catharsis should be achieved using magnesium citrate or polyethylene glycol 3350 (Golytely); if the patient is comatose, enemas may be required.

Most patients should be monitored in the intensive care unit for at least 24 hours or until they are hemodynamically stable. The need for more invasive intravascular monitoring with arterial lines, central venous catheters is decided on a case-by-case basis. Urine output should be monitored hourly.

Endoscopy should be done as soon as the patient is hemodynamically stable, and is both diagnostic and potentially therapeutic. Active bleeding, or stigmas of a recent bleed, such as a platelet plug on a varix leads directly to sclerotherapy or banding. This will control bleeding in approximately 90% of patients.

Should Patients Receive Concomitant Pharmacologic Therapy?

Opinion is divided as the highest risk time for rebleeding is in the following week. Administration of terlipressin or octreotide may reduce the risk of this early rebleed, but there are no randomized trials in support.

Balloon Tamponade

This is reserved for patients in whom the acute bleeding is not controlled by endoscopic therapy (i.e. 10% or less of all patients). Management requires a strict protocol as outlined above, and the tube should not be left in place for longer than necessary to move to the next level of treatment. Pressure on the mucosa from the tamponade leads to further damage and the risk of early rebleeding.

Decompression

This may be required for the patient who has required balloon tamponade or for the patient who rebleeds soon after endoscopic therapy, particularly from gastric varices. A TIPS will usually control the bleeding.

Prevention of Recurrent Variceal Bleeding

Decisions are based on the evaluation outlined above, which should be completed within 48–72 hours after an acute bleed. The principles for prevention of rebleeding can be summarized as:

- First-line treatment with pharmacologic and endoscopic therapy
- Second-line treatment with variceal decompression
- Liver transplantation for end-stage liver disease.

First-line treatment of prevention of rebleeding is initially the same irrespective of the severity of the underlying liver disease and involves a combination of pharmacologic and endoscopic therapy. This treatment buys time to evaluate the liver disease fully, educate the patient about the disease and assess the likely course and the chance of reversibility of the underlying liver disease.

First-Line Treatment Using Pharmacologic and Endoscopic Therapy

Properly implemented, this will reduce the risk of rebleeding from 75–80% to 25–30%. Endoscopic therapy is based on band ligation, which should aim to obliterate esophageal varices over 4–6 weeks (usually with three to three ligation sessions).[21] Patients should be started on a noncardioselective β-blocker (propranolol or nadolol) at a dose sufficient to produce β-blockade.[11] The objective is to obtain a 20% reduction in HVPG or an HVPG of no >12 mm Hg (1.6 kPa), but this is impractical for all patients; a target of reducing the pulse rate by 20% is usually sufficient.

Multiple trials have compared sclerotherapy to TIPS for primary therapy,[1] but no advantage was shown by going directly to TIPS.

Second-Line Therapy to Prevent Recurrent Bleeding

This should be considered for patients who rebleed through the above primary therapy. The decision to move to second-line treatment can be difficult due to timing, severity of the rebleeding, and hepatic status. The severity and rate of progression of the underlying liver disease are the major factors in the decision. Does the patient need a transplant now, or is he or she likely to need a transplant in the next few years? If so, the decision for the best bridge to transplantation depends upon current liver function: if well-preserved hepatic function (Child's A or B), decompression may be preferable to transplantation, but if poor (Child's C) the bridge to transplantation is shorter and the rebleeding may be the event that leads to transplantation.

The other major dilemma is the severity of the rebleed and its timing during the course of first-line treatment. How much rebleeding is acceptable during first-line treatment? For the patient who is rebleeding early because of failure to obliterate varices, there should be an expeditious move towards decompression. For the patient who has had an initial successful obliteration of varices and has a minor rebleeding episode 1–2 years later, it may be reasonable to repeat the endoscopic therapy.

Decisions on optimal decompression should be based on outcomes from available studies. Data show that TIPS is the preferred option for decompression in most patients.

Variceal Decompression

Surgical decompression to prevent recurrent bleeding is associated with rebleeding rates of <10%, but is used relatively infrequently because of the use of endoscopic therapy and transplantation, and more recently TIPS.

Each type of surgical shunt has a bleeding control of >90%. The difference between the types of shunts lies in the rate of encephalopathy. Total shunts are associated with a higher rate of encephalopathy than partial or selective shunts.

Data from the many randomized controlled trials that have compared surgical shunts show that:[22]

- Bleeding is controlled in 90% of patients after operative decompression.

- Encephalopathy occurs in 10–15% of patients after a distal splenorenal shunt, 10–20% of patients after a partial shunt, and 30–40% of patients after a total shunt.
- Survival is not significantly different for any of the shunt procedures.

Data on surgical shunts in previous uncontrolled series supported these findings. The operative mortality rate was 5% or less and bleeding control was excellent. The risk of complications and death is related to the underlying liver disease. Patients who have well-maintained liver function do well with any type of decompressive procedure, at least in the short-term.

Total portosystemic shunts have been championed by Orloff and colleagues,[23] who have had an excellent outcome overall. A 30-year experience showed an improved survival and bleeding control at every time point. Orloff attributes much of his success to overall patient care, rehabilitation, and intensive follow-up. Another series of total portosystemic shunts from Stipa documented excellent bleeding control, but a 50% rate of encephalopathy and liver failure.

Partial shunts have been championed in the 1990s by Sarfeh and colleagues,[24] building on the work of Bismuth and Johansen. Bleeding was controlled in over 90% of patients, with shunt stenosis occurring in 10–20%. These series have also documented maintenance of portal perfusion in over 80% of patients if the graft is reduced to 8 mm in diameter. The encephalopathy rate was approximately 15% in these uncontrolled series.

Selective shunts controlled bleeding in over 90%, with encephalopathy in the 10–15% range.[25] Various modifications of selective shunting have involved portal-azygos disconnection or pancreatic disconnection and the ability to maintain selectivity has been evaluated; selectivity is best achieved in patients who have nonalcoholic portal hypertension. Survival in these series is primarily determined by the severity of the underlying liver disease. The only place for DSRS is in patients with rebleeding and good liver function when a TIPS cannot be placed.

Decompression of varices has evolved in the past two decades such that TIPS is now the procedure of choice. Technical improvements, primarily with covered stents but also in technique, have led to safer and better outcomes.[15] A randomized trial comparing TIPS to DSRS[26] showed no significant difference in bleeding control (10% vs 5%), survival (60%), or any episode of encephalopathy (50%) at 5 years. The rate of transplant in the two groups was similar (< 10%). Transjugular intrahepatic portosystemic stenting patients required significantly more reintervention (80% vs 10%), but was marginally more cost-effective at 5 years [27] Another trial comparing TIPS to 8 mm portacaval H-graft surgical shunt [28] showed some longer-term benefit for the surgical procedure. In conclusion, TIPS emerges as the optimal therapy for decompression.

Effect of the Treatment of Portal Hypertension on Subsequent Liver Transplantation[29]

First-line treatment has no impact on subsequent liver transplantation, but there may be some thickening around the gastroesophageal junction from endoscopic therapy. No data have documented an increased rate of PVT with endoscopic therapy.

Decompressive procedures may, however, have an impact on subsequent transplantation. Careful placement of a TIPS is important because if it is placed too far down the portal vein or extrudes into the suprahepatic inferior vena cava, it may be technically challenging to remove the stent at the time of transplant. The effect of surgical shunts on subsequent liver transplant has been extensively reviewed; in summary, although the transplant procedure may be more complex and entail a higher blood loss, the overall outcome is not influenced by the presence of a previous surgical shunt.

An overall scheme for the management of variceal bleeding can be summarized in an algorithm (Flowchart 54.1). The absolute ordering of therapies may differ between centers depending upon available expertise, but all centers should have in common general concepts of therapy for:

- Prophylaxis
- Acute bleeding
- Preventing recurrent hemorrhage.

MANAGEMENT OF EXTRAHEPATIC PORTAL VEIN THROMBOSIS

The management of patients with variceal bleeding secondary to extrahepatic PVT differs in important aspects from that of those with cirrhosis. As these patients have a normal liver, the emphasis is on controlling the bleeding. In addition, the etiology of the PVT should be identified as this may indicate the need for other hematologic management. Clinical evaluation of these patients follows the same principles outlined above. Angiography is more important for this group of patients than for cirrhotics because accurate identification of the vessels that are still open will dictate further therapy. Cavernous

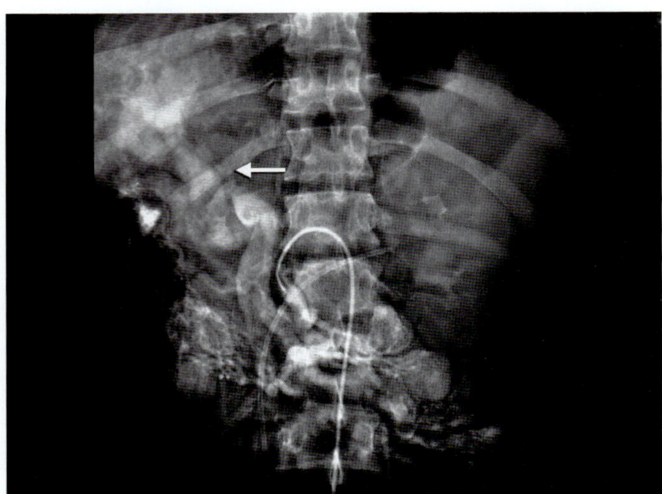

Fig. 54.12: Portal vein thrombosis with cavernous transformation (arrow) and several larger collateral veins carrying portal blood to the low pressure sinusoids.

transformation of the portal vein can produce a confusing picture on Doppler ultrasound, particularly if there is one dominant large collateral mimicking the portal vein. The picture can usually be clarified with adequate angiography (Fig. 54.12), and the patency or occlusion of the superior mesenteric and splenic veins are key factors in management decisions. Liver biopsy is often required to document a normal liver.

Management of this group of patients is initially by endoscopic therapy, but if the varices are not readily obliterated and there is rebleeding, there should be a low threshold for proceeding to definitive decompression.[30] Of these patients, 80% have a patent splenic vein and are ideal candidates for a distal splenorenal shunt. Bleeding is controlled by the shunt, and portal perfusion is maintained through cavernous transformation to the normal liver. An alternative surgical decompression is with the meso-Rex bypass from the superior mesenteric to left intrahepatic portal vein.[31]

Total portosystemic shunts have been used in patients with PVT using either central splenorenal or mesocaval shunts. The classic mesocaval shunt used for PVT divides the inferior vena cava just above its bifurcation and swings the inferior vena cava up in an end-to-side fashion to the superior mesenteric vein.[32] The long-term outcome of such total shunts is controversial. Portosystemic encephalopathy has been documented at 10–20 years in this group of patients,[33] as confirmed by other reports, but other investigators[34] have found no late development of portosystemic encephalopathy.

Devascularization procedures may be indicated for this group of patients if there are no shuntable vessels. The operation should follow the same principles as those outlined above for extensive gastroesophageal devascularization. An added caveat is that splenectomy may unmask an underlying myeloproliferative disorder in adult patients who have PVT. A normal platelet count in the face of massive splenomegaly should trigger a careful hematologic evaluation before proceeding to splenectomy.

ASCITES

Ascites is a sign of "decompensation" in liver disease and so has a much more sinister significance than variceal bleeding. Like variceal bleeding, ascites need careful evaluation and management.

Pathogenesis

Ascites results from a combination of:[35]

- Portal hypertension
- Altered renal sodium and water handling
- Hypoalbuminemia.

It forms as a "hepatic lymph" from the surface of the liver as a result of fluid exuding from the damaged, high venous pressure sinusoids of cirrhosis. The kidney's role in pathogenesis is through reduction in renal blood flow, decreased glomerular filtration, and decreased effective plasma volume. Hypoalbuminemia decreases the intravascular oncotic pressure and further contributes to ascites formation.

Evaluation

This requires analysis of ascitic fluid obtained by paracentesis and assessment of renal function. Ascitic fluid should be examined for cell count, culture and total protein, and albumin content. Measurement of the serum:ascites albumin gradient can help differentiate the etiology of ascites. Renal function is assessed primarily from urine and serum electrolytes and blood urea nitrogen and serum creatinine. Further management requires a 24-hour urine creatinine clearance.

Management

Ascites is managed initially by dietary sodium restriction and diuretics. Spironolactone counters the secondary hyperaldosteronism of chronic liver disease, blocks tubular sodium reabsorption, and allows diuresis. Once sodium reabsorption has been adequately blocked by an aldosterone antagonist, further diuresis may be required using a loop diuretic such as furosemide (frusemide). The goal should be a gentle diuresis.

If ascites is refractory to medical management, the next line of therapy is paracentesis. Large-volume paracentesis can be performed with minimal risk, and the patient who requires this once a month may find this treatment very acceptable. If large-volume paracentesis is needed on a weekly basis, other therapeutic interventions should be considered.

The primary surgical treatment for intractable ascites is liver transplantation because the patient has "decompensated" liver disease. However, for patients who are not transplant candidates or for those awaiting transplant, other interventions may be indicated. Peritoneovenous shunts have largely disappeared from the repertoire of options for these patients because they thrombose easily, carry the risk of infection, and have been shown to precipitate variceal bleeding. Transjugular intrahepatic portosystemic stenting is a decompressive option for those with intractable ascites as it decompresses the sinusoids and can greatly improve matters.[36]

BUDD-CHIARI SYNDROME

Budd-Chiari syndrome encompasses a group of disorders characterized by hepatic venous outflow obstruction. The severity of the syndrome may vary from mild nonspecific upper abdominal symptoms to a fulminant course with severe hepatic necrosis. Most patients present with a subacute form that is progressive over weeks to months.

Etiology

There is usually some other underlying pathology that leads to hepatic vein thrombosis.[37] The most common etiologies are summarized in Table 54.6. The vast majority reflect an underlying hematologic disorder, polycythemia vera being the most common.[38] Other conditions such as tumors causing pressure on the hepatic veins are important to identify because of their exceedingly poor prognosis. Membranous webs of the suprahepatic vena cava are uncommon in the United States or Europe, but are a frequent cause of Budd-Chiari syndrome in the Far East.

Table 54.6 Causes of Budd-Chiari syndrome.

Cause	*Proportion of cases (%)*
Myeloproliferative disorder	50
Idiopathic	20
Tumor	10
Estrogen use, pregnancy	10
Hypercoagulable state	5
Paroxysmal nocturnal hemoglobinuria	5

Pathophysiology

This is the same regardless of etiology. The sequence of outflow obstruction, sinusoidal dilatation and congestion, hepatocyte necrosis from the increased pressure and progressive liver damage produces the syndrome. The process may involve only one or two of the three main hepatic veins, leading to differential involvement of the liver lobes. The extent of involvement dictates the degree of liver damage. If only one hepatic vein is initially involved, the symptoms may be relatively mild and simply lead to scarring and fibrosis of that lobe. However, the sequence then usually repeats itself, involving one of the other main hepatic veins and leading to progressive liver damage and scarring. The caudate lobe of the liver is spared from this damage because it has a separate drainage with vessels passing directly into the inferior vena cava and may therefore undergo considerable hypertrophy.

Clinical Presentation

This is usually subacute with relatively mild symptoms and signs of ascites, hepatomegaly, and right upper quadrant abdominal pain. Other stigmas of chronic liver disease are usually absent, and standard liver tests are only minimally abnormal. As Budd-Chiari syndrome is uncommon, the diagnosis is frequently missed. Patients are often thought to have a gynecologic or gastrointestinal malignancy or an intra-abdominal inflammatory process. An awareness of the syndrome together with a high index of suspicion when a patient presents with atypical ascites can lead to the correct diagnosis.

Investigation

This depends upon the use of appropriate laboratory studies, radiologic imaging, and liver biopsy.[38] Laboratory studies are often minimally disturbed in Budd-Chiari syndrome, disproportionately so relative to the damage frequently seen on biopsy. Analysis of the ascites usually shows a serum:ascites albumin gradient >1.1 g/dL and a white cell count that is usually <100/mm^3.

Doppler ultrasound can usually readily visualize the three major hepatic veins and show a characteristic phasic flow pattern. Inability to demonstrate these veins or to show phasic flow should raise a suspicion of hepatic vein occlusion. The portal vein should be imaged both

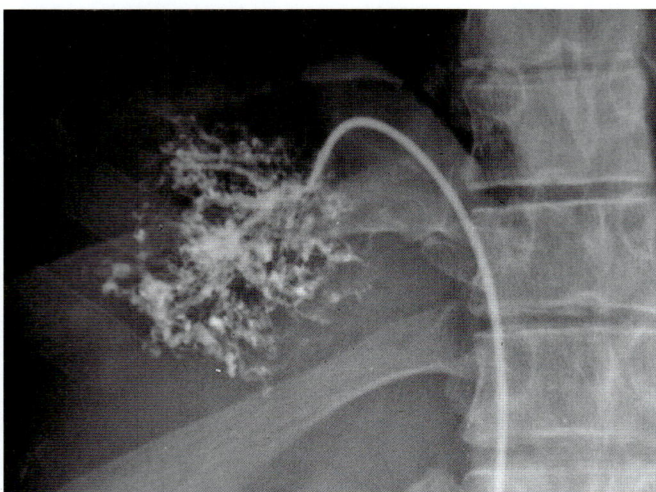

Fig. 54.13: Spider's web of Budd–Chiari syndrome as the sinusoids attempt to decompress to the liver capsule.

for patency and for any dampening of portal flow suggestive of sinusoidal obstruction. Other radiologic imaging techniques such as hepatic scintigraphy, CT, and MRI have been used, but although they can contribute to the diagnosis of Budd-Chiari syndrome, they are not first-line diagnostic modalities. Hepatic venography best performed through a transjugular approach will show the classic appearance of the "spider's web," which reflects the multiple collaterals attempting to drain the obstructed sinusoids (Fig. 54.13).

Liver biopsy should be carried out concurrent with hepatic venography. Biopsies should be taken through all three hepatic veins or at their occluded locations. If this is not possible, differential biopsies of the right and left lobes should be made percutaneously. The axiom that "no patient is too sick to biopsy" is important, as further management decisions are based on biopsy findings. The essential features on liver biopsy are:

- Centrilobular congestion
- Hepatocellular necrosis
- The degree of lobular collapse
- These injuries may lead ultimately to fibrosis and cirrhosis.

It is essential to look for an underlying hematologic disorder, which may be compounded by the development of portal hypertension and splenomegaly. Routine hematologic evaluation (including a blood smear) should be augmented with bone marrow examination, leukocyte alkaline phosphatase measurement, platelet aggregometry, and specific tests for protein C, protein S, antithrombin III, and factor V Leiden.

Flowchart 54.2: Evaluation and management of Budd–Chiari syndrome. (OLT: Orthotopic liver transplantation).

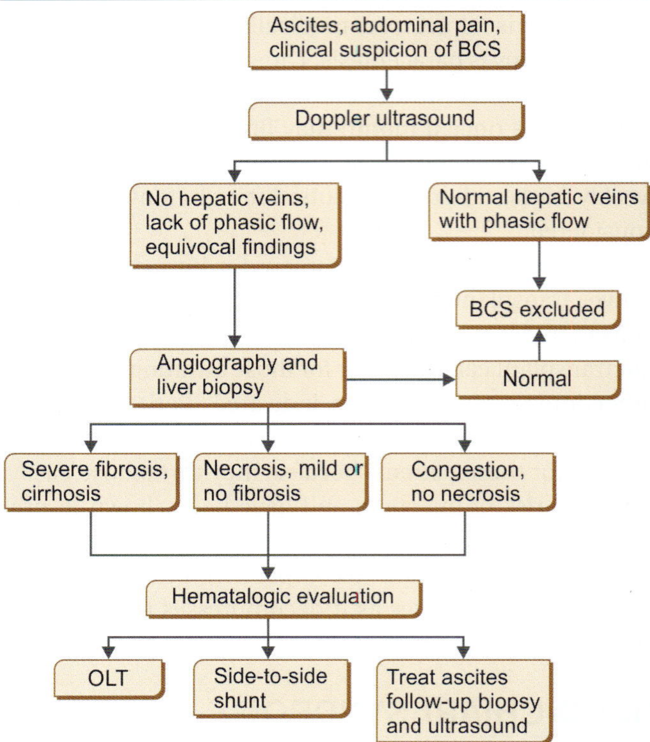

Management

The management of Budd-Chiari syndrome is dictated by the liver biopsy findings and is summarized in Flowchart 54.2. The options are:

- Nonsurgical management
- Surgical decompression
- Liver transplantation.

If the liver biopsy shows congestion but no histologic evidence of ongoing necrosis, symptomatic management of the ascites and treatment of any underlying hematologic disorder will suffice, with a repeat liver biopsy approximately 3 months later to ensure that there is no further liver damage.

If the biopsy shows an acute injury with ongoing hepatocellular necrosis, sinusoidal decompression is indicated. This procedure usually requires a side-to-side portosystemic shunt, thereby using the open portal vein as a decompressive route from the obstructed sinusoids. This can be achieved by:

- Transjugular intrahepatic portosystemic stenting[15,39]
- Side-to-side portacaval shunt[40]
- Mesoatrial shunt if the inferior vena cava is obstructed

Full assessment is needed to determine the best option to achieve sinusoidal decompression. Evaluation of the inferior vena cava with venography and pressure measurements is key in making this decision.

Liver transplantation is indicated for patients with advanced disease, usually those who have had repeated thrombotic episodes with progressive fibrosis and cirrhosis.[41,42] Transplant is technically difficult in these patients because of the massive collaterals to the diaphragm, which make hepatectomy hazardous.

Management of the hematologic disorder must parallel the therapy for liver damage. It is important that the hepatologist, the surgeon, and the hematologist all work together in evaluating these patients and making appropriate combined treatment decisions.

REFERENCES

1. Hahn M, Massen O, Nenki M, et al. De eckshe fistel zwischen der unteren hohlvene and der pfortaden und folgen fr den organismus. Arch fr Exp Pathol Pharmakol. 1893;32: 162-210.
2. Whipple AO. The problem of portal hypertension in relation to the hepatosplenopathies. Ann Surg. 1945;122:449-56.
3. Rosch J, Hanafee W, Snow H, et al. Transjugular intrahepatic portacaval shunt. An experimental work. Am J Surg. 1971;121:588-92.
4. Starzl TE, Demetris AJ, Van Thiel D. Liver transplantation (1). N Engl J Med. 1989;321:1014-22.
5. Vianna A, Hayes PC, Moscoso G, et al. Normal venous circulation of the gastroesophageal junction. A route to understanding varices. Gastroenterology. 1987;93:876-89.
6. Gupta TK CL, Groszman RJ. Pathophysiology of portal hypertension. In: LaBreque D (Ed). Clinics in Liver Disease. Philadelphia: WB Saunders; 1997. pp. 1-12.
7. Boyer T. Natural history of portal hypertension. In: LaBreque D (Ed). Clinics in Liver Diseases—Portal Hypertension, Vol 1. Philadelphia: WB Saunders; 1997. pp. 31-44.
8. Pugh RN, Murray-Lyon IM, Dawson JL, et al. Transection of the oesophagus for bleeding oesophageal varices. Br J Surg. 1973;60:646-9.
9. North Italian Endoscopic Club for the Study and Treatment of Esophageal Varices. Prediction of the first variceal hemorrhage in patients with cirrhosis of the liver and esophageal varices. A prospective multicenter study. N Engl J Med. 1988;319:983-9.
10. Burns P, Taylor K, Blei AT. Doppler flowmetry and portal hypertension. Gastroenterology. 1987;92:824-6.
11. D'Amico G, Pagliaro L, Bosch J. The treatment of portal hypertension: a meta-analytic review. Hepatology. 1995;22: 332-54.
12. Lebrec D, Nouel O, Corbic M, et al. Propranolol—a medical treatment for portal hypertension? Lancet. 1980;ii:180-2.
13. Stiegmann GV, Goff JS, Michaletz-Onody PA, et al. Endoscopic sclerotherapy as compared with endoscopic ligation for bleeding esophageal varices. N Engl J Med. 1992; 326:1527-32.
14. Colapinto RF, Stronell RD, Gildiner M, et al. Formation of intrahepatic portosystemic shunts using a balloon dilatation catheter: preliminary clinical experience. Am J Roentgenol. 1983;140:709-14.
15. Boyer TD, Haskal ZJ. The role of transjugular intrahepatic portosystemic shunt (TIPS) in the management of portal hypertension: update 2009. Hepatology. 2010;51:306.
16. Orloff MJ, Orloff MS, Orloff SL, et al. Three decades of experience with emergency portacaval shunt for acutely bleeding esophageal varices in 400 unselected patients with cirrhosis of the liver [see comments]. J Am Coll Surg. 1995;180:257-72.
17. Sarfeh IJ, Rypins EB, Mason GR. A systematic appraisal of portacaval H-graft diameters. Clinical and hemodynamic perspectives. Ann Surg. 1986;204:356-63.
18. Warren WD, Zeppa R, Fomon JJ. Selective trans-splenic decompression of gastroesophageal varices by distal splenorenal shunt. Ann Surg. 1967;166:437-55.
19. Sugiura M, Futagawa S. Esophageal transection with paraesophagogastric devascularizations (the Sugiura procedure) in the treatment of esophageal varices. World J Surg. 1984;8:673-9.
20. de Franchis R, Primignani M, Arcidiacono PG, et al. Prophylactic sclerotherapy in high-risk cirrhotics selected by endoscopic criteria. A multicenter randomized controlled trial. Gastroenterology. 1991;101:1087-93.
21. Laine L, Cook D. Endoscopic ligation compared with sclerotherapy for treatment of esophageal variceal bleeding. A meta-analysis. Ann Intern Med. 1995;123:280-7.
22. Orozco H, Mercardo MA. Rise and downfall of the empire of portal hypertension surgery. Arch Surg. 2007;142:219-21.
23. Orloff MJ, Isenberg JI, Wheeler HO, et al. Emergency portacaval shunt versus rescue portacaval shunt in a randomized controlled trial of emergency treatment of acutely bleeding esophageal varices in cirrhosis. J Gastrointest Surg. 2010;14:1782-95.
24. Sarfeh I, Rypins E. Partial versus total portacaval H-graft diameters. Ann Surg. 1986;204:356-62.
25. Henderson JM, Gilmore GT, Hooks MA, et al. Selective shunt in the management of variceal bleeding in the era of liver transplantation. Ann Surg. 1992;216:248-54.
26. Henderson JM, Boyer TD, Kutner MH, et al. and the DIVERT Study Group. Distal splenorenal shunt versus transjugular intrahepatic portal systematic shunt for variceal bleeding: a randomized trial. Gastroenterology. 2006;130(6):1643-51.
27. Boyer TD, Henderson JM, Heerey AM, et al. Divert Study Group. Cost of preventing variceal rebleeding with transjugular intrahepatic portal systemic shunt and distal splenorenal shunt. J Hepatol. 2008;48(3):407-14.
28. Rosemurgy AS, Frohman HA, Teta AF, et al. Prosthetic H-graft portacaval shunts vs transjugular intrahepatic portasystemic stent shunts: 18-year follow-up of a randomized trial. J Am Coll Surg. 2012;214:445-53.
29. Bismuth H, Adam R, Mathur S, et al. Options for elective treatment of portal hypertension in cirrhotic patients in the transplantation era. Am J Surg. 1990;160:105-10.

30. Warren WD, Henderson JM, Millikan WJ, et al. Management of variceal bleeding in patients with noncirrhotic portal vein thrombosis. Ann Surg. 1988;207:623-34.
31. Lautz TB, Keys LA, Melvin JC, et al. Advantages of the meso-Rex bypass compared with portosystemic shunts in the management of extrahepatic portal vein obstruction in children. J Am Coll Surg. 2013;216:83-9.
32. Clatworthy HW, Wall T, Watman RN. A new type of portal to systemic venous shunt for portal hypertension. Arch Surg. 1955;71:588-96.
33. Voorhees AB Jr, Chaitman E, Schneider S, et al. Portal-systemic encephalopathy in the noncirrhotic patient. Effect of portal-systemic shunting. Arch Surg. 1973;107:659-63.
34. Alvarez F, Bernard O, Brunelle F, et al. Portal obstruction in children. II. Results of surgical portosystemic shunts. J Pediatr. 1983;103:703-7.
35. Epstein M. Deranged sodium homeostasis in cirrhosis. Gastroenterology. 1979;76:622-35.
36. Ochs A, Rossle M, Haag K, et al. The transjugular intrahepatic portosystemic stent-shunt procedure for refractory ascites [see comments] [published erratum appears in N Engl J Med 1995;332:1587]. N Engl J Med. 1995;332:1192-7.
37. Henderson JM, Warren WD, Millikan WJ Jr, et al. Surgical options, hematologic evaluation, and pathologic changes in Budd-Chiari syndrome. Am J Surg. 1990;159:41-8; discussion 48-50.
38. Valla D, Casadevall N, Lacombe C, et al. Primary myeloproliferative disorder and hepatic vein thrombosis. A prospective study of erythroid colony formation *in vitro* in 20 patients with Budd-Chiari syndrome. Ann Intern Med. 1985;103:329-34.
39. Blum U, Rossie M, Haag K, et al. Budd-Chiari syndrome: technical, hemodynamic, and clinical results of treatment with transjugular intrahepatic portosystemic shunt. Radiology. 1995;197:805-11.
40. Orloff MJ, Girard B. Long-term results of treatment of Budd-Chiari syndrome by side to side portacaval shunt. Surg Gynecol Obstet. 1989;168:33-41.
41. Bismuth H, Sherlock D. Portosystemic shunting versus orthotopic liver transplantation for the Budd-Chiari syndrome. Ann Surg. 1992;214:581-9.
42. Halff G, Todo S, Tzakis AG, et al. Liver transplantation for the Budd-Chiari syndrome. Ann Surg. 1990;211:43-9.

55

Gallbladder and Biliary Tree

Thomas M van Gulik, Dirk J Gouma

Key Points

- Only 50% of individuals have "normal" biliary anatomy. An understanding of the common anomalies of the ducts and arteries is vital to perform a safe cholecystectomy.
- About 10% of the population of the United States have gallstones. Cholesterol is the major component, while bilirubinate predominates in those with hemolysis (black pigment stones) or cholangitis (brown pigment stones).
- Gallbladder stones are frequently "silent" (asymptomatic) but can give rise to one of four clinical syndromes: biliary colic, acute cholecystitis, chronic cholecystitis, and gallstone dyspepsia.
- Bile duct stones are associated with gallbladder stones in 10–15% of patients. They are less likely to be silent and can cause acute cholangitis, obstructive jaundice or acute pancreatitis. About 750,000 cholecystectomies are performed annually in the United States for the symptoms or complications of cholelithiasis, mostly (>95%) by the laparoscopic route.
- Bile duct injury is more common with laparoscopic than open cholecystectomy (0.5% vs. 0.1% of operations), in particular after single incision laparoscopic procedures (SILC). Application of the critical view of safety (CVS) helps to prevent bile duct injury.
- Carcinoma of the gallbladder is related to gallstones, is more common in women and has a better prognosis when discovered incidentally in a cholecystectomy specimen.
- Cholangiocarcinoma is less common and most frequently occurs at the hepatic duct confluence (hilar cholangiocarcinoma), typically giving rise to painless obstructive jaundice.
- Curative resection of (hilar) cholangiocarcinoma usually encompasses resection of the extrahepatic bile ducts in combination with major liver resection including segment 1 of the liver.
- The mainstay of palliative treatment of (hilar) cholangiocarcinoma consists of endoscopic or percutaneous biliary drainage.

INTRODUCTION

In recent years, considerable attention has focused on nonoperative or minimally invasive surgical techniques for the management of symptomatic cholelithiasis. Advances in the treatment of gallstone disease have made it essential for general surgeons to understand the biochemistry and anatomy of the biliary tract. The management of gallstone disease has been revolutionized by the development of laparoscopic cholecystectomy and related procedures, such as endoscopic retrograde cholangiopancreatography (ERCP). This new technology continues to evolve, and its broad application to the management of gallstone disease represents one of the greatest advances in modern surgery and also one of its greatest challenges. Laparoscopic cholecystectomy has rapidly become the preferred treatment for patients with symptomatic gallstone disease. Laparoscopic methods have shortened hospital stay and return to employment, thereby reducing the direct and indirect costs of gallstones. Although concerns persist regarding the incidence of bile duct injury and appropriate mechanisms for credentialing, laparoscopic cholecystectomy has evolved as the gold standard of surgical care. Nevertheless, understanding the appropriate indications for percutaneous or endoscopic treatment of gallstones is essential to manage high-risk patients who might be poor candidates for operation.

SURGICAL ANATOMY OF THE BILIARY TREE

Embryology and Development of the Biliary Tract

The liver, gallbladder, and bile ducts arise during the fourth week of gestation as a ventral bud from the most caudal

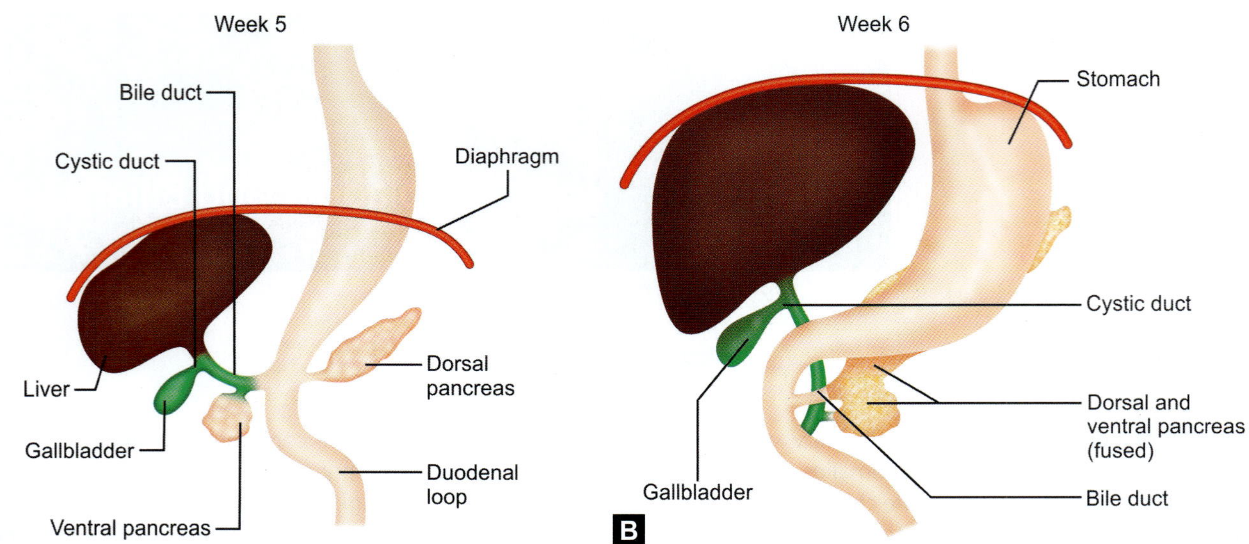

Figs. 55.1A and B: Early development of the foregut. The extrahepatic biliary tree rotates relative to the duodenum between weeks 5 and 6 of gestation. As a result, the common bile duct courses through the ventral pancreas posterior to the duodenum. The gallbladder then develops as a true diverticulum of the bile duct.

part of the foregut (Figs. 55.1A and B).[1] As a result, the common bile duct (CBD) remains associated with the ventral pancreas, which develops into the uncinate process of the pancreas in the adult. Counterclockwise rotation of the foregut causes the CBD to cross behind the first portion of the duodenum and course through the uncinate process, draining into the dorsal duodenal lumen. A small caudal portion of the hepatic diverticulum expands to form the gallbladder, with its stalk becoming the cystic duct. Initially, the extrahepatic biliary tree is occluded with endodermal cells, but is later canalized to form the bile ducts.

Congenital Anomalies of the Gallbladder and Bile Ducts

Most congenital anomalies of the biliary tree result from failure of the extrahepatic biliary tract to canalize. Persistent occlusion of the bile ducts by endoderm may explain extrahepatic biliary atresia, which occurs at the rate of 1 in 20,000 births. These defects are typically recognized during the evaluation of a jaundiced neonate. Developmental defects in the gallbladder are rare and usually lack clinical importance. Anomalies may range from complete agenesis of the gallbladder to hypoplasia, complete duplication of the gallbladder, gallbladder diverticulum, or a septated gallbladder (Fig. 55.2).[2] Furthermore, variations in the position of the gallbladder relative to the liver may also occur. The gallbladder may be totally embedded within the liver substance (known as an intrahepatic gallbladder) or may be floating on a long pendulous mesentery. Most of these anatomic variations are of interest only to surgeons and embryologists.

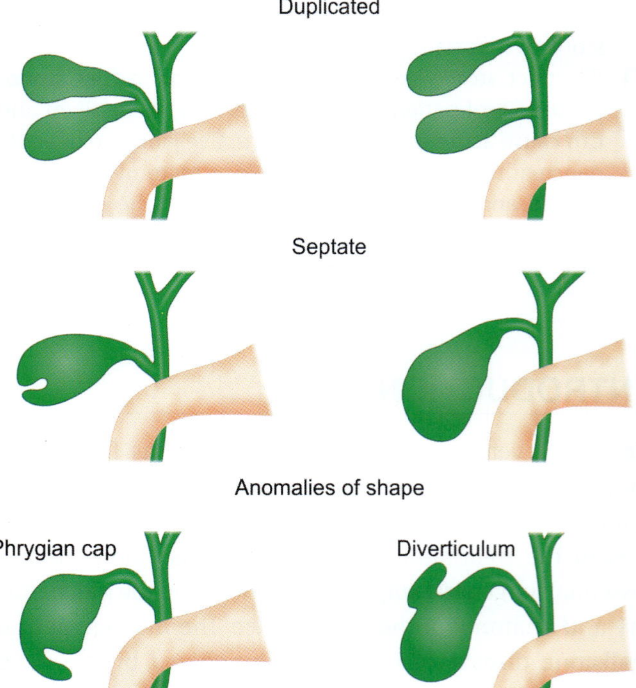

Fig. 55.2: Developmental anomalies of the gallbladder.

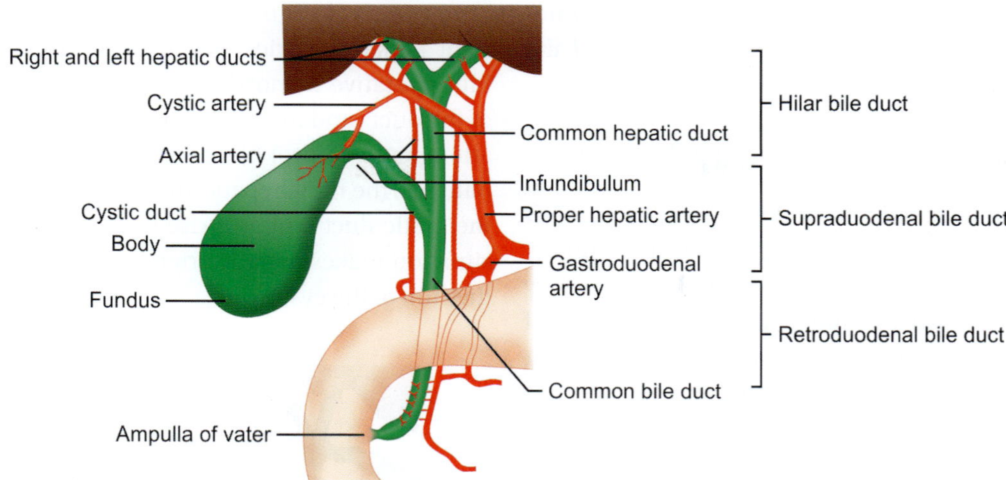

Fig. 55.3: Anatomy of the porta hepatis. The extrahepatic bile duct is divided into three separate anatomic regions—hilar (or proximal), supraduodenal (or mid), and retroduodenal (or distal) bile duct.

Anatomy of the Biliary Tree

The gallbladder develops as a musculomembranous sac lying in a fossa beneath the liver (Fig. 55.3).[2] The gallbladder fossa marks the location of the anatomic division of the right and left hepatic lobes (Cantlie's line). The gallbladder consists of three anatomic regions: the fundus, body and infundibulum (neck), from which bile drains through crescentic mucosal folds known as the spiral valves of Heister into the cystic duct. The capacity of the average gallbladder is 30–50 mL. The gallbladder receives its blood supply from the cystic artery, which is typically a branch of the right hepatic artery. This vessel is subject to wide anatomic variation in up to 25% of individuals.

The right and left main bile ducts drain the right and left hepatic lobes and join at the confluence to form the common hepatic duct. At the entrance of the cystic duct, this structure becomes the CBD, which drains into the duodenum through the ampulla of Vater. The extrahepatic bile ducts pass through the hepatoduodenal ligament anterior to the portal vein and lateral to the arterial structures. The blood supply to the common duct arises from two vessels oriented at the 3 and 9 o'clock positions relative to the duct. These vessels derive their nutrient flow from the right hepatic artery (38% of total flow) and gastroduodenal artery (60%) (Fig. 55.4).[3]

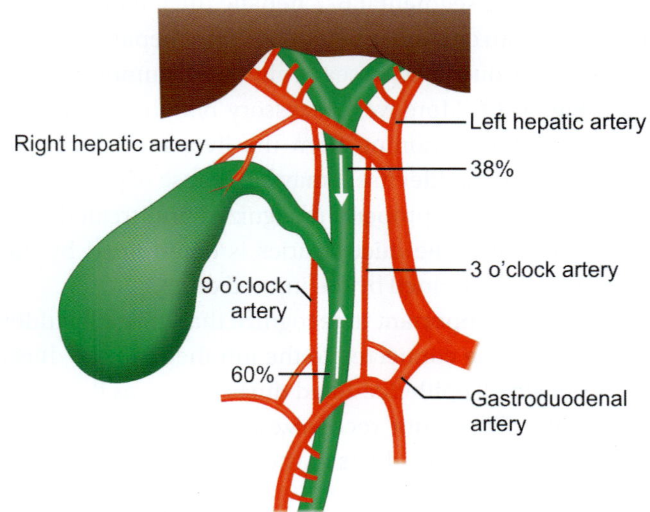

Fig. 55.4: Distribution of blood supply to the extrahepatic biliary tree. The right hepatic artery supplies 38%, and the gastroduodenal artery supplies 60% of blood flow to the common duct.

Microscopic Anatomy of the Gallbladder

Histologically, the gallbladder consists of four layers:

1. Mucosa
2. Fibromuscular layer
3. Perimuscular connective tissue
4. Serosa

The gallbladder is lined by a single layer of columnar epithelial cells that absorb water from the bile and secrete mucus. The mucosa is based on a layer of connective tissue stroma and is surrounded by a fibromuscular layer of smooth muscle, which is responsive to cholecystokinin (CCK); contraction empties the gallbladder following meals. A perimuscular layer containing inflammatory cells and a serous peritoneal layer cover the inner layers, except over the hepatic surface of the gallbladder fossa. The function of the gallbladder is to store and concentrate bile (x10).

In response to CCK secreted by fat entering the duodenum, it contracts with concomitant relaxation of the sphincter of Oddi.

Anatomic Variation of the Biliary Tree

Variations in the development of the hepatic ducts, CBD and cystic duct are so common that "normal" biliary anatomy is found in only 50% of individuals.[4] Accessory hepatic ducts are also common, and an awareness of their potential location is of great importance to prevent bile duct injury during cholecystectomy. Bile duct injuries frequently occur as a result of failure to appreciate the ductal anatomy, whether normal, altered by inflammation or anomalous from birth. Important anatomic variants (Figs. 55.5A to D) that often contribute to this complication are the presence of a short cystic duct, a cystic duct draining into a segmental 6/7 hepatic duct, a cystic duct that drains into or crosses behind the right hepatic duct, or a spiral cystic duct that passes behind the common hepatic duct (Fig. 55.6). Moreover, accessory bile ducts, such as segmental ducts draining from the liver into the cystic duct or the gallbladder itself, may be a cause of postoperative bile leak if not properly recognized and treated. The severity of these bile duct injuries is determined by the amount of liver drained by the injured duct.

Lastly, it is important to recognize that the gallbladder may normally be connected to the intrahepatic bile ducts by way of small, epithelial-lined ducts known as the ducts of Luschka. When not recognized and oversewn intraoperatively, these tiny ducts may cause postoperative bile leaks and bile peritonitis.

Similarly, variations in the location of the cystic and right hepatic arteries can lead to vascular injuries and intraoperative hemorrhage, which obscures the location of the ducts and may predispose to bile duct injury during attempts to control bleeding (Fig. 55.7).[5] In up to 12% of patients, the right hepatic artery may cross directly behind the cystic duct and give rise to a short cystic artery. This situation makes hepatic arterial injury more likely during division of the cystic duct.

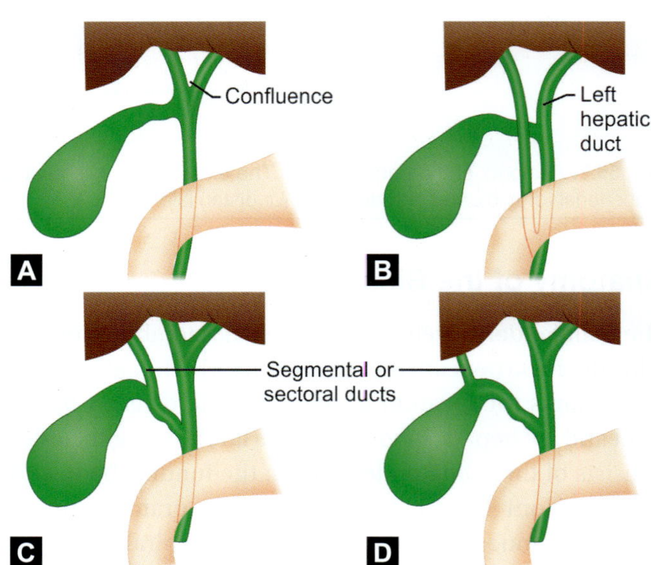

Figs. 55.5A to D: Anatomic variation in the cystic duct and accessory ducts to the gallbladder. The cystic duct can arise directly from the hilar confluence (A) as well as from the left hepatic duct. Anomaly (B) requires the cystic duct to cross behind the right hepatic duct before reaching the gallbladder. Accessory segmental (C) and sectoral (D) ducts may also enter the gallbladder directly from the hepatic parenchyma.

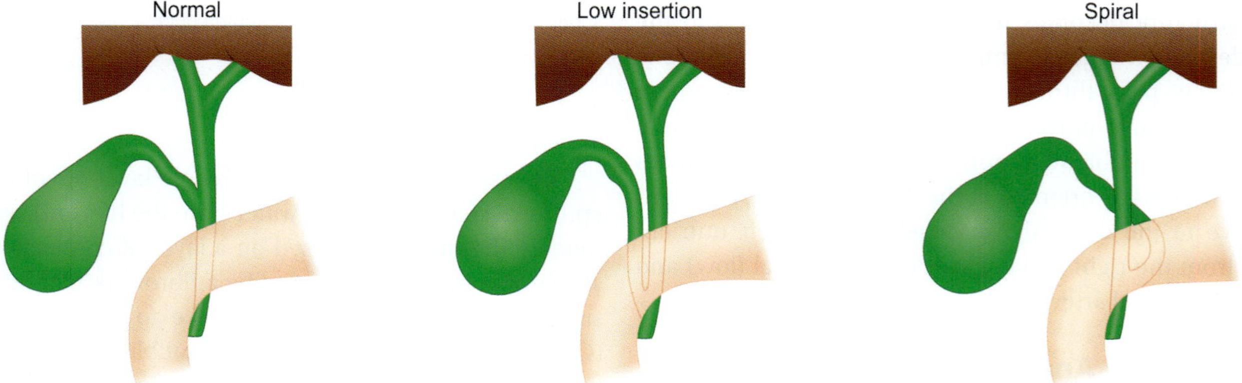

Fig. 55.6: Variations in length and disposition of the cystic duct. The cystic duct has a "normal" relationship with the common duct in 75% of individuals, but may also arise distally and share a common wall with the hepatic duct (20%) or pass spirally behind the common duct to enter the gallbladder (5%). The spiral arrangement places the common duct at greater risk for inadvertent injury during cholecystectomy.

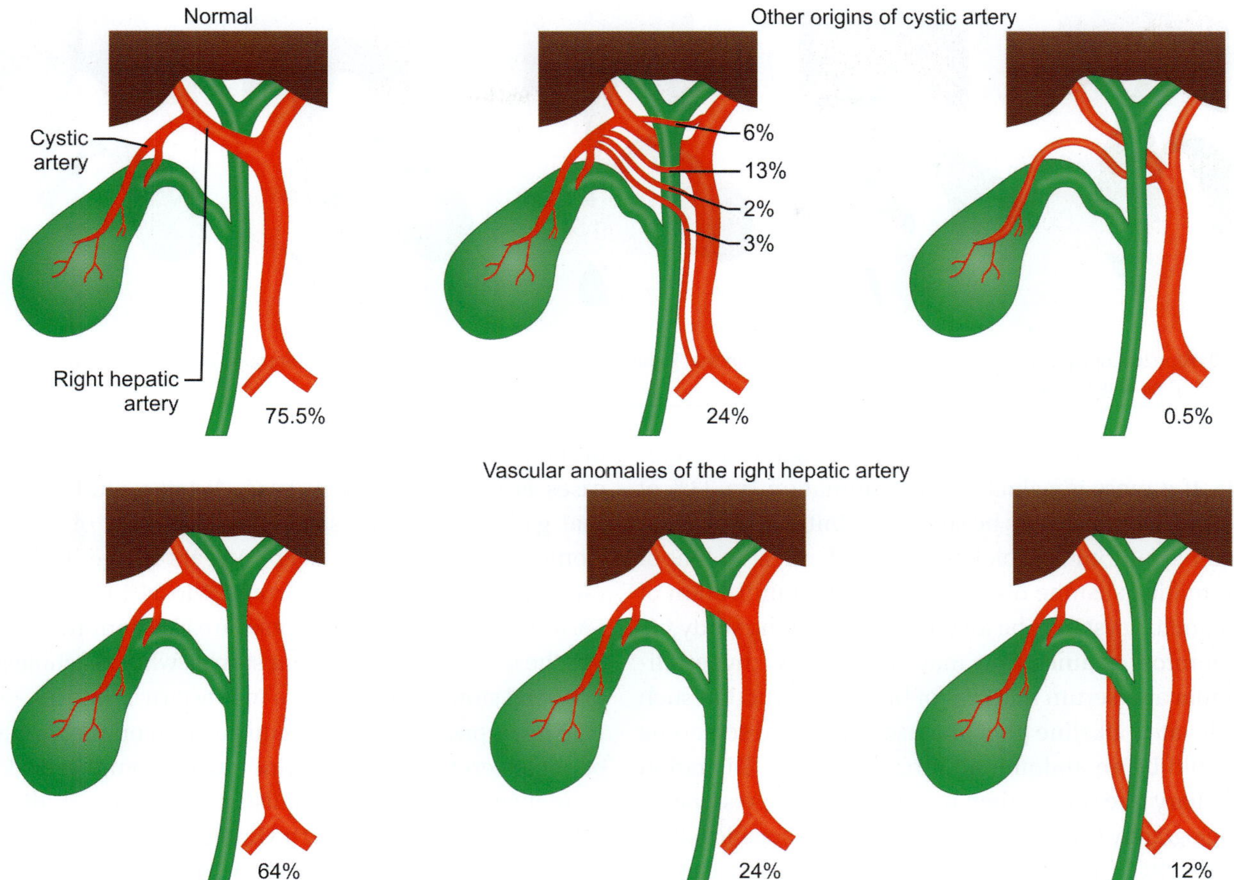

Fig. 55.7: Vascular anomalies of the porta hepatis. The cystic artery "normally" arises from the right hepatic artery to the right of the bile duct, but may also arise from the left (6%) or proper (2%) hepatic arteries as well as the gastroduodenal (3%) artery before crossing the common hepatic duct and entering the gallbladder. Vascular anomalies of the right hepatic artery may cause it to be misidentified as the cystic artery.

CONGENITAL ANOMALIES OF THE BILIARY TRACT

Biliary Atresia

Biliary atresia is covered in Chapter 125, "Gastrointestinal Surgery in Children".

Choledochal Cyst

Choledochal cysts are congenital malformations of the biliary tree characterized by extrahepatic ductal dilatation in over 90% of cases. Although rare worldwide, they are more common in Japan than in North America and Western Europe. Surgical management of choledochal cyst disease is based upon the anatomic classification first proposed by Alonzo-Lej in 1959 (Fig. 55.8).[6]

Histologically, choledochal cysts are thick-walled fibrotic dilatations of the extrahepatic biliary tree with usually discontinuous columnar epithelium. They are thought to form as a result of reflux of pancreatic secretions into the CBD because of an anomalous union of the pancreatic and bile ducts, which creates a long common channel. Reflux of trypsin into the common duct damages the duct and produces ductal dilatation.

Patients with choledochal cysts have an increased risk of malignant degeneration of the biliary epithelium and the development of cholangiocarcinoma, in addition to recurrent cholangitis and gallstone formation. The incidence of bile duct cancer increases with age and exceeds 10% in patients over 20 years of age.[7]

Patients are divided into two distinct groups based on the presenting symptoms. The first group comprises infants who present within the first 6 months of life with symptoms of bile duct obstruction suggestive of biliary atresia. Approximately, 50% of choledochal cysts are recognized before the patient is 10 years of age. The second, adult form of presentation occurs in people over 2 years of age and is characterized by abdominal pain (78% of cases),

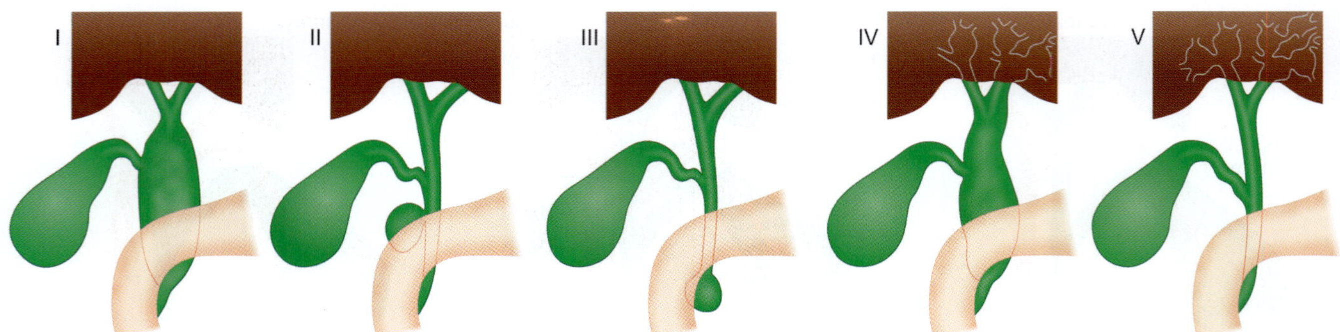

Fig. 55.8: Alonzo-Lej classification of choledochal cysts with the Todani modification. Type I is the most common. Type III is known as a choledochocele. Type V is Caroli's disease.

jaundice (43%), and occasionally cholangitis or pancreatitis. If a mass is palpable on examination (in 33% of cases), the diagnosis may be suspected initially. However, the adult symptom complex is almost identical to that of symptomatic gallstone disease, and the first indication of a choledochal cyst may be an abnormal imaging study.[8]

Laboratory examination may reveal direct hyperbilirubinemia and serum markers of biliary obstruction such as an elevated alkaline phosphatase. The initial screening test should be an abdominal ultrasound scan. Dilatation of the biliary tree should then prompt magnetic resonance cholangiography (MRC) to visualize the extrahepatic biliary tree. The ERCP or transhepatic cholangiography can be performed to aid in preoperative planning of the type of resection. Modern surgical management stresses resection of the cyst with either choledocho- or hepaticojejunostomy to minimize the risks of malignant degeneration of the cyst lining and postoperative cholangitis, as well as stricture.[8,9]

Anomalous pancreaticobiliary ductal junction (APBDJ) occurs when union of the main pancreatic duct and CBD occurs before the ducts enter the duodenal wall. Anomalous pancreaticobiliary ductal junction is often associated with choledochal cyst formation and pancreaticobiliary reflux and can give rise to intermittent abdominal pain, jaundice, and cholangitis. The anomaly is confirmed at ERCP or magnetic resonance cholangiopancreatography (MRCP). Because of the increased risk of malignant transformation, resection of the gallbladder and extrahepatic bile ducts is usually advised.[10,11]

PATHOPHYSIOLOGY OF GALLSTONES

Incidence of Gallstones

The incidence of gallstones varies throughout the world, as a result of ethnic, dietary, and poorly understood demographic factors.[12] In the United States, approximately 10% of the population has gallstones and up to 1 million new cases are diagnosed each year. Autopsy studies suggest that gallstones are present in at least 20% of American women and 8% of men over 40 years of age. In Europe, rates of cholelithiasis range from 8% to 34% in women and 5% to 13% in men.[13,14] Gallstones are also common in Asia, but these are usually pigment stones, whereas cholesterol or mixed stones predominate in Western countries.

The impact of genetic predisposition on the formation of cholesterol gallstones cannot be overemphasized. The incidence of cholesterol gallstones in Pima Indians, a tribe from the southwestern United States, has been well characterized: in women aged 25–34 years it is in excess of 70%.[15] By contrast, the incidence of gallstones in Africa is reported to be <5%.[16]

Classification of Gallstones

Biliary calculi can be classified according to their:

- Composition (cholesterol, mixed, or pigment stones)
- Location within the gallbladder or bile ducts
- Site of origin

The clinical syndrome associated with gallbladder calculi appears to be virtually identical regardless of stone composition. The management of bile duct stones, however, may be quite different depending upon their composition.

Gallstone Composition

Gallstones reside within the gallbladder, extrahepatic biliary tract, or intrahepatic ductal system. Most gallstone patients in Western countries have gallbladder stones, whereas intrahepatic stones are endemic in Southeast Asia. Gallbladder stones may be small and multiple or single and moderately large. Despite wide variation in their color, size and shape, these calculi can be simply grouped as either cholesterol or pigment stones.

Pure cholesterol stones are relatively uncommon and have a characteristic appearance, tending to be yellow with multiple facets. Most patients in the United States have mixed gallstones that contain a small amount of calcium, bile salt, and protein in addition to cholesterol. In the United States, cholesterol and mixed gallstones account for approximately 60–70% of all calculi. Pigment gallstones occur in a diverse group of clinical settings and are characterized by high concentrations of calcium and bilirubin and low concentrations of cholesterol (<10%). "Black" pigment stones are typically tarry in appearance and form exclusively in the gallbladder. They are common in patients who have cirrhosis and hemolytic disorders. "Brown" pigment stones are soft and crush easily. These stones form in association with endemic biliary tract infection and often arise within the extrahepatic biliary tree.

Location and Site of Origin

Most patients with calculous disease have gallbladder calculi. These stones may be cholesterol, mixed, or pigment stones. Bile duct stones are generally classified as either primary (stones forming de novo in the CBD) or secondary (arising in the gallbladder and passing into the CBD through the cystic duct). Epidemiologic evidence suggests that CBD stones are usually of gallbladder origin in Western countries.[17]

Calcium bilirubinate and pigment stones form anywhere within the bile ducts and constitute the largest fraction of primary ductal stones; most of these patients have biliary bacterial infection and stasis. Intrahepatic stones are uncommon in Western countries, whereas the incidence of hepatolithiasis is highest in Southeast Asia.

Factors Predisposing to Gallstone Formation

The three specific events leading to cholesterol gallstone formation comprise hepatic secretion of cholesterol saturated bile, nucleation, and stone growth. In addition, changes in gallbladder absorptive function and contractility contribute to early cholesterol gallstone formation. The formation of pigment gallstones is promoted by excessive bilirubin production, disorders of bile acid and calcium metabolism, and gallbladder stasis combined with bacterial infection.

Several etiologic factors can increase the risk of gallstone formation. The incidence increases linearly with age. Although there is some evidence that genetic factors predispose to gallstone formation, the importance of a family history of gallstones is not well defined. The clinical axiom that the typical patient who has gallstones is "female, fat, fertile, and forty" is based on strong scientific evidence. Some studies have suggested that multiple pregnancies increase the risk of gallstones, while incomplete emptying of the gallbladder and stasis of bile are important contributing factors to gallstone formation in pregnant women.[18] The incidence is also higher in women on the oral contraceptive pill.

Morbidly obese patients have an intrinsic, increased risk of cholelithiasis. The explanation is probably altered hepatic lipid metabolism with increased secretion of biliary cholesterol relative to phospholipids and bile salts, resulting in cholesterol-saturated bile. Numerous studies indicate that gallstones may be a complication of both operative and nonoperative treatment for morbid obesity. Over 25% of obese patients who undergo vertical banded gastroplasty had previously required cholecystectomy for gallstones.[19]

The inherent association between obesity and gallstone formation, coupled with the observation that rapid weight loss causes the hepatic secretion of cholesterol-saturated bile, has led to considering prophylactic cholecystectomy during bariatric surgery, although this remains a matter of debate. Warschkow and coworkers showed in a meta-analysis that the rate of patients needing a subsequent cholecystectomy because of symptomatic biliary disease after laparoscopic gastric bypass without concomitant cholecystectomy is 6.8%.[20] Prophylactic cholecystectomy during bariatric surgery should, however, be avoided in patients without cholelithiasis. A recent report of weight-loss induced gallstone formation indicates that prophylactic oral therapy with ursodiol effectively prevents cholelithiasis after gastric bypass. Obese patients appear to be more resistant to oral dissolution therapy with bile acids than patients of normal weight.

An increased risk of gallstone formation has been reported as a consequence of diseases that alter biliary metabolism or decrease gallbladder motility. Therefore, hyperlipidemia, diabetes mellitus, cystic fibrosis, short bowel syndrome, and resection of the terminal ileum have all been associated with an increased risk of cholelithiasis. In addition, total parenteral nutrition has been associated with an increased risk of gallstone formation in both adults and children.

DIAGNOSIS OF CHOLELITHIASIS

Natural History

Defining the natural history of gallstone disease has become more important in recent years because of the emergence of minimally invasive technologies. Previously, definitive treatment for gallstone disease was reserved for patients who had definite symptoms because of the morbidity and mortality rates of surgical management. Following increased patient acceptance of laparoscopic operations, cholecystectomy rates have been increasing rapidly, reaching 750,000 operations annually in the United States alone. The economic importance of this phenomenon is underscored by the frequency with which this disease occurs throughout the world.

It is necessary to understand the natural history of asymptomatic gallstones to avoid overtreating the large number of asymptomatic patients who have a minimal risk of developing complications. Longitudinal studies indicate that gallstones become symptomatic at a lower rate than originally thought, with <20% of initially asymptomatic patients requiring operation for symptoms or complications of cholelithiasis over a 20-year period. Therefore, prophylactic cholecystectomy cannot be endorsed for all asymptomatic patients. However, the clinical course for patients who have cholelithiasis is not predictable once symptoms begin to occur.[21] Minor episodes of biliary colic may resolve or progress to any of the numerous complications of gallstones. As a result of the uncertain course of symptomatic stones, surgical intervention is widely advocated once symptoms develop.

Laboratory Studies

The presence of gallstones in the gallbladder does not necessarily produce any hematologic or biochemical abnormalities. Patients who have symptomatic stones may manifest laboratory evidence of inflammation and abnormal liver function. Most patients with symptoms but without acute inflammation of the gallbladder have a normal white blood cell count. An elevated white blood cell count is generally observed in patients who have acute cholecystitis or cholangitis. Leukocytosis associated with fever and right upper quadrant tenderness is excellent clinical evidence for acute cholecystitis, whereas the addition of jaundice suggests acute cholangitis.

Evaluation of a patient with abnormal liver function tests must determine whether the underlying disease process is cholestatic, hepatocellular, or hemolytic. Jaundice in a patient who has gallstones does not necessarily signify choledocholithiasis; other disease processes such as acute hepatitis, ischemic liver injury, hemolytic anemia, and intrahepatic cholestasis must be excluded. The typical pattern of liver enzymes in a patient with extrahepatic bile duct obstruction includes a serum alkaline phosphatase level more than two to three times normal in the presence of aminotransferase levels < 300 U/L (5 μkat/L).[22] The degree of elevation in serum bilirubin depends upon the duration of CBD obstruction.

Diagnostic Imaging Studies

Several diagnostic studies are available to evaluate patients with suspected cholelithiasis. It is important to understand the sensitivity, specificity, and limitations of each of them to maximize the diagnostic accuracy. This is a particularly relevant consideration in the modern era of cost containment.

Although less used nowadays, supine and upright abdominal films may be obtained when patients present with acute abdominal pain to exclude other diagnoses such as pneumoperitoneum resulting from a perforated viscus. On occasion, plain radiographs may establish the diagnosis of gallstones when appreciable amounts of calcium are present, a finding in only 10–25% of patients. When present on plain radiographs, gallstones appear as an incomplete ring density in the right upper abdominal quadrant. The calcified silhouette of a gallbladder is pathognomic of a porcelain gallbladder, and air within the biliary tree is evidence of a *cholecystenteric* fistula.

Ultrasonography

Ultrasound scanning is established as the diagnostic test of choice for patients with uncomplicated gallstone disease. It has numerous advantages including ease of performance, independence from patient compliance and gastrointestinal function, and avoidance of radiation exposure. Furthermore, ultrasonography allows routine evaluation of the liver, CBD, and pancreas in addition to the gallbladder. The accuracy of identifying gallstones exceeds 95%.[23] Classically, gallstones appear as intraluminal echogenic foci with acoustic shadowing that move as the patient changes position. Ultrasonography reveals the number of gallstones, size, and shape of the gallbladder, and thickness of the gallbladder wall. It may support the clinical suspicion of acute cholecystitis by revealing gallbladder wall thickening, pericholecystic fluid, and a sonographic Murphy's sign (defined as right upper quadrant tenderness produced by pressure from the ultrasound probe on the inflamed gallbladder). In addition, dilatation of the intra- and extrahepatic biliary ducts may indicate the presence of common duct stones or obstruction, although bowel gas may obscure the ductal calculi themselves.

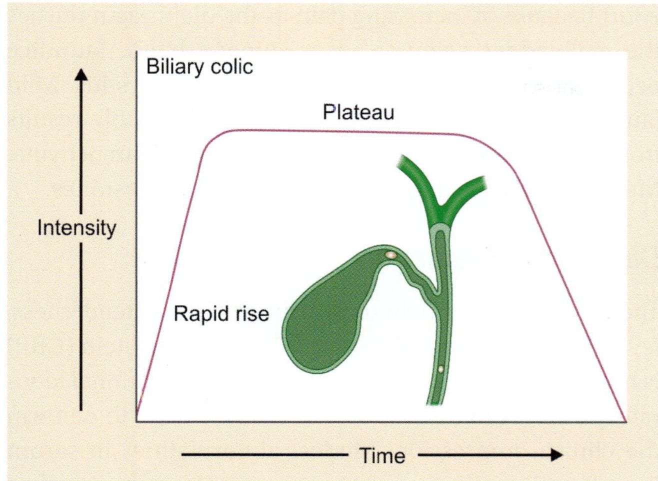

Fig. 55.9: Intensity of biliary colic with time. Impaction of a gallstone in the cystic duct leads to prolonged painful contraction of the obstructed gallbladder and a profile of pain represented diagrammatically in this figure.

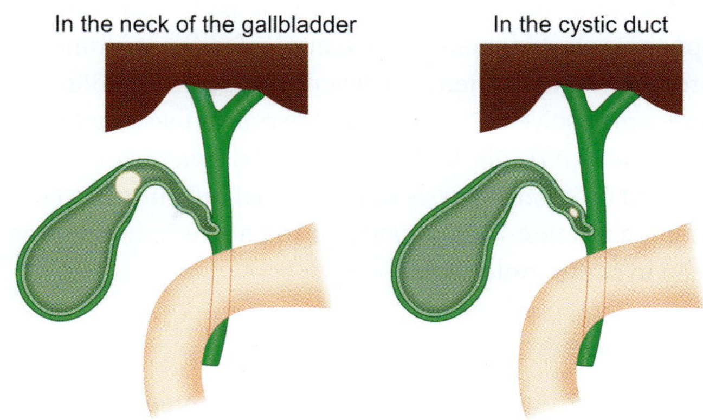

Fig. 55.10: Impacted gallstone. Impaction of a gallstone in the neck of the gallbladder or cystic duct obstructs the gallbladder and initiates the cascade of events leading to acute cholecystitis.

Computed Tomography

In general, CT scanning is not a good screening test for the identification of gallstones, although it will reveal the presence of calcified stones. In this context, the sensitivity of CT scanning does not approach that of ultrasonography. The low sensitivity of CT, coupled with the necessary radiation exposure and higher cost, makes it unjustifiable as a routine study in patients suspected of having uncomplicated gallstone disease.

Cholangiography: ERCP and Percutaneous Transhepatic Cholangiography

Endoscopic retrograde cholangiopancreatography is an important modality for both the diagnosis and therapy of complicated gallstone disease.[24] The advent of laparoscopic cholecystectomy has created enormous interest in defining the role of preoperative ERCP in patients with suspected CBD stones. This is discussed in more detail later in this chapter.

Percutaneous transhepatic cholangiography (PTC) is an additional radiologic procedure that can be of great diagnostic and therapeutic benefit in the management of complicated biliary disease, but it is rarely needed for the routine management of gallstones.

Magnetic resonance imaging (MRI) including cholangiopancreatography (MRCP) is generally not applied for detection of gallstone disease but is useful for the diagnosis of CBD stones and has partly replaced ERCP.

CLINICAL SYNDROMES ASSOCIATED WITH GALLBLADDER STONES

Biliary Colic

The classic symptom of patients with cholelithiasis is intermittent right upper quadrant pain, commonly known as biliary colic. The pain results from cystic duct obstruction and distension of the gallbladder. In contrast to the waxing and waning pattern of other colic syndromes, biliary colic is often described as sudden in onset with a steady increase in intensity. The pain reaches a peak and persists for a variable period of time, up to 24 hours, before its gradual resolution (Fig. 55.9). Although the classic location is in the right upper quadrant, pain may be localized to the midepigastrium, the back or the inferior edge of the right scapula. Biliary colic typically begins postprandially and is particularly common in the evening after a large meal. Although fatty foods are widely believed to exacerbate biliary colic, any type of meal can precipitate an attack.

Acute Cholecystitis

Pathogenesis

The inciting event for the development of acute cholecystitis is cystic duct obstruction. The obstruction is usually caused by a stone becoming impacted in the cystic duct or, less commonly, in Hartmann's pouch (Fig. 55.10). The pathogenesis of cholecystitis is not well understood, but it is probably a consequence of combined mechanical, chemical, and infectious processes.[25] Gallbladder distension eventually leads to ischemia and chemical irritation of the mucosa because of the local release of lysolecithin and other factors. Although the initial pathologic process appears to be biochemical, bacterial infection is ultimately present in most patients with acute cholecystitis. Bile cultures are positive in 75% of cases. The commonest organisms are *Escherichia coli, Klebsiella* spp, and *Enterococcus* spp. Current opinion suggests that bacterial infection is a consequence rather than a cause of the acute inflammation seen in acute cholecystitis.

Incidence

Acute cholecystitis has traditionally accounted for 20% of all patients who undergo cholecystectomy.[26] Recent studies suggest that acute cholecystitis is increasingly an indication for cholecystectomy. Analysis of 42,474 cholecystectomies showed a 35% incidence of acute cholecystitis.[27] This trend is particularly evident in hospitals that provide care for the indigent. In one such institution, the proportion of patients requiring cholecystectomy for acute cholecystitis increased from 33% to 49% over an 8-year period. Possible explanations for the growing incidence of acute cholecystitis in the United States include alterations in healthcare reimbursement, reallocation of healthcare resources, limited access for an increasing segment of the population and physician attitudes to operative treatment, especially for elderly patients in the United States; all these factors may have reduced the number of operations performed for biliary colic alone.

Clinical Syndrome

Symptomatically, the pain of acute cholecystitis is similar to that of biliary colic. However, acute cholecystitis is longer in duration and lasts from one to several days, in contrast to biliary colic, which resolves spontaneously within 24 hours. As the gallbladder becomes progressively distended, the adjacent parietal peritoneum becomes inflamed, which results in the perception of well-localized pain. Associated symptoms include anorexia, nausea, emesis, and fever. Although most patients who have cholecystitis have an elevated temperature and leukocytosis, fever may be absent in the elderly or immunocompromised patient. Abdominal examination reveals tenderness and guarding over the fundus of the gallbladder in the right upper quadrant. A palpable mass in the right upper quadrant may be appreciated in 20% of patients with acute cholecystitis. This finding results from the presence of a distended gallbladder or adherent omentum. The classic physical finding of Murphy's sign is the arrest of inspiratory effort because of increasing pain as the diaphragm pushes the gallbladder against the examiner's hand. Jaundice occurs in <15% of patients with acute cholecystitis. Mild jaundice in cases of acute cholecystitis probably results from contiguous inflammation of the hepatic parenchyma. Marked jaundice suggests the presence of CBD stones.

Diagnostic Evaluation

The combination of right upper quadrant pain, tenderness, fever, leukocytosis, and elevated C-reactive protein (CRP) is highly suggestive of acute cholecystitis. Additional laboratory and radiologic studies should be used to confirm the clinical impression. Modest abnormalities in serum liver function tests are not unusual. However, marked elevations of alkaline phosphatase and bilirubin suggest a diagnosis of cholangitis rather than acute cholecystitis. As the presence of gallstones is the only information required in a patient who has a straightforward clinical presentation of acute cholecystitis, ultrasound scanning has become the diagnostic procedure of choice in this clinical setting. The differential diagnosis of acute cholecystitis includes other important causes of right-sided abdominal pain, such as peptic ulcer disease, acute appendicitis, gastric ulcer, acute pancreatitis, viral hepatitis, acute alcoholic hepatitis, pneumonia, and myocardial ischemia.

Management

The treatment of acute cholecystitis has evolved over the past 20 years.[25] Although early cholecystectomy is currently favored, initial therapy used to consist of hospitalization, intravenous hydration, and antibiotic therapy. Cholecystectomy was deferred for 6–8 weeks to allow inflammation to subside. This approach was challenged by a number of prospective, randomized studies that compared delayed and early cholecystectomy for acute cholecystitis.[28] Early cholecystectomy was associated with a lower risk of bile duct injuries, shorter total hospital length of stay, and improved operative outcomes.

As 75% of patients who have acute cholecystitis improve rapidly with antibiotic therapy, it is theoretically possible to "relax" the time frame for early cholecystectomy. However, delay often means performing cholecystectomy during the subacute phase of the disease. In place of the edema that may facilitate dissection in early acute cholecystitis, subacute cholecystitis is characterized by increased vascularity and early fibrosis, which makes dissection more difficult. Although "early" cannot be defined

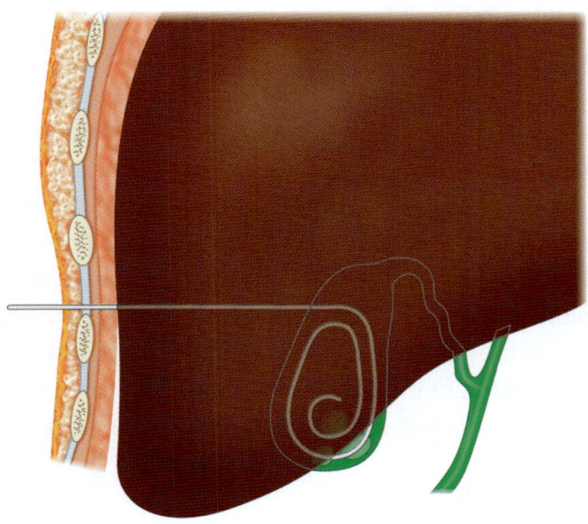

Fig. 55.11: Percutaneous cholecystostomy tube placed transhepatically for evacuation of the gallbladder.

precisely, cholecystectomy performed shortly after the diagnosis of acute cholecystitis will avoid operations during the subacute phase. The routine use of the laparoscopic approach also in an emergency context supports the policy of early cholecystectomy in acute cholecystitis.

Occasionally, cholecystectomy may be associated with excessive operative mortality in patients with medical comorbidities. In this clinical setting, cholecystostomy under local anesthetic or (preferably) percutaneous catheter drainage (Fig. 55.11) of the gallbladder may be lifesaving.[29] Alternatively, subtotal cholecystectomy leaving a strip of gallbladder wall adjacent to the liver or leaving a portion of the neck of the gallbladder avoids a full dissection in Calot's triangle.

Chronic Cholecystitis

Chronic cholecystitis is the result of inflammatory changes in the gallbladder wall caused by the mere presence of gallstones. Histologically, only minimal evidence of chronic mural inflammation may be present. Rokitansky-Aschoff sinuses in the gallbladder wall may become prominent because of elevated intraluminal pressure. The gallbladder may vary in size between contracted and enlarged; and its size depends upon the balance between mural fibrosis and ductal obstruction. Typically, the gallbladder wall is thickened, but the mucosa itself is intact and there is a variable degree of inflammatory cell infiltrate. Previous bouts of acute or subacute cholecystitis are not necessary preludes to a clinical syndrome of chronic cholecystitis. Symptoms of chronic cholecystitis are those of long-standing biliary colic with recurrent bouts of postprandial pain. Patients often complain of moderate-to-severe bouts of pain in the right upper quadrant or epigastrium, which typically radiate to the right scapula. Ultrasound examination reveals cholelithiasis and a thickened gallbladder wall. Depending upon the severity of the inflammatory process, the diagnosis may also be suggested by the presence of a small contracted gallbladder.

Atypical presentations of gallstone disease are not uncommon. Rather than the classic symptoms of biliary colic, these include chronic upper abdominal discomfort, dyspepsia, flatulence, and heartburn. The precise physiologic basis for these symptoms in the setting of gallstones remains unclear. Nonetheless, cholecystectomy is often curative. There may be tiny calculi in the resected gallbladder that have been missed on imaging or mild degrees of chronic cholecystitis or one of the cholecystoses, namely adenomyosis (diverticular disease) or cholesterosis. Xanthogranulomatous cholecystitis is an uncommon inflammatory condition characterized by a destructive inflammatory process featuring lipid-laden macrophages.

Choledocholithiasis

Detection

Between 10% and 15% of patients who have stones in the gallbladder also have stones in the CBD. The incidence of CBD stones increases with age and reaches 50% in patients over the age of 65 years. Most CBD stones form in the gallbladder and pass through the cystic duct into the CBD. Although CBD stones are often asymptomatic, they can be a cause of obstructive jaundice, cholangitis, or biliary pancreatitis. Patients with ductal stones may present with abdominal pain and back pain that is intermittent and episodic in nature. A suspicion of CBD stones before operation (e.g. previous jaundice or a dilated duct on ultrasonography) should prompt evaluation to confirm the diagnosis and achieve stone removal if possible.

Although there is considerable controversy about the optimal and most cost-effective way to accomplish this goal, most surgeons recommend ERCP.[30] Endoscopic sphincterotomy and lithotomy can result in clearance of the duct in most cases. If CBD stones are recognized at the time of open or laparoscopic cholecystectomy, they should be removed. The experience with laparoscopic removal of common duct stones varies, and occasionally a surgeon may opt to defer stone removal to the endoscopist postoperatively because this can usually be achieved with ERCP. Stones are inadvertently left in the bile duct in approximately 1–5% of patients undergoing cholecystectomy, and they require removal at a later date. The options for the treatment of missed CBD stones include endoscopic retrieval, percutaneous removal using lithotripsy, or baskets and surgical intervention.

Clinical Syndromes

Obstructive jaundice: Patients with CBD stones may present with jaundice as the only manifestation. In this setting, the onset of jaundice is likely to be acute, rather than progressive, as might be noted with malignant obstruction. Likewise the gallbladder is not usually palpable because the bile duct obstruction is seldom complete (Courvoisier's law). Careful evaluation should exclude other types of jaundice including hepatocellular disturbances and other causes of extrahepatic biliary obstruction.[22] Ultrasonography, CT scan, or MRI/MRCP should demonstrate an obstructed biliary tree with evidence of intra- and extrahepatic bile duct dilatation. Appropriate therapeutic options include endoscopic extraction of the CBD stones, percutaneous manipulation by the radiologist and, ultimately, surgical CBD exploration.

Biliary pancreatitis: The relationship between gallstones and acute pancreatitis was first recognized >100 years ago,[31] but it was Acosta and Ledesma in Argentina who showed that transient blockage of the ampulla of Vater by a migrating stone initiates the cascade of events culminating in acute pancreatitis.[32] Multiple small gallstones and a patent cystic duct are among the factors that predispose to gallstone pancreatitis.[33] The pathophysiology of biliary pancreatitis has been the subject of considerable investigation in recent years.

Acute cholangitis: This common presentation of ductal stones is covered later in this chapter.

COMPLICATIONS OF CHOLECYSTITIS

Perforation

Gallbladder perforation occurs in approximately 3–10% of patients with acute gallbladder inflammation. Traditionally, gallbladder perforation has been classified as acute, subacute, or chronic.

Acute free perforation of the gallbladder is uncommon and typically occurs in patients who are immunosuppressed or who have systemic vascular disease.[18] The fundus is the least vascularized portion of the gallbladder and the most common site of perforation. These patients generally present with an acute abdomen, and aggressive intervention is essential. Precise preoperative diagnosis is unusual, and the diagnosis is usually secured at the time of operation for an acute abdomen. Long-standing gallstone disease and repeated episodes of inflammation lead to scarring, fibrosis, and adhesions between the gallbladder and contiguous structures. Diffuse peritoneal contamination after perforation is usually minimized by these adjacent adhesions. Gallbladder perforation with pericholecystic fluid or abscess is often suspected on an ultrasound or CT scan. Optimal treatment includes cholecystectomy when feasible, in addition to wide drainage of the right upper quadrant.

Gallstone Ileus

Chronic perforation with formation of a cholecystoenteric or cholecystocutaneous fistula represents the commonest type of gallbladder perforation. As a result of its close anatomic proximity, the gallbladder typically develops a fistula into the duodenum. A cholecystoduodenal fistula develops when a gallstone erodes through the gallbladder and passes directly into the duodenum. This process is frequently silent and the patient may be asymptomatic. Small stones may traverse the length of the gastrointestinal tract and pass unnoticed in the feces. However, stones >2 cm in diameter are likely to become impacted in the terminal ileum the narrowest portion of the intestinal tract. The impacted stone produces a mechanical small bowel obstruction referred to as gallstone ileus. This complication should be suspected in elderly women who present with small bowel obstruction in the absence of a previous laparotomy or femoral hernia. Diagnostic findings include an intact gallbladder with pneumobilia and some dilatation of small bowel loops; sometimes a calcified calculus is visible within the bowel lumen. Appropriate treatment includes resuscitation, nasogastric decompression, and early operation.[34] The goal of operation to correct the bowel obstruction and remove the gallstone is best accomplished by "milking" the gallstone in a retrograde manner and creating an enterotomy, through which it can be removed. As most of these patients are elderly and frail, definitive surgical treatment of the biliary-enteric fistula is best delayed until a later date.

Empyema

Empyema of the gallbladder is a severe form of acute cholecystitis that occurs primarily in the elderly.[35] The main distinction between empyema and uncomplicated acute cholecystitis is the presence of pus within the gallbladder lumen. In addition to complaining of right upper quadrant pain, these patients appear septic, with a high fever and marked leukocytosis. Percutaneous drainage of the gallbladder or early cholecystectomy is mandatory after adequate resuscitation to prevent gram-negative sepsis or perforation. "Neglected" empyema carries an excessively high mortality rate.

Emphysematous Cholecystitis

The presence of gas within the wall of the gallbladder is an unusual complication in patients with cholecystitis. It occurs most frequently in elderly men, and 40% of patients have diabetes mellitus. The classic finding of gas within the gallbladder wall results from infection with gas-producing organisms, usually *Clostridium perfringens.* These patients have evidence of severe sepsis requiring urgent surgical intervention.

Mucocele

Whereas acute obstruction of the cystic duct typically causes acute cholecystitis, chronic cystic duct obstruction is associated with a mucocele (hydrops) of the gallbladder. It is generally believed that gradual insidious obstruction of the cystic duct leads to distension of the gallbladder with sterile mucus or a clear transudate. These patients often present with a massively distended gallbladder, but little or no pain. The diagnosis may be suspected on plain films by the presence of a shadow in the right upper quadrant. Cholecystectomy is curative.

Complications of Gallbladder Disease in Specific Settings

Acute Acalculous Cholecystitis

Acute acalculous cholecystitis accounts for <5% of all cases of cholecystitis.[36] This clinical entity is most commonly observed in critically ill patients following trauma or burns, or postoperatively. The precise pathogenesis is unclear and numerous etiologies have been proposed. The two most important predisposing factors are as follows:

1. Biliary stasis as a consequence of decreased gallbladder stimulation, ampullary spasm or obstruction, or cystic duct obstruction
2. Increased viscosity of bile as a result of dehydration or multiple transfusions

The combination of these factors leads to altered prostaglandin metabolism, which triggers a sequence of events that result in acute gallbladder inflammation.

The diagnosis of acute acalculous cholecystitis is often difficult. The key to expeditious diagnosis is a high index of suspicion. In critically ill patients, the development of fever, right upper quadrant pain and tenderness, leukocytosis, mild liver function test abnormalities or worsening sepsis should provoke consideration of this entity. However, given the frequency of multisystem dysfunction in critically ill patients, it may be difficult to recognize the signs classically associated with acute acalculous cholecystitis. Many of these patients have had recent operations or are obtunded, making the physical examination unreliable. In addition, laboratory examination is not generally helpful. In critically ill patients, fever, leukocytosis, and elevated bilirubin levels are too nonspecific to establish a diagnosis of acalculous cholecystitis.

Ultrasonography can be invaluable in supporting the clinical impression. It has several advantages in an intensive care unit setting. In addition to being both sensitive and specific, it is portable, a considerable advantage for critically ill and often unstable patients. Several ultrasound criteria have been defined to establish the diagnosis of acute acalculous cholecystitis. These include the presence of:

- Gallbladder wall thickening of > 4 mm
- Echogenic bile sludge
- Gallbladder distention
- Pericholecystic fluid in the absence of ascites
- Subserosal edema
- A sonographic Murphy's sign

Cholecystectomy or percutaneous puncture and drainage of the gallbladder may be required to establish or refute the diagnosis of acalculous cholecystitis. Caution is advised in managing acute acalculous cholecystitis conservatively because gangrene and perforation of the gallbladder are more common and may necessitate early cholecystectomy rather than percutaneous drainage.

Cirrhosis and Gallstones

For reasons that are unclear, alcohol consumption may slightly reduce the risk of developing cholesterol gallstones. However, cirrhosis of the liver is associated with a statistically significant increased risk of developing pigment gallstones.[37] Although the exact cause of pigment gallstone formation in cirrhotics is unknown, altered bile acid metabolism has been implicated as an important factor. The mortality and morbidity rates following cholecystectomy in patients who have cirrhosis are increased. Usually, technical difficulties arise as a consequence of bleeding secondary to portal hypertension (with potential varices in the gallbladder wall), coagulopathy, thrombocytopenia, and hypersplenism. Indications for operative intervention should be stringent, and careful consideration should be given to the perioperative risk in individual patients. Operation should be undertaken only in patients who are symptomatic and have an acceptable operative risk. Although cirrhosis is not an absolute contraindication to laparoscopic cholecystectomy, appropriate judgment must be exercised in patient selection. Much of the operative bleeding problem can be prevented by subtotal cholecystectomy, in which the posterior wall of the gallbladder is cauterized and left in situ. This technique avoids inadvertent dissection into the substance of the liver in patients who have clotting factor abnormalities.

CHOLECYSTECTOMY

Perspective

The cost of treating gallstones in the United States exceeds $5 billion. Despite enormous effort to identify nonoperative treatments, the mainstay of therapy for symptomatic gallstones remains cholecystectomy, either laparoscopically or by the open technique.

Open Cholecystectomy

As gallstones affect so many patients, cholecystectomy has become the most common general surgical procedure in the United States. Indications include the following:

- Biliary colic
- Acute and chronic cholecystitis
- Complications of gallstone disease

Patients scheduled for elective cholecystectomy are typically admitted to the hospital on the day of operation. Numerous studies have shown that same-day admission (SDA) policies have not adversely affected complication rates or outcomes. The SDA policies have shortened the duration of hospitalization after cholecystectomy and improved its cost-effectiveness. Also, laparoscopic cholecystectomy is widely performed as a day case procedure.[38,39]

Laparoscopic Cholecystectomy

Although laparoscopic cholecystectomy was only first reported in 1988,[40] it has rapidly become the standard of care for patients who have symptomatic gallstone disease. More than 95% of all cholecystectomies are being accomplished laparoscopically. The advantages of laparoscopic cholecystectomy include reduced postoperative pain, improved recovery, faster recuperation, an improved cosmetic result, shortened hospital stay, and a lower cost.

Although laparoscopic cholecystectomy has been rapidly embraced, lingering questions about its safety remain. Unresolved issues include the need to train and credential surgeons adequately as well as to identify the indications and contraindications to laparoscopic cholecystectomy, the incidence of bile duct injuries and cost-effectiveness. Moreover, old controversies, such as the role of intraoperative cholangiography and the timing of cholecystectomy in patients who have acute cholecystitis, have reemerged.[28,41]

Technical Details

Whether cholecystectomy is performed laparoscopically or by open operation, adequate exposure of the porta hepatis is critical to its safe performance. General considerations applicable to both laparoscopic and open techniques include clear identification of the structures in the triangle of Calot with application of the CVS, and exclusion of additional biliary tract pathology such as CBD stones.[42]

Open Cholecystectomy

Open cholecystectomy is typically undertaken through a right subcostal incision 3 cm below the right costal margin. Placing laparotomy sponges above the right lobe of the liver enhances exposure of the porta hepatis. The hepatic flexure is packed inferiorly, and an automatic retractor is placed to improve exposure. Two techniques are available for open cholecystectomy:

- Antegrade method
- Retrograde method

Retrograde cholecystectomy begins with dissection in the triangle of Calot to identify the cystic duct, as it enters the infundibulum of the gallbladder. This region may demonstrate considerable edema and inflammation in the presence of acute cholecystitis, raising the chance of inadvertent CBD, or hepatic duct injury. Under this circumstance, antegrade ("fundus-first") cholecystectomy is generally safer. This procedure starts at the fundus, dividing the peritoneal attachments of the gallbladder to the liver and mobilizing the gallbladder from the gallbladder fossa. Electrocautery minimizes troublesome bleeding that otherwise obscures the biliary anatomy. Once identified, the cystic duct is mobilized and divided and the cystic duct stump is suture ligated. The cystic artery is similarly divided and ligated. Abdominal closure is achieved in

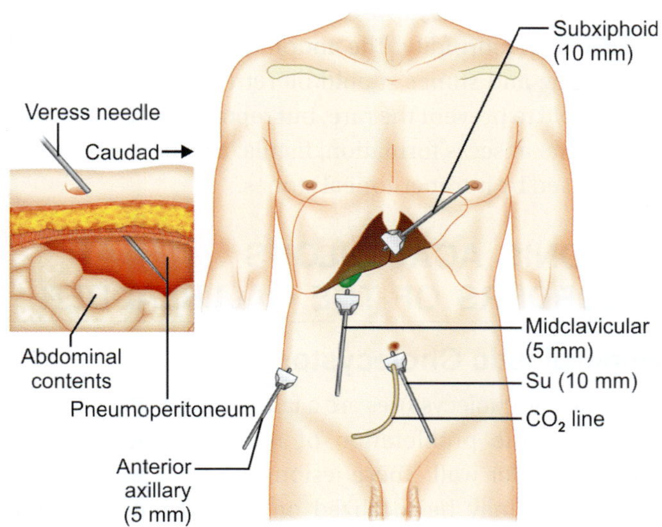

Fig. 55.12: Laparoscopic cholecystectomy showing the position of trocars in the four-port technique. After insufflation with the Veress needle, ports are placed in the umbilicus, anterior axillary, midclavicular, and subxiphoid locations. (SU: Subumbilical).

standard fashion. The routine use of suction drains is no longer supported, but many surgeons leave a drain to the area if the dissection has been bloody or there is any sign of bile leak. In the presence of severe inflammation, subtotal cholecystectomy should be considered.

Laparoscopic Cholecystectomy

The key to laparoscopic cholecystectomy is to create a satisfactory pneumoperitoneum and to apply the CVS.[43]

Two methods of peritoneal entry are routinely used:

1. Open method of trocar placement
2. Veress needle method

In the Veress needle method, the anterior abdominal wall is retracted and a blunt needle is inserted through the umbilicus into the peritoneal cavity. In the open method, a longitudinal or transverse incision is made beneath the umbilicus and the linea alba is divided under vision to prevent bowel injury. Once the laparoscope has been introduced, generally three additional trocars and ports are inserted under direct vision (Fig. 55.12). Thereafter, the principles of safe cholecystectomy are the same as those used for open retrograde cholecystectomy. The cystic duct and artery must be clearly visualized with application of the CVS. In this technique, the neck of the gallbladder is dissected off the liver bed exposing Calot's triangle to achieve conclusive identification of these two structures. Anatomic variation in the position of ductal and arterial structures must be sought to avoid ductal injury and vascular compromise or hemorrhage. Initial recommendations included routine cholangiography to define the ductal anatomy. However, as experience with laparoscopic cholecystectomy has accumulated, selective cholangiography has been advocated more recently.[41] There is still an ongoing discussion on the use of routine cholangiography, which has been shown to reduce the risk of bile duct injury.[44]

The MRCP is usually performed to provide information on the morphology of the biliary system. When the information has not been obtained with MRCP, the indications for cholangiography during laparoscopic cholecystectomy include the following:

- CBD dilatation
- A history of jaundice or hyperamylasemia
- Abnormal liver function tests
- Palpable ductal stones

It is essential that surgeons who carry out laparoscopic cholecystectomy are adept at intraoperative cholangiography.

Indications to convert to open cholecystectomy: These include the following:

- Inability to achieve CVS or failure to progress with dissection
- Marked inflammation with adhesions to adjacent viscera
- Hemorrhage that cannot readily be controlled
- Suspected bile duct injury
- The discovery of unexpected pathology such as gallbladder carcinoma

Opening the abdomen during the performance of laparoscopic cholecystectomy should not be considered a complication, but is rather the exercise of safe surgical judgment. Approximately, 3–6% of elective cases and up to 26% of procedures for acute cholecystitis are converted to open cholecystectomy.

Laparoscopic cholecystectomy for acute cholecystitis: Laparoscopic cholecystectomy is carried out routinely for acute cholecystitis, but conversions to open cholecystectomy are more frequent than for routine cholecystectomy. The combination of adhesions, distension of the gallbladder, and limited visualization of structures in the triangle of Calot makes this procedure more challenging. Generally, numerous adhesions may be found between the hepatic flexure, omentum, and the fundus of the gallbladder. The duodenum may also be involved and is at risk of inadvertent injury if insufficient care is exercised at this stage of the operation. Judicious use of electrocautery is appropriate. The distended edematous gallbladder is difficult to grasp with laparoscopic instruments. Percutaneous drainage of the gallbladder may help to obtain a firm grasp on the gallbladder and facilitate subsequent dissection of the cystic duct and artery.[28]

Indications and contraindications: The most frequent indication for laparoscopic cholecystectomy is recurrent biliary colic. Acute cholecystitis increases the risk of conversion to open cholecystectomy and is technically more demanding, but does not contraindicate safe cholecystectomy. Other clinical settings in which caution must be exercised include cirrhosis, portal hypertension and pregnancy. The role of laparoscopic cholecystectomy in patients with CBD stones remains unclear and depends on local expertise with laparoscopic CBD exploration.

Postoperative morbidity and mortality rates: Technical difficulties during laparoscopic cholecystectomy include the potential complications of open cholecystectomy in addition to problems with peritoneal insufflation (pneumoperitoneum). Introducing carbon dioxide into the abdomen has been associated with hypotension, bradycardia, cardiac arrhythmias, acidosis, and hypercapnia. Although the pathophysiology of these intraoperative disturbances has not been clearly elucidated, they are probably related to gas emboli, vasovagal reactions, and the absorption of carbon dioxide.[45] Awareness of these complications is important in patients with pre-existing cardiopulmonary disease, in whom invasive intraoperative monitoring may be required.

Complications related to trocar placement include subcutaneous emphysema, abdominal wall bleeding and hematoma and serious injuries to the bowel, bladder, or vessels. The major complications of laparoscopic cholecystectomy include bleeding, bile leakage from the cystic duct stump and bile duct injury. The true incidence of major hemorrhage is indeterminate because most such cases can now be managed laparoscopically without the need for laparotomy. Numerous reports in the literature suggest that the risk of bile duct injury during open cholecystectomy is 0.1–0.5%. Shortly after the introduction of laparoscopic cholecystectomy, the incidence of bile duct injury appeared to be ten times as high as with open cholecystectomy. More recent reports indicate, however, that the true incidence of bile duct injury associated with laparoscopic cholecystectomy is approximately 0.5%.[46] A higher incidence of ductal injury has been reported in minilaparoscopic cholecystectomy including single incision laparoscopic surgery.[47]

Spillage of the gallbladder contents is not uncommon during laparoscopic cholecystectomy. Considerable experience suggests, however, that this is rarely the source of infectious morbidity. The abdomen should be irrigated free of bile and stones should be retrieved as completely as possible to prevent the rare, but reported, occurrence of abdominal abscess formation, fistula, and bowel obstruction caused by intraperitoneal stones.

CHRONIC ACALCULOUS DISORDERS OF THE GALLBLADDER

Hyperplastic Cholecystoses

Hyperplastic cholecystoses are a family of disorders characterized by the proliferation of normal components of the gallbladder wall. These lesions are benign, and their distribution may be localized or generalized along the gallbladder wall. Gallstones are present in up to 50% of patients. The spectrum of disease includes cholesterosis and adenomyosis, both of which may produce small benign gallbladder polyps.

Cholesterosis describes the histologic finding of cholesterol ester and lipid deposition within the gallbladder epithelium. Although no linkage has been identified with systemic disorders of cholesterol metabolism, most patients have a statistically significant increased amount of cholesterol in their bile when compared with normal patients without gallstones. The classic example of cholesterosis is the "strawberry gallbladder", characterized by yellowish mucosal protrusions laden with cholesterol on the surface of the gallbladder. Occasionally, focal accumulations of lipid and cholesterol produce sessile "cholesterol polyps" up to 4 mm in diameter. These lesions are not neoplastic, but may mimic gallbladder cancer.

Adenomyosis and Gallbladder Polyps

Adenomyosis is a spectrum of disorders characterized by localized or generalized hyperplasia of the mucosa and muscular layers of the gallbladder. Adenomyomas are typically sessile lesions located in the fundus and <1 cm in diameter. These lesions are benign and not thought to be premalignant.

The frequency of biliary tract symptoms in patients with hyperplastic cholecystoses and small polyps remains poorly defined. Most authors suggest that symptoms result from the presence of unrecognized small stones. There is little evidence that oral dissolution agents are beneficial, and cholecystectomy is generally reserved for individuals with symptoms and gallstones. Gallbladder polyps are occasionally an incidental finding during routine abdominal ultrasonography. Given the potential for early gallbladder cancer, a rational algorithm is required for the treatment of these patients. For patients with concomitant gallstones, cholecystectomy should be performed and the surface of the gallbladder should be inspected both at the time of operation and later in the pathology laboratory. For asymptomatic patients with gallbladder polyps identified incidentally, lesions <10 mm in diameter may be followed by repeated ultrasound examinations because 94% of small polyps are benign.[48] Cholecystectomy is advised in patients with lesions >10 mm in diameter. If during exploration there is any suspicion of malignancy conversion to an open procedure should be performed to allow a more radical resection.

Porcelain Gallbladder

Porcelain gallbladder is thought to be a complication of recurrent attacks of gallstone disease. Most patients with a porcelain gallbladder are asymptomatic at the time of detection. Often, evaluation is prompted because a suspicious mass is noted on physical examination or a calcified mass in the right upper quadrant is incidentally discovered on chest radiography. Since porcelain gallbladder is associated with carcinoma of the gallbladder, cholecystectomy is advised.

BENIGN BILIARY STRICTURES

Etiology

Classically, operative injury to the bile duct has accounted for >80% of biliary strictures. More specifically, 95% of iatrogenic strictures occur as a consequence of cholecystectomy. Two factors are largely responsible for this fact:

1. Anatomic variability of structures in the porta hepatis
2. Technical misadventures

The porta hepatis is the region with the greatest anatomic variation in the body. Anomalous insertion of the cystic and common ducts and variations of the intrahepatic ductal drainage and arterial anatomy exist in up to 50% of patients and lead to misidentification of structures during operation.[49] The impact of anatomic variability on bile duct injuries cannot be underestimated. In up to 30% of cases in which bile duct injury occurs, anomalous anatomy is noted only after the bile duct is injured. Poor exposure and acute inflammation compound this situation and add to the perioperative bile duct injury rate.

Technical difficulty in the control of hemorrhage during laparoscopic cholecystectomy and the inability to identify clearly the cystic duct lead to inadvertent bile duct injury or postoperative ischemia with stenosis.

A second type of biliary stricture develops after operative exploration or repair of the bile duct. The technique and experience of the surgeon, severity of ductal fibrosis and inadequacy of ductal blood supply contribute to the substantial rate of postoperative stenosis. Interruption of the common duct arteries by division of the duct or thermal injury by electrocautery sets the stage for ischemic stenosis during the healing phase. Higher rates of stricture recurrence ranging between 12% and 39% result from biliary-enteric anastomoses carried out to manage previous strictures.[50]

Although 80% of bile duct strictures are a consequence of injury or previous biliary reconstruction, 20% of benign biliary strictures are caused by diseases that incidentally involve the bile duct. Injury can occur during antrectomy for peptic ulcer disease. Dividing a chronically scarred duodenum places the bile duct at risk of injury when the position of the ampulla relative to the pylorus is unclear. Additional causes of biliary stricture include hepatic resection with injury to the remaining ducts, pancreatectomy and right upper quadrant abdominal trauma. As the common duct courses through the pancreas for nearly 4 cm, both acute and chronic pancreatitis can produce bile duct stenosis and obstruction of varying severity. Most patients with jaundice during acute pancreatitis experience complete resolution as the inflammatory process subsides. By contrast, CBD stricture secondary to chronic pancreatitis may require endoscopic or surgical intervention. Failure to correct biliary obstruction in this setting can lead to biliary cirrhosis.

Clinical Features

As most biliary strictures are caused by operation, the presence or absence of a bile leak and sepsis dominates the postoperative clinical presentation. Only 10–21% of bile duct injuries are recognized intraoperatively. Of the remaining patients, 25% become symptomatic within the first week and the remaining 40% are found after 30 days. As many as 20% of patients who have biliary stricture may present after 1 year, when the signs and symptoms of biliary stenosis can be subtle. As a result, the clinical consequences of biliary stricture fall into three categories:

1. Postoperative biliary fistula
2. Bile duct obstruction and jaundice
3. Delayed presentation with recurring cholangitis and slow progression to biliary cirrhosis

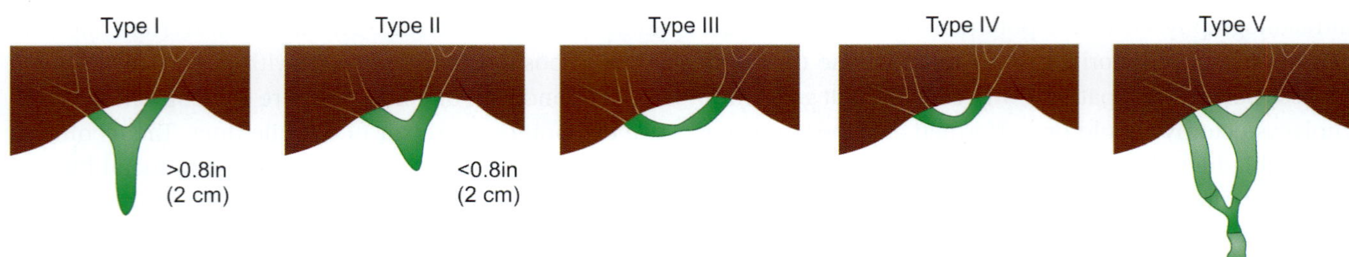

Fig. 55.13: Bismuth classification of benign biliary strictures. Types I–III are classified by the length of common hepatic duct that is injured. Type IV strictures involve the hilar confluence, while type V includes the right hepatic duct as well.
Source: Adapted from Pitt.[51]

The constellation of symptoms depends upon the degree of associated sepsis and the severity of injury in the porta hepatis. Complex bile duct injuries associated with a major vascular insult, abscess formation, and hepatic resection have a much poorer long-term prognosis.

Classification

Several classification systems have been suggested for bile duct injuries and postoperative strictures. In the Bismuth system, biliary strictures are classified according to their proximity to the hilar confluence (Fig. 55.13).[50] The anatomic location of the bile duct injury determines the technical difficulty of the subsequent repair. Proximal lesions involve dissection and anastomosis of progressively smaller biliary radicals, with high rates of postoperative stenosis. Level 1 lesions in the distal CBD are technically less demanding and the success rates of repair approach 100%.

The Strasberg classification of BDI is more complete and divides BDI into five groups (A to E), in which the E class corresponds to a complex bile duct injury with complete transection of the hepatic duct. Recently, the ATOM classification has been proposed by the European Association for Endoscopic Surgery (EAES), which combines all information on bile duct injuries during cholecystectomy and provides guidelines for effective therapy.[46]

Management of Bile Duct Injury

To develop a therapeutic algorithm, the clinical management of bile duct injury can be divided into three groups. In general, these patients are ideally managed by a multidisciplinary team with expertise in surgery, interventional radiology, and therapeutic endoscopy.[51]

Intraoperative Recognition

Injury to the bile duct may occur during challenging cases, but it has also been reported, however, during "the easiest case I've ever done". Operative bile duct injuries differ greatly in their severity and include:

- Clip injuries to the common duct
- Avulsion or leakage of the cystic duct
- Lateral ductotomy
- Electrocautery burns
- More severe injuries such as complete transection or resection of the duct with or without concomitant major vascular involvement

Failure to identify the cystic duct clearly or observation of bile during dissection of the porta hepatis mandates cholangiography or immediate conversion to open cholecystectomy. Misidentifying the cystic duct may lead to resection of a portion of the common duct and ligation of the right hepatic artery. This scenario produces a difficult reconstruction even under optimal circumstances. When such a devastating lesion is discovered intraoperatively, the emotional impact upon the operating surgeon is enormous. The medicolegal aspects are equally intimidating. Under these circumstances, it is best for the surgeon to consult a more composed or experienced colleague.

In the presence of normal caliber ducts, durable repair of the injured biliary tree is especially challenging. Most operative lesions are found in the proximal common hepatic duct (43%) and hilum (23%), where reconstruction is most difficult. In fact, the larger (and technically simpler) distal CBD is injured in < 34% of cases.[50] If the operating surgeon is not experienced in bile duct reconstruction, drainage of the biliary tree and subhepatic space alone is acceptable interim therapy. Under these circumstances, the patient should be transferred to a referral center where definitive therapy can be undertaken by a trained team of surgeons, gastroenterologists, and interventional radiologists.

For immediate bile duct reconstruction to be successful, certain anatomic factors must be considered. Of these, the anatomic location of the lesion within the biliary tree, length of injured bile duct and extent of vascular involvement

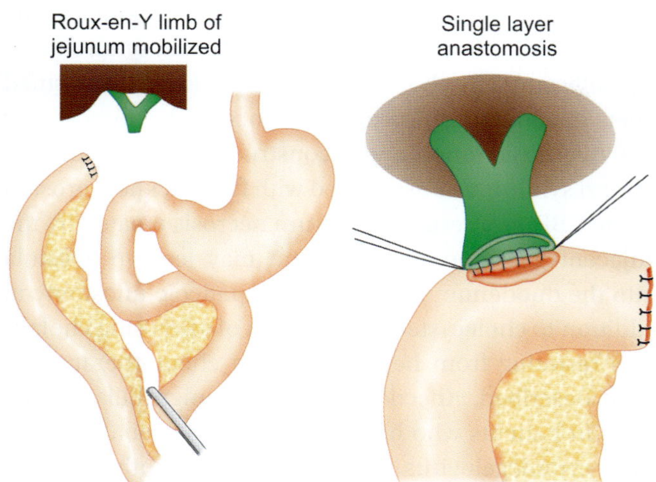

Fig. 55.14: Surgical technique for creating a Roux-en-Y hepaticojejunostomy for bile duct injury. A 40–60 cm Roux-en-Y limb of jejunum is mobilized and a single-layer interrupted anastomosis is sewn in a mucosa-to-mucosa fashion.

are most important and must be determined, preferably by intraoperative cholangiography, before deciding upon the method of reconstruction. Lesions amenable to simple maneuvers are scarce. A simple lateral injury of the bile duct or avulsion of the cystic duct stump may be repaired primarily over a T-tube. Similarly, transection of the CBD may be repaired in an end-to-end fashion and splinted with a T-tube providing that the duct is not shortened >1 cm and placed under tension.

Minimal injuries are, however, unusual and these simple methods of repair are inadequate in the face of extensive ductal injury. Depending upon the level of the lesion, biliary-enteric anastomosis with a 40–60 cm Roux-en-Y jejunostomy is the best strategy to establish bile flow into the gastrointestinal tract and minimize postoperative stricture formation (Fig. 55.14). The use of a defunctioned (Roux) limb of jejunum also decreases enteric reflux into the biliary tree and prevents cholangitis. If an anastomotic leak develops, the resulting biliary fistula is usually well controlled by operatively placed drains and a high-output small bowel fistula is avoided. Success rates following either Roux-en-Y choledochojejunostomy or hepaticojejunostomy are 88–100% if an adequate mucosa-to-mucosa anastomosis can be constructed.[51] When in the case of complete transection of the hepatic duct, PTC and biliary drainage (PTBD) has been performed preoperatively, the transhepatic drain may be used across the anastomosis to relieve pressure and to permit postoperative cholangiography.

Early Postoperative Recognition

Patients who have sustained bile duct injuries that are not recognized intraoperatively often present within the first 7–10 days after operation. Depending upon the nature of the injury, their complaints may range from painless jaundice to an acute abdomen with bile peritonitis, persistent right upper quadrant pain possibly radiating to the shoulder, slow resolution of ileus, low-grade fever, and increasing liver function tests. If a drain has been left at operation, sustained losses of >100 mL bile per day require investigation. Given these complaints, a careful search for an unrecognized bile duct injury is extremely important because delayed diagnosis is associated with death as a result of biliary peritonitis. Numerous studies are available to secure the diagnosis of bile duct injury. Although jaundice may be a consequence of retained stones or a bile duct injury, bilious drainage from the wound or operatively placed drains is clear-cut evidence of a biliary fistula. In addition to an elevated white blood cell count (WBC) and CRP, laboratory evidence typically includes an elevated total bilirubin in the 2–6 mg/dL (34.2–102.6 μmol/L) range and an elevated alkaline phosphatase. Although an ultrasound scan is an effective and low-cost screening test for right upper quadrant fluid collections, abdominal CT gives more accurate anatomic localization of a bile duct injury based on the pattern of duct dilatation and the extent of intra-abdominal biloma. Ductal dilatation in the absence of free fluid is consistent with inadvertent ligation or clipping of the CBD. The MRCP is useful to visualize the intrahepatic and extrahepatic bile ducts in relation with the level of injury.

Patients who have a suspected bile duct leak should be hydrated and placed on intravenous antibiotics specific for biliary pathogens, such as ampicillin/gentamicin, mezlocillin/metronidazole, or piperacillin/tazobactam. Following laboratory examination, CT is needed to look for a subhepatic fluid collection or ascites. The extent of ductal dilatation may suggest the location of injury, especially if abdominal plain films reveal surgical clips in that region of the porta hepatis. If an obvious fluid collection is identified by CT scan, a percutaneous drain should be placed and inspected for bile.

Small accessory ducts between the liver and gallbladder (foramina of Luschka) can produce these findings and such leaks typically close with conservative therapy alone. If a tangential injury to the duct or a cystic duct stump leak is suspected, then ERCP can be both diagnostic and therapeutic.[52] In this setting, placement of a biliary endoprosthesis may be all that is required to manage the ductal injury and leak. If a major transection of the bile duct is suspected, ERCP is usually not helpful, because it merely demonstrates the distal segment of the duct. Most lesions are located in the proximal biliary tree and are inaccessible to drainage through the distal duct. For this reason, PTC is better at delineating the injury. It also permits transhepatic drainage and the placement of catheters that can be used to identify the bile ducts during surgical repair. In patients who have a transected duct and a "biloma", placement of a transhepatic catheter allows precise definition of the injury and provides resolution of the inflammatory process before definitive surgical management.[53] Placement of transhepatic catheters helps the surgeon identify the duct at the time of repair. Once adequate internal or external drainage is assured, there is no urgency to reconstruct the bile duct in the early postoperative period. Ultimately, a Roux-en-Y hepaticojejunostomy is the best reconstruction for most patients who have a bile duct injury.[51]

Delayed Recognition

Nearly half the patients with bile duct injury present in a delayed fashion without signs of biliary fistula or peritonitis. These patients are evaluated semielectively. Following injury, 40% of strictures do not become clinically evident for at least 1 month and much longer delays in diagnosis are common. Given the indolent course of some bile duct strictures, chronic obstruction is responsible for most symptoms, such as progressive asymptomatic jaundice, recurring cholangitis or liver failure. The presence of a biliary stricture is suggested by recurring cholangitis in a patient who has had a previous operation in the porta hepatis. Under these circumstances, the cholangitis is usually mild and responds rapidly to intravenous antibiotics. A less dramatic type of presentation arises in the outpatient setting in an asymptomatic patient with elevated serum alkaline phosphatase and bilirubin levels. If untreated, obstructing lesions gradually progress to secondary biliary cirrhosis with ultimately pruritus, portal hypertension, variceal hemorrhage, and liver failure. It takes an average of 48 months for cirrhosis to become clinically evident after injury.

Other Causes of Biliary Stricture

Common bile duct obstruction occasionally occurs as a result of contiguous inflammation from chronic gallstone disease. In the absence of choledocholithiasis, compression of the bile duct can occur from a large stone impacted in the infundibulum or from severe inflammation in the gallbladder itself. This clinical entity, Mirizzi syndrome, is typically cured by cholecystectomy, preferably performed open depending on local experience with laparoscopic bile duct exploration and reconstruction.[54] On occasion, Mirizzi syndrome is associated with full-thickness erosion of the CBD as a result of pressure necrosis created by the adjacent gallstone. This problem may lead to a fistula into the duodenum and requires hepaticojejunostomy in addition to cholecystectomy. A form of sclerosing cholangitis resulting from hepatic infusion chemotherapy has been described. Anecdotal cases of benign biliary strictures in patients who have HIV infection probably result from cytomegalovirus infection. More recently, autoimmune cholangitis has been identified as a cause of biliary stricture, typically characterized by elevated plasma Ig-G4 levels and microscopically, by lymphocyte and plasma cell infiltrates.[55]

EVALUATING BILIARY OBSTRUCTION

Diagnostic Imaging

The diagnosis of benign biliary stricture must be made definitively before selecting the method of treatment. The differential diagnosis for biliary obstruction or cholangitis includes the following:

- Retained or primary common duct stones
- Primary sclerosing cholangitis
- Cholangiocarcinoma
- Pancreatic or ampullary carcinoma
- Benign biliary stricture, whether iatrogenic or secondary to severe chronic pancreatitis

In an era of successful nonsurgical means of ductal drainage, missing a diagnosis of cholangiocarcinoma may delay curative surgical resection if balloon dilatation is attempted instead. Benign strictures in the region of the confluence may be especially difficult to distinguish from a small hilar cholangiocarcinoma.[56]

Improvements in noninvasive imaging have made anatomic localization of biliary strictures and exclusion of malignancy far more accurate.[57] In a patient with bile duct obstruction, abdominal ultrasonography and CT are complementary tests. Ultrasound studies reveal intra- and extrahepatic biliary dilatation, confirm the absence of the gallbladder, and suggest the level of obstruction. Computed tomography is more sensitive than ultrasound in detecting a tumor within the bile duct and allows high-resolution imaging of small (2 cm) lesions within the pancreatic head and ampulla, which may be obscured by bowel gas during ultrasonography. Computed tomography scan also suggests the presence of cholangiocarcinoma when a mass is seen in association with the bile duct, although its sensitivity (44%) and specificity (78%) are not ideal.[58]

Once the location of bile duct obstruction is suspected from noninvasive studies, satisfactory operative planning requires some form of cholangiography. Traditionally, ERCP and PTC have been the preferred methods. Percutaneous transhepatic cholangiography allows definition of the bile ducts proximal to the lesion, prevents contamination of the obstructed biliary tree with enteric contents during ERCP cannulation of the ampulla, and permits catheters to be placed so that the surgeon can identify the hepatic ducts intraoperatively.

Magnetic Resonance Cholangiopancreatography

MRCP is a useful methodology for investigating the biliary tree. It has the distinct clinical advantage of being noninvasive, so avoiding the periprocedural risks of cholangitis, hemobilia, and pancreatitis associated with PTC and ERCP. Single-shot MRCP detects common duct stones in 73% of cases and compression and dilatation of the biliary tree in 100%.[59] Its wide applicability and high resolution are finding an increasing role in the management of biliary pathology, especially in patients with contrast allergies or high-risk medical conditions. In a prospective evaluation of patients with a biliary-enteric anastomosis and postoperative biliary obstruction, MRCP correctly diagnosed anastomotic stenosis in 100% of cases and showed stones as small as 5 mm in diameter.[60]

Is the Stricture Malignant?

Differentiating between a benign and a malignant stricture remains a challenge despite the recent availability of new diagnostic modalities such as bile cytology and endoscopic brushing.[56] The hypocellular nature of bile duct tumors frequently prevents accurate cytologic examination and definitive preoperative diagnosis. The presence of bile duct carcinoma may be suspected by the appearance of a mass in association with the bile duct.

Despite advances in nonoperative methodology, such as biliary cytology, tumor marker (CA19-9) levels and endoscopic brushing, it is difficult to exclude malignant disease preoperatively. A study by Kurzawinski and associates showed that only one third of those with known bile duct cancers had positive bile cytology.[61] Endoscopic brush cytology represents a substantial improvement over bile cytology alone in the diagnosis of malignant biliary obstruction. Sensitivity is increased to 63% and specificity approaches 100%.[62] If there is a high suspicion that a bile duct stricture is malignant, as in those patients who have weight loss (50%) or back pain in addition to jaundice, contast-enhanced CT scan may reveal encasement of the vascular structures and secure the diagnosis. The final determinant for diagnosis and treatment of apparently resectable bile duct cancer remains surgical resection.

Elective Surgical Reconstruction

Endoscopic treatment with one or more stents or percutaneous balloon dilatation is considered as initial treatment. Failure of these nonoperative methods leaves surgical biliary-enteric bypass as the ultimate treatment in patients with extrahepatic benign strictures and acceptable risk factors.[57] Successful long-term biliary reconstruction, defined as the absence of cholangitis, jaundice, or subsequent intervention, may be anticipated in up to 100% of good-risk patients with Bismuth level I injuries and technically sound mucosa-to-mucosa anastomoses.

Percutaneous transhepatic drains may be placed preoperatively to facilitate identification of the bile ducts. The fibrotic duct should be resected to exclude malignancy, but unnecessary dissection must be avoided to prevent ductal ischemia, which promotes postoperative stricture formation. A 40–60 cm Roux-en-Y jejunostomy is then created to minimize enteric reflux into the biliary tree. Some authors advocate fashioning a subcutaneous jejunostomy by the Hutson loop technique to permit subsequent percutaneous endoscopic evaluation of the Roux limb. Although the concept is attractive, we have had patients who have developed external biliary fistulas from the Roux loop under these circumstances and cannot recommend the procedure routinely. The biliary bypasses that now have the best long-term patency are choledocho- and hepaticojejunostomy. Alternatively, for distal strictures, a choledocho-duodenostomy may be undertaken although complications of the closed end of the bile duct (sump syndrome) have been reported. The choice of suture material has not been shown to affect the anastomotic stricture rate. However, we prefer a monofilament absorbable suture, such as PDS 4-0, in the belief that a permanent foreign body in the duct may serve as a nidus for choledocholithiasis.

Using these techniques, the success rate of primary repair of biliary strictures can be 83–88%.[50,51] Hilar lesions, on the other hand, may require special operative procedures to assure drainage of both the left and the right hepatic ducts. Hepaticojejunostomy using the left biliary trunk (Hepp–Couinaud technique) was originally described to permit biliary reconstruction when the proximal common hepatic duct is short or the left and right ducts are separated.[63] In these circumstances, the left hepatic duct is usually intact because it resides under Glisson's capsule in the hilar plate and is not exposed during cholecystectomy. The left duct is also of adequate caliber to permit a satisfactory anastomosis, unlike the right, which may be substantially smaller and also less accessible. In lesions extending more proximally along the left hepatic duct, the round-ligament approach offers access to construct a segment 3 ductal anastomosis.

Nonoperative Dilatation

Nonsurgical dilatation of biliary strictures began in the early 1980s.[64] Since that time, balloon dilatation using endoscopic or radiologic techniques has gained widespread acceptance as a safe and effective alternative to surgical reconstruction. However, the necessity for repeated intervention to maintain biliary patency and the uncertain long-term rate of postdilatation stricture has delayed establishment of firm guidelines for its use. Davids and colleagues have shown that an average of five sessions of ERCP is required within the first year to maintain biliary patency.[65] In this nonrandomized retrospective study, patients who had benign biliary strictures received either surgical bypass or endoscopic treatment with dilatation followed by stenting. Overall, the results were identical, 83% of surgical and endoscopic patients having a good outcome. The post-treatment stricture rate was equal at 17%, but the dilatation group developed strictures more rapidly (at 3 ± 11 months vs. 40 ± 11 months, $p < 0.04$) and became symptomatic with cholangitis, cholestasis and stent migration. Given the necessity for repeated intervention, the ERCP group developed a higher total complication rate during the period of study (35 vs. 26%).

Pitt and associates have addressed the indications for operative and nonoperative therapy of benign strictures.[51] Despite this being a retrospective analysis, patients in the operative and percutaneous transhepatic balloon dilatation (PTBD) groups were well matched in terms of their strictures and risk factors. The mean number of PTBD sessions per patient was 3.9, and stents were placed after dilatation and changed every 3–4 months. As a result of long-term stricture formation in the PTBD group, an initial 100% procedural success fell to 55% after 5 years, significantly lower than the operative success rate of 88%. The cumulative complication rate of PTBD was 35% as a result of hemobilia, pancreatitis, and cholangitis caused by repeated intervention. This fact increased the duration of stay and total cost to the levels seen in the operative group.

Long-term success with nonoperative therapy remains difficult to evaluate because follow-up periods in the available studies are short. Given the apparent tendency of benign strictures to recur after dilatation, expandable metal stents (e.g. Wallstent) have been placed to evaluate their long-term efficacy.[66] Although placement was successful in 100% of patients, only 60% had good patency at 9 months and these nonremovable stents occluded after 3–55 months, limiting future treatment options. Permanent biliary stents stimulate scar formation within the duct, which extends far beyond the original stricture and makes definitive surgical repair far more difficult.

Dilatation may be appropriate initial therapy for patients who have intrahepatic or extrahepatic biliary strictures. If stenting is considered, removable devices are preferable if the patient has long-term life expectancy and future surgical therapy might be considered. Nonoperative dilatation is best for patients who have an increased operative risk because of cirrhosis, ascites, cardiopulmonary disease, renal failure, and a technically difficult surgical bypass. Anastomotic strictures following previous biliary-enteric bypass are successfully treated by initial dilatation and long-term placement of a removable stent.

Medicolegal Implications

The morbidity of bile duct injuries remains a source of considerable consternation to patients and surgeons alike. The frequency of ductal and vascular anomalies in the porta hepatis makes laparoscopic cholecystectomy less straightforward and routine, despite it being a relatively common surgical procedure. Bile duct injuries occur in approximately 0.5% of laparoscopic cholecystectomies. This reality makes it incumbent upon surgeons to have a thorough preoperative discussion with patients about the risks of operating on the biliary tract. Although no amount of preparation with the family can prevent all lawsuits, the consent discussion removes the shock associated with a major complication after what is perceived to be a routine operation. It also fulfills the legal mandate for full disclosure of all relevant risks before invasive treatment. In addition to the emotional toll that these devastating injuries have upon the surgeon, the legal costs are enormous.

MISCELLANEOUS BENIGN INFLAMMATORY LESIONS

Sclerosing Cholangitis

A number of disease entities are characterized by a progressive, inflammatory, fibrotic process that involves either the intrahepatic and/or extrahepatic biliary tract. In most cases, jaundice and recurrent cholangitis are the clinical hallmarks regardless of etiology. Treatment should be instituted early to reduce the sequelae of biliary cirrhosis and liver failure or the development of a superimposed malignancy.

Etiology

Sclerosing cholangitis can occur as an idiopathic disorder and is often associated with ulcerative colitis. Evidence suggests that alterations in immune function are important etiologic factors. Recently, several patients with HIV infection have been reported to have the clinical and radiologic features of sclerosing cholangitis. Another variant has been described in patients with suppurative cholangitis. Similarly, a sclerosing process of the bile ducts has been described in patients after liver transplantation and in patients receiving intra-arterial hepatic infusions of cytotoxic chemotherapy as treatment for liver metastases. Typically, these lesions are characterized by areas of alternating fibrosis and inflammation, and often create a histologic picture indistinguishable from scirrhous adenocarcinoma of the bile duct.

Management

Treatment options are based on the presumed etiology as well as the location and extent of the disease and the patient's clinical course. For many years, a surgical biliary bypass was performed for patients who had extrahepatic primary sclerosing cholangitis. The developments of new and efficacious immunosuppressive agents coupled with refinements in liver transplantation have led to an evolution of our management of these patients.

ACUTE CHOLANGITIS

Etiology

Cholangitis develops in the presence of bile duct obstruction and biliary infection (bactibilia).[67] Most typically cholangitis occurs in patients with CBD stones, but it can also occur in those with biliary strictures (both benign and malignant), after biliary reconstructive procedures and after intubation or manipulation of the bile duct. The pathogenesis of cholangitis includes biliary obstruction with increased intraluminal pressure and reflux of bacteria into the hepatic veins and through the lymphatics into the systemic circulation. The bacteriology of cholangitis is evolving, although gram-negative organisms continue to be the most common pathogens.

Clinical Features

In 1877, Charcot described the clinical triad that bears his name: fever, jaundice, and right upper quadrant pain. These are the predominant symptoms observed in patients who have biliary sepsis or cholangitis. All three components are present in only 25% of patients who have documented cholangitis. Initial clinical and laboratory assessment generally confirm the presence of sepsis and jaundice. Blood culture is important to look for the infecting organism; septicemia may cause mental confusion. Important anatomic information can be gleaned by imaging studies to define the degree of biliary dilatation and the level of the obstruction. This information helps to identify the etiology and select the appropriate therapy.

Management

In most cases, therapy should be instituted concurrently with diagnostic evaluation. Intravenous hydration and monitoring of fluid resuscitation are essential, particularly in the elderly frail patient. Antibiotic therapy should be started as soon as possible, with coverage directed against gram-negative rods and gram-positive anaerobes while awaiting the results of blood or bile culture. Ideally, adequate serum levels should be obtained before manipulation of the biliary tract. Although many patients require some form of biliary decompression during the course of their disease, patients can frequently be temporized with antibiotics alone. Ultimately, the decision to proceed with endoscopic, percutaneous or surgical drainage of the biliary tract is based upon the patient's anatomy, severity assessment, and local expertise.[68] Outcome is determined by the nature of the obstruction much more than by the manner in which biliary decompression is accomplished.

TUMORS OF THE GALLBLADDER AND BILIARY TRACT

Perspective

Neoplasms of the gallbladder and bile ducts are relatively uncommon. Patients in the United States with carcinomas of the gallbladder or extrahepatic biliary tract account for only 7% of the total number of patients with colorectal malignancies. Tumors of the gallbladder or extrahepatic biliary tract account for fewer than 5,000 deaths each year in the United States.[69]

Gallbladder cancer is commoner in parts of the world where the incidence of cholelithiasis is exceptionally high, such as in certain countries of South America. The clinicopathologic features of gallbladder cancer are unusual in that most lesions are asymptomatic and are discovered at the time of cholecystectomy. This fact presents specific management issues and challenges for the surgeon.

Although bile duct tumors tend to be small in size, their location and anatomic relationship to vital structures frequently preclude surgical extirpation. During the past 20 years, remarkable advances in related fields have had an enormous impact on the management of patients with bile duct cancer (cholangiocarcinoma). The treatment of extrahepatic biliary tract carcinomas should include a multidisciplinary approach employing endoscopic, radiologic, and surgical expertise.

Other than small polyps in the gallbladder, benign tumors of the gallbladder and extrahepatic biliary tract are rare. Such lesions are frequently discovered at the time of cholecystectomy and warrant no further therapy. Benign tumors of the bile duct are observed in <0.05% of all patients undergoing biliary tract operations. The inability to make a precise histologic diagnosis or the associated finding of jaundice frequently leads to surgical extirpation and/or biliary bypass for patients who have benign biliary lesions.[56]

GALLBLADDER CARCINOMA

Incidence and Etiology

Carcinoma of the gallbladder is the commonest cancer arising from the hepatobiliary tract, accounting for two thirds of all biliary tract cancer. Although it is the fifth commonest cancer in the gastrointestinal tract, it accounts for only 2–4% of all gastrointestinal malignancies; between 5,000 and 7,000 new cases of gallbladder cancer are diagnosed each year in the United States. The gravity of this diagnosis is underscored by the fact that approximately 6,500 patients die from gallbladder cancer annually in the United States. Worldwide, the incidence of this disease increases with age. The highest incidence of gallbladder cancer is found in South American and American Indians and Alaskan natives, in whom the incidence is 6–10 times that in non-Indian populations.[70]

The association between cholelithiasis and carcinoma of the gallbladder has been well described. It is, therefore, not surprising that cancer of the gallbladder is more common in women. Gallstones have been documented in over 70% of patients with carcinoma of the gallbladder. Whether the number and size of gallstones are risk factors for gallbladder cancer remains unclear. Gallbladder carcinoma has also been noted to occur with increasing frequency in patients who have adenomas, congenital abnormalities characterized by biliary dilatation and porcelain gallbladder.

Considerable evidence suggests that the chronic presence of gallstones induces alterations in epithelial morphology that appear premalignant. Dysplastic epithelium has been observed adjacent to invasive cancer and provides support for the hypothesis that chronic inflammation is an important etiologic factor in the development of gallbladder cancer. A number of potential carcinogens have been identified, including dimethylnitrosamine and chemical analogs of bile salts.

Pathology

Most malignant tumors that involve the gallbladder are adenocarcinomas (80%); the remainders are squamous cell carcinomas, mixed tumors with glandular and squamous components and rarely lymphoma, sarcoma, melanoma, or carcinoid. Most gallbladder tumors are scirrhous (fibrotic), although up to 15% are papillary in nature.[71] Often, the gallbladder is grossly thickened, firm, and densely adherent to the liver.

Carcinomas of the gallbladder tend to spread through local extension and invasion as well as through the lymphatics. Although 25% of patients have evidence of lymph node metastasis at the time of operation, regional node involvement is noted at the time of autopsy in over 70% of patients with gallbladder cancer. Direct extension into the liver occurs from local invasion and growth along biliary ducts, veins, and lymphatics and is reported in approximately 35% of patients at the time of cholecystectomy and in 90% at autopsy. Most patients eventually develop peritoneal metastases and succumb before the appearance of pulmonary disease.

Staging

As with other tumors, a staging system for gallbladder carcinoma has been developed based on postoperative histology and the clinical extent of tumor:

- *Tis*: Intramucosal disease or carcinoma in situ
- *T1a*: Submucosal invasion into lamina propria

- *T1b*: Invasion into muscular layer
- *T2*: Invasion through muscular layer into perimuscular connective tissue or into serosa
- *T3*: Either extension into the liver (< 2 cm) or beyond the serosal layer into one adjacent organ or structure
- *T4*: Advanced disease with either extension into the liver (> 2 cm) and/or into several adjacent organs or structures

Clinical Features

Typically, patients who present with gallbladder cancer have symptoms indistinguishable from those with uncomplicated gallstone disease. Right upper quadrant pain is generally the predominant complaint (60–80% of cases); other symptoms are nausea and emesis, weight loss and jaundice. These complaints tend to be nonspecific and rarely help to establish the diagnosis. Diagnostic evaluation is generally focused on confirming or excluding gallstone disease as the etiology of the symptoms. A change in long-standing and previously stable symptoms may indicate gallbladder malignancy. Nonspecific tumor markers of gastrointestinal malignancies, such as carcinoembryonic antigen (CEA) and CA 19-9, may be elevated in patients with gallbladder carcinoma, but few data show that biochemical detection is correlated with clinical stage or prognosis. A preoperative diagnosis of gallbladder cancer is made in < 10% of patients.

Management

Surgical extirpation of the gallbladder and surrounding tissues continues to be the mainstay of treatment for patients who have gallbladder cancer.[72] The recognition that carcinoma of the gallbladder tends to be locally invasive with involvement of regional lymph nodes has provided the basis for a rational approach to this disease when it is recognized intraoperatively. Therapeutic options include simple cholecystectomy, cholecystectomy with regional lymphadenectomy and wedge resection of the gallbladder bed (part of segment 4/5) plus more radical procedures including (extended) right hemihepatectomy.[73]

The long-term benefits of such radical procedures are not well established. Not infrequently the surgeon is in the uncomfortable position of being informed by the pathologist that the gallbladder contains carcinoma several days after the patient has left the hospital, although such delayed diagnosis can be minimized by opening the gallbladder during operation and submitting any suspicious areas to frozen-section examination. The dilemma is whether or not to offer the patient another operation to perform an extensive resection as suggested above. These decisions should be governed by the pathologic staging of the tumor and the overall medical status of the patient. Simple cholecystectomy suffices for Tis and T1a tumors, whereas in T1b tumors, cholecystectomy in combination with wedge resection of the gallbladder bed and lymphadenectomy of the hepatoduodenal ligament is advised.

Providing palliation is an important measure for a patient who has obstructive jaundice secondary to unresectable gallbladder cancer. Endoscopic or percutaneous stenting usually provides adequate biliary drainage. Rarely the surgeon may be compelled to perform a biliary-enteric bypass. Recent studies suggest a possible benefit of chemotherapy.[74]

The relative rarity of gallbladder cancer has made careful prospective analysis of any protocol difficult to implement and interpret.

Outcome

The long-term survival of aggressive surgery (extensive resection in combination with surrounding organs) is unclear and controversial, partly given the fact that such operations are associated with high morbidity and mortality.[69] In relation to this, 5-year survival rates of 7–87% are reported, with a morbidity rate of 40–57% and a mortality rate of 0–6%. Extended liver resection in combination with resection of other organs is not recommended on a routine basis.[75]

Factors associated with improved survival include occult lesions found incidentally plus a favorable histologic type, grade, and pathologic stage of the carcinoma.

CHOLANGIOCARCINOMA

Incidence and Etiology

Cholangiocarcinoma of the extrahepatic bile duct is a rare malignancy found in 0.01–0.50% of all autopsies. It accounts for only one third of extrahepatic biliary tract malignancies. For reasons that are not entirely clear, the disease is five times more common in Japan than in the United States.[76]

The lesion occurs with increased frequency in patients with gallstones, although the relationship is not nearly as well defined as it is for gallbladder cancer. The development of bile duct carcinoma in patients with pre-existing sclerosing cholangitis has been well described, but <10% of patients who have bile duct tumors have an antecedent history of ulcerative colitis. As with gallbladder cancer, chronic infection of the biliary tract with typhoid, *Clonorchis sinensis, Giardia lamblia,* and other microbes and/or parasites has been linked to the development of bile duct cancer. Other conditions causally associated with these tumors include exposure to industrial chemicals and toxins as well as congenital choledochal cysts.

Pathology

As a result of their location, cholangiocarcinomas tend to be relatively small at the time of diagnosis. They cause jaundice early on because of partial or complete biliary obstruction. Most bile duct tumors are adenocarcinomas, although adenomas, cystadenomas, and granular cell tumors have all been reported. The lesions are usually flat scirrhous tumors that are quite fibrotic. Occasionally, bile duct tumors are papillary in nature and these patients have an improved prognosis. Local lesions are found in approximately 60% of cases, with diffuse cholangiocarcinomas found in <10% of cases. Approximately, one third of all cases of cholangiocarcinoma have invaded the liver or regional lymph nodes at the time of diagnosis. Distant metastases do not develop early, being present in <5% of patients at the time of diagnosis.[77]

Cholangiocarcinomas are classified by their location within the ductal system. Lesions in the area of the confluence of the hepatic bile duct and upper common hepatic duct (hilar cholangiocarcinoma, HCCA) account for at least >50–60%. Middle third lesions comprise approximately 15–20%, lower third lesions represent 15%, and diffuse cholangiocarcinomas account for <10%.

Clinical Features

Patients typically present with jaundice in the absence of pain. In addition, many of them complain of pruritus, dark urine, and light-colored stools (i.e. symptoms consistent with biliary obstruction). Other than scleral icterus and cutaneous jaundice, there are few physical findings.[78]

Patients who have tumors of the bile duct have the classic laboratory profile of obstructive jaundice. Hyperbilirubinemia is quite pronounced, and serum values tend to be considerably higher than for patients who have CBD stones or benign strictures. The value of serum tumor markers in the diagnosis of cholangiocarcinoma is unclear, although there is evidence that some bile duct tumors contain CEA, CA 19-9, and small c-Ha-ras p21 antigen reactants.

Biliary imaging studies and cross-sectional studies play a key role in the diagnostic evaluation and staging of patients with presumed bile duct cancer. Traditionally, ultrasonography and CT scanning have been the first procedures used for patients with obstructive jaundice. The MRCP is a noninvasive technique providing information on the site of biliary stenosis.[79] These modalities are useful and accurate in recognizing biliary dilatation within both the intrahepatic and extrahepatic biliary systems. A more precise definition of the site of obstruction and an "anatomic roadmap" can be obtained using direct cholangiography. Although ERCP can be helpful in some patients, PTC is generally more definitive in elucidating ductal anatomy in patients with resectable bile duct tumors. Delineation of both intra- and extrahepatic biliary anatomy as well as identification of the site of obstruction then permits the formulation of a comprehensive operative or nonoperative approach. The advent and development of endoscopic ultrasound (EUS) and MR technology have provided a new approach to evaluating these patients.[80] MR technology allows definition of the biliary tract (MRCP) and vasculature simultaneously. Recent experience suggests that this test, particularly when coupled with EUS, may shortly become the new gold standard for the evaluation of patients who have suspected biliary malignancy.[81]

Management

Patients with obstructive jaundice have alterations in their immune competence and renal function that place them at increased risk for wound infection, pneumonia, and postoperative death.[82] This relationship between obstructive jaundice and postoperative sepsis suggested that preoperative drainage might reduce the morbidity and mortality rates of operations for bile duct tumors. A recent trial, however, showed that preoperative biliary drainage had no beneficial effects in patients with distal bile duct carcinoma undergoing subtotal pancreatoduodenectomy.[83] In HCCA, however, often requiring extensive liver resection, the presumptive advantages of preoperative biliary drainage are the treatment of segmental cholangitis, definition of proximal extent of the tumor, and improvement of function and regenerative capacity of the (future) remnant liver.[84] In these patients, preoperative complete drainage of at least the ductal system of the future remnant liver is strongly advised. Preoperative biliary drainage can be achieved by percutaneous transhepatic biliary drainage (PTBD) or by endoscopic placement of one or more biliary stents. Percutaneous catheters may facilitate intraoperative identification of the intrahepatic segmental bile ducts in patients with proximal lesions.

Intraoperative strategies and management depend upon the location of the tumor and are discussed below.

Proximal bile duct tumors: Since the initial description by Klatskin in 1965, the management of patients with HCCA has been viewed as challenging. Surgical resection offers the only hope of cure.[85] A more extensive surgical approach has been advocated in the past decade, in which hilar resection was combined with large liver resections for the majority of HCCA to achieve R0 resection. Radical resection of HCCA encompasses excision of the liver hilum en bloc with (extended) hemihepatectomy including the caudate lobe, excision of the portal vein bifurcation when involved, and complete lymphadenectomy of the hepatoduodenal ligament.[86] R0 resection of HCCA is the most important prognostic determinant for long-term survival.

The goals of preoperative investigation should be to establish a diagnosis, define the biliary anatomy, and determine the extent of disease. HCCA is usually classified according to proximal infiltration of the tumor into the proximal segmental ducts using the Bismuth–Corlette system (types I–IV) . Specific criteria for unresectability include distant metastases, evidence of intraperitoneal metastases, diffuse hepatic involvement, multifocal or diffuse disease throughout the biliary tract or bilateral involvement of major vascular structures. The use of staging laparoscopy in the workup of patients with HCCA is under debate.

The scirrhous nature of these lesions and their intimate relationship with the major vascular structures contained within the hepatoduodenal ligament frequently make diagnosis difficult, while establishing a tissue diagnosis can be extremely challenging. Cholangioendoscopy can be employed to assess the lesion and provide an opportunity for directed biopsy, but the technique requires considerable expertise. The size of the ducts makes this procedure difficult and often limits the ability to obtain an adequate sample. In many cases, the surgeon must make the decision based upon cholangiographic and gross findings at the time of laparotomy, often without the benefit of a confirmed histologic diagnosis. After a thorough regional and general examination, the hilum should be carefully assessed for resection. Cholecystectomy may be performed if the gallbladder is in place because this will facilitate visualization and palpation of the hepatic bile duct bifurcation and associated structures (right portal vein, right hepatic artery). The distal bile duct is then divided and reflected in a cephalad direction, thereby separating the portal vein and hepatic artery from the duct. This maneuver allows the surgeon to assess the relationship of the tumor to the vein and branches of the hepatic artery to determine the presence or absence of invasion. In case of tumor invasion into the portal vein, resection of the portal vein bifurcation is undertaken followed by end-to-end reconstruction.[87] For biliary reconstruction, end-to-side anastomoses of the segmental ducts and a Roux-en-Y jejunal loop are constructed.

Conceptually, total hepatectomy and replacement of the liver with a liver graft is an attractive alternative in the treatment of HCCA, since the entire hepatic pedicle including the portal vein bifurcation and hepatic arteries is removed with the liver. Although selected series have shown a benefit of this strategy in combination with extensive chemotherapy, this approach is currently considered experimental.

Mid and distal bile duct tumors: Although cancers that arise in the mid and distal portion of the bile duct share some features with the proximal lesions, their unique anatomic relationships are largely responsible for differing management strategies. Unlike proximal bile duct tumors for which curative resection is technically difficult, mid and distal bile duct tumors are often amenable to resection with a radical pancreatoduodenectomy [pylorus preserving proximal pancreatoduodenectomy (PPPP) or Whipple's procedure]. The frequency with which curative resection is undertaken for patients with middle and distal bile duct tumors has increased steadily over the past several years and exceeds 60% in most series. In those patients in whom curative resection is not appropriate, internal biliary drainage can generally be achieved endoscopically or surgically by a hepaticojejunostomy.

Role of nonoperative management: The ability to intubate the biliary tract, either endoscopically or percutaneously, has greatly facilitated the management of patients with unresectable cholangiocarcinoma. The decision to proceed with placement of an endoscopic[88] or percutaneous biliary endoprosthesis[89] should be made at a multidisciplinary conference.

Radiation and chemotherapy: Most patients who die as a result of cholangiocarcinoma succumb to local recurrence and ensuing cholangitis. Failure to achieve local control has been the primary problem identified with surgical resection for proximal cholangiocarcinoma.

Anecdotal experiences suggest that local control and long-term survival may be enhanced with radiation therapy, although data from prospective, randomized, controlled studies are lacking. Whether systemic chemotherapy has a role in the management of patients with cholangiocarcinoma has not been well defined; several limited studies have failed to demonstrate any benefit. More recently, the use of the combination of gemcitabine and cisplatin has shown a benefit in terms of improved progression-free survival in patients with unresectable disease.[74]

Outcome

Owing to advances in perioperative and operative management in combination with a more aggressive surgical approach, the prognosis of proximal bile duct tumors has improved over the last two decades. The ultimate outcome of these patients is determined by the location and extent of disease, the histology and the operation performed. Patients with proximal bile duct tumors have a more favorable cancer-specific survival after resection than those with distal bile duct tumors, although location was not an independent prognostic factor.[90]

REFERENCES

1. Moore KL. The digestive system. The developing human: clinically-oriented embryology. Philadelphia, PA: WB Saunders;1982:231-7.
2. Cheslyn-Curtis S. Anatomy of the biliary tract. In: Carter D, Russell RCG, Pitt HA, Bismuth H (Eds). Hepatobiliary and pancreatic surgery. London: Chapman & Hall Medical; 1996. pp. 256-60
3. Strasberg SM, Helton WS. An analytical review of vasculobiliary injury in laparoscopic and open cholecystectomy. HPB (Oxford). 2011;13(1):1-14.
4. Vakili K, Pomfret EA. Biliary anatomy and embryology. Surg Clin North Am. 2008;88(6):1159-74.
5. Strasberg SM, Gouma DJ. "Extreme" vasculobiliary injuries: association with fundus-down cholecystectomy in severely inflamed gallbladders. HPB (Oxford). 2012;14(1):1-8.
6. Alonzo-Lej F, Revor WB, Pessagno DJ. Congenital choledochal cyst, with a report of 2, and an analysis of 94 cases. Surg Gynecol Obstet Int Abstr Surg. 1959;108:1-30.
7. Mabrut JY, Bozio G, Hubert C, et al. Management of congenital bile duct cysts. Dig Surg. 2010;27(1):12-8.
8. Chijiiwa K, Koga A. Surgical management and long-term follow-up of patients with choledochal cysts. Am J Surg. 1993;165:238-42.
9. De Vries JS, De Vries S, Aronson DC, et al. Choledochal cysts: age of presentation, symptoms, and late complications related to Todani's classification. J Pediatr Surg. 2002; 37:1568-73.
10. Alexander LF. Congenital pancreatic anomalies, variants, and conditions. Radiol Clin North Am. 2012;50:487-98.
11. Tashiro S, Imaizumi T, Ohkawa H, et al. Todani, Pancreaticobiliary maljunction: retrospective and nationwide survey in Japan. J Hepatobiliary Pancreat Surg. 2003;10:345-51.
12. Stinton LM, Shaffer EA. Epidemiology of gallbladder disease: cholelithiasis and cancer. Gut Liver. 2012;6(2):172-87.
13. Acalovschi M, Dumitrascu D, Caluser I, et al. Comparative prevalence of gallstone disease at 100-year intervals in a large Romanian town; a necropsy study. Dig Dis Sci. 1987;32:354.
14. Sama C, Morselli Labate AM, Taroni F, et al. Epidemiology and natural history of gallstone disease. Semin Liv Dis. 1990; 10:149.
15. Sampliner RE, Bennett PH, Comess LJ, et al. Gallbladder disease in Pima Indians: demonstration of high prevalence and early onset by cholecystography. N Engl J Med 1970;283:1358.
16. Biss K, Ho KJ, Mikkelson B, et al. Some unique biologic characteristics of the Masai of East Africa. N Engl J Med. 1971;284:694-9.
17. Saharia PC, Zuidema GD, Cameron JL. Primary common bile duct stones. Ann Surg. 1977;185:598.
18. Roslyn JJ, Thompson JE, Darvin H, et al. Risk factors for gallbladder perforation. Am J Gastroenterol. 1987;82:636-40.
19. Deitel M, Petrov I. Incidence of symptomatic gallstones after bariatric operations. Surg Gynecol Obstet. 1987;164:397.
20. Warschkow R, Tarantino I, Ukegjini K, et al. Concomitant cholecystectomy during laparoscopic Roux-en-Y gastric bypass in obese patients is not justified: a meta-analysis. Obes Surg. 2013;23(3):397-407.
21. Cuccihiaro G, Watters CR, Rossitch JC, et al. Deaths from gallstone; incidence and associated clinical factors. Ann Surg. 1989;209:149.
22. Frank BB. Clinical evaluation of jaundice: a guideline of the Patient Care Committee of the American Gastroenterological Association. JAMA. 1990;263:2050-51.
23. Cooperberg PL, Burhenne HJ. Real-time ultrasonography. Diagnostic technique of choice in calculous gallbladder disease. N Engl J Med. 1980;302:1277.
24. Cotton PB. Endoscopic treatment for bile duct stones. Surgical Rounds. 1990:43-6.
25. Kimura Y, Takada T, Strasberg SM, et al. Current terminology, etiology, and epidemiology of acute cholangitis and cholecystitis. J Hepatobiliary Pancreat Sci. 2013;20(1):8-23.
26. Hermann RE. The spectrum of biliary stone disease. Am J Surg. 1989;158:171.
27. Roslyn JJ, Binns GS, Hughes EX, et al. Open cholecystectomy: a contemporary analysis of 42,474 patients. Ann Surg. 1993;218:129.
28. de Mestral C, Rotstein OD, Laupacis A, et al. Comparative operative outcomes of early and delayed cholecystectomy for acute cholecystitis: a population-based propensity score analysis. Ann Surg. 2014;259(1):10-5.
29. Gurusamy KS, Rossi M, Davidson BR. Percutaneous cholecystostomy for high-risk surgical patients with acute calculous cholecystitis. Cochrane Database Syst Rev. 2013;8: CD007088.

30. Dasari BV, Tan CJ, Gurusamy KS, et al. Surgical versus endoscopic treatment of bile duct stones. Cochrane Database Syst Rev. 2013;9:CD003327.
31. Opie EL. The etiology of acute hemorrhagic pancreatitis. Bull Johns Hopkins Hosp. 1901;12:182.
32. Acosta JM, Ledesma CL. Gallstone migration as a cause of acute pancreatitis. N Engl J Med. 1974;290:484-7.
33. Carr-Locke DL. Biliary pancreatitis. Can J Gastroenterol. 2003;17(3):205-8.
34. Mallipeddi MK, Pappas TN, Shapiro ML, et al. Gallstone ileus: revisiting surgical outcomes using National Surgical Quality Improvement Program data. J Surg Res. 2013;184(1):84-8.
35. Thornton JR, Heaton KW, Espiner HJ, et al. Empyema of the gallbladder—reappraisal of a neglected disease. Gut. 1983; 24:1183.
36. Barie PS, Eachempati SR. Acute acalculous cholecystitis. Gastroenterol Clin North Am. 2010;39(2):343-57.
37. Coelho JC, Slongo J, Dambroski Silva A, et al. Prevalence of cholelithiasis in patients subjected to liver transplantation for cirrhosis. J Gastrointest Liver Dis. 2010;19(4):405-8.
38. Akoh JA, Watson WA, Bourne TP. Day case laparoscopic cholecystectomy: reducing the admission rate. Int J Surg. 2011;9(1):63-7.
39. Keulemans Y, Eshuis J, de Haes H, et al. Laparoscopic cholecystectomy: day-care versus clinical observation. Ann Surg. 1998;228(6):734-40.
40. DuBois F, Icard P, Berthelot G, et al. Coelioscopic cholecystectomy. Preliminary report of 36 cases. Ann Surg. 1990; 211:60.
41. Törnqvist B, Strömberg C, Persson G, et al. Effect of intended intraoperative cholangiography and early detection of bile duct injury on survival after cholecystectomy: population based cohort study. BMJ. 2012;11:345:e6457.
42. Wu YV, Linehan DC. Bile duct injuries in the era of laparoscopic cholecystectomies. Surg Clin N Am. 2010;90(4): 787-802.
43. Strasberg SM, Brunt LM. Rationale and use of the critical view of safety in laparoscopic cholecystectomy. J Am Coll Surg. 2010;211(1): 132-8.
44. Buddingh KT, Nieuwenhuijs VB, van Buuren L, et al. Intraoperative assessment of biliary anatomy for prevention of bile duct injury: a review of current and future patient safety interventions. Surg Endosc. 2011;25(8):2449-61.
45. Wittgen CM, Andrus CH, Fitzgerald SD, et al. Analysis of the hemodynamic and ventilatory effects of laparoscopic cholecystectomy. Arch Surg. 1991;126:997.
46. Fingerhut A, Dziri C, Garden OJ, et al. ATOM, the all-inclusive, nominal EAES classification of bile duct injuries during cholecystectomy. Surg Endosc. 2013; DOI 10.1007/ s00464-013-3081-6
47. Thakur V, Schlachta CM, Jayaraman S. Minilaparoscopic versus conventional laparoscopic cholecystectomy a systematic review and meta-analysis. Ann Surg. 2011;253(2): 244-58.
48. Koga A, Watanabe K, Fukuyama T, et al. Diagnosis and operative indications for polypoid lesions of the gallbladder. Arch Surg. 1988;123:26-9.
49. Ellis H. Anatomy of the gallbladder and bile ducts. Surgery (Oxford). 2011;29(12):593-6.
50. Millis JM, Tompkins RK, Zinner MJ, et al. Management of bile duct strictures: an evolving strategy. Arch Surg. 1992; 127:1077-84.

Additional references appear in the online version of this book.

56

Pancreas

Richard M Charnley, Robin CN Williamson

Key Points

- Preoperative imaging of the pancreas has been revolutionized by the modern imaging techniques of computed tomography (CT), magnetic resonance pancreatography, and endoscopic ultrasound (EUS).
- Gallstones and then alcoholism are the most frequent causes of acute pancreatitis worldwide. The necrotizing type of acute pancreatitis is often complicated by pseudocyst formation or infected pancreatic necrosis. Management of these complications has improved with minimally invasive techniques.
- Indications for operation in chronic pancreatitis are pain, obstructive complications, and suspicion of cancer. Resection of an inflammatory mass with duct obstruction provides good symptomatic relief.
- Pancreatic ductal adenocarcinoma is the predominant type of pancreatic tumor. Resectability is low at 20% and overall 5-year survival is 3%. Periampullary tumors carry a much better prognosis.
- Cystic tumors of the pancreas are more common than previously recognized. Mucinous tumors are premalignant. Resection is often indicated, although small cysts may be kept under surveillance.
- Functioning neuroendocrine tumors, notably insulinoma and gastrinoma, are diagnosed when they are still small because of the syndromes associated with hormonal hypersecretion. Resection gives good results. The nonfunctioning variant is seldom identified until large and potentially metastatic.

SURGICAL ANATOMY

Embryologic Development

The pancreas develops from two separate buds. The ventral bud arises from the hepatic diverticulum, which is destined to form the liver and biliary tree. The dorsal bud arises from the opposite (dorsal) surface of the primitive duodenum. Rotation combined with rapid growth of the bile duct and duodenal wall carries the ventral pancreas into a dorsal position behind the superior mesenteric vessels. The two pancreatic buds begin to fuse during the 6th week (Fig. 56.1). Fusion of the right leaf of the dorsal mesentery with the posterior abdominal wall dictates the retroperitoneal position of the pancreas.

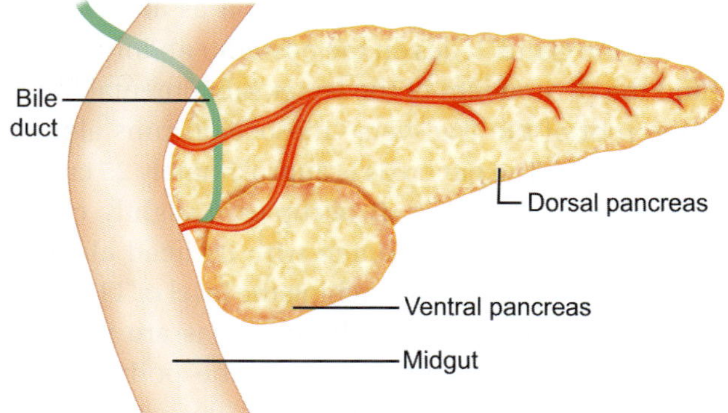

Fig. 56.1: Normal embryologic development of the pancreas from dorsal and ventral buds, which fuse during weeks 6–7 of intrauterine life.

The ventral pancreas only gives rise to the lower part of the head of pancreas and its uncinate process; the dorsal pancreas constitutes the rest of the adult gland. The duct of the ventral pancreas retains its common site of drainage with the bile duct via the major duodenal (pancreatic) papilla, but the duct of the dorsal pancreas drains separately via the minor (accessory) papilla. When the ducts fuse, most of the pancreatic secretion drains via the main pancreatic duct (of Wirsung), whereas the terminal portion of the original dorsal duct (of Santorini) either atrophies or persists as a patent channel that reaches the minor papilla. Failure of fusion of the ducts results in pancreas divisum (Figs. 56.2A and B).

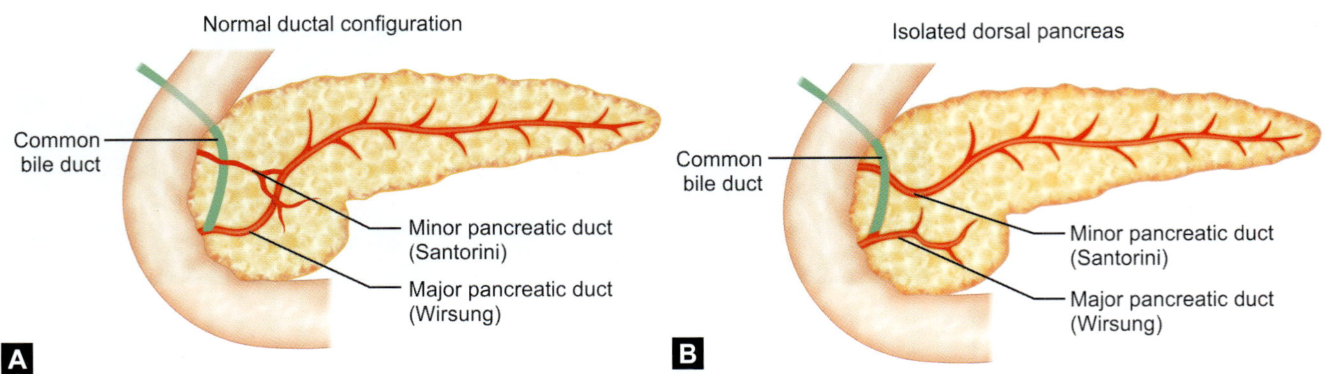

Figs. 56.2A and B: Development of the pancreatic ductal tree. (A) The common pattern in adults is achieved by a communication between the ducts of the dorsal and ventral pancreas so that most exocrine secretion drains via the major pancreatic papilla. The duct of Santorini and the accessory papilla are only present in a proportion of normal individuals. (B) In pancreas divisum or isolated dorsal pancreas, most exocrine secretion drains through the accessory papilla, which may be relatively narrow.

Gross morphologic development of the pancreas is generally complete by the 8th week of gestation, but functional differentiation into endocrine and exocrine tissue lags behind. Secretory acini begin to bud from the terminal ducts during the third intrauterine month, when islets can also be recognized. Trypsin and insulin can be detected midway through pregnancy, but exocrine and endocrine functions are immature at birth and continue to develop through the 1st year of postnatal life.

Anatomic Relationships

The adult pancreas shows no external trace of either its dual embryologic origin or its dual function as an endocrine and exocrine gland. It lies on the posterior abdominal wall behind the peritoneum of the lesser sac (omental bursa), and the root of the transverse mesocolon runs along its inferior border. The pancreas is approximately 25 cm long and weighs nearly 100 g. It occupies a slightly oblique position in the upper abdomen with its head alongside the L2 vertebra and its tail reaching the level of T12.

The component parts of the pancreas are the head, with its uncinate process, the neck, the body, and the tail (Fig. 56.3). The head of pancreas lies snugly in the C-shaped loop of the duodenum. It is intimately adherent to the bowel from just beyond the pylorus to the end of the third part of the duodenum (D_3), and there is a common blood supply. The proximity of the head of the pancreas to the duodenum explains why pancreatic inflammation and tumors can affect duodenal patency. It is possible to separate the pancreas from the duodenum by tedious dissection, but there is a risk of duodenal ischemia. The terminal portion of the bile duct runs through the head

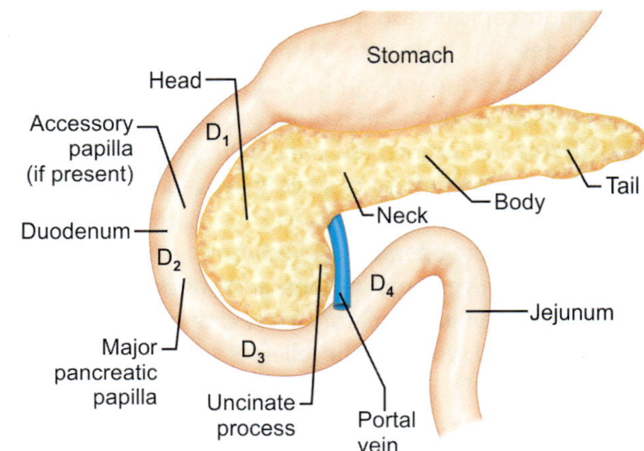

Fig. 56.3: Major relationships and component parts of the pancreas. D_1, D_2, D_3, and D_4 represent the four parts of the duodenum.

of pancreas in a tunnel and is commonly affected by pancreatic pathology. The uncinate process extends medially from the lower part of the head behind the superior mesenteric artery (SMA) and vein.

The neck of pancreas blends imperceptibly with the head at the level of the gastroduodenal artery (to the right of the midline) and with the body to the left of the portal vein (PV). It has a crucial posterior relationship with the origin of the PV from the junction of the splenic and superior mesenteric veins (SMVs). Identification of the PV tunnel is an important part of most pancreatic resections, and direct invasion of the vein is a common cause of irresectability in pancreatic cancer. The neck lies on the body of L1 and can be fractured against the spine in blunt abdominal trauma.

The body of the pancreas lies behind the stomach, separated by the lesser sac, but the two organs can become adherent in pancreatitis or if there is a penetrating gastric ulcer. The posterior relations of the body of pancreas are from medial to left lateral: the aorta, the left crus of the diaphragm, the left renal vessels, the left adrenal, and the left kidney. The splenic artery runs along its superior border, and the splenic vein is plastered against its posterior surface; these vessels can become encased or thrombosed in pancreatic cancer or chronic pancreatitis. Mobilization of the body of pancreas requires incision of the peritoneum along its upper and lower borders.

The tail of pancreas lies within the hilum of the spleen. It is relatively mobile and is at some risk of injury during mobilization of the spleen for a splenectomy. As the pancreas tapers toward its tail, it is related posteriorly to the splenic artery and vein, and their branches.

Pancreatic Ducts

Like the backbone of a fish, the main pancreatic duct increases in diameter as it runs from the tail (1 mm) to the head (3 mm). In the neck of the pancreas, it usually lies eccentrically toward the posterior aspect and superior border. As the duct turns downwards to enter the head, it "dives" more deeply into the pancreatic tissue. The major pancreatic papilla is situated on the medial wall of the descending duodenum about 10 cm distal to the pylorus; when present, the minor (accessory) papilla lies 1–2 cm proximal.

The duct of Wirsung is usually joined by the common bile duct as the two ducts pierce the medial wall of the duodenum to form a short common channel. Each duct has its own integral sphincter, but in addition, the common channel (ampulla of Vater) is surrounded by circular muscle (the sphincter of Oddi). Anomalous patterns of ductal union are quite common, and the length of the common channel varies. Sometimes the bile duct and pancreatic duct open separately on the apex of the major papilla. Rarely there may be a long common channel exceeding 15 mm in length so that the anomalous pancreatobiliary ductal junction lies above the sphincter of Oddi.

Vascular and Nerve Supply

The pancreas has a rich blood supply, and the proximity of several important vessels constitutes much of the risk of pancreatic surgery. As befits a junctional organ (foregut and midgut), it is supplied by both the celiac artery and the SMA. The arterial supply to the head of pancreas comes from the anterior and posterior pancreaticoduodenal arcades, supplied above from the gastroduodenal artery and below from the inferior pancreaticoduodenal artery, this being the first branch of the SMA. The body and tail of pancreas are supplied by numerous branches of the splenic artery, which runs along the superior border in a sinuous fashion. One early branch of the splenic artery, the dorsal pancreatic artery, runs behind the proximal body of pancreas to reach its lower border, where it continues in either direction as the transverse pancreatic artery to supply the tail of pancreas and anastomose (to the right) with the gastroduodenal artery. Anatomical anomalies of the hepatic arteries are common (such as the right hepatic artery arising from the SMA in 12% of individuals). Preoperative identification of the course of the hepatic arteries, usually on CT, is very important.

The venous drainage of the left pancreas mirrors the arterial arrangement, with numerous tributaries entering the wide-bore splenic vein. Fortunately for the surgeon, there are no veins running directly from the neck of pancreas into the front of the PV. Typically the inferior mesenteric vein enters the splenic vein just before it reaches the SMV, but often the three vessels join at the same point; the inferior mesenteric vein can nearly always be spared when ligating the splenic vein during a distal pancreatectomy. The spleen is usually included in this resection because it has a common blood supply, but it is sometimes possible (in a case of chronic pancreatitis without splenic vein thrombosis) to separate the body and tail of pancreas from the splenic vessels and therefore preserve the spleen. The left gastric (coronary) vein enters the PV just above the neck of pancreas. The middle colic vein(s) joins the terminal segment of the SMV and can be used as a guide to the PV tunnel at operation. The right pancreas is drained by a number of short thin-walled pancreaticoduodenal veins.

The pancreas is located close to the cisterna chyli and has a complex system of lymphatic drainage, making carcinomas of the gland difficult to eradicate. Lymph nodes lie in the anterior and posterior duodenopancreatic grooves of the head of pancreas and also surround the bile duct and PV within the free edge of the lesser omentum; these can be directly involved by adenocarcinoma of the head. The body and tail of pancreas drain initially to lymph nodes lying along the superior border of the pancreas and at the splenic hilum. Lymphatic vessels run alongside the hepatic and splenic arteries to reach the celiac nodes and along the inferior pancreaticoduodenal artery to reach the superior mesenteric nodes.

The pancreas has a dual autonomic innervation. The sympathetic supply is relayed from the thoracic sympathetic chain on each side via the splanchnic nerves and the celiac plexus. There are efferent (vasomotor) fibers and afferent fibers conveying pain sensation. This pattern is clinically relevant when considering nerve blocking procedures for relief of pancreatic pain. The parasympathetic supply to the pancreas derives from the vagus nerves and is secretomotor to the acinar tissue; there may also be vagal afferents. There is a complex intrinsic system of nerves within the pancreas involving several different chemical neurotransmitters.

Microscopic Anatomy

The exocrine pancreas is a compound gland; acinar cells comprise about 80% of the pancreatic volume. The terminal ductules are lined by centroacinar cells and surrounded by acinar cells, which secrete the pancreatic juice. The ductules unite to form intra- and then interlobular ducts, which join the main pancreatic duct. The large ducts are lined by columnar and mucous cells.

The endocrine pancreatic tissue (2% by volume) is organized into islets of Langerhans, which are scattered throughout the gland with a relative preponderance in the left pancreas. There is a close anatomic relationship between acinar and islet cells.

APPLIED PHYSIOLOGY

Exocrine Function

The pancreas is an active gland. The acinar tissue synthesizes up to 20 g of protein per day, and the ductal cells secrete alkaline juice rich in bicarbonate (approximately 2.5 L per day). Enzyme secretion is stimulated by cholecystokinin (CCK) and ductal secretion by secretin; the autonomic nerve supply modulates this activity. Pancreatic juice is clear and watery and has a pH of 7.5–8.5 and a bicarbonate concentration of 25–150 mEq/L (25–150 mmol/L) depending upon flow rates. The principal enzymes capable of splitting protein, fat, and carbohydrate are mostly secreted in an inactive zymogen form. Duodenal enterokinase converts trypsinogen into trypsin, with the release of trypsinogen activation peptide (TAP), and trypsin then catalyzes the release of all the other active enzymes. The pancreas is the major source of lipase and amylase in the gastrointestinal (GI) tract; pancreatic and salivary amylases represent different isoamylases.

Circulating levels of amylase, lipase, and trypsin are increased in acute pancreatitis, and TAP can be detected in the urine. Phospholipase A2 is thought to play an important pathophysiologic role by damaging membrane phospholipids and liberating lysolecithin. Mechanisms that protect against autodigestion of the pancreas include the intraduodenal activation of trypsinogen and the presence of a trypsin inhibitor within the pancreas and of protease inhibitors, such as α_1-antitrypsin and α_2-macroglobulin, within the plasma. These protective mechanisms can be overwhelmed in severe acute pancreatitis.

The exocrine secretion of the pancreas has cephalic (vagal) and postprandial (hormonal) phases that are triggered by eating and are then followed by an interdigestive phase. Inhibition of CCK secretion by an increasing content of pancreatic enzymes in the jejunal lumen provides a negative feedback loop. Besides stimulating enzyme secretion, CCK has a trophic role in maintaining pancreatic growth; exogenous CCK causes hypertrophy and hyperplasia of the gland.

Endocrine Function

Several different peptide hormones are synthesized by the various types of normal pancreatic islet cell. In addition, certain "ectopic" hormones, such as gastrin and adrenocorticotropin, can be synthesized by neoplastic islet cells. Insulin, the most important pancreatic hormone, is elaborated by β cells, which constitute at least two-thirds of the islet cell mass. Proinsulin is cleaved within the Golgi apparatus to insulin and C-peptide. Insulin promotes glucose uptake by most tissues in the body. Diabetes mellitus may be caused by surgical diseases, such as chronic pancreatitis and pancreatic carcinoma, and as a consequence of surgical operation. In selected patients, such as those who have diabetic renal failure, diabetes mellitus may be cured by pancreatic or islet transplantation.

Other notable hormones elaborated by islet cells are as follows:

- Glucagon, which increases blood glucose levels and therefore acts as an insulin antagonist
- Somatostatin, which inhibits exocrine pancreatic secretion and has a wide range of secretory and motility functions outside the pancreas
- Pancreatic polypeptide (PP; precise role uncertain).

The intimate relationship between endocrine and exocrine tissue in the pancreas may have functional importance. Acinar cells are exposed to high levels of islet hormones, such as insulin and somatostatin, and possess high-affinity surface receptors. Insulin potentiates the secretory response to CCK, whereas CCK and secretin have an insulinotropic effect. Peri-insular acinar cells may become atrophic in diabetes mellitus, and chronic pancreatitis can interfere with insulin release. The exocrine and endocrine pancreases have complementary roles in digestion and the use of nutrients.

INVESTIGATION

Preoperative Imaging of the Pancreas

Conventional Radiography

Plain abdominal radiographs are of extremely limited value in pancreatic disease and should not be relied upon for diagnosis. In acute pancreatitis, they may show localized ileus (the so-called "sentinel loop") while in chronic pancreatitis pancreatic calcification may be seen, but a CT scan is essential for planning treatment.

Transabdominal Ultrasound

Real-time high-resolution ultrasound can often provide excellent anatomic definition of the pancreas, bile duct, and adjacent blood vessels. It may demonstrate swelling of the gland, related fluid collections (pseudocysts), and is extremely useful as the first investigation in a patient who has obstructive jaundice to confirm the presence of extrahepatic biliary dilatation and often the likely cause, whether gallstone or tumor. Ultrasound images of the whole pancreas, however, may be difficult to obtain mainly due to intra-abdominal gas, and ultrasound should not be relied upon to exclude pancreatic disease.

Computed Tomography

A CT scan is the single most useful investigation for the pancreatic surgeon. The CT scan should be carried out on a multidetector scanner using intravenous and oral contrast with care to obtain images in the precontrast, arterial, and portal venous phases as a pancreas protocol scan.[1] In patients with extrahepatic biliary obstruction with no duct stones on ultrasound, a pancreas protocol CT is the imaging investigation of choice to determine the cause of the obstruction and provide valuable information about stage of disease and resectability of a potential tumor. Tumors are easily missed on nonprotocolized scans. In acute pancreatitis, CT provides valuable prognostic information and is essential to decide when to intervene surgically, radiologically, or endoscopically. Lack of perfusion with contrast indicates ischemia or necrosis. In chronic pancreatitis, CT is essential in all patients to provide invaluable information about an inflammatory mass, calcification, a pseudocyst, and involvement of adjacent viscera.

Magnetic Resonance Imaging

Magnetic resonance imaging (MRI) is increasingly used in the preoperative assessment of pancreatic and biliary disease. In terms of pancreatic imaging, it is not as accurate as CT and fails to identify calcification. Both the bile duct and the pancreatic duct, however, can be delineated by magnetic resonance cholangiopancreatography (MRCP), which is totally noninvasive. It provides accurate information about the cause and level of biliary obstruction and is very useful if CT fails to show the cause of an obstruction. Some clinicians will use MRCP in all patients with biliary obstruction, but the main advantage of MRCP is to avoid endoscopic retrograde cholangiopancreatography (ERCP) in patients without an endoscopically treatable obstruction.[2] Pancreatic MRI is also used in the differentiation of solid and cystic lesions, in the imaging of neuroendocrine tumors, the long-term follow up of cysts, and screening of high-risk individuals.

Biliary Scintigraphy

Hepatobiliary iminodiacetic acid scanning is now rarely used in relation to pancreatic disease, but may be useful to assess a stenosis at a biliary–enteric anastomosis.

Endoscopic Ultrasound

This is a technique whereby ultrasound images are obtained using an ultrasound transducer mounted on the tip of an upper GI endoscope. When the endoscope is passed into the stomach or duodenum, high-resolution ultrasound images of the pancreas and extrahepatic bile duct can be obtained. Endoscopic ultrasound is used for staging of pancreatic biliary tumors following CT, including assessment of vascular invasion and lymph node involvement; identification of small neuroendocrine tumors of the pancreas; diagnosis of bile duct stones and microlithiasis; and characterization of pancreatic cysts. Endoscopic ultrasound-guided fine-needle aspiration (FNA) cytology is one of the most accurate techniques for pancreatic tissue biopsy. Therapeutic EUS is used for drainage of pancreatic collections, including infected pancreatic necrosis. Although complications may occur with EUS, the risk of complications is significantly lower than with ERCP and therefore EUS is indicated in many instances in which an ERCP would previously have been used.[3]

Positron Emission Tomography

Positron emission tomography (PET) scan is a technique whereby functional three-dimensional images can be obtained following intravenous injection of a radiolabeled biologically active molecule, the most commonly used being fluorodeoxyglucose. Positron emission tomography scan is most commonly used to identify whether a mass on CT may be tumor or whether metastases are present in a patient who is already known to have a primary tumor. If PET is combined with CT or MRI, the images complement each other to provide functional information about lesions seen on CT or MRI. In pancreatic cancer, PET–CT is significantly more sensitive in detecting metastatic disease than conventional CT imaging, but its overall accuracy and its role in the management of pancreatic cancer are yet to be determined.[4]

Endoscopic Retrograde Cholangiopancreatography

Over the past 30 years, endoscopic retrograde cholangiopancreatography has assumed a dominant role in pancreatic imaging. Because of the relatively high risk of severe complications (acute pancreatitis, hemorrhage, perforation, and infection) and the evolution of other techniques (MRCP and EUS), however, ERCP has been almost totally superseded in terms of diagnosing pancreatic and biliary pathology.[5] The only reasons, therefore, for doing a diagnostic ERCP would be either to obtain tissue from a previously identified suspicious biliary or pancreatic ductal lesion or to perform biliary and/or pancreatic manometry in a patient with a compelling history of sphincter of Oddi dysfunction. By contrast, therapeutic ERCP is an essential procedure in many types of pancreatic pathology. In those patients with bile duct stones, ERCP may allow stone extraction by means of an endoscopic sphincterotomy. In chronic pancreatitis, ERCP may be used for duct drainage, transpapillary cyst drainage, stricture dilatation, and stone removal. In patients with obstructive jaundice, ERCP is used for stone extraction, stenting strictures—benign and malignant—either for preoperative biliary decompression or as a permanent alternative to an operative bypass. Finally, pancreas divisum may be treated by endoscopic pancreatic sphincterotomy via the minor duodenal papilla.

Percutaneous Transhepatic Biliary Drainage

Sometimes ERCP is technically difficult or impossible because of papillary fibrosis, a previous Billroth II gastrectomy or duodenal stenosis. In such patients who have obstructive jaundice, percutaneous transhepatic biliary drainage (PTBD) provides a useful alternative method for displaying the bile duct that can be decompressed through a percutaneous route. The intrahepatic insertion has its own potential complications of bleeding, bile leakage, and cholangitis.

Angiography

Because of the accuracy of contrast-enhanced CT in demonstrating vascular involvement in pancreatic disease, there is now little role for visceral angiography in diagnosis or for staging tumors although it is still used in some patients for localizing an insulinoma (by arterial injection of calcium combined with venous sampling). Therapeutic celiac and superior mesenteric angiography, however, is essential for treatment of bleeding complications of acute and chronic pancreatitis and for the management of hemorrhagic complications of pancreatic surgery.

Intraoperative Imaging of the Pancreas

Laparoscopy

Preoperative laparoscopy has become less important in staging pancreatic cancer because the accuracy of CT has increased. The chance of finding disease at laparoscopy that would render an otherwise resectable patient, unresectable is only about 10% although more likely in those with tumors of the body and tail of pancreas. Laparoscopy (with laparoscopic ultrasound) does, however, have a major role in obtaining a tissue diagnosis from the pancreas (*see* below in section on Pancreatic Biopsy) and in laparoscopic pancreatic resection (*see* section on pancreatic resection).

Intraoperative and Laparoscopic Ultrasonography

Direct application of an ultrasound probe to the surface of the pancreas provides high-resolution images, but experience is needed to interpret them. Intraoperative ultrasonography is invaluable in pancreatic surgery and is generally used to identify small pancreatic tumors or liver metastases, demonstrate involvement of the PV, target tumors for biopsy, and assess the pancreas in chronic pancreatitis surgery.

Pancreatic Function Tests

The pancreas has a considerable functional reserve. At least 80% of the gland must be destroyed before the patient becomes overtly diabetic or develops clinical evidence of exocrine failure. Alternative mechanisms are available for protein and carbohydrate digestion, so the clinical picture of exocrine insufficiency is dominated by steatorrhea, which is often accompanied by abdominal pain and excessive flatus as colonic bacteria degrade the undigested fat.

Exocrine function testing has become simpler in recent years. The traditional tests that require an indwelling duodenal tube provide the most accurate data, but are difficult to carry out and unpleasant for the patient, whereas those that require fecal fat analysis are unpopular in the laboratory. Now the most commonly used test is estimation of fecal elastase. Elastase is a pancreatic enzyme that is not absorbed from the GI tract, and its presence is therefore representative of pancreatic function. Few other tests are now used to evaluate exocrine dysfunction. Endocrine pancreatic function testing relies on a standard oral glucose tolerance test (using a 75-g oral loading dose) supplemented by random estimations of blood glucose levels and measurement of glycosylated hemoglobin (HbA1c), which gives a long-term assessment of diabetic control.

When possible, endocrine and exocrine pancreatic function should be measured before and after an operation for chronic pancreatitis. Major pancreatic resection (pancreatoduodenectomy or distal pancreatectomy) has been shown to cause diabetes in approximately 25% of patients, and it is important to warn patients of this possibility. Lesser resections such as head resection for chronic pancreatitis are less likely to cause diabetes, but patients with pancreatitis in the remnant are at risk of further deterioration of pancreatic function.[6]

Pancreatic Biopsy

Unresectable patients: There is a definite role for pancreatic biopsy in patients not undergoing resectional surgery. An accurate tissue diagnosis may justify the use of aggressive treatments, such as chemotherapy and radiotherapy. Biopsy may refine the use of these treatments by identifying the occasional case of lymphoma or endocrine cancer.

In many patients biliary drainage is necessary, and this is usually carried out by ERCP and endoscopic stent placement. Biliary brushing using an endoscopic cytology brush is a good technique for achieving a tissue diagnosis and should always be done. It has a sensitivity rate of 60–80% in pancreatic cancer.

If biliary brushings are negative, needle biopsy of the pancreatic tumor or liver metastases is indicated. For needle biopsy of the pancreas, several techniques are available, the choice depending on local expertise. In the authors' practice, EUS-guided biopsy, by FNA or core biopsy, is the first choice technique and has a sensitivity in cancer of 85% (which is improved by the presence of an in-room cytopathologist).[7] If this first biopsy is negative and a further attempt is required, a percutaneous or laparoscopic pancreatic biopsy would be done. The percutaneous ultrasound-guided route is also used for liver metastases.

Resectable patients: In fit patients who have a resectable pancreatic mass suspicious of tumor, surgical resection is usually inevitable and preoperative biopsy should not be carried out. Insisting on a positive biopsy before pancreatic resection is likely to delay operation.[8] Due to sampling error (tumors contain areas of inflammation and fibrous tissue), a "negative" result does not exclude cancer. Another concern is the risk of complications, which although low may involve acute pancreatitis, a pancreatic fistula, and the possibility of tumor dissemination along the needle track, all of which would complicate or might prevent operation.

Operative confirmation of the diagnosis should always be obtained before completing the operation if unresectable disease is found at laparotomy. It is simple and safe to sample an involved lymph node or a secondary deposit in the liver or omentum; otherwise, the primary tumor itself should be sampled.

CONGENITAL ANOMALIES OF THE PANCREAS

Annular Pancreas

Annular pancreas is rare and is seen once in every 7,000 autopsies. It is thought to arise from fixation of the tip of the ventral pancreas to the duodenal wall before rotation of that organ, so that the descending duodenum becomes encircled by a ring of pancreatic tissue. The rich supply of PP cells within the annulus may indicate an origin from the ventral bud. Annular pancreas commonly presents in a neonate who has other congenital anomalies, such as duodenal atresia or stenosis, Down's syndrome, or intestinal malrotation. Duodenal obstruction causes bile-stained vomiting in the first few days of life. The classic "double bubble" sign on plain abdominal radiograph may be supplemented by contrast studies and an ultrasound scan. Simple division of the constricting ring of pancreatic tissue is unwise because of the possibility that there may be an associated intrinsic duodenal narrowing and the risk of developing pancreatic fistula. Duodenoduodenostomy is the most satisfactory form of bypass. Annular pancreas may come to light in older children who undergo surgical exploration for duodenal stenosis or malrotation. The condition may predispose to pancreatitis, both acute and chronic.

Heterotopic Pancreas

Small foci of ectopic pancreatic tissue are sometimes seen in the wall of the stomach, duodenum, or jejunoileum, or even further afield (liver, mediastinum). Nodules of ectopic exocrine tissue within a Meckel's diverticulum can lead to invagination and intussusception of a Meckel's diverticulum. The vast majority of patients who have heterotopic pancreas are completely asymptomatic, but bleeding, ulceration, inflammation, and malignant degeneration have been described.

Congenital Pancreatic Cysts

The pancreas is occasionally involved in generalized polycystic disease, but less often than the liver and kidney. Cysts of the pancreas and other viscera including the cerebellum are part of von Hippel–Lindau disease and certain other rare congenital syndromes (*see* below in section on cystic tumors of the pancreas). Small degenerative cysts are seen in cystic fibrosis, when complete exocrine failure is associated with progressive, but painless dilatation of the pancreatic ductal tree. Solitary cysts of the pancreas have been reported in young children and occasionally lead to biliary or duodenal obstruction. More often, they are found incidentally on abdominal CT scans.

Pancreas Divisum

Malfusion of the dorsal and ventral pancreatic ducts is a common anomaly that is seen in approximately 5% of ERCP examinations, but its clinical importance is debatable. Types seen are as follows:

- The commonest variant (type 1) in which there is complete failure of fusion so that the dorsal pancreas drains entirely via the duct of Santorini (*see* Fig. 56.2B)
- In the type 2 variant, the type 1 arrangement is associated with agenesis of the ventral duct
- Type 3 represents a forme fruste, in which there is a tenuous communication between the dorsal and ventral systems.

Pancreas divisum results in most of the exocrine secretion reaching the duodenum via the accessory papilla, so narrowing of this orifice could give rise to a functional obstruction and predispose to pancreatitis.

Pancreas divisum is an unconvincing explanation for chronic upper abdominal pain. The anomaly may protect against acute pancreatitis caused by lodgment of a calculus at the major papilla, but appears to be linked with recurrent attacks of acute "idiopathic" pancreatitis; a few of these patients may eventually develop chronic pancreatitis.

Magnetic resonance cholangiopancreatography before and after secretin is now the definitive confirmatory test for pancreas divisum. Magnetic resonance cholangiopancreatography is carried out as a baseline and then after intravenous secretin injection.[9] Widening of the main pancreatic duct and development of a Santorinicele (dilatation of the accessory duct just proximal to the minor papilla), often accompanied by pain, following secretin is indication that there is delayed secretion at the minor papilla.

Treatment of pancreas divisum should only be carried out in the presence of confirmatory evidence from a secretin MRCP and matching symptoms. Endoscopic accessory sphincterotomy by ERCP is the treatment of choice, but this is a challenging procedure and should only be carried out by an experienced ERCP practitioner. Restenosis is a risk. Operative accessory sphincteroplasty should then be considered. The accessory papilla may be tiny and is approached by a transduodenal incision, using intravenous secretin and irrigation of the duodenal lumen with methylene blue to help localize it in case of difficulty (the secretin will wash away the methylene blue at the papilla). Following insertion of a lacrimal probe, the papilla is divided for about 10 mm, and fine sutures are used to appose the ductal and duodenal mucosae (Fig. 56.4).

Anomalous Pancreatobiliary Ductal Junction

An anomalous pancreatobiliary ductal junction is particularly common in the Japanese population. It is diagnosed at ERCP when the common pancreatobiliary channel exceeds 15 mm in length as follows:

- In the type 1 anomaly, the two ducts join at a right angle, and this arrangement predisposes to choledochal cyst (and cholangiocarcinoma)
- In the type 2 anomaly, the two ducts join at an acute angle, and this arrangement may predispose to carcinoma of the gallbladder.

Because the point of ductal union lies above the sphincter of Oddi, pancreatic juice may reflux into the bile duct and vice versa. The presence of high amylase levels

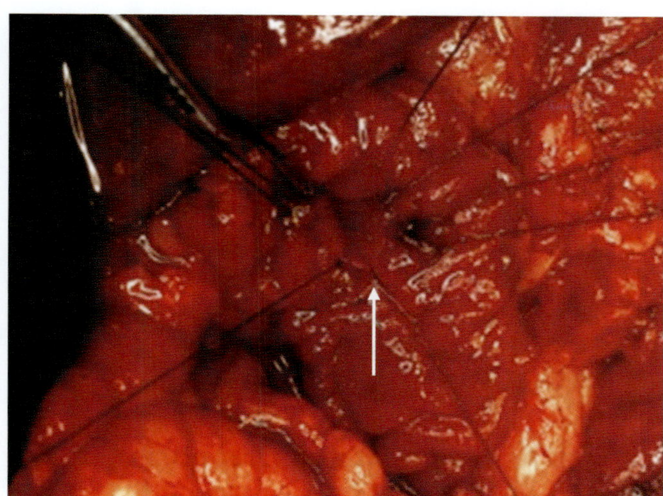

Fig. 56.4: Accessory sphincteroplasty in an elderly woman who had recurrent acute pancreatitis secondary to pancreas divisum. The previously tiny orifice of the accessory pancreatic duct has been incised (arrow) and sutured to the duodenal mucosa.

in the bile could account for the increased risk of biliary neoplasia, whereas bile reflux could explain an increased incidence of pancreatitis.

ACUTE PANCREATITIS

Acute pancreatitis is a common cause of the "acute abdomen" worldwide. Etiology, however, varies from country to country. The sex incidence is approximately equal, but gallstones are more common in women and alcoholism more common in men. Acute pancreatitis is often seen in elderly patients and has an overall mortality rate of approximately 5%.[10] Most deaths occur in one of two settings:

- During the initial period of hypovolemic shock (especially in the elderly)
- After ≥2 weeks of a septic illness that leads to multiorgan failure in those who have infected pancreatic necrosis.

Treatment remains largely supportive, and intervention is confined to those patients with extensive and usually infected necrosis. In approximately three of every four patients who have acute pancreatitis, the course is "benign," but the fourth patient develops one or more serious complications and is at risk of death.

Etiology and Pathology

Gallstones and alcohol consumption are the leading causes among a multitude of reported factors. In several Western countries including the UK, gallstones account for one-half to two-thirds of attacks of acute pancreatitis, the actual incidence reflecting the diligence of the search. Biliary sludge can be identified in up to two-thirds of those initially thought to have idiopathic disease.[11] Acute biliary pancreatitis is more common in those individuals with small gallstones and a long common pancreatobiliary channel. Lodgment of a stone at the papilla (even transiently), so allowing reflux of bile along the pancreatic duct, is the likely pathogenesis.[12]

Acute pancreatitis is a complication of alcoholism, but although it can be precipitated by an alcoholic binge there is nearly always a history of chronic alcohol abuse. Therefore, most affected patients have some degree of pre-existing chronic pancreatitis. The pathogenesis may include pancreatic hypersecretion, direct cellular toxicity, and a disturbed microcirculation in the pancreas.

Postoperative pancreatitis has been reported after many different procedures, the most common being ERCP but also surgical procedures in the vicinity of the papilla that can cause papillary edema or ductal overdistension. Hyperamylasemia is common after ERCP, but clinical pancreatitis only occurs in 2–3%. Pancreatic ischemia secondary to a low cardiac output is the probable mechanism involved in the fulminating acute pancreatitis (and likewise acute acalculous cholecystitis) that can follow cardiopulmonary bypass, whereas drugs and infection may be the causes after organ transplantation.

Acute pancreatitis is occasionally the presenting feature of a neoplasm of the pancreas or the periampullary region. The diagnosis should become evident during investigation of "idiopathic" pancreatitis by abdominal ultrasound, CT, and EUS.

A wide variety of microorganisms and parasites have been incriminated as causes of acute pancreatitis. Acute pancreatitis can complicate salmonella enteritis, mumps, coxsackievirus infection, and roundworms in the pancreatobiliary tree, and it also occurs in patients who have AIDS. Scorpions can cause pancreatitis in Trinidad. Many different drugs have been implicated as causes of acute pancreatitis (often on tenuous grounds), including tetracyclines, thiazides, anti-inflammatory drugs, corticosteroids, immunosuppressants, and antiepileptic agents.

Acute pancreatitis is associated with hyperlipidemia, whether familial or linked with gallstones or alcoholism. Hyperparathyroidism and hypothermia are occasional causes. In China, a heavy meal of cold rice can provoke pancreatitis, as can refeeding a patient who has anorexia nervosa.

Table 56.1 Morphological features of acute pancreatitis.[13]

Pathologic state	*Description*
Interstitial edematous pancreatitis	Acute inflammation without necrosis
Necrotizing pancreatitis	Inflammation with pancreatic parenchymal necrosis and/or peripancreatic necrosis
Acute peripancreatic fluid collection	Peripancreatic fluid associated with interstitial edematous pancreatitis but no associated with peripancreatic necrosis; occurs within 4 weeks of onset with no definable wall encapsulating the collection
Pancreatic pseudocyst	Encapsulated collection of fluid with a well-defined wall, usually outside the pancreas with little or no necrosis; usually occurs >4 weeks after the onset of acute pancreatitis
Acute necrotic collection	A collection containing variable amounts of both fluid and necrosis associated with necrotizing pancreatitis
Walled-off necrosis	A maturing encapsulated collection of pancreatic and/or peripancreatic necrosis with a well-defined wall; occurs >4 weeks after onset of necrotizing pancreatitis

There remains a group of patients for whom there is no recognizable cause of acute pancreatitis and whose disease must therefore be labeled as idiopathic, but thorough investigation should reduce the proportion of patients in this group to <10%.

Whatever the trigger, there is likely to be a common pathway for the subsequent pathologic changes of acute pancreatitis that lead to autodigestion of the gland. Escape of activated enzymes into the interstitium is a critical step, mediated by conversion of trypsinogen to trypsin by lysosomal cathepsin B and overexpression of heat shock protein 70, which results in acinar cell injury and cell death. Pancreatic edema is prominent at first, and the disease may "stabilize" at this stage with variable degrees of acute inflammatory infiltration. If the disease progresses, the pancreas becomes hemorrhagic and then necrotic. Necrosis may be extensive, in which case bacterial infection is likely to supervene. Fluid collections are related to the severe local inflammation; there may be blood-stained ascites in hemorrhagic disease plus considerable sequestration of fluid in the retroperitoneal tissues. Fat necrosis in and around the pancreas is explained by the release of lipolytic enzymes. Many different terms have been used to define the various pathologic conditions in acute pancreatitis, and these have been helpfully updated recently (Table 56.1).[13]

Dysfunction of distant organs, such as the heart, lungs, and kidneys, is thought to be caused by the release of inflammatory mediators such as bradykinin and cytokines, plus the effects of circulating trypsin and phospholipase A_2. Several different cytokines may be involved, including interleukins 1 and 6, tumor necrosis factor, and platelet activating factor (PAF), and these activate neutrophils to cause tissue damage. Pancreatic perfusion is impaired as acute pancreatitis worsens, and this leads to the production of reactive oxygen metabolites.

Clinical Assessment and Diagnosis

Clinical Presentation

The typical patient who has acute pancreatitis develops upper abdominal pain of rapid onset that radiates to the back and to the rest of the abdomen. It is constant and usually causes nausea and vomiting. The patient may have known gallstones or a history of alcohol abuse, and the attack may follow a heavy meal or heavy alcohol consumption. The patient is often distressed with a tachycardia and shows evidence of dehydration or even shock. The temperature is often subnormal unless there is concomitant biliary infection. There may be cyanosis or icterus. The abdominal signs are those of peritonitis, which may be localized to the epigastrium or generalized. Occasionally, there is bruising at the umbilicus (Cullen's sign) or in the flanks (Grey Turner's sign) in a patient who has severe pancreatitis with retroperitoneal hemorrhage. A pleural effusion, especially on the left side, may be diagnosed clinically or radiologically at an early stage.

Acute pancreatitis can be subdivided into interstitial edematous pancreatitis and necrotizing pancreatitis.[13] The majority of patients have interstitial edematous pancreatitis with diffuse enlargement of the pancreas on CT due to inflammatory edema. There may also be peripancreatic fluid. In most patients, the symptoms settle within the 1st week. In necrotizing pancreatitis, necrosis of the pancreas and/or peripancreatic tissues occurs. These changes develop over several days, and early CT scan may therefore underestimate the degree of necrosis.

Pancreatic and peripancreatic necrosis may remain sterile or become infected. Those patients with extensive necrosis are more likely to develop infected necrosis. Infected necrosis is less likely within the first 2 weeks following onset of the original symptoms and in many cases does not occur until 4–6 weeks after onset.

Initial Investigation

The diagnosis of acute pancreatitis depends upon a serum amylase level that is at least three times the upper level of normal for the laboratory plus acute onset of upper abdominal pain. Many other pancreatic enzymes can be measured in the blood (including lipase), but none has proved superior to amylase in routine practice. Serum lipase or urinary amylase levels (which stay elevated for longer) may help confirm the diagnosis if hyperamylasemia does not reach diagnostic levels or if diagnosis is delayed.

Leukocytosis is nearly always present. Blood urea, electrolytes, glucose, calcium, and liver function tests should also be performed to obtain baseline values and detect early complications. Similarly, arterial blood gas analysis provides an early warning of hypoxia. Plain abdominal radiographs may show a localized ileus. An ultrasound scan is useful to detect gallstones, but overlying bowel gas frequently obscures the pancreas. A contrast-enhanced CT scan detects changes in over 90% of patients: diffuse pancreas enlargement, blurring of the tissue planes, and decreased contrast enhancement.

Differential Diagnosis

Acute pancreatitis can be confused with other causes of peritonitis, many of which require urgent intervention. Acute cholecystitis can cause a similar radiation of pain, tenderness, and guarding in the upper abdomen. Acute cholangitis is identified by high fever, chills, and marked derangement of liver function tests; urgent endoscopic sphincterotomy is indicated. A perforated peptic ulcer may be suggested by a history of indigestion, and free gas is often present on an erect chest radiograph. Strangulating small bowel obstruction can be associated with an elevated serum amylase, and if the level of obstruction is high there may be little to find on abdominal radiographs; abdominal colic and vomiting are prominent symptoms. A leaking abdominal aneurysm will sometimes cause diagnostic difficulties if back pain is prominent. Medical conditions, such as basal pneumonia with pleurisy and myocardial infarction, may produce overlapping clinical features; a thorough history and physical examination combined with relevant tests (chest radiograph, cardiac enzymes, and electrocardiogram) should provide the correct diagnosis.

If the diagnosis is in doubt, an urgent CT scan is mandatory and might prevent unnecessary surgery. Peritoneal lavage is rarely necessary, but if serious doubt remains it is safer to proceed to laparoscopy (or rarely laparotomy) to exclude a treatable condition. Laparoscopy/laparotomy evidence of acute pancreatitis includes free fluid, patches of fat necrosis on the omentum and mesentery (Fig. 56.5), and pancreatic inflammation.

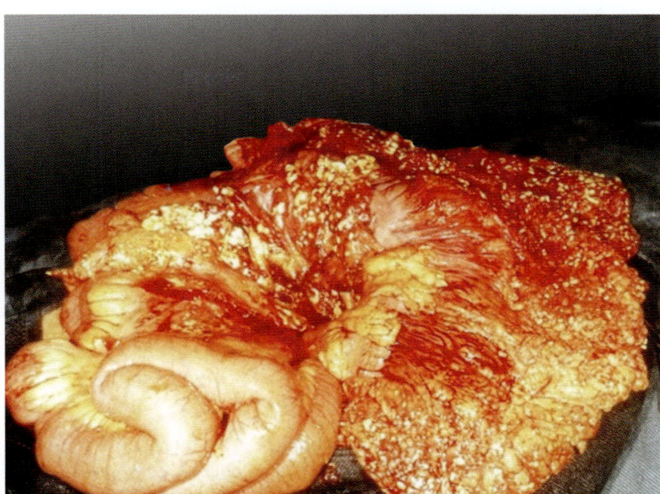

Fig. 56.5: Severe acute pancreatitis. Florid fat necrosis is seen within the greater omentum at laparotomy.

Early Prediction of Severity

It is important to identify patients who have a severe attack of acute pancreatitis as soon as possible after admission to hospital to allow vigilant management in an intensive care setting. Clinical examination on admission is neither sensitive nor specific, although by 48 hours it can offer quite an accurate differentiation between mild (edematous) and severe (hemorrhagic or necrotizing) disease. Age over 55 years and body mass index >30 are also important risk factors. A number of complex scoring systems are based upon the acquisition of clinical and laboratory data over the first 24–48 hours. According to the Ranson or Modified Glasgow systems (Table 56.2),[14,15] a patient who has three or more positive criteria has severe acute pancreatitis, and nearly all the deaths occur in this group of patients. The Apache II classification for severity of disease provides a similarly useful assessment based upon cardiorespiratory function and basic laboratory parameters of illness. Useful comparisons of scoring systems are available.[16]

These multiple scoring systems are cumbersome, and it takes time to acquire a full set of data. The ideal single marker should be simple to measure on a daily basis, and C-reactive protein is the best candidate. It has excellent

Table 56.2 Prediction of severity in acute pancreatitis.

	Scoring system	
Factor	*Modified Glasgow*[15]	*Ranson*[14]
Age	–	> 55 years
White blood cell count	> 15,000/mm³ (15 × 10⁹/L)	> 16,000/mm³ (16 × 10⁹/L)
Blood glucose	> 180 mg/dL (10 mmol/L), no diabetic history	> 200 mg/dL (11.2 mmol/L)
Lactate dehydrogenase	> 600 U/L	>700 U/L
AST		>250 U/dL
AST/ALT	> 100 U/L	
Blood urea	49 mg/dL (16 mmol/L), no response to intravenous fluids	> 5 mg/dL (1.8 mmol/L) within 48 hours
PaO_2	< 60 mm Hg (7.8 kPa)	< 60 mm Hg (7.8 kPa) within 48 hours
Serum calcium	< 8 mg/dL (2 mmol/L)	< 8 mg/dL (2 mmol/L) within 48 hours
Serum albumin	< 3.2 g/dL (32 g/L)	
Hematocrit decrease		> 10% within 48 hours
Base deficit		> 4 mEq/L (4 mmol/L) within 48 hours
Fluid sequestration		> 6 L within 48 hours

More than three positive criteria according to the Modified Glasgow[15] or Ranson[14] criteria constitute a severe attack.
(AST: Aspartate aminotransferase; ALT: Alanine aminotransferase; PaO_2: Partial pressure of arterial oxygen).

sensitivity and specificity to allow distinction between mild and severe disease, but again there is a delay of 48 hours or so before peak values are reached.[17] An early CT scan with contrast enhancement shows the extent of tissue necrosis and therefore the risk of septic complications, but CT criteria should supplement rather than replace the clinical criteria of severity. A scoring system for the severity of CT changes in acute pancreatitis is in use in many centers.[18] The presence of organ failure on admission is an important prognostic factor in acute pancreatitis but if corrected within 48 hours, those patients with transient organ failure revert to the less severe group.[19]

Complications

It is appropriate to consider the complications of acute pancreatitis before treatment because management is largely supportive and is concerned with the detection and eradication of these complications. Approximately one-third of patients who have fatal acute pancreatitis die within the 1st week, one-third during the 2nd and 3rd weeks, and one-third thereafter. The causes of early death are dominated by adult respiratory distress syndrome (ARDS) and renal failure and the causes of late death by sepsis and multiorgan failure in patients with infected pancreatic necrosis.[20]

Early (Medical) Complications

The early complications of acute pancreatitis comprise metabolic derangements and organ dysfunction. Hypocalcemia is a feature of all but the mildest attack, and magnesium levels may also fall. There may be transient hyperglycemia, but acute diabetes mellitus is rare. Raised levels of serum triglycerides in the blood are quite common, especially in alcoholic disease, and can lead to a spurious (dilutional) hyponatremia. Transient jaundice may be caused by associated gallstones or an edematous head of pancreas, but marked jaundice and fever indicate acute cholangitis.

A pleural effusion is the commonest respiratory complication, and it may be associated with atelectasis, basal pneumonia, and ARDS. The pulmonary injury is thought to be caused by circulating phospholipase A_2 together with other pancreatic enzymes, free fatty acids, kinins, and activated complement. Early hypoxia is common, and routine arterial blood gas measurement is essential. Respiratory failure also occurs later in those who have necrotizing pancreatitis. Reductions in renal blood flow and glomerular filtration rate may also be related to phospholipase A_2 and can herald renal failure. Acute GI bleeding is generally caused by stress ulceration of the stomach and duodenum. Later, intestinal involvement combined with pancreatic insufficiency may lead to progressive malnutrition. There may be disseminated intravascular coagulation (DIC) secondary to the release of proteolytic enzymes, sepsis, or hepatic dysfunction.

Late (Surgical) Complications

The late complications of acute pancreatitis are the consequences of pancreatic necrosis, namely pseudocyst formation and infected pancreatic necrosis and the complications that result from these (i.e. hemorrhage, mesentericoportal thrombosis, pancreatic fistula, abscess, and generalized sepsis). Acute fluid collections develop adjacent to the pancreas in about 50% of patients with acute pancreatitis, but the large majority subside spontaneously as the attack settles and the fluid is reabsorbed. These only require treatment if they compromise respiration. In <10% of patients, a mature pseudocyst develops requiring treatment. Approximately 15–20% of patients develop necrotizing pancreatitis, with necrosis of the pancreas and surrounding retroperitoneal fat. Generally, the necrotic tissue is sterile at first, but the onset of bacterial infection, usually at 2–6 weeks after disease onset, often coincides with clinical deterioration. Pseudocyst and infected necrosis management are considered later in this chapter.

Management

Supportive Measures

Supportive measures are the mainstay of treatment of acute pancreatitis because of the paucity of specific measures. The initial requirement is adequate intravenous fluid replacement with crystalloid (isotonic saline) and colloid (plasma expanders and sometimes blood). There is a suggestion from retrospective studies that larger quantities of intravenous fluids given very early in the acute attack may reduce complications. Sequestration into the retroperitoneal tissues combined with vomiting and pooling in the gut means that several liters of fluid are required in a severe attack, and replacement should be monitored by central venous and urethral catheters. Inotropic drugs should be used with caution and only if hypotension persists after fluid replenishment. The patient need not be kept "nil by mouth," and a nasogastric tube is only necessary to treat symptomatic gastric distension or ileus. Intravenous administration of a proton pump inhibitor may help prevent gastric erosions.

There is continuing controversy regarding early administration of antibiotics in acute pancreatitis. In mild or moderate pancreatitis, antibiotics should be withheld until there is a clear indication of infection. Many clinicians give prophylactic broad-spectrum antibiotics in severe acute pancreatitis, but the supporting evidence is sparse. Broad-spectrum antibiotics allow proliferation of resistant bacteria and fungi. The use of antibiotics should therefore be restricted to treatment of proven infection.[21] In case of proven infection, those antibiotics of benefit in pancreatic infection include third-generation cephalosporins, piperacillin–tazobactam, ciprofloxacin and imipenem/meropenem with metronidazole. Selective decontamination of the gut has also been advocated, but evidence is not supportive.[22]

Many attacks of acute pancreatitis subside within a few days, but patients who have a severe attack need early nutritional support to correct their rapidly developing catabolic state. Depriving patients of oral nutrition was previously thought to be necessary in acute pancreatitis to avoid "stimulating the pancreas." This policy is not now believed to be appropriate; in fact, even a small quantity of enteral nutrition has been shown to protect the GI tract from translocation of bacteria across the intestinal mucosa. Patients should therefore be started on food early in the course of acute pancreatitis, the route of delivery depending on what can be tolerated and starting with the least invasive route, i.e. food by mouth. If not tolerated, other routes are considered: fine bore nasogastric tube or nasojejunal tube. Finally if tube feeding cannot be achieved, it is reasonable to resort to parenteral nutrition, although enteral feeding should be re-established as soon as possible.

Supportive management embraces the vigilant detection and treatment of the early complications of the disease. Arterial hypoxemia requires supplemental oxygen by mask, progressing to full mechanical ventilation if respiratory failure ensues. Aspiration of pleural effusions, diuretic therapy for fluid overload, or antibiotic treatment of pulmonary infection may also be beneficial. Hypocalcemia should be corrected by intravenous calcium gluconate. Renal failure is treated by hemofiltration or full hemodialysis according to circumstances. Peritoneal lavage has no benefit. Hyperglycemia may require insulin administration. Bleeding as a result of a systemic coagulopathy requires appropriate hematologic support.

Specific Drug Therapy

Many different agents have been used to treat acute pancreatitis. They act either by inhibiting the secretion and activation of enzymes or by improving pancreatic perfusion and reticuloendothelial activity. Despite a sound pathophysiologic basis and promising results in experimental models of pancreatitis, agents such as low molecular weight dextran, glucagon, aprotinin, fresh frozen plasma, anticholinergic and anti-inflammatory drugs, gabexate mesilate, calcitonin, octreotide (somatostatin analog) and lexipafant (a PAF antagonist) have all failed to influence the course of the human disease in a reproducible manner.

Endoscopic Retrograde Cholangiopancreatography and Endoscopic Sphincterotomy

For those patients with acute pancreatitis and coexistent cholangitis, ERCP with endoscopic sphincterotomy is an important therapy and should be carried out as soon as possible to provide drainage to the infected bile duct.

The idea that a gallstone impacted at the ampulla of Vater might perpetuate the attack of acute pancreatitis has led several groups to investigate this concept in randomized controlled trials. Several studies have randomized patients with predicted severe acute pancreatitis (without cholangitis) to early ERCP and sphincterotomy versus no ERCP. The trials have had conflicting results, but a recent review concluded that there was no role for routine early ERCP/ endoscopic sphincterotomy in predicted severe acute biliary pancreatitis in the absence of cholangitis.[23] Due to the early onset of extensive duodenal edema, ERCP can be extremely challenging in severe acute pancreatitis after the first 48–72 hours.

Surgical Operations

Laparoscopy or laparotomy should be considered in four circumstances:

- Diagnostic laparotomy is very occasionally needed for patients who have peritonitis and an equivocal serum amylase, though an urgent CT scan and laparoscopy should reduce the need for such intervention.
- Therapeutic laparotomy with partial or even total pancreatectomy has been advocated as a last-ditch measure in patients who have fulminant disease, but this is only mentioned to warn surgeons of the high mortality rate of operation in this situation: severe venous hemorrhage is the major risk, and such early operation should never be attempted.
- Prophylactic operations mostly comprise removal of the causative gallstones to prevent a further attack; cholecystectomy should be carried out once the attack has settled, but during the same admission to prevent another attack. The laparoscopic route is appropriate, but the procedure is more difficult in the early aftermath of acute pancreatitis and on-table cholangiography (or previous ERCP) should be carried out to visualize any ductal stones, which must also be removed.
- There is a clear-cut role for intervention in the management of complications, such as a pseudocyst and infected pancreatic necrosis, but as seen below this is not always surgical.

INFECTED PANCREATIC NECROSIS

Necrotizing pancreatitis may be suspected on first admission from the clinical features, such as shock with generalized peritonitis, hypoxia, and an excessive fluid requirement, by more than three positive Ranson or Glasgow criteria of severity (*see* Table 56.2) and by the contrast-enhanced CT appearances of marked pancreatic swelling and ischemia. Such patients need to be admitted to an intensive therapy unit, where early complications such as respiratory or renal failure, hypocalcemia, and DIC require vigorous treatment.

Unless there is an early clinical resolution and the patient is ready for discharge within 2 weeks, a repeat contrast-enhanced CT should be carried out at 2 weeks to ensure ongoing resolution of necrosis. In patients requiring persistent hospitalization, careful monitoring to detect infection is essential. The onset of infection within the necrotic peripancreatic and pancreatic tissues is heralded by clinical deterioration with fever, increasing leukocytosis, and elevated C-reactive protein, and usually progressive organ failure. Continued assessment by contrast-enhanced CT scan is essential (Figs. 56.6A and B). Intervention is indicated in patients with signs of infection or persistent extensive necrosis, particularly if this is tracking posteriorly, inferiorly, or towards the diaphragm. In the past, conventional treatment for infected necrosis has been necrosectomy by open operation using one of a variety of techniques, including open necrosectomy with closed lavage, open drainage, planned staged relaparotomies with repeated lavage, and open necrosectomy with closed packing.[24] Open necrosectomy has been associated with relatively high mortality and often clinical deterioration following operation. Minimally invasive (percutaneous) retroperitoneal necrosectomy was introduced in 2000 following several reports of treatment of infected necrosis with radiological drainage.[25] The various techniques of percutaneous necrosectomy, characterized by radiological access into the necrosis cavity, followed by endoscopy of the necrosis cavity differ only in the surgical detail (Figs. 56.7A to C). Early reports suggested that open necrosectomy could be avoided, and a randomized trial showed that the percutaneous approach (as part of a step-up approach from percutaneous drainage) was superior.[26] Interestingly, some patients avoided necrosectomy as they were treated successfully by the initial wide-bore tube drainage. Endoscopic transgastric necrosectomy evolved as expertise was gained in the transgastric drainage of pancreatic pseudocysts, first by direct puncture and then under EUS guidance.[27] Infected collections were also drained, and with dilatation of the opening into the necrosis cavity even large pieces of solid necrosis could be removed (Figs. 56.8A to D).[28]

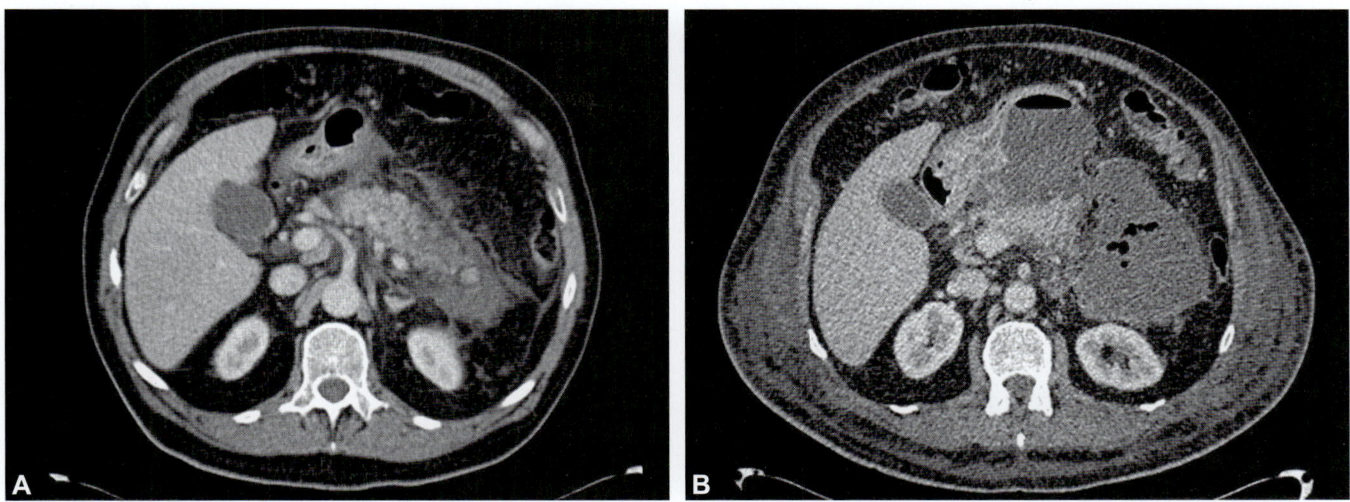

Figs. 56.6A and B: Severe acute pancreatitis with necrosis. (A) Computed tomography scan showing necrotizing pancreatitis, (B) which has progressed in 14 days to walled-off necrosis containing gas, highly suspicious of infection.

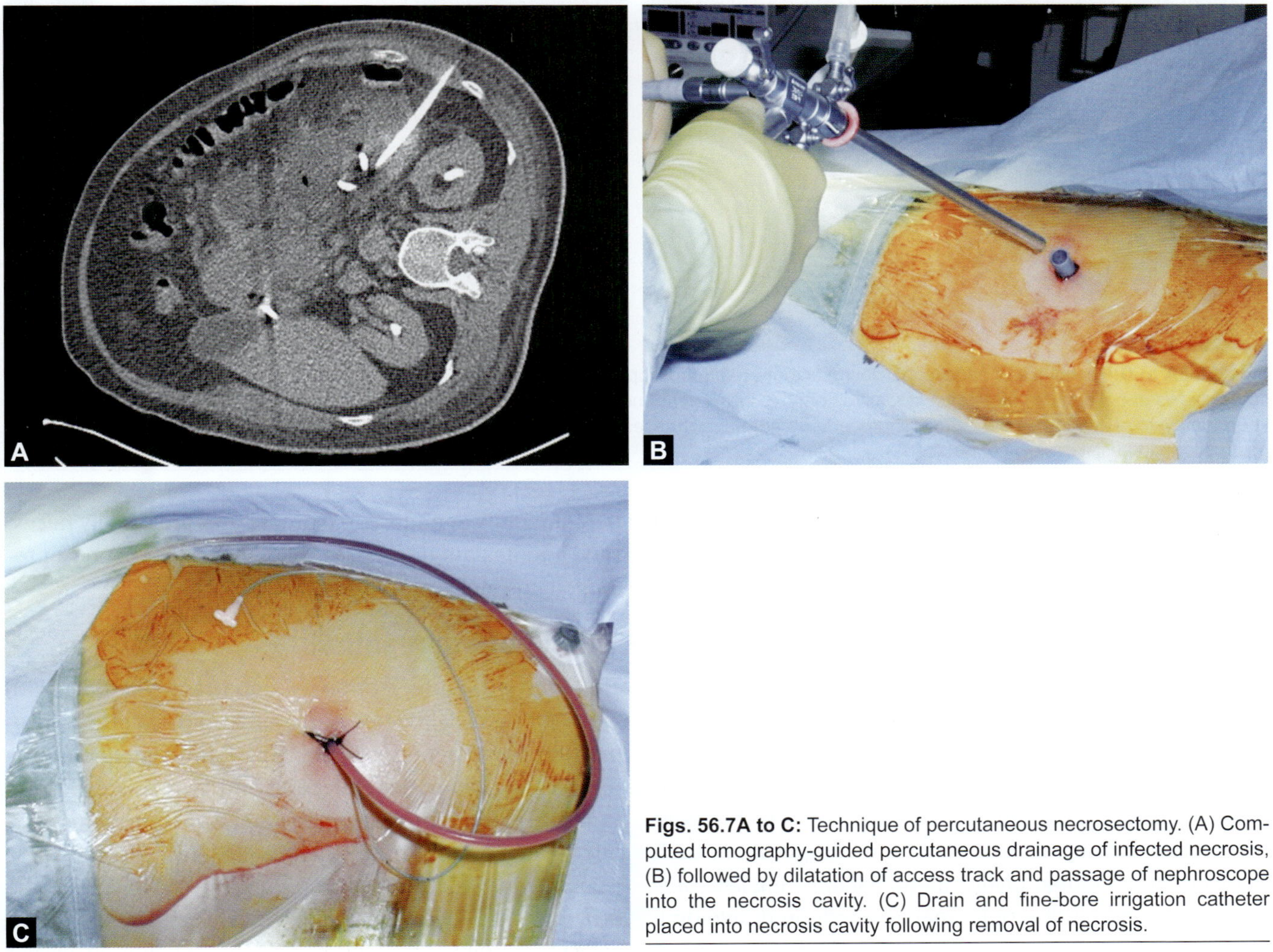

Figs. 56.7A to C: Technique of percutaneous necrosectomy. (A) Computed tomography-guided percutaneous drainage of infected necrosis, (B) followed by dilatation of access track and passage of nephroscope into the necrosis cavity. (C) Drain and fine-bore irrigation catheter placed into necrosis cavity following removal of necrosis.

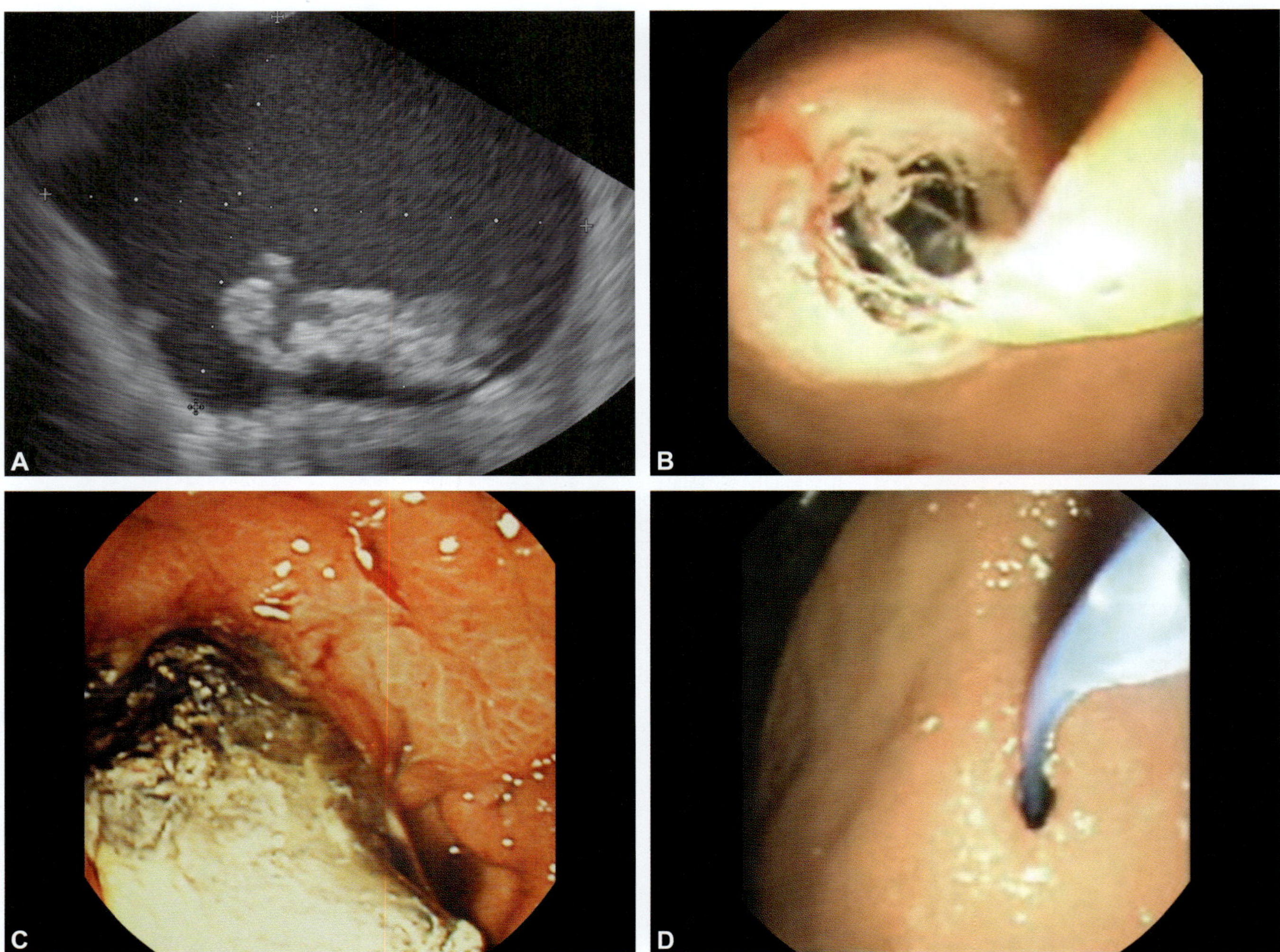

Figs. 56.8A to D: Technique of endoscopic necrosectomy. (A) Endoscopic ultrasound image of necrosis surrounded by infected fluid. (B) Endoscopic views of balloon dilatation of cystogastrostomy, (C) removal of necrotic tissue, (D) and insertion of stent at the end of the procedure to keep the cystogastrostomy open. Several procedures are usually necessary to remove all the solid tissue. The cavity may be entered with a gastroscope to assist removal of necrosis.

With good radiological and endoscopic support, almost all patients with infected pancreatic necrosis can be managed percutaneously or endoscopically, and this is now the authors' preferred practice. Patients with clinically suspicious and radiologically confirmed (on CT) infected necrosis are assessed for either percutaneous (under CT guidance) or endoscopic (under EUS guidance) drainage, depending on the anatomy of the necrosis. In Newcastle upon Tyne open necrosectomy is no longer offered as primary treatment, although occasional patients still require open necrosectomy as treatment for a complication, such as bleeding or colonic involvement. Establishing safe percutaneous and endoscopic management and avoiding open necrosectomy if possible has resulted in a marked reduction in mortality rates from 34% to 15%. Repeat percutaneous or endoscopic procedures are usually necessary, and it is not unusual for patients to experience a prolonged hospital stay.

Timing of Intervention

The timing of intervention is important. Patients with clear-cut signs of infected necrosis should undergo appropriate (percutaneous or endoscopic) drainage depending on the anatomy of the collection and available expertise. In those patients with extensive necrosis but no signs of infection, drainage may be delayed to allow maturation of a collection, which will often reduce the complexity of the procedures. However, in those with extensive extrapancreatic necrosis, drainage should be considered earlier rather than later to avoid extensive tracking of fluid either inferiorly towards the pelvis or superiorly to the chest; fistulation of collections is a difficult clinical problem. Drainage is made on clinical and radiological grounds. Fine-needle aspiration of suspected infected necrosis is not usually necessary as most such collections will undergo drainage anyway. Once drainage has been done (all collections should be adequately drained with the use of multiple drains if necessary), irrigation of the necrotic cavities is usually necessary. Regular CT surveillance of the abdomen should also be carried out to ensure that drainage has been successful and that the necrosis is dispersing.

The operation of open necrosectomy is usually very demanding because the tissues are very inflamed and there is a risk of bleeding from mesenteric and PV tributaries if the main channels are thrombosed. Formal pancreatic resection is not appropriate, but the operation entails debridement of necrotic tissue that may inadvertently include the removal of nonviable pancreas as well as the surrounding fat because distinguishing between the two can be very difficult. It is necessary to open the retroperitoneum widely to explore the pancreatic bed via the transverse mesocolon and to follow the necrotizing process upwards toward the diaphragm, downwards into the paracolic gutters, and forwards into the root of the small bowel mesentery. This process of "pancreatic sequestrectomy" must be radical and thorough, but it puts the mesenteric vessels at risk. Necrosectomy is followed by insertion of large bore drains into the necrosis cavity, and postoperatively these are irrigated continuously with large volumes of saline. If the pancreatitis is caused by gallstones then cholecystectomy can be carried out at the same time as necrosectomy if feasible.

The problem with necrosectomy is that complete separation of necrotic from viable tissue may not be possible at the time of the first operation. Therefore, repeat procedures may be necessary, which may result in the need for a laparostomy (open abdomen); this is associated with a risk of damage to the intestine and hence a higher mortality. The preferred minimally invasive techniques (percutaneous and endoscopic) avoid many of these problems.

Complications

The complications of infected pancreatic necrosis include hemorrhage, which may occur as a consequence of arterial or venous erosion, especially in a coagulopathic patient. Bleeding may be into the peritoneal cavity, down the abdominal drains or into the upper GI tract in the presence of erosive gastroduodenitis. Urgent visceral angiography is

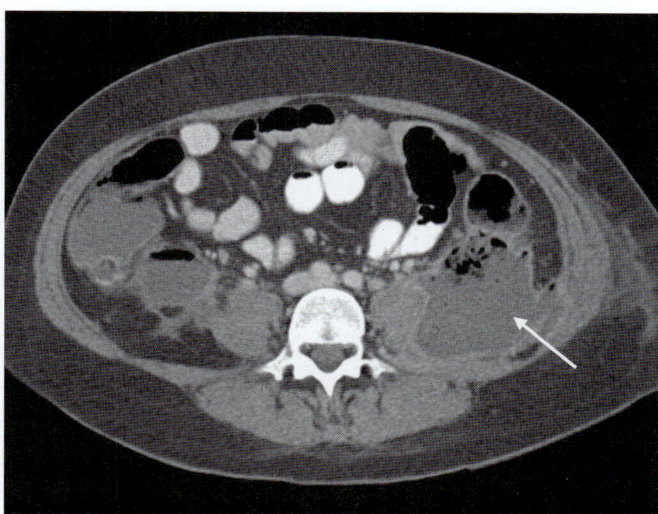

Fig. 56.9: Computed tomography showing extrapancreatic necrosis (arrowed) involving descending colon.

the preferred method of treatment as laparotomy is fraught with difficulty. Intestinal ischemia follows thrombosis of mesenteric vessels and usually presents as colonic necrosis affecting the ascending and transverse colon; occasionally the entire colon and/or the small bowel are involved. Colonic fistulation may occur spontaneously or as a complication of treatment (Fig. 56.9). Following necrosectomy by whichever technique, a pancreatic fistula may develop after one or more operations for infected necrosis, but it does not lead to skin excoriation unless it is mixed with intestinal contents or bile. Nearly all pancreatic fistulas eventually close spontaneously after the patient recovers from the severe attack; octreotide therapy may speed up this process. Duodenal obstruction may arise from compression by an inflamed head of pancreas, but it is best to wait for resolution than rush into doing a gastroenterostomy (which is only occasionally necessary).

Infected pancreatic necrosis is responsible for nearly all deaths in acute pancreatitis after the 1st week. Adverse factors include the extent of pancreatic and extrapancreatic necrosis, bacterial contamination, and pancreatic ascites; colonic necrosis also implies a grave prognosis. The overall mortality rate in patients with infected necrosis has reduced significantly with the advent of minimally necrosectomy to approximately 15–20%.

RECURRENT ACUTE PANCREATITIS

Approximately 15% of patients admitted to hospital with acute pancreatitis have had a documented previous episode. Although recurrent attacks tend to be less severe

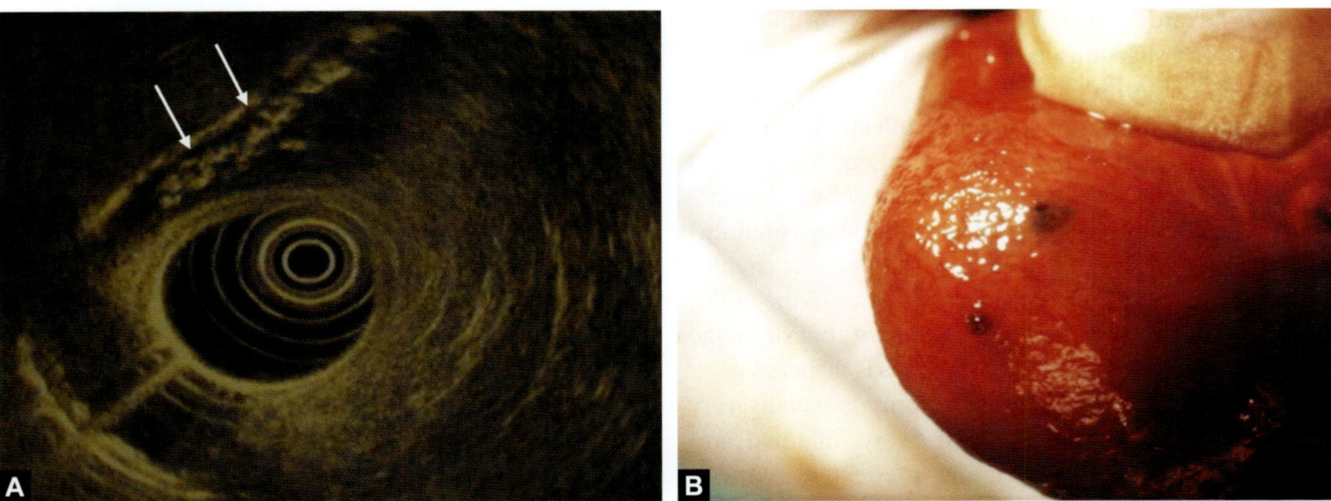

Figs. 56.10A and B: Recurrent acute pancreatitis. (A) Microlithiasis seen on endoscopic ultrasound (arrows) (B) and in a cholecystectomy specimen. The operation successfully prevented any further attacks.

than the initial attack, there is still a risk of complications and even death. Gallstones may already have been diagnosed or may come to light on reinvestigation, in which case cholecystectomy should be carried out as soon as the patient recovers and before leaving hospital. Alcoholic pancreatitis is often recurrent, but pancreatic imaging may reveal a pseudocyst or a dilated pancreatic duct that is amenable to surgical treatment.

In Newcastle upon Tyne, we have a three-phase algorithm for investigating patients with recurrent acute pancreatitis. The first phase involves a detailed history (to rule out alcohol excess, family of history pancreatitis, relevant drug history); simple blood tests (such as serum calcium and fasting lipids); and a repeat abdominal ultrasound to recheck the gallbladder for gallstones. If these phase 1 noninvasive tests are all normal, we stop investigations unless a further attack of pancreatitis occurs. After the second attack, phase 2 investigations are carried out as follows: MRCP to check for pancreas divisum and duct abnormalities of the pancreas; duodenoscopy to check the papilla for an ampullary tumor; and EUS to check the gallbladder and bile duct for microlithiasis (biliary sludge) (Figs. 56.10A and B). Phase 1 and 2 tests will identify the cause in over 90% of patients with recurrent acute pancreatitis. If all these tests are negative, we consider ERCP (which is only of value to check for sphincter of Oddi dysfunction) if the patient experiences further attacks. The risk of ERCP-induced pancreatitis, however, is increased fivefold in those patients with suspected sphincter of Oddi dysfunction, so it should only be carried out after careful discussion and patient counseling.

PANCREATIC PSEUDOCYSTS

A true cyst possesses an epithelial lining, whereas a false cyst or pseudocyst does not. In the pancreas, true cysts are either congenital or neoplastic. Pseudocysts are false cysts that complicate acute or chronic pancreatitis. Traumatic pseudocyst is the occasional consequence of an injury to the pancreas, especially in children. Disruption of a pancreatic duct leads to the slow accumulation of fluid rich in amylase in close proximity to the gland. This collection causes increasing abdominal pain within 1–2 weeks of the injury and a raised serum amylase. A cystic collection is seen on an ultrasound or a CT scan. These cysts are at risk of bleeding and infection and should be drained at an early stage, usually by operative cystojejunostomy (Fig. 56.11).

It was previously thought that most cystic disease of the pancreas was seen in connection with pancreatitis, and this is certainly the case for symptomatic cysts. With the advent of axial imaging by CT and MR for many abdominal conditions, incidental pancreatic cysts, mainly neoplastic cysts, have been more frequently recognized. Acute and chronic pancreatitis are each associated with pseudocyst formation in about one-third of cases. The distinction between acute and chronic pseudocysts becomes blurred in alcoholic disease in which there is nearly always preexisting disease of the gland, which may be exacerbated by an acute attack.

Acute Pancreatitis Pseudocyst

Acute pancreatitis pseudocysts develop after an attack of acute pancreatitis, i.e. in association with a gland that was

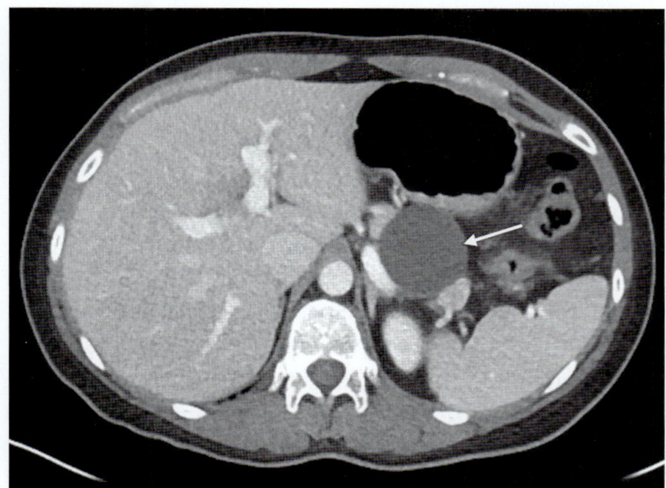

Fig. 56.11: Pseudocyst of the body of the pancreas. Acute pancreatitis resulted in necrosis of the body of the pancreas with pancreatic duct disruption and pseudocyst. The pseudocyst (arrow) was initially treated by endoscopic drainage but recurred several years later, and a distal pancreatectomy was then carried out with a good result.

previously normal. Acute fluid collections are commonly seen adjacent to the pancreas on early ultrasound or CT scans, but most of these resolve spontaneously. Persisting cysts tend to enlarge and develop a "capsule" from the surrounding viscera and omentum. Acute pseudocysts generally occupy the lesser sac, though they can occur within the greater or lesser omentum or even remote from the pancreas. A substantial proportion is associated with central gland pancreatic necrosis, following pancreatic duct disruption where the main pancreatic duct may terminate in the pseudocyst (Fig. 56.11).

The typical patient has a moderately severe attack of acute pancreatitis, which begins to settle, but pain recurs usually after the 4th week and there is a renewed elevation of serum amylase. An epigastric mass may eventually be palpable. There may be nausea and some vomiting caused by compression of the gastric outlet or mild jaundice caused by compression of the bile duct. Serial scans show an increasing cystic collection behind the stomach. The patient is usually in reasonably good health at this stage so there is no urgency to intervene, although some nutritional support may be required. The traditional policy has been to wait for 5–6 weeks for the cyst to develop a mature capsule. Large symptomatic pseudocysts are best drained internally. Techniques include endoscopic drainage (EUS-guided); laparoscopic cystogastrostomy (usually stapled); and open cystogastrostomy. Needle aspiration of a pseudocyst under ultrasound or CT guidance is simple but inadequate because of the 70% recurrence rate due to communication with the pancreatic duct. The endoscopic technique is done by accessing the pseudocyst under EUS guidance via the stomach and then dilating up the opening using an endoscopic dilating balloon. Plastic stents are then placed across the opening to allow fluid to drain. If there is any necrosis in the cavity, seen by EUS, infection is likely to develop due to gastric bacteria entering the cavity, and it is important to repeat the procedure within 2 weeks to ensure the necrotic material has passed. If not, the cavity should be irrigated endoscopically and the necrosis removed.

The laparoscopic approach is also transgastric, as in the traditional open operation. Operative approaches have the advantage of allowing removal of associated gallstones from the biliary tree and extraction of the necrotic debris that is nearly always found in these acute pseudocysts. An operation remains an appropriate means to ensure rapid and complete drainage of a large cyst in a patient whose general condition allows the necessary 5–6-week period of delay while the cyst wall matures. Cystogastrostomy is satisfactory provided that the cyst is closely applied to the posterior wall of the stomach (verified by preoperative scanning). There is a low incidence of complications, such as hemorrhage and gastric fistula. Internal drainage into a Roux loop of jejunum (cystojejunostomy) can also be carried out and will achieve better drainage if the pseudocyst is remote from the stomach or has a mainly inferior component. Comparison of cyst treatment by different techniques emphasizes the fact that local expertise is important. The results of endoscopic, laparoscopic, and open drainage are similar, but the endoscopic approach is likely to require more than one procedure.[29]

Chronic Pancreatitis Pseudocyst

Two types of pseudocyst can complicate chronic pancreatitis (Table 56.3). The first or postnecrotic type follows an acute exacerbation of underlying inflammatory disease and is associated with at least some exacerbation of pain and hyperamylasemia; it contains necrotic debris. The second, which is two or three times more common in our experience, develops insidiously and may be regarded as a retention cyst of the pancreas that follows obstruction of a duct. These insidious cysts are nearly always intrapancreatic and contain clear grayish fluid. They commonly have a communication with the pancreatic duct.

Chronic pseudocysts may be found incidentally on investigation of a patient with chronic pancreatitis or may contribute to abdominal pain and obstructive jaundice.

Table 56.3 Pseudocysts in pancreatitis.

Type	Underlying disease	Site	Necrotic debris	Communication with duct	Spontaneous resolution	Need for intervention
Acute (postnecrotic)	Acute pancreatitis	Extrapancreatic	Yes	Uncommon	Common	Only if persists
Chronic (postnecrotic)	Chronic pancreatitis	Extrapancreatic with or without intrapancreatic	Yes	Uncommon	Unusual	Yes
Chronic (insidious)	Chronic pancreatitis	Intrapancreatic	No	Common	Rare	Yes (unless small)
Traumatic	Pancreatic injury	Extrapancreatic	Yes	Rare	Unusual	Yes

Table 56.4 Complications of chronic pancreatic pseudocysts.

Complication	Consequence or cause
Rupture	Pancreatic ascites
	Pleural effusion
Hemorrhage	From coincident varices
	From arterial pseudoaneurysm
Fistula	Internal from spontaneous rupture (rare)
	External following percutaneous intervention
Infection	Spontaneous
	Iatrogenic (following intervention)
Obstruction	Gastric outlet (vomiting)
	Esophagus (dysphagia)

Small cysts (<3–4 cm diameter) can usually be left alone, but larger cysts often dominate the clinical presentation and may even be palpable. They are prone to several complications (Table 56.4), which occur in about one-third of cases, and for this reason they are best treated if symptomatic. Percutaneous drainage is less attractive than open drainage because of the likelihood of creating a chronic fistula, though the transgastric route is sometimes feasible. Endoscopic cystogastrostomy or cystduodenostomy may be appropriate in the first instance, but the lesser sac is likely to be patent (unlike with acute cysts) so there is a gap between the stomach and the cyst; and there may be varices in the gastric wall secondary to portal hypertension (shown on CT and EUS). In addition, many of these patients have other changes of chronic pancreatitis including stricture formation and duct disruption that may need treatment in their own right.

The surgical procedure of choice is cystojejunostomy Roux-en-Y. About 20% of chronic pseudocysts are multiple, and the same Roux loop can be used to drain the cysts together with the main pancreatic duct or combined with a duodenum-preserving resection of the head of the pancreas (*see* below in section on Chronic Pancreatitis) and/or the bile duct (if dilated). There is little need for open drainage into the stomach or duodenum, especially if endoscopic expertise is available to deal with the few chronic cysts that abut onto these organs. Many chronic cysts can be included in a proximal or distal pancreatectomy carried out for inflammatory disease with or without calcification. Generally, resection is appropriate for smaller cysts and those confined to the body or tail of pancreas, whereas a drainage procedure is preferred for large cysts and those in the head of pancreas. An infected cyst or a ruptured cyst with pancreatic ascites may be managed with drainage, but it is usually better to do a formal resection for a cyst that led to the development of an external pancreatic fistula or an arterial pseudoaneurysm. Less than 5% of chronic pseudocysts are associated with arterial erosion, but this should always be searched for on a CT angiogram. In addition, splenic vein thrombosis commonly accompanies pseudocyst formation in the left pancreas. Differentiation from a cystic neoplasm is important.

CHRONIC PANCREATITIS

Chronic pancreatitis is a debilitating disease that is linked with national patterns of alcohol consumption, at least in Western countries where its incidence is increasing. Part of the increase may reflect better diagnosis of this insidious condition with modern imaging techniques. Pain is the usual indication for intervention, though other patients develop complications of the disease or are suspected of harboring a cancer. Specific intervention in the form of endoscopic or surgical procedures is appropriate for a minority of patients with obstructive jaundice, duodenal obstruction, or an inflammatory mass in the head of the pancreas with pancreatic duct obstruction. Management also includes care of nutrition, diabetes, chronic pain, and psychosocial issues.

Etiology and Pathology

In many countries, alcoholism is the leading cause of chronic pancreatitis, and it is responsible for 70–80% of cases in the USA and the UK. The quantity and duration of alcohol consumption correlates with the development of chronic pancreatitis. The amount of alcohol required to cause chronic pancreatitis varies, and there is emerging evidence to suggest that unidentified genetic factors may be responsible for one individual having a different threshold to alcohol than another. Persistent ethanol abuse increases the protein concentration of pancreatic juice, leading to protein plugs, which block the ducts and eventually calcify. Precipitation of calcium carbonate is usually prevented by lithostatin (pancreatic stone protein). The liver usually appears remarkably normal in most patients with chronic alcoholic pancreatitis.

The next most common cause is idiopathic, and this appears to be a distinct entity. These patients should not be labeled as "alcoholic." Less common causes of chronic pancreatitis include hypercalcemia, hyperlipidemia, gallstones, pancreatic tumors, and pancreas divisum. Hereditary pancreatitis is being increasingly recognized and must be suspected in patients with a family history of pancreatitis or diabetes.[30] It is inherited as an autosomal dominant condition with penetrance of 80%, with over 80% of affected individuals developing clinical pancreatitis before the age of 20 years. Point mutations have been identified in the cationic trypsinogen gene (PRSS1) located on chromosome 7. Example mutations are named R122H, N29I, and A16V. The R122H mutation results in the elimination of a failsafe self-destruct mechanism, which prevents the rapid accumulation of large concentrations of active trypsin so resulting in autodigestion of the pancreas. Mutations in the SPINK1 gene are also an important cause of genetic pancreatitis. Cystic fibrosis is a rarer genetic cause. Patients with hereditary pancreatitis are usually more susceptible to acute attacks of pancreatitis secondary to alcohol, and these patients and their relatives should avoid alcohol at all costs. Hereditary pancreatitis carries a substantially increased risk of pancreatic cancer.[31] Tropical pancreatitis is a very common cause in Southern India but is rarely seen elsewhere. It is thought to be due to a combination of nutritional and genetic factors. Other rare causes include recurrent gallstone pancreatitis.

Autoimmune pancreatitis is a rare but increasingly recognized cause of chronic pancreatitis. It is associated with raised levels of IgG4, and its presentation often mimics that of pancreatic cancer in the head of the pancreas, though pancreatic duct dilatation is often absent. Extrapancreatic involvement is not uncommon. Specialist management is required, and treatment with corticosteroids will usually lead to resolution of complications, including extrapancreatic manifestations.[32]

About 10–20% of patients with chronic pancreatitis have no known etiology and can be labeled as idiopathic. More of these than previously are thought to be related to genetic or autoimmune causes (not just IgG4-related disease but also associated with primary biliary cirrhosis, sclerosing cholangitis, or Sjögren's syndrome). Nonalcoholic patients are often unfairly accused (by healthcare professionals) of alcohol abuse, a label that they resent intensely.

Repeated attacks of acute pancreatitis can lead to focal areas of necrosis and progressive fibrosis, which results in ductal strictures, acinar destruction, cyst formation, and stone deposition. The pathologic changes of chronic pancreatitis are those of chronic inflammatory infiltration and parenchymal fibrosis, which gradually replaces the acinar tissue. The intralobular ducts become distorted and contain eosinophilic proteinaceous material and calcareous deposits. Even in advanced disease, the changes are often surprisingly patchy. Nerve trunks may be prominent and likewise islet cell tissue, which is relatively preserved. Ultimately there is diffuse acinar atrophy and scarring throughout the pancreas.

Clinical Assessment and Diagnosis

Clinical Presentation

The typical patient is a man is his late 30s or 40s who has been drinking heavily for at least 10–15 years before being admitted with acute abdominal pain and a raised serum amylase. This presentation may be a full-blown attack of acute pancreatitis, or it may resolve rapidly and subsequent investigation reveals early ductal changes with or without calcification and exocrine insufficiency. The first attack is followed by repeated attacks of pain, which gradually become more frequent but less severe, culminating in constant pain within 2–5 years. Other patients develop an insidious onset of daily pain, and the diagnosis is only reached after prolonged investigation. A few patients have little or no pain and present with obstructive jaundice or a pseudocyst seen on imaging. Genetic pancreatitis is often diagnosed late because of its presentation at a young age. If this is a possibility, then specific investigations should be done early.

The dominant symptom of chronic pancreatitis is abdominal pain, which is situated deep in the epigastrium and bores through to the back between the shoulder blades. It may be eased by sitting up and leaning forwards. It is usually aggravated by eating, which may explain why weight loss is such a marked feature of end-stage disease. There may be associated nausea and vomiting. Exocrine insufficiency is suggested by the passage of loose bulky stools and excessive flatus, but overt diabetes mellitus is seldom present until the later stages of the disease.

Investigation

Blood tests are of limited value. The serum amylase is not elevated unless the patient has either acute-on-chronic pancreatitis or a pseudocyst. Computed tomography is essential and may show swelling or atrophy of the pancreas, dilatation of the pancreatic duct (or bile duct), pancreatic calcification, necrosis, and pseudocyst formation (intrapancreatic and extrapancreatic). Endoscopic retrograde cholangiopancreatography is no longer necessary in the assessment of patients (but may be used for therapy). Magnetic resonance cholangiopancreatography, however, may show additional ductal changes such as ductal irregularity affecting a segment of the main pancreatic duct or its side branches, but it is only used as a guide to specific intervention. Endoscopic ultrasound should be used in selected patients but is essential if the changes of chronic pancreatitis on CT are in doubt or if cancer is suspected, in which case EUS-guided biopsy should be done. Investigation must also include a careful evaluation of exocrine and endocrine function, dietary assessment, and a social and drug history.

Differential Diagnosis

Other causes of abdominal and back pain, such as gallstones, duodenal ulcer with posterior penetration, carcinoma of the stomach, and disease of the thoracic spine can usually be diagnosed by appropriate investigations. It is more difficult to rule out carcinoma of the pancreas in a patient who has a pancreatic mass, especially in the presence of obstructive jaundice and the absence of calcification. Computed tomographic assessment is vital with review of images by a pancreatic radiologist. Endoscopic ultrasound with FNA is usually recommended. If a mass is suspicious for malignancy and there is no contraindication to operation, resection of the mass may be the best way to establish the diagnosis and resolve the problem, whether inflammatory or neoplastic.

Complications

Complications of chronic pancreatitis are frequent and have a major impact on management. Pseudocysts occur in at least one-third of patients who are considered for surgical treatment. Small cysts may be left alone, but large cysts require interventional treatment in their own right. Obstructive jaundice develops in up to 20% of patients, usually due to inflammation and/or scarring in the head of pancreas. Unless it resolves spontaneously with normalization of serum alkaline phosphatase, some form of biliary drainage is needed. Endoscopic stenting used to be a temporary solution, but use of removable expandable metal stents means that benign biliary strictures may be treated adequately without operation. Duodenal stenosis is much less common than biliary stenosis and denotes severe disease of the pancreatic head; duodenal stenting is not a good treatment, and gastrojejunostomy is an option unless there is an indication for a major resection. Thrombosis of the splenic vein is quite common with left-sided pancreatitis, and the resultant esophagogastric varices are an occasional source of upper GI hemorrhage; distal pancreatectomy with splenectomy is usually appropriate. Much less often, the SMV and even the main PV become narrowed or even occluded as a consequence of right-sided disease. This complication usually precludes safe resection of the pancreatic head. Hemorrhage may also result from an arterial pseudoaneurysm, in which case CT angiography followed by angiographic embolization may be life-saving.

Some of the complications of chronic pancreatitis are linked to pseudocyst formation. Rupture of a cyst into the peritoneal cavity can lead to pancreatic ascites, which can be differentiated from the ascites of liver disease by its high-amylase content. The site of ductal rupture can usually be seen on CT, which will guide the clinician as to whether an attempt at ERCP stenting is likely to be successful in stopping the leakage (which it often is). In pancreatic ascites associated with duct disruption, management by ERCP, total parenteral nutrition (TPN), and intravenous octreotide infusion for 10 days usually produces resolution. If ERCP is not successful, operation may be necessary; it usually entails Roux loop drainage of the duct and associated pseudocyst or distal pancreatectomy up to the point of the fistula.

The link between chronic pancreatitis and pancreatic carcinoma is not clear, but the conditions are related. The differential diagnosis can be extremely difficult (*see* section on Differential Diagnosis), and most cancers in the head and neck of pancreas give rise to distal obstructive pancreatopathy. There are common etiologic associations, such as cigarette smoking and alcohol consumption. The evidence suggests that chronic pancreatitis is a premalignant condition and that patients with chronic pancreatitis have on average an approximately 10% chance of developing pancreatic malignancy. The risk, however, appears to be particularly increased in those patients with onset of pancreatitis early in life and in those with hereditary pancreatitis, which conveys a lifetime risk of malignancy of over 30%.[31]

Management

Medical Management

A multidisciplinary approach to the management of chronic pancreatitis is essential. Nonoperative measures are appropriate for patients with mild or moderate chronic pancreatitis without complications and are directed toward pain relief and controlling pancreatic insufficiency. Patients should stop alcohol consumption and cigarette smoking completely and should be offered appropriate counseling. Pain may require the regular use of analgesics, avoiding opiates when possible because of the problem of a spiraling dose, tolerance, and subsequent addiction. Nonsteroidal anti-inflammatory drugs can be a useful adjunct. Octreotide treatment has proved disappointing. Pancreatic enzyme therapy is extremely important and helps prevent weight loss and improve general nutritional health in those who have exocrine impairment. Enteric-coated preparations, such as Creon 40000 and Nutrizym, help prevent denaturation of the enzymes by gastric acid; ranitidine or omeprazole may be similarly beneficial. Pancreatic enzyme therapy should also theoretically relieve pain by feedback inhibition of exocrine secretion, but in practice it is of very limited benefit in established chronic pancreatitis, although it may be of value in those with minimal change disease. Diabetes mellitus should be controlled by dietary means, oral hypoglycemic agents or insulin, as necessary. A celiac plexus block may help interrupt the cycle of pain, but the effect is unpredictable and the improvement is usually short-lived. Chemical splanchnicectomy is best carried out by percutaneous injection of a neurolytic agent, such as 50% alcohol, under CT guidance, but again the results are disappointing. Thoracoscopic splanchnicectomy is an alternative, but the results have also been short-lived and disappointing.[33]

Endoscopic Management

The rationale of endoscopic therapy of the pancreas in chronic pancreatitis is to improve pancreatic drainage by pseudocyst drainage, stricture dilatation, and stone removal. Endotherapy for chronic pancreatitis includes the following:

- Endoscopic ultrasound-guided transgastric pseudocyst drainage
- Pancreatic sphincterotomy alone for a short stricture close to the papilla
- Pancreatic sphincterotomy followed by extracorporeal shock-wave lithotripsy to disperse ductal stones combined with stent insertion
- Dilatation of pancreatic duct strictures combined with short-term stent insertion across an area of duct disruption.

Technical success rates have been reported in at least 80% of patients and prolonged pain relief may be achievable, but generally multiple procedures are necessary and the results are unpredictable.[34] There is concern that an indwelling stent may cause duct damage and, in addition, pancreatic stents tend to occlude after a few months. Pain relief on stenting can be used to predict the likelihood of success with surgical drainage, but it is uncertain that endotherapy is a necessary intermediate step.

Surgical Management

Surgical management of chronic pancreatitis is reserved for patients with complications. Some patients with chronic pancreatitis benefit from major surgery, but expectant therapy is adequate for most patients. Operation to treat intractable pain or to preserve pancreatic function depends on the caliber of the main duct and the distribution of disease in the pancreas; the appropriate selection of these patients is paramount. The required operation varies between patients: one operation does not fit all. A patient with pain and a dilated pancreatic duct (>7 mm in diameter) with or without ductal calculi is likely to benefit from drainage, which works by decompressing the pancreatic duct and/or by relieving the pancreatic capsular hypertension. If the duct is not dilated, duct drainage is unlikely to be effective. An inflammatory mass in the head of the pancreas is often a major contribution to the pain, and resection of the head may then be important.

The commonest drainage procedure, longitudinal pancreaticojejunostomy (a modified Puestow or Partington–Rochelle procedure) involves exposure of the gland, opening of the entire length of the pancreatic duct to the ampulla of Vater, and anastomosis to a Roux-en-Y loop of jejunum. This procedure has disadvantages. Pancreatic head tissue is left in situ. If this is inflammatory, as it often is, a neuroinflammatory pain is likely to persist, and biliary obstruction or thrombosis of the PV can develop. A better result can be obtained if part of the head is excised in addition to the lateral pancreaticojejunostomy (as described by Frey; Fig. 56.12). Alternatively, a duodenum-preserving resection of the head of the pancreas, as described by Beger, may be done. This is a similar procedure, but with a more extensive resection of the head of the pancreas and requires exposure of the PV. It has similar results to the Frey procedure in terms of pain relief and therefore

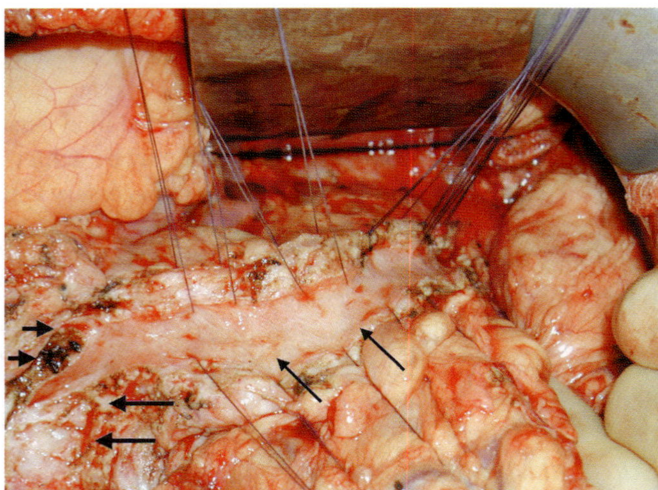

Fig. 56.12: Duodenum-preserving resection of head of pancreas with longitudinal pancreatojejunostomy: Frey procedure. The mass in the head of the pancreas has been resected (bold arrows) and the pancreatic duct laid open from the tail of the pancreas to the papilla (thin arrows—duct held open by stay sutures). A Roux-en-Y loop of jejunum will be anastomosed longitudinally to the cut edges of the pancreas.

has no distinct advantages.[35] These duodenum-preserving resection procedures provide good relief from recurrent attacks of pain. For a mass in the head of the pancreas with duct dilatation, the authors prefer a Frey procedure with removal of as much inflammatory tissue as possible combined with a longitudinal pancreaticojejunostomy (Fig. 56.12). A biliary drainage procedure (supraduodenal or intrapancreatic) may be done during the same operation. Pancreatoduodenectomy has no advantage in chronic pancreatitis, although it may be necessary if there is duodenal stenosis or if pancreatic cancer is suspected. Distal pancreatectomy may be carried out for disease confined to the tail of the pancreas, and this is the only one of these procedures that is commonly attempted laparoscopically if the degree of inflammation is minimal. In our experience 10–20% of patients who have a partial pancreatectomy proceed to a completion pancreatectomy within about 3 years because of unrelenting pain, and it makes little difference whether the right or left part of the gland has been removed on the first occasion.[36] For patients with diffuse chronic pancreatitis and no pancreatic duct dilatation (so-called small duct disease), surgical treatment is often unrewarding. There is no duct to drain, and unless the disease is focal (e.g. confined to the tail), the only reliable surgical option is a total pancreatectomy. Total pancreatectomy relieves pain in only about 50% of individuals with constant pain because autonomic pathways are damaged; it renders the patient a brittle diabetic and is seldom indicated. If total pancreatectomy is unavoidable in a patient with good glucose tolerance, islet autotransplantation (using a PV catheter) should be considered.

Choice of Treatment

Chronic pancreatitis is a curiously unpredictable disease. Some patients have no pain, whereas others are afflicted by one of the most severe pains known to man and become addicted to narcotic drugs. The tendency is for the pain to continue for many years and then gradually diminish as the patient develops exocrine and endocrine failure. Nonoperative measures may render life more palatable during this extended process, but surgical intervention should be considered before the patient requires opiates on a regular basis. In addition, pancreatic duct disruption can result in persistent inflammation (often extrapancreatic) and early resection, and/or drainage can prevent progression of inflammation and reduce the chances of complications such as biliary obstruction or portal/mesenteric vein occlusion. When possible, major resections should be avoided in patients who continue to abuse alcohol, but a timely operation can help rehabilitate someone who is trying to stop drinking but has crippling pain. Although intractable pain is the commonest reason for surgical referral, the development of complications and a suspicion of cancer are more clear-cut indications for operation. In addition, those patients who experience recurrent flare-ups of pain and who have an obstructed dilated pancreatic duct often combined with an inflammatory mass in the head of the pancreas (often without a major component of continuous chronic pain), tend to do very well from a head resection and drainage procedure; this procedure should be considered early in this group of patients.

Preoperative up-to-date imaging is invaluable, and decision making can usually be made according to preoperative information. Assessment of the disease at operation remains very important, and the final choice of procedure should depend upon the detailed findings at operation, including assessment by intraoperative ultrasound.

Endoscopic management is rarely a final treatment. Multiple treatments are almost always necessary, and if a patient is fit for operation and anatomically there is a surgical option, then that is what is indicated since the short- and long-term results of resection and drainage are superior to those of multiple endoscopic procedures.[37]

CARCINOMA OF THE PANCREAS

Perspective

Carcinoma of the exocrine pancreas accounts for over 90% of pancreatic tumors and remains an unresolved oncologic challenge. Despite improvements in perioperative care and adjuvant therapy, the outcome of the disease has scarcely improved over the last 40 years. In the USA, pancreatic cancer is now the fourth leading cause of cancer death for men and the fifth for women. Its incidence has increased threefold since the 1930s and is now approximately 9.5/100,000 per year in the USA. Over 6,000 people die from pancreatic cancer in the UK each year. Excluding small tumors confined to the pancreatic head, pancreatic cancer is virtually incurable. Regardless of therapy, median survival is <6 months from diagnosis.[38] The overall survival rate after 1 year is about 15% and after 5 years <3%. At initial presentation, approximately 90% patients have metastases. Early diagnosis is required to make an impact upon these depressing figures.

Epidemiology

Demographic Factors

More than 80% of pancreatic cancers occur in individuals aged between 60 and 80 years. In affluent countries in which there is a high overall incidence, men are affected nearly twice as often as women (1.5–2.0:1), whereas in low incidence areas the rates for men and women are similar. Pancreatic cancer is commoner in urban areas, but (unlike other GI cancers) socioeconomic status has a negligible effect. Racial groups at higher risk include New Zealand Maoris, native Hawaiians, and African Americans (14.4/100,000 per year). Throughout the USA, African Americans have incidence rates that are 1.5–2.0 times higher than those of the white population; Connecticut is the one exception. As this trend is not mirrored in African populations, environmental factors must play a part in the etiology of the disease.

Risk Factors

A variety of occupations have been implicated in the causation of pancreatic cancer. Chemical plant workers, atomic energy workers, and radiologists may have an increased risk, but none of the links are proved. Cigarette smoking clearly predisposes to pancreatic cancer,[39] and there is also a positive correlation with per capita consumption of fats. The only other definite known risk factor is a positive family history for pancreatic cancer.[40]

There are known familial predisposition syndromes, many of which are linked to other cancers, which predispose to pancreatic cancer including hereditary pancreatitis, Peutz–Jeghers syndrome, familial atypical multiple mole melanoma, cystic fibrosis, familial breast and ovarian syndrome (BRCA2 gene), hereditary nonpolyposis colorectal cancer, ataxia telangiectasia, Li–Fraumeni syndrome, and familial adenomatous polyposis. Familial pancreatic cancer is a known syndrome of families with two or more first-degree relatives who have been diagnosed with pancreatic cancer that is not associated with a known cancer syndrome.[41] It is thought that approximately 5% of all pancreatic cancers have a familial link.

Diabetes mellitus is difficult to evaluate as a risk factor because glucose intolerance may be a consequence of pancreatic cancer, but there is now evidence that diabetes is both a risk factor for pancreatic cancer and a presenting symptom.[42] This phenomenon is probably a result of profound insulin resistance rather than islet cell destruction, because resection may improve the endocrine function of the remaining gland.

Although chronic pancreatitis and pancreatic cancer may simply coexist, chronic pancreatitis does itself predispose to subsequent malignancy.[43] K-Ras mutations at codons 12 and 13 have been identified in up to 95% of pancreatic cancers, and similar mutations have been identified in patients with chronic pancreatitis and ductal hyperplasia, thereby providing a genetic basis for the potential progression of chronic pancreatitis to pancreatic cancer.[44] Inactivation of p53, p16, and DPC 4 genes may also play an important part in pancreatic carcinogenesis.

Pathology

Ductal adenocarcinoma of the pancreas is the most common malignant tumor of the pancreas and comprises approximately 80% of malignant pancreatic tumors. The majority of cases, approximately 70%, arise within the head or uncinate process of pancreas, 20–25% in the body and tail, and the remainder involves the whole pancreas. While cancers in the head of pancreas tend to present with obstructive jaundice, those arising in the body and tail are generally more advanced at the time of diagnosis and less likely to be resectable. Carcinomas of the ampulla, lower bile duct, and duodenum also tend to present with jaundice (or in the case of a duodenal lesion, with anemia or duodenal obstruction). For this reason as well as more favorable biology, they have a better prognosis than ductal carcinoma.

There is now strong evidence that many pancreatic cancers begin as precursor lesions known as pancreatic intraepithelial neoplasia (PanIN). In the same way that adenomas of the colon may progress to carcinoma, PanINs, are also thought to progress in a stepwise fashion from normal mucosa to PanIN 1a, PanIN 1b, PanIN 2, PanIN 3, and finally to invasive carcinoma. Different tumor promoter genes and tumor suppressor genes are involved in this process.[45] The majority of PanINs are asymptomatic, and only PanIN 3 is associated with a radiological lesion in some patients. Once invasion has occurred, however, disease progression tends to be more rapid than for most tumors, and early invasion is the rule.

Less common types of pancreatic cancer include acinar cell carcinoma, which often presents as a larger tumor and carries a better prognosis than ductal carcinoma. Adenosquamous is a mixed type with squamous differentiation, but also carries a poor prognosis.

Despite occupying only a small volume of the gland, pancreatic ductal tissue gives rise to approximately 90% of pancreatic tumors. Pancreatic cancer spreads by direct invasion and has a propensity for both perineural invasion and rapid lymphatic permeation. These cancers present late with approximately 60% being metastatic at the time of diagnosis, 20% showing lymph node involvement, and < 15% being confined to the pancreas.

Pancreatic cancer involves many different gene mutations. The most common of these is a mutation of the K-ras oncogene, which occurs in over 90% of pancreatic cancers and is also present in precursor lesions. It can also be identified in pancreatic juice. The HER-2 oncogene is also overexpressed in pancreatic cancers. Pancreatic cancers also tend to have mutations in tumor suppressor genes including p 53, p16, and SMAD4. They also demonstrate aberrant expression of various growth factors including epidermal growth factor, transforming growth factor β, and vascular endothelial growth factor. This fact is important in regard to targeted therapy.

Duct cell carcinoma is characterized immunohistochemically by its expression of carcinoembryonic antigen (CEA), carbohydrate antigen (CA) 19-9, and the keratins 7, 8, 18, and 19. Histologically, these tumors are mucinous adenocarcinomas that elicit an intense desmoplastic reaction. Hemorrhage and fat necrosis are often seen plus acinar atrophy with duct obstruction.

Clinical Assessment and Diagnosis

Clinical Presentation

As for most cancers, the size and stage of the tumor at presentation profoundly influences outcome. Worldwide reports have shown resectability rates of only 10–20%. Tumors <2 cm in size have a reported 5-year survival of 37%,[46] but identification at this stage is exceptional. Unfortunately, the first symptoms of the tumor—malaise, anorexia, weight loss, change in bowel habit, and epigastric discomfort—are nonspecific. Pain is common, but it is often a dull ache that is only elicited upon direct questioning. In left-sided tumors, the pain may be altered by position, being worst when recumbent and eased by sitting forward. The classic severe, penetrating pain is a late symptom and may herald extracapsular extension of the tumor. The timing of obstructive jaundice reflects the precise site of the tumor within the head of pancreas, but once present it progresses relentlessly with time. A recent onset of diabetes mellitus should be regarded with suspicion, as should a sudden increase in the insulin requirement of a diabetic. Courvoisier's law states that a palpable gallbladder in obstructive jaundice is seldom the result of gallstones because the biliary obstruction is less complete when caused by stones and gallstone disease causes some fibrosis of the gallbladder wall, so preventing distension. Pancreatic cancer may also present with acute pancreatitis, and thromboembolic complications are also common (as originally described by Trousseau).

Diagnosis and Staging

The diagnosis of a patient suspicious of having a pancreatic cancer goes hand-in-hand with assessment of the patient and the suspicious lesion for possible resection. Imaging is the mainstay of assessing resectability, but clinical assessment is also extremely important since patients may harbor unresectable disease that is not suspected on imaging. Abdominal ultrasound is usually the first investigation in patients with jaundice, but when pancreatic cancer is in any way suspected, a full multidetector, contrast-enhanced pancreas protocol CT scan should be carried out; this will identify over 90% of patients at presentation. Preoperative identification of distant metastases is absolutely vital since such patients will usually survive <12 months following resectional surgery. Computed tomography is extremely accurate in identifying unresectable disease in the form of liver (or lung) metastases, enlarged lymph nodes outside the boundaries of resection, and the presence and extent of vascular invasion (Fig. 56.13). In a recent international consensus statement, invasion of the coeliac axis, hepatic artery or SMA is considered as a contraindication to resection.[47] Invasion of < 180° of the circumference of the SMV or PV is considered as resectable disease, but > 180°

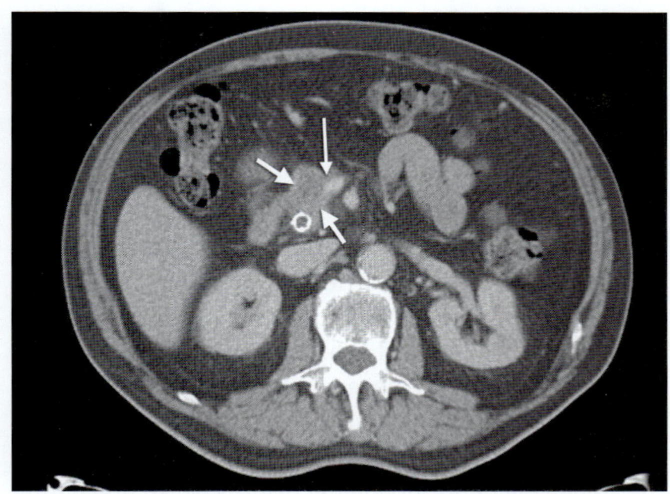

Fig. 56.13: Irresectable pancreatic cancer. Portal venous phase computed tomography of carcinoma of the head of the pancreas (bold arrows) with 360° constriction of the superior mesenteric vein (thin arrow) rendering the tumor irresectable. A metal biliary stent is also present.

invasion is borderline resectable. Magnetic resonance imaging offers no advantage over CT scanning.

If CT shows a clearly resectable tumor, other imaging investigations have little more to offer in terms of staging. However, in those patients with a lower biliary stricture and no mass, a small malignant tumor is still a distinct possibility. The most accurate second-line investigation is EUS, which has excellent resolution for small lesions of the pancreas and extrahepatic bile duct. In cases of borderline venous invasion on CT and equivocal lymph node involvement, EUS is also extremely accurate, although it is less accurate for arterial involvement.[48] Endoscopic ultrasound has the added advantage of tissue biopsy by EUS-guided FNA or core biopsy. It is the authors' policy in unresectable or borderline resectable disease to perform EUS with tissue acquisition. Laparoscopy with laparoscopic ultrasound is also used for staging purposes and is particularly valuable for identifying peritoneal and small liver metastases missed by CT. The value of preoperative laparoscopy in pancreatic cancer surgery is much less than previously because of the improved accuracy of multidetector CT. Only approximately 10% of patients will benefit from a laparoscopy. It is not therefore used routinely but selectively, particularly in those patients with high tumor markers but apparently resectable disease on CT. Positron emission tomographic scanning is not used routinely in staging of pancreatic malignancy but may be of use in those patients with equivocal lesions outside the pancreas on CT. Endoscopic retrograde cholangiopancreatography is no longer a standard imaging investigation in pancreatic cancer and certainly has very little role in confirming the diagnosis, although biliary brushing of a suspicious stricture may be appropriate. Endoscopic ultrasound has superseded ERCP in the diagnosis of pancreatic pathology. Serologic tumor markers have been used in the screening, diagnosis, and follow up of pancreatic cancer; CA 19-9 and CEA are often elevated, but they do not provide sufficient diagnostic accuracy to be used as a true screening test. They may help differentiate between benign and malignant disease particularly if markedly elevated.

Surgical Management

Preoperative Preparation

Patients who are deeply jaundiced do not tolerate major operations well. The obstructed liver fails to synthesize albumin and certain clotting factors (II, V, VII). Although coagulopathy can be easily reversed with vitamin K, jaundice combined with dehydration and hypoproteinemia predisposes patients to renal failure, sepsis, and poor healing. Biliary decompression has therefore become widely accepted as essential management in all jaundiced patients undergoing pancreatic resection. Biliary drainage is not without complications, however. An important randomized trial in patients with bilirubin < 250 µg/L compared immediate operation with biliary drainage followed by delayed operation.[49] Endoscopic retrograde cholangiopancreatography failed to achieve drainage in 25%, had a complication rate of 40%, and in addition 10% of patients experienced recurrent jaundice before resectional operation could be achieved. In those patients who underwent immediate operation, the incidence of any complication was 40% compared with 74% in those who had drainage followed by delayed operation. Fit patients with bilirubin < 250 µg/L should therefore be considered for resection without biliary drainage, and pancreatic surgical centers should make this possible logistically. Those patients with bilirubin > 250 mg/L or who are clearly unfit for immediate resection should undergo endoscopic drainage in the first instance.

Surgical Decision Making and Resectability

The decision about whether or not to operate for pancreatic cancer can be extremely challenging. Surgical resection often gives poor results with early recurrence, which is very disappointing for patients and their families. On the other hand, surgical resection provides the only hope of a cure and, in many patients, improved quality of life even if they eventually die of the disease. The mortality rate of a pancreatoduodenectomy is much lower than in previous decades and is now quoted at 2–3%.[50] Hospital stay may be as little as 7 days, although the median is nearer 14 days. The rate of complications has scarcely fallen, however. Clinical teams are just better at dealing with complications, many of which are treated by interventional radiology. A prolonged hospital stay with eventual recovery is commoner than before; this is very worthwhile if it results in good quality of life but disappointing if there is early recurrence. Selection of patients, including preoperative anesthetic assessment, is therefore very important.[50]

The only cure for pancreatic cancer is resection, but surgeons should be realistic. Symptomatic pancreatic cancer arising in the neck, body, or tail of pancreas is almost always unresectable. The few left-sided lesions that are resectable have usually presented as incidental tumors on imaging carried out for a different reason. In patients with tumors in the head of pancreas, there is a real chance of a curative resection, so patients with a suspicious lesion at this site should be put forward for resection even in the absence of positive histology. In some patients, it may be difficult to obtain a tissue diagnosis, but in the presence of a mass on CT or EUS and no suspicion of pancreatitis resection is advised.[8] The size of a mass is not a factor in resectability. Occasionally large, well-differentiated ductal carcinomas may be resectable, and neuroendocrine tumors often present as larger resectable lesions. Enlarged local lymph nodes within the plane of resection[51] are not a contraindication to operation, but proven metastatic disease (nodal, peritoneal, or liver) outside the resection plane indicates unresectable disease.

Patients with arterial involvement (SMA or hepatic artery) do badly from resection, and there is no indication for arterial resection (occasionally this may be necessary if the remainder of the resection has already been carried out). In patients with involvement of the PV/SMV, there are now also clear international consensus guidelines regarding resectability.[47] Patients with < 180° involvement of the PV/SMV should be considered resectable so long as it is considered that microscopic clearance (also known as an R0 resection) can be achieved. That may require resection of several centimeters of vein. The SMV may be particularly thin-walled, and SMV resection is not recommended more distally than the first jejunal branch. Occasionally patients have involvement of the dorsal pancreatic space without vascular involvement. For this reason, it is essential that patients undergoing pancreatoduodenectomy for malignant tumors undergo a wide resection of the dorsal pancreatic space removing all connective, lymphoid, and neural tissue up to the SMV and SMA, clearing tissue from the right side of the SMA.

"Curative" Operations

Pancreatoduodenectomy: This operation, also known as Whipple's procedure, is carried out for malignant tumors of the head of pancreas, ampulla, lower bile duct, and duodenum. The classical Whipple's includes an antrectomy, but this is only necessary when tumor clearance cannot be achieved otherwise. The preferred resection is pylorus-preserving proximal pancreatoduodenectomy. The advantage of preserving the pylorus lies in preventing enteric gastric reflux and theoretically reducing postoperative ulceration. The additional perigastric nodal clearance in the classical Whipple's has been shown to offer no additional survival advantage. If a classical Whipple's is necessary, it is advisable to drain the stomach into a separate loop of bowel to avoid bile reflux and gastritis.

The extent of lymphadenectomy necessary in pancreatoduodenectomy for pancreatic cancer has been the subject of a recent international consensus document.[51] Extended lymphadenectomy (i.e. skeletonization of the coeliac axis, SMA, hepatic artery, and PV and clearance of para-aortic nodes) confers no survival advantage, puts the patient at risk of severe diarrhea, and is not appropriate. A standard lymphadenectomy resects all peripancreatic nodes, nodes to the right of the porta, nodes to the right of the SMA, and the hepatic artery nodes (nodal station 8a).

For distal pancreatectomy for malignant disease, radical clearance of the primary tumor is essential. This is achieved by an adequate resection margin of the neck of the pancreas, division of the splenic artery at its origin and splenic vein at the PV, and resection of the connective and nodal tissue anterior to the renal vessels and left suprarenal gland. The spleen is mobilized and also resected (although it may be preserved in nonmalignant cystic tumors and chronic pancreatitis). A cuff of stomach may also be resected if involved. Again, extended lymphadenectomy is not appropriate, but all lymph nodes to the left of the PV and coeliac axis are removed.[51]

Total pancreatectomy is sometimes necessary in operations for pancreatic malignancy, most commonly when a tumor involves the head and neck of the pancreas (or is multifocal) and the remnant would be too small or difficult to achieve a pancreatic anastomosis.

Palliative Procedures

For 80% of patients with pancreatic cancer who cannot undergo resection, palliative procedures are frequently required. Palliation has three objectives:

- To treat or prevent jaundice
- To maintain gastric outflow
- To control pain

Most unresectable patients will require palliation of jaundice and can be treated adequately by self-expanding metal stents, usually placed endoscopically. Stents partially covered with a synthetic membrane are preferred as they reduce tumor ingrowth and allow anchoring of the stent to the bile duct. If endoscopic stent placement is not possible, percutaneous placement by the transhepatic route (PTBD) is also a safe option. Endoscopic and percutaneous procedures are much safer than previously, although complications can still occur; these include pancreatitis (an appreciable complication of ERCP but less common after PTBD), bleeding, duodenal perforation, biliary infection, stent migration, and bile peritonitis (after leakage from percutaneous liver puncture).

Because metallic stents tend to remain patent for at least 18 months, operative palliation by surgical bypass is practiced less often nowadays. However, if a pancreatic tumor is found to be unresectable at operation, a biliary enteric anastomosis should be carried out. The most efficient type of anastomosis is an end-to-side choledochojejunostomy. A cholecystectomy is done and then the bile duct is divided approximately 1 cm below the hilum of the liver. The distal end is oversewn and a Roux loop of jejunum is mobilized in an antecolic fashion (positioned to avoid tumor ingrowth) and anastomosed to the divided bile duct. If the pancreatic mass is bulky or close to the liver hilum, it is usually safer to opt for an endoscopic or percutaneous metal stent postoperatively rather than struggle with a biliary anastomosis.

Gastric outlet obstruction is uncommon at the time of presentation of pancreatic cancer, but if it does occur, it can be treated effectively by a surgical gastroenterostomy (which can be done via minilaparotomy or laparoscopy). A laparoscopic gastroenterostomy, for technical reasons, is usually done to the anterior surface of stomach and this usually results in less efficient gastric emptying. In the authors' experience, a dependent gastroenterostomy using the dependent part of the greater curve of the stomach (after detaching the greater omentum, close to the stomach) results in superior gastric emptying. If palliative surgery is being carried out for biliary obstruction, a gastroenterostomy should also be performed (usually onto the same Roux loop) to avoid future gastric outlet problems (Fig. 56.14).

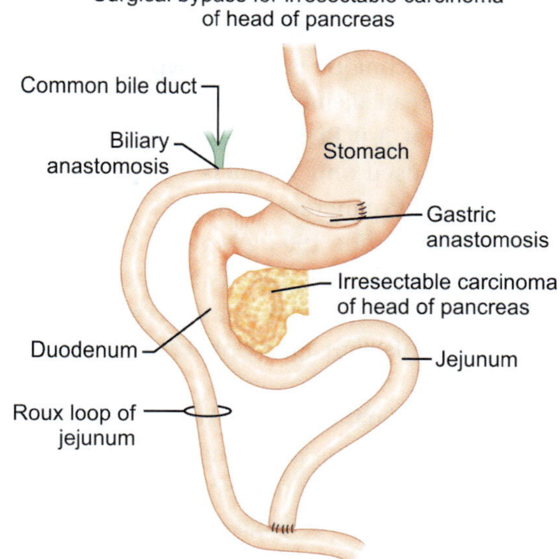

Fig. 56.14: The authors' preferred technique of surgical bypass for irresectable carcinoma of the head of pancreas. The bile duct is divided well above the "leading edge" of tumor after removal of the gallbladder. A single antecolic Roux loop of jejunum is created for biliary and gastric anastomosis.

At the same time as performing a palliative surgical procedure, a celiac plexus block (with alcohol or phenol) is carried out at operation to relieve pain if this is technically feasible.

Patients with pancreatic cancer should also receive specific advice about diet, pain control, and management of vomiting and other GI symptoms. They should be referred early to a multidisciplinary palliative care team experienced in dealing with such symptoms.

Complications of Pancreatic Resection

The operative mortality for pancreatoduodenectomy is now <5% in high-volume centers. Mortality in the UK fell from 10% in the 1990s to 4% in the following decade following centralization of pancreatic services (unpublished NHS data, 2013). The most common complications are sepsis (usually related to leakage at the pancreatic anastomosis—also the commonest cause of death), hemorrhage, delayed gastric emptying, and cardiopulmonary events. Much effort has been focused on prevention of pancreatic leakage by modification of the anastomotic technique, use of the stomach rather than jejunum for drainage, use of pancreatic duct stents, and the use of octreotide to reduce pancreatic leakage. Octreotide has been shown to reduce the magnitude of leakage rather than the overall rate.[52] The authors' chosen technique is: a two-layer duct-to-mucosa, end-to-side pancreaticojejunostomy (inner layer of 5/0 PDS and outer layer of 3/0 PDS) with an indwelling silastic pancreatic stent used only in ducts <3 mm in diameter. In those with a soft pancreas or narrow pancreatic duct, subcutaneous octreotide 100 μg is given 3 times a day for 7 days. Evidence suggests that using abdominal drains may not be necessary in those patients with low risk of leakage, i.e. patients with a hard pancreas or duct >5 mm in diameter.[53]

Management of pancreatic leakage is conservative in most cases. Many patients simply have a biochemical leak rather than a clinical leak, and no specific action is needed. In patients with clinical leakage (such as manifested by pyrexia, increased white cell count/CRP) but no abdominal signs, it is the authors' policy to instigate the following leak treatment: reduce oral intake to fluids only; intravenous octreotide infusion 50 μg/h; TPN; and intravenous antibiotics if clinically indicated. An abdominal CT scan is carried out to ensure that there are no undrained collections. Leak treatment is continued for at least 5 days or until clinical improvement allows oral feeding. It is unusual to require reoperation, but in the presence of peritoneal signs reoperation should not be delayed. Completion pancreatectomy may be necessary.

Hemorrhage may occur intraoperatively or postoperatively. Intraoperative hemorrhage is avoided by careful attention to vascular anatomy, care with dissection around major blood vessels, and attention to ligatures and suturing. An experienced assistant is essential. Postoperative hemorrhage can usually be treated adequately. Early hemorrhage within the first 5 days usually represents inadequate hemostasis at operation or a surgical tie being dislodged; reoperation is indicated. Postoperative hemorrhage later than 5 days is usually associated with pancreatic leakage and is most commonly the result of erosion of an artery by pancreatic enzymes leaking around the vessels and forming a pseudoaneurysm. The stump of the gastroduodenal artery is the usual culprit. The patient presents either with intraluminal hemorrhage (with the pseudoaneurysm leaking into the anastomotic defect) or intraperitoneal hemorrhage caused by rupture of the pseudoaneurysm. It is not unusual for the patient to have a "herald bleed." Any postoperative hemorrhage, be it intraluminal or into an abdominal drain, should be investigated immediately by upper GI endoscopy, CT angiography, and celiac axis angiography with embolization and/or arterial stenting.

Surgical Outcomes

Despite marked improvements in postoperative mortality rates, median long-term survival for patients undergoing resection is only of the order of 15 months. Long-term survival after resection is approximately 15% at 5 years. Surgical treatment is unfortunately not very successful at clearing microscopic tumor. Microscopic resection margin involvement is much more common than previously thought (over 70% in many contemporary series). This fact has been shown by a more meticulous approach to histopathological analysis of pancreatic surgical specimens.[54] Margin involvement is undoubtedly due to the infiltrative nature of the disease. Imaging might be expected to predict more accurately those patients with positive margins, but currently this is not the case. A more radical resection does not offer a better prognosis.[51]

Adjuvant Therapy

Many clinical trials of adjuvant chemotherapy and chemoradiotherapy have been carried out in pancreatic cancer resection patients. Only two trials included an observation arm compared to chemotherapy alone. Both of these trials (ESPAC1 and CONKO1) show a clear survival advantage to systemic chemotherapy.[55,56] In the ESPAC 3 study, there were no significant differences between adjuvant 5-fluorouracil (FU) and adjuvant gemcitabine, although gemcitabine had an improved safety profile. Currently there are no control data supporting adjuvant radiotherapy, but nevertheless it is typical for patients in some centers, particularly in the USA, to receive adjuvant chemotherapy and radiotherapy following resection for pancreatic cancer.

Neoadjuvant Therapy

The rationale for neoadjuvant therapy (preoperative treatment) is that it allows early introduction of systemic treatment and downstaging of a borderline resectable tumor so that it becomes resectable, thereby giving the patient an improved chance of having an R0 resection. However, if the patient does not respond, such treatment may delay operation needlessly. At least two neoadjuvant pancreatic cancer trials have closed early because of inadequate patient recruitment and without any conclusive findings. An important meta-analysis concluded that neoadjuvant treatment offered no benefit compared to adjuvant chemotherapy in patients with resectable tumors.[57] Further trials are expected.

CYSTIC TUMORS OF THE PANCREAS

Perspective

Pancreatic cystic neoplasms are an important group of tumors that have been increasingly recognized over recent years. The increase in axial imaging for a variety of symptoms has led to the identification of many more of these lesions at an asymptomatic stage. In the past, most cystic lesions of the pancreas have been labeled as pseudocysts. The distinction is essential because drainage of a cystic tumor is totally inappropriate. Patients with a pseudocyst almost always have a history of acute pancreatitis or evidence on imaging of chronic pancreatitis. In the absence of pancreatitis therefore, a cystic lesion of the pancreas should be assumed to be neoplastic. The recognition of the histological type of a pancreatic cystic tumor is important because mucinous lesions are usually premalignant and resection may be indicated, depending on a variety of factors. Nonmucinous lesions can often be ignored unless the patient's symptoms warrant resection. Assessment of a pancreatic cyst therefore focuses on determining whether a lesion is mucinous and if so, whether resection is appropriate.

Investigations

Computed tomography and/or MR are the first-line imaging investigations of choice. The histological nature of a pancreatic cystic lesion can often be strongly suspected on axial imaging by an experienced pancreatic radiologist. Endoscopic ultrasound, often with FNA for cytology and biochemistry (amylase, CEA, and CA19-9) is used in specific cases in which it might change management. Increased fluid CEA is indicative of a mucinous lesion, while fluid amylase is increased in pseudocysts and intraductal papillary mucinous neoplasms (IPMNs). Measurement of serum tumor markers CEA and CA19-9 is also important.

Serous Cystadenoma

Serous cystadenomas of the pancreas are slow-growing tumors that are either macrocystic (single large cyst) or microcystic (made up of many small cysts in a spongiform pattern). They mainly occur in the elderly. Serous cystadenoma is not a premalignant condition and should be left alone if possible. The only indication for resection is for symptoms that the patient cannot tolerate, but resection for this condition is unusual (Fig. 56.15).

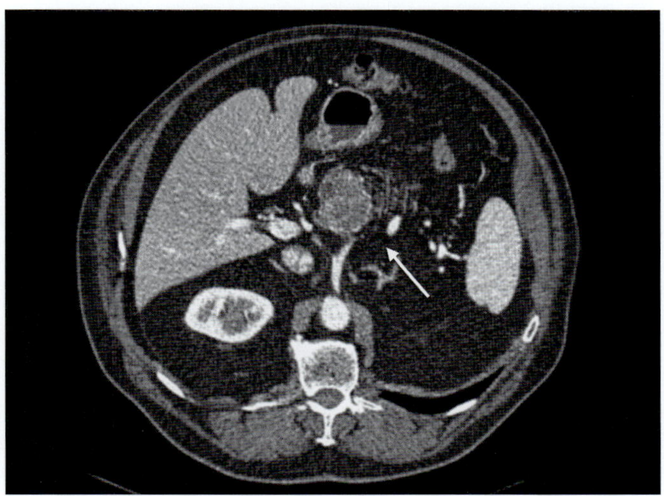

Fig. 56.15: Serous cystadenoma of head of pancreas (arrow). Characteristic honeycomb pattern is seen. The cyst did not require resection.

Mucinous Cystic Neoplasms

Mucinous cystic neoplasms (MCNs) are rare tumors that mainly occur in middle-aged women. The tumor occurs as a unilocular or multilocular cyst filled with viscid mucin. The cyst wall may be calcified. Histologically, it is characterized by an ovarian-type stroma. Mucinous cystic neoplasms are premalignant, but the likelihood of malignancy is < 15% and zero in MCNs < 4 cm in diameter without mural nodules (that are well seen on EUS). Mucinous cystic neoplasms tend to progress in terms of size and dysplasia and therefore should be removed in young patients (who comprise the majority). If an MCN contains solid elements in the wall of the cyst or its lumen, this is highly suspicious of malignancy and represents a likely mucinous cyst adenocarcinoma. Most MCNs arise in the distal pancreas in young women and are resected by distal pancreatectomy with splenic preservation (Fig. 56.16); the laparoscopic approach should be considered. In more proximal lesions, a parenchyma-sparing resection (middle pancreatectomy) should be considered (Figs. 56.17A and B). Resection of MCN is usually curative.[58]

Intraductal Papillary Mucinous Neoplasm

Intraductal papillary mucinous neoplasms of the pancreas are lesions of the duct system of the pancreas, usually arising in the head of the pancreas. The epithelium of the duct forms papillary projections into the duct and produces mucin, which causes intraluminal cystic dilatation of the pancreatic duct system. At endoscopy, mucin may be seen extruding from the duodenal papilla. An intraductal

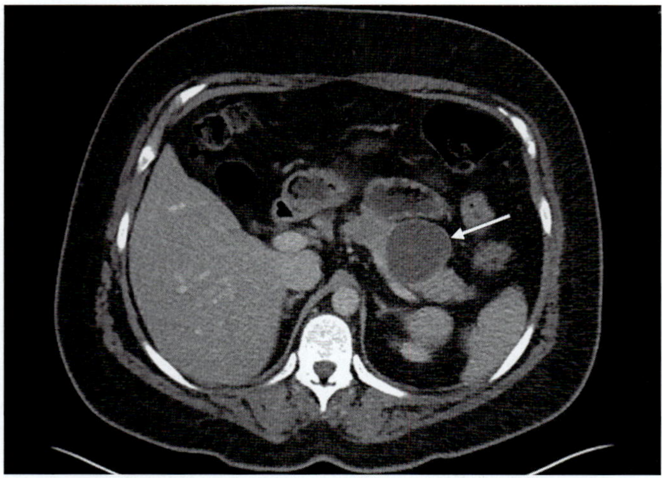

Fig. 56.16: Mucinous cystic neoplasm. A 33-year-old woman presented with nonspecific upper abdominal pain and was found to have this 5-cm cyst in the tail of the pancreas. A mucinous cyst was suspected and a distal pancreatectomy done with good recovery. Histology showed a mucinous cystic neoplasm with low-grade dysplasia.

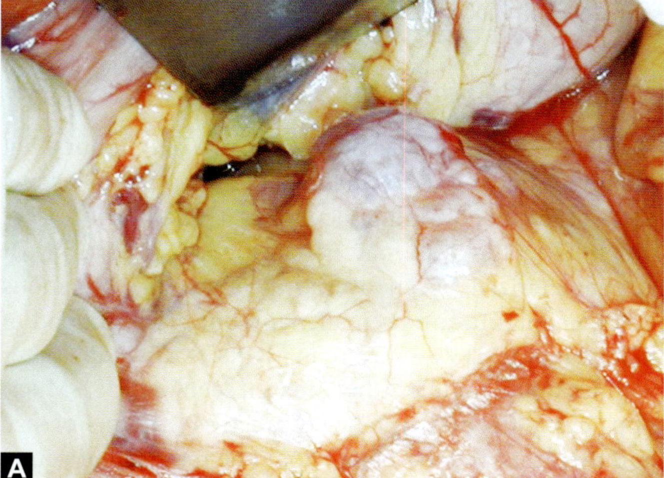

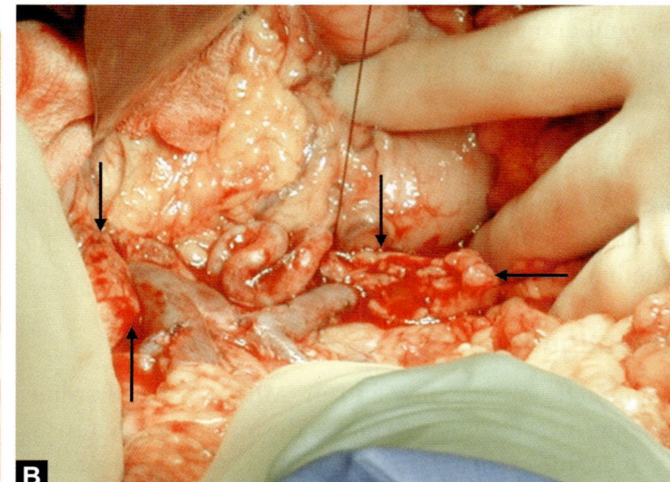

Figs. 56.17A and B: Mucinous cystic neoplasm (A) in proximal body of pancreas resected by a middle pancreatectomy. Arrows in (B) show cut ends of neck (on left) and body (on right) of pancreas prior to pancreaticojejunostomy anastomoses to neck and body.

papillary mucinous neoplasm may arise from the main pancreatic duct (main duct IPMN), and this is usually associated with main duct dilatation. In main duct IPMN, the risk of malignancy is high (mean 43%)[59] and surgical resection is strongly recommended (Figs. 56.18A and B). If the lesion arises from branch ducts (branch duct IPMN), the risk of malignancy is nearer 10%. In branch duct IPMN, the presence on CT or MR of one or more of the following five worrisome features is an indication for EUS assessment: cyst >3 cm; thickened/enhancing cyst walls; main duct size 5–9 mm; nonenhancing mural nodule; and abrupt change in caliber of pancreatic duct with distal pancreatic atrophy.[59] Following EUS assessment, operation should be considered if any of the following is present: (1) definite mural nodule(s), (2) main duct features suspicious for involvement, (3) cytology suspicious or positive for malignancy. If there is no clear-cut evidence of worrisome features, patients should enter a surveillance program, which is best carried out with MR to avoid irradiation. There is evidence that IPMNs will slowly progress, and therefore imaging surveillance of IPMN should be for life, although at increasing intervals and dependent on size.[59]

Solid Pseudopapillary Tumor of the Pancreas

A solid pseudopapillary tumor of the pancreas is a very rare tumor, usually occurring in young women aged 10–25 years. It is a well-circumscribed, solid-cystic lesion of the pancreas that presents as a mass lesion. The lesion is best described as a low-grade malignancy. Surgical resection is usually curative, but rarely metastases have been reported (Fig. 56.19).

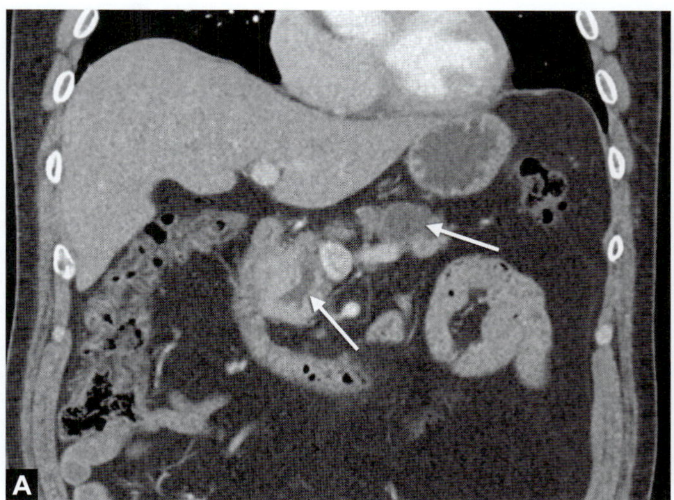

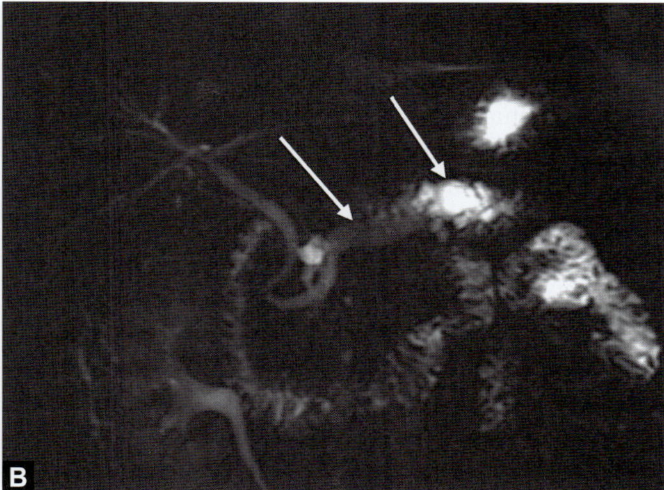

Figs. 56.18A and B: Main duct intraductal papillary mucinous neoplasm. Computed tomography and magnetic resonance imaging of same patient showing cystic dilatation (arrows) affecting the main duct of the head and body of pancreas. The patient underwent total pancreatectomy.

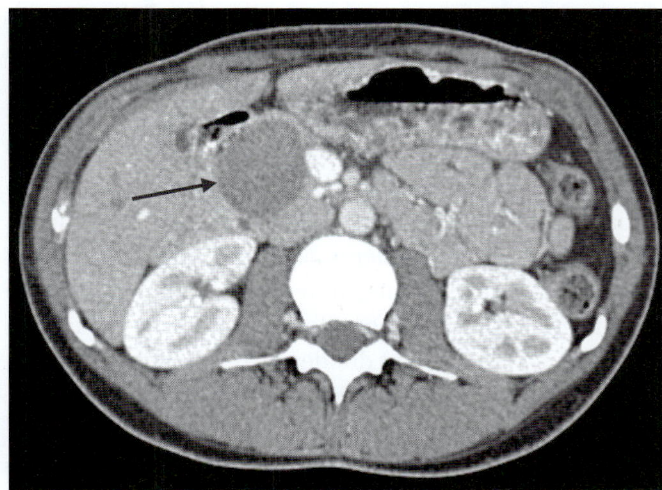

Fig. 56.19: Solid pseudopapillary tumor presented as a lump in the head of the pancreas (arrow) in a 19-year-old woman. It was resected as pancreaticoduodenectomy. The patient is doing well 8 years following surgery.

Other cystic lesions include cystic degeneration of a ductal carcinoma and a cystic neuroendocrine tumor of the pancreas. The differential diagnosis of cystic lesion should always consider these possibilities.

PERIAMPULLARY TUMORS

Perspective

The term "periampullary tumor" refers to neoplasms that arise from the ampulla and its immediate vicinity (including distal cholangiocarcinoma and primary duodenal carcinoma) but excludes pancreatic head tumors. Carcinoma of the distal common bile duct and carcinoma of the ampulla each account for approximately 5% of pancreatobiliary tumors. Most patients are over 65 years of age, and men are affected slightly more often than women.

Carcinoma of the Ampulla

Ampullary cancer is about 12 times less common than pancreatic cancer. Considering its small surface area, however, this particular area of the GI tract must have an increased susceptibility to malignant change, secondary perhaps to exposure to pancreatic, biliary, and duodenal secretions. It is probable that all ampullary cancers arise in pre-existing adenomas; the frequency of a focus of malignancy in adenomas of the papilla approaches 25%. In addition, areas of severe dysplasia can be found in contiguous or distant areas of the lesion in approximately 80% of ampullary carcinomas that arise in a papillary adenoma. These observations support the adenoma–carcinoma sequence in papillary tumors, a situation similar to that in the large bowel. A villous adenoma of the papilla should therefore be regarded as a premalignant lesion that requires aggressive management to avoid the subsequent development of cancer.

Ampullary tumors can arise from the inner (biliary) or the outer (duodenal) aspect of the ampulla, and they usually project into the duodenum. Microscopically, the tumor is composed of atypical tall columnar epithelial cells, which have a faintly eosinophilic or clear cytoplasm. Ampullary carcinoma may invade locally into the duodenum, pancreas, and common bile duct. As invasion progresses, the tumor tends to become more poorly differentiated and anaplastic. Perineural invasion may also be present. Ampullary tumors metastasize to both anterior and posterior lymph nodes of the pancreatic head, to hepatoduodenal nodes, and finally to para-aortic nodal tissue. Lymphatic spread is found in approximately 50% of resected ampullary tumors.

Assessment before treatment is important; all patients should undergo a pancreas protocol CT and EUS. An apparently small endoscopic lesion may invade the lower bile duct or pancreas or be associated with malignant nodes. If deep endoscopic biopsies are benign and there is no spread on EUS outside the ampulla, open operation can usually be avoided. Endoscopic snare excision or diathermy ablation (usually after endoscopic sphincterotomy) is then the treatment of choice. If deep biopsies are still benign and there is no evidence of spread but the lesion is too large for endotherapy, open ampullectomy can be carried out (via a duodenotomy) with re-implantation of the pancreatic and bile ducts. A more extensive lesion or one with malignancy on biopsy warrants a pancreatoduodenectomy.

Following pancreatoduodenectomy, 5-year survival rates that approach 50% have been reported for patients with ampullary cancer.[60] This figure contrasts sharply with survival for patients with pancreatic ductal cancer and emphasizes the need to identify these tumors preoperatively. It can be difficult to decide whether to carry out a transduodenal ampullectomy rather than a formal pancreatoduodenectomy. Although complications may be fewer after local resection, many apparently benign lesions contain foci of malignant change and unsuspected lymph node metastases; long-term survival in this group of patients would be unlikely without a formal resection and lymphadenectomy. In addition, as preoperative biopsy has a high sampling error, pancreatoduodenectomy is recommended for all patients whose preoperative biopsy shows malignancy and also in the majority of patients whose biopsy shows high-grade dysplasia. The results of a randomized trial have recommended chemotherapy following resection for ampullary carcinoma.[61]

Carcinoma of the Bile Duct

Primary neoplasms of the extrahepatic biliary tree are uncommon and occur in <0.5% of autopsy examinations (*see* Chapter 55, "Gallbladder and Biliary Tree"). Distal bile duct cancers, classed here as periampullary cancers, are even less common. Bile duct tumors are typically small, firm, well-circumscribed lesions that involve the full thickness of the duct wall. These tumors are adenocarcinomas and have varying degrees of differentiation. Local spread is common at the time of presentation; lymph node and hepatic metastases occur later in the disease process. Operative treatment is the mainstay of treatment for distal bile duct tumors, whether intentionally curative or to provide palliation. Radical resection can produce long-term cure, and the prognosis is more favorable than that of pancreatic exocrine cancer. It may be difficult to differentiate a lower bile duct cancer from a pancreatic cancer. The principles of investigation and surgical management are the same, but adjuvant therapy options may differ.

Carcinoma of the Duodenum

Adenocarcinoma of the duodenum is another uncommon malignancy that accounts for approximately 5% of periampullary tumors or 0.5/100,000 population per year. As in the large intestine, duodenal cancers are thought to begin as small neoplastic polyps that develop through a dysplastic stage into invasive carcinomas. Patients with familial polyposis coli are at particular risk of developing duodenal adenoma and carcinoma, and as this is the second most common malignancy in these patients, endoscopic screening is mandatory.

A personal series of 22 duodenal cancers showed an equal sex incidence, with a median age at presentation of 60 years.[62] Many patients reported vague symptoms of pain, anemia, and intermittent vomiting, but 12 were jaundiced. A pre-existing villous adenoma was seen in 11 patients and adjacent duodenal dysplasia in 13, which seemingly supports the adenoma–carcinoma sequence. Seventeen patients underwent "curative" resection with one hospital death at 25 days; the 5-year survival rate thereafter was 40%.

In general, treatment of periampullary duodenal cancers is pancreatoduodenectomy, but small lesions in the fourth part of the duodenum may be amenable to duodenal resection with duodenojejunostomy. Unresectable lesions should be treated by bypass, with gastroenterostomy and biliary bypass if necessary. Less commonly, carcinoid tumors, gastrinomas, and sarcomas arise in the duodenum, whereas another rare tumor, a somatostatinoma, can arise at the major papilla in patients who have neurofibromatosis.

ENDOCRINE TUMORS OF THE PANCREAS

Perspective

Over recent years, there has been an increased recognition of pancreatic endocrine tumors as a result of improved diagnostic technique and better understanding of the clinical syndromes. These tumors are derived from the diffuse neuroendocrine system of the pancreas and are no longer classified as benign or malignant. Neuroendocrine cells are characterized by the biosynthesis and secretion of either biogenic amines or polypeptide hormones, such as insulin, gastrin, glucagon, vasoactive intestinal polypeptide (VIP), or PP. In addition, neuroendocrine tumors have similar morphologic and cytochemical characteristics.

Pancreatic neuroendocrine tumors are very uncommon, but occur more frequently than previously thought, the incidence being 2.2 cases per 100,000 population per year.[63] Nonfunctioning tumors are much the most common type; insulinomas account for over 70% of functioning tumors, whereas gastrinomas account for 20% and the rarer tumors only 5%.

In general, pancreatic endocrine tumors are slow-growing and of indeterminate malignancy. Often it is difficult to establish malignant potential on histologic grounds, and a definitive diagnosis of cancer is only made when there is infiltration of adjacent structures or metastatic spread to regional lymph nodes or the liver. Similarly, prolonged follow-up may be required to establish the benign nature of a tumor because metastases may appear some years after removal of the primary.

Insulinoma

Insulinomas occur with an equal gender incidence and mostly between the ages of 30 and 60 years. Nesidioblastosis is a distinct condition that affects neonates and is characterized by persistent hyperinsulinemic hypoglycemia as a result of generalized b-cell hyperplasia or focal adenomatosis.

Pathology

Most insulinomas are benign, with malignancy occurring in only 4–16%. Virtually all insulinomas arise within the pancreas from the b cells of the pancreatic islets; only 1% are ectopic. At least 90% are solitary and measure 2–50 mm in diameter. Multiple insulinomas should prompt a search for multiple endocrine neoplasia type 1 (MEN 1), in which gastroenteropancreatic tumors are associated with hyperparathyroidism and pituitary tumors. Malignant insulinomas tend to be larger, and one-third of malignant lesions have metastasized by the time of diagnosis.

Clinical Presentation and Diagnosis

Symptoms of an insulinoma are intermittent and are caused by hypoglycemia, which develops during fasting or after severe exercise. The onset of hypoglycemia can be rapid, but is more often gradual. Neuroglycopenia presents oddly with confusion, automatism, epileptic seizures, or transient paralysis. This wide range of bizarre symptoms may lead to patients being labeled as psychiatrically disturbed. As eating relieves the symptoms, many patients have gained weight.

A diagnosis of insulinoma can be established by demonstrating Whipple's triad, namely:

- Hypoglycemic attacks occurring in the fasting state
- Blood glucose levels under 36 mg/dL (2 mmol/L) during the attack
- Relief of symptoms by the administration of glucose.

This triad forms the basis of the fasting test, which is the most useful provocative test. The diagnosis is clinched by demonstrating hypoglycemia with simultaneous elevation in blood insulin levels [>7.0 mU/L (50 pmol/L)] and C-peptide of >2.5 ng/mL (normal <2 ng/mL). A sulfonylurea screen should also be negative.

Localization of the Tumor

Localization of an insulinoma preoperatively is important so that the surgeon can plan the procedure to remove it and counsel the patient accordingly. It is now very unusual not to be able to identify an insulinoma preoperatively. Computed tomography and MR are the first investigations of choice (tumors are hypervascular and seen in the arterial phase), but the most accurate technique is EUS, which can image the whole pancreas. Detection of insulinomas is facilitated by the fact that these tumors are hypoechoic on EUS compared to the normal pancreas. Endoscopic ultrasound will also show the relationship of the tumor to the pancreatic duct and major vessels. If these tests fail to localize a tumor, we proceed to selective pancreatic arteriography and calcium arterial stimulation with hepatic venous sampling.[64] A small dose of calcium is injected into each artery (gastroduodenal or splenic), and the insulin concentration of hepatic venous blood is measured; it should only increase when calcium is injected into an artery supplying tumor tissue. Although less invasive than portal venous blood sampling, it gives a less precise anatomic location of the tumor. Preoperative localization is important, but localization at operation even more so.

Management and Outcome

Surgical removal of the tumor represents the only prospect of cure and should be carried out whenever possible. The tumor can be removed by either enucleation or pancreatic

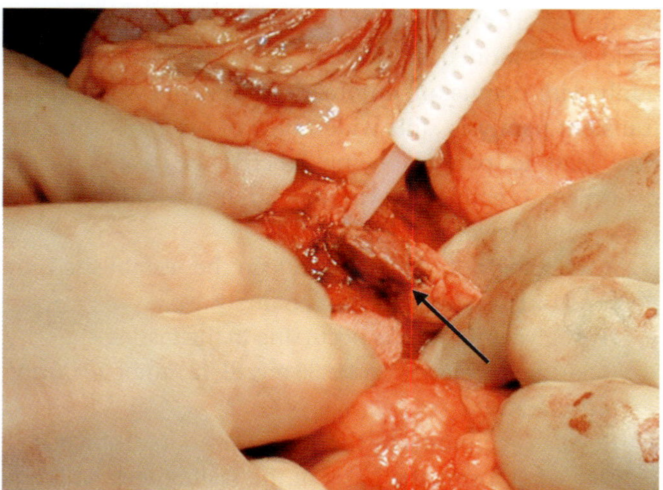

Fig. 56.20: Insulinoma. Enucleation of insulinoma from head of pancreas. The lesion (arrow) was easily palpable at operation.

resection. Even in the presence of liver metastases, excision of the primary tumor has a place to reduce hypoglycemic symptoms, in combination with adjuvant therapy to the liver (such as embolization and/or chemotherapy). Medical treatment with diazoxide can control symptoms (it inhibits insulin release from tumor cells), but the response is variable and side effects are common; its use should be restricted to patients who are unfit for general anesthetic.

Preoperative localization procedures can give the operating surgeon an idea of the site of tumor, but a detailed examination of the pancreas at operation is the final determinant. The pancreas must be fully exposed to allow thorough inspection and palpation. The tumor is palpable in at least 90% of cases. Multiple tumors should be excluded by careful inspection and palpation of the whole gland with intraoperative ultrasound. If the tumor cannot be found, blind resection is not generally advised and a further attempt at localization is recommended after an interval of 6–12 months.

The surgical procedure of choice for a solitary insulinoma is usually enucleation because it preserves the maximum normal pancreatic parenchyma (Fig. 56.20). The cavity should be inspected for damage to the pancreatic duct, which results in a postoperative pancreatic fistula if unrecognized. If there is any suggestion of a duct leak, a Roux-en-Y loop should be brought up and anastomosed to the cavity. A drain should be placed close to the relevant area. If a tumor is located in the tail of the gland, distal pancreatectomy (with splenic conservation if possible) is an appropriate alternative. It is very unusual to require a pancreatoduodenectomy for a benign insulinoma, and this should be avoided whenever possible. Some surgeons recommend laparoscopic exploration and resection. Laparoscopic distal pancreatectomy is a standard procedure, but laparoscopic enucleation is difficult.

The most common complication is a pancreatic fistula, which occurs in 10–20% of operations.[65] More rarely, acute pancreatitis and pseudocyst formation occur. Laparoscopic resections appear to have a higher incidence of positive margins and postoperative leakage. The operative mortality rate for insulinomas is low, and cure is usually achieved. In one recent series of 198 patients, mortality was zero and recurrence was 3%. Without operative excision, insulinomas can prove fatal; death results from intractable hypoglycemia.

Gastrinoma

In 1955, Zollinger and Ellison postulated a causal relationship between recurrent ulcer disease, gastric hypersecretion, and non-b cell pancreatic endocrine tumors.[66] Gastrinomas represent 20–25% of functioning pancreatic endocrine tumors. They are reported at a rate of 1/1000 patients with duodenal ulcer disease. They generally present between 30 and 50 years of age, but can occur at the extremes of age. Between 60% and 70% of tumors arise in men.

Pathology

Gastrinomas are usually small tumors <2 cm in diameter. Typically, they are oval or round lesions and have a smooth, tan appearance. Most gastrinomas occur in the pancreas, but a previously unrecognized group of patients has recently been described who have small (1–2 mm diameter) tumors in the duodenum. Although gastrinomas may also arise in other organs (e.g. stomach or jejunum), 89% are found to be in the "gastrinoma triangle,"[67] which is bounded by the junction of the cystic duct and common bile duct above, the junction of the second and third parts of the duodenum below, and the junction of the neck and body of pancreas medially. At least 60% of gastrinomas show malignant behavior. Approximately one-third of gastrinoma patients have the autosomal dominant syndrome of MEN 1, and the gastrinoma is very likely to be malignant in these patients.

Clinical Presentation and Diagnosis

The usual clinical presentation of gastrinoma is peptic ulceration, which is often multiple and atypical in site, occurring in the esophagus, distal duodenum, and upper jejunum. Complications, which used to occur in a high proportion of patients, include perforation, pyloric stenosis, hemorrhage, and fistula. As a result of the introduction of H_2-receptor antagonists and proton pump inhibitors, patients have a more prolonged presentation of chronic abdominal pain and the duration of ulcer symptoms before diagnosis now averages 4–5 years. Diarrhea occurs in up to 60% of patients and is caused by acid inactivating pancreatic lipase in the proximal jejunum and causing mucosal irritation.

Patients with gastrinoma are sometimes on long-term ulcer therapy, and the diagnosis goes undetected. In addition, it is now accepted that patients who have the Zollinger-Ellison syndrome succumb more often to the malignant nature of the disease than to ulcer complications. Early detection of gastrinoma is vital to allow localization and surgical resection.

The clinician should be alerted to the diagnosis of Zollinger-Ellison syndrome when one of the following occurs:

- Peptic ulcer disease in a young patient
- Virulent peptic ulcer disease
- Peptic ulcer disease occurring at an unusual site, such as in the third or fourth parts of the duodenum
- Stomal ulceration following a gastric operation for peptic ulcer
- Persistent unexplained diarrhea
- A family history of peptic ulcer or diarrhea.

The combination of an elevated fasting gastrin and an elevated basal gastric acid output is essential to diagnose gastrinoma. An elevated gastrin level is also seen in patients who have achlorhydria or renal failure, in patients after vagotomy, and in those who take H_2-receptor antagonists. Gastric hypersecretion in association with the gastrinoma syndrome is usually >1 L and contains over 100 mEq (100 mmol) of acid after a 12-hour overnight collection. In practice, a 1-hour basal acid output is sufficient, and the value should exceed 10 mEq/h (10 mmol/h) or less following gastrectomy.

Tumor Localization

Computed tomography and MR are the imaging investigations of choice, but small tumors may be missed, particularly those in the duodenum, which are usually associated with MEN 1. Endoscopic ultrasound can provide high-resolution images of the pancreatic parenchyma and duodenum and should be carried out by an experienced practitioner. A combination of CT scanning and selective arterial secretin injection and hepatic vein sampling probably gives the highest detection rate.[68] Intraoperative ultrasound can also visualize tumors, though they are often easily palpable at laparotomy. Finally, intraoperative endoscopy with transillumination of the duodenal wall has been advocated to detect duodenal microadenoma.

Management and Outcome

Surgical excision of the tumor with resultant cure is certainly feasible for a single localized and resectable tumor. Surgical cure can be defined as resection of all gastrinoma tumors so that the patient is rendered eugastrinemic, requires no antiulcer medication, and has no evidence of recurrent disease on long-term follow up. Pancreatic tumors can be enucleated or excised locally, taking care to avoid damage to the pancreatic duct. Pancreatoduodenectomy should be considered for a gastrinoma in the head of pancreas that is too deeply placed for safe enucleation, especially if adjacent involved nodes confirm the malignant nature of the tumor.

If there are multiple tumors (as in MEN 1 syndrome) or local metastases, cure is very unlikely. Palliative surgery, including radical debulking of liver metastases, may lead to a survival benefit in a small number of patients, but such high-risk operations should be confined to those who have symptomatic disease (Fig. 56.21). Gastric hypersecretion can usually be controlled by omeprazole (a dose as high as 120 mg daily may be required), thereby reducing the need

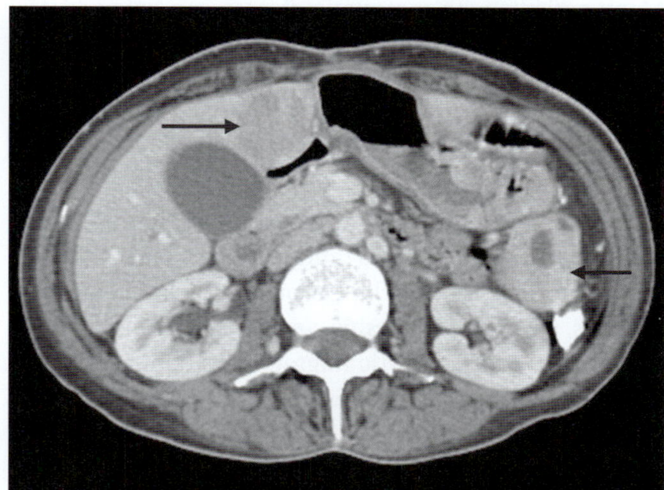

Fig. 56.21: Gastrinoma. Primary tumor in tail of pancreas (arrow), with one of three liver metastases (arrow). All macroscopic disease was resected by distal pancreatectomy and liver resection with good recovery, but liver metastases recurred within 2 years.

for total gastrectomy; the long-term effects of this drug are not yet established, however, and there may still be a role for less extensive acid-reducing operations.

Chemotherapy, which is usually based on 5-FU, has been used in patients with metastatic disease. Response rates as high as 60% have been reported (but also as low as 5%). Somatostatin and its long-acting analog octreotide relieve symptoms, but the original claims that hepatic metastases regress on this treatment have not been substantiated. Hepatic artery embolization or selective internal radiotherapy may provide good palliation in selected patients, but both these treatments require a patent PV and considerable expertise.

In patients who have Zollinger-Ellison syndrome in association with MEN 1 syndrome, omeprazole has been suggested as the first-line therapy because most patients were thought to have multiple malignant tumors of the pancreas that would require treatment by total pancreatectomy. It is increasingly recognized, however, that MEN 1 gastrinomas are often extrapancreatic and of indeterminate malignant potential. Patients should therefore undergo localization procedures to ascertain whether or not the tumor is amenable to surgical therapy.

Generally, the prognosis is excellent in patients in whom the tumor can be excised and the syndrome controlled, even if there are small metastatic deposits in regional lymph nodes. If there are metastases to the liver or extra-abdominal sites, however, the 5-year survival rate is only 20%. This figure contrasts with 5-year survival rates >80% for patients who have a single resectable lesion.[69] Many patients with metastatic disease can enjoy several years of good-quality life despite a large tumor bulk.

Rare Functioning Tumors

Glucagonoma

Glucagonomas constitute approximately 1% of all pancreatic endocrine tumors and can also occur in the MEN 1 syndrome. The clinical picture includes diabetes mellitus, weight loss, glossitis, angular stomatitis, anemia, depression, and necrolytic migratory erythema (a severe skin rash localized to the lower abdomen and legs that is characterized by superficial epidermal destruction and a tendency to migrate).

The diagnosis is made by detecting an elevated fasting level of glucagon in patients who have the typical clinical picture. Glucagonomas are usually large (>4 cm in diameter), located in the tail of the pancreas, and easily visible on CT or ultrasound scans. Approximately 70% are malignant, so formal resection is necessary usually by distal pancreatectomy. Surgical debulking in the presence of metastatic disease may provide good palliation for this slow-growing tumor. Chemotherapy or hepatic artery embolization are other useful options.

VIPoma

VIPomas comprise 3–5% of all pancreatic endocrine tumors. They cause watery diarrhea, which precipitates hypokalemia and either hypochlorhydria or achlorhydria. Abdominal pain and marked weight loss may also be present. Between 10% and 20% of VIPomas are found in an extrapancreatic site (retroperitoneal sympathetic chain or adrenal medulla), and 50–75% are malignant. The diagnosis is made when an elevated fasting plasma concentration of VIP coincides with a typical clinical picture. The lesion should be localized by CT and angiography.

All patients who have VIPomas should undergo operation and resection of the pancreatic tumor whenever possible. Debulking may provide useful palliation in those with metastatic disease, and the cytotoxic drug streptozocin may be used as an adjunct. Response to therapy and early recurrence can be identified by serial determinations of VIP. Patients with benign tumors are invariably cured, whereas those with malignant VIPomas have an average survival time of 12 months.

Somatostatinoma

Somatostatin is secreted by the D cells of the pancreas and inhibits the release of all known gut hormones; it decreases gastric emptying and slows intestinal transit. Patients with a somatostatinoma may have diabetes mellitus, diarrhea, steatorrhea, and gastric hypochlorhydria. Most somatostatinomas are solitary and located in the pancreatic head. They should be removed by surgical resection, and 50% are malignant.

Pancreatic Parathyroid Hormone-Related Peptide-Secreting Tumor (PTHrPoma) (Ectopic Hypercalcemia Syndrome)

Ectopic production of the polypeptide parathyroid hormone-related peptide (PTHrP), which has activity similar to that of parathyroid hormone, may occur from a pancreatic islet cell tumor. The resulting syndrome is similar to that resulting from hypercalcemia secondary to parathyroid adenoma or hyperplasia. Surgical excision of the pancreatic tumor is the treatment of choice.

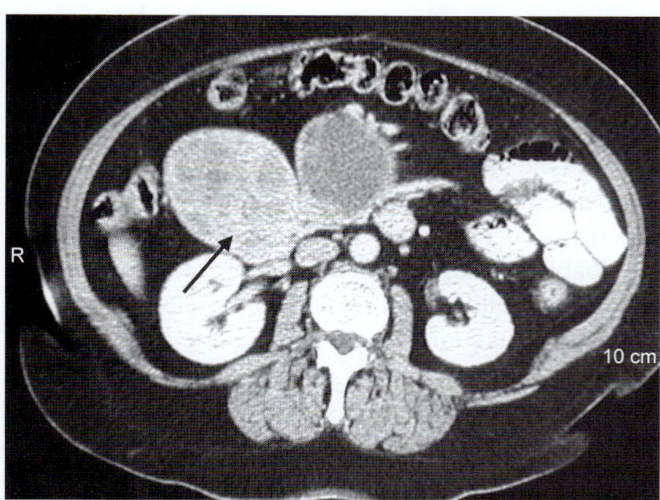

Fig. 56.22: Nonfunctioning pancreatic neuroendocrine tumor. Large bilobed lesion (arrow) arising from the head of the pancreas. The major vessels were pushed aside by the tumor rather than invaded, and a pancreaticoduodenectomy was carried out. The patient was alive and free of recurrence 10 years following surgery.

NONFUNCTIONING ENDOCRINE TUMORS

Pathology

With increased axial imaging, the number of incidental neuroendocrine tumors of the pancreas has increased dramatically. The majority are nonfunctioning. They become symptomatic due to their size, therefore may present as large tumors with invasion of local structures (Fig. 56.22). Immunohistochemistry usually shows at least one peptide (e.g. insulin, glucagon, PP, C-peptide) in addition to the general markers for neuroendocrine tumors (e.g. neuron-specific enolase, chromogranin, synaptophysin), but circulating hormone levels are normal. Elevated serum neuropeptides, particularly chromogranin A, are usually present. Nonfunctioning tumors are equally distributed through the pancreas.

Clinical Presentation and Diagnosis

Nonfunctioning tumors are generally much larger (>5 cm in diameter) than functioning tumors at the time of diagnosis, and patients present with the symptoms and signs of a mass, which may even be palpable. If the tumor arises in the head or neck of pancreas, it may enlarge sufficiently to cause partial obstruction of the bile duct, pancreatic duct, or duodenum. This process causes jaundice, pancreatic duct obstruction, or vomiting. Erosion into the duodenum or stomach can cause severe GI bleeding, or there may be spontaneous hemorrhage into the abdominal cavity.

Most of these tumors are malignant and show evidence of local invasion or metastasis (nodal or hepatic). Localization is usually straightforward, and CT scan is the modality of choice. Occasionally, asymptomatic tumors are picked up by screening a patient who has MEN 1. Some of these neoplasms show calcification, a few are clearly cystic and some of the larger ones have areas of central necrosis.

The diagnosis of a neuroendocrine tumor should be suspected if the tumor is large, but the patient remains in relatively good health, if it is situated in the head of pancreas, but jaundice is either absent or minimal, and if there is evidence of calcification or vascularity on imaging. Fasting neuropeptides may be elevated. As with any pancreatic mass, preoperative biopsy is only required if it is clearly irresectable.

Management and Outcome

Although diagnostic delay frequently means that these tumors are large by the time of presentation, surgical resection is the best treatment if possible. In the case of a tumor of the tail of pancreas, operation may be indicated even in the presence of metastases. It is the relatively indolent progress of the malignancy that justifies palliative resection, and this situation is very different to that seen for the common type of pancreatic ductal carcinoma. Resection usually entails a distal pancreatectomy with or without a splenectomy for lesions of the left pancreas and a pancreatoduodenectomy with or without an antrectomy for lesions of the right pancreas. A curative resection rate of about 50% can be anticipated in this disease, depending on tumor stage,[70] but the operation is often difficult because of the substantial size and vascularity of the tumors. Chemotherapy can relieve symptoms in those who have irresectable disease.

PRINCIPLES OF PANCREATIC SURGERY

All operations on the pancreas are major undertakings, but few are emergencies, except in the context of abdominal trauma or infected pancreatic necrosis. Generally, there is time to prepare the patient first with appropriate counseling, assessment of any cardiorespiratory disease, correction of anemia, and gross malnutrition and usually in the context of chronic pancreatitis measurement of endocrine and exocrine functions. Special precautions must be considered in those who have obstructive jaundice (*see* above in section on surgical management under Carcinoma of the Pancreas) or those undergoing splenectomy.

Operative Approach to the Pancreas

A bilateral subcostal or "rooftop" incision provides excellent access for all pancreatic operations and causes less respiratory embarrassment afterwards than a vertical incision. Laparotomy starts with examination of the adjacent viscera that may be affected in pancreatic disease, including the gallbladder, liver, bile duct, spleen, stomach, and colon. The head of the pancreas is examined after wide mobilization of the second and third parts of the duodenum (Kocher's maneuver). The neck, body, and tail of the pancreas are exposed by entering the lesser sac through the greater omentum, outside the gastroepiploic arcade; incision of the peritoneum along the upper and lower borders allows examination of the posterior surface. The uncinate process is relatively inaccessible, but can be exposed by identifying the right-hand border of the SMV as it runs towards the tunnel behind the neck of the pancreas. Delineation of this tunnel is the key step in nearly every pancreatic resection. The SMV is identified below the pancreas by retracting the second part of the duodenum laterally and the transverse colon inferiorly, so opening up the angle between these structures within which lies the vein. It can also be found by following the middle colic vein towards its termination and by dissecting the underlying areolar tissue with great care. The easiest approach to the PV is to divide the bile duct that is usually required if the PV is being exposed. Intraoperative investigations of the pancreas—biopsy and operative ultrasound—are considered earlier in this chapter.

Pancreatic Sphincter Procedures

Transduodenal Sphincteroplasty

Surgical division of the sphincter of Oddi—transduodenal sphincteroplasty—may be indicated for stenosis of the major pancreatic papilla that causes recurrent acute pancreatitis or for sphincter of Oddi dysfunction. Selection of appropriate patients may be assisted by ERCP manometry, a morphine-prostigmine (Nardi) provocation test, or MRCP evidence of prolonged pancreatic duct dilatation with intravenous secretin.[71] Pancreatic sphincteroplasty can be carried out in patients who have mild-to-moderate chronic pancreatitis and a dominant stricture near the papilla if an endoscopic approach has failed. The papilla is approached through a longitudinal duodenotomy, and the pancreatic duct is cannulated after biliary sphincteroplasty, if necessary giving intravenous secretin (1 unit/kg) to locate the orifice of the pancreatic duct. The common septum between the terminal portions of the bile duct and pancreatic duct is then incised for about 10 mm, and fine absorbable sutures are used to coapt the mucosae. The operation should produce a double-barreled appearance with both ducts sutured widely open.

Accessory Pancreatic Sphincterotomy or Sphincteroplasty

Accessory pancreatic sphincterotomy or sphincteroplasty can be achieved endoscopically, though considerable expertise is required, or by a transduodenal approach using secretin to locate the tiny papilla. The procedure may be indicated for recurrent acute pancreatitis in pancreas divisum.

Pancreatic Drainage Procedures

The distinction between acute and chronic pancreatic pseudocysts is discussed earlier in this chapter, together with the wide variety of possible drainage techniques (i.e. radiologic, endoscopic, laparoscopic, and open operation). The choice may rest in part upon the local availability of expertise. Most cysts that fail to resolve within 4–6 weeks of an attack of acute pancreatitis and most cysts over 5 cm in diameter in patients who have chronic pancreatitis require drainage.

Cystogastrostomy

Cystogastrostomy is appropriate for the typical retrogastric pseudocyst that develops after an attack of acute pancreatitis, although many of these are now dealt with endoscopically. The anterior wall of the stomach is opened and the posterior wall is then incised for about 5 cm to open into the cyst cavity. The fluid contents are evacuated and any particulate debris is freed. A running suture is used to oversew the margins of the cystogastrostomy. An almost identical procedure can be carried out laparoscopically, although some surgeons prefer to use a linear stapler to enlarge the cystogastrostomy opening.

Cystojejunostomy

For many patients who have acute or chronic pancreatitis, a cystojejunostomy (Roux-en-Y) is a better option than a cystogastrostomy, particularly if the pseudocyst is prominent inferiorly. The anterior wall of the cyst is opened and a biopsy is taken to confirm its inflammatory nature, followed by a side-to-side anastomosis in two layers to the Roux loop. In a patient with recent acute pancreatitis, the lesser sac is usually obliterated, so the cyst is approached through the transverse mesocolon; all necrotic debris is removed.

Longitudinal Pancreaticojejunostomy

The suitable patient for longitudinal pancreaticojejunostomy has painful chronic pancreatitis and a pancreatic duct of at least 8 mm diameter (*see* Fig. 56.12). Operative ultrasound allows complete assessment of the parenchyma and duct system of the pancreas. Dissection around the head of the pancreas is often difficult due to inflammation and venous collaterals, the extent of which should be checked preoperatively on an up-to-date CT. The main pancreatic duct is then identified (by ultrasound) and opened following aspiration with a needle. The duct should be opened from tail to head, with division and under-running of the gastroduodenal artery as it crosses the neck of the pancreas. It is the authors' preference to ensure that all inflammatory tissue is removed from the head of the pancreas (modified Frey procedure) rather than purely providing drainage. All pancreatic calculi are removed and all areas of inflammation and loculated cysts should be drained before the long side-to-side anastomosis is created between the filleted pancreas and a retrocolic Roux loop of jejunum.[72]

Pancreatic Resections

Distal Pancreatectomy

Indications for distal pancreatectomy include chronic pancreatitis localized to the body and tail of the pancreas, and also neuroendocrine and cystic tumors and the occasional resectable ductal cancer. Although splenectomy is included in a conventional distal pancreatectomy, it may be possible to preserve the spleen in pancreatitis patients who do not have gross inflammation. The simplest technique is to ligate the splenic vessels adjacent to the tail of the pancreas and leave the spleen to survive on the short gastric and left gastroepiploic vessels (Warshaw operation).[73] This is a good procedure, but the spleen may occasionally end up being removed anyway if it is ischemic at the end of the operation. It is also possible in some chronic pancreatitis patients with little active inflammation to preserve the splenic artery and vein by dissecting the pancreas off these vessels, a dissection that is facilitated by the harmonic scalpel. This conservative distal pancreatectomy is not appropriate for malignant tumors or severe chronic pancreatitis, especially if there is an associated pseudocyst or splenic vein thrombosis.[74]

Many surgeons begin a conventional distal pancreatectomy by mobilizing the spleen and then proceeding towards the midline, but this technique usually results in damage to the spleen and bleeding. It is therefore the authors' preference to identify the PV tunnel, divide the neck of the pancreas, and dissect the gland in a retrograde fashion. The standard distal resection usually incorporates 50–70% of the gland; insulin may only be needed thereafter if the remnant is diseased. There is no foolproof method to secure the pancreatic stump, and there is a risk of postoperative pancreatic fistula of about 10% whichever technique is used. In cases of chronic pancreatitis where there is disease in the remnant, closure of the duct in the neck of the pancreas may result in a fistula and is not advised. An end-to-side anastomosis of the neck of the pancreas to the first loop of jejunum will prevent this complication. Adequate drainage is important. Octreotide is not used routinely.

Laparoscopic resection of the left pancreas is now a standard procedure in patients with cystic and neuroendocrine tumors of the body and tail of the pancreas. The benefits are reduced pain and length of hospital stay. Long-term outcomes are similar to those of laparotomy.[75] Robotic surgery for the pancreas is currently in its infancy.

Proximal Pancreatectomy

Resection of the pancreatic head is indicated for carcinoma of the pancreas, periampullary cancers, and selected patients with chronic pancreatitis. As previously discussed (in sections on Carcinoma of the Pancreas, Cystic Tumors of the Pancreas, Periampullary Tumors, and Chronic Pancreatitis), the pylorus-preserving proximal pancreatoduodenectomy (PPPP) modification is appropriate for many cancers and most cases of chronic pancreatitis.

Proximal pancreatoduodenectomy can be subdivided into two phases—resective and reconstructive—each lasting 2.5–3 hours on average. The operation starts by excluding the presence of distant metastases (with biopsy if needed) and then dissecting the PV and SMV. Clear-cut PV invasion is usually an indication to abandon the resection, but sometimes malignant involvement of the right border of the vein is only found at a late stage. The surgeon can then choose between accepting a palliative resection and proceeding to a localized resection of up to 4 cm or so of PV with an end-to-end reconstruction.[76] Cure may yet be thwarted by encasement of the origin of the SMA. Histologic studies show that adherence of tumor to the PV frequently does not imply actual invasion of the vein wall.

In a standard PPPP, the pancreas is divided in front of the PV, the duodenum is divided 3–5 cm beyond the pylorus, the bile duct is divided above the entry of the cystic duct with removal of the gallbladder, and the jejunum is divided 20–30 cm distal to the ligament of Treitz. When operating for cancer, it is advisable to send tissue from the pancreatic resection margin for frozen section examination to ensure adequate clearance. Increasing recognition that retroperitoneal invasion is common supports the removal of the tissue overlying the inferior vena cava behind the head of pancreas. In chronic pancreatitis, the objective is simply to remove all or most of the inflammatory mass by the safest means available.

There are many different methods for reconstructing the upper GI tract after pancreatoduodenectomy. The most important anastomosis is the pancreatojejunostomy because leakage at this point can cause lethal postoperative complications (pancreatic fistula, sepsis, and hemorrhage). Pancreatic leakage is related to a variety of factors, but the most crucial of these is pancreatic consistency (increased leakage with a soft pancreas) and pancreatic duct diameter (increased leakage with a narrow duct).[53] In those patients with a narrow duct, an indwelling silastic stent is usually used. Leakage is also related to reduced cardiopulmonary function.[50] The biliary–enteric anastomosis is usually straightforward in a patient who has malignant biliary obstruction, and in a wide duct it is the authors' practice to use a continuous 3/0 PDS anastomosis. In those patients with a normal caliber bile duct, the authors feel strongly that the anastomosis should be done with interrupted sutures, such as 5/0 PDS.

At the end of every pancreatoduodenectomy, care must be taken to ensure good hemostasis and at least two tube drains should be left to the region of the pancreatic anastomosis. If the preoperative serum albumin is low [<3.0 g/dL (30 g/L)], then some form of enteral feeding tube should be considered. The operative mortality rate of pancreatoduodenectomy should not exceed 5%, but complication rates of at least 30% are generally reported.

Total Pancreatectomy

Removal of the entire pancreas for carcinoma of the head of pancreas fails to improve the 5-year survival rate[12] and should be reserved for two groups of patients:

- Those who are already insulin-requiring diabetics
- Those who have a positive pancreatic resection margin on frozen section examination.

There is a role for total pancreatectomy as the ultimate treatment for chronic pancreatitis, especially for those who have endocrine failure or recurrence of intractable pain after less extensive operations. Technically, total pancreatectomy is a combination of proximal and distal resections. It is usually possible to preserve the pylorus and sometimes to preserve the spleen, especially in a completion distal pancreatectomy. Subsequent follow-up is important, particularly to optimize exocrine and endocrine replacement therapy. There is a worrying incidence of late deaths, especially among alcoholics who continue to drink.

ORGANIZATION OF PANCREATIC SERVICES

In the past, pancreatic surgeons have worked as general surgeons with an interest in the pancreas. By and large, this meant that in each hospital there would be one or two surgeons with an interest in pancreas, and in each hospital fairly small volumes of pancreatic operations were taking place. Experience was therefore diluted and specialist expertise, particularly in radiology, pancreatic endoscopy, and pathology, was restricted to a few large hospitals. It became apparent that surgical outcomes in smaller hospitals were unsatisfactory. In the UK in the early 2000s, a centralization process took place for upper GI surgery (esophagogastric on the one hand and hepatopancreatobiliary on the other) that became known as Improving Outcomes Guidance.[77] Each pancreatic center was expected to serve a population of at least 2 million. Each center would have a multidisciplinary pancreatic team consisting of at least four pancreatic surgeons and also gastroenterologists (with ERCP and EUS expertise), radiologists, pathologists, oncologists, anesthetists, dieticians, and specialist nurses, all with a specialist interest in the pancreas. Patients with suspected pancreatic or periampullary tumors would be referred to the pancreatic center for confirmation of diagnosis and specialist care. Surgical treatment and specialist endoscopic and radiological management would only be delivered at the pancreatic center, while palliative care, including chemotherapy, would be given locally. This centralization process has now been operating in the UK for 10–15 years and has also been adopted by several other countries. Since then it has become apparent that a strong relationship exists between increasing hospital (institutional) volume and reduced operative mortality for major resections, as well as between hospital volume and long-term survival.[78] Although data on surgeon volume are less consistent than those for hospital volume, improved outcomes are seen in units with higher individual surgeon volumes. Patients are seen quicker and a multidisciplinary approach is applied to each patient. Resection rates have doubled across the UK, and mortality from pancreatic resection has reduced from 10% to 4%.

REFERENCES

1. Catalano C, Laghi A, Fraioli F, et al. Pancreatic carcinoma: the role of high-resolution multislice spiral CT in the diagnosis and assessment of resectability. Eur Radiol. 2003;13: 149-56.
2. Sica GT, Braver J, Cooney MJ, et al. Comparison of retrograde cholangiopancreatography with MR cholangiopancreatography in patients with pancreatitis. Radiology. 1999; 210:605-10.
3. Oppong K, Raine D, Nayar M, et al. EUS-FNA versus biliary brushings and assessment of simultaneous performance in jaundiced patients with suspected malignant obstruction. J Pancreas (Online). 2010;11(6):560-7.
4. Serrano OK, Chaudhry MA, Leach SD. The role of PET scanning in pancreatic cancer. Advances Surg. 2010;44:313-25.
5. Mallery JS, Baron TH, Dominitz JA, et al. Complications of ERCP. Gastrointest Endosc. 2003;57:633-8.
6. Jalleh RP, Williamson RCN. Pancreatic exocrine and endocrine function after operations for chronic pancreatitis. Ann Surg. 1992;216:656-62.
7. Hewitt MJ, McPhail MJ, Possamai L, et al. EUS-guided FNA for diagnosis of solid pancreatic neoplasms: a meta-analysis. Gastrointest Endosc. 2012;75(2):319-31.
8. Asbun HJ, Conlon K, Fernando-Cruz L, et al. When to perform a pancreatoduodenectomy in the absence of positive histology? A consensus statement by the International Study Group of Pancreatic Surgery. Surgery. 2014;155:887-92.
9. Manfredi R, Brizi MG, Costamagna G, et al. Pancreas divisum and santorinicele: assessment by dynamic magnetic resonance cholangiopancreatography during secretin stimulation. Radiol Med. 2002;103:55-64.
10. MP Ellis, JJ French, RM Charnley. Acute pancreatitis and the influence of social deprivation. Br J Surg. 2009:96:74-80
11. Lee SP, Park HZ. Biliary sludge as a cause of acute pancreatitis. N Engl J Med. 1992;326:589-93.
12. Armstrong CP, Taylor TV, Jeacock J, et al. The biliary tract in patients with acute gallstone pancreatitis. Br J Surg. 1985;72: 551-5.
13. Banks PA, Bollen TL, Dervenis C, et al. Classification of acute pancreatitis - 2012: revision of the Atlanta classification and definitions by international consensus. Gut. 2013;62:102-11.
14. Ranson JHC, Rifkind KM, Turner JW. Prognostic signs and nonoperative peritoneal lavage in acute pancreatitis. Surg Gynecol Obstet. 1976;143:209-19.
15. Blamey SL, Imrie CW, O'Neill J, et al. Prognostic factors in acute pancreatitis. Gut. 1984;25(12):1340-6.
16. Taylor SL, Morgan DL, Denson KD, et al. A comparison of the Ranson, Glasgow and APACHE II scoring systems to a multiple organ scoring system in predicting patient outcome in pancreatitis. Am J Surgery. 2005;189:219-22.
17. Puolakkainien P, Valtonen V, Paananen A, et al. C-reactive protein (CRP) and serum phospholipase A2 in the assessment of the severity of acute pancreatitis. Gut. 1987;28:764-71.
18. Balthazar EJ, Robinson DL, Megibow AJ, et al. Acute pancreatitis: value of CT in establishing prognosis. Radiology. 1990;174(2):331-6.
19. Johnson CD, Abu-Hilal M. Persistent organ failure during the first week as a marker of fatal outcome in acute pancreatitis. Gut. 2004;53:1340-4.
20. Corfield AP, Cooper MJ, Williamson RCN. Acute pancreatitis: a lethal disease of increasing incidence. Gut. 1985;26: 724-9.
21. Working Group IAP/APA Acute Pancreatitis Guidelines. IAP/APA evidence-based guidelines for the management of acute pancreatitis. Pancreatology. 2013;13(4):1-15.
22. Luiten EJ, Hap WC, Lange JF, et al. Controlled clinical trial of selective gut decontamination for the treatment of severe acute pancreatitis. Ann Surg. 1995;222:57-65.
23. van Geenen EJ, van Santvoort HC, Besselink MG, et al. Lack of consensus on the role of endoscopic retrograde cholangiography in acute biliary pancreatitis in published meta-analyses and guidelines: a systematic review. Pancreas. 2013;42:774-80.
24. Bassi C, Butturini G, Falconi M, et al. Outcome of open necrosectomy in acute pancreatitis. Pancreatology. 2003; 3(2):128-32.
25. Carter CR, McKay CJ, Imrie CW. Percutaneous necrosectomy and sinus tract endoscopy in the management of infected pancreatic necrosis: an initial experience. Ann Surg. 2000;232(2):175-80.
26. van Santvoort HC, Besselink MG, Bakker OJ, et al. A step-up approach or open necrosectomy for necrotizing pancreatitis. N Engl J Med. 2010;362:1491-502.
27. Baron TH, Thaggard WG, Morgan DE, et al. Endoscopic therapy for organized pancreatic necrosis. Gastroenterology. 1996;111:755-64.
28. Charnley RM, Lochan R, Gray H, et al. Endoscopic necrosectomy as primary therapy in the management of infected pancreatic necrosis. Endoscopy. 2006;38:925-8.
29. Melman L, Azar R, Beddow K, et al. Primary and overall success rates for clinical outcomes after laparoscopic, endoscopic, and open pancreatic cystogastrostomy for pancreatic pseudocysts. Surg Endosc. 2009;23(2):267-71.
30. Charnley RM. Hereditary pancreatitis. World J Gastroenterology. 2003;9:1-4.
31. Lowenfels AB, Maisonneuve P, DiMagno EP, et al. Hereditary pancreatitis and the risk of pancreatic cancer. International Hereditary Pancreatitis Study Group. J Natl Cancer Inst. 199719;89(6):442-6.
32. Sugumar A, Chari ST. Autoimmune pancreatitis. J Gastroenterol Hepatol. 2011;26(9):1368-73.

33. Maher JW, Johlin FC, Heitshusen D. Long-term follow-up of thoracoscopic splanchnicectomy for chronic pancreatitis pain. Surg Endosc. 2001;15:706-9.
34. Nguyen-Tang T, Dumonceau JM. Endoscopic treatment in chronic pancreatitis, timing, duration and type of intervention. Best Pract Res Clin Gastroenterol. 2010;24:281-98.
35. Izbicki JR, Bloechle C, Broering DC, et al. Extended drainage versus resection in surgery for chronic pancreatitis. A prospective randomized trial comparing the longitudinal pancreaticojejunostomy combined with local pancreatic head excision with the pylorus-preserving pancreatoduodenectomy. Ann Surg. 1998;228:771-9.
36. Fleming WR, Williamson RCN. Role of total pancreatectomy in the treatment of patients with end-stage chronic pancreatitis. Br J Surg. 1995;82:1409-12.
37. Cahen DL, Gouma DJ, Laramee P, et al. Long-term outcomes of endoscopic versus surgical drainage of the pancreatic duct in patients with chronic pancreatitis. Gastroenterology. 2011;141:1690-5.
38. Rosewicz S, Wiedenmann B. Pancreatic carcinoma. Lancet. 1997;349(9050):485-9.
39. The Health Consequences of Smoking: A Report of the Surgeon General. Atlanta, GA: US Department of Health and Human Services. Department of Health and Human Services, Centers for Disease Control and Prevention, National Center for Chronic Disease Prevention and Health Promotion, Office on Smoking and Health; 2004.
40. Li D, Xie K, Wolff R, et al. Pancreatic cancer. Lancet. 2004; 363(9414):1049-57.
41. Klein AP, Brune KA, Petersen GM, et al. Prospective risk of pancreatic cancer in familial pancreatic cancer kindreds. Cancer Res. 2004;64(7): 2634-8.
42. Teich N. Pancreatic cancer. Cause and result of diabetes mellitus. Gastroenterology. 2008;134:344-5.
43. Lowenfels AB, Maisonneuve P, Cavallani G. Pancreatitis and the risk of cancer. N Engl J Med. 1993;328:1433-7.
44. Rivera J, Werner J, Adrie C, et al. Analysis of K-ras oncogene mutations in chronic pancreatitis with ductal hyperplasia. Surgery. 1997;121:42-9.
45. Hruban RH, Adsay NV, Albores-Saavedra J, et al. Pancreatic intraepithelial neoplasia: a new nomenclature and classification system for pancreatic duct lesions. Am J Surg Pathol. 2001;25:579-86.
46. Tsuchiya R, Tsunoda T, Yamaguchi T. Collective review of small carcinomas of the pancreas. Ann Surg. 1986;203:77-81.
47. Bockhorn M, Uzunoglu FG, Adham M, et al. Borderline resectable pancreatic cancer: A consensus statement by the International Study Group of Pancreatic Surgery (ISGPS). Surgery. 2014;155:977-88.
48. Mansfield SD, Sen G, Oppong K, et al. Comparison of multislice computed tomography and endoscopic ultrasonography with operative and histological findings in suspected pancreatic and periampullary malignancy. Br J Surg. 2008;95:1512-20.
49. Van der Gaag NA, Rauws EAJ, van Eijck CHJ, et al. Preoperative biliary drainage for cancer of the head of the pancreas. N Engl J Med. 2010;362:129-37.
50. Ausania F, Snowden CP, Prentis JM, et al. Effects of low cardiopulmonary reserve on pancreatic leak following pancreaticoduodenectomyBr J Surg. 2012;99(9):1290-4.

Additional references appear in the online version of this book.

57

Spleen

James ML Williamson, Robin CN Williamson

Key Points

- The spleen has important hematologic and especially immunologic functions. It should therefore not be removed without good cause. Splenectomized patients require immunization and may require life-long antimicrobial prophylaxis against encapsulated bacteria.
- Postsplenectomy sepsis is a rare but lethal disease, so splenectomized patients need urgent medical attention for all but the most trivial infections.
- The main indications for splenectomy are traumatic rupture and hypersplenism, in which splenomegaly is associated with low counts of red cells, platelets, and/or white cells in the peripheral blood.
- Splenectomy may be indicated for splenic involvement by lymphoma or other neoplasms, and it may be included as part of a gastric or pancreatic resection.
- There are potential alternatives to splenectomy in both the elective and emergency context.

INTRODUCTION

The spleen is a unique and fascinating organ that combines hematologic and immunologic functions. Hematologic function includes hemopoiesis and hemofiltration, which allows removal of older erythrocytes from the circulation. Immunologic function provides both innate and acquired immunity by producing antibodies and allowing T-cell maturation. The immunologic function is probably the more important in adult life, and awareness of this fact has led to an increased use of splenic preservation techniques. Organ removal for diagnostic purposes, radical cancer resection, or traumatic injury has been questioned in the light of improvements in radiologic imaging, pathologic assessment, and spleen-preserving techniques plus the expanding role of expectant management in abdominal trauma. Most elective splenectomies are now performed either to relieve the effects of hypersplenism or because the organ is infiltrated by a diffuse neoplastic process.

SURGICAL ANATOMY

Embryologic Development

The spleen develops in utero at day 12, when the splanchnic mesodermal plate forms from condensations of mesenchyme within the dorsal mesogastrium.[1] Rotation of the stomach carries it to the left of the midline and leads to the development of a retrogastric pouch of peritoneum, the lesser sac, or omental bursa. Incomplete mesodermal fusion is responsible for the persistence of accessory spleens or splenunculi; these are very common and can be found in approximately 15–20% of the population.[2,3] Markedly less common is polysplenia, in which the main bulk of the spleen is divided into two or more distinct entities; this condition is sometimes associated with situs inversus. Splenic agenesis is rare, but can occur either alone or in conjunction with congenital anomalies of the heart.

Anatomic Relationships

The spleen lies beneath the left cupola of the diaphragm against the 9th, 10th, and 11th ribs. It is covered by a fibrous capsule of connective tissue and is completely invested by peritoneum. Its posterolateral attachment to the left kidney (the lienorenal ligament) is relatively bloodless. By contrast, its anteromedial attachment to the stomach (via the gastrosplenic ligament) contains the short gastric vessels (or vasa brevia) plus the left gastroepiploic branches of the splenic artery and vein. The gastrosplenic ligament can be short and tight, so that there is a risk of injury to the greater curve of the stomach when ligating and dividing the vasa brevia. The other organ at potential risk of injury during splenectomy is the tail of pancreas, which lies deeply within the splenic hilum.

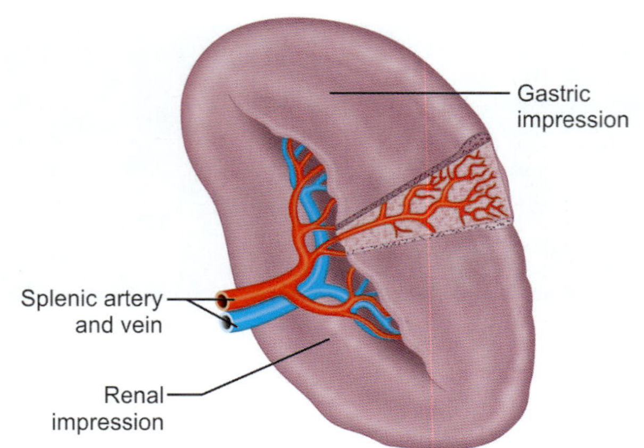

Fig. 57.1: Anatomy of the splenic artery. The vessel divides into its major branches before entering the substance of the spleen, and segmental end-arteries supply transverse sections of the organ.

The normal adult spleen weighs about 150 g, but it declines in size in old age. The organ has to be at least three times the normal size to become palpable in the left hypochondrium. An enlarged spleen can be confused with the left lobe of the liver or the left kidney; all three move on respiration. A splenic mass lies further laterally than the liver and may have a palpable notch. It can be differentiated from an enlarged left kidney because it is uniformly dull to percussion and cannot be felt in the loin.

Blood Supply

The splenic artery supplies the stomach, greater omentum, and left pancreas (body and tail) in addition to the spleen. If the splenic artery (and/or vein) is ligated alongside the body of the pancreas, the spleen will generally remain fully viable (and/or uncongested) provided that the short gastric and left gastroepiploic vessels are preserved. However, if the arterial supply to the spleen is critically compromised, part or all of the organ can undergo infarction leading to subsequent atrophy. The arterial supply to the spleen is segmental with division of the splenic artery into its terminal branches outside the organ. These vessels supply small transverse segments that have relatively little blood flow between them (Fig. 57.1). Between three and seven segments may be found, each with its own arterial supply and venous drainage. It is the presence of these segmental end arteries that makes partial splenectomy feasible. The blood entering the spleen is discharged into the red pulp and courses slowly along the splenic cords as the blood cells are squeezed through tiny pores into the venous sinuses.[4] There is therefore, a delayed microcirculation (open system) allowing time for splenic phagocytosis, but there can also be a more rapid transit of blood through the closed sinuses of the red pulp. The rapid-transit circulation takes approximately 1–2 minutes and the slow-transit circulation 30–60 minutes.

Blood leaves the spleen by segmental veins that unite to form the splenic vein. The splenic vein contributes up to 40% of the portal venous blood flow, and splenic vein thrombosis can lead to the development of gastric fundal varices (*see* Chapter 54, "Portal Hypertension"). The optimal management of splenic vein thrombosis, from acute pancreatitis for example, is not fully known; anticoagulation may play a role in allowing the vessel to recanalize in acutely symptomatic patients.[5,6]

Structure

The spleen consists of three functional compartments: the red pulp, white pulp, and marginal zone.[7] The whole organ is invested with a capsule of collagen from which trabecula pass deeply through the pulp and give rise to the supporting reticular framework. Most of the organ appears to be red pulp on naked-eye examination, with small islands of lymphoid aggregates constituting the white pulp.[1] The red pulp comprises large blood-filled cavities lined by endothelium containing splenic cords formed by a reticulum of fibroblasts and dendritic cells, which subsequently drain into sinuses. The white pulp is distributed along the central arteriole branching from the splenic artery; it comprises lymph follicles or malpighian bodies, which develop a germinal center after antigenic stimulation. T cells form a lymphoid sheath around this central arteriole (periarteriolar lymphoid sheath), and also surround B-cell follicles in a thin layer (Fig. 57.2).[1,7] This thin layer is comprised of a light central zone—the "germinal center" and area of B-cell selection—and a dark outer layer—the "mantle zone" containing dominantly proliferating small B-cell lymphocytes. The marginal zone, containing memory B cells, is the extreme periphery of the white pulp in direct contact with the perifollicular area.[7]

APPLIED PHYSIOLOGY

Normal Splenic Function

Normal splenic function is summarized in Table 57.1.

Hematologic Function

The human spleen plays a minor role in hemopoiesis, which is normally confined to the middle weeks of fetal life, but can be reactivated in childhood if the marrow

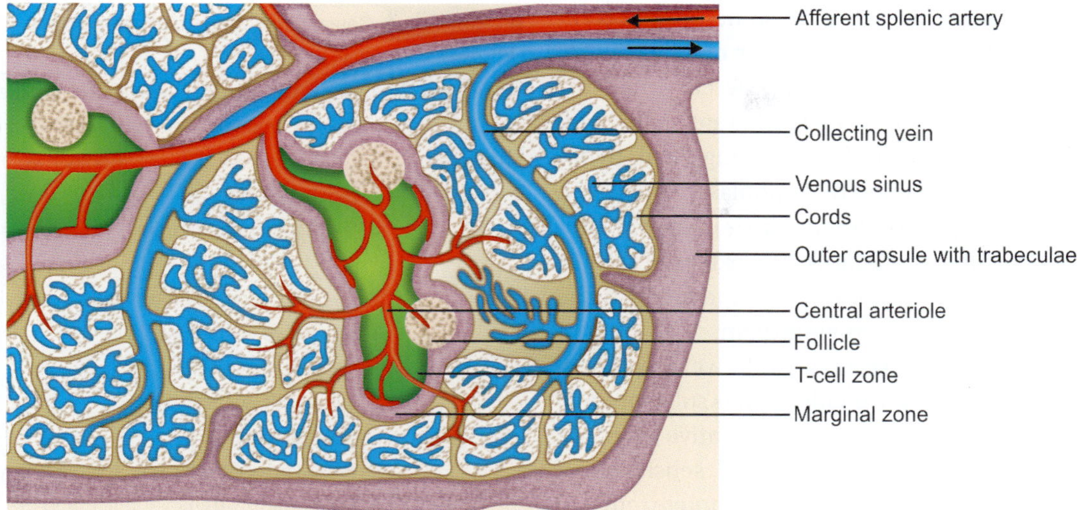

Fig. 57.2: Schematic representation of the spleen. The afferent splenic artery branches into central arterioles, which are sheathed by white pulp. These white pulp areas consist of the T-cell zone (periarteriolar lymphoid sheath), arterioles, and B-cell follicles. The arterioles end in cords in the red pulp, where the blood runs into venous sinuses that collect into the efferent splenic vein.

Table 57.1 Hematologic and immunologic functions of the spleen.

Hematologic	
Hemapoiesis	Normal during fetal life
	Compensatory in childhood
	Abnormal in adult (myeloid metaplasia)
Red cell maturation	Molding of reticulocytes
	Removal of intracellular inclusions
Red cell destruction	Effete and damaged cells
Storage	Iron, platelets, factor VIII (blood)
Filtration of particles	Debris, bacteria
Immunologic	
Humoral immunity	Antibody production
Cell-mediated immunity	T-cell maturation
Opsonin synthesis	Tuftsin
	Factor P
Lymphopoiesis	Suppressor T cells
	Memory B cells
Leukocyte storage	T and B cells

capacity is exceeded. Splenic hemopoiesis in adults is only seen in myeloproliferative disorders and leads to the production of abnormal red cell forms. The spleen makes a unique contribution to the maturation of red cells, molding the reticulocytes into biconcave discs and removing surface pits and nuclear fragments. It also extracts senescent and abnormal cells from the circulating blood via phagocytosis and is involved in recycling of iron.[1,6] It is estimated that each circulating red blood cell traverses the spleen 1000 times per day. Although the human spleen does not possess the reservoir capacity for blood that is seen in some other mammalian species, it is an important storage site for iron and platelets.[1,7]

Immunologic Function

Being the largest lymphoid organ in the body, the spleen makes an important contribution to both humoral and cell-mediated immunity.[8] Antigens are filtered by the dendritic cells in the white pulp and are presented to immunocompetent cells in the germinal centers of the follicles. Immunoglobulins, notably IgM, are produced by plasma cells, and the germinal centers become hyperplastic. The spleen produces some lymphocyte subsets, but most of the white cells it contains derive from the bone marrow. Circulating monocytes are converted into fixed macrophages within the red pulp, and these cells account for the powerful phagocytic activity of the spleen. Phagocytosis is enhanced by the splenic production of the opsonins, tuftsin, and factor P (properdin). Poorly opsonized bacteria, especially some encapsulated bacteria (e.g. *Streptococcus pneumoniae*), can only be cleared in the spleen.[6]

HYPOSPLENISM AND ASPLENIA

Causes

Asplenia (absence of the spleen) is generally the result of surgical resection. Congenital asplenia is rare and usually associated with other severe anomalies of the cardiac, gastrointestinal, and genitourinary systems. Hyposplenism should be regarded as an acquired condition, potentially associated with several diseases and sometimes accompanied by reduction in spleen size.[6] Four main causes of acquired hyposplenism should be considered: celiac disease, sickle cell disease, bone marrow transplant (with graft-versus-host disease), and HIV. Congenital hyposplenism may be accompanied by hypoplastic anemia in Fanconi's syndrome. Overwhelming sepsis is an ever-present threat among surviving infants. The extent of splenic malfunction can be determined by isotope scans using sulfur colloid labeled with technetium-99m.

In 1979, some 35,000 patients underwent splenectomy in the United States;[9] the incidence has subsequently fallen, primarily thanks to a more conservative management of traumatic injuries and increased sensitivity of radiologic diagnosis.[10] Attempts to avoid complete removal of the spleen may still be associated with some loss of function, but ligation of segmental arteries with partial splenectomy may allow some compensatory hypertrophy of the remnant and recovery of normal splenic function.

Acquired hyposplenism is seen in three quarters of patients with untreated celiac disease (gluten enteropathy). The spleen may be overloaded with circulating immune complexes that result from increased absorption of dietary antigens through the atrophic jejunal mucosa. Splenic function can improve with the institution of a gluten-free diet. Other diseases of the intestinal mucosa that can lead to hyposplenism are listed in Table 57.2. Patients with sickle cell disease can develop progressive hyposplenism following repeated episodes of segmental infarction.[6] Functional hyposplenism occurs in some 15–40% of patients with allogenic bone marrow transplantation; patients with associated reduction of splenic size and chronic graft-versus-host disease should receive long-term antibiotic prophylaxis.[11,12] Functional hyposplenism has a prevalence of 36% in patients who are HIV positive;[13] in addition the virus can decrease the activity of tuftsin, while depletion of IgM memory B cells has been reported in patients with a low CD4 T-cell count (<300 cells per μL).[14,15] Thus, the incidence of pneumococcal disease is >100 times greater in the HIV-positive population. Antiretroviral therapy may restore the pool of IgM memory B cells and decrease the incidence of pneumococcal infection.[15]

Table 57.2 Causes and effects of hyposplenism.

Causes	
Congenital	Asplenia (usually associated with other anomalies)
	Splenic hypoplasia in Fanconi's syndrome
Acquired	Celiac disease
	Sickle cell disease
	Dermatitis herpetiformis
	HIV
	Systemic lupus erythematosus
	Ulcerative colitis
	Crohn's disease
	Lymphangiectasia
Iatrogenic	Splenectomy
	Partial splenectomy and splenic artery ligation
	Bone marrow transplantation and graft-versus-host disease
Effects	
Red cell abnormalities	Of shape (e.g. target cells)
	Of surface (e.g. craters and pits)
	Cytoplasmic inclusions (e.g. Howell–Jolly bodies)
Platelet abnormalities	Increased number (thrombocytosis)
	Abnormal function (thrombocytopathia)
White cell abnormalities	Increased number (leukocytosis)
	Abnormal function (postsplenectomy sepsis)

Effects

Hematologic

The hematologic effects of hyposplenism are characterized by the appearance of defective red cells that would normally be eliminated from the peripheral blood. Target cells and burr cells are seen, together with surface craters and pits and a variety of red cell inclusions: Howell-Jolly bodies (nuclear remnants), Heinz bodies (denatured hemoglobin), and Pappenheimer bodies (iron granules). Counting the proportion of pitted red cells allows an assessment of residual splenic function.[16] Thrombocytosis, caused by increased production of platelets rather than their prolonged survival, usually develops within 1 week of splenectomy and may persist for years. Leukocytosis results from a transient rise in neutrophils and a sustained rise in lymphocytes and eosinophils.

Immunologic

The immunologic effects of hyposplenism are greatest in neonates. After splenectomy, IgM levels remain low for up to 4 years, whereas IgA and IgG levels usually return to normal. Low plasma tuftsin levels impair neutrophil phagocytosis, while low factor P levels interfere with complement activation. There is also a loss of helper T-cell function. The net result is a failure to opsonize and then phagocytose encapsulated bacteria, leading to an increased risk of postsplenectomy sepsis. Tuftsin deficiency may be the critical factor.[16]

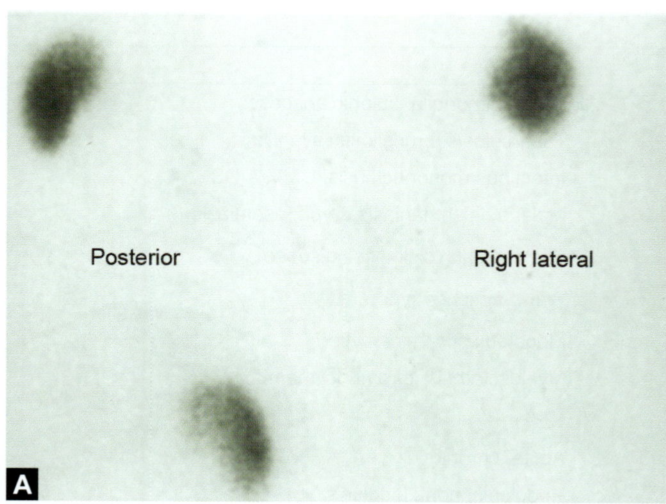

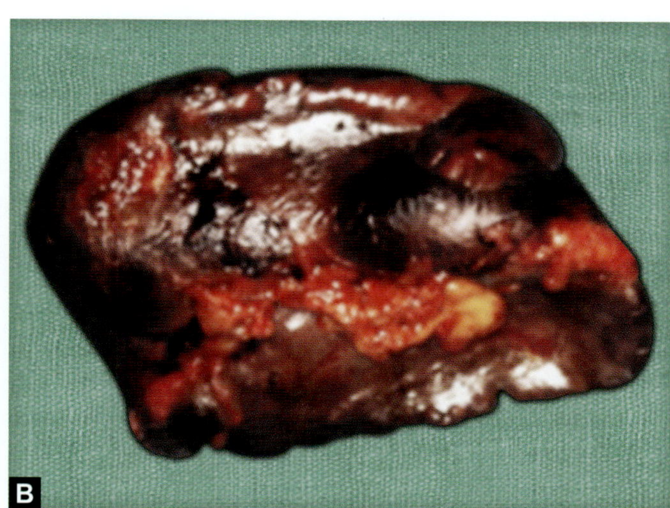

Figs. 57.3A and B: Splenectomy for idiopathic thrombocytopenic purpura in a 30-year-old man. (A) Platelet kinetic studies show accumulation of indium-labeled platelets on splenic scintigrams. (B) The resected spleen is of normal size.

Table 57.3 Major causes and effects of hypersplenism.

Causes	
Primary splenomegaly	*Secondary splenomegaly*
Parasitic infestations (e.g. malaria, kala-azar)	Portal hypertension (generalized or left-sided)
Lymphoma (Hodgkin's and non-Hodgkin's)	
Leukemia (chronic lymphatic, hairy cell)	
Hematologic disease (e.g. spherocytosis)	
Miscellaneous causes (e.g. Felty's syndrome, Gaucher's disease)	
Effects	
Anemia	
Leukopenia	
Thrombocytopenia	
Pancytopenia	

Overwhelming Postsplenectomy Infection

The term overwhelming postsplenectomy infection (OPSI) defines fulminating sepsis, meningitis, or pneumonia triggered mainly by *S. pneumoniae* (50–90% of cases), *Neisseria meningitidis,* and *Haemophilus influenzae* type b in hyposplenic patients.[17] The infection rate in splenectomized patients is >50 times that of the general population.[6] Although the infection risk is greatest in the first few years after splenectomy, the risk is permanent; cases of OPSI have been documented some 20–40 years after splenectomy.[6] Overwhelming postsplenectomy infection is a medical emergency that requires prompt diagnosis and treatment to reduce the mortality rate of 50–70%.[18]

HYPERSPLENISM

Causes

Hypersplenism is strictly defined as the combination of splenomegaly and decreased numbers of circulating blood cells, whether red blood cells, leukocytes, or platelets. Although the spleen tends to enlarge as a consequence of its excessive work in destroying abnormal cells, this is not invariable; for example, in immune (idiopathic) thrombocytopenic purpura (ITP) the spleen is generally of normal size (Figs. 57.3A and B). Any type of chronic splenomegaly can lead to hypersplenism, whether primary in nature (i.e. intrinsic splenic disease) or secondary to portal hypertension causing splenic congestion (Table 57.3).

Effects

Anemia, leukopenia, and thrombocytopenia occur either singly or in a combined form as pancytopenia. The reduced cell count results first from pooling in the enlarged spleen; up to 50% of the red cells and up to 90% of the platelets, granulocytes and lymphocytes can be sequestered in a massive spleen. If the bone marrow can compensate by increased cell synthesis the peripheral blood count remains normal, but myeloproliferative disease leads to cytopenias. There is also an element of increased cell destruction in many types of hypersplenism. Thus, the abnormal red cells of hereditary spherocytosis are preferentially destroyed by the spleen, whereas in other conditions immune mechanisms are responsible: antiplatelet antibodies in ITP, antired cell antibodies in certain

Table 57.4 Causes of primary splenomegaly.

	Type of cause	*Examples*
Infections and infestations	Bacteremia	SBE, salmonella, splenic abscess
	Specific bacterial	Tuberculosis, brucellosis, syphilis
	Viral	Infectious mononucleosis, CMV, AIDS
	Protozoal	Malaria, leishmaniasis, trypanosomiasis
Hematologic	Congenital hemolytic	Thalassemia, sickle cell disease
	Acquired hemolytic	Warm-antibody type
	Secondary to chronic anemia	Megaloblastic, microcytic
	Myeloproliferative disease	Myelosclerosis, thrombocythemia
	Polycythemia vera	
Neoplastic	Leukemias	Acute, chronic
	Lymphomas	Hodgkin's, non-Hodgkin's
	Myelomatosis	
	Rare	Primary sarcoma, secondary carcinoma, hemangioma
Cystic	Congenital	Solitary cyst, polycystic disease
	Traumatic	Delayed splenic rupture
	Parasitic	Hydatid
Miscellaneous	Storage disease	Gaucher's disease, histiocytosis X
	Amyloidosis	
	Autoimmune	Rheumatoid arthritis, SLE
	Granulomatous	Sarcoidosis

(CMV: Cytomegalovirus; SBE: Subacute bacterial endocarditis; SLE: Systemic lupus erythematosus).

acquired hemolytic anemias and an antinuclear factor in Felty's syndrome (i.e. splenomegaly in rheumatoid arthritis). Abnormal cells or cells trapped in the spleen for a prolonged period become susceptible to phagocytosis.

SPLENOMEGALY

Causes

Primary splenomegaly results from a wide variety of different conditions (Table 57.4) and is termed massive splenomegaly when splenic weight exceeds 1,500 g.[19] Transient enlargement is a feature of several infections, especially viral. Human immunodeficiency virus (HIV) infection is an increasingly common cause secondary to repeated opportunistic infection or the development of lymphoma; thrombocytopenia is seen in 5–15% of HIV-positive patients irrespective of their clinical status.[20] Chronic infections such as tuberculosis can lead to persistent enlargement of the spleen. Worldwide, malaria and kala-azar (leishmaniasis) are two of the commoner causes of splenomegaly. In endemic areas, patients can develop a massive spleen and hypersplenism without evidence of active malaria but with raised antibody titers (tropical splenomegaly). The splenomegaly of schistosomiasis can be aggravated by liver involvement and portal hypertension.

An enlarged spleen can accompany many different types of anemia: the megaloblastic anemia of vitamin B_{12} or folate deficiency, congenital hypoplastic anemia in children, the sideroblastic anemia that can precede frank leukemia and (less often) the microcytic anemia of iron deficiency anemia. An enlarged spleen is commonly seen in hemolytic anemias, both congenital and acquired, and in the myeloid metaplasia that accompanies myelosclerosis.

Marrow replacement in leukemia, myeloma, or lymphoma also leads to splenomegaly, but in both Hodgkin's and non-Hodgkin's lymphoma there may be direct tumor involvement of the spleen.[19,21] Sometimes, unexplained splenomegaly is the first sign of an occult lymphoma that might not become manifest for months or years. Secondary splenomegaly accompanies portal hypertension, which may be either generalized or limited to the left side of the portal venous tree (Table 57.5). Left-sided (sinistral)

Table 57.5 Causes of splenomegaly secondary to portal hypertension.

Generalized portal hypertension	*Left-sided portal hypertension*
Hepatic	*Compression or occlusion of the splenic vein*
Alcoholic cirrhosis	
Posthepatic cirrhosis	
Primary or secondary biliary cirrhosis	Acute pancreatitis
Hemochromatosis	Chronic pancreatitis
Prehepatic (portal vein occlusion)	Pancreatic pseudocyst
Congenital (atresia, malformation)	Carcinoma of pancreas
Acquired (infection, malignant invasion)	Spontaneous
Posthepatic	
Budd-Chiari syndrome	
Congestive cardiac failure	

hypertension results from compression or occlusion of the splenic vein. Chronic pancreatitis with or without pseudocyst formation and tumors of the body and tail of pancreas are the commonest causes of splenic vein thrombosis.[5]

Presentation and Investigation

Splenomegaly may be detected incidentally in a patient without any symptoms, e.g. in chronic malaria, rheumatoid arthritis, or sarcoidosis. A massive spleen causes discomfort in the left hypochondrium, but pleuritic pain and a pleural rub indicate capsular inflammation from splenic infarction. Infarction is commonest in sickle cell disease, chronic myeloid leukemia, and myelofibrosis. An enlarged spleen can usually be differentiated from a gastric, pancreatic, colonic, or renal mass by careful palpation. There may be concomitant hepatomegaly, lymphadenopathy, anemia, purpura (e.g. in blood dyscrasias), ascites, and stigmata of chronic liver disease (e.g. in cirrhosis). Splenomegaly is often associated with an increased plasma volume, causing dilutional anemia.[21]

Most primary splenomegalies are either infective or neoplastic in origin. Malarial parasites may be seen in a peripheral blood film and Leishman-Donovan bodies in a marrow smear. Hematologic disease is investigated by a full blood count and bone marrow aspiration, plus biopsy of any enlarged lymph node. Infectious mononucleosis (glandular fever) causes atypical lymphocytes in the peripheral blood, and serologic tests are positive (Paul-Bunnell, Epstein-Barr virus titers). Tuberculosis may be manifest on chest radiography.

Scanning (ultrasound, CT, MRI) will confirm the splenic nature of the mass and shows its size and consistency

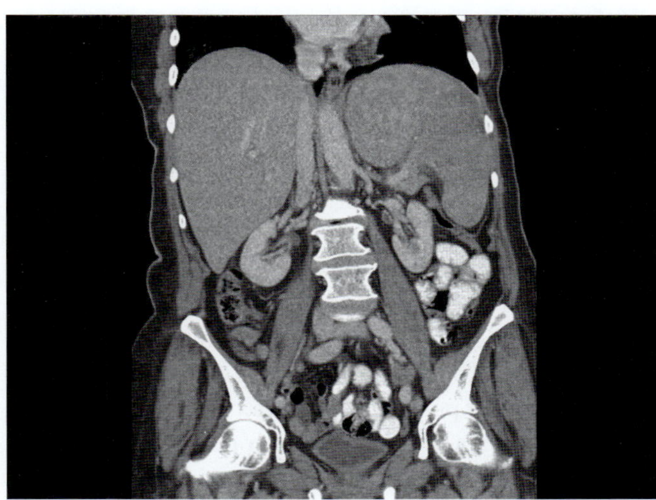

Fig. 57.4: Massive splenomegaly (with associated perihilar lymphadenopathy) in an 80-year-old with B-cell lymphoma. Note heterogenous areas and areas of low density.

(solid or cystic) (Fig. 57.4). CT (with or without intravenous contrast) is currently the most useful modality and plays a crucial role in the management of splenic trauma.[22] CT can also detect the presence of accessory spleens, although it may not be as accurate as diagnostic laparoscopy.[23] Angiography helps to distinguish between compression and occlusion of the splenic vein. Isotope scanning using sulfur colloid labeled with technetium-99m gives some indication of splenic size and vascularity; filling defects suggest splenic infarction. Red cell survival is measured by labeling the patient's cells with chromium-51 and observing both the disappearance of radioactivity from the blood and its accumulation within the spleen. Similar techniques using indium-111 are available for investigating thrombocytopenia (*see* Fig. 57.3). Splenic biopsies are gaining popularity for tissue diagnosis as an alternative to splenectomy. Biopsy should be performed under radiological guidance with an 18-gauge needle. Average sensitivity is 87% and complication rate 2.2% (bleeding and pain), in line with both renal and hepatic biopsy.[24]

INDICATIONS FOR SPLENECTOMY (TABLE 57.6)

Ruptured Spleen

The spleen is the organ most commonly injured in blunt abdominal trauma, usually following road traffic accidents. Commonly a blow or crushing injury to the left lower rib cage or upper abdomen results in splenic laceration; alternative mechanisms include a fall onto a protruding object (e.g. a bicycle handlebar). The incidence of splenic injury is between 0.17% and 1.3% of all traumatic injuries presenting to hospital.[25,26] It is frequently a part of multiple trauma and often associated with fractured ribs and damage to other abdominal viscera.[26] Penetrating injuries are much less common except in military situations or in areas of endemic urban violence. If the spleen is enlarged (e.g. in malaria or lymphoma), it may rupture following a relatively trivial injury. Spontaneous rupture can occasionally complicate the splenic enlargement of infectious mononucleosis, portal hypertension, histiocytic medullary reticulosis or polycythemia vera.

Capsular tears of the spleen can occur during operations such as hiatal hernia repair, whether open or laparoscopic, or during mobilization of the splenic flexure during colonic resection. They usually result when an omental adhesion is pulled off the surface of the organ or from the overenthusiastic use of a retractor. Ruptured spleen has also been reported as a complication of colonoscopy, either via direct trauma or excessive traction on the splenocolic ligament; the reported incidence is 0.00005–0.017%.[27] The bleeding from a capsular tear can be very persistent, but the temptation to remove the spleen for a simple capsular tear should be resisted (*see* below for alternatives to splenectomy).

Classically, a ruptured spleen leads to hemoperitoneum and hypotensive shock, but a delayed presentation hours or even weeks later is not particularly uncommon. The patient develops either a subcapsular hematoma (Fig. 57.5) or (at a later stage) a post-traumatic pseudocyst, which can secondarily rupture into the peritoneal cavity. There is an increasing tendency to manage splenic trauma expectantly, especially in patients without other serious abdominal injuries who are hemodynamically stable. Approximately two thirds of patients with splenic injuries can be treated without operation, with success rates of 90%.[28] Vigilant clinical observation and serial scans are required, with operation reserved for unstable patients or failure of conservative management. Embolization therapy for splenic lacerations is increasingly used to decrease the

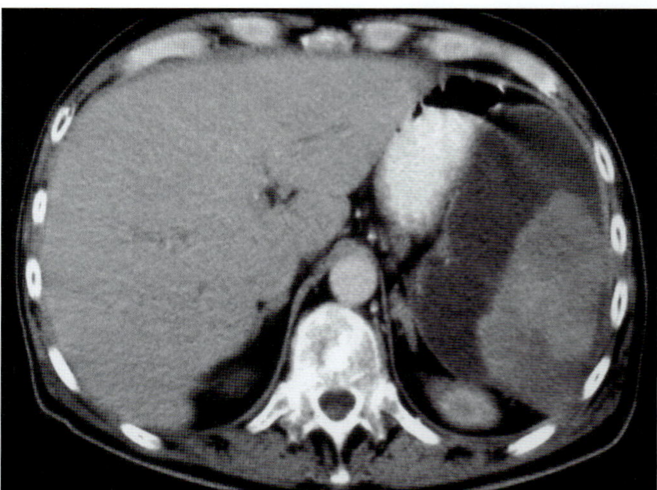

Fig. 57.5: CT showing large perisplenic hematoma in a young man involved in a road traffic accident. Conservative management proved successful.

Table 57.6 Indications for splenectomy.

Traumatic rupture	*With other viscera*
Immediate Iatrogenic Delayed Spontaneous	Gastrectomy for cancer Distal pancreatectomy *Secondary splenomegaly* Bleeding varices with splenic vein thrombosis Conventional splenorenal shunt
Cytopenias with or without pain	*Infections*
Hemolytic anemias (congenital or acquired) Immune thrombocytopenic purpura Neutropenia (Felty's syndrome, hairy cell leukemia) Tropical splenomegaly (parasitic) Myelosclerosis (sometimes)	Tuberculosis Hydatid cyst Splenic abscess
Neoplastic	*Diagnosis and/or staging*
Lymphomas Chronic leukemias Massive hemangioma (rare) Secondary carcinoma (rare)	Hodgkin's disease Unexplained splenomegaly *Miscellaneous* Splenic artery aneurysm Nonparasitic splenic cyst Torsion of a wandering spleen

morbidity and mortality rates associated with emergency splenectomy.[29] The management of a ruptured spleen is considered fully in Chapter 40, "Abdominal, Urologic and Perineal Injuries".

Hypersplenism

The treatment of hypersplenism varies widely according to the cause, and nonoperative measures are often effective. For example, in lymphoma the spleen diminishes in size with the appropriate chemotherapy. Corticosteroids often induce a remission in autoimmune hemolytic anemia and ITP, although splenectomy is indicated for those who do not respond or relapse. In myeloproliferative disorders such as myelosclerosis, it is important to determine whether there is sufficient hematopoietic reserve in the bone marrow to cope after removal of the spleen; however, the outcome is not fully predictable.[30] Recurrent cycles of infarction and pain tend to favor splenectomy in this condition, as does the development of portal hypertension and variceal hemorrhage.

The most common hematologic diseases requiring splenectomy are hereditary spherocytosis and ITP (*see* below).[31] Hereditary elliptocytosis is seldom of much clinical importance, while progressive splenic infarction usually obviates the need for splenectomy in sickle cell disease. In thalassemia major, splenectomy is occasionally indicated for a massive spleen causing pain or for recurrent hemolysis requiring repeated blood transfusion. Thrombotic thrombocytopenic purpura is a rare and potentially lethal disease in which the use of plasmapheresis, corticosteroids, and antiplatelet drugs may avoid or at least delay the necessity to remove the spleen. Splenectomy can improve the anemia of pyruvate kinase deficiency, a rare congenital defect of red cells.

During splenectomy for hypersplenism, a search should be made for splenunculi; if found they should be removed to prevent late recurrence of symptoms and the occasional need for reoperation.[32]

Hereditary Spherocytosis

Hereditary spherocytosis is the commonest type of congenital hemolytic anemia and is inherited as an autosomal dominant disorder. An abnormality of the red cell membrane leads to formation of small round cells, which are relatively rigid and therefore at increased risk of disruption during their passage through the channels in the splenic pulp. These cells also show increased osmotic fragility. Patients present during childhood or adult life with mild or moderate anemia, prehepatic jaundice, and splenomegaly. Pigment gallstones have usually formed by the time the patient reaches adult life, and chronic leg ulcers are an occasional complication. Investigations reveal anemia (generally normocytic), 10–20% reticulocytosis, increased (unconjugated) serum bilirubin levels, and increased hemolysis of cells on exposure to saline. Splenectomy is nearly always curative.[2] It should be performed after the age of 5 years (to reduce the risk of infection), but before complications develop such as gallstones or hypoplastic crises leading to profound anemia and severe constitutional symptoms.[31]

Immune Thrombocytopenic Purpura

Immune thrombocytopenic purpura is characterized by a low platelet count, reduced platelet lifespan and plentiful megakaryocytes in the bone marrow. The spleen is seldom enlarged. Immune thrombocytopenic purpura can be either idiopathic or secondary to drug treatment, viral infection (including AIDS), systemic lupus erythematosus or lymphoma. There may be:

- An acute onset (especially in children) with ecchymosis and bleeding
- An insidious onset (especially in adults), with an increased tendency to bruise and menorrhagia

Treatment is required if the platelet count falls below 50×10^9/L. Prednisolone (60 mg/day) improves the platelet count and averts the risk of hemorrhage in 75% of patients. Splenectomy is indicated for the remaining 25% and for those who relapse or develop the chronic form of the disease. Once the splenic vessels have been ligated at operation, platelets may be transfused to improve hemostasis.

Splenectomy produces a sustained remission in about 80% of patients with ITP, especially those with less severe forms of the disease and those who responded initially to corticosteroids.[2] The platelet count increases within 24 hours of operation and reaches a peak at 1–2 weeks; if it remains high at 1–2 months, the patient is likely to be cured. Patients with secondary ITP are less likely to respond to splenectomy and may require prolonged corticosteroids or immunosuppressive therapy.[31] Splenectomy appears to be safe for patients who are HIV positive, and it may ameliorate the thrombocytopenia.[20]

Lymphoma and other Neoplasms

The requirement for splenectomy for lymphoma has diminished with improved radiological accuracy and tissue biopsy (whether lymph-node or splenic). Its diagnostic

Table 57.7 Clinical staging and treatment outline in Hodgkin's disease.

Clinical stage		*Treatment*
I	Single lymph node group or extranodal site	Megavoltage radiotherapy
II	Two or more lymph node groups or lymph node group(s) plus extranodal site on the same side of the diaphragm	Radiotherapy ± chemotherapy
III	Lymph node groups on both sides of the diaphragm with or without localized extranodal or splenic disease	Wide-field radiotherapy ± chemotherapy
IV	Diffuse involvement of extranodal organs (e.g. liver, spleen, lung, marrow, skin, bone)	Multiagent chemotherapy
A	Denotes no constitutional symptoms (e.g. IIA, IIIA)	
B	Denotes constitutional symptoms	

role should be balanced against the risk of postsplenectomy sepsis. Splenectomy may be indicated in the following situations:[21,33]

- *Diagnostic*: To diagnose unexplained splenomegaly in the absence of an enlarged lymph node for biopsy or to differentiate between lymphoma and splenic marginal zone lymphoma.
- *Symptomatic*: To relieve pain or pressure symptoms caused by a massive spleen.
- *Hypersplenism*: Lymphoma is a common cause of splenomegaly requiring splenectomy.
- *Staging*: Use of staging laparotomy for Hodgkin's disease has declined sharply since the advent of CT (*see* below).

Hodgkin's Disease

Hodgkin's disease typically presents with unilateral cervical lymphadenopathy in middle-aged men, but axillary, mediastinal, or inguinal nodes may be enlarged either at first or later. Constitutional symptoms (so-called "B" symptoms) may develop early or late and include fever, malaise, anorexia, pruritus, and weight loss. The disease progresses to involve many different organs of the body, including the liver, spleen, bone marrow, pleura, meninges, skin, and genitourinary tract. The diagnosis is usually obtained by excisional biopsy of an enlarged node providing an adequate specimen to allow assessment of the nodal architecture as well as the cell types. The clinical stages of Hodgkin's disease are shown in Table 57.7 and each stage is subdivided into A and B according to the absence or presence of constitutional symptoms. Routine assessment includes a detailed physical examination, chest radiography, urinalysis, blood count, marrow aspiration, and CT of the chest and abdomen; lymphangiography is seldom performed nowadays. Rarely nowadays, staging laparotomy in selected patients with early (stage I or II) disease allows splenectomy, liver biopsy and lymph-node sampling and can lead revision of the clinical staging (to stage III or IV); the technique is described below (*see* Table 57.7).

Non-Hodgkin's Lymphoma

Non-Hodgkin's lymphoma comprises a diverse group of malignant tumors of the immune system. Like Hodgkin's disease, it tends to present with lymphadenopathy, but the first manifestation may be extranodal. Organs commonly involved are the skin, central nervous system, gastrointestinal tract, and tracheobronchial tree. Constitutional symptoms can again develop with progressive disease, especially in patients with histiocytic disease. There is a bewildering variety of classifications for non-Hodgkin's lymphomas, most of which present with stage III or IV disease. Chemotherapy is the mainstay of treatment, with little role for staging laparotomy. Irradiation is confined to a minority of patients with localized nodal disease or selected extranodal sites (bone and mediastinum).

Leukemia

Patients who have certain types of leukemia may be suitable for splenectomy, especially in the presence of pain and hypersplenism. The value of splenectomy in chronic myeloid leukemia is unclear unless there is recurrent painful infarction or troublesome cytopenia. It is seldom required in chronic lymphatic leukemia unless chemotherapy is contraindicated because of a low white cell count. Splenectomy used to be a popular treatment for hairy cell leukemia, but its role has declined since the advent of α-interferon therapy. However, many affected patients have hypersplenism, and in these patients splenectomy provides useful remission.

Primary Tumors

Many different types of primary tumor have been reported in the spleen, both benign and malignant, but all are rare.[21,34] Benign tumors include hemangioma, lymphangioma and fibroma. Intrinsic malignancies may be primary (lymphoma, sarcoma) or secondary (carcinoma, melanoma).

Splenectomy Combined with Other Visceral Resections

Splenectomy remains a part of the conventional distal pancreatectomy procedure, which is accomplished with ligation of the splenic artery and vein close to the midline. This procedure is appropriate for carcinoma of the body and tail of pancreas and for most cases of chronic pancreatitis, especially those complicated by pseudocyst or splenic vein thrombosis. With a relatively normal pancreas, it is often possible to dissect the pancreas away from the splenic artery and vein, dividing the numerous vascular tributaries and preserving the spleen.[5] Such a procedure may be particularly appropriate when resecting a small neuroendocrine tumor (*see* Chapter 56, "Pancreas"). All patients scheduled for distal pancreatectomy should receive prophylactic immunization against encapsulated bacteria in case splenectomy is required.

Splenectomy as a Part of Portal Decompression

If surgical decompression of the portal vein is required for bleeding gastroesophageal varices, splenectomy may not necessarily be indicated even if there is hypersplenism. In practice, the hypersplenism associated with cirrhosis is seldom very severe. Secondary splenomegaly is likely to recede and cytopenia to improve if a successful portasystemic shunt is achieved.

Splenectomy is an integral part of a conventional lienorenal shunt procedure, but in a distal splenorenal (Warren) shunt procedure the spleen is left in situ to act as a conduit for blood draining from the gastric veins (*see* Chapter 54, "Portal Hypertension"). Segmental portal hypertension secondary to splenic vein thrombosis is effectively managed by splenectomy, as is the occasional case of generalized portal hypertension complicated by a hyperdynamic splenic circulation and massive splenomegaly. Lastly, splenectomy is a frequent concomitant of gastric devascularization procedures for bleeding varices.

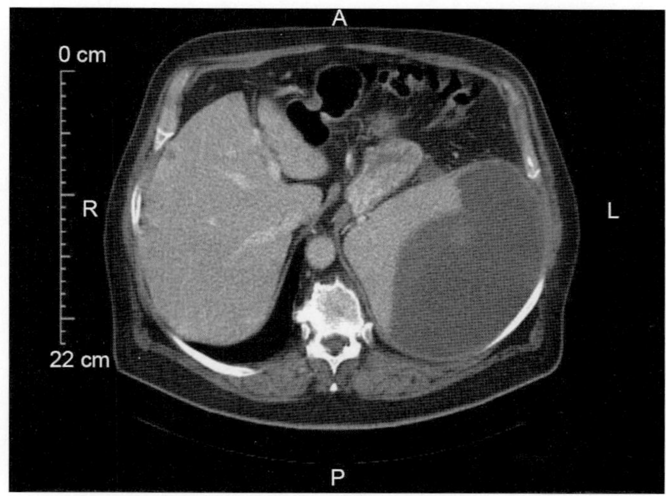

Fig. 57.6: CT showing a massive 20-cm simple cyst in a patient with left upper quadrant pain.

Other Indications for Splenectomy

Splenic Abscess

Splenic abscess is rare, but potentially lethal. Generally the infection is blood-borne, but it can follow delayed splenic rupture or an infected pseudocyst in the pancreatic tail. In systemic sepsis there are likely to be abscesses elsewhere in the body; some of these patients are intravenous drug abusers. There is hectic fever and leukocytosis. Plain abdominal radiography may show gas in the spleen, and ultrasonography or CT can also be diagnostic. High-dose antibiotic therapy should be started immediately and should be modified according to the results of blood cultures.[35] Gram-positive cocci are often isolated, but many other organisms have been reported. Urgent splenectomy is usually required for a localized abscess of the spleen, although percutaneous drainage may be safer in the critically ill patient.[35]

Splenic Cysts

As with splenic abscesses, splenic cysts are also very uncommon. They may be congenital, either in isolation or associated with polycystic disease involving the liver and kidneys. Congenital cysts are dermoid, endothelial, or epidermoid (epithelial) in origin (Figs. 57.6 and 57.7). Pseudocysts arise from infarction, either spontaneously or following embolization or ligation of the splenic artery, and from delayed rupture of the spleen. Echinococcal (hydatid) cysts may be associated with peripheral eosinophilia, calcification in the wall, positive serologic tests

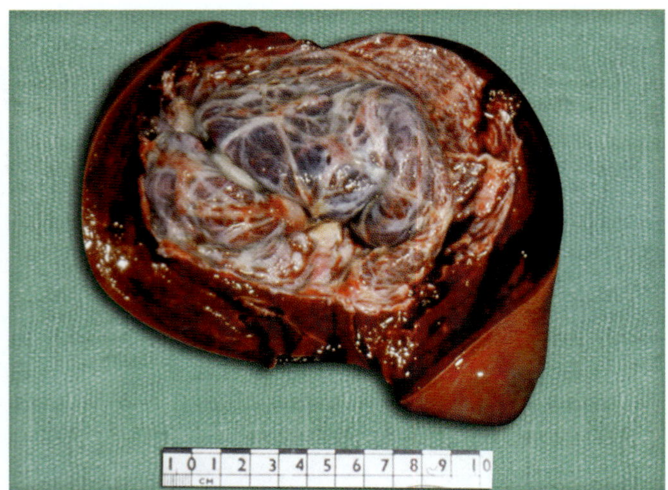

Fig. 57.7: Epidermoid (epithelial) cyst of the spleen. The cut surface of a splenic cyst showing the squamous epithelium of the cyst and its trabecular pattern.

and evidence of hydatid disease in the liver or elsewhere in the body. Calcification can also occur in congenital splenic cysts. Most symptomatic splenic cysts require splenectomy, but local excision or marsupialization may suffice for simple (congenital) cysts provided that neoplasia and hydatid disease can be firmly excluded.[34]

Splenic Artery Aneurysm

The splenic artery is the commonest visceral artery to undergo aneurysmal dilatation, with an incidence of up to 0.8%[36] (*see* Chapter 82, "Aneurysmal Disease"). There is an increased risk of rupture for aneurysms >2 cm in diameter, with associated mortality rates of 10–40% (and up to 75% in pregnancy).[37] There has been a move toward endoluminal treatment, in the form of embolization or stent grafts, but operative ligation, via an open or laparoscopic approach, can be employed, especially in the emergency setting. There are three distinct syndromes:

1. Young women who have congenital aneurysms may sustain a rupture during pregnancy and therefore require a prophylactic operation—generally the aneurysm affects the distal vessel and is best treated by splenectomy.
2. Elderly patients who have calcified atherosclerotic aneurysms and no symptoms (who can be left alone) or who develop splenic vein thrombosis and portal hypertension as a result of aneurysmal compression (for whom splenectomy is indicated).
3. Development of a false aneurysm of the splenic artery as a result of chronic pancreatitis, especially in the presence of a pseudocyst—treatment options include distal pancreatectomy with splenectomy or transcatheter embolization in the presence of active bleeding.

Wandering Spleen

This rare condition is largely confined to women. The mass may descend into the pelvis, and the long pedicle is liable to undergo torsion.[37] Ectopic and accessory spleens can be localized by radionuclide scans.

SPLENECTOMY

Preoperative Preparation

The principles are to correct anemia and coagulation deficiencies, treat any infection and immunize the patient against encapsulated bacteria before undertaking an elective splenectomy. The management priority for a patient with ruptured spleen is to restore the circulating blood volume. Thereafter management depends upon the grade of rupture and the experience of the operating surgeon; while splenectomy is the simplest definitive management of traumatic injuries, spleen-preserving measures can be employed in certain situations (*see* below).[23] In thrombocytopenia, corticosteroids or immunoglobulin therapy may help to improve the platelet count preoperatively; platelet transfusions should be delayed intraoperatively until after ligation of the splenic artery. All patients should be immunized against pneumococcus, meningococcus, and *H. influenzae* type B, 2–4 weeks in advance of an elective splenectomy.

Techniques

Elective "Open" Splenectomy

An upper midline or left subcostal laparotomy incision is appropriate, or rarely, a thoracoabdominal approach in massive splenomegaly. Ligation of the splenic artery alongside the body of pancreas reduces the flow of blood to an enormous spleen with or without intra-arterial injection of 1 mL 1:10,000 epinephrine (adrenaline) immediately beforehand.[38] Previous episodes of splenic infarction may give rise to extensive vascular adhesions to the diaphragm, and these need careful separation.

The spleen is mobilized by dividing the posterior leaf of the lienorenal ligament. The short gastric vessels are generally ligated and divided before dealing first with the

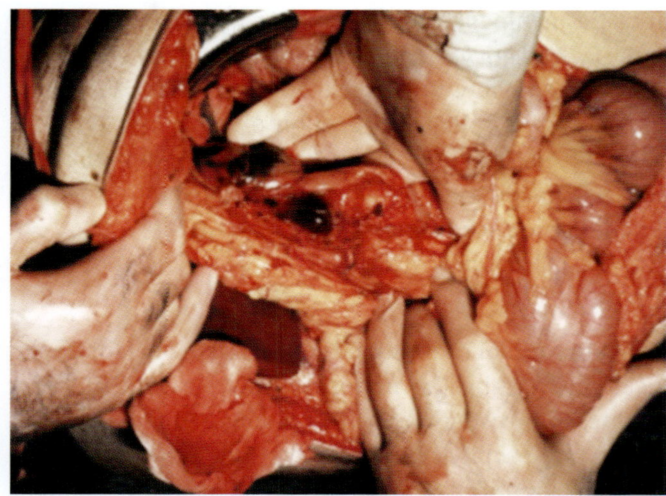

Fig. 57.8: Splenunculi. Exposure of two splenunculi during a splenectomy in a patient who has chronic myeloid leukemia and hypersplenism.

splenic artery and then the splenic vein. Care must be taken to avoid injury to the greater curve of the stomach, pancreatic tail, and left colic flexure. During operations for hematologic disease a careful search must be made for splenunculi (*see* Fig. 57.8), which can be anticipated in 15–30% of patients and could otherwise enlarge and lead to eventual recurrence. It is customary to place a drain to the splenic bed and to leave a nasogastric tube in place at the end of the operation.

Staging Laparotomy for Hodgkin's Disease

A long midline incision is employed. Splenectomy is combined with liver biopsy (both wedge and needle core) and a thorough abdominal exploration. Any abnormal lymph nodes are sampled, and routine nodal biopsies are taken from the para-aortic region and the root of the small bowel mesentery. Metal clips placed adjacent to any diseased nodes assist subsequent localization for radiotherapy. Radiation damage to the ovaries is minimized by oophoropexy. Bone marrow aspiration can be performed under the same anesthetic.

Laparoscopic Splenectomy

Laparoscopic splenectomy has become increasingly utilized over the last two decades and is now the preferred approach for elective splenectomy because of shorter hospital stay and enhanced postoperative recovery.[23] It is usually reserved for small or moderate-sized spleens, notably in ITP. Morcellation of the spleen is necessary for extraction through a small incision, so the technique is inappropriate for neoplastic disorders such as Hodgkin's disease in which an assessment of the splenic architecture is important. Hemorrhage from the splenic vessels and overlooking an accessory spleen are potential drawbacks. However, the rate of detection of accessory spleens is the same by open and laparoscopic techniques,[39] and higher with laparoscopy than with preoperative CT.[23]

Emergency Splenectomy

In a shocked patient with a massive hemoperitoneum, it may be easier to palpate than visualize the ruptured spleen intraoperatively. Prompt delivery into the wound is necessary if the spleen is bleeding profusely, and this can be done by digital dissection of the lienorenal ligament. In a more stable situation, gentle mobilization under direct visualization is preferable because it may allow an alternative procedure to total splenectomy (*see* below).

Effects and Early Complications

Nearly all patients show an increase in their platelet count within a few days of a splenectomy, reaching a peak at 1–2 weeks, but often persisting for several weeks or months. It is not clear that this thrombocytosis increases the risk of deep vein thrombosis or pulmonary embolus; full anticoagulation is generally unnecessary, but antiplatelet therapy with dipyridamole or aspirin is a sensible precaution if the platelet count increases above $1{,}000 \times 10^9$/L. Patients have a risk of splenic and portal vein thrombosis of approximately 3.3%, regardless of open or laparoscopic approach.[40] The incidence is higher in myeloproliferative disorders and hereditary hemolytic anemia and lower in autoimmune thrombocytopenia and trauma. Most cases present between 8 and 12 days. Treatment of symptomatic patients with heparin and warfarinization leads to complete resolution in two thirds of patients and partial resolution in 13%. In the remaining 20%, there is persistent occlusion, portal hypertension, or cavernous transformation of the vein.[40] There is an associated leukocytosis after splenectomy resulting from a transient increase in neutrophils and a sustained increase in lymphocytes and eosinophils. Abnormal red blood cells are seen in the peripheral blood for several weeks, including target cells and Howell–Jolly bodies.

Patients with preoperative thrombocytopenia have an increased risk of hemorrhage following splenectomy.[2] Minor degrees of oozing from the raw surface of the splenic bed can produce a left subphrenic collection, causing pain, fever, leukocytosis, and a left pleural effusion;[41] abdominal drains do not necessarily prevent this complication. Symptomatic collections should be aspirated percutaneously under ultrasonographic guidance. Left basal collapse should respond to physiotherapy with or without antibiotics. There is a small risk of a gastric or pancreatic fistula, but this may close spontaneously if satisfactory drainage is instituted. Although the complication rate is higher in patients with massive spleens (>1,500 g in weight), careful attention to detail can make splenectomy relatively safe in such circumstances.[19,24,38,42]

Postsplenectomy Sepsis

Incidence

Postsplenectomy sepsis or OPSI is now recognized as a dangerous long-term complication, but its incidence varies widely between series, depending upon the age of the patient and the reason for removal of the spleen. The overall incidence of postsplenectomy sepsis is about 4%, but it ranges from 1% to 2% (or less) when the spleen is removed for trauma or iatrogenic injury, through 8% for acquired hemolytic anemia or portal hypertension, to over 10% for lymphoreticular tumors or thalassemia.[17] The risk is clearly greatest in young children, but sepsis is also an occasional cause of death in healthy adults.[18] Most cases occur within 2 years of splenectomy; however, overwhelming infection can rarely develop 20 or more years after a splenectomy. Even at the lowest estimate, the risk is 50 times that of the normal population.

Features

The typical infection starts insidiously with few if any localizing signs, but the patient rapidly deteriorates. High fever is accompanied by malaise, vomiting, extreme prostration, and ultimately circulatory collapse; disseminated intravascular coagulation is a terminal feature. Death follows within 24–48 hours unless the infection can be arrested by broad-spectrum antibiotics given intravenously in high dose. Bacteria can be visualized on Gram or Wright stain while awaiting blood culture, and this allows specific rather than empiric therapy. A real-time PCR (polymerase chain reaction) test can also be used to allow simultaneous identification of the three main encapsulated bacteria for OPSI. In at least half the reported cases, the pneumococcus (*S. pneumoniae*) has been implicated, so penicillin is an important part of the aggressive antibiotic therapy needed. Other encapsulated organisms involved include meningococcus (*N. meningitidis*), *H. influenzae* type B, *Escherichia coli*, and *Staphylococcus aureus*.[18,43] This susceptibility to encapsulated bacteria is explained by the loss of splenic production of opsonins. Mortality rates of 50–70% have been reported,[7,9,43] and bilateral adrenal hemorrhage may be seen at autopsy (Waterhouse-Friederichsen syndrome).

Prevention

The best form of prevention is the avoidance of total splenectomy, e.g. by the nonoperative treatment of lesser injuries or by using salvage techniques at operation. Education and prophylaxis of patients should help to reduce the incidence of OPSI. In children, splenectomy should be delayed, where possible, until the age of 6–12 years.[7]

Education

Since up to 84% of splenectomized patients are unaware of their increased susceptibility to severe sepsis,[44] provision of proper education prevents infectious complications.[7,44] Patients should be advised to seek urgent medical attention if they have any signs of acute febrile illness, especially if there are signs of rigors or systemic symptoms.[45] Animal bites should receive prompt treatment and any foreign travel should be covered for endemic infections. There is no consensus regarding antimicrobial prophylaxis for dental work.[7]

Antibiotic Prophylaxis

The use of antibiotics for the prevention of OPSI is not evidence based. In children, who are at greatest risk, it is customary to give penicillin V (250 mg/day) for at least 2 years. There are problems with patient compliance and the development of penicillin-resistant organisms in long-term treatment. The actual effectiveness of antibiotic prophylaxis is unknown: antibiotics may only reduce and not eliminate the risk of OPSI.[7] Life-long antibiotic therapy is recommended for high-risk groups, but low-risk patients should be counseled as to the risks and benefits of prophylaxis, especially where there are compliance issues.[45] They should be advised to carry an emergency course of antibiotics to use as required.

Vaccine Prophylaxis

All splenectomized patients and those with functional hyposplenism should receive pneumococcal vaccination,

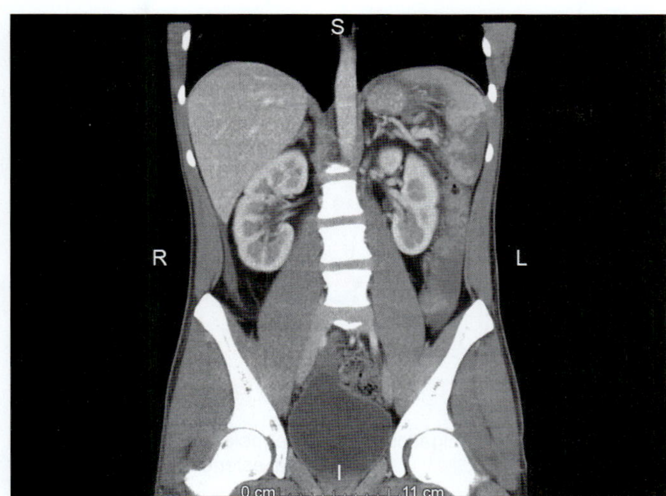

Fig. 57.9: CT of young man with right upper quadrant pain following a road traffic accident. A grade 2 splenic laceration can be seen, with associated hematoma. Nonoperative management proved successful.

H. influenzae type b conjugate vaccine, and meningococcal vaccine to minimize their risk of OPSI.[7] Influenza immunization should be undertaken yearly[45] and is associated with a 54% reduction in risk of death.[46] Whenever possible, the vaccines should be given at least 2 weeks before operation because the antibody response is better in the presence of an intact spleen. If splenectomy has not been anticipated, vaccination should take place 2 weeks later;[7] however, antibody titers reach scarcely half the level of those that can be achieved with the spleen in situ. The pneumococcal vaccination is based on the production of opsonizing anticapsular antibodies by means of a T-cell independent mechanism, but only provides temporary protection; revaccination is recommended after 5 years, although the serological response declines more rapidly.[45]

SPLEEN-PRESERVING OPERATIONS

Alternatives to Emergency Splenectomy

The possibility of preserving all or part of the spleen depends upon the extent of damage both to the organ itself and to the adjacent viscera. In an unstable patient with major laceration of the spleen, the priority is to save life; the spleen should be delivered and removed as soon as possible, and measures can then be taken to counter postsplenectomy sepsis (*see* above). With less severe injuries, and particularly in children, consideration should be given to avoiding total splenectomy by one of the following means.

Nonoperative Management

In the absence of shock, patients with suspected splenic injury should undergo ultrasonography and/or CT to assess the degree of organ damage (*see* Figs. 57.5 and 57.9). A policy of vigilant observation and limited blood transfusion may then avoid the need for laparotomy. The need for >2 units of blood, the likelihood of other internal injuries and especially any sign of renewed bleeding are indications for prompt laparotomy. Splenic trauma is discussed further in Chapter 40, "Abdominal, Urologic and Perineal Injuries".

Topical Applications

Unless the spleen is clearly injured beyond repair, it should be gently mobilized at laparotomy and carefully inspected. Bleeding from simple lacerations and capsular tears can generally be controlled by the application of pressure combined with electrocautery or a hemostatic agent such as gelatin sponge, fibrin glue, thrombin, and microfibrillar collagen (Fig. 57.10).[23,47]

Splenorrhaphy

More extensive injuries necessitate the removal of any devitalized splenic tissue followed by an attempt at repair. Simple suture of the laceration may be supported by the use of Teflon buttresses, a tongue of omentum, or a topical hemostatic agent. The spleen can also be wrapped in omentum or an absorbable (polyglycolic acid) mesh (*see* Fig. 57.10).[23]

Arterial Ligation and Embolization

Ligation of the main splenic artery outside the splenic hilum may lessen blood flow and increase the likelihood of splenic salvage.[48] The spleen will survive on the collateral circulation supplied by the short gastric arteries. Peripheral splenic branch embolization and main splenic artery embolization are two methods of radiological control of hemorrhage that may avoid the need for laparotomy.[29] The immunologic function of the organ is impaired by experimental ligation of the main splenic artery, however.

Partial Splenectomy

Partial splenectomy is feasible because of the segmental nature of the blood supply. The upper or lower pole of the organ can be removed using a finger-fracture technique followed by suture of the stump.

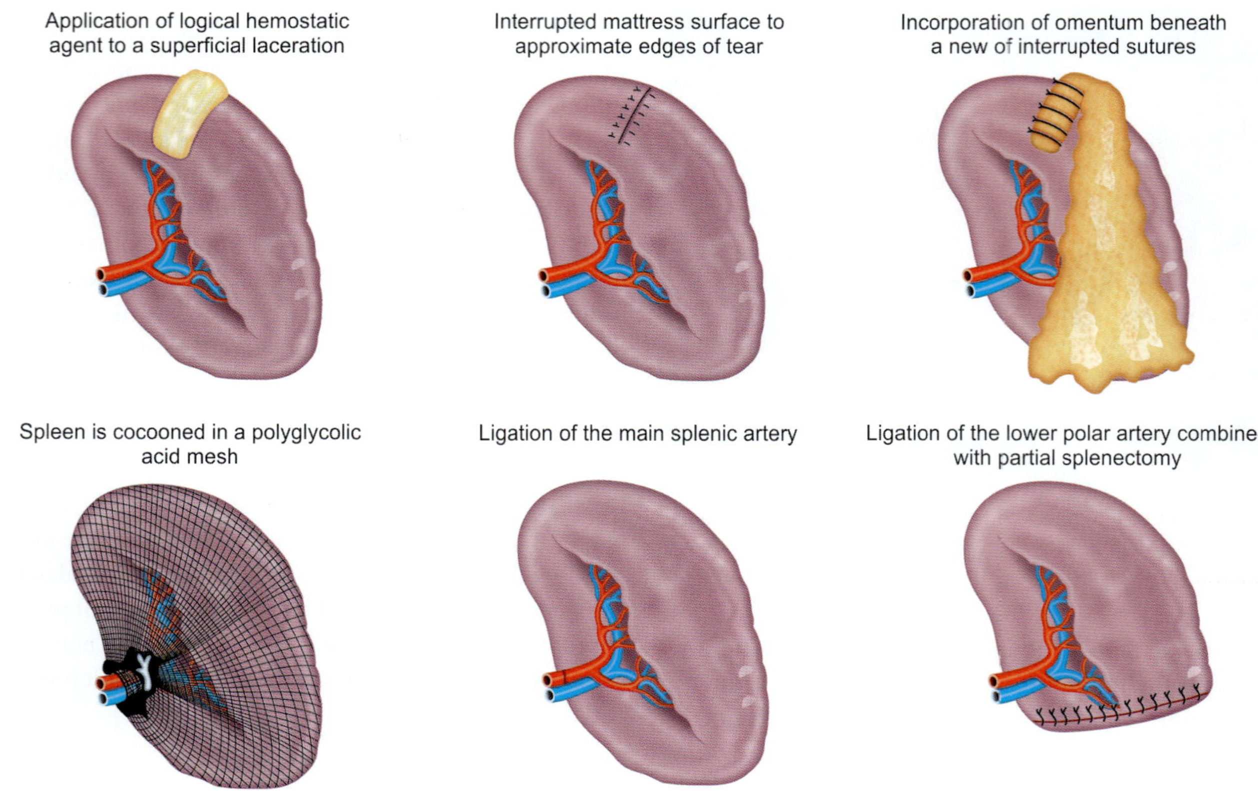

Fig. 57.10: Techniques of splenic conservation.

Autotransplantation

The relatively low risk of postsplenectomy sepsis after splenectomy for trauma may reflect seeding of splenic cells within the peritoneal cavity (splenosis).[49] Plasma tuftsin levels are higher in patients with emergency as opposed to elective splenectomy, and they correlate with residual splenic function as assessed by the pitted red cell count.[16] Following total splenectomy, attempts have been made to retain some immunologic function by replacing nests of splenic tissue within an omental pocket or artificial mesh. At least 20–30 cm^3 of splenic tissue may need reimplanting to preserve adequate tuftsin activity. Although viable, these explanted cells are of doubtful functional value; there have been several reports of postsplenectomy sepsis.[43]

Alternatives to Elective Splenectomy

The need for staging laparotomy that includes splenectomy has progressively declined with improved imaging techniques and the use of splenic biopsy.[29] It has also been recognized that splenectomy may not be advantageous during radical gastrectomy for carcinoma or invariably necessary during distal pancreatectomy for benign disease. Likewise, removal of the spleen is seldom performed nowadays during portasystemic shunting for generalized portal hypertension.

In tropical splenomegaly, splenectomy will reverse the risk of cytopenia and avoid the increased risk of splenic rupture at the expense of reducing the immune response to a parasite. If a malarial spleen does not decrease in size with long-term proguanil therapy, subtotal splenectomy may be accomplished with minimal morbidity (in the absence of portal hypertension), but there may be some risk of regrowth and recurrence of symptoms. Similar concepts have been applied to the treatment of the hypersplenism of myeloproliferative disease or portal hypertension, for which partial splenectomy may be achieved either surgically or by arterial embolization to produce a 40% infarction.[50] Complications of partial splenic embolization include shoulder tip pain, fever, pleural effusion, and ischemic pancreatitis.

Simple splenic cysts may be amenable to cure by marsupialization into the peritoneal cavity or even by stripping the cyst lining from the parenchyma.[34] If there is any question of hydatid disease, splenectomy is strongly preferred.

REFERENCES

1. Mebius RE, Kraal G. Structure and function of the spleen. Nat Rev. 2005;5:606-16.
2. Musser G, Lazar G, Hocking W, et al. Splenectomy for haematologic disease: the UCLA experience with 306 patients. Ann Surg. 1984;200:40-5.
3. Mortelé KJ, Mortelé B, Silverman SG. CT features of the accessory spleen. AJR. 2004;183:1653-7.
4. Redmond HP, Redmond JM, Rooney BP, et al. Surgical anatomy of the human spleen. Br J Surg. 1989;76:198-201.
5. Riva N, Donadini MP, Dentali F, et al. Clinical approach to splanchnic vein thrombosis: risk factors and treatment. Thromb Res. 2012;130:S1-3.
6. Acosta S, Alhadad A, Svensson P, et al. Epidemiology, risk and prognostic factors in mesenteric venous thrombosis. Br J Surg. 2008;95:1245-51.
7. Di Sabatino A, Carsetti R, Corazza GR. Post-splenectomy and hyposplenic states. Lancet. 2011;378:86-97.
8. Llende M, Santiago-Delpin EA, Lavergne J. Immunobiological consequences of splenectomy: a review. J Surg Res. 1986;40:85-94.
9. Dickerman JD. Splenectomy and sepsis: a warning. Pediatrics. 1979;64:938-40.
10. Rose AT, Newman MI, Debelak J, et al The incidence of splenectomy is decreasing: lessons learned from trauma experience. Am Surg. 2000;66:481-6.
11. Cuthbert RJ, Iqbal A, Gates A, et al. Functional hyposplenism following allogenic bone marrow transplantation. J Clin Pathol. 1995;48:257-59.
12. Kulkarni S, Powles R, Treleaven J, et al. Chronic graft versus host disease is associated with long-term risk for pneumococcal infections in recipients of bone marrow transplants. Blood. 2000;95:3683-86.
13. Grotto HZ, Costa FF. Hyposplenism in AIDS. AIDS. 1991; 5:1538-40.
14. Corazza GR, Zoli G, Finaldi L, et al. Tuftsin deficiency in AIDS. Lancet. 1991;337:12-13.
15. D'Orsogna LK, Krueger RG, McKinnon EJ, et al. Circulating B-cell subpopulations are affected differently by HIV and antiretroviral therapy. AIDS. 2007;21:1747-52.
16. Zoli G, Corazza GR, D'Amato G, et al. Splenic autotransplantation after splenectomy: tuftsin activity correlates with residual splenic function. Br J Surg. 1994;81:716-8.
17. Hansen K, Singer DB. Asplenic-hyposplenic overwhelming sepsis: postsplenectomy sepsis revisited. Pediatr Dev Pathol. 2001;4:105-21.
18. Holdsworth RJ, Irving AD, Cuschieri A. Postsplenectomy sepsis and its mortality rate: actual versus perceived risks. Br J Surg. 1991;78:1031-8.
19. Taner T, Nagorney DM, Tefferi A, et al. Splenectomy for massive splenomegaly. Ann Surg. 2012;00:1-6.
20. Alonso M, Gossot D, Bourstyn E, et al. Splenectomy in human immunodeficiency virus-related thrombocytopenia. Br J Surg. 1993:80:330-3.
21. Shimizu-Kohno K, Kimura Y, Kiyasu J, et al. Malignant lymphoma of the spleen in Japan: a clinicopathological analysis of 115 cases. Pathol Int. 2012;62:577-82.
22. Murken DR, Weis JJ, Hill GC, et al. Radiographic assessment of splenic injury without contrast: is contrast truly needed? Surgery. 2012;152:676-84.
23. Koshenkov VP, Pahuja AK, Németh ZH, et al. Identification of accessory spleens during laparoscopic splenectomy is superior to preoperative computed tomography for detection of accessory spleens. J Soc Laparoendosc Surg. 2012;6: 387-91.
24. McInnes MDF, Kielar AZ, Macdonald DB. Percutaneous image-guided biopsy of the spleen: systematic review and meta-analysis of the complication rate and diagnostic accuracy. Radiology. 2011;260:699-708.
25. Garber BG, Mmath BP, Fairfull-Smith RJ, et al. Management of adult splenic injuries in Ontario: a population based study. Can J Surg. 2000;43:283-8.
26. Brady RRW, Bandari M, Kerssens JJ, et al. Splenic trauma in Scotland: demographics and outcomes. World J Surg. 2007;31:2111-6.
27. Singla S, Keller D, Thirunavukarasu P, et al. Splenic injury during colonoscopy—a complication that warrants urgent attention. J Gastrointest Surg. 2012;16:1225-34.
28. Renzulli PR, Schnüriger B, Schoepfer AM, et al. Management of blunt injuries to the spleen. Br J Surg. 2010;97: 1696-703.
29. Dasgupta N, Matsumoto, Arslan B, et al. Embolization therapy for traumatic splenic lacerations. Cardiovasc Int Radiol. 2010;35:795-806.
30. Wilson RE, Rosenthal DS, Moloney WC, et al. Splenectomy for myelo-proliferative disorders. World J Surg. 1985;9:431-6.
31. Dawson AA, Jones PF, King DJ. Splenectomy in the management of haematological disease. Br J Surg. 1987;74:353-7.
32. Rudowski WJ. Accessory spleens: clinical significance with particular reference to the recurrence of idiopathic thrombocytopenic purpura. World J Surg. 1985;9:422-30.
33. Martin P, Rutherford S, Leonard JP. Splenic lymphomas: is there still a role for splenectomy? Oncology (Williston Park). 2012;26:204-6.
34. Morgenstern L, Rosenberg J, Geller SA. Tumors of the spleen. World J Surg. 1985;9:468-76.
35. Herman P, Oliveira e Silva A, Chaib E, et al. Splenic abscess. Br J Surg. 1995;82:355.
36. Williamson JML, Sherman DIN, Canelo R. Operative ligation of multiple splenic artery aneurysms. Int Surg. 2008; 93:261-4.
37. Gunning KA, Rosenberg IL. Symptomatic wandering spleen. Br J Surg. 1993;80:93.
38. Shaw JHF, Clark M. Splenectomy for massive splenomegally. Br J Surg. 1989;76:395-7.
39. Winslow ER, Brunt LM. Perioperative outcome of laparoscopic versus open splenectomy: a meta-analysis with an emphasis on complications. Surgery. 2003;134:647-53.
40. Krauth M-T, Lechner K, Neugebauer EAM, et al. The postoperative splenic/portal vein thrombosis after splenectomy and its prevention—an unresolved issue. Haematologica. 2008;93:1227-32.
41. Ellison EC, Fabri PJ. Complications of splenectomy. Etiology, prevention and management. Surg Clin North Am. 1983;63:1313-30.

42. Letoquart J-P, La Gamma A, Kunin N, et al. Splenectomy for splenomegaly exceeding 1000 grams: analysis of 47 patients. Br J Surg. 1993;80:334-5.
43. Zarrabi MH, Rosner F. Serious infections in adults following splenectomy for trauma. Arch Int Med. 1984;144:1421-4.
44. Brigden ML, Pattullo AL, Brown G. Pneumococcal vaccine administration associated with splenectomy: the need for improved education, documentation, and the use of a practical checklist. Am J Hematol. 2004;5:25-9.
45. Davies JM, Lewis MPN, Wimperis J, et al. Review of guidelines for the prevention and treatment of infection in patients with an absent or dysfunctional spleen: prepared on behalf of the British Committee for Standards in Haematology by a Working Party of the Haemato-Oncology Task Force. Br J Haematol. 2011;155:308-17.
46. Langley JM, Dodds L, Fell D, et al. Pneumococcal and influenza immunization in asplenic persons: a retrospective population based cohort study 1990-2002. BMC Infect Dis. 2010;10:219-6.
47. Kram HB, del Junco T, Clark SR, et al. Techniques of splenic preservation using fibrin glue. J Trauma. 1990;30:97-101.
48. Büyükünal C, Danismend N, Yeker D. Spleen-saving procedures in paediatric splenic trauma. Br J Surg. 1987;74: 350-2.
49. Pearson JA, Johnson D, Smith KA, et al. The born-again spleen. Return of splenic function after splenectomy for trauma. N Engl J Med. 1978;298: 1389-92.
50. Alwmark A, Bengmark S, Gullstrand P, et al. Evaluation of splenic embolization in patients with portal hypertension and hypersplenism. Ann Surg. 1982; 196:518-24.

Case Study: 58
Biliary Injury Following Laparoscopic Cholecystectomy

James ML Williamson, Robin CN Williamson

THE PROBLEM

Although the incidence of biliary injury following laparoscopic cholecystectomy is small, ranging between 0.33% and 0.5%, it is associated with considerable morbidity and often requires complex management. Biliary injuries can be identified intraoperatively (often with the use of cholangiography), over the next few days or some weeks to months later. Presentation is often related to the severity of injury, with unrecognized or inadequately treated injuries resulting in bile duct stricture and associated cholestasis and ultimately liver failure. All iatrogenic injuries should be discussed with a hepatopancreatobiliary unit and management is typically multimodal, with interventional radiology, endoscopic and operative interventions all being considered as therapeutic.

THE TYPICAL CASE

A 33-year-old woman underwent and elective laparoscopic cholecystectomy for symptomatic gallstones—she had had three episodes of acute cholecystitis and was experiencing recurrent episodes of biliary colic. Previous investigations, in the form of blood tests and ultrasonography, had not detected any evidence of jaundice or common bile duct stones. At operation there were adhesions covering the gallbladder, which was thickened. These adhesions were divided prior to retraction of the gallbladder to expose Calot's triangle, which was obscured with dense inflammatory adhesions. Calot's triangle was explored and anomalous ductal anatomy identified—the cystic duct was identified to be entering the right hepatic duct—the cystic artery appeared in a standard position. The cystic duct was clipped and divided and then the cystic artery clipped and also divided in a standard fashion. The gallbladder was then excised from the gallbladder fossa with diathermy, placed into a retrieval bag and removed from the patient. The remained of the operation was completed without incidence and included copious irrigation and aspiration of the operative field.

Review of the patient on the first postoperative day revealed that she was complaining of significant right upper quadrant abdominal pain. This was confirmed on examination, which detected signs of localized peritonism, although she was afebrile. Routine blood tests only revealed a slight elevation in inflammatory markers, but no derangement of liver function tests. An urgent ultrasound was arranged, which showed a large subhepatic collection; a radiological drain was subsequently placed and bile aspirated. Over the next few days, the intraabdominal tube continued to drain between 200 and 300 mL of bile daily; despite this the patient continued to improve clinically, although she became profoundly depressed, and her inflammatory markers settled. In view of the ongoing bile leak, she was transferred to a regional hepatopancreatobiliary unit.

Following transfer she was investigated with endoscopic retrograde cholangiopancreatography (ERCP); this showed a normal left hepatic duct and common bile duct, but a complete transection of the right hepatic duct (Fig. 58.1). There was extravasation of bile from the right hepatic duct into the subhepatic biloma—part of the contrast, however, did flow retrogradely into the proximal duct and showed no other injury. The images from the ERCP were reviewed at a multidisciplinary meeting and management options considered. It was thought that radiological or endoscopic stenting would not resolve the injury and that operative intervention, in the form of hepaticojejunostomy, would offer the best chance of successful resolution. At laparotomy, the presence of the subhepatic collection was confirmed and a low bifurcation of the right and left hepatic ducts noted, with subsequent complete transection of the right hepatic duct. It was thought that this low bifurcation was misinterpreted as the cystic duct entering the right hepatic duct. A hepaticojejunostomy was performed onto the right hepatic duct only via a Roux limb. The patient made an uncomplicated recovery and showed no evidence of hepatic dysfunction at discharge from long-term follow-up some 3 years later.

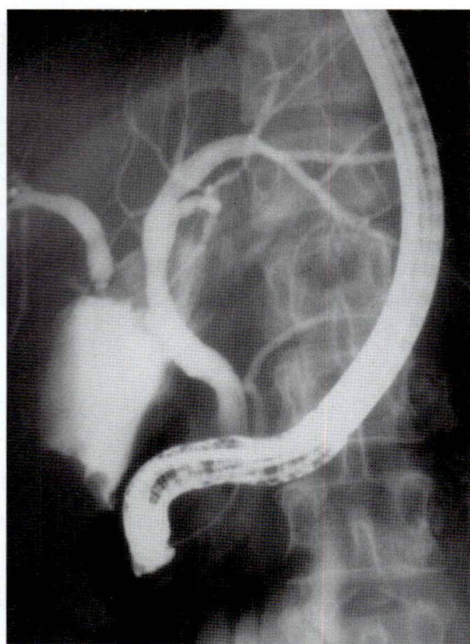

Fig. 58.1: ERCP outlining a normal left hepatic duct and common bile duct. There is complete transection of the right hepatic duct; extravasation of bile can be seen (forming a subhepatic biloma), although some contrast re-enters the right hepatic duct to flow retrogradely into the proximal duct. (ERCP: Endoscopic retrograde cholangiopancreatography).

DIAGNOSTIC DILEMMAS

This case illustrates how misidentification of structures during laparoscopic cholecystectomy can result in significant biliary injury. Although Calot's triangle was explored cautiously, the aberrant anatomy (low bifurcation of the common hepatic duct) was misinterpreted as a cystic duct entering the right hepatic duct. A second section of the right hepatic duct must have been divided to allow extraction of the gallbladder, but this was not noted during the operation suggesting that there was considerable chronic inflammation within the Calot's triangle to distort findings. Intraoperative cholangiography or ultrasonography was not considered; while this may not have prevented the injury, it may have detected it. Likewise, conversion to open operation was not performed. It is likely, therefore, that the operating surgeon was confident that they had correctly identified the anomalous anatomy.

The presence of postoperative pain following an atypical laparoscopic cholecystectomy should raise the possibility of a postoperative complication. Sterile bile may produce limited symptoms, but can cause local peritoneal irritation as in this case. Urgent blood tests should be performed to look for signs of infection and to check that there is not any signs of biliary obstruction. In terms of further investigation, dilemmas exist regarding the benefits of each imaging modality with the desire for repeat laparoscopy. Ultrasonography and computed tomography should detect any perihepatic collections and, as in this case, facilitate drainage. ERCP and magnetic resonance imaging should produce higher resolution imaging of the biliary tree than either CT or ultrasonography, with magnetic resonance cholangiopancreatography highlighting the biliary tree proximal to any areas of transection or clipping that may not be shown on ERCP (although images may be disrupted by the presence of clips). Laparoscopy allows direct visualization of the operative field and this can facilitate irrigation and drain placement (for simple leaks) or the conversion to an open procedure and subsequent repair of any injury. In this case, the management dilemmas relate to the management of a persistent bile leak and are discussed below.

MANAGEMENT OPTIONS

The presence of some bile in the drain immediately following cholecystectomy does not necessarily indicate ductal injury; bile can leak from patent ducts of Luschke (which are more patent in acute inflammation), although this tends to be < 50 mL and settles over a couple of days or so. Given the ERCP findings, the management options in this case relate to the timing and which intervention to perform to facilitate repair of the right hepatic ductal injury. The presence of the drain did stabilize the patient's condition to an extent, but was not a long-term satisfactory solution. The complete transection of the right hepatic duct meant that ERCP and stenting was deemed unsuitable—even percutaneous transhepatic antegrade stenting was thought not to be possible, given the nature of the injury (and loss of ductal tissue). Thus, the only method of repair was thought to be operative.

In terms of operative repair, four main techniques were considered and discussed. A simplistic end-to-end repair of the ductal injury could have been performed—this would have been technically challenging, given the presence of nondilated ducts and missing segment of duct. However, this end-to-end anastomosis was not performed as it is associated with a high risk of stricturing in part due to localized tissue ischaemia resulting from the repair. The second relatively simple intervention considered was to tie off the right hepatic duct. The bile leak would stop once the duct was closed, but there would be resultant atrophy of the whole right side of the liver and possible infection of the stagnant bile. This technique, which can be usefully employed for isolate segment VI ductal leakage, was therefore not performed. The last two methods considered involved hepaticojejunostomies: one to both ducts and one to only the right hepatic duct. As the left hepatic duct was in continuity with the rest of the biliary tree, no advantage was seen in anastomosing this duct to the jejunum. Therefore, the hepaticojejunostomy was performed to the right hepatic duct only, via a Roux limb. This method of repair is recommended to provide the best long-term results and can be altered slightly by tacking one end of the Roux limb to the underside of the abdominal wall and placing marking clips around the site. This provides an "access limb", which can be entered percutaneously under radiological guidance, should an anastomotic stricture form and require dilatation.

The timing of intervention should also be considered in cases of biliary injury. This, in part, is dependent on the type of injury sustained and its resulting symptoms. All cases should be discussed at a multidisciplinary meeting and the entirety of the biliary tree assessed prior to any definitive repair. Early repair of complex injuries is preferable, but if this is not possible then operation should be delayed for several weeks to allow inflammation and fibrosis to subside. During this period, biliary flow needs to be controlled by other means.

FURTHER READING

1. Biffl WL, Moore EE, Offner PJ, et al. Routine intraoperative laparoscopic ultrasonography with selective cholangiography reduces bile duct complications during laparoscopic cholecystectomy. J Am Coll Surg. 2001;193:272-80.
2. Bismuth H, Franco D, Corlette MB, et al. Long term results of roux-en-Y hepaticojejunostomy. Surg Gynecol Obstet. 1978;146:161-7.
3. Gurusamy KS, Davidson BR. Surgical treatment of gallstones. Gastroenterol Clin North Am. 2010;39:229-44.
4. Nordin A, Grönross JM, Mäkisalo H. Treatment of biliary complications after laparoscopic cholecystectomy. Scand J Surg. 2011;100:42-8.
5. Stewart L, May LW. Bile duct injuries during aparoscopic cholecystectomy; factors that influence the results of treatment. Arch Surg. 1995;130:1123-9.
6. Strasberg SM, Hertl M, Soper NJ. An analysis of the problem of biliary injury during laparoscopic cholecystectomy. J Am Coll Surg. 1995;180:101-25.
7. Williamson JML. Traumatic injuries to the biliary tree. Br J Hosp Med. 2013;74:138-43.

Case Study: 59
Intraoperative Detection of Hepatic Metastases During Pancreatic Insulinoma Enucleation

James ML Williamson, Ian M Pope

THE PROBLEM

Although insulinomas are rare, with an incidence of 1–4 per million, they are the most common functioning pancreatic neuroendocrine tumor. The vast majority of insulinomas arise from β cells within the islets of Langerhans, but they can arise from ectopic pancreatic tissue. Approximately 5% of cases are associated with multiple endocrine neoplasia (MEN) type 1, the rest being sporadic. Most insulinomas are small (<2 cm) when detected, and over 90% of sporadic lesions are benign. Patients present with symptoms of insulin excess resulting in hypoglycemia, and the neurological symptoms (neuroglycopenia) can result in ataxia, malcoordination, slurred speech, lethargy, confusion, blurred vision, paralysis, seizures, and ultimately coma. In fasting patients, the presence of Whipple's triad is diagnostic for insulinomas and comprises: (i) symptoms and signs of hypoglycemia, (ii) concomitant plasma glucose level of 45 mg/dL (2.5 mmol/L) or less, and (iii) reversibility of symptoms with administration of glucose. Biochemical diagnosis is based on a low fasting glucose and elevated fasting serum insulin, C-peptide and proinsulin. Computed tomography provides the mainstay of imaging, which can be combined with magnetic resonance imaging, endoscopic ultrasound (with sensitivity of 43–90% depending on the location of lesion), and octreotide scanning. Angiography with percutaneous transhepatic pancreatic vein catheterization (and selective venous sampling) is seldom performed.

Operative resection is advocated since in benign tumors it is curative; recurrence is uncommon (approximately 3%) and tends to occur with histologically more aggressive lesions (grade 2). Metastatic disease presents a therapeutic challenge: isolated hepatic lesions should be resected, but when clearance is not possible debulking of tumor mass (whether synchronous or metachronous) can improve both symptoms and survival. Tumors are relatively insensitive to nonoperative measures such as chemotherapy and radiotherapy, although hepatic ablation can be used to treat lesions that are not suitable for hepatectomy.

THE TYPICAL CASE

A 38-year-old previously healthy man was investigated for a 3-year history of progressive neuroglycopenia. The patient was unaware of his hypoglycemic symptoms and merely complained of tingling in his hands, feet, lips, and poor coordination. He was lethargic and tired easily; decreased exercise tolerance was associated with weight gain. There was no family history of endocrine disease. The diagnosis of insulinoma was confirmed biochemically with low blood glucose (32.4 mg/dL = 1.8 mmol/L), and elevated serum insulin (225 pmol/L; normal = 14.3–122 pmol/L), C-peptide (678 pmol/L; normal = 0.26–0.63 pmol/L), and proinsulin (272 pmol/L; normal = 6.4–9.4 pmol/L). He had normal serum calcium and prolactin levels. Urgent computed tomography revealed a solitary 1.8 cm enhancing lesion in the pancreatic head, consistent with an insulinoma (Fig. 59.1), with no evidence of lymphadenopathy or metastases. These findings were confirmed on subsequent

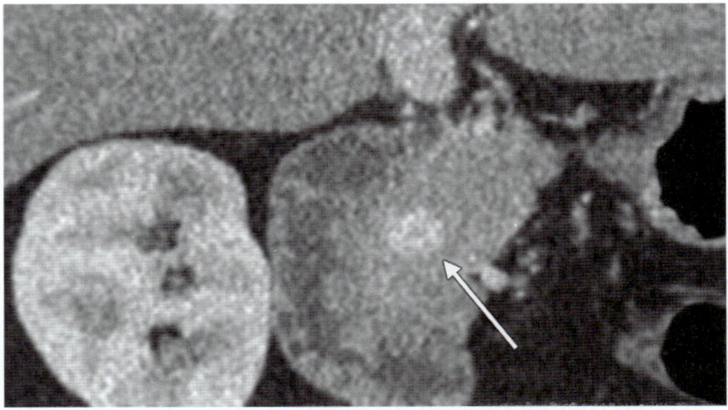

Fig. 59.1: Enlarged CT scan shows a solitary enhancing lesion just under 2 cm in diameter (arrow) in the head of pancreas, close to the medial wall of duodenum and in front of common bile duct. No metastases were seen.

magnetic resonance imaging and endoscopic ultrasound (EUS). Although EUS localized the lesion with difficulty, it showed that the insulinoma was sitting just above the confluence of the pancreatic and biliary ducts, with no ductal invasion. Given these findings, the patient was listed for enucleation of the pancreatic head insulinoma.

At laparotomy no pancreatic or hepatic lesions were visible or palpable, but two lymph nodes were identified at the superior border of the pancreatic neck adjacent to the portal vein, measuring 2 cm and 1 cm, respectively. Intraoperative ultrasonography (IOUS) revealed a poorly defined lesion within the pancreatic head, but it was difficult to identify its relationship to the pancreatic duct. An incidental 2 cm lesion with segment VII of the lesion was also detected on IOUS. Frozen-section histological examination of a Trucut biopsy revealed necrotic material only, and subsequent wedge incision biopsy confirmed necrotic debris but with associated neuroendocrine cells; thus, a metastasis could not be excluded. After considering the management options (*see* below), it was decided to proceed to synchronous resection of both the insulinoma and metastasis. An uncomplicated hepatic wedge resection of the segment VII lesion was combined with a Whipple's pancreatoduodenectomy and feeding jejunostomy, with drains to the pancreatic anastomosis and subhepatic space. The patient was transferred to the high dependency unit postoperatively and made a steady recovery, with no amylase in the drains by day five. Histological examination confirmed a solitary pancreatic pT1N0M0 insulinoma (grade 1 neuroendocrine tumor, Ki67 index <2%) and a necrotic liver nodule (consistent with a previous liver abscess) with no evidence of malignancy (Fig. 59.2).

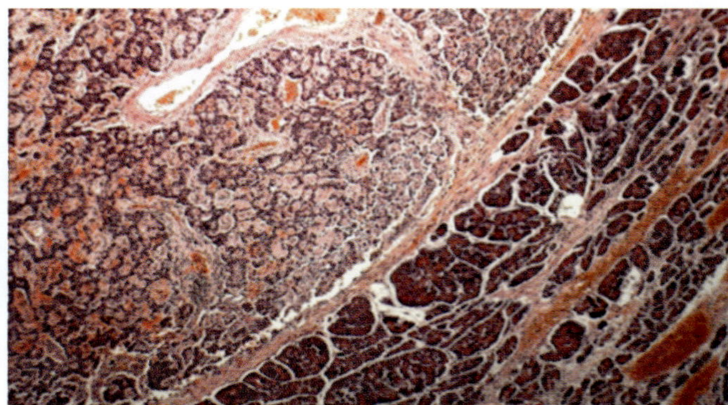

Fig. 59.2: Histological image showing a grade 1 (benign) pancreatic insulinoma (x 400 magnification). No mitoses are present, and the Ki67 index is <2%.

DIAGNOSTIC DILEMMAS

These were twofold: first, planning the operative resection and second, how to manage an incidental liver lesion detected intraoperatively. Enucleation is advocated for most pancreatic insulinomas given that over 90% of sporadic lesions are benign and that cross-sectional imaging and EUS should detect any metastatic deposits. Enucleation risks incomplete excision of the lesion and is associated with more complications than a formal pancreatic resection (fistula rates of up to 30%), but it does preserve parenchyma and avoid postoperative pancreatic insufficiency. The location of the insulinoma (deep within the head of the pancreas) and the close proximity of the pancreatic duct further impacted on the type of resection planned. The concerns regarding a formal proximal pancreatoduodenectomy, with its associated operative risks, mainly relate to performing the anastomosis in a soft pancreas with an undilated duct.

The routine use of intraoperative ultrasound detected an incidental hepatic lesion and thus presented the problem on how best to proceed with the operation. Although the insulinoma was both sporadic and measured <2 cm (both of which facts meant that it was unlikely to be associated with a metastasis), the frozen section results could not exclude hepatic spread. Three main options were available: (1) curtailing the operation and further counseling of the patient; (2) pancreatic resection alone with further postoperative investigation of the hepatic disease (and potentially subsequent resection); and (3) combined pancreatic and hepatic resection. The patient had not been consented for a liver resection and not been prepared for this step (with regard to anesthetic preparation, minimal fluid resuscitation and lowering of central venous pressure). Nevertheless, given his age, the isolated nature of the hepatic lesion and his unawareness of the hypoglycemic symptoms, the decision was reached to proceed to synchronous resection.

MANAGEMENT OPTIONS

These reflected the intraoperative dilemma posed by the incidental hepatic lesion. Abandoning the operation would allow full assessment of the nature of the liver lesion including confirmation of the frozen-section results and possible octreotide imaging. If the liver lesion proved to be definitely malignant, then a full discussion with the patient could involve both operative and nonoperative management options; reoperation could be planned as either a synchronous or staged resection. Resection of hepatic metastases is indicated where possible in insulinoma because of the relative inefficiency of medical treatment and the fact that excision confers the best chance of cure. Since the neuroglycopenia meant that at least resection of the primary lesion was desirable, the key question concerned synchronous or staged resection of his hepatic disease.

The decision to perform a synchronous hepatic resection is complex: the benefits of excision (chiefly a single operation) must be weighed against the potential increased morbidity and mortality. Adding a liver resection to a proximal pancreatoduodenectomy does confer an additional risk to the patient, with a postoperative complication rate of up to 44%. Excision of the primary alone would have allowed him to recover from the pancreatic operation and then consider all options for the presumed metastatic disease. In retrospect, as the histology was benign, excision of the primary lesion was all that would have been required.

FURTHER READING

1. Bettini R, Partelli S, Boninsegna L, et al. Tumor size correlates with malignancy in nonfunctioning pancreatic endocrine tumor. Surgery. 2011;150:75-82.
2. Crippa S, Zerbi A, Boninsegna L, et al. Surgical management of insulinomas: short- and long-term outcomes after enucleations and pancreatic resections. Arch Surg. 2012;147:261-6.
3. Falconi M, Mantovani W, Crippa S, et al. Pancreatic insufficiency after different resections for benign tumours. Br J Surg. 2008;95:85-91.
4. Gaujoux S, Gonen M, Tang L, et al. Synchronous resection of primary and liver metastases for neuroendocrine tumours. Ann Surg Oncol. 2012;19:4270-77.
5. Jensen RT, Cadiot G, Brandi ML, et al. ENETS consensus guideline for the management of patients with digestive neuroendocrine neoplasms: functional pancreatic endocrine tumor syndromes. Neuroendocrinology. 2012;95:98-119.

Case Study: 60
Bleeding into an Incidental Hepatocellular Adenoma Following Minor Blunt Trauma

James ML Williamson

THE PROBLEM

Hepatocyte proliferation resulting in hepatocellular adenoma is strongly associated with hormonal contraceptive use, which increases the incidence from 1 per million to 3–4 per 100,000. The patient will often be a nulliparous young woman who has taken the oral contraceptive pill for some months or years for menorrhagia or dysmenorrhea. Hepatocellular adenomas have spontaneous rupture rates of 12–20%; risk is related to size, rupture being unusual in those <4 cm in diameter. Management of bleeding adenomas is dependent on cardiovascular stability to permit expectant management plus imaging, if necessary on a serial basis. Arterial embolization or resuscitative laparotomy will be required for ongoing hemorrhage.

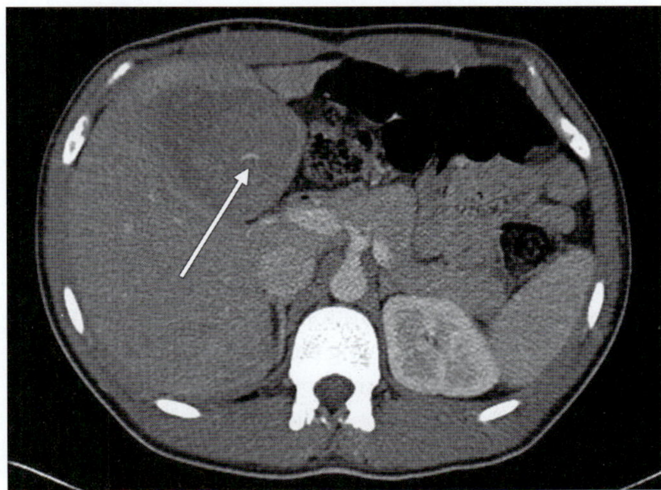

Fig. 60.1: Contrast-enhanced CT showing a 7-cm mixed echogenicity lesion in segment IV of the liver with associated bleeding point (arrow).

THE TYPICAL CASE

A 20-year-old woman in previous good health presented with right upper quadrant pain 6 hours after falling down a flight of three stairs. Her only relevant history was that she was taking norethisterone (progesterone-based oral contraceptive) for menorrhagia for 2 years and had a tendency to bruise easily; there was nothing to suggest platelet dysfunction. She was hemodynamically stable, but had tenderness on palpation in the right upper quadrant, without peritonism, masses, or bruising. Initial hematological investigations were unremarkable, and urgent computed tomography (CT) demonstrated a 7-cm mixed-attenuating lesion within the right lobe of the liver. This lesion was associated with an enhancing vessel, which suggested active bleeding into the mass, but no other signs of parenchymal disruption (Fig. 60.1). A triple-phase hepatic CT showed active extravasation of contrast into the mass, which was either a simple hematoma or a bleed into an existing hepatic lesion (adenoma or focal nodular hyperplasia). Hepatic angioplasty identified no active bleeding point, while the appearances were suggestive of hepatocellular adenoma. Pain settled with conservative management, and there was only transient derangement of liver function tests. She was advised to stop her oral contraceptive. Subsequent magnetic resonance imaging (MRI) confirmed the likely diagnosis of hepatic adenoma, which was supported by regression of the lesion on cross-sectional imaging (Fig. 60.2). She remains under surveillance.

DIAGNOSTIC DILEMMAS

Hepatic trauma is becoming increasingly common, with an annual incidence of 2.95 per 100,000 people. Blunt trauma typically affects the right lobe of the liver and is usually caused by road traffic collisions (with associated deceleration injuries) or by direct impact. Given the current trend toward conservative management of traumatic abdominal injuries, any stable patient in whom organ trauma is suspected should undergo urgent CT to identify and classify the extent of damage. In the present case, the appearances on cross-sectional imaging were atypical for liver trauma and raised a diagnostic conundrum: the mixed heterogeneous mass with an active bleeding point could have represented either a simple hematoma or a bleed into a pre-existing lesion. The position of the mass

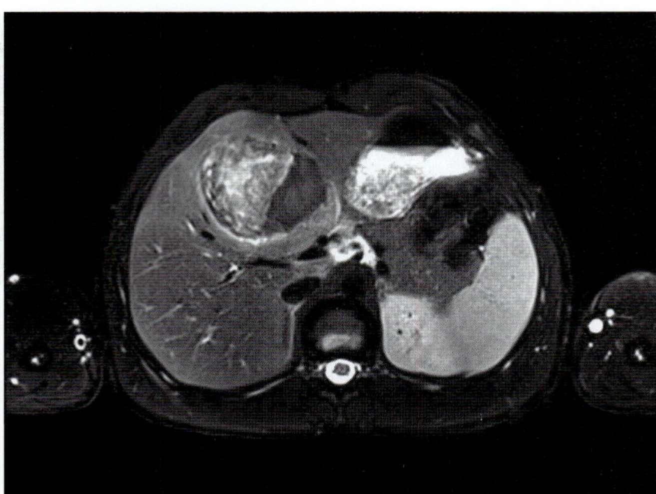

Fig. 60.2: MRI showing mixed-echogenicity lesion in segment IV of the liver, with probable hemorrhage into underlying hepatocellular adenoma.

deep within segment IV of the liver, combined with the lack of parenchymal disruption and its atypical appearance, indicated an underlying pathology.

The patient's history of minor bleeding and her norethisterone therapy raised the possibility of a proliferative disorder resulting in hepatocellular adenoma or focal nodular hyperplasia. Although adenomas can bleed spontaneously, especially in those with a known bleeding tendency, in this particular patient the bleeding was precipitated by abdominal trauma. Her stable condition gave time for cross-sectional imaging followed by hepatic angiography.

MANAGEMENT OPTIONS

The management of liver trauma depends on the patient's general condition and the severity of the injury. Cardiovascular status dictates whether urgent CT can be performed or whether an urgent laparotomy is required. Patients with minor hepatic injuries can be managed conservatively in 83–97% of cases, hematomas often being amenable to hepatic angioembolization. Unstable patients, or those in whom conservative management has failed, should proceed to laparotomy and damage-control surgery. In the reported case, expectant management in the initial situation was successful and hemorrhage stopped spontaneously.

Subsequent management options for hepatocellular adenoma relate to the risk of bleeding and the likely risk of malignant alteration, while location of the lesion also plays a role. The overall risk of malignant transformation is 4.2%, being generally greater in lesions measuring over 5 cm in diameter (although smaller lesions have been known to progress to carcinoma). High-risk groups include those with a history of androgen or anabolic steroid intake, male gender, or glycogen storage disease. Discontinuation of oral contraceptives is recommended in all patients, but this may not abort the risk of malignant transformation. Thus, patients who are managed conservatively require surveillance imaging.

Present guidelines recommend that all lesions >5 cm in diameter should be resected, even though this policy means that 95% of patients may be exposed to unnecessary operative intervention. Potentially, biopsy of the lesion can be performed to detect mutations in the β-catenin gene, although the benefits need to be balanced against the risks of bleeding or tumor seeding during the procedure. Mutations to the β-catenin signaling pathway, which regulates hepatocyte activity, can lead to hyperproliferation and subsequent malignant transformation. Immunohistochemical markers that reveal an increased risk of cancer include several hepatocyte nuclear factors: 1α, β-catenin-activated, inflammatory, and unclassified.

Minimally invasive procedures, such as percutaneous radiofrequency or microwave ablation, are being explored as alternatives to operation, as they have very low morbidity and mortality rates. Arterial embolization provides a novel alternative for adenomas, as it results in tumor regression with limited complications; this reduction in tumor size is correlated with a reduction in bleeding risk and malignant transformation.

FURTHER READING

1. Burch JM, Moore EE. Injuries to the liver, biliary tract, spleen and diaphragm. In: Souba WW, Fink MP, Jurkovich GJ, et al. (Eds). ACS Surgery: Principles and Practice. New York, NY: WebMD Professional Publishing; 2006.
2. Corsnier H, Thibaud E, Duflos C, et al. Norethisterone-induced hepatic adenomas can cause life-threatening bleeding in girls with inherited platelet disorders. Fertil Steril. 2010;94:2329e1-e3.
3. Kapp N, Curtis KM. Hormonal contraceptive use among women with liver tumors: a systemic review. Contraception. 2009;80:387-90.
4. Moore EE, Cogbill TH, Jurkovich GJ, et al. Organ injury scaling: spleen and liver (1994 revision). J Trauma. 1995;38:323-4.
5. Stoot JHMB, Coelen RJS, de Jong MC, et al. Malignant transformation of hepatocellular adenomas into hepatocellular carcinomas: a systemic review including more than 1600 adenoma cases. HPB. 2010;12:509-22.
6. Williamson JML, Rees JRE, Streets CG, et al. Management of liver trauma. Br J Hosp Med. 2013;74(8):432-8.

Part 3C: Coloproctology
(Chapters 61 to 66)

61

Inflammatory Colorectal Conditions

Neil Borley, Neil Mortensen

Key Points

- The distinction between ulcerative proctocolitis and Crohn's disease is important because it may affect management. It can also be difficult, requiring the examination of multiple biopsies, or even impossible, in which case the colitis is labeled "indeterminate".
- Operative treatment of ulcerative colitis may be required in three settings: acute fulminant disease, chronic ill health, and for the treatment or prevention of carcinoma. Proctocolectomy with pouch formation is usually appropriate, but panproctocolectomy with ileostomy or even subtotal colectomy with ileorectal anastomosis is still indicated for certain subgroups.
- Crohn's disease is a panintestinal disorder with a particular propensity to fistula formation; obstructive symptoms are less frequent with colonic than small-bowel disease. As with ulcerative colitis, there is an increased risk of colonic carcinoma.
- Perianal lesions in Crohn's disease comprise recurrent abscesses and fistulas and fissures that are slow to heal. Conservative management options include drainage of pus, fistulotomy or the use of setons, advancement flaps to cover skin defects, and a defunctioning stoma.

ULCERATIVE COLITIS

Ulcerative colitis emerged as a distinct disease entity in the second half of the 19th century,[1] when it became clear that it was an inflammatory colitis not caused by primarily an infective process. It had a high associated mortality rate, with acute severe colitis being fatal. With the widespread introduction of corticosteroid treatment, administered both topically and as intensive intravenous therapy,[2-4] the mortality rate was reduced and the appropriate use of acute total colectomy and ileostomy[5] also had an effect. Since the establishment of these principles of treatment, operative and medical therapies have continued to improve, particularly with the recognition of the concept of joint medical and surgi-cal team management of the disease.

Epidemiology

The pattern of individuals affected has remained unchanged for the past 25 years. The disease is two to three times more common in Caucasian Anglo-Saxon than other populations, and the annual incidence rate varies from just under 2 to 6/100,000 population. It most commonly presents in the third decade of life, although it can occur in any age group, but it is extremely rare among neonates. There is a slightly higher incidence in females than in males (1.4:1).

Etiology

The precise etiology remains unclear.

Molecular Mechanisms

The processes surrounding mucosal inflammation and failure of repair are complex. A range of proinflammatory cytokines are involved including those promoting inflammation [interleukin 6 (IL-6), IL-13, IL-17, IL-18, and tumor necrosis factor alpha (TNF-α)], those affecting Th1 polarization (IL-2, IL-12, interferon gamma (IFN-γ)], and those which act to suppress inflammation in normal circumstances (IL-10, IFN) variations in the levels of which have all been shown to be related to active disease. Changes in growth factor release such as vascular endothelial growth factor, transforming growth factor beta, and endothelial growth factor may affect mucosal barrier integrity and repair. Variations in the signaling of the toll-like receptor (TLR) pathways may also be involved.

The serum of ulcerative colitis contains a range of antibodies not normally found in serum, including cytotoxic anticolonocyte forms.[6] It is not clear, however, whether they are a primary phenomenon associated with the disease pathogenesis or epiphenomena caused by the release of colonic and luminal antigens into the circulation from the breakdown of the mucosal barrier, once the disease has become established.

Genetic Factors

There is a 35% incidence in first-degree relatives, which suggests a genetic component, and it has long been recognized that there is an association with HLA type B27.

Multiple genetic loci have been associated with the development of ulcerative colitis in linkage and genome-wide association studies and many are shared with the risk of developing Crohn's disease, especially those related to IL-23/Th-17 transduction and signaling among the "IBD2" locus on chromosome 12 and ECM1, but the precise interaction of the various sites and many of the proteins coded for remain unclear. Also, there is evidence of involvement of genes related to mucosal barrier function.[7]

Bacterial Action

Although there is no evidence that bacteria play any role in the pathogenesis of ulcerative colitis, they are important as:

- There may be changes in the colonic bacterial flora during attacks
- An episode of infective diarrhea in a patient who has pre-existing disease may precipitate an acute attack and complicate both the diagnosis and the management.

Pathology

Ulcerative colitis (or, more accurately, proctocolitis as the rectum is almost invariably involved) is primarily a disorder of the colonic mucosa, although in more severe episodes of inflammation and fulminant colitis, diffuse inflammation is seen throughout the colonic wall beneath the ulcerated mucosa.

There are several disease patterns:

- Isolated proctitis
- Distal or left-sided colitis
- Total colitis

The disease almost always occurs in the rectum where it may be limited, which gives rise to an isolated proctitis (40% of cases). Proximal spread occurs, with the mucosa characteristically involved as a continuous colitis. The inflammation characteristically has a sharp cutoff between diseased and unaffected proximal colon. The next most common pattern of involvement (35% of cases) affects the colon distal to the splenic flexure (distal or left-sided colitis). In 25% of patients, there is additional involvement of the more proximal large bowel (i.e., total colitis). True isolated right-sided or proximal colitis is rare, although effective control of rectosigmoid disease by topical corticosteroid enemas during an episode of acute colitis can mimic it.

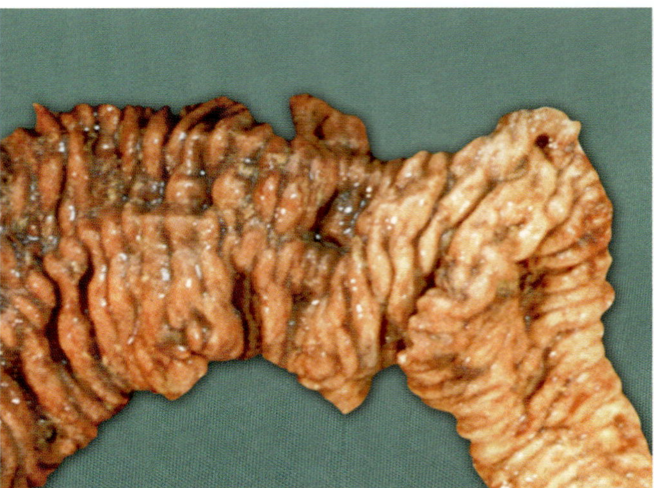

Fig. 61.1: Moderately severe active ulcerative colitis. The mucosa is friable and edematous with patchy hemorrhage.

The macroscopic changes in the mucosa may be mild, particularly during periods of quiescence, with little more than edema and congestion of the mucosal vasculature. With progressively more severe inflammation, the mucosa becomes friable and bleeds with minimal trauma (contact bleeding; Fig. 61.1). Submucosal hemorrhage and mucosal sloughing give rise initially to punctate ulceration, which readily becomes confluent during more severe attacks. Loss of most of the colonic mucosa in one area with only residual islands of edematous colonocytes and regenerative tissue gives rise to the appearance of pseudopolyposis (Fig. 61.2), characteristic of severe disease.

In mild colitis, the mucosa is infiltrated predominantly by neutrophils. Breakdown of the mucosa at the crypt bases gives rise to crypt abscesses (Figs. 61.3 and 61.4). If this inflammation is sufficiently severe, the muscularis propria may undergo myocytolysis (Fig. 61.5), which results in the external appearance of hyperemia with serosal proteinaceous exudate and wall thinning during acute severe attacks.

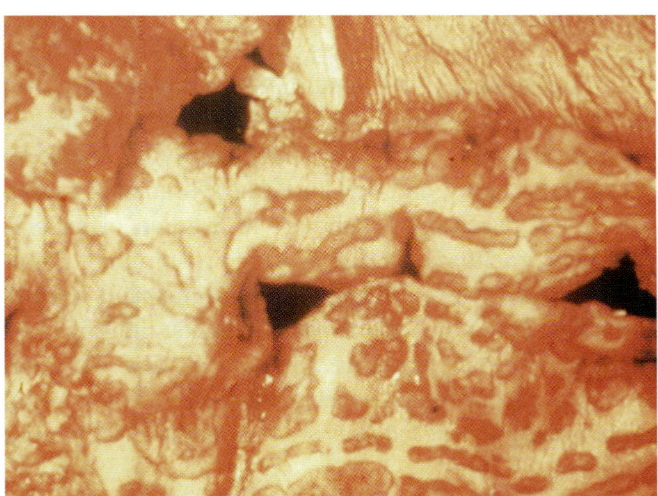

Fig. 61.2: Colonic pseudopolyposis in ulcerative colitis. The majority of colonic mucosa is replaced with inflammatory exudate, which leaves regenerative islands of tissue that appear superficially like polyps.

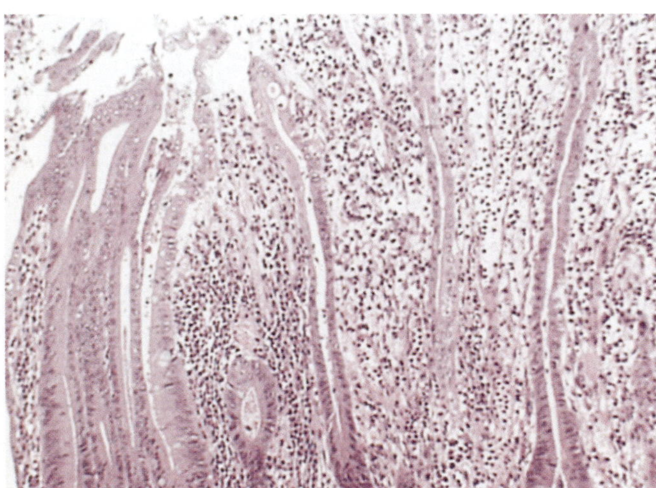

Fig. 61.3: Mucosal goblet cell depletion and crypt distortion. The crypts are tall and distorted with only occasional goblet cells among the epithelial cells.

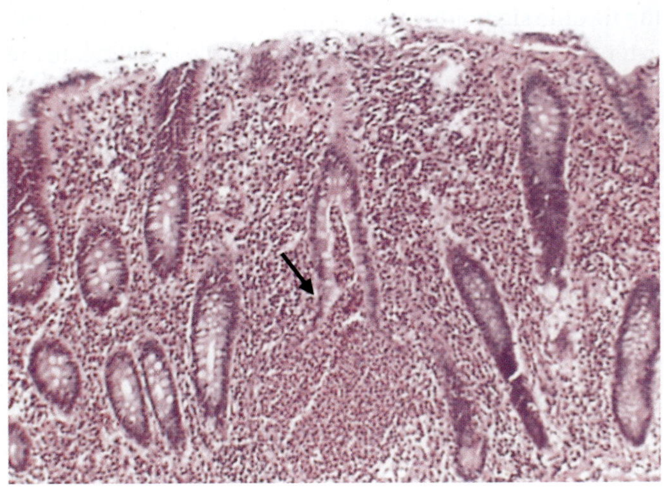

Fig. 61.4: Crypt abscess formation in ulcerative colitis. The central crypt is clearly ruptured at the base (arrow) with resultant abscess formation.

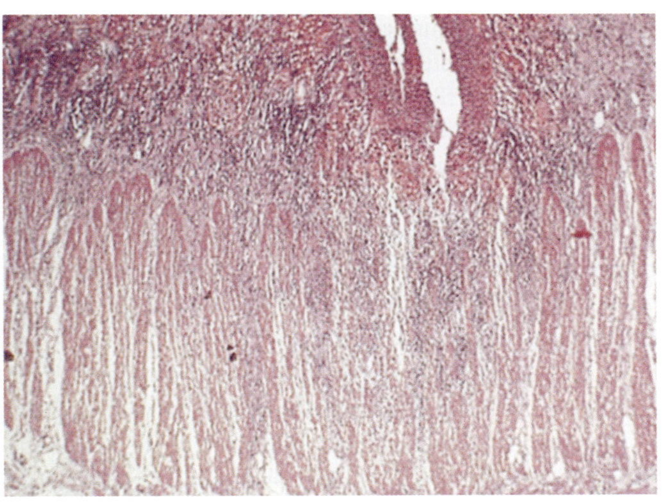

Fig. 61.5: Myocytolysis of muscularis propria. The bundles of smooth muscle are infiltrated with acute inflammatory cells and are undergoing focal myocytolysis.

The extent of macroscopic disease does not always accurately reflect the microscopic changes present in the mucosa, and biopsy changes consistent with mild disease can be found in bowel that appears colonoscopically normal.

Differentiation from Crohn's Disease

Ulcerative colitis must be differentiated from colonic Crohn's disease because the treatments offered may be very different. The main difficulties in distinguishing between ulcerative colitis and Crohn's disease occur either in long-standing colitis, in which marked regeneration and chronic lymphoid cell accumulation, or in the setting of fulminant disease. Transmural inflammation that involves lymphoid aggregates is pathognomonic of Crohn's disease. Granulomas deep in the wall are diagnostic of Crohn's disease, but granulomas may also occur in ulcerative colitis in response to crypt rupture with spillage of mucin into the submucosal tissue (Fig. 61.6).

Macroscopically, discontinuous inflammatory changes (skip lesions) are highly suggestive of Crohn's disease, although this should not be confused with cecal changes

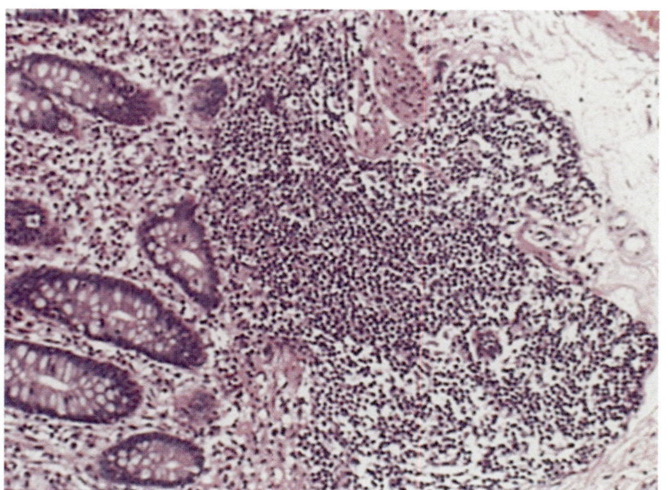

Fig. 61.6: Crypt abscess granuloma. A crypt abscess and a poorly formed macrophage granuloma can be seen.

that can be seen. Although it may occur in the presence of defecatory frequency in ulcerative colitis, perianal disease, such as fistula or chronic fissure, is suggestive of Crohn's disease. The presence of internal fistulation and multiple isolated fibrous strictures is strongly suggestive of Crohn's disease being extremely rare in ulcerative colitis.

Diagnosis based on colonoscopic biopsy alone can be very difficult. Biopsies that contain mucosa only are common, and the presence of regenerative changes caused by topical corticosteroid or immunomodulatory therapy can give rise to bizarre appearances.

A definitive diagnosis is not always possible, particularly on the basis of isolated biopsies early in the course of the disease. The diagnosis may need to be revised in the light of subsequent clinical and pathologic findings, and a label of indeterminate colitis may be used until the complete picture is clear (*see* below). However, a label of indeterminate colitis can give rise to problems in clinical management, and the diagnosis should be reviewed if it is used for >10% of all patients who have inflammatory colitis.

Clinical Features

Ulcerative colitis exists as a spectrum of disease, both in severity and location around the colon, but several distinct clinical entities are recognized under the Montreal Classification (E1/2/3). Any of the types of disease may run an acute relapsing or chronic active course, but isolated left-sided or distal colitis is characteristically more resistant to treatment and more prone to relapse.

Proctitis (E1)

With involvement of the rectum, the symptoms are predominantly of colonic inflammation, such as bloody mucoid diarrhea. Rectal irritation usually gives rise to frequency, urgency, and tenesmus (the sensation of incomplete rectal evacuation), although in a group of patients who have proctitis constipation is the predominant symptom during attacks. Urgency is an important feature and often dominates the lives of patients, limiting their social and working patterns. Diarrhea alone is not common, but can be the presenting feature in a small group of patients. Systemic features are uncommon with limited disease.

Abdominal examination is almost always unremarkable, but rectal palpation usually reveals a soft, velvety mucosa with excess mucus and blood seen on the glove. Proctoscopy reveals the inflamed rectal mucosa, and the upper limit may be seen with the rigid or, more usually, the flexible sigmoidoscope. If there is any doubt about the extent of disease, colonoscopy is advisable to delineate the degree of proximal involvement.

Left-Sided Colitis (E2)

Symptoms of colonic irritation are the most troublesome complaints. As a result of the larger area of involved colon, the symptoms can be more difficult to control, particularly with topical therapy, although high-penetration foam enemas may be effective against disease as far proximal as the splenic flexure. Marked bleeding can be a problem, but frank anemia is usually only a feature in severe or recurrent attacks.

Total Colitis/More Extensive Disease (E3)

Colitis may be present from the outset, but limited or distal disease can spread to involve the more proximal colon with time. Involvement of the whole colon has a marked effect on the clinical picture of the disease. In addition to the symptoms of distal involvement, anergia, fatigue, and anorexia tend to be features when the disease is active as a result of the load of disease activity in the entire colon. Weight loss is common and attributable to a combination of:

- Reduced calorie intake during attacks
- Raised metabolic rate from the inflammatory process
- Protein loss in the diarrhea during chronic or recurrent attacks.

Tenderness of the involved colon is more common in total colitis than in other forms, but marked tenderness should raise a suspicion of more severe colonic inflammation than indicated by the symptoms.

Acute Fulminant Colitis

For acute fulminant colitis see "Acute Severe Colitis (Toxic Colitis and Megacolon)," below.

Chronic Colitis

Following long-standing or intermittent inflammation, the involved colon may undergo characteristic changes, which can produce clinical features that are not solely the result of inflammation. Repeated regeneration of the colonic mucosa following inflammation eventually leads to loss of the mucosal folds and haustral pattern. Together with a degree of fibrosis of the wall, the colon may be featureless and shortened and is referred to as the "drainpipe" or "hosepipe" colon. A consequence may be decreased fluid reabsorption and soft stools in the absence of inflammation. If there is severe fibrosis, particularly in one segment of colon, a postinflammatory stricture may develop that may lead to obstructive symptoms. It may be difficult to exclude a malignant stricture that has developed after chronic colitis, and endoscopic and histologic assessment is usually required once the diagnosis of stricture is made.

Diagnosis

Although biopsies are usually diagnostic, sometimes a combination of clinical, radiologic, endoscopic, and histopathologic features may be needed to make the diagnosis. Rarely, a diagnosis of ulcerative colitis may not be established with certainty even after total colectomy.

Radiology

The prime role of radiology in ulcerative colitis is to monitor rather than diagnose the disease. The features of the acute disease on the plain abdominal radiograph are well recognized and include:

- Mucosal thickening ("thumbprinting")
- Loss of haustrations
- Blurring of the mucosal border.[8]

Findings on the plain abdominal radiograph correlate well with disease extent, particularly in the differentiation between left-sided and total colitis. The severity of mucosal ulceration can be assessed from the plain radiograph,[9,10] particularly when air is introduced to improve visualization of the mucosa.[11] Colonoscopy, however, is the baseline investigation of choice for the diagnosis and assessment of disease including distribution and severity other than in acute severe colitis. A plain abdominal radiograph can be carried out easily, which makes it an effective method of imaging to monitor disease progress, particularly if acute fulminant colitis is suspected where endoscopy is contraindicated. The features of complicated acute severe colitis ("toxic colonic dilatation") include:

- Colonic diameter larger than 5 cm
- Predominantly air-filled colon
- Wall thinning
- Presence of free intra-peritoneal gas.

Contrast studies have a relatively limited role in common clinical practice. A single-contrast enema may help to delineate the extent of the disease on diagnosis, but it is less sensitive than colonoscopy and the risk of perforation caused by pressurization of the colon during the procedure makes it an undesirable investigation during an acute attack. They have also been superseded by colonoscopy for surveillance of chronic or long-standing disease and the diagnosis of malignancy other than patients who cannot tolerate endoscopic assessment or for the assessment of colonic shortening or strictures.

Contrast-enhanced computed tomogram scanning is probably the optimum investigation for the assessment of acute severe colitis, especially for the identification of complications the assessment of extent of colonic involvement by disease. Labeled leukocyte scans correlate well with colonic disease extent, but the benefits of this investigation over those of endoscopy (*see* below) are limited.[12]

Endoscopy

Endoscopy is more useful than contrast radiology in delineating disease extent, and this may be enhanced with additional narrow band imaging techniques.[13] Subtle changes in the mucosa can be identified, and biopsies can be taken throughout the colon. The characteristic findings are:

- Hyperemic hemorrhagic mucosa with contact bleeding
- Bloody purulent mucus in the lumen
- Pseudopolyposis in established severe cases.

The risk of perforation during endoscopy is maximal during acute attacks; the greater the number of biopsies taken, the higher the risk.

Endoscopy is ideal to monitor long-standing disease because the extent can be accurately assessed (Figs. 61.7 to 61.11) and it allows screening for malignant change (*see* further).

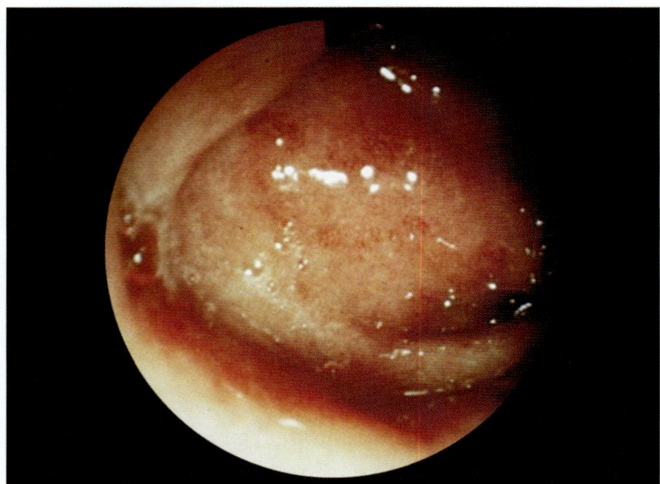

Fig. 61.7: Mild colitis. The mucosa is slightly edematous. There is a blurred vascular pattern and mild erythema.
Source: Reproduced with permission from Silverstein FE, Tytgat GNJ. Gastrointestinal Endoscopy, 3rd edition. London: Mosby–Wolfe; 1997.

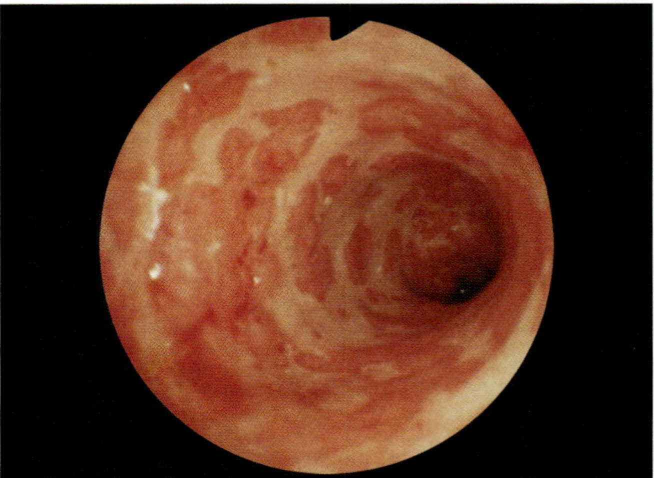

Fig. 61.8: Moderate colitis. The mucosa has aphthous ulceration and there is marked erythema and friability.
Source: Reproduced with permission from Silverstein FE, Tytgat GNJ. Gastrointestinal Endoscopy, 3rd edition. London: Mosby–Wolfe; 1997.

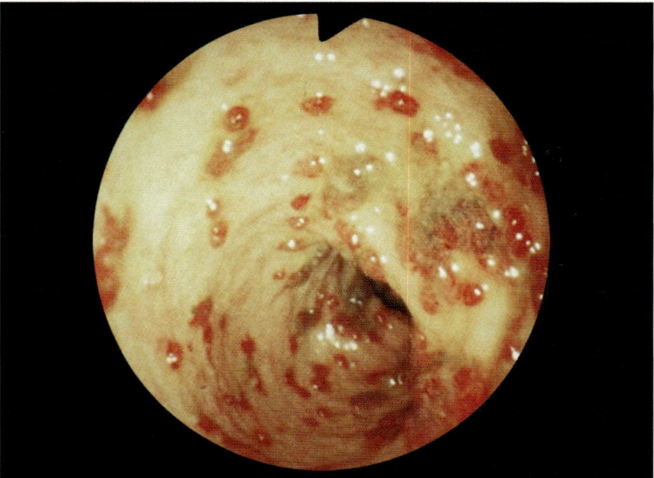

Fig. 61.9: Severe colitis. The mucosa has been almost completely lost with islands of surviving epithelium among a covering of acute inflammatory exudate.
Source: Reproduced with permission from Silverstein FE, Tytgat GNJ. Gastrointestinal Endoscopy, 3rd edition. London: Mosby–Wolfe; 1997.

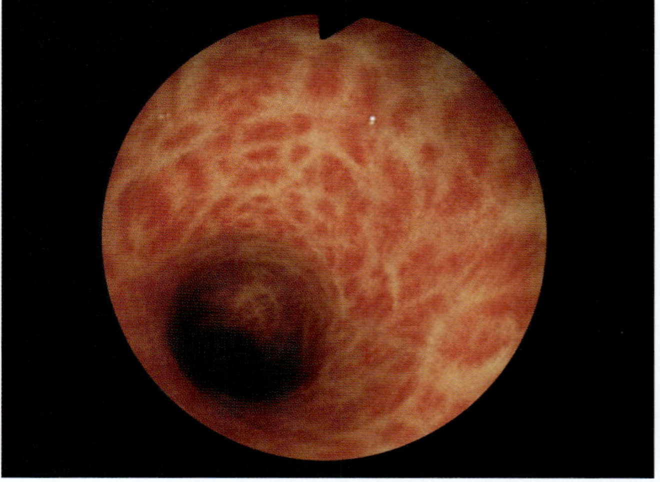

Fig. 61.10: Healing colitis. The epithelium has been restored and a flattened mucosa with a lace-like pattern indicates the sites of previous inflammation.
Source: Reproduced with permission from Silverstein FE, Tytgat GNJ. Gastrointestinal Endoscopy, 3rd edition. London: Mosby–Wolfe; 1997.

Cecal Patch Lesion or Periappendiceal Inflammation

Although the primary site of disease involvement runs from distal to proximal in typically continuous fashion, it is relatively common for a "patch" of mucosal inflammation to exist in the cecal mucosa particularly in the periappendiceal mucosa in the absence of total colitis.[14] Focal cryptitis and mucosal-based nonspecific inflammation is typical of this "lesion".

Backwash Ileitis

Mild inflammatory change such as villous atrophy and mucosal edema in the terminal ileum may be seen in up to a quarter of patients in association with pan colitis, but hardly ever in left-sided disease. It may be caused by reflux of altered colonic fluid and bacterial flora into the terminal ileum when inflammation extends as far as the ascending colon and cecum, but may also represent mild intrinsic ileal inflammation as part of the colitis process.

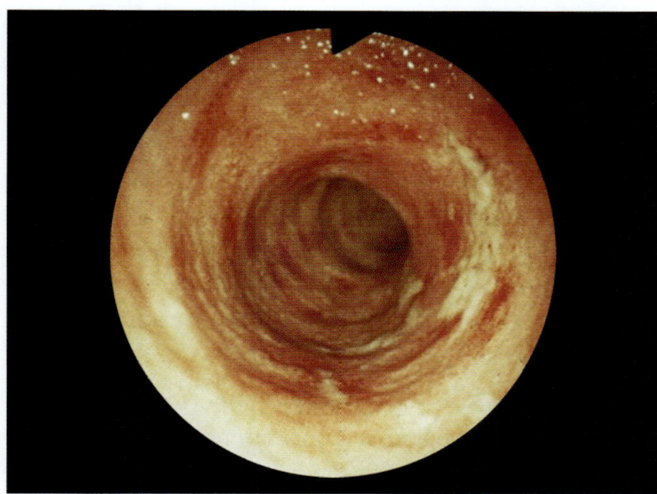

Fig. 61.11: Chronic colitis. The descending colon is characteristically featureless and tubularized with loss of haustrations and mucosal folds. *Source*: Reproduced with permission from Silverstein FE, Tytgat GNJ. Gastrointestinal Endoscopy, 3rd edition. London: Mosby–Wolfe; 1997.

Histopathology

Biopsies alone from acute colitis are not always diagnostic of the disease. Crypt distortion and destruction with a neutrophil mucosal infiltrate indicates disease activity, but is not diagnostic. In partially treated disease, particularly with topical corticosteroid therapy or after cyclosporin A treatment, the histopathologic features can be extremely difficult to interpret, and the use of biopsy to assess disease activity is often inaccurate.

Biopsies play a considerably greater role in screening for malignant change in chronic disease (*see* below).

Antinuclear Cytoplasmic Antibodies

The presence of antinuclear cytoplasmic antibodies (ANCAs) in patients who have ulcerative colitis has been clearly demonstrated,[16-18] with a perinuclear distribution (p-ANCA) in a fine granular "snowdrift" appearance.[17] Perinuclear ANCA is also found in other systemic conditions, notably some necrotizing vasculitides, and although the particular type of p-ANCA in ulcerative colitis appears to differ from that present in these other conditions, there is a similar pattern present in some cases of Crohn's disease and it has no routine role in clinical practice as a useful discriminator between the conditions.

There is some evidence for an association between disease activity in the colon of patients who are p-ANCA positive and the level of p-ANCA, which may indicate that it is a predictor of colonic disease severity[19], and it may be a marker for developing pouchitis following restorative colectomy, although the evidence is unclear.[20,21]

PRINCIPLES OF MANAGEMENT

The management of ulcerative colitis may involve several specialties so a multidisciplinary team (MDT) approach is ideal, particularly when operative management is being considered and the regular meeting of an "IBD MDT" is now commonplace. The various options for management are complementary and not exclusive. The disease has a considerable effect on the lifestyle of patients. Their decisions and responses may be highly subjective, being complicated by the personal experiences of others and their own preconceptions and fears. If possible, following initial diagnosis and management, clinical nurse specialists, stoma therapists, nutritionists, patient support groups, and fellow patients should be involved. These may all help educate the patient and their family and to make any discussion focusing on the difficult future decisions about operative management easier and more objective.

Medical Management

The principles of medical therapy are to reduce and prevent the underlying inflammatory process in the colonic mucosa.[22]

Corticosteroid therapy: Disease within the range of topical delivery methods responds to corticosteroids in the form of prednisolone suppositories, enemas, and (high retention) foam enemas, although they are rarely the first line of treatment for disease up to the splenic flexure.[23] Acute exacerbations of distal disease may need to be controlled this way but although there may be reduced toxicity with topical corticosteroid therapy, systemic effects may result in part from absorption of corticosteroids across the inflamed mucosa.

Systemic corticosteroid therapy is usually reserved for severe distal diseases, slowly responsive distal disease, or total colitis. Parenteral routes are preferred initially, especially for acute or toxic colitis, because high loading doses can be given this way and the onset of action is more rapid. Treatment can normally be switched over to the oral route once the disease has been brought under control, with a progressively reducing regimen. Budesonide is a corticosteroid available in enema and oral form and has effects equivalent to those of prednisolone given by a similar route.[24] The pharmacokinetics of budesonide also confer the advantage of a much lower endogenous cortisol suppression than that with prednisolone therapy.[25]

Longer-term maintenance therapy with corticosteroid is not commonly used because of the side effects, such as osteoporosis, disordered protein metabolism, and truncal obesity, but budesonide may offer the opportunity for such prevention as the side effect profile is reduced.

Salicylic acid derivatives: 5-aminosalicylic acid (5-ASA), which is effective in both acute and relapsing disease, is the drug of first choice for acute exacerbations. It may be given both rectally and orally, as well as by foam enema, with excellent retention properties,[26] and has the benefit of offering a corticosteroid-sparing effect with a reduction in corticosteroid dose in responsive patients. The beneficial results, particularly in distal colitis, have been confirmed by meta-analysis.[27] Oral and topical 5-ASA compounds have a protective effect against relapse[28,29] when used over the longer term, and there may be a reduction in the risk of malignant change. Their use can be limited by bone marrow toxicity, but this is rare.

Cyclosporin A: Cyclosporin A is a second-line therapy for acute ulcerative colitis, especially if the disease is of short duration. Its acts by interfering with lymphocyte activation and is a potent immunosuppressive. Although not common, the serious nature of its side effects, such as bone marrow suppression and nephrotoxicity, limit its use to acute attacks resistant to conventional therapy. It is administered either as a foam enema or intravenously. There is considerable evidence that many patients can avoid early colectomy if cyclosporin is added to standard therapy that has failed to induce remission[30,31] and that colectomy following cyclosporin administration may be equivalent to corticosteroid therapy alone.[32] Debate continues, however, as to whether the ultimate rate of operative intervention is altered[33], and a course of several months maintenance therapy is usual for those who do respond, with its main use being as a bridge to introduction of other immunomodulator therapy.

Azathioprine and 6 mercaptopurine (6-MP): The antimetabolites azathioprine and 6-MP have been largely replaced by the immunomodulators anti-TNF-α and cyclosporin as the medical treatment of choice in corticosteroid-resistant attacks but may still have an occasional place as third-line treatment or if immunomodulators are contraindicated (e.g. renal disease, hypertension, hypocholesterolemia); they are more widely used in maintenance therapy. Oral cyclosporin maintenance therapy can be used to act as a bridge until azathioprine therapy begins to take effect (usually 2–4 months). Before treatment the patient's thiopurine methyltransferase (TPMT) level or genotype should be assessed since low levels of TPMT activity are associated with a high risk of drug-related complications, particularly myelosuppression.

Antitumor necrosis factor α (Anti-TNF-α): This family of immunomodulators is commonly used as the second line therapy of choice in patients failing to respond to first line therapy in acute attacks, although the relatively slower speed of onset of action may limit their use in the most pressing situations of acute severe colitis.

Supportive measures: Nutritional support may be necessary in severely ill patients. Total parenteral nutrition may help to maintain the nutritional state of patients who are preparing to undergo operation or in whom prolonged treatment has led to nutritional compromise. There is no evidence that total parenteral nutrition reduces attack severity or duration or lessens the complications associated with operative management. Colonic mucosal nutrition has been suggested as an important factor in supporting the colonic mucosa during attacks, and the use of diets or foam enemas that contain butyrate and omega-3 fatty acids has been advocated, but their success is yet to be proved.[34]

Long-term dietary adjustments may be necessary in chronic colitis. Antidiarrheal agents, such as codeine phosphate, loperamide or diphenoxylate, may be useful for mildly symptomatic cases, but should not be used for long term and do not change the course of the disease. Antibiotics also do not alter the course of disease.

Operative Management

Indications: Operative management has three clear objectives:

- Save the life or prevent the continued deterioration of a patient with acute colitis who has failed/is failing to respond to medical therapy
- Cure the symptoms of a patient who has chronic or relapsing intermittent disease
- Treat or prevent the complications of recurrent or long-standing disease (e.g. carcinoma of colon).

It can also be argued that operative management offers a cure for patients who have acute colitis, in whom medical therapy palliates but does not ultimately control the disease.

Elective versus urgent operation: The timing of operation can be difficult. For those patients who have peritonitis, massive hemorrhage or obvious rapidly worsening acute severe ("fulminant" or "toxic") colitis, an emergency operation is appropriate. For elective indications, timing is a matter of patient preparation as much as operative need. This should include psychological and physical preparation of the patient with appropriate counseling from stoma and other clinical specialists to enable the correct choice of procedure and to build patient cooperation.

The timing of operative intervention for episodes of severe acute colitis is more difficult. With close cooperation between physicians and surgical staff, a salvage colectomy in a very sick patient may be avoided. A 5-day regimen of aggressive treatment with high-dose intravenous methylprednisolone and rectal prednisolone can be used together with serial plain abdominal radiographs to assess the patient's response to treatment. Failure of first-line treatment can be followed by the use of cyclosporin or anti-TNF-α therapy.[33]

The disadvantage of prolonged medical therapy that ultimately fails is the adverse effect that immunosuppression can have on the mortality and morbidity rates. The duration for a trial of medical therapy should therefore be clearly defined to ensure that a colectomy is carried out without undue delay. Corticosteroids may mask the severity of the disease; however, close clinical and radiologic monitoring is necessary.

Several clinical features predict those patients who ultimately need operative management. These can be used to select those patients who should be offered acute colectomy if second-line medical therapy fails to induce remission. Such indicators include:

- Failure to respond to intravenous immunomodulators within 48 hours
- Stool frequency exceeding eight per day
- C-reactive protein concentration over 45 mg/L.[35]

Total Proctocolectomy (Panproctocolectomy)

Indications: Total proctocolectomy is indicated for patients who prefer complete disease control and who do not wish to risk the possible complications associated with a restorative operation. Occasionally, it may be the preferred option of the surgeon for technical reasons, including situations in which there is inadequate sphincter function to permit reconstruction, such as in the elderly and those who have damaged sphincters or poor results on physiologic testing. In addition, it may be necessary to excise the anal canal for actual or potential malignancy low in the rectum. Patients who have a foreshortened mesentery, obesity or a mesenteric vascular injury during the operation may require proctocolectomy and ileostomy. Patients who have had a temporary ileostomy following acute colectomy and who have become familiar with their stoma may opt for a conver-sion to proctocolectomy (completion proctectomy) if the rectal stump remains troublesome.

Technical considerations: Abdominal colectomy is performed as for any benign condition, with the vascular pedicles being taken as close to the colonic wall as convenient. Laparoscopic resection is relatively straightforward, although chronic inflammatory change may be associated with omental wrapping of the left colon in particular, making mobilization more challenging than normal. The rectal dissection is kept close to the serosal perimuscular plane. The mesorectum and the middle rectal pedicles, such as may exist, can be deliberately preserved using a "periserosal" plane of excision to minimize the risk of pelvic autonomic nerve dysfunction, particularly in men,[36] although in experienced hands the mesorectum may be safely excised in the mesorectal plane. The anus is excised in the intersphincteric plane to optimize healing of the perineal wound.

Subtotal Colectomy with Ileorectal Anastomosis

Indications: Subtotal colectomy with ileorectal anastomosis is carried out less frequently than total proctocolectomy because of the risks of persistent symptoms from the retained inflamed rectum and of malignant change that increases over time. The procedure is usually reserved for the elderly for whom pouch formation is inappropriate and ileostomy is either impractical or refused. It is also occasionally used for prepubertal children during their schooling and adolescence as a temporizing measure before pouch or ileostomy formation. Ileorectal anastomosis may also be preferred for patients who have ulcerative colitis, a quiescent rectum and inoperable metastatic colon cancer. Continued close surveillance of the rectal remnant is necessary in older patients to identify malignant change, and this requires a compliant and motivated patient who has appropriate medical support. The rate of completion proctectomy and conversion to an ileostomy is approximately 35% for patients with persistent symptoms and less than this for reasons of personal choice.

Kock Pouch

The Kock pouch (Fig. 61.12) was designed as a reservoir formed from the terminal ileum together with a valved outlet, which prevents spontaneous pouch emptying.[37] The pouch is emptied by self-catheterization of the valve.

Indications: The indications for the Kock continent ileostomy are similar to those for the conventional Brooke ileostomy (so called because Bryan Brooke first described primary mucocutaneous suturing of an everted, spouted ileostomy), but in patients who wish to minimize the social and psychological effects of permanently wearing a stoma appliance. The patient must have good understanding and motivation because the intubation needed to empty the pouch requires dexterity and care. The benefits of needing to wear only a small, discreet covering for activities such as swimming and sexual intimacy make this attractive to patients. In particular, it may be used for patients who:

- Are not suitable for, or who do not wish to consider, ileoanal pouch construction
- Have already undergone completion proctectomy, but wish to be rid of their Brooke ileostomy
- Require excision of an ileoanal pouch for whatever reason.

The Kock pouch is associated with a higher rate of complications than a conventional Brooke ileostomy, primarily related to poor valve function, fistula, stomal stenosis, and retraction[38] and has a higher pouch-related complication rate and higher long-term failure rate than ileoanal pouch formation.

Technical considerations: The pouch is formed from terminal ileum by doubly (or trebly) folding the bowel to form a reservoir of suitable volume. A section of the efferent limb is then intussuscepted into the pouch to form a 5-cm-long nipple valve, which prevents spontaneous pouch emptying. The formation of the valve is a major determinant for the functional result of the pouch. The valve construction may be reinforced with synthetic material, such as a polypropylene mesh strip,[39] or the nipple valve may be stapled to the pouch[40] to reduce valve slippage and dysfunction.

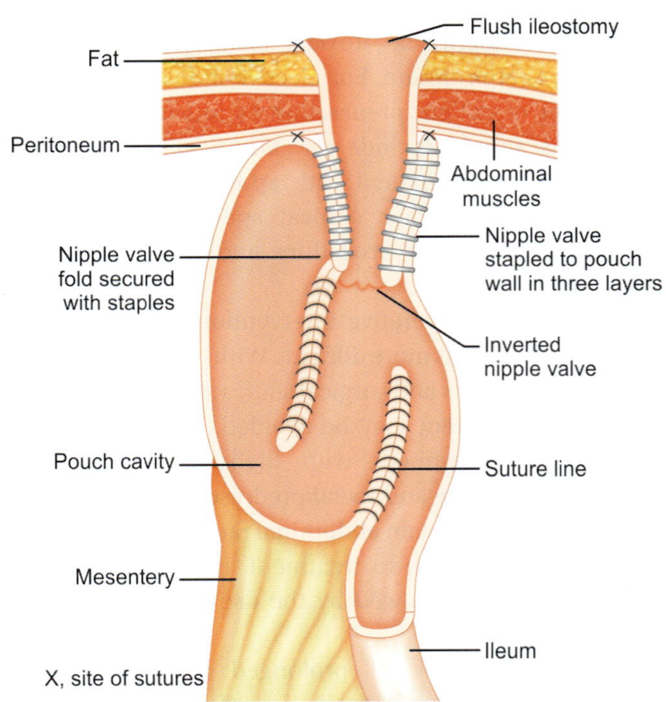

Fig. 61.12: Continent ileostomy (Kock pouch).

Ileoanal (Pelvic) Pouch with Ileopouch–Anal Anastomosis

Indications: Since the first suggestions that a pouch formed from ileum could be anatomized to the anal canal to use the endogenous sphincters and avoid an external stoma of any kind, the ileoanal pouch has undergone many revisions. It is now considered by most surgeons to be the operation of choice for most patients who require operation for ulcerative colitis. Informed consent requires discussion of this option when advising a patient on operative management. There are, however, important considerations in patient selection to produce the good functional results that have popularized the ileoanal pouch.

It is important to exclude a diagnosis of Crohn's disease as far as possible, because recurrence of Crohn's disease in the pouch is often associated with a poor outcome and a high conversion rate to a permanent ileostomy.[41] There is some evidence that the results with particular groups of patients who have Crohn's disease and have been offered an ileoanal pouch are similar to those for ulcerative colitis,[42] but the indications are limited and not widely accepted. Other important considerations are:

- Evaluation of the anal sphincter to demonstrate good physiologic function
- Previous or current use of corticosteroids, as this may influence the choice of procedure or the decision to form a defunctioning ileostomy proximal to the pouch
- The patient's age, social and domestic arrangements (would a pouch or a permanent ileostomy be preferable?)
- Psychologic and physical preparation of the patient.

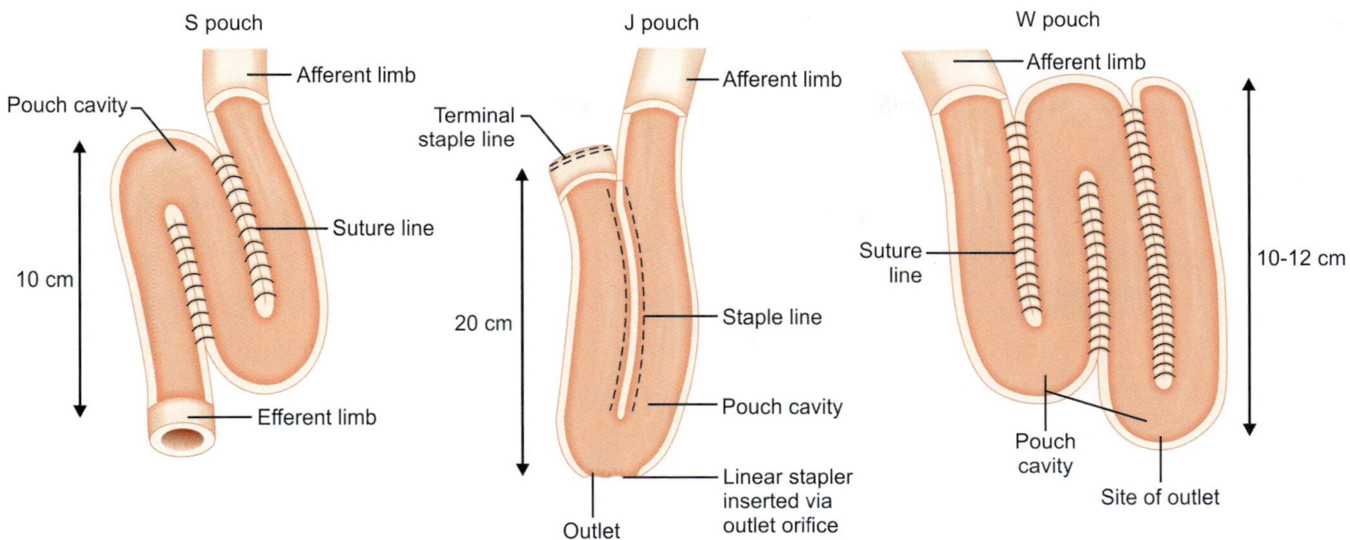

Fig. 61.13: S, J and W ileal pouches. The common methods of pouch construction offer different sizes of reservoir, although only the J pouch is usually made using mechanical staplers. There is little obvious advantage to anyone type of pouch.

Although most patients are extremely satisfied with the functional outcome of pouch operations, some may have unrealistically high expectations so careful preoperative counseling is essential. Patient support groups and previous patients are invaluable sources of information and advice for potential pouch patients.

Technical considerations: For elective procedures, the operation consists of total proctocolectomy or completion proctectomy in those patients who have previously undergone acute colectomy. The rectal dissection may be in the mesorectal or close rectal/periserosal plane to optimize preservation of the pelvic autonomics, and the upper anal canal is mobilized. There are several issues regarding the details of technique in forming the pelvic pouch.

A. *Preservation of the anorectal mucosa:* No clear evidence indicates that preservation of a cuff of the muscularis propria of the rectum with stripping of the mucosa down to the dentate line conveys any benefit in terms of retaining the sensation of rectal fullness. Transection at the anorectal junction is an easier technique, and the results appear to be similar or better in terms of function.[43]

B. *Pouch construction:* The first pouch design was the original S pouch with a triple fold of terminal ileum. The initial length of the efferent limb was long, which often caused obstructive outflow problems. The S pouch is still used, but with a considerably shorter efferent limb. The double (J pouch) or fourfold (Nicholls W) pouches are now the most popular (Fig. 61.13).

The advantage of including more folds of ileum is that the functional volume of the pouch is increased. There is good evidence that the volume of the pouch as well as its compliance are important to obtain good function,[44,45] but the evidence that design makes a marked difference to function is poor.[46--48] The increased length of ileum needed for the multiply folded pouches occasionally poses technical difficulties in mobilizing sufficient ileum to form the pouch and position it in the pelvis without tension. This can be troublesome in obese or tall male patients. There is no clear evidence that a stapled pouch construction is superior to a hand-sewn one. The J pouch is often easier to form with stapling devices, while the W version lends itself more to hand-sewn formation.

C. *Anastomotic technique:* Two options exist for pouchanal anastomosis. The anorectal junction may be transected at the level of the pelvic floor with a transverse stapling device (Fig. 61.14), and a conventional end-to-end circular staple gun is inserted into the anal stump with the anvil secured in the orifice of the pouch (Fig. 61.15). This comprises the double stapling technique.

Alternatively, the mucosa of the anorectal junction and anal transition zone can be dissected free from the muscularis propria, and a hand-sewn anastomosis to the anus can be fashioned (Fig. 61.16). Theoretically, this mucosectomy removes all columnar epithelium, and thus avoids the risk of recurrent inflammation or the development of malignant change in the columnar epithelial remnant.

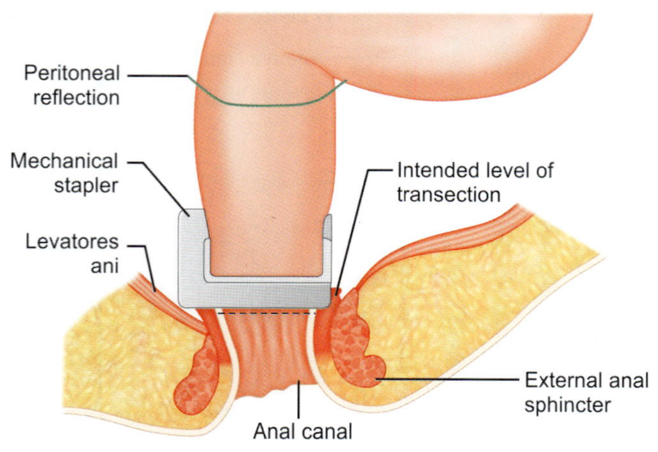

Fig. 61.14: Stapled rectal transection.

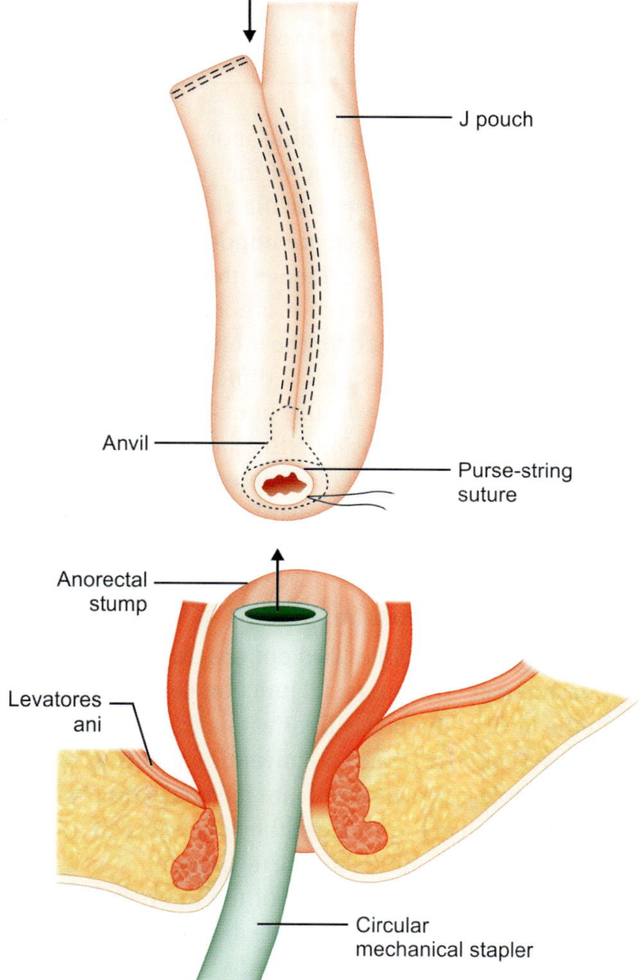

Fig. 61.15: Endoanal stapled pouch–anal anastomosis.

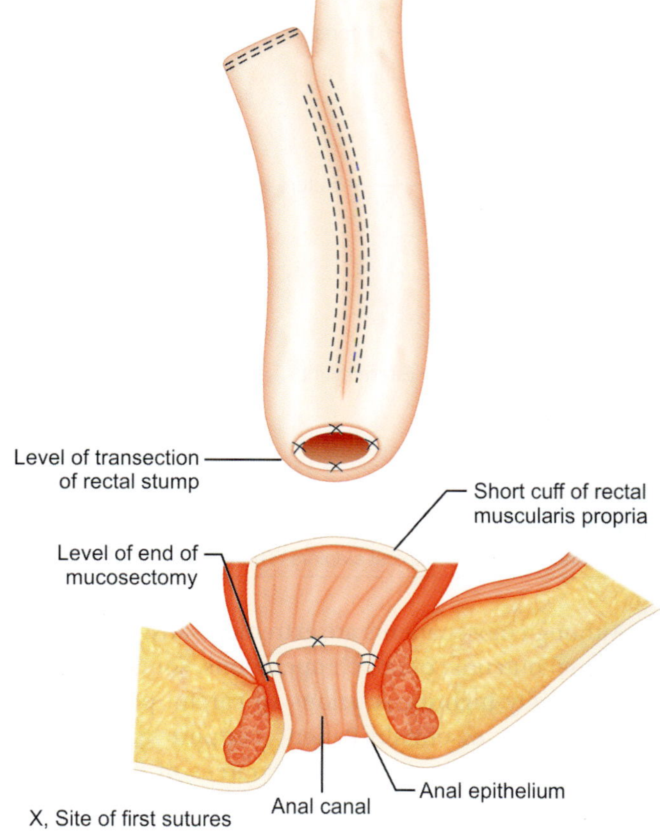

Fig. 61.16: Hand sewn pouch–anal anastomosis showing the level of mucosectomy.

The double stapling may be technically easier, and since the only instrument introduced into the anal canal is the stapling device, this avoids the need to retract the anus. This omission may help to prevent sphincter injury that may detract from pouch function, and preservation of the mucosa of the anal transition zone may also contribute to improved function by preserving fine submucosal nerve endings involved in sensation during sampling of the pouch contents. Overall, the balance of evidence favors the stapled technique in most surgeons' hands, but there is a lack of large controlled trials,[49] particularly in younger patients who have good-to-excellent documented preoperative sphincter function.

D. *Laparoscopic pouch surgery:* Rectal resection (proctectomy) and ileal pouch–anal anastomosis is, in many respects, an operation ideally suited to laparoscopic surgery. Patients are often relatively young, potentially placing a greater value on cosmetic impact, undergoing surgery for a benign condition with a modest lifetime risk of further surgery. Visualization of the rectal dissection is usually very good to the pelvic floor,

Table 61.1 Pouch function following restorative proctocolectomy.

Parameter	Normal range	
	Double stapled	*Mucosectomy*
Frequency of emptying/day	3–8	3–8
Frequency of nocturnal emptying	0–2	0–2
Incidence of urgency of evacuation (% of cases)	<10	<10
Night leakage (% of cases)	10	20–30
Discrimination of flatus (% of cases)	>60	>60

From McGuire et al.[54]

Table 61.2 Causes of pouch dysfunction.

Prepouch
Bacterial overgrowth as a result of poor pouch inlet function
Adhesions
Small bowel dysmotility
Food intolerance
Pouch
Pouchitis
Peripouch or pelvic sepsis
Small pouch volume
Pouch dysmotility
Postpouch
Pouch–anal stenosis
Sphincter complex dysfunction
Pouch-perineal fistula
Inflammation of residual columnar epithelium
Anal fissure

although the transection at the anorectal junction using current semiangled endoscopic stapling devices is a challenge, particularly in the male pelvis, due to limitation of the placement of the device flush with the pelvic floor. The mini Pfannenstiel incision may need to be enlarged to allow the placement of a conventional "open" transverse linear stapler to ensure there is no element of retained rectal wall. Functional outcomes and complications are, however, probably no different between laparoscopic and open pouch formation.[50]

E. *Defunctioning loop ileostomy:* Pouch formation is often accompanied by the construction of a proximal diverting loop ileostomy. There is no difference in the risk of pouch-related complications with and without stoma formation, and the belief that some complications, notably pelvic sepsis, may be more severe in the absence of a protective stoma is debatable.[51] The ileostomy is not without complications (*see* below) and requires a further hospital admission and procedure for closure. Ileostomy is still widely used in situations in which the operation is technically difficult or the pouch has been created in a semiurgent situation in the presence of systemic immunosuppression or malnutrition. Most surgeons advocate a selective and liberal use of defunctioning.

Pouch Dysfunction and Pouchitis

Most ileoanal pouches have good function that is acceptable to most patients. Variations in dietary intake and daily routine influence pouch output, both in frequency and content, but most patients can expect results similar to those given in Table 61.1.[52-54]

The broad term pouch dysfunction includes both patients who have unacceptable function and those who have additional symptoms that may indicate a pathologic process occurring in relation to the pouch. Although some patients do have function at the extremes of the normal range, symptoms of excessive frequency, urgency, and leakage may indicate pathology, particularly if the symptoms are new. Pain in the abdomen, pelvis or perineum, bloody and mucoid stools and systemic upset should always raise the suspicion of an underlying problem. Conditions that give rise to symptoms of pouch dysfunction are listed in Table 61.2, but one problem may be linked to another (e.g., pouch outlet obstruction that causes stasis and bacterial overgrowth) and a methodical approach to the clinical problems is necessary.[55]

Investigation of pouch dysfunction should include a careful history to determine the exact pattern of symptoms and their relationship to food and pouch evacuation. A digital examination of the pouch and careful inspection of the perineum is required, if necessary under general anesthetic, if severe pain is present from sepsis or stenosis. Rigid or flexible pouchoscopy is carried out, and a full pattern of biopsies of the pouch and prepouch ileum is obtained. Endoluminal ultrasound, anal physiology studies and MRI scanning may be required to differentiate between the possible causes.

The term pouchitis has in the past been a source of confusion because it was used to refer to a range of symptoms of pouch dysfunction. A uniformly agreed-upon definition of pouchitis is still lacking, but several have been proposed.[56,57] The term is generally taken to identify a group of patients who have a syndrome of malaise, bloody diarrhea and systemic upset together with endoscopic evidence of pouch inflammation and histologic evidence of acute inflammation on biopsy. Using these definitions, the incidence of pouchitis is in the region of 10–20%. It is likely that there is more than one cause for the clinical

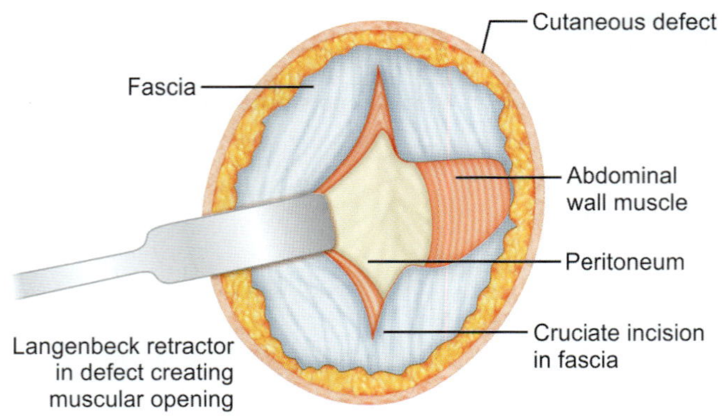

Fig. 61.17: Creation of a snug body wall defect.

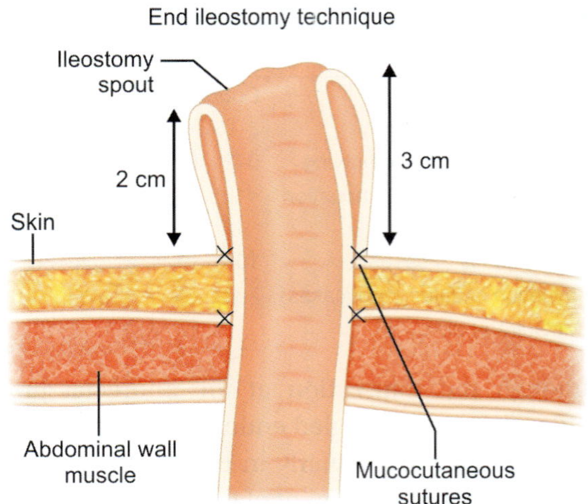

Fig. 61.18: Positioning of the sutures to ensure a down-pointing ileostomy spout.

syndrome. Bacterial overgrowth may be directly involved in some cases, but no evidence shows a relationship between bacterial counts and symptoms except when there are episodes of infective diarrhea. Colonic phenotypic change, which occurs in the vast majority of pouches, may render the pouch liable to inflammation similar to that of ulcerative colitis, and it is widely accepted that a marked proportion of cases represent a form of recurrence of the underlying disease process in the pouch.

Most episodes of pouchitis respond well to metronidazole. Occasionally, alternative antibiotics, topically administered corticosteroids or 5-ASA compounds may be tried. It is only rarely that the pouch needs to be defunctioned via a loop ileostomy, and the excision rate for pouchitis is <5%.[52]

Principles of Ileostomy

Whether formed as an end or loop stoma, permanent or temporary, the main principles of ileostomy formation are the same. Successful rehabilitation of the patient requires adherence to these principles:

- The orifice of the stoma should be well clear of the skin surface, ideally protruding 2 or 3 cm to allow the contents to discharge "out" into an appliance
- The stoma is sited within the surface marking of the rectus abdominis muscle on the summit of the infraumbilical fat mound, away from skin creases or disturbed skin
- Avoidance of bony prominences is essential if the stoma appliance is to fit securely; care should always be taken to avoid sitting the stoma beneath pendulous folds of the abdomen so that it is visible and easy to access for the patient.

Preoperative marking of the stoma site with the stoma therapist avoids many difficulties that the surgeon may not anticipate in a supine patient and should be attempted for all cases, especially those that are elective.

Types of Ileostomy and Techniques

End: The end or Brooke ileostomy is often technically easier to form than a loop stoma, except in obese patients. A circle of skin is excised. The rectus fascia is incised for approximately 3 cm vertically (Fig. 61.17). The rectus muscle fibers are separated (not divided), and the posterior sheath is incised to accommodate an aperture through which the ileum and associated mesentery will fit snugly. Although often said to be typically "two fingers" in diameter, the size varies according to body habitus and care should be taken not to over-widen the defect in the elderly or those with little abdominal musculature as this may result in an excessive rate of (para)stomal hernia in the long term. Once the ileum has been delivered and any staples or excess tissue removed, the spout is formed by the placement of sutures, which will evert the spout once tightened. A method of suturing to produce a downward-pointing stoma is shown in Figure 61.18. Suturing full thickness of skin should be avoided as the needle may "drive" in implants of ileal mucosa, which can secrete mucus.

Loop: The body wall defect for the loop stoma is formed in the same way as that for an end ileostomy, but is slightly larger. The difficulty is to create an adequate spout on the proximal end (Fig. 61.19). It is important to mark clearly the proximal end, especially if the abdomen is closed before the stoma is opened. A soft bridge or rod may be inserted either subcutaneously or resting on the skin to

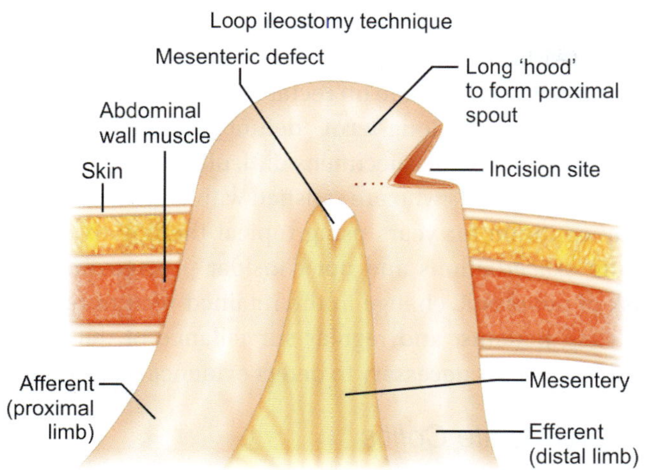

Fig. 61.19: Opening of a loop ileostomy to provide a proximal spout.

support the loop, and the lumen is opened at the 9 o'clock position (i.e., 5–10 mm above the skin surface). Protrusion of the spout is then achieved as for the end stoma, except that to encourage eversion of the spouted afferent limb, sutures are placed from the ileal wall to the subserosa and thence to the abdominal skin at the 12 o'clock position, but sutures are placed either side of the afferent limb, through the ileal wall midway between this 12 o'clock suture and "bridge" of wall tissue between the two limbs, with the subserosal bite being placed close to the edge of the mesenteric fat of the afferent limb and thence to the abdominal wall skin at the 3 and 9 o'clock positions. This will encourage folding of this section of wall under the afferent limb to enhance the spouting without recourse to manipulation of the spout by instruments.

Complications: The complications are shown in Table 61.3. Although rarely life-threatening, the incidence of stoma associated complications is high. Poor operative technique is often a factor, particularly in retraction (undue tension on the ileum), prolapse and herniation (inappropriately large defects) and infarction and stenosis (ischemia).[58,59]

Table 61.3 Complications of end ileostomy.

Early complications	*% of cases*
Stomal sepsis	<5
Stomal ischemia	5–10
Retraction	<5
Hemorrhage	<5
Late complications	
Stenosis	10
Prolapse	5–10
Peristomal dermatitis	10–30
Parastomal herniation	5–15
Psychosexual dysfunction	25

Table 61.4 Complications of ileoanal pouch formation.

Early complications	*% of cases*
Small bowel obstruction	10
Pelvic sepsis	8–10
Pouch hemorrhage	2–4
Late complications	
Pouch dysfunction (includes "pouchitis")	10–30
Pouch–anal stricture	<10
Pelvice autonomic dysfunction	<5

Complications of Operative Management for Ulcerative Colitis

The complications of ileoanal pouch formation are shown in Table 61.4.[53]

Special Problems

Ulcerative colitis and pregnancy: The fertility rate of women who have ulcerative colitis is similar to that of women who do not have ulcerative colitis.[61] This rate includes those who have undergone operative management. Those who have undergone colectomy, with ileostomy formation, tend to have a higher rate of fertility than preoperatively, probably attributable to higher sexual activity because of enhanced general health and libido.[62] Those who have had a proctectomy with or without a pouch have a reduced fertility rate, presumably on account of tubal occlusion secondary to pelvic adhesions, and this may be taken into consideration when planning the timing of surgery. Pregnancy appears to have little effect on the course of the disease, although occasional exacerbations have been noted in the third trimester.[63] The effect of the disease on the pregnancy is less clear. Some evidence indicates an increased rate of preterm delivery and low birth weight.[64,65] A related issue in pregnancy is the role of medical therapy. Cyclosporin is contraindicated in the first trimester of pregnancy, but has been shown to be nonteratogenic in a range of species;[66] 5-ASA compounds are safe in pregnancy.[67]

Acute Severe Colitis (Toxic Colitis and Megacolon)

Toxic or fulminant colitis characteristically occurs in the setting of total colitis, particularly at the onset of the disease. Any flare-up of ulcerative colitis in any distribution, however, can become acutely life threatening. Acute severe colitis is associated with a profound systemic upset including a persistent pyrexia, a tachycardia disproportionate to the fever, greatly raised erythrocyte sedimentation rate, anemia, systemic hypotension, and a colonic diameter >6 cm on plain abdominal radiography. Extreme local irritation may be a feature, and results in copious diarrhea and grossly bloody stool. Close observation of patients who have a severe attack is necessary, including daily blood tests and plain abdominal radiography. Symptoms of a sudden, unexpected reduction in stool frequency or abdominal distention are highly suggestive of toxic colonic dilatation.

In cases of acute toxic dilatation, a rapid progression of the disease leads to thinning of the colonic wall, dilatation, and potential ischemic perforation. The mortality rate associated with fecal peritonitis in perforation has been shown to exceed 30%,[68] since many patients are on large doses of parenteral immunosuppressives at the time of operative management. The role of acute operative intervention is discussed below, but the essence of treatment is to identify the situation as it develops and to carry out emergency acute colectomy, which may be lifesaving.

Management of the Rectal Stump

Following acute colectomy or colectomy when the rectal stump has been retained, there is a risk of proctitis in the isolated rectum. The cause may be:

- Recurrence of intrinsic colitis
- Bacterial stasis with overgrowth and secondary mucosal inflammation
- Mucosal hyponutrition, caused by lack of short chain fatty acids (hydroxybutyrate and acetoacetate) normally present in feces due to bacterial action from which the rectal mucosa derives a substantial proportion of its nutritional requirements.

Its ready accessibility means that topical treatment to the rectum is relatively easy. Corticosteroid or 5-ASA enemas are usually sufficient to control any episodes of active disease, and fatty acids enemas can be prepared and administered regularly to control symptoms due to nutritional deficiency. Systemic therapy is usually not necessary, and only rarely is completion proctectomy indicated for resistant disease or bleeding. The diagnosis of proctitis can be made on rectal biopsy, but the changes associated with long-term defunctioning can make interpretation of the specimens difficult.

Many patients who are satisfied with an end ileostomy may continue for years using topical therapy to control acute exacerbations and not consider proctectomy. The risk of neoplastic change in the retained rectum remains in such patients, and regular surveillance of the stump with biopsies is necessary to detect evidence of dysplasia.

Indeterminate Colitis

If the histopathologic features are unclear despite the clinical picture, a diagnosis of indeterminate colitis may be necessary. Some pathologists add a caveat indicating the probable definitive diagnosis (e.g. indeterminate colitis—probably Crohn's disease), but this diagnosis raises several important issues. Ablation of the rectum and anus is the usual operative treatment of choice for widespread colonic Crohn's disease, but renders the patient ineligible for a reconstructive pouch operation. Equally, ileoanal pouch construction in the presence of Crohn's disease can lead to severe complications that necessitate excision and conversion to an end ileostomy. If the diagnosis is uncertain based upon preoperative biopsies and clinical features, it is reasonable to leave the rectum *in situ* and form an end ileostomy. This policy allows full histopathology of the excised specimen and does not preclude any definitive or reconstructive operation later.

If the diagnosis remains uncertain, the risks and benefits of the possible options should be presented to and fully discussed with the patient. The rate of ileopouchanal anastomosis failure when there is a diagnosis of indeterminate colitis may be up to twice that of pouches for confirmed ulcerative colitis.[69] In this context it is important to use comparisons of ileopouch-anal anastomosis for Crohn's or indeterminate colitis with other operations for the same disease.

Cancer and Ulcerative Colitis

There is little evidence that the primary disease mechanism in ulcerative colitis is itself a neoplastic process in the colon or rectum. The risk of neoplastic change in colitis, however, has long been recognized. It is likely to be related to the increased cell division rate in the colonic mucosa, which increases the risk of acquiring the genetic mutations necessary for malignant change. The overall cumulative risk may be as high as 10% after 20 years of active disease.[70] Several features of the disease are markers of an increased risk of malignant change, including:

- Early age of onset
- Severe episode of colitis at presentation
- The presence of total colitis
- Chronic active disease
- Associated primary sclerosing cholangitis.

Although dysplasia occurs in ulcerative colitis and is probably a precursor to frank malignant change, there are several problems associated with this finding. A diagnosis of dysplasia may be difficult, particularly in the presence of regenerative change in the colonic mucosa on biopsy. Mucosal biopsies have a low sensitivity to the presence of dysplasia, a sensitivity that rises only as increasing numbers of biopsies are obtained. Some evidence suggests that malignant change can occur in areas that showed no evidence of dysplasia despite thorough biopsies, indicating possible spontaneous malignant change. It has been suggested that aneuploidy of the colonocytes on biopsy may be a more sensitive and reliable marker for potential future malignant change, but this is unproved[71-73] and entails an expensive program if carried out routinely.

Dysplasia-associated lesions or masses DALMs are areas of mucosal dysplasia with a heaped, nodular or firm consistency that occur in ulcerative colitis. They are most readily located in the mucosa of colectomy specimens after fixation, but can be identified at endoscopy, particularly with chromoendoscopy. Although the lesions probably occur in <5% of patients who have ulcerative colitis and dysplasia,[74] they are endoscopically impossible to differentiate from early invasive tumors and are associated with a greater than normal risk of high-grade dysplasia or synchronous malignancy elsewhere in the colon.

Surveillance mechanisms: Currently, colonoscopy with mucosal biopsy remains the only accepted way of screening for (pre)malignant change. It is not clear when to start surveillance, but it is usually considered to be after 10 years of active disease. Most recent guidance (British Society of Gastroenterology Guidelines for the Management of Inflammatory Bowel Disease in 2011) recommends division of patients into those at low, medium or high risk according to extent of disease, activity, a diagnosis of Crohn's colitis, coexisting family history, presence of PSC and presence of dysplasia. This can be used to determine interval (1, 3 or 5 years). The usual procedure has been a full colonoscopy with widespread dyespraying to identify areas of possible concern as preferable to random biopsies, although biopsies of any suspicious areas or polypoid lesions should be undertaken.

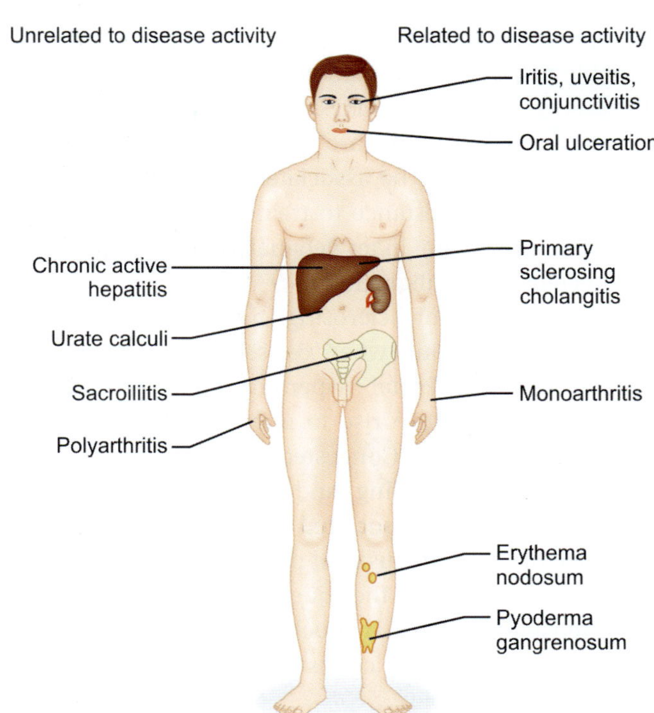

Fig. 61.20: Extraintestinal manifestations of ulcerative colitis.

When to recommend colectomy is unclear. The presence of malignant change is an absolute indication. High-grade dysplasia confirmed by two independent pathologists, particularly at two or more sites, indicates a need for prophylactic colectomy in an otherwise healthy, low surgical-risk patient. There is some debate about whether low-grade dysplasia is associated with a markedly increased risk of carcinoma, particularly in older patients.[75,76]

Extraintestinal manifestations: The extraintestinal manifestations of ulcerative colitis are shown in Figure 61.20. Some are trivial and self-limiting, but many can be extremely troublesome. If present, pyoderma gangrenosum can be widespread, severe and cause considerable skin loss. Although mild cases rarely cause scarring, more severe cases can do so and secondary infections can be highly dangerous.

The arthritis associated with ulcerative colitis is only rarely destructive or deforming, but can be highly symptomatic and leads to considerable incapacity.

In general, the symptoms of extraintestinal manifestations that are relieved by medical therapy, including corticosteroids, also respond to proctocolectomy.

Sclerosing Cholangitis

Sclerosing cholangitis is one of the most important extraintestinal manifestations of ulcerative colitis. It can be a progressive, highly symptomatic disorder and has a variable response to treatment. At worst, it can be fatal. There is evidence that it may act as a marker for a subtype of colitis following a more aggressive clinical course. In particular, it may be associated with a higher risk of relapse, greater resistance to treatment, a higher risk of pouchitis developing in an ileoanal pouch[77] and a higher risk of colorectal malignancy.[78]

The presence of sclerosing cholangitis also needs to be borne in mind when considering reconstructive proctocolectomy. Portal hypertension associated with liver disease may give rise to marked problems during any pelvic dissection. Congested pelvic varices may lead to troublesome bleeding and increase the morbidity and mortality rates associated with the procedure. The presence of caput medusae of peristomal veins or stomal varices should raise the question of marked portal hypertension. An ileoanal pouch with mucosectomy is the preferred procedure for colitis associated with sclerosing cholangitis, if feasible.

COLONIC CROHN'S DISEASE

Epidemiology and Etiology

Isolated colonic disease forms approximately 25% of all cases of Crohn's disease and has a similar age and sex distribution to that of ileal or ileocolic disease.

The precise etiology of Crohn's disease remains unknown. Infectious agents, autoimmune reactions precipitated by viral infections, food allergies and responses to luminal antigens have all been proposed. Mutations in NOD2 (IBD protein1) on chromosome 16 are strongly associated with the development of Crohn's disease, possibly influencing the production of proinflammatory cytokines, but numerous other loci have been associated with Crohn's disease. No evidence suggests that colonic and small bowel Crohn's disease do not have the same cause.

Pathology

Colonic Crohn's disease exhibits the same general pathologic features as that in the small bowel. It is a panintestinal disorder, with transmural inflammation in the form of lymphoid aggregates, granulomas and fissuring ulceration. Chronic inflammatory cell infiltrates are usually present, but also occur in long-standing and partially treated ulcerative colitis. The difficulties in diagnosis between the two conditions are discussed in "Differentiation from Crohn's Disease" (*see* above). Anal disease is common with Crohn's colitis and the absence of marked rectal inflammation (rectal sparing) is highly suggestive of Crohn's disease, provided no topical rectal treatment has been used.

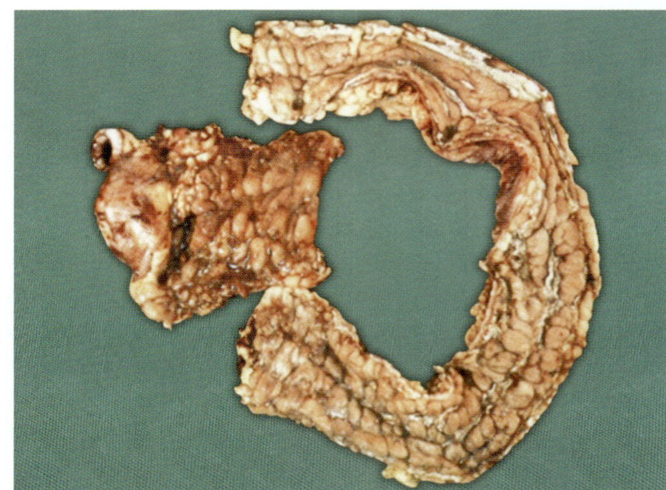

Fig. 61.21: Colonic Crohn's disease. Longitudinal ulceration and cobblestoning of the mucosa can be seen throughout the colon.

The macroscopic appearance of Crohn's colitis is very similar to that in the ileum. The wall is thickened with excess fat deposition in the epiploic fat, although fat wrapping is much less marked than in the small bowel. The serosal appearance is of a bluish discoloration with spiral neovascularization on the serosa. Internally, the mucosa is often grossly thickened and heaped up with a similar appearance to that of small bowel cobblestoning (Fig. 61.21). As at other sites in the gastrointestinal tract, the disease is often discontinuous, which gives rise to skip lesions; it may affect all, one part or several segments of the colon. Generally, the proximal ascending colon and cecum are most commonly affected, but distal colonic (rectal) disease or a pancolitis are not uncommon.

Clinical Features

Classifications

The features and presentations of Crohn's disease are varied and several classifications have been proposed; a widely used one is the Montreal Classification. It identifies location (L1, L2, L3) and behavior (B1, B2, B3) alongside age of onset, which can vary the typical clinical presentations (A1, A2, A3).

Inflammatory Features (B1)

So-called inflammatory symptoms may be marked in the colon. Occasionally, Crohn's colitis may present as an acute fulminant colitis with rapidly progressive symptoms of fever, tachycardia and bloody diarrhea and even toxic dilatation, as seen with acute fulminant ulcerative colitis (*see* above). In these circumstances, the diagnosis may only be made on pathologic examination of the colectomy specimen. More commonly, the colitis of Crohn's disease presents as altered bowel habit, usually diarrhea, which is often bloody and occasionally associated with abdominal pain. The symptoms tend to be slower and more insidious in onset and more persistent rather than intermittent as in ulcerative colitis; if associated with disease elsewhere in the gastrointestinal tract, it may be an obvious diagnosis. Isolated Crohn's colitis, however, may be difficult to distinguish from ulcerative colitis on clinical grounds.

Fistulizing/Penetrating Features (B3)

Colonic fistulation is rarer in Crohn's colitis than in small bowel Crohn's disease. Colocutaneous fistulas are uncommon, but colovaginal, colovesical, and coloenteric fistulas occur more frequently. Recurrent urinary tract infections or persistent vaginal discharge should always raise the possibility of a fistula. The presence of a fistula in colitis is almost diagnostic of Crohn's disease rather than ulcerative colitis, provided malignant and iatrogenic causes have been excluded.

Fibrostenosing/Stricturing Features (B2)

Although no evidence suggests that the disease process and pathologic changes in the wall of affected colon are any different to those of affected ileum, symptoms of stricturing are less common in colonic disease (perhaps because the colon has a greater initial diameter). If obstructive symptoms develop when luminal size reaches a certain cross-sectional area, it may take longer or more severe disease to cause sufficient wall thickening and luminal narrowing to reach this critical size, and therefore make colonic disease less likely to cause obstructive symptoms. The differential diagnosis of a malignant stricture is important to exclude since the two may coexist.

Diagnosis

The problems of diagnosis are covered above in the section on ulcerative colitis, yet colonic Crohn's disease is more accessible to the physician than ileal disease and so the imaging used for diagnosis differs slightly.

Radiology

Cross-sectional imaging is the radiological investigation of choice, although usually for the evaluation and assessment of disease extent/response to treatment rather than for diagnosis. Contrast-enhanced CT or CT colonography may give valuable information about the extent of disease, especially where endoscopic evaluation is impossible due to stricture formation. CT colonography is relatively contraindicated in acute severe colitis or where perforation is suspected. Single-contrast barium enema is hardly ever used now but is very occasionally useful to demonstrate the colonic origin of fistulas where CT is inconclusive. MR scanning is less useful for colonic disease than ileal disease but has a role when the radiation of repeated CT examinations makes its use valuable.

Endoscopy

Colonoscopy offers the best assessment of disease. The endoscopic appearances of Crohn's colitis are easily recognized (Fig. 61.22), and the extent and severity of disease and any luminal narrowing can be assessed. Biopsy may help to confirm clinical suspicion, but is rarely diagnostic alone.

Management

The management of colonic Crohn's disease follows the same broad principles as that of small bowel disease. However, some differences arise because of the functional differences between colon and ileum and the availability of the rectal route for topical treatment.

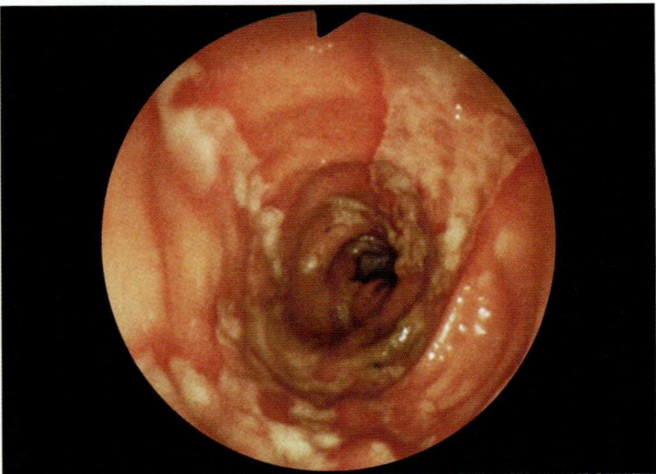

Fig. 61.22: Endoscopic appearance of Crohn's colitis. The colonic mucosa is grossly thickened with deep longitudinal ulcerations.
Source: Reproduced with permission from Silverstein FE, Tytgat GNJ. Gastrointestinal Endoscopy, 3rd edition. London: Mosby–Wolfe; 1997.

Medical Treatment

Corticosteroids: Topically administered corticosteroids are highly effective, particularly for distal disease exacerbations. Conventional or foam retention enemas are both used with a low risk of side effects, but the systemic absorption of active corticosteroid from the inflamed mucosa in widespread Crohn's colitis can be marked. Parenteral corticosteroids are used for resistant episodes.

5-Aminosalicylic acid: 5-Aminosalicylic acid enemas are also highly effective in Crohn's colitis. They offer the opportunity to reduce the corticosteroid dose either topically or parenterally, as in ulcerative colitis (corticosteroid-sparing effect), and may offer a degree of disease control if used when the colitis is in remission. Whether there is a marked reduction in relapses is unclear, but several studies indicate a possible role for maintenance therapy given the relatively low incidence of systemic side effects.

Anti-TNF-α therapy: Anti-TNF-α antibody therapy has a very similar role in Crohn's colitis to that in ulcerative colitis, being used mainly as salvage therapy in acute attacks not responding to therapy with corticosteroids and immunomodulators, but can be used as maintenance therapy in resistant cases to avoid the need for surgery with appropriate imaging surveillance and clinical reassessment. It has a specific role in the treatment of fistulizing disease, with evidence that particularly perianal fistulation may be successfully closed by treatment.[79]

Nutritional and supportive: Isolated Crohn's colitis does not pose the same difficulties of nutrition associated with severe chronic small bowel disease. There is a decreased likelihood of chronic malabsorption because the colon does not have a prime role in nutrient absorption, but active colitis can lead to fluid and salt depletion. Parenteral nutrition is less likely to be needed to support the patient's nutritional status. Occasionally, chronic active colitis renders the patient anorexic, which leads to reduced nutritional input in a situation in which the overall metabolic demands may be increased; parenteral nutrition may have a role in these circumstances. Severe perianal disease, particularly with complex fistulation and sepsis, may have a profoundly catabolic effect. Anemia is slightly more common than in small bowel disease because of bleeding, and blood transfusions may be required in colonic Crohn's disease. Nutritional therapy with elemental, polymeric or specific enteric diets may have some role in treating Crohn's colitis, but the evidence for efficacy is less compelling than in small bowel disease.

Operative Management

Indications: Operative intervention in Crohn's colitis is marginally less common than that in ileal disease, probably because of the lower rate of obstructive symptoms.[80] Hemorrhage, either persistent or acute and uncontrolled, is a rare indication, although more common in colonic than in small bowel disease. Free perforation of colonic disease is also rare. The most common indications for operation are symptoms uncontrolled by medical therapy or acute colitis resistant to medical therapy. Colonic disease is frequently associated with perianal disease (*see* below), and occasionally the alteration of stool consistency and frequency caused by the colonic disease results in sufficient deterioration in the perianal disease for colonic resection or diversion to be required.

Technical principles: Operative management of colonic Crohn's disease may be divided into procedures designed to:

- Conserve bowel
- Remove involved bowel.

Many of the technical principles of operative management for colonic Crohn's disease are the same as those for ileal disease. Those segments of the colon that possess a mesentery are likely to have a thickened friable mesentery, which (like that of affected small bowel) is prone to bleeding and requires careful handling. Tissue planes may be difficult to find or open, and careful blunt dissection often helps reduce the risk of an inadvertent colotomy. No evidence suggests that any type of anastomosis or colotomy closure is superior to any other, whether in single or two layers, although the avoidance of nonabsorbable braided sutures seems reasonable in a chronic inflammatory disorder.

Macroscopic Disease Clearance

Total colectomy: The operation of choice for widespread colonic and rectal Crohn's disease with perianal involvement is panproctocolectomy and permanent ileostomy. In the acute setting the rectal dissection may be deemed too hazardous to complete, and total colectomy with preservation of the rectal stump is carried out instead. The rectal disease is often amenable to topical treatment, but persistent symptoms from the rectal stump make completion proctectomy likely. Reconstructive operative management after colectomy for Crohn's disease was generally considered to be contraindicated. Recent evidence suggests, however, that there may be a group of patients who have Crohn's disease in whom ileoanal pouch construction is not associated with a high risk of recurrent disease in the pouch (*see* above).[42] It may be appropriate to offer these selected patients ileopouch–anal anastomosis after counseling about the risks.

Segmental colectomy: If disease is localized to one segment or half of the colon, total colectomy is often inappropriate because it is almost certain to commit the patient to a permanent ileostomy, which may be avoidable, at least temporarily. The risk of recurrence, as indicated below, is marginally less than that for ileal or ileocolic disease. A limited resection may result in delay of the formation of a permanent ileostomy for many years, until recurrence forces a completion colectomy.

Bowel Preservation

Split ileostomy: There is good evidence that small particulate matter in the fecal stream may help to perpetuate active inflammation.[81] Several studies showed that diversion of the fecal stream is associated with an improvement in both the clinical and endoscopic features of active inflammation.[82,83] These studies, however, also showed that restoration of the fecal load on the colon is associated with prompt recurrence of symptoms and inflammatory changes. The diversion of the fecal stream, although not a permanent solution, may have a temporizing role in the treatment of acute active colonic disease. In patients for whom resectional operative management is either too hazardous or is considered to be inappropriate for other reasons, formation of a diversionary stoma may allow the disease to settle sufficiently for medical control to be regained or for the patient to be prepared more thoroughly for definitive operative management.[84]

Strictureplasty: Strictureplasty may be used for strictures at a previous ileocolic anastomosis, but its role in the management of isolated colonic strictures is less clear since the risk of an occult malignancy may make resection more preferable. Colonic length and preservation do not have the same high priority as in the small bowel. Recent studies suggest that palliation of obstructive Crohn's disease strictures in the colon can be achieved with balloon dilatation for 2 years or more, although perforation of the bowel occurs in 10% of cases.

Special Problems

Appendix and Crohn's disease: The appendix may feature in Crohn's disease in several ways.

Acute exacerbations of undiagnosed ileocolic Crohn's disease may present as right iliac fossa pain in a young adult, which mimics acute appendicitis. The presence of a mass in the right iliac fossa may further confound the diagnosis, and ultrasound imaging may not necessarily differentiate between the two. If a laparoscopy is carried out before appendectomy, the diagnosis may become clear and a midline laparotomy may be preferred. If the diagnosis is made following a right iliac fossa incision, extension of the incision may allow sufficient access to perform an ileocolic resection. If there is any doubt, however, conversion to a midline approach offers the best exposure. Ileocolic Crohn's disease that presents acutely and is diagnosed at laparotomy should be resected even if there is no free perforation, because symptoms are likely to continue with medical treatment.

The appendix may be involved with ileocolic Crohn's disease and is occasionally the site of origin of fistulation or perforation. Management of these complications should follow the same system as for ileocolic disease.

Rarely, Crohn's disease is found isolated in the appendix with no evidence of associated ileal or colonic disease. The diagnosis may be made at appendicectomy for appendicitis or on histopathologic examination of a specimen. In these circumstances there is good evidence that the clinical course of the disease is considerably more benign than that of other forms of the disease.[85] The rates of fistula formation, recurrence and complications associated with isolated appendiceal Crohn's disease are very low.

Finally, acute ileitis, a self-limiting inflammation of the terminal ileum, often caused by *Yersinia enterocolitica,* may mimic appendicitis. At operation, the normal appendix is removed and the ileum is left intact.

Recurrence: The risk of recurrence in Crohn's disease is difficult to assess. In all studies of recurrence, isolated colonic disease is generally associated with a marginally lower recurrence rate than that in ileal disease, but this is by no means clear. Using life table analysis, the risk of recurrence after resection appears to rise from around 25% at 5 years to 40% at 20 years after operative management.[86] Smoking is associated with an increased risk of colonic recurrence, as it is for ileal disease.

Cancer risk: Evidence suggests that patients who have Crohn's colitis have a very similar risk of developing adenocarcinoma of the colon, as do those who have ulcerative colitis. The risk appears to be highest for those who have pancolitis and is around 10% at 20 years after the onset of symptoms.[87] The actual risk of cancer is difficult to assess because the rate of colectomy for symptomatic disease is higher for Crohn's disease than for ulcerative colitis, and a larger proportion of people who have Crohn's colitis undergo colectomy within 20 years of developing the disease. Colonic strictures should always be investigated for malignancy and resection should be considered. The implications for screening are less certain than those for chronic ulcerative colitis. It seems prudent to say that patients who have long-standing colonic Crohn's disease should undergo screening colonoscopy and biopsy, but interpretation of the histology of the biopsies may be even more difficult than it is in chronic ulcerative colitis.

PERIANAL CROHN'S DISEASE

Etiology

The perianal changes associated with Crohn's disease, which can be marked, usually result from active disease at the site. Abscesses and fissures occur and are usually caused by active chronic inflammation. The histopathologic changes in the perianal tissues are similar to those in the colon or small bowel, with the presence of lymphoid aggregates and granulomas being almost diagnostic. "Simple" abscesses and fistulas may occur as in conventional cryptoglandular sepsis.

Clinical Features

The inflammation of Crohn's disease in the perineum can manifest in a range of ways and with varying severity. Features range from simple abscesses to recurrent sepsis and multiple, complex, nonhealing fistulas. The presence of perianal Crohn's disease has a strong association for colonic Crohn's disease. The secondary changes that result from the inflammation are often characteristic and may be the presenting clinical feature.

Primary Lesions

The initial lesion is often nonhealing fissuring ulceration of the anus and lower rectum. The chronic inflammation and scarring then lead to the development of submucosal and, less frequently, higher or complex fistulas. Occasionally, the ulceration develops into a deep cavitating destructive lesion, which may bore into the anal sphincters or the ischiorectal fat. The presence of chronic inflammation results in edematous, swollen perianal tissue, which has a characteristic bluish discoloration. This appearance should always suggest the diagnosis. The symptoms of anal irritation predominate, pain being more characteristic of abscess development. Loss of continence does not necessarily imply permanent damage to the anal sphincter because involvement in the inflammatory process may compromise function, which can be restored by controlling the sepsis. Altered bowel habit suggests active colonic or small bowel disease.

Secondary Lesions

If the sinuses or fistulas undergo partial healing, secondary perianal abscesses may develop and are the usual cause of perianal pain. Skin tags are a common secondary phenomenon. Recurrent urinary tract infections, pneumaturia, or the passage of feces or excessive mucus vaginally indicate the presence of a complex fistula.

Diagnosis

Biopsy

If the diagnosis is suspected, careful biopsies should be taken to confirm it. The absence of granulomas and lymphoid aggregates does not exclude the diagnosis, but their presence is highly relevant. Patients who have recurrent perianal sepsis and no firm diagnosis should always have a biopsy taken from the surrounding tissue, including any skin tags, in an attempt to diagnose a case of Crohn's disease presenting with perianal disease. Examination and biopsy under anesthetic are often necessary.

Endoscopy

The role of colonoscopy is to identify the presence and extent of colorectal disease. It helps to delineate the distribution of the disease and is useful to evaluate the presence of strictures. Although not the best way to visualize fistulous tracts, sigmoidoscopy may help delineate the severity of rectal involvement and may indicate the need for rectal excision to control the symptoms. Cystoscopy is the preferred method to establish the presence of urethral or bladder involvement in a complex fistula because cystography has a lower sensitivity. Computed tomography may show an air-fluid level in the bladder.

Imaging

Contrast: Contrast examinations are useful to delineate the tracts involved in complex fistulas and sinuses. Sinography and fistulography may reveal more extensive disease than suspected clinically and indicate involvement above or below the level of the levator ani muscles. They are invasive, however, and can be uncomfortable for the patient.

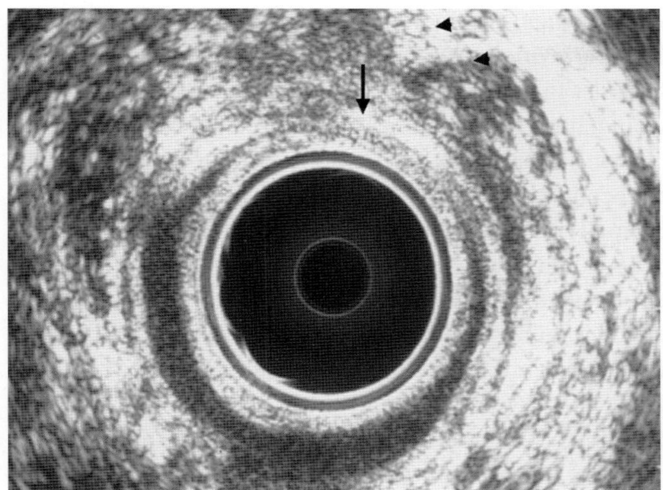

Fig. 61.23: Endoanal ultrasound image of sphincter injury secondary to perianal disease. The internal sphincter is grossly attenuated anteriorly (arrow); this is accompanied by spotty abnormalities in the external sphincter (arrowhead), probably caused by sepsis or a fistula.

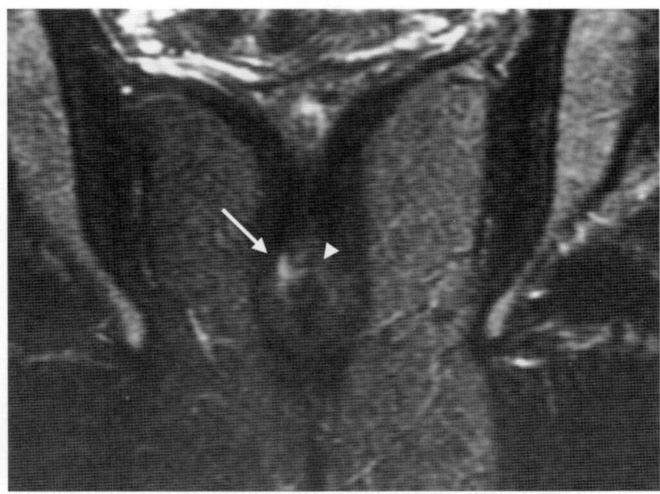

Fig. 61.24: Anal fistula in Crohn's disease. The anatomy of the fistula is well demonstrated in this MRI with the track (arrow) passing deep to the external anal sphincter (arrowhead).

Endoanal ultrasound: Endoanal ultrasound is a relatively noninvasive and highly accurate method to assess the integrity of the anal structures, particularly the sphincter complex (Fig. 61.23). It is an invaluable tool in identifying sphincter injuries before planning treatment and in assessing incontinence related to perianal Crohn's disease.[88]

Magnetic resonance imaging: Pelvic MRI is a highly sensitive and noninvasive method for delineating the limit of pelvic sepsis and fistulation (Fig. 61.24). The involved tissue can be reliably identified, and the proximal extent of fistulas can be identified.[89] Recent advances in technology now permit the use of endoanal coils, which allow the production of highly detailed views of the rectum and anus as well as the surrounding tissue.[90]

Assessment of the Problem

Assessment of the problem is both clinical and anatomic. Although extensive disease is usually symptomatic, it can be surprisingly pain free provided there is no acute sepsis in the region of the anal canal. The severity of the patient's symptoms is an important guide as to how aggressive therapy needs to be. Accurate recording of the state of the sepsis and the tissue involved allows correct treatment planning. Imaging should be combined with clinical examination, usually under anesthetic, together with proctosigmoidoscopy. Weak hydrogen peroxide solution can be gently injected into the external opening of a fistula; frothing bubbles on the mucosa indicate the internal opening of the tract. It is important to identify high fistulas, atypical fistulas such as urethral or bladder fistulas and involvement of the sphincter complex.

Management

Goals

Management is aimed at the minimal intervention needed to control the patient's symptoms and dangerous or destructive lesions. Several basic rules apply:

- If there is acute sepsis adequate drainage must be established
- Chronic sepsis should be controlled and allowed to drain freely
- Asymptomatic fistulas other than to the urinary tract do not require treatment
- Tissue should be preserved whenever possible
- Any operation should be the least invasive for satisfactory palliation.

Medical Management

Anti-inflammatory and immunosuppressive therapy can be highly effective provided that all active sepsis is controlled. If there is proximal disease, reduction in stool frequency and alteration of the consistency may make a considerable difference to the perianal symptoms. Topical anti-inflammatory therapy to the perianal disease may be effective, particularly if irritative symptoms predominate. Antibiotics such as ciprofloxacin and metronidazole have a role in controlling sepsis, and there is some evidence for the use of metronidazole as a disease-modifying agent.

Conservative Operative Management

Setons: The mainstays of operative management are procedures to control sepsis. Careful examination is necessary with probing to identify all superficial fistulas. Although superficial tracts can be curetted or laid open and lightly packed, as with any other perianal sepsis, if there is any doubt about involvement of the sphincter complex a seton should be used. Setons may be cutting or loose, although in Crohn's disease the advantage of the loose seton is that the sepsis is well controlled and there is no risk of sphincter injury; as a result it is more commonly used (Fig. 61.25). Whatever the situation, great care must be taken not to injure tissue unnecessarily and to avoid reducing the volume of perianal tissue unduly because this may cause incontinence.

Defunctioning Stoma

If the perianal sepsis is severe or slow to respond to conservative operative management, a defunctioning stoma may be used. This maneuver has the advantage of diverting the fecal stream, which reduces symptoms and allows the lesion to heal without prejudicing the options for definitive operative management.

Definitive Operative Management

Fistulotomy: Fistulotomy has a role in controlling simple intersphincteric or low trans-sphincteric fistulas and can be used successfully for quiescent rectal disease. The risk of damage to vital structures, particularly if the anatomy may be distorted through scarring and recurrent sepsis, limits its use. It is best reserved for those surgeons who have a wide experience in its use.

Advancement flaps: The principles of advancement flaps are to provide coverage with unaffected mucosa or skin to assist in the healing of damaged or scarred areas that would heal spontaneously only slowly. For the internal opening of a fistula, particularly an anterior one, a flap of rectal mucosa provides a highly vascular flap that can be made to stretch to cover the defect with relative ease (Figs. 61.26A and B). The flap may include all or a partial thickness of internal anal sphincter. It may be raised either via the vagina or, more conveniently, directly via the anus with minimum retraction. The flap provides a particularly good closure of the rectal defect because it acts like a curtain to exclude all fecal material from the area and prevents the high-pressure implantation of feces that may cause a fistula to recur. An endorectal advancement flap is only completely effective if all underlying sepsis has

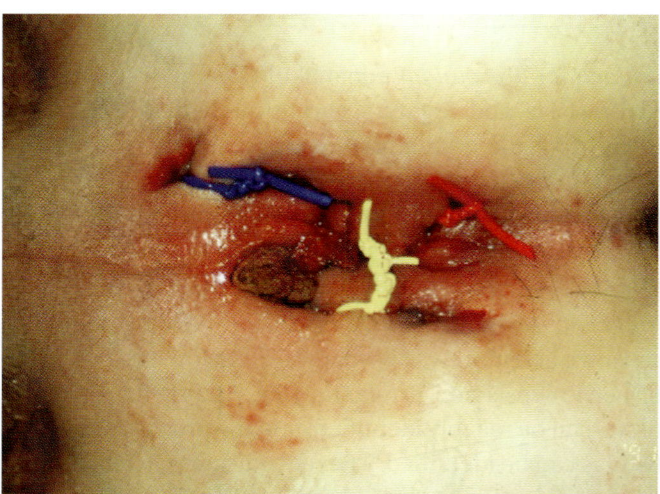

Fig. 61.25: Setons in the control of perianal sepsis in Crohn's disease.

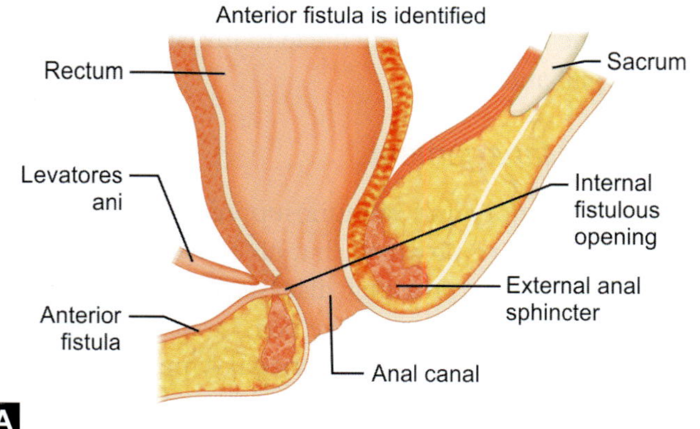

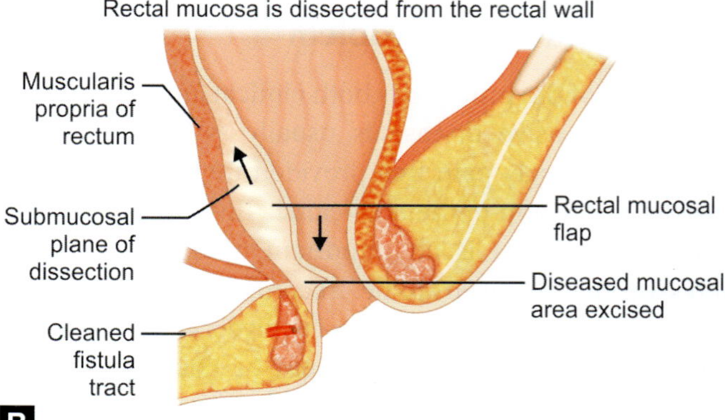

Figs. 61.26A and B: Rectal advancement flap in the treatment of an anterior fistula. The fistula is identified and cleaned. The mucosal defect and surrounding damaged mucosa are excised and a flap of rectal mucosa is dissected from the rectal wall in sufficient length and circumference to advance the flap comfortably over the fistulous defect.

been eradicated and the rectal mucosa used is itself free from Crohn's disease. It is best combined with procedures aimed at dealing with the external or vaginal end of the fistula simultaneously. It can be formed as a simple V of mucosa, a broad flap or even a circumferential sleeve of mucosa to match the size and extent of the defect that needs coverage. When used in these circumstances, the advancement flap can provide very good results and can greatly enhance the rate of healing.[91]

Myocutaneous advancement flaps are another form of flap that may be used in the treatment of perianal Crohn's disease, usually in the context of proctectomy and wide fistula excision. Occasionally, radical resection and debridement leaves such a large defect that the area requires coverage once all sepsis has settled. This goal can be achieved with a pedicled gluteal flap from the buttock, which has the advantage of excellent vascularity.

Proctectomy: The ultimate control of perianal symptoms is proctectomy. If there is widespread colonic Crohn's disease, this may form part of a panproctocolectomy. The indications for proctectomy in perianal Crohn's disease are given in Table 61.5. Proctectomy does have associated problems, however. If there is colonic disease that is not resected, the output of the end colostomy may be more fluid than that of a standard colostomy and this may pose difficulties. In this case a panproctocolectomy is more appropriate. The perineal wound may also be a problem, particularly if the rectum is severely involved. In such cases, it may be necessary to:

- Perform a wide excision of all areas of sepsis and fistulas leaving the wound open rather than attempt primary closure
- Raise a defunctioning loop colostomy before proctectomy to allow the sepsis to settle.

Table 61.5 Indications for proctectomy in Crohn's disease.
Active proctocolitis failing to respond to medical therapy
Severe intractable perianal disease involving fistulation to the rectum
Actual or potential malignant change in the rectum
Recurrent or life-threatening rectal hemorrhage

Special Considerations

Management of complex fistulas: The management of complex fistulas follows the same broad principles as that for any other perianal disease:

- Sepsis must be controlled
- Drainage is achieved
- Full planning is necessary, including imaging.

Labio-vaginal and scrotal fistulas: Labio-vaginal fistulas caused by perianal Crohn's disease are almost always low in the vagina and frequently involve the perineal body. Rectoscrotal fistulas may track more subcutaneously, but the loose connective tissue of the superficial perineal pouch allows considerable extension of the sepsis and can lead to distressing multiple tracks as far forwards as the base of the penis. For labio-vaginal disease, it is essential to plan any operative intervention carefully. Not all fistulas require operative management, and the close relationship of the sphincter complex and the perineal body means that scrupulous care is necessary in reconstructing the anterior anatomy of the anorectal junction to minimize the risk of incontinence. The labial or vaginal end of the track can be left open to heal by secondary intention.

Urethral fistula: Fistulation to the urethra is uncommon, even in severe perianal Crohn's disease. The site is usually the bulbous or membranous urethra. General management follows the simple rules for eradicating sepsis. Given the small numbers reported, there is no clear consensus about the best approach for operative management. Simple division and curettage of the fistula via the perineal approach have been used, as has a full thickness rectal advancement flap, both with success. The role for more extensive procedures, such as combined abdominoperineal approaches with omental, gracilis or other tissue interposition flaps, is uncertain. A suprapubic catheter cystostomy is required to divert the urinary stream, but fecal diversion is not necessarily required.[92]

Unhealed perineal wound: Following proctectomy or proctocolectomy, the perineal wound may fail to heal. The rate of nonhealing is higher than that for other indications for proctectomy such as malignancy.[93] There may be several causes, all of which should be sought before the assumption is made that there is active Crohn's disease in the perineal remnant. Retained foreign bodies such as suture materials may act as a nidus of sepsis, and any retained mucosa may be actively inflamed and generate purulent mucus. The perineal wound may be the external opening of an enteroperineal fistula from residual involved bowel or the opening of a chronic pelvic abscess. If there is any doubt, examination under anesthetic should be carried out and imaging to exclude sepsis may be required.

If these causes have been excluded, simple wound toilet and debridement may suffice to heal the wound. Regular debridement of excessive granulation tissue and shaving the hair from the surrounding perineal skin alone may heal the wound. There is a tendency for the perineal skin to close over an incompletely healed sinus and then recurrently break down. The use of a small pack or wick may allow the sinus to heal into an ulcer. The ulcer may then spontaneously close over.

REFERENCES

1. Wilks S, Moxon W. Lectures on Pathological Anatomy, 2nd edition. Philadelphia: Lindsay and Blakiston; 1875. pp. 408-9.
2. Truelove SC. The management of ulcerative colitis. Curr Med Drugs. 1967;7:3-15.
3. Truelove SC. Medical management of ulcerative colitis. Br Med J. 1968;2:539-42.
4. Truelove SC, Jewell DP. Intensive intravenous regimen for severe attacks of ulcerative colitis. Lancet. 1974;1:1067-70.
5. Brooke BN. The management of an ileostomy including its complications. Dis Colon Rectum. 1993;36;512-6.
6. Khoo UY, Bjarnason I, Donaghy A, et al. Antibodies to colonic epithelial cells from the serum and colonic mucosal washings in ulcerative colitis. Gut. 1995;37;63-70.
7. Lees CW, Barrett J, Parkes M, et al. New IBD genetics: common pathways with other diseases. Gut. 2011;60:1739-53.
8. Bartram CI. Radiology in the current assessment of ulcerative colitis. Gastrointest Radiol. 1977;1:383-92.
9. Almer S, Bodemar G, Franzen L, et al. Plain X-ray films and air enema films reflect severe mucosal inflammation in acute ulcerative colitis. Digestion. 1995;56:528-33.
10. Buckell NA, Williams GT, Bartram CI, et al. Depth of ulceration in acute colitis: correlation with outcome and clinical and radiologic features. Gastroenterology. 1980;79:19-25.
11. Bartram CI, Preston DM, Lennard Jones JE. The "air enema" in acute colitis. Gastrointest Radiol. 1983;8:61-5.
12. Kolkman JJ, Falke TH, Roos JC, et al. Computed tomography and granulocyte scintigraphy in active inflammatory bowel disease. Comparison with endoscopy and operative findings. Dig Dis Sci. 1996;41:641-50.
13. Esaki M, Kubokura N, Kudo T, et al. Endoscopic findings under narrow band imaging colonoscopy in ulcerative colitis. Dig Endosc. 2011;23(suppl 1):140-2.
14. D'Haens G, Geboes K, Peeters M, et al. Patchy cecal inflammation associated with distal ulcerative colitis: a prospective endoscopic study. Am J Gastroenterol. 1997;92:1275-9.
15. Silverstein FE, Tytgat GNJ. Gastrointestinal Endoscopy, 3rd edition. London: Mosby-Wolfe; 1997.
16. Romas E, Paspaliaris B, d'Apice AJ, et al. Autoantibodies to neutrophil cytoplasmic (ANCA) and endothelial cell surface antigens (AECA) in chronic inflammatory bowel disease. Aust NZ J Med. 1992;22:652-9.
17. Rump JA, Scholmerich J, Gross V, et al. A new type of perinuclear anti-neutrophil cytoplasmic antibody (p-ANCA) in active ulcerative colitis but not in Crohn's disease. Immunobiology. 1990;181:406-13.
18. Rump JA, Worner I, Roth M, et al. p-ANCA of undefined specificity in ulcerative colitis: correlation to disease activity and therapy. Adv Exp Med Bioi. 1993;336:507-13.
19. Abad E, Tural C, Mirapeix E, et al. Relationship between ANCA and clinical activity in inflammatory bowel disease; variation in prevalence of ANCA and evidence of heterogeneity. J Autoimmun. 1997;10:175-80.
20. Sandborn WJ, Landers CJ, Tremaine WJ, et al. Antineutrophil cytoplasmic antibody correlates with chronic pouchitis after ileal pouch-anal anastomosis. Am J Gastroenterol. 1995;90:740-7.
21. Esteve M, Mallolas J, Klaassen J, et al. Antineutrophil cytoplasmic antibodies in sera from colectomised ulcerative colitis patients and its relation to the presence of pouchitis. Gut. 1996;38:894-8.
22. American Gastroenterological Association Institute Medical Position Statement on corticosteroids, immunomodulators, and infliximab in inflammatory bowel disease. Gastroenterology. 2006;130(3):935-9.
23. Frei P, Bioedermann L, Manser CN, et al. Topical therapies in inflammatory bowel disease. Digestion. 2012;86 (suppl 1):36-44.
24. De Cassan C, Fiorino G, Danese S. Second-generation corticosteroids for the treatment of Crohn's disease and ulcerative colitis: more effective and less side effects? Dig Dis. 2012;30(4):368-75.
25. Spencer CM, McTavish D. Budesonide. A review of its pharmacological properties and therapeutic efficacy in inflammatory bowel disease. Drugs. 1995;50:854-72.
26. Campieri M, Corbelli C, Gionchetti P, et al. Spread and distribution of 5-ASA colonic foam and 5-ASA enema in patients with ulcerative colitis. Dig Dis Sci. 1992;37:1890-7.
27. Marshall JK, Irvine EJ. Rectal corticosteroids versus alternative treatments in ulcerative colitis: a meta-analysis. Gut. 1997;40:775-81.
28. D'Albasio G, Pacini F, Camarri E, et al. Combined therapy with 5-aminosalicylic acid tablets and enemas for maintaining remission in ulcerative colitis: a randomized double-blind study. Am J Gastroenterol. 1997;92:1143-7.
29. Feagan BG, Chande N, Macdonald JK. Are there any differences in the efficacy and safety of different formulations of oral 5-ASA used for induction and maintenance of remission in ulcerative colitis? Evidence from Cochrane reviews. Inflamm Bowel Dis. 2013;19(9):2031-40.
30. Mañosa M, Cabré E, Garcia-Planella E, et al. Decision tree for early introduction of rescue therapy in active ulcerative colitis treated with steroids. Inflamm Bowel Dis. 2011 Dec;17(12):2497-502.
31. Sharkey L, Bredin F, Nightingale A, et al. The use of Cyclosporin A in acute steroid-refractory ulcerative colitis: long term outcomes. J Crohns Colitis. 2011;5(2):91-4.
32. Fleshner PR, Michelassi F, Rubin M, et al. Morbidity of subtotal colectomy in patients with severe ulcerative colitis unresponsive to cyclosporin. Dis Colon Rectum. 1995; 38:1241-5.
33. Kobayashi T, Naganuma M, Okamoto S, et al. Rapid endoscopic improvement is important for 1-year avoidance of colectomy but not for the long-term prognosis in cyclosporine A treatment for ulcerative colitis. J Gastroenterol. 2010;45(11):1129-37.

34. Steinhart AH, Hiruki T, Brzezinski A, et al. Treatment of left-sided ulcerative colitis with butyrate enemas: a controlled trial. Aliment Pharmacol Ther. 1996;10:729-36.
35. Travis SP, Farrant JM, Ricketts C, et al. Predicting outcome in severe ulcerative colitis. Gut. 1996;38:905-10.
36. Berry AR, de Campos R, Lee EC. Perineal and pelvic morbidity following perimuscular excision of the rectum for inflammatory bowel disease. Br J Surg. 1986;73:675-7.
37. Koch M. Intra-abdominal reservoir in patients with permanent ileostomy. Arch Surg. 1969;99:223-31.
38. Nessar G, Fazio VW, Tekkis P, et al. Long-term outcome and quality of life after continent ileostomy. Dis Colon Rectum. 2006;49(3):336-44.
39. Ecker KW, Hildebrandt U, Haberer M, et al. Biomechanical stabilization of the nipple valve in continent ileostomy. Br J Surg. 1996;83:1582-5.
40. Fazio VW, Tjandra JJ. Technique for nipple valve fixation to prevent valve slippage in continent ileostomy. Dis Colon Rectum. 1992;35:1177-9.
41. Grabler SP, Hosie KB, Keighley MR. Randomized trial of loop ileostomy in restorative proctocolectomy. Br J Surg. 1992;79:903-6.
42. Panis Y, Poupard B, Nemeth J, et al. Ileal pouch/anal anastomosis for Crohn's disease. Lancet. 1996;347:854-7.
43. Annibali R, Oresland T, Hulten L. Does the level of stapled ileoanal anastomosis influence physiologic and functional outcome? Dis Colon Rectum. 1994;37:321-9.
44. Nicholls RJ, Moskowitz RL, Shepherd NA. Restorative proctocolectomy with ileal reservoir. Br J Surg. 1985; 72(suppl): S76-9.
45. Oresland T, Fasth S, Akervall S, et al. Manovolumetric and sensory characteristics of the ileoanal J pouch compared with healthy rectum. Br J Surg. 1990;77:803-6.
46. Allan RN, Keighley MR, Rhodes M, et al., (Eds). Inflammatory Bowel Diseases, 3rd ed. Glasgow: Churchill Livingstone; 1998.
47. Hallgren T, Fasth S, Nordgren S, et al. Manovolumetric characteristics and functional results in three different pelvic pouch designs. Int J Colorectal Dis. 1989;4:156-60.
48. Oresland T, Fasth S, Nordgren S, et al. A prospective randomized comparison of two different pelvic pouch designs. Scand J Gastroenterol. 1990;25:986-96.
49. Seow Choen F, Ho YH, Goh HS. The ileo-anal reservoir: results from an evolving use of stapling devices. J R Coli Surg Edinb. 1994;39:13-6.
50. Singh P, Bhangu A, Nicholls RJ, et al. A systematic review and meta-analysis of laparoscopic vs open restorative proctocolectomy. Colorectal Dis. 2013;15(7):e340-51.

Additional references appear in the online version of this book.

62A

Benign Neoplasms of the Large Bowel

Vanessa W Hui, Jose G Guillem

Key Points

- Familial adenomatous polyposis is an autosomal dominant disorder. Families should be identified, so that prophylactic resection can be offered before malignancy develops.
- Adenomatous colonic polyps are a precursor to colorectal cancer.
- Pedunculated polyps should be treated by endoscopic polypectomy and require rigorous histopathological scrutiny with follow-up.
- Sessile polyps need total excision by EMR or ESD (endoscopic mucosal resection or endoscopic submucosal dissection) and rigorous histopathological examination with follow-up.
- Families with histories consistent with Lynch syndrome require genetic counseling and colonoscopic surveillance.

ADENOMA

Epidemiology

Colorectal polyps may be classified as adenomatous, hyperplastic and/or serrated, or miscellaneous (which includes mucosal, inflammatory, juvenile, hamartomatous, and nonmucosal polyps). Populations with the highest incidence of colonic polyps and cancers are in Western Europe, North America, and Australia. There appears to be a strong correlation between geographic prevalence of adenomas and CRC, as both adenoma and cancer frequencies increase when populations migrate from low- to high-risk areas. In addition, the prevalence of adenomatous polyps correlates well with CRC risk. Though hyperplastic polyps were traditionally seen as benign lesions, the World Health Organization (WHO) and expert panels have recently acknowledged their malignant potential.[1,2]

Pathogenesis

Genetics

Since the initial proposal of the adenoma-carcinoma sequence suggesting the cause of sporadic CRC as a result of accumulated mutations in specific oncogenes and tumor-suppressor genes (Fig. 62A.1), it has been shown that a multitude of genes and their products interact in numerous complex pathways in order to drive the progression to cancer. Whole-genome sequencing and subsequent cancer genome landscaping have allowed us to assess the frequency of specific mutations in individual cancers. In CRC, the number of nonsynonymous mutations can range from <50 to >250, depending on the particular characteristics of the tumor. While we have focused our research on the handful of mutated genes commonly seen in a large proportion of CRC, it appears that the mutations that are actually driving CRC development appear in $<5\%$ of the tumors. As such, not all genetic mutations contribute equally to cancer, if at all. However, our knowledge to date suggests that there are three general molecular pathways that can lead to genomic instability and a resultant CRC.[3,4]

The chromosomal instability pathway, which results from a mutated oncogene or tumor-suppressor gene such as *APC, TP53, DCC, SMAD4, K-ras, BRAF,* and *PIK3CA*, is responsible for most sporadic CRC. In particular, *APC* is the gatekeeper of the *Wnt* (Wingless) signaling pathway and a somatic *APC* mutation results in the constitutive activation of the oncoprotein β-catenin and the *Wnt* pathway, leading to mucosal cell hyperproliferation and early phases of CRC. Familial polyposis syndrome (FAP) is a consequence of a germline *APC* mutation on chromosome 5.[5]

Microsatellites are highly repetitive DNA sequences that were historically thought to be "junk" DNA, but have

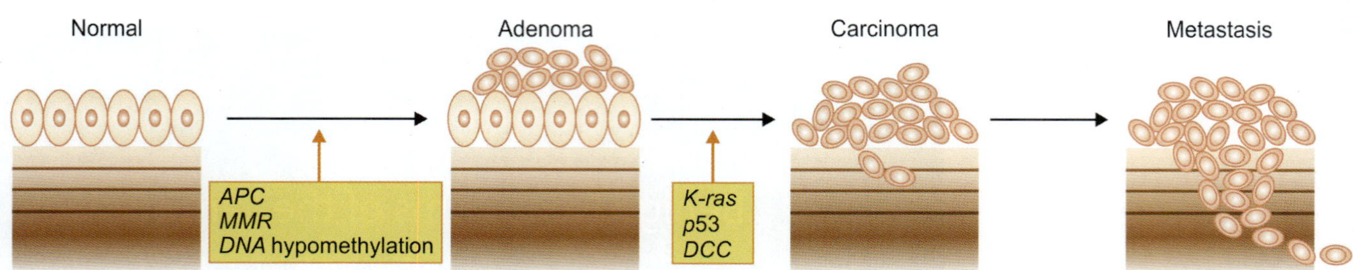

Fig. 62A.1: Adenoma-to-carcinoma sequence. (APC: Adenomatous polyposis coli gene; DCC: Deleted in colorectal carcinoma gene; K-ras: Kirsten rat sarcoma gene; MMR: DNA mismatch repair genes; p53: tumor suppressor protein of TP53 gene).

since been found to provide a high degree of polymorphism in genetic linkage studies. In normal tissue, DNA errors during the replication process are corrected by mismatch repair (MMR) genes such as *MLH1, MSH2, MSH6,* and *PMS2.* An accumulation of such errors leads to microsatellite instability and gene insertions/deletions, eventually leading to colorectal neoplasia. A germline mutation in one of the four MMR genes results in Lynch syndrome and an accelerated development to CRC.[5]

Hypermethylation of CpG islands in DNA promoter regions reduces gene expression and leads to CRC via epigenetic silencing, as it occurs upstream from the gene in question and does not require a mutation in the gene itself. Epigenetic silencing of MMR gene can also lead to loss of MMR protein function and sporadic CRC development. Known as the CpG island methylator phenotype (CIMP) pathway, this appears to be the main driving force in the progression of serrated lesions into carcinoma.[2,5]

Recent research has suggested that germline mutations in the proofreading domains of DNA polymerases POLE and POLD1 are associated with colorectal adenoma and cancer development. Currently, there are ongoing analyses of approximately 20,000 transcripts from the human genome in order to determine the timing as well as the specific mutations driving the progression to CRC.[3,4,6]

Clinical Features and Diagnosis

Adenoma Detection

Five-year survival after resection of a CRC localized to the bowel wall is approximately 90%, while it is about 70% and 12% for patients with nodal and distant metastasis, respectively.[7] Therefore, early screening and detection are the keys to curative treatment and prolonging survival. Fecal occult blood tests (FOBTs), sigmoidoscopy, and colonoscopy are the main methods used in order to detect CRC at an earlier curative stage.

Fecal occult blood test can be performed as a guaiac or fecal immunochemical test. Compliance is better with both tests than the more invasive endoscopy screening programs.[8,9] However, endoscopic screening has been shown to be four to eight times better than FOBT at detecting colorectal neoplasia.[8] Currently, the United States Multi-Society Task Force (US MSTF) on CRC does not endorse the substitution of a high-quality colonoscopy with FOBT.[10]

Though flexible sigmoidoscopies have been shown to significantly reduce CRC mortality (26% per the Prostate, Lung, Colorectal, and Ovarian Cancer Screening trial), this benefit remains only limited to the distal colon.[11,12] As such, average-risk patients should still undergo a full colonoscopic surveillance at 10-year intervals, assuming that the baseline colonoscopy was adequately completed and that all visible polyps that were completely removed were benign.[10]

Indications for colonoscopy include rectal bleeding or melena, adenoma on flexible sigmoidoscopy, history of CRC or inflammatory bowel disease (IBD), and family history of CRC or adenomatous polyps. Colonoscopic polypectomy of adenomas results in a 51% reduction in CRC mortality in 10-year follow-up and supports recommendations for early screening, detection, and removal of adenomas to prevent CRC.[13] Patients may benefit from an interval colonoscopy to ensure complete removal of the polyp, since as many as 27% of interval cancers develop at or adjacent to the previous polypectomy site.[10] Patients with multiple adenomas, adenomas ≥1 cm in diameter, and adenomas with villous tissue or severe dysplasia are also at increased risk of developing synchronous or metachronous CRC. Close colonoscopic surveillance and complete polyp resections greatly reduce CRC incidence in such cases.[10,13]

New endoscopic technologies such as narrow band imaging, chromoendoscopy, and magnification endoscopy may be used to identify suspicious lesions during colonoscopy, but do not influence surveillance intervals.

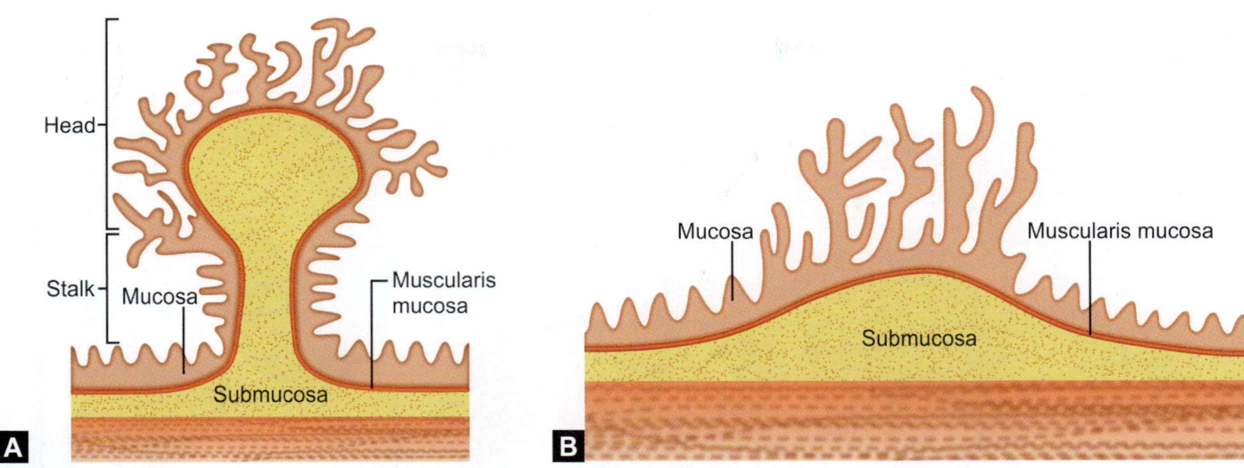

Figs. 62A.2A and B: Polyp morphology. (A) Pedunculated polyp. (B) Sessile polyp.

Computed tomography (CT) colonography and barium enema have been used as adjuncts or alternatives to screening and surveillance in patients who are unable to complete a colonoscopy. Though CT colonography may detect 90% of adenomatous lesions measuring 1 cm and greater, they are less sensitive to smaller lesions.[14] Therefore, it is not currently used as a surveillance tool.

Adenoma Management

Although most colorectal polyps are <1 cm in diameter, large adenomas may develop, especially on the right side. In the rectum and distal sigmoid colon, most diminutive polyps are non-neoplastic. In the rest of the colon, however, approximately two-thirds of diminutive polyps are adenomas. There are two main polyp configurations:

- Pedunculated, which attaches to the intestinal wall by a stalk (Fig. 62A.2A)
- Sessile, which has a broad-base attachment to the wall (Fig. 62A.2B)

Adenomas are classified as tubular, tubulovillous, or villous according to their histologic appearance (Figs. 62A.3A to C). Tubular, Tubulovillous, or villous adenomas comprise approximately 87%, 8%, and 5% of sporadic adenomas, respectively.[15] The malignant potential of adenomas is related to the size (polyps ≥1 cm) and the presence of villous histology (> 25% dysplastic villous component). For adenomas >1 cm, the malignant risk is approximately 3%. This risk increases to about 17% in villous adenoma > 1 cm.

Although pedunculated polyps are easily removed, sessile polyps may require advanced endoscopic techniques such as endoscopic mucosal resection (EMR) and endoscopic submucosal dissection (ESD). Both methods typically mandate a submucosal injection of a lifting agent such as saline in order to lift the mucosa away from the rest of the bowel wall. In this manner, the sessile polyp may be removed in a piecemeal fashion via EMR while minimizing the risk of perforation. ESD, however, uses diathermic knives to perform an en-bloc resection of the polyp. A retrospective study comparing both techniques showed that though ESD has higher perforation rates and longer procedure times, it has a lower polyp recurrence rate than EMR (2 vs. 14%, respectively).[16] Both techniques may necessitate the use of argon plasma coagulation to fulgurate residual adenomatous tissue as well as short-term endoscopic follow-up to ensure completeness of the removal.

Perforation is rare (<1–3%), but is the most significant complication following a polypectomy, and can result from pressures from a looped colonoscope and/or pneumatic pressures as well as thermal injury.[17] While innovative techniques such as endoscopic clipping have demonstrated some success in avoiding major abdominal surgery, surgical resection and/or closure remains the mainstay of management for iatrogenic perforation. Primary or delayed bleeding is more common following a polypectomy and may be managed with observation, endoscopic intervention (manual pressure, coagulation by injection or thermal probe, hemoclip), and possibly surgery, depending on the degree of hemorrhage. For incompletely removed polyps or those not amenable to endoscopic resection, surgical oncologic resection should be considered given the approximately 18% risk of invasive carcinoma in these cases.[18]

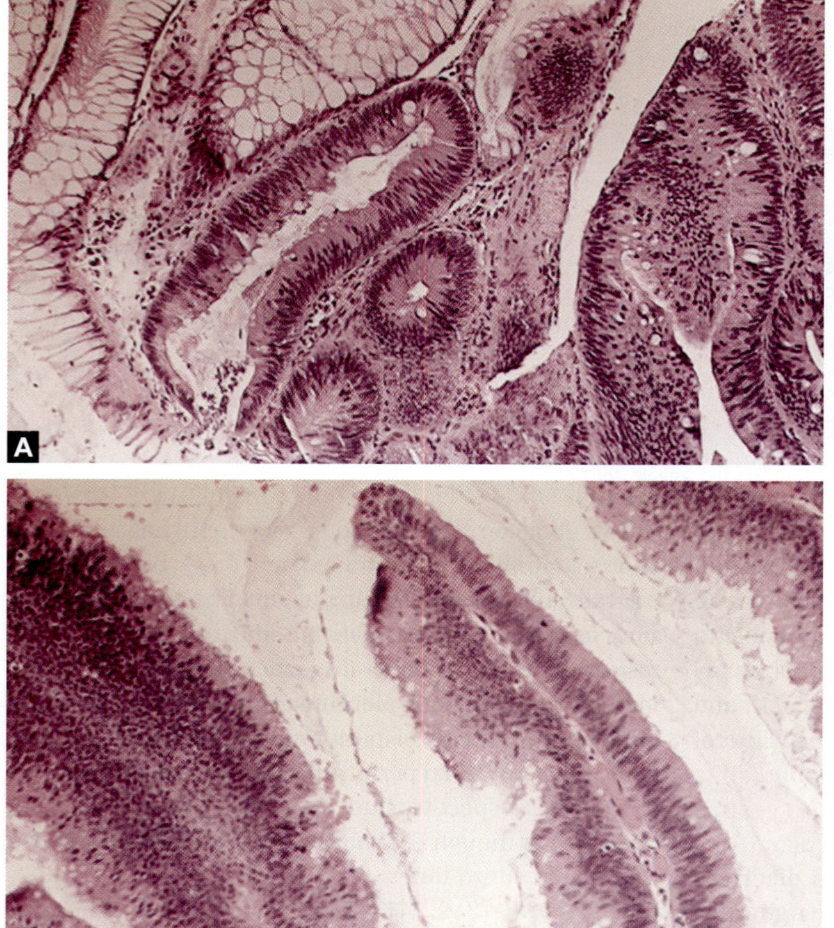
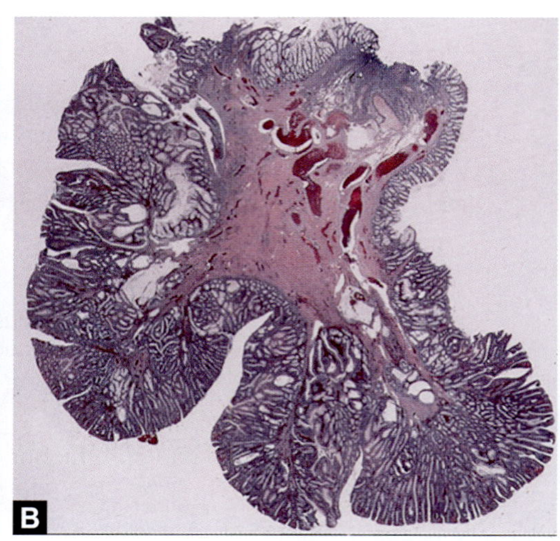

Figs. 62A.3A to C: Adenoma histologies. (A) Tubular adenoma. Branching tubules embedded in lamina propria surrounded by adenomatous epithelium. (B) Tubulovillous adenoma. Adenomatous polyp with both tubular and villous characteristics. (C) Villous adenoma. Thin plates of lamina propria surrounded by adenomatous epithelium.
Source: Courtesy of Stephen S Sternberg and Satish Tickoo.

Follow-Up

Colonoscopy is the preferred examination method following removal of an initial adenoma. According to the US MSTF recommendations: (1) patients with 1–2 small (< 10 mm) TAs without dysplasia should undergo repeat colonoscopy in 5–10 years; and (2) patients with 3–10 adenomas, an adenoma ≥ 1 cm in diameter or who have a family history of CRC should undergo surveillance colonoscopy 3 years after polypectomy. A follow-up colonoscopy may be necessary after piecemeal removal of large sessile lesions, malignant polyps, numerous polyps (> 10), or a technically unsatisfactory examination. The complete US MSTF recommendations for surveillance and screening intervals are listed in Table 62A.1.[10,19]

Malignant Polyp

A malignant polyp is a protrusion from the colorectal mucosa that contains cancer. The degree of invasion by this malignant focus is histologically defined by Haggitt levels, with level 1 defined as invasion through the muscularis mucosa but limited to the head of a pedunculated polyp, level 2 defined as the invasion extending into the polyp neck, level 3 defined as invasion into the polyp stalk, and level 4 defined as invasion into the submucosa of the bowel wall below the stalk of a pedunculated polyp. When a patient has a malignant polyp excised by polypectomy, the decision to carry out a colectomy in order to eradicate possible residual primary and/or nodal disease is weighed against the morbidity and mortality of the surgery. Important considerations include the resected polyp margin status, degree of cellular differentiation, vascular or lymphatic invasion, and completeness of excision (Fig. 62A.4). Favorable pathologic characteristics include:

- Haggitt level 1–3
- Negative resection margins
- Well differentiated
- Absent lymphatic and vascular invasion.

Table 62A.1 2012 US Multi-Society Task Force Recommendations for Surveillance and Screening Intervals in Individuals with Baseline Average Risk.

Baseline colonoscopy: most advanced finding(s)	*Recommended surveillance interval (y)*	*Quality of evidence supporting the recommendation*	*New evidence stronger than 2006*
No polyps	10	Moderate	Yes
Small (< 10 mm) hyperplastic polyps in rectum or sigmoid	10	Moderate	No
1–2 small (< 10 mm) tubular adenomas	5–10	Moderate	Yes
3–10 tubular adenomas	3	Moderate	Yes
> 10 adenomas	< 3	Moderate	No
One of more tubular adenomas ≥ 10 mm	3	High	Yes
One or more villous adenomas	3	Moderate	Yes
Adenoma with HGD	3	Moderate	No
Serrated lesions			
Sessile serrated polyp(s) < 10 mm with no dysplasia	5	Low	NA
Sessile serrated polyp(s) ≥ 10 mm	3	Low	NA
OR			
Sessile serrated polyp with dysplasia			
OR			
Traditional serrated adenoma			
Serrated polyposis syndromeo[a]	1	Moderate	NA

Note: The recommendations assume that the baseline colonoscopy was complete and adequate and that all visible polyps were completely removed.

NA: Not applicable.

[a] Based on the World Health Organization definition of serrated polyposis syndrome with one of the following criteria: (1) at least 5 serrated polyps proximal to sigmoid, with 2 or more ≥ 10 mm; (2) any serrated polyps proximal to sigmoid with family history of serrated polyposis syndrome; and (3) > 20 serrated polyps of any size throughout the colon.

Source: Reprinted with permission from Elsevier Lieberman DA, Rex DK, Winawer SJ, et al. Guidelines for colonoscopy surveillance after screening and polypectomy: a consensus update by the US Multi-Society Task Force on Colorectal Cancer. Gastroenterology. 2012;143(3):844-57.

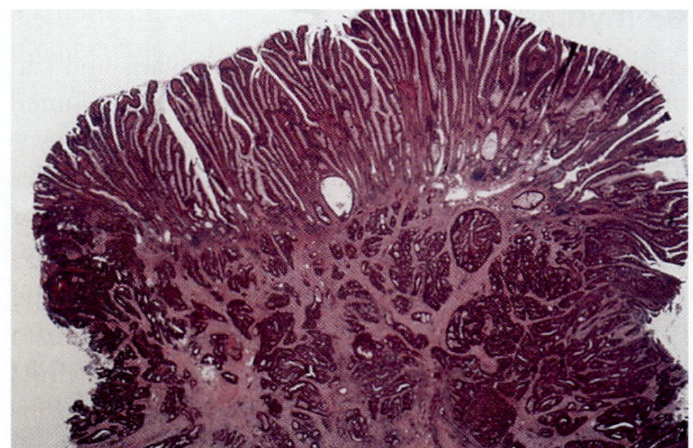

Fig. 62A.4: Adenocarcinoma in villous adenoma. The submucosa is invaded by adenocarcinoma.
Source: Courtesy of Stephen S Sternberg and Satish Tickoo.

These factors are considered along with the operative risk, lesion location, and patient life expectancy. Patients with a pathologically favorable adenoma following a complete endoscopic excision may not need to undergo surgical resection, as the risk of lymph node metastasis is <1% for pedunculated polyps with Haggitt levels 1–3.[15] However, patients with a sessile or Haggitt level 4 lesion and/or high-risk histologic features have a higher risk of nodal disease and are not ideal candidates for the treatment by endoscopic excision alone.

Repeat endoscopic evaluation of the polypectomy site should be carried out shortly thereafter to access the completeness of excision. If recurrent tumor is found, the patient should be counseled regarding surgical resection. Identification of the polyp site at the time of polypectomy by injecting permanent markers such as India ink may be useful, as the area of concern may not be readily palpable at the time of surgery.

Adenoma Prevention

The use of resistant starch as a form of dietary fiber supplement has been shown to be ineffective in preventing CRC.[20] Aspirin and nonsteroidal anti-inflammatory drugs (NSAIDs) have been shown to prevent the formation of colorectal adenomas and reduce the incidence of CRC.[21,22] However, the adequate dose for adenoma/carcinoma prevention remains unclear, as doses from such trials have ranged from 81 to 1200 mg daily.

There are several ongoing trials looking into such chemopreventive measures in FAP patients. In particular, the CHIP study is an international clinical trial evaluating the use of celecoxib, a COX-2 inhibitor, to prevent adenoma formation in FAP teens.[23] Randomized controlled trials assessing the effects of other chemopreventive drugs such as sulindac and eflornithine in adenoma and cancer prevention in the FAP population are currently in progress.[24-26]

OTHER COLORECTAL POLYPS

Hyperplastic Polyps

Hyperplastic polyps (HP) are usually small (2–5 mm in diameter), plaque-like, and have the same color as normal mucosa. They are the most common polyp found in the rectum and are rarely symptomatic (Fig. 62A.5A). Hyperplastic polyps are now considered part of the morphologic spectrum of serrated adenomas/polyps. Patients with a considerable HP burden should be evaluated for serrated polyposis, as these patients may have an increased risk of CRC.[1,2]

Juvenile Polyps

Juvenile or retention polyps are hamartomas, which are disorganized growths of normal tissue. Most are commonly seen in childhood, though can be observed in infancy and adulthood. They are typically pedunculated, spheroid, 1–5 cm in diameter, and may be multilobulated. Juvenile polyps typically have an eroded surface, with reactive epithelium containing inflammatory cells and dilated cystic spaces filled with mucus (Fig. 62A.5B]). An abundance of juvenile polyps should raise suspicion for a hereditary CRC syndrome.[27]

Inflammatory Polyps

Inflammatory polyps are almost always multiple, segmental, or diffuse and usually seen in patients with IBD (especially in ulcerative colitis, UC). They have also been found in patients with bacillary dysentery, amebic colitis, schistosomiasis, ischemic colitis, and near ureterosigmoidostomies where a mix of urinary and fecal material initiates localized inflammation of the mucosa. Inflammatory polyps can be divided into three groups:

- Pseudopolyps produced by contiguous ulcerations isolating an island of residual inflamed mucosa
- Undermining ulcerations giving rise to polypoid inflamed mucosal tags
- Mature inflammatory polyps derived from repeated repair and regeneration of mucosal tags (Fig. 62A.5C)

Operative treatment in the setting of IBD is aimed at the exclusion of malignancy as well as symptomatic management. Patients with inflammatory polyps are considered to be at moderate risk of developing CRC and are recommended to undergo colonoscopy every 1–3 years, should the frequency or severity of polyps progress.[28]

Lipomas

Historically, the incidence of colonic lipomas is < 1%. Lesions > 3.5 cm can become symptomatic, causing obstruction or bleeding via ulceration and necrosis. Lipomas arise from deposits of adipose tissue in the bowel wall, are more common in the cecum and right colon, and have no malignant potential (Fig. 62A.6). Lipomas that arise in the subserosa tend to grow outward into the peritoneal cavity, while those arising in the submucosa tend to grow into the lumen.

Such submucosal lipomas can form a lead point, causing intussusception and obstruction. A lipoma can be removed endoscopically, with the greatest success for complete removal achieved for smaller pedunculated lesions. Histologic examination reveals mature adipose tissue without atypia. Often these lesions may be found as incidental masses during laparotomy, and a partial colectomy is performed to confirm the diagnosis and exclude carcinoma.[29]

Leiomyomas

Leiomyomas arise from the colonic muscularis and can remain in the bowel wall or grow into the bowel lumen or peritoneal cavity. On histologic examination, leiomyomas consist of spindle-shaped cells arranged in bundles (Fig. 62A.7). Colonic leiomyomas usually form rubbery nodules and are asymptomatic, but may present with abdominal pain, bleeding, perforation or obstruction. They can present as benign small yellow-white or as sessile polyps. They are also typically found incidentally during endoscopy or surgery. Small lesions may be considered for polypectomy or transanal excision (TAE) for rectal leiomyomas.[15,29]

POLYPOSIS SYNDROMES

Lynch Syndrome

Definition and Features

Lynch syndrome, also known as hereditary nonpolyposis colorectal cancer, is an autosomal dominant condition that predisposes patients to colorectal adenocarcinoma and extracolonic malignancies located in the endometrium, ovary, and urologic tract, among others. It is characterized

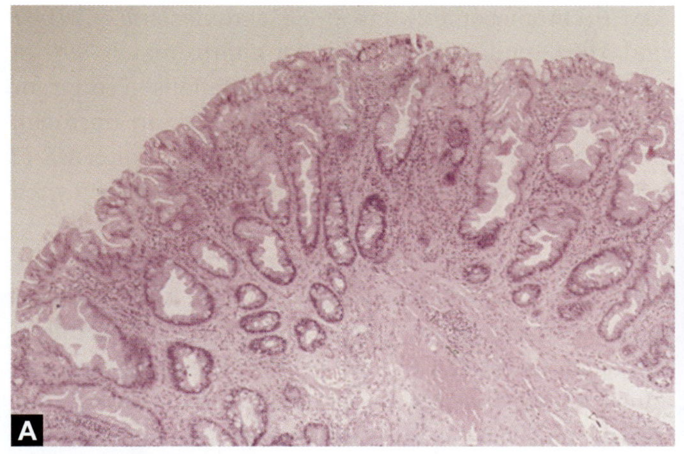

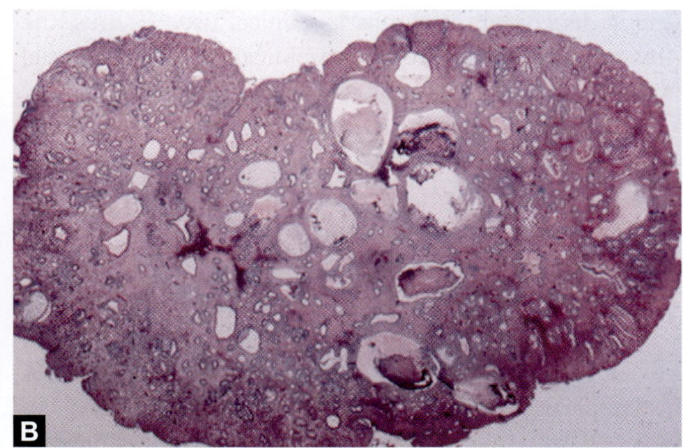

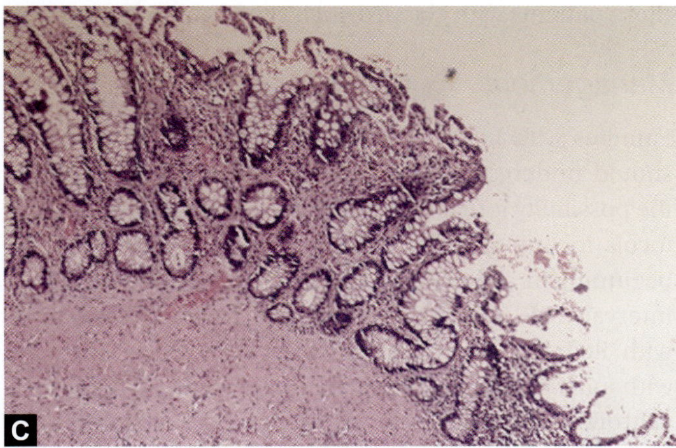

Figs. 62A.5A to C: Other polyps with malignant potential. (A) Hyperplastic polyp. There are elongated nonbranching mucosal crypts. (B) Juvenile polyp. There are multiple mucus-filled cysts in this macroscopic view. (C) Inflammatory polyp. Inflamed and regenerative mucosa enclosing a core of muscularis mucosae and submucosa.
Source: Courtesy of Stephen S Sternberg and Satish Tickoo.

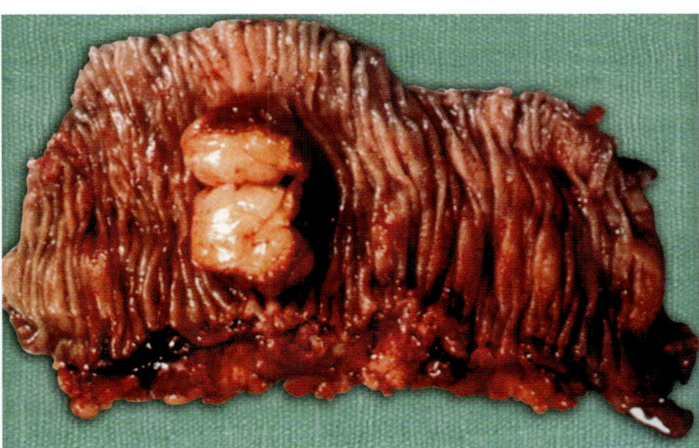

Fig. 62A.6: Lipomatous polyp. The opened specimen of the large bowel shows tumor composed of mature adipose tissue located in the splenic flexure.
Source: Courtesy of Stephen S Sternberg and Satish Tickoo.

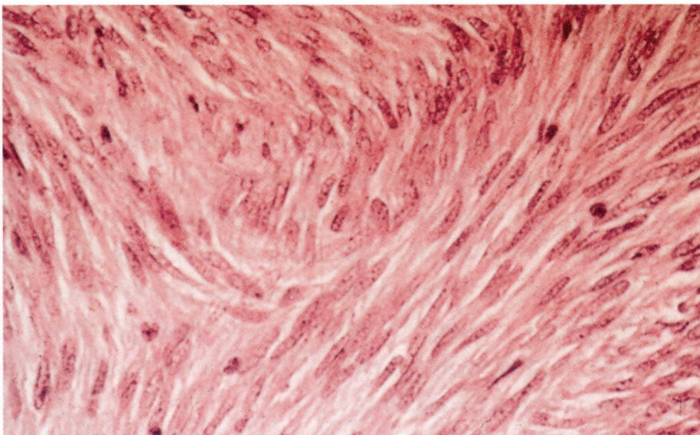

Fig. 62A.7: Leiomyosarcomatous polyp. The elongated cells grow in fascicles. A leiomyomatous polyp would show more smooth muscle characteristics and less mitotic activity.
Source: Courtesy of Stephen S Sternberg and Satish Tickoo.

by early age of cancer onset (40s), right-sided predominance of CRC, and multiple synchronous as well as metachronous CRC.[30] On histology, the CRC associated with this syndrome is often mucinous with signet-ring cells, a Crohn's-like reaction and significant tumor-infiltrating lymphocytes.

Lynch syndrome is the most common hereditary CRC syndrome and accounts for approximately 3% of the estimated annual incidence of CRC.[30,31] While the revised Bethesda guidelines are commonly used to identify patients who may benefit from tumor microsatellite instability testing, its complexity limits its clinical use.[31,32] Thus, the Amsterdam criteria II are used to clinically identify potential families with Lynch syndrome and require:

- At least three family members with a Lynch-syndrome associated cancer (CRC or cancer of the endometrium, small bowel, ureter, or renal pelvis), one of whom is a first-degree relative to the other two
- At least two successive generations represented
- At least one individual younger than 50 years at diagnosis
- FAP should be excluded in CRC cases
- Tumors should be verified by pathologic examination.

People with Lynch syndrome generally tend not to develop polyposis. They form adenomas at about the same rate as the general population, but at a younger age. Adenomas in the setting of Lynch syndrome are more likely to undergo malignant transformation than adenomas in the general population.[30,33]

The average age at diagnosis of the index CRC among Lynch patients is 45 years. Approximately 70–80% of Lynch CRC are located proximal to the splenic flexure (compared to 30% of sporadic CRC). The risk of developing adenoma by age 60 in Lynch patients ranges from 48% to 68% with a 22–35% risk of CRC development. As such, even when surveillance recommendations are followed, patients with Lynch syndrome tend to have a high rate of interval CRC.[30,33]

In addition to CRC, patients with Lynch syndrome are at 30–70% risk of developing extracolonic tumors including cancers of the endometrium, ovary, stomach, small bowel, urinary tract, hepatopancreatobiliary tract, brain, prostate, breast, and skin. Though female patients have a very high risk of developing endometrial cancer, their prognosis is good as 10-year survival following surgery is about 80%.[31] Patients also have a 6–10% risk of urologic tract carcinoma and are almost six times more likely to develop gastric cancer.[34,35] Patients with Muir-Torre syndrome are said to be at risk of Lynch-associated cancers as well as sebaceous neoplasms.

Genetics

As aforementioned, mismatch repair (MMR) genes are responsible for correcting errors of DNA replication. Alterations in these genes result in the inability to repair insertions or deletions within microsatellites, which can lead to instability of the genetic material and consequent malignant transformation.

The MMR genes associated with Lynch syndrome include *MLH1* (chromosome 3), *MSH2* (chromosome 2), *MSH6* (chromosome 2), and *PMS2* (chromosome 7). *MLH1* and *MSH2* mutations account for approximately 80% of all Lynch kindred, whereas *PMS2* mutations account for only 5%.[35] Germline mutation of *EPCAM*, an upstream neighbor of the *MSH2* gene, has been shown to alter *MSH2* expression and is now selectively tested during Lynch syndrome workup.[31,36]

The diagnosis of familial colorectal cancer syndrome X (FCC X) is made when patients with family histories meeting Amsterdam criteria II do not have a detectable germline mutation. In FCC X, CRC may be more left-sided, have less mucin and with well to moderate cell differentiation. They also present with CRC at a later average age (55 years) than those patients with classic Lynch syndrome.[37]

Management

Families with histories consistent with Lynch syndrome should undergo genetic counseling and be informed of the possibility for genetic testing. Current surveillance protocols include a complete colonoscopy every 1–2 years beginning at age 20–25 years, given the increased risk of interval CRC. The risks and benefits of a total colectomy with ileorectal anastomosis (IRA) should be discussed with individuals who develop CRC, given the risks of metachronous lesions. Upper endoscopies are recommended in Lynch families from countries with a high incidence of gastric cancer every 1–2 years beginning at 30–35 years old, with additional screening for and eradication of *Helicobacter pylori* in order to minimize the risks of neoplasia. Women may be offered gynecologic examinations with 1- to 2-year transvaginal ultrasound and aspiration biopsy beginning at age 35–40 years to detect premalignant and early disease, provided that they understand the risks and benefits of such procedures. Prophylactic bilateral oophorectomy and hysterectomy may be considered in those who have completed childbearing age or are postmenopausal. Surveillance recommendations for urologic tract cancers include an annual urine cytology/analysis starting at 25–30 years old.[31,38-40]

Familial Adenomatous Polyposis

Features

Familial adenomatous polyposis is the second most common hereditary CRC syndrome and is characterized by 100 or more adenomatous polyps throughout the colon and rectum (Fig. 62A.8). A germline *APC* mutation is responsible for the development of such adenomas

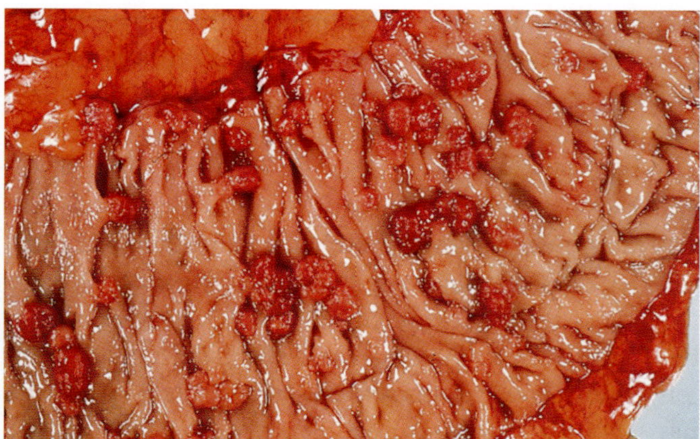

Fig. 62A.8: Colon from a patient with familial adenomatous polyposis. *Source:* Courtesy of Stephen S Sternberg and Satish Tickoo.

and the CRC risk invariably reaches to near 100% by age 50, if the colon remains intact.[41] As such, individuals at risk are screened with flexible sigmoidoscopy starting at age 10–15 years. Prophylactic colon resection should be recommended for FAP patients with uncontrolled polyposis, as surveillance colonoscopies with polypectomy will be inadequate to ensure the absence of carcinoma.[40]

Recognized extracolonic manifestations of FAP include epidermoid cysts, lipomas, supernumerary teeth, aggressive fibromatosis (also known as desmoid disease), osteomas of the jaw or skull, thyroiditis, juvenile nasopharyngeal angiofibromas, and congenital hypertrophy of the retinal pigment epithelium (CHRPE). Patients with FAP have a higher risk of stomach and duodenal malignancies due to the development of extracolonic polyps in these organs. Other less common tumors associated with FAP include adrenal adenoma, medulloblastoma as well as cancers of the gallbladder and bile duct, pancreas, urinary bladder, and testes. Familial adenomatous polyposis patients, especially females, are at increased risk of developing papillary thyroid carcinoma.[41,42] The lifetime prevalence of hepatoblastomas in FAP patients is approximately 1–2% and most typically present in young boys ages 0–4.[43]

Similarly, attenuated FAP (aFAP) is resultant from a germline *APC* mutation and is a variant of classic FAP. The aFAP phenotype is not as striking, as patients typically have >10 and <100 colonic adenomas by ages 40–50. Nevertheless, aFAP patients are at an increased risk of developing CRC and the associated extracolonic malignancies, relative to the general population. As such, surveillance and surgical recommendations for patients with aFAP are guided by symptomatology as well as polyp burden.[41]

Genetics

While there are at least 1,000 genetic variants on the *APC* gene responsible for FAP, there appears to be a genotype-phenotype correlation that dictates the severity of polyposis and extracolonic manifestations. For example, the most common genotype is a five-base deletion beginning at codon 1309 and is responsible for the classical FAP presentation. This deletion, in addition to mutations within codons 1249–1549, results in polyposis at an earlier age and worse survival. In addition, patients with genotypes within such cluster regions have a higher risk of rectal involvement that may require surgical removal. Further, desmoid disease has recently been shown to be most severe in patients with mutations near the 3′-end of the *APC* gene. Current studies are attempting to further delineate various aspects of the FAP genotype–phenotype relationship.

Though FAP is typically inherited in an autosomal dominant manner, approximately 10–30% of patients develop adenomatous polyposis as a result of a de novo mutation. Further, there is a small subgroup diagnosed based on physical presentation alone, as not all *APC* mutations can be identified at this time. Mutations along the 5′-end (codons 1–157), exon 9, and the 3′-end (codons 1595 and greater) of *APC* are typically responsible for the aFAP phenotype.[41,44,45]

Management

Individuals belonging to a FAP family can be genetically tested to determine if they have an *APC* mutation. If the mutation associated with the FAP phenotype in a particular family is known, at-risk relatives who test negative for the mutation have an average risk of developing CRC and should be screened accordingly. It is unclear how these people should be followed, but it may not be unreasonable to perform one endoscopic examination before age 20 and then another between 26 and 30 years, if the initial examination is not concerning for FAP or aFAP phenotype. These individuals are then offered screening as practiced for the average-risk population.

At-risk relatives who test positive for an *APC* mutation should undergo a baseline colonoscopy beginning at age 10–12 years and then every 1–2 years thereafter. Prophylactic surgery should be considered when the polyposis becomes unmanageable. If a patient has already had surgery, they should undergo an endoscopic examination of their rectum or ileal pouch every 6 months to 2 years, depending on the extent of polyp burden. They should also undergo upper endoscopies every 1-3 years beginning at age 20-25 years. In addition, annual thyroid ultrasounds and abdominal ultrasounds should be offered in order to detect thyroid cancer as well as hydronephrosis related to desmoid disease.[42,46]

If an *APC* mutation is not detected in affected individuals, other conditions such as MAP should be considered. If other differential diagnoses can be eliminated, then the test is considered uninformative and all at-risk relatives should undergo endoscopic screening according to guidelines for patients afflicted with FAP as commercial testing may not be able detect all syndrome-causing mutations at this time.

People at risk by virtue of their pedigree who have not undergone molecular tests should undergo annual flexible sigmoidoscopy beginning at age 10-12 with plans for a full colonoscopy to assess the rest of the colon. If FAP phenotype has not been expressed by age 44, these individuals may be able to reduce the frequency of colonoscopic surveillance.[40,47] However, affected individuals are still strongly encouraged to undergo genetic evaluation and testing in order to assist in providing accurate screening recommendations for other at-risk family members.

Surgical Options

Nearly all persons with FAP develop CRC by ages 40-50 years if the colon is left in place. Symptoms typically manifest by age 20 and carcinoma is detected by 35 years of age. However, malignant changes can occur as early as 15-20 years of age.[41,46] The timing and type of prophylactic surgery in those with FAP who are < 20 years old are often influenced by the schooling calendar and the patient's self-image. Generally, if the polyps are small and there is no evidence of dysplasia, prophylactic surgery is scheduled between high school and college. Possible surgical options include:

- Total proctocolectomy and ileal pouch anal anastomosis (IPAA)
- Total abdominal colectomy and IRA
- Proctocolectomy and ileostomy
- Proctocolectomy and Kock pouch.

Restorative proctocolectomy with IPAA and total abdominal colectomy with a restorative IRA are the two most commonly performed options. The decision to carry out a particular surgery is influenced by patient age, polyp density in the rectum, patient compliance for lifelong rectal stump surveillance, patient acceptance of risk of rectal cancer versus inferior function, and pouch-associated complications. Proponents of rectal preservation argue that the risk of rectal cancer is not prohibitive and that proctectomy may result in autonomic nerve dysfunction. Those in support of proctectomy argue that the lifetime risk of rectal cancer is unacceptable and rectal preservation commits the patient to lifelong endoscopic surveillance. Patients for whom genetic testing is not available or possible and who have either a phenotype of excessive (> 1,000) colon polyps or > 30 rectal polyps at the time of colectomy have an increased risk of developing rectal cancer and should strongly consider a restorative proctocolectomy, as their cumulative risk of developing rectal cancer remains high. Patients for whom genetic testing results are available and who have a severe polyposis phenotype (at least 500 polyps), are younger than 25 years old at the time of surgery, and have mutations within codons 1250-1464 on the *APC* gene should consider a restorative proctocolectomy, given the likelihood of rectal involvement.[45,48]

Restorative proctocolectomy with IPAA: When possible, a temporary diverting ileostomy should accompany a restorative proctocolectomy with an IPAA. The rectal dissection is carried out close to the fascia propria of the rectum to preserve the nervi erigentes, which provide parasympathetic innervation to the hindgut. An ileal pouch reservoir is constructed from the distal ileum and is anastomosed within the anal canal to the dentate line via a hand-sewn anastomosis after a mucosectomy. Reconstruction can also be carried out with a double-stapled technique, but this approach, while associated with improved function, potentially leaves behind rectal mucosa at risk of developing adenomatous polyps or cancer at the anastomotic site. The neorectal reservoir can be constructed in various configurations including J, S, and W pouches. The apex of the pouch should reach a point 5 cm below the upper border of the pubic symphysis in order to ensure a tension-free anastomosis to the dentate line. Adequate length can be achieved by mobilizing the small bowel mesentery from the retroperitoneum up to the level of the duodenum, with division of the visceral peritoneum on either side of the ileal mesentery as well as division of noncritical arcade vessels to form windows in a foreshortened small bowel mesentery. Unless not technically possible because of mesentery and/or thick abdominal wall precluding a Brooke-like ileostomy, a temporary diverting ileostomy should always be created in order to protect the IPAA. It can be closed as early as 3 months following a water-soluble contrast study demonstrating anastomotic integrity.

Total abdominal colectomy with an IRA: Total abdominal colectomy with an IRA removes at-risk colon, but leaves the rectum in place for reservoir function. This operation is an option for patients with good sphincter function and rectal sparing of polyps, who are compliant with regular screening proctoscopies and understand the risk of metachronous rectal cancer. The risk of requiring a subsequent proctectomy for rectal cancer or polyp burden ranges from 10% to 60% over a 20-year period.[48] Proctoscopic examination of the entire rectal remnant should be carried out every 6 months. Oral or rectal NSAIDs may be prescribed to decrease or prevent adenoma formation in the remaining rectum.

Proctocolectomy with ileostomy: Proctocolectomy with ileostomy removes all at-risk colorectal tissue and manages gastrointestinal output with a permanent ileostomy. In the absence of a rectal cancer, dissection is carried out close to the rectum and along the intersphincteric plane so as to protect the hypogastric and sympathetic nerves in the pelvis. Disadvantages of this operation include incontinence of gas and stool and a permanent stoma. Most people, particularly young patients, are hesitant to accept this operation as a prophylactic measure. The operation is specifically indicated if a coexisting rectal cancer precludes curative resection with a restorative procedure.

Proctocolectomy with a Kock ileostomy: Proctocolectomy with a Kock continent ileostomy involves the construction of an ileal pouch with a valve formed by intussuscepting the terminal ileum into the pouch. This pouch is then emptied intermittently by intubation. This technique eliminates the need for a permanent stoma and is an option for patients who desire bowel continuity without a stoma but are not candidates for an IPAA. However, it is not commonly performed due to high complication and reoperation rates.

Desmoid Tumors

Desmoids, or aggressive fibromatosis, are nonmalignant lesions that occur in 10–25% of people with FAP.[49] Though they do not metastasize, they are life-threatening because they can invade and compress vital organs. They commonly develop in the small bowel mesentery, retroperitoneum or within the abdominal wall, but can occur in other parts of the body. Desmoid disease can be categorized into four stages:

- Stage I (asymptomatic, < 10 cm maximum diameter and not growing)
- Stage II (mildly symptomatic, < 10 cm maximum diameter and not growing)
- Stage III (moderately symptomatic, or bowel/ureteric obstruction, or 10–20 cm or slowly growing)
- Stage IV (severely symptomatic, septic complications such as fistula and abscess, or > 20 cm or rapidly growing)

Five-year survival for patients with stages I and II disease is 95–100% and 76–89% for stages III–IV. Patients who have stage IV disease and other risk factors such as severe pain, desmoid diameter > 10 cm, and need for parenteral nutrition have an estimated 5-year survival of only 53%.[50]

The exact cause of desmoids is unclear. As aforementioned, patients with mutations within the 3′-end of the *APC* end appear to have a higher propensity for desmoid disease. Familial adenomatous polyposis patients who have undergone a colectomy have a higher rate of mortality from desmoid complications than those with an intact colon and rectum, supporting the theory that surgery triggers a fibromatotic response. High estrogen levels also seem to perpetuate the growth of desmoid tumors.[50-52]

For this reason, though radical excision for desmoids may temper the disease, surgery remains controversial given the risk of complications such as bleeding, significant bowel resection leading to short bowel syndrome as well as the high likelihood of recurrence. Procedures such as intestinal bypass or ureteral stenting may be necessary in the event of bowel or ureteral obstruction. Medical management and prevention of desmoid disease include the use of NSAIDs such as sulindac, antiestrogens such as tamoxifen and selective estrogen receptor modulators, targeted therapies such as imatinib or interferon, doxorubicin-based cytotoxic therapies, and radiation. In addition, sorafenib may be used as off-label therapy for truncal or extremity desmoids.[53] In individualized cases, surgical resection may be considered for symptomatic, isolated abdominal desmoids, especially for disease limited to the abdominal wall.[50]

Gastroduodenal Tumors

Since gastroduodenal tumors are common in people with FAP, upper gastrointestinal surveillance is a standard part of management. Though the lifetime risk of gastric cancer in FAP patients is 1%, duodenal adenomas have been found in 50–90% of FAP patients and duodenal polyposis is associated with an increased risk of periampullary malignancies.[46] According to the Spigelman classification, duodenal polyp burden can be categorized into mild (stage I), moderate (stage II), and severe (stages III/IV) disease. Current practice is to screen the upper digestive tract at the time of FAP diagnosis. Polypectomy and histologic examination are recommended, though removal of all disease is unlikely given the floridity and sessile nature of these polyps. Recommended surveillance intervals based on polyp burden are every 5, 3, and 1–2 years for stages I, II, and III disease, respectively. Surgery is recommended for stage IV disease and options may range from a local duodenotomy with polypectomy and/or ampullectomy to a pancreaticoduodenectomy. While ursodeoxycholic acid as a chemopreventive drug for duodenal adenoma prevention has not demonstrated an effect, other preventive studies using anti-inflammatories such as curcumin as well as celecoxib with or without eflornithine are in progress.[54-56]

MUTYH-Associated Adenomatous Polyposis

MUTYH-associated adenomatous polyposis is an autosomal recessive syndrome resulting from biallelic mutations in the base excision repair gene *MUTYH* and is similar to aFAP in terms of colonic phenotype. An estimated 2% of the general population are monoallelic carriers of a mutated *MUTYH* gene, but the prevalence of MAP is unclear. Patients with MAP tend to develop proximal CRC and have a 4% lifetime risk of developing duodenal cancer. Extracolonic manifestations are similar to FAP and include osteomas, desmoids, CHRPE, and thyroid cancer. They also may be at increased risk of developing ovarian, bladder, sebaceous gland, and breast tumors. Screening colonoscopies should begin by age 25–30 years with 1–3 year intervals based on findings and recommendation for prophylactic colorectal surgery in cases of uncontrolled polyposis. Screening upper endoscopies are recommended by age 30–35 years with 3–5-year intervals based on findings. The exact risk of developing such malignancies in those with a monoallelic *MUTYH* mutation is unclear, though some have suggested that their risk is higher than the general population but lower than those with biallelic mutations.[41,46]

Peutz-Jeghers Syndrome

Features

Peutz-Jeghers syndrome is an autosomal dominant disorder characterized by hamartomatous polyposis with a resultant increased risk of gastrointestinal cancers and mucocutaneous melanin pigmentation. It was first described by Peutz in 1921, and its inheritance was delineated by Jeghers in 1959. PJS predisposes patients to an almost 40% risk of developing CRC as well as an increased risk of developing other gastrointestinal cancers. Polyps occur in 90–100% of affected individuals and are found in the small intestine, colon and stomach (in decreasing order of frequency). Polyp sizes range from 1 mm to 3 cm in diameter, may be sessile or pedunculated in morphology and typically become symptomatic by the second or third decade of life. Presenting symptoms include obstruction due to intussusception, abdominal pain, hematochezia, and anal extrusion of a polyp. Microscopically, the polyps are frond-like with muscularis mucosae extending into arborizations covered with normal epithelium (Fig. 62A.9). Mucocutaneous pigmentation of the lips, buccal mucosa, and periorbital area is the other defining feature of PJS and typically appears during childhood, but they may also appear on other parts such as forearms, palms, soles, digits, and perianal area. The diagnostic criteria for a clinical diagnosis of PJS require two of the three of the following findings:

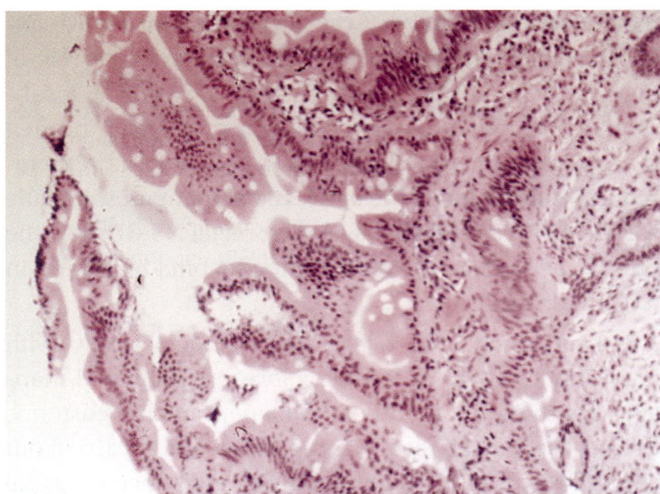

Fig. 62A.9: Hamartomatous polyp. Normal mucosal elements cover a scaffolding of muscularis mucosae. This is typical in a patient who has Peutz–Jeghers syndrome.
Source: Courtesy of Stephen S Sternberg and Satish Tickoo.

- Two or more Peutz-Jeghers-type hamartomatous polyps of the small bowel
- Mucocutaneous hyperpigmentation of the mouth, lips, nose, eyes, genitalia, or fingers
- Family history consistent with autosomal dominant inheritance

In addition to intestinal polyps, PJS is associated with a 45–50% lifetime risk of breast, 18–21% risk of ovarian, 11–36% risk of pancreatic and 29% risk of gastric cancer. Patients with PJS are also at increased risk of testicular and lung cancers.[40,57]

Genetics

A germline mutation in *LKB1/STK11* on the short arm of chromosome 19, a gene that encodes a serine/threonine kinase, is responsible for the manifestations of PJS. Such germline mutations are found only in about 50% of clinical cases suspicious for PJS, and a negative genetic test does not preclude patients who fulfill the clinical criteria from a diagnosis of PJS and appropriate genetic counseling.[40,57]

Management

Current screening guidelines for PJS include:

- Esophagogastroduodenoscopy and colonoscopy every 2–3 years, beginning in late teens
- Biannual breast examination with annual mammogram and magnetic resonance imaging (MRI) from age 25 years
- Magnetic retrograde cholangiopancreatography and/or endoscopic ultrasound every 1–2 years from age 25 to 30 years
- Annual pelvic examination and Pap smear for females from age 18 years, with consideration for and transvaginal ultrasound
- Annual testicular examination from age 10 years
- Small bowel visualization with CT enterography baseline at ages 8–10 years and every 2–3 years thereafter.[40]

Juvenile Polyposis

Features

A juvenile polyp is an isolated hamartoma or disorganized growth of normal tissue that is typically seen in childhood and is not usually associated with an increased CRC risk. Juvenile polyposis syndrome (JPS) is an autosomal dominant condition characterized by multiple juvenile polyps of the gastrointestinal tract that predisposes affected individuals to cancers of the colon and rectum, stomach, pancreas, and small bowel. The term juvenile refers to the polyp, not necessarily the patient's age at the time of presentation. The WHO criteria for JPS diagnosis include any one of the following findings:

- At least three to five juvenile polyps in the colon and rectum
- Juvenile polyps throughout the gastrointestinal tract or
- Any number of juvenile polyps with a family history of JPS.[27]

Genetics

Juvenile polyposis syndrome is caused by a germline mutation of the *SMAD4, BMPR1A*, or *ENG* genes whose proteins interact in the transforming growth factor-beta signaling pathway and has variable penetrance. Patients with *SMAD4* mutations appear to have a higher frequency of gastric polyposis and hereditary hemorrhagic telangiectasias (HHT). Hereditary hemorrhagic telangiectasia, or Osler-Weber-Rendu syndrome, increases the risk of epistaxis, gastrointestinal bleeding, mucocutaneous telangiectasia as well as life-threatening potential for hemorrhage secondary to HHT-associated arteriovenous malformations in the lungs and brain.[58] Congenital cardiac, gastrointestinal, central nervous system, vascular, genitourinary or soft tissue defects have been noted in affected individuals.[27,59]

Management

Patients with JPS have a lifetime 40–50% risk of developing CRC and about a 21% risk of developing gastric cancer if multiple polyps are present.[40] As such, the screening guidelines for JPS include:

- A baseline colonoscopy beginning at age 15 years, with a repeat at 1–3 year intervals, depending on the presence of polyps
- A baseline upper endoscopy beginning at age 15 years, with a repeat at 1–3 year intervals, depending on the presence/absence of polyps[27,40]

Any juvenile polyp with adenomatous changes should be completely removed and examined histologically to rule out dysplasia and carcinoma. Definitive surgical resection depends upon the location and severity of polyp burden as well as the feasibility of long-term endoscopic surveillance. Though there is a 10–15% risk of small bowel and pancreas cancer development, there are currently no additional recommendations regarding screening and surveillance of these sites in JPS patients.[27,40]

Serrated Polyposis Syndrome

Serrated polyps are so named due to their saw-toothed appearance of epithelial crypts in the intestinal mucosa. Serrated polyposis syndrome (SPS), previously known as hyperplastic polyposis syndrome, is characterized by the presence of serrated colorectal lesions and is associated with an increased risk of CRC. The WHO criteria for establishing a diagnosis of SPS include any one of the following:

- At least five serrated polyps proximal to the sigmoid colon with two or more of these being > 10 mm
- Any number of serrated polyps proximal to the sigmoid colon in an individual who has a first-degree relative with SPS
- >20 serrated polyps of any size distributed throughout the colon.[1]

Polyp burden in patients with SPS can range from few to hundreds and typically present with CRC by ages 50–60 years. No known genetic mutation has been identified thus far, though the epigenetic CIMP pathway appears to be the major force driving CRC development.[1,2]

REFERENCES

1. Snover DC, Ahnen D, Burt RW, et al. Serrated polyps of the colon and rectum and serrated polyposis. In: Bosman FT, Carneiro F, Hruban RH, et al. (Eds). Classification of Tumours of the Digestive System. Lyon: IARC Press; 2010. pp. 160-5.
2. Rex DK, Ahnen DJ, Baron JA, et al. Serrated lesions of the colorectum: review and recommendations from an expert panel. Am J Gastroenterol. 2012;107(9):1315-29.
3. Wood LD, Parsons DW, Jones S, et al. The genomic landscapes of human breast and colorectal cancers. Science. 2007;318(5853):1108-13.
4. Vogelstein B, Papadopoulos N, Velculescu VE, et al. Cancer genome landscapes. Science. 2013;339(6127):1546-58.
5. Markowitz SD, Bertagnolli MM. Molecular origins of cancer: molecular basis of colorectal cancer. N Engl J Med. 2009; 361(25):2449-60.
6. Palles C, Cazier JB, Howarth KM, et al. Germline mutations affecting the proofreading domains of POLE and POLD1 predispose to colorectal adenomas and carcinomas. Nat Genet. 2013;45(6):713.
7. Howlader N, Noone A, Krapcho M, et al. (2013). SEER Cancer Statistics Review, 1975-2010, National Cancer Institute. Bethesda, MD. [online] http://seer.cancer.gov/csr/1975_2010/. Based on November 2012 SEER data submission. [Accessed June 5, 2013].
8. Hol L, van Leerdam ME, van Ballegooijen M, et al. Screening for colorectal cancer: randomised trial comparing guaiac-based and immunochemical faecal occult blood testing and flexible sigmoidoscopy. Gut. 2010;59(1):62-8.
9. Quintero E, Castells A, Bujanda L, et al. Colonoscopy versus fecal immunochemical testing in colorectal-cancer screening. N Engl J Med. 2012;366(8):697-706.
10. Lieberman DA, Rex DK, Winawer SJ, et al. Guidelines for colonoscopy surveillance after screening and polypectomy: a consensus update by the US Multi-Society Task Force on Colorectal Cancer. Gastroenterology. 2012;143(3):844-57.
11. Schoen RE, Pinsky PF, Weissfeld JL, et al. Colorectal-cancer incidence and mortality with screening flexible sigmoidoscopy. N Engl J Med. 2012;366(25):2345-57.
12. Atkin WS, Edwards R, Kralj-Hans I, et al. Once-only flexible sigmoidoscopy screening in prevention of colorectal cancer: a multicentre randomised controlled trial. Lancet. 2010;375(9726):1624-33.
13. Zauber AG, Winawer SJ, O'Brien MJ, et al. Colonoscopic polypectomy and long-term prevention of colorectal-cancer deaths. N Engl J Med. 2012;366(8):687-96.
14. Johnson CD, Chen MH, Toledano AY, et al. Accuracy of CT colonography for detection of large adenomas and cancers. N Engl J Med. 2008;359(12):1207-17.
15. Beck DE, Roberts PL, Rombeau JL, et al. (Eds). The ASCRS Manual of Colon and Rectal Surgery. New York: Springer Science+Business Media, LLC; 2009.
16. Saito Y, Fukuzawa M, Matsuda T, et al. Clinical outcome of endoscopic submucosal dissection versus endoscopic mucosal resection of large colorectal tumors as determined by curative resection. Surg Endosc. 2010;24(2):343-52.
17. Kim JS, Kim BW, Kim JI, et al. Endoscopic clip closure versus surgery for the treatment of iatrogenic colon perforations developed during diagnostic colonoscopy: a review of 115,285 patients. Surg Endosc. 2013;27(2):501-4.
18. Bertelson NL, Kalkbrenner KA, Merchea A, et al. Colectomy for endoscopically unresectable polyps: how often is it cancer? Dis Colon Rectum. 2012;55(11):1111-6.
19. Cunningham D, Atkin W, Lenz HJ, et al. Colorectal cancer. Lancet. 2010;375(9719):1030-47.
20. Mathers JC, Movahedi M, Macrae F, et al. Long-term effect of resistant starch on cancer risk in carriers of hereditary colorectal cancer: an analysis from the CAPP2 randomised controlled trial. Lancet Oncol. 2012;13(12):1242-9.
21. Cuzick J, Otto F, Baron JA, et al. Aspirin and non-steroidal anti-inflammatory drugs for cancer prevention: an international consensus statement. Lancet Oncol. 2009;10(5): 501-7.
22. Burn J, Gerdes AM, Macrae F, et al. Long-term effect of aspirin on cancer risk in carriers of hereditary colorectal cancer: an analysis from the CAPP2 randomised controlled trial. Lancet. 2011;378(9809):2081-7.
23. ClinicalTrials.gov. (2006). A Phase III Placebo-Controlled Trial Of Celecoxib In Genotype Positive Subjects With Familial Adenomatous Polyposis (CHIP). Bethesda, MD: National Libary of Medicine. Available at: http://www.clinicaltrials.gov/ct2/show/NCT00585312. NLM Identifier: NCT00585312. [Accessed June 5, 2013].
24. ClinicalTrials.gov. (2006). Genetic Events Leading to APC-Dependent Colon Cancer in High-Risk Families: a Clinical Trial of COX and EGFR Inhibition in Familial Polyposis Patients. Bethesda, MD: National Libary of Medicine. Available at: http://clinicaltrials.gov/ct2/show/NCT01187901. NLM Identifier: NCT01187901. [Accessed March 22, 2013].
25. ClinicalTrials.gov. (2006). Phase III Trial of the Safety and Efficacy of Eflornithine Combined With Sulindac Compared to Eflornithine, Sulindac as Single Agents in Patients With Familial Adenomatous Polyposis and Attenuated Familial Adenomatous Polyposis. Bethesda, MD: National Libary of Medicine. Available at: http://clinicaltrials.gov/ct2/show/NCT01483144. NLM Identifier: NCT01483144. [Accessed March 22, 2013].
26. ClinicalTrials.gov. (2006). A Double Blind Placebo-Controlled Trial of Eflornithine and Sulindac to Prevent Recurrence of High Risk Adenomas and Second Primary Colorectal Cancers in Patients With Stage 0–III Colon Cancer, Phase III–Preventing Adenomas of the Colon With Eflornithine and Sulindac (PACES). Bethesda, MD: National Library of Medicine. Available at: http://clinicaltrials.gov/ct2/show/NCT01349881. NLM Identifier: NCT01349881. [Accessed March 22, 2013].
27. Offerhaus GJA, Howe JR. Juvenile polyposis. In: Bosman FT, Carneiro F, Hruban RH, et al. (Eds). Classification of Tumours of the Digestive System. Lyon: IARC Press; 2010. pp. 166-7.
28. Cairns SR, Scholefield JH, Steele RJ, et al. Guidelines for colorectal cancer screening and surveillance in moderate and high risk groups (update from 2002). Gut. 2010;59(5): 666-89.

29. Miettinen M, Fletcher CDM, Kindblom LG, et al. Mesenchymal tumours of the colon and rectum. In: Bosman FT, Carneiro F, Hruban RH, et al. (Eds). Classification of Tumours of the Digestive System. Lyon: IARC Press; 2010. pp 181-2.
30. Lynch HT, Lynch PM, Lanspa SJ, et al. Review of the Lynch syndrome: history, molecular genetics, screening, differential diagnosis, and medicolegal ramifications. Clin Genet. 2009;76(1):1-18.
31. Vasen HF, Blanco I, Aktan-Collan K, et al. Revised guidelines for the clinical management of Lynch syndrome (HNPCC): recommendations by a group of European experts. Gut. 2013;62(6):812-23.
32. Umar A, Boland CR, Terdiman JP, et al. Revised Bethesda Guidelines for hereditary nonpolyposis colorectal cancer (Lynch syndrome) and microsatellite instability. J Natl Cancer Inst. 2004;96(4):261-8.
33. Peltomaki P, Offerhaus GJA, Vasen HFA. Lynch syndrome. In: Bosman FT, Carneiro F, Hruban RH, et al. (Eds). Classification of Tumours of the Digestive System. Lyon: IARC Press; 2010. pp. 152-55.
34. Watson P, Vasen HF, Mecklin JP, et al. The risk of extra-colonic, extra-endometrial cancer in the Lynch syndrome. Int J Cancer. 2008;123(2):444-9.
35. Win AK, Lindor NM, Young JP, et al. Risks of primary extracolonic cancers following colorectal cancer in lynch syndrome. J Natl Cancer Inst. 2012;104(18):1363-72.
36. Kempers MJ, Kuiper RP, Ockeloen CW, et al. Risk of colorectal and endometrial cancers in EPCAM deletion-positive Lynch syndrome: a cohort study. Lancet Oncol. 2011;12(1):49-55.
37. Steinhagen E, Markowitz AJ, Guillem JG. How to Manage a Patient with Multiple Adenomatous Polyps. Surg Oncol Clin N Am. 2010;19:711-23.
38. Kalady MF, McGannon E, Vogel JD, et al. Risk of colorectal adenoma and carcinoma after colectomy for colorectal cancer in patients meeting Amsterdam criteria. Ann Surg. 2010;252(3):507-11; discussion 511-3.
39. Palomaki GE, McClain MR, Melillo S, et al. EGAPP supplementary evidence review: DNA testing strategies aimed at reducing morbidity and mortality from Lynch syndrome. Genet Med. 2009;11(1):42-65.
40. National Comprehensive Cancer Network. NCCN Clinical Practice Guidelines in Oncology: Colorectal Cancer Screening. Available at: http://www.nccn.org/professionals/physician_gls/pdf/colorectal_screening.pdf. [Accessed June 5, 2013].
41. Patel SG, Ahnen DJ. Familial colon cancer syndromes: an update of a rapidly evolving field. Curr Gastroenterol Rep. 2012;14(5):428-38.
42. Steinhagen E, Hui VW, Levy RA, et al. Results of a prospective thyroid ultrasound screening program in adenomatous polyposis patients. Am J Surg. 2014. pii: S0002-9610(14)00264-5.
43. Groen EJ, Roos A, Muntinghe FL, et al. Extra-intestinal manifestations of familial adenomatous polyposis. Ann Surg Oncol. 2008;15(9):2439-50.
44. Newton KF, Mallinson EK, Bowen J, et al. Genotype-phenotype correlation in colorectal polyposis. Clin Genet. 2012; 81(6):521-31.
45. Sinha A, Tekkis PP, Rashid S, et al. Risk factors for secondary proctectomy in patients with familial adenomatous polyposis. Br J Surg. 2010;97(11):1710-5.
46. Jasperson KW, Tuohy TM, Neklason DW, et al. Hereditary and familial colon cancer. Gastroenterology. 2010;138(6): 2044-58.
47. Talbot IC, Burt RW, Jarvinen H, et al. Familial adenomatous polyposis. In: Bosman FT, Carneiro F, Hruban RH, et al. (Eds). Classification of Tumours of the Digestive System. Lyon: IARC Press; 2010. pp. 120-5.
48. Nieuwenhuis MH, Bulow S, Bjork J, et al. Genotype predicting phenotype in familial adenomatous polyposis: a practical application to the choice of surgery. Dis Colon Rectum. 2009;52(7):1259-63.
49. Giardiello FM, Burt RW, Jarvinen H, et al. Familial adenomatous polyposis. In: Bosman FT, Carneiro F, Hruban RH, et al. (Eds). Classification of Tumours of the Digestive System. Lyon: IARC Press; 2010. pp. 147-51.
50. Quintini C, Ward G, Shatnawei A, et al. Mortality of intra-abdominal desmoid tumors in patients with familial adenomatous polyposis: a single center review of 154 patients. Ann Surg. 2012;255(3):511-6.

Additional references appear in the online version of this book.

62B

Malignant Neoplasms of the Large Bowel

Rohin Mittal, Benjamin Perakath

Key Points

- Colorectal cancer (CRC) is the third most common cancer in either men or women. Factors associated with CRC development include aging, cigarette smoking, obesity, sedentary lifestyle, a diet high in red meat, as well as vitamin and mineral deficiencies.
- Sporadic colorectal carcinogenesis is the consequence of complex molecular interactions among a variety of genes and gene products.
- A screening program that allows identification and endoscopic removal of precancerous polyps can reduce deaths from CRC.
- Genetic predispositions to large bowel neoplasia include Lynch syndrome, classic or attenuated familial adenomatous polyposis, MUTYH-associated polyposis (MAP), Peutz-Jeghers syndrome (PJS), juvenile polyposis, and serrated polyposis.
- Anatomic considerations and patterns of lymph node spread govern the extent of bowel resection and lymph node clearance for carcinoma of the colon and rectum.
- The role of neoadjuvant chemotherapy, chemoradiation therapy (CRT), and adjuvant chemotherapy for rectal cancer is ever-evolving, with several ongoing clinical trials attempting to assess (1) a nonoperative approach for patients with a clinical complete response following neoadjuvant therapy, (2) the optimal sequence and timing of CRT and surgery, and (3) survival benefits of the newer targeted therapies.
- Early short-term data suggest equivalency between minimally invasive techniques such as laparoscopic and robotic-assisted colorectal resections and open surgery in terms of obtaining an adequate oncologic resection. Currently, large clinical trials are in progress to assess the benefits of minimal access techniques over the conventional open approach.

COLORECTAL CARCINOMA

Incidence and Risk Factors

Worldwide, colorectal cancer is the third most common cancer in men after lung and prostate cancer, and the second most common cancer in women after breast cancer. It accounts for about 10% of all new cancers diagnosed, and 8% of all cancer-related mortality.[1] Even though both incidence and mortality rates for colorectal cancer have shown a declining trend, about 1,234,000 people were diagnosed to have colorectal cancer worldwide in 2008 and 608,000 died from it. Incidence rates are higher in men than in women, with a sex ratio of 1.4:1. The primary histologic type is adenocarcinoma. Carcinogenesis occurs over many years and is influenced by various factors, both environmental and genetic.

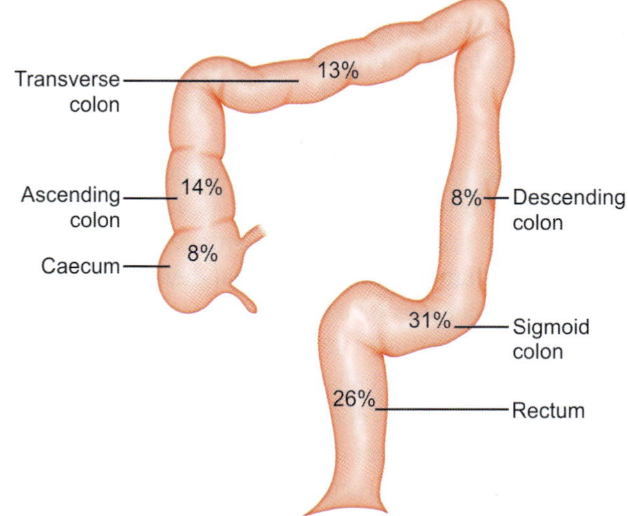

Fig. 62B.1: Distribution of colon and rectal cancer.

Most large bowel cancers arise in the sigmoid colon and rectum (Fig. 62B.1).[2] Right-sided colon cancer is becoming more common, while left-sided colorectal cancer is becoming less common. These trends are explained in part by early detection and treatment of lesions within reach of the rigid or flexible sigmoidoscope.

Geography and Diet

Worldwide, there is a 10-fold geographic variation in the incidence and age-adjusted death rate from large bowel cancer. The highest incidences of colorectal cancer are in Australia (46/10,000 population), New Zealand, Western and Southern Europe, and North America (34.1/10,000). The lowest rates are seen in developing countries, such as Africa (except Southern Africa) (3.5/10,000), and South Central Asia (4.3/100,000).[1] The incidence of colorectal cancer among immigrants from low-risk to high-risk countries converges to that of their adopted country, suggesting a strong influence by environmental factors.

Dietary habits play an important role in the development of colorectal cancer. A diet high in fruits, vegetables, and fiber has a protective role,[4,5] while a diet rich in red meat, animal fat, and cholesterol increases the risk.[6]

Alcohol and Smoking

Moderate (2–3 drinks a day) to heavy consumption (4 or more drinks a day) of alcohol is associated with an increased risk of colorectal cancer development.[7] Cigarette smoking is a significant risk factor for both development of colorectal cancer and mortality from colorectal cancer.[8]

Physical Activity and Obesity

There is an inverse relationship between physical activity and risk of colorectal cancer. Obesity, particularly abdominal adiposity, is associated with a 1.5 times elevated risk of developing colorectal cancer and also an increased likelihood of dying from colorectal cancer.[9]

Age

The incidence of colorectal cancer in the general population begins to rise after the age of 40 years. In the USA between 2007 and 2009, the percentage of the population younger than 40 years of age that developed invasive colorectal cancer was 0.08%. The incidence increased to 0.75–0.94% for those aged 40–59 years, 0.98–1.4% for those aged 60–69 years, and 3.80–4.19% for those aged 70 years and above.[10] However, recent reports have indicated that the incidence of colorectal cancer in younger patients is on the rise.[11] Colon and rectal cancer appears to present at an earlier age in Asian countries.[12,13]

Family History and Genetics

A family history of colorectal cancer is a risk factor for the disease. The absolute cumulative risk of developing colorectal cancer between age 40 and 75 years for men and women who have affected first-degree relatives is 9.6% and those with affected second-degree relatives is 4.7%.[14] It is also suggested that risk conferred by colorectal cancer in siblings may be higher than that by parents. People with a family history of colorectal adenomas may also be at a higher risk of developing colorectal adenomas and also malignancy. Data on this are still evolving and remain unclear.[15] The incidence is even higher for patients who carry genetic mutations associated with familial adenomatous polyposis (FAP) and hereditary nonpolyposis colorectal cancer (HNPCC). Without treatment, all patients with FAP develop colorectal cancer. Penetrance of the cancer phenotype among patients who have HNPCC is 80%.

Disease History

Adenomatous polyps may undergo malignant transformation; the risk increases with the size and the percentage of villous component. A personal history of large (>1 cm) or multiple adenomatous polyps also increases the future risk of colorectal cancer. Hamartomatous polyposis syndromes, including Peutz–Jeghers syndrome and juvenile polyposis, are also associated with colorectal cancer. Individuals who have developed one colorectal cancer have an increased risk of developing synchronous and metachronous lesions. In large studies, the risk of synchronous lesions is about 3.8–3.9%[16,17] and that for metachronous lesions is 3.1–3.4% at 10 years.[18,19] There is increasing evidence that diminutive polyps, previously considered innocuous, can harbor malignant potential[20] by turning into adenomatous polyps and following the adenoma-carcinoma sequence.

Inflammatory bowel disease has been recognized since the 1920s as one of the diseases that increases the risk of developing colorectal cancer. Colorectal carcinoma caused by ulcerative colitis accounts for approximately 1% of all cases of colorectal cancer. A population-based study of Swedish patients with a diagnosis of ulcerative colitis found that the incidence of colorectal cancer was 5.7 times the expected rate. Age and extent of disease at diagnosis were strong and independent risk factors for the development of colorectal cancer. The absolute risk of colorectal cancer 35 years after diagnosis was 30% for patients who had pancolitis at diagnosis and 40% for those who had a diagnosis of ulcerative colitis before 15 years of age. The ratios of observed-to-expected cases of colorectal cancer were 1.7, 2.8, and 14.8 for patients who have ulcerative proctitis, left-sided colitis, and pancolitis, respectively.

Epidemiologic studies in the USA and in the UK have shown a 4–20-fold increased risk of colorectal cancer among patients with Crohn's disease compared to the general population. In another Swedish study of Crohn's disease, the overall relative risk of large bowel cancer was 2.5. The relative risks of Crohn's disease of the terminal ileum only, terminal ileum and colon, and for the colon alone were 1.0, 3.2, and 5.6, respectively. Epidemiologic studies have shown that women who have recovered from breast, uterine, or ovarian cancer have about twice the expected risk of developing colorectal cancer.

Therapeutic Interventions

Ureterosigmoidostomy and pelvic irradiation are both associated with large bowel cancer. A 100–500-fold increase in the incidence of colon carcinoma has been reported at the site of ureterocolonic anastomosis. Patients who receive pelvic radiation are at risk of developing malignancy within the radiation field. An increased incidence of large bowel cancer has been observed in patients who have received pelvic irradiation to treat gynecologic and prostatic neoplasms. Children receiving abdominal radiation are also at risk of developing intestinal malignancies, mainly colorectal.[21]

There have been reports for and against an association between cholecystectomy and colorectal cancer. A recent meta-analysis concluded that while there is a small observed association, it may be due to a publication bias. Even if this were a real effect, the risk to any individual was very small.[22]

DIAGNOSIS OF COLORECTAL CANCER

Screening

Colorectal cancer mortality rate has been reduced by the detection and treatment of early stage colorectal cancers and by the identification and removal of precancerous lesions. Colorectal cancer screening should be initiated at 50 years (45 years in African Americans) in patients at average risk of developing colorectal cancer. A cancer prevention test like colonoscopy (every 10 years) is preferred to a cancer detection test like an annual fecal immunochemical test for occult blood testing. Computed tomography (CT) colonography every 5 years is an alternative to patients who refuse colonoscopy.[23]

Screening should be more aggressive in patients with a positive family history of colorectal malignancy or advanced adenoma, and in whom HNPCC and FAP have been ruled out. In patients with a single first-degree relative diagnosed with colorectal cancer or advanced adenoma at age <60 years or two first-degree relatives with colorectal cancer or advanced adenoma, screening should begin at 40 years or 10 years younger than the youngest affected relative. The recommended screening test is a colonoscopy every 5 years. In patients with a single first-degree relative diagnosed to have colorectal cancer or advanced adenoma at age ≥ 60 years, the screening protocol is the same as for average risk individuals.[23]

Clinical Diagnosis

History, physical examination, and diagnostic tests are all important in the diagnosis of colorectal cancer. Symptoms include abdominal pain, gastrointestinal blood loss, a change in bowel habit, abdominal distension, and anemia. Systemic symptoms like fever, loss of weight and appetite, and cachexia may be present. Patients with metastatic disease may present with jaundice, ascites, or other symptoms based on the site of metastasis. Specific questions pertaining to family history of colorectal cancer must be asked. Masses are sought on abdominal and digital rectal examination. Presence of a left supraclavicular lymph node, umbilical nodule, ascites, or a Blumer's shelf on digital rectal examination indicates probable metastatic disease.

Colonoscopy is the investigation of choice for diagnosing colorectal carcinoma. It provides information on the site of the primary and the presence of synchronous lesions, and it allows biopsy of the lesion. Computed tomography, magnetic resonance imaging (MRI), or positron emission tomography (PET) scans of the abdomen and pelvis help in staging the disease. Colorectal cancer is occasionally diagnosed on imaging performed for other indications. In emergency situations, such as complete colonic obstruction or colonic perforation, extensive diagnostic testing may delay a necessary operation. In these cases, the diagnosis of colorectal cancer may be suspected on preoperative imaging, but is confirmed only at operation and on postoperative histopathology.

Staging

The purpose of staging is to define the extent of disease. Accurate staging also facilitates communication between caregivers, provides information about prognosis, and guides therapy. In 1926, Lockhart-Mummery reported a staging system for rectal cancer using depth of tumor invasion and lymph node involvement as prognostic

Table 62B.1 Dukes classification of rectal cancer.

Dukes classification	*Definition*
A	Growth limited to wall of the rectum
B	Extension of growth to extrarectal tissues, but no metastases in regional lymph nodes
C	Metastases in regional lymph nodes

Table 62B.2 TNM classification of colon and rectal tumors.

T – Primary tumor	
TX	Primary tumor cannot be assessed
T0	No evidence of primary tumor
Tis	Carcinoma in situ: intraepithelial or invasion of lamina propria
T1	Tumor invades submucosa
T2	Tumor invades muscularis propria
T3	Tumor invades through muscularis propria into pericolorectal tissue
T4a	Tumor penetrates to the surface of the visceral peritoneum
T4b	Tumor directly invades or is adherent to other organs or structures
N – Regional lymph nodes	
NX	Regional lymph nodes cannot be assessed
N0	No regional lymph node metastasis
N1	Metastasis in 1–3 regional lymph nodes
N1a	Metastasis in 1 regional lymph node
N1b	Metastasis in 2–3 regional lymph nodes
N1c	Tumor deposit(s) in the subserosa, mesentery, or nonperitonealisedpericolic or perirectal tissues without regional node metastasis
N2	Metastasis in 4 or more regional lymph nodes
N2a	Metastasis in 4–6 regional lymph nodes
N2b	Metastasis in 7 or more regional lymph nodes
M – Distant metastasis	
M0	No distant metastasis
M1	Distant metastasis
M1a	Metastasis confined to one organ or site (e.g., liver, lung, ovary, nonregional node)
M1b	Metastasis in more than one organ/site or the peritoneum

factors. Dukes subsequently proposed several staging systems based on Lockhart-Mummery's classification. The classification published in 1932 is the one most commonly identified as the Dukes classification (Table 62B.1). The principles of the Dukes system were subsequently extended to include carcinomas of the colon and distant metastatic disease. The tumor node metastasis (TNM) classification is now widely used to stage colorectal cancers.[24] In this system T indicates depth of tumor invasion, N represents lymph node status, and M indicates distant metastasis (Table 62B.2). The Dukes and TNM staging systems are compared in Table 62B.3.

Table 62B.3 Comparison of the TNM and the Dukes staging systems.

TNM stage	*T*	*N*	*M*	*Dukes system*
0	Tis	N0	M0	
I	T1/T2	N0	M0	A
II	T3/T4	N0	M0	B
III	Any T	N1/N2	M0	C
IV	Any T	Any N	M1	D*

*Although the original Dukes classification did not include a stage D, metastatic disease is now referred to as Dukes D.

Table 62B.4 Prognostic factors in colorectal cancer.

- Stage of disease
- Perforation
- Obstruction
- Poor differentiation
- Mucinous/signet ring histology
- Lymphovascular invasion
- Perineural invasion
- Elevation of carcinoembryonic antigen
- Resection (R) status of tumor
- Circumferential margin
- DNA aneuploidy
- Allelic loss

Prognostic Factors

The most important prognostic factor is disease stage, which is determined by the depth of penetration of the bowel wall, the lymph node status, and the presence of distant metastases. In addition, other factors (Table 62B.4) may impair survival.

Investigation

Patients with colorectal cancer need a total colonic examination to look for synchronous lesions plus imaging to stage the disease and measurement of tumor markers to help prognosticate and follow up the patient.

A complete evaluation of the colon and rectum by colonoscopy is recommended. If a lesion is detected by barium enema on screening (Fig. 62B.2), colonoscopy is carried out to obtain tissue for pathologic examination (Figs. 62B.3 and 62B. 4). For colon cancers, CT is used to identify the primary tumor, its relationship to neighboring structures, and metastases (Figs. 62B.5 and 62B.6). In rectal cancers, transrectal ultrasound (TRUS) and MRI are useful for preoperative local staging (Figs. 62B.7 and 62B.8). These techniques accurately predict depth of tumor invasion in about 75% of cases. The accuracy of prediction of mesorectal lymph node involvement in rectal cancer by MRI and TRUS is 79 and 65%, respectively.[25] Magnetic

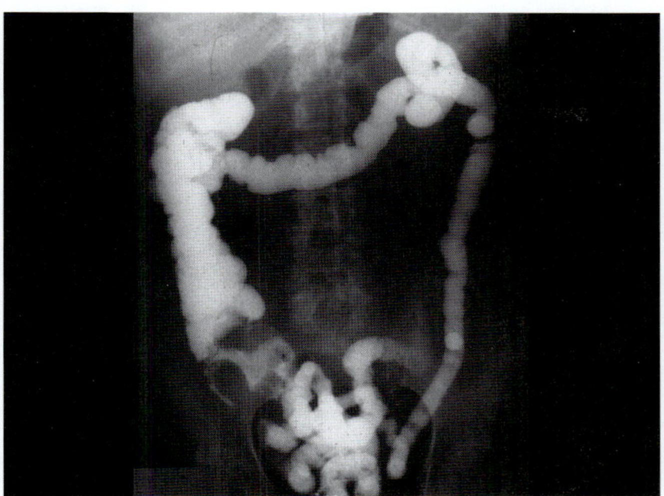

Fig. 62B.2: Barium enema appearance of an annular carcinoma of the proximal ascending colon.

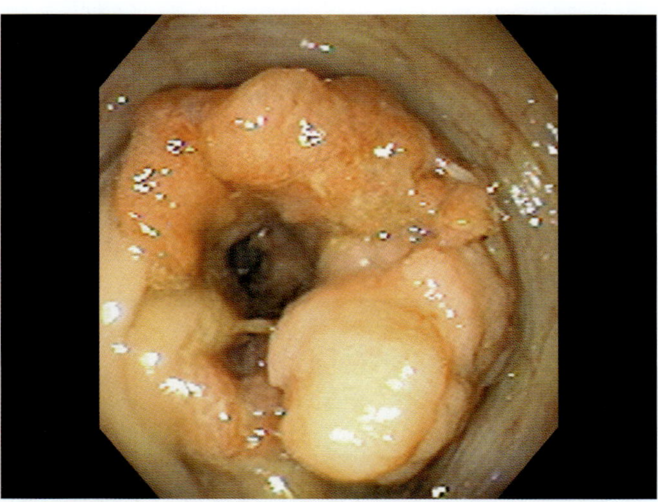

Fig. 62B.3: Colonoscopic appearance of an annular near-obstructing colon carcinoma.
Source: Courtesy of Surinder K Batra.

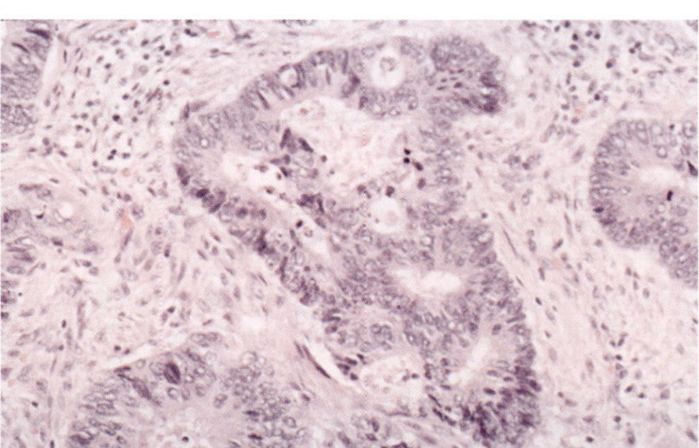

Fig. 62B.4: Moderately differentiated adenocarcinoma with malignant glands composed of columnar epithelium with hyperchromatic nuclei and characteristic central necrosis.
Source: Courtesy of Dario V Caccamo.

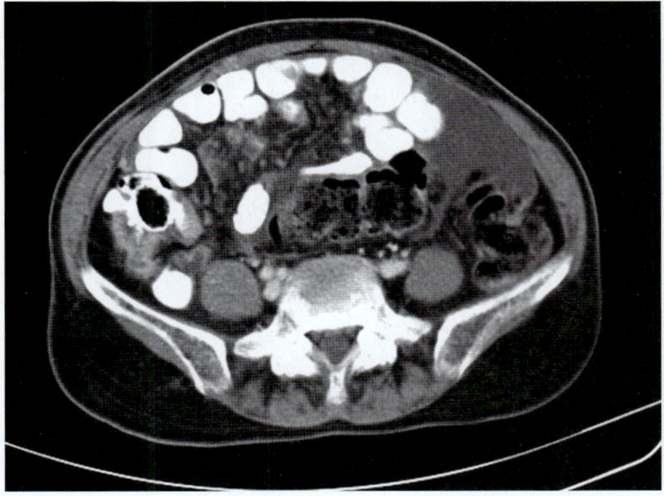

Fig. 62B.5: Computed tomography scan showing a growth in the caecum. Note the ascites, which indicates peritoneal disease.

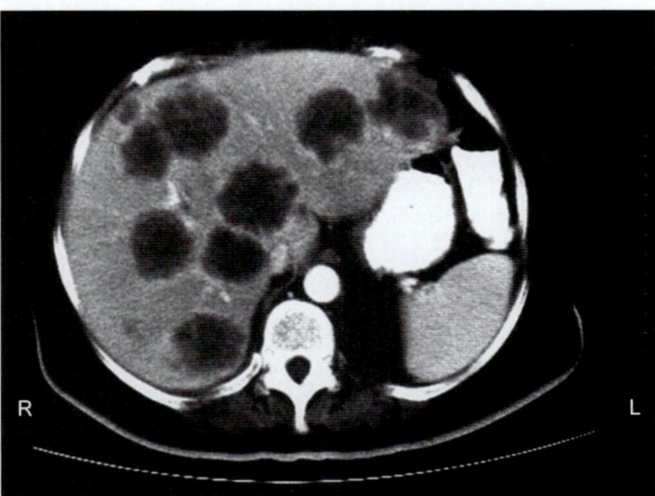

Fig. 62B.6: Computed tomography scan showing multiple liver metastases from colorectal cancer.

resonance imaging (MRI) also helps to predict involvement of the circumferential resection margin (CRM) in advanced rectal cancers,[26] therefore aiding the selection of patients for neoadjuvant therapy. Staging for metastatic disease can be achieved by a CT/MRI of the abdomen and a CT of the thorax. Positron emission tomography scans are only used in patients with metastatic disease, in whom a curative resection of the metastasis might otherwise be feasible, to look for other occult metastasis.[27]

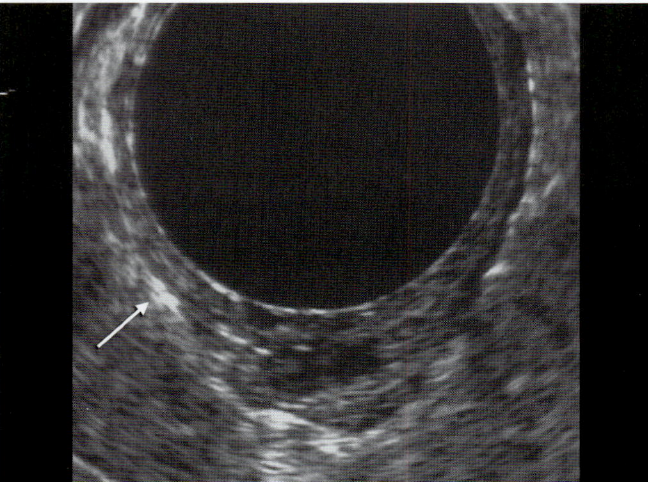

Fig. 62B.7: Transrectal ultrasound of a low rectal cancer showing invasion through the muscularis mucosae (arrow) into the muscularis propria. The outer border of the tumor is scalloped, consistent with invasion through the muscularis propria. The ultrasonic stage is uT3N0. The pathologic stage after resection was pT3N0.

Carcinoembryonic antigen (CEA) is an antigen extracted from colon cancer tissue that is present in primitive endoderm, but absent from normal adult intestinal mucosa. An elevated serum CEA level may be found in patients with colorectal cancer; however, the test is not specific. Elevated serum CEA levels are also found in smokers and benign and malignant conditions of other organs, including the stomach, pancreas, biliary tract, lung, breast, prostate, cervix, uterus, and ovary. Carcinoembryonic antigen is not recommended as a screening tool to detect early cancer, but levels may be useful in follow-up after colorectal cancer resection. A sudden or persistent rise from the normal range after resection suggests tumor recurrence. Markedly elevated (>25 ng/mL) serum CEA levels are highly suggestive of metastatic disease, especially hepatic metastasis. Carbohydrate antigen (CA) 19-9 is another marker that can be used in colorectal cancer. A high level of CA 19-9 can indicate the presence of liver metastasis,[8] and a fall in levels after therapy can provide prognostic information.[29]

MANAGEMENT OF COLORECTAL CANCER

Surgery, chemotherapy, and radiation therapy are the primary methods used to treat colorectal cancer.

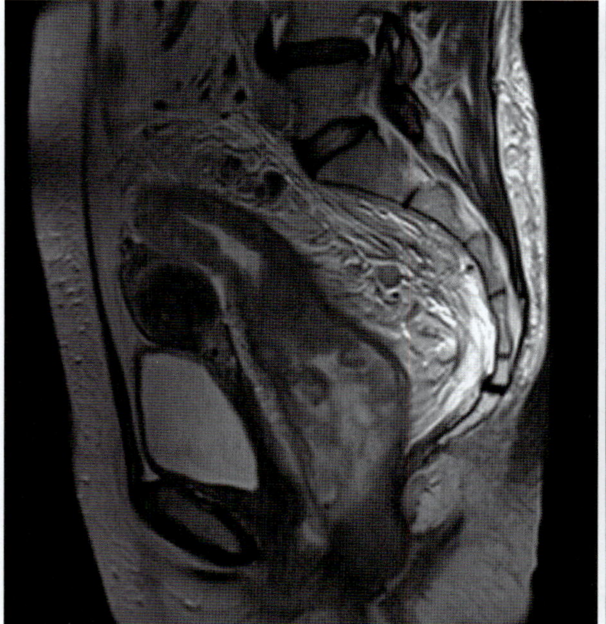

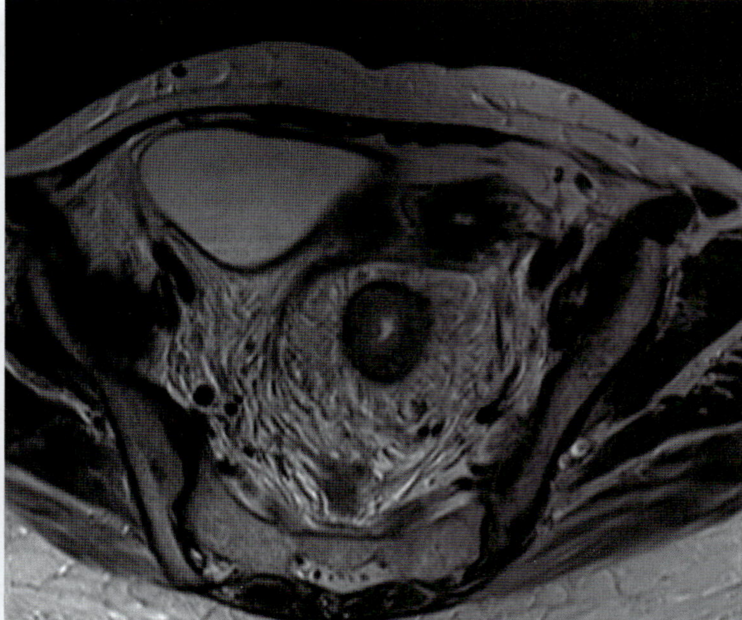

Fig. 62B.8: Magnetic resonance imaging scan showing an upper and midrectal growth. Note that the tumor does not reach the circumferential margin, and that there are mesorectal nodes present.

Table 62B.5 Five-year survival in colonic and rectal tumors.

Stage	Colon cancer	Rectal cancer
I	74.0	74.1
IIA	66.5	64.5
IIB	58.6	51.6
IIC	37.3	32.3
IIIA	73.1	74.0
IIIB	46.3	45.0
IIIC	28.0	33.4
IV	5.7	6.0

A curative resection is carried out when the tumor together with contiguous tissue including the regional lymph nodes is resected en-bloc with no known tumor remaining either locally or at distant sites.

A palliative *resection* is carried out when the tumor is resected, but there is disease remaining locally or at a distance. A palliative *operation*, such as laparotomy with biopsy or with fecal diversion (stoma or internal bypass) alone, is one in which the primary cancer is not removed. Local excision means removal of the carcinoma without regional lymphadenectomy.

Table 62B.5 shows the survival rates of colon and rectal cancer patients.[30]

Surgery is the mainstay of management of colon cancer. All patients in whom a curative resection is possible should undergo operation. Options for patients in whom a curative resection is not possible include chemotherapy, palliative debulking, internal bypass, or a colostomy. In some patients with advanced metastatic disease, just comfort care is advisable.

In stages III and IV colon cancer, adjuvant chemotherapy is advisable. Chemotherapy with oxaliplatin and 5-fluorouracil (5FU) is the current standard treatment.[31]

Patients with rectal cancer are staged preoperatively with a TRUS or an MRI. All patients found to have locally advanced, nonmetastatic disease (T3-4 or node-positive disease) are candidates for preoperative neoadjuvant therapy prior to rectal resection. Adjuvant chemotherapy is advisable for all patients with stages III and IV rectal cancer.

Neoadjuvant Therapy in Rectal Cancer

Indications for neoadjuvant therapy in rectal cancer are outlined in Table 62B.6.[32] Radiotherapy is the mainstay of neoadjuvant therapy for rectal cancer, which can be delivered as long-course radiotherapy (5040 Gray in 28 fractions) or as short-course radiotherapy (25 Gray in 5 fractions). In

Table 62B.6 Indications for neoadjuvant therapy in rectal cancer.

- Threatened circumferential resection margin (<2 mm)
- T3 disease
- N1 disease
- Mobile T4 disease
- Low rectal cancers

the long-course group, concurrent chemotherapy is added by way of infusional, bolus, or oral 5FU derivatives.

Neoadjuvant therapy in rectal cancer has been shown to significantly reduce local recurrence rates and thereby improve outcomes.[32,33] It also may allow for sphincter-saving operations, thus avoiding a permanent colostomy.[32,33] There are recent data emerging on nonoperative management of patients who have a complete clinical response to chemoradiotherapy.[34]

Operative Management

Before operation, reversible risk factors such as anemia, dehydration, electrolyte imbalance, malnutrition, diabetes, hypertension, and cardiopulmonary disease are treated. If a stoma is a possibility, an appropriate site is marked before the operation. Surgical preparation includes intravenous antibiotics effective against aerobic and anaerobic enteric organisms administered before the skin incision, blood typing, and prophylaxis against deep vein thrombosis. The patient is counseled about the operation and postoperative recovery, and enhanced recovery after surgery guidelines, if in place, should be followed.[35] Bowel preparation is not routinely recommended for colonic surgery. The role of bowel preparation in rectal cancer surgery is under intense surveillance, with proponents for and against it. A recent Cochrane review on the subject has suggested a selective use of bowel preparation in rectal surgery.[36]

The operation is carried out under general endotracheal anesthesia. A Foley catheter or a suprapubic catheter is placed in the bladder, and a nasogastric tube is placed in the stomach. If access to the perineum is needed, the patient is positioned in modified Lloyd Davies position on "Allen" stirrups. The abdomen is prepared with povidone-iodine or chlorhexidine. The perineum is similarly prepared if a rectal operation is planned. Stents may be inserted for ureteral identification in operations where the lesion is closely related to the ureter.

General Operative Principles

A general laparotomy is carried out, and the liver, omentum, parietes, viscera, ovaries, and retroperitoneum are

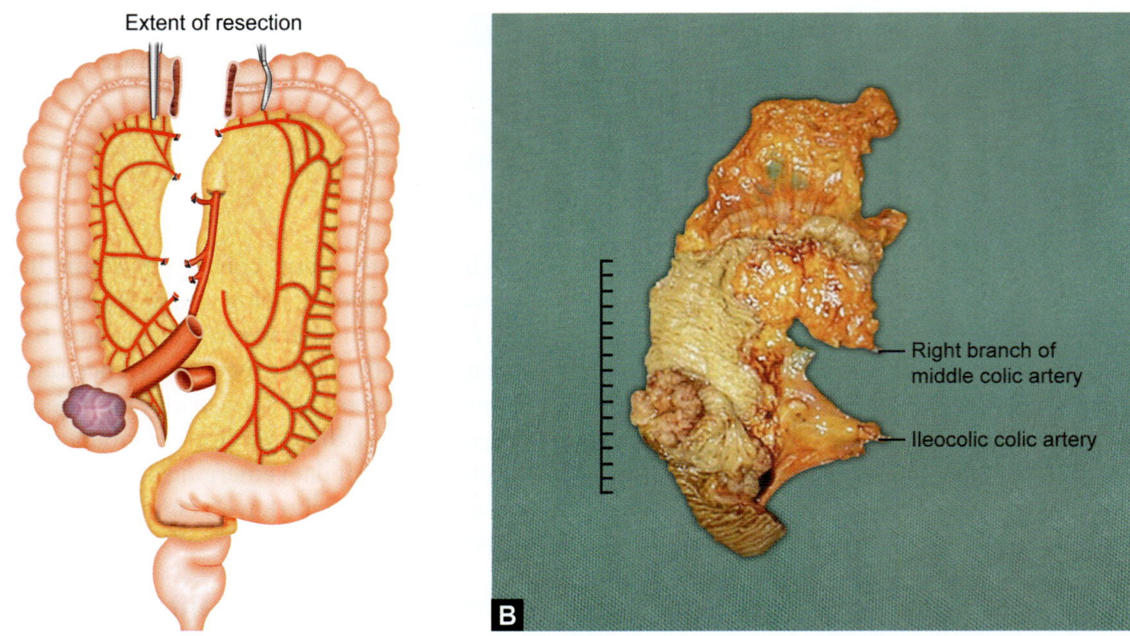

Figs. 62B.9A and B: Right hemicolectomy. (A) Extent of resection. (B) Operative specimen.

examined for metastases. The primary tumor(s) is not manipulated except to confirm its presence and to determine its resectability. A prophylactic oophorectomy to avoid ovarian metastases is a reasonable precaution in postmenopausal women.

Operations for Colonic Cancer

Carcinoma of the right colon: Right hemicolectomy is the standard method of treating right-sided colon carcinoma uncomplicated by FAP, HNPCC, or colitis (Figs. 62B.9A and B). The extent of resection is determined by the lymphatic drainage. Resection lines are approximately the same whether the carcinoma is in the cecum, the ascending colon, or the hepatic flexure. The ileocolic, right colic, and right branch of the middle colic arteries and veins are divided close to their origin. For cancer in the hepatic flexure or proximal transverse colon, the bowel is divided at the distal transverse colon with ligation of both branches or the main trunk of the middle colic vessels. The omentum attached to the proximal transverse colon is removed with the specimen. Bowel continuity is restored by an ileocolic anastomosis.

Carcinoma of the transverse colon: Two alternative operations are commonly carried out in the elective setting, and neither has been shown to be superior to the other. In the extended right colectomy, the margins of resection are the distal ileum and the descending-sigmoid colon junction. The left colic artery is included in the resection (Fig. 62B.10A). In transverse colectomy alone, the middle colic vessel is ligated, and the ileocolic and right colic vessels are preserved (Fig. 62B.10B).

Carcinoma of the splenic flexure: The resection lines for a carcinoma of the splenic flexure are the colon just beyond the hepatic flexure proximally and the descending-sigmoid colon junction distally. The vascular structures included in the resection are the left branch of the middle colic vessels and the ascending and descending branches of the left colic vessels (Fig. 62B.10C). An alternative approach is an extended right hemicolectomy with an ileosigmoid anastomosis.

Carcinoma of the descending colon: Carcinoma of the descending colon is treated by a left hemicolectomy (Fig. 62B.10D). The inferior mesenteric artery (IMA) is divided at its origin, and the left colic and sigmoid vessels are included in the resection. The inferior mesenteric vein is divided at the lower border of the pancreas. Proximally, the colon is divided at the junction of the proximal two-thirds and the distal one-third of the transverse colon. Distally, the resection line is at the junction of the sigmoid colon and the rectum. The omentum attached to the distal transverse colon is removed with the specimen.

Carcinoma of the sigmoid colon: For lesions in the sigmoid colon, the bowel is divided proximally at the mid-descending colon and distally at the rectosigmoid junction. The inferior mesenteric vessels are ligated, and the left colic vessels as well as the sigmoid branches are resected (Figs. 62B.11A and B). Left hemicolectomy is preferred by

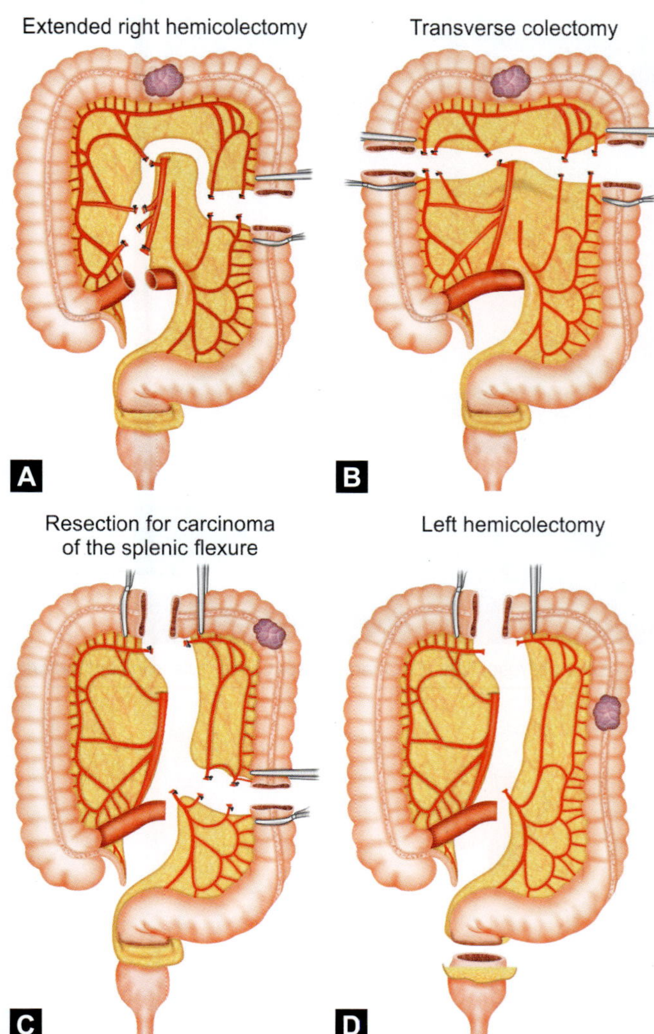

Figs. 62B.10A to D: Different types of colectomy for cancer of the transverse and descending colon. (A) Extent of resection in extended right hemicolectomy. (B) Extent of resection for transverse colectomy. (C) Extent of resection for carcinoma of the splenic flexure. (D) Left hemicolectomy for carcinoma of the descending colon.

some surgeons. In either case, the anastomosis must be tension free and the anastomosed bowel well perfused.

Other types of colon cancer: When synchronous cancers are located on the right and left sides of the colon, a subtotal colectomy with ileorectal anastomosis is carried out (Fig. 62B.12). An unresectable near-obstructing colonic cancer can be bypassed (Fig. 62B.13), thereby avoiding a stoma.

Operations for Rectal Cancer

Curative surgical options include radical resection and local procedures. The primary goal of rectal cancer surgery is to remove the tumor with clear margins (distal, proximal, and circumferential). Inadequate resection results in local cancer recurrence, which is a devastating complication that may produce pelvic pain, ureteric, intestinal and lymphovascular obstruction, bleeding, profuse mucous discharge, fecal incontinence, or symptoms from sciatic nerve root invasion. Most patients who develop local recurrence die from it. Technically, radical proctectomy is difficult because the rectum is surrounded by neighboring structures within the narrow confines of the pelvis.

Operations for carcinoma of the rectum include:

- Abdominoperineal excision (Fig. 62B.14A)
- Anterior resection of rectum and sigmoid colon (AR) with restoration of intestinal continuity (Fig. 62B.14B)
- Extended Hartmann's resection (Fig. 62B.15), and
- Local procedures

Abdominoperineal resection: Abdominoperineal resection (APR) as described by Miles in 1908 is the standard against which all other procedures are compared with regard to the cancer-specific end points of survival and local recurrence (*see* Fig. 62B.14A). The operation was designed to take into account the possibility of lymphatic spread in all directions: upward accompanying the superior rectal vessels, lateral along the middle rectal vessels, and downward toward the inguinal nodes. Abdominoperineal resection achieves the greatest possible distal margin of resection by removing the anus in continuity with the rectum. For rectal tumors, the direction of lymphatic spread nearly always follows the IMA to the aorta. Therefore, the IMA is ligated near the take-off of the left colic artery. Inferior mesenteric artery ligation at the aorta (high ligation) is advocated by some surgeons to maximize lymph node clearance. Others prefer IMA ligation distal to the origin of left colic artery on the premise that high ligation does not confer a survival benefit. The bowel is divided at the junction between the sigmoid and descending colon. After the rectum is mobilized, the entire sphincter mechanism is removed with a cuff of levator ani muscle, ischiorectal fat, and perianal skin, by a perineal operator. Specific complications of APR include injury to neighboring structures including ureter, urethra, prostate, vagina, presacral veins, and urogenital nerves as well as perineal wound and colostomy complications.

Extralevator APR is a technique whereby an attempt is made to obtain a cylindrical specimen by consciously dividing the levator muscles as far laterally as possible. The abdominal operation stops at the level of the coccyx posteriorly, the seminal vesicles anteriorly, and the so called "lateral ligaments" laterally. The perineal operation is best done with the patient in the prone jack-knife position. This position provides better ergonomics and vision, and

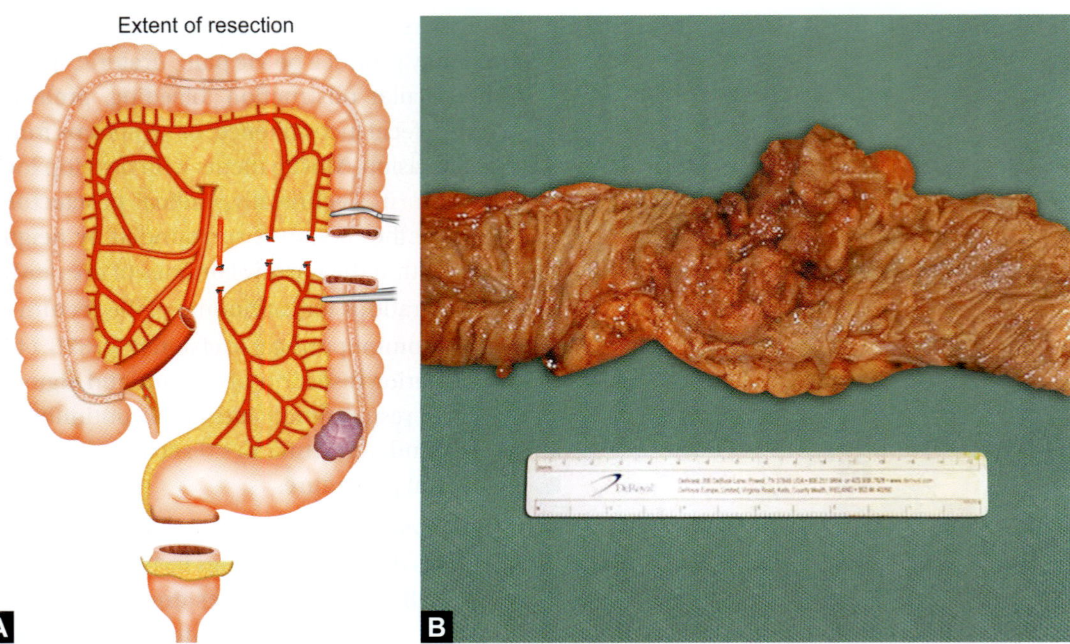

Figs. 62B.11A and B: Sigmoid colectomy for carcinoma of the sigmoid colon. (A) Extent of resection. (B) Operative specimen (rule is in centimeters).

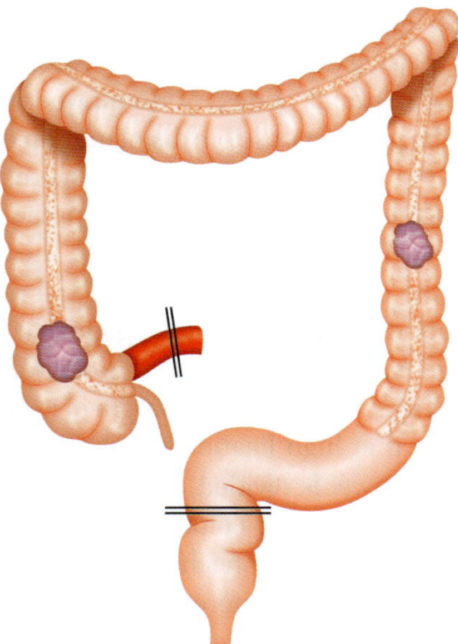

Fig. 62B.12: Extent of resection for subtotal colectomy.

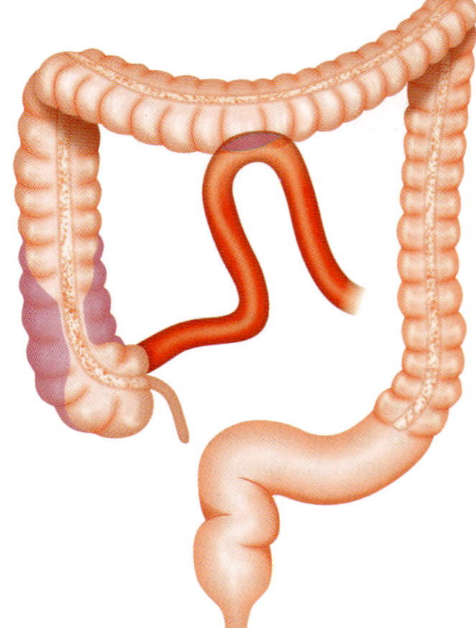

Fig. 62B.13: Bypass of unresectable colon carcinoma.

allows for a wider excision of the sphincter complex and the levator muscles. Recent data have indicated that these benefits may translate to a lower CRM positivity and local recurrence rates.[37]

Anterior resection: Anterior resection with sphincter preservation is carried out for most cancers of the upper and mid rectum. Rectal mobilization is identical to that carried out for APR. However, distal to the tumor, the rectum is transected and an anastomosis is created between the descending colon and the distal rectal cuff or anal canal. While a temporary loop ileostomy for fecal diversion was the norm for anterior resections, it is used selectively by most colorectal surgeons nowadays in low rectal or coloanal anastomosis. Local pelvic recurrence, a major complication of rectal cancer surgery, is associated with factors shown in Table 62B.7. Of these, the surgeon has direct control in determining intestinal and lymphatic margins of resection.

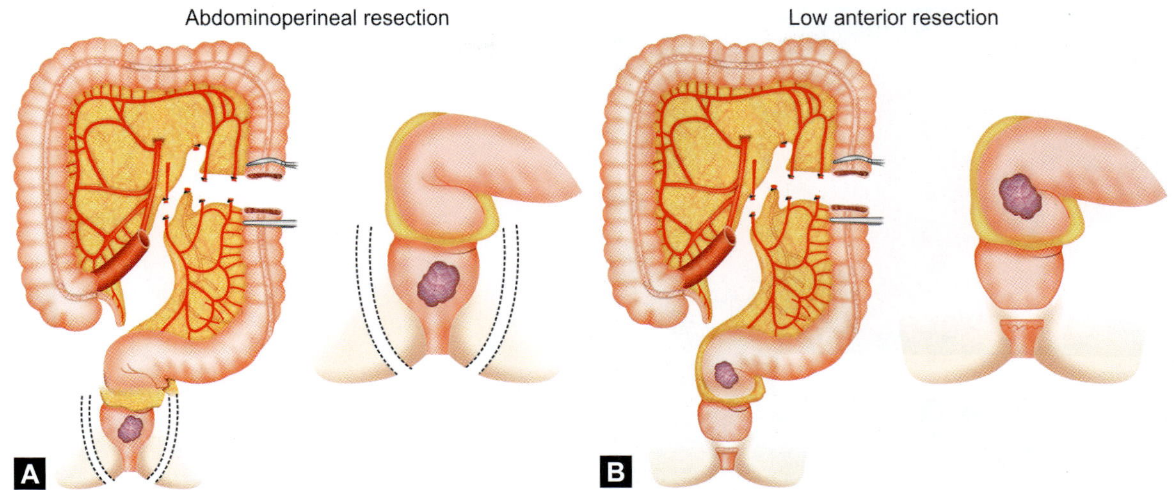

Figs. 62B.14A and B: Resection for carcinoma of the rectum.

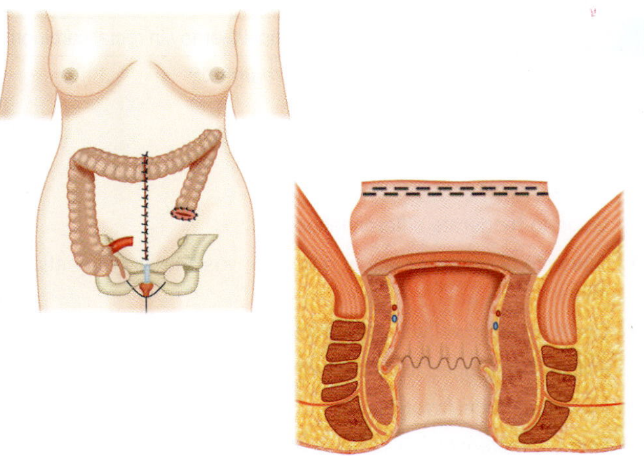
Fig. 62B.15: Extended Hartmann's operation for carcinoma of the rectum. Left, location of incision and ostomy; right, Hartmann's pouch. The proximal end of the divided bowel is brought out as an end colostomy. The stapled distal rectal pouch is shown diagrammatically.

Resection margins have evolved since the advent of restorative operations. Pathologic studies have demonstrated microscopic tumor spread in the intestinal wall distal to the visible tumor border. These observations led to early recommendations for a 5 cm distal margin of resection for rectal cancer. Subsequent studies have challenged this rule, citing the facts that distal intramural spread rarely exceeds 1 cm and that when distal spread is >1 cm the prognosis is poor. Although a precise value has not been defined, a distal margin of resection of 2 cm below the tumor in the nonfixed specimen is generally considered adequate distal clearance for anterior resection (Fig. 62B.16). In practical terms, this policy means that most tumors 6 cm or more from the anal verge or 2–3 cm from

Table 62B.7	Factors studied related to local recurrence after anterior resection for rectal carcinoma.
Depth of invasion and lymph node positivity	
Tumor differentiation	
Distal margin of resection	
Mesorectal tumor deposits	
Lateral margin of resection	
Iliac nodes	
Lower half of rectum	
Surgeon experience	

the anorectal junction are suitable for restorative resection. However, there is emerging evidence that smaller distal resection margins may be acceptable in these patients.[38]

Discovery of minute foci of adenocarcinoma in the mesorectum several centimeters distal to the visible lower edge of rectal cancers has led to the recommendation that cancers of the rectum should be excised with the mesorectum intact with its investing fascia, a technique referred to as total mesorectal excision (TME). When TME is carried out, local recurrence rates as low as 3.3% at the anastomosis or within the pelvis are reported. For tumors of the upper rectum, a 5 cm distal margin with tumor-specific mesorectal excision results in a low rate of local recurrence and good 5-year survival rates.

Inadequate surgical resection in rectal cancer may occur at the circumferential margin. For low rectal cancers, this problem is apt to occur deep in the pelvis when the distal rectum is cleared of pararectal tissue before division or the mesorectum thins out. An extralevator approach to APR may help in reducing positive circumferential margin.[37]

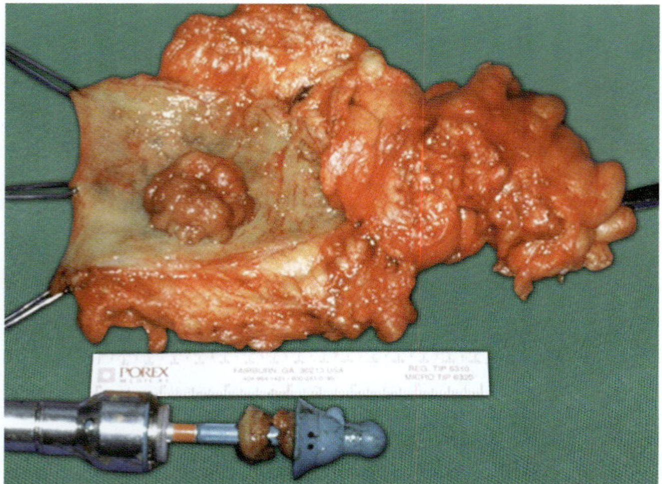

Fig. 62B.16: Operative specimen after anterior resection for low rectal cancer. The anastomosis was created using a double-stapled technique.

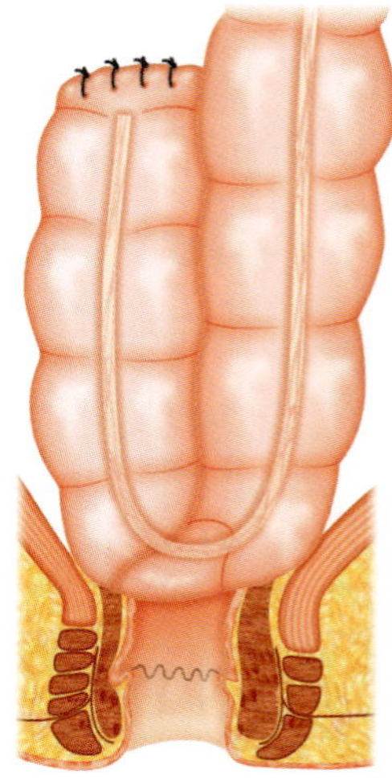

Fig. 62B.17: Colonic J-pouch reservoir in situ in pelvis.

Metastases can occur in nodes on the lateral pelvic sidewall associated with the iliac and the obturator vessels. In a nonrandomized study comparing wide iliopelvic lymphadenectomy to conventional pelvic lymphadenectomy, stage for stage the cumulative 5-year survival rate was better among patients who had received lateral node dissection; however, complications were greater. As there are no randomized trials demonstrating the effectiveness of lateral pelvic lymph node dissection, the data are insufficient to justify this technique at present.[39]

Methods of reconstruction after anterior resection include anastomosis to the distal rectum or anus using either a straight tube of colon or a reservoir, such as a colonic J-pouch (Fig. 62B.17). Recent studies suggest that short-term functional results are better when a reservoir is used.

Local procedures: Local treatment of rectal cancer is attractive because it offers the opportunity to avoid a major operation, but it is only appropriate for selected patients. Techniques include local excision, transanal endoscopic microsurgery, electrocoagulation, and contact radiotherapy. Selection criteria for local therapy in the treatment of rectal cancer are shown in Table 62B.8.

Table 62B.8 Selection criteria for local therapy in rectal carcinoma.

Tumor characteristics favoring local treatment
• Mobile
• <3 cm in diameter
• Exophytic rather than ulcerated
• Good-to-moderate differentiation
• Absence of colloid or signet ring cells, vascular or lymphatic invasion
• Confined to bowel wall (by endoluminal ultrasound)
• Palpable or judged to be below the peritoneal reflection
• No lymph nodal involvement
Patient characteristics favoring local treatment
• Unfit for major surgical procedure
• Unwilling to undergo major surgical procedure
• Extensive distant metastases

Management of locally advanced rectal cancer: Approximately 5% of patients with rectal cancer have locally advanced (T4) tumor, with direct invasion into other organs, such as the vagina, uterus, bladder, prostate, or sacrum. It is important to recognize contiguous involvement to other structures because exenteration or partial sacral resection may be required for surgical cure. With en-bloc resection, 5-year survival rates of 50% may be possible. The major morbidity of wide excisional procedures in these cases must be balanced against the possibility of long-term cure.

Management of liver metastases: In patients with metastases confined to the liver, operative resection combined with the other modalities of treatment offers the best chance of cure, with 5-year survivals ranging from 24% to 58%.[40,41] Criteria for offering an operation in these cases include documented absence of extrahepatic disease,[42] operable liver lesions, adequate functional liver remnant, and patient fitness for surgery.

Extrahepatic disease is ruled out with the help of a PET-CT scan.[43] Patients with liver-only metastasis may present either synchronously with the primary tumor or in a metachronous fashion, after completing treatment of the primary tumor. The ideal sequencing of appropriate chemotherapy, radiotherapy and surgery in these patients is not established and is a matter of much debate.

Adjuvant Therapy for Colorectal Cancer

The initial trials in adjuvant therapy for colorectal cancer revealed that treatment with 5-fluorouracil (5-FU) combined with levamisole significantly reduced the risk of cancer recurrence and the overall death rate in patients with stage III colon cancer. Later trials revealed that postoperative 5-FU and leucovorin for 6 months prevent tumor relapse and improve survival of patients with stage III colon cancer compared with control patients treated with surgery alone. Recent trials have shown that the addition of oxaliplatin to regimens containing 5-FU and leucovorin (FOLFOX) significantly improve disease-free and overall survival in stage III colon cancer,[31] and this is therefore the current preferred treatment of colorectal cancer. Other chemotherapeutic agents used in colorectal cancer include irinotecan and capecitabine. Monoclonal antibodies like bevacizumab (targeting the vascular endothelial growth factor receptor) and cetuximab (targeting the epidermal growth factor receptor) are increasingly being used in the metastatic setting. The value of adjuvant therapy in the treatment of stage II colon cancer is not clear at present, and management is individualized.

Follow-Up of Colorectal Cancer

Follow-up after operation for colorectal carcinoma is individualized, taking into consideration the risk of recurrent disease and metachronous cancer as well as the age and general health of the patient. Most recurrences after operation for cure of colorectal carcinoma occur within 2 years. Common sites of recurrence are the liver, lungs, primary tumor bed, peritoneum, and lymph nodes. In general, patients are followed up every 3–6 months for 2 years, then every 6 months for 2 years, then yearly. Specific inquiries are made concerning weight loss, change in bowel habit, bleeding, or pain. The abdomen is examined for tenderness, masses, or lymphadenopathy. The perineum is examined if the patient has been treated by APR. Digital rectal examination and flexible sigmoidoscopy are carried out for patients who have undergone restorative surgery for rectal cancer. Colonoscopy is carried out at 1 year and is repeated at 3–5-year intervals thereafter if no abnormalities are found. The value of the CEA level is controversial, but it is usually measured. For a single elevation higher than 10 ng/dL or two persistent elevations, further investigations, such as colonoscopy and chest, abdominal and pelvic CT are carried out to look for recurrent disease. Magnetic resonance imaging and positron emission scanning can be considered if other tests are negative.[44] The NICE guidelines from UK suggest a CT scan of the chest, abdomen, and pelvis at least twice in the first 3 years of follow-up.[45]

Management of Recurrent Cancer

Patients in whom recurrent tumor is found may be considered for surgery, chemotherapy or radiation for either cure or palliation.

Patients who have isolated local recurrences may be eligible for surgical resection, including pelvic exenteration. Major resective surgery is not offered if disease is so widespread that there is no chance for cure. Resection of recurrent colorectal cancer may result in improved survival in selected cases. In a few selected patients, surgical palliation may be achieved by internal bypass or a stoma.

Intraoperative irradiation is being used at some institutions to treat locally advanced and locally recurrent rectal cancer. Radiotherapy as palliation for intractable pain or bleeding may be given in select cases.

Chemotherapy may be offered to some patients with metastatic disease. In others with advanced recurrent disease, no further intervention is feasible, and these patients are treated with supportive care alone.

Laparoscopic Operations

Laparoscopic and laparoscopy-assisted colectomy for colorectal cancer offers the advantages of faster return to normal activity and diet, reduced hospital stay, reduced postoperative pain, and better cosmesis. However, there have been concerns about a suboptimal cancer operation. A number of large, randomized controlled trials have, however, shown that oncological outcomes with laparoscopic surgery are similar to those of open operation.[46-49] This fact has led to a large proportion of surgeons embracing laparoscopic colorectal resections as standard procedure for colorectal cancers.

OTHER LARGE BOWEL MALIGNANCIES

Carcinoid of the Large Bowel

Carcinoid tumor (Fig. 62B.18) is the most common neuroendocrine tumor of the gut, and the estimated incidence is 7 per million. Carcinoid tumors of the lower gastrointestinal tract are found in the appendix, rectum and colon.

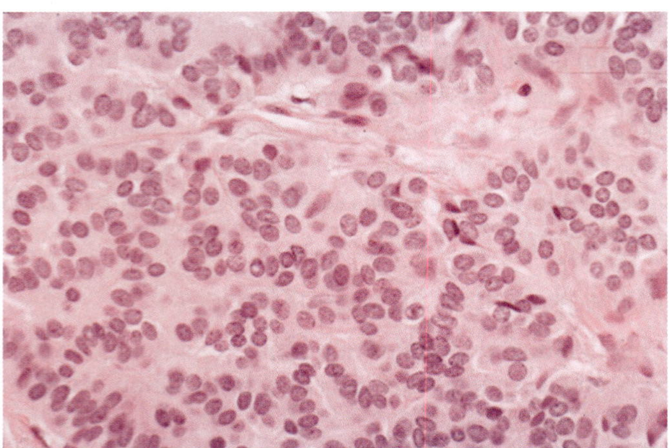

Fig. 62B.18: Carcinoid tumor composed of chords and ribbons of uniform neoplastic cells with round nuclei and characteristically finely granular chromatin.
Source: Courtesy of Dario V Caccamo.

They have malignant potential, and metastases occur most commonly in the liver. When liver metastases are present, hormone production by tumor cells may cause the carcinoid syndrome, which is characterized by flushes, diarrhea, bronchial obstruction, and right-sided heart failure.

Therapy for carcinoid tumors is multidisciplinary and may include operation for excision or debulking and symptomatic control using somatostatin analogs and chemotherapy. Appendiceal carcinoids comprise 35–44% of all carcinoids, making them the most common carcinoid tumor. The probability of metastatic disease is related to tumor size. Carcinoid tumors of the appendix < 1 cm in diameter rarely metastasize and simply require appendectomy for treatment. Lesions >2 cm in diameter are treated by a right hemicolectomy because of a high risk of metastases. The appropriate management of appendiceal carcinoids 1–2 cm in diameter is controversial because a few cases of regional metastases have been reported with tumors of this size.

Rectal carcinoids comprise 12–15% of carcinoid tumors. As they are of hindgut origin, they are not associated with the carcinoid syndrome. The two findings associated with malignancy are tumor invasion into or beyond the muscularis propria and a diameter of 2 cm or more. The risk of metastases is about 6% for tumors < 2 cm in diameter but 83% for tumors >2 cm in diameter. Local excision or fulguration is considered adequate treatment of rectal carcinoids <1 cm in diameter. For tumors 1–2 cm in diameter, an initial full-thickness transanal excision is recommended. Proctectomy may be considered if there is invasion of the muscularis propria. For tumors >2 cm in diameter or showing invasion through the bowel wall (T3/T4), the prognosis is poor even with radical surgical treatment, and treatment recommendations are therefore individualized.

Colonic carcinoids constitute about 7% of all carcinoids. In most reports, colonic carcinoids are discovered at an advanced stage with symptoms that are indistinguishable from those of adenocarcinoma. Most tumors are found in the right side of the colon and are diagnosed in the sixth decade of life. Right-sided colon carcinoids are of midgut origin and may therefore be associated with the malignant carcinoid syndrome; surgical resection is the primary method of treatment.

Primary Colorectal Lymphoma

Primary colorectal lymphomas (Figs. 62B.19A to C) comprise 0.2% of colorectal malignancies. Most large intestinal lymphomas are of the B-cell phenotype. The most common complaint is abdominal pain; other presenting features may be indistinguishable from those of adenocarcinoma. Most tumors are found in the cecum and are diagnosed in the fifth decade of life.

Treatment of primary colorectal lymphomas is chemotherapy. Chemotherapy with CHOP regimen (cyclophosphamide, doxorubicin, vincristine, and prednisone) with rituximab results in a good response in most cases. The role of surgical resection in such cases is debatable. However, in the absence of disseminated disease, surgical resection is usually performed. Curative resection results in 5-year survival rates of 44–60%.

Colorectal Stromal Tumors

Stromal tumors are rare and comprise 0.1% of colorectal cancers. The histogenesis of these spindle cell and epithelioid stromal tumors is controversial. In the past, most of these tumors were thought to arise from the smooth muscle of the intestinal wall. However, recent evidence has shown that most mesenchymal tumors of the gastrointestinal tract lack conclusive ultrastructural or immunohistochemical evidence of smooth muscle differentiation. Therefore, the term leiomyosarcoma has gradually been replaced with "stromal tumor" (Fig. 62B.20). The interstitial cell of Cajal is now believed to be the cell of origin of these tumors.[50] Most of these tumors occur in the fifth and sixth decades of life. Common signs and symptoms are abdominal pain, gastrointestinal bleeding, and abdominal

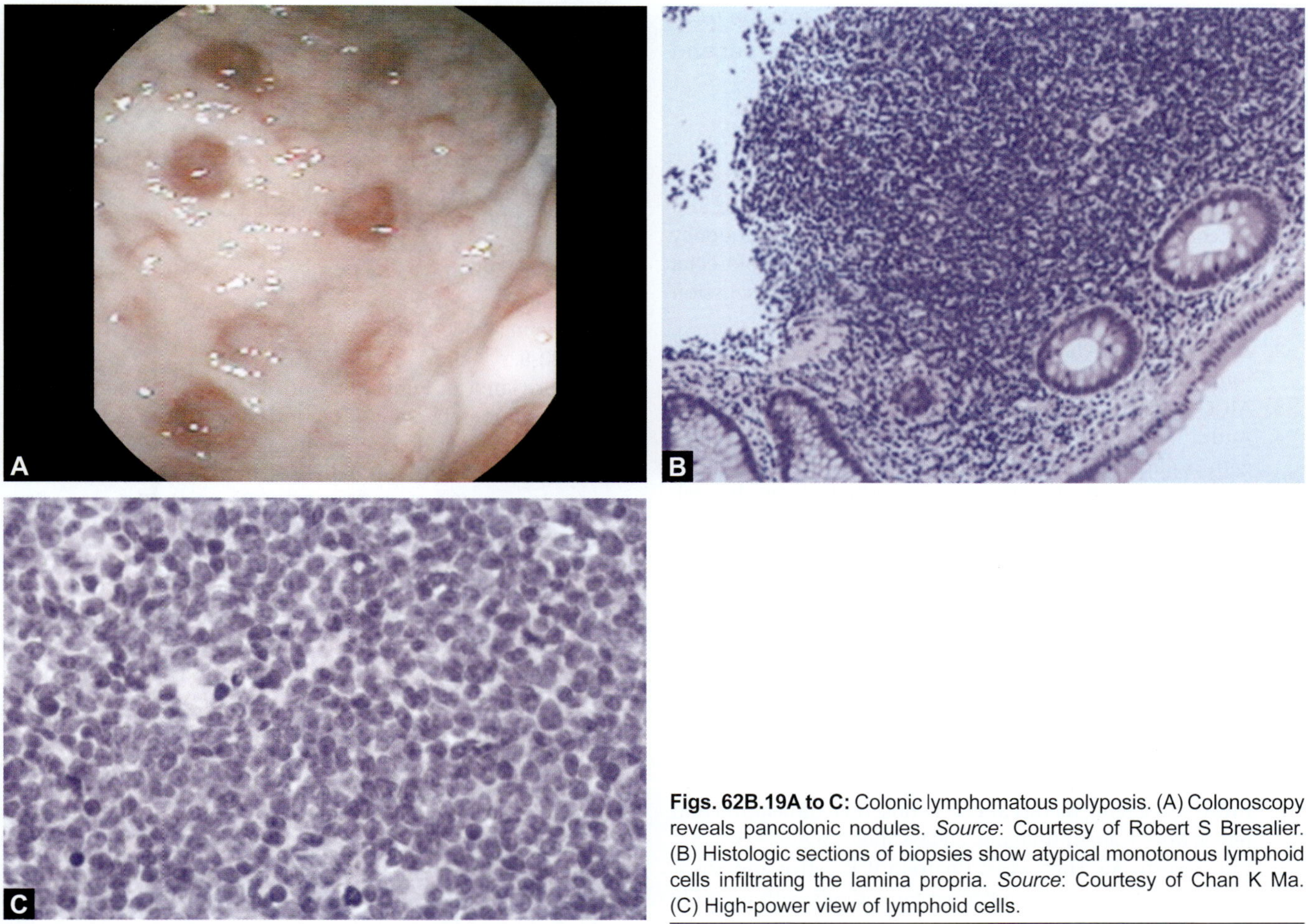

Figs. 62B.19A to C: Colonic lymphomatous polyposis. (A) Colonoscopy reveals pancolonic nodules. *Source*: Courtesy of Robert S Bresalier. (B) Histologic sections of biopsies show atypical monotonous lymphoid cells infiltrating the lamina propria. *Source*: Courtesy of Chan K Ma. (C) High-power view of lymphoid cells.

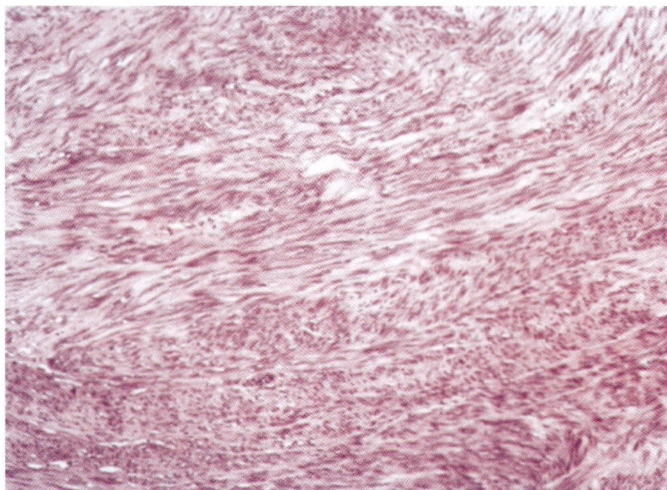

Fig. 62B.20: Colonic stromal tumor. A microscopic section reveals a spindle cell neoplasm composed of cells with a moderate degree of nuclear atypia.
Source: Courtesy of John R Goldblum.

mass. These tumors are characterized by the presence of CD117 antigen. Various other markers like CD 34 and DOG1 can assist in diagnosis.

At present operative treatment offers the best chance for cure. Five-year survival rates are as high as 50% after curative resection. Adjuvant therapy with imatinib is needed for patients with high-risk features. Adverse prognostic indicators include a high histologic grade, the presence of metastases, and noncurative treatment. Late recurrence after operation is common.

Patients with initial unresectable disease may be treated with neoadjuvant imatinib to downsize the tumor and make it resectable.

REFERENCES

1. Abdalla EK, Vauthey JN, Ellis LM, et al. Recurrence and outcomes following hepatic resection, radiofrequency ablation, and combined resection/ablation for colorectal liver metastases. Ann Surg. 2004;239(6):818-25; discussion 25-7.
2. A comparison of laparoscopically assisted and open colectomy for colon cancer. N Engl J Med. 2004;350(20):2050-9.
3. AJCC Cancer Staging Manual: Springer; 2010.
4. Andre T, Boni C, Navarro M, et al. Improved overall survival with oxaliplatin, fluorouracil, and leucovorin as adjuvant treatment in stage II or III colon cancer in the MOSAIC trial. J Clin Oncol. 2009;27(19):3109-16.
5. Aune D, Chan DS, Lau R, et al. Dietary fibre, whole grains, and risk of colorectal cancer: systematic review and dose-response meta-analysis of prospective studies. BMJ. 2011;343:d6617.
6. Botteri E, Iodice S, Bagnardi V, et al. Smoking and colorectal cancer: a meta-analysis. JAMA. 2008;300(23):2765-78.
7. Bouvier AM, Latournerie M, Jooste V, et al. The lifelong risk of metachronous colorectal cancer justifies long-term colonoscopic follow-up. Eur J Cancer. 2008;44(4):522-7.
8. Brown G. Staging rectal cancer: endoscopic ultrasound and pelvic MRI. Cancer Imaging. 2008;8 Spec No A:S43-5.
9. Butterworth AS, Higgins JP, Pharoah P. Relative and absolute risk of colorectal cancer for individuals with a family history: a meta-analysis. Eur J Cancer. 2006;42(2):216-27.
10. Bystrom P, Berglund A, Nygren P, et al. Evaluation of predictive markers for patients with advanced colorectal cancer. Acta Oncol. 2012 Sep;51(7):849-59.
11. Chaput U, Alberto SF, Terris B, et al. Risk factors for advanced adenomas amongst small and diminutive colorectal polyps: a prospective monocenter study. Dig Liver Dis. 2011;43(8):609-12.
12. Dong H, Tang J, Li LH, et al. Serum carbohydrate antigen 19-9 as an indicator of liver metastasis in colorectal carcinoma cases. Asian Pac J Cancer Prev. 2013;14(2):909-13.
13. Edge SB, Byrd DR, Compton CC, et al. (Eds). AJCC (American Joint Committee on Cancer) Cancer Staging Manual, 7th edition. New York: Springer; 2010. p.143.
14. Fedirko V, Tramacere I, Bagnardi V, et al. Alcohol drinking and colorectal cancer risk: an overall and dose-response meta-analysis of published studies. Ann Oncol. 2011;22(9): 1958-72.
15. Ferlay J SH, Bray F, Forman D, et al. GLOBOCAN 2008 v2.0, Cancer Incidence and Mortality Worldwide: IARC CancerBase No. 10 [Internet]. Lyon, France: International Agency for Research on Cancer; 2010. Available from: http://globocan.iarc.fr.
16. Fernandez-Esparrach G, Ayuso-Colella JR, Sendino O, et al. EUS and magnetic resonance imaging in the staging of rectal cancer: a prospective and comparative study. Gastrointest Endosc. 2011;74(2):347-54.
17. Giacomobono S, Gallicchio R, Capacchione D, et al. F-18 FDG PET/CT in the assessment of patients with unexplained CEA rise after surgical curative resection for colorectal cancer. Int J Colorectal Dis. 2013;28(12):1699-705.
18. Guenaga KK, Matos D, Wille-Jorgensen P. Mechanical bowel preparation for elective colorectal surgery. Cochrane Database Syst Rev. 2009(1):CD001544.
19. Gupta S, Bhattacharya D, Acharya AN, et al. Colorectal carcinoma in young adults: a retrospective study on Indian patients: 2000-2008. Colorectal Dis. 2010;12(10 Online): e182-9.
20. Habr-Gama A, Perez RO, Nadalin W, et al. Operative versus nonoperative treatment for stage 0 distal rectal cancer following chemoradiation therapy: long-term results. Ann Surg. 2004;240(4):711-7; discussion 7-8.
21. Herbertson RA, Lee ST, Tebbutt N, et al. The expanding role of PET technology in the management of patients with colorectal cancer. Ann Oncol. 2007;18(11):1774-81.
22. Imperiale TF, Ransohoff DF. Risk for colorectal cancer in persons with a family history of adenomatous polyps: a systematic review. Ann Intern Med. 2012;156(10):703-9.
23. Jarvinen R, Knekt P, Hakulinen T, et al. Dietary fat, cholesterol and colorectal cancer in a prospective study. Br J Cancer. 2001;85(3):357-61.
24. Jayne DG, Thorpe HC, Copeland J, et al. Five-year follow-up of the Medical Research Council CLASICC trial of laparoscopically assisted versus open surgery for colorectal cancer. Br J Surg. 2010;97(11):1638-45.
25. Jiang HY, Zhou YB, Zhang DF. Meta-analysis of extralevator abdominoperineal excision and conventional abdominoperineal excision for low rectal cancer. Chin J Gastrointest Surg. 2013;16(7):622-7.
26. Lacy AM, Delgado S, Castells A, et al. The long-term results of a randomized clinical trial of laparoscopy-assisted versus open surgery for colon cancer. Ann Surg. 2008;248(1):1-7.
27. Lacy AM, Garcia-Valdecasas JC, Delgado S, et al. Laparoscopy-assisted colectomy versus open colectomy for treatment of non-metastatic colon cancer: a randomised trial. Lancet. 2002;359(9325):2224-9.
28. Lassen K, Soop M, Nygren J, et al. Consensus review of optimal perioperative care in colorectal surgery: Enhanced Recovery After Surgery (ERAS) group recommendations. Arch Surg. 2009;144(10):961-9.
29. Latournerie M, Jooste V, Cottet V, et al. Epidemiology and prognosis of synchronous colorectal cancers. Br J Surg. 2008;95(12):1528-33.
30. Lee JE, Chan AT. Fruit, vegetables, and folate: cultivating the evidence for cancer prevention. Gastroenterology. 2011; 141(1):16-20.
31. Min KW, Leabu M. Interstitial cells of Cajal (ICC) and gastrointestinal stromal tumor (GIST): facts, speculations, and myths. J Cell Mol Med. 2006;10(4):995-1013.
32. Mulder SA, Kranse R, Damhuis RA, et al. Prevalence and prognosis of synchronous colorectal cancer: a Dutch population-based study. Cancer Epidemiol. 2011;35(5):442-7.

33. Mulder SA, Kranse R, Damhuis RA, et al. The incidence and risk factors of metachronous colorectal cancer: an indication for follow-up. Dis Colon Rectum. 2012;55(5):522-31.
34. Nakamura T, Watanabe M. Lateral lymph node dissection for lower rectal cancer. World J Surg. 2013;37(8):1808-13.
35. Nath J, Wigley C, Keighley MR, et al. Rectal cancer in young adults: a series of 102 patients at a tertiary care centre in India. Colorectal Dis. 2009;11(5):475-9.
36. National Institute for Health and Care Excellence. [The diagnosis and management of colorectal cancer]. [CG131]. London: National Institute for Health and Care Excellence; 2011.
37. Nordlinger B, Guiguet M, Vaillant JC, et al. Surgical resection of colorectal carcinoma metastases to the liver. A prognostic scoring system to improve case selection, based on 1568 patients. Association Francaise de Chirurgie. Cancer. 1996;77(7):1254-62.
38. Nottage K, McFarlane J, Krasin MJ, et al. Secondary colorectal carcinoma after childhood cancer. J Clin Oncol. 2012;30(20):2552-8.
39. Pahlman L, Bujko K, Rutkowski A, et al. Altering the therapeutic paradigm towards a distal bowel margin of <1 cm in patients with low-lying rectal cancer: a systematic review and commentary. Colorectal Dis. 2013;15(4):e166-74.
40. Ponz de Leon M, Marino M, Benatti P, et al. Trend of incidence, subsite distribution and staging of colorectal neoplasms in the 15-year experience of a specialised cancer registry. Ann Oncol. 2004;15(6):940-6.
41. Poston GJ, Adam R, Alberts S, et al. OncoSurge: a strategy for improving resectability with curative intent in metastatic colorectal cancer. J Clin Oncol. 2005;23(28):7125-34.
42. Reid FD, Mercer PM, Harrison M, et al. Cholecystectomy as a risk factor for colorectal cancer: a meta-analysis. Scand J Gastroenterol. 1996;31(2):160-9.
43. Renehan AG, Tyson M, Egger M, et al. Body-mass index and incidence of cancer: a systematic review and meta-analysis of prospective observational studies. Lancet. 2008; 371(9612):569-78.
44. Rex DK, Johnson DA, Anderson JC, et al. American College of Gastroenterology guidelines for colorectal cancer screening 2009 [corrected]. Am J Gastroenterol. 2009;104(3): 739-50.
45. Sauer R, Becker H, Hohenberger W, et al. Preoperative versus postoperative chemoradiotherapy for rectal cancer. N Engl J Med. 2004;351(17):1731-40.
46. Sebag-Montefiore D, Stephens RJ, Steele R, et al. Preoperative radiotherapy versus selective postoperative chemoradiotherapy in patients with rectal cancer (MRC CR07 and NCIC-CTG C016): a multicentre, randomised trial. Lancet. 2009 Mar 7;373(9666):811-20.
47. Siegel R, Naishadham D, Jemal A. Cancer statistics. CA Cancer J Clin. 2013;63(1):11-30.
48. Siegel RL, Jemal A, Ward EM. Increase in incidence of colorectal cancer among young men and women in the United States. Cancer Epidemiol Biomarkers Prev. 2009;18(6):1695-8.
49. Troisi RJ, Freedman AN, Devesa SS. Incidence of colorectal carcinoma in the U.S.: an update of trends by gender, race, age, subsite, and stage, 1975-1994. Cancer. 1999;85(8):1670-6.
50. Wiering B, Krabbe PF, Jager GJ, et al. The impact of fluor-18-deoxyglucose-positron emission tomography in the management of colorectal liver metastases. Cancer. 2005; 104(12):2658-70.

63

Anal Canal

Andrew J Malouf, Michael D Cadogan, Laurence A Webber, David C C Bartolo

Key Points

- Some 4 cm long, the anal canal comprises the anal margin, pecten, and (above the dentate line) anal transitional zone. Endoluminal ultrasound can now be used to supplement digital examination and proctoscopy.
- Fecal incontinence (FI) is common, socially disabling, and often the legacy of obstetric injury to the internal and external anal sphincters (IAS and EAS). Physiologic studies assess sphincter function, anorectal sensation, rectal compliance, and pudendal nerve conduction. Surgical options include sphincter repair, sacral nerve stimulation, and dynamic graciloplasty.
- Rectal prolapse can be occult (internal) or overt (external). Obstructed defecation and FI are frequent concomitants. Full-thickness prolapse is usually treated by either transabdominal rectopexy or perineal resection. Solitary rectal ulcer is normally a manifestation of prolapse.
- Hemorrhoids represent distal displacement of the anal cushions. Depending on their size, injection, banding, and operative excision can be effective. Constipation predisposes to both hemorrhoids and anal fissure.
- Anorectal abscess and anal fistula share common etiologic factors, notably anal gland infection and Crohn's disease. Fistulas above the dentate line are managed by a seton to preserve sphincter integrity. Pilonidal sepsis in the natal cleft may require excision of infected tissue with or without primary closure.
- Neoplasms generally comprise squamous, basal cell, or cloacogenic carcinomas in the anal canal proper or very low rectal adenocarcinomas that encroach from above. Chemoradiation is a valid alternative to abdominoperineal excision (APE) for epidermoid tumors.
- Anal pathology is common in male homosexuals with or without HIV and includes fissure and fistula, opportunist infections, and unusual neoplasms such as lymphoma and Kaposi's sarcoma.

SURGICAL ANATOMY

Embryology

The proximal anal canal lining derives from hindgut endoderm and the distal portion from ectoderm. The primitive cloaca becomes divided by a septum into an anterior urogenital sinus and a posterior anorectal canal. The latter fuses with an ectodermal pit (proctodeum) to establish continuity between hindgut and exterior.

Epithelium

The adult anal canal is 3.0–4.5 cm in length, depending on gender and body habitus, and is encircled by internal and external sphincters (Fig. 63.1). The area below the dentate line, the pecten, has a modified squamous epithelium that lacks skin appendages and is pale. Beyond the anal verge, the anal margin is keratinized squamous epithelium bearing

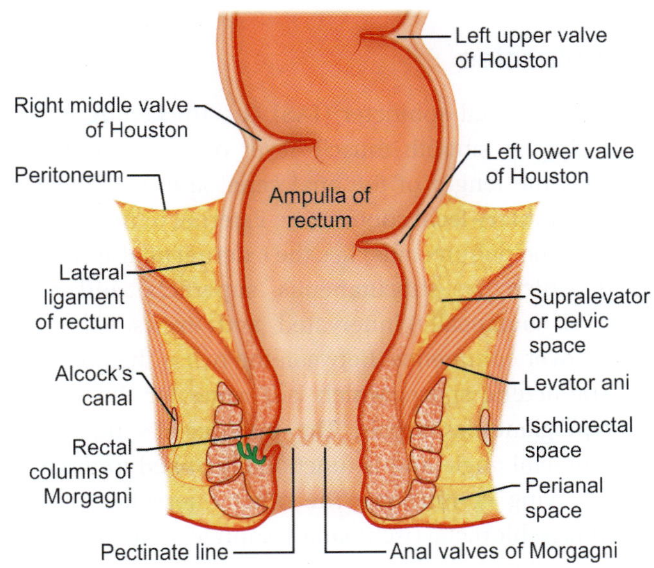

Fig. 63.1: Anal sphincters and surrounding perianal tissues.

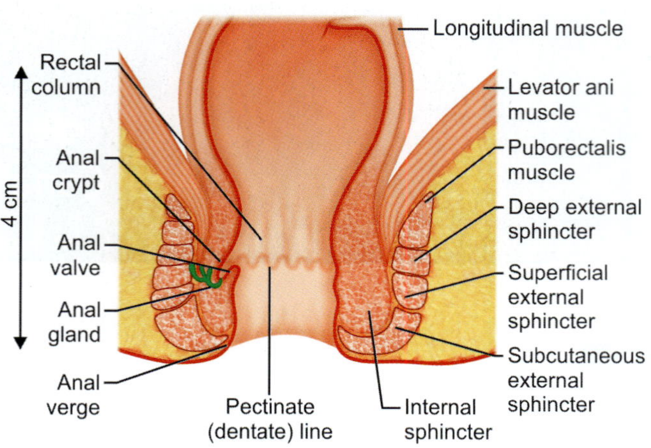

Fig. 63.2: Anal transition zone and surrounding musculature.

normal appendages. Above the dentate line, the anal transitional zone (ATZ) has plum-colored mucosa and contains a mixture of transitional, squamous, columnar, endocrine and glandular cells, plus melanocytes (Fig. 63.2).

Mucosa above the dentate line is supplied by autonomic nerves and is insensitive to pain. Below the dentate line, the supply is provided by spinal nerves, which are highly sensitive to pain. The upper anal canal contains longitudinal anal cushions, which are joined distally by small horizontal anal valves. Anal sinuses form above these valves, and into these sinuses drain 3 to 12 mucus-secreting anal glands, the bodies of which lie submucosally within the internal anal sphincter (IAS) or in the intersphincteric space between IAS and the external anal sphincter (EAS).

Anal Muscles

The internal anal sphincter (IAS) is a thickening of the inner circular smooth muscle layer of the rectum that encircles the length of the anal canal and is associated with involuntary fecal continence. External to this muscle (distal to the puborectalis) lies the external anal sphincter (EAS), which has subcutaneous, superficial and deep parts, is somatically innervated and exerts voluntary control over continence. Between the two is the potential intersphincteric space, which is a route for the spread of cryptoglandular sepsis. The puborectalis maintains the anorectal angle and is functionally linked to the EAS in preserving continence. The other anorectal spaces–perianal, ischiorectal (ischioanal), supralevator, postanal–are shown in Figure 63.1; they are also important in the development of anorectal abscesses.

Vascular Supply

The upper anal canal is supplied by the inferior mesenteric artery (the artery of the hindgut) and the lower third by systemic inferior rectal arteries, which are branches of the internal pudendal arteries. The middle rectal arteries are branches from the anterior division of the internal iliac arteries. They are variable branches, less constant in the female pelvis (as they may be replaced by the uterine and vaginal branches), and they may also supply the prostate in the male. The dentate (pectinate) line lies at the level of the anal valves. It represents the junction between endodermal and ectodermal parts and is the lymphatic watershed. Proximally, lymphatics drain via the middle rectal vessels to the internal iliac and then para-aortic nodes. Distally, lymphatics drain along cutaneous pathways to the inguinal nodes.[1]

PHYSIOLOGY

Defecation

A complex combination of anatomy and physiology allows the cortically controlled act of passage of stool from the rectum. The rectum acts as a reservoir for stool, and its distensible walls can expand to increase capacity. This process allows for small increases in intraluminal pressure in response to large changes in rectal volume. Either defecation or incontinence will occur if rectal pressure increases rapidly and exceeds anal pressure. Stool characteristics are important because marginal continence may allow leakage of liquid stool, while solid stool may be controlled without difficulty.

Sensation includes intrinsic and extrinsic components. Intrinsic components within the distal anal canal are thought to be important in distinguishing liquid from solid and gas. Extrinsic receptors within the rectal wall and/or puborectalis sense rectal distension and initiate the events that lead to defecation. Evidence for the presence of pressure receptors outside the rectal wall includes the fact that continence and sensation are maintained after rectal resection and coloanal anastomosis, provided the puborectalis muscle remains intact.

Tonic IAS contraction achieves most resting anal tone, aided by the anal cushions. Voluntary EAS contraction is recruited when intra-abdominal pressure increases. The loss of anorectal angulation with puborectalis relaxation, the propagation of mass colonic contraction waves into the rectum, and reflex IAS relaxation are all integrated parts of coordinated defecation.

Rectal distension by stool triggers the sampling or rectoanal inhibitory reflex. Relaxation of the IAS plus simultaneous contraction of the EAS allows rectal contents to reach the upper anal canal, where sensory fibers distinguish between liquid, solid, and gas and can send a signal that the rectum is full and defecation should continue. At this point the individual determines whether defecation or passage of flatus is socially appropriate. If so, the puborectalis muscle relaxes, the anorectal angle straightens and the EAS relaxes, decreasing anal pressure. With Valsalva's maneuver intra-abdominal pressure is transmitted to the rectum, and defecation occurs as intrarectal pressure overcomes anal canal pressure. If an individual chooses not to defecate, voluntary contraction of the EAS and puborectalis increases the anal pressure and narrows the anorectal angle to maintain continence.

Anorectal Physiologic Testing

In complex cases advanced physiologic testing will supplement a thorough history and examination and assist diagnosis and treatment. The four most common techniques are:

1. *Anal manometry*: Pressures can be recorded within the distal rectum and anal canal by balloon systems, water-perfused catheters, or solid-state microtransducers. Most systems use water-perfused multiple-port catheters and are interpreted using standard software programs. Manometry defines the length of the anal canal or high pressure zone. Normal resting pressure (a measure of IAS function) ranges from 40-80 cm H_2O (3.9-7.8 kPa). Anal squeeze pressure (a measure of EAS function) ranges from 80–160 cm H_2O (7.8-15.7 kPa). Anal sensation is also evaluated by inflating an attached balloon with saline. The minimal sensory threshold and maximum tolerated volume can be identified, as well as the presence or absence of the normal rectoanal inhibitory reflex.
2. *Endoanal ultrasonography (EUS)*: EUS is easy to perform and provides the best visualization of anal musculature and perianal structures. The anal structures appear as a series of concentric rings. The IAS (smooth muscle) produces a dark ring, the EAS (striated muscle) produces a mixed echogenic or gray ring, while the puborectalis looks similar to the EAS but is found more cephalad and is "U" shaped because it has no anterior component. Defects in the sphincter muscles are easily identified as breaks in the muscular rings. Anal masses such as abscesses, cysts, or lymph nodes are also readily seen.
3. *Electromyography (EMG)*: EMG was commonly used in the past to evaluate anal sphincter defects and look for muscle denervation, but it has been largely replaced by EUS and manometry, which are less painful and provide reliable results. However, pudendal nerve terminal motor latency (PNTML) remains an important tool for evaluation. It measures the time required for a nerve impulse to travel along the pudendal nerve and cause contraction of EAS. The study is performed with two electrodes placed on the gloved index finger. The proximal electrode near the fingertip stimulates the pudendal nerve adjacent to the distal rectal wall, while the second electrode at the base of the finger records EAS contraction. Prolonged PNTML (>0.2 ms) is found in pudendal neuropathy, which is usually secondary to prolonged labor or rectal prolapse causing hypotonia of the sphincter muscles and incontinence. Abnormal PNTML predicts a poor response to sphincter repair.
4. *Defecography*: Defecating proctography assesses the ability to evacuate stool and is important in the evaluation of chronic constipation. A semisolid barium paste is instilled into the rectum, and the patient is then asked to evacuate it. The anorectal angle is measured during squeeze and strain. With squeeze the puborectalis muscles should contract and narrow the anorectal angle. With strain and evacuation, the anorectal angle should widen in response to relaxation of the puborectalis. Paradoxic puborectalis contraction is readily identified as narrowing of the anorectal angle during attempts at defecation. The presence or absence of a rectocele and/or intussusception (telescoping of the sigmoid colon into the rectum) can be identified by defecography. Since both of these entities can exist in the absence of symptoms, they should only be corrected in symptomatic patients.

CLINICAL FEATURES

Symptoms

The history of anal problems includes features of general health and comorbidity and symptoms related to gastrointestinal conditions that may present with anal pathology, such as inflammatory bowel disease (IBD). Change of bowel habit should be noted, as well as pelvic and abdominal pain and bloating. The history of bowel function may suggest obstructed defecation or other functional bowel disorders or indicate chronic stool looseness associated with incontinence. Constitutional symptoms of pyrexia, weight loss, lethargy, and arthralgia suggest chronic inflammation, sepsis, or an immunocompromised state. Diet and drug intake is important, especially the use of laxatives and motility agents. Information concerning sexual preference, anal receptive intercourse, intravenous drug abuse, previous blood transfusions, and HIV status (if known) should be requested.

Anorectal symptoms of bleeding, discharge, pain, and tenesmus are of vital importance. Fecal and urinary continence requires assessment, and a history should be sought of previous anorectal pathology, peranal prolapse, and anorectal or abdominal operations. A detailed obstetric history is important, in particular difficult or forceps vaginal deliveries and episiotomies. Any concomitant neurologic disease should be noted.

Signs

Examination is carried out in the left lateral or knee-chest position. Inspection with the buttocks gently separated may reveal perianal cutaneous lesions, such as warts and neoplasms, skin tags, fistulas or pilonidal disease, and scarring from a previous operation. Perianal soiling, discharge, and excoriation and anal contour are assessed. There may be erythema, induration, tenderness, or discharge associated with sepsis or anocutaneous ulceration. Straining may reveal perineal descent or hemorrhoidal, mucosal or full-thickness rectal prolapse (FTRP). Eversion of the anal verge may show the distal end of an anal fissure. An opportunity presents to discriminate between a chronic fissure with exposed IAS and the sentinel tag and linear fissuring that can develop with chronic excoriation due to minor leakage. This distinction is fundamental when considering therapeutic options.

Digital anorectal examination should be gentle, and adequate lubricant should be used. An assessment is made for mass lesions, induration and tenderness, polyps, ulceration, prostatic size and tenderness, puborectalis spasm, and rectocele. Sphincter and perineal body bulk, sphincter spasm, and resting pressure and squeeze pressure should be assessed. High digital examination may reveal pelvic tenderness, a mass, or the bogginess of a pelvic collection. The glove is examined for blood, mucus, and pus on removal, the stool is assessed and fecal occult blood testing may be carried out. Vaginal, cervical, and uterine examinations are sometimes appropriate.

Proctosigmoidoscopy usually confirms digital findings, and mucosal visualization allows an assessment of anal cushions and hemorrhoids and exclusion of proctitis. Abnormal lesions are biopsied, and swabs are taken for culture if indicated. Minor therapeutic procedures can be carried out, such as banding of hemorrhoids or mucosal prolapse. On sigmoidoscopy, if the subject is asked to bear down, occult rectal prolapse or solitary rectal ulcer may be evident. Occult or complete prolapse may also be demonstrated on examination during straining in the squatting position or sitting on a commode.

Table 63. 1 Causes of fecal incontinence

Cause category	*Examples*
Sphincter injury	Obstetric, surgical, accidental
Neurologic	Central (e.g., tumor, trauma, cerebrovascular accident, demyelination), peripheral (e.g., tumor, diabetes mellitus, cauda equina lesion, disc injury and surgery, diabetes, demyelination)
Anorectal	Hemorrhoids, rectal prolapse, inflammatory bowel disease, fistula, tumor, resection (loss of reservoir), fecal impaction, diarrhea, or liquid stool
Congenital	Spina bifida, meningocele, imperforate anus operations, Hirschsprung's disease
Idiopathic	
Miscellaneous	Behavioral, dementia, mental retardation

Endoluminal ultrasound and anorectal manometry to assess sphincter anatomy and function are especially helpful in patients with FI. Colonoscopy and barium enema complement clinical assessment, when appropriate. Severe perianal pain or tenderness requires examination under anesthesia (EUA).

FECAL INCONTINENCE

Fecal incontinence is common and socially disabling. Incontinence to flatus or feces affects up to 11% of adults and occurs frequently (daily or weekly) in 2%. It is commoner in females as a result of obstetric sphincter damage and is more prevalent with increasing age.[1,2] Incontinence is either:

- Passive, in which losses occur without patient awareness, and this is usually associated with IAS dysfunction
- Associated with urge, in which losses result from an inability to suppress defecation and are frequently associated with external anal sphincter (EAS) dysfunction.

Etiology

The etiology of FI is often multifactorial (Table 63.1). Incontinence may occur with disruption to one or more of several factors that are involved in maintaining normal anorectal continence, including:

- IAS and EAS function
- Anorectal sensation

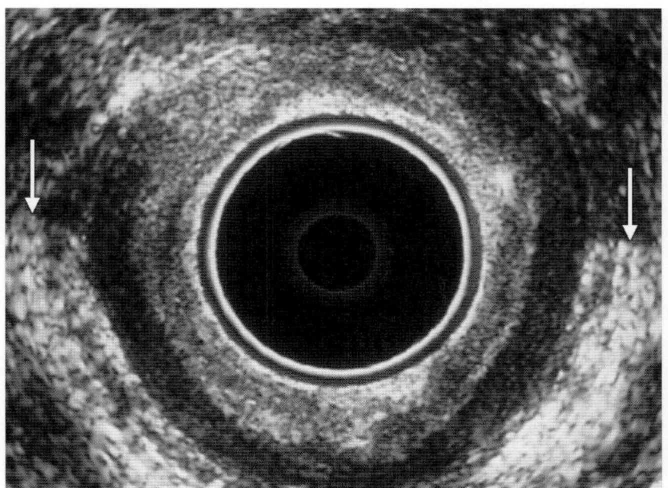

Fig. 63.3: Endoluminal ultrasound showing a large anterior external anal sphincter (EAS) disruption from a forceps-assisted vaginal delivery. Arrows show the extent of the EAS defect.

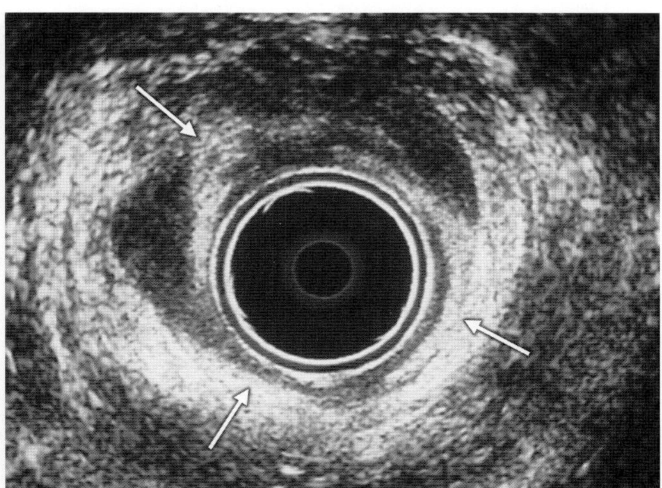

Fig. 63.4: Endoluminal ultrasound showing extensive internal anal sphincter disruption secondary to anal dilatation (arrows).

- Rectal capacity and compliance
- Stool consistency
- The rectoanal inhibitory reflex.

Of these, sphincter function is of greatest importance. Although both sphincters are tonically active at rest, the IAS contributes approximately 80% of resting anal tone. The EAS is recruited when continence is threatened during periods of raised intra-abdominal pressure with coughing or straining or when unplanned IAS relaxation occurs. Reduced anal sensation may inhibit the regular anorectal sampling of solids, liquids, and flatus. Rectal reservoir size and compliance may be reduced after operation, irradiation, or in IBD. Copious liquid stool can produce incontinence, even in the presence of normal motor and sensory anorectal function.

Most surgical referrals relate to obstetric sphincter injuries or iatrogenic sphincter injuries from previous operation, or are idiopathic. The commonest cause in healthy women is unrecognized sphincter damage during childbirth.[3] After a first vaginal delivery, 13% of women develop incontinence or urgency, and studies have shown that 30% of women have structural sphincter defects on ELUS (Fig. 63.3) after vaginal delivery. Third-degree tears that involve one or both sphincters complicate 0.5–2.0% of vaginal deliveries, and many defects are unrecognized at the time of delivery. Forceps use is the usual predisposing factor, but primiparous delivery, birth weight over 4 kg, occipitoposterior delivery presentation, and a prolonged second stage of labor are all associated. Immediate repair is frequently inadequate; 85% of patients have persisting structural sphincter defects on ELUS, and 50% remain symptomatic.[2] Increasing evidence points toward structural childbirth trauma as being more important than neurologic factors in the development of FI, although the role of pudendal denervation by childbirth stretching or entrapment, possibly exacerbated by defecatory straining, is likely to explain the atrophic degeneration found in some patients with incontinence. The role of the menopause in the onset of incontinence is poorly understood since it is fairly common to see women with marked sphincter defects sustained during delivery that only become symptomatic at or after the menopause.

Fistula operations account for many iatrogenic cases of FI, usually for high or multiple fistulas or recurrent procedures for complex disease. Anal dilatation for fissure produces incontinence in up to 20% of patients and has largely been abandoned in adult practice (Fig. 63.4).

Lateral sphincterotomy (LS) results in a much lower incidence of FI.[4] Posterior sphincterotomy through a fissure base may produce a keyhole (gutter) deformity and fecal leakage, and it is not associated with as high a cure rate as LS. Minor soiling is not uncommon after hemorrhoidectomy and may reflect reduced anal sensation or loss of the anal cushions. Such soiling does not usually require operative management. Low anterior resections and coloanal anastomoses may also produce varying degrees of FI because of:

- Reduced capacity and compliance of the neorectum (which may be improved by using small colonic J pouches)
- Loss of coordinated IAS function because of interference with local intramural nerve pathways.

Table 63.2 Cleveland Clinic scoring system of fecal incontinence

Frequency of incontinence					
Incontinence type	*Never*	*Rarely (< 1/month)*	*Sometimes (> 1/month, < 1/week)*	*Usually (> 1/week, < 1/day)*	*Always (> 1/day)*
Solids	0	1	2	3	4
Liquids	0	1	2	3	4
Flatus	0	1	2	3	4
Use of pad	0	1	2	3	4
Lifestyle alteration	0	1	2	3	4

Continence score is determined by adding points for all five parameters and total score is out of 20. A continence score of 0 = perfect continence and of 20 = complete incontinence.

The etiology of incontinence in elderly women is often unclear, but frequently there is an associated unrecognized obstetric sphincter injury. The late onset has been attributed to progression of nerve damage, but may be related to changes of the normal aging process:[5] with increasing age, the IAS generates a lower pressure and its thickness and fibrous component increase, pudendal nerve latencies increase, and rectal and anal sensory thresholds increase.[6] Approximately 10% of women who present with idiopathic incontinence, however, have no apparent structural damage, and the only currently identifiable factor is nerve damage. Histologic sphincter assessment in these patients shows an innervation–denervation injury with atrophy that may be caused by pudendal nerve injury.

History

It is important to identify what a patient means when describing incontinence. Incontinence to solids, liquids, and flatus should all be assessed, as well as frequency of episodes, the need to wear pads, and the impact on lifestyle. The history often suggests etiologic factors. Inadvertent fecal seepage suggests reduced anal sensation or IAS dysfunction. Urgency suggests EAS dysfunction, and coexisting urinary incontinence may indicate a neuropathy. Details of previous anorectal operations and trauma and a full obstetric history are important. To standardize assessment, formal continence scoring systems should be used, such as that shown in Table 63.2.

Examination

General assessment includes abdominal and peripheral neurologic examinations. The perineum is assessed for soiling, scarring, signs of present or past sepsis or fistulation, anal contour, and perineal descent. Straining may demonstrate FTRP, mucosal rectal prolapse, or prolapsing hemorrhoids. Anocutaneous reflex testing assesses perineal sensory innervation. Digital assessment of sphincter integrity includes an assessment of both resting and squeeze tone, although the correlation with physiologic evaluation is unclear.[7] In lower motor neuron injuries, e.g., from lumbar disc and spinal causes, the cough reflex may be absent and the patient will be unable to contract the sphincter, whereas with higher injuries, the cough reflex will be intact and again sphincter contraction will not be possible.

Anterior sphincter defects can often be palpated or seen, and perineal body bulk is assessed. Associated rectoceles, fecal impaction, and mass lesions should be identified. All patients require proctoscopy and sigmoidoscopy to identify locally correctable lesions and exclude other pathology. Stool consistency and internal prolapse are assessed. Celiac disease, pancreatic insufficiency, and diabetes need to be considered in the differential diagnosis.

Investigation

Ideally, all patients who have symptomatic FI are assessed using anorectal physiology studies and ELUS. Defecography is reserved for those in whom rectal prolapse or internal intussusception is suspected, but remains clinically occult.

Physiologic studies incorporate several tests that assess IAS and EAS function and morphology, anorectal sensation and local reflex integrity, rectal capacity and compliance, and pudendal nerve terminal motor latency. Manometry measures maximum resting anal pressure (reflecting IAS function) and maximum voluntary contraction and cough anal pressures (assessing EAS function). The rectoanal inhibitory reflex provides an assessment of local neural pathways, and rectal balloon inflation is used to evaluate rectal sensation and compliance. Sensation is further quantitatively assessed using anal mucosal electrical stimulation. Pudendal nerve terminal motor latency records the time to muscular contraction after pudendal nerve stimulation and may be prolonged in idiopathic FI.

As it measures the fastest conducting neurons, it is a very unreliable test that has shown very poor correlation both with function and outcome following surgical repair.

An ELUS provides high-resolution images of both sphincters. Dissection studies show close image correlation with anatomy. Sphincter defects are identified with a high degree of accuracy.

Management

The causes of FI are usually identified by a combination of history and investigations, and specific treatment depends on the etiologic factors identified. Clearly remediable benign anorectal lesions should be corrected. A FTRP requires surgical repair for cure. Active IBD and radiation proctitis are managed medically in most cases. Perianal skin tags, prolapse of hemorrhoids or mucosa, and anal and low rectal polyps may all contribute to postdefecation soiling, and many patients find improvement after surgical removal of such lesions. Minor perianal soiling may need no treatment other than diligent perianal hygiene.

Many patients can be managed conservatively, and this is a worthwhile initial regimen for all of them. Of the patients who fail to respond, those who have a documented anatomic sphincter defect are best managed by direct overlapping surgical repair, which results in a long-term successful outcome in about 50% of cases.[8] For those who have neurogenic or idiopathic incontinence, postanal repair may be considered in the knowledge that the initial results may not be maintained, but temporary improvement may at least be achieved in up to 75% of patients. Some surgeons suggest carrying out an anterior sphincter repair if patients fail to respond to a postanal repair. The role of stimulated graciloplasty is yet to be defined, but should be considered for patients who have had previous unsuccessful attempts at surgical cure; long-term results have yet to be reported. Sacral nerve stimulation,[9] artificial bowel sphincters,[10] and injection sphincter augmentation[11] are currently being studied and are possible future treatment options. A permanent defunctioning stoma is used as an end-stage operative alternative.

Neurological diseases of varying types damage the nerve supply to the anal sphincter and cause incontinence. Obstetric injury from a large baby or forceps delivery is associated with two injuries that may coexist to varying degrees. First, delivery may be accompanied by tearing of the anal sphincter and anal canal. Second, the nerves supplying the anal sphincter can also be damaged. Evidence of nerve damage includes changes in the muscle histology with fiber hypertrophy, large motor units and fiber grouping, EMG changes, and the findings on histochemistry consistent with denervation.

When nerves are damaged, repairing denervated muscle serves little purpose. While the results of sphincter repair may be good, in the past the success rates of sphincter repair were greatly exaggerated. With modern methods of reporting that allow better collection of data, early outcomes have been shown to deteriorate with time. Some patients may have reported better outcomes because they were happy to have had some help from a sympathetic clinician.

Furthermore, if the nerve supply to the sphincter is damaged, there is a high probability that there will also be interference with the normal functioning of the rectum and possibly the colon. This is because the nerve supply to the left colon arises deep in the pelvis where it is susceptible to damage by the delivering infant's head. Thus, rectal sensation and colonic motility are altered together with co-ordination between anal muscles and the rectum. In addition, altered anal sensation and rectal awareness can compromise effective continence and defecation. Given the complexity of the pathophysiology, it is not surprising that successful therapeutic avenues are challenging.

Sacral neuromodulation (SNS) goes some way toward addressing the complexity in that the mechanism of successful action appears to be multimodal. There have been local effects on rectal awareness and urgency in some studies on sphincter function plus central effects as seen on PET and functional MRI studies of the brain. Thus, SNS addresses multiple aspects of the continence and defecatory mechanism.

Tan et al. published a meta-analysis of studies published between 1995 and 2008 on SNS for FI.[12] Outcomes evaluated were functional, physiological, and quality of life. A random-effects model was used and sensitivity analyses performed. Subgroup analyses were performed on age and sphincter status. Thirty-four studies were included, reporting on 944 patients undergoing peripheral nerve evaluation; 665 underwent permanent SNS. Weekly incontinence episodes and incontinence scores were significantly reduced with SNS, while the ability to defer defecation increased. Quality-of-life indices improved following SNS, and mean anal pressures increased significantly ($p < 0.001$). Results remained consistent on sensitivity analysis. The under-56 years age group showed smaller functional but greater physiological and quality-of-life improvements. Results were similar between sphincter-intact and impaired subgroups. The complication rate was 15% for permanent SNS, with 3% resulting in permanent explanation.

The great advantage of SNS over normal surgical approaches is the trial stage using a temporary wire attached to a stimulator. Success rates vary between 50% and 80%. Unfortunately, for reasons that are unclear, not all positive temporary outcomes translate into permanent ones, once the definitive implant has been inserted. There may be a placebo benefit or variability of the stimulation site. Some advocate multiple lead testing, which may lead to better permanent site selection.

The indications for SNS have spread. Initially, it was used in patients with intact anal sphincters. Success was then reported in patients with sphincter defects. Indeed, if the divided sphincter does not contract, then SNS is a logical choice. Comparable outcomes have been achieved with SNS and sphincter repair in appropriately selected patients. It may therefore be worth trying SNS in patients with FI of most etiologies, including those with poor function after rectal reconstruction or prolapse procedures and those with diabetes or neurological disease.

The mechanism of action of SNS continues to be the subject of ongoing debate. Some studies report improvement in sphincter pressures while others do not. Others describe altered rectal awareness possibly allowing earlier perception of the need to defecate. Improved urgency is an important outcome reported in some studies. Newer evidence of the central responses indicates that the benefits are subtle and multifactorial.

The crossover studies by LeRoi et al. are fascinating since in the off periods persisting benefits are seen in terms of elevated sphincter pressures significantly above pressures before implantation.[13] Thus, the benefits of SNS may not be "on-off" but could represent some form of training or long-term modulation. However, loss of benefit with time is becoming increasingly reported. The mechanisms are still obscure, but may include changes around the stimulation leads with loss of function.

Sacral neuromodulation has been used in constipation, but the success rates are not impressive and the definition of constipation was too weak in Kamm's series.[14] Patients with constipation underwent percutaneous nerve evaluation (PNE) and 73% proceeded to implantation. Sixty-three percent achieved a 50% improvement, with stool frequency rising from 2.3 to 6.6 evacuations a week. The problem is referral of patients for the treatment of constipation when they only evacuate once a month. Finally, on an intention-to-treat basis, only just under two thirds achieved an improvement of 50%. Clearly, more work needs to be done to define and explore how to use SNS in severe constipation. The work of Dinning et al. sheds some insight into the complexity of the responses in constipation. In 8 patients with severe slow-transit constipation, they studied propagating waves in the colon using a long multiport manometer tube. S3 stimulation induced a significant increase in pan-colonic propagating sequences compared with baseline measurements. Conversely, S2 stimulation produced an increase in retrograde wave sequences.

Michelsen in 2008 showed that SNS in FI not only induced changes in the left colon that could be explained by pre-sacral nerve stimulation of the long colonic nerves but also resulted in changes to the right colon that must be vagally induced.[15] These data provide strong evidence that the mechanism of action is central as much as peripheral. Precisely that is predominant is unknown. Studies using transcranial mapping with electromagnetic stimulation and positron emission tomography (PET) have shown changes in the frontal cortex that change with the duration of stimulation, possibly reflecting learning or an altered response in the brains of incontinent subjects. Laurberg's group used PET to record indices of regional cerebral blood flow (CBF) before and after 30 minutes of continuous stimulation. They repeated this procedure after 2 weeks of continued stimulation, before and 30 minutes after arrest of the stimulation. The initial stimulation activated a region of the contralateral frontal cortex that normally is active during focused attention. After 2 weeks of stimulation, this activation had been replaced by activity in parts of the ipsilateral caudate nucleus, a region of the brain thought to be specifically involved in learning and reward processing. They concluded that sacral nerve stimulation induced changes in cerebral activity consistent with an effect on afferent projections of the vagus. The initial activation of the frontal cortex may reflect focused attention, whereas the subsequent activation of the caudate nucleus may reflect recruitment of mechanisms involved in learning and reward processing. These changes may contribute to the improved continence, which is an acquired result of the stimulation. There is evidence that the effect of SNS is mediated by modulation of afferent projections, and SNS has been shown to induce propagating pressure waves throughout the colon in patients with severe slow-transit constipation. A study by Sheldon showed that SNS improves symptoms of FI and reversibly reduces corticoanal excitability without changes of anorectal manometry measures.[16] Indeed, functional brain imaging shows that the therapeutic effect of SNS is associated with activity in several brain centers in patients with urinary retention. Direct and indirect stimulation of regions of the central nervous system is known to change measures of CBF and glucose consumption. Vagal nerve stimulation is a therapeutic approach to several neurological disorders that takes advantage of the abundance of afferent projections in the vagus nerve. Other approaches include deep brain stimulation, transcranial magnetic stimulation, and electroconvulsive therapy. The most consistent observation is an increase in PET, functional MRI, and single-photon emission CT indices of CBF in the frontal cortices, including orbitofrontal and superior and medial frontal cortices, and anterior cingulate, with variable changes in other brain regions and some evidence of decreased indices of CBF) after prolonged stimulation.

Percutaneous/Transcutaneous Stimulation

The tibial nerve can be stimulated using either transcutaneous or percutaneous (PCTNS) methods. The nerve contains sensory and motor fibers. Whether it contains nerve fibers below the S1 root is unclear. Perhaps its mode of action is to spread stimulation through the sacral nerve plexus, but central effects are also important. An attractive feature of transcutaneous stimulation is that since the benefits appear to last beyond stimulation with SNS, the technique could be applied at night while the subject is sleeping, thus helping a much wider population; it is also cheaper than expensive sacral nerve implants.

Duelund-Jacobsen et al. from Aarhus reported 342 patients of whom 158 had idiopathic FI.[17] One-hundred twenty nine had an active implant and 108 responded to an enquiry. Ninety-nine had the active implant and 75 were satisfied with the function. Thus, on an intention to treat basis, only 51% of patients implanted in this series are satisfied. These figures appear to follow the path of sphincter repair where better results were reported initially than were actually the case in the longer term. It is imperative to provide patients with realistic outcomes. The Aarhus group took 87 patients for PNE and followed them through to implantation, but at a median 39 months only 35% were satisfied on an intention to treat basis if one starts with PNE compared to the final outcome. This is important when putting into context what outcome might be expected in an incontinent patient. Importantly, incontinence scores and bowel habit diaries did not necessarily correlate with patient satisfaction. Thus, there is no reliable scoring method at present.

The same group studied alternative pacemaker settings to assess whether patient satisfaction could be improved.[18] Higher-frequency settings of 310 Hz/210 microseconds (μs) improved patient satisfaction in a small study of 15 patients.

Given the fall-off in success rates, the selection of patients after PNE needs to be more stringent to avoid subsequent disappointment in the future. Following an initial successful PNE, if there is loss of function with the definitive implant, there are a number of actions that can be taken. The device and lead integrity should be checked. If there is loss of sensation, lead replacement may be required especially if there is high impedance on testing.

Nonoperative Management

Nonoperative measures are successful in 40–60% of cases. Loose and liquid stools can be made firmer using bulking agents, and bowel transit can be slowed by using antidiarrheal agents, such as codeine phosphate or loperamide. Low-fiber diets can be helpful. Glycerine or bisacodyl suppositories frequently improve late post-defecation soiling by improving the completeness of rectal evacuation. Morning phosphate enemas can be helpful in more resistant cases. The use of well-fitted and absorbent incontinence pads reduces major accidents. Biofeedback conditioning, pelvic floor physical therapy, and anorectal electrostimulation have all been used with varying success, but long-term data are lacking and the techniques are time-consuming and demanding.

Operative Management

Patients with persisting FI after correction of simpler remediable causes and a trial of conservative measures are classified into those with and without anatomic sphincter defects. Sphincter disruptions should be reconstituted using a layered overlapping repair at the site of injury, which is almost always anterolateral, except in iatrogenic injury after sphincterotomy and fistulotomy or accidental trauma. Postoperative confinement of the bowels, i.e., induced constipation with drugs or a low residue diet, does not alter results. Overall, good results from overlapping repair can be expected in about 75% of patients,[19] and the addition of levatorplasty appears beneficial.[20] Failure to respond is commoner in the presence of coexisting pudendal neuropathy,[21] but age itself does not adversely affect outcome.[22] Some patients with a poor outcome have persisting sphincter defects on ELUS. Repair improves

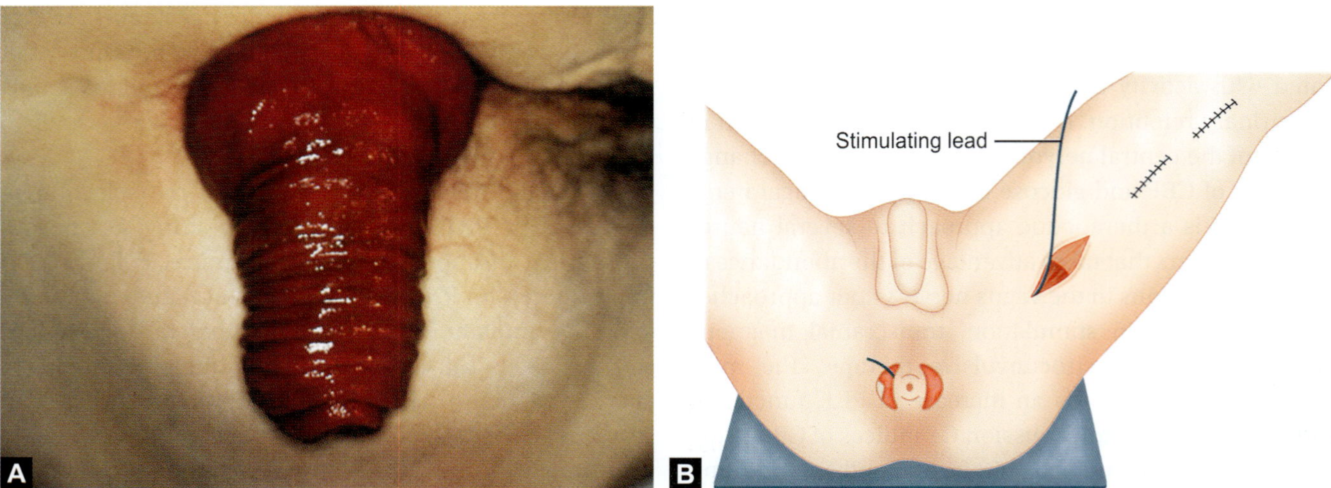

Figs. 63.5A and B: Dynamic graciloplasty. (A) Operative view of gracilis muscle mobilization upon its neurovascular supply following division of its tendon insertion onto the medial tibia. (B) The muscle is then wrapped around the anus and secured to the appropriate ischial tuberosity. Stimulating electrodes are then tracked subcutaneously to a stimulating device, which is implanted via a separate incision into the abdominal wall.

mean resting pressure, increases anal canal length, and, most importantly, increases maximum squeeze pressures. The long-term results of overlapping repair, however, appear to deteriorate with time, with about half of patients having a good clinical outcome at a minimum follow-up of 5 years. The procedure can be repeated if necessary.

The traditional approach for idiopathic or neurogenic incontinence has been *postanal repair* with the aim of restoring the normal anorectal angle, which is obtuse in many patients. Although initial reports suggested high success rates, the long-term results are poor, with 3–5-year continence rates of only 25–34%.[23] Similarly disappointing long-term results have been reported following total pelvic floor repair, which combines postanal repair with anterior sphincter plication and levatorplasty.[24]

Dynamic graciloplasty has a limited role in the management of FI of all etiologies for which other treatment modalities and in particular sacral nerve stimulation have failed. In the past such FI was frequently managed by permanent diversion as a last resort. The gracilis muscle is transposed and wrapped around the anal canal, using various configurations, and its tendon is attached to the ischial tuberosity. The muscle is attached via leads to an implantable stimulator and is stimulated over several weeks to convert it from a type 2 skeletal muscle to a fatigue-resistant type 1 muscle (Figs. 63.5A and B). Improved or normal continence is achieved in up to 81% of patients,[25,26] and is accompanied by a resultant improvement in lifestyle. The procedure is more cost-effective than the long-term use of pads or defunctioning colostomy. The associated morbidity rate is up to 50%, although most associated problems are minor and resolve to result in an excellent functional outcome. The continence of those patients who fail to respond can be restored by a second contralateral graciloplasty. Long-term continence and success rates are unfortunately sustained in only about half the operated patients.

Artificial bowel sphincters have a role, but to date the failure rates have been high, with over 50% failing after the first operation followed by long-term failures related to device degeneration with cuff and balloon rupture. With the gracilis overall long-term results may be disappointing, but if it is initially successful then the only ongoing issue is replacement of the stimulator every 7 years or so.

Fecal diversion with a *stoma* is the last-resort procedure, with the usual long-term complication rate approaching 50%.

RECTAL PROLAPSE

Rectal prolapse is a rectorectal intussusception that with time prolapses outside the anal canal. Associated predisposing anatomic features include a deep pouch of Douglas, lack of mesorectal fixation, weak or atonic sphincters, redundant rectosigmoid, and levator diastasis.[27] Sphincter histology shows marked denervation and myopathic features, which possibly result from pudendal nerve entrapment or stretching from repeated defecatory straining or childbirth trauma. A generalized pelvic floor dysfunction is frequently present on defecating proctography.

Prolapse is classified as internal, external, or mucosal (Fig. 63.6):[28]

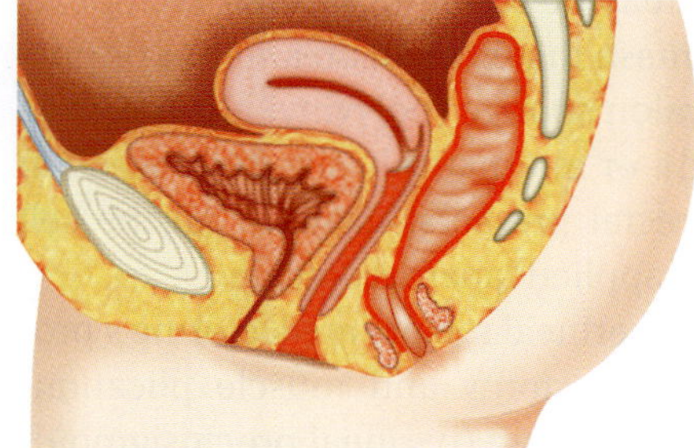

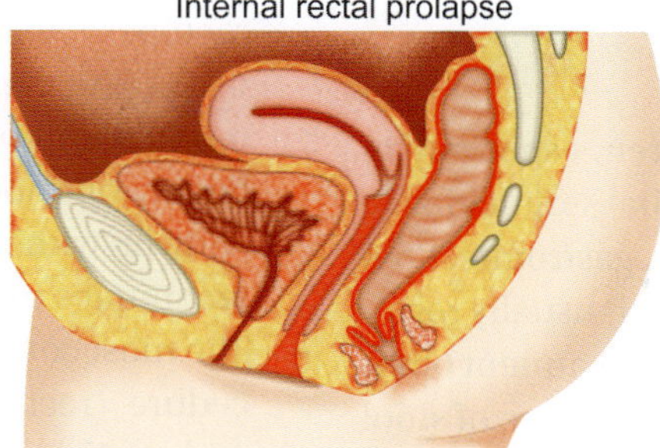

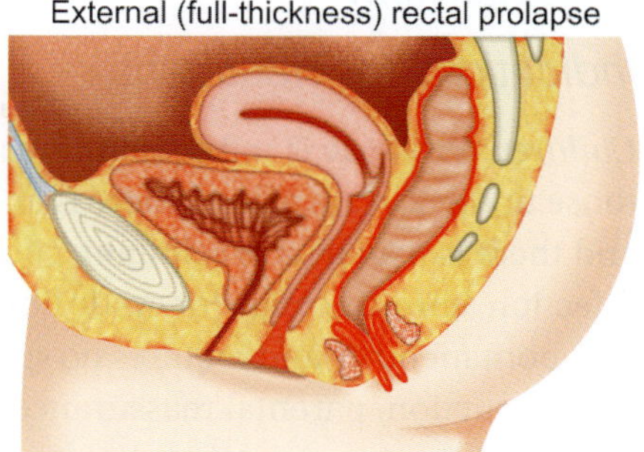

Fig. 63.6: Rectal prolapse.

- *Internal prolapse* (occult, hidden, or concealed prolapse) is an intussusception of the upper rectum that does not reach the anal verge and may be a precursor of external prolapse
- In *external prolapse* (complete rectal prolapse, FTRP, overt rectal prolapse, or procidentia) the intussusception extends beyond the anal verge with full-thickness circumferential rectal protrusion
- In *mucosal prolapse*, the underlying rectal musculature remains *in situ*, with only overlying mucosa prolapsing distally, sometimes beyond the anal verge; it presents with minor soiling, pruritus ani, or bright rectal bleeding secondary to trauma.[29]

Full-thickness rectal prolapse occurs predominantly in adult females, with a female-to-male ratio of up to 6:1 and a peak incidence in middle age. There is no association with multiparity. The most common presentation is impaired fecal continence from associated sphincter laxity. Patients often describe a postdefecation mass protruding from the anal verge, for which digital reduction is sometimes required. Constipated straining or obstructed defecation is common. Soiling occurs frequently without warning or knowledge. Urgency is uncommon. Complications include proctitis with rectal ulceration and bleeding from repeated trauma, irreducibility, and, rarely, infarction with necrosis.

Evaluation

The history includes details of continence, defecation, constipation, and straining. Often a postdefecation prolapse or "lump" is described. Symptoms of other colorectal disease, such as bleeding, distension, and change in bowel habit, should be sought. Obstetric details and previous anorectal pathology and perianal, pelvic or sphincter operations are important. Diet, the use of laxatives, and motility agents and concomitant urinary incontinence and neurologic disease are assessed. General medical health is also assessed and may influence the operative options for a particular patient.

Abdominal examination is usually normal, but may show a loaded left colon. On rectal examination, the presence of any perineal excoriation, mucous discharge, fecal soiling, and scarring from previous operation or sepsis is noted. Full-thickness rectal prolapse patients often have a patulous anus. Digital examination is used to assess resting and squeeze pressures, exclude mass lesions, and identify rectoceles. The leading point of an intussusception may be felt during anal digitation on straining. Straining may deliver a FTRP with a palpable lateral circumferential sulcus. Occult lesions may be revealed by examination while straining in the squatting position or sitting on a commode.

Proctoscopy and sigmoidoscopy exclude other local lesions. Straining with a rigid sigmoidoscope placed at 7–10 cm may show the apex of an elusive prolapse. The entire colon should be visualized by colonoscopy or barium enema to exclude proximal disease. Among patients who have constipation, transit studies identify a group of people who have delayed colonic transit as a contributing factor. Resection gives superior results to rectopexy alone for this group by reducing the debilitating postoperative deterioration of constipation that frequently occurs.[30] Defecating proctography is helpful if the diagnosis remains in doubt, and it also delineates associated functional pelvic floor disorders, such as puborectalis spasm and perineal descent. Endoluminal ultrasound assesses sphincter integrity in those who have impaired continence or a history of obstetric trauma. In patients who have both impaired continence and a sphincter defect, the prolapse should be corrected first because it improves continence in many patients by relieving rectoanal inhibition caused by the prolapse bulk within the anal canal. Those patients who do not improve should be offered sphincter repair.[31]

Management

Indications for Treatment

Children: Prolapse is infrequent in children, especially in those under 2 years of age. There is an equal sex incidence and there is usually a precipitant, such as gastrointestinal infection, chronic cough, or cystic fibrosis. It usually resolves spontaneously and requires no special treatment other than reduction, parental reassurance, and the use of stool softeners. Even recurrent prolapse usually resolves spontaneously. Rarely, a rectopexy is necessary. The results are good.

Mucosal prolapse: Symptoms of minor soiling, bleeding, and pruritus are amenable to minimally invasive procedures, such as band ligation or submucosal sclerosant injection to promote fibrosis. Mucosal excision under general anesthetic produces excellent results for large or persistent lesions.

Adults and the elderly: As the natural history of FTRP is frequent progression to the complications of incontinence and constipation, all patients should be offered surgical repair. The appropriate treatment of internal prolapse is less clear, however, because the natural history is less well defined.

Choice of Operation

Many factors influence the choice of procedure in any patient. These include:

- Type and degree of prolapse
- Associated anatomic abnormalities
- Sphincter integrity and function
- Continence
- Presence of slow transient constipation or obstructed defecation; and
- Age, medical condition, and previous attempts at repair.

Management should be based on an attempt to restore normal physiology. Continence restoration depends on restoring a positive gradient between sphincter and rectal pressures and can be achieved in patients who have very poor sphincter function. An effective operation allows sphincter recovery by prolapse elimination, while maintaining a compliant rectal reservoir to avoid high rectal pressures.

Many prolapse operations are described and can broadly be divided into transabdominal and perineal approaches:

- *Transabdominal* procedures incorporate some form of rectopexy, which may be a simple sutured rectopexy, use of prosthetic mesh materials in an anterior or posterior position, Ivalon sponge (polyvinyl alcohol, now largely outmoded), or alternatively sigmoid resection with or without rectal presacral fixation. All the sell techniques can be applied laparoscopically.
- The most common perineal repairs are Delorme's procedure (rectal mucosectomy and muscle plication) and an Altemeier procedure (perineal proctosigmoidectomy); Thiersch encirclement is infrequently used nowadays.

Transabdominal approaches: In general, in healthy patients an abdominal approach gives the best opportunity to restore normal anatomy, provides the best functional results, and results in the lowest recurrence rates. Randomized study has shown better functional and physiologic outcomes for incontinent patients having resection rectopexy compared with those treated with perineal proctosigmoidectomy.

Resection rectopexy results in the lowest recurrence rate (<2%) of all prolapse operations and is favored for those patients who have slow-transit constipation. Complication rates of 20–30% have been reported in most series.[32] Resection reduces postoperative constipation and avoids the rectosigmoid angulation that may occur with fixation procedures. Continence is restored in 40–85% of cases. Those patients whose continence fails to improve may be considered for sphincter repair or graciloplasty.

The major drawback of resection is the theoretic risk of anastomotic leakage. Using this technique, we reported no anastomotic complication and no deaths among 118 patients.[33] Compared with sutured, meshed and Ivalon (polyvinyl alcohol) sponge rectopexy, resection gives superior results in terms of rectal emptying and anorectal function. Sphincter pressures increase appreciably after resection and suture rectopexy, but not after any form of implant operation. The most marked pressure increases follow resection. Postresectional constipation is uncommon.

Rectopexy alone results in constipation rates of up to 43%, and the constipation is often refractory to treatment. Implants, especially Ivalon (polyvinyl alcohol), induce intense fibrosis, reduce rectal compliance, and may adversely affect continence and cause constipation.

Despite advantages, abdominal procedures all carry the risks of any laparotomy. In young men in particular, there is the risk of sexual and bladder dysfunction. There is also the long-term risk of adhesive small bowel obstruction.

Perineal approaches: Many patients with FTRP are elderly and frail, in whom an abdominal approach is associated with high morbidity and mortality rates. In this situation, Delorme's procedure is most commonly used, although the Altemeier procedure is also advocated.

Delorme's procedure involves minimal dissection, can be carried out under regional or even local anesthetic, is a short operation, avoids a laparotomy, has no resultant risk of full-thickness anastomotic dehiscence, and can be readily repeated. It is especially effective for low internal prolapse. It has acceptable complication rates of 6–25%, and many of the complications reflect the frequent selection bias for frail elderly patients.[34,35] However, there is less improvement in incontinence (31%) when compared to abdominal procedures.[36] There are also much higher recurrence rates of up to 25% and a higher incidence of postoperative urgency. In general, however, it is an excellent albeit short-term alternative to an abdominal procedure for elderly infirm patients.

Peripheral rectosigmoidectomy known as the Altemeier procedure has lower complication and recurrence rates than those of the Delorme's procedure, and it allows levatorplasty and simultaneous enterocele and rectocele repair.[37] It does, however, involve anastomosis of the sigmoid colon to the anus, removes the compliant rectum, carries a risk of anastomotic dehiscence, and results in less improvement in incontinence than abdominal procedures.

Thiersch loops are quickly placed under local anesthetic and produce little trauma. However, there is a short-term failure rate of up to 80%; resultant constipation is common, and inflammation and erosion may occur. These loops have a limited role as a temporizing measure for patients who have limited life expectancy or severe comorbidity.

SOLITARY RECTAL ULCER

The term solitary rectal ulcer is misleading; the lesion is not always solitary, and is not always ulcerated. Solitary rectal ulcer syndrome (SRUS) is a chronic benign syndrome that predominantly affects young adults with equal gender incidence; it is associated with localized specific histologic features of the rectum and symptoms of obstructed defecation. Its annual incidence is estimated at 1 in 100,000 population, but is probably much greater.

Characteristically, there is disordered and obstructed defecation, anal pain, rectal bleeding, and mucous discharge. The clinical picture may be diverse and represent a spectrum of disorders.[38] Frequent unproductive straining is almost universal and is associated with a constant desire to defecate and feelings of incomplete evacuation. Bleeding and passage of mucus occur in almost all cases; bleeding sometimes leads to anemia and, rarely, is massive. Difficulty initiating defecation is common. Most patients complain of tenesmus, and pain occurs in 20% of patients as a deep-seated pelvic ache.[39] About 50% of patients have some degree of FI. There is an association with the abdominal symptoms of irritable bowel syndrome plus a high prevalence of psychoneurosis.

Although poorly understood, the etiology is thought to relate to disordered rectal evacuation that leads to straining. A paradoxic rise in puborectalis activity has been shown on straining with SRUS, whereas straining normally inhibits activity.[40] This spasm is not unique to SRUS, however. It and many of the clinical symptoms are also features of other functional evacuation disorders, such as idiopathic constipation, idiopathic megarectum, and neurogenic incontinence.

Defecating proctography shows varying degrees of associated prolapse, from complete to anterior rectal bulging, in up to 90% of cases. The lesions are always on the redundant migratory part of the rectal wall. Rectal induration and ulceration are thought to be secondary to the trauma of mucosal prolapse onto the sphincter complex. Typically, visible mucosal lesions occur anteriorly 7–10 cm from the anal verge. Ulceration occurs in up to 70% of cases, but other findings are of mucosal nodularity or erythema. Microscopically, the muscularis mucosae are thickened, smooth muscle fibers extend into the lamina propria, and there is associated fibrosis and a polymorph infiltrate. The muscularis propria is also thickened because of excess collagen deposition.[41] Ectopic mucosal glands may be histologically confused with the picture of adenocarcinoma.

Apart from inconstant perineal descent, there are few physical signs. Digital examination may reveal anterior rectal wall nodularity. At sigmoidoscopy, there is frequently rectal mucus and localized mucosal edema and reddening, often with ulceration, and generally with prolapse of the lesion. Lesions are anterior in over 90% of cases. Biopsy excludes neoplasia and confirms the diagnosis. Defecating proctography may show an underlying prolapse or a failure of normal puborectalis relaxation during defecation.

Management

Management is mainly conservative with fiber supplementation (30–40 g/day) and avoidance of straining. This regimen leads to symptomatic improvement in up to 73%

of patients, although symptom relief and ulcer healing may take several months. Up to 21% of lesions have been shown endoscopically to heal completely. Other non-operative treatments include corticosteroid and sucralfate enemas and local anesthetics. Patients who have ulcerated lesions are less likely to respond than those who have polypoid lesions. More recently, biofeedback has been advocated; it has resulted in short-term success in up to 100% of patients and lower recurrence rates than other conservative regimens. Long-term studies are required.

Patients who have associated FTRP benefit from rectopexy that improves symptoms in up to 60% of cases. It is unlikely to improve symptoms if FTRP cannot be shown preoperatively. Rectopexy carried out for symptoms in the absence of physical changes of solitary ulceration is ineffective and therefore contraindicated.

COLITIS CYSTICA PROFUNDA

Colitis cystica profunda is a rare benign entity that has many similarities, both clinically and histologically, with SRUS, and many investigators consider the two conditions to be analogous or part of a spectrum of disease.[42] The lesions are thought to result from repeated trauma of anterior mucosal prolapse, and this process is possibly exacerbated by straining. Support for this hypothesis is provided by the association of all forms of rectal prolapse with SRUS and the observation of similar pathology in patients with functional pelvic floor disorders. Lesions can be segmental or diffuse, but localized anterior rectal lesions within 15 cm of the anal verge are most common. Lesions are more commonly polypoid and sessile and less commonly ulcerated than in SRUS.

Symptoms usually include excessive rectal mucus, bleeding, and disordered defecation. Diagnosis is assisted by ELUS, which shows multiple submucosal cysts and intervening echorefringent fibrosis.[43] An ELUS excludes muscular infiltration and lymph node involvement; the main differential diagnosis is mucosecretory carcinoma. Deep biopsy of the lesions establishes the diagnosis and reveals whole submucosal cysts and obliteration of the fibroblastic lamina propria.

Management

Conservative management is satisfactory for most patients and includes patient re-education about bowel habit with avoidance of straining, a high-fiber diet, and bulk laxatives. Operation is reserved for selected patients and usually involves a local excision of affected mucosa.

DESCENDING PERINEUM SYNDROME

Descending perineum syndrome is a functional pelvic floor disorder that is characterized by a loss of normal pelvic floor muscle tone. It is more common in women, but rare before 20 years of age. It is thought to be related to obstetric pudendal nerve injury or chronic defecatory straining. Muscle weakness leads to pelvic floor ballooning and descent as intrapelvic pressure increases on straining. This process results in anterior rectal protrusion into the lumen, which impedes rectal emptying.

Patients report feelings of rectal obstruction, straining, and incomplete rectal emptying. Frequently patients learn to support the pelvic floor digitally to assist defecation. Intractable tenesmus and a perineal dragging sensation are common, as are rectal blood and mucus. Incomplete rectal emptying leads to further straining, which produces further nerve traction and progressive EAS and puborectalis denervation. This sequence may ultimately lead to incontinence.[44]

During straining the anal canal should not descend >2 cm below a line joining the ischial tuberosities. In descending perineum syndrome at rest, the perineum lies at a lower level than this and descends even further on straining.

However, gross perineal descent in isolation does not always produce symptoms. Digital examination may reveal a lax sphincter, and EMG may show abnormal muscle tone. An anterior rectal prolapse may be seen on proctoscopy, and in intractable cases a solitary rectal ulcer may develop. Proctography and in particular MRI proctography as illustrated above have provided imaging that is an aid to diagnosis.

Management

Management of descending perineum syndrome is difficult, and symptoms commonly persist. Mainstays of treatment are stool softening and bulking agents and avoidance of further straining. Suppositories and enemas may improve rectal emptying. Associated mucosal prolapse or prolapsing hemorrhoids may require band ligation or injection. Caution is required when surgically excising hemorrhoidal tissue, because such tissue may be making an appreciable contribution to the patient's residual continence.

HEMORRHOIDS

Hemorrhoids are caused by distal displacement of the anal canal cushions, which are normal anatomic structures thought to play a role in maintaining continence.[45] Varying definitions and patient understanding of the term have led to a reported incidence of 4.4–80%.[46] Hemorrhoids occur equally in males and females, and there is a peak incidence in people aged 45–75 years.

The pathophysiology of hemorrhoids is poorly understood. Anal cushions consist of redundant rectal mucosa, arterioles, venules, and arteriovenular malformations supported by elastic connective tissue and smooth muscle. There are usually three cushions. They begin development in early embryonic life, aid anal expansion during defecation, and enable the IAS to produce a watertight seal on contraction. The arterial supply comes from terminal superior rectal arterial branches, and there are inconstant contributions from the inferior and middle rectal arteries; this rich supply explains the bright red bleeding that is so often associated. Anatomically, degeneration of the fibroelastic and smooth muscle supporting structure is the only constant finding in the prolapsing cushions of hemorrhoids. The vascular spaces are not altered in number, size or structure.

It is unclear why anal cushions prolapse, but many factors have been associated, including defecatory straining, constipation, and pregnancy (through constipation, increased circulating blood volume with venous dilation and engorgement and hormone-mediated connective tissue laxity).[47] Other factors are the absence of valves in hemorrhoidal and draining vessels, increased intra-abdominal pressure resulting in vascular engorgement, acute or chronic diarrhea, the erect posture, and inheritance; a family history is present in about 50% of cases.

Classification

Most patients have three hemorrhoids, usually in the right anterior, right posterior and left lateral positions of the anal canal. Smaller secondary hemorrhoids often occur between these. External hemorrhoids occur distal to the dentate line and can be seen easily on inspection. Internal hemorrhoids occur above the dentate line and are best appreciated at anoscopy. Internal hemorrhoids can be classified as shown in Table 63.3.

Table 63.3 Classification of internal hemorrhoids

Classification	*Criteria*
First degree	Anal cushion enlargement with painless bleeding, but no prolapse
Second degree	Prolapse on defecation with spontaneous reduction
Third degree	Prolapse spontaneously or with defecation and requires manual reduction
Fourth degree	Irreducible prolapse

Clinical Presentation

The most common presentations are bleeding on defecation and prolapse. Pruritus and minor soiling are common as a result of exteriorized mucosal exudation or the passage of small amounts of liquid rectal content through the anus. Bleeding is usually bright red, limited in quantity and associated with straining and especially with the passage of firm-to-hard stools. Fresh blood drips into the pan or smears the stool surface. Bleeding is intermittent and not mixed with the stool; often there are variable periods of resolution. It is sometimes spontaneous and profuse, and retained ampullary blood can lead to the passage of dark blood or clots. Occasional patients present with anemia. Acute severe pain heralds the complications of acute thrombosis, strangulation or infarction. Burning, throbbing or dragging pain accompanies hemorrhoidal engorgement with prolapse. Rarer complications include tissue necrosis with pyemia.

Examination and Diagnosis

The history and abdominal examination are necessary to identify other causes of rectal bleeding. Anorectal examination includes assessment for soiling and excoriation, anal skin tags, and signs of external prolapse. Gentle anal eversion may demonstrate coexisting fissures, and straining may demonstrate prolapse.

Proctoscopy excludes other anal lesions and allows an assessment of the internal anal cushions on instrument withdrawal. All patients require at least rigid sigmoidoscopy to exclude higher rectal and rectosigmoid pathology. If there is doubt about the bleeding site or bowel habit has changed, if the patient is aged over 40 years or bleeding does not cease with appropriate hemorrhoidal treatment, entire colonic assessment by double-contrast barium enema or colonoscopy is indicated.

Management

After exclusion of other pathology, treatment is tailored to symptom severity. External hemorrhoids usually only require treatment for acute thrombosis or local irritation caused by trapping of stool of fecal fluid. Symptomatic internal hemorrhoids are best managed conservatively at first. More than 80% of patients respond to medical management, banding, injection, or coagulation.

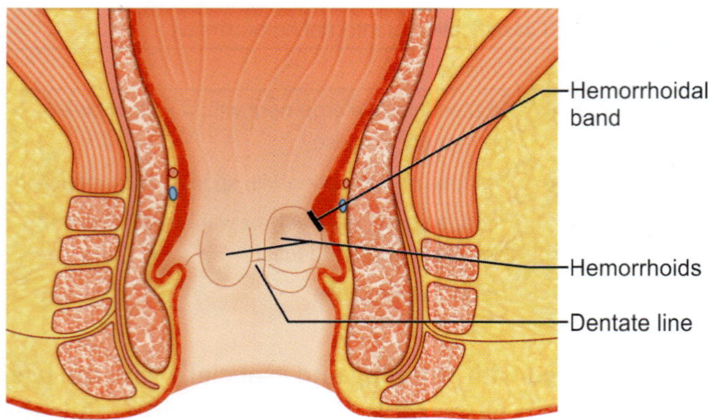

Fig. 63.7: Hemorrhoidal banding: Note that band placement is above the dentate line at the proximal portion of the lesion.

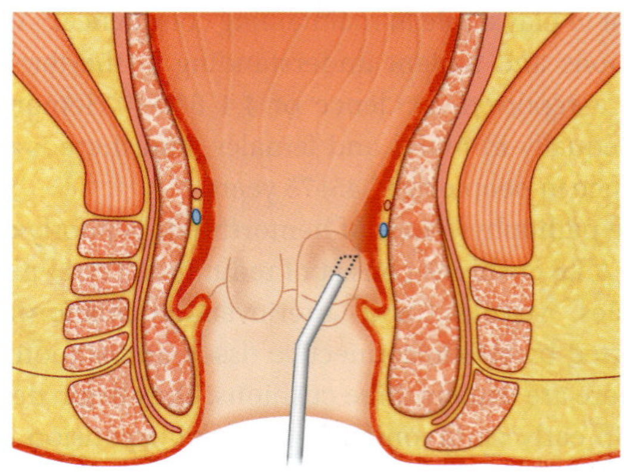

Fig. 63.8: Sclerosant injection of hemorrhoids: Note that injection is submucosal, above the dentate line and at the proximal portion of the hemorrhoid.

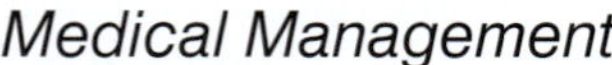

Medical Management

Many patients require no treatment. When bleeding is minimal and intermittent, exclusion of serious underlying pathology and an explanation of the natural history of the disorder may be all that is required. Advice to avoid straining and promptly to reduce prolapsed hemorrhoids may provide adequate symptom relief. Patients should be advised to increase dietary fiber and fluids, and bulk laxatives may be helpful. Topical agents may reduce discomfort and bleeding, but may merely provide a lubricant action.

Operative Management

Patients who have persistent symptoms despite medical treatment should be offered intervention, either:

- Outpatient procedures aimed to produce mucosal adherence and prevent prolapse and bleeding or
- Operative hemorrhoidectomy.

The most common outpatient procedures include rubber band ligation, injection sclerotherapy, and infrared photocoagulation, and there are conflicting reports of their relative effectiveness. Other less commonly used procedures include cryotherapy, bipolar diathermy, laser photocoagulation and direct current electrotherapy.

Band ligation: Band ligation is the preferred method for most symptomatic hemorrhoids because it is more effective than injection sclerotherapy in comparative trials.[48] Bands are placed under direct vision to the proximal portion of the prolapsing cushion onto insensitive mucosa (Fig. 63.7). Pain sensation is variable above the dentate line and before releasing a band it is necessary to check that mucosal purchase has not produced pain. Incorrect placement almost immediately causes incapacitating pain that worsens and necessitates band removal. Other complications of banding include vasovagal reactions, urinary retention, reactionary and secondary hemorrhage, and, rarely, infection or impairment of continence. Discomfort is not uncommon but usually controllable with simple analgesics. Patients should be warned of minor bleeding when the ischemic tissue separates after 3–10 days. Three cushions can be banded in one sitting. For larger or prolapsing lesions, repeat banding at intervals of 6–8 week may be required. Wechter and Luna reported complications in 14% of cases in a meta-analysis of 8060 patients treated by band ligation. The most common complications were pain (5.8%), hemorrhage (1.7%), and treatment failure or recurrence (2.8%).[49] As a result of bleeding and infection risks, banding should probably be avoided in anticoagulated or immunosuppressed patients.

Injection sclerotherapy: Injection sclerotherapy is less effective than banding, but it is useful for persistent bleeding associated with minimal prolapse on proctoscopy.[50] Using a Gabriel needle, 3–5 mL of 5% phenol in almond or arachis oil are injected submucosally above the dentate line at the proximal portion of the anal cushions (Fig. 63.8). Deeper injection can cause perirectal fibrosis, rectal ulceration, perirectal sepsis, urethritis or hematospermia complicated by impotence or sepsis. Although popular, there is little evidence that sclerotherapy is any better than simple dietary adjustment with increased fiber intake and avoidance of defecatory straining.

Infrared coagulation: Infrared coagulation is less useful if prolapse is present. Burn depth is proportional to the duration of application. A fullness and aching similar to that following banding may occur.

Surgical hemorrhoidectomy: Hemorrhoidectomy is the most definitive of all treatments and has a reported recurrence rate of <3% in a patient group that is overall more symptomatic than patients treated by nonoperative measures. It may be offered if symptoms persist despite conservative measures and is the procedure of choice if there are appreciable external hemorrhoidal components that are not controlled because of inability to deal with sensitive skin below the dentate line.

Several techniques are described, and there is little between them with regard to efficacy. All techniques remove offending prolapsed cushions while maintaining adequate skin bridges between resected specimens and preserving the underlying IAS. Pedicles can be ligated or diathermy resected, and wounds can be left open or closed, with little apparent difference in long-term results. Complications include anal pain, urinary retention, bleeding, and fecal impaction. Mazier[51] reported late complications of heavy bleeding in 2% of cases, anal stenosis in < 1%, and abscess and fistula in < 0.1% over a 25-year period.

Painful Prolapsed and Thrombosed Internal Hemorrhoids

Painful prolapsed and thrombosed internal hemorrhoids can be managed conservatively with bed rest and elevation, ice packs, salt baths, and topical and oral analgesics, but symptoms usually take several days to abate and subsequent hemorrhoidectomy is often required. We advocate emergency hemorrhoidectomy under antibiotic cover, but because of edema, added care must be taken to preserve skin bridges and avoid stenosis.

Thrombosed external piles or perianal hematomas produce acutely painful lesions at the anal verge. The natural history is subsidence over several days as the clot organizes, which often results in an anal skin tag. Pain usually starts to ease within 48 hours, and if the patient is seen after this time nonoperative measures are probably indicated. Before this, surgical incision and evacuation of the hematoma under local anesthetic achieves immediate pain relief by releasing clot under tension.

Stapled hemorrhoidectomy has the advantage that the sensitive anorectal region is not injured and so in most there is little post-operative pain. The principle is that removing a redundant cuff of distal rectal mucosa and often deeper layers suspends the hemorrhoidal plexus and deals with the prolapse. The major disadvantage is it is less effective than ligation excision in dealing with very large hemorrhoids. In randomized trials, the differences are small.[52]

Hemorrhoidal dearterialization has gained popularity in recent times. The principle is to identify the main hemorrhoidal artery using a Doppler probe and then encircle it to interrupt the vascular supply to the hemorrhoid. The problem with the method is it does little for the prolapse that frequently requires attention; in consequence, the excision will invariably cause pain that in turn defeats the objective, which is to ligate the artery in an insen sitive area.

ANAL FISSURE

An anal fissure is a linear tear or ulcer in the anal mucosa and occurs distal to the dentate line. Most are primary, but secondary fissures are caused by IBD (especially Crohn's disease), trauma, operation or infection. There is a slight male predominance. Lesions occur at any age, with a peak in the third and fourth decades. Constipated stool is the most common predisposing factor and is thought to produce a mechanical tear. Diarrhea may also be a factor by producing an alkaline chemical burn. This type of fissure should be differentiated from the classic fissure as it produces linear ulcers around the full circumference of the anus and is the result of burning or excoriation. A new diagnosis of fissure is rare in the over fifties, and great caution should be exercised when confirming the diagnosis and considering treatment options such as sphincterotomy in older patients. It is far more likely that anal linear ulceration is the consequence of fecal leakage and irritation. In such a patient, a sphincterotomy with invariably make them worse. Moreover, it is important not to descend down a cascade to operative treatment when topical relaxants and botulinum toxin fails as the sphincter is almost certainly hypotonic in such cases.

Although the precise etiology is unknown, fissures are associated with IAS overactivity and increased resting anal pressure, which may prevent healing as a result of hypoperfusion. Patients who have fissures have reduced transcutaneous anal oxygen partial pressures, with levels correlating inversely with anal pressure. This ischemic concept is supported by the fact that transcutaneous oxygen partial pressures are increased after sphincterotomy and correlate with fissure healing. Fissures also occur at sites of vascular watershed.

Fissures can be acute or chronic. Acute fissures are superficial, show little induration and have sharply defined margins and a smooth base. There is no associated skin tag formation or hypertrophic anal papilla. With chronicity, the edges become raised and there is the classic triad of:

- A sentinel skin tag
- Anal ulcer
- Hypertrophic anal papilla.

With chronicity, the whitish transverse IAS fibers become visible in the base, which is usually deeper than in acute ulcers. Undermined edges may lead to mucus and stool trapping, and partial healing by bridging may lead to superficial abscess formation.

Patients usually present with pain on and immediately after defecation, which may last some hours and is often described as tearing. Bleeding occurs in almost all cases as smearing on the toilet paper or stool surface. Constipation is exacerbated by fear of defecatory pain. The pain of acute ulcers may be intense, but surprisingly it is sometimes insidious in onset. In contradistinction, the pain of excoriation with linear fissuring is normally post-defecatory. Unhealed fissures give rise to chronic, intermittent or continuous symptoms that may vary with the clinical appearance of the fissure, which may range from a crack to an incompletely drained abscess. Systemic and bowel-related symptoms suggest a secondary fissure that might suggest IBD.

Gentle anal eversion usually exposes the distal end of a fissure on straining. Fissures are mostly posterior in the midline; anterior midline fissures occur in only up to 10% of cases in men and 20% in women. Laterally placed or multiple fissures are usually secondary to other pathology, such as IBD or anorectal sexually transmitted disease (STD). Primary fissures do not extend proximal to the dentate line, and such lesions suggest possible idiopathic HIV-related or STD-related ulceration.

Anal fissures are often too painful for office evaluation and require EUA. Underlying sepsis must be excluded. Fissures may require biopsy, and in immunocompromised patients or if an infectious etiology is suspected, this is combined with bacterial and viral biopsy cultures and serology. Sigmoidoscopy must be undertaken at some stage in the management to exclude other pathology.

Management

Medical Management

Up to 85% of acute fissures and nearly 50% of chronic fissures can be successfully managed nonoperatively. The principles are to avoid constipation and relieve IAS spasm by means of high-fiber diets and stool softeners, combined with topical local anesthetic and other measures. Initiation of treatment should progress stepwise from simple measures related to stool and defecatory habits through the pharmacological options and onto operation if indicated. When successful, healing usually occurs within 6 weeks. Anal dilators do not influence healing rates. The knowledge that nitric oxide is the principal inhibitory neurotransmitter to the IAS has led to the use of nitric oxide donors to reduce anal tone. Topical application of 0.2% glyceryl trinitrate ointment q12h or q8h reduces anal pressure and achieves healing in up to two-thirds of chronic fissures.[53] Early recurrence occurs in approximately one-third of cases, but longer term results are not available. Another limitation of treatment with glyceryl trinitrate is a high incidence of headaches, which may be overcome by the use of topical pharmacologic agents, such as diltiazem which is a calcium channel blocker that leads to IAS relaxation.[54]

A newer pharmacological approach to sphincter relaxation to aid mucosal perfusion and healing is injection of botulinum A toxin. In terms of efficacy, there has been extensive study and analysis in recent years, both comparing botulinum A toxin with topical treatments such as nitrates and with surgical sphincterotomy. Reviews are mixed: some trials have shown dramatic healing results such as those published by Brindisa with a 92% healing rate at 2 months in 50 patients treated with toxin compared with 70% in 50 patients treated with topical nitrate ointment.[55] Meta-analysis of 75 randomized trials including 5031 patients demonstrated no significant advantage for botulinum A toxin over other proven pharmacological therapies.[56] There is heterogeneiety of study results, potentially attributable to site of injection and dose of toxin given. Newer studies are showing improvement with anterior injection away from the scarred posterior muscle (which is thought to limit diffusion of toxin and decrease efficacy). Side effects are generally limited to minor incontinence of flatus and fecal leakage in the early period after injection in some studies. Given its reasonable efficacy and low side effect profile, botulinum A toxin is perhaps best used as a second-line medical therapy after trial of medical management and nitrates/CCB prior to definitive surgical therapy if required.

Operative Management

Lateral sphincterotomy is the preferred surgical option following failed medical treatment because of its high success and low complication rates. Anal dilatation has been largely abandoned because of the risk of producing incontinence; so too has posterior midline sphincterotomy, with or without ulcer excision, because of postoperative soiling rates of up to 25% from the resultant keyhole deformity.

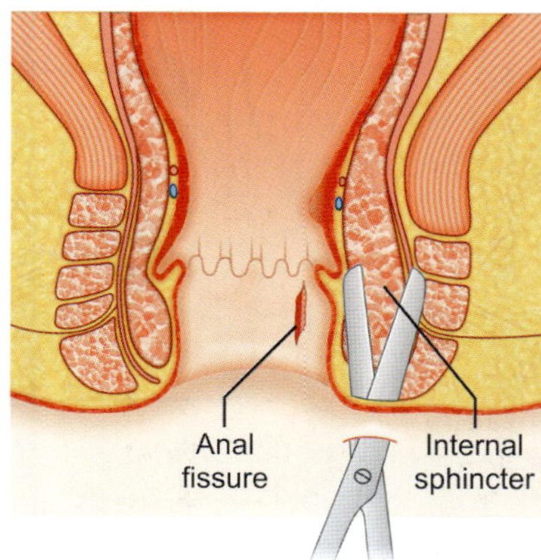

Fig. 63.9: Lateral sphincterotomy: Note that division should not extend proximal to the dentate line.

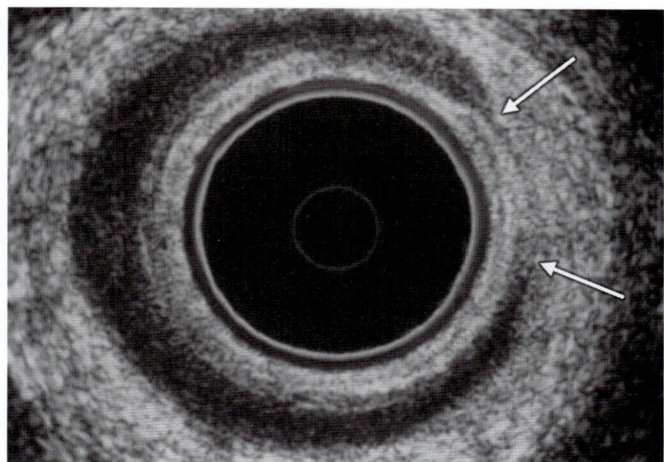

Fig. 63.10: Endoluminal ultrasound showing a defect of the distal internal anal sphincter at 3 o'clock following lateral sphincterotomy for anal fissure (arrows).

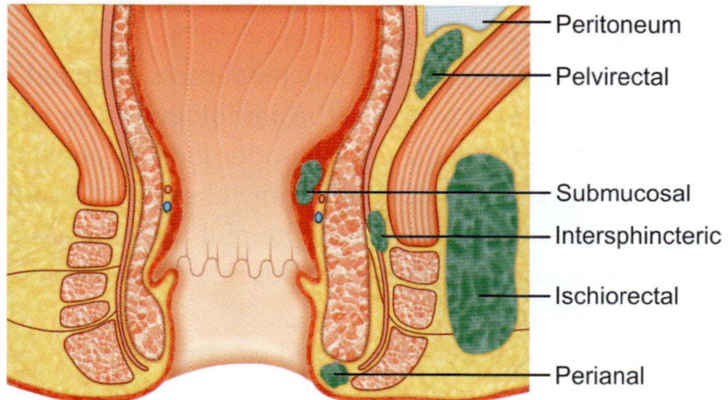

Fig. 63.11: Sites of anorectal abscess formation.

Lateral sphincterotomy works by decreasing anal canal tone and improving local tissue perfusion. There appears to be no benefit (and indeed it is illogical) to divide the IAS beyond the most proximal level of the fissure. Division should not continue proximal to the level of the dentate line because this increases the risk of postoperative incontinence (Figs. 63.9 and 63.10). Lateral sphincterotomy is successful in over 95% of cases; FI is rare and occurs in <1% of cases in most series.[57] Flatus incontinence varies widely (from 0% to 30%) in different series.

More recently, increasing experience with flap repair of fissures is being reported, without the risk of impairing continence. The main indications are failed LS or an increased likelihood of postoperative incontinence. The latter group of patients includes those who have IBD, who have had obstetric injuries and previous anal dilatation, and those in whom preoperative anal resting pressure is not increased or is low. Patients who have marked pruritus or diarrhea are more likely to have less successful results after LS and should also be considered. Although the series are small, good results have been reported with both V-Y advancement and rhomboid island fiaps.[58]

ANORECTAL ABSCESS

Anorectal sepsis is a common surgical emergency and presents as an acute abscess or a chronic anal fistula. Anorectal abscess has a recurrence rate of up to 48%.[59] There is a male predominance (2.4:1), and it is most common in people aged between 30 and 50 years. Abscesses are classified according to which of a number of potential anorectal tissue spaces they occupy, such as perianal, ischiorectal, submucosal, intersphincteric, high intermuscular and pelvirectal (Fig. 63.11). More than one space may be occupied simultaneously.

Most anorectal abscesses originate in the anal glands situated in the intersphincteric space. Duct obstruction predisposes to infection, which in turn leads to abscess formation, commencing in the intersphincteric plane.

Sepsis spreads vertically, horizontally or circumferentially, and this dictates the ultimate site and presentation of an abscess (Figs. 63.12 and 63.13). Distal intersphincteric spread produces a perianal abscess. Horizontal spread through the EAS forms an ischiorectal abscess. These two types comprise approximately 80% of all anorectal abscesses. Cephalad intersphincteric spread leads to a high intermuscular abscess and, if it perforates the levator complex, to a pelvirectal (supralevator) abscess. Medial extension through the IAS produces a submucosal abscess. Circumferential spread may occur in the intersphincteric,

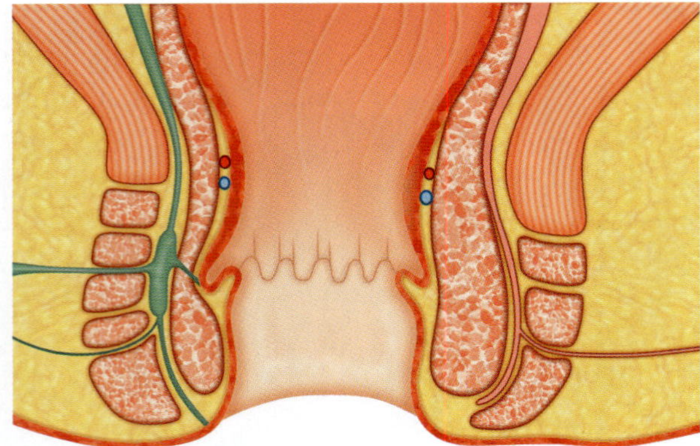

Fig. 63.12: Possible directions of spread of anorectal sepsis from a diseased anal gland in the intersphincteric space. Tracking leads to distant extension and collections, and fistulation: Note the internal opening at the level of the dentate line.

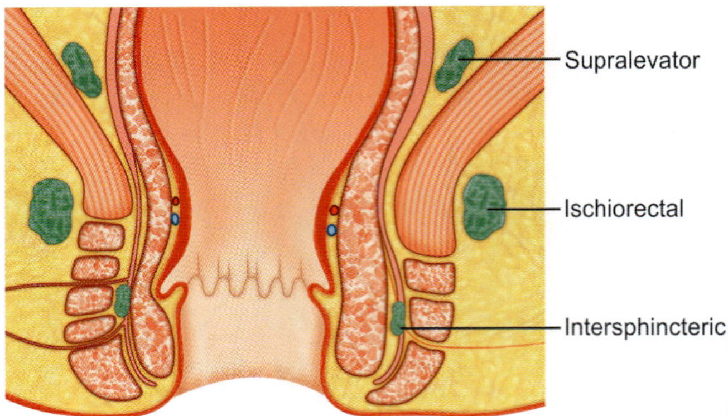

Fig. 63.13: The three possible circumferential routes for tracking horseshoe anorectal sepsis.

ischiorectal or supralevator compartments to form horseshoe abscesses (*see* Fig. 63.10). Of these, posterior ischiorectal spread is the most common.

Approximately 20% of abscesses have other etiologies, the most common being IBD, particularly Crohn's disease. A perianal fistula can antedate Crohn's disease diagnosis by many years. Other causes are septic anal fissure, anorectal cancer, infected perianal hematoma or complicated internal hemorrhoid, recent hemorrhoidectomy, foreign body (e.g., fish bone) and tuberculosis. Abscesses also complicate several anorectal STDs, particularly in immunocompromised patients with HIV infection. In addition, perianal skin sepsis can lead to perianal abscesses. Abscesses sometimes arise in septicemic patients and diabetics.

Clinical Presentation

The site of an abscess largely determines its mode of presentation. Superficial *perianal* abscesses usually present with a short history of progressive pain at the anal verge. Defecation is painful. There is localized tender induration and heat, with or without fluctuation and spreading cellulitis and, rarely, overlying skin necrosis and crepitation.

Ischiorectal abscesses tend to present later with more diffuse buttock pain and tenderness and pronounced pain on sitting. Constitutional symptoms are not uncommon because of the development of large amounts of pus in the loose areolar ischiorectal fat. Deep ischiorectal abscesses are often insidious, especially in diabetics and the immunocompromised. They infrequently produce appreciable induration or fluctuation and often present with pyrexia, constitutional upset, and little pain, so creating diagnostic confusion.

Submucosal abscesses present with anal pain and irritability and voiding difficulties. They are palpable digitally as tender mucosal elevations.

Diagnosis is usually obvious, but tenderness often indicates the need for EUA to define the pathology accurately. If diagnostic doubt remains, ELUS under local or general anesthetic is highly sensitive for anorectal sepsis. CT and particularly MRI can be extremely helpful in delineating the anatomy of complex high intermuscular or pelvirectal abscesses and fistulae.

Cultures grow either gut-related organisms, such as *Bacteroides fragilis, Escherichia coli,* and *Streptococcus faecalis,* or skin-derived organisms, such as *Staphylococcus aureus* or skin-derived *Bacteroides* spp. Abscesses growing gut-related organisms are more often associated with an underlying fistula than those from which skin organisms are cultured.[60] Occasionally, *Mycobacterium tuberculosis,* or *Actinomyces* spp. are identified.

Management

Abscesses require prompt surgical drainage, usually under general anesthetic. Incisions are placed over areas of greatest fluctuance as close as possible to, but outside, the sphincter complex. It is imperative that drainage is early and adequate. Delay and small incisions put the patient at risk of necrotizing fasciitis particularly if they are diabetic or immunocompromised. Pus is sent for culture, and atypical lesions should be biopsied. All loculi of pus are broken down digitally, and the cavity is curetted and lavaged. Saucerization maintains drainage, and usually a small wick into a generous incision is sufficient. Maintenance antibiotics are unnecessary in the absence of cellulitis.

Postoperative care includes analgesia, stool softeners, sitz baths, and daily loose packing until healing from the base prevents premature wound closure.

Previous anorectal sepsis is strong evidence of an underlying fistula. Internal openings may be identified before drainage by gentle abscess pressure while examining the anal mucosa for exuded pus. Associated superficial fistulas can be opened at the same time as drainage. In the main, for most abscesses, it is preferable simply to drain and address associated fistulas at a later stage since the majority do not recur. In recurrent abscess, a fistula if identified can be drained with a snug vessel loop as a seton.

If no fistula is identified, the patient is followed up as an outpatient with proctoscopy. If pus culture produces skin-derived organisms, proctoscopic surveillance is adequate because the risk of fistulation is low. If gut-derived organisms are cultured, the risk of fistulation is higher; some surgeons advocate early repeat EUA to identify and treat any such tracts before recurrent abscess formation. Most patients are managed expectantly with proctoscopic surveillance.

Crohn's abscesses are almost always associated with fistulas, which may be multiple. Initial operation is conservative and aimed primarily at symptom relief and drainage of pus. All but the most superficial fistulas are managed by seton placement. A full course of metronidazole and medical therapy with corticosteroids and azathioprine, if clinically indicated, may improve outcome.

Horseshoe Fistulas

Abscesses perforating the EAS anteriorly and posteriorly enter the deep preanal and postanal spaces and may spread extensively into the ischiorectal spaces (*see* Fig. 63.13). This pattern of spread produces anterior and posterior horseshoe abscesses, which often contain large quantities of pus in diffuse perirectal fat planes. Associated fistulas are usually trans-sphincteric, but may open above the dentate line, and management can be difficult. The authors advocate posterior midline drainage, stopping short of the sphincters and initial seton management of any fistula.

ANAL FISTULA

An anal fistula is an abnormal communication between the mucosa of the anal canal and the perianal skin. Sometimes no internal or external opening can be identified. There is a male predominance of up to 4 to 1 and an annual incidence of I in 10,000; fistula is most common in people aged between 20 and 50 years. Secondary fistulas may be multiple and complex, particularly in Crohn's disease and hidradenitis suppurativa, but most are cryptoglandular (idiopathic or nonspecific) and single. They are caused by cryptoglandular sepsis and abscess formation from anal duct blockage. Recent evidence suggests epithelialization from one or both fistula tract ends, leading to chronicity, may be commoner than previously thought.[61] Other causes of secondary fistulas include ulcerative colitis, anorectal malignancy, tuberculosis, actinomycosis, pilonidal disease, trauma, foreign body, previous anorectal operation or irradiation, lymphogranuloma venereum, pelvic sepsis, presacral dermoids, and rectal duplications. Some of these conditions manifest by anal duct obstruction and others by direct infiltration or invasion.

Most lesions start as intersphincteric abscesses, which may perforate the sphincters and spread transversely, longitudinally or circumferentially in the intersphincteric, extrasphincteric, or supralevator planes (*see* Figs. 63.11 to 63.13). The relationship of the primary tract to the EAS is paramount to surgical treatment. Parks and coworkers[62] divided fistulas into four main groups: intersphincteric, trans-sphincteric, suprasphincteric, and extrasphincteric. These groups can be further subdivided according to the presence and course of associated secondary tracts. Superficial fistulas not involving the sphincter complex at all (up to 16% of cases) and fistulas associated with fissure bridging are not included in this classification.

Intersphincteric fistulas comprise up to 56% of all anal fistulas. They lie in the intersphincteric plane and enter the anal canal by crossing the IAS at the level of the dentate line; they do not cross the EAS at any point. Most are simple, and continence is usually not at risk with fistulotomy. Some have a high blind intersphincteric tract, a high tract opening into the rectum, a high tract with no perineal opening or a high tract perforating the levators with a pelvic extension. Primary pelvic disease can produce intersphincteric spread of sepsis to the anal verge.

Trans-sphincteric fistulas comprise up to 21% of anal fistulas. They cross both the IAS at the dentate level and the EAS at various levels to enter the ischiorectal space. The tracts may be solitary or complicated by a high blind ischiorectal tract that may pierce the levators, but rarely enters the rectum higher up.

Suprasphincteric fistulas (4% of anal fistulas) track up the intersphincteric plane above the puborectalis and

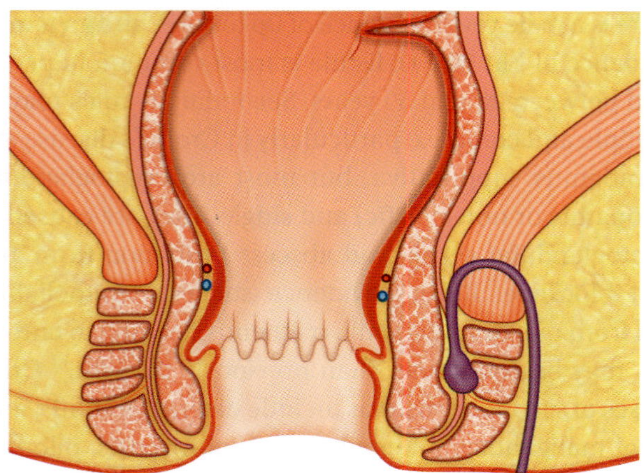
Fig. 63.14: Suprasphincteric fistula.

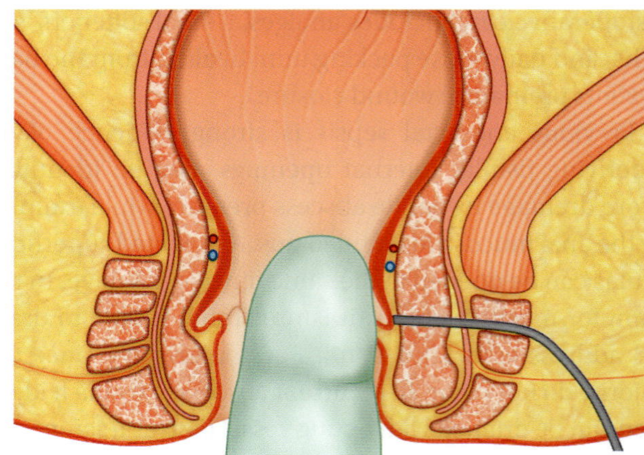
Fig. 63.15: Fistula tract probing against a palpating finger in the anal canal to aid localization of an internal opening.

then down through the levators and ischiorectal fossa to reach the skin (Fig. 63.14). They may have blind upward extensions.

Extrasphincteric fistulas (3% of cases) lie completely external to the sphincter complex and pass from perianal skin through ischiorectal fat and levators into the rectum or sigmoid colon. Secondary tracts may pass through both sphincters to enter the anal canal.

Clinical Presentation

Patients with anal fistulas present with intermittent pain and purulent, often bloodstained, perianal discharge. Pain frequently escalates and then eases with the spontaneous discharge of pus. There is often a history of past anorectal abscess drainage. Perineal examination identifies external openings and signs of sepsis. Digital anorectal examination often identifies tract induration and course. Mucosal indentation or induration may represent an internal opening. Supralevator induration suggests a high extension of sepsis. Proctoscopy may reveal the internal opening, and sigmoidoscopy excludes other underlying pathologies.

Goodsall's rule indicates the most likely position of an internal opening based on the position of identified external openings in relation to a horizontal line transecting the mid anus. Those openings anterior to the line usually enter the rectum radially, whereas those posterior to the line enter in the midline posteriorly, following a curved tract. An exception to the rule is the long anterior tract with an external opening over 3 cm from the anal verge, which may be an anterior extension of a posterior horseshoe fistula and enter in the posterior midline. Fistulas associated with Crohn's disease, malignancy, and atypical mycobacterial infection may also produce exceptions to the rule.

A EUA complements outpatient assessment and identifies the anatomy in most cases. Tract massage can identify an internal opening as a bead of pus. In simpler tracts, probes passed against a "feeling" finger in the anal canal traverse their entire length (Fig. 63.15). If difficulty is encountered, an injection of hydrogen peroxide or methylene blue dye through the external openings while visualizing the canal may reveal internal openings by bubbling or dye extravasation. Dye has the disadvantages of staining anal and peri fistulous tissues. If an internal opening is not found, the external opening should be laid open to identify the characteristic granulation tissue lining a tract, which can then be re-probed. All secondary tracts must be identified and drained.

High, multiple or complex tracts can be challenging. The several techniques used to aid anatomic definition are variably successful. Fistulography results in low internal opening pick-up and high false-positive rates, and it risks dissemination of sepsis. It has a role in defining extrasphincteric tracts, but these are uncommon. CT provides poor resolution of the sphincters and levators and has not added appreciably to assessment. ELUS is helpful for distal fistulas, particularly when combined with peroxide instillation to produce echo-rich bubbles. MRI identifies up to 86% of primary tract courses, secondary tract extensions and abscesses and 90% of horseshoeing. Although promising, particularly for the complex lesions of Crohn's disease, MRI is expensive and its impact on clinical management is yet to be demonstrated.

Management

Treatment is tailored to individuals, and decisions about sphincter division are based on the risk of producing incontinence. Conservatism is required in the elderly, especially women, and in those who have pre-existing impairment of continence, complex and recurrent fistulas, anterior lesions or Crohn's disease. Management aims to eradicate all septic foci while preserving sphincter function. This goal requires precise anatomic assessment, drainage of all tracts and collections, eradication of the anal gland itself, curettage of granulation tissue, and postoperative wound drainage. The tracts may require biopsy to identify the primary cause.

The emphasis is on sphincter preservation. Any muscle above the dentate line should be left intact and managed by seton placement or flap repair. The IAS below the dentate line and the lowermost fibers of the EAS can usually be safely divided, but decisions depend on surgeon experience and pre-existing patient continence risk factors. If there is concern about inducing incontinence, conservatism with seton placement with referral to a specialist center is always preferred. Postoperative care includes sitz baths and daily loose pack to prevent premature skin closure.

Superficial and intersphincteric fistulas do not involve the EAS and are managed by fistulotomy and healing by secondary intention. Low trans-sphincteric fistulas are usually dealt with by fistulotomy, but the decision is based on the factors noted above.

High trans-sphincteric fistulas should be managed initially by seton placement combined with laying open the part of the tract outside the EAS. *IAS division to the level of the tract and curettage to the intervening portion may be required but not invariably.* Secondary extensions are identified, curetted and drained. Fistulectomy (coring out the fistulous tract) has been used with moderate success, but has not been widely adopted.

Suprasphincteric and extrasphincteric fistulas are difficult to treat and are best managed in tertiary referral centers. Fistulotomy leads to total inconti, and seton placement with intersphincteric drainage and anal gland curet is the treatment of choice. Healing is usually prolonged.

Setons

The objective of a seton is the control or cure of fistula with sphincter preservation. Several materials can be used including silk, nylon, and plastic vascular loops. Most are placed loosely to promote drainage, which promotes healing over time by eradication of sepsis (Fig. 63.16). More than one seton can be placed simultaneously. All extensions and secondary tracts must be drained.

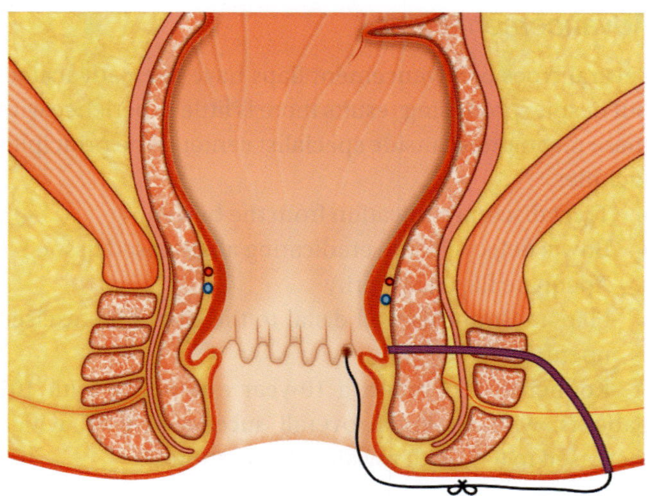

Fig. 63.16: Loose seton placement through a trans-sphincteric fistula to promote drainage.

Setons can be removed after several months, and fistula healing has been reported in up to 78% of cases.[63] Failure or ongoing sepsis requires repeat EUA to identify missed extensions and other pathology. Persisting fistulas may require repeated seton placement. Other options include fistula "control" with long-term draining setons placed indefinitely (often for some years), placement of a tight seton or, rarely, fistulotomy. The full continence rate for those patients ultimately requiring fistulotomy for failed setons is 32%, compared with 83% for patients managed with setons alone.

Cure requires that the track be laid open. If there is adequate muscle above the track, then this should be possible. For many, our approach has been to lay open the whole of the track as far as the sphincter. The anal lining from the internal opening is cut open and thereafter a snug simple seton is placed with a single reef knot. We believe that avoiding multiple knots leaves the patient much more comfortable and able to tolerate the seton for prolonged periods. This illustration shows the result of a snug seton placed around half the sphincter and left for several months. Only a tiny lay-open was required.

Less commonly inserted than loose setons, tight (or cutting) setons are sequentially tightened around the sphincters to produce a semicontrolled staged fistulotomy. The muscle heals by fibrosis behind the seton as it slowly cuts through. Setons are tightened at 1–6-week intervals, but the regimens vary considerably and there is no standardized way of assessing tightness. The results vary, with up to 62% of patients reporting some degree of incontinence after cut-through.[64]

Advancement Flaps

Several types of advancement flaps have been advocated, but despite promising results there is little experience with these techniques outside specialist centers. The principles include:

- Tract discommunication from the bowel
- Bowel defect closure eradicating all diseased tissue
- Adequate flap vascularity
- Flap anastomosis well distal to the site of the excised opening.

Kodner et al.[65] report a 10-year experience with 107 patients, with an initial overall success of 84%, which increased to 94% with revisional operation.

Anal Fistula Plugs

Fistula plugs using collagen-derived material have been reported to heal fistulas in high numbers of patients. A fistula plug of this material is drawn into the track and sutured in place. Initially the success rates were said to be very high, but recent randomized trials have been abandoned because of the poor success rates of plugs compared to advancement flaps.

Lift Procedure

The principle of the lift procedure is to isolate the fistula track in the inter-sphincteric space and ligate it. In principle, this should allow the sepsis to heal. The long-term results are not known.[66]

RECTOVAGINAL/ANOVAGINAL FISTULA

The term rectovaginal fistula usually includes anovaginal fistulas, which actually account for the majority. Together they comprise 5% of all anorectal fistulas. Obstetric injuries cause 50–90% of cases, and fistulation complicates 0.1% of vaginal deliveries, as a result of full-thickness tears or pressure necrosis. Inflammatory bowel disease, particularly Crohn's disease, in which fistulas may be complex and difficult to treat, is another common cause. The other common etiology in surgical practice is surgical operation, particularly ileal pouch construction, pelvic anastomoses, and anal and vaginal procedures.

Clinical Presentation

The clinical presentation of rectovaginal fistulas depends on the etiology. The most common symptom is the passage of flatus or feces through the vagina, which is often associated with a purulent vaginal discharge and irritation. Approximately 50% of patients have some degree of incontinence. Rectal bleeding, mucous discharge, diarrhea, tenesmus, and abdominal pain are usually symptoms of the primary pathology causing fistulation (Table 63.4).

Table 63.4 Causes of anovaginal and rectovaginal fistulas

Cause category	*Examples*
Obstetric	Full-thickness rectal tear, pressure necrosis
Inflammatory bowel disease	Crohn's disease, ulcerative colitis
Operative	Pouch surgery, anastomoses, anal and vaginal operations, sphincter repair
Neoplastic	Rectal carcinoma, anal carcinoma, genital tract carcinoma
Infective	Diverticular disease, pelvic sepsis, cryptoglandular sepsis, tuberculosis, actinomycosis, AIDS related, lymphogranuloma venereum
Radiation injury	
Trauma	Foreign body, violent injury
Fecal impaction	
Idiopathic	
Congenital	

The history suggests the diagnosis. Previous pelvic irradiation is documented, as is traumatic vaginal delivery. General examination may reveal abdominal signs related to a predisposing cause. Perineal examination combined with proctoscopy, rigid sigmoidoscopy, and vaginoscopy successfully identifies most fistulas. Biopsies are recommended. Sphincter integrity is assessed, particularly postpartum, because of a high incidence of associated injury. Multiple fistulas suggest Crohn's disease. Vaginal and rectal contrast studies or colonoscopy may be indicated depending on the history and physical findings. Manometry and ELUS are required for all cases.

Small low fistulas are the most difficult to identify because the openings may be hidden within the anal or hymenal valves. Digital examination to palpate tract induration is helpful, although occult lesions are usually identified on probing at EUA. Other techniques to aid identification include:

- Tract instillation of peroxide and observing for bubbling at the other end
- Rectal air insufflation after filling the vagina with water and looking for bubbling
- Rectal instillation of methylene blue with a tampon in the vagina to confirm that a communication is present.

Management

Management depends on the etiology, symptoms, and site of the fistula. The principles include fistula excision and the interposition of well-vascularized tissue between the vagina and bowel.[67] Attempts at repair should be avoided in the presence of inflammation or sepsis, which should be treated first. In IBD, prior treatment with immunomodulating agents like 6-mercaptopurine or methotrexate or the biologic agents adalimamab or infliximab may modify the inflammatory response and increase the chances of success. Associated sphincter defects need repair to maintain or restore function. Those repairs combined with levatorplasty achieve better functional results compared with sphincter repair alone.

Temporary fecal diversion may be required for severely symptomatic patients or uncontrolled perineal sepsis, but it is used only for selected complex cases. Repair should not be delayed in women of childbearing age, and cesarean section should be preferred following repair to avoid risking repeat trauma.

Crohn's fistulas may benefit from optimal medical treatment with cyclosporine, 6-mercaptopurine and metronidazole. One series reported fistula closure in 44% of cases and moderate improvement in another 44% of 16 patients treated with oral cyclosporine. Other investigators have shown no ongoing benefit. Medical treatment may have a role in optimizing a patient's condition before operation. If there is a rectal or anal neoplasm, treatment should be directed at the primary tumor.

High fistulas are generally managed by resection and interposition of healthy tissues, such as omentum, gracilis, or a rectus abdominis flap between bowel and vagina. A proximal defunctioning colostomy may be required.

Radiation proctitis usually involves the whole rectum, and low anterior resection is required.

Fistulating sigmoid tumors and diverticular disease require resection down to healthy well-vascularized rectum. Cancers also require en-bloc resection of the affected parts of the posterior vaginal wall. Most procedures are successful, but previous irradiation may lead to poor bladder and rectal function. If sphincter function is inadequate, APE of the rectum and anus may be more appropriate.

Low fistulas are most commonly obstetric in origin or caused by Crohn's disease. Obstetric cases frequently have a history of a tear or episiotomy that may not have been recognized as full thickness at the time of repair. Patients are usually symptomatic within a few days, but urgent repair is not advised in the presence of edema and inflammation. Occasionally, EUA is required to confirm the diagnosis. Sphincters are sometimes disrupted and may require repair at the time of fistula operation. If the sphincters are intact, several direct surgical approaches have been described, all of which produce similar results. A transrectal advancement flap, in which the mucosa and muscle are separately closed in layers, is the one most commonly used. Transvaginal layered closure is also commonly used, but transperineal operations are less frequently employed. With any of these techniques ultimate success rates of 88–100% have been reported.[68] Initial surgical failure is often followed by success with a repeat operation. Antibiotic cover is necessary.

Several pedicled transposition grafts have been used, including omentum, gracilis, sartorius, gluteus maximus, rectus abdominus, and bulbospongiosus muscles, for complex or multiply recurrent fistulas. Patients who have severe active anorectal Crohn's disease and symptomatic anovaginal fistulas usually require proctectomy.

The management of rectovaginal fistulas can pose a major challenge even for the most experienced coloproctologist. Failure is common, and many may require multiple procedures to achieve success.

PERIANAL INFECTIONS

Hidradenitis Suppurativa

Hidradenitis suppurativa is a chronic acneiform apocrine gland infection associated with recurrent sepsis and abscess formation, and frequently with extensive sinus formation, fistulation and scarring. There is a 2:1 male predominance. The estimated prevalence is about 1 in 300.

Hidradenitis suppurativa develops only after puberty and is most common in people aged between 16 and 40 years. Although the most frequently affected sites are the axilla and groin, the hair-bearing anogenital region is involved in up to 30% of cases.

Hidradenitis suppurativa develops as a result of apocrine sweat gland obstruction with keratinous plugs. The obstruction leads to glandular dilatation and bacterial overgrowth, leucocyte infiltration, and eventual duct destruction. Acute infections present as anogenital abscesses or cellulitis. Recurrence is common after simple drainage and results from the establishment of a chronic low-grade infection. Chronic sepsis and recurrent attacks produce extensive fibrosis, which often results in a complex array of fistulas and sinuses or multiple painful nodules with surrounding inflammation and cellulitis. Chronicity is associated with the development of a thin serous discharge from multiple subcutaneous sinuses. Cultures usually grow anaerobic gram-positive cocci and asaccharolytic *Bacteroides* spp. Rarely, chronic cases are complicated by squamous cell carcinoma (SCC).

The diagnosis is usually obvious, but clinical differences may aid differentiation from other causes of fistulas. Cryptoglandular fistulas enter the anal canal at the dentate line and produce suppurative discharge. Hidradenitis tracts are often eccentric, subcutaneous and drain thin serous fluid. The conditions often overlap. Apocrine gland involvement on histology confirms the diagnosis. *It has overlap with Crohn's disease and the two may coexist.*

Management

Acute abscesses are drained and deroofed, but sepsis recurs in up to 83% of cases. Quiescent limited disease can be cured by local excision and primary closure. Chronic and more extensive disease rarely responds to conservative measures, and radical excision is usually required. Maintenance low-dose prophylactic antibiotics do not alter disease course. Smaller wounds are primarily closed. Larger wounds are usually healed by secondary intention; although this prolongs the surgical morbidity, recurrence rates are low. Split skin grafts and rotation flaps have been used to accelerate healing with variable success. Extensive deroofing of individual tracts has also proved successful.[69] Uncommonly, temporary colostomy is required when there are extensive debridement defects.

It is important to note that cases may be associated with Crohn's disease elsewhere, although this may not be apparent initially.

Perianal Tuberculosis

Perianal tuberculous abscess and fistulation are rare, but their incidence is increasing in immunocompromised patients and those who have AIDS. They occur rarely in populations in whom tuberculosis is endemic, especially Asian and African migrants. They affect <2% of patients who have pulmonary tuberculosis,[70] but when present, there is frequently tuberculosis elsewhere.

Abscesses are managed according to general principles. If tuberculosis is suspected, suitable Gram staining may show acid-fast bacilli. Laboratory culture takes 6 weeks and is difficult to achieve. Less than 4% of anal fistulas culture *M. tuberculosis.* Biopsies show caseating granulomas. Patients require antituberculous therapy.

Perianal Actinomycosis

Perianal actinomycosis is a rare chronic granulomatous bacterial infection. It is most common in the ileocecum and rectosigmoid, but also occurs in the anal region. Predispositions may include intrauterine device usage and HTV infection.[71] Lesions produce local inflammation with abscesses and fistulation. Infection spreads insidiously through tissue planes, mimicking tumor infiltration and anorectal Crohn's sepsis. Strictures or luminal masses simulate obstructing carcinomas.

Patients present with anorectal abscesses or fistulas and may be pyrexial. Mucosal irregularity is typical, with bowel wall thickening, reactive adenopathy, sinus tracts and peri- anorectal fascial thickening. Diagnosis is rarely achieved preoperatively, but Actinomyces *israelii* is frequently grown anaerobically and identified histologically. Sulfur granules are characteristic.

Successful treatment combines operation and long-term antibiotics. Operation achieves drainage and excision of affected tissues and provides tissue for histology and culture. A favorable outcome is reported with various penicillin regimens continued for up to 6 months, including penicillin or amoxicillin alone or in combination and penicillin combined with tetracycline or amoxicillin. Initial doses can be given intravenously.

PILONIDAL DISEASE

Sacrococcygeal pilonidal disease is common and occurs in the natal cleft 3–8 cm dorsal to the anus. The peak incidence is between 16 and 20 years, and the condition is uncommon in those over 40 years of age. It is more common in dark, coarse-haired Caucasians, and there is a male predominance of 3 to 1. Patients present because of pain, persistent discharge or abscess formation.

Despite a long-standing belief in a congenital origin, recent work favors an acquired etiology. Bascom has described a sequence that ultimately culminates in chronic abscess formation.[72] A negative subcutaneous natal cleft pressure produced by local shear forces, which is thought to stretch and enlarge normal cleft follicles to produce pits, is critical to the pathogenesis. Pit stretching causes inflammation, which occludes follicle openings. A negative subcutaneous pressure and pressure within closed follicles force follicular keratin into subcutaneous fat to produce an acute abscess. Spontaneous or surgical drainage results in a chronic abscess, which has no epithelial lining and is not a cyst. Tract epithelialization, however, occurs in up to 10% of long-standing cases and may extend up to 2 cm.

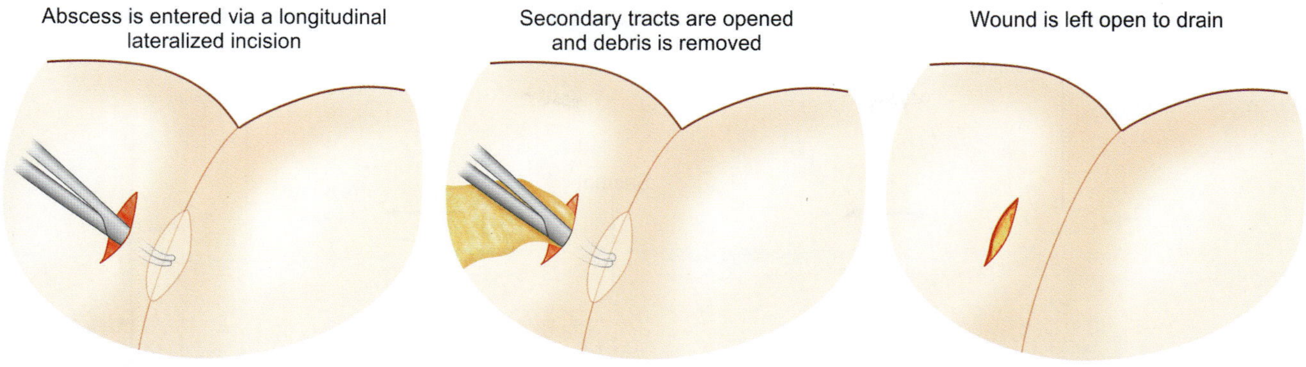

Fig. 63.17: Bascom procedure for pilonidal sinus.

Deep to this, tracts are replaced by chronic granulation tissue. Hair shafts are present in about 50% of abscesses and are probably a secondary phenomenon, being drawn by negative intergluteal pressure into existing sinus tracts; they potentiate chronic sepsis and discharge. Sinus tract blockage places pus and secretion under pressure, which leads to the development of secondary tracts, with lateral rupture creating secondary openings. These tracts may be complex. All these mechanisms are exacerbated in the obese buttock and by prolonged sitting or vibration, hence "jeep disease."

Patients present with natal cleft pain. Pain can be acute and fulminating, with acute abscess formation, or recurrent, cyclic and chronic, with intermittent exacerbation and spontaneous drainage of chronic abscesses. The diagnosis is usually clinically apparent, with one or more midline pits, and often tenderness, induration and redness or secondary sinus and abscess formation. Differential diagnoses include congenital dimples, midline epidermoid cysts, and coccygeal spurs.

Treatment depends on clinical presentation. Minimally symptomatic or intermittently and mildly symptomatic lesions that do not affect lifestyle may not require operative intervention. However, most patients fit into one of three broad categories: acute pilonidal abscess, chronic pilonidal abscess, and complex pilonidal disease.

Acute Pilonidal Abscess

Acute pilonidal abscess is exquisitely tender, erythematous, edematous, and hot. Simple drainage is appropriate, rather than definitive operation, with vertical drainage through the point of maximal fluctuance, away from the midline if possible, and with curettage to the base. All secondary tracts are identified and laid open, but no attempt is made to excise the complete abscess complex. Removal of overlying skin promotes ongoing drainage and basal wound healing. A general anesthetic is preferable because local anesthetic infiltration is extremely painful. Perioperative antibiotic prophylaxis is required. Initial daily loose saline-soaked gauze packing and sitz baths promote healing, which takes an average of 5–6 weeks, but may be protracted. Between 40% and 80% of patients are cured by this approacht. A chronic abscess requiring further operation develops in the remainder of patients.

Chronic Pilonidal Abscess

Chronic pilonidal abscess is the most common presentation of pilonidal disease and results from previous spontaneous or surgical drainage of an acute abscess. The optimal treatment is not clear. Most surgeons carry out complete sinus and abscess excision incorporating all secondary tracts, with either primary layered closure obliterating dead space, or beveled or marsupialized margins with healing by secondary intention. General anesthetic and antibiotic cover are required. The reported results vary enormously. Excision and marsupialization result in recurrence rates as low as 6% with healing in 4 weeks on average, but series generally report poorer figures. Primary closure results in primary healing in up to 90% of cases at 2 weeks, but a recurrence rate of approximately 25%. It does, however, avoid the need for daily dressings and the risk of protracted healing.

As a result of the change in the perceived etiology of pilonidal disease, less radical operation is increasingly advocated. Avoidance of midline and deep natal cleft incisions minimizes slow and nonhealing wounds by preventing sheering cleft stresses. En-bloc excision down to the sacrum is frequently associated with slow or nonhealing and should not be used.

Bascom advocates drainage and pit excision (Fig. 63.17). Abscesses are entered via a longitudinal lateralized incision and, after opening all secondary tracts, curettage and

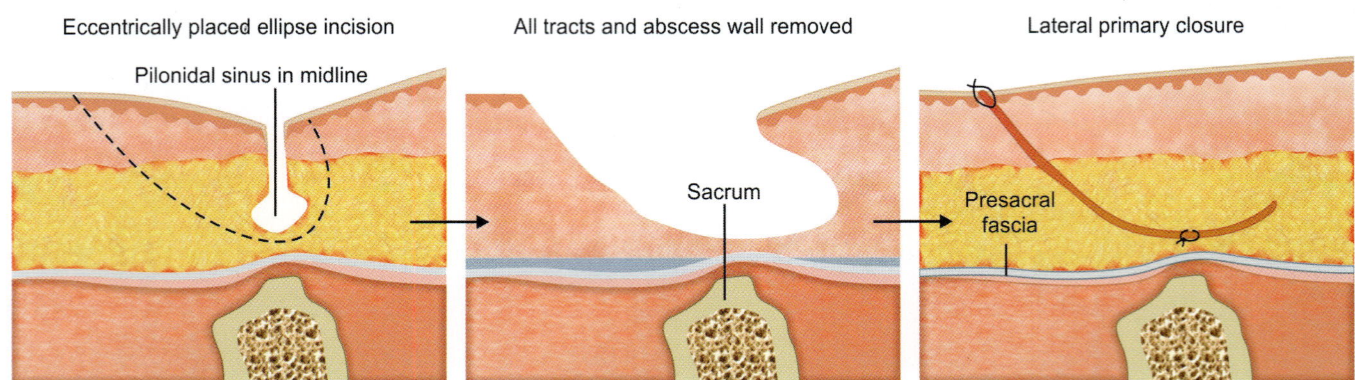

Fig. 63.18: Karydakis procedure for pilonidal sinus.

removal of granulation tissue, hair, and debris, the midline pits are excised with primary closure. The large lateral wound is left open to drain, and patients return to normal sitting and showering immediately. Bascom reports a mean healing time of 3 weeks and recurrence or epithelial inclusion cyst in only 5% of 184 patients.[73]

Karydakis advocates a more extensive excisional procedure, removing all tracts plus the abscess wall in an eccentrically placed ellipse crossing the midline, with elevation of an adipocutaneous flap, which is primarily closed laterally (Fig. 63.18). He reports recurrence in <1% of 6545 cases with an 8.5% complication rate, but this figure has not been reproduced by others.[74]

Complex Pilonidal Disease

Complex pilonidal disease is difficult to manage, often being characterized by multiple sinus openings, previous surgical attempts at repair and large postoperative nonhealing natal cleft ulcers. Extensive midline tissue excision is inappropriate and prolongs morbidity, usually as a result of large nonhealing wounds.

Multiple plastic procedures using buttock rotation flaps have been described. Bascom advocates cleft closure by transferring a donor buttock skin flap across the midline to the recipient buttock and closing the defect following complete pilonidal complex excision. Although this procedure is more complex than other procedures and requires experience, he reports:

- Wound healing in all of 35 patients within 3 months
- No appreciable functional or cosmetic defects
- No recurrences at follow up after 6–84 months.

Full-thickness Z-plasty requires extensive fat mobilization and produces a suture line across the midline of the natal cleft. Split skin grafts are seldom satisfactory because of local sepsis, trauma and ooze; they are not recommended.

ANAL AND PERIANAL WARTS

Anal and perianal warts (condylomata acuminata) are caused by human papillomavirus (HPV) infection of stratified squamous epithelium. Of over 50 types of HPV identified, benign exophytic warts are generally associated with HPV-6 and -11, whereas HPV-16 and -18 are more often associated with severe forms of dysplasia and invasive SCC.

The incidence of anal and perianal warts is increasing. They are most common in male homosexuals. Transmission requires epithelial trauma and is almost always sexual, but anal coitus is not necessary. Rarely, close contact alone allows clinical infection. Vertical transmission also occurs. The incubation period is usually between 1 and 6 months.

The warts present with pruritus, discharge or bleeding. Pain is uncommon. The lesions present a clinical appearance of pink papillary growths, which are usually multiple. Confluence may encircle the anus and extension can occur onto the vulva or scrotum. The diagnosis is usually obvious. Rare differential diagnoses include condylomata lata (a secondary manifestation of syphilis) and SCC. Spirochetes on darkfield examination and invasion on biopsy clarify the diagnosis. Histologically, there is prickle cell hyperplasia, but with orderly epithelial maturation and sharp demarcation between normal and abnormal epithelium. Electron microscopy shows the virus. It is important to notify pathologists of previous podophyllin treatment, which may increase the epithelial mitotic rate and result in an appearance that mimics carcinoma in situ.

Disease extent should be accurately assessed because warts can extend into the anal canal or lower rectum or onto the external genitalia. The vulva, vagina and cervix must be assessed in women because recurrence is likely if all lesions are not treated.

Management

All treatments are associated with high recurrence rates, and none completely eradicate the virus. Topical agents are useful first-line treatments for limited disease confined to the perianal skin. The commonest agent used is 15% podophyllin resin in compound benzoin tincture. It is very irritating and should not be applied to the anal canal. It is applied directly to the warts, and the area should be washed several hours later. Multiple weekly applications are usually required. Bichloroacetic acid can be used similarly, but is less caustic and can be directly applied to anal canal warts, which turn white almost immediately.

Physical obliteration is required if the response to podophyllin is inadequate, perianal involvement is extensive or the anal canal or lower rectum are involved. The treatment of choice for limited disease is scissor excision. This technique avoids diathermy use except to control occasional persistent bleeding points, and it preserves intervening healthy skin and mucosa. Subcutaneous infiltration of anesthetic with epinephrine (adrenaline) splays warts from each other because there is normal skin even between large lesions. The wounds heal rapidly, but if they are extensive a two-stage procedure separated by 1 month may be appropriate. Alternatively, electrocoagulation and fulguration can be used, but diathermy burns may compromise skin bridges and cause pain and weeping. These techniques are less satisfactory for large and confluent lesions, which may heal slowly and result in anal stenosis.

Carbon dioxide laser ablation produces aerosolized viral particles and requires special filter masks and smoke evacuators.[75] It may be helpful for intra-anal lesions. Circumferential submucosal excision is occasionally needed for confluent upper canal lesions, which cannot be removed individually. These lesions are seldom larger than 2 cm in diameter and are closed primarily.

Six-week intramuscular autologous vaccination injections have recently been reported, resulting in complete remission in 84% of patients with no recurrence at 6 months.[76] Only 5% of patients had no benefit, and there were no complications. Similar results with α-interferon have been reported, although both techniques require further investigation before being widely adopted.

Most series report recurrence rates of 25–50%. Patients should be counselled for this eventuality, and regular follow-up is required. Sexual transmission should be discussed and abstinence advocated during treatment. Sexual contacts should be screened.

Anal Warts in Patients Who Have HIV Infection

Anal warts in patients with HIV infection grow quickly and extensively, tend to involve mucosa and have greater neoplastic potential. Nevertheless, aggressive treatment in patients who have early-stage HIV infection appears to be well tolerated and gives reasonable results for both perianal and intra-anal lesions. In late-stage infection, however, nonhealing is common and conservative symptomatic measures are recommended.

Anal Warts in Children

Despite some series concluding frequent nonsexual transmission, others report sexual abuse in up to 60–90% of cases. Lesions in children under 1 year of age may represent vertical transmission. Abuse must be strongly considered at any other age. Phage typing may be useful.

Neoplastic Potential

Anal neoplasia, ranging from anal intraepithelial neoplasia (AIN) to invasive SCC, is being increasingly associated with anal warts. AIN is frequently identified in the warts of homosexual males and predisposes to invasive SCC. Human papillomavirus infection occurs in up to 70% of AIN and up to 60% of anal cancers; these facts explain the higher incidence of anal neoplasia in homosexual men.[77]

Buschke-Löwenstein Tumor

A Buschke-Löwenstein tumor, or giant condyloma acuminatum, presents as an extensive perianal exophytic, pale, warty mass that frequently extends into the anal canal. It can involve large areas of the perineum. It has little metastatic potential, but is locally aggressive and often produces multiple sinuses or fistulas. There is growing consensus that rather than undergoing malignant transformation, it may represent a verrucous carcinoma.

Treatment is usually by wide local excision, often with split skin grafting, rotation flap repair or anoplasty. When extensive, a defunctioning stoma may be necessary to promote perianal healing.

PRURITUS ANI

Pruritus ani (or perianal itching) occurs in up to 5% of the population, is more common in males, with a male-to-female ratio of 4 to 1, and is most common between the ages of 30 and 60 years. It may be a manifestation of a generalized medical problem or dermatosis, but more frequently reflects a local disorder; often no cause is identified. Many perianal afflictions produce irritation and leakage, and soiling and itch can accompany almost any benign or malignant anorectal pathology. Benign dermatologic conditions may be present, including contact dermatitis from topical agent sensitization, psoriasis, lichen planus, and neurogenic dermatitis. Many infections and infestations may also be present, including warts, *Candida albicans* or dermatophyte infestation, and, often in children, *Enterobius vermicularis (threadworm)* infestation. Recent antibiotic use encourages monilial overgrowth. Local irritation may also result from excessive efforts at wiping and scratching. Any lesion increasing stool looseness or defecation frequency may produce leakage and irritation, as may any degree of sphincter dysfunction or incontinence. Hemorrhoids, mucosal prolapse, anal polyps, and skin tags can all cause leakage and itch.

Idiopathic pruritus most commonly results from minor fecal soiling, which itself results from subtle IAS dysfunction producing excessive relaxation with rectal distention.[78] Scratching, inappropriate topical applications, and overzealous cleansing of the skin increase skin sensitivity and perpetuate a vicious circle. Dietary factors, such as caffeine, alcohol, and spicy irritant foods, may exacerbate this process. High-fiber diets increase flatus production and therefore the number of IAS relaxations.

The history relates to the etiologic factors discussed above, as well as to recent overseas travel and contact with children (suggesting *E. vermicularis* infestation) or pets. Generalized itch or skin eruptions should be sought. A general skin examination is followed by a detailed perianal assessment. Minor perianal soiling is the most common finding, often with skin tags or prolapsing hemorrhoids, mucosa, rectum or polyps. Skin lesions or fistulation may be seen. Perianal excoriation and ichthyosis are common, as are superficial perianal radial fissures. The anus may gape as a result of poor tone. Gentle anal wiping with a moistened swab may confirm minor leakage that is not otherwise seen. Sphincter integrity is assessed and anorectal lesions are sought on proctosigmoidoscopy. Skin scrapings may be helpful in the diagnosis if candidal infection is suspected. Perianal swabs and stool microscopy may reveal ova, cysts or parasites, and STD serology may be appropriate. Manometry and ELUS are appropriate for those patients who have sphincter dysfunction.

Management

Treatment is dictated by the clinical findings. In secondary pruritus, any identified pathology is treated. The most common causes are hemorrhoidal and mucosal prolapse, for which banding or injection sclerotherapy usually suffice. Prolapsing polyps are excised, and FTRP requires definitive repair. Primary dermatologic conditions are managed in liaison with a dermatologist. Threadworms require treatment with piperazine or mebendazole.

The management principles for primary pruritus are leakage reduction, improved perianal hygiene and prevention of further perianal skin injury. Topical agents should be suspended, but short-term topical hydrocortisone may initially help break the itch cycle. Prolonged use (>2 weeks) can produce skin atrophy and fungal infection. Foods producing excessive flatus should be avoided; reducing fiber, caffeine, and alcohol intake sometimes produces similar benefit. Antimotility agents, such as loperamide, can be helpful if stools are frequent or loose.

Soaps, powder and other irritants should be avoided around the anus. The anus should be cleansed at least daily and dabbed rather than wiped dry with cloth. Toilet paper use should be minimized. Ideally it should be soft, but strong to minimize residual particulate debris. Use of a bidet or a moistened soft cloth or cotton wool ball is less irritant. Tight-fitting synthetic underwear should be avoided. Nocturnal itch may respond to nocturnal antihistamines. Scratching and rubbing should be strongly discouraged.

Secondary pruritus usually responds to treatment of the underlying cause. Most cases of idiopathic pruritus improve to some extent, but long-standing pruritus ani may be particularly difficult to control and is rarely completely eradicated.

ANAL NEOPLASIA: A PERSPECTIVE

Location

Anal tumors are uncommon and anal cancer is rare, comprising only 1–5% of all large bowel malignancies. Over 80% of cases are squamous cell or epidermoid carcinomas (SCC), and approximately 10% are adenocarcinomas. Rarer tumors include malignant melanoma, sarcoma, lymphoma, and carcinoid. The increasing incidence of HIV infection has led to an increased incidence of anal cancer of all types, especially in males. Some 70% of squamous tumors arise from above the dentate line. Tumors in this location are more common in women than in men with a male-to-female ratio approaching 1 to 2. Half of the remaining tumors occur between the dentate line and anal verge. Both these tumors and tumors of the perianal skin are more common in men, and their incidence is increasing, particularly among individuals with HIV infection.

Etiology

There is a strong correlation between anal SCC and HPV-16 and, to a lesser extent, HPV-18, -31 and -33, and herpes simplex virus (HSV) type 2. Cigarette smoking has been associated with anal malignancy, and chronic anal inflammation (e.g., Crohn's disease) has been associated with an increase in incidence of up to tenfold. Although previously thought to be a factor, anal receptive intercourse itself may not predispose to cancer when factors such as smoking and chronic anogenital infection are taken into account. An increased incidence of up to 200-fold has been reported in renal transplant recipients on maintenance immunosuppression. The disproportionately high incidence among male homosexuals, particularly those who have HIV infection, may reflect both the high incidence of HPV infection and HIV immunosuppression; HIV appears to act as a promoter rather than an initiator of dysplasia. Daling and associates[79] showed that the incidence of SCC in homosexual and bisexual men is 25–50 times higher than that in heterosexual men. More generally, there has also been an association with poor anal hygiene. The premalignant lesions of Bowen's disease, bowenoid papulosis, and AIN may all progress to invasive SCC.

ANAL MARGIN TUMORS

Bowen's Disease and Bowenoid Papulosis

Bowen's disease and bowenoid papulosis are squamous carcinomas in situ, similar to and often coexisting with AIN. Although occurring in the anogenital region, they are more common on the extremities and trunk. Bowen's disease appears as erythematous plaque-like lesions, which can be scaly, crusted or nodular, with irregular edges and occasional pigmentation. Bowenoid papulosis more often produces multiple discrete papules and may occur in younger patients.[80] Histologically the basement membrane is intact, there is loss of epithelial polarity and an inflammatory infiltrate is present. Characteristic bowenoid cells have large hyperchromatic nuclei with vacuoles, which produce a halo effect.

Reports that Bowen's disease is associated with a long-term risk of other visceral and cutaneous malignancies have not been supported. Lesions can progress to frankly invasive SCC, however, particularly when associated with HIV infection. Oliver and Labow note an association between Bowen's lesions and HPV infection and suggest close follow-up for HPV-associated anogenital carcinomas.

Bowen's disease lesions are adequately treated by wide local excision. Split skin grafting or rotation flap repair may be necessary. Clear margins are necessary to prevent recurrence.

Extramammary Paget's Disease

Paget's disease is extremely rare and presents in regions of abundant apocrine glands, such as the axilla and perianal skin. The intraepithelial tumor presents as pale or erythematous skin, often with crusting, ulceration or scaling. Characteristic pagetoid cells, which have abundant vacuolated cytoplasm and a pale staining nucleus, are seen on histology. Paget's disease may be associated with invasive carcinomas of skin appendages, such as apocrine glands, and occasionally with rectal carcinoma or a concurrent breast carcinoma. Sigmoidoscopy and breast examination should be performed.

The lesions are managed by wide local excision that ensures histologic clearance to prevent recurrences. Associated apocrine adenocarcinomas require radical local excision, but tend to behave aggressively. Long-term follow-up is needed because of the risk of cancer.

Basal Cell Carcinoma

Basal cell carcinoma is a rare tumor with a good prognosis. It presents as an indurated and ulcerated lesion with raised edges. The lesions grow slowly and metastasize seldom and late. Wide local excision is usually curative. Local recurrences can occur and should be treated by repeat adequate wide local excision.

Squamous Cell Carcinoma

Squamous or epidermoid carcinomas are the most common anal margin malignancy, but represent only 15–30% of all squamous anal cancers. The average age at presentation is 55–60 years. Patients whose tumors carry HPV DNA are on average 9 years younger than those whose tumors do not carry this DNA. Most of the tumors are well differentiated, produce keratin and behave biologically like SCCs found elsewhere on the skin.

About half of patients present with pain and bleeding, and an ulcerating mass is identified in about 25% of cases. Pruritus and discharge are common. High lesions can involve the sphincters, causing FI and tenesmus, but these manifestations are more common with anal canal tumors, as is anovaginal fistulation. Bowel habit may change, but this is not common. Patients may present with secondary inguinal lymphadenopathy. Squamous cell carcinoma may be an unexpected histologic finding on a hemorrhoidectomy specimen. In approximately 60% of cases there are associated perianal conditions, such as warts, chronic fistula or radiation damage. These findings are associated with < 10% of anal canal SCCs.

The lesion is usually a raised everted malignant ulcer with associated induration and tenderness. Tumors of the pecten may not be visible externally. Sphincter spasm is common, proximal tumor extension is variable and perianal abscess or fistula formation is sometimes present. Inguinal lymphadenopathy, mostly ipsilateral, is present in up to one-third of cases, but only 50% of the time is it the result of metastatic spread. Needle aspiration cytology is usually adequate to diagnose metastases in the inguinal lymph nodes. Distal metastatic spread is usually late and related to the size of the primary tumor.

Diagnosis is obtained on histology. Local assessment is frequently best achieved with EUA to assess size, infiltration of adjacent structures and nodal involvement, and to allow biopsy of lesions that are often tender. Sigmoidoscopy should be carried out. ELUS may be helpful.

Management

Treatment depends on the size and local infiltration of the lesions and the presence of inguinal metastatic disease. The depth of invasion may determine prognosis. Small mobile lesions without deep infiltration and with clinically uninvolved groin nodes are usually treated by wide local excision or radiotherapy. Five-year survival rates are mostly above 70–80% overall, with rates up to 100% in highly selected series.[81] Some cases require split skin grafting or local flap closure.

Larger lesions, poorly differentiated lesions, and lesions that involve the sphincters or inguinal nodes are best managed by chemoirradiation, with or without local surgical resection or subsequent salvage anal resection. Irradiation techniques include radium implantation and external beam delivery. Therapeutic node dissection is beneficial only if clinically detectable disease persists after combined modality treatment. Despite variations in protocols and tumor details, overall 5-year survival rates for all comers using this technique vary between 50% and 85%.[82]

As <20% of patients develop groin nodal metastases, and node dissection causes appreciable morbidity, so prophylactic dissection is not recommended. Whereas synchronous groin metastases are a poor prognostic factor, therapeutic dissection of metachronous nodes can result in 5-year survival rates of up to 80%.

The traditional radical APE is unnecessary and now uncommonly used. It is usually reserved for persistent or recurrent disease, and results in 5-year survival rates of about 50%.

Verrucous Carcinoma

Verrucous carcinomas are large exophytic warty lesions that occur in the anal canal or perianal skin. They have little metastatic potential, but are locally invasive and often form multiple sinuses or fistulas. The giant condyloma acuminatum or Bushke-Löwenstein tumor may represent a verrucous carcinoma.

Treatment is usually by wide local excision, often with split skin grafting, rotation flap repair or anoplasty. When extensive, a defunctioning stoma may be necessary to promote perianal healing.

ANAL CANAL TUMORS

Squamous Cell/Cloacogenic Carcinoma

Anal canal cancers arise in the portion of the anus that extends from the puborectalis to either the dentate line or anal verge depending on which definition is used. This segment incorporates some 70–85% of epidermoid anal cancers, most occurring in the ATZ, and 30–50% of these are basaloid histologically. Epidermoid tumors comprise several morphologic types, including keratinizing SCC, nonkeratinizing SCC, basaloid (cloacogenic) carcinomas, mucoepidermoid carcinomas and SCC with mucus microcysts. Morphologic type does not appear to alter prognosis,[83] and all tumors are managed in the same way. Anal canal epidermoid cancers are in general more poorly differentiated, more locally advanced and more likely to have metastasized at presentation; they have a worse prognosis than anal margin tumors. Prognosis depends on histologic grade, tumor size, depth of invasion, and overall staging.

Most patients present with bleeding, pain, or tenesmus. Extensive lesions may protrude through the anus, but lesions are usually felt digitally as tender, indurated masses that are ulcerated and have everted edges. The findings are confirmed at proctoscopy, but biopsy is often difficult because of pain and tenderness. Over 80% of lesions are larger than 2 cm in diameter at diagnosis, and up to 76% are initially misdiagnosed as benign.

Local assessment usually requires EUA because the lesions are often painful. Proximal and distal margins, depth of penetration, mobility and associated pelvic lymphadenopathy are assessed, and targeted biopsies are taken. Rigid sigmoidoscopy is carried out to exclude higher lesions. Endoluminal ultrasound aids identification of deep penetration and pelvic nodal disease; CT and MRI give better definition of tumor infiltration.

Management of squamous cell and cloacogenic carcinomas are both chemo-and radiosensitive. Chemoirradiation has become the treatment of choice, giving the best survival rates while preserving the sphincters. Operation is reserved for failures.

Local excision: Local excision is not generally recommended, but is helpful for selected elderly patients who have small favorable tumors. The reported 5-year survival rate is 55% for superficial well-differentiated lesions that are <2 cm in diameter and lie distal to the dentate line.

Abdominoperineal excision of the rectum and anus: The historic standard, APE, results in a 50–60% 5-year survival rate, but has the added morbidity of a pelvic and perineal operation and a permanent stoma; in addition the locoregional recurrence rates are up to 40%. Extensive pelvic lymphadenectomy does not improve the results. Synchronous inguinal lymphadenopathy requires block dissection. Prophylactic node dissection is not indicated.

Radiotherapy alone: Modem cobalt source generators and linear accelerators enable greater dose delivery to deeper structures with less superficial toxicity and enhanced tumoricidal effect. James *et al.* describe local control rates with interstitial radiation alone of 47%. When combined with external beam irradiation, the 5-year survival rate was 66%, with most patients maintaining sphincter function.[84] Green et al. quote a 75% 3-year survival rate using high-dose external beam irradiation alone.[85]

Chemoirradiation: Nigro and associates showed no residual tumor in 22 of 24 APE specimens resected after chemoirradiation using mitomycin-C and 5-fluorouracil. Five-year survival rates were 83%. Numerous modifications of dosage and cycling have followed, with consistently good results. Nigro modified his practice to excise the primary tumor site after treatment, but subsequently omitted APE if the anal canal looked and felt normal. Current regimens combine external beam irradiation to the tumor bed and draining pelvic and inguinal lymph nodes with intravenous 5-fluorouracil and mitomycin-C, the course being completed in 31 days. Severe toxicity is uncommon and usually results from hematologic suppression by mitomycin-C. An APE is used for salvage for persistent or recurrent disease. Cummings and coworkers[86] showed local tumor control rates of 90% versus 56% when comparing the effects of chemoirradiation with historic controls treated by radiotherapy alone. The United Kingdom Co-ordinating Committee on Cancer Research (UKCCCR) trial[87] randomized 585 patients to chemoirradiation or irradiation alone. Chemoirradiation was superior, resulting in a local failure rate of 36% compared with 59% for irradiation alone. Although there was a decreased anal cancer mortality rate, no overall survival advantage was demonstrated.

Inguinal recurrence rates of 15–25% in nonirradiated lymph nodes fall to as low as 2.6% after prophylactic irradiation. Therefore prophylactic inguinal irradiation is indicated.

Summary

In general, anal canal epidermoid carcinoma is primarily managed with chemoirradiation, with operation reserved for patients who fail to respond. About 70% of patients show a complete response and 20% a partial response; there is little or no effect in about 10% of patients. Those who fail to respond require APE for tumor salvage. It is unclear in responders what to do with the tumor scar, but it appears that APE is not required and local scar excision is more appropriate, thereby preserving the sphincters.

Adenocarcinoma of the Anal Canal

The most common adenocarcinoma of the anal canal is a very low rectal adenocarcinoma with distal spread into the anal canal. True anal canal adenocarcinoma is rare. It can arise from the glandular cells of the ATZ, but more commonly arises from the anal glands and ducts at the level of the dentate line. Sometimes it arises in anorectal duplications and is mucinous; other tumors arise in chronic perianal fistulas or abscesses. Unlike colorectal adenocarcinomas there is an association with HPV DNA, similar to that of HPV-16 and epidermoid carcinoma.

Adenocarcinomas have a poor prognosis and show aggressive spread to both inguinal and pelvic nodes with invariable sphincter involvement. For these reasons APE is the usual treatment, although preoperative radiotherapy to both the primary and draining nodal regions has been advocated. Small good-prognosis tumors have been successfully managed by electrocoagulation or local excision, with or without external beam radiotherapy.

Carcinoma in an Anorectal Fistula

Adenocarcinomatous change in chronic perianal fistulas or abscesses is rare. It has been reported in longstanding perianal Crohn's disease. The tumors may contain or discharge mucus, and involved tracts may be several centimeters from the anal verge. Some evidence suggests that the tumors develop in lower hindgut duplications, because normal rectal mucosa can be shown to line tracts adjacent to the carcinomas. There are no large series, but treatment is usually by APE and the prognosis is poor.

OTHER TUMORS OF THE ANAL REGION

Malignant Melanoma

Anal malignant melanoma is a rare aggressive tumor and comprises <1% of all melanomas and <1% of malignant anal tumors. It is most common in the ATZ, but also occurs in the pecten, perianal skin or rectal mucosa, where melanocytes are found. It is usually occult and identified by chance, but lesions may present with bleeding, a mass or anal pain. The tumor metastasizes early to liver, lung and brain, and, once it is symptomatic, distant metastases are invariably present. More than 75% of patients have inguinal lymphadenopathy on presentation.

Although occasionally amelanotic, the lesions are usually pigmented and can mimic a hemorrhoid or thrombosed external pile. They can be sessile or pedunculated, but ulceration is uncommon. Histologically, giant cells help distinguish melanoma from other poorly differentiated anal cancers. Identification of tumor cell melanin, S-100 protein, or melanosomes confirms the diagnosis.

The prognosis is extremely poor, with 5-year survival rates being universally <10%. Survival correlates best with tumor depth. Lesions deeper than 2 mm are uniformly fatal before 5 years. Multiple therapies have been advocated, including local resection with or without nodal dissection, cryotherapy, APE, radiotherapy, and chemotherapy. Treatment type does not correlate with survival,[88] with dismal results for all but the thinnest lesions. Treatment should therefore be aimed at symptom palliation for all but the thinnest melanomas. Asymptomatic lesions that are inadvertently identified should be managed by wide local excision, which is likely to be therapeutic as well as diagnostic in the absence of metastatic disease. There is no indication for prophylactic inguinal node dissection.

Sarcomas

Sarcomas are extremely rare and occur at an average age of 60 years. Most are leiomyosarcomas. They present with bleeding, pain, change in bowel habit or a perianal mass and occur in the muscularis propria, with mucosal involvement in only one-third of cases. Proctoscopy shows a submucosal tumor projecting into the anal canal. Tumors spread locally and hematogenously to liver and lungs. Nodal involvement is uncommon. Sphincters are frequently involved. ELUS assesses local tumor characteristics.

Not all stromal mural neoplasms are malignant. Sarcomatous behavior correlates with muscularis propria location, size, nuclear atypia, and tumor necrosis, but mitotic activity is the primary indicator. Malignant behavior is unpredictable, and tumors can recur or metastasize several years after treatment.[89] High-grade lesions, lesions larger than 6 cm in diameter, and previous incomplete local excision are poor prognostic factors. Diagnosis is achieved on excisional biopsy. Most of these tumors show microscopic infiltration of the advancing border despite macroscopic circumscription.

The optimal treatment is unknown, but the standard treatment is APE, with long-term survival rates up to 50% at 10 years. Lesions <2.5 cm in diameter and confined to the bowel wall can be managed by wide local excision, although high recurrence rates have been reported in small series. Radical excision has not been shown to produce superior results to wide local excision. Adjuvant chemotherapy and radiotherapy are thought to be ineffective.

Lymphoma

Lymphomas are rare and usually occur in immunocompromised patients, especially those who have HIV infection, and especially in those who have AIDS (see below). Outcomes of treatment are better in patients who do not have AIDS. Such patients can tolerate multi agent chemotherapy regimens better than those who have AIDS.[90]

Carcinoid

Cells of neuroectodermal origin contained within the ATZ may give rise to anal canal carcinoids. These tumors are rare and generally do not secrete active peptides and neurotransmitters. Lesions <2 cm in diameter may be amenable to wide local excision, but lesions greater than 2 cm in diameter behave more aggressively and should be managed by APE.

ANAL AND PERIANAL DISEASE ASSOCIATED WITH HIV INFECTION AND AIDS

Perspective

Patients who have HIV infection and AIDS are prone to other anorectal diseases. Many have more than one disease, and over 60% have more than one concurrent

STD.[91] Stool should be cultured, and any lesions are biopsied and cultured for viral agents.

The HIV-and AIDS-associated pathologies are classified into three categories:

- Common generally occurring pathology, such as hemorrhoids and fissures
- That encountered in high-risk individuals, especially homosexuals practicing anal receptive intercourse (mostly STDs, such as HPV infection and gonorrhea)
- HIV-associated pathology, such as atypical opportunistic infections, non-Hodgkin's lymphoma (NHL), and Kaposi's sarcoma.

The most common anorectal pathologies in *AIDS* and HIV-positive patients are perianal sepsis (>50%), warts (35%), anorectal ulcers (33%), hemorrhoids (17%), invasive anorectal carcinoma (17%), and polyps (11%).

Surgeons have been hesitant about carrying out anorectal operations in patients with HIV infection because of the aggressive behavior of the conditions involved, poor wound healing and frequent wound sepsis. Moenning et al. reported morbidity, mortality, and nonhealing rates of 62%, 6%, and 48%, respectively. Wound healing rates following surgical treatment of only 25% have been reported in patients with AIDS. A direct correlation between wound healing and absolute leukocyte or CD4 T cell count has been reported. Selective intervention, based on accurate diagnosis, however, can result in high rates of complete or partial wound healing, but more importantly it achieves appreciable symptom relief without resulting in excessive morbidity or mortality rates. Beck redefines the primary therapeutic goal in patients who have HIV infection as symptom relief. Secondary goals are resolution of underlying pathology and wound healing. Marked symptomatic improvement can be achieved surgically, even in the presence of incomplete healing.

Benign Anal Fissures

Benign anal fissures are common in people who have HIV infection and AIDS and may relate to chronic diarrhea or trauma from anal receptive intercourse. Any patient who has HIV infection and appreciable anal pain requires EUA to exclude undrained pus. Benign fissures need differentiation from the more aggressive idiopathic AIDS-related ulceration and the myriad of anorectal infective and neoplastic ulcerations. Fecal continence is assessed because of the risk of sphincter damage with aggressive anal receptive intercourse, rectal noncompliance from infective disorders and the frequency of diarrhea. If sphincter integrity is questioned, anorectal physiology testing is carried out before considering sphincterotomy.

Benign fissures are initially treated conservatively with bulk laxatives and topical anesthetics and vasodilators. Lateral sphincterotomy may be required for pain relief for those fissures that fail to respond. Although this procedure often replaces the fissure with a second nonhealing sphincterotomy wound, the symptom relief can be dramatic.

Perianal Sepsis

Perianal sepsis is common in all stages of HIV infection, especially AIDS. As a result of immunosuppression and the risks of septicemia and Fournier's gangrene, immediate abscess drainage is imperative. Sepsis may relate to cryptoglandular abscesses or deep invasion of idiopathic or STD-related ulceration. Abscesses can be subtle and present only as pain and erythema. All cases require EUA. The emphasis is on surgical drainage using small incisions over the point of maximal fluctuance and maintained drainage, frequently using mushroom-tipped catheters until the induration resolves. Biopsies are required to exclude a masquerading inflammatory submucosal lymphoma and erosive anal tumors with abscess or fistula formation. Pus is sent for culture (including acid-fast bacilli). All procedures require a full course of broad-spectrum antibiotics.

Anal Fistulas

Anal fistulas are frequently multiple and complex in HIV patients, especially those with AIDS. In otherwise asymptomatic patients, simple low intersphincteric fistulas are usually treated by standard fistulotomy.

All other types of fistulas require insertion of long-term draining setons, which minimize recurrent sepsis and prevent creation of surgical wounds that may not heal. Such setons have been shown to be effective in resolving pain.

Hemorrhoids

Hemorrhoids in people with HIV infection and AIDS are managed using conservative measures if at all possible. Those who fail to respond may benefit from injection sclerotherapy. Nonresponders are considered for band ligation, but this carries a considerable septic risk and patients need close monitoring.[92] Surgical hemorrhoidectomy is avoided in all but the early stages of disease because of the risks of wound sepsis and nonhealing. Thrombosed external piles can be incised or excised in the early stage of disease, but are otherwise managed conservatively. Chronic diarrhea predisposes to hemorrhoidal prolapse and requires treatment.

Kaposi's Sarcoma

Kaposi's sarcoma is the most common AIDS-related malignancy and occurs in up to 43% of homosexual and bisexual males who have AIDS.[93] It may be related to the newly identified sexually transmitted opportunistic virus, human herpesvirus 8 (Kaposi's sarcoma-associated herpes virus). The most common site is the skin, but anorectal involvement also occurs. The lesions are frequently widespread throughout the skin, mucosa, viscera, and lymph nodes, and are usually asymptomatic. Although they can cause appreciable morbidity, the lesions are rarely fatal. Characteristic anorectal lesions are violet-to-red nodules, plaques or polyps. The lesions may bleed, but serious bleeding is uncommon. Perforation is rare. Occasionally, bulky lesions cause obstruction.

Presentation of Kaposi's sarcoma may be incidental or as a nodule on rectal examination or sigmoidoscopy. The purple coloration results from the vascularity, red blood cell extravasation, and hemosiderin formation. Most lesions are submucosal and require deep biopsy, which is safe despite the vascularity.

Small slowly progressing lesions are observed or treated with zidovudine. Progressive symptomatic accessible lesions are treated with intralesional vinblastine sulfate or interferon, and less accessible lesions by radiotherapy, chemotherapy, or immunomodulation. Operation is used only for biopsy or complications of massive hemorrhage, perforation or obstruction.

Cytomegalovirus Infection

Cytomegalovirus (CMV) infection is a ubiquitous DNA virus infection among homosexuals and those who have AIDS. More than 90% of healthy homosexual males are seropositive, and >95% of AIDS patients develop active CMV infection. Primary infections usually become latent, so relapse is common after treatment. Cytomegalovirus ileocolitis is the most common intestinal manifestation, but symptomatic CMV proctitis is common and presents with tenesmus, diarrhea, weight loss, anemia, melena, or hematochezia.

The proctosigmoidoscopic appearance varies from submucosal hemorrhage and patchy erythema to multiple wide deep ulcers. Biopsies show vasculitis plus intranuclear and intracytoplasmic CMV inclusion bodies. Typical purplish "smudge" cells are highly suggestive of pathogenicity. Viral cultures of biopsies are sometimes positive. The serology is frequently positive, but this finding does not establish invasive disease.

Treatment of CMV infection is with the antiviral agents foscarnet and ganciclovir. Ganciclovir has a structure similar to that of aciclovir, but is 50 times more effective against CMV. Foscarnet can produce irreversible renal failure, and ganciclovir can cause bone marrow suppression. Both drugs are virostatic; therefore relapse is common after cessation, and lifelong treatment may be required. Operation is sometimes required for refractory disease, hemorrhage or perforation.

Lymphoma

Extranodal lymphomas occur in up to 10% of patients with HIV infection and are mostly high-grade NHLs. They are aggressive and often fatal. After the stomach, the anorectum is the most common site in the gastrointestinal tract. Diagnosis may be difficult because most present as extraluminal lesions and a deep diffuse mass, sometimes with overlying induration. Discrete anorectal masses sometimes occur. Larger lesions may ulcerate. Some patients present with the constitutional symptoms of fever, weight loss and night sweats. The lesions are frequently misdiagnosed as perianal abscesses; in one series up to 10% of suspected perianal abscesses undergoing drainage were NHLs. Biopsy of all HIV anorectal lesions is therefore mandatory. Specimens are sent fresh for immunostaining, histopathology and culture.

The tumors are frequently very aggressive. Definite treatment strategies are not clearly defined, and the outcome is poor irrespective of treatment type. Surgical excision does not adequately control the disease and is not recommended. Aggressive multimodal chemotherapeutic regimens are poorly tolerated and associated with a high incidence of opportunistic infections. The complications of sepsis, bleeding, and incontinence or persistence of lesions may require stomal diversion.

Anal Neoplasia

There are no large reported series of SCC treatment in patients with HIV infection and AIDS, but the prognosis is universally poor and treatment is aimed at symptom palliation. Cure may be achieved for a few early tumors. In otherwise asymptomatic HIV patients, the standard

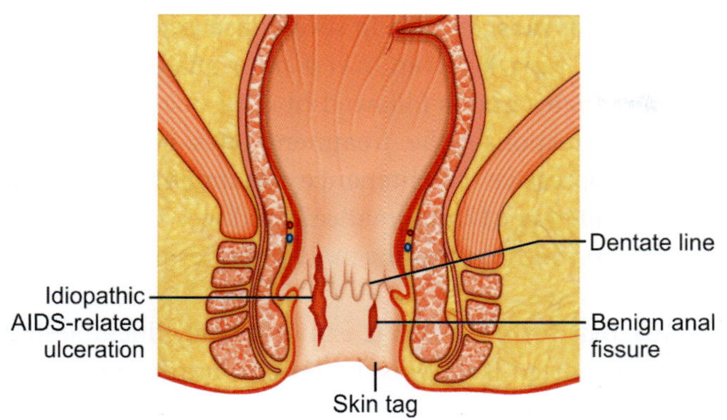

Fig. 63.19: Comparison of idiopathic AIDS-related ulceration and benign anal fissure: Idiopathic AIDS-related ulceration frequently extends proximal to the dentate line, is undermining and may erode through the sphincter muscle. A benign anal fissure is located more distally and has an associated anal skin tag.

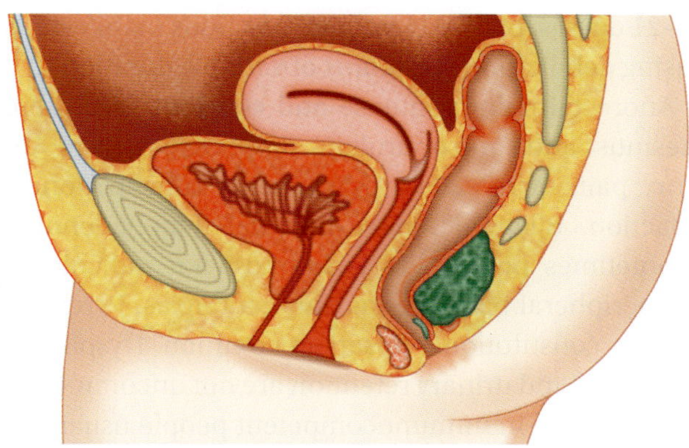

Fig. 63.20: Deeply cavitating idiopathic AIDS-related ulceration: This condition promotes pocketing and local sepsis and leads to muscle erosion and perforation, with deep space abscess formation.

chemoirradiation seems appropriate but is poorly tolerated; regimens are frequently shortened or modified. Pare and Gottesman advocate APE rather than trial chemoirradiation because of the high morbidity rates.[94] In symptomatic patients who have HIV infection or AIDS, local tumor control is the treatment aim and radiotherapy seems logical, although data are lacking. Chemotherapy is poorly tolerated. A diverting stoma may be required.

Bowen's Disease

The presentation and histology of Bowen's disease in patients with HIV infection and AIDS are the same as in the general population. There have been reports of progression under observation to frankly invasive SCC in immunocompromised homosexual males with HIV infection. In general, the lesions are treated by wide local excision.

Anorectal Ulceration

Idiopathic anal ulceration specific to AIDS is common and troublesome. The lesions need to be differentiated from benign anal fissures, neoplastic ulcerations, and a myriad of infectious ulcerations, of which HSV is the most common cause. Despite extensive investigation, no etiology is identified in up to 50% of all ulcerations in this group of patients; these ulcerations are termed idiopathic. Approximately 80% are posterior midline, but the site can be eccentric and the ulcers are often multiple. Most ulcerations have several typical features (Fig. 63.19). They frequently have a purplish hue. They occur more proximally in the anal canal than benign fissures and frequently extend proximal to the dentate line. They lack the sentinel tag of benign fissures, and resting tone is usually reduced in contrast to the IAS hypertonicity of benign fissures. Deep basal erosion into muscle suggests idiopathic ulceration.

Ulcers associated with AIDS are frequently locally aggressive and appear as a deep broad-based erosion with overhanging edges. There is submucosal spread and often invasion into or through the sphincters. Undermining hinders drainage from resultant cavities, promoting secretion and fecal pooling, sepsis, abscess formation, and severe pain. Collections under tension may perforate the EAS and result in the formation of ischiorectal abscesses (Fig. 63.20).

The lesions require EUA and biopsy, viral culture, and darkfield examination. Pus is drained, and cavitating ulcers are deroofed. Sphincterotomy may be required if sphincter erosion is present. Ulcer injection with long-acting anesthetic and depot methylprednisolone gives good-to-excellent pain relief in up to 95% of cases, although repeat injections may be required.

SEXUALLY TRANSMITTED INFECTIONS

Herpes Simplex Viral Proctitis

Up to 95% of male homosexuals are infected with HSV at some stage, and 6–30% of homosexuals who have rectal symptoms have positive cultures for HSV. Almost all herpetic anorectal disease is caused by HSV-2. Anal herpes simplex is common in patients with HIV infection and AIDS, and its incidence is increasing.

Clinical Presentation

Spread is direct from the skin to the mucosa, most commonly by anal receptive intercourse. An incubation period of 4–21 days is followed by acute infectious manifestations causing debilitating symptoms of variable duration.

Anorectal pain is intense and constant, and there is tenesmus and mucopurulent discharge. Severe defecatory pain may lead to psychogenic constipation with impaction. Bilateral tender inguinal lymphadenopathy is sometimes present, as is lumbosacral radiculopathy with peripheral paresthesias and neuralgias. Pyrexia and systemic constitutional upset are common. Dyspareunia, impotence, and urinary retention are not uncommon. The clinical course in immunocompetent people usually lasts 7–10 days, and infective recurrences are usually mild. In the immunocompromised, and particularly in patients who have AIDS, the clinical course is much more aggressive and is characterized by the appearance of large persistent lesions and severe and repetitive outbreaks. Cell-mediated responses appear to be important in controlling the severity of mucocutaneous outbreaks. Neural invasion occurs and a poorly understood latency state results, leading to recurrence rates of >80% after a first infection, despite high antibody titers. Recurrences are usually in the same distribution as first episodes.

There is usually exquisite tenderness on anorectal examination, which is best carried out using local or general anesthetic. Acute lesions present as multiple small round pale vesicles in the anogenital and anorectal regions, often with a red halo and frequently confluent; they present in varying stages of vesicle formation with ulceration and scaling. Clear vesicle fluid is highly contagious from the first vesicle appearance to complete re-epithelialization. Confluent ulcers can extend into the sacrococcygeal region in a butterfly distribution. The diagnosis is suggested by the typical vesicles and is confirmed on viral culture in over 90% of suspected cases. Scrapings with Giemsa stains and histology show characteristic nucleated giant cells and ground-glass nuclear inclusions. Crypt abscesses occur in 50% of cases. Proctosigmoidoscopy shows mucopus with friable mucosa, diffuse ulceration, and, sometimes, vesicles and pustules. Rectal involvement is usually limited to the lower 10 cm.

Management

Management involves treatment of the acute infection and reduction in the number of and extent of symptomatic recurrences. For acute infection, the antiviral agent aciclovir shortens the clinical course, reduces severity, and suppresses HSV-2 infection in most patients. Oral aciclovir 200–400 mg five times daily for 10 days gives better results than 5% topical aciclovir and has become the standard treatment for most lesions. In severe disease, intravenous aciclovir at 5 mg/kg given over 1 hour q8h is used until the pain abates and is followed by a 10-day oral course. Despite a response, the treatment does not eradicate HSV. Suppressive maintenance treatment with oral aciclovir 400 mg q12h dramatically reduces symptomatic recurrences, without causing major long-term side effects, for up to 4 years.

Aciclovir-resistant HSV-2 is increasingly documented and is suspected if there is a failure to improve or if the cultures remain positive after 1 week of an adequate dose of aciclovir. This condition is treated with second-line newer antiviral agents, such as foscarnet or vidarabine,[95] but resistance occurs and the relapse rates are high on cessation. There is a strong association between HSV-2 infection and subsequent HIV infection, and all patients should be tested for HIV.

Chlamydial Proctitis

Chlamydia are small obligate intracellular pathogens related to bacteria. Chlamydial proctitis is the most common STD in the USA, and the incidence is increasing in both males and females. It is present in 15% of asymptomatic homosexuals. Of 15 known immunotypes, types D and K are responsible for chlamydial proctitis and types L1–3 for lymphogranuloma venereum.

Anal receptive intercourse or oroanal transmission is followed by an incubation period of < 10 days. Other STDs, especially gonorrhea, may be present. Rectal infection presents with pain, tenesmus, mucoid, or bloody discharge and constitutional upset. Inguinal nodes may be enlarged and matted, but less so than in the enormous nodal inflammatory response of lymphogranuloma venereum. Sigmoidoscopy shows nonspecific granular proctitis with friability, but rarely ulceration. Late extraluminal strictures or masses can occur. Histology shows crypt abscesses with infectious granulomas and giant cells. Granulomas may lead to a mistaken diagnosis of Crohn's disease. Microimmunofluorescent antibody titer is the most sensitive diagnostic modality. Immediate biopsy culture inoculation confirms the diagnosis, but is difficult to achieve.

Management

Infective episodes generally respond to oral tetracycline or erythromycin at 500 mg q6h for 7–10 days. Alternative regimens include oral doxycycline or Vibramycin. Late rectal strictures can extend as far proximally as the splenic flexure. Treatment principles include the exclusion of other causes, such as ischemia, IBD or carcinoma, and symptomatic management. Asymptomatic strictures require no specific treatment. For symptomatic lesions a 3-week course of erythromycin, tetracycline, or doxycycline is worthwhile. If there is no response, a sphincter-saving resection or a diverting proximal stoma may be required. There are limited reports of balloon dilatation.

Gonococcal Proctitis

Neisseria gonorrhoeae, a gram-negative intracellular diplococcus, is present in up to 55% of screened homosexual males. Isolated rectal involvement occurs in half of them, and most patients are asymptomatic. The higher incidence in males reflects anoreceptive transmission. In females, autoinoculation from the vagina is the prominent transmission mode, and gonococcal proctitis in the absence of cervical or urethral infection occurs in only 6% of cases. The incubation period of 5–7 days is followed by a rectal inflammatory response of varying intensity, often with cryptitis. The most common symptom is viscous yellow mucopurulent anal discharge, often with pruritus, severe tenesmus, and sometimes bright red rectal bleeding. Hematogenous dissemination in severe disease can produce peripheral manifestations, such as arthritis, endocarditis, pericarditis, and meningitis.

The diagnosis is suspected from the history of a mucopurulent discharge combined with ulcerating proctitis at sigmoidoscopy. Mucopus expression from anal crypts by sigmoidoscopic pressure is considered to be a sensitive clinical sign. The anal canal itself is classically uninvolved. Direct sigmoidoscopic pus sampling improves culture yield from blind rectal swabbing from 34% to 79%. Thayer-Martin or Stuart's culture media are used. Gram stains are unreliable and result in high false-positive rates. Empiric treatment is commenced on clinical suspicion.

As a result of a large increase in the number of penicillinase-producing strains, cefotaxime 250 mg intramuscularly followed by doxycycline 100 mg orally q12h for 7 days has become the preferred treatment to traditional procaine penicillin and oral probenecid. Other regimens include spectinomycin and cefotaxime with probenecid. Recurrence is common, with long-term failure rates of 35%.[96] Therefore, careful follow-up is required with repeat cultures at 3 months, and all contacts must be treated. Cure rate of 95% can be expected with this regimen.

Lymphogranuloma Venereum

Lymphogranuloma venereum is caused by serotypes L1–3 of *Chlamydia trachomatis* and is transmitted by oro-anal or anal receptive intercourse. An incubation period of up to 1 month is followed by the appearance of anorectal vesicular lesions, which resolve quickly, while intense inguinal lymphadenopathy develops and progresses to form an extensive tender indurated mass with overlying erythema. Acute infection causes pain and tenesmus, and constitutional symptoms are common. Unlike chlamydial proctitis, ulceration is frequent and the pronounced mucosal friability resembles that of Crohn's disease. Pronounced inguinal lymphadenopathy helps in differentiation. The lesions can be aggressive; if untreated, they fistulate into the bladder or vagina, form abscesses, or produce late rectal strictures. Chronic node inflammation can produce lower limb lymphedema. Complement fixation testing or microimmunofluorescent antibody titers confirm the diagnosis.

Treatment is with tetracycline 500 mg orally q6h or doxycycline 100 mg q12h for 21 days. Treatment of late rectal strictures is as for late chlamydial strictures.

REFRENCES

1. Kamm MA. Obstetric damage and faecal incontinence. Lancet. 1994;344:730-3.
2. Sultan AH, Kamm MA, Bartram CI, et al. Anal sphincter trauma during instrumental delivery. Int J Gynecol Obstet. 1993;43:263-70.
3. Sultan AH, Kamm MA, Hudson CN, et al. Anal sphincter disruption during vaginal delivery. N Engl J Med. 1993; 329:1905-11.
4. Hoffman DC, Goligher JC. Lateral subcutaneous internal sphincterotomy in the treatment of anal fissure. Br Med J. 1970;3:673-5.
5. Jameson JS, Chia YW, Kamm MA, et al. Effect of age, sex, and parity on anorectal function. Br J Surg. 1994;81:1689-92.
6. Jorge JM, Wexner SD. Etiology and management of fecal incontinence. Dis Colon Rectum. 1993;36:77-97.
7. Keating JP, Stewart PJ, Eyers AA, et al. Are special investigations of value in the management of patients with faecal incontinence? Dis Colon Rectum. 1997;40:896-901.
8. Malouf AJ, Norton CS, Engel AF, et al. Long term results of overlapping anterior anal sphincter repair for obstetric trauma. Lancet. 2000;355:260-5.
9. Matzel KE, Stadelmaier U, Hohenfellner M, et al. Electrical stimulation of sacral spinal nerves for treatment of faecal incontinence. Lancet. 1995;346:1124-7.
10. Wong WD, Jensen LL, Bartolo DCC, et al. Artificial anal sphincter. Dis Colon Rectum. 1996;39:1345-5l.
11. Kumar D, Benson M. GAX collagen injections: a novel treatment for faecal incontinence. Gut. 1997;40(Suppl 1):A52.
12. Tan E, Ngo NT, Darzi A, et al. Meta-analysis: sacral nerve stimulation versus conservative therapy in the treatment of faecal incontinence. Int J Colorectal Dis. 2011;26(3):275-94.
13. Leroi AM, Parc Y, Lehur PA, et al. the Study Group. Efficacy of sacral nerve stimulation for fecal incontinence: results of a multicenter double-blind crossover study[Randomized Controlled Trials]. Ann Surg. 2005;242:662-9.

14. Kamm MA, Dudding TC, Melenhorst J, et al. Sacral nerve stimulation for intractable constipation. Gut. 2010;59:333-40.
15. Michelsen HB, Christensen P, Krogh K, et al. Sacral nerve stimulation for faecal incontinence alters colonic transport. Br J Surg. 2008;95:779-84.
16. Sheldon R, Kiff E S, Clarke A, et al. Sacral nerve stimulation reduces corticoanal excitability in patients with faecal incontinence. Br J Surg. 2005;92:1423-31. doi: 10.1002/bjs.5111.
17. Duelund-Jacobsen J, van Wunnik B, Buntzen S, et al. Functional results and patient satisfaction with sacral nerve stimulation for idiopathic faecal incontinence. Colorectal Dis. 2001;14:753-9.
18. Duelund-Jacobsen J, Dudding T, Bradshaw S, et al. Randomized double-blind crossover study of alternative stimulator settings in sacral nerve stimulation for faecal incontinence. Br J Surg. 2012;99:1445-52.
19. Manning PC, Pratt JH. Faecal incontinence caused by laceration of the perineum. Arch Surg. 1964;88:569-76.
20. Setti Carraro P, Nicholls RJ. Postanal repair for faecal incontinence after rectopexy. Br J Surg. 1994;81:305-7.
21. Engel AF, Kamm MA, Sultan AH, et al. Anterior anal sphincter repair in patients with obstetric trauma. Br J Surg. 1994; 81:1231-4.
22. Simmans C, Birnbaum EH, Kodner IJ, et al. Anal sphincter reconstruction in the elderly: does advancing age affect outcome. Dis Colon Rectum. 1994;37:1065-9.
23. Yoshioka K, Hyland G, Keighley MRB. Physiological changes after pestanal repair and parameters predicting outcome. Br J Surg. 1988;75:1220-4.
24. Keighley MRB, Korsgen S. Long term results and predictive parameters of outcome following total pelvic floor repair. Dis Colon Rectum. 1996;39:A15.
25. Sielezneff I, Malouf AJ, Bartolo DCC, et al. Dynamic graciloplasty in the treatment of patients with faecal incontinence. Br J Surg. 1999;86:61-5.
26. Baeten CGMI, Gerdes BP, Adang EMM, et al. Anal dynamic graciloplasty in the treatment of intractable fecal incontinence. N Engl J Med. 1995;332:1600-5.
27. Hull T, Milsom J. Pelvic floor disorders. Surg Clin North Am. 1994;74:1399-413.
28. Jacobs LK, Lin YJ, Orkin BA. The best operation for rectal prolapse. Surg Clin North Am. 1997;77:49-70.
29. Malouf AJ, Bartolo DCC. Rectal prolapse. In: Sackier M, Wexner SD (Eds). Protocols in General Surgery; Laparoscopic Colorectal Surgery. New York: John Wiley & Sons; 1999. pp. 159-87.
30. Sioroudhis L, Ropert A, Gosselin A, et al. Constipation after rectopexy for rectal prolapse. Where is the obstruction? Dig Dis Sci. 1993;38:1801-8.
31. Browning GGP, Parks AG. Postanal repair for neuropathic faecal incontinence: correlation of clinical result and anal canal pressures. Br J Surg. 1983;70:101-4.
32. Luukkonen P, Mikkonen U, Jarvinen H. Abdominal rectopexy with sigmoidectomy vs. rectopexy alone for rectal prolapse: a prospective, randomized study. Int J Colorectal Dis. 1992;7:219-22.
33. Bartolo DCC. Rectal prolapse. Br J Surg. 1996;83:3-5.
34. Oliver GC, Vachon D, Eisenstat TE, et al. Delorme's procedure for complete rectal prolapse in severely debilitated patients: an analysis of 41 cases. Dis Colon Rectum. 1994;37:461-7.
35. Tobin SA, Scott IHK. Delorme operation for rectal prolapse. Br J Surg. 1994;81:1681-4.
36. Plusa SM, Charig JA, Balaji V, et al. Physiological changes after Delorme's procedure for full-thickness rectal prolapse. Br J Surg. 1995;82:1475-8.
37. Williams JG, Rothenberger DA, Madoff RD, et al. Treatment of rectal prolapse in the elderly by perineal rectosigmoidectomy. Dis Colon Rectum. 1992;35:830-4.
38. Ho YH, Ho JMS, Parry BR, et al. Solitary rectal ulcer syndrome: the clinical entity and anorectal physiological findings in Singapore. Aust N Z J Surg. 1995;65:93-7.
39. Nicholls J. Rectal prolapse and the solitary rectal ulcer syndrome. In: Kamm MA, Lennard Jones JE (Eds). Constipation. Petersfield: Wrightson Biomedical Publishing; 1994. pp. 289-97.
40. Womack NR, Williams NS, Holmfield JHM, et al. Pressure and prolapse—the cause of solitary rectal ulceration. Gut. 1987;28:1228-33.
41. Kang YS, Kamm MA, Engel AF, et al. Pathology of the rectal wall in solitary rectal ulcer syndrome and complete rectal prolapse. Gut. 1996;38:587-90.
42. Levine DS. 'Solitary' ulcer syndrome. Are 'solitary' rectal ulcer syndrome and 'localised' colitis cystica profunda analogous syndromes caused by rectal prolapse? [Review]. Gastroenterology. 1997;592:243-53.
43. Valenzuela M, Alvarez-Cienfuegos E, Caballero F, et al. Colitis cystica profunda: imaging, diagnosis and conservative treatment: report of two cases. Dis Colon Rectum. 1996;39:587-90.
44. Sagar PM, Pemberton JH. Anorectal and pelvic floor function. Relevance to continence, incontinence, and constipation. Gastroenterol Clin North Am. 1996;25:163-82.
45. Loder PB, Kamm MA, Nicholls RJ, et al. Haemorrhoids: pathology, pathophysiology and aetiology [Review]. Br J Surg. 1994;81:946-54.
46. Johanson JF, Sonnenberg A. The prevalence of hemorrhoids and chronic constipation: an epidemiologic study. Gastroenterology. 1990;98:380-6.
47. Medich DS, Fazio VW. Hemorrhoids, anal fissure, and carcinoma of the colon, rectum, and anus during pregnancy. Surg Clin North Am. 1995;75:77-88.
48. Gartell PC, Sheridan RJ, McGinn FP. Outpatient treatment of haemorrhoids: a randomised clinical trial to compare rubber band ligation with phenol injection. Br J Surg. 1985;72:478-9.
49. Wechter DG, Luna GK. An unusual complication of rubber band ligation of hemorrhoids. Dis Colon Rectum. 1987;30: 137-40.
50. Sim AJW, Murie JA, MacKenzie I. Three year follow-up study on the treatment of first and second degree haemorrhoids by sclerosant injection or rubber band ligation. Surg Gynecol Obstet. 1983;157:534-6.

Additional references appear in the online version of this book.

64

Diverticular Disease and Other Conditions of the Large Bowel

David E Beck

Key Points

- About one-third of the population in developed countries have acquired colonic diverticula by the age of 60 years, predominantly in the sigmoid colon; most are symptom free. Lack of dietary fiber and resultant stool bulk leads to increased luminal pressure and mucosal "blow-outs" through the muscle coat.
- Operative treatment may be required either for acute diverticulitis and its complications—peritonitis, abscess formation, and occasionally hemorrhage—or for chronic diverticulitis in the presence of fistula or stricture. Carcinoma is the important differential diagnosis. Resection is performed in one of the two stages according to circumstances.
- Ischemic colitis is usually found in arteriopaths, but it may develop "spontaneously" in renal transplant patients or those with systemic hypotension. The watershed area at the junction of midgut and hindgut (around the splenic flexure) is commonly affected. Alternative outcomes are resolution, gangrene, and delayed fibrotic stricture.
- Colorectal infections of surgical importance include pseudomembranous colitis and actinomycosis, while amebic colitis and Chagas' disease are tropical infestations.

DIVERTICULAR DISEASE

Incidence

Diverticulosis is an acquired condition, and the incidence of colonic diverticular disease has increased during this century.[1] Cruveilhier[2] in 1849 detailed the first pathologic description of diverticular disease. Over the next several years, isolated reports of colonic diverticula and related complications appeared in the literature. Subsequent autopsy and barium enema studies in the early 1900s reported a 5% incidence of diverticulosis in patients older than 40 years.[3] Since then, numerous studies conducted in industrialized nations have demonstrated an increasing prevalence of diverticulosis and its complications. The incidence of diverticulosis increases with age and reaches a peak in the sixth, seventh, and eighth decades of life. It is now reported that at least 30% of the population older than 60 years and as many as 50% of those who are 80 years of age have diverticulosis.[4-6] Diverticular disease almost never presents as a surgical emergency due to complications in Africa and India.

Colonic diverticula are false diverticula composed of mucosal pouches that protrude through the colonic musculature alongside any of the three taeniae. Typically, diverticula are located along the mesenteric side of the two antimesenteric taeniae. The mucosa escapes through the colonic musculature defect created by the vasa recta, small arteries that supply blood to the mucosa (Fig. 64.1). In 95% cases of diverticulosis, the sigmoid colon is involved, and it may be the only affected segment in 65% of cases. Cecal or right-sided diverticula are not as common, occurring in 6–7% of those patients who have diverticulosis.[7] These right-sided diverticula were once thought to represent true diverticula, but recent evidence suggests that they too are false diverticula.[1]

Pathogenesis

Several theories have been postulated to explain the increasing prevalence of diverticulosis.[8] Factors potentially predisposing to the development of colonic diverticula include the following:

- Decreased colonic wall strength
- Increased intraluminal pressure
- Decreased stool bulk
- Lack of dietary fiber

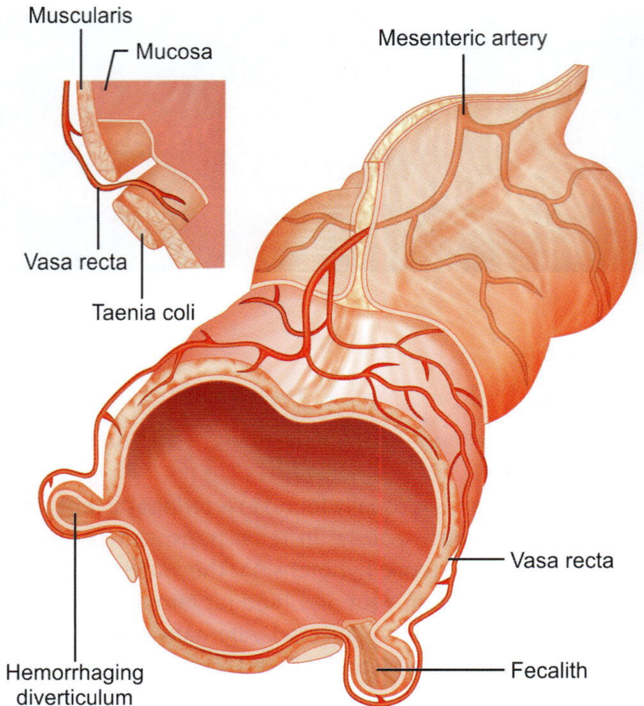

Fig. 64.1: Anatomy of colonic diverticulosis. The diverticulum occurs as mucosa protrudes through the musculature defect associated with the vasa recta. A fecalith trapped in a diverticulum may injure a vasa recta, resulting in injury.

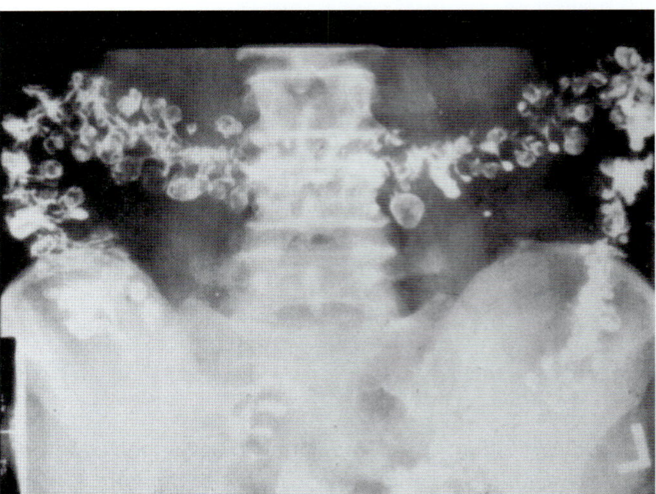
Fig. 64.2: Diverticulosis.

Table 64.1 Complications of diverticulitis.

Acute	*Chronic*
Peridiverticular inflammation	*Fistula:* Colovesical, colocutaneous, coloenteral, colovaginal
Peridiverticular abscess or phlegmon	Obstruction
Intra-abdominal or pelvic abscess	
Generalized peritonitis and hemorrhage	

No well-controlled studies have determined whether one or a combination of several factors leads to the development of diverticular disease. Painter and Burkitt[9] noted that an increase in diverticulosis correlated directly with industrialization, which leads to more refined foods and a decreased fiber consumption. Based on Laplace's law in which pressure = tension/radius, they postulated that decreased stool bulk results in a decreased colonic diameter and subsequently increased intraluminal pressure. A colon containing small stool is not distended, creating narrow segments with increased intraluminal pressure, which causes the mucosa to herniate through defects in the colonic musculature. They suggested that increasing dietary fiber might prevent diverticulosis.

Others reporting from industrialized nations reviewed dietary fiber intake and changes in stool weight for healthy patients and those who had diverticulosis and found wide variability with no significant difference between the two groups.[9,10] Clearly other factors may be involved.[10,11] Several authors have shown that the colonic wall is weakened in patients who have diverticulosis, and colonic wall tensile strength is related to the age of the patient and to changes in the colonic connective tissue.[1,10,12]

Diagnosis and Treatment

Most people who have diverticulosis remain symptom free, but as many as 10–20% develop symptoms such as infection (diverticulitis), fistula, obstruction, or hemorrhage. The inflammatory complications of diverticulitis involve a spectrum of infections (Table 64.1). Asymptomatic diverticula are occasionally documented on colonoscopy or barium enema studies obtained for other reasons (Fig. 64.2). Minimal involvement begins with peridiverticular inflammation. The infectious process may progress to a peridiverticular abscess or phlegmon. Toxicity increases as an intra-abdominal or pelvic abscess forms. Generalized peritonitis results from a free peritoneal perforation.[13] Evaluation and management can be divided into acute and chronic presentations (Table 64.1).

Acute Diverticulitis

Peridiverticular Inflammation

Inspissated stool, a fecalith trapped within a diverticulum, produces thinning of the diverticular wall, resulting in a localized contained microperforation with infection or peridiverticular inflammation. The patient typically seeks treatment for acute left lower abdominal discomfort. The abdominal examination reveals minimal lower abdominal tenderness with no appreciable mass. The patient may have low-grade fever and does not usually have a tachycardia. No further diagnostic evaluation is needed.

Management consists of broad-spectrum oral antibiotics—trimethoprim-sulfamethoxazole (cotrimoxazole), and metronidazole or doxycycline—and a fiber-restricted diet. Follow-up clinical examination should include flexible sigmoidoscopy and barium enema or colonoscopy after the inflammation has resolved (at least 3–4 weeks) to exclude other pathology.

Peridiverticular Abscess and Phlegmon

The patient may complain of moderate-to-severe left lower abdominal pain and anorexia. Abdominal examination reveals a tender mass (representing the inflamed colon) and voluntary guarding in the lower abdomen. Rebound tenderness or Rovsing's sign may also be present. The infection is localized by the adjacent structures, the abdominal wall, mesentery, omentum, small bowel, bladder, or retroperitoneal fat. Pyrexia, tachycardia, and leukocytosis are usually present. An upright chest radiograph and flat and upright abdominal radiographs exclude the presence of free intraperitoneal air or intestinal obstruction. Urinalysis excludes urinary tract infection, fecaluria, and ureterolithiasis.

The patient is best treated with hospitalization, intestinal rest, intravenous fluids, and intravenous antibiotics (e.g. ampicillin sodium-sulbactam sodium or gentamicin and clindamycin). Nasogastric decompression is generally unnecessary except for persistent emesis or obstruction.

A water-soluble contrast enema or CT scan is useful to confirm the diagnosis in atypical presentations.[14] Recently, experienced ultrasonographers have been able to identify acute diverticulitis, but this examination is operator-dependent and not as reproducible as CT or contrast enemas.

Intra-Abdominal or Pelvic Abscess

Occasionally, a patient who has a peridiverticular abscess will not improve and will develop a persistent fever, prolonged ileus, or sustained leukocytosis.[1] This clinical picture represents more than a small, contained infection. Usually, an intra-abdominal or pelvic abscess has developed. A CT scan of the abdomen and pelvis with intraluminal contrast will define the walled-off cavity. The abscess appears as a fluid-filled, often loculated collection, which may contain gas.

Ultrasonography may reveal subphrenic or pelvic abscesses, but is not useful for other intra-abdominal locations of pus. Ultrasound scan offers a portable, inexpensive, real-time method to guide percutaneous drainage of these abscesses and is particularly useful for unstable patients in the intensive care unit; CT-directed drainage of abscesses is preferred in most other cases. Percutaneous drainage allows resolution of the inflammation and a delayed one-stage operative resection. If the abscesses cannot be localized by CT or ultrasound scan or be safely drained percutaneously, operative exploration and drainage are necessary. A two-stage procedure is preferred with resection of the involved colon, colostomy, and drainage of the abscess cavity (Hartmann's procedure) as the first stage. Increasingly, resection, primary anastomosis, and protective colostomy are being used.

Generalized Peritonitis

Generalized peritonitis occurs when inflamed colon or abscess freely perforates into the peritoneal cavity. The patient usually complains of severe diffuse abdominal pain with anorexia and vomiting. The toxic patient is tachycardic, pyrexial, and dehydrated. Severe tachycardia and hypotension are signs of septic shock, which may accompany free perforation.

On examination, the abdomen is diffusely tender and there is involuntary guarding. Rebound and percussion tenderness are also usually present, and severe leukocytosis develops. An upright chest radiograph and an acute abdominal series may reveal free intraperitoneal air.

The first step in the management of peritonitis is volume replacement with intravenous fluids. Treatment also includes insertion of a nasogastric tube and urinary catheter and administration of intravenous antibiotics. Operative management should follow the correction of metabolic abnormalities. Operative treatment commonly involves resection of the involved colonic segment, colostomy (Hartmann's operation), abdominal irrigation, and drainage of any abscesses (Fig. 64.3C). A newer variation of operative management is laparoscopic lavage. Myers et al. described laparoscopic peritoneal lavage in 100 patients with perforated diverticulitis.[15] Conversion was required in eight patients, and the group experienced 4% morbidity and 3% mortality rates. Two patients required drainage of pelvic abscesses, and two others developed recurrent diverticulitis within 84 months. Since then, 11 series have been published, two prospective and nine retrospective. The studies vary significantly in disease presentation,

Table 64.2 Classification of acute perforative diverticulitis.

Hinchey stage[17]	Description	Incidence[18](%)	Mortality rate[10](%)	
			Staged resection	Primary resection
I	Pericolic or mesenteric abscess	3–31	0	5
II	Walled-off pelvic abscess	10–63	8	5
III	Generalized purulent peritonitis	17–62	17	8
IV	Generalized fecal peritonitis	2–24	64	28

operative techniques, and management of perforations. Surgeons have used two to five trocars and irrigated with 1-25 L of fluid. Some surgeons advocate mobilization of tissues, whereas others do not. All managed perforations differently: some not at all, and some with sutures, patch, or fibrin glue. The results to date indicate that mortality and morbidity are low at 2% and 17%, respectively. By comparison, Hartmann's procedure has a reported mortality rate of 10-28% and high risks for postoperative surgical site infections (20%), fistula formation (16%), and cardiovascular complications (25%). With laparoscopic lavage, failure occurred in 6% of patients in the reported series.[16] Prospective trials are currently underway, which will help define patient selection and thus which patients will benefit from this procedure.

Patients who have acute diverticulitis and perforation may present with a wide range of disease. Several classification systems have been proposed to grade these presentations and allow comparison between series. The system described by Hinchey et al.[17] (Table 64.2) is the most widely used. The incidence of the various stages varies in different series depending upon referral patterns and the surgeon's indication for operation. The surgeon who operates early and frequently on patients with acute diverticulitis will have more patients who have inflammation (Hinchey category 1), whereas those who wait may have to operate on fewer patients, but among those who come to operation there may be a higher percentage of category II or III patients.[18] Silvis and Keeman[19] reviewed several studies to determine patients' outcome relative to their stage of disease and operation performed. The mortality rates compiled by these authors are listed in Table 64.2. The retrospective nonrandomized nature of available studies does not control selection bias, which may be a factor in the lower mortality rate reported for primary resection (Table 64.2).

Chronic Diverticulitis

Diverticular Fistulas

A peridiverticular abscess may erode into an adjacent viscus, causing a fistula. The most common fistula involves the bladder (a colovesical fistula).[20] Colovesical fistulas usually occur in men, because in women the uterus is normally interposed between the colon and the bladder. Patients typically complain of urinary frequency, dysuria, pneumaturia, fecaluria, or hematuria.

Intravenous antibiotics are administered, and a urinary catheter is used during the acute infection. After the infection has been treated, the suspected colovesical fistula is confirmed. Several procedures have been used to identify colovesical fistulas, including cystoscopy, barium enema, and CT scan. Sigmoidoscopy is necessary to exclude inflammatory bowel disease or cancer. Once the fistula has been defined, patients may undergo bowel preparation and elective one-stage colonic resection with closure of the fistula. A section of bladder does not need to be removed if the attachment is caused by benign fibrosis rather than malignancy. A urinary catheter should remain in place for 5–7 days. Most surgeons obtain a cystogram before catheter removal. If the clinical picture suggests a colovesical fistula, but the fistula cannot be identified by preoperative test, operative intervention is indicated for patients who are fit for operation.

Other fistulas include colocutaneous, coloenteral, and colovaginal fistulas:

- Colocutaneous fistulas with minimal contamination can be managed conservatively; they will usually close, allowing for elective colonic resection; if contamination from a colocutaneous fistula is difficult to control, a diverting colostomy or ileostomy is performed, and once the inflammation has subsided, the involved colonic segment is resected.
- Coloenteric fistulas are uncommon and usually present with persistent diarrhea after resolution of diverticulitis; a barium upper gastrointestinal series with small bowel follow-through, barium enema, or flexible sigmoidoscopy may reveal the fistula site, and operative treatment entails elective resection of the involved small and large bowel and primary anastomosis.
- Colovaginal fistulas result in feculent drainage from the vagina and generally occur only in women who have previously undergone hysterectomy; vaginal

inspection reveals reactive granulation around the fistula, and elective operative resection of the involved colonic segment with primary anastomosis resolves the condition.

Colonic Obstruction

Colonic obstruction results from chronic fibrosis and inflammation in the sigmoid colon. It may be difficult to differentiate a diverticular stricture ("diverticuloma") from carcinoma, ischemic strictures, or inflammatory bowel disease. The obstruction may be partial or complete. Complete obstruction requires correction of electrolyte and fluid imbalances and operative intervention. A two-stage operation consisting of primary resection and end colostomy is usually preferred. Partial obstruction generally allows careful preoperative bowel preparation with one-stage elective resection and primary anastomosis. If carcinoma cannot be excluded, an oncologic resection should be performed.

Operative Procedures for Diverticulitis

Emergency Operations

In 1907, Mayo et al.[21] recommended the use of a temporary diverting colostomy and subsequent elective resection of the involved segment of the colon for the treatment of acute diverticulitis. Since then a wide range of operations have been used to treat the condition. The first operations emphasized irrigation of the peritoneal cavity, drainage of infection, and diversion of the fecal stream. Smithwick[22] in 1942 was a proponent of a three-stage procedure designed to decrease the morbidity and mortality rates of operative interventions for diverticulitis. First, the patient underwent a diverting colostomy and drainage of intra-abdominal infection. The second stage involved resection of the diseased segment. The diverting transverse colostomy was not closed until the final stage. Smithwick believed that this policy would protect the anastomosis performed in the proximity of the previously inflamed colon. However, three-stage procedures were associated with high mortality rates (29–32%)[23] because the perforated diseased segment remained after the initial fecal diversion. Colonic content could and did continue to contaminate the peritoneal cavity through the perforation.

Alternatively, the procedure of exteriorization was used to create a colostomy and remove the inflamed segment from the peritoneal cavity. However, the toxins in the inflamed colon remain a source of sepsis with access to the bloodstream. The exteriorized segment develops a malodorous serositis and produces dermatitis; these are difficult problems for even an experienced enterostomal therapist to control. Exteriorization requires sufficient mobilization of the colonic mesentery so that the diseased segment can be resected, and it is not generally recommended.

A two-stage procedure has several advantages:

- The initial procedure removes the infected colon and diverts the fecal stream with a colostomy; removing the septic focus during the initial operation reduces the mortality rate to 10–12% (from 20–25% when left behind).
- The final stage closes the colostomy.

To minimize the morbidity and mortality rates associated with additional operations (i.e. the third stage), the two-stage procedure has become the preferred operative approach. Several variations of resectional procedures have been described, including the following:

- Hartmann's procedure of operative excision, end-descending colostomy, and rectal stump closure
- Operative excision, end-descending colostomy, and mucous fistula
- Paul-Mikulicz procedure (double-barrel colostomy)
- Operative excision and primary closure with or without a protective colostomy or ileostomy[24]

Hartmann's procedure entails the removal of the inflamed sigmoid colon, closure of the rectal stump, and a descending colostomy. It removes the involved diverticular segment and facilitates the second stage of the procedure. During the second stage, closure of the colostomy usually requires no further resection of the distal segment. This colostomy takedown can often be accomplished with laparoscopic techniques.[25] If a mucous fistula is used or the distal rectal segment is longer than 15 cm, residual diverticulosis may be a source of recurrent symptoms. This retained segment of the colon often proves difficult to resect during colostomy closure because of pericolonic fibrosis remaining after the inflammation resolves. Because of comorbidity or personal choice, up to 25% of patients retain a colostomy after Hartmann's operation.

One-stage procedures for acute diverticulitis have a limited role.[26] Exploration of the abdominal cavity may reveal a mesenteric abscess or limited inflammatory reaction in the left lower quadrant, allowing the infected colon and involved mesentery to be resected with minimal contamination. Intraoperative colonic washout of the remaining colon and rectum with saline may allow a primary anastomosis, which may be protected with a diverting colostomy or ileostomy. Increasingly, laparoscopic techniques are being used in the management of

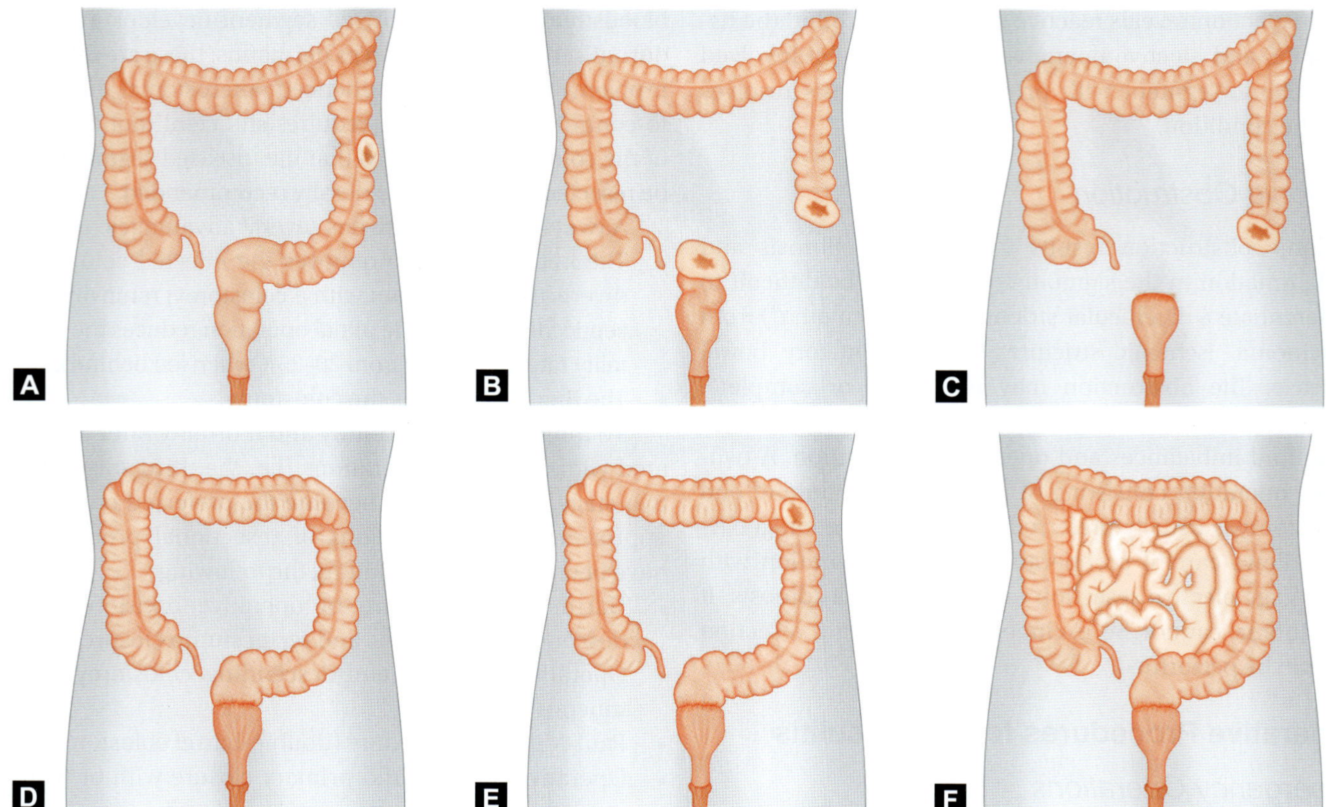

Figs. 64.3A to F: Operative treatment of diverticulitis. (A) Exteriorization; (B) resection end colostomy; (C) resection, end colostomy, oversew rectum (Hartmann's); (D) resection, primary anastomosis; (E) resection, primary anastomosis, diverting loop colostomy; and (F) resection, primary anastomosis, diverting loop ileostomy. (Adapted with permission from Opelka.[1])

diverticular disease, but their use in emergency procedures often requires advanced techniques and increased skills. Operative options are summarized in Figures 64.3A to F.

Elective Resection for Diverticulitis

Most patients who have diverticulitis do not require operative intervention. Elective resection is recommended for patients who have required hospitalization for repeated (more than three or four) attacks of moderate-to-severe diverticulitis. Treatment of acute attacks typically consists of intravenous antibiotics and intestinal rest. Repeated attacks of diverticulitis increase the risk of a complication from diverticular disease. Emergency operation for complicated diverticular disease is associated with higher morbidity and mortality rates than a one-stage elective colon resection. Therefore, elective resections are recommended for patients who have recurrent attacks.

Ouriel and Schwartz,[27] in 1983, recommended elective resection for young patients (<40 years) after their first marked attack of diverticulitis, having noted that younger patients more frequently required readmission during the follow-up period (55% of cases); 23% of patients had a serious complication and 45% of medically managed patients eventually required elective resection. Diverticulitis is less common in young patients but is associated with more complications than in older patients, and early elective operative intervention is recommended.

Elective resection is recommended in several less common situations (e.g., when radiographic or endoscopic studies cannot exclude carcinoma). Persistent urinary tract symptoms after attacks of diverticulitis also indicate possible fistula formation and suggest a need for elective resection. Immunosuppressed and transplant patients who have mild diverticular symptoms have a high incidence of complicated diverticulitis and should be considered for elective sigmoid resection.

Recent advances in laparoscopic surgery have extended the use of this technology into the area of colonic surgery.[28,29] Laparoscopic-assisted colon resection has evolved into a standardized operative technique. Initial learning curves have established criteria for the following:

Flowchart 64.1: Algorithm for the management of lower gastrointestinal hemorrhage.

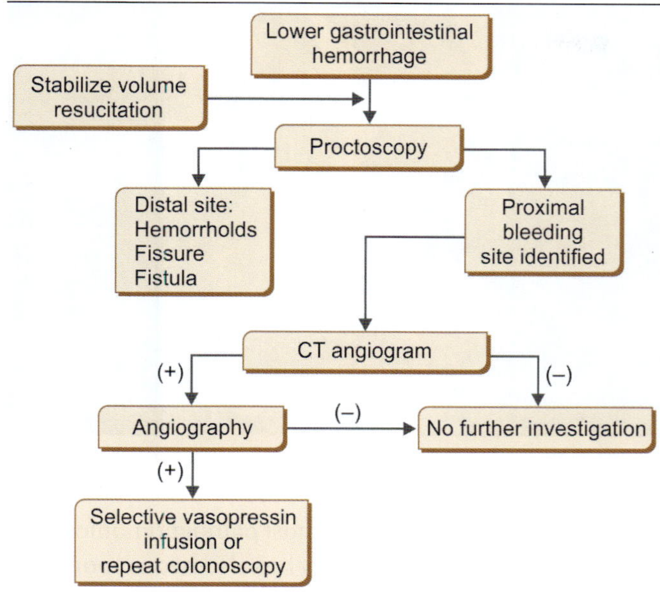

- Appropriate patient selection
- Better operative logistics
- Awareness of the dangers and pitfalls of laparoscopic surgery.

The left or sigmoid colon can be resected and delivered through a small incision. The anastomosis is performed intracorporeally or extracorporeally using standard or double-staple techniques. Most laparoscopic studies suggest a quicker return of intestinal function, decreased use of postoperative narcotics, and shorter duration of hospital stay.[28,30] The concomitant use of enhanced recovery techniques in many of these studies has made it difficult to ascribe all of the documented advantages to the use of laparoscopy alone.

Diverticular Hemorrhage

Diverticular bleeding (Flowchart 64.1) occurs in 5–15% of patients with diverticulosis, and the average age of patients with bleeding is 65 years. Elderly patients with diverticular hemorrhage have associated cardiac, pulmonary, and renal dysfunction, which contribute to the reported mortality rate of up to 20%.

Diverticular hemorrhage may be brisk, but is often self-limited.[31] The bleeding stops spontaneously with supportive management in 70–95% of cases.[1] Recurrent episodes of hemorrhage requiring a second admission to hospital occur in 25% of patients. After the second episode of diverticular hemorrhage, the chance of a third event increases to 50%.

Classic diverticular bleeding is painless. However, the cathartic effect of intracolonic blood can cause mild crampy abdominal pain. Painless lower gastrointestinal bleeding may also arise from colonic angiodysplasia, carcinoma, and Meckel's diverticulum. Marked abdominal pain associated with bleeding suggests an etiology such as ischemic colitis, whereas diarrhea suggests an inflammatory bowel or infectious etiology.

The precise mechanism of diverticular hemorrhage is unknown. The vascular anatomy of the vasa recta and the mucosal blood supply was outlined in the late 1800s, and the relationship between the vasa recta and the neck of the diverticulum was displayed in 1917 (*see* Fig. 64.1).[32] In 1976, Meyers et al.[33] defined the bleeding sites as the ruptured vasa recta in the diverticulum. They noted structural changes located eccentrically in the vasa recta at the site of rupture, intimal thickening with thinning of the media, and the absence of any acute or chronic inflammation, and stated that these vascular changes were typically the result of focal injury. It is generally accepted that thinning of the media in the vasa recta predisposes to intraluminal rupture, whereas focal injury may result from trauma related to a fecalith.

Past reports indicate that nearly 70% of patients had bleeding diverticula in the right colon.[1] However, within the past 20 years, the use of selective mesenteric angiography and endoscopy has revealed that angiodysplasias of the colon are an important alternative cause of lower gastrointestinal hemorrhage: 80% of angiodysplasias are located in the right colon, and at least 50% of patients who have angiodysplasia have diverticulosis.[34] The discovery of angiodysplasia as a source of lower gastrointestinal bleeding has created uncertainty in identifying the precise etiology in individual patients. Data from several reports further complicate the incidence of diverticular hemorrhage by attributing bleeding to angiodysplasias seen on angiography without actual contrast extravasation. Evaluation and management of gastrointestinal bleeding is discussed further in Chapter 73, "Upper and Lower Gastrointestinal Hemorrhage".

Conclusion

Diverticulosis is an increasing healthcare problem. The incidence of diverticular disease continues to increase in industrialized nations. Diverticular disease is common among the elderly population, which is itself increasing. Complications of the disease include diverticulitis, fistula, obstruction, and hemorrhage. Early diagnosis and treatment may decrease the need for emergency resection. Identification of patients for elective colon resection before diverticular complications develop can limit operative treatment to a one-stage procedure.

PNEUMATOSIS CYSTOIDES INTESTINALIS

Pneumatosis cystoides intestinalis is a rare condition in which the bowel submucosa or subserosa contains cystic pockets of gas. Although it can occur in all sections of the gut, it is most common in the small intestine. The colon is involved in 36% of collected series.[35] The male-to-female ratio has varied from 3.5 to 11, and the peak incidence is between 30 and 50 years of age.[35,36]

The three proposed etiologies for this condition are mechanical, pulmonary, and bacterial.[37] The mechanical theory suggests that gastrointestinal gas is forced by distal obstruction through mucosal defects into the submucosal lymphatics (Fig. 64.4). The gas is then distributed distally in the submucosa by peristalsis.[38] Pneumatosis cystoides intestinalis has been associated with chronic pulmonary disease; it has been postulated that severe coughing ruptures alveoli and produces pneumomediastinum,[39] and that this gas dissects down the retroperitoneum and along perivascular spaces to the bowel wall and accumulates in subserosal locations. Artificial ventilation and asthma have also been associated with pneumatosis. However, the higher hydrogen content of the cystic gas argues against a pulmonary etiology. The bacterial theory suggests that intraluminal bacteria produce submucosal gas.[40]

A number of associated conditions have been described with pneumatosis cystoides intestinalis, including pulmonary disease, inflammatory conditions of the bowel (e.g. enterocolitis, diverticulitis, Crohn's disease, and ulcerative colitis), trauma, and immunosuppression (e.g. due to transplant and chemotherapy).

Symptoms associated with pneumatosis cystoides intestinalis are related to the associated conditions or are nonspecific. Manifestations vary from no symptoms in patients in whom the condition is an incidental finding to severe symptoms including partial intestinal obstruction, diarrhea, constipation, and intestinal bleeding.[41]

Radiographically, the cysts can be seen on plain abdominal radiographs as radiolucent clusters along the bowel wall. A direct communication between the cysts and the lumen has never been demonstrated. Another radiologic finding is bilateral retroperitoneal air that does not move with patient repositioning. Identification of the cysts in asymptomatic individuals is almost pathognomonic of the disease. Computed tomography has also been reported to be useful in evaluating patients who have suspected pneumatosis cystoides intestinalis.[41]

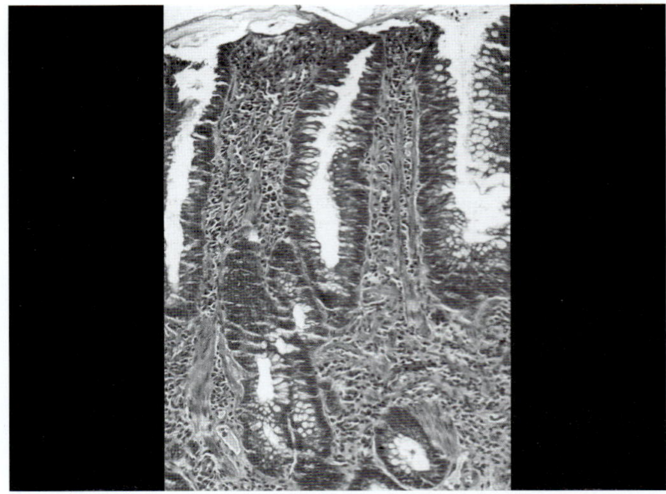

Fig. 64.4: Pneumatosis cystoides intestinalis.

Asymptomatic pneumatosis does not require treatment and may spontaneously resolve.[40] Treatment based on gas exchange was suggested in 1973.[42] Administration of high concentrations of oxygen by face mask washes out nitrogen from the lungs and increases the concentration of oxygen in the cysts. The oxygen in the cysts is either metabolized or resorbed by diffusion over 3–5 days. However, it has been suggested that this therapy works due to the toxic effect of oxygen on anaerobic gut bacteria.[43]

Another therapeutic option is administration of an elemental diet for 2 weeks. Operation is indicated when pneumatosis cystoides intestinalis is associated with the following:

- Necrosis of the bowel or sepsis
- Severe complications (volvulus, obstruction, hemorrhage)[40,44]
- A primary disease (e.g., Crohn's disease).

COLONIC ISCHEMIA

Although the colon has a generous overlapping blood supply, any interruption in blood flow produces ischemia. Potentially vulnerable anatomic locations for ischemic disease include "Griffith's point" at the splenic flexure [junction of the superior mesenteric artery (SMA) and the inferior mesenteric artery (IMA)] and "Sudeck's critical point" at the mid-sigmoid colon (junction of the IMA and hypogastric vasculature). This latter "point" remains controversial.

Table 64.3 Classification of ischemic colitis.

I. Interruption of flow in large vessels
A. After ligation during aortic surgery
B. Injury secondary to angiographic, blunt, or penetrating trauma
C. Spontaneous thrombosis of large vessels
II. Intrinsic small-vessel disease
III. Low-flow state in the critically ill
IV. Spontaneous ischemic colitis without demonstrable vessel occlusion
A. Self-limiting without sequelae
B. With subsequent stricture obstruction
V. Miscellaneous
A. Secondary to luminal obstruction
B. Young adults
C. Renal allograft recipients

Etiology and Pathophysiology

Interruption in blood flow to the colon can occur in several ways.[45] A useful scheme is presented in Table 64.3.

The incidence of colonic ischemia (endoscopic or clinical) after an aortic operation varies from 1% to 2% for elective cases to as high as 60% during emergency aneurysmectomy.[45,46] During aneurysmectomy, the IMA is usually routinely ligated, although in some patients it will have already thrombosed. Sigmoid or left colonic ischemia occurs in these circumstances if the collateral circulation from the SMA via the marginal artery is insufficient to supply the oxygen demands of the left colon. The adequacy of colonic circulation can also be compromised by large fluid shifts and the use of vasoactive drugs. Measurement of the IMA stump pressure in patients who have a patent IMA, identification of Doppler signals on the bowel surface, and measurement of intraluminal pH have all been used to predict which patients have the highest risk for developing ischemia after IMA ligation.[47,48] Sudden occlusion of the IMA can also occur as a result of angiographic trauma with subintimal dissection or as a result of either blunt or penetrating abdominal trauma (Table 64.3).

Atheromatous narrowing or occlusion of the IMA is not unusual. However, in most cases this occurs gradually and the collateral circulation from the SMA can compensate for the decrease in flow through collateral circulation via the marginal artery. If the IMA becomes acutely thrombosed or occluded with embolus and the collateral circulation is inadequate, the clinical picture is similar to that found after IMA ligation during operations for aortic aneurysm.

Any of the connective tissue diseases that produce inflammation in the small arteries (intrinsic small-vessel disease) can result in colonic ischemia. This condition has been described in polyarteritis nodosa, systemic lupus erythematosus, rheumatoid arthritis, dermatomyositis, primary amyloidosis, and Degos' disease. These diseases can cause ischemia in the small and large bowel. Colonic ischemia due to small-vessel disease has also been described in patients who have diabetes mellitus and chronic renal failure.

Spontaneous ischemic colitis in people who were previously well was described in the 1960s.[49,50] The ischemia occurs without any demonstrable vessel occlusion on angiography. The pathologic changes seen in the colon are identical to those reproduced in the laboratory with vessel occlusion; the presumption is that this entity is due to decreased flow to the colon. The spectrum of disease varies from mild submucosal edema to frank full-thickness necrosis. Most cases are the milder self-limiting variety that is typically seen in middle-aged or elderly patients.

In younger patients, the clinical syndrome is identical to that of the spontaneous ischemic colitis seen in the older age group. As most these reported cases occur in women, some authors have proposed an association between this form of ischemic colitis and the use of oral contraceptives.[51]

Ischemic colitis has also been reported in approximately 1–2% of renal allograft recipients.[52-54] Another variant of ischemic colitis occurs in patients who are severely ill with conditions that cause either hypotension, decreased cardiac output, or peripheral vasoconstriction, with a decreased flow to the end-organ (low-flow states). This group of patients appears to have a higher incidence of full-thickness necrosis and a preponderance of right-sided colonic involvement.

The mortality rate associated with colonic infarction is extremely high (57% in a group of 17 patients).[55] A very high index of suspicion for full-thickness necrosis and a readiness to intervene early are needed for this group of patients.

Diagnosis

Mild colonic ischemia usually presents with diffuse and bloody diarrhea. Patients who have frank colonic infarction frequently develop acidosis, glucose intolerance, renal failure, obvious sepsis, and abdominal distension or tenderness.

A diagnosis of postoperative ischemia can be made with flexible sigmoidoscopy performed at the bedside. If the symptoms are not explained by flexible sigmoidoscopy, a colonoscopy is occasionally required to rule out more proximal disease. The endoscopic appearance of colonic ischemia may range from submucosal edema with hemorrhage and ulceration to the dusky blue color of the mucosa of infarcted bowel. The submucosal edema produces the radiological feature called "thumbprinting." Frank gangrene mandates immediate operation and resection. Patients who have "just" mucosal edema and hemorrhage may be watched closely. The endoscopy is repeated in 24 hours, and operation is recommended if the lesion appears to be progressive. This approach should enable the surgeon to intervene before perforation occurs. Some authors suggest that flexible endoscopy is carried out routinely after aortic aneurysm resections because endoscopic findings may precede the development of symptoms.[56] The hope is that early recognition facilitates more effective and timely treatment of this condition, which is associated with a 40% mortality rate.

Patients who have spontaneous ischemic colitis typically present with a sudden onset of usually mild, crampy lower abdominal pain, mostly on the left side. Often bloody diarrhea is noted within 24 hours of the onset of pain. On physical examination, the left lower quadrant is tender to palpation. There is often an accompanying fever or tachycardia. The diagnosis can be made with CT scanning, barium enema, or endoscopy. Endoscopy can be carried out in the office or at the bedside, and the pathology can be viewed directly. A barium enema study performed soon after the onset of the pain will show a typical thumbprinting pattern, which is the result of submucosal edema and hemorrhage. A barium enema is contraindicated if there are peritoneal signs, sepsis, or a strong suspicion of bowel necrosis. This serious clinical picture is, however, unusual. The increasing availability of CT scanning has made this the most common current method of diagnosis. CT findings of ischemia include the thickened bowel wall and pericolonic fat stranding together with gas in the wall of the bowel.

There are three possible outcomes of ischemic colitis:

1. Resolution of the process is the most common clinical course—typically, the symptoms will subside over a few days to a week or so and recovery will be complete without any sequelae; repeat episodes are rare.
2. Progression to full-thickness necrosis—unusual, especially if there is no evidence of gangrenous bowel at the first examination; in one experience it occurred only twice in 174 patients.[50]
3. Evolution to an ulcerative stage, which may eventually result in stricture formation—during the ulcerative stage, the endoscopic and radiographic findings may mimic those of Crohn's disease; occasionally, the early phases of this disease are unnoticed or undiagnosed and the patient presents with a stricture.

The differential diagnosis of a chronic stricture includes inflammatory bowel disease or malignancy. If the strictured area can be adequately examined, is asymptomatic, and biopsies can be taken to rule out malignancy, no resectional procedure needs be done. If the stricture cannot be completely examined endoscopically or it is causing symptoms, a resection is indicated.

Ischemic colitis may also be associated with a complete or partial bowel obstruction. In one series, 10% of patients who had colonic ischemia had an associated carcinoma and another 10% had another condition that potentially interfered with colonic motility.[49] When ischemic colitis occurs in association with the tumor, the ischemic area is usually proximal to the tumor and may or may not be associated with obstruction. It has been speculated that colonic blood flow can decrease as a consequence of increased intraluminal pressure, hyperperistalsis with increased muscular spasm and resultant diminution in blood flow in the colonic wall, or a decrease in aortic blood pressure and vena caval return during straining at stool in the presence of an obstructive lesion.[57] Knowledge of this association is important so as to avoid using ischemic bowel for an anastomosis.

Management

If the diagnosis of ischemic colitis is made early, conservative therapy is warranted. Mild cases can be managed as outpatients, with a clear liquid diet, close observation, and possibly antibiotics.[58] More severe cases require hospitalization, bowel rest, nasogastric suction, and optimizing blood flow to the mucosa (intravenous hydration and optimization of cardiac output). If the patient is taking digoxin, a serum level should be checked because toxic digoxin levels can have a marked vasoconstrictive effect on the visceral circulation.

Some surgeons use parenteral antibiotics (such as second- or third-generation cephalosporins) because of the suggestion that colonic ischemia may allow colonic bacterial transmigration.[59] Ischemia caused by arteritides may respond to corticosteroid treatment.

Specific indications for operation include peritonitis, perforation, sepsis, and failure of nonoperative therapy.[59] At operation, a wide resection of nonviable colon is performed. Primary anastomosis is usually unsafe due to the potential for postoperative progression of the ischemia.

A double-barrel stoma or end-stoma and separate mucous fistula is safer and allows postoperative assessment of the bowel viability.

The mortality rate for ischemic colitis in renal transplant patients may be as high as 70%. Diagnostic maneuvers should be initiated at the first suspicion of ischemia in these high-risk patients, and operative management should be aggressive once the diagnosis has been made (resection of any compromised bowel with an end-stoma). Primary anastomosis after resection is ill advised in these cases.

COLORECTAL INFECTIONS

Pseudomembranous Colitis

Pseudomembranous colitis is a consequence of overgrowth of *Clostridium difficile* and its toxin.[60] Although up to 40% of newborns may harbor this organism and its toxin without harm, a potentially lethal enterocolitis can develop in older children and adults, usually after antibiotic administration.[61] The *C. difficile* toxin affects the large bowel mucosa, producing watery diarrhea, fever, and leukocytosis. Symptoms may develop during or several weeks after antibiotic administration. Severe cases may progress to a toxic megacolon.

Endoscopy is helpful to support the diagnosis. Macroscopic findings vary from normal mucosa to mild inflammation to characteristic white or yellow adherent plaque-like membranes on inflamed mucosa. In at least 50% of antibiotic-associated colitis cases, there are no membranes, and involvement of the large bowel may be patchy or segmental.[62] A confirmatory diagnosis of *C. difficile* colitis is made by tissue culture assay of a stool sample for *C. difficile* toxin. Overgrowth of other organisms has been associated with *C. difficile*-negative colitis.[63]

Treatment starts with discontinuing the antibiotics, which resolves the diarrhea in most patients. If antibiotics must be continued or the diarrhea persists, specific therapy is indicated:

- The initial drug of choice is metronidazole 250–500 mg orally qd for 10 days.[63]
- A more costly alternative is vancomycin 250–500 mg orally qd for 10 days.
- Fidaxomicin 200 mg bid for 10 days.
- Other options include bacitracin.

Failure of the primary course of therapy or recurrence is usually treated with an additional or longer course of therapy or an alternative drug. Another option is fecal microbial transplantation.[64,65] The technique seeks to reestablish colonic flora that inhibit *C. difficile*. Donor material is usually obtained from a close relative and is tested for infectious organisms and then administered to the colon with an enema or colonoscopic instillation.

A small percentage of patients with severe *C. difficile* infection will require emergency operation for toxic megacolon, with or without bowel perforation. The most common operation performed is total colectomy with end ileostomy. A meta-analysis of 31 studies from 1989 to 2011 (1433 patients) documented a 30-day mortality rate of 41% and a high morbidity rate.[66] Death is more likely to occur with preoperative intubation, acute renal failure, multiple organ failure and shock requiring vasopressors.

Due to the high mortality and morbidity rates, alternatives to operation have been explored. One is loop ileostomy followed by antegrade colonic lavage and irrigation.[67] After the ileostomy is created, a Malecot catheter is placed in the efferent limb of the ileostomy and high-volume polyethylene glycol/electrolyte solution is infused to clear the *C. difficile*. The fluid is collected via a rectal drainage tube. Postoperatively, patients then receive antegrade Vancomycin flushes (500 mg in 500 mL of lactated Ringer's q 8 hours) via the Malecot catheter along with intravenous Metronidazole (500 mg q 8 hours) for 10 days. This method was associated with a 19% mortality rate.

Actinomycosis

Actinomycosis is caused by *Actinomyces israelii,* a non-acid-fast organism. This organism can cause proctitis, abscesses, and fistulas. The infection can also occur in the ileocecal region. The diagnosis can be confirmed by identifying characteristic "sulfur" bodies with club-shaped rays in sinus discharges. The infection is treated with penicillin.

Other Bacterial Colitis

Escherichia coli Colitis

Infectious diarrhea resulting from *E. coli* infection is generally a self-limiting diarrheal syndrome, but the *E. coli* 0157:H7 strain produces a severe and potentially life-threatening hemorrhagic colitis.[68] Patients develop crampy abdominal pain and watery diarrhea that progresses to bloody mucorrhea and potentially a hemolytic uremic syndrome.[69] Endoscopically, there are scattered ulcerations in the colon, with edema and occasionally a dusky mucosa. Diagnosis is confirmed by stool culture. Treatment is supportive because antimicrobial agents have not been shown to modify the disease. Symptoms typically last 4–7 days.[70]

Salmonella Colitis

Infection with salmonella usually results in a self-limited secretory diarrheal illness due to small bowel involvement, but colitis can also occur. Endoscopic findings are nonspecific and include scattered edema and ulceration. Diagnosis is confirmed by stool or blood culture. Supportive therapy is indicated, and operation is necessary only for intestinal perforation. Chloramphenicol remains the drug of choice.

Shigella Colitis

Shigella spp. are virulent gram-negative rods that invade the small bowel and colonic mucosa and cause a characteristic illness known as bacillary dysentery. They are spread by ingestion of contaminated food and water and through person-to-person contact. The symptoms and physical findings vary according to the anatomic location of the infection.

Shigella spp. first infect and invade the small bowel, causing crampy abdominal pain, high fever, and large volumes of watery diarrhea. Usually within 2 days, the infection moves on to the colon. Colonic involvement corresponds with the development of more severe lower abdominal pain, the onset of bloody mucoid diarrhea, urgency, and tenesmus.[71] There is often marked abdominal tenderness in the lower quadrants at this stage. Frequently, the clinical presentation mimics that of acute appendicitis.[72]

Shigellosis should be suspected whenever an acute diarrheal illness producing bloody mucoid stools lasts longer than 2 days. The diagnosis is made by stool culture of a fresh specimen or immunofluorescent antibody labeling. Sigmoidoscopy often reveals inflamed, ecchymotic, friable, or ulcerated mucosa.

In most cases the illness is self-limited, lasting an average of 1 week.[73] However, untreated patients shed viable organisms for up to 1 month after symptoms resolve. Antibiotic treatment shortens the clinical illness and limits the duration of active shedding of the organisms. For these reasons, most authors recommend antibiotic treatment with ampicillin, tetracycline, ciprofloxacin, or trimethoprim-sulfamethoxazole.[71,74] Since Shigella spp. develop antibiotic resistance rapidly, it is important to check culture sensitivities.[75] Antimotility agents are contraindicated. Symptomatic patients and screened asymptomatic carriers should be treated until proven cured by repeat stool cultures.

Postdysentery irritable bowel syndrome can be a problem in some patients after elimination of the pathogen.

Amebic Colitis

It is estimated that more than 10% of the earth's population is infested with the intestinal protozoan parasite *Entamoeba histolytica.* In certain subpopulations, especially immigrants, institutionalized patients, promiscuous homosexual men, and patients with AIDS, the infestation rate is substantially higher.[68,76,77] In some studies, the incidence in institutionalized patients such as the mentally retarded is greater than 70%.[78] The disease is limited to a mild dysentery in most patients who develop symptoms. However, in a small percentage of patients, fulminant amebic colitis ensues, and these patients may require operation.[68,79]

The adult parasite or trophozoite populates the colon. Both trophozoites and an encysted form of the organism are intermittently shed in the stool. Although trophozoites quickly die outside the body, the cysts do not. Infection occurs when these cysts find their way into food or drinking water, usually via asymptomatic carriers. The ingested cysts release their trophozoites in the small bowel, and these then populate the colon. In general, they survive by feeding on bacteria and superficial mucosal cells. In a small percentage (<5%) of patients, the amebae invade the colonic wall and may disseminate to the liver, resulting in the formation of an amebic liver abscess. In 60–70% of cases, there is a pancolitis; in the remaining patients, infection is localized to one or several segments of the colon.[80] The most commonly involved colonic segments, in descending order of frequency, are the cecum, the ascending colon, the rectum, and the sigmoid colon.[81]

Clinical Features

Most symptomatic patients have mild disease manifested by diarrhea (sometimes bloody), mild abdominal pain, and tenderness. There may be tenesmus and a mild leukocytosis. In contrast, patients with severe disease usually have frankly bloody diarrhea as well as severe abdominal pain and marked tenderness. In such cases, fever, tachycardia, dehydration, and other evidence of systemic toxicity also tend to be present.[82]

Diagnosis

The diagnosis is confirmed by identification of motile trophozoites containing ingested red blood cells (hemocytophagia) in fresh stool. Multiple samples are submitted, and special preparation of the specimens is carried out by the laboratory. The detection rate can be as high as 92%.[81]

A number of serologic tests can be used to diagnose amebic infection, including the indirect hemagglutination test (which is the most sensitive), the indirect immunoelectrophoresis test, and an enzyme-linked immunosorbent assay (ELISA). Using these tests, antibodies or antigens can be detected in 82–91% of patients who have amebic colitis. A positive test result is not necessarily indicative of acute disease because the antibodies may persist for years after eradication of infection and asymptomatic carriers may test positive.[80] In addition, the antibody tests may be negative early in acute infection and should be repeated after 5–7 days if initially negative.[77]

Endoscopic evaluation without bowel preparation should be performed on all patients. Sigmoidoscopy is sufficient for most patients because distal disease is present in up to 85%.[68] Findings vary: diffuse erythema and mild nonspecific changes may be all that is found. The "classic" findings are round ulcerations ("flask-shaped" on microscopic section), 0.2–2 cm in diameter, covered with a yellow exudate and with normal-appearing mucosa between ulcers.[82] The ulcer has a small mucosal opening with a wider base in the submucosa or muscularis propria. Biopsies of the ulcer margins should be examined for pathology. Examination of endoscopically obtained stool and mucus samples for trophozoites will document amebic infection in up to 85% of cases.[82,83]

Management

Metronidazole (750 mg orally q 8 hours for 10 days) is the treatment of choice for most patients because it provides amebicidal concentrations both systemically and in the bowel lumen. Patients with severe colitis who cannot tolerate oral agents must be given intravenous dehydroemetine or emetine, the only parenterally administered drugs that provide adequate tissue and luminal drug concentrations. Adverse cardiac effects are often associated with both these agents, so frequent electrocardiograms are advisable during a course of treatment and the duration of treatment should be limited to 2 or 3 days. Oral metronidazole should be substituted for these drugs as soon as possible.[82] A course of iodoquinol, 650 mg orally qd for 3 weeks, is necessary after completion of primary therapy to ensure full eradication of amebic cysts from the colonic lumen.[80] Asymptomatic carriers need receive only iodoquinol 650 mg orally qd for 20 days.[82] A follow-up stool examination should be obtained after treatment has ended.[74]

From 3–11% of symptomatic patients develop fulminant colitis, which can perforate and require operation.[68,79,83] These patients present with severe bloody diarrhea, fever, and diffuse abdominal tenderness. Toxic dilatation of the colon may be present.[68] Most authorities agree that segmental or total abdominal colectomy with diverting ileostomy or colostomy is necessary in these gravely ill patients. Despite such operative treatment, the mortality rate of fulminant disease ranges from 66% to 83%.[68]

Ameboma

An inflammatory mass known as an ameboma may develop and can be difficult to distinguish from a carcinoma. This lesion has a fibrous outer wall and contains hyperplastic lymphatic tissue, acute inflammatory cells, trophozoites, and necrotic debris.[84] The most common location is the cecum, followed by the sigmoid colon. This granulomatous lesion may also cause an acute inflammatory reaction or a chronic fibrous stricture, most commonly found in the anus, rectum, or sigmoid colon. Rare complications include complete obstruction, severe hemorrhage, or intussusception with the ameboma forming the leading edge.

An ameboma is usually found on barium enema or endoscopy. In the absence of perforation or complete obstruction, it should be treated nonoperatively as most resolve with appropriate amebicidal therapy.[80] Those that do not resolve must be reevaluated and biopsied to avoid missing a neoplasm. Although uncommon, anorectal abscesses and fistulas have been reported.[84]

Chagas' Disease

Chagas' disease is caused by the protozoan *Trypanosoma cruzi*.[85] Most new infections in humans are acquired from insect vectors, but recently transmission by transfusion and transplantation has become an important source of infection.[86,87] The disease is endemic in Central and South America, and almost all of the cases seen in the United States are in immigrants from these areas.[88]

Clinical Features

The acute phase of the disease lasts 2–4 months and is usually a mild illness. Symptomatic chronic Chagas' disease develops in 10–30% of patients.[89] The heart is most frequently affected, followed by the gastrointestinal system. The gastrointestinal manifestations, mainly megacolon and megaesophagus, usually become evident many years after the acute infection.[90] The most commonly involved segments of bowel are the sigmoid colon and rectum.[91]

Intestinal dilatation is thought to result from the destruction of the autonomic nerve plexuses of the intestinal wall that occurs during the acute phase of infection. Microscopically, there is marked destruction of Auerbach's myenteric and Meissner's submucosal plexuses.[92]

The most common presenting symptoms of megacolon are progressive constipation and obstipation. Sigmoid volvulus occurs in 10–27% of patients who have megacolon.[93,97]

Diagnosis

Contrast enema usually reveals a markedly dilated sigmoid colon and rectum. The acute phase of the disease is diagnosed by detecting parasites on blood smears. The diagnosis of chronic infection depends upon detecting antibodies using complement fixation tests or ELISA, because parasites are no longer detectable on blood smears.[89,90] More recently, however, the polymerase chain reaction has proven to be an effective and highly sensitive method for detecting chronic infection.[95,96]

Management

The results of medical treatment for patients who have chronic infection have generally been disappointing. However, recent studies show that treatment of early chronic infection with benznidazole is effective in producing negative seroconversion in 55% of cases.[97]

Controversy exists about the best operation for chagasic megacolon. Most agree that rectosigmoid resection is necessary. If more proximal colon is dilated, that should also be resected. A variety of different techniques can be used to restore distal continuity, including low colorectal anastomoses, coloanal anastomoses, or a modified two-stage Duhamel procedure.[91,92] Dehiscence of the anastomosis has been a marked problem with all techniques involving immediate anastomosis and has led many surgeons to recommend two- or three-stage procedures.[91,94,98] Currently, the most popular technique is the modified two-stage Duhamel procedure. There is, however, increasing use of laparoscopic techniques for the treatment of this disease.[99]

REFERENCES

1. Opelka FG. Diverticular disease. In: Beck DE (Ed). Handbook of Colorectal Surgery. St. Louis: Quality Medical Publishing; 1997. pp. 217-33.
2. Cruveilhier J. Traite Anat Pathol Paris 1849;1:593-5.
3. Heller SN, Hackler LR. Changes in the crude fiber content of the American diet. Am J Clin Nutr. 1978;31:1510-4.
4. Gordon PH. Diverticular disease of the colon. In: Gordon PH, Nivatvongs S (Eds). Principles and Practice of the Surgery for the Colon, Rectum, and Anus. St. Louis: Quality Medical Publishing; 1992. pp. 739-97.
5. Parks TG. Natural history of diverticular disease of the colon. Clin Gastroenterol. 1975;4:53-69.
6. Morson BC. Pathology of diverticular disease of the colon. Clin Gastroenterol. 1975;4:37-52.
7. Rankin FW, Brown PW. Diverticulitis of the colon. Surg Gynecol Obstet. 1930;50:836-47.
8. Ryan P. Changing concepts in diverticular disease. Dis Colon Rectum. 1983;26:12-8.
9. Painter NS, Burkitt DP. Diverticular disease of the colon: a deficiency disease of Western civilization. Br Med J. 1971;2:450-4.
10. Arfwidsson S. Pathogenesis of multiple diverticula of the sigmoid colon in diverticular disease. Acta Chir Scand. 1964; 63(Suppl 342):1-68.
11. Eastwood MA. Colonic diverticulosis. Medical and dietary management. Clin Gastroenterol. 1975;4:85-97.
12. Whiteway J, Morson BC. Pathology of the ageing diverticular disease. Clin Gastroenterol. 1985;14:829-46.
13. Chappus CW, Cohn I. Acute colonic diverticulitis. Surg Clin N Am. 1988;68:302-13.
14. Hulnick DH, Megibow AJ, Balthazar EJ, et al. Computed tomography in the evaluation of diverticulitis. Radiology. 1984;152:491-5.
15. Myers E, Hurley M, O'Sullivan GC, et al. Laparoscopic peritoneal lavage for generalized peritonotis due to perforated diverticulitis. Br J Surg. 2008;96(1):97-101.
16. Hass E. Laparoscopic lavage: new standard for acute perforated diverticulitis? Vancoover, CA: ASCRS Annual Meeting; May 2011.
17. Hinchey, EJ, Schaal PGH, Richards GK. Treatment of perforated disease of the colon. Adv Surg. 1978;12:86-109.
18. Gordon PH. Diverticular disease of the colon. In: Gordon PH, Nivatvongs S (Eds). Principles and Practice of Surgery for the Colon, Rectum and Anus. St. Louis: Quality Medical Publishing; 1999. pp. 975-1043.
19. Silvis R, Keeman JN. Complicated diverticulitis in acute surgery. Neth J Surg. 1988;409:117-20.
20. Corman ML, ed. Colon and rectal surgery, 2nd ed. Philadelphia: Lippincott; 1989. pp. 665-702.
21. Mayo WJ, Wilson LB, Griffin HZ. Acquired diverticulitis of the large intestine. Surg Gynecol Obstet. 1907;5:8-15.
22. Smithwick RH. Experiences with surgical management of diverticulitis of sigmoid. Ann Surg. 1942;115:969-85.
23. Bonello JC, Howerton RA. Single-stage resection without coloctomy in acute diverticulitis. Semin Colon Rectal Surg. 1990;1:81-6.
24. Greif JM, Fried G, McSherry CK. Surgical treatment of perforated diverticulitis of the sigmoid colon. Dis Colon Rectum. 1980;23:483-7.
25. Beck DE. Minimally invasive surgery. In: Beck DE (Ed). Handbook of Colorectal Surgery. St. Louis: Quality Medical Publishing; 1997. pp. 79-104.
26. Marshall SF. Earlier resection in one stage for diverticulitis of the colon. Am Surg. 1963;29:337-46.

27. Ouriel K, Schwartz SI. Diverticular disease in the young patient. Surg Gynecol Obstet. 1983;156:1-5.
28. Beart RW. Laparoscopic colectomy: status of the art. Dis Colon Rectum. 1994;37(Suppl 2):S47-9
29. Bruce CJ, Coller JA, Murray JJ, et al. Laparoscopic resection for diverticular disease. Dis Colon Rectum. 1996;39:S1-6.
30. Senagore AJ, Duepree HJ, Delaney CP, et al. Cost structure of laparoscopic and open sigmoid colectomy for diverticular disease. Dis Colon Rectum. 2002;45(4):485-90.
31. Opelka FG, Timmcke AE. Management of bleeding diverticulosis. Semin Colon Rectal Surg. 1990;1:109-15.
32. Drumond H. Sacculi of intestine. Br J Surg. 1917;4:407-13.
33. Meyers MA, Alonso DR, Gray GF, et al. Pathogenesis of bleeding colonic diverticulosis. Gastroenterology. 1976;71:577-83.
34. Boley SJ, DiBiase A, Brandt U, et al. Lower intestinal bleeding in the elderly. Am J Surg. 1979;137:57-64.
35. Jamart J. Pneumatosis cystoides intestinalis: a statistical study of 919 cases. Acta Hepato Gastroenterol. 1979;26:419-22.
36. Stone HH, Webb HW, Kovalchik MT III. Pneumatosis intestinalis of Infancy. Surg Gynecol Obstet. 1970;130:806-12.
37. Reyna R, Soper RT, Condon RE. Pneumatosis intestinalis: report of twelve cases. Am J Surg. 1973;125:667-71.
38. Koss LG. Abdominal gas cysts (pneumatosis cystoides intestinorum homlnis): analysis with report of a case and critical review of literature. Arch Pathol. 1952;53:523-49.
39. Keyting WS, McCarver RR, Kovarik JL, et al. Pneumatosis intestinalis: a new concept. Radiology. 1961;76:733-41.
40. Gordon PH. Misellaneous entities. In: Gordon PH, Nivatvongs S (Eds). Principles and Practice of Surgery of the Colon, Rectum, and Anus. St. Louis: Quality Medical Publishing; 1992. pp. 1054-9.
41. Caudill JL, Ross BS. The role of computed tomography in the evaluation of pneumatosis intestinalis. J Clin Gastroenterol. 1987;9:223-6.
42. Forgacs P, Wright PH, Wyatt AP. Treatment of intestinal gas cysts by oxygen breathing. Lancet. 1973;1:579-82.
43. Down RHL, Castleden WM. Oxygen therapy for pneumatosis coli. Br Med J. 1975;1:493-4.
44. Galandiuk S, Fazio VW. Pneumatosis cystoides intestinalis: review of the literature. Dis Colon Rectum. 1986;29:358-63.
45. Haglhara PF, Ernst CB, Griffen WO Jr. Incidence of ischemic colitis following abdominal aortic reconstruction. Surg Gynecol Obstet. 1979;149:571-3.
46. Johnson WC, Nabseth DC. Visceral infarction following aortic surgery. Ann Surg. 1974;180:312-8.
47. Bulkley GB, Zuidema GD, Hamilton SR, et al. Intraoperative determination of small intestinal viability following ischemic injury: a prospective, controlled trial of two adjuvant methods (Doppler and fluorescein) compared with standard clinical judgement. Ann Surg. 1981;193:628-37.
48. Ernst CB, Hagihara PF, Daugherty ME, et al. Inferior mesenteric artery stump pressure: a reliable index for safe IMA ligation during abdominal aortic aneurysmectomy. Ann Surg. 1978;187:641-6.
49. Boley SJ, Schwartz S, Lash J, Sternhill V. Reversible vascular occlusion of the colon. Surg Gynecol Obstet. 1963;116:53-60.
50. Marston A, Pheils MT, Thomas ML, et al. Ischaemic colitis. Gut. 1966;7:1-15.

Additional references appear in the online version of this book.

Case Study: 65
Synchronous Colonic Cancer with Liver Metastases and Threatened Obstruction

James ML Williamson, Jeremy JT Tate

THE PROBLEM

The incidence of synchronous colorectal carcinoma (one or more primary cancers detected at time of initial presentation) is approximately 2–5% for sporadic cancers, increasing to 10–20% in patients with polyposis conditions or ulcerative colitis. Some 25% of patients with any primary colorectal cancer present with hepatic metastases. Hepatic resection of colorectal liver metastases (CRM) offers the best chance of long-term survival and is often performed before removal of the colonic primary tumor. Advances in chemotherapy (and portal vein embolization) have increased the numbers of patients suitable for operative intervention; thus all patients with CRM should be discussed at a hepatopancreatobiliary multidisciplinary meeting. However, the colonic primary may present with obstructive symptoms that demand operative relief and thus preclude neoadjuvant chemotherapy. Patients with synchronous colonic lesions should be assessed for either an extended colonic resection or two separate resections, balancing possible diarrhea against the risk of two anastomoses.

THE TYPICAL CASE

A 53-year-old man was investigated for altered bowel habit and iron deficiency anemia with both upper and lower gastrointestinal endoscopy. Gastroscopy showed esophagitis, while colonoscopy detected two malignant-looking masses (at 40 cm from the anus and within the ascending colon) plus multiple colonic polyps. Each probable cancer was tattooed and biopsied; histopathological examination revealed moderately differentiated tubulovillous adenocarcinoma. Urgent computed tomography (CT) confirmed two synchronous lesions: a 10 cm annular tumor in the ascending colon and a 4 cm semiannular tumor in the proximal sigmoid colon. Each carcinoma was associated with localized lymphadenopathy, and five low-attenuation lesions were seen in segments V, VI, VII, and VIII of the liver; an incidental lung lesion was also noted. Before further investigation could be performed to clarify the disease burden, the patient was admitted as an emergency with abdominal pain and distension, nausea, and absolute constipation.

Examination revealed gross painless abdominal distension, with scanty but nonobstructive bowel sounds and an empty rectum. Colonic obstruction was suspected at the level of the sigmoid lesion, and management options were considered. He was treated conservatively with nasogastric intubation, catheterization, and intravenous fluids pending urgent repeat CT, which then confirmed the two primary tumors and hepatic metastases but did not show actual colonic obstruction. He began to pass flatus, so supportive measures were withdrawn as his symptoms resolved. He then completed his staging investigations: both magnetic resonance imaging (MRI) and CT positron emission scanning (PET) showed bilobar liver disease, with CTPET confirming no other sites of signal uptake apart from the known colonic tumors (Fig. 65.1). The patient was discharged and was commenced on neoadjuvant chemotherapy with a view to downstaging his metastatic disease to allow hepatic resection and subtotal colectomy.

DIAGNOSTIC DILEMMAS

This case illustrates some of the difficulties in managing patients with advanced colorectal cancer and how acute obstruction can impact on decision making. This patient has two colonic primary cancers (with multiple polyps in between) that are locally resectable plus bilobar liver disease and a further indeterminate lung lesion. The nature of this lung lesion (and the presence of any further extra-colonic deposits) is crucial to determine the extent of metastatic disease and thus the appropriate therapeutic options. Moreover, the extent of hepatic disease will greatly influence the management of these metastases by helping to decide whether operative resection is a viable

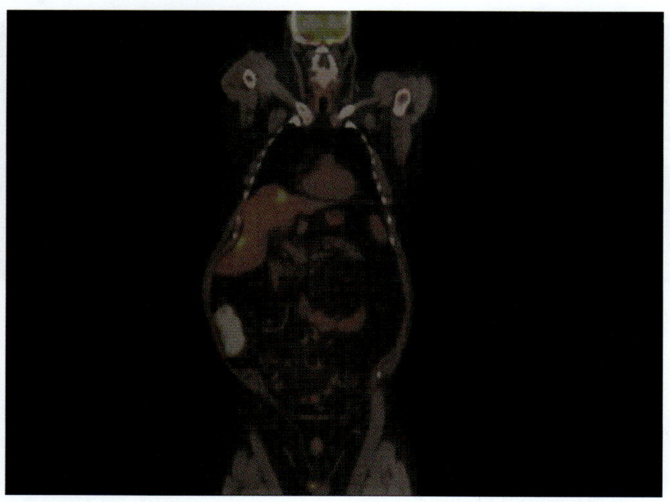

Fig. 65.1: Computed tomography positron emission scanning (CTPET) showing high signal uptake in both lobes of the liver, consistent with metastatic colorectal cancer.

option (with or without portal vein embolization to ensure a functional liver remnant) or whether chemotherapy is needed first to reduce the liver burden. Further assessment of the liver, in the form of a hepatobiliary contrast MRI, is performed to detect the extent of disease laparoscopy, and laparoscopic ultrasound is an alternative technique that can also show unsuspected peritoneal deposits. Computed tomography PET can detect signal uptake from active disease at distant sites to clarify the extent of tumor spread. If this lung lesion proved to be a metastatic deposit, then a palliative approach would be pursued. To prevent future obstruction, either colonic resection or chemotherapy and possible stenting of the colonic lesions should be considered. As the lung lesion was inactive on CTPET, however, intervention was refocused on the hepatic metastases, but the extent of liver disease on MRI was thought to preclude liver resection.

The ongoing management of this patient relates to how his liver metastases respond to chemotherapy and whether these will become suitable for operative resection or other local therapies such as radiofrequency ablation. The threatened colonic obstruction will also influence management and may require endoscopic or operative intervention.

MANAGEMENT OPTIONS

This case highlights two separate dilemmas: first, the management of the two primary colorectal cancers and their metastases and second, the management of subacute colonic obstruction. Several options are available for treating liver metastases, with an increasing emphasis on the role of resection, but the main question revolves on whether to treat them before or after the primary tumor(s). The extent of liver metastases in this patient made hepatic resection unsuitable initially, although neoadjuvant chemotherapy could reduce the disease burden sufficiently to permit liver resection with or without preoperative portal vein embolization (to stimulate growth of the intended liver remnant). Likewise, chemotherapy might also reduce the size of the colonic lesions and facilitate operative resection. The advantage of early treatment of the metastases has to be balanced against the risk of progression of the colonic lesions.

The alternative strategy for this patient would be (1) primary colonic resection, probably by means of subtotal colectomy given the multiplicity of neoplasms (although two separate resections with anastomosis could be performed) and then (2) treat the metastatic disease with chemotherapy, holding further interventions on the liver in reserve should the metastases respond. The disadvantage of starting with colectomy is that it delays the treatment of his liver disease until the patient has recovered from operation. Some patients with synchronous colonic and liver metastases can have simultaneous resections, but this option was not possible in the present case.

The management of acute colonic obstruction in this context raises some further issues for debate, which primarily concern the need for emergency operation. Both laparoscopic and open intervention can be considered, either to defunction the bowel via a loop ileostomy or to carry out subtotal colectomy with or without an ileocolic anastomosis and covering ileostomy; primary anastomosis may be unsafe in the context of obstruction. Again, although these procedures would relieve the obstruction, they would delay any subsequent chemotherapy. Colonic stenting would be a suitable alternative, decompressing the large bowel and allowing early chemotherapy. Colonic stenting is gaining in favor as the intervention of choice for left-sided obstructing lesions, although it is not without technical problems. In the patient under discussion, resolution of obstructive symptoms with purely conservative measures negated the need for any further intervention in this regard.

FURTHER READING

1. Abbott AM, Parsons HM, Tuttle TM, et al. Short-term outcomes after combined colon and liver resection for synchronous colon cancer liver metastases: a population study. Ann Surg Oncol. 2013;20:139-47.
2. Brouquet A, Nordlinger B. Surgical strategies to synchronous colorectal liver metastases. Dig Dis. 2012;30(S2):132-6.
3. Ghazal A-H A, El-Shazly WG, Bessa SS, et al. Colonic endoluminal stenting devices and elective surgery versus emergency subtotal/total colectomy in the management of malignant obstructed left colon cancer. J Gastrointest Surg. 2013;17:1123-9.
4. Lam AK-Y, Carmichael R, Buettner PG, et al. Clinicopathological significance of synchronous carcinoma in colorectal cancer. Am J Surg. 2011;202:39-44.
5. Rahbari NN, Lordick F, Fink C, et al. Resection of the primary tumour versus no resection prior to systemic therapy in patients with colon cancer and synchronous unresectable metastases (UICC stage IV): SYNCRONOUS - a randomised controlled multicentre trial (ISRCTN30964555). BMC Cancer. 2012;12:142-53.
6. Yoon JW, Lee SH, Ahn SH, et al. Clinical characteristics of multiple primary colorectal cancers. Cancer Res Treat. 2008;40:71-4.

Case Study: Obstructive Defecation Successfully Managed by Colostomy Irrigation after Salvage Abdominoperineal Excision of the Rectum 66

MRB Keighley

THE PROBLEM

A 42-year-old woman presented with rectal bleeding, mucous discharge, annoying skin tags, and a short history of straining. She had third-degree hemorrhoids, but the possibility of rectal intussusception was raised. She underwent a PPH (procedure for prolapse and hemorrhoids), a stapled hemorrhoidectomy, with disastrous results. Almost immediately she developed perineal pain, tenesmus, and the sensation of a lump obstructing defecation. A proctogram showed a large recto-rectal intussusception and failure to evacuate, associated with a rectocele and cystocele.

When all conservative measures to control symptoms failed, she underwent a STARR (stapled transanal rectal resection) procedure 9 months later. The rectal pain and obstructive defecation continued unabated. The gynecologists treated the genital prolapse by vaginal hysterectomy, plus transvaginal tape with anterior and posterior colporrhaphy. The genital prolapse was improved, but the rectal pain and obstructive defecation persisted. She then had a robotic-assisted ventral rectopexy and a transvaginal mesh. The mesh eroded the rectal wall, necessitating its removal by laparotomy and an end colostomy.

After colostomy construction, her symptoms improved so much that she decided to have an abdominoperineal excision of the rectum (APER) because she had diversion proctitis. The APER was complicated by pelvic bleeding, transient bladder dysfunction, and some delay in perineal wound healing. Worst still, the colostomy became unmanageable owing to pancaking of feces at the exit of the stoma.[1]

It was suggested that she might discuss colostomy irrigation, but the response was that she would be psychologically unsuitable and the stoma care nurse did not seem to know how to order the equipment. Our resourceful patient made her own enquiries. Far from being psychologically unsuitable, she robustly learned to irrigate. She was asymptomatic and employed full time even though it took her about 50 minutes to irrigate. It transformed her life.

THE TYPICAL CASE

Obstructive defecation syndrome (ODS) may be primary or secondary.

In primary ODS, the child or adolescent is usually simply labeled as having constipation. This problem causes embarrassment when the person hogs the toilet while everyone else in the household wants to go. There may be coexisting emotional factors and psychiatric illness such as eating disorders, sexual abuse as a child, and attention seeking behavior. These people are often manipulative, and although they have lived with the condition all their life, now seek immediate attention preferably by an operation, which in the mind of the patient has magical power. There is often somatization.

Secondary ODS may be secondary to anorectal or gynecological pathology such as rectocele, prolapse, intussusception, solitary ulcer, fissure, or hemorrhoids. Obstructive defecation syndrome may also complicate colorectal surgery, classically after low anterior resection (anterior resection syndrome), rectopexy or even pouch surgery. Symptoms may even occur for the first time after hemorrhoidectomy, and stapled procedure for prolapse and hemorrhoids is no exception. Likewise, ODS may also occur for the first time after gynecologic procedures, both abdominal and vaginal hysterectomy and prolapse operations.

DIAGNOSTIC DILEMMAS

Whenever a patient presents for the first time with symptoms of ODS, it is essential to take a thorough history: find out when symptoms started; what were the precipitating factors; are there any unspoken fears and past emotional issues that are hidden? Is there a simple cause? One cannot stress too much the importance of the history and physical examination. Are the real facts being communicated? What about the person's appearance? Are there signs of chronic straining such as perineal descent at rest as well as on straining; is there visible pathology on the perineum? Is there a deficient sphincter from previous trauma; is there a rectal prolapse; can you detect any gynecologic prolapse, especially is there a rectocele? The rigid anoscopy and sigmoidoscopy are critical to make an accurate assessment. Is there a chronic fissure; are there hemorrhoids and, if so, do they prolapse; is there any evidence of an incomplete rectal intussusception during straining on sigmoidoscopy?

Investigation is a real difficulty in these patients. Dynamic studies of highly intimate acts such as defecation are not possible. All that we have to assess patients is artificial and subject not only to observer variation but also the willingness of the patient to cooperate. Thus, the dynamic video proctographic studies are subject to enormous variation. In the near perfect setting of placing the patient on a thunder-box through which the radiologist, who is no longer in the room but at a distant site, can direct their X-rays over an ethically acceptable time of low-dose screening, all depends on the patient's willingness to cooperate, which may be deliberately compromised if the patient is manipulative and determined to have their operation tomorrow.

MANAGEMENT OPTIONS

If ODS can be managed conservatively, this is the best policy. The present case history only highlights all that can go wrong with operative therapy. The results of surgical treatment are poor. Long-term reports from independently assessed outcomes provide dismal reading in terms of the effectiveness of rectocele repair, the STARR procedure, and various suspensory procedures. Serious consideration should be given to evacuation therapy with suppositories or self-administered rectal washouts, or even colonic irrigation. Such therapies must be part of a whole package of behavioral therapy including diet, toileting habits, and pelvic floor relaxation during defecation. This is all part of a whole person retraining program, the success of which is hugely influenced by the personality of the therapist.

TAKE-HOME MESSAGE IN THIS CASE

In this case everything failed until a colorectal nurse who proved to be a good communicator painstakingly taught this frustrated person, who was desperate to become a valued member of society again, to manage her impossible stoma by colostomy irrigation.

Colostomy irrigation is only practiced by about 5% of all patients with a permanent stoma in the United Kingdom.[2] I have assessed the role of colostomy irrigation in India. The infrequent use of irrigation is the same as in the United Kingdom: very few patients do it. This fact is rather surprising, especially as being ritually clean is very important in their society and all patients have to purchase their appliances.

This author is of the view that colostomy irrigation is a forgotten art. In the past, there were some pioneers of colorectal surgery who insisted that all patients having a permanent colostomy for rectal cancer should be taught irrigation before they left the hospital.[3] My colleagues of that era tell me that once a patient had been taught irrigation they never reverted to stoma appliances: no fear of flatus during the dinner party and none of the psychosexual compromise of wearing a device during sexual intimacy.

The Muslim community with a stoma in India is often not understood by the imam. Like many Hindus and Sikhs, they do not feel able to pray because they consider themselves unclean. Muslims in Western society are better understood by the religious leaders and change their appliances before prayers.[4] Hindus, especially those of high caste, also feel the need to change appliances before religious ritual both at home and in Western society.[5] Were Asians to become more aware about the impact of colostomy irrigation on their sense of cleanliness, this inexpensive daily ritual would gain much greater acceptance. We have data to suggest that feeling unclean, clothing compromise, sexual intimacy, body image, and quality of life are better in those practicing colostomy irrigation than in other stoma patients.[6]

REFERENCES

1. Redmond C, Cowin C, Perrin A. Survey of patients' experiences with pancaking-quantitative research amongst colostomists. Colorectal Dis. 2013;15(suppl.1):15.
2. Luke D, Ebanks A, Bowley DM. Colostomy irrigation can enhance quality of life after abdominoperineal excision of the rectum. Colorectal Dis. 2012;14:783-8.
3. Holzer B, Matzel K, Schiedeck T, et al. Do geographic and educational factors influence the quality of life in rectal cancer patients with a permanent colostomy? Study group of quality of life in rectal cancer. Dis Colon Rectum. 2005;48:2209-16.
4. Albar AA. Permanent diversion stomas: "guidelines foe Muslim physicians and patients." J Family Community Med. 1995;2:21-6.
5. Black PK. Cultural and religious beliefs in stoma care nursing. Brit J Nurs. 2009;18:790-3.
6. Keighley MRB, Nagomy I, Mitchell C, et al. Religious and cultural factors impacting on adjustment to a stoma amongst Indian and British subjects: sexual intimacy is the greatest morbidity. Colorectal Dis. 2014;16(suppl 2):12.

67

Peritoneum and Retroperitoneum

Graeme W Couper

Key Points

- Primary peritonitis is rare, accounting for 1% of cases of peritonitis. The most common form is spontaneous bacterial peritonitis (SBP), which occurs almost exclusively in patients with large-volume ascites in liver cirrhosis.
- Secondary peritonitis is the commonest form, with appendicitis and perforated diverticular disease being the two most frequent causes.
- Tertiary peritonitis has been defined as the persistence or recurrence of intra-abdominal infection following apparently adequate therapy of primary or secondary peritonitis or occurring after any operation for secondary bacterial peritonitis.
- Intra-abdominal adhesions generally follow laparotomy, with rates as high as 95% reported in some series. They are the commonest cause of small bowel obstruction, accounting for 60%–70% of cases.
- Pseudomyxoma peritonei (PMP) classically originates from a perforated appendiceal mucinous tumor. Patients should be offered treatment in high-volume centers of specialist peritoneal surface malignancy. Mortality rates of 2% and median survival rates of 196 months (16.3 years) have been reported.
- Iliopsoas abscess (IPA) is classified into primary and secondary according to the mechanism of spread. Primary IPA is often seen in immunosuppressed patients or those predisposed to infections, in whom an occult infectious process somewhere in the body results in hematogenous spread to the muscle. Secondary IPA occurs when infection is present in organs adjacent to the psoas muscle. Historically spinal tuberculosis was a major cause of IPA, but the reduced incidence of TB in developed nations has seen a change in the source of infection. Secondary IPA now accounts for up to 80% of cases in some modern series.
- There are two main types of retroperitoneal fibrosis. Idiopathic retroperitoneal fibrosis (RPF), with no identifiable cause, accounts for over 70% of cases. Secondary forms can be due to benign or malignant conditions.
- Sarcomas comprise a third of retroperitoneal tumors, with two histological subtypes predominating, namely liposarcoma (70%) and leiomyosarcoma (15%).

INTRODUCTION

Although many conditions could be included in this chapter, several will have already been covered in sections relating to specific organs. This chapter will therefore limit the discussion to conditions relating specifically to the peritoneum and retroperitoneum. It will include conditions that may present on an acute surgical "take" or present in a surgical clinic. To help organize the conditions of surgical relevance, it is first important to understand the anatomy of the peritoneum and retroperitoneum.

ANATOMY

The peritoneum develops from the mesoderm of the trilaminar embryo. As the mesoderm differentiates, the lateral plate mesoderm splits to form two layers (separated by an intraembryonic celom), which later develop into the visceral and parietal peritoneum. The potential space between these two layers is the peritoneal cavity, and in the adult it is filled with approximately 50–100 mL of peritoneal fluid.

As the embryo develops, the abdominal organs grow into the abdominal cavity from structures in the abdominal wall. In this process they become enveloped in a layer of peritoneum along with the supplying blood vessels, lymphatics, and nerves forming the mesentery. The parietal peritoneum derives its blood supply from the arteries in the abdominal wall, with venous drainage into the systemic circulation. The visceral peritoneum blood supply is from the mesenteric and celiac arteries, with drainage into the portal venous system.

Table 67.1 Anatomical classification of abdominal structures.

Location	Intraperitoneal	Retroperitoneal	Infraperitoneal/Subperitoneal
Gastrointestinal tract	Stomach, 1st part of the duodenum, jejunum, ileum, caecum, appendix, transverse colon, sigmoid colon, rectum (upper 1/3)	Duodenum 2nd, 3rd, and 4th parts, ascending colon, descending colon, rectum (middle 1/3)	Rectum (lower 1/3)
Solid organs/urinary system	Liver, spleen, tail of pancreas	Head and body of pancreas Kidneys, adrenal glands, proximal ureters	Urinary bladder, distal ureters
Reproductive system	In women: uterus, fallopian tubes, ovaries	Gonadal blood vessels	
Major vessels		Inferior vena cava, aorta	

The intraperitoneal space has two subdivisions. The greater sac (or general cavity of the abdomen) is connected by the epiploic foramen (also known as the omental foramen or foramen of Winslow) to the lesser sac. The greater sac contains the lesser omentum (gastrohepatic ligament) extending from the lesser curve of the stomach to the liver and the greater omentum (gastrocolic ligament) extending from the greater curve of the stomach and looping down in front of the intestines before curving back upward to attach to the transverse colon. The structures within the abdomen are classified as intraperitoneal, retroperitoneal, or infraperitoneal depending on whether they are covered with visceral peritoneum and whether they are attached by mesenteries (Table 67.1).

PERITONITIS

Peritonitis is defined as inflammation of the peritoneal cavity and is classified as primary, secondary, or tertiary. Sclerosing peritonitis is a rare fibrosing form with an often fatal outcome. The major risk factor of sclerosing peritonitis is peritoneal dialysis treatment, but it can also occur following renal or liver transplantation or in association with certain drug treatment such as beta-blockers.

Primary Peritonitis

Primary peritonitis is a diffuse infection of the peritoneal cavity that occurs in the absence of another source of infection and without disruption of the gastrointestinal tract. It is rare and accounts for only 1% of all cases of peritonitis.[1] The most common form is spontaneous bacterial peritonitis (SBP), first described in 1963 by Kerr and colleagues.[2] SBP occurs almost exclusively in patients with large-volume ascites in liver cirrhosis. Ascites of other causes present in low volume rarely give rise to SBP. Bacterial translocation is the most common cause of SBP, and three factors have been implicated in cirrhotics: (1) alteration in gut microflora, (2) increased gut permeability, and (3) impaired immunity.[3] Other contributory factors in cirrhosis with ascites are thought to include bacteremia secondary to compromised host defenses, intrahepatic shunting of colonized blood, and defective bactericidal activity within the ascitic fluid.

In-hospital mortality for the first episode of SBP ranges from 10% to 50% depending on various risk factors.[3] Symptoms include fevers, chills, nausea, vomiting, general malaise, abdominal pain, and worsening ascites.[4] Spontaneous bacterial peritonitis may present with hepatic encephalopathy, and in the absence of a clear precipitant all patients should undergo paracentesis. If the fluid contains bacteria or large numbers of polymorphonuclear leukocytes (>250 cells/mm^3), infection is confirmed and antibiotic therapy is commenced. The most common pathogens are *Escherichia coli, Klebsiella pneumoniae,* and *Enterobacteriaceae*. In 25% of cases, gram-positive cocci are involved, principally *Streptococci* and *Enterococci*. Treatment is with broad-spectrum intravenous antibiotics such as a third-generation cephalosporin and/or a fluoroquinolone.

Primary peritonitis may occur in children without predisposing disease, but it is especially associated with postnecrotic cirrhosis and nephrotic syndrome.[5] In prepubertal girls, transfallopian spread may be the route of infection as suggested by the simultaneous presence of pneumococci in vaginal secretions and peritoneal fluid. The change in vaginal secretions from alkaline to acidic may have a protective inhibitory effect on bacterial growth after puberty.[5]

Tuberculous peritonitis can result from direct entry into the peritoneal cavity of tubercle bacilli (from the lymph nodes, intestine, or genital tract) or more commonly by hematogenous spread from remote foci of tuberculosis, typically in the lung. It may complicate end-stage renal or liver disease, which further adds to the diagnostic difficulty. It may only become clinically evident after the initial focus has completely healed and be of gradual onset. Typical symptoms include fever, weight loss, malaise, night sweats, and abdominal distension. The findings at

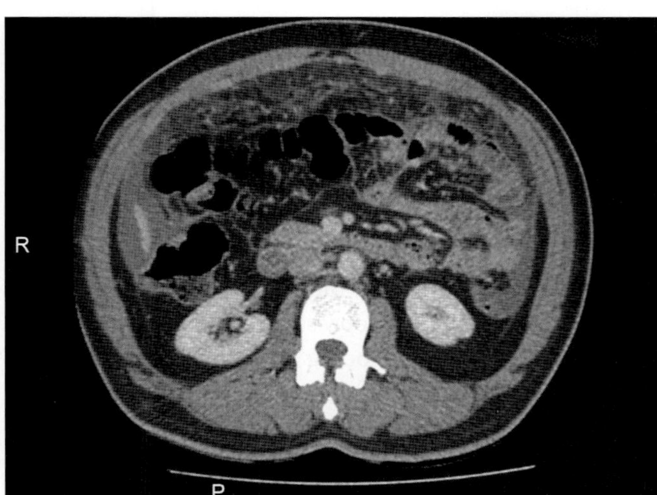

Fig. 67.1: CT image of patient with tuberculous peritonitis.
Source: Image courtesy of Mr. de Beaux, Consultant Surgeon, Royal Infirmary of Edinburgh.

laparotomy or laparoscopy consist of multiple nodules scattered over the peritoneal surface and omentum. Adhesions and a variable amount of peritoneal fluid are usually present (Fig. 67.1). Treatment is for 6 months with first-line antituberculous drugs (isoniazid, rifampicin, ethambutol, and pyrazinamide) in uncomplicated cases.[6]

Secondary Peritonitis

Secondary peritonitis is the most common form of peritonitis encountered by the surgeon. Acute appendicitis is the most frequent cause of intra-abdominal infection in the Western world. It is associated with a lower mortality, lower morbidity, and shorter duration of hospital stay than other intra-abdominal infections.[7] A nonoperative course has been advocated in patients with early, nonperforated appendicitis.[8] A study of 252 men were randomized to antibiotic therapy or appendicectomy. In the antibiotic group treated with intravenous antibiotics for 2 days followed by oral treatment for 10 days, 86% improved without operation, but 18 patients required operation within 24 hours. The rate of recurrence of symptoms of appendicitis among the 111 patients treated with antibiotics was 14% during the 1-year follow-up. Laparoscopic appendectomy is now the standard surgical technique for acute appendicitis, but may not be appropriate for patients who have diffuse peritonitis due to difficulties in performing an adequate peritoneal lavage.

Colonic perforations are the second commonest cause of secondary peritonitis in Western countries, with colonic diverticulitis the most frequent disease process resulting in perforation.[9] Perforated diverticulitis is usually managed by a two-stage approach. As the first stage, Hartmann's procedure involves drainage of any abscess, colonic resection, and formation of an end colostomy. The colostomy is closed and a definitive anastomosis is performed at a later stage. Resection with primary anastomosis has been advocated in patients with less severe disease and those with early contamination who are in better physiologic condition. Perforated colon cancer, ischemic colitis, and foreign body perforations can also result in intra-abdominal infection from a colonic source.

Secondary peritonitis caused by peptic ulcer perforation is now much less common in Western society due to the discovery and eradication of *Helicobacter pylori*.[10] Gastroduodenal perforations have decreased considerably in Western countries due to the widespread adoption of medical therapies for peptic ulcer disease. Operative management principally entails closure with an omental patch performed at either open operation or laparoscopically. It is essential that patients with perforated duodenal ulcers receive eradication for *H. pylori* as ulcer healing occurs quicker with eradication and ulcer recurrence at follow-up endoscopy at 12 months is reduced from 29.6% to 6.1%.[11] Resective approaches are usually reserved for patients with perforations due to gastric cancer.

Antibiotic regimens must be effective against both gram-negative enteric aerobic and anaerobic bacteria. A review of prospective randomized studies of antibiotic regimens for secondary peritonitis of gastrointestinal origin in adults from the Cochrane Colorectal Cancer Group concluded that 16 antibiotic regimens had similar rates of clinical success.[12] There was no difference in mortality rate between any of these regimens. The appropriate duration of treatment for intra-abdominal infections remains controversial. Antibiotics may either be stopped once fever and leukocytosis have resolved and gastrointestinal function has returned or be continued for a specific period. Switching from intravenous to oral antibiotics has not been shown to affect outcomes in patients with complicated appendicitis.[13] The authors of this study question whether continued antibiotics are needed in patients once gastrointestinal function has returned.

Tertiary Peritonitis

Tertiary peritonitis has been defined as the persistence or recurrence of intra-abdominal infection following apparently adequate therapy of primary or secondary peritonitis or occurring after any operation for secondary bacterial peritonitis.[14,15] The major risk factors include malnutrition, a high APACHE II (Acute Physiology and Chronic Health Evaluation) score, the presence of organisms resistant to antimicrobial therapy and organ system failure. Patients with tertiary peritonitis have a significantly longer ICU stay (21.8 +/- 14.9 vs 8.5 +/- 7.9 days), more advanced organ dysfunction and higher ICU mortality rates (64% vs 33%) than patients with uncomplicated secondary peritonitis.[14] The most common infecting organisms in patients with tertiary peritonitis are *Enterococcus* spp. *Candida albicans, Staphylococcus epidermidis,* and *Enterobacter* spp. Management should include the provision of appropriate physiologic support, the administration of antimicrobial therapy, and intervention to control the source of contamination. However, infectious foci are rarely amenable to percutaneous drainage and may be poorly localized at laparotomy.[14] Compared with secondary peritonitis, antibiotic-resistant organisms and bacteremia are seen more commonly and mortality is greater in patients with tertiary peritonitis. Early recognition and effective intervention are critical to achieving a successful outcome.[15]

INTRA-ABDOMINAL ABSCESS

Intra-abdominal abscesses can complicate many illnesses including diverticulitis, pancreatitis, and appendicitis, or they may occur during the postoperative period, often as a result of anastomotic breakdown or inadequate peritoneal lavage in secondary peritonitis. Intra-abdominal abscesses can be either visceral (e.g. hepatic or splenic) or nonvisceral (e.g. pelvic or subphrenic) and intraperitoneal or retroperitoneal. Nonvisceral abscesses generally arise following resolution of diffuse peritonitis or as a result of a visceral perforation or anastomotic breakdown that has successfully walled itself off. Visceral abscesses commonly arise via hematogenous or lymphatic dissemination of bacteria to a solid organ.

Patients may present with mild abdominal pain and localized tenderness in the region of the infection, which may be associated with an abdominal mass. The patient is often pyrexial, anorexic, and has a leukocytosis. Abscess localization is achieved using either ultrasound or CT. Treatment consists of two steps: source control is the principal step, antimicrobial therapy to cover the often polymicrobial infection the second. Historically, surgical exploration was performed alongside debridement and drainage of the infected cavity. Modern image-guided procedures have been developed that complement surgical drainage techniques. These procedures have proved comparable to surgical techniques in terms of adequate drainage of the cavity and mortality rates. Complex multiloculated abscesses may still require laparotomy and formal drainage.

PERITONEAL ADHESIONS

Intra-abdominal adhesions most commonly occur following open operation, with rates as high as 95% reported in some series.[16,17] They represent the commonest cause of intestinal obstruction, being responsible for 60–70% of patients presenting with obstruction of the small bowel.[18,19] Surgery of the colon and rectum is particularly associated with a high risk of adhesion-related problems.[18] The risks of readmission directly related to adhesions in the 5 years following laparotomy are 15.4% for panproctocolectomy, 8.8% for total colectomy, and 10.6% for ileostomy operations. Appendectomy was associated with a lower rate of readmission (0.9%), but still contributed over 7% of the total readmission rate for lower abdominal surgery. Gynecological operations also carry a high risk of postoperative adhesions. Other reported risk factors include age younger than 60 years, previous laparotomy within 5 years, peritonitis, multiple laparotomies, emergency surgery, omental resection, and penetrating abdominal trauma, especially gunshot wounds.[17,20-22] Postoperative adhesions represent an appreciable workload to healthcare providers. A 10-year follow-up study of 29,790 patients who underwent open abdominal or pelvic operations in 1986 in Scotland reported that 34.6% were readmitted a mean of 2.1 times over the next 10 years for a disorder directly or possibly related to adhesions.[23] Over 22% of all readmissions occurred in the first year after the initial operation.

An excellent guideline on the diagnosis and management of adhesive small bowel obstruction was published following a consensus conference during the 1st International Congress of the World Society of Emergency Surgery and 9th Peritoneum and Surgery Society meeting in Bologna, July 1–3, 2010.[24] The resulting Bologna Guidelines are essential reading for all surgeons involved in the management of patients presenting with an acute surgical abdomen.

The initial investigation for adhesive small bowel obstruction is a plain abdominal X-ray (Fig. 67.2). The typical features are distended, centrally placed small bowel loops, multiple air-fluid levels, and the absence of gas in the colon. A plain abdominal film has a sensitivity and specificity ranging from 65% to 80%.[25]

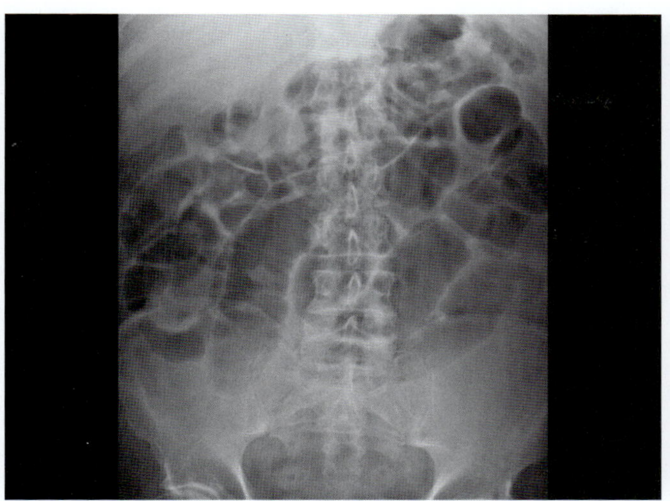

Fig. 67.2: Plain abdominal X-ray of patient with small bowel obstruction. This was due to adhesions from a previous laparotomy for perforated appendicitis.

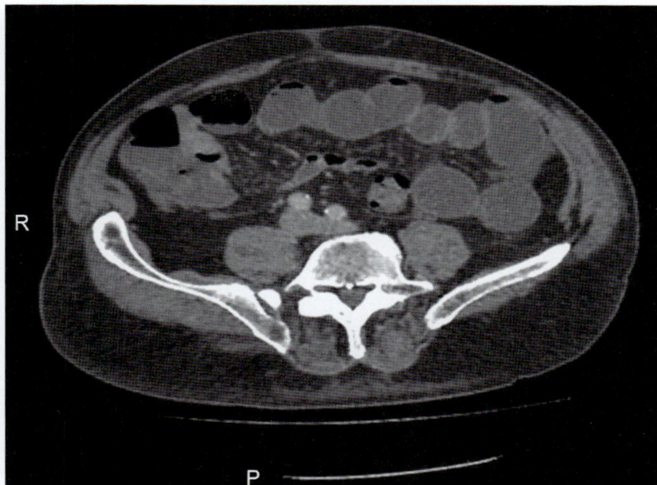

Fig. 67.3: CT image of patient with small bowel adhesive obstruction. This was not evident on initial plain abdominal X-ray and was due to adhesive obstruction from a previous laparotomy for splenic trauma.

When plain films are inconclusive, CT scan should be the next investigation[26] (Fig. 67.3). CT can confirm the presence of obstruction and also the presence of strangulation or ischemia.[27] Typical features of ischemia are reduced enhancement of the small-bowel wall, mural thickening, mesenteric fluid, congestion of small mesenteric veins, and ascites. In a study of 142 patients, CT correctly diagnosed the presence of ischemia in 23 out of 24 patients undergoing operation for small bowel obstruction.

Water-soluble contrast medium is safe and reduces the need for operation, the time to resolution of obstruction, and length of hospital stay.[24] About 50–150 mL of an agent such as Gastrografin may be administered either orally or via a nasogastric tube. An abdominal radiograph performed after at least 4 hours can accurately predict the likelihood of resolution of small bowel obstruction.[28] The appearance of the contrast agent in the colon within 24 hours of administration predicts resolution of obstruction with a sensitivity of 96–97% and specificity of 96–98%.[29,30]

In the absence of any signs of strangulation, patients with an adhesive small bowel obstruction can be managed safely with nonoperative treatment, and nasogastric tube decompression should be attempted for 24–48 hours.

Historically, intestinal obstruction refractory to conservative treatment was managed by laparotomy. It is widely recognized that repeated laparotomies can increase adhesion formation and increase the likelihood of further adhesive obstruction, with approximately 10–30% of patients requiring further laparotomy for recurrent bowel obstruction.[31] In an attempt to reduce this likelihood, laparoscopic adhesiolysis is now widely performed in specialized units. In a meta-analysis of four retrospective studies, laparoscopic adhesiolysis was associated with a reduced overall complication rate, a reduced prolonged ileus rate and reduced pulmonary complication rate when compared to laparotomy.[32] No significant differences existed with respect to intraoperative bowel injury, wound infection rate or mortality.

In addition to an increasing rate of minimally invasive primary operations and a laparoscopic approach to any subsequent small bowel obstruction, there are a number of adhesion-reduction agents available in the form of site-specific and broad-coverage barriers and solutions.[33] The POPA study randomized 181 patients with small bowel obstruction undergoing laparotomy, adhesiolysis, and bowel resection if required to either the addition of icodextrin 4% solution (Adept, Shire Pharmaceuticals, UK) before abdominal closure or immediate closure. After a mean follow-up period of 41.4 months, the small bowel obstruction recurrence rate was 2.19% (2/91) in the icodextrin groups versus 11.11% (10/90) in the control group ($p < 0.05$). The trial concluded that the use of icodextrin 4% solution in small bowel obstruction is safe and reduces intra-abdominal adhesion formation and the risk of reobstruction. This area of surgical research is a space to watch!

PSEUDOMYXOMA PERITONEI

Pseudomyxoma peritonei (PMP) is a rare condition caused by tumor-cell production of mucin or gelatinous ascites that fills the abdominal cavity.[34] The incidence of

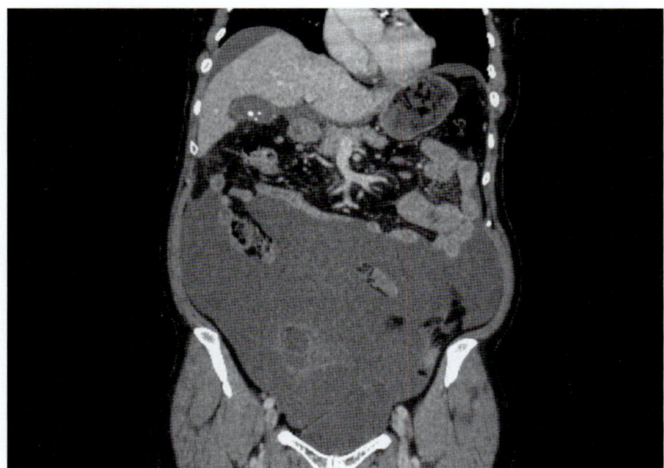

Fig. 67.4: CT image of patient with pseudomyxoma peritonei.
Source: Image courtesy of Dr. Patel, Consultant Radiologist, Royal Infirmary of Edinburgh.

PMP is approximately 2 per million per year. Classically it originates from a perforated appendiceal mucinous tumor.[35] It is slightly more common in women than men (male:female ratio = 9:11). The median age at presentation is about 50 years, with a range of 20–75 years. Left untreated, the tumors will generate increasing amounts of mucin and eventually compress vital intra-abdominal organs. The disease rarely spreads through the lymphatic system or through the bloodstream. Patients generally present with suspected acute appendicitis or a new-onset hernia or during investigation of an ovarian mass with increasing abdominal girth (the ovary is a common site for spread). More recently, with the widespread availability of cross-sectional imaging, many patients present with a CT diagnosis of mucinous ascites, often supported by image-guided biopsy[35] (Fig. 67.4).

Patients should be offered treatment in high-volume centers for specialist peritoneal surface malignancy. Optimal therapy is complete macroscopic tumor removal [complete cytoreduction surgery (CRS)] combined with heated intra-operative intraperitoneal chemotherapy, commonly mitomycin C. Operation entails combined peritonectomy and visceral resection of involved organs. Peritonectomy includes right and left parietal peritonectomy, pelvic peritonectomy, and bilateral subdiaphragmatic peritonectomy. In addition, sometimes other "organs" need to be removed such as the greater gallbladder, spleen, liver capsule, stomach, colon, and rectum. Bilateral oophorectomy and hysterectomy may be required in women.[35] When complete cytoreduction cannot be achieved maximal tumor debulking is performed, but this is associated with a much poorer prognosis. A recent retrospective analysis of 2,298 patients undergoing CRS for PMP in 16 specialized units reported a treatment-related mortality of 2% and a major operative complication rate of 24%. The median survival rate was 196 months (16.3 years) and the median progression-free survival rate 98 months (8.2 years), with 10- and 15-year survival rates of 63% and 59%, respectively.[36] In contrast, 5- and 10-year predicted survival was 34% and 23% in patients who had major tumor debulking in another published study.[35]

ILIOPSOAS ABSCESS

First described by Mynter in 1881 as "psoitis," an iliopsoas abscess (IPA) is a collection of pus involving the iliopsoas muscle compartment.[37] A classical triad of pain, fever, and limp was originally described but is often not present. The psoas and iliacus muscles (considered as the iliopsoas muscle) insert into the lesser trochanter of the femur via a common tendon and function as the main hip flexors. The psoas major arises from the transverse processes and the lateral aspects of the vertebral bodies between T12 and L5. Its anatomical relations include the sigmoid colon, appendix, jejunum, ureters, kidneys, abdominal aorta, pancreas, spine, hip joints, and iliac lymph nodes.

IPA is classified into primary and secondary according to the mechanism of spread. Primary IPA is often seen in immunosuppressed patients or those predisposed to infections such as diabetics, the elderly, patients on steroids, patients with malignancies, and alcoholics.[38] In these patients there is a probable occult infectious process within the body resulting in hematogenous spread to the muscle. *Staphylococcus aureus* is the most common pathogen, occurring in over 88% of cases.[39]

Secondary IPA occurs when infection is present in organs adjacent to the psoas muscle. Historically spinal tuberculosis was a major cause of IPA, but the reduced incidence of TB in developed nations has seen a change in the source of infection. The diagnosis of TB, however, must always be considered in patients who have emigrated from regions where TB is prevalent (Fig. 67.5). Secondary IPA accounts for up to 80% of cases in some modern series.[40,41] The origins of the infective focus are often the gastrointestinal or urinary tract. Crohn's disease is the commonest cause of secondary IPA,[41-43] and it carries a greater possibility of gram-negative organisms, anaerobes, or polymicrobial infection, so initial empirical coverage should include antibiotics with a wide antimicrobial spectrum. CT is generally used to diagnose IPA[41] (Fig. 67.6).

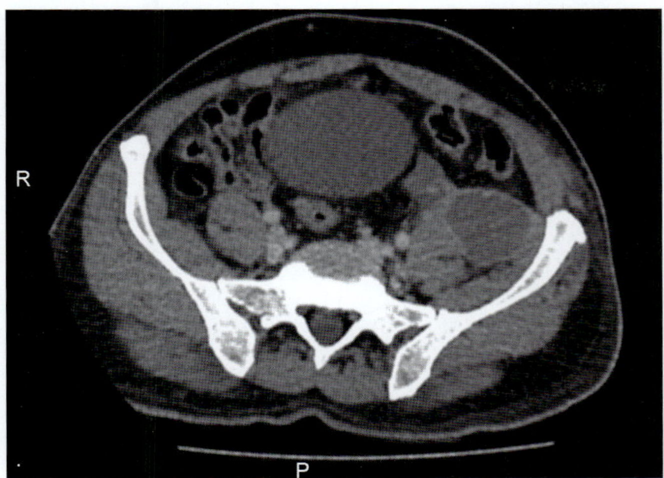

Fig. 67.5: CT image of patient presenting with a left groin swelling. Differential diagnosis was of a left inguinal hernia. Diagnosis is of iliopsoas abscess secondary to TB. The abscess was drained and the patient received anti-tuberculous treatment.
Source: Image courtesy of Mr. Lamb, Consultant Surgeon, Royal Infirmary of Edinburgh.

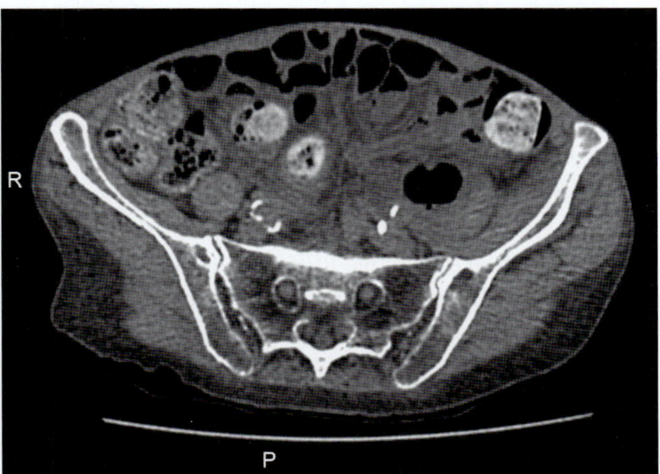

Fig. 67.6: CT image of patient with iliopsoas abscess secondary to perforated sigmoid diverticular disease. The patient also has left-sided hydronephrosis. Treatment included insertion of a left ureteric stent and a Hartmann's procedure.

Initial management involves broad-spectrum antibiotics plus consideration of percutaneous drainage of larger collections. Success rates reported in the literature for percutaneous drainage range from 40% to 90%.[41,44,45] In patients with an underlying gastrointestinal tract cause, open surgical management is often required. The overall mortality rate for IPA is 5%.[40,41] Advanced age, positive blood cultures, and isolation of *E. coli* may be associated with an unfavorable outcome.[40]

RETROPERITONEAL FIBROSIS

Retroperitoneal fibrosis is a rare disease that can lead to extensive fibrosis that entraps the ureters, vessels, and/or other abdominal organs. It appears as a dense fibrous plaque that usually arises at or just below the level of the aortic bifurcation or sacral promontory.[46] This fibrosis surrounds the aorta and inferior vena cava and spreads through the retroperitoneum in a perivascular distribution. The fibrosis often extends laterally and may involve the ureters, especially in the middle third, as well as the psoas muscles. There are two main types. Idiopathic RPF, with no identifiable cause, accounts for over 70% of cases and is probably linked to systemic autoimmune diseases with involvement of a vasculitic process of small and medium retroperitoneal vessels. Its prevalence is estimated at 1.4 cases per 100,000, and it usually affects men in the fifth to seventh decades of life.[47] There is a two to three times male predominance.[48] No ethnic differences have been described.

Secondary forms can be due to either benign or malignant conditions. Benign causes include aortic aneurysm, drugs (e.g. ergo dopamine agonists), infection, hemorrhage, irradiation, and immunologic disorders such as primary biliary sclerosis, glomerulonephritis, rheumatoid arthritis, systemic lupus erythematosus polyarteritis nodosa, ankylosing spondylitis, orbital pseudotumor, fibrosing mediastinitis, and Hashimoto's thyroiditis. Malignant causes include Hodgkin's disease and other lymphomas, sarcomas and numerous carcinomas including colon, kidney, bladder, prostate, cervix, breast, lung, and stomach.

The clinical presentation may be varied, including both localized and systemic symptoms. Pain is the most common symptom, affecting over 90% of patients and involving the abdomen, lower back and the flanks, often radiating to the groin. Other symptoms include edema of the lower limbs, scrotal or testicular swelling, hydrocele or varicocele, and decreased urinary excretion. Retroperitoneal fibrosis often leads to ureteral obstruction, with impaired renal function reported in 80–100% of cases. Involvement of the abdominal vasculature may cause deep venous thrombosis or mesenteric ischemia. In untreated patients intestinal obstruction affects the small bowel in 3.4% and the large bowel in 2%. Systemic symptoms such as fatigue, weight loss, anorexia, and low-grade fever probably reflect the systemic inflammatory nature of the disease.

Inflammatory markers such as C-reactive protein or erythrocyte sedimentation rate may not help to differentiate idiopathic RPF from secondary RPF or to monitor treatment.

CT is the imaging technique of choice. It provides more information on urinary tract involvement than MRI. Distinguishing between idiopathic RPF and malignant RPF can be difficult on imaging, so histological assessment is often required.[49,50] Samples can be obtained by CT-guided needle biopsy or open biopsy, but both techniques risk hemorrhage. Because of an increased fluorodeoxyglucose (18F-FDG) uptake in active RPF, 18F-FDG positron emission tomography is also considered an effective imaging modality to assess the extent and features of RPF and to look for recurrence.[51]

The aim of the treatment is to relieve ureteral obstruction and prevent progression of inflammation. Patients who are prescribed methysergide should be taken off this medication immediately. Surgical treatment consists of multiple deep retroperitoneal biopsies to exclude malignancy, ureterolysis, and lateral transposition of the ureters. The ureters may be wrapped in omentum or transplanted into the peritoneal cavity and a posterior peritoneal flap closed behind them. Alternatively, a polytetrafluoroethylene (Gor-Tex) sheet can be placed between the ureters and the retroperitoneum.

Retroperitoneal fibrosis can cause iliocaval venous occlusion. Such patients can be managed conservatively, but venous bypass is an option for those with symptoms of chronic venous obstruction or those in whom medical treatment has failed.[52] Corticosteroids are used in the active inflammatory stage, but their benefit during the fibrotic stage is unclear. More recently, tamoxifen and immunosuppressive drugs such as azathioprine and cyclophosphamide have been used therapeutically.[53,54]

RETROPERITONEAL TUMORS

Most retroperitoneal tumors are primary lymphoproliferative (Hodgkin's and non-Hodgkin's lymphoma), parenchymatous epithelial tumors (renal, adrenal or pancreas), or metastatic in origin.[55] In contrast to other sites within the body, soft tissue lesions in the retroperitoneum are more likely to be sarcomas than benign lesions. Two histological subtypes predominate, namely liposarcoma (70%) and leiomyosarcoma (15%). Benign pathologies encountered in the retroperitoneum include benign neurogenic tumors (schwannomas, neurofibromas), paragangliomas (functional or nonfunctional), fibromatosis, renal angiomyolipomas, and benign retroperitoneal lipomas.

Presentation tends to be late as there is room to expand within the loose connective tissue of the retroperitoneum. Symptoms relate to the pressure effects on adjacent organs or direct invasion. Patients often present with abdominal swelling, early satiety, abdominal discomfort, or a palpable mass.[56] Although the gastrointestinal and urinary tracts are often displaced, they are rarely invaded; thus gastrointestinal or urinary symptoms are unusual.[57] CT and MRI are the imaging modalities of choice, with positron emission tomography useful in the assessment of sarcomas (Fig. 67.7). Many benign lesions are discovered as an incidental finding during imaging for unrelated symptoms.

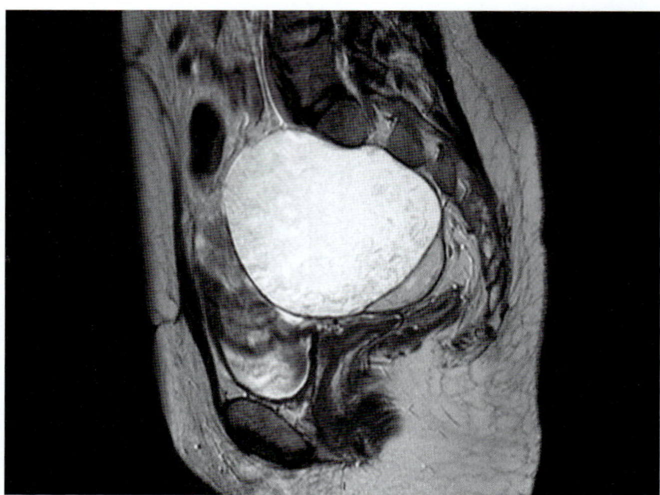

Fig. 67.7: MRI of patient with retroperitoneal mature cyst teratoma.

Fine needle aspiration cytology may help differentiate between primary or metastatic carcinoma, lymphoproliferative, or mesenchymal tumors. Needle core biopsy can give a more definitive diagnosis, but it risks seeding of the tumor.

REFERENCES

1. McWhinnie DL. The peritoneum and peritonitis. In: Morris PJ, Malt RA (Eds). Oxford Textbook of Surgery, vol 1. Oxford: Oxford University Press; 1994. pp. 1161-4.
2. Kerr DNS, Pearson DT, Read AE. Infection of ascetic fluid in patients with hepatic cirrhosis. Gut. 1963;4:394-8.
3. Weist R, Krag A, Gerbes A. Spontaneous bacterial peritonitis: recent guidelines and beyond. Gut. 2012;61:297-310.
4. Lata J, Stiburek O, Kopacova M. Spontaneous bacterial peritonitis: a severe complication of liver cirrhosis. World J. Gastroenterol. 2009;15(44):5505-10.
5. Johnson CC, Baldessarre J, Levison ME. Peritonitis: update on pathophysiology, clinical manifestations, and management. Clin Infect Dis. 1997;24:1035-47.
6. Sanai FM, Bzeizi KI. Systematic review: tuberculous peritonitis—presenting features, diagnostic strategies and treatment. Aliment Pharmacol Ther. 2005;22(8):685-700.
7. Merlino JI, Malangoni MA, Smith CM, et al. Prospective randomized trials affect the outcomes of intraabdominal infection. Ann Surg. 2001;233:859-66.

8. Styrud J, Eriksson S, Nilsson I, et al. Appendectomy versus antibiotic treatment in acute appendicitis. A prospective multicenter randomized controlled trial. World J Surg. 2006;30:1033-7.
9. Malangoni MA, Inui T. Peritonitis—the Western experience. W J Emerg Surg. 2006;1:25.
10. Marshall BJ, Warren JR. Unidentified curved bacilli in the stomach of patients with gastritis and peptic ulceration. Lancet. 1984;i:1311-5.
11. El-Nakeeb A, Fikry A, Abd El-Hamed TM, et al. Effect of Helicobacter pylori eradication on ulcer recurrence after simple closure of perforated duodenal ulcer. Int J Surg. 2009;7(2):126-9.
12. Wong PF, Gilliam AD, Kumar S, et al. Antibiotic regimens for secondary peritonitis of gastrointestinal origin in adults. Cochrane Database Syst Rev. 2005;2:CD005539.
13. Taylor E, Berjis A, Bosch T, et al. The efficacy of postoperative oral antibiotics in appendicitis: A randomized prospective double-blinded study. Am Surg. 2004;70:858-62.
14. Nathens AB, Rotstein OD, Marshall JC. Tertiary peritonitis: clinical features of a complex nosocomial infection. World J Surg. 1998;22(2):158-63.
15. Malangoni MA. Evaluation and management of tertiary peritonitis. Am Surg. 2000;66(2):157-61.
16. Menzies D, Ellis H. Intestinal obstruction from adhesions: how big is the problem? Ann R Coll Surg Engl. 1990;72:60-3.
17. Luijendijk RW, de Lange DC, Wauters CC, et al. Foreign material in postoperative adhesions. Ann Surg. 1996;223:242-8.
18. Parker C, Ellis H, Moran BJ, et al. Postoperative adhesions: ten-year follow-up of 12,584 patients undergoing lower abdominal surgery. Dis Colon Rectum. 2001;44:822-30.
19. Ellis H. The magnitude of adhesion related problems. Ann Chir Gynaecol. 1998;87:9-11.
20. Parker C, Wilson MS, Menzies D, et al. The SCAR-3 study: 5-year adhesion related readmission risk following lower abdominal surgical procedures. Colorectal Dis. 2005;7:551-8.
21. Tortella BJ, Lavery RF, Chandrakantan A, et al. Incidence and risk factors for early small bowel obstruction after celiotomy for penetrating abdominal trauma. Am Surg. 1995;61:956-8.
22. Stewart RM, Page CP, Brender J, et al. The incidence and risk of early postoperative small bowel obstruction: a cohort study. Am J Surg. 1987;154:643-7.
23. Ellis H, Moran BJ, Thompson JN, et al. Adhesion-related hospital readmissions after abdominal and pelvic surgery: a retrospective cohort study. Lancet. 1999 May 1;353(9163):1476-80.
24. Catena F, Di Saverio, Kelly MD, et al. Bologna guidelines for diagnosis and management of adhesive small bowel obstruction (ASBO): 2010 Evidence-based guidelines of the World Society of Emergency Surgery. World J Emerg Surg. 2011;6:5.
25. Thompson William M, et al. Accuracy of abdominal radiography in acute small-bowel obstruction: Does reviewer experience matter? AJR 2007;188:W233-8.
26. Obuz F, Terzi C, Sokmen S, et al. The efficacy of helical CT in the diagnosis of small bowel obstruction. Eur J Radiol. 2003;48(3):299-304.
27. Zalcman M, Sy M, Donckier V, et al. Helical CT signs in the diagnosis of intestinal ischemia in small-bowel obstruction. AJR Am J Roentgenol. 2000;175(6):1601-7.
28. Abbas S, Bissett IP, Parry BR. Oral water soluble contrast for the management of adhesive small bowel obstruction. Cochrane Database Syst Rev. 2007;18(3):CD004651.
29. Abbas SM, Bissett IP, Parry BR. Meta-analysis of oral water-soluble contrast agent in the management of adhesive small bowel obstruction. Br J Surg. 2007;94(4):404-11.
30. Branco BC, Barmparas G, Schnüriger B, et al. Systematic review and meta-analysis of the diagnostic and therapeutic role of water-soluble contrast agent in adhesive small bowel obstruction. Br J Surg. 2010;97(4):470-8.
31. Landercasper J, Cogbill TH, Merry WH, et al. Long-term outcome after hospitalization for small-bowel obstruction. Arch Surg. 1993;128:765-70.
32. Li MZ, Lian L, Xiao LB, et al. Laparoscopic versus open adhesiolysis in patients with adhesive small bowel obstruction: a systematic review and meta-analysis. [Review] Am J Surg. 2012;204(5):779-86.
33. Catena F, Ansaloni L, Di Saverio S, et al. P.O.P.A. study: prevention of postoperative abdominal adhesions by icodextrin 4% solution after laparotomy for adhesive small bowel obstruction. A prospective randomized controlled trial. World Society of Emergency Surgery. J Gastrointest Surg. 2012;16(2):382-8.
34. Qu Z, Liu L. Management of pseudomyxoma peritonei. World J Gastroenterol. 2006;12(38):6124-7.
35. Youssef H, Newman C, Chandrakumaran K, et al. Operative findings, early complications, and long-term survival in 456 patients with pseudomyxoma peritonei syndrome of appendiceal origin. Dis Colon Rectum. 2011;54(3):293-9.
36. Chua TC, Moran BJ, Sugarbaker PH, et al. Early- and long-term outcome data of patients with pseudomyxoma peritonei from appendiceal origin treated by a strategy of cytoreductive surgery and hyperthermic intraperitoneal chemotherapy. J Clin Oncol. 2012;30(20):2449-56.
37. Mynter H. Acute psoitis. Buffalo Med Surg J. 1881;21:202-10.
38. Bagul NB, Abeysekara AMS, Jacob S. Primary psoas abscess due to Streptococcus milleri. Ann Clin Microbiol Antimicrob. 2008; 7:7.
39. Gruenwald I, Abrahamson J, Cohen O. Psoas abscess: case report and review of the literature. J Urol. 1992;147:1624-6.
40. Navarro Lopez V, Ramos JM, Meseguer V, et al. GTI-SEMI Group. Microbiology and outcome of iliopsoas abscess in 124 patients. Medicine. 2009;88(2):120-30.
41. Tabrizian P, Nguyen SQ, Greenstein A, et al. Management and treatment of iliopsoas abscess. Arch Surg. 2009;144(10):946-9.
42. Ricci MA, Rose FB, Meyer KK. Pyogenic psoas abscess: worldwide variations in etiology. World J Surg. 1986;10:834.
43. Agrawal SN, Dwivedi AJ, Khan M. Primary psoas abscess. Dig Dis Sci. 2002;47:2103-5.

44. Hamano S, Kiyoshima K, Nakatsu H, et al. Pyogenic psoas abscess: difficulty in early diagnosis. Urol Int. 2003;71(2): 178-83.
45. Cantasdemir M, Kara B, Cebi D, et al. Computed tomography-guided percutaneous catheter drainage of primary and secondary iliopsoas abscesses. Clin Radiol. 2003;58(10): 811-5.
46. Kottra JJ, Dunnick NR. Retroperitoneal fibrosis. Radiol Clin North Am. 1996;34:1259-75.
47. Uibu T, Oksa P, Auvinen A, et al. Asbestos exposure as a risk factor for retroperitoneal fibrosis. Lancet. 2004;363(9419): 1422-6.
48. Koep L, Zuidema GD. The clinical significance of retroperitoneal fibrosis. Surgery. 1977;81(3):250-7.
49. Amis ES Jr. Retroperitoneal fibrosis. AJR. 1991;157:321-9.
50. Mulligan SA, Holley HC, Koehler RA, et al. CT and MR imaging in the evaluation of retroperitoneal fibrosis. J Comput Assist Tomogr. 1989;13:277-81.

Additional references can be found in the online version of this book.

68

Appendix

Peter Lamb

Key Points

- Appendectomy remains the gold standard for acute appendicitis because nonoperative treatment with antibiotics has a high recurrence rate.
- Laparoscopic appendectomy results in a more rapid return to normal activities than open appendectomy, but there may be a higher risk of postoperative abscess formation.
- A nonoperative approach is appropriate for most patients with appendix mass or abscess, with radiological drainage if required. Other underlying disease should be excluded, but interval appendectomy is only indicated for patients with recurrent symptoms.

INTRODUCTION

Despite being a vestigial structure in humans, the appendix has great clinical importance: acute appendicitis remains the most common abdominal surgical emergency that requires operation. Other rare but important conditions of the appendix include appendiceal carcinoid and appendiceal carcinoma.

SURGICAL ANATOMY

The vermiform appendix is a diverticulum of the cecum, arising from its posteromedial surface about 2 cm below the ileocecal valve. It is of variable length (from 2 to 20 cm) and position; with the tip most commonly lying in a retrocecal or pelvic site (Fig. 68.1). The appendiceal artery, a branch of the ileocolic artery, runs within the free edge of the mesoappendix. This is a triangular mesenteric fold originating from the posterior leaf of peritoneum from the terminal ileum. Lymphatic drainage is along the appendiceal and ileocolic arteries toward the superior mesenteric lymph nodes.

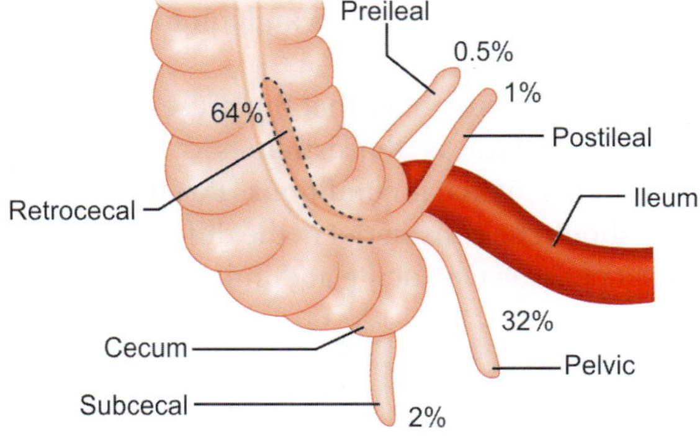

Fig. 68.1: The anatomical position of the tip of the appendix.

ACUTE APPENDICITIS

The incidence of acute appendicitis is 7–10% in the United Kingdom and North American population. Although it is often thought of as a disease of childhood, appendicitis can develop at any age, with a peak incidence in the third decade and a male to female ratio of 1.5:1.

Pathophysiology

Acute appendicitis develops secondary to blockage of the lumen commonly by a fecolith, enlarged lymphoid tissue within the appendix wall, worms, or tumors of the cecum or appendix. Obstruction leads to bacterial infection and inflammation of the appendix wall and adjacent tissues, often including the omentum. The inflammation may remain localized or progress to gangrenous appendicitis and perforation. This in turn can lead to a localized appendiceal mass or abscess, or more generalized contamination with peritonitis.

Clinical Features

The classic presentation of acute appendicitis is of 6–12 hours' central abdominal pain, which migrates to the right iliac fossa and is exacerbated by movement. It is not simply a pain and is usually accompanied by systemic upset; nausea, vomiting, and, in particular, anorexia are common. On clinical examination, patients often have low-grade pyrexia, appear flushed, and exhibit signs of localized peritonitis in the right iliac fossa. Clinical evidence of peritoneal inflammation is best elicited by percussion tenderness rather than with traditional rebound tenderness, which is poorly tolerated by the patient. Rovsing's sign, demonstrated by pain in the right lower quadrant on palpation of the left lower quadrant, is an unreliable sign. Although the point of maximal tenderness may be over McBurney's point (two-third of the way along a line from umbilicus to anterior superior iliac spine), this can vary with the position of the appendix. A retrocecal appendix can lead to tenderness in the right loin or even right upper quadrant, whereas a pelvic appendix may be associated with a history of diarrhea and minimal abdominal tenderness.

It is important to remember that the presentation can vary widely, particularly at the extremes of age and in patients with other medical conditions. For this reason, appendicitis should be considered in the differential diagnosis for most patients with acute abdominal pain.

DIAGNOSIS OF ACUTE APPENDICITIS

Acute appendicitis remains a condition in which the decision to operate is usually based solely on clinical assessment. A classic history and the presence of peritonism in the right iliac fossa are highly predictive of acute appendicitis. Although most senior surgeons will make an assessment based on experience, formal clinical scoring systems have been developed to aid the diagnosis of appendicitis. The best known is the Alvarado score, which allocates points for elements of the clinical history, examination, and blood results (Table 68.1).[1] It is reported to be reliable at ruling out appendicitis below a score of 5, but a score of 7 tends to overpredict appendicitis, particularly in children and females.[2]

Table 68.1 The Alvarado scoring system for the diagnosis of appendicitis.[1]

Abdominal pain migrating to the right iliac fossa	(1 point)
Anorexia	(1 point)
Nausea/vomiting	(1 point)
Right iliac fossa tenderness	(2 points)
Rebound tenderness in right iliac fossa	(1 point)
Pyrexia > 37.3	(1 point)
Raised serum white cell count (WCC > 10000)	(2 points)
Increase in neutrophils within the WCC	(1 point)

(A score of 5 or 6 is in keeping with a diagnosis of acute appendicitis. A score of 7 or 8 indicates probable appendicitis, and a score of 9 or 10 indicates very probable appendicitis).

Differential Diagnosis

Many abdominal emergencies must be considered in the differential diagnosis of acute appendicitis, depending on the age and sex of the patient.

Children

In children the most common conditions that mimic appendicitis are gastroenteritis and mesenteric adenitis. It is important to consider the diagnosis of appendicitis even in younger children; although the incidence is lower in the under-fives, the perforation rate is higher, partly due to delays in diagnosis.

Young Adults

In young adults, the most common differentials include mesenteric adenitis, gynecological diseases, gastroenteritis, right-sided urinary tract problems, and distal small bowel disease (including Meckel's diverticulitis). Gynecological disorders constitute an important group as lower abdominal pain in young women is a common presentation, and removal of a normal appendix is most frequent in this group. Pelvic inflammatory disease and complications of ovarian cyst may be difficult to differentiate on clinical grounds, although they are often associated with less gastrointestinal upset. Patients with pelvic inflammation generally have a longer history and may demonstrate cervical excitation and discharge on pelvic examination. A ruptured ovarian follicle is a normal part of ovulation occurring midcycle (mittelschmerz), and such pain is associated with less systemic upset. Torsion of an ovary requires urgent intervention and should be suspected if there is a sudden onset of severe pain. It is essential to rule out a ruptured ectopic pregnancy, although it must be remembered that acute appendicitis can occur during early pregnancy also.

Older Patients

In addition to an exacerbation of pre-existing abdominal problems, other acute gastrointestinal diagnoses such as diverticulitis, cecal cancer, large bowel obstruction, closed

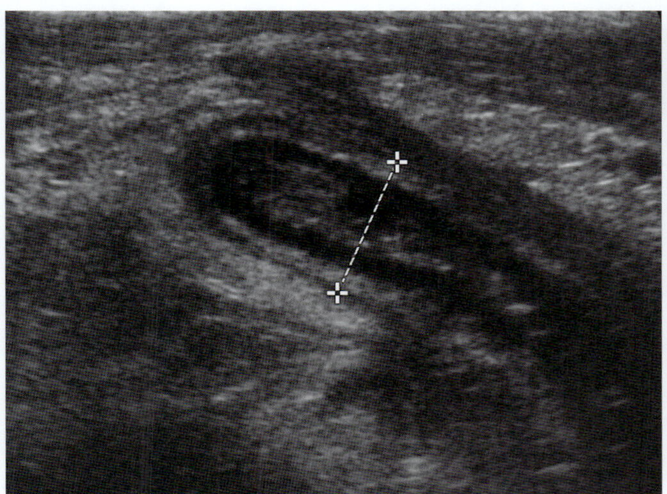

Fig. 68.2: Transabdominal ultrasound showing an acutely inflamed appendix.
Source: Dr. Judith Anderson, Royal Infirmary of Edinburgh.

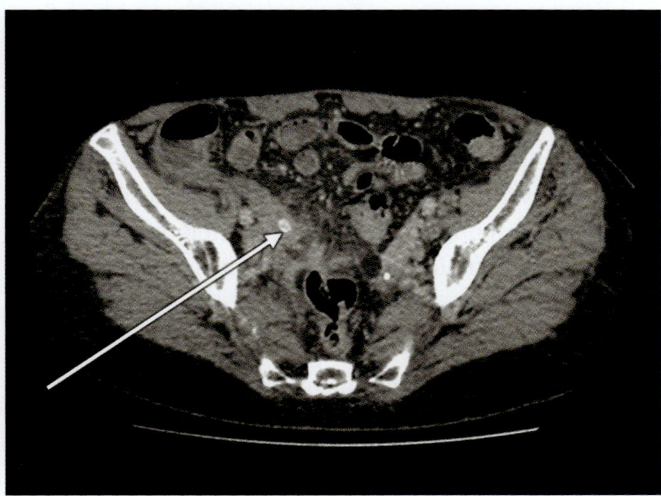

Fig. 68.3: Contrast enhanced computed tomography (CT) scan showing acute appendicitis with a fecolith in the distal appendix (arrow).

loop small bowel obstruction, perforated peptic ulcer disease, and cholecystitis should be considered. Nonsurgical diagnoses such as urinary tract conditions and lower lobe pneumonia can also cause diagnostic confusion.

Investigations

Many patients with appendicitis will have a moderate leukocytosis with a relative increase in neutrophils. C-reactive protein may be more accurate than white cell count and can be used in combination to aid in the diagnosis of appendicitis.[3] Urinalysis should be performed as a routine; red cells and white cells may be present in appendicitis when the inflamed appendix is in contact with the urinary tract. The presence of organisms on microscopy is more suggestive of urinary tract infection. Patients who are unwell with right flank pain should undergo urgent radiological investigation to exclude an obstructed kidney and to differentiate this from retrocecal appendicitis. All women of child-bearing age should undergo a urinary pregnancy test, with selective use of serum BHCG.

Ultrasonography

Transabdominal ultrasound is commonly used for patients with suspected appendicitis. The criterion for diagnosis of acute appendicitis is visualization of a noncompressible appendix that has a maximal outer diameter of 6–7 mm (Fig. 68.2). Despite a systematic review reporting a sensitivity of 0.86 in published series, in most units ultrasound scanning is not accurate enough to exclude appendicitis.[4] The main role of ultrasound scan is to exclude other pathology, particularly gynecological diagnoses in young women. It may also identify secondary features of appendicitis such as free fluid and aperistaltic bowel in the right iliac fossa. In patients with a high clinical suspicion of appendicitis, operation should not be delayed waiting for the availability of such imaging, or as a result of false reassurance following a "normal" ultrasound scan.

Computed Tomography (CT)

There has been a move toward using cross-sectional imaging, primarily CT, in assessing patients with suspected appendicitis (Fig. 68.3). It has been reported to have an accuracy of 98% and to be costeffective.[5] In North America it has even been proposed that CT should form a routine part of the assessment of adult patients with lower abdominal pain.[6] Standard surgical practice in the UK is still to proceed directly to laparoscopy for most patients with clinical suspicion of appendicitis. There should be a low threshold for using CT imaging to confirm the diagnosis in older patients, where the risk of malignant pathology is more likely, and when the risks of laparoscopy are increased due to comorbidities or previous abdominal surgery. If laparoscopic equipment is not available, then traditional appendectomy via a small right iliac fossa incision remains appropriate.

OPERATIONS FOR APPENDICITIS

In patients who are clinically well and have mild signs, emergency operation in the middle of the night is not indicated and should be deferred to a dedicated emergency theater list in the morning. The incidence of perforation in this group is no higher than if they are taken to theater for early exploration.[7,8] Intravenous antibiotics may be given once a decision has been made to operate. The risk of morbidity is increased if the appendix perforates; therefore when appendicitis is suspected, intervention (usually laparoscopy) remains best surgical practice.

Open Appendectomy

A transverse (Lanz) incision has replaced the historical, more vertical, gridiron incision. It is made over the point of maximum tenderness, usually centered over McBurney's point. The muscle layers are then sequentially split, lateral to the rectus sheath, in the direction of the muscle fibers until the peritoneum is identified and opened. Palpation of the patient's abdomen once they are anesthetized may reveal a lump or fullness, and the incision should be centered there.

Once the peritoneal cavity has been entered, any peritoneal fluid should be sampled for culture. An inflamed appendix is often identified by palpation and can be mobilized from inflammatory adhesions with blunt dissection. If the appendix is not easily identified, as can be the case with an inflamed retrocecal organ, then the cecum should be mobilized into the wound and the convergence of the teniae coli used to identify the base of the appendix. The appendix is then mobilized into the wound so that the appendiceal artery can be ligated, usually within the mesoappendix adjacent to the appendix base. Sometimes it can be necessary to dissect in retrograde fashion from the tip of the appendix to its base. The appendix is ligated close to its base, and a purse-string suture can be used to invert the appendix stump, although simple ligation is adequate.[9] If the appendix has perforated at its base, formal repair of the cecal pole is required. Peritoneal lavage should be performed but an abdominal drain is not required unless there is an established abscess cavity.

If the appendix is normal, further examination should include: terminal ileum to exclude an inflamed Meckel's diverticulum or Crohn's ileitis, small bowel mesentery for lymph nodes, the pelvis to rule out tubo-ovarian pathology, and sigmoid colon for diverticulitis. If no abnormality is identified, removal of the appendix is appropriate to avoid diagnostic confusion in the future. The presence of free bile suggests a perforated peptic ulcer, small bowel or gallbladder. In this situation, unless the source is easily accessible it is best to convert to a midline incision.

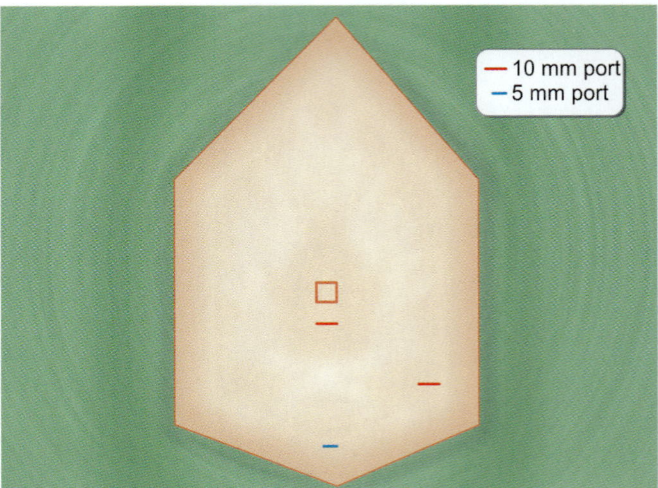

Fig. 68.4: Port positions for laparoscopic appendectomy.

Laparoscopic Appendectomy

A number of port positions have been described for laparoscopic appendectomy. One technique is to place working ports at the umbilicus (10 mm) and in the suprapubic region (5 mm), with the camera port in the left iliac fossa (10 mm) (Fig. 68.4). A 5 mm left iliac fossa port can be used if a 5 mm camera is available, or if the umbilicus is used as the camera port. Occasionally an additional 5 mm right iliac fossa port may be required for retraction, such as for an obese patient with a retrocecal appendix. More recently the role of single-port laparoscopic appendectomy has been evaluated. Although this technique is feasible, it does not appear to improve pain or cosmesis compared with standard laparoscopic appendectomy.[10]

The technical steps of laparoscopic appendectomy mirror those of open operation. The mesoappendix can be divided with diathermy at the level of the appendix, tied in continuity with ligatures or controlled by clips. The appendix is usually ligated at its base with a preformed ligature. An alternative, but expensive, technique is to fire a laparoscopic stapler across the base of the appendix. It is important to ensure that the whole appendix has been mobilized to prevent leaving a long stump and risking recurrent symptoms.[11]

The appendix should be removed from the abdomen in a retrieval bag, along with any fecoliths, to avoid wound contamination. Peritoneal lavage is vital in contaminated cases to prevent postoperative abscess. In the author's hospital it is standard practice to leave a drain in the pelvis to remove residual lavage fluid in the immediate postoperative period (this is often removed within

24 hours). If conversion to open operation is required, then the laparoscope can be used to allow accurate placement of the incision.

Laparoscopic versus Open Appendectomy

As laparoscopic skills have developed, laparoscopic appendectomy has been widely adopted as the standard of care. It has also been extensively studied and compared to open appendectomy. A recent Cochrane systematic review of 67 studies has reported that laparoscopic appendectomy results in less pain, faster recovery and lower incidence of wound infection.[12] Laparoscopic appendectomy was recommended, particularly for young female, obese, and working patients. The Cochrane review did report an increase in intra-abdominal abscesses (odds ratio 1.87) when compared to an open approach. The reason for this is not clear, but it could reflect a failure to adequately drain lavage fluid, as already discussed, or poor patient selection.

The Normal Appendix at Laparoscopy

In general, a normal appendix should not be removed at a first laparoscopy if a definite alternative diagnosis for the patient's symptoms is identified. If a normal appendix is seen and there is no other cause for the patient's symptoms, there are two arguments for removing the appendix. First, there is a small incidence of inflammation within a macroscopically normal appendix, although the clinical significance is debatable,[13] and second, to avoid diagnostic confusion in the future. The patient should be counseled about the options preoperatively. In someone with recurrent episode of right iliac fossa pain, it is logical to remove the appendix.

Postoperative Complications

The most common postoperative complication is wound infection, occurring in about 10% of patients following open appendectomy, although less following laparoscopic surgery. All patients should receive a single dose of prophylactic broad-spectrum antibiotics against the risk of wound infection. For perforated appendicitis, a treatment course of intravenous antibiotics is appropriate, with conversion to the oral route once patients are tolerating diet. Washing out the wound prior to skin closure with saline or antiseptic solution is also commonly practiced.

Infected intra-abdominal collections are a less common but potentially serious complication of appendectomy. Local collections around the cecum often present with abdominal discomfort and a failure to progress postoperatively. They can be diagnosed by ultrasound or CT and are usually treated with antibiotics, with radiological drainage reserved for larger collections. A pelvic abscess can present in a more delayed fashion with lower abdominal discomfort, swinging pyrexia, and diarrhea. Digital rectal examination may raise suspicion of the presence of a pelvic abscess. CT is usually required for diagnosis, and a percutaneous radiological drain should be placed if possible. If this is not possible and a trial of antibiotics is unsuccessful, then formal surgical drainage is required. Rectal examination and digital rupture through the rectal wall into the abscess cavity is rarely indicated now.

The length of hospital stay following appendectomy depends on the patient's acute condition and any comorbidity. Laparoscopic appendectomy is associated with a more rapid return to normal activities than open operation.[12] However, oral diet and early mobilization are well tolerated by most patients, regardless of the surgical approach.[14] Discharge can be within 24 hours for routine cases, but those with perforated appendicitis or comorbidity often have a more protracted recovery.

The mortality of appendicitis is associated with patient age and delay in diagnosis. The Royal College of Surgeons of England reported a mortality of 0.24% and morbidity of 7.7% in 6596 patients undergoing open appendectomy between 1990 and 1992.[15]

Long-Term Effects of Appendectomy

The main long-term complication after appendectomy is adhesional small-bowel obstruction. This complication has been evaluated in a cohort study in Sweden with population-based matched controls.[16] The overall risk of reoperation for adhesional small-bowel obstruction 30 years after open appendectomy was 1.3%, compared with 0.21% in the nonoperated control group. A higher risk was associated with patients who had undergone appendectomy for other conditions, or for a perforated appendix.

Another, somewhat controversial, long-term consideration is the risk of tubal infertility after appendectomy. It had been reported that the increased risk of tubal infertility following perforated appendicitis was as high as 4.8 in nulliparous women.[17] A more recent historical cohort study found no effect on fertility.[18]

NONSURGICAL TREATMENT OF APPENDICITIS

There is no doubt that on occasion acute appendicitis can settle spontaneously, as some patients report similar previous episodes.[19] There are also some patients with localized signs who will recover with antibiotic treatment. This fact has been demonstrated by a number of randomized trials comparing antibiotic treatment versus appendectomy in patients with suspected appendicitis.[20-23] The difficulty with nonoperative treatment was highlighted by a recent trial, which found that despite CT assessment 18% of patients were found at operation to have unexpected complicated appendicitis.[23] Importantly, 12% of patients treated with antibiotics required appendectomy within 30 days and a further 26% developed recurrent symptoms requiring operation within one year. A Cochrane review of five randomized trials reported that only 73% of patients treated with antibiotics were cured (including recurrence within one year) within two weeks without major complication, compared to 97% of patients who underwent early appendectomy.[24]

At present, operative treatment remains the standard treatment for acute appendicitis. Antibiotic treatment might be used as an alternative treatment in specific patients, with localized signs and factors that favor a nonoperative approach. Regular clinical review is important as early operation is indicated if there is a failure to improve.

TREATMENT OF ATYPICAL PRESENTATIONS OF APPENDICITIS

Appendix Mass/Abscess

An appendix mass develops when the presentation of acute appendicitis is delayed and the inflamed appendix becomes contained by omentum and small bowel (Fig. 68.5). Patients usually present with 7–10 days of right iliac fossa pain and a tender fullness in this region. An appendix mass should be managed nonoperatively with antibiotics. If an abscess is present, the patient is often systemically unwell with increased abdominal tenderness (Fig. 68.6A), and radiological drainage is usually first-line treatment (Fig. 68.6B). If operation is required, then the residual appendix should be removed with any associated fecoliths.

A recent meta-analysis reported that nonoperative treatment of appendix mass or abscess is associated with

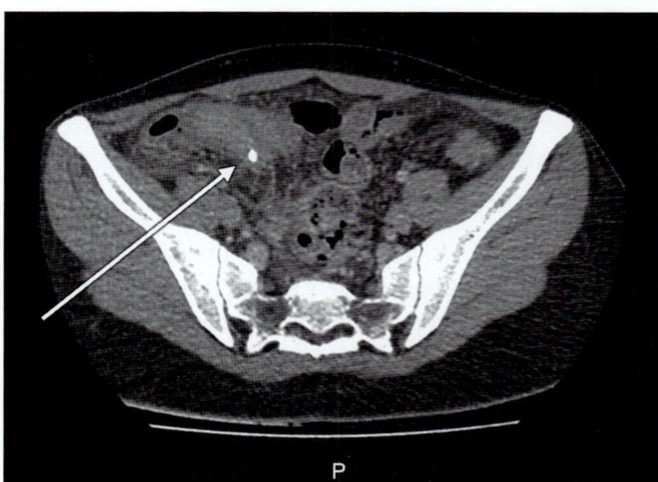

Fig. 68.5: Contrast enhanced computed tomography (CT) scan showing an appendix mass with a fecolith (arrow).

fewer complications than acute appendectomy.[25] Radiological drainage can occasionally lead to the development of a fistula (Fig. 68.6C); however, this will usually resolve spontaneously providing there is no other underlying pathology. Once an appendix mass or abscess has been treated, further investigations including CT and colonoscopy should be performed to exclude alternative diagnoses such as Crohn's disease or cecal carcinoma. Providing other conditions are excluded, then routine interval appendectomy is no longer recommended other than for the small group of patients who develop troublesome recurrent symptoms.[26]

Appendicitis in Pregnancy

The assessment of patients with right lower quadrant pain during pregnancy is something many trainee surgeons find difficult due to concern about missing appendicitis but also the risks of unnecessary operation. It is important to remember that the incidence of appendicitis in pregnancy is similar to that in the general population. The preoperative diagnosis of appendicitis can be difficult, and a low threshold for surgical intervention has traditionally been recommended, as perforated appendicitis is associated with an increased rate of fetal loss and maternal morbidity. The reported rates of fetal loss are 3.4%, 12.1%, and 7.3% for simple, complicated and negative appendectomy, respectively.[27] The negative appendectomy rate is higher than in the general population and the risk associated with a negative appendectomy[28] has led to an increase in preoperative investigation. The American College of Radiology recommends that MRI can be used

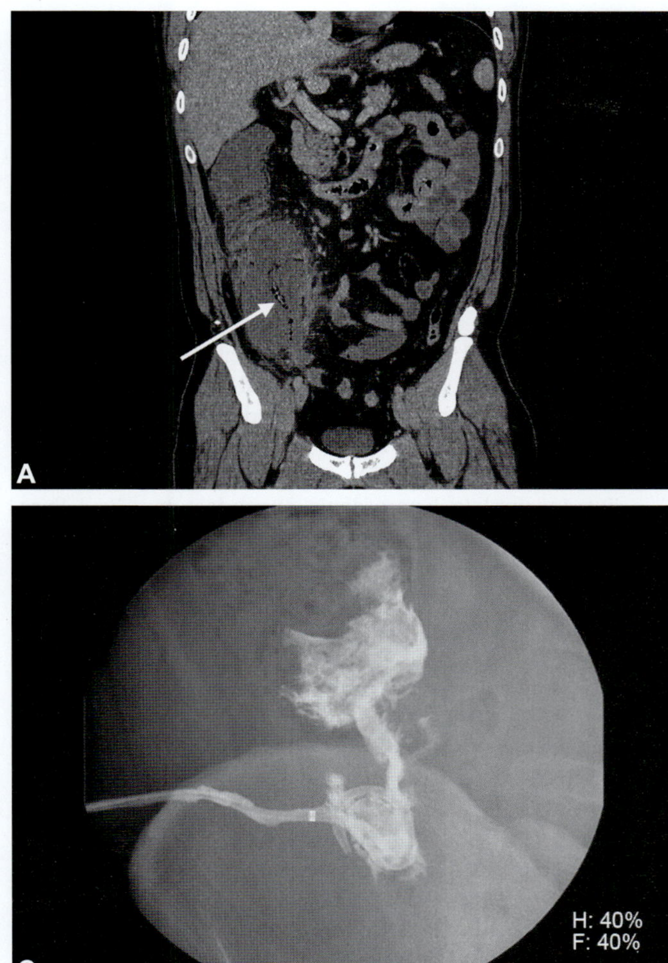

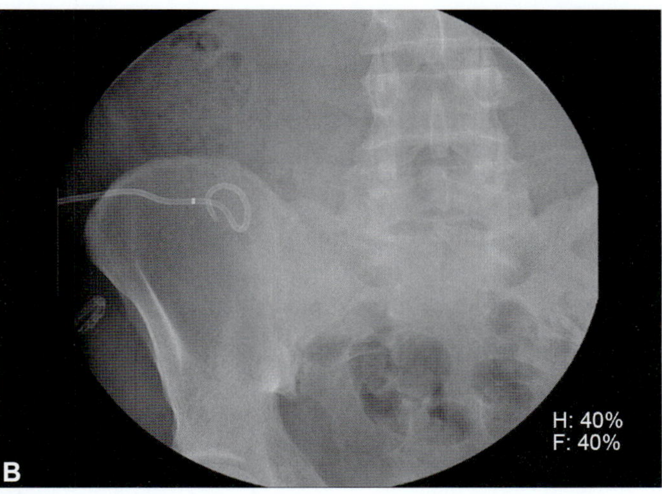

Figs. 68.6A to C: (A) Coronal image of a contrast enhanced computed tomography (CT) scan showing an appendix abscess with the appendix lying within it (arrow); (B) Radiologically guided drainage of the appendix abscess shown in (A); (C) Tubogram performed 4 weeks after drain placement in (B) showing a fistulous connection to the cecal pole at the site of previously perforated appendix.
Source: Dr. Fergus Perks, Royal Infirmary of Edinburgh.

to exclude appendicitis if ultrasound examination cannot identify a normal appendix. If emergency access to such imaging is available it is recommended, but it should not delay operation in patients with a high clinical suspicion of appendicitis.

Many studies have demonstrated laparoscopic appendectomy to be safe during pregnancy. However, a large observational study has reported a higher risk of fetal loss for laparoscopy compared to open operation (odds ratio 2.3),[28] and this has influenced the findings of a subsequent systematic review.[27] This fact does not contraindicate laparoscopic appendectomy in pregnancy, but it does indicate a need for further research. The Society of American Gastrointestinal and Endoscopic Surgeons (SAGES) continue to recommend laparoscopic appendectomy as the treatment of choice for pregnant patients.[29]

The assessment of pregnant patients should involve senior general and obstetric surgeons. A reasonable approach is to use laparoscopy in the first trimester or when despite imaging the diagnosis is in doubt. There should be a low threshold for converting to open operation. In later pregnancy open surgery may be preferred when the diagnosis is confirmed. If the appendix is normal at laparoscopy, it should not routinely be removed.

TUMORS OF THE APPENDIX

Neuroendocrine Tumors

Carcinoid tumors account for 50% of tumors of the appendix. They are usually found incidentally on histopathology after an operation for acute appendicitis. They are most commonly located at the tip, with only 10% involving the base of the appendix. Current guidelines recommend that small (<1 cm), completely excised carcinoids of the appendix that are well differentiated with no evidence of lymphovascular invasion can be regarded as cured. A right hemicolectomy is recommended for patients with tumor invasion at the appendix base, and for tumors >2 cm.

For patients with tumors >2 cm, the 5-year mortality is almost 30%.[30]

Epithelial Tumors of the Appendix

Epithelial tumors of the appendix account for about 1% of colorectal tumors in the United States each year. Patients with invasive adenocarcinoma of the appendix require right hemicolectomy for management of the primary tumor. Often tumors are mucinous in nature, and although many are noninvasive, they have frequently ruptured at the time of presentation, leading to peritoneal dissemination. Rupture can produce pseudomyxoma peritonei. In this condition, there are multiple peritoneal implants of gelatinous material that microscopically are made up of nests of tumor cells. Patients may present acutely as "appendicitis" or with abdominal distension secondary to intra-abdominal tumor. Traditionally patients were managed with palliative debulking surgery, but cytoreductive surgery combined with intraperitoneal chemotherapy has led to long-term survival for many patients in specialist units, and is now recommended.[31] Some appendiceal tumors are very aggressive, leading to death within 2 years of diagnosis.

Other Benign Tumors

A number of rare benign tumors of the appendix have been reported, including neurofibromas and leiomyomas. Appendectomy is recommended, both to confirm the diagnosis and as treatment.

REFERENCES

1. Alvarado A. A practical score for the early diagnosis of acute appendicitis. Ann Emerg Med. 1986;15:557-64.
2. Ohle R, O'Reilly F, O'Brien KK, et al. The Alvarado score for predicting acute appendicitis: a systematic review. BMC Med. 2011;28(9):b139.
3. Yu CW, Juan LI, Wu MH, et al. Systematic review and meta-analysis of the diagnostic accuracy of procalcitonin, C-reactive protein and white blood cell count for suspected acute appendicitis. Br J Surg. 2013;100(3):322-9.
4. Terasawa T, Blackmore CC, Bent S, et al. Systematic review: computed tomography and ultrasonography to detect acute appendicitis in adults and adolescents. Ann Intern Med. 2004;141(7):537-46.
5. Rao PM, Rhea JT, Novelline RA, et al. Effect of computed tomography of the appendix on treatment of patients and use of hospital resources. N Engl J Med. 1998;338:141-6.
6. Krajewski S, Brown J, Phang PT, et al. Impact of computed tomography of the abdomen on clinical outcomes in patients with acute right lower quadrant pain: a meta-analysis. Can J Surg. 2011;54(1):43-53.
7. McLean AD, Stonebridge PA, Bradbury AW, et al. Time of presentation, time of operation, and unnecessary appendectomy. Br Med J. 1993;306:307.
8. Surana R, Quinn F, Puri P. Is it necessary to perform appendectomy in the middle of the night in children? Br Med J. 1993;306:1168.
9. Engstrom L, Fenvo G. Appendectomy: assessment of stump invagination: a prospective, randomised trial. Br J Surg. 1985;72:971-2.
10. Lee WS, Choi ST, Lee JN, et al. Single-port laparoscopic appendectomy versus conventional laparoscopic appendectomy: a prospective randomized controlled study. Ann Surg. 2013;257(2):214-8.
11. Milne AA, Bradbury AW. 'Residual' appendicitis following incomplete laparoscopic appendectomy. Br J Surg. 1996;83:217.
12. Sauerland S, Jaschinski T, Neugebauer EA. Laparoscopic versus open surgery for suspected appendicitis. Cochrane Database Syst Rev. 2010;(10):CD001546.
13. Wang Y, Reen DJ, Puri P. Is a histologically normal appendix following emergency appendectomy always normal? Lancet. 1996;347:1076-9.
14. Salam IMA, Fallouji MA, El Ashaal YI, et al. Early patient discharge following appendectomy: safety and feasibility. J R Coll Surg Edinb. 1995;40:300-2.
15. Baigrie RJ, Dehn TCB, Fowler SM, et al. Analysis of 8651 appendicectomies in England and Wales during 1992. Br J Surg. 1995;82:933.
16. Andersson REB. Small bowel obstruction after appendectomy. Br J Surg. 2001;88:1387-91.
17. Mueller BA, Daling JR, Moore DE, et al. Appendectomy and the risk of tubal infertility. N Engl J Med. 1986;315:1506-7.
18. Andersson R, Lambe M, Bergstrom R. Fertility patterns after appendectomy: historical cohort study. BMJ. 1999 Apr 10;318(7189):963-7.
19. Barber MD, McLaren J, Rainey JB. Recurrent appendicitis. Br J Surg. 1997;84:110-12.
20. Eriksson S, Granstrom L. Randomised controlled trial of appendectomy versus antibiotic therapy for acute appendicitis. Br J Surg. 1995;82:166-9.
21. Styrud J, Eriksson S, Nilsson I, et al. Appendectomy versus antibiotic treatment in acute appendicitis. A prospective multicentre randomized controlled trial. World J Surg. 2006;30:1033-7.
22. Hansson J, Korner U, Khorram-Manesh, et al. Randomised clinical trial of antibiotic therapy versus appendectomy as primary treatment of acute appendicitis in unselected patients. Br J Surg. 2009;96:473-81.
23. Vons C, Barry C, Maitre S, et al. Amoxicillin plus clavulanic acid versus appendectomy for treatment of acute uncomplicated appendicitis: an open-label, non-inferiority, randomised controlled trial. Lancet. 2011;377(9777):1573-9.

24. Wilms I, de Hoog D, de Visser. Appendectomy versus antibiotic treatment for acute appendicitis. Cochrane Database Syst Rev. 2011 Nov 9;(11):CD008359.
25. Simillis C, Symeonides P, Shorthouse AJ, et al. A meta-analysis comparing conservative treatment versus acute appendectomy for complicated appendicitis (abscess or phlegmon). Surgery. 2010;147(6):818-29.
26. Deakin DE, Ahmed I. Interval appendectomy after resolution of adult inflammatory appendix mass—is it necessary? Surgeon. 2007;5(1):45-50.
27. Walsh CA, Tang T, Walsh SR. et al. Laparoscopic versus open appendectomy in pregnancy: a systematic review. Int J Surg. 2008;6:339-44.
28. McGory ML, Zingmond DS, Tillou A, et al. Negative appendectomy in pregnant women is associated with a substantial risk of fetal loss. J Am Coll Surg. 2007;205(4):534-40.
29. Society of American Gastrointestinal and Endoscopic Surgeons (SAGES). Guidelines for diagnosis, treatment, and use of laparoscopy for surgical problems during pregnancy, 2011. Available at: http://www.sagescms.org.
30. Boudreaux JP, Klimstra DS, Hassan MM. The NANETS consensus guideline for the diagnosis and management of neuroendocrine tumors. Pancreas. 2010 Aug;39(6):753-66.
31. Sugarbaker PH. New standard of care for appendiceal epithelial neoplasms and pseudomyxoma peritonei syndrome. Lancet Oncol. 2006;7:69-76.

69

Small Bowel

John H Robertson, Hugh M Paterson

Key Points

- Pathology of the small intestine is frequently encountered by the general surgeon in both the emergency and elective setting and can present in any age group.
- Disease may affect the small bowel primarily (e.g. Crohn's disease) or through secondary involvement with adjacent intra-abdominal structures (e.g. diverticular disease of the colon with abscess formation).
- The length and the enormous surface area of the small intestine allow it to fulfill its prime purpose of nutrient absorption while also enabling it to perform important immune functions.
- The past decade has seen huge advances in diagnostic tools for small bowel investigation, including magnetic resonance imaging, capsule endoscopy, and enteroscopy. Consequently, laparoscopy and laparotomy have a decreasing role in the primary investigation of small intestinal disease.
- Small intestinal pathology can be managed by a variety of techniques: interventional radiological (CT angiography and embolization), endoscopic (interventional enteroscopy), and operative (both open and laparoscopic).
- Crohn's disease with its preferential involvement of the small intestine remains an important condition. The medical management of Crohn's disease has seen major advances in recent years.
- Small bowel conditions of surgical importance include congenital and acquired diverticula, radiation enteritis, intussusception, bacterial and other microbiological infections, celiac disease, blunt and penetrating trauma, intestinal failure, and the emergence of small bowel transplantation.
- Fistula of the small intestine is most commonly iatrogenic or due to Crohn's disease. Successful management requires control of sepsis, adequate nutrition, defining the anatomy of the fistula and planned surgical intervention in those that do not close spontaneously.
- Cancer of the small intestine is rare, given the size of the organ.

INTRODUCTION

The small intestine is the most important part of the gastrointestinal tract. Without sufficient length to permit proper digestive and absorptive function, adequate enteral nutrition cannot be achieved. The surgeon has a key role in manipulating this process, whether by timely intervention to prevent the downward spiral of intra-abdominal sepsis caused by intestinal fistulae, through progress in the establishment of small intestinal transplantation, or in therapeutic weight loss achieved by bariatric surgery techniques of duodenal switch and gastric bypass procedures. Failure to achieve adequate enteral nutrition as a consequence of inadequate intestinal length is associated with appreciable morbidity and mortality.

In addition to its critical role in processing enteral nutrients, the small intestine has key immunological functions. The enormous surface area of the small intestine facilitates absorption of nutrients but simultaneously exposes the body to pathogens and toxins. The small intestine immune system in health prevents these agents from entering the blood and lymphatic systems; by contrast, dysregulated immune responses between gut stimuli and host underpin the pathophysiology of inflammatory bowel disease.

Small bowel pathology frequently presents to the general surgeon in both the emergency and elective setting. The range of investigation modalities has grown in the past decade with important advances in radiological imaging and continuing development of interventional radiological and endoscopic techniques. For those patients requiring operation, minimally invasive techniques and implementation of the principles of enhanced recovery offer restoration to health with minimal physiological derangement for the patient.

SURGICAL ANATOMY

Embryology

At the beginning of the third week of embryologic development, the alimentary canal is supported by a dorsal mesentery containing three gut arteries supplying the foregut, midgut, and hindgut. The midgut is that portion supplied by the superior mesenteric artery (SMA) that will develop into the intestine running from the distal duodenum to the distal transverse colon in the adult.[1] During the fifth week, rapid elongation of the midgut causes it to bend ventrally in the midplane and form a primary loop. This loop consists of a cephalic and a caudal portion. The cephalic segment forms the proximal small bowel while the caudal segment develops into the final 2 feet of the ileum, the cecum and the proximal colon as far as the distal transverse colon. As the midgut grows, it becomes too large for the abdominal cavity and herniates into the umbilical cord. At this point, it undergoes a counterclockwise rotation of 90° around the axis of the SMA. A further 180° counterclockwise rotation is associated with return of the midgut loops to the abdomen at around the 10th week of gestation. From the 12th week on, the final fixation of the colon and its mesentery to the retroperitoneum takes place.[2]

Regression of the omphalomesenteric (vitelline) duct, a tube joining the midgut to the yolk sac, generally occurs during the 5th to 7th week. Persistence of this duct results in a Meckel's diverticulum or other vitelline duct remnant anomaly.[3] Failure of proper return of the midgut to the abdomen may result in malrotation (Fig. 69.1), omphalocele and mesenteric anomalies (*see* Chapters 124, "Abdominal Wall Deformities", and 125, "Gastrointestinal Surgery in Children").

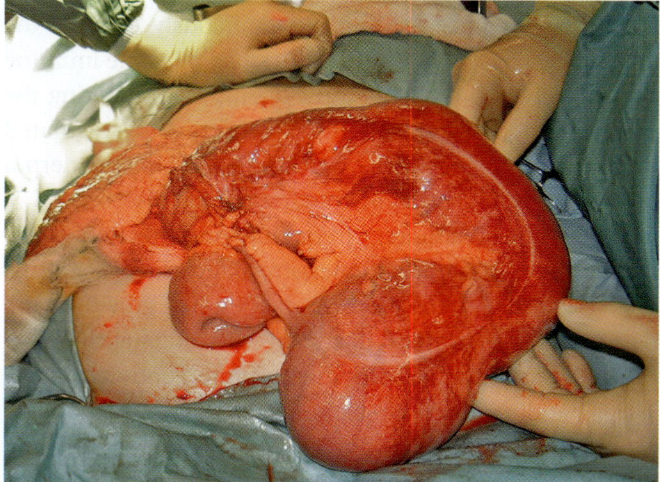

Fig. 69.1: Malrotation of the large intestine. At laparotomy, the cecum and ascending colon are seen to lie to the left of the midline.

Gross Anatomy

The small intestine extends from the pylorus to the ileocecal valve and has a variable overall length ranging from 3 to 9 m. It consists of the duodenum, jejunum, and ileum. The duodenum begins at the pylorus and extends to the duodenojejunal flexure, where it is supported by the ligament of Treitz. The jejunum compromises the proximal 40% of the small intestine and the ileum the remainder; here is no obvious demarcation between them.[4] The small intestine tends to decrease in luminal diameter and mucosal thickness as it extends distally.

Duodenum

The duodenum is 25 cm long, commences at the pylorus, forms a C-shape around the head of the pancreas and terminates at the duodenojejunal flexure at the ligament of Treitz. Anatomically the duodenum can be divided into four sections:

- First part or duodenal bulb (D1), which arises from the pylorus and is 5 cm in length. It lies upon the liver pedicle (portal vein, common bile duct, and hepatic artery).
- Second part (D2) that descends around the head of the pancreas and is crossed by the attachment of the transverse mesocolon.
- Third or transverse part (D3) curves under the uncinate process of the pancreas and is crossed by the superior mesenteric vessels. Posteriorly lie the aorta, inferior vena cava and the vertebral column.
- The fourth or ascending part (D4) runs in the retroperitoneum to the ligament of Treitz, whence it becomes the intraperitoneal jejunum.

These anatomical relationships have important clinical relevance. Most peptic ulcers occur in the first part of the duodenum and are strongly associated with *Helicobacter pylori* infection.[5] Anterior ulceration results in perforation into the peritoneal cavity and clinical presentation with peritonitis. The relationship of the duodenal bulb and the gastroduodenal artery means that posterior ulceration results in major hemorrhage (Figs. 69.2A to C) (*see* Chapter 48, "Peptic Ulcer Disease").

The second part of the duodenum is intimately related to the pancreatic head, sharing a common blood supply. Thus, resection of the second part of the duodenum usually mandates inclusion of the head of the pancreas, that is,

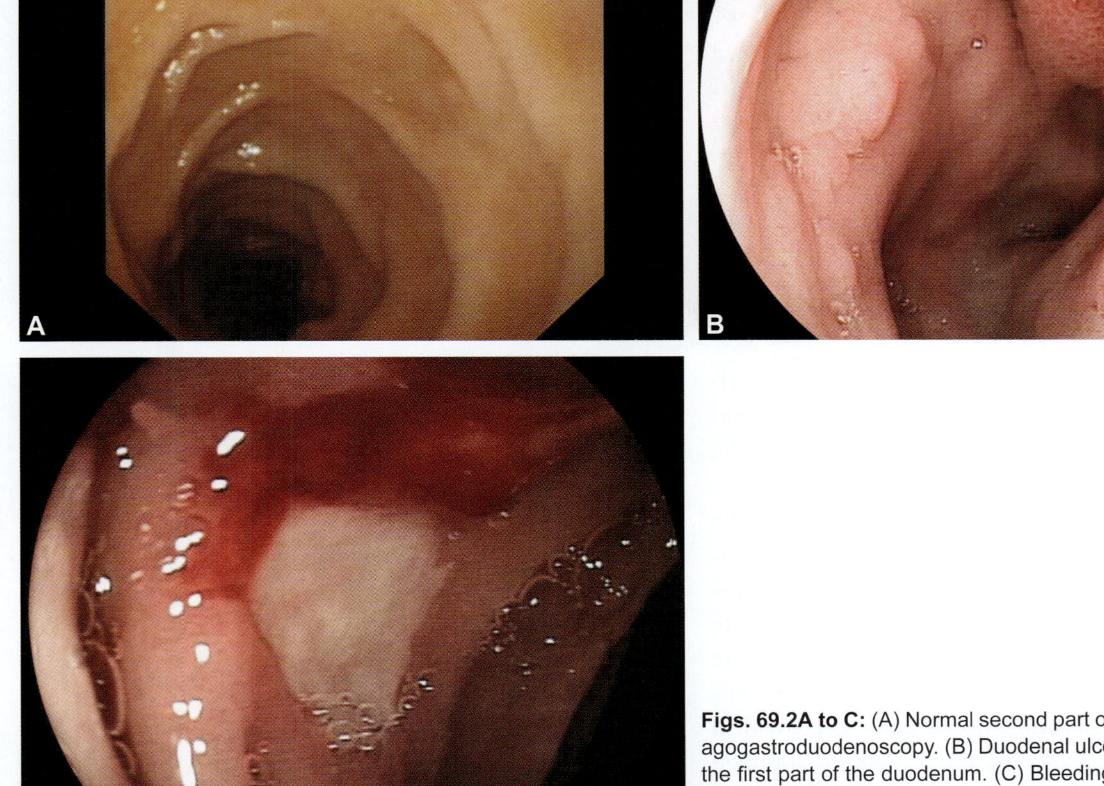

Figs. 69.2A to C: (A) Normal second part of duodenum seen at esophagogastroduodenoscopy. (B) Duodenal ulcer seen in anterior aspect of the first part of the duodenum. (C) Bleeding duodenal ulcer—posterior aspect of first part of duodenum. Gastroduodenal artery lies behind ulcer.

pancreatoduodenectomy—Whipple's procedure. Mobilization of the second part of the duodenum (Kocher's maneuver) involves dissecting the duodenum from the inferior vena cava and the perirenal (Gerota's) fascia. The anatomical arrangement of the relatively fixed retroperitoneal duodenum and the mobile intraperitoneal jejunum makes the duodenal-jejunal junction susceptible to injury in deceleration blunt trauma.

Jejunum and Ileum

The jejunum begins at the ligament of Treitz and occupies the upper left quadrant of the abdomen. The jejunum has a larger circumference than the ileum due to the thicker *valvulae conniventes* or circular folds of mucosa.[6] The ileum courses toward the right lower quadrant of the abdomen and generally contains more fat in the mesentery than the jejunum. Unlike the retroperitoneal duodenum, the jejunoileum is entirely intraperitoneal. The mesentery, which is a large peritoneal fold containing the blood vessels, nerves and lymphatics, suspends the small intestine from the posterior abdominal wall. The root of the mesentery is attached to the retroperitoneum from the left of the second lumbar vertebra and passes obliquely down toward the right sacroiliac joint.

Blood Supply

The duodenum receives its blood supply from branches of the celiac artery and the SMA. The celiac artery divides into three branches—the splenic, common hepatic, and left gastric artery. The hepatic artery usually gives off the gastroduodenal artery, which in turn bifurcates into the anterior and posterior branches of the superior pancreaticoduodenal artery. These branches form anastomoses with anterior and posterior branches of the inferior pancreaticoduodenal artery. The inferior pancreaticoduodenal artery is a branch of the SMA.

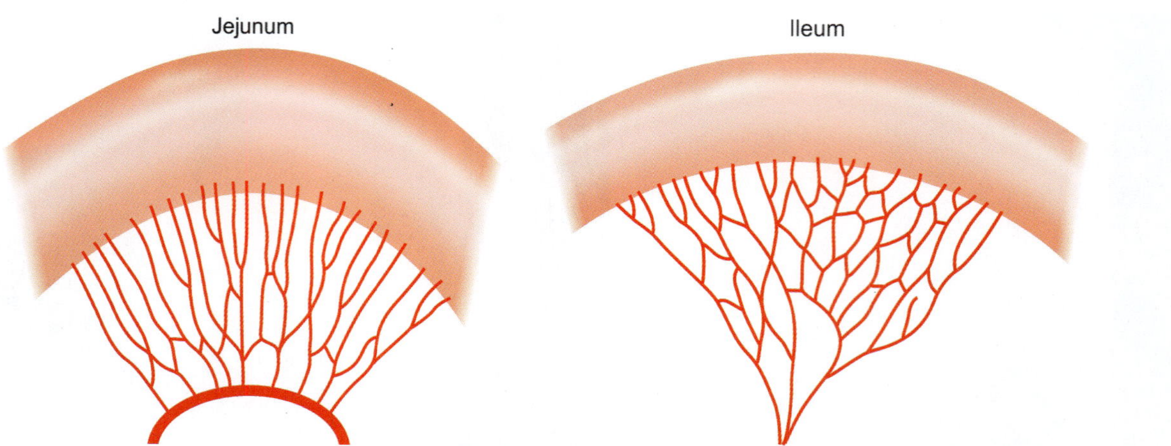

Fig. 69.3: Small intestinal vasculature. Compared with the ileum, jejunal arcades are simpler with long vasa recta.

The blood supply to the entire jejunum and ileum arises from the SMA. The SMA arises from the aorta behind the pancreas and crosses over the uncinate portion of the pancreas and duodenum to enter the mesentery. A variable number of jejunal and ileal branches arise from the left side of the SMA to supply blood to the small intestine. These arteries in turn form a complex series of arterial arcades. Small straight arteries, the vasa recta, arise from these arcades to approach and bifurcate about the intestine, giving off small branches that enter the intestinal wall. These tiny vessels anastomose extensively within the wall of the intestine itself (Fig. 69.3). Venous drainage parallels the arterial circulation. The jejunal and ileal veins drain into the superior mesenteric vein, which joins the splenic vein behind the neck of the pancreas to form the portal vein. The small bowel lymphatics follow the vascular supply and drain toward the origin of the superior mesenteric trunk.

Innervation

The small intestine receives afferent fibers from both the parasympathetic and sympathetic divisions of the autonomic nervous system:

- Parasympathetic preganglionic fibers arising from the celiac division of the vagus nerve synapse with the intrinsic neural plexuses of the intestine.
- Sympathetic innervation derives from the preganglionic fibers arising from the ninth and tenth thoracic segments of the spinal cord, which then synapse in the superior mesenteric ganglion.

There are also afferent fibers of both parasympathetic and sympathetic divisions, but pain appears to be derived from sympathetic afferents only.

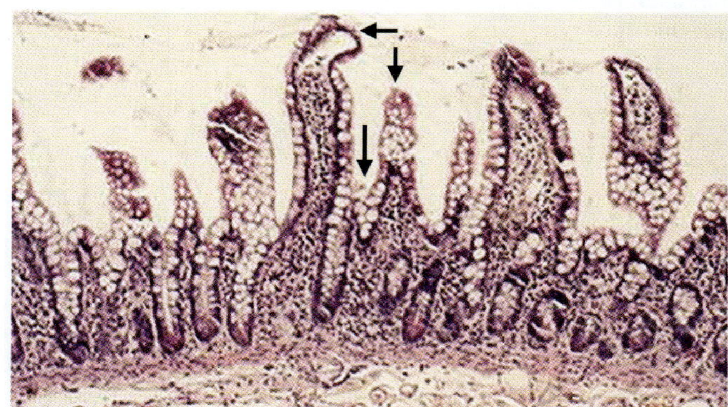

Fig. 69.4: Intestinal villi. Small bowel mucosa with villi (large arrows) and crypts (small arrow) of Lieberkühn.

Histology

The small intestinal wall consists of four layers: mucosa, submucosa, muscularis, and serosa.

Mucosa provides the critical absorptive membrane between the nutrient-containing luminal contents and the intestinal blood supply. It has a number of specialized features that allow it to function as a superb absorptive surface. Grossly, the mucosa is characterized by transverse folds (valves of Kerckring or plicae circulares), which pleat the mucosa and maximize the surface area in contact with intestinal contents. These folds are greatest in height and most numerous in the proximal small bowel and become less numerous and shorter in an aboral gradient.

The mucosa is divided into three layers: epithelium, lamina propria and muscularis mucosa.

The columnar cells of the epithelium represent the true absorptive interface with the lumen. The epithelial surface has fingerlike projections, known as villi (Fig. 69.4).

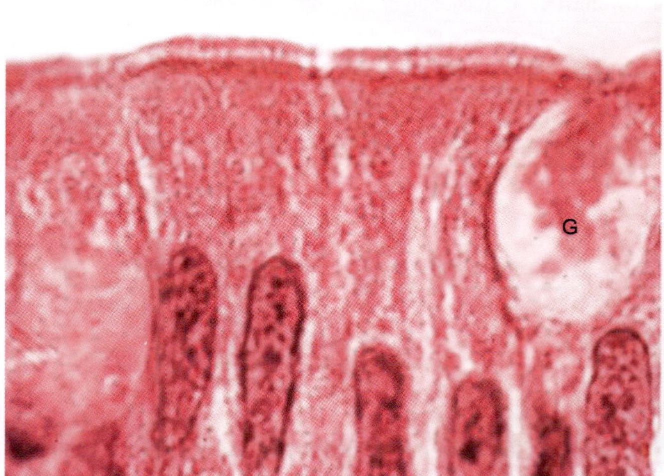

Fig. 69.5: Brush border. Epithelial cells with microvilli (brush border). Note the goblet cell (G).

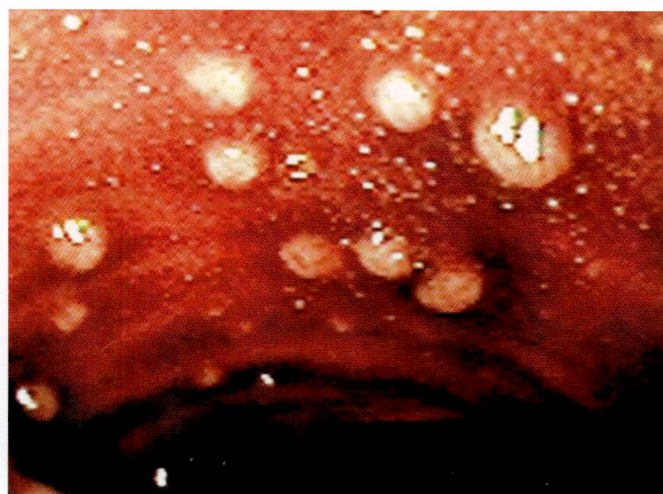

Fig. 69.6: Peyer's patches. Lymphatic nodules in the terminal ileum.

Between each protruding villus are "valleys" known as the crypts of Lieberkűhn. The striated luminal borders of the columnar absorptive cells contain numerous microvilli and are yet another adaptation that markedly increases the absorptive abilities of the epithelial cells. Microvilli give rise to the so-called "brush border" appearance (Fig. 69.5). This brush border is rich in digestive enzymes. There are several other cells in the epithelial layer—mucus-secreting goblet cells, enterochromaffin cells, Paneth cells, and other undifferentiated cells. The epithelial layer is mitotically very active, with repopulation of the epithelial cells approximately every 3 days.

Deep to the epithelial layer is the lamina propria, a connective tissue layer containing blood vessels and lymphatics. There are many plasma cells, which are active sites of immunoglobulin synthesis and facilitate the important immune function of the small intestine. A thin slip of muscle, the muscularis mucosae, separates the mucosa from the submucosa.

The submucosa is a strong connective tissue layer containing nerves, vessels, and aggregates of lymphoid tissue (Peyer's patches). These lymphatic nodules are most prominent in the terminal ileum (Fig. 69.6). Meissner's plexus is the submucosal neural bundle. The muscularis propria contains two distinct layers of smooth muscle:

- An outer longitudinal layer
- An inner circular layer

The myenteric nerve plexus is located between these two muscle layers. The serosa is the outermost layer and is a peritoneal surface that covers the entire length and circumference of the small intestine.

APPLIED PHYSIOLOGY

Digestion and Absorption

The small intestinal epithelium is essentially a large semipermeable membrane with critical absorptive and secretory functions. It plays the key role in the body's absorption of water, electrolytes, and nutrients. In addition, the epithelial surface reabsorbs the salivary, gastric, pancreaticobiliary and intestinal fluids that facilitate digestion of these nutrients. There are functionally active, specialized areas responsible for the absorption of specific nutrients along the entire length of the small intestine.

Water and Electrolytes

Between 5 and 10 L of water enter the small bowel daily but only 500 mL passes through the ileocecal valve into the colon. Small pores between epithelial cells are thought to allow the transfer of water and water-soluble substances across the cell membrane by simple diffusion. Jejunal pores are larger (7–9 Å) than those in the ileum (3–4 Å), accounting for more efficacious water absorption in the proximal small intestine.[7] Osmotic pressures are generated from the active transport of sodium, glucose, or amino acids into cells.

Conversely, sodium is actively transported from the interior of cells into the intercellular spaces via a sodium-potassium ATPase pump located on the basolateral membrane of the cell. This process results in the intracellular movement of potassium. The movement of sodium by active transport also facilitates the transport of glucose, amino acids, and oligopeptides into the absorptive epithelial cells.

Calcium absorption occurs in the proximal small intestine by active transport and depends upon the presence of parathyroid hormone and vitamin D. The small intestine also absorbs iron, usually in very small amounts. However, absorption may be appreciable if iron stores are depleted.

Carbohydrates

Carbohydrates comprise 30–40% of the typical diet in developed countries. The two major forms are polysaccharides and disaccharides. Digestion begins with salivary amylase, and absorption is generally completed within the proximal 1–1.5 m of the small intestine. Salivary and pancreatic amylases are extremely efficient at digesting starch into oligosaccharides within minutes of their secretion into the duodenal lumen. Surface enzymes located in the brush border of the luminal surface hydrolyze oligosaccharides, reducing them to monosaccharides. Eventually, most ingested carbohydrate is broken down to and absorbed as glucose. Glucose and the other monosaccharides are too large to be absorbed by passive diffusion and are taken up by a specific active transport system mediated by the sodium-potassium ATPase pump.[8]

Proteins

Protein digestion begins in the stomach under the action of activated pepsins. However, pancreatic proteases are responsible for the bulk of protein digestion. These consist of the following:

- Endopeptidases (trypsin, chymotrypsin, and elastase)
- Exopeptidases (carboxypeptidase A and carboxypeptidase B)

These enzymes digest peptide links and depend upon activation by enterokinases produced by the duodenal mucosa (Flowchart 69.1).[9] Approximately half of protein absorption takes place in the duodenum and it is normally completed by the mid-jejunum. The relative rarity of protein malabsorptive states, even following extensive small intestinal resection, attests to the efficiency of the process.

Fats

The process of lipid digestion and absorption is quite complex. Like that of protein and carbohydrate digestion and absorption, it relies upon the coordinated activity of gastric, pancreatic, biliary, and small intestinal functions. However, unlike carbohydrate and protein absorption, lipid absorption depends upon several unique physical and biochemical processes that allow lipids to enter epithelial cells.

Flowchart 69.1: Activation of pancreatic proteases.

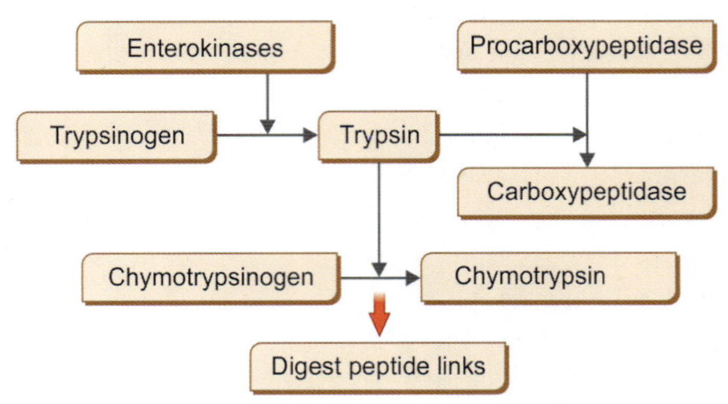

Dietary fat consists mainly of triglycerides. The predominant fatty acid components are palmitic, stearic, oleic, and linoleic fatty acids. Digestion and absorption of triglycerides relies on four major events:

- Secretion of digestive enzymes
- Fat emulsification
- Enzymatic hydrolysis of ester linkages
- Solubilization of lipolytic products with bile salt micelles.

Fat in the duodenum results in the secretion of cholecystokinin and secretin, which stimulates secretion of pancreatic digestive enzymes and promotes gallbladder emptying. Bile salts emulsify fats during the initial phase of digestion. Micelles are formed and represent the most critical aspect of fat absorption. Fats are enveloped in a bilayer bile salt disc. Once in contact with the brush border of the epithelial cell, lipids diffuse across the membrane quite rapidly; this process is not energy dependent. After lipid absorption, triglyceride resynthesis and re-esterification take place within the cytoplasm of the intestinal epithelial cells. The final step in triglyceride absorption is the formation of chylomicrons, which are crucial for transport across the cell membrane.

INTESTINAL ADAPTATION

The small intestine has a remarkable ability to adapt. The small bowel can, therefore, compensate for extensive resection or disease before intestinal failure occurs. However, dependence on parenteral nutrition is likely if total gut length comprises <1 m of small intestine or <50 cm of small intestine with the colon in situ. Adaptation appears to be dependent on enteral feeding. Villous adaptation due to hypertrophy and hyperplasia greatly increases absorptive capacity. A competent ileocecal valve is important in slowing transit time.

Absorptive problems can result in various conditions. Fat malabsortion, for example, secondary to bile deficiency, results in fat secretion in feces (steatorrhea). With the inability to absorb fat, patients can suffer from essential fatty acid deficiency and deficiencies in fat soluble vitamins A, D, E, and K. Bile salt absorption occurs in the terminal ileum, and malabsorption leads to diarrhea. This condition can be idiopathic but is frequently associated with Crohn's disease (due to active ileal disease or following ileal resection). The distal ileum is also responsible for vitamin B_{12} absorption; therefore, following ileal resection patients will require vitamin B_{12} supplementation. Duodenal resection can result in calcium, iron, folate, and magnesium deficiencies.

INVESTIGATION

Historically, the anatomy of the small intestine, inaccessible to inspection other than by laparotomy, made investigation difficult. However, the last decade has seen major progress in radiological and endoscopic techniques to provide the surgeon with a wide variety of diagnostic tools.

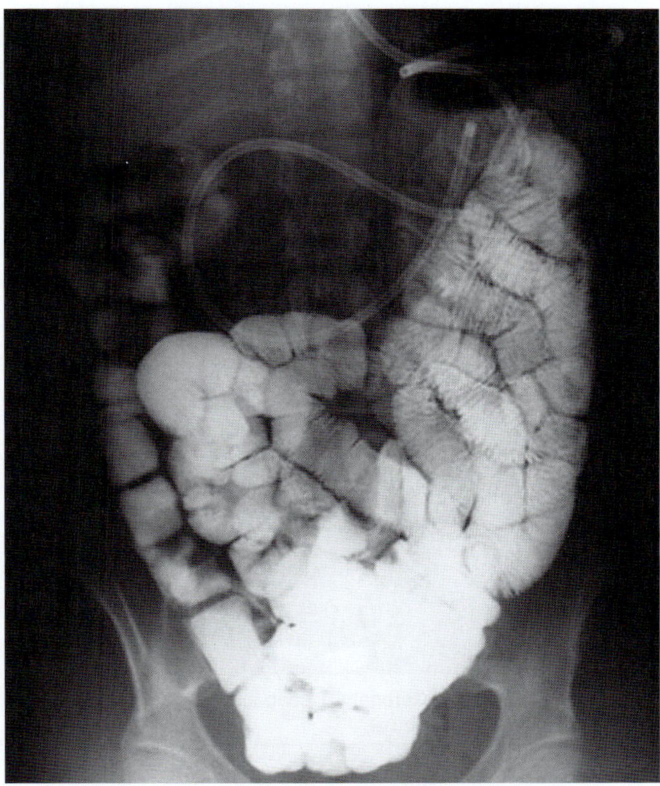

Fig. 69.7: Enteroclysis. Contrast is infused directly into the small intestine.

Radiological Investigation and Therapeutic Intervention

Radiological techniques are frequently used as the primary investigation for small bowel pathology. Despite increasing clinical reliance on cross-sectional imaging by computed tomography (CT), there remains a role for less advanced techniques. Plain abdominal radiographs may be used to confirm a diagnosis of small bowel obstruction. Contrast radiographs (Fig. 69.7) using barium can be useful in demonstrating mucosal detail or stricture in some situations. Water-soluble contrast studies may be helpful in the management of adhesional small bowel obstruction.[11] Ultrasound scanning is useful in inflammatory bowel disease, but remains highly user-dependent;[10] it has the benefit of avoiding patient exposure to radiation.

Contrast-enhanced CT plays a major role in the investigation of small bowel disease; it is particularly useful in the emergency setting, where it is often more readily available and easier to interpret than other techniques. Primary small bowel lesions and their extent (Figs. 69.8A and B) can be identified and important information about the status of the mesenteric vasculature determined. CT is excellent for characterization of intramural and extraluminal abnormalities and can define the relationship of small bowel pathology with adjacent organs, for example in fistulating Crohn's disease or invasive malignancy. CT angiography (Fig. 69.9) is valuable for localizing GI hemorrhage at rates as low as 0.3 mL/min and is more readily available than formal mesenteric angiography.[13] CT is less good at demonstrating abnormalities at mucosal level, and the cumulative burden of radiation in some patients should not be overlooked. These shortcomings are addressed by magnetic resonance (MR) small bowel imaging (Fig. 69.10), which offers the advantages of not exposing the patient to ionizing radiation, superb contrast resolution of disease including mucosal abnormalities, multiphasic imaging and better tolerated contrast agents compared to CT.[12]

Interventional radiological techniques in the small intestine are less well established. Angiography and selective embolization of bleeding vessels is described, though infarction of bowel in the territory of the vessel may necessitate operation. Radiolabelled red blood cell scans are more sensitive than angiography and have a secondary role in the investigation of blood loss or in chronic hemorrhage. Indium-labeled white cell radionucleotide scans were used previously to investigate inflammatory bowel

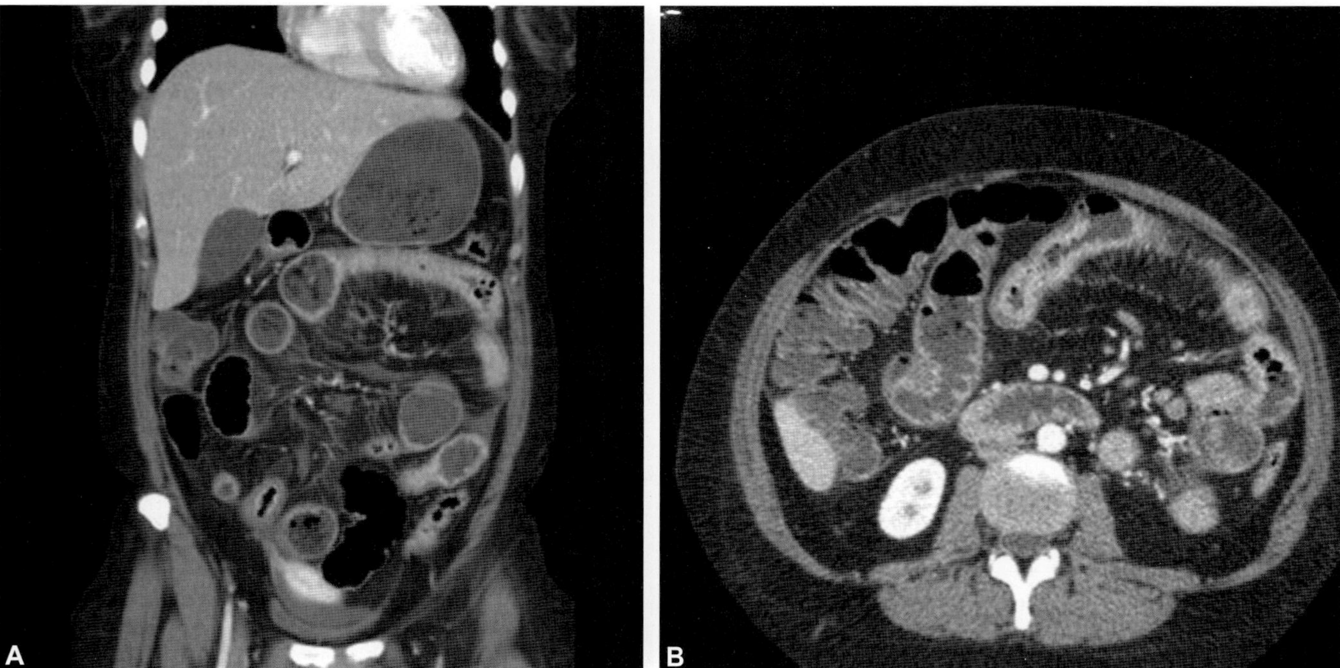

Figs. 69.8A and B: (A) Coronal CT scan showing a strictured segment of small bowel in Crohn's patient. (B) Axial CT scan of same patient showing strictured small bowel.

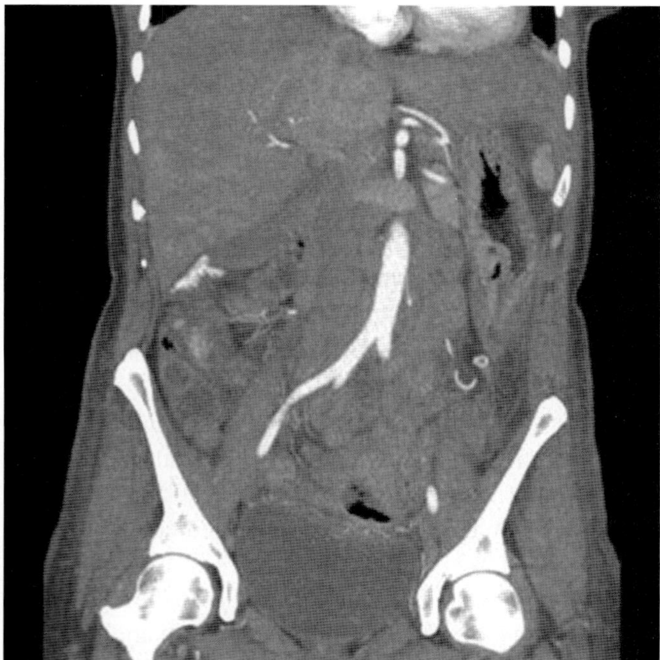

Fig. 69.9: CT angiography showing bleeding source in right hypochondrium.

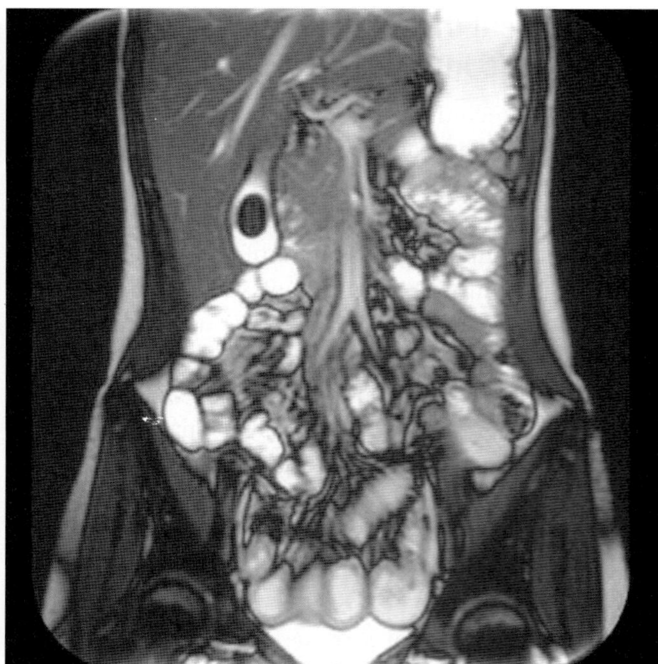

Fig. 69.10: MR of small bowel showing contrast within the small bowel. MR is being used more frequently to image the small bowel. Key features that favor MR over other imaging modalities are that it is noninvasive, radiation free, and can identify active disease.

disease of the small intestine but have now been superseded by other techniques. Positron emission tomography scanning in combination with CT scanning has an increasing role in the staging of small bowel tumors.[14]

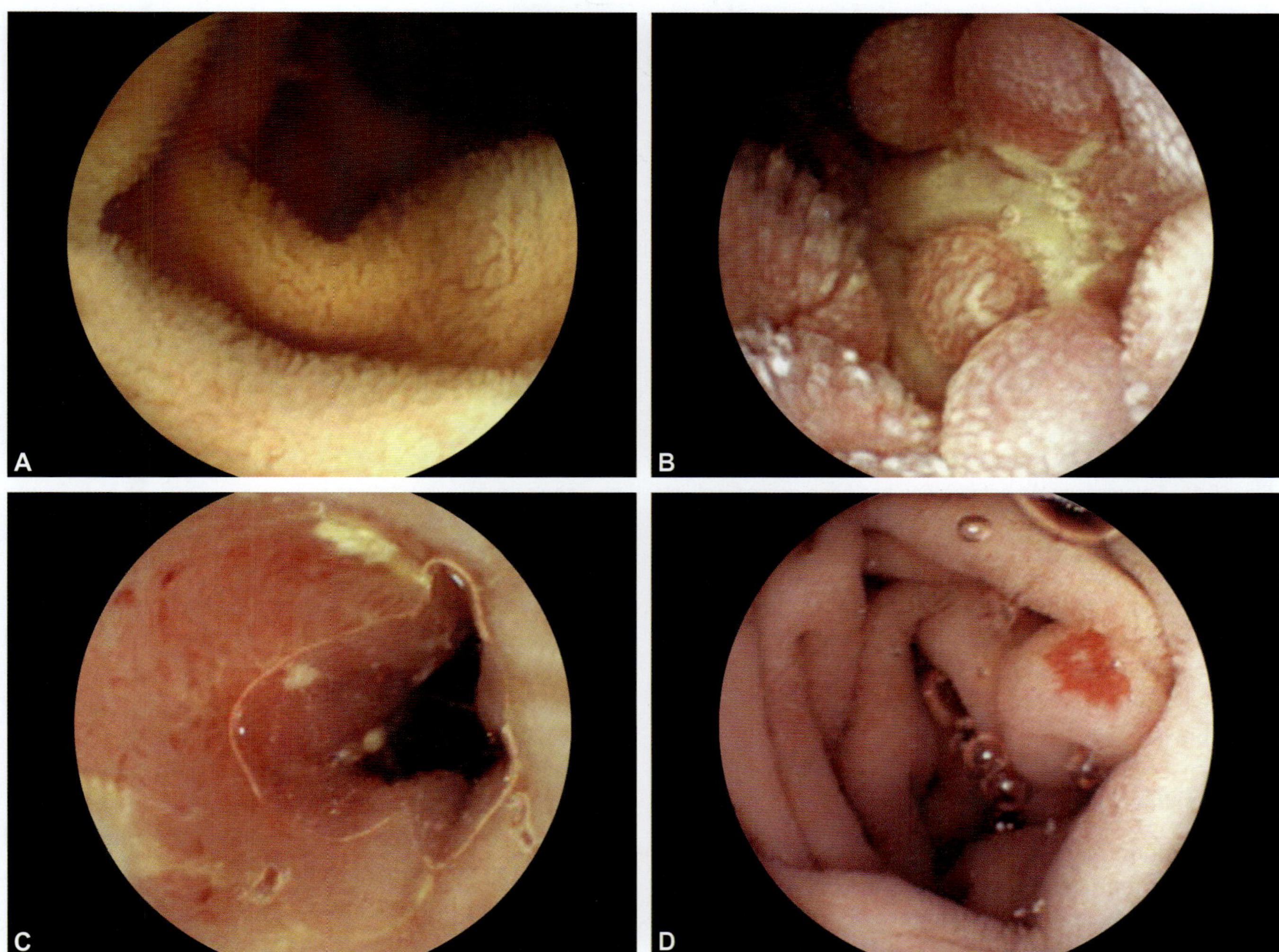

Figs. 69.11A to D: Capsule video endoscopy of the small bowel. (A) Normal small bowel showing villi and plicae circulares. (B) Cobblestone appearance seen in the small bowel in Crohn's disease. (C) Small aphthous ulcers seen in the small bowel in a Crohn's disease patient. There is confluent circumferential inflammation. (D) Arteriovenous malformation found during the investigation of a patient with iron deficiency anemia with a normal upper gastrointestinal endoscopy and colonoscopy.

Endoscopic Investigation and Therapeutic Intervention

Upper gastrointestinal endoscopy is well established in diagnosis and treatment of duodenal pathology, and colonoscopy can be used to investigate the terminal ileum. Until recently, direct visualization of the small bowel in between was limited. Over the past decade capsule endoscopy, in which a wireless miniature camera is swallowed by the patient, has become established in the diagnosis of obscure gastrointestinal bleeding, inflammatory bowel disease, neoplasia and malabsorption disorders[15] (Figs. 69.11A to D). It may be augmented by double balloon enteroscopy, which uses a push-and-pull technique that effectively shortens the intestine by alternate inflation and deflation of balloons fitted over the endoscope, and permits biopsy of any part of the small bowel.

Enteroscopy can also be used intraoperatively (Fig. 69.12), for example, in the management of multiple small bowel polyps in Peutz–Jeghers syndrome or in localization of obscure GI hemorrhage.

Laparoscopy and Laparotomy

In difficult diagnostic circumstances, the surgeon may require recourse to operative intervention for diagnosis and therapy. Laparoscopy is a minimally invasive technique allowing direct visualization of the small bowel and the ability to obtain biopsies. Laparoscopic techniques may be used to resect diseased small bowel, particularly in

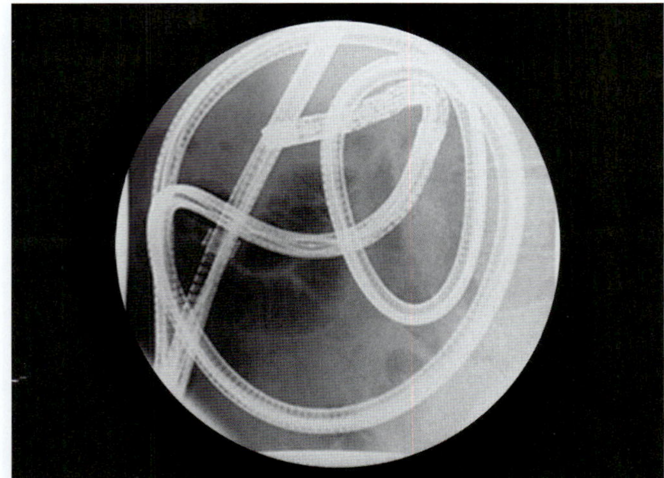

Fig. 69.12: Enteroscopy. An enteroscope has been passed well into the coils of the small intestine in a patient who has a jejunal arteriovenous malformation.

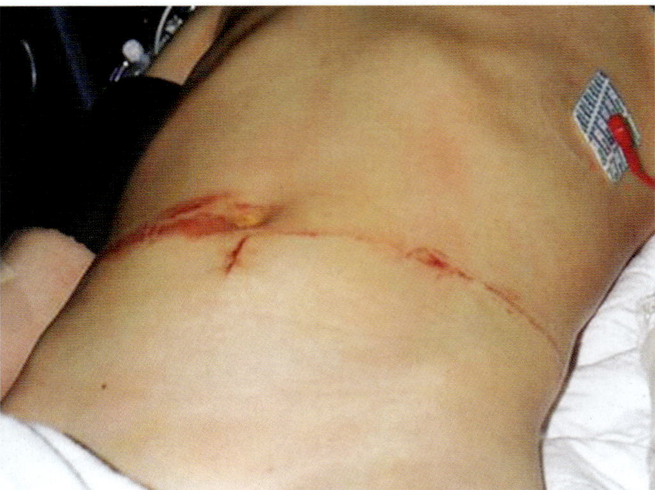

Fig. 69.13: Seat belt injury. Note the abdominal wall ecchymoses caused by the lap belt.

Crohn's disease of the terminal ileum. When laparoscopy is not possible due to intra-abdominal adhesions or other technical reasons, laparotomy allows definitive examination by both palpation and direct inspection of the small bowel.

TRAUMA

It is paramount to consider an occult abdominal injury in the multiply injured trauma patient (*see* Chapter 40, "Abdominal, Urologic and Perineal Injuries"). Since the small intestine fills a large portion of the abdominal cavity, injury is highly likely in blunt or penetrating abdominal injury.

The clinical sign of ecchymoses in the seat belt distribution across the abdominal wall signifies a high-energy injury in motor vehicle accidents and is associated with an increased incidence of abdominal injury (Fig. 69.13).[16] Deceleration injuries occur to organs that are tethered in the peritoneal cavity.[17] Most commonly injured are the liver and spleen, but the small bowel particularly near the duodenal-jejunal flexure can also be involved. High and low-velocity penetrating abdominal trauma may cause small bowel injury in multiple locations, and the surgeon attending such a case should have a high index of suspicion.

The management of the trauma patient should follow established ATLS resuscitation principles. Clinical examination is unreliable in patients with head injury, in the intubated patient and in the patient with drug or alcohol intoxication. Small intestinal injury in the hemodynamically normal patient can be diagnosed through CT.[18] In the hemodynamically unstable patient, small intestinal injury may only be established at laparotomy. Special consideration needs to be given to surgical repair of small bowel injury in the trauma patient. Resection and primary anastomosis can safely be deployed in the hemodynamically stable patient. In the multiply-injured patient with hemodynamic instability, the principles of damage-limitation surgery apply and small bowel injuries should be controlled by the simplest method available. Following full resuscitation and patient optimization, delayed resection and anastomosis may be performed.

SMALL BOWEL OBSTRUCTION

Small bowel obstruction is one of the most common emergency presentations to the general surgeon (Fig. 69.14). By far the commonest etiologies are adhesions from previous abdominal surgery or abdominal hernia. While adhesional small bowel obstruction may resolve with conservative treatment, 30–40% will require surgical intervention. Small bowel obstruction secondary to hernia will almost invariably need surgical intervention. Small bowel obstruction is covered in more detail in Chapter 75, "Intestinal Obstruction".

Intussusception

Intussusception is the invagination of intestine upon itself. It is most common during infancy and early childhood and is usually a primary phenomenon with no underlying abnormality of the bowel. In adults, intussusception is almost always secondary to a tumor. It commonly affects the ileocecal region. Symptoms are obstructive with vomiting and abdominal pain. Rectal bleeding ("red currant jelly" stool) may be seen, and abdominal examination may reveal a mass. Ultrasound scanning is useful for diagnosis in children. In the adult, diagnosis is usually established by CT scan (Figs. 69.15A and B).

In children the intussusception may be reduced radiologically by contrast enema (see Chapter 125, "Gastrointestinal Surgery in Children").

If reduction is not achieved, surgical intervention is required. Laparoscopic intervention has been used to try and reduce the intussuscepted section. However if the intestine shows evidence of ischemia or has a more sinister etiology, laparotomy with resection is the best surgical management.

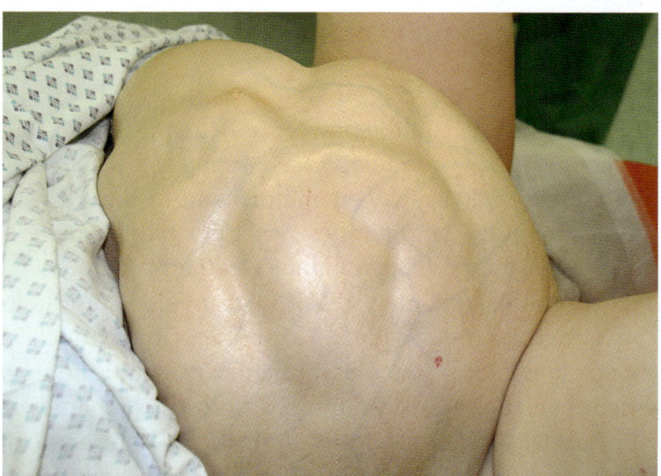

Fig. 69.14: Patient presenting with small bowel obstruction with visible peristalsis of distended intestine.

CROHN'S DISEASE

Crohn's disease was first described in Mt Sinai Hospital, New York in 1932 as a "regional ileitis".[19] It is a chronic granulomatous inflammatory disease that may affect any part of the gastrointestinal tract from the mouth to the anus.[20] Despite recent advances in both medical and surgical management of Crohn's disease, the cause of the condition is unknown and there is no cure. Approximately, two thirds of patients with Crohn's disease have ileal involvement: 45% have ileocecal involvement, 20% have terminal ileal involvement alone and 5% have extensive small bowel disease. The inflammation in Crohn's disease is characteristically transmural in nature and frequently discontinuous in distribution, a pattern termed as "skip lesions."

Etiology

Crohn's disease has a prevalence in Western society of 100 cases per 100,000 population and an annual incidence of 7 cases per 100,000. The peak age of onset is 15–25 years of age. The incidence has increased in the developed world over recent decades but has now reached a plateau.[21] There is no association with social class.

The exact cause of Crohn's disease is unknown. A complex interaction between genetic and environmental factors is thought to activate the inflammatory process. The interaction of gut content and intestinal epithelial cells in susceptible individuals produces a dysregulated innate and adaptive immune response leading to chronic

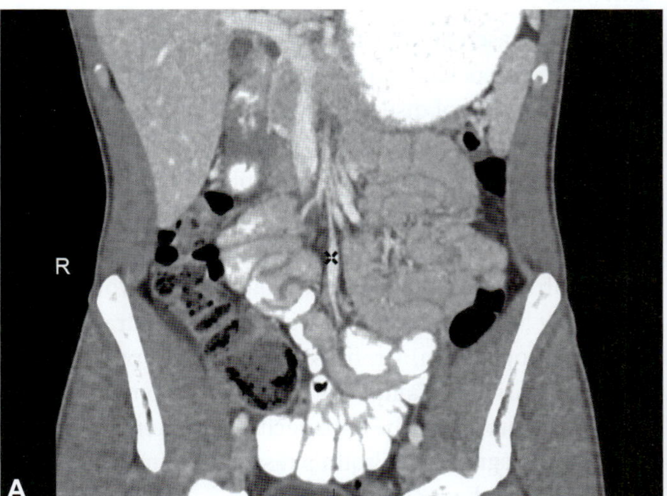

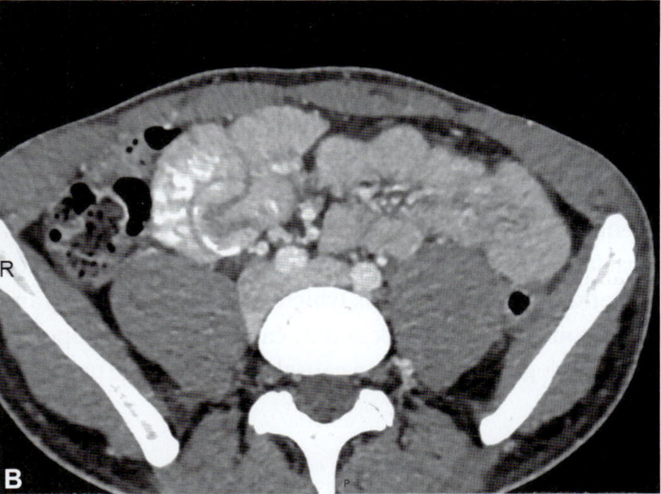

Figs. 69.15A and B: These coronal (A) and axial (B) CT scan images demonstrate small bowel intussusception in a patient presenting acutely with abdominal pain.

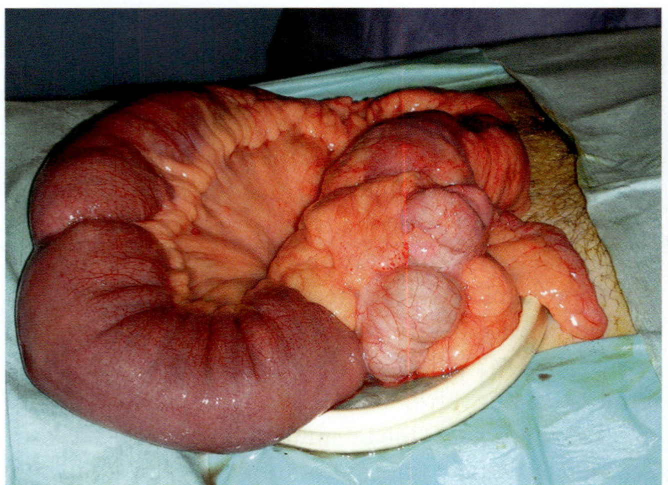

Fig. 69.16: Macroscopic Crohn's disease seen at laparotomy. Note the fat wrapping of the ileum and the chronic inflammation with resultant proximal ileal dilatation.

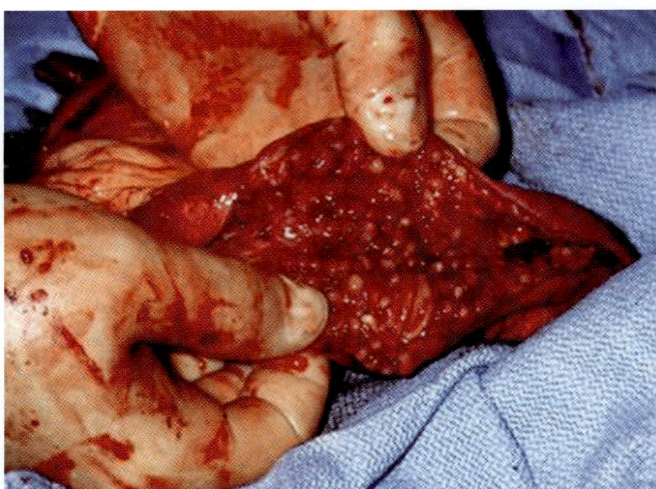

Fig. 69.17: Stricturing disease in neoterminal ileum.

mucosal inflammation. Research over the next decade is likely to identify key mediators of this response as therapeutic targets.

Evidence for a genetic susceptibility to Crohn's disease is supported by a 10% prevalence in first degree relatives and 40% concordance in monozygotic twins. Early onset disease has a higher familial prevalence. Genome analysis has identified over 30 risk loci for Crohn's disease, some of which overlap with ulcerative colitis. These loci code for proteins involved in cellular innate immunity, and mutations in specific genes are associated with greatly increased risk of Crohn's disease: for example, CARD15 mutations can increase the risk for Crohn's disease up to 40-fold, and NOD2 mutations predispose to ileocolic Crohn's disease and a fibrostenotic disease pattern.

Environmental factors are also implicated. Smoking is associated with an increased incidence of Crohn's disease and is strongly associated with disease recrudescence. A number of dietary factors have been implicated in Crohn's disease without conclusive proof of a single etiological agent; an elemental diet improves symptoms and remains a useful therapeutic maneuver in refractory patients. Mycobacterium paratuberculosis which is known to cause granulomatous intestinal infection in cattle has been proposed as an etiological agent, but a causal link is yet to be proven.[22]

Pathology

Crohn's disease tends to be discontinuous, with segmental involvement or "skip lesions." Grossly the serosal aspect of the intestine demonstrates an extension of mesenteric fat around the surface of the bowel (fat wrapping), with wall thickening and a prominent vascular pattern (Fig. 69.16). The mesentery is usually edematous and thickened with enlarged matted lymph nodes. Strictures may be of variable length from a few millimeters to many centimeters. Transmural fissures may result in fistulation into adjacent structures or formation of abscesses. On the mucosal aspect, longitudinal deep fissuring ulcers, cobblestoning, strictures, fistulas, and intramural abscesses are characteristic (Fig. 69.17). Histologically, the cardinal features are of transmural mononuclear inflammation, fissuring ulcers, and noncaseating granulomas.

Clinical Features

Crohn's disease can affect any part of the gastrointestinal tract and is associated with extraintestinal manifestations. The presentation of disease can vary from abdominal pain to a perianal abscess or fistula. Disease patterns are locus- and phenotype specific, for example, small/large bowel disease or fistulating or stenosing disease. A typical presentation is persistent diarrhea, fever and right lower quadrant pain, with or without anorexia, nausea, and vomiting. A mass may be palpable in the right lower quadrant. In the pediatric population, Crohn's patients may present with failure to thrive or failure to reach developmental milestones. Symptoms can be nonspecific and intermittent, and hence the diagnosis of Crohn's disease is often delayed in comparison with ulcerative colitis.

The clinical course is unpredictable, but is characterized by waxing and waning of symptoms, frequently with

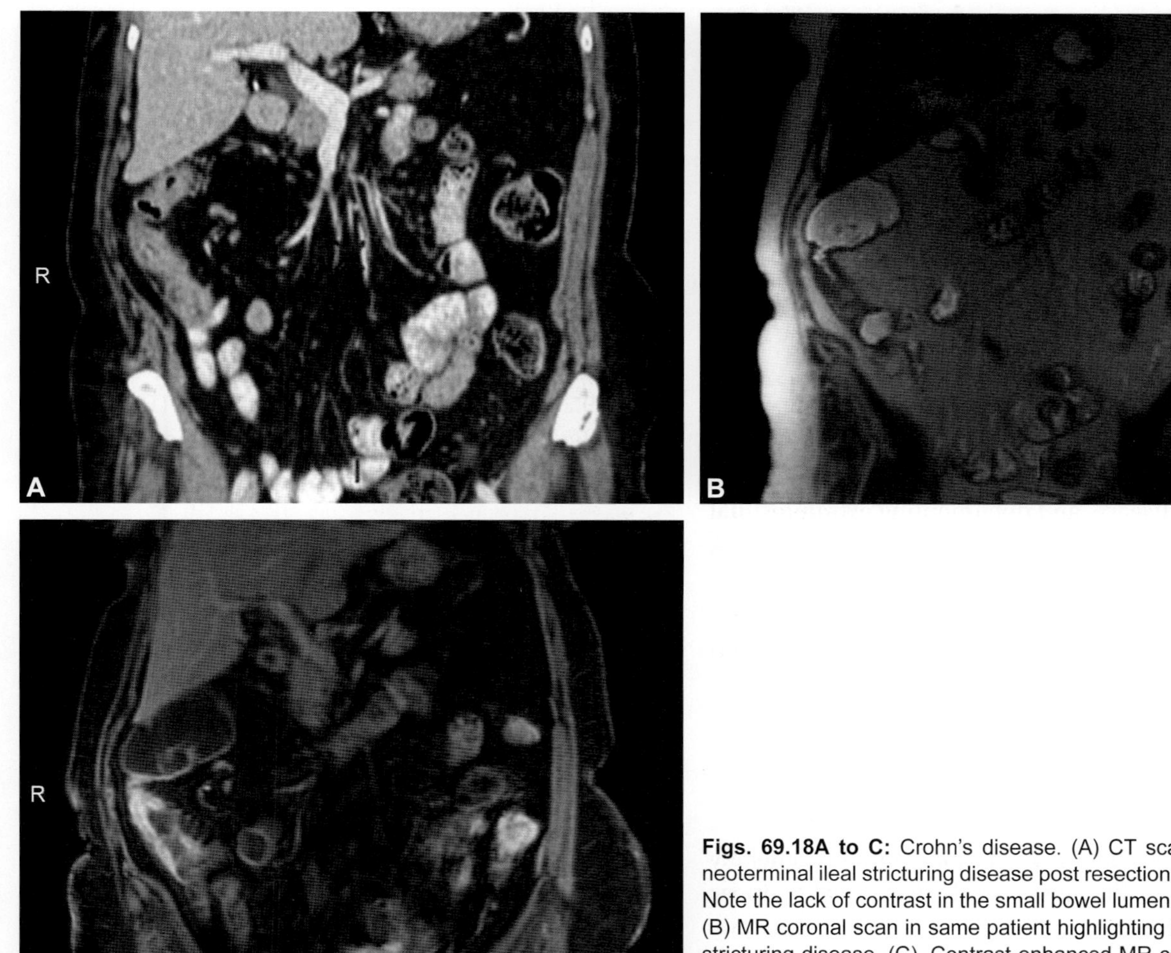

Figs. 69.18A to C: Crohn's disease. (A) CT scan coronal image of neoterminal ileal stricturing disease post resection for Crohn's disease. Note the lack of contrast in the small bowel lumen in the affected area. (B) MR coronal scan in same patient highlighting the neoterminal ileal stricturing disease. (C). Contrast-enhanced MR coronal scan in same Crohn's patient showing active disease in the neoterminal ileum.

a progressive shortening of the relatively asymptomatic intervals. Weight loss, fatigue, and anemia often ensue. If the disease is limited to the small intestine, recurrent postprandial pain, abdominal distension, nausea, and vomiting tend to be more prominent. With repeated inflammation injury to the bowel wall and increasing fibrosis, the lumen becomes progressively narrower (Figs. 69.18A to C) resulting in obstructive symptoms.

In other patients, transmural enteric inflammation leads to complications of perforation. Although free perforation with diffuse peritonitis is rare, localized perforation with abscess formation or fistulous communication to adjacent structures is common. If the colon is also involved, internal fistulas and perianal disease may complicate the clinical picture.

The extraintestinal manifestations of Crohn's disease are rheumatological, ophthalmic, and dermatological conditions. Two common patterns of arthritis may occur:

- A migratory polyarthritis that primarily affects large joints—symptoms often resolve with treatment of the associated intestinal activity.
- An ankylosing spondylitis variant that appears to behave more independently of the bowel involvement.

Ophthalmologic disease, including episcleritis, uveitis, and conjunctivitis, occurs in 1–10% of patients. Pyoderma gangrenosum and erythema nodosum are among the associated cutaneous manifestations. Although clinically important, liver disease is uncommon; liver function test abnormalities are often noted as a result of a mild pericholangitis, fatty liver, or sclerosing cholangitis. In rare patients, the kidneys are involved with amyloidosis and progressive renal failure.

Many other systemic derangements occur in patients who have small bowel Crohn's disease as a result of the primary disease activity itself. Terminal ileal disease (or resection) can result in fat malabsorption, increased oxalate absorption and hyperoxaluria, resulting in a tendency to form renal stones. Similarly, an increased incidence of cholelithiasis is caused by impaired enterohepatic circulation.

Inadequate food intake from anorexia and malabsorption causes a variety of complex multifactorial nutritional deficiencies including protein-losing enteropathy and specific vitamin (e.g., vitamin B_{12}) malabsorption. Inflammatory bowel disease patients are also at increased risk of developing deep venous thrombosis and pulmonary emboli.

Investigations

Crohn's disease can present with vague symptoms. Investigations are targeted at establishing the diagnosis, assessing nutritional status, identifying sepsis, mapping the extent of the disease, and documenting extraintestinal manifestations. Although inflammatory markers such as ESR and CRP may be elevated, there are no specific diagnostic tests. Malnourished patients may have a low albumin. Anemia may be a feature secondary to chronic blood loss and specific vitamin deficiencies.

Celiac serology can be used to exclude celiac disease. Stool cultures are useful in excluding an infective etiology. There is an emerging role in Crohn's disease for fecal calprotectin, a protein found in the cytosol of neutrophils.[23]

Radiographic evaluation of the small bowel is generally the most important diagnostic study. Historically, upper gastrointestinal contrast radiology was used to demonstrate mucosal edema, ulceration, internal fistulas, or stenoses characteristic of Crohn's disease (Fig. 69.19). This has now been superseded by other imaging modalities. In the emergency setting, ready access to CT scanning makes this the modality of choice. Computed tomography is accurate in identifying segments of thick-walled bowel and can often localize strictures. It is of considerable value in delineating complications of Crohn's disease, such as intra-abdominal abscess and fistula. In the elective setting, magnetic resonance (MR) small bowel imaging (enterolysis) with contrast is becoming the imaging modality of choice. It can demonstrate good mucosal detail including short strictures, and it removes the concern regarding cumulative radiation exposure in this relatively young group of patients. As described above, enteroscopy (Figs. 69.20A and B) and capsule endoscopy (Figs. 69.21A to F) give excellent information as to the extent and

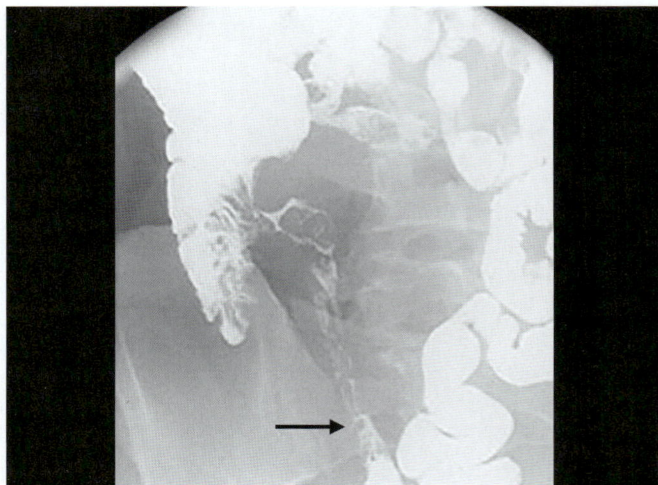

Fig. 69.19: Terminal ileal Crohn's disease. The terminal ileum is ulcerated and narrowed (arrow).

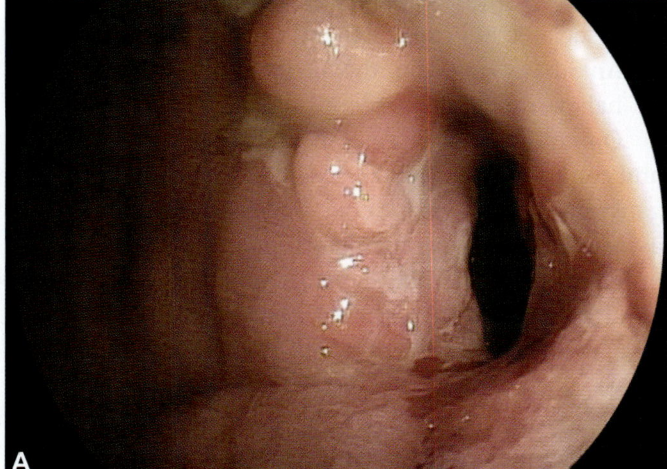

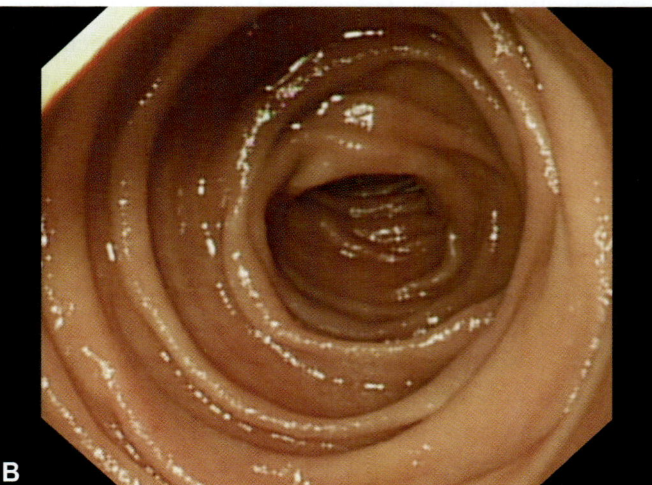

Figs. 69.20A and B: Enteroscopic appearances of small bowel in Crohn's patient showing pseudopolyps and stricturing (A) and jejunum in a healthy individual (B).

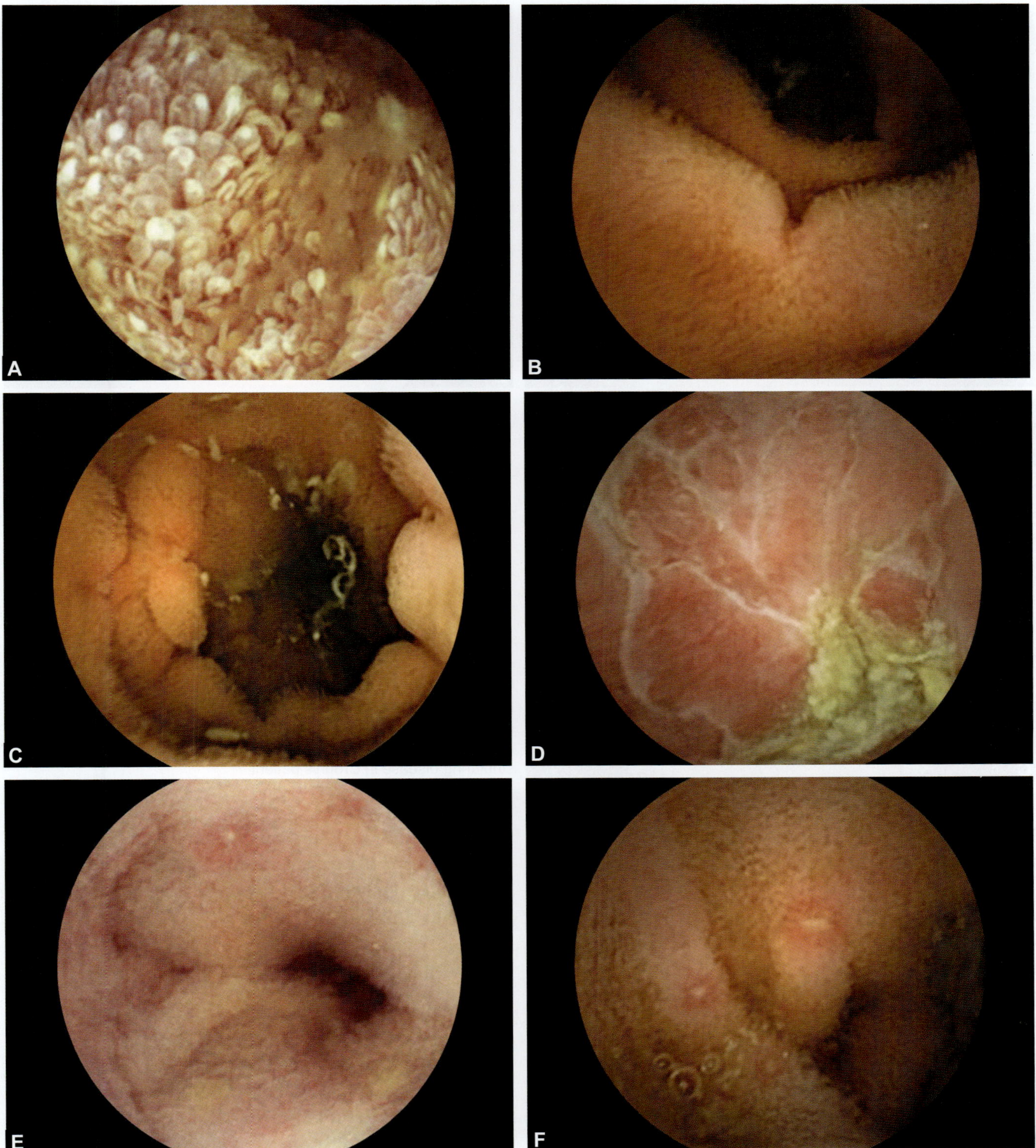

Figs. 69.21A to F: Capsule video endoscopy in Crohn's disease. Early changes in disease process (A) to (C). Severe disease seen in (D) to (F). (A) Villous edema—early inflammation associated with mild Crohn's disease. (B) Early Fissuring ulcers causing distortion of the plicae circulares. (C) Pseudopolyps associated with Crohn's disease. (D) Severe confluent Crohn's disease. (E) Aphthous ulceration. (F) Aphthous ulceration.

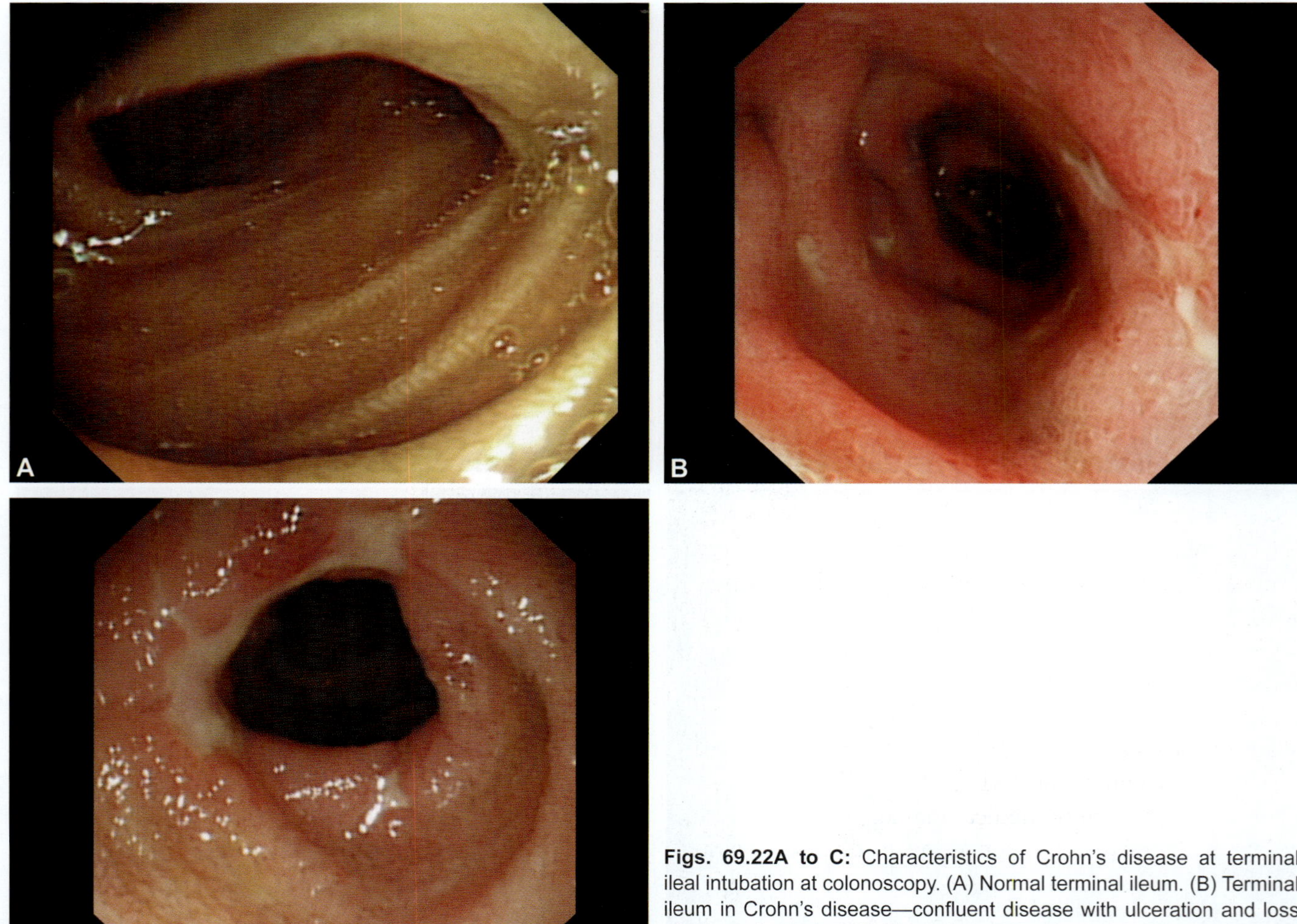

Figs. 69.22A to C: Characteristics of Crohn's disease at terminal ileal intubation at colonoscopy. (A) Normal terminal ileum. (B) Terminal ileum in Crohn's disease—confluent disease with ulceration and loss of plicae circularae. (C) Ulceration of the terminal ileum causing early stricturing disease in Crohn's patient.

location of small bowel disease, but may be of limited use in the patient with established intestinal strictures.

Colonoscopy with intubation of the terminal ileum may be diagnostic (Figs. 69.22A to C), and assessment of colonic involvement is vital for surgical planning. Careful inspection of the perianal region combined with rigid proctoscopy and anoscopy are indicated if there are anorectal symptoms.

Management

The management of the Crohn's patient can be very challenging. Patients with severe disease may present with chronic malnutrition exacerbated by acute systemic sepsis on a therapeutic background of potent and long-term immunosuppression. Furthermore, the past decade has seen a significant expansion of therapeutic agents. Selection of best medical management and appropriate choice and timing of surgical intervention requires careful evaluation and discussion, ideally within the framework of a multidisciplinary meeting with gastroenterology, radiology, and pathology colleagues.

Medical Management

The aim of medical management of Crohn's disease embraces those medications used to induce remission and those used to maintain remission. Management is also guided by disease severity. Corticosteroids have been used for many years as the mainstay of treatment, particularly in inducing remission. However, corticosteroids have potent and disabling long-term side effects that can be particularly problematic in the younger age groups commonly affected by Crohn's disease, including osteoporosis, avascular necrosis of the femoral head, cataracts, diabetes, and Cushingoid appearance. Accordingly, long-term treatment with corticosteroids should be avoided. Budesonide, a corticosteroid with a high first-pass metabolism, is associated with fewer systemic side effects than other steroids and is used to treat terminal ileal and right-sided disease. Recent data suggest that mesalazine is ineffective in Crohn's disease. Immunomodulators such as azathioprine, 6-mercaptopurine or methotrexate can be used to induce and maintain remission and are increasingly used earlier, particularly in patients with aggressive disease.

The biggest advance in the management of Crohn's disease in the past decade is the introduction of biological agents. Infliximab,[24,25] a mouse chimeric monoclonal antibody against tumor necrosis factor-α, and the newer agent adalimumab,[26,27] a fully human monoclonal antibody, may be used both to induce and maintain remission. It is postulated that early treatment with these agents can alter the disease course, reducing the morbidity associated with recurrent hospital admission and surgery, particularly in patients exhibiting a phenotype of aggressive or fistulating disease, but this remains to be proven. There are concerns about long-term immunosuppression with these agents. A further strategy in attempting to alter disease course is by autologous stem cell transplantation, currently under evaluation in a clinic trial (ASTIC).[28]

The ultimate goal of medical management is to tailor therapy to the individual according to disease severity, distribution, drug side effects, complications, and impact on lifestyle.

Operative Management

Given that the condition is incurable, the guiding principle for surgeons dealing with Crohn's disease is to operate only for complications and to try and preserve gut length where possible. Within 10 years of diagnosis of Crohn's disease of the small bowel, 66% of patients have undergone operative management. With concomitant colonic involvement, the operative rate increases to 90% at 10 years. Half will require a further operation within this time-frame, so the potential for multiple operations must be borne in mind at each intervention.

Of fundamental importance is thorough preoperative evaluation and preparation. The surgeon must carefully consider the following factors:

- Disease mapping—what are the surgical targets, and which parts of the gut are affected?
- Patient factors—dehydration, coagulation abnormalities, anemia and comorbid conditions should be optimized.
- Nutritional status—if deficient, consider how it can be improved prior to operation by enteral or parenteral feeding. In the emergency patient in whom optimization is not possible, consider how it will impact on surgical strategy and whether anastomosis is prudent.
- Intra-abdominal sepsis—preoperative CT-guided drainage and patient stabilization followed by semielective surgery is usually preferable.
- Concurrent medical therapy—preoperative high-dose corticosteroids adversely affect surgical outcomes; consideration should be given to dose reduction or withdrawal if disease severity allows.[29]
- Stomas—patient discussion, siting, and avoidance of incisions at potential sites.

The main indications for surgery in small bowel Crohn's disease are as follows:[30]

- Obstruction
- Abscess
- Fistula
- Perforation
- Failure of medical management.

Obstruction is the most common indication for operation in patients with Crohn's enteritis. With recurrent local inflammation, rigid scar tissue is laid down in the bowel wall and medical therapy becomes ineffective. The current treatment of choice in primary surgical intervention for terminal ileal disease is laparoscopic ileocolic resection with primary anastomosis.[31,32] There is no convincing evidence that the method of anastomosis influences recurrence rates.[33] When possible, all grossly involved intestine is resected back to bowel of normal appearance, but this should be kept to a minimum to prevent short gut syndrome. Ileocolic resection and anastomosis is associated with higher anastomotic dehiscence rates compared to similar resections in other patient groups. Patient factors are mainly to blame, and in the patient with poor nutrition and recent treatment with high-dose corticosteroids, consideration should be given to formation of a temporary stoma, to be reversed at a later date when the patient has recovered, rather than risk the disaster of anastomotic failure in a patient with little physiological reserve.

One of the most important therapeutic advances in the operative management of small bowel Crohn's disease has been the application of *strictureplasty* to treat patients with diffuse jejunoileitis who have multiple strictures, avoiding extensive resection to preserve gut length. The technique consists of making a longitudinal incision on the antimesenteric border of the stricture and closing the

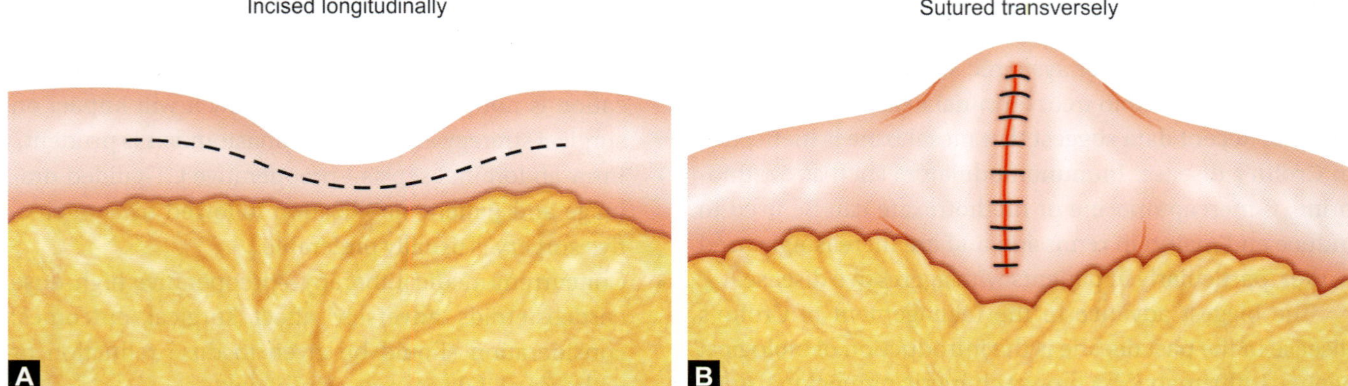

Figs. 69.23A and B: Strictureplasty. The stricture is incised longitudinally and then closed transversely. This procedure is analogous to a pyloroplasty procedure.

defect in a transverse manner analogous to pyloroplasty (Figs. 69.23A and B).

Abscesses result from transmural ulceration with containment by the parietes (intra-abdominal abscess), retroperitoneal tissues (psoas abscess), adjacent viscus (interloop abscess) or the leaves of the mesentery (intra-mesenteric abscess). Fever, neutrophilia and a mass are usually present, but the concomitant use of immuno-suppressants can mask the diagnosis. Patients who have an intra-abdominal abscess and who are toxic or chronically ill may benefit from preliminary operative or CT-directed drainage, but a definitive operation to resect the site of perforation will generally be required.

Penetrating ulcers can also result in *fistula* formation rather than abscess (Fig. 69.24). Fistulas may be enterocutaneous, enteroenteric, enterovesical, ileoduodenal, ileosigmoid, ileovaginal, or ileoperineal. Except for enteroenteric fistulas, all these usually require operative management. The surgical principle here is to resect the diseased segment of bowel responsible; the secondarily involved viscus can usually be simply repaired, unless it is also affected by Crohn's disease. Thus in the relatively commonly encountered situation of terminal ileal disease fistulating into the sigmoid colon, preoperative colonoscopy is essential.

Free *perforation* with diffuse peritonitis occurs in approximately 2% of patients and requires resection of the diseased intestinal segment.

Operation is also indicated in acute or chronic *failure of medical treatment*, particularly in patients dependent on corticosteroids for disease control. Intestinal hemorrhage and carcinoma are rare complications of small bowel Crohn's disease that also require operative treatment.

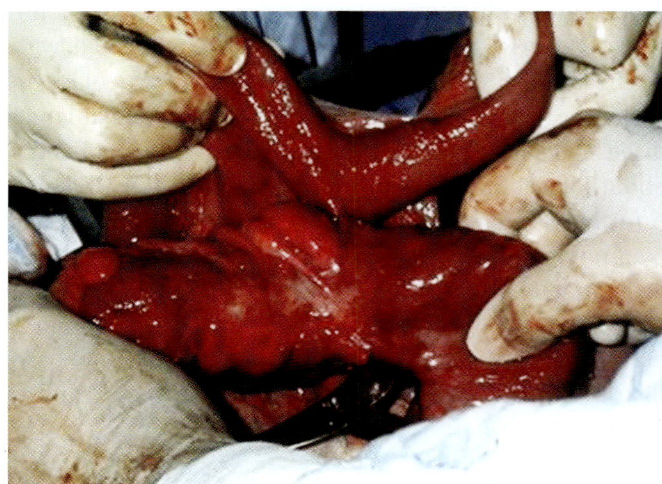

Fig. 69.24: Ileosigmoid fistula as a result of Crohn's disease.

Definitions of and methods used to detect recurrence affect the reported incidence of recurrent disease following complete resection of (usually) terminal ileal disease. If recurrence is defined by the presence of microscopic disease on a mucosal biopsy, most patients will have recurrent disease within 1 year of operation. The role of medication postoperatively in Crohn's patients as prophylaxis against disease relapse remains under investigation, but it is clear that the greatest risk of relapse is in patients who continue to smoke.

INTESTINAL FAILURE

Intestinal failure is the inability of the bowel to maintain adequate protein, nutrient, fluid, and electrolyte balance.[34] It comprises a variety of disorders. Three types of intestinal failure are defined:

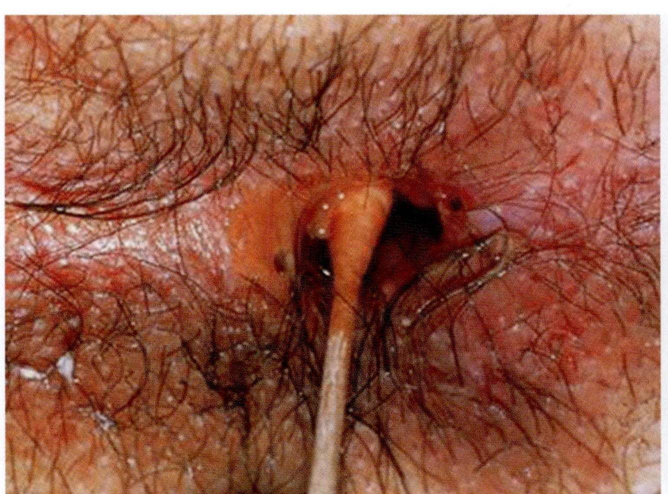

Fig. 69.25: Enterocutaneous fistula to the perineal skin.

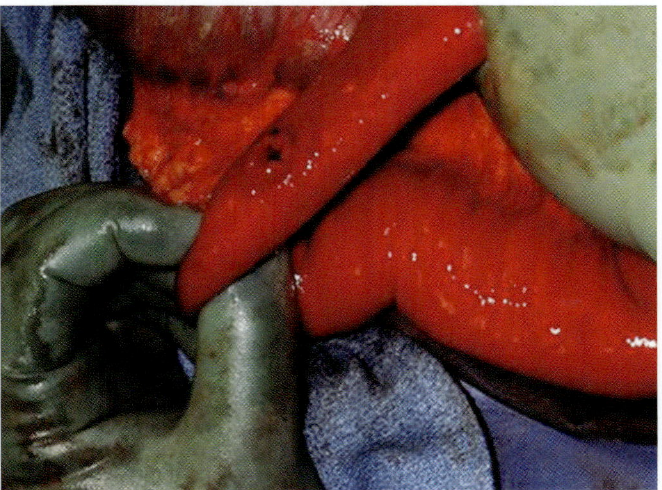

Fig. 69.26: Penetrating small bowel injury requiring a laparotomy. A missed injury to the small intestine can result in a fistula.

- Type I failure is common, short term and self-limiting (e.g., postoperative ileus): It requires fluid and nutritional support for < 28 days.
- Type II failure is associated with metabolically unstable patients in hospital and requires prolonged parenteral nutrition over weeks or months until the intestinal failure resolves or is corrected by surgical intervention. It is often associated with sepsis and renal impairment and usually requires intensive care support. Both type I and type II intestinal failure should recover intestinal function with appropriate supportive management.
- Type III intestinal failure is a chronic condition and comprises stable patients unable to maintain adequate nutrition without parenteral feeding.

Intestinal Fistula

The commonest surgical condition associated with type II intestinal failure is intestinal fistula of which the commonest causes are iatrogenic (an injury sustained at the time of laparotomy) and Crohn's disease, either as a result of the disease process itself or as a postoperative complication.

A small bowel loop may fistulate to the skin [enterocutaneous fistula (Fig. 69.25)] or to an adjacent organ (e.g., enterovesical fistula). Fistulae may result from a leaking intestinal anastomosis or an inadvertent enterotomy that occurs during lysis of adhesions. It can also follow undetected intestinal injury from penetrating trauma (Fig. 69.26). Other pathological processes of the small intestine that cause full-thickness erosion of the intestinal wall, such as malignancy or radiation enteritis, can also give rise to fistulas.

Management

After an enterocutaneous fistula is diagnosed, the first step is stabilization of the patient. The principles of management are SNAPPP.

- S—Control of sepsis
- N—Nutritional support
- A—Define anatomy of fistula
- P—Protect skin
- P—Protect patient's psyche
- P—Planned definitive procedure.

Aggressive diagnosis and management of intra-abdominal sepsis is the first priority in these patients. Uncontrolled sepsis can quickly escalate to multiorgan failure and death. Drainage of sepsis by minimally invasive techniques, usually insertion of a percutaneous drain under CT-guidance, is preferable to avoid the "second hit" of laparotomy in an unstable patient, but in some cases, effective drainage may only be achieved by operation. The goal is to achieve a "controlled" fistula in a stable patient. Appropriate fluid and electrolyte management is essential, particularly for high-output fistulas. Once metabolic disorders have been corrected, prompt attention must be directed toward early institution of nutritional support. This usually entails total parenteral nutrition (TPN), but it may be possible to use elemental nutrition for some patients with distal fistulas (*see* Chapter 25, "Nutritional Support"). When parenteral nutrition is required, securing reliable central venous access by means of a dedicated tunneled line is vital. The role of somatostatin and its analogs in the management of enterocutaneous fistula

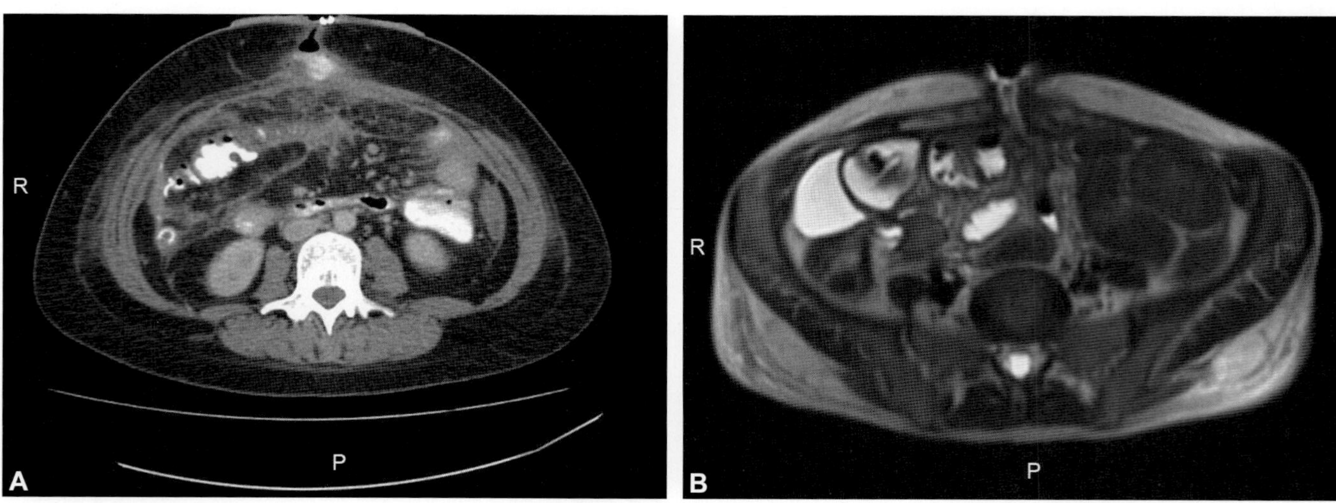

Figs. 69.27A and B: Enterocutaneous fistula seen on CT scan (A) and on MR scan (B).

has been controversial. However, recent evidence from meta-analysis would suggest that in enterocutaneous fistula these drugs increase the likelihood of fistula closure and reduce time to closure, with no effect on mortality.[35] Proton pump inhibitors are also advantageous in reducing gastric hypersecretion and reducing the acidity of fistula effluent.[36] Unless there is a component of obstruction, a nasogastric tube is generally unnecessary and adds to the patient's physical and emotional discomfort. Similarly, although relatively short courses of intravenous antibiotics may be helpful to control systemic septic manifestations, prolonged courses only serve to select for resistant micro-organisms. Early and prompt attention must be directed to the skin because excoriation and damage of the abdominal wall soft tissue may complicate later operative intervention. Adequate pouching of the fistula markedly contributes to the patient's comfort.

Subsequent management and expectations depend upon the clinical circumstance. Most enterocutaneous fistulas result from technical errors during operation and frequently heal with nonoperative management. However, a number of factors predict poor spontaneous closure rates including a completely disrupted anastomosis, the presence of a foreign body, irradiated bowel, malnutrition, and distal obstruction. Even if adverse factors are present and complete healing is not expected, nonoperative management generally remains the preferred initial approach for a controlled fistula, with reoperation planned for a more favorable time.

The timing of operation is crucial. Early reoperation, within the first week, can usually be performed safely. However, patients go on to develop an obliterative peritoneal reaction that makes subsequent operation extremely hazardous, with a high risk of further iatrogenic injury and recurrent fistulation. Assuming the patient is stable, delaying the reoperation by several months will markedly improve the ease of operation and patient outcome. Home TPN is very useful in this situation.

Patients who have primary small intestinal disease such as Crohn's disease, radiation enteritis or malignant fistula rarely respond to nonoperative management. However, they still benefit from a period of nutritional support, correction of fluid and electrolyte abnormalities, and appropriate preoperative preparation and planning.

Patients requiring operation must have a thorough workup to facilitate planning of the operative approach. Radiological imaging–contrast CT scanning and MRI is useful to define anatomy (Figs. 69.27A and B).

The preferred operative procedure is resection of the fistula and diseased bowel with a primary anastomosis. Direct closure of the fistula should not be performed because breakdown is virtually inevitable.

Most enterocutaneous fistulas that are not associated with adverse features close with conservative management. Better understanding of fluid and electrolyte management and the use of TPN has markedly lowered the high mortality rates that used to be reported. However, morbidity rates remain high and prolonged hospitalization continues to be common.

Short Bowel Syndrome

Type III intestinal failure is an irreversible condition due to inadequate functional intestine. Short bowel syndrome refers to the sequelae brought about by removal of an extensive amount of small intestine. It is difficult to determine exactly how much small intestine must be left in a specific case to avoid short bowel syndrome. Multiple factors are involved including the function of the remaining bowel and the age of the patient. However, the syndrome may be anticipated if more than 80% of the small intestinal length is resected.

After intestinal resection, the small intestine undergoes intense *compensatory hyperplasia*, which has been detected as early as 48 hours after jejunal resection. The small intestine dilates, lengthens, and thickens. The intestinal villi undergo hypertrophy. These adaptations result in a greater absorptive surface area and prolongation of intestinal transit time. The compensatory process may continue for 1 or 2 years before adaptation is maximal. A wide variety of factors is believed to mediate intestinal growth and adaptation, including growth hormone, thyroxine and local factors such as exposure of the intestinal mucosa to specific luminal nutrients and pancreaticobiliary secretions.

Etiology

Any disease process that results in massive small bowel resection may result in short bowel syndrome. Common causes in adults include:

- Acute mesenteric ischemia
- Crohn's disease with diffuse jejunoileitis
- Radiation enteritis
- Necrotizing enterocolitis, intestinal atresia, and midgut volvulus are frequent causes in infants.

Management

Prevention of short bowel syndrome requires avoidance of extensive small bowel resection. Historically, a high-risk group were patients with type II intestinal failure and uncontrolled sepsis, in whom repeated emergency surgery led to further complications and loss of intestinal length. Therefore, good management of type II intestinal failure is essential in minimizing progression to type III. Although massive enteric resection may be unavoidable in acute mesenteric thrombosis, early diagnosis of mesenteric vascular disease and attempted revascularization may be appropriate. Second-look laparotomies should be used liberally in this scenario so that bowel of questionable viability is given every opportunity to recover. Conservative resection should be used for patients who have Crohn's disease, with appropriate use of strictureplasty rather than resection for patients who have diffuse jejunoileitis.

Initial management of short bowel syndrome consists of intravenous hydration, fluid and electrolyte management and establishment of TPN.

Reliable venous access with a tunneled silastic catheter is essential for long-term TPN, which can usually be administered at home. As intestinal adaptation progresses and the medical regimen is optimized, patients will achieve good fluid and electrolyte balance and adequate caloric intake for weight maintenance.

A wide variety of complications frequently occurs with long-term parenteral nutrition (*see* Chapter 25, "Nutritional Support"). These include:

- Catheter-related problems, such as occlusion or infection.
- Hepatic dysfunction and failure, which may be the most common serious complication associated with long-term TPN.

In addition, the small bowel itself undegoes marked mucosal atrophy (as in starvation). These problems highlight the need for aggressive treatment to wean the patient back to enteral feeding as early as possible. Enteral nutrients stimulate hypertrophy of intestinal villi and should be instituted early. "Out of circuit" sections of bowel should be placed back in continuity as soon as possible to maximize the available absorptive surface.

Intestinal adaptation allows many patients to be successfully weaned from TPN with its attendant morbidity. However, some patients have insufficient residual bowel to allow a return to exclusive enteral feeding.

Operative techniques have been used with the goal of lengthening the intestine or slowing small bowel transit time including reversed small bowel segments, colonic interposition, construction of valves, use of recirculating loops, and retrograde electrical pacing; none is entirely satisfactory. Small intestine transplantation has now evolved to the point that it should be considered in this patient group (*see* Chapter 120, "Small Bowel and Multivisceral Transplantation"). However, an intestinal transplant is associated with considerable and is mainly indicated in patients with secondary complications of home parenteral nutrition. Current criteria in the United Kingdom to be considered for intestinal transplantation are patients with irreversible intestinal failure in whom there is increasing difficulty obtaining venous access, progressive liver disease or life-threatening sepsis associated with parenteral nutrition catheters.

RADIATION ENTEROPATHY

Radiotherapy has an established role in the curative and palliative treatment of various malignancies. Recent advances in treatment algorithms (gynecological cancers,[37] urological cancers,[38,39] and rectal cancer[40,41]) and in radiation delivery have tried to maximize the therapeutic benefit of radiotherapy in cancer management while simultaneously reducing adverse effects. Small bowel radiation injury predominantly occurs during radiation therapy for pelvic tumors, and it causes major complications that may not become clinically apparent for many years or even decades.

Pathology

Ionizing radiation causes molecular disruption. Rapidly dividing cells, such as those in the intestinal mucosa, are highly susceptible to the cytotoxic effects of radiation. Acutely, the mucosa is denuded because of the loss of normal epithelial cells. In addition, mitotic activity of undifferentiated epithelial cells is inhibited, with subsequent mucosal atrophy and loss of intestinal villi. There is also a submucosal inflammatory response that damages small intramural vessels. Intimal fibrosis ensues, resulting in an obliterative endarteritis.

The mucosal injury is usually self-limiting and re-epithelialization will occur. However, excessive damage to the connective tissue in the submucosa can ultimately lead to stenosis and the symptoms of intestinal obstruction. Along with submucosal fibrosis, there continues to be a progressive sclerosis of blood vessels. Chronic ischemia may lead to nonhealing ulcers that bleed or penetrate deeply into adjacent organs. Submucosal thickening often causes narrowing of the intestinal lumen, which progresses slowly over many years. Carcinoma is also a potential long-term complication of radiation therapy.

Presentation and Diagnosis

The small intestine is radiosensitive and easily injured during radiation therapy for gynecologic or other pelvic tumors. During the acute phase of radiation injury, the clinical picture is that of acute radiation enteritis.[42] Damage and symptoms are generally dose related. Patients complain of crampy abdominal pain, nausea, anorexia, and watery diarrhea. With continued irradiation, the symptoms may become so severe that hospitalization is necessary. The abdomen is generally mildly to moderately tender on physical examination.

Conversely, the late complications of radiation therapy are usually not self-limited, and a thoughtful diagnostic and therapeutic approach is necessary. The clinical picture may be that of chronic malabsorption, intestinal stricturing with obstructive symptoms, fistula formation, and overt necrosis.

Symptoms may start insidiously and progress slowly and relentlessly over relatively long periods of time.[43] The history of previous abdominal or pelvic radiation may be remote, and the etiology and nature of the symptoms may elude both the patient and their primary care physician. Malabsorption may result in weight loss, diarrhea, and a variety of nonspecific abdominal complaints. Strictures present with intermittent and progressive obstructive symptoms, characterized by frequent unscheduled admissions with overt small bowel obstruction. Complete bowel obstructions can be particularly dangerous because these patients already have chronic intestinal ischemia from the associated radiation-induced vascular insufficiency. Fistulation may occur, often to the vagina, bladder or perineum.

Management

The management of acute radiation enteritis is generally supportive and aimed at relieving symptoms. Analgesics or antispasmodics are used to treat abdominal pain. Diarrhea is controlled with opiates or standard antidiarrheal agents. Severe cases may require intravenous rehydration and bowel rest. Operative management is rarely needed.

On the other hand, the late complications of radiation therapy present a major management challenge, often causing major morbidity or even death. Partial small bowel obstruction frequently responds to intestinal decompression and intravenous hydration. However, complete or repetitive obstruction generally requires operative correction. Although obstruction is the most common indication, operative intervention is also indicated for bleeding, perforation or the development of a fistula.

Operative procedures to treat the complications of radiation enteritis are generally difficult, time-consuming, and risk complications. Contrast CT or MR abdomen/pelvis examination helps to delineate the affected site(s) and facilitate preoperative planning.

Several technical points need to be emphasized:

- Dissection must be particularly meticulous, as an enterotomy is likely to break down after repair because of chronic radiation-induced ischemia.

- Generous resection is required to remove all of the thickened diseased bowel and allow an anastomosis between healthy nonirradiated bowel ends.
- The distal anastomosis should generally be to the upper abdominal colon, which is well out of the radiation field (e.g., hepatic flexure).
- Despite the general preference for resection, bypass still seems advisable for cases of a "frozen pelvis" in which the risks of excessive bleeding, injury to adjacent structures or need for extensive resection with development of a short bowel syndrome seem inevitable.

Outcome

The probability of developing small intestinal complications as a result of radiation therapy depends upon a number of factors:

- The higher the total dosage or the individual fractions, the higher the probability of clinical injury to the small intestine, although marked injury can occur at dosages in the range of 40 Gy, a total dose of 65 Gy is associated with a very high rate of radiation enteritis.
- Concomitant use of chemotherapy and patient factors such as diabetes mellitus, hypertension, and previous surgery increase the risk of complications.
- Adhesions of the small bowel into the pelvis or previous pelvic inflammatory disease allow the same loop of intestine to be irradiated with each fraction.

The increased use of preoperative radiotherapy[40,41] has the advantage of allowing the patient to be positioned so that the small intestine falls safely out of the radiation field. If the possibility of postoperative therapy exists, surgical maneuvers to exclude small bowel from the pelvis such as an omental pedicle or an absorbable mesh sling between the dependent coils of small intestine and the freshly operated pelvis minimizes small bowel radiation toxicity.

INFECTIVE ENTERITIS

A wide variety of pathogens can cause infective enteritis.[44] Bacterial infections may be caused by elaborated enterotoxins or direct invasion of the microorganism itself into the mucosal coat. Viruses and other microbes also cause diarrhea and debilitation. This section focuses on pathogenic micro-organisms of particular surgical relevance (*see* Chapter 17, "Geographic Factors Influencing Surgical Practice").

Acute Infective Enteritis

Acute infectious enteritis can cause acute abdominal symptoms easily confused with appendicitis. Certain bacterial infections, most notably *Yersinia enterocolitica* and *Campylobacter jejuni* infection, cause acute ileal inflammation with an associated acute mesenteric lymphadenitis. There is commonly a history of nausea and vomiting in conjunction with marked right lower quadrant tenderness. It may be very difficult to differentiate the findings at laparoscopy/laparotomy from those seen with Crohn's disease. Excision of a mesenteric lymph node with appropriate culture will usually be diagnostic of the specific infectious etiology.

Typhoid Fever

Typhoid fever is a febrile illness caused by *Salmonella* species, usually *Salmonella typhi.* It is characterized by fevers, delirium, splenomegaly, and abdominal pain. The micro-organism penetrates the small intestinal mucosa and enters the mesenteric lymphatics and bloodstream. The bacteria are then sequestered in the macrophages and monocytes of the reticuloendothelial system. This process results in swollen lymph nodes and enlargement of the intestine, liver, and spleen.

As a result of the systemic nature of the illness, a wide variety of organ systems may become involved with inflammatory change. However, the major complications remain intestinal perforation and hemorrhage. It has been estimated that approximately 3% of patients who have typhoid fever develop an intestinal perforation, most commonly of the distal ileum. Blood and stool cultures are usually diagnostic.

Tuberculosis

Any portion of the gastrointestinal tract may be involved with tuberculosis. Gastrointestinal tract involvement remains common in developing countries, but there has also been a marked increase in the incidence of tuberculosis in developed countries related to the AIDS epidemic. The major pathogen is *Mycobacterium tuberculosis.*

The ileocecal area is the most common site of intestinal involvement. The gross appearance is that of ulceration, often with associated fibrosis. Much like Crohn's disease, there may be strictures, fistula formation, stenotic bowel, and matted mesenteric lymph nodes. The classic histologic finding is of caseating granulomas.

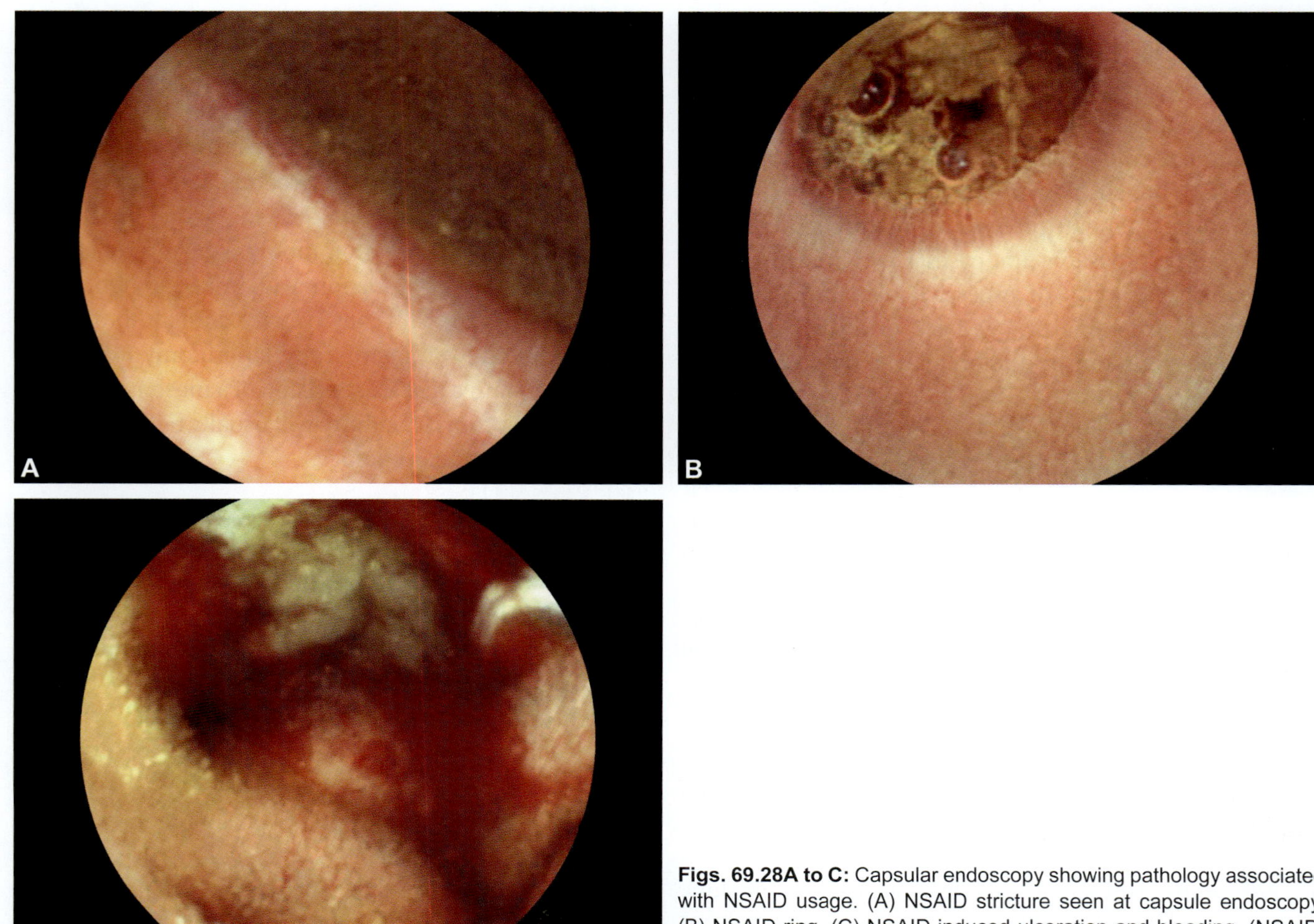

Figs. 69.28A to C: Capsular endoscopy showing pathology associated with NSAID usage. (A) NSAID stricture seen at capsule endoscopy. (B) NSAID ring. (C) NSAID-induced ulceration and bleeding. (NSAID: Nonsteroidal anti-inflammatory drug).

The commonest symptom is chronic nonspecific abdominal pain. A right lower quadrant mass may be evident on physical examination. Complications include hemorrhage, perforation, obstruction, fistulation, and chronic malabsorption. Most uncomplicated cases are cured by standard antituberculous treatment. Fistulas often respond to medical management, but stenotic segments causing obstruction require operative resection.

ULCERATION AND BLEEDING

Small intestinal bleeding, remote from conventional gastroscopy and colonoscopy, is a major diagnostic and therapeutic challenge. A wide variety of etiologies may be responsible for small intestinal bleeding. Meckel's diverticulum is the commonest etiology in children. Small bowel ulceration in adults is more complex and can be associated with a variety of specific etiologies including bacterial infections, Behcet's disease or Crohn's disease. Small bowel ulceration may be caused by concomitant medications such as nonsteroidal anti-inflammatory drugs (NSAIDs) (Figs. 69.28A to C) and enteric-coated potassium tablets. Benign ulceration may be produced by a wide variety of infectious agents such as cytomegalovirus and inflammatory conditions such as celiac sprue. Symptoms can be vague. In the elective setting, patients may present with recurrent abdominal pain similar to irritable bowel syndrome. Iron-deficient anemia is the most likely trigger to extensive small bowel investigation particularly when upper gastrointestinal and colonic investigation is negative. Chronic ulceration may lead to fibrosis, stricture, and small bowel obstruction. In the emergency setting, patients may present with vigorous bleeding requiring the full range of endoscopic (enteroscopy and capsule endoscopy) and radiological techniques (CT angiography and labeled red cell scans) to aid localization before surgical intervention is undertaken.

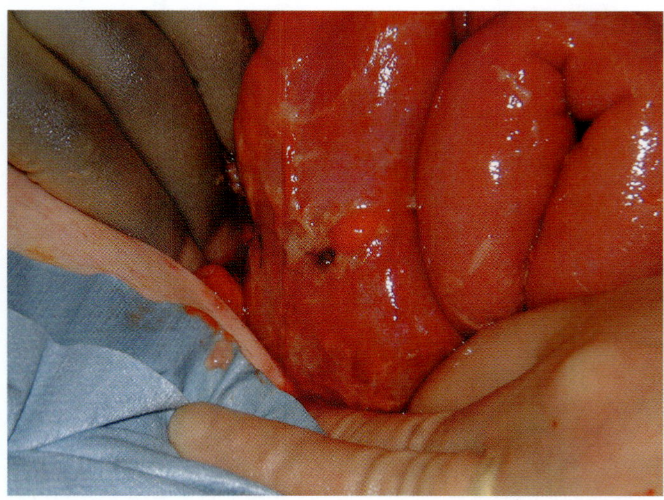

Fig. 69.29: Laparotomy findings for a small bowel perforation in the jejunum secondary to NSAID use.

Management

Small intestine ulcerations associated with NSAIDs or other medications can result in perforation (Fig. 69.29). The treatment of nonperforated ulcers is conservative, ceasing NSAIDs. Ulcerations complicated by obstruction or hemorrhage require operative resection. In the emergency situation, CT angiography can be used to identify the bleeding source. Interventional radiology with coil embolization can be used to secure hemostasis. The development of transmural ischemic necrosis and perforation are potential drawbacks of this technique, though at least localization is then unequivocal.

Laparotomy may be required for a patient who has massive bleeding that defies preoperative identification. However, it is notoriously difficult to identify the bleeding site at the time of laparotomy, so every attempt should be made to reach the diagnosis preoperatively. When this is not possible, enterotomy to allow intraoperative enteroscopy allows visualization of the entire length of the small (and large) intestine.

CELIAC DISEASE

Celiac disease is an increasingly common autoimmune disease affecting the small bowel. The condition affects between 1 in 105 and 1 in 1,750 people in the United States.[45] Presenting symptoms include abdominal pain, fatigue (from anemia) diarrhea, and failure to thrive in children. Celiac disease is due to abnormal host response to gliadin, a gluten protein. Dietary gluten simulates an inflammatory process mediated by T cells leading to disruption of small bowel mucosa and villous architecture with consequent malabsorption. Diagnosis is based on serological detection of appropriate A-gliadin titres and villous atrophy in duodenal biopsies from four quadrants in the second part of the duodenum. Treatment is through dietary modification and gluten avoidance.[46] Celiac patients may present to the surgeon for investigation of anemia. Given the increasing incidence and awareness of this disease, in anemic patients the second part of the duodenum should be routinely biopsied for exclusion of celiac disease. Longstanding untreated celiac disease increases the risk of small bowel adenocarcinoma and small bowel lymphoma, particularly enteropathy-associated T-cell lymphoma. The risk returns to baseline with dietary modification.[47]

DIVERTICULAR DISEASE

Diverticulosis of the small bowel is thought to be relatively uncommon, as most cases are asymptomatic. However, ileojejunal diverticulosis can produce life-threatening complications.

Small intestinal diverticula can be classified in various ways:

- True diverticula represent herniations of all layers of the intestinal wall and are generally congenital.
- Conversely, false diverticula are acquired herniations of the mucosa and submucosa through the muscular wall of the small intestine.

False diverticula are thought to occur secondary to pulsion of the intestinal lining through weaknesses in the small intestine where blood vessels penetrate the intestinal wall.

Duodenal Diverticula

Duodenal diverticula appear to be the most common small bowel diverticula. Most occur in the second portion of the duodenum along the medial or pancreatic border. Unlike jejunoileal diverticulosis, duodenal diverticula are usually solitary (Fig. 69.30).

Most patients with duodenal diverticula are asymptomatic. When symptoms do occur, they are generally thought to be related to obstruction of the neck of the diverticulum with resultant distension of the diverticular pouch. Symptoms caused by the subsequent inflammatory reaction may mimic those of other upper abdominal disorders such as cholecystitis or pancreatitis. Alternatively, there may be direct compression of the contiguous

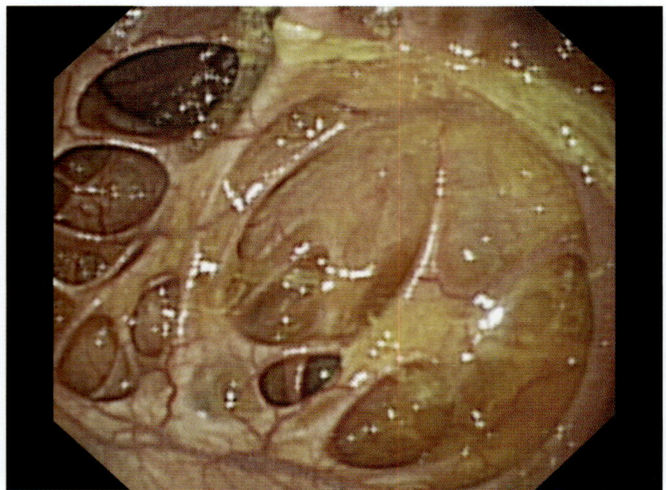
Fig. 69.30: Duodenal diverticulum seen during upper GI endoscopy.

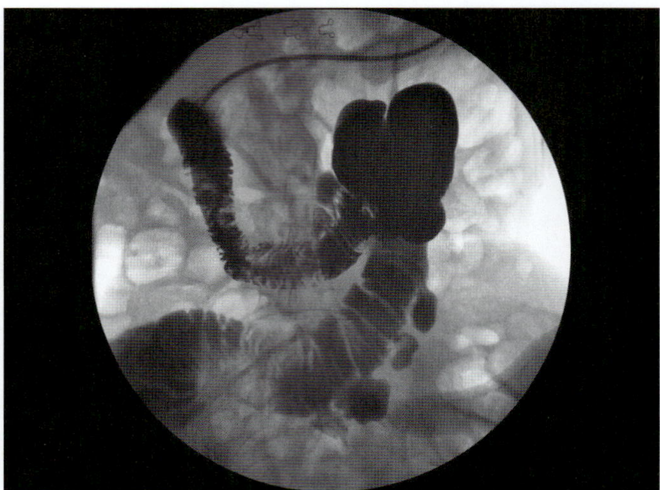
Fig. 69.31: Jejunal diverticulae seen on small bowel enema.

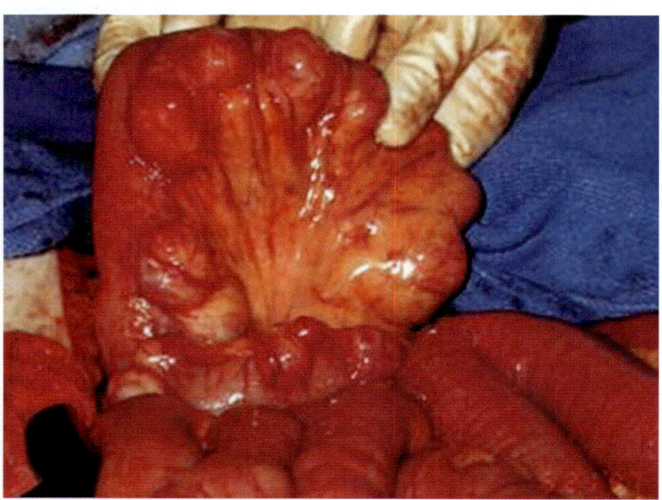
Fig. 69.32: Jejunal diverticulosis. Incidental jejunal diverticula seen during a laparotomy.

common bile duct or pancreatic duct by the diverticulum, resulting in jaundice or pancreatitis. Rarely, the inflammatory response may progress to perforation or result in gastrointestinal hemorrhage.

Although duodenal diverticula can be the clear cause of acute abdominal crises, the relationship between diverticular disease of the duodenum and chronic abdominal symptoms is less certain. Duodenal diverticula most commonly come to attention as an incidental finding on radiographic studies or at the time of laparotomy for another condition. They can be very difficult to treat operatively because of their frequent close anatomic relationship to the pancreas and common bile duct.

A wide variety of operative procedures have been advocated to treat symptomatic duodenal diverticula. Resection has usually been associated with high morbidity and mortality rates because of pancreaticobiliary complications. These diverticula should therefore be left alone unless operative treatment is necessary for a defined complication.

Jejunoileal Diverticula

Jejunoileal diverticula occur in approximately 1% of the population.

- They are usually incidental findings on small bowel contrast examinations.[15]
- They are most frequently identified in people aged 50–70 years.
- They seem to be substantially more common in the proximal jejunum than further distally (Fig. 69.31).

The diverticula usually occur on the mesenteric border (Fig. 69.32) as a result of herniation of the mucosa and submucosa through an attenuated thin-walled muscular layer. Some affected patients have chronic abdominal pain. However, it seems likely that the pain results from disordered motility of the small bowel with resultant diverticulosis rather than from the diverticula per se.

A few patients have clinically important problems related to jejunoileal diverticula. Diverticular inflammation and ulceration may result in localized or free perforation and erosion into mesenteric vessels with massive hemorrhage. Operative treatment is generally straightforward and consists of resecting the diseased small bowel segment.

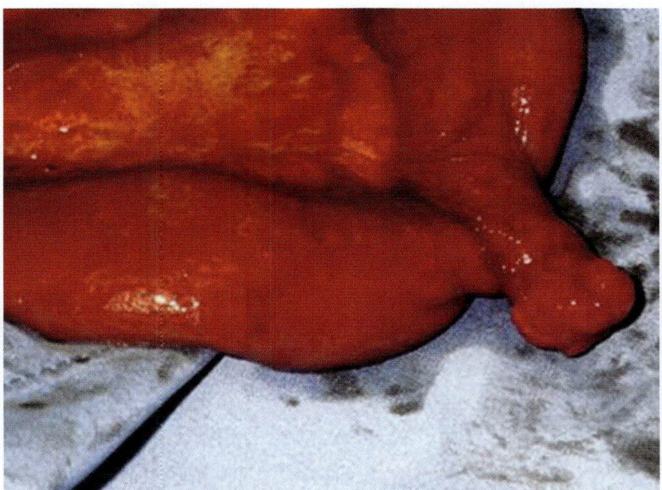

Fig. 69.33: Meckel's diverticulum. An asymptomatic diverticulum seen during a laparotomy.

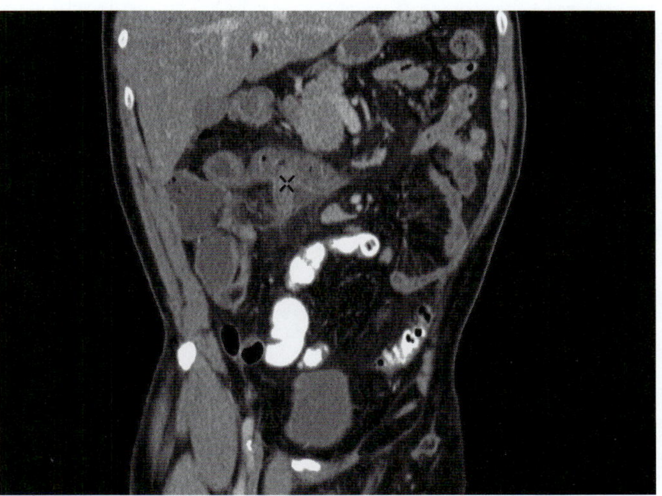

Fig. 69.34: Inflamed Meckel's diverticulum on CT scan marked with a cross seen in patient with vague abdominal pain and raised inflammatory markers.

Meckel's Diverticulum

A Meckel's diverticulum is a true diverticulum of congenital origin occurring in approximately 2% of the population. It results from failure of obliteration of the omphalomesenteric duct, which embryologically connects the gut to the yolk sac. The diverticulum arises from the antimesenteric border, usually approximately 0.6 m from the ileocecal valve. A Meckel's diverticulum may contain ectopic mucosa, usually gastric, but pancreatic, duodenal, or intestinal mucosa may also be present.

Most Meckel's diverticula are asymptomatic and are incidental findings at the time of laparotomy for other conditions (Fig. 69.33). A symptomatic Meckel's diverticulum usually presents in childhood as the source of massive gastrointestinal bleeding, intestinal obstruction or acute right lower quadrant pain (when it may be confused with appendicitis). Ulceration is usually associated with ectopic gastric mucosa, which can lead to either massive hemorrhage or perforation. Obstruction may result from intussusception of the diverticulum or twisting of the small bowel about the axis of a fibrous band connecting the diverticulum to the abdominal wall (*see* Chapter 125, "Gastrointestinal Surgery in Children").

Meckel's diverticulum may be diagnosed by contrast CT or MR scan (Fig. 69.34). Technetium 99 m scanning will reveal those diverticula containing ectopic gastric mucosa. Meckel's diverticulum may be found incidentally at laparotomy, and in adults it is then best left alone. However, resection is appropriate in children or patients for whom the diverticulum may complicate later diagnosis (e.g., Crohn's disease). Symptomatic diverticula can be treated by diverticulectomy or segmental small bowel resection with primary anastomosis. In the emergency setting, CT angiography can assist in the identification of a bleeding source in massive hemorrhage.

MESENTERIC VASCULAR DISEASE

The small intestine has a rich blood supply, receiving approximately 25% of the cardiac output at rest. Although the SMA supplies the whole length of the small intestine, collateral flow is available from both the celiac and inferior mesenteric arteries. This anatomic arrangement helps to prevent intestinal ischemia when the SMA is diseased.

Acute Occlusion of the SMA

Acute SMA occlusion is the commonest cause of small bowel ischemia. The occlusion may be caused by embolism or thrombosis. Most emboli originate in the heart. Clot may form in the left heart from atrial fibrillation or ventricular thrombus complicating a myocardial infarction. The SMA is vulnerable to blood-borne emboli because it is a large-caliber vessel that has an acute-angle take-off from the aorta. Acute thrombosis occurs in the setting of chronic atherosclerotic narrowing of the SMA origin, perhaps complicated by a low-flow state.

Emboli usually lodge where the SMA narrows at the level of its first major branch, the middle colic artery, allowing for continued perfusion through the first jejunal branches (Fig. 69.35). The proximal jejunum is therefore

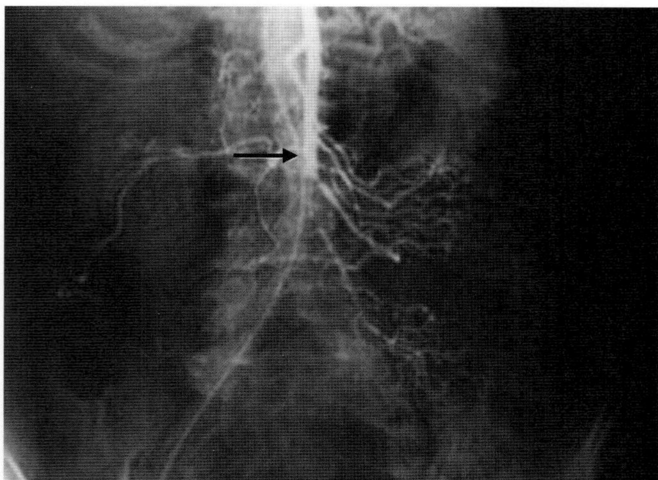

Fig. 69.35: Embolus to the SMA. Flow is preserved to several proximal jejunal branches. There is an acute cutoff of flow in the superior mesenteric artery (arrow) caused by the embolus.

generally spared, but the remaining small bowel and ascending colon become profoundly ischemic. Smaller emboli may lodge more distally, creating segmental ischemia. Acute thrombosis occurs at the origin at the SMA when there is a pre-existing atherosclerotic stenosis. Ischemia therefore tends to extend from the ligament of Treitz to the midtransverse colon.

Clinically, the classic presentation is severe abdominal pain that seems out of proportion to the findings on physical examination. The pain may be diffuse or focal and is commonly associated with vomiting and sweating. As a result of the nonspecific nature of the presentation, the diagnosis is commonly missed unless a high level of suspicion is maintained.

As ischemia progresses, small intestinal necrosis becomes evident. There is usually a dramatic leukocytosis, with the development of a metabolic acidosis. Contrast CT scan and elevated serum lactate levels may be of help but establishing a diagnosis early can be difficult and requires a low threshold for exploratory laparotomy.[48] The goal is to make the diagnosis before ischemic necrosis of the intestine develops.[49] Sudden onset of abdominal pain in a patient who has a history of cardiac disease such as atrial fibrillation or other stigmata of severe atherosclerotic disease should heighten suspicion. Mesenteric angiography will differentiate between embolism, thrombosis and nonocclusive ischemia. After completing the diagnostic phase, the angiography catheter may be left in the SMA to permit the infusion of vasodilating agents. This can be helpful in the nonocclusive ischemia setting.

The definitive management of an SMA embolus is arteriotomy with embolectomy. Thrombotic disease is usually treated by an aortomesenteric bypass (*see* Chapter 95, "Mesenteric Ischemia"). After the blood flow has been restored, the intestinal viability is assessed. Standard criteria for bowel viability have classically been:

- Presence of mesenteric arterial pulsations
- "Pinking up" of the bowel
- Presence of peristalsis

Thrombolysis of the clot medically and interventional radiological vascular techniques are being used more frequently.[49] Clearly necrotic bowel should be resected, but it may be difficult to assess the viability of some bowel segments. A second-look laparotomy after 24–48 hours when the patient has been stabilized can be extremely useful.

Mesenteric Vein Thrombosis

Mesenteric vein thrombosis usually involves small venous channels and causes segmental small intestinal ischemia. Although many cases are idiopathic, mesenteric vein thrombosis also occurs with hypercoagulable states, such as deficiencies of antithrombin III, protein C or protein S. Other predisposing conditions include the use of oral contraceptives, portal hypertension, and sepsis.

Clinically, the affected intestinal segment becomes massively edematous with hyperemia and submucosal hemorrhage. With progression, venous stasis may lead to arterial occlusion and frank bowel necrosis. The clinical presentation is usually nonspecific, with vague abdominal pain, nausea, and abdominal distension. Symptoms may progress over a period of weeks until it is apparent that the patient has an acute abdominal catastrophe. Plain abdominal radiographs may show intramural edema, and there is generally a marked leukocytosis. CT scanning to evaluate abdominal symptoms has markedly changed the diagnosis and management of patients who have mesenteric vein thrombosis. CT can reveal the diagnosis of clot in the superior mesenteric vein, allowing anticoagulation before the onset of irreversible intestinal ischemia. For patients presenting with an acute abdomen, the diagnosis is usually made at the time of exploratory laparotomy.

If the diagnosis is made before the onset of peritoneal signs, anticoagulation with heparin is indicated. Careful clinical observation is required to watch for the development of overt necrosis requiring urgent laparotomy. When the diagnosis is made intraoperatively in a patient with an acute abdomen (Fig. 69.36), the treatment is

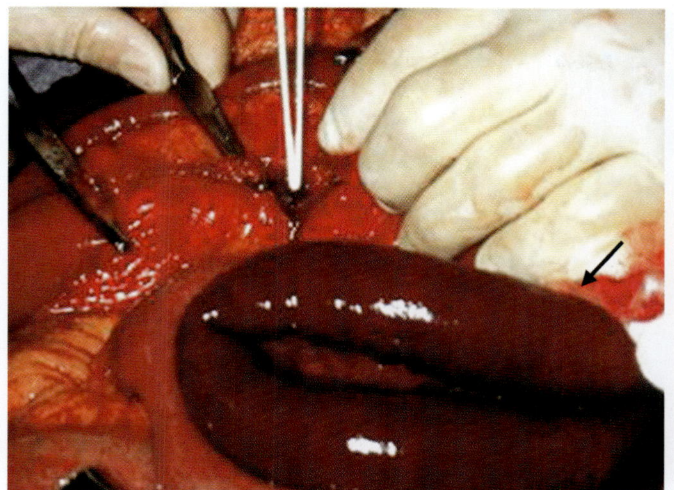

Fig. 69.36: Segmental small bowel ischemia secondary to mesenteric vein thrombosis. Arrow marks the affected bowel.

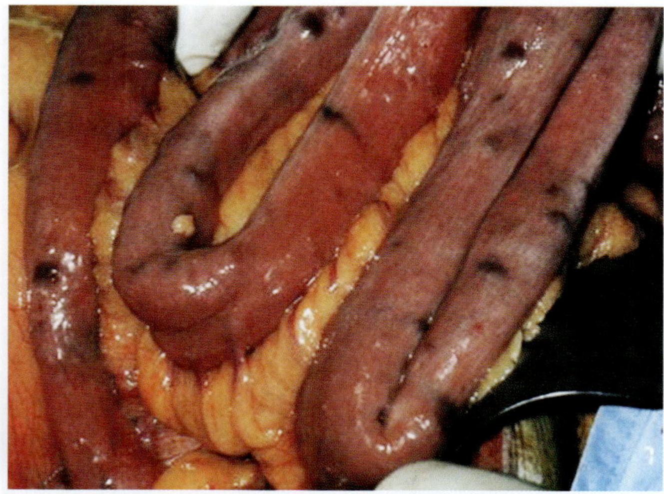

Fig. 69.37: Chronic mesenteric ischemia from occlusion of the SMA with extensive collateral formation (particularly in the abdominal wall) in a patient with an ectatic aorta.

immediate anticoagulation and resection of the segment of affected bowel, usually with primary anastomosis. Anticoagulation with warfarin should continue for at least 3 months. Appropriate investigations should be performed to assess for the presence of a hypercoagulable state that may require chronic long-term anticoagulation.

Nonocclusive Mesenteric Ischemia

Nonocclusive mesenteric ischemia usually occurs in association with low-flow states, such as congestive heart failure, myocardial infarction, arrhythmia, hypovolemia or sepsis, or after cardiac operations. These low-flow states can result in prolonged mesenteric (splanchnic) vasoconstriction causing marked resistance to intestinal blood flow. Like other causes of mesenteric ischemia, patients frequently complain of severe abdominal pain out of proportion to physical findings. Again, a high index of suspicion is required to make this diagnosis as the presentation is frequently nonspecific. Angiography may be diagnostic and will rule out the presence of obstructing lesions in the major visceral arteries.

Management consists of correcting the low-flow state as soon as possible. Angiography is not only diagnostic, but allows therapeutic infusion of vasodilating agents to reverse the intense mesenteric vasoconstriction that can accompany low-flow states. The development of peritonitis is an indication for laparotomy with resection of the gangrenous intestine. Involvement is frequently patchy (Fig. 69.37). Second-look procedures are often helpful for reassessing areas of questionable viability.

Chronic Intestinal Ischemia

Chronic mesenteric ischemia, or intestinal angina, usually occurs in patients who have known widespread atherosclerotic disease. There is generally a history of postprandial abdominal pain that begins shortly after eating. As eating causes abdominal pain, most patients avoid food and marked weight loss follows. An occult malignancy is therefore frequently suspected. Physical examination is generally normal except for the manifestations of diffuse vascular disease. The diagnosis is suspected on the basis of postprandial abdominal pain, fear of eating, and weight loss.

The diagnosis is confirmed by CT angiography (Figs. 69.38A and B), which demonstrates atherosclerotic narrowing at the orifices of the major mesenteric vessels and can show collateral vessel formation. It is generally believed that severe involvement of at least two of the mesenteric vessels is required to cause intestinal ischemia because of the presence of rich collateral flow between the celiac artery, SMA, and inferior mesenteric artery. However, clinical symptoms should be critically assessed as some patients can be asymptomatic even with severe disease in all three major mesenteric arterial trunks.

Patients who have disabling intestinal ischemia are generally candidates for visceral arterial revascularization. The standard approach is bypass to one or more of the visceral vessels or perform endarterectomy. Promising results have been reported with angioplasty in selected cases, but long-term durability remains to be established.

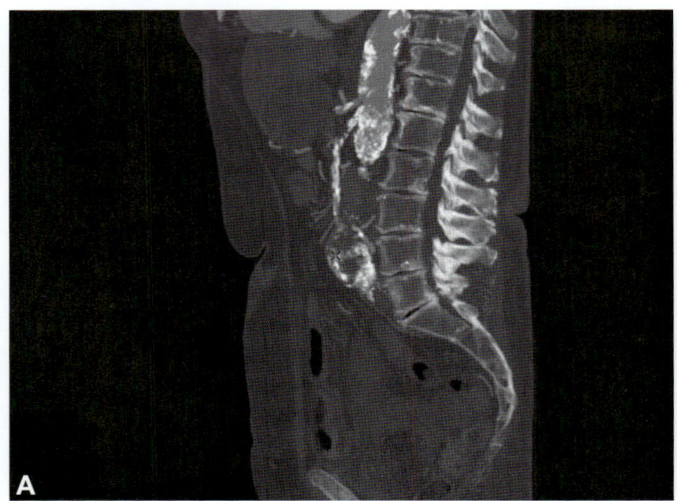

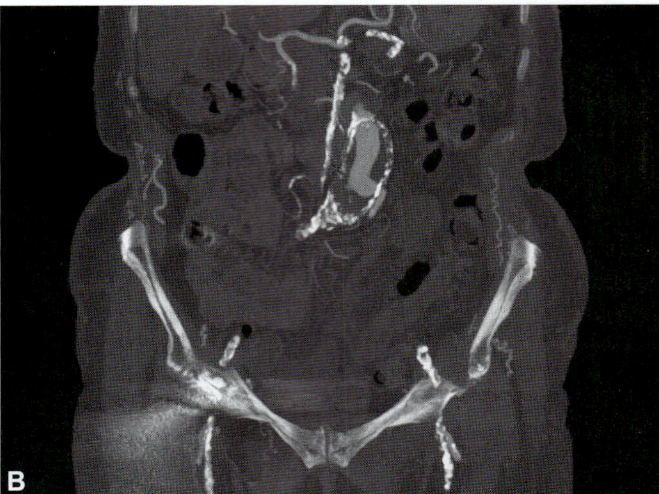

Figs. 69.38A and B: CT angiography. (A) Sagittal CT scan showing narrowing and occlusion of the SMA near its origin from the aorta. (B) Coronal CT scan showing occlusion of the SMA. This scan also shows the extensive collateral circulation secondary to chronic ischemia, particularly laterally in the abdominal wall.

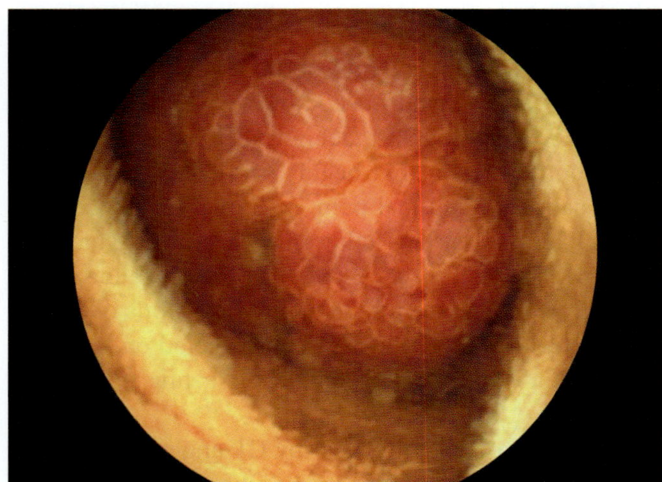

Fig. 69.39: Peutz-Jeghers small bowel polyp seen on capsule endoscopy.

SMALL BOWEL TUMORS

Small bowel neoplasms are uncommon: Only 1–2% of all malignant gastrointestinal tumors are found in the small intestine.

Benign Tumors

Hamartomas (Peutz–Jeghers Syndrome)

Peutz-Jeghers syndrome is an autosomal dominant disorder characterized by multiple intestinal hamartomas and pigmented spots on mucocutaneous surfaces. The classic melanin spots are noted about the lips or buccal mucosa, but may also be noted on the extremities, face or perianal mucosa. The polyps are generally numerous and are up to 3 cm in diameter, with larger polyps frequently becoming pedunculated. Although polyps may be found in the stomach and large intestine, they are most frequent in the small intestine, notably the jejunum.

Diagnosis is suggested by the presence of the characteristic pigmentation. Gastrointestinal contrast studies and small bowel capsule endoscopy will demonstrate numerous polyps (Fig. 69.39). A polyp may serve as a lead point for intussusception or result in gastrointestinal blood loss. Treatment is reserved only for very large or symptomatic polyps on a selective basis. However, patients who have Peutz-Jeghers syndrome are at increased risk for developing small and large bowel adenocarcinoma and other extraintestinal malignancies such as breast, duodenal, and genital tumors.

Adenoma

Adenomatous polyps may be found anywhere in the small intestine, but are most commonly noted in the duodenum. This preponderance may be because the duodenum is routinely visualized at the time of diagnostic upper endoscopy. Adenomas occur either sporadically or as a result of genetic mutations (e.g., familial adenomatous polyposis or FAP). As in the large intestine, they may be tubular (Fig. 69.40A), villous (Fig. 69.40B), or a combination of these histologic types. Endoscopic surveillance in FAP patients may reveal severe dysplastic change in one or more larger polyp which may then necessitate pancreatoduodenectomy.

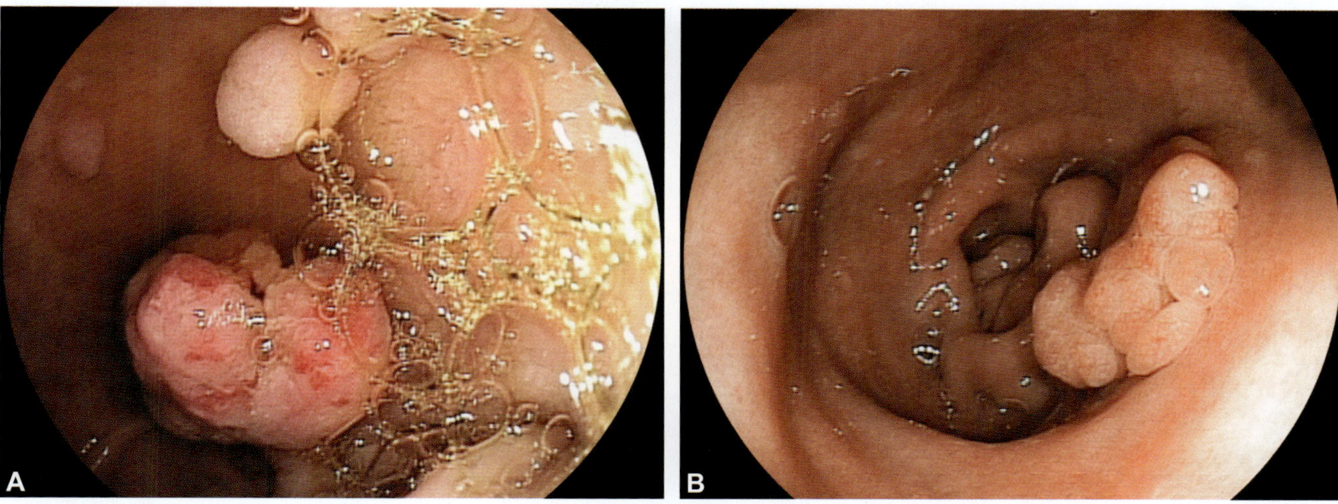

Figs. 69.40A and B: Duodenal polyps seen on upper GI endoscopy. (A) Adenomas—multiple pedunculated polyps seen in the duodenum of a patient with familial adenomatous polyposis. (B) Villous polyp. These polyps are associated with higher malignant potential.

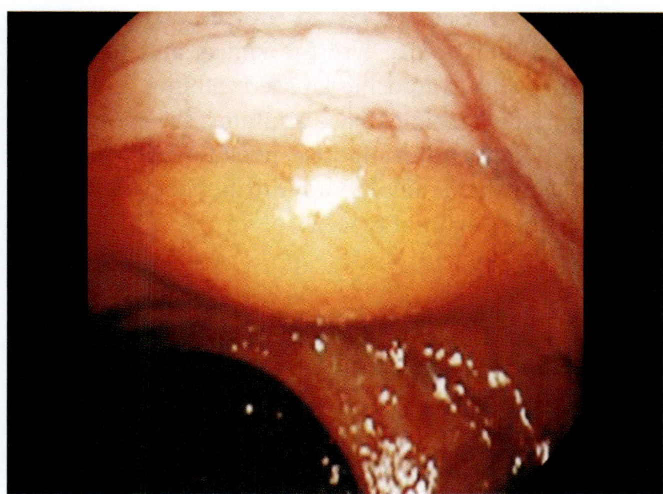

Fig. 69.41: Submucosal lipoma.

Most adenomas are asymptomatic. However, larger lesions may serve as a lead point for intussusception, causing obstructive symptoms or overt intestinal obstruction. Adenomas can cause chronic gastrointestinal blood loss or present with massive hemorrhage. Adenomatous polyps have the potential to degenerate into adenocarcinoma. The risk appears to be low for tubular adenomas and highest for villous lesions. Endoscopic resection of adenomatous polyps is therefore advised when feasible.

Leiomyoma

Leiomyomas are common benign neoplasms that arise from the smooth muscle of the intestinal wall and occur in any part of the small intestine. They may undergo central necrosis with ulceration of the mucosa and subsequent hemorrhage. Alternatively, there may be abdominal pain and obstructive symptoms from a mass effect or intussusception. Segmental resection is required for symptomatic lesions.

Lipoma

Like adenomas and leiomyomas, lipomas are relatively common benign small bowel neoplasms (Fig. 69.41). They seem to be most commonly noted in the ileum and are occasionally multiple. They are usually soft well-circumscribed lesions that indent locally when probed with the biopsy forceps ("pillow" sign) and have a characteristic appearance on CT scans. Treatment is only required for symptomatic lesions that cause intestinal obstruction.

Other Benign Lesions

A host of other benign lesions have been described in the small intestine, including fibromas, schwannomas, neurilemomas, lymphangiomas, and hemangiomas. Operative excision is generally reserved for symptomatic lesions.

Intermediate Tumors

Villous Adenoma

Adenomatous polyps are relatively common in large series of benign small intestinal neoplasms. Villous adenomas (Fig. 69.40B) present a special problem in both diagnosis and treatment because of their considerable malignant potential. Management is complicated by their sessile nature and propensity to occur in the duodenum.

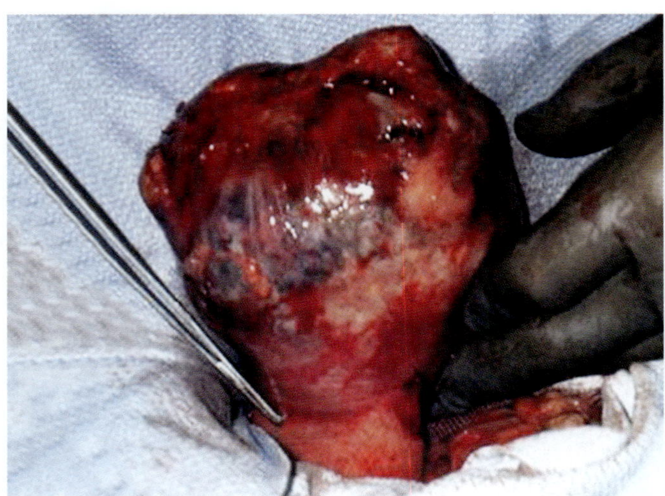

Fig. 69.42: Gastrointestinal stromal tumor. Note the exophytic growth pattern.

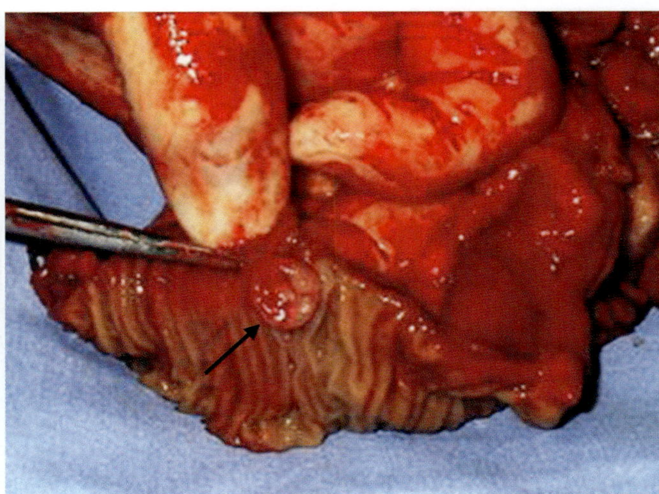

Fig. 69.43: Ileal carcinoid tumor (arrow).

The diagnosis is generally made endoscopically. Although endoscopic biopsies may disclose only the presence of a villous adenoma, many such lesions harbor invasive carcinoma. Villous adenomas must therefore be completely excised. Occasionally, duodenal lesions are removed endoscopically, but many require local excision using a transduodenal approach. Periampullary villous adenomas create special problems with avoiding injury to the orifice of the pancreatic and common bile duct. Pancreatoduodenectomy is generally required if there is malignancy.

Gastrointestinal Stromal Tumors

Gastrointestinal stromal tumors are spindle cell neoplasms of varying malignant potential (Fig. 69.42). Gastrointestinal stromal tumors commonly grow exophytically, often becoming large masses (10 cm or more) prior to clinical detection. They may invade adjacent organs by direct extension, ulcerate the mucosa, resulting in bleeding or perforate into the peritoneal cavity.

The tendency to grow in an extraluminal fashion makes obstruction a less common presentation than with other small intestinal tumors. CT scanning is the most helpful diagnostic modality for determining the size of the tumor and its relation to adjacent structures. Treatment is by small bowel resection with adequate margins. Involved adjacent organs should be resected en bloc when possible. The risk of recurrence is related to tumor size, mitotic rate, and location. Malignant potential is related to the expression of the *c-KIT* oncogene, which encodes a transmembrane tyrosine kinase receptor. In malignant GIST tumors, there is a mutation in the *c-KIT* gene or in the α-gene of platelet-derived growth factor receptor causing upregulation of tyrosine kinase and tumor cell growth. Imatinib, a tyrosine kinase inhibitor, and sunitinib, a multiple tyrosine kinase inhibitor, are used to treat GIST tumors as adjuvant and neoadjuvant therapies. Chemotherapy and radiotherapy are ineffective treatment modalities in this tumor type.

Gastrinoma

These tumors are commonly found in the wall of the duodenum or pancreas. They can be associated with the multiple endocrine neoplasia type I syndrome. The lesions are usually very small (< 1 cm diameter) and often defy preoperative imaging studies. Resection is curative.

Carcinoid Tumor

Carcinoid tumors are neuroendocrine tumors arising from gut enterochromaffin cells. The commonest sites in the gastrointestinal tract are the appendix, rectum, and small intestine. Approximately, one third of patients have multiple tumors. Unlike appendiceal carcinoid tumors, small bowel carcinoid tumors are frequently symptomatic and are much more likely to cause carcinoid syndrome. Grossly, the typical carcinoid tumor is a firm, yellow submucosal nodule (Fig. 69.43).

Carcinoid tumors can be asymptomatic, but they can also be associated with dramatic symptoms caused by local or systemic disease. Although the primary tumors are usually quite small, the involved intestinal segment may develop a severe desmoplastic reaction in the mesentery that results in obstruction or even intestinal ischemia. Serotonin and other physiologically active peptides secreted by small intestine carcinoid tumors are safely metabolized by the liver to the breakdown product 5-hydroxyindoleacetic acid (5-HIAA), which is then excreted in the urine. Liver metastases, however, have direct access to the systemic circulation for their vasoactive byproducts. These patients may have the symptoms of carcinoid syndrome—flushing, intractable diarrhea, and bronchospasm. Likewise bronchial carcinoids can secrete vasoactive kinins directly into the systemic circulation and cause carcinoid syndrome.

Many intestinal carcinoid tumors are incidental findings at the time of laparotomy for other conditions. However, carcinoid tumors can grow indolently over many years and ultimately metastasize to regional nodes and distant sites. CT scan may demonstrate a prominent mesenteric reaction, nodal metastases or liver involvement. Urinary 5-HIAA and blood chromogranin A help to establish the diagnosis.

Carcinoid tumors <1 cm in diameter and identified incidentally at the time of operation require local excision only. However, carcinoid tumors >2 cm in diameter require small bowel resection with adequate lymphatic clearance. Patients frequently have large bulky lymph nodes at the origin of the ileocolic artery, precluding safe resection of all nodal disease. However, palliative small bowel resection can provide long periods of symptomatic relief from this indolent tumor. Similarly, liver resection of a manageable number of metastases may provide relief from the carcinoid syndrome. Standard chemotherapy is of limited benefit, but subcutaneous injections of the long-acting somatostatin analog octreotide can be an effective treatment for the symptoms of carcinoid syndrome.

The outlook for patients who have incidental carcinoid tumors or carcinoid tumors that have not yet metastasized is excellent. However, most symptomatic carcinoid tumors are metastatic at presentation. The outlook is then poor, although approximately 30–40% of patients who have metastatic disease survive at least 5 years. Well-timed palliative operative procedures can therefore lead to long periods of high-quality survival.

Malignant Tumors

Adenocarcinoma is the most common primary malignant neoplasm of the small intestine (Table 69.1).[50]

Adenocarcinoma

Adenocarcinoma accounts for approximately 50% of the malignant tumors noted in the small intestine. The frequency of occurrence is highest in the proximal small intestine, within about 25 cm of the duodenojejunal flexure in either direction, and diminishes distally. The duodenum is much the most frequent site for adenocarcinoma, particularly the second part.

Table 69.1 Most common location of each histologic tumor.[50]

Tumor	*Duodenum*	*Jejunum*	*Ileum*	*Total (%)*
Adenocarcinoma	13	10	6	29 (40)
Carcinoid	1	4	13	18 (25)
Lymphoma	2	9	7	18 (25)
Sarcoma	2	4	2	8 (10)
Total (%)	18 (25)	27 (37)	28 (38)	73 (100)

Etiology: Most adenocarcinomas of the small intestine probably arise from adenomatous polyps. This transformation has been particularly well demonstrated in the duodenum, where villous adenomas have been noted to undergo progression to malignancy while being observed without operative intervention over a period of time. Patients who have familial adenomatous polyposis have a substantially increased risk of developing duodenal adenocarcinoma and require regular screening. Patients with long-standing Crohn's disease also appear to have a higher incidence of small intestinal adenocarcinoma. Adult coeliac disease (enteropathy-associated T-cell lymphoma) and Peutz–Jeghers syndrome are other risk factors.

Pathology: Morphologically, adenocarcinomas of the small intestine may be polypoid, ulcerated, annular, or flat. Like their large bowel counterparts, they penetrate through the intestinal wall, ultimately metastasizing to regional lymph nodes and hematogenously to distant sites.

Clinical Features: The clinical course is frequently nonspecific and consists of abdominal pain, weight loss, obstructive symptoms, and anemia. As a consequence of the relative infrequency of small bowel neoplasms, many other diagnoses are considered. Some adenocarcinomas present more dramatically with gastrointestinal hemorrhage, perforation or overt small bowel obstruction. Periampullary duodenal adenocarcinomas commonly produce jaundice.

Diagnosis: MR small bowel or contrast CT scan (Fig. 69.44) are the imaging modalities of choice. CT scanning provides information on local and metastatic spread. Upper GI endoscopy and colonoscopy may allow access to proximal and distal lesions, respectively. Advances in enteroscopy have markedly improved diagnostic assessment of suspicious lesions.

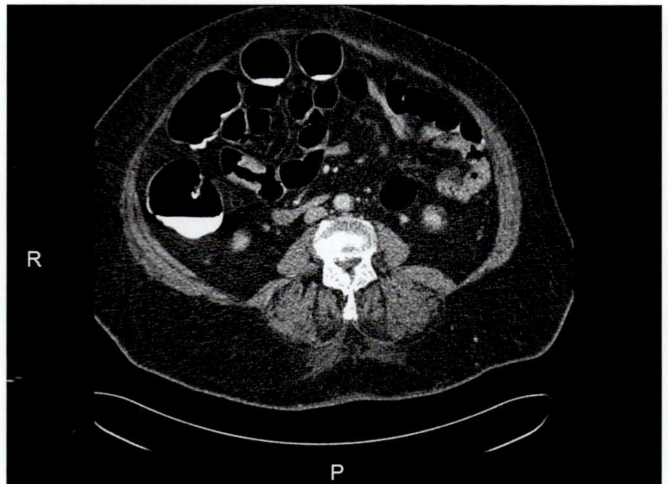

Fig. 69.44: Small bowel carcinoma diagnosed during a CT colonography. Note the shouldering of the tumor.

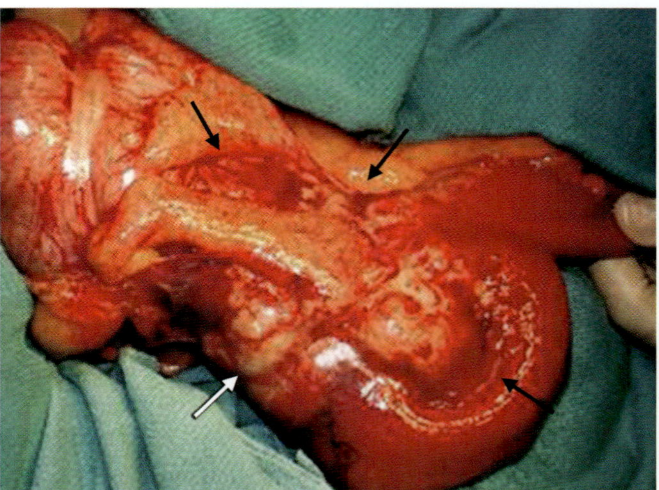

Fig. 69.45: Terminal ileal lymphoma found at laparotomy (arrows outline the tumor).

Management: Treatment of adenocarcinoma of the small intestine is by wide operative resection with appropriate lymphadenectomy. Involved adjacent organs, such as other small intestinal loops, should be resected en bloc. Duodenal carcinomas require pancreatoduodenectomy. Many patients present with metastatic disease, but still require palliative resection or bypass.

Outcome: Overall 5-year survival for adenocarcinoma is generally poor in the range of 10–20%, which reflects the fact that most patients present with locally advanced or metastatic disease. However, the prognosis for node-negative patients is reasonably good, and 50% or more of these cases are cured by surgical resection.

Lymphoma

The small bowel is the commonest site for primary gastrointestinal tract lymphoma. The small intestine may also be a secondary site of lymphoma involvement in patients who have diffuse systemic disease. Primary lymphoma of the gastrointestinal tract implies an absence of peripheral lymphadenopathy, with the disease process confined to a specific site along the gastrointestinal tract.

Etiology: Primary small intestinal lymphoma arises from the lymphatic tissue of the submucosa. The ileum is particularly rich in submucosal lymphatic tissue, explaining the propensity for lymphomas to form in the ileum (Fig. 69.45).

Primary lymphomas occur sporadically in older patients, usually without evidence of distant disease. Celiac disease or immune deficiency states such as AIDS may predispose to the development of lymphoma. As with other primary small bowel neoplasms, the symptoms commonly consist of crampy abdominal pain, weight loss, anemia, and fatigue. An abdominal mass may be palpable. Patients may present with diffuse peritonitis caused by perforation or overt obstruction from intussusception.

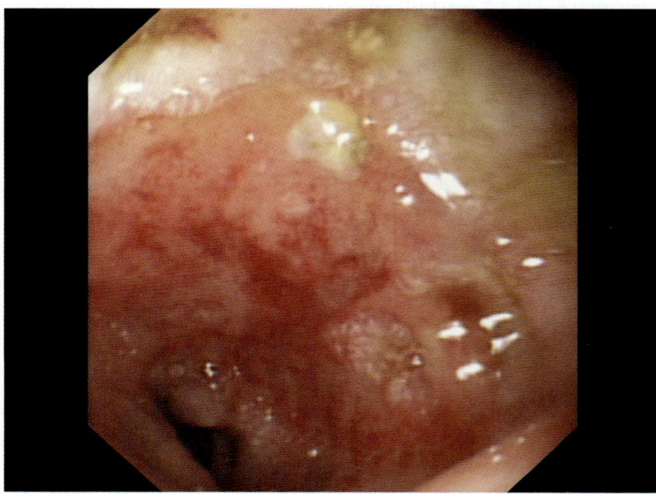

Fig. 69.46: Lymphoma seen in the jejunum during enteroscopy. The patient had a history of night sweats, abdominal pain, fatigue, and weight loss. CT scan had shown an abdominal mass and enteroscopy enabled tissue biopsies to be obtained.

Diagnosis: Contrast CT scan establishes the diagnosis of primary small intestinal lymphoma and provides information on local mesenteric adenopathy. The presence of hepatosplenomegaly, involved nodes at distant sites or multiple segments of involved bowel suggest secondary rather than primary lymphoma. Endoscopy can be used for investigation and diagnostic purposes (Fig. 69.46).

Management: Disease localized to a segment of small intestine and its draining lymph nodes should be treated by small bowel resection with appropriate lymphadenectomy. Adjuvant chemotherapy is required in most cases.

REFERENCES

1. Ellis H. Clinical Anatomy, 10th edition. London:Blackwell Publishing; pp. 70-99.
2. Moore KL. The Developing Human: Clinically Oriented Embryology, 4th edition. Philadelphia, PA: WB Saunders; 1988. pp. 217-43.
3. Hyman NH, Le Leiko NS, Dolgin S. The curious umbilicus: a clue to the cause of abdominal pain. J Pediatr Gastroenterol Nutr. 1991;13:90-1.
4. Gosling JA, Harris PF, Humpherson JR, et al. Human Anatomy, 2nd edition. London: Gower Medical Publishing; 1990. pp. 41-63.
5. Suerbaum S, Michetti P. Helicobacter pylori infection. N Engl J Med 2002;347(15):1175-86.
6. Black S, Marrone GC. Anatomy and embryology of the small intestine. In: Zuidema GD, Nyhus LM (Eds). Surgery of the Alimentary Tract, 3rd edition. Philadelphia: WB Saunders; 1991. pp. 227-36.
7. Jones RS. The small intestine: physiology. In: Sabiston DC (Ed). Textbook of Surgery, 13th edition. Philadelphia, PA: WB Saunders; 1986. pp. 901-5.
8. Simmons RL, Steed DL. Basic Science Review for Surgeons. Philadelphia, PA: WB Saunders; 1992. pp. 234-41.
9. Mason GR, Kahrilas PJ, Otterson MF, et al. The digestive system. In: O'Leary JP (Ed). The Physiologic Basis of Surgery, 2nd edition. Baltimore, MD: Williams and Wilkins; 1996. pp. 406-40.
10. Choi H-K, Chu K-W, Law W-L. Therapeutic value of gastrograffin in adhesive small bowel obstruction after unsuccessful conservative treatment. Ann Surg. 2002;236(1):1-6.
11. Strobel D, Goertz RS, Bernatil T. Diagnostics in inflammatory bowel disease: ultrasound. World J Gastroenterol. 2011;17(27):3192-7.
12. Laing CJ, Tobias T, Rosenblum DI, et al. Acute gastrointesinal bleeding: emerging role of multidetector CT angiography and review of current imaging techniques. Radiographics. 2007;27(4):1055-70.
13. Amzallag-Bellenger E, Oudjit A, Ruiz A, et al. Effectiveness of MR enterography for the assessment of small-bowel disease beyond Crohn's disease. Radiographics. 2012;32(5):1423-44.
14. Cronin CG, Scott J, Kambadakone A, et al. Utility of positron emission tomography/ CT in the evaluation of small bowel pathology. Br J Radiol. 2012;85(1017):1211-21.
15. Lee NM, Eisen GM. 10 Years of capsule endoscopy: an update expert. Rev Gastroenterol Hepatol. 2010;4(4):503-12.
16. Chandler CF, Lane JS, Waxman KS. Seatbelt sign following blunt trauma is associated with increased incidence of abdominal injury. Am Surg. 1997;63:885-8.
17. Dischinger PC, Cushing BM, Kerns TJ. Injury patterns associated with direction of impact: drivers admitted to trauma centres. J Trauma. 1993;35:454-9.
18. Donohue JH, Federle MP, Griffiths BG, et al. Computed tomography in the diagnosis of blunt intestinal and mesenteric injuries. J Trauma. 1987;27:11-17.
19. Crohn BB, Ginzburg L, Oppenheimer GD. Regional ileitis: a pathologic and clinical entity. JAMA. 1932;99:1323-32.
20. Farmer RG, Hawk WA, Turnbull RB. Clinical pattern in Crohn's disease: a statistical study of 615 cases. Gastroenterology. 1975;68:627-35.
21. Satsangi J, Sutherland LR. Inflammatory Bowel Diseases. Amsterdam: Elsevier; 2003.
22. Sartor RB. Does mycobacterium avium subspecies paratuberculosis cause Crohn's disease? Gut. 2005;54:896-8.
23. Tibble J, Teahon K, Thjodleifsson B, et al. A simple method for assessing intestinal inflammation in Crohn's disease. Gut. 2000;47:506-13.
24. Hanauer SB, Feegan BG, Lichtenstein GR, et al. Maintenance infliximab for Crohn's disease: the ACCENT I randomised trial. Lancet. 2002;359:1541-9.
25. Sands BE, Anderson FH, Bernstein CN, et al. Infliximab maintenance therapy for fistulating Crohn's disease. N Engl J Med. 2004; 350:876-85.
26. Hanauer SB, Sandborn WJ, Rutgeerts P, et al. Human antitumour necrosis factor monoclonal antibody (adalimumab) in Crohn's disease: the CLASSIC-I trial. Gastroenterology. 2006;130(2);323-33.
27. Sandborn WJ, Hanauer SB, Rutgeerts P, et al. Adalimumab for maintenance treatment of Crohn's disease: results of the CLASSIC II Trial. Gut. 2007;56(9):1232-9.
28. Hawkey CJ. Stem cells as treatment in inflammatory bowel disease. Dig Dis. 2012;30(Suppl 3):134-9.
29. Ismael H, Horst M, Farooq M, et al. Adverse effects of preoperative steroid use on surgical outcomes. Am J Surg. 2011;201(3):305-8.
30. Fazio VW. Crohn's disease of the small bowel: operative tactics and techniques. Hepatogastroenterology. 1990;37(1):56-62.
31. Bemelman WA, Slors JF, Dunker MS, et al. Laparoscopic assisted vs. open ileocolic resection for Crohn's disease. A comparative study. Surg Endosc. 2000;14(8):721-5.
32. Lawes DA, Motson RW. Avoidance of laparotomy for recurrent disease is a long term benefit of laparoscopic resection for Crohn's disease. Br J Surg. 2006;93(5):607-8.
33. McLeod RS, Wolff BG, Ross S, et al. Recurrence of Crohn's disease after ileocolic resection is not affected by anastomotic type: results of a multicenter, randomized, controlled trial. Dis Colon Rectum. 2009;52(5):919-27.
34. Lal S, Teubner A, Shaffer JL. Review article: intestinal failure. Ailment Pharmacol Ther. 2006;24(1):19-31.
35. Rahbour G, Siddiqui MR, Ullah MR, et al. A meta-analysis of outcomes following use of somatostatin and its analogues for the management of enterocutaneous fistulas. Ann Surg. 2012;256(6):946-54.
36. Bleier JI, Hedrick T. Metabolic support of the enterocutaneous fistula patient. Clin Colon Rectal Surg. 2010;23(3): 142-8.
37. Randall ME, Ibbott GS. Intensity-modulated radiation therapy for gynaecologic cancers: pitfalls, hazards and cautions to be considered. Semin Radiat Oncol. 2006;16(3):138-43.

38. Denham JW, Wilcox C, Lamb DS, et al. Rectal and urinary dysfunction in the TROG 03.04 RADAR trial for locally advanced prostate cancer. Radiother Oncol. 2012;105(2): 184-92.
39. Webster GJ, Stafford J, Rodgers J, et al. Comparison of adaptive radiotherapy techniques for the treatment of bladder cancer. Br J Radiol. 2013;86(1021).
40. Peeters KC, Marijnen CA, Nagteggaal ID, et al. The TME trial after a median follow-up of 6 years: increased local control but no survival benefits in irradiated patients with respectable rectal carcinoma. Ann Surg. 2007;246(5);693-701.
41. Sebag-Montefiore D, Stephens R, Steele R, et al. Preoperative radiotherapy or selective postoperative chemoradiotherapy in patients with rectal cancer? (MRC CR07 Trial and NCIC-CTG C016): a multicentre, randomised trial. Lancet. 2009;373(9666):811-20.
42. Novak JM, Collins JT, Donowitz M, et al. Effects of radiation on the human gastrointestinal tract. J Clin Gastroenterol. 1979;1:9-21.
43. Galland RB, Spencer J. The natural history of clinically established radiation Enteritis. Lancet. 1985;i:1275-86.
44. Gorbach SL. Infectious diarrhea and bacterial food poisoning. In: Sieisenger MH, Fordtran JS (Eds). Gastrointestinal Disease, 5th edition. Philadelphia, PA: WB Saunders; 1993. pp. 1128-73.
45. Rewers, MJ. Epidemiology of celiac disease: what are the prevalence, incidence and progression of celiac disease? Gastroenterology. 2005;128(4suppl1): S47-51.
46. Kupper C. Dietary guidelines and implementation for celiac disease. Gastroenterology. 2005;128(4 Suppl 1): S121-7.
47. Ludvigsson JF, Leffler DA, Bai JC, et al. The Oslo definitions for celiac disease and related terms. Gut. 2013;62(1):43-52.
48. Evennett NJ, Petrov MS, Mittal A, et al. Systematic review and pooled estimates for the diagnostic accuracy of serological markers for intestinal ischaemia. World J Surg. 2009;33(7): 1374-83.
49. Sreenarasimhaiah J. Diagnosis and management of intestinal ischaemic disorders. BMJ. 2003;326(7403):1372-6.
50. Cunningham JD, Aleali R, Aleali M, et al. Malignant small bowel neoplasms: histopathologic determinants of recurrence and survival. Ann Surg. 1997;225(3):300-6.

70

Abdominal Wall Hernia

Andrew de Beaux, Bruce R Tulloh

Key Points

- Hernias of the abdominal wall are common and may exploit natural openings or surgical incisions in association with a defect in collagen metabolism.
- Mesh repair of a hernia is associated with a lower recurrence rate than non-mesh repairs, even in small hernias.
- The majority of inguinal hernias will become symptomatic with time, but asymptomatic hernias can be safely managed by a watch and wait strategy.
- All femoral hernias should be repaired because of their high risk of incarceration/strangulation.
- The incidence of incisional hernia can be reduced by careful surgical closure of the abdominal wall fascia with a small-stitch, small-bite technique.
- In open incisional hernia repair, the sublay technique is recommended, with the onlay approach suggested as an alternative, but the inlay repair is condemned except in exceptional circumstances.
- Laparoscopic ventral and incisional hernia repair reduces the wound morbidity of the open approach. However, the role of defect closure, mesh fixation technique, and size of mesh overlap required as the hernia defect increases in size remain controversial.

GENERAL CONSIDERATIONS

Definitions

A hernia is defined as an abnormal protrusion of the contents of a cavity through a weakness in its wall, taking with it all the linings of the cavity, although these may be markedly attenuated. Hernias can be described as reducible, incarcerated, or strangulated. A reducible hernia is one in which the contents of the hernial sac can be manually returned to the abdomen, while, conversely, the contents of an irreducible or incarcerated hernia cannot be so returned. A strangulated hernia occurs when the vascular supply to the contents contained within the hernia is compromised, resulting in ischemic and gangrenous tissue. The clinical presentation and treatment of a strangulated hernia are considered in Chapter 75, "Intestinal Obstruction". This chapter addresses hernias of the abdominal wall in adults. For a consideration of the different types of hernia in children, *see* Chapter 124, "Abdominal Wall Deformities".

Etiology of Hernias

Multiple factors contribute to the development of hernias. In essence, hernias can be considered design faults, either anatomical or through inherited collagen disorders, although these two etiological factors probably work together in most patients. Anatomical design faults can be considered at any site where internal structures exit through an opening in the wall of the cavity that exist for blood vessels, bowel, spermatic cord, or esophagus, for example. Since not every individual develops a groin hernia, other factors must be important. The fascia and surrounding tissues that cover muscle and hold its bundles together are complex, living structures. Fascia and tendon are made up of type I and type III collagen: type I, imparts the strength to the fascia or tendon, and type III provides elastic recoil following stretch when the tissues have been loaded. The type I to III collagen ratio varies between individuals, with an average value of 5, but is constant in all the fascia of a particular individual. The current concept is that most hernias are a disease of collagen metabolism, in particular the type I to III collagen ratio.[1] The lower this ratio, the more likely the individual is to develop a hernia, and indeed, a recurrence of a hernia following repair.

Prosthetic Mesh

Mesh repair is considered the best technique for most hernias. Meshes are either synthetic (manmade) or biological (preparations from animal or human tissue). Most

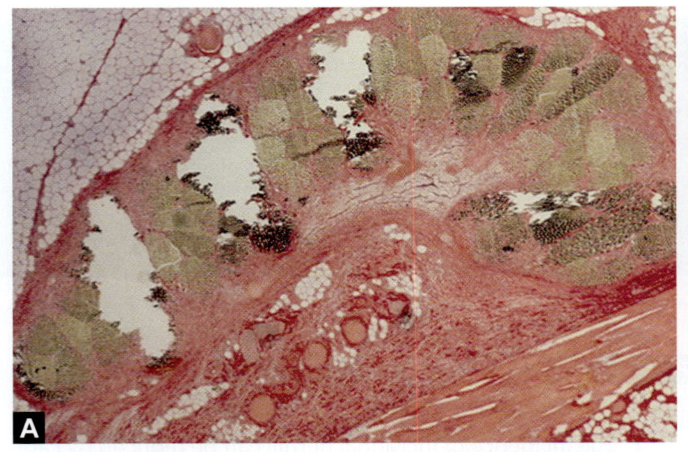

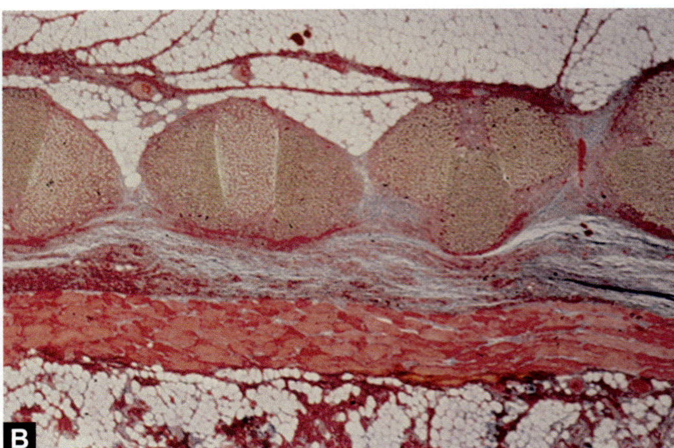

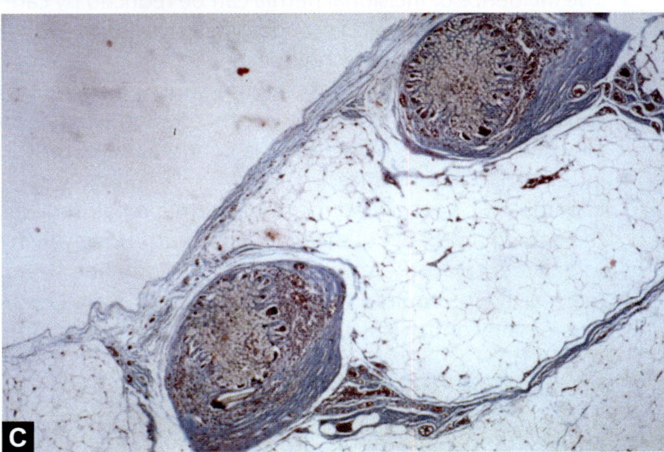

Figs. 70.1A to C: (A) Micrograph of a macropore mesh of <0.5 mm pore size showing scar plate formation and contraction/distortion of the mesh. (B) Micrograph of a macropore mesh of 0.8 mm pore size showing minimal scar bridging and no distortion of the mesh. (C) Micrograph of a macropore mesh of 3 mm pore size showing scar net formation and no contraction/distortion of the mesh.
Source: Micrographs courtesy of Covidien, UK.

synthetic meshes are woven from either polypropylene or polyester fibers. Biological meshes are typically animal collagen, either from skin, bowel, or pericardium. Biological meshes tend to be much more expensive and are thus reserved for specialist use.

The current trend in developed countries is to use mesh that is lightweight (polypropylene <50 g/m^2) with large pores or spaces between the mesh fibers. A pore size of at least 1 mm in diameter is thought to be important to minimize bridging of the scar tissue around each fiber and thus mesh contraction as the scar plate matures[2] (Figs. 70.1A to C). In developing countries, the cost of commercial hernia mesh can be prohibitive. There is current interest in the use of "industrial" mesh such as mosquito netting as a cheap but effective alternative.

Traditional meshes placed within the abdominal cavity have a high rate of adhesion to omentum and bowel. This process can result in bowel fistulation or make subsequent laparotomy more difficult, with increased risk of bowel perforation, and thus the need for bowel resection during the process of re-entering the abdominal cavity.[3] A number of tissue-separating meshes are available in which the intra-abdominal side of the mesh is coated with a product to minimize adhesion formation. Although such coatings do reduce adhesion formation, they do not prevent it. The main points of adhesion appear to be the edge of the mesh and the points of fixation, whether sutures, tacks, or staples.

The other important considerations are (1) the use of mesh "augmentation" of a repair, where mesh reinforces the re-approximated fascia and (2) mesh "bridging," when the fascial layers cannot be approximated and the mesh is used to bridge the gap in the fascia. In general, bridging is associated with a higher hernia recurrence rate, especially when biological mesh is used.

INGUINAL HERNIA

Anatomy

The inguinal canal is approximately 4 cm in length, located just above the inguinal ligament between the internal and external rings. It allows passage of the spermatic cord into the scrotum along with the testicular and cremasteric vessels and the ductus deferens. The superficial ring is a triangular opening in the aponeurosis of the external

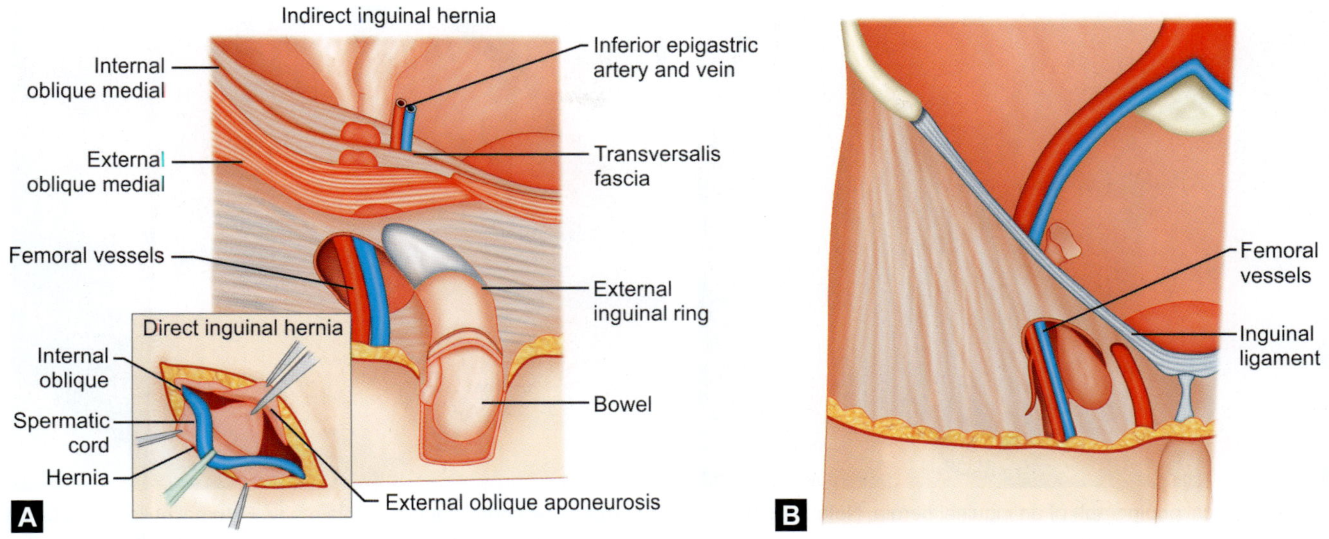

Figs. 70.2A and B: Anatomy of inguinal and femoral hernias.

oblique, lying about 1 cm above the pubic tubercle. The deep ring is a U-shaped condensation of the transversalis fascia and it lies about 1 cm above the inguinal ligament, midway between the pubic tubercle, and the anterior superior iliac spine. The transversalis fascia is the fascial envelope of the abdomen, and the competency of the deep inguinal ring depends on the integrity of this fascia. The anterior boundary of the inguinal canal comprises mainly the external oblique aponeurosis, with the conjoined muscle laterally. The posterior boundary is formed by the fascia transversalis and the conjoint tendon medially (internal oblique and transversus abdominis). The inferior epigastric vessels lie posteriorly and medially to the deep inguinal ring. The superior boundary is formed by the conjoined muscles (internal oblique and transversus) and the inferior boundary by the inguinal ligament.

An indirect hernia travels down the canal on the outer (lateral and anterior) side of the spermatic cord (Figs. 70.2A and B). A direct inguinal hernia comes out directly forward through the posterior wall of the inguinal canal. While the neck of an indirect hernia is lateral to the epigastric vessels, the direct hernia emerges medial to these vessels, except in the saddlebag or pantaloon type, which has both a lateral and a medial component.

Etiology

The pathogenesis of groin hernias is multifactorial. It was initially believed that persistence of a patent processus vaginalis into adult life was the predisposing factor for inguinal hernia formation. However, postmortem studies have shown that 15–30% of adult males without a clinically apparent inguinal hernia have a patent processus vaginalis.[4] Similarly, review of the contralateral side in infantile inguinal hernias reveals a patent processus vaginalis in 60% of neonates and a contralateral hernia in only 10–20%.[5] During 20 years of follow-up after infantile hernia repair, only 22% of men will develop a contralateral hernia. So the problem of indirect inguinal hernia is not simply one of a congenital defect. The high frequency of indirect inguinal hernia in middle-aged and older people suggests that a pathological change in connective tissue of the abdominal wall may be a contributory factor,[1] as discussed earlier.

Diagnosis

The history of a swelling in the groin that goes away on lying down is typical of an inguinal hernia. Asymmetry of the groin on inspection is usually obvious (Fig 70.3). Sometimes, the diagnosis of a hernia or the precise nature of a swelling in the groin or scrotum is unclear on clinical grounds, and ultrasound scanning, or CT/MRI may be useful. Herniography (injection of contract material into the abdominal cavity) may be helpful if the above investigations are not available.

Management

In developed countries, the open Lichtenstein mesh repair is the current gold standard against which other techniques are compared.[6,7] However, there is still a role for the suture or darn techniques, in which tension in the repair is avoided or minimized.[8] Laparoscopic repair is becoming the standard technique in many centers.

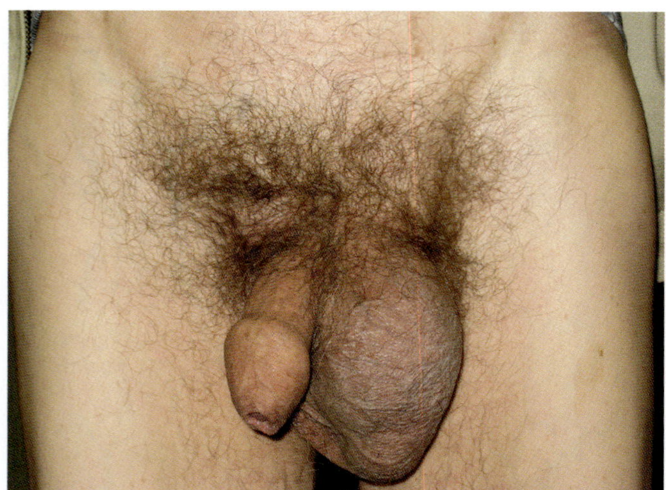

Fig. 70.3: Clinical photograph of an inguinal hernia. Note the swelling of the right groin of an associated right inguinal hernia—a common finding consistent with a generalized collagen disorder.

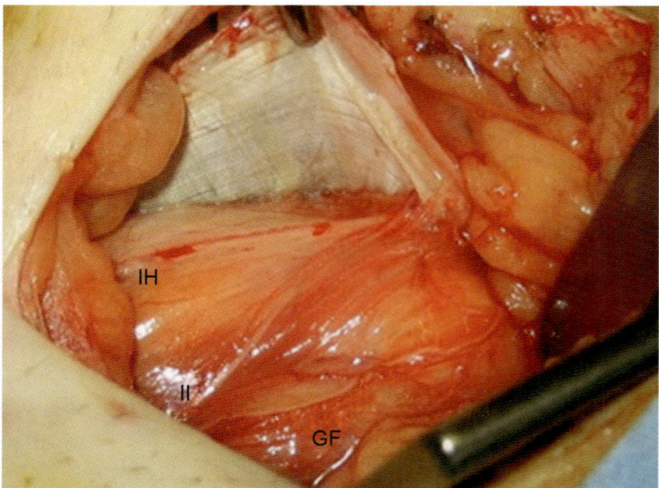

Fig. 70.4: Open right inguinal hernia repair. External oblique has been opened. Medial is to the right of the picture. Note the iliohypogastric (IH), ilioinguinal (II) that splits into two branches, and the small genitor-femoral nerve lying inferiorly.
Source: Clinical photograph courtesy of Mr Martin Kurzer, London, UK.

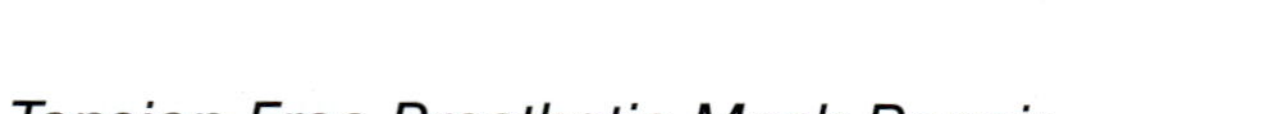

Tension-Free Prosthetic Mesh Repair

This procedure can usually be performed under local anesthesia through a groin skin-crease incision. Care should be taken to avoid damage to the nerves, in particular the iliohypogastric, ilioinguinal, and genitofemoral nerve (Fig. 70.4). There remains debate as to whether these nerves should be identified in every case and/or divided in every case, and what to do when attempting nerve preservation if a nerve is divided. However, current opinion is in favor of nerve preservation where possible. Indirect hernial sacs lie anterolaterally to the cord structures, and dissection should be done with care. The sac may be simply inverted into the abdominal cavity or suture-ligated at the level of the deep ring and redundant peritoneum excised. To prevent postoperative hydrocele formation, complete scrotal sacs are transected at the midpoint of the canal, with the distal section left in place and open. This technique minimizes damage to the testicular vessels. In the event of a large direct hernia, the sac (transversalis fascia) is invaginated with a plicating suture to achieve a flat surface over which to lay the mesh. Typical mesh size is 11 cm × 6 cm, but this will vary depending on the size of the patient and the size of the hernial defect. The mesh is fish-tailed and placed snug laterally around the cord structures (Fig 70.5). The mesh can be secured by absorbable sutures or glue, but a watch should be kept for the nerves and there is no need to insert sutures into the pubic tubercle. Unrestricted activity is encouraged, and patients are expected to return to their normal activity 2–7 days after operation.

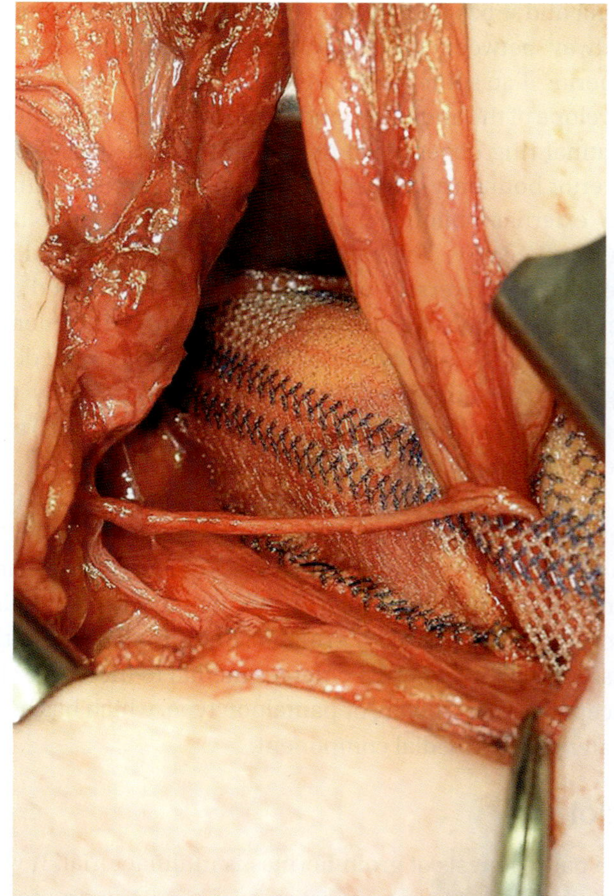

Fig. 70.5: Left inguinal hernia repair. Mesh in place, fish-tailed laterally to create a new deep ring. Cord structures and ilioinguinal nerve intact. Mesh lying flat and "tension" free.

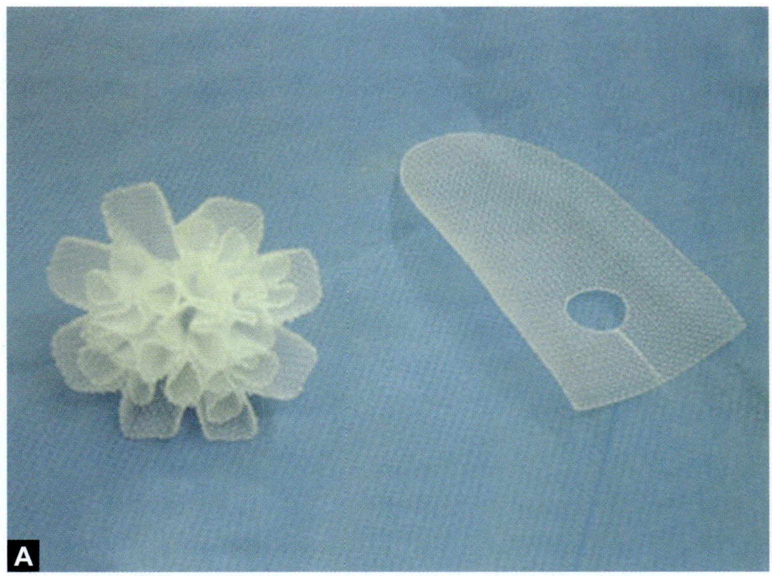

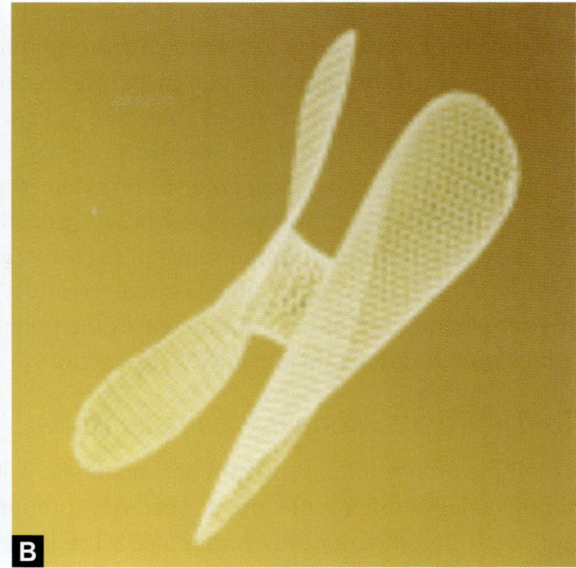

Figs. 70.6A and B: (A) Typical plug prosthesis. (B) Prolene hernia system.

In the past few years, there has been an explosion in different mesh types for the open repair of inguinal hernias. The plug and patch utilizes a cone-shaped mass of mesh that can be inserted, tip side inward, into either the deep or superficial rings, depending on the type of hernia (Fig 70.6A). A flat mesh is then placed over the plug akin to the Lichtenstein technique. The Prolene hernia system comprises two flat meshes secured together by a small cylinder of mesh (Fig. 70.6B). The aim is to insert one mesh into the preperitoneal space while the other is secured as for the Lichtenstein technique. There is also the open preperitoneal approach with the Kugel patch.

Laparoscopic Repair

The alternative to an open operation is a laparoscopic approach. Although a variety of laparoscopic repairs have been described, they can be categorized in general according to the approach used to expose the defect. Three exposures are used: the intraperitoneal approach; the transabdominal preperitoneal prosthetic (TAPP) repair; and the totally extraperitoneal prosthetic (TEP) repair.

Intraperitoneal Repair

In the intraperitoneal repair with an onlay graft, the prosthesis is placed within the peritoneal cavity. Compared to the TAPP and TEP approaches, it has the advantages of being less time-consuming to perform and requiring less dissection of the preperitoneal space. It has the disadvantages of leaving the prosthetic material exposed within the peritoneal cavity and having a higher recurrence rate. It is the authors' view that this operation is very much a procedure of last resort, when other open or laparoscopic techniques have failed. It is possible that when better nonstick meshes become available, combined with glue fixation, this technique may gain in popularity.

Transabdominal Preperitoneal Prosthetic Repair

Transabdominal preperitoneal prosthetic repair is one of the most popular approaches used for laparoscopic herniorrhaphy, particularly in Europe. The abdomen is insufflated with carbon dioxide, and the laparoscope is introduced through an umbilical incision. Two accessory trocars, placed well above and slightly medial to the anterior superior iliac spines, are used to provide access for the dissecting instruments and the stapler. An incision is then made in the pelvic peritoneum several centimeters above the hernia defect, typically in line with the level of the anterior iliac spine, and the peritoneum is peeled away to expose the hernial defect. The peritoneum is dissected bluntly away from the abdominal wall, allowing the hernial sac to be inverted and dissected free of adherent tissue. The dissection is carried just across the midline, well laterally and inferiorly, to allow mesh of approximately 10 cm × 15 cm is be inserted so that it covers the entire myopectineal orifice. Some surgeons fix the mesh in place with staples, sutures or glue although there is little evidence to support such practices. The peritoneum is closed over the mesh with staples or sutures. This approach has the advantage of permitting inspection of the abdomen in general, and of the opposite side in particular, enabling bilateral repairs to be performed if necessary. In addition, exposure is usually excellent. The disadvantage is that a wider dissection is required to accommodate the mesh than is used in the intraperitoneal onlay procedure. In addition, the intra-abdominal incision presents the possibility of injury to intraperitoneal structures, and a second peritoneal incision in the groin increases the potential for adhesion formation and late bowel obstruction.

Totally Extraperitoneal Prosthetic Repair

Totally extraperitoneal prosthetic repair is a laparoscopic adaptation of the open posterior preperitoneal approach first described by Annandale.[9] The laparoscope is introduced into the preperitoneal space through an infraumbilical incision. Direct hernial sacs usually reduce with ease, but an indirect hernial sac may need more work. The key landmark here is the vas (ductus deferens). The indirect hernial sac lies above and lateral to the vas, taking the dissection away from the iliac vessels and thus preventing their inadvertent injury. A mesh of minimum size 10 cm × 15 cm is used to cover all the inguinal and femoral hernia orifices, ensuring good cover laterally and superomedially. As with TAPP repairs, there is now good evidence that suturing, tacking or stapling of mesh does not reduce the risk of hernia recurrence but is a cause of postoperative chronic pain.[10] The authors do occasionally tack the mesh, mainly in a patient with a very large direct hernial defect. Tacks are only placed medial to the inferior epigastric vessels and superior to the pubic bone. More recently, the authors have attempted laparoscopic closure of large direct inguinal hernias with a nonabsorbable suture rather than using tacks. The TEP approach avoids the risks of entering the peritoneal cavity and subsequent intraperitoneal adhesion formation.

There is little evidence to support TEP as opposed to TAPP, and the technique used is largely down to the individual surgeon. The authors' preference is the TEP approach, with the TAPP approach reserved for recurrence after a previous TEP or open preperitoneal operation.

Complications

Complications of herniorrhaphy include recurrence, urinary retention, ischemic orchitis and testicular atrophy, wound infection, and nerve injuries (neuromas of the ilioinguinal or genitofemoral nerves). A wide variation in recurrence rates is reported in the literature, depending on both the surgical technique employed and the method and length of follow-up (questionnaire, physical examination, etc.). In general, papers comparing mesh to suture repair note lower recurrence rates in the mesh group, but this is not always the case. There has been a suggestion that mesh repairs in the groin can affect fertility in males.[11] This is a very controversial area, as the occurrence of a hernia per se in the young is associated with reduced fertility. There is no convincing evidence to support the view that a mesh repair affects fertility except when there is obviously direct trauma to the vas or vessels to the testicle.

The complication that is becoming the benchmark for comparing hernia repairs is the incidence of chronic pain, rather than recurrence rate. Risk factors for chronic pain include nerve damage, preoperative pain in the hernia, young age, pain at other sites of the body, postoperative complications, and psychosocial features.[12] Pain response to a standardized heat stimulus appears to be a useful tool in assessing the risk of postoperative chronic pain.[13]

Suture, Mesh, or Laparoscopic Repair?

The operation performed is the end result of a discussion between the patient and the surgeon, and the surgical options available will depend on local circumstances. Nevertheless, the 2004 report of NICE (the UK National Institute for Clinical Excellence) commented on 37 randomized controlled trials that compared laparoscopic with open mesh repair of inguinal hernias in a total of 5,560 participants.[14] In summary, the results showed that laparoscopic repair as compared to open repair was associated with less acute pain and thus a quicker return to daily activities and work, fewer wound complications such as hematoma, seroma, and infection, and a lower risk of chronic pain. There was a similar recurrence rate and a similar risk of major vessel, bowel, or bladder injury. However, the laparoscopic repair took longer to perform and was a more expensive option. The financial cost of laparoscopic operation has to be set against the price of open operation for the patient and society, namely more acute and chronic pain, more time off work, and more wound complications. In addition, many centers now report that laparoscopic repairs, whether unilateral or bilateral, can be performed more quickly than open repairs.[15]

The Asymptomatic Hernia

Traditional teaching was that once an inguinal hernia was detected, it merited repair to prevent hernia-related complications unless the patient was not fit for operation. However, increasing awareness of complications following hernia repair, particularly chronic pain, has questioned this approach. Two randomized trials have reported similar results.[16] In essence, chronic pain on follow-up is similar between the operation groups and the "watchful waiting" group. Both studies noted that by 7 years, most in the watchful waiting group cross over to the operation arm because of increasing symptoms as follow-up continues. However, the risk of incarceration or strangulation is much lower than previously thought. Thus, following informed consent, either operation or watchful waiting may be appropriate for an asymptomatic hernia. The younger the patient or the less fit the patient on presentation, then perhaps the earlier operation should be offered, with suitable informed consent of the risks, benefits, and alternatives.

FEMORAL HERNIA

Femoral hernia represents the third commonest type of primary hernia. It accounts for approximately 20% of hernias in women and 5% in men, strangulation being the initial presentation in 40% of cases.

Anatomy

The femoral canal occupies the most medial compartment of the femoral sheath, extending from the femoral ring above to the saphenous opening below. It contains fat, lymphatic vessels, and the lymph node of Cloquet. It is closed above by the septum crurale, a condensation of extraperitoneal tissue pierced by lymphatic vessels, and below by the cribriform fascia. The femoral ring is bounded anteriorly by the inguinal ligament and posteriorly by the iliopectineal (Cooper) ligament, the pubic bone and the fascia over the pectineus muscle. Medially, the boundary is the edge of the lacunar ligament, while laterally it is separated from the femoral vein by a thin septum (*see* Fig. 70.1).

Diagnosis

The presentation of a femoral hernia is similar to that of an inguinal hernia. On examination, the femoral hernia sac typically lies lateral and below the pubic tubercle, as opposed to that of an inguinal hernia, which is superior and medial to the tubercle). A femoral hernia often presents as an emergency, with a painful red, firm swelling in the groin. Infected lymph nodes in the groin can present in a similar manner and it is important to differentiate from these two diagnoses as the latter rarely requires an operation (Fig. 70.7).

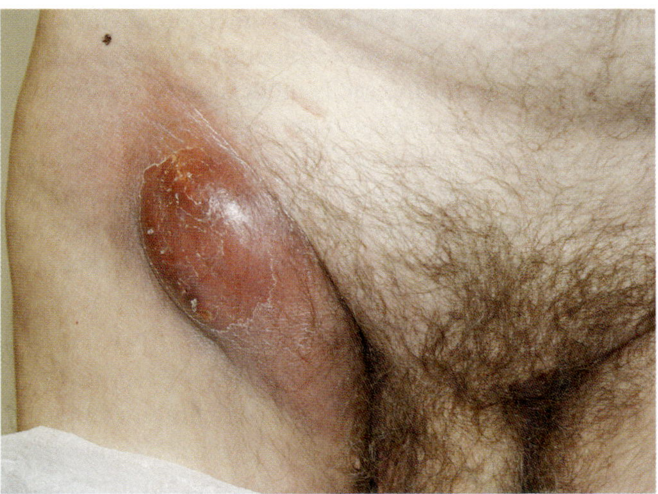

Fig. 70.7: Clinical image of infected inguinal lymphadenopathy—not to be confused with a strangulated groin hernia.

Management

The treatment of femoral hernia is surgical repair due to the invariable presence of incarceration and the high associated risk of strangulation. Several open operative approaches have been described as well as the laparoscopic approach.

The Low Approach (Lockwood)

The low approach is based on a groin-crease incision and dissection of the femoral hernia sac below the inguinal ligament. The anatomical layers covering the sac are peeled away, and the sac is opened to inspect its contents. Once empty, the neck of the sac is pulled down and ligated as high as possible and redundant sac is excised. The neck then retracts through the femoral canal, and the canal is closed with a plug or cylinder of polypropylene mesh, anchored to the inguinal ligament and iliopectineal ligament with nonabsorbable sutures. Suturing of the iliopectineal ligament to the inguinal ligament may result in tension due to the rigidity of these structures and may predispose to recurrence. Moreover, the low approach is unsuitable for a strangulated femoral hernia because of the difficulty in safely reducing a knuckle of small bowel through the tight femoral ring.

Transinguinal Approach (Lotheissen)

Techniques of femoral repair that open the posterior inguinal wall for exposure and repair should rarely be used. This technique usually involves ligation and division of the inferior epigastric vessels at the medial border of the internal inguinal ring followed by incision of the transversalis fascia to expose the extraperitoneal space and the femoral hernia sac. The sac is reduced, and the defect is closed by either suture (as in the original description) or, increasingly, mesh. However, the need to incise the natural fascial barrier in Hesselbach's triangle for exposure results in this technique being inferior to either the low or high approach, both of which leave the inguinal floor intact.

High Approach (McEvedy)

The high approach was classically based on a vertical incision made over the femoral canal and continued upward above the inguinal ligament. This approach has now been replaced by a transverse incision. The anterior rectus sheath is divided, the rectus muscle is retracted medially and the preperitoneal space is entered. The femoral hernia sac is identified medial to the iliac vessels and is reduced by traction. If the hernia is incarcerated, the sac may be released by incising the insertion of the iliopubic tract into Cooper's ligament at the medial margin of the femoral ring. The sac is then opened, the contents are dealt with appropriately and the sac is ligated at its neck. The hernioplasty may then be completed by either suturing the iliopubic tract to the posterior margin of Cooper's ligament or by insertion of a prosthetic mesh, either as a sheet covering the whole of the myopectineal opening or as a mesh plug. The high approach is particularly useful in the presence of strangulated femoral hernias, as it is easy to convert to a laparotomy for bowel resection.

Laparoscopic Approach

The laparoscopic approach is the same as for inguinal hernias and may employ the TAPP or TEP technique. The femoral ring is easily seen during either of these approaches and, indeed, visualization of the whole of the myopectineal opening is frequently quoted as one of the advantages of laparoscopic herniorrhaphy. The use of the laparoscopic approach is more technically challenging in emergency cases, especially if strangulation is present, but is a good approach in expert hands.

VENTRAL HERNIAS

After groin hernias the next most common group comprises ventral hernias. The European Hernia Society classification[17] divides these into primary ventral hernias and incisional hernias, which are anatomically ventral but which arise secondary to a previous operation. The most common primary ventral hernias are, in descending order of frequency, umbilical, epigastric, paraumbilical, and Spigelian.[2] Parastomal hernias are classified separately, even though they can be considered as a variety of incisional hernia. By convention, the ventral hernia group also includes lumbar hernias (which protrude dorsolaterally) but does not include obturator hernias into the thigh), sciatic and gluteal hernias (protruding into the buttock), or rectus divarication, which is not a hernia at all. Nevertheless, these will also be discussed briefly in this section.

Some ventral hernias are traumatic in origin, reflecting either an injury-related defect in the musculofascial layers (a rupture in the truest sense) or a bulge secondary to traumatic abdominal wall denervation.

ADULT UMBILICAL AND PARAUMBILICAL HERNIAS

Definitions

From a clinical point of view these two conditions are virtually identical, although an important anatomical detail defines them: true umbilical hernias protrude through the dilated umbilical ring, while paraumbilical hernias arise through a defect in the linea alba adjacent to, but separate from, the true umbilicus. Paraumbilical hernias generally have an elliptical defect because they begin as a transverse split in the decussating fibers of the linea alba, while true umbilical hernia defects remain circular in shape. The typical paraumbilical hernia appears as an eccentric swelling in the umbilicus with a crescentic skin depression, while true umbilical hernias protrude centrally and retain their round shape (Figs. 70.8A and B). True adult umbilical hernias are commonly seen during pregnancy, after which they often resolve completely, and also in patients with cirrhosis and ascites who have both weak collagen and raised intra-abdominal pressure as etiological factors. In these cases, the hernia represents a reopening of the true umbilical ring.

Clinical Presentation

Adult umbilical and paraumbilical hernias are frequently symptomatic, producing intermittent abdominal pain and tenderness. The pain may be caused by pinching of extraperitoneal fat, traction on the falciform ligament or colic from intermittent intestinal obstruction. These hernias tend to enlarge over time and may progress to intertrigo and skin ulceration when very large. Because of the unyielding fibrous margins of the defect, both types of hernia are prone to acute incarceration, obstruction, and/or strangulation.

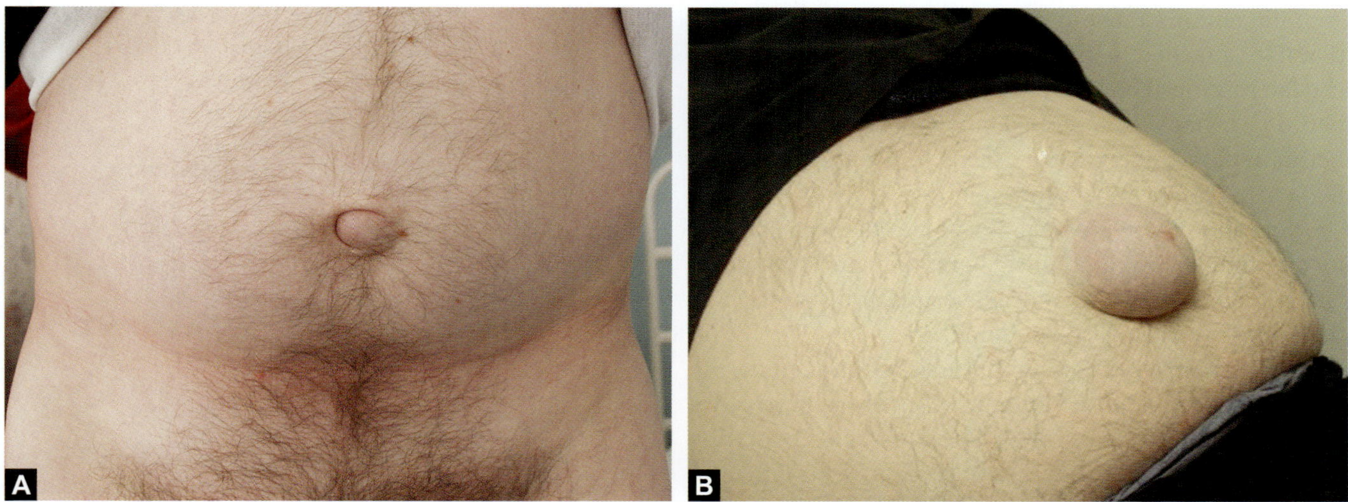

Figs. 70.8A and B: Clinical images of (A) paraumbilical hernia showing the crescentic umbilical slit and (B) umbilical hernia noting the thin overlying skin.

Management

There are many options. With the increasing popularity of laparoscopic surgery and the introduction in recent years of new mesh devices specifically for umbilical/paraumbilical hernia repair, a surgeon may be overwhelmed by choice. The best approach for any individual umbilical/paraumbilical hernia depends on the hernia size and contents, the patient's body habitus and general fitness as well as their wishes, and the surgeon's training and experience.

Nonoperative

Although the only effective treatment is operative repair, not all patients require an operation. Small asymptomatic hernias can be managed expectantly as long as the patient is counseled about the small risk of incarceration/strangulation.

Open Repair with Sutures

A case can be made for using mesh for all umbilical/paraumbilical hernia repairs because of evidence that it is associated with a lower recurrence rate than using sutures alone.[18] However, a balance must be struck between the risks and benefits of each approach. A suture repair is a reasonable option, and widely practiced, for hernias with small defects—certainly <2 cm in maximum size, and the smaller the better. Suturing options include direct edge-to-edge fascial closure, overlapping closure (as in the classic Mayo repair) and a suture-darn. For each of these procedures, the initial exposure is the same: a curved periumbilical incision is made for optimum cosmesis, then deepened to define the neck of the sac and the margins of the defect. It is useful to divide through the neck some distance above the linea alba in order to leave a small cuff that is easy to close. While not necessary in terms of repair strength, closing the emerging sac does help to separate the repair from the intraperitoneal contents. This maneuver is certainly important if mesh is to be used, and probably important for a suture darn.

Open Repair with Mesh

Mesh repair should be planned for all hernias with defects larger than about 2 cm in diameter, but also if there is appreciable divarication of the rectus muscles. Divarication indicates a thin and attenuated linea alba, which will not hold sutures under tension and thus requires mesh for reinforcement.

For large hernias, an ellipse of skin may need to be removed and this may be oriented either transversely or vertically. Orientating it along the midline provides excellent access if multiple defects are present or if an extensive laparotomy is anticipated. The umbilicus itself may need to be sacrificed, and preoperative planning will allow skin flaps to be preserved for subsequent umbilical reconstruction. Once the incision has been made, it is deepened to isolate the sac and define the margins of the defect.

Small sacs may be reduced intact; others can be opened and the contents reduced. If the defect is of such size that primary facial closure is anticipated to be impossible and mesh is likely to be left exposed centrally across a fascial gap, the authors recommend preserving as much sac as possible (attached to the fascial margins of the defect) for use later as mesh coverage. The technique utilizing these peritoneal "flaps" is described in the section on incisional hernia repair. If there are no plans to use the peritoneal flaps as part of the repair, they may be excised.

Nowadays there are several varieties of mesh suitable for an umbilical/paraumbilical hernia repair: flat meshes, "plug-&-patch" devices and bilayer mesh disks. Each of these mesh repairs will be outlined:

1. *Flat mesh repairs*: Simple flat meshes strengthen the repair by providing a framework for collagen ingrowth. Thus an expansive mesh-tissue interface, created by providing a generous mesh overlap all around the defect, is important. They work best as reinforcement after primary fascial closure, rather than bridging a fascial gap. These meshes generate dense adhesions if exposed to the abdominal contents, so the peritoneum at the very least must be closed. Ideally fascial closure should be achieved over the mesh as well to exclude it from the subcutaneous space:
   a. Flat meshes may be placed in one of several planes. The extraperitoneal plane is quite easy to develop with predominantly blunt dissection just deep to the rectus sheaths, but only for several centimeters around the umbilicus. Thus, an extraperitoneal flat mesh repair is limited to small-to-moderate-sized hernias in which a few centimeters of overlap are all that are required, and the fascial defect is still small enough to close primarily over the mesh. For larger defects, the retromuscular space is preferred, for two reasons: first, because larger meshes can be used and second because the linea alba can be incised longitudinally in both directions, thus converting the original round umbilical defect into an ellipse and facilitating fascial closure. The retromuscular mesh repair is described in detail in the section on incisional hernia.
   b. The third plane in which flat mesh can be used is the subcutaneous plane. In these repairs, the fascial defect is closed and a flat mesh is laid over this onto the anterior surface of the rectus sheaths and linea alba. This "onlay" repair is relatively quick and easy compared to the extraperitoneal and retromuscular repairs, and for these reasons it is widely practiced. However, the mesh is at risk of exposure and contamination in the event of overlying wound infection or breakdown.

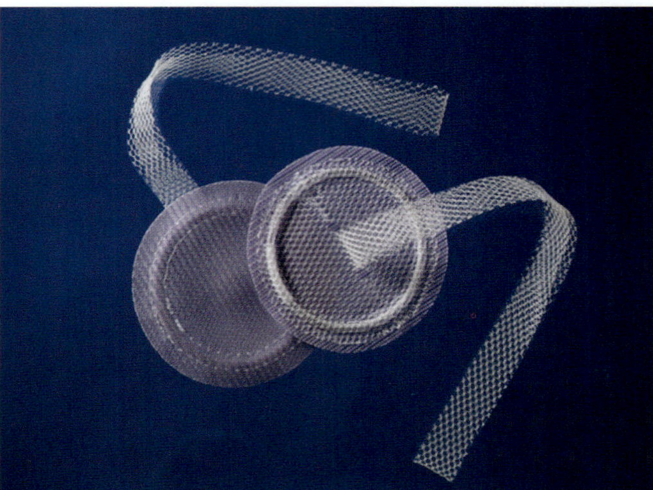

Fig. 70.9: Bilayer mesh for the repair of small ventral hernias and port sites.

2. *"Plug-&-Patch" devices*: These are three-dimensional prostheses comprising two mesh discs separated by a short cylindrical connecter (*see* Fig. 70.4B). The mesh prosthesis is positioned through the defect so that one mesh flange lies deep and one superficial to the fascia. The mesh is not suitable for intraperitoneal use, so the deep flange must lie in the extraperitoneal or retromuscular plane. Results are satisfactory.[19]
3. *Bilayer mesh disks*: These are designed for intraperitoneal placement. The mesh disk is pushed into the abdominal cavity then pulled back by the attached tab(s) with the hope that it will resume its broad flat shape, neatly abutting the undersurface of the abdominal wall (Fig. 70.9). Here, the bilayer is important, as the surface facing the intra-abdominal contents must resist adhesions, while the surface pulled against the abdominal wall should promote tissue ingrowth and mesh incorporation. This is a relatively quick and easy repair, but adhesive bowel obstructions, mesh infection, and recurrences from imperfect deployment have been reported.[20]

Laparoscopic Repair

The technique is straightforward in principle, and indeed laparoscopic umbilical hernia repair is commonly regarded as a good training operation. The principles of a laparoscopic ventral hernia repair are outlined in Box 70.1, and the current controversies with this approach are discussed below.

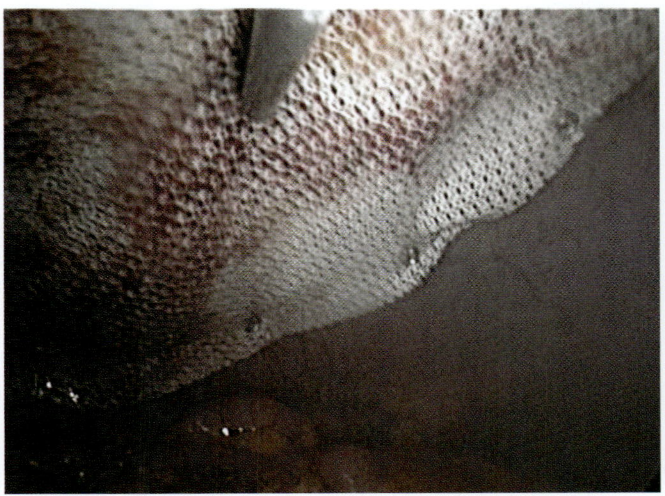

Fig. 70.10: Laparoscopic view of mesh secured to the anterior abdominal wall using the double crown technique.

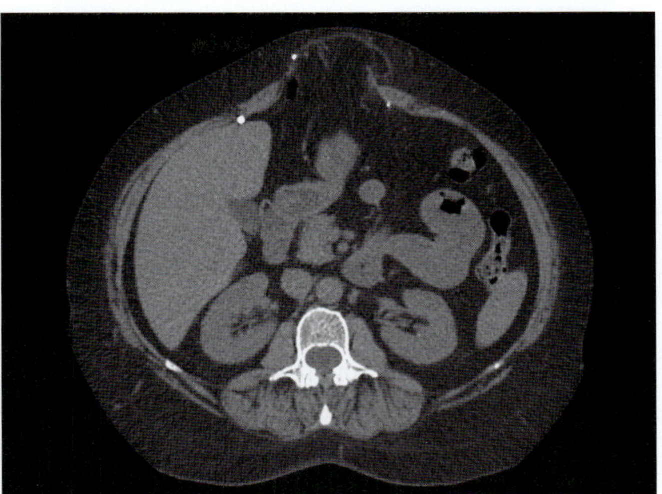

Fig. 70.11: CT scan demonstrating mesh migration into the old hernia sac. Note the sac that has been pulled out and dragged into the old sac by the mesh slippage.

Box 70.1 Essential steps of a laparoscopic ventral hernia repair.

The camera port is placed well laterally in the abdomen to keep clear of the zone of repair. Smaller working ports are placed above and below the camera port, aiming for a 60°–90° working angle between them (*see* Fig. 70.5). Hernial contents are reduced using a combination of internal traction and external pressure as required, and the defect may be enlarged by incising the linea alba to facilitate this. Often the falciform ligament and median umbilical fold need to be taken down to provide the smooth, firm fascial base for optimal mesh fixation. The defect(s) can be closed with sutures prior to mesh placement as long as no undue tension is introduced. Special mesh designed specifically for intraperitoneal use is then introduced through a port and drawn up onto the peritoneal surface of the abdominal wall with pretied sutures passed to the outside. Positioning of the mesh with adequate overlap of the defect(s) in all directions is crucial to achieving a successful repair. The mesh is then fixed to the abdominal wall by staples, spiral tacks, or transfascial sutures around the edges of the mesh, close enough together to prevent bowel herniation between the mesh and the abdominal wall (Fig. 70.10). It is useful to place fixation centrally, such as around the margins of the defect or into the rectus sheaths either side of the midline, in addition to around the periphery of the mesh to help the mesh conform to the three-dimensional curvature of the abdominal wall.

Current Controversies with Laparoscopic Ventral Hernia Repair

1. *Case selection*: It is difficult to justify the complexity and expense of a laparoscopic repair for small hernias that might do just as well with an open approach via a small incision, especially if this is achievable under local anesthesia. However, the presence of multiple defects, for which a single large piece of mesh would suffice, and obese patients, in whom one would prefer to avoid a sizeable skin incision, tip the balance in favor of a laparoscopic approach. Defects larger than about 8 cm in diameter are better done open because it is difficult to prevent the unsupported mesh from slowly migrating into the defect (Fig. 70.11). Open repair is also preferred if there is plenty of redundant skin to be excised anyway to achieve a neat result.
2. *Closing the defect*: The early descriptions of laparoscopic ventral and incisional hernia repair were of a tension-free patch that simply bridged the defect and relied on mesh fixation and peripheral tissue ingrowth for strength. Bridging repairs are prone to mesh migration and postoperative bulging.[21] Suturing the defect and then adding mesh as reinforcement would overcome this problem and are strongly advocated by some,[22] but doing so necessarily introduces tension. Current expert opinion is that this technique should only be employed when approximation is possible without undue tension, that is, defects up to about 3 cm in diameter or elliptical defects (e.g. in the midline).
3. *Choice of mesh*: Numerous products are available, and surgeons have their own preferences related to mesh science, handling, and cost. The chosen mesh should have a low propensity for forming adhesions within the peritoneal cavity, and it is helpful if the mesh is transparent (so its positioning over the defect can be readily monitored), thin and flexible (so it can easily be put down a laparoscopic port) and robust (so that it is not easily damaged during deployment). Finally, its cost should be a consideration.

4. *Mesh fixation*: Early experience was of using transfascial sutures to fix the mesh to the abdominal wall, but it has been found that these do not prevent mesh migration and are associated with abdominal wall pain, presumably due to somatic nerve entrapment.[23] The advent of laparoscopic tacking devices has reduced reliance on sutures,[24] although many surgeons still use them for mesh positioning. However, tacks and staples may also injure nerves and vessels. Absorbable tacks may reduce the incidence of long-term abdominal wall pain.[25] Tissue glues have not found a place in intraperitoneal mesh fixation because it is widely agreed that fixation needs to be to the underlying muscular-fascial layer rather than just the peritoneum.

Complications

For open repair, these include seroma, hematoma, and infection. Suction drains may be employed in the retromuscular and subcutaneous planes to prevent fluid collections. Superficial wound infection can be treated in the usual way, but deep mesh infection is a serious problem and usually necessitates removal of the mesh, leading to inevitable hernia recurrence.

After laparoscopic repair, early postoperative severe pain is very common. It usually settles within the first week and is thought to be due to parietal peritoneal irritation from the adjacent mesh. Seroma is also very common, filling the space previously occupied by the hernial sac, but is usually transient and rarely of clinical significance. The most serious complication is an occult bowel injury, reported in approximately 1.5% of laparoscopic repairs.[26] Because the diagnosis is often delayed, sepsis may be well established on presentation. Definitive treatment is likely to involve laparotomy and removal of the mesh combined with bowel repair or stoma formation, and it may be associated with a prolonged and stormy postoperative course.

The only consistent finding in studies comparing open and laparoscopic repairs has been that laparoscopic repair is associated with fewer wound complications. Recurrence rates are similar, ranging from 5% to 29% depending on the hernia characteristics, whether or not the defect was closed laparoscopically, and length of follow-up.[27,28]

EPIGASTRIC HERNIA

These arise through a fascial defect anywhere along the linea alba from the xiphoid process to the umbilicus. The true prevalence is difficult to establish, but autopsy studies have suggested a prevalence of up to 10% in the general population.[29] Epigastric hernia is more common in males, with a ratio of approximately 4:1, and it usually arises in young-to-middle adult life. Those hernias arising close to the umbilicus are sometimes referred to as supraumbilical hernias.

Clinical Features

Patients are often asymptomatic, but epigastric hernia can produce vague epigastric discomfort, sharp at times, often more related to posture and physical activity than eating or gastrointestinal function. As the contents usually comprise preperitoneal fat or omentum, incarceration and/or strangulation generally results in no more than localized pain and tenderness.

The classic examination finding is a soft midline mass, although the emerging hernia may push to one side and lie distinctly off-center. It is generally irreducible as the herniating fatty material assumes a "mushroom" shape, expanding into the subcutaneous space after emerging through the small fibrous defect. In obese patients, palpation of the mass may be difficult, and confirmation of the diagnosis by ultrasound or computed tomography (CT) is helpful.

Management

Small epigastric hernias sometimes resolve without treatment, presumably through spontaneous strangulation and infarction. Involvement of bowel is rare because the defects tend to be small, so the decision for surgical intervention depends on the presence and severity of symptoms. They may be repaired by open or laparoscopic approaches.

Open Repair

Small solitary defects may be approached with either a midline or transverse incision. Note that the defect will be in the midline, even if the hernial swelling is not. Transverse incisions following Langer's lines heal neatly, but if the defects are large or multiple, or when intraperitoneal access may be required such as in the emergency setting when a strangulated viscus is suspected, a midline incision is preferred. The hernial sac is dissected free of the surrounding tissues, the margins of the defect are clearly defined and the contents are either resected or reduced intact.

The smaller the defect, the more successful a primary repair with nonabsorbable sutures will be. The repair can be edge-to-edge closure, overlapping fascial closure, or a tension-free darn, but irrespective of the technique used at least 1 cm of linea alba should be exposed all around before suturing begins. Some surgeons prefer a vertical repair and others a horizontal orientation, but this will depend on the shape of the defect. The most appropriate direction of repair will be that resulting in the least tension. As defects become larger, and especially if they arise through the thinned and attenuated linea alba that is associated with divarication of the rectus muscles, the more important it is to employ prosthetic mesh. The techniques for mesh repair are identical to those described earlier for umbilical/paraumbilical hernias. The cutoff size of defect above which mesh repair becomes mandatory is not defined, but experts commonly agree that it is unwise to rely on a suture repair alone for defects > 2 cm in minimum dimension.

Laparoscopic Repair

As for umbilical hernias, laparoscopy is suitable for all but the smallest and largest hernias. Epigastric hernias may not be visible on initial laparoscopy, as they lie in the root of the falciform ligament, but even if the defect can be clearly seen it is mandatory to take down the falciform ligament, expose the fibrous margins of the defect and take care to remove all the fatty hernial contents. If these steps are not taken, a lump may still be palpable postoperatively to the dismay of the patient. This phenomenon is one variety of "pseudorecurrence" described after laparoscopic ventral hernia repair.[21]

Complications

As for umbilical hernia repair, complication rates are low and most of them are related to the incision. A large review from the Danish hernia registry found low morbidity and mortality rates but a high readmission rate, mostly because of wound problems,[30] and others have found persistent pain to be an issue with these hernias as well, even in the absence of recurrence.[31] The Danish hernia registry recently reported a clinical recurrence rate of 15%.[32] In some of these cases, the recurrence may represent the persistence of a second hernia or area of weakness overlooked at the initial procedure.

SPIGELIAN HERNIA

These hernias represent approximately 2% of all ventral hernias and are most commonly seen in patients over the age of 50, although they have been reported in neonates, children, and younger adults.[33] They arise through the Spigelian fascia, which is the fused aponeuroses of the transversus abdominis and internal oblique muscles that extends between these muscle bellies and their insertion into the rectus sheath. Hernias can protrude through the Spigelian fascia anywhere along its length from the costal margin to the groin, although they are most commonly seen just below the level of the umbilicus where the crescent-shaped aponeurosis is at its widest. It used to be said that they arose just below the arcuate line, through a weak point where the posterior rectus sheath became deficient, but more recent laparoscopic evidence has shown that the majority protrude above the arcuate line (Figs. 70.12A and B). They are often small and contain no more than extraperitoneal fat, but can become very large indeed and entrap omentum and bowel.

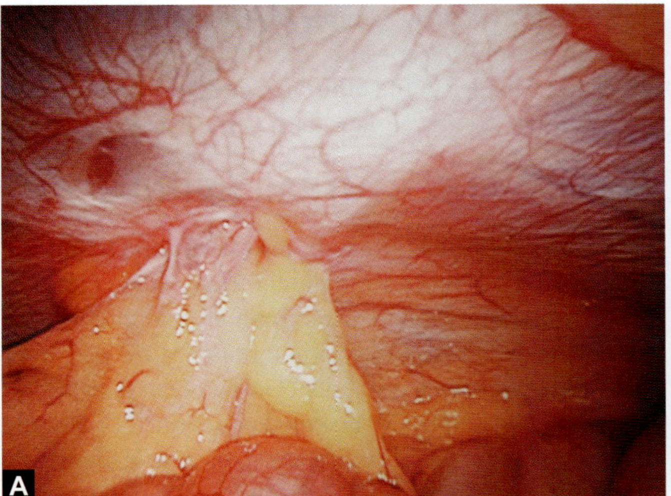

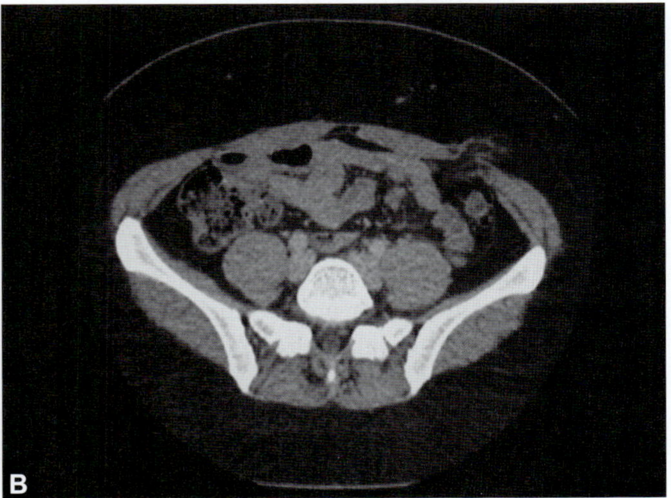

Figs. 70.12A and B: (A) Laparoscopic view of the LIF showing a Spigelian hernia arising above the arcuate line. (B) CT scan of an interstitial Spigelian hernia.

Clinical Features

Patients typically present with intermittent pain and swelling at the lateral margin of the rectus sheath. A mass may or may not be palpable, and is more likely in the older population as the hernias tend to be larger in this group. Ultrasound and CT scan may miss small hernias if they reduce spontaneously when the patient is supine for the examination. Laparoscopy will miss those that comprise entirely extraperitoneal fat, and so a high index of suspicion is required if the small hernias are to be picked up.

Management

Operation can be performed open or laparoscopically. Open repair may involve sutures alone for small defects, or employ mesh that is conveniently placed in the space deep to external oblique. It is important to remember that when cutting down onto the hernia, nothing will be seen until the external oblique layer has been incised. Open repair is arguably better for the very small Spigelian hernias (which may not be visible laparoscopically) and the very large ones (because the defects are difficult to control laparoscopically).

Laparoscopic repair can be done using intraperitoneal mesh as described for umbilical and epigastric hernia repair. Care must be taken when tacking the mesh low or laterally in the abdomen to avoid injury to intercostal and iliofemoral nerves and vessels. Alternatively, a totally extraperitoneal approach may be used, although this is only feasible in the minority of cases in which the hernia lies below the arcuate line.

LUMBAR HERNIA

Most lumbar hernias arise either through the inferior lumbar triangle (of Petit), bounded by the iliac crest and the free edges of external oblique and latissimus dorsi, or the superior lumbar triangle (of Grynfeltt) that is bounded by the 12th rib, sacrospinalis and the posterior border of the internal oblique muscle. While these represent congenital "weak spots," most lumbar hernias are acquired in association with another process such as raised intra-abdominal pressure, trauma, or intra-abdominal infection tracking posteriorly.[34]

Clinical Features

Patients usually present with a dorsal swelling that may be intermittent and cause local discomfort. Occasionally, they present with incarceration or established bowel obstruction.

Management

The CT scanning confirms the diagnosis. Open operation has been the standard approach, and mesh repair has been advocated, as it is not always easy to obtain direct fascial closure. Laparoscopy is generally successful as well, and the authors favor a transabdominal preperitoneal technique. With the patient in a semilateral tilt, a standard laparoscopy is performed and then the peritoneum over the hernia is incised to enter the extraperitoneal plane. This plane is easy to open widely, and the dissection can continue posterior to the paraspinal muscles. The contents of the sac can be reduced and the defect closed, then covered with mesh. The peritoneum can then be tacked or sutured back in place to exclude the mesh from the peritoneal cavity.

OBTURATOR HERNIA

These hernias pass from the pelvis into the thigh through the obturator foramen. They are most commonly seen in elderly women, but occasionally a small obturator defect is found incidentally at laparoscopy in younger patients. The defect is small with fibrous margins, so it is not surprising that these hernias are difficult to diagnose and classically present with a small bowel obstruction. Some may also be responsible for nonspecific pelvic pain. A swelling cannot be palpated in the thigh but may sometimes be felt on rectal examination. Thus, the diagnosis is usually made at laparotomy for obstruction, although nowadays CT scanning will also identify the hernia.[35] If obturator hernia is diagnosed electively, it should be repaired, and this can be done at laparotomy or laparoscopy. In the authors' experience, the totally extraperitoneal approach provides excellent views and exposure. The obturator defect cannot be closed because of the obturator nerve and vessels that pass through it, so a cautious darn or mesh is required.

SCIATIC AND GLUTEAL HERNIA

These pelvic hernias protrude into the buttock and are the rarest of all hernias mentioned here. Sciatic hernias pass through the lesser sciatic foramen and gluteal hernias through the greater sciatic foramen. Like obturator hernias they may be a cause of pelvic pain, but usually present for the first time with bowel obstruction. CT scanning should make the diagnosis, but most have been found and treated at laparotomy. Both transabdominal and transgluteal approaches have been described, as well as laparoscopic extraperitoneal mesh repairs.

RECTUS DIVARICATION

Also known as diastasis recti, this is no more than a stretched and thinned linea alba and is usually a consequence of central obesity, although it may also arise after pregnancy. The patient presents with a sausage-shaped bulge in the upper midline, most noticeable when they sit up from a lying position as the rectus muscles contract and the unsupported linea alba bulges forward (Fig. 70.13). Although it may look alarming, it is not a true hernia as there is no neck, no sac, and no risk of incarceration or strangulation. Patients often describe local discomfort, but it is debatable whether this can be attributed to the divarication. Repair is technically possible by reapproximating the muscles in the midline, and this may even be done laparoscopically, but results are disappointing. Recurrence is common, especially if obesity is the underlying cause, and discomfort may not be relieved. Thus surgical correction is not generally offered except perhaps as a cosmetic procedure.

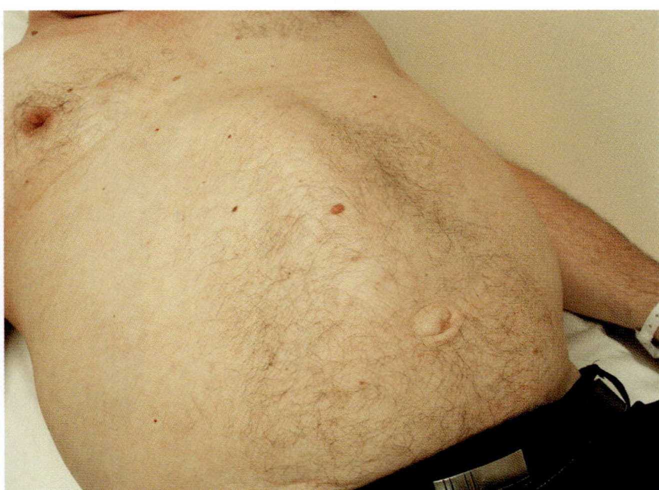

Fig. 70.13: Clinical image showing diversification of the recti as the patient attempts a sit up. Note the small paraumbilical hernia also.

INCISIONAL HERNIA

These are iatrogenic hernias arising through one or more defects in the musculofascial layers of the abdominal wall in relation to a previous surgical incision. Incisional hernias are said to arise in up to 30% of laparotomy incisions and approximately 5% of laparoscopic port-site incisions. Predisposing to their development are as follows:

- Patient factors: obesity; generally poor healing due to malnutrition, chronic disease, immunosuppression or steroid therapy; chronic cough
- Wound factors (local tissue ischemia, wound infection)
- Surgeon factors (closure technique, suture material, suture placement).

Early separation of the musculofascial layers in the early postoperative period can pass unnoticed if the overlying skin wound has healed securely. Some of the most troublesome incisional hernias are those that follow a laparostomy ("open abdomen"), when epithelialization has closed a large defect in the abdominal wall but there is only a thin layer of skin overlying the small bowel and the abdominal muscles are widely retracted and often deficient.

Clinical Features

Incisional hernias typically appear as a reducible swelling in the region of a laparotomy scar. They may be single or multiple, and may be localized to one area or involve the whole length of the incision (Figs. 70.14A to C). They may lie directly beneath the scar or protrude to one side. These hernias tend to increase steadily in size with time, and the overlying skin may become thin and atrophic. Because many incisional hernias are wide necked, they carry a low risk of bowel obstruction or strangulation, but these problems are more likely when the fibrous defect is relatively small and the sac relatively large. Symptoms of nonobstructive colicky abdominal pain are common and may reflect coexistent intestinal adhesions.

Management

The only definitive treatment is operative repair, but in those patients with asymptomatic hernias, especially if the defect is wide, and in those for whom the risks of operation are judged to be prohibitive, conservative management may be best. In such cases, the wearing of an abdominal binder or belt may prevent the hernia from becoming problematic.

For most incisional hernias, both open and laparoscopic surgical options are available. A number of principles apply, irrespective of the technique used:

- The repair should deal with the whole length of the previous incision
- Approximation of the musculofascial layers should be done with minimal tension
- Prosthetic mesh reinforcement should be used to reduce the risk of recurrence

Using mesh in a frankly contaminated field, for example, fecal soiling from bowel injury during the dissection, is contraindicated because of the risk of postoperative mesh infection.

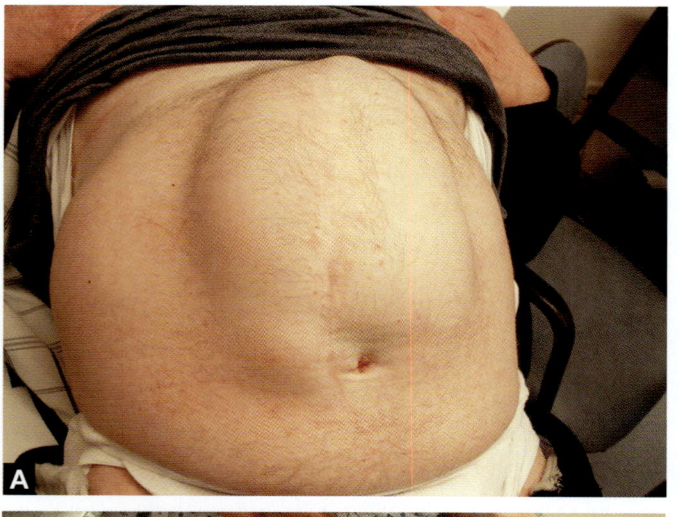

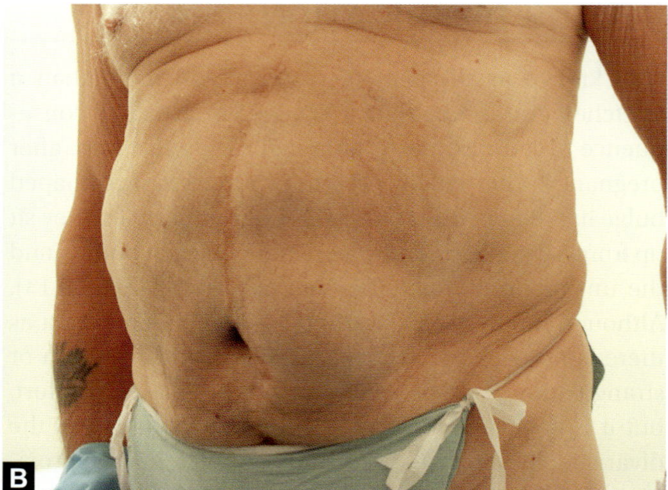

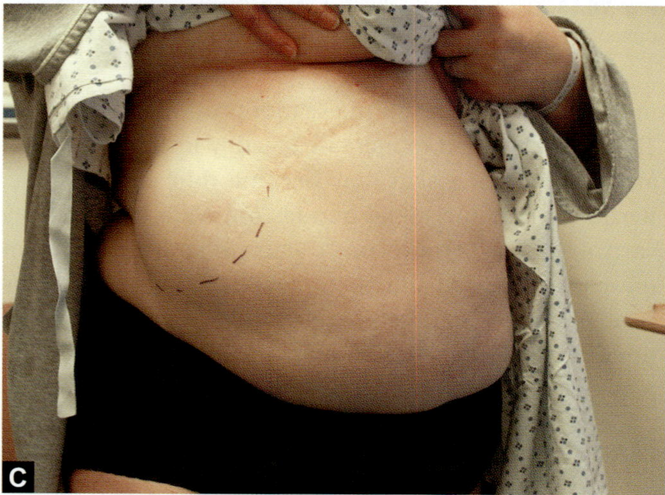

Figs. 70.14A to C: Clinical images of incisional hernias of (A) the whole of the incision, (B) multiple defects, and (C) part of the incision.

In a clean-contaminated field, such as after an elective bowel resection, mesh may be used if it is deployed in a separate anatomical plane to the contamination, such as in the extraperitoneal/retromuscular space; appropriate systemic antibiotics are given before mesh placement, and meticulous surgical technique is used to prevent hematoma.

Open Repair

Simple suture techniques without the use of prosthetic mesh are not recommended because of the high risk of recurrence. However, a suture repair may be the only option in the presence of gross contamination in which it can be regarded as a temporary solution and there can be a plan to return for a formal mesh repair at a later date in the event of recurrence.

The previous scar is excised over the full length of the incision so as to reveal any unsuspected defects. The hernial sac, its neck and the margins of the defect, are fully exposed. The sac can be opened, contents reduced, local adhesions divided and any redundant sac excised to allow safe reclosure of the layers of the abdominal wall.

Mesh Repair

As for other ventral hernia repairs, mesh is better used to reinforce a fascial repair than to bridge a fascial gap. Bridging may be used if the defect is too large for fascial closure but is best avoided. Reinforcing mesh in an open incisional hernia repair may be used in several positions as shown in Figure 70.15:

- The *retromuscular* or "sublay" position, between the rectus muscle and the posterior sheath. This mesh position is preferred by many surgeons because:
  - It is an avascular space that can be developed widely for large hernias.

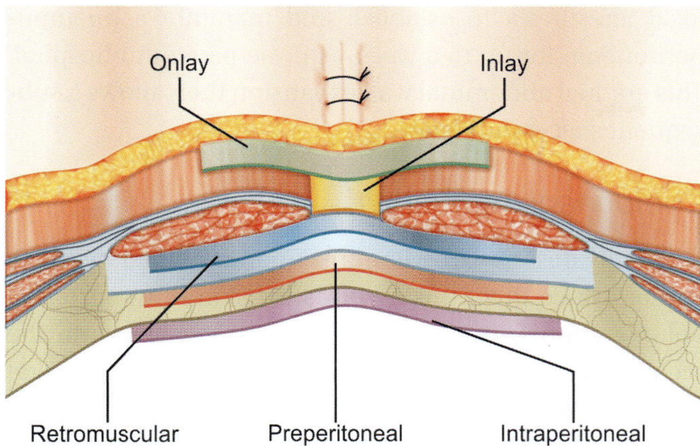

Fig. 70.15: Locations of the abdominal wall that mesh can be placed. Current accepted terms are onlay, inlay, sublay, preperitoneal and IPOM (intraperitoneal onlay mesh).

- The mesh lies against well-vascularized muscle that encourages native tissue ingrowth and discourages infection.
- The mesh can be excluded from the subcutaneous space, which reduces the risk of mesh contamination in the event of wound breakdown.

  In hernias arising laterally in the abdominal wall, or through transverse incisions, this plane may be extended into the space between the external and internal oblique layers.[36]

- The *subcutaneous* on "onlay" position, over the anterior rectus sheath and external oblique aponeurosis. This mesh position is popular because it is an easier space to develop than the retromuscular space and can be extended very widely, but to do so requires elevation of skin and subcutaneous tissue that divides perforating nerves and vessels and thus risks neuralgia, seroma formation, and wound edge necrosis.
- The *"inlay"* position, in which the mesh is sutured edge-to-edge with the fascia on each side to bridge a gap. This position is mentioned only to condemn it. Mesh repairs derive their strength from tissue ingrowth, and this requires a broad overlap of mesh on a healthy, well-vascularized bed. Edge-to-edge apposition does not achieve this result, but leaves the strength of the repair to rely solely on the suture material attaching the mesh.
- Intraperitoneal mesh is occasionally used at open repair. This is the usual mesh position in laparoscopic repair and requires special mesh with a low adhesion profile to lie within the peritoneal cavity. At open operations it is used most commonly as a last resort when the abdominal wall is deficient (e.g., after multiple previous repairs) or to bridge an unclosable fascial gap.

Although there is no good evidence to show that sublay is better than onlay (or vice versa), the retromuscular sublay repair is the expressed preference of many hernia surgeons, including the authors. The procedure will be described in some detail.

The sublay operation begins by excising the old scar and performing a laparotomy. Adhesions tend to be maximal at the neck, so entering the abdominal cavity through the fundus of the hernia sac is usually straightforward. It is helpful to mobilize adhesions from the underside of the anterior abdominal wall for some distance, but generally an extensive abdominal adhesiolysis is not required unless there is a history suggesting episodes of obstruction. The retromuscular space is entered at the margin of the defect and the space is developed in all directions. Care must be taken to avoid the inferior epigastric vessels that traverse the space in the lower abdomen; these should be lifted up with the rectus muscle. Watch also for the arcuate line, below which the space is purely extraperitoneal. From here the space can be developed across the midline and behind the pubic arch, over the bladder. Superiorly, the posterior rectus sheaths are divided on either side immediately deep to the linea alba to expose the root of the falciform ligament. This maneuver creates a common space across the midline and allows dissection to extend up behind the xiphisternum if necessary. If the space needs to be extended laterally, then the lateral aspects of the rectus sheath can be incised to enter either the plane between external and internal oblique[36] or the extraperitoneal space.[37] Care must be taken at the edge of the rectus sheath to avoid damaging intercostal nerves and vessels, as they run from the plane between internal oblique and transverses into the rectus muscle.

Once the sac has been dealt with and the plane established, the posterior rectus sheath is closed with an absorbable suture. This closure is not usually difficult as the dissection allows advancement of the layers and reduction of tension across the wound. The mesh is cut to size, aiming to have at least a 6-cm overlap in all directions. This mesh is fixed at several points to the posterior rectus sheath with interrupted absorbable sutures or tissue glue. This fixation is purely to hold the mesh in position until tissue ingrowth occurs. A suction drain is often left anterior to the mesh, and the anterior fascia is closed over it. Any redundant skin is excised to minimize subcutaneous dead space. Further drains may be placed to the subcutaneous space.

Laparoscopic Repair

As with primary ventral hernias, incisional hernias are increasingly being repaired by the laparoscopic placement of mesh. The principles of the operation are as for laparoscopic umbilical hernia repair (*see* Box 70.1), but there are some important differences that make a laparoscopic incisional hernia repair considerably more complex:

- Possible intra-abdominal adhesions from previous surgery. These can make the initial trocar insertion difficult, as well as exposure of the defect. An iatrogenic bowel injury is a potential disaster.
- Possible multiple defects which, if sufficiently large or close together, may be difficult or impossible to close prior to mesh placement.
- Possible loss of working space once the hernia is reduced. If this situation is anticipated, the repair should be done open from the start.
- Potential danger in tacking the mesh for laterally placed hernias, such as Spigelian hernias and incisional hernias arising through appendicectomy or stoma closure scars. Tacks placed inferiorly and laterally may injure intercostal or pelvic nerves and vessels. The bladder is also at risk with repair of pelvic hernias, and tacks should not be placed into the diaphragm for fear of injuring the lung and/or coronary vessels.

Large Hernias and Loss of Domain

Very large incisional hernias require careful planning before treatment begins. If the volume of the sac is >25% of the volume of the abdominal cavity—and this can be calculated from CT scan images[38]—then there is likely to be an issue with loss of abdominal domain when the hernia is repaired. The problem is that the contents of the hernia, which have been outside the abdominal cavity for a long time, will not fit back inside: or if they do, the repaired abdominal wall will be under a great deal of tension. The high intra-abdominal pressure can lead to visceral compression and pulmonary complications secondary to limitation of diaphragmatic descent with respiration. A tight abdomen can lead to wound breakdown and failure of the repair. A number of special techniques may be used to aid in the repair of large incisional hernias.

Progressive Preoperative Pneumoperitoneum

This technique has been available for a long time, and several reports attest to its usefulness with giant hernias.[38] Modern techniques utilize a Veress needle placed under local anesthesia to establish and maintain a pneumoperitoneum for up to a week with the patient in hospital. This gradual abdominal wall expansion then allows a subsequent successful repair.

Component Separation

Originally described by Ramirez[39] and modified by many authors since then, this involves incision of the external oblique aponeurosis just lateral to its insertion into the rectus sheath, all the way from the groin to the costal margin. The relaxing incision allows the rectus apparatus and linea alba to advance toward the midline and thus permits midline fascial closure. It may be augmented by mesh in the retromuscular space or as an onlay in the subcutaneous space. The technique can be carried out laparoscopically, but is only suitable for midline defects; wound seroma and skin necrosis are recognized complications because of the wide elevation of skin flaps required. Nevertheless this is a very useful technique for large hernias with a difficult abdominal closure. Novitsky and colleagues have devised a "posterior" modification in which the transversus layer is divided instead in order to reduce wound complications.[37]

Peritoneal Flap ("Mesh Sandwich") Technique

This technique was first reported in France, but has been described in the English literature recently.[40] Here, the peritoneal flaps are preserved, one attached to the posterior wound margin and the other to the anterior margin. The posterior flap is used to span the fascial gap and close the peritoneal cavity, which allows a standard sublay flat mesh repair in the retromuscular space. The remaining anterior flap of preserved peritoneum is then used to provide fascial closure over the mesh and exclude it from the subcutaneous plane, which prevents mesh exposure in the event of wound infection or breakdown. This technique is suitable for hernias arising in transverse and oblique incisions. However, it does require the presence of a useable sac.

Prevention of Incisional Hernia

The incidence of incisional hernia may be reduced by improving the patient's general condition preoperatively where possible, that is, correcting anemia, maximizing cardiac and respiratory function and correcting nutritional deficiencies. Closing the fascial layers with slowly absorbable sutures of adequate gauge is as strong as using nonabsorbable material,[41] and there is evidence that meticulous fascial closure using multiple small bites of a 2/0 suture is as effective as, or better than, large mass-closure bites of heavy (no. 1 gauge suture material).[42] It makes no difference whether the abdominal fascia is closed with interrupted or continuous sutures, but if a continuous suture is used the tissue bites must not be too near the fascial edge nor pulled too tight, or they may cut out. It has been shown that the optimal ratio of suture length to overall wound length is 4:1.[43] If a lower suture-to-wound-length ratio is used, the suture bites are too far apart or too tight and the converse applies if a higher ratio is used.

Bringing drain tubes out through the surgical wound rather than through a separate stab incision is associated with a higher incidence of postoperative incisional hernia.

Laparoscopic port-site hernias are more common through larger incisions. Because of the risk of bowel entrapment, some surgeons recommend that laparoscopic incisions > 12 mm in diameter should be closed by deep fascial suture, especially in the infracolic compartment, around the umbilicus and single-port entry wounds.

A recent meta-analysis has shown that placing mesh prophylactically into the retromuscular space at the time of abdominal closure can significantly lower the incidence of later incisional hernia.[44] There is a risk of mesh infection, especially in contaminated operations such as bowel resections, but with careful technique and appropriate antibiotics the published rates of mesh infection are very low. As a result, the use of prophylactic mesh is gaining in popularity, and a number of randomized trials in this area are ongoing.

PARASTOMAL HERNIA

Herniation adjacent to an emerging stoma occurs in up to 100% of cases, and the use of alternative techniques, such as extraperitoneal tunneling or siting it lateral to the rectus muscle, does not appear to affect the incidence.[45]

Clinical Features and Indications for Operation

Some parastomal herniation is subclinical, picked up incidentally on cross-sectional imaging, but most patents report a bulge at the site of their stoma. The hernia can interfere with fitting of stoma bags and lead to leakage, particularly if it is associated with stomal retraction due to traction on the emerging bowel loop within the sac. Pain is common, whether from intermittent bowel obstruction from loops within the sac or from stomal obstruction, and renal impairment may follow if the stoma is draining an ileal conduit. Operative repair of parastomal hernia is complex and associated with a high rate of recurrence, but nevertheless it is indicated when symptoms are distressing enough to justify the risks.

Surgical Options

Open techniques have been available for a long time. In the days before mesh repair, stomal relocation was better than fascial repair alone, but it required a full laparotomy and the new stoma carried the same risk of herniation as the original one. Mesh repairs proved more secure, and the risk of infection was reduced when the mesh was placed in the retromuscular sublay position, or intraperitoneally as originally described by Sugarbaker.[46] When mesh was "keyholed" to allow it to be passed around the emerging stomal limb, some recurrences arose through the defect in the mesh and cases of mesh erosion and fistulation were reported.[47] The Sugarbaker repair avoided this by parietalizing the stomal limb behind a sheet of intact mesh instead. Unfortunately, recurrence rates after open repair, even with mesh, still occur in at least 20%.[48] Newer biologic meshes, introduced in an attempt to further reduce problems of potential mesh infection, have not proved superior.[49]

Laparoscopic approaches have also been developed, and both keyhole and modified Sugarbaker techniques are described.[50,51] Laparoscopic repair is judged to be safe, affords identification of other hernia defects, and is associated with better short-term outcomes than open.[52] The laparoscopic Sugarbaker technique has a lower recurrence rate and less risk of mesh erosion and fistula formation than the keyhole repair, so at present it should be regarded as the procedure of choice[45] (Figs. 70.16A to C).

Complications

Whichever approach or technique is used, parastomal hernia repair is a major operation. Problems may be encountered with intra-abdominal adhesions, particularly within the sac where access may be difficult. Unplanned enterotomy leads to contamination of the operative field, which precludes the use of mesh. Damage to the conduit can lead to a urinary or fecal fistula. Mesh adjacent to an emerging stomal limb may cause erosion and fistulation. Finally, even in the best of hands, recurrence rates of around 15% are common.[45]

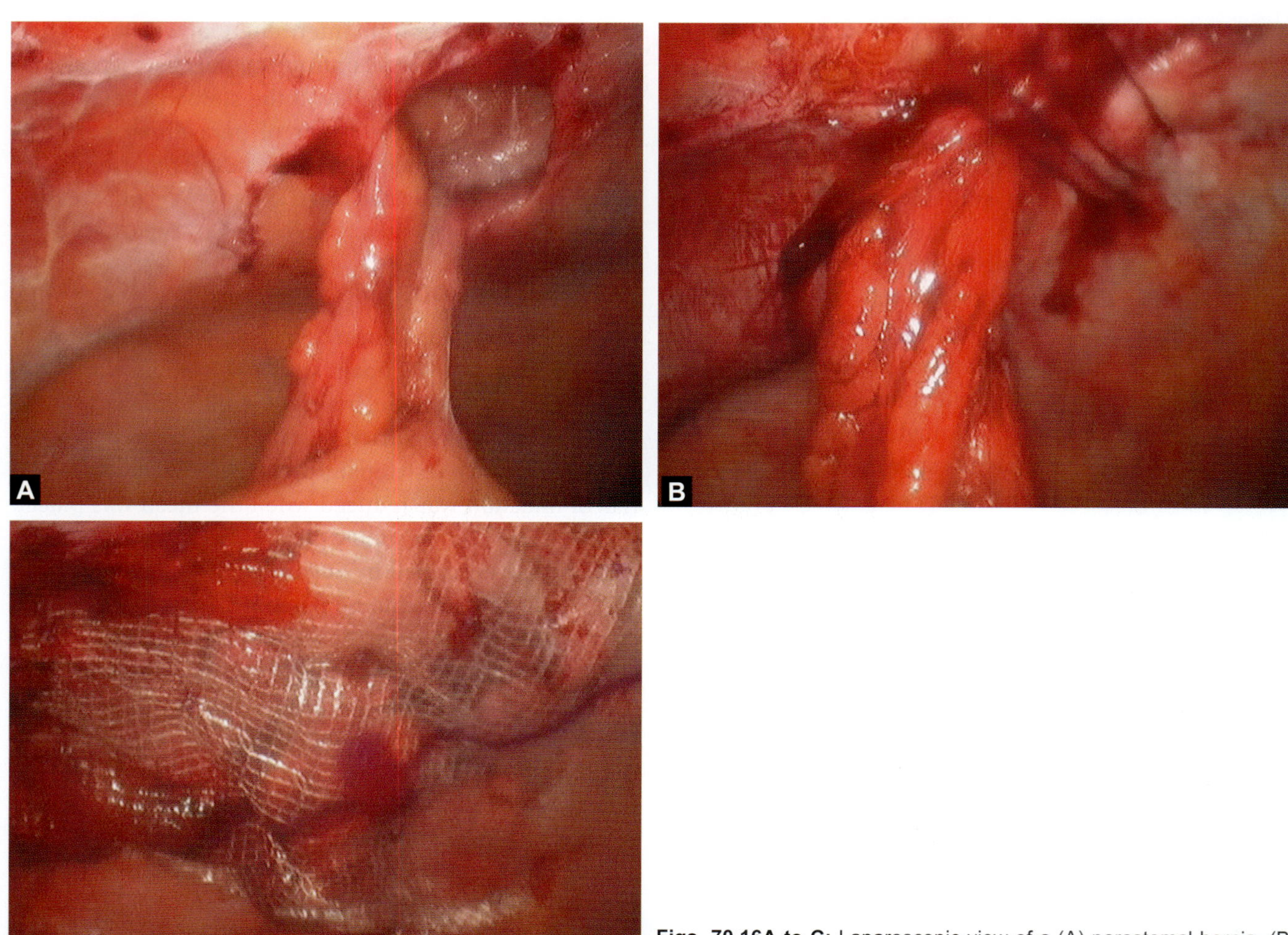

Figs. 70.16A to C: Laparoscopic view of a (A) parastomal hernia, (B) same parastomal hernia following closure of the defect, (C) Sugarbaker parastomal hernia repair—note parietalization of the conduit.

Prevention

Much interest has been generated in the use of prophylactic mesh at the time of initial stoma formation. A systemic review published in 2012 analyzed 27 studies, of which only three were suitable for inclusion. Nevertheless the evidence was compelling that prophylactic mesh reduces the subsequent herniation rate from around 50% to around 12%, with minimal mesh-related morbidity.[53] The evidence suggests that prophylactic mesh placement is current best practice.

TRAUMATIC HERNIA

Types

These hernias arise through nonanatomic defects caused by injury. They can be classified into three types:

1. Hernias through abdominal stab wound sites: These are effectively incisional hernias, akin to port-site hernias after laparoscopy.
2. Hernias protruding through splits or tears in the abdominal muscles following blunt trauma (Fig. 70.17A).
3. Abdominal bulging secondary to muscle atrophy that occurs as a result of nerve injury or other traumatic denervation. Similar to the lumbar pseudo-hernia incurred by subcostal nerve damage during open nephrectomy, this can arise following chest or abdominal injury with damage to the intercostal nerves (Fig. 70.17B).

Clinical Features

Traumatic hernias present as any other hernia. The key to the etiology is in the history and the nonanatomic location of the hernia.

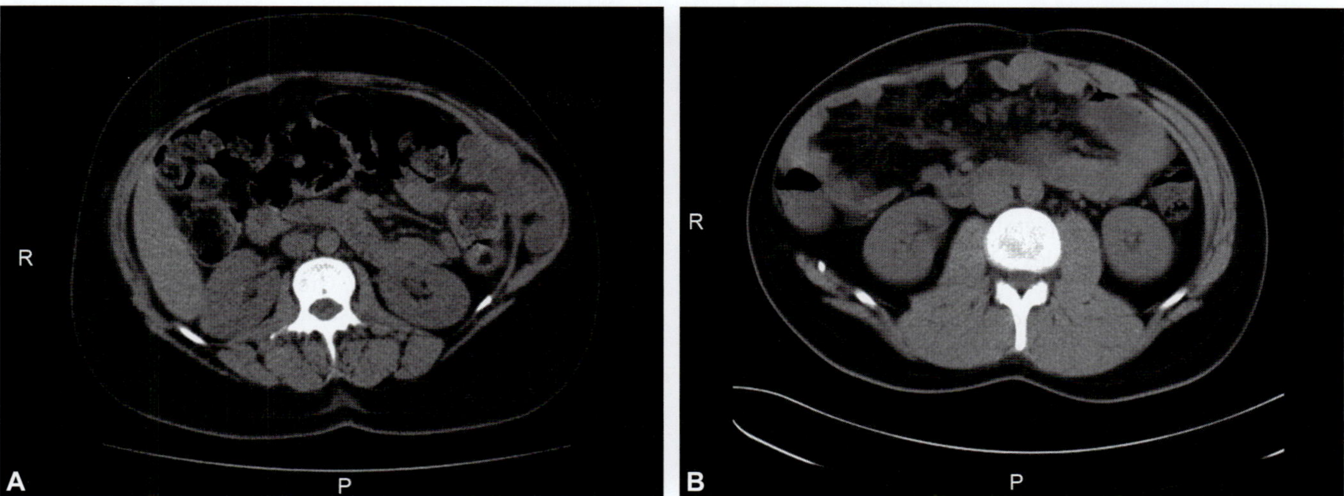

Figs. 70.17A and B: (A) CT scan showing rupture of the left transversus abdominis and internal oblique layers following a motor vehicle accident, with interstitial herniation of bowel (B). CT scan showing a right-sided chest injury with intercostal nerve injury causing atrophy of the right abdominal wall musculature.

Management

Operative repair may be justified if the hernia is sufficiently symptomatic, or if investigations suggest a narrow neck and hence a risk of obstruction or strangulation. True traumatic hernias are straightforward to repair using open or laparoscopic techniques, as for other ventral hernias. Early repair after blunt trauma can be made difficult by tissue hyperemia and edema, so a delayed repair is preferred if possible. Diffuse abdominal bulges are more difficult to correct and require some form of plication of the stretched musculofascial layer with mesh reinforcement in an attempt to prevent further bulging in the future.

REFERENCES

1. Junge K, Klinge U, Rosche R, et al. Decreased collagen typeI/III in patients with recurring hernia after implantation of alloplastic prostheses. Langenbeck's Arch Surg. 2004;389:17-22.
2. Klinge U, Klosterhalfen B. Modified classification of surgical meshes for hernia repair based on the analyses of 1,000 explanted meshes. Hernia. 2012;16:251-8.
3. Holm JA, de Wall LC, Steyerberg EW, et al. Intraperitoneal polypropylene mesh hernia repair complicates subsequent abdominal surgery. World J Surg. 2007;31:423-9.
4. Hughson W. The persistence or performed sac in relation to oblique inguinal hernia. Surg Gynecol Obstet. 1925;41:610-4.
5. Schier F. Laparoscopic inguinal hernia repair—a prospective personal series of 542 children. J Pediatr Surg. 2006; 41:1081-4.
6. Lichtenstein IL, Shulman AG, Amid PK, et al. The tension-free hernioplasty. Am J Surg 1989; 157:188–93.
7. van Veen RN, Wijsmuller AR, Vrijland WW, et al. Long term follow up of a randomized clinical trial of non-mesh versus mesh repair of primary inguinal hernia. Br J Surg 2007;94: 506–10.
8. Kucuk HF, Siker HE, Kurt N, et al. Lichenstein or darn procedure in inguinal hernia repair: a prospective randomised comparative study. Hernia. 2010;14:357-60.
9. Annandale T. Case in which a reducible oblique and direct inguinal and femoral hernia existed on the same side and were successfully treated by operation. Edinb Med J. 1876;27:1087-9.
10. Taylor C, Layani L, Liew V, et al. Laparoscopic inguinal hernia repair without mesh fixation, early results of a large randomized clinical trial. Surg Endosc. 2008;22:757-63.
11. Fitzgibbons RJ. Can we be sure polypropylene mesh causes infertility. Ann Surg. 2005;241:559-61.
12. Franneby U, Sandblom G, Nordin P, et al. Risk factors for long-term pain after hernia surgery. Ann Surg. 2006;244:212-9.
13. Aasvang EK, Gmaehle E, Hansen JB, et al. Predictive risk factors for persistent postherniotomy pain. Anaesthesiology. 2010;112:957-69.
14. National Institute for Clinical Excellence. Laparoscopic surgery for inguinal hernia repair. Technology Appraisal Guidance 83. London: NICE, 2004. Available from www.nice.org.uk/TA083guidance. [Accessed November 5, 2014.]
15. Duff M, Mofidi R, Nixon SJ. Routine laparoscopic repair of primary unilateral inguinal hernias—a viable alternative in the day surgery unit? Surgeon. 2007;5:209-12.
16. Chung L, Norrie J, O'Dwyer PJ. Long term follow up of patients with a painless inguinal hernia from a randomized trial. Brit J Surg. 2011;98:596-9.
17. Muysoms FE, Miserez M, Berrevoet F, et al. Classification of primary and incisional abdominal wall hernias. Hernia. 2009;13:407-14.

18. Arroyo A, García P, Pérez F, et al. Randomized clinical trial comparing suture and mesh repair of umbilical hernia in adults. Br J Surg. 2001;88(10):1321-3.
19. Polat C, Dervisoglu A, Senyurek G, et al. Umbilical hernia repair with the prolene hernia system. Am J Surg. 2005; 190(1):61-4.
20. Tollens T, Den Hondt M, Devroe K, et al. Retrospective analysis of umbilical, epigastric and small incisional hernia repair using the Ventralex™ hernia patch. Hernia. 2011;15: 531-40.
21. Tse G, Stutchfield BM, Duckworth AD, et al. Pseudo-recurrence following laparoscopic ventral and incisional hernia repair. Hernia. 2010;14:583-7.
22. Franklin ME Jr, Gonzalez JJ Jr, Glass JL, et al. Laparoscopic ventral and incisional hernia repair: an 11-year experience. Hernia. 2004;8:23-7.
23. Le Blanc KA. Laparoscopic incisional hernia repair: are transfascial sutures necessary? A review of the literature. Surg Endosc. 2007;21:508-13.
24. Brill JB, Turner PL. Long-term outcomes with transfascial sutures versus tacks in laparoscopic ventral hernia repair: a review. Am Surg. 2011; 77: 458-65.
25. Cavallaro G, Campanile FC, Rizzello M, et al. Lightweight polypropylene mesh fixation in laparoscopic incisional hernia repair. Minim Invasive Ther Allied Technol. 2013;22:283-7.
26. Sharma A, Khullar R, Soni V, et al. Iatrogenic enterotomy in laparoscopic ventral/incisional hernia repair: a single center experience of 2,346 patients over 17 years. Hernia. 2013;17:581-7.
27. Banerjee A, Beck C, Narula VK, et al. Laparoscopic ventral hernia repair: does primary repair in addition to placement of mesh decrease recurrence? Surg Endosc. 2012;26: 1264-8.
28. Ballem N, Parikh R, Berber E, et al. Laparoscopic versus open ventral hernia repairs: 5 year recurrence rates. Surg Endosc. 2008;22:1935-40.
29. Ponten JE, Somers KY, Nienhuijs SW. Pathogenesis of the epigastric hernia. Hernia. 2012;16:627-33.
30. Bisgaard T, Kehlet H, Bay-Nielsen M, et al. A nationwide study on readmission, morbidity, and mortality after umbilical and epigastric hernia repair. Hernia. 201;15:541-6.
31. Erritzøe-Jervild L, Christoffersen MW, Helgstrand F, et al. Long-term complaints after elective repair for small umbilical or epigastric hernias. Hernia. 2013;17:211-5.
32. Helgstrand F, Rosenberg J, Kehlet H, et al. Reoperation versus clinical recurrence rate after ventral hernia repair. Ann Surg. 2012;256:955-8.
33. Skandalakis PN, Zoras O, Skandalakis JE, et al. Spigelian hernia: surgical anatomy, embryology, and technique of repair. Am Surg. 2006;72:42-8.
34. Stamatiou D, Skandalakis JE, Skandalakis LJ, et al. Lumbar hernia: surgical anatomy, embryology, and technique of repair. Am Surg. 2009;75:202-7.
35. Stamatiou D, Skandalakis LJ, Zoras O, et al. Obturator hernia revisited: surgical anatomy, embryology, diagnosis and technique of repair. Am Surg. 2011;77:1147-57.
36. Stumpf M, Conze J, Prescher A, et al. The lateral incisional hernia: anatomical considerations for a standardized retromuscular sublay repair. Hernia. 2009;13:293-7.
37. Novitsky YW, Elliott HL, Orenstein SB, et al. Transversus abdominis muscle release: a novel approach to posterior component separation during complex abdominal wall reconstruction. Am J Surg. 2012;204:709-16.
38. Tanaka EY, Yoo JH, Rodrigues AJ Jr, et al. A computerized tomography scan method for calculating the hernia sac and abdominal cavity volume in complex large incisional hernia with loss of domain. Hernia. 2010;14:63-9.
39. Ramirez OM, Ruas E, Dellon AL. Components separation method for closure of abdominal-wall defects: an anatomic and clinical study. Plast Reconstr Surg. 1990;86:519-26.
40. Malik A, Macdonald AD, de Beaux AC, et al. The peritoneal flap hernioplasty for repair of large ventral and incisional hernias. Hernia. 2014;18:39-45.
41. Bloemen A, van Dooren P, Huizinga BF, et al. Randomized clinical trial comparing polypropylene or polydioxanone for midline abdominal wall closure. Br J Surg. 2011;98:633-9.
42. Harlaar JJ, van Ramshorst GH, Nieuwenhuizen J, et al. Small stitches with small suture distances increase laparotomy closure strength. Am J Surg. 2009;198:392-5.
43. Millbourn D, Cengiz Y, Israelsson LA. Effect of stitch length on wound complications after closure of midline incisions: a randomized controlled trial. Arch Surg. 2009;144:1056-9.
44. Bhangu A, Fitzgerald JE, Singh P, et al. Systematic review and meta-analysis of prophylactic mesh placement for prevention of incisional hernia following midline laparotomy. Hernia. 2013;17(4):445-55.
45. Hotouras A, Murphy J, Thaha M, et al. The persistent challenge of parastomal herniation: a review of the literature and future developments. Colorectal Dis. 2013;15:202-14.
46. Sugarbaker PH. Peritoneal approach to prosthetic mesh repair of parastomal hernias. Ann Surg. 1985;201:344-6.
47. Steele SR, Lee P, Martin MJ, et al. Is parastomal hernia repair with polypropylene mesh safe? Am J Surg. 2003;185:436-40.
48. Hansson BM, Slater NJ, van der Velden AS, et al. Surgical techniques for parastomal hernia repair: a systemic review of the literature. Ann Surg. 2012;255:685-95.
49. Slater NJ, Hansson BM, Buyne OR, et al. Repair of parastomal hernias with biologic grafts: a systematic review. J Gastrointest Surg. 2011;15:1252-85.
50. Le Blanc KA, Bellanger DE. Laparoscopic repair of parastomy hernias: early results. J Am Coll Surg. 2002;194:232-9.

Additional references appear in the online version of this book.

71 Case Study: Appendicitis: Perils of Delayed Operation

James ML Williamson, Robin CN Williamson

THE PROBLEM

Acute appendicitis is one of the most common causes of an acute abdomen, with a lifetime incidence of 7–9%. It can occur at almost any age, but is most frequent in children and young adults. Typically patients complain of vague central abdominal pain (from visceral receptors) that shifts to the right iliac fossa when the parietal peritoneum becomes inflamed. Associated symptoms include nausea, anorexia, alteration of bowel habit, and pyrexia. Typical examination reveals tenderness in the right iliac fossa with rebound tenderness, a positive Rovsing sign or frank peritonism. Retrocecal appendicitis may cause loin pain, while abdominal tenderness may be less prominent due to the presence of the overlying cecum. Luminal obstruction results in rapid deterioration and perforation with purulent peritonitis.

The diagnosis of acute appendicitis is usually clinical, with a wide range of differential diagnoses present among women of reproductive age. Investigations will often reveal an elevated C-reactive protein (CRP) or white cell count (WCC), appendiceal thickening on ultrasonography or inflammation on computed tomography (CT). The standard treatment for appendicitis is appendectomy (either open or laparoscopic). Patients with perforation are at risk of postoperative abscess formation and wound infection and, as such, generous lavage is advocated with the judicious use of a drainage tube. Operative delay is likely to result in progression of disease, with an increased risk of complications and the very occasional death in a really neglected case.

THE TYPICAL CASE

A 31-year-old obese woman presented with a 3-day history of right lower quadrant pain with some radiation to the back. The pain was exacerbated by moving the right leg and was associated with anorexia and two episodes of vomiting. Her pain had not improved despite 36 hours of co-amoxiclav prescribed by her general practitioner for a presumed urinary tract infection. There were no gynecologic or urinary symptoms and no relevant past medical history. Examination revealed no pyrexia, but guarding and tenderness in the right iliac fossa (Rovsing sign negative). Urinalysis was unremarkable, WCC was 8.9×10^9/L (normal < 10.8), and CRP was mildly elevated at 33.4 mg/L (normal < 5). No definitive diagnosis was reached, although the possibility of retrocecal appendicitis was considered, and the patient was admitted for overnight observation. Next morning she was still complaining of lower abdominal and back pain and had tenderness in the right iliac fossa and loin on examination. As she was afebrile and not overtly peritonitic, it was felt that a diagnosis of appendicitis was unlikely. Further investigation in the form of ultrasonography and CT was considered, and the patient was commenced on triple antibiotic therapy (amoxicillin, gentamicin, and metronidazole).

In the subsequent 36 hours taken to perform CT, she had an isolated temperature spike of 38°C, with associated tachycardia (100 bpm). Her pain was controlled with regular analgesia including morphine. Computed tomography confirmed a distended appendix with surrounding inflammatory change consistent with acute appendicitis; no evidence of perforation was seen. The patient was then reviewed with regard to operation. As the abdomen was soft with little tenderness, and as the emergency operating theater was in heavy demand that evening, she was listed for laparoscopic appendectomy the following morning (5 days after admission and 8 days from onset of symptoms). At operation, a very inflamed, adherent, and perforated retrocecal appendix was removed with difficulty in piecemeal fashion. Copious lavage was followed by placement of an abdominal drain. She received another 3 days of intravenous antibiotics before going home in ostensible good health.

The patient returned 4 months later with a 3-week history of intermittent pain in the right iliac fossa (as before). There was local tenderness but no fever, although WCC (12×10^9/L) and CRP (39 mg/L) were raised. Computed tomography showed stranding in the right iliac fossa, inflammation between the cecum and psoas, and a 3-cm fluid collection nearby. Despite recommencement of triple antibiotic therapy, the pain persisted and the inflammatory markers deteriorated over the next 48 hours (WCC 14×10^9/L, CRP 288 mg/L). Laparotomy via a Lanz incision now revealed a small abscess cavity containing a lump with a mucosa-lined lumen, although the cecum had healed. The lump was excised and was found to be the tip of the appendix showing lymphoid hyperplasia. The second operation was curative.

DIAGNOSTIC DILEMMAS

The differential diagnosis for right lower quadrant pain in women of menstruating age is widespread and requires careful elucidation of the clinical features. In the absence of gynecologic or urinary symptoms, a diagnosis of appendicitis must always be entertained. In the present case no clear diagnosis was reached initially, and the patient was admitted for observation and further clinical review. However, there were several suggestive features of appendicitis: (1) pain and tenderness in the right iliac fossa; (2) exacerbation of pain on moving the right leg (psoas sign); (3) the gastrointestinal upset (vomiting, anorexia); (4) radiation of pain to the back (consistent with retrocecal appendicitis); (5) the lack of gynecologic symptoms and negative urinalysis to suggest alternative diagnoses; and (6) a raised CRP in the absence of clear-cut infection. Given these features, there was a choice of options: whether to proceed directly to laparoscopy (and appendectomy), or whether to observe the patient with or without radiological investigation. Clinical experience will influence the decision, and in this case overnight observation was chosen.

Next morning the patient continued to complain of abdominal pain, although the symptoms were not thought to be diagnostic. The same options existed: operation, observation, or imaging. The decision process was not fully logical, in that antibiotics were commenced while waiting for radiological investigation. Most surgeons would avoid this step until a clinical diagnosis of appendicitis was made, when antibiotic therapy would act as a bridge to appendectomy. The patient's condition deteriorated during the wait for CT, and perforation probably occurred during this time. The next dilemma concerned the timing and type of operation. The overnight delay meant a more difficult procedure next day, and with greater confidence the surgical team should have insisted on operation that same day once the emergency theater was available; potentially a second operating theater could have been opened or the patient operated upon during the night. Moreover, given the difficulties at laparoscopy, it might have been better to convert to laparotomy to facilitate complete removal of the appendix.

The final dilemma revolves around the management of a patient with right iliac fossa pain following appendectomy. A postoperative collection should be sought by ultrasound or CT scan. A small abscess may respond to antibiotics alone, but it generally requires percutaneous or operative drainage (as in this case). The retrieval of the appendix tip supported the decision to operate and demonstrated the inadequacy of the previous laparoscopic procedure.

MANAGEMENT OPTIONS

Young women with pain in the right lower quadrant of the abdomen present a common diagnostic challenge. The crucial question is: "Does this patient have appendicitis?" In patients with peritonism, the answer should be reached by prompt operation. In the absence of peritonism, the situation is less well defined, and here clinical observation should be supplemented with biochemical and hematologic markers plus radiologic investigation. Numerous scoring systems exist—Alvarado, Fenyö, RIPASA, Mantrels, and Tzanakis—to predict the likelihood of appendicitis, but none are 100% accurate. Radiologic investigation can decrease the negative appendectomy rate from 26% (range 16–47%), when based on clinical and laparotomy findings alone, to 6–10% when imaging is performed. It is not entirely diagnostic, however: ultrasonography has a sensitivity rate of 86% and a specificity rate of 81%, while CT has a sensitivity rate of 94% and a specificity rate of 95%. Magnetic resonance imaging is not usually considered as a first-line investigation for the diagnosis of appendicitis, but may be considered in pregnancy and in children.

The established treatment of appendicitis is appendectomy, whether open or laparoscopic, and this remains one of the most commonly performed operations in the world. Antibiotics alone can be tried in the early stages of the disease, but even when they achieve resolution of symptoms there is a 14–35% readmission rate. There has been a trend toward laparoscopic intervention as this is associated with less pain, an earlier return to full activity, a reduction in wound infection rates, and a lower risk of postoperative ileus. However, the laparoscopic technique is associated with higher rates of intra-abdominal abscess formation (possibly owing to the use of intraoperative irrigation), bleeding, and postoperative urinary tract infection. Both operative modalities should be covered with broad-spectrum antibiotics for between 1 and 3 doses to decrease the incidence of postoperative wound infection and intra-abdominal abscess formation.

Once the diagnosis has been made, operative intervention should be undertaken with minimal delay. There is little difference in complication rate between appendectomy within 12 hours of presentation or within 24 hours, although this may not take into account the time of onset of symptoms. A previous review by Humes and Simpson[3] noted that the risk of perforation after 36 hours of symptoms is between 16 and 30%, and this increases by 5% every 12 hours. The mortality rate associated with nonperforated appendicitis is 0.8 per 1,000, but this increases to 5.1 per 1,000 in perforated disease.

FURTHER READING

1. Ansaloni L, Catena F, Coccolini F, et al. Surgery versus conservative antibiotic treatment in acute appendicitis: a systematic review and meta-analysis of randomized controlled trials. Dig Surg. 2011;28:210-11.
2. Gaitini D. Imaging acute appendicitis: state of the art. J Clin Imaging Sci. 2011;1:49.
3. Humes DJ, Simpson J. Acute appendicitis. BMJ. 2006;333: 530-4.
4. Li X, Zhang J, Sang L, et al. Laparoscopic versus conventional appendectomy—a meta-analysis of randomized controlled trials. BMC Gastroenterol. 2010;10:129.
5. Ruffolo C, Fiorot A, Pagura G, et al. Acute appendicitis: what is the gold standard of treatment? World J Gastroenterol. 2013;19:8799-807.
6. Sauerland S, Lefering R, Neugebauer EA. Laparoscopic versus open surgery for suspected appendicitis. Cochrane Database Syst Rev. 2004;18:CD001546.
7. Teixeira PG, Demetriades D. Appendicitis: changing perspectives. Adv Surg. 2013;47:119-40.
8. Terasawa T, Blackmore CC, Bent S, et al. Systematic review: computed tomography and ultrasonography to detect acute appendicitis in adults and adolescents. Ann Intern Med. 2004;141:537-46.

Case Study: 72
Surgical Management of the Acute Abdomen—The Role of Laparoscopy

Andrew de Beaux

THE PROBLEM

One of the most exciting aspects of emergency surgery lies in the management of patients presenting with an acute abdomen. Here, the process of history, examination, investigation, and treatment may not run in such an organized manner as elective surgery. In a sense, the process is the same; it is just that the diagnostic steps are broken up into a number of smaller chunks. Recognizing that the patient is unwell and starting resuscitation are as important as determining why the patient is unwell. Indeed, sometimes the pathological diagnosis is only made at the time of operation, yet the two key steps beforehand are to recognize that the patient is ill and that urgent/emergency surgery is required to make them better.

THE TYPICAL CASE

A 78-year-old man was brought in to the accident and emergency department acutely unwell. The history was poor for the current event, but he had become more unwell over the last 24 hours until his collapse at home. He was tachycardic, with atrial fibrillation, hypotension and tachypnea, and he was complaining of a sore abdomen. He had signs of peritonitis maximal in the right iliac fossa. White cell count was normal, but arterial lactate was elevated at 4.3 mmol/L and base deficit was 10. He was able to give a history of a myocardial infarction several years before, although his recent exercise tolerance was good and he was able to live independently with minimal social support.

A decision was made that a computed tomographic (CT) scan was appropriate, as the differential diagnosis included ischemic bowel (perhaps from an atrial embolus) as well as acute appendicitis. The CT scan was performed in both the arterial and portal venous phases. There was no evidence of bowel ischemia, but the appendix appeared thickened and edematous, with a small amount of free fluid in the abdominal cavity (Fig. 72.1).

DIAGNOSTIC DILEMMAS

I have a rather simplistic approach to the acute abdomen that embraces three questions. (1) Is the patient unwell? If physiologically well, then there is time for a period of watch and review as well as more leisurely investigations. If the patient is unwell, then resuscitation needs to commence, asking question (2): does the patient require surgical intervention or not? If operation is considered necessary to correct the problem, question (3) relates to the timing of operation: whether now, later today following optimization or perhaps never if the patient is unfit for operation and/or the pathology is not survivable. The last option can be a difficult decision, as it may need to be made quite quickly while there may not be much history from the unwell patient. Here, relatives, friends of the patient, perhaps the family doctor, past medical notes if available, and also help from the anesthetist or critical care doctors are all useful in making the right decisions.

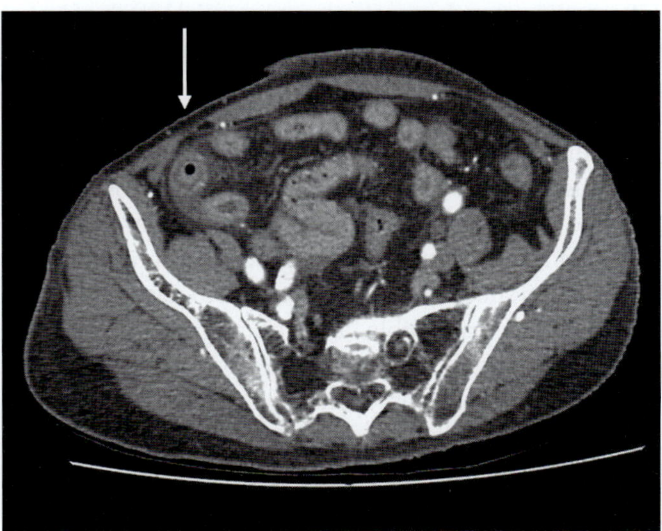

Fig. 72.1: Computed tomographic scan of the abdomen—thickening and edema seen in the appendix in the right flank.

MANAGEMENT OPTIONS

It is more difficult to make clear algorithms for the acute abdomen as compared to elective surgery. However, there are some general points.

Except in the case of ongoing hemorrhage, it is rare that a patient with an acute abdomen needs to go to theater within an hour of presentation. Oxygen administration, fluid resuscitation, analgesia, antibiotics, and blood sugar control are some of the important preliminary steps. They may be taken in the admission ward, or may require the benefit of invasive monitoring within a critical care environment.

Older surgeons will talk about the need to proceed with surgery in cases of peritonitis, especially if free gas under the diaphragm is evident on the erect chest X-ray. While I believe that this policy is correct in general, I find that in my own practice I undertake more preoperative CT scans than I did in the past. This fact reflects partly improved access to CT scanning, especially out of hours, but partly the experience from seeing a number of patients operated for peritonitis in which prior knowledge of the pathology would have supported a plan of terminal care. Most patients with an acute abdomen will present with a short history. However, there may be a history of a longer prodromal illness, e.g. with weight loss and a general deterioration in health plus evidence of anemia or deranged liver function tests. These findings, particularly in the older patient, then raise the specter of cancer and perhaps inoperable cancer, which may alter the decision to operate. Similarly, in cases of suspected bowel ischemia, CT scanning may demonstrate a substantial length of bowel infarction in the mid and hind gut distribution with or without liver, spleen, or renal infarcts, for which operative treatment is unlikely to have a successful outcome.

In the present case, the CT scan suggested acute appendicitis as the cause of the peritonitis and a laparoscopy was planned for the same day following several hours of resuscitation. At laparoscopy, the findings were of fibrinous material centered subumbilically and toward the right iliac fossa. The appendix was visible, and although perhaps thicker than usual, it was a similar color to the cecum and did not appear inflamed. The ascending colon was also easily seen and appeared normal. The small bowel was then inspected in a retrograde direction from the cecum. A small Meckel's diverticulum was evident but appeared normal. About one meter from the cecum, a 5-cm segment of small bowel was thickened with more obvious fibrous material clinging to the bowel and the mesentery. On closer inspection, there was a perforation in the small bowel close to the mesenteric border. The operation was converted to a laparotomy though an 8-cm right transverse incision, and a limited small bowel resection with primary anastomosis was performed. In view of the location of the incision, the appendix was removed as well. Pathology confirmed mild serosal inflammation on the appendix plus evidence of more marked peritonitis on the small bowel with a perforation as described, although the small bowel was otherwise normal histologically. The cause of the perforation was not clear, but in view of the findings, it was thought likely to have resulted from a fish bone or perhaps a small chicken bone. The patient made an uneventful recovery and was discharged from the hospital 6 days later.

There is an increasing trend toward laparoscopy in the acute abdomen, especially when the working diagnosis is acute appendicitis. While my own laparoscopic skills do not always allow correction of the pathology found, laparoscopic inspection of the abdomen can be particularly valuable when, as in this case, the suspected organ of disease was actually normal. Once the pathology is found, then a small incision can be made at the optimum spot to deal with the pathology encountered. However, a timely operation is at least as important as the approach to operation, which itself depends upon the local skills available.

FURTHER READING

1. Green G, Shaikh I, Fernandes R, et al. Emergency laparotomy in octogenarians: a 5-year study of morbidity and mortality. World J Gastrointest Surg. 2013;5:216-21.
2. Macaluso CR, McNamara RM. Evaluation and management of acute abdominal pain in the emergency department. Int J Gen Med. 2012;5:789-97.
3. Solis CV, Chang Y, De Moya MA, et al. Free air on plain film: do we need a computed tomography too? J Emerg Trauma Shock. 2014;7:3-8.
4. Steinbach C, Stockmann M, Jara M, et al. Accidentally ingested toothpicks causing severe gastrointestinal injury: a practical guideline for diagnosis and therapy based on 136 case reports. World J Surg. 2014;38:371-7.

73

Upper and Lower Gastrointestinal Hemorrhage

Raymond SY Tang, Francis KL Chan, Joseph WY Lau

Key Points

- Peptic ulcers and erosions in the stomach and duodenum account for 75% of cases of upper gastrointestinal (GI) hemorrhage. Certain stigmas can predict those patients at risk of rebleeding and thus likely to need surgical management.
- Combination endoscopic therapies and high-dose intravenous proton pump inhibitor infusion after endoscopic hemostasis are the cornerstones of treatment of ulcer bleeding in those with high-risk stigmas.
- Bleeding from gastroesophageal varices is associated with high rates of rebleeding and mortality.
- Endoscopic variceal ligation is the mainstay of treatment for esophageal variceal bleeding. For bleeding gastric varices, endoscopic variceal obturation with glue or placement of transjugular intrahepatic portosystemic shunt is the first-line therapy.
- Bleeding from beyond the duodenojejunal flexure comprises 10–20% of acute GI hemorrhage. Colonic diverticula and colonic angiodysplasia are common causes of lower GI bleeding.
- Gastrointestinal bleeding of obscure origin generally originates from the small intestine. Small bowel capsule endoscopy and balloon-assisted deep enteroscopy have increased the diagnostic and therapeutic options for patients with overt obscure GI bleeding.
- Endoscopy is the optimal investigation almost irrespective of the source of bleeding.

INTRODUCTION

Acute gastrointestinal (GI) bleeding is a common abdominal emergency and a major cause of morbidity and mortality. Bleeding from the upper GI tract is about four times as common as bleeding from the lower GI tract. Peptic ulcers and gastroduodenal erosions account for 75% of upper GI bleeding, whereas other causes such as varices, esophagitis, gastritis, and Mallory-Weiss syndrome each account for 5-15% (Fig. 73.1).[1] Despite improvement in endoscopic hemostasis and other therapeutic modalities, the mortality rate from GI bleeding has not changed significantly in the last few decades and has remained around 5-10%. This fact most likely reflects the increasing proportion of elderly patients with multiple comorbidities compromising the GI bleeding population and the growing use of antiplatelet agents, anticoagulants, and nonsteroidal anti-inflammatory drugs (NSAIDs).[2-4]

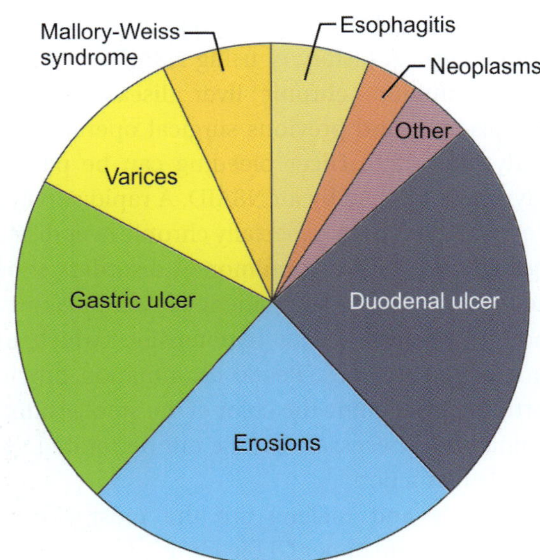

Fig. 73.1: Causes of upper gastrointestinal bleeding.
Source: Data from Silverstein, Gilbert DA, Tedesco FJ, Buenger NK, Persing J. The National ASGE survey on upper gastrointestinal bleeding I. Study design and baseline data. Gastrointest Endosc. 1981; 27:73-9.

In the last several decades, the epidemiology and management of peptic ulcer disease (PUD) have undergone marked changes. The discovery of *Helicobacter pylori* (HP) in the 1980s and the availability of effective eradication therapy have led to decline in recurrent PUD and its complications.[5,6] While the prevalence of HP-associated ulcers declines, NSAIDs and low-dose aspirin have emerged as increasingly important causes of PUD and its complications.[7,8] Over the last 2 decades, endoscopic therapy and acid suppression with proton pump inhibitors (PPIs) have become the mainstay of management of bleeding peptic ulcer, while the role of emergency surgery has decreased.[3,4,9] In centers in which expertise is available, angiographic embolization is an alternative for patients who do not respond to repeated endoscopic therapy.

In patients with acute lower GI bleeding, the initial management would include urgent colonoscopy after rapid bowel purge. Angiography or operation may be required for definitive management if the bleeding source cannot be identified on endoscopy or the patient does not respond to endoscopic hemostasis.

The availability of small bowel capsule endoscopy and balloon-assisted deep enteroscopy has increased the diagnostic and therapeutic options for patients with GI bleeding of obscure origin. Angiography or intraoperative enteroscopy may still be required in selected patients, while operation is often reserved for definitive management when the pathology is identified or the patient does not respond to endoscopic hemostasis.

DIAGNOSIS

The history and past history are crucial in the evaluation of GI hemorrhage. A history of using NSAIDs or aspirin, alcohol consumption, chronic liver disease, previous bleeding episodes, and previous surgical operations are particularly important. Ulcer bleeding can be painless, especially when induced by an NSAID. A rapid survey for signs of associated illness, especially chronic liver disease, bleeding diathesis, and cardiopulmonary disorders, should be carried out promptly. The patient should be assessed for orthostatic tachycardia or hypotension, which may indicate subclinical shock. Rectal examination provides an opportunity to examine the color of the stool. Abdominal examination is necessary to rule out perforated ulcer or intestinal obstruction.

Hematemesis and melena are the most common presentations of acute upper GI bleeding.

- Melena is a black, sticky, and distinctively foul-smelling stool that may be either liquid or semisolid. The odor, once experienced, is impossible to be mistaken for anything else. The black discoloration of stool is a result of bacterial degradation of hemoglobin when blood passes through the GI tract. It must not be confused with the dark-colored stool of patients who are taking iron supplements or bismuth therapy.
- Hematemesis and coffee-ground vomiting point to bleeding from the upper GI tract. Except in the case of Mallory-Weiss syndrome, when fresh blood often mixes with vomitus, hematemesis may indicate more severe blood loss than in patients who present with melena alone.
- Hematochezia, the passage of bright red or maroon blood rectally, can be a manifestation of profuse upper GI bleeding or bleeding from a lower intestinal source.

Symptoms of hypovolemia such as tachycardia, pallor, sweating, mental confusion, and oliguria indicate massive blood loss and a high risk of death. However, GI blood loss may be occult (i.e. detected only by chemical testing).

INITIAL MANAGEMENT

Patients presenting with GI bleeding should be assessed and resuscitated promptly. Resuscitation of a hemodynamically unstable patient begins with obtaining adequate intravenous access using large-bore venous cannulas. The intravenous volume should be replenished with normal saline or a plasma expander while blood is being cross-matched for transfusion. Close monitoring of vital signs, urine output, and central venous pressure is mandatory. The amount and rate of intravenous fluid given should be governed by the rate of bleeding, age of the patient, and the presence of cardiopulmonary disease. Complete blood count, electrolytes, liver function tests, clotting profile, and blood cross-matching should be obtained. The initial hemoglobin concentration or hematocrit may not reflect the actual amount of blood loss due to hemoconcentration. Hemoglobin levels often drop further after volume replacement with saline or a plasma expander during resuscitation. Low initial hemoglobin may indicate a chronic condition such as gastric ulcer, which has been bleeding slowly in an occult fashion.

Blood should be transfused for patients with evidence of ongoing bleeding, symptomatic anemia, or chronic cardiac diseases at risk of impaired tissue oxygenation. However, the transfusion threshold for hemodynamically stable patients is less well defined. For instance, a UK National Audit in 2010 reported a twofold increase in rate of rebleeding and a 28% increase in mortality rate in upper GI bleeding patients transfused within 12 hours of admission.[10] A large randomized trial in 2013 compared a restrictive transfusion strategy (transfusion to 7 g/dL) to a liberal transfusion strategy (transfusion to 9 g/dL) in 921 patients with acute upper GI bleeding and reported less rebleeding and higher survival at 6 weeks in the restrictive transfusion group.[11] The difference in survival was mainly noted in patients with Child-Pugh class A and B cirrhosis. In patients with peptic ulcer bleeding, there was a trend toward less rebleeding and a significant reduction in need of emergency surgery.

Coagulopathy should be corrected by administration of appropriate blood components. Patients with GI bleeding who are also on antithrombotic drugs present unique clinical challenges. For instance, double antiplatelet therapy with aspirin and clopidogrel is often needed for coronary drug-eluting stents, and newer generations of anticoagulants without antidote are increasingly used for thromboembolic diseases. The decision to withhold or resume antithrombotic drugs in patients with GI bleeding should be both individualized and multidisciplinary, balancing between the rebleeding risk and the thromboembolic risk.[4,12]

UPPER GI BLEEDING

History and physical examination are seldom sufficiently useful for identifying the source of bleeding; investigations are therefore necessary for most cases of GI bleeding. Current or recent use of aspirin or NSAIDs may suggest bleeding from peptic ulcer. Stigmas of chronic liver disease suggest bleeding from gastroesophageal varices, but peptic ulcer and portal hypertensive gastropathy are more common causes of bleeding in patients with cirrhosis.

Assessment

Risk Stratification

Several scores of risk stratification have been published and are helpful in predicting the need for intervention in patients with acute upper GI bleeding. For instance, the Rockall score includes both pre-endoscopy clinical parameters and endoscopic findings to predict mortality in acute upper GI bleeding.[13] The Glasgow Blatchford score is calculated on the basis of clinical parameters alone.[14]

Endoscopy

Endoscopy allows identification of the cause of bleeding and provides important prognostic information based on endoscopic stigmas of bleeding. In an early meta-analysis of patients with upper GI bleeding, endoscopic therapy was shown to reduce rate of recurrent bleeding, use of operation, and mortality.[15]

Timely endoscopy is important. Patients with hemodynamic instability and evidence of active bleeding should be offered urgent endoscopy, while those who are stable after initial resuscitation can generally undergo endoscopy within 24 hours.[16-18]

During endoscopy, patients should be closely monitored for changes in blood pressure, pulse, electrocardiogram, and oxygen saturation as their condition can change rapidly. Facilities for resuscitation, including endotracheal intubation and defibrillation, should always be available. The endoscopy assistant should watch the patient's condition closely and keep the airway clear by oropharyngeal suction. Oxygen via nasal cannula may be useful for patients who have cardiopulmonary insufficiency.

Patients should be placed in a left lateral position so that blood in the stomach pools in the fundus and the greater curve. Because most cases of bleeding arise from lesions on the lesser curve, distal antrum, and the duodenum, an adequate examination in these areas should be possible by passing the endoscope along the lesser curve without disturbing the pool of blood (Fig. 73.2). Turning the patient to the right shifts the blood and clots into the distal stomach allowing better visualization of the fundus and greater curve. Irrigation using the Water Pik system facilitates examination of bleeding lesions covered by blood clots. When the stomach is filled with blood clot, gastric lavage with an overtube might be helpful to improve the view. A large 3.7-mm channel therapeutic endoscope allows the use of large-caliber accessories such as a 10°F heat probe. A dual-channel therapeutic endoscope with

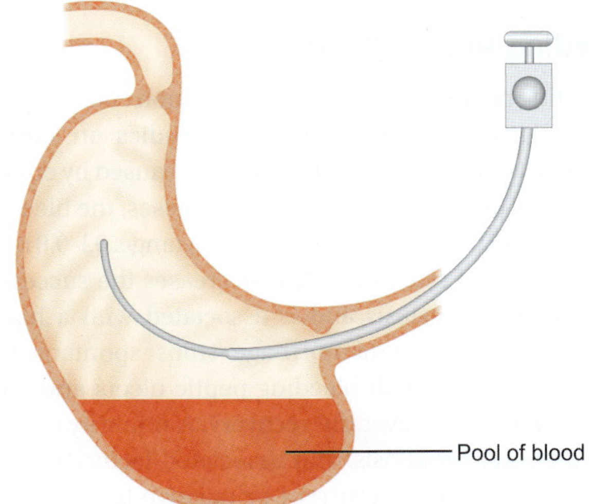

Fig. 73.2: The endoscope passes above the pool of blood in the fundus and the body of the stomach when the patient is lying in a left lateral position.

Table 73.1 Outcome of bleeding peptic ulcers based on endoscopic appearance. Data collected from prospective trials in which patients did not receive endoscopic therapy.

Type	*Endoscopic appearance*	*Prevalence (%)*	*Rebleeding (%)*	*Operation (%)*	*Death (%)*
Ia	Active spurting	18 (4–26)	55–88	35 (20–69)	
Ib	Active oozing		10–27		11 (0–23)
IIa	Protuberant vessel	17 (4–35)	43–50	34 (0–56)	11 (0–21)
IIb	Adherent clot	17 (0–49)	22–35	10 (5–12)	7 (0–10)
IIc	Flat pigmented spot	20 (0–42)	8–10	6 (0–10)	3 (0–10)
III	Clean base	42 (19–52)	3–5	0.5 (0–3)	2 (0–3)

Sources: Data from Forresth JAH, Finlayson NDC, Shearman DJC. Endoscopy of upper gastrointestinal bleeding. Lancet. 1974;ii:394-7; Laine L, Peterson WL. Bleeding peptic ulcer. N Engl J Med. 1994;331:717-27; and Kovacs TO, Jensen DM. Complications of peptic ulcer disease. In: Dimarino AJ, Jr, Benjamin SB (Eds). Gastrointestinal Disease: An Endoscopic Approach. Thorofare, NJ: Slack; 2002. pp. 411-38.

one 2.8-mm and one 3.7-mm channel allows better suction and irrigation, even when the endoscopic accessories are in place. The endoscopic appearance of peptic ulcers and varices predicts the risk of rebleeding.

Radiologic Studies

Plain radiograph such as an erect chest x-ray would be an initial step in ruling out free air under the diaphragm if a perforated peptic ulcer is suspected (although combined bleeding and hemorrhage is very uncommon). An abdominal X-ray would be useful in looking for dilated bowel loops if intestinal obstruction is suspected. If plain radiographs are negative but clinical suspicion of perforation or intestinal obstruction remains, computed tomography (CT) should be considered, especially in patients with postsurgical GI anatomy. The use of barium studies in diagnosing upper GI bleeding has declined markedly since the advent of endoscopy.

Bleeding Peptic Ulcer

A bleeding peptic ulcer is the most common cause of acute upper GI tract bleeding. Histologic studies on surgical specimens demonstrate that bleeding is caused by erosion of an artery at the ulcer base.[19] In most cases, the bleeding artery is small (mean diameter = 0.7 mm; range: 0.1–0.8 mm). A larger arterial size (> 1.5 mm) decreases the success of endoscopic hemostasis and is associated with a higher mortality rate.[20] The hemorrhage stops spontaneously in 80% of patients with bleeding peptic ulcers and these patients have an uneventful recovery. A minority of cases have a poorer prognosis, and associated factors in these cases are as follows: recurrent or massive hematemesis; age > 60 years; presence of comorbid illness; onset of GI bleeding after hospital admission for another medical condition; and coagulopathy.[21,22]

The appearance of ulcers at endoscopy provides important information on the risk of rebleeding. Large ulcers (>2 cm) are more likely to rebleed. The stigmas of hemorrhage from peptic ulcer were first classified by Forrest and colleagues (Table 73.1; Figs. 73.3A to D).[23] An ulcer may be actively bleeding from an arterial spurter or a pulsatile vessel at the ulcer base (class Ia) or just continuously oozing (class Ib). A nonbleeding ulcer can present as a "visible" or protuberant vessel (class IIa), an adherent clot (class IIb), or a flat-pigmented spot (class IIc). A clean base nonbleeding ulcer is classified as Forrest class III. Studies have shown repeatedly that the risk of rebleeding, requirement for operation, and risk of death may be predicted by the presence of these stigmas (Table 73.1).[24,25] Large ulcers are more likely to have one or more of these stigmas.

Medical Therapy

Multiple pharmacologic agents have been studied in the management of nonvariceal upper GI bleeding. Currently, there is no convincing evidence that vasoactive agents such as somatostatin or octreotide will stop active ulcer bleeding. It has been suggested that once bleeding stops and initial clotting occurs, suppression of gastric acidity may prevent dissolution of the clot as proteolytic enzymes function poorly in a high-pH environment. Acid suppression medications such as H_2-receptor antagonists (H_2RA) and PPIs have been extensively evaluated in this context. The use of intravenous H_2RAs is limited by their ineffectiveness in maintaining a sustained high gastric pH due to rapid development of tolerance within 12 hours of infusion.[25]

Studies have evaluated high-dose intravenous PPI use before endoscopy and after successful endoscopic hemostasis. Data from a recent meta-analysis of 6 randomized

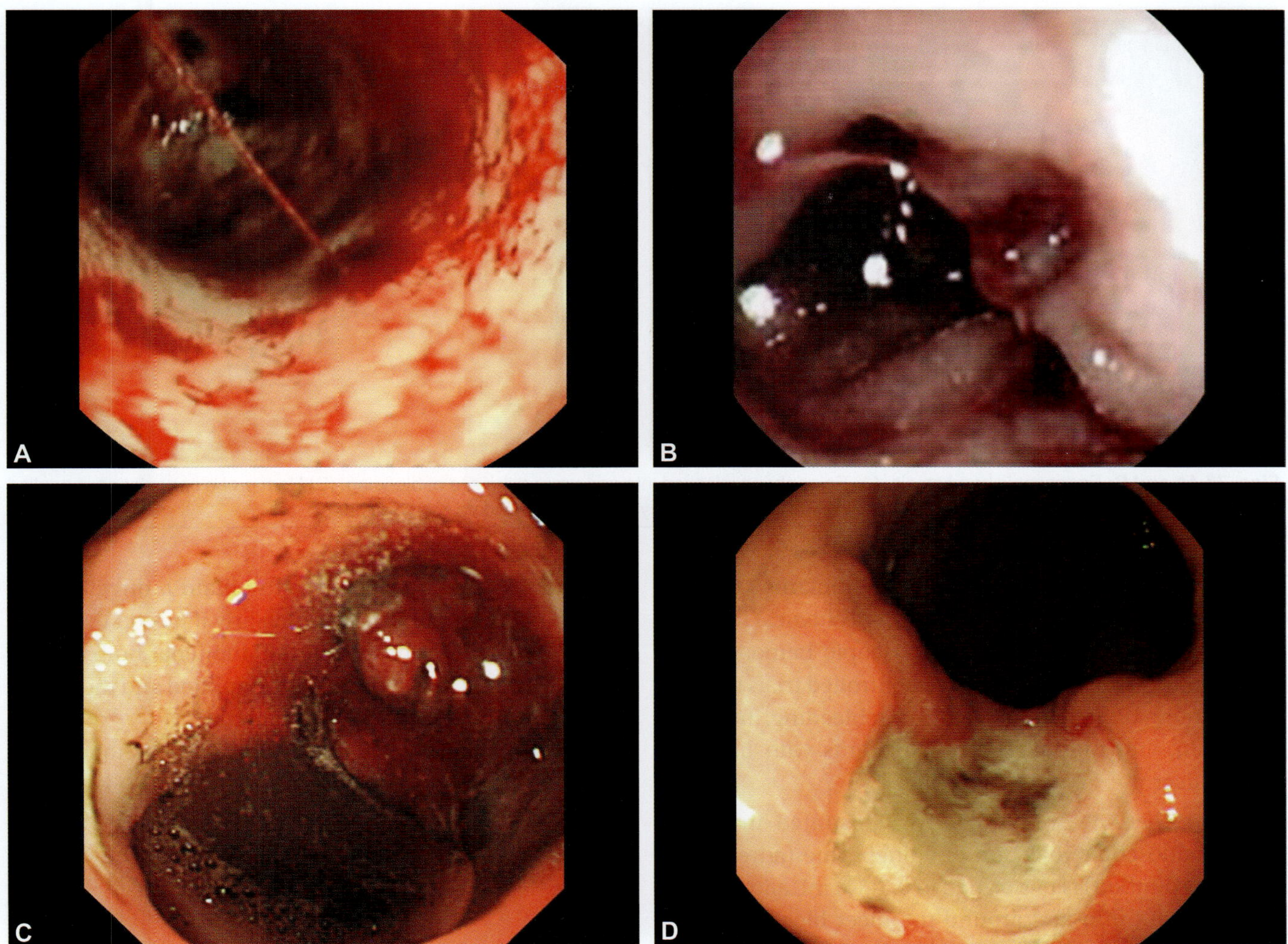

Figs. 73.3A to D: Stigmas of hemorrhage in bleeding peptic ulcers. (A) A jet of blood is seen spurting across the endoscopic field. (B) A protuberant vessel is clearly visualized in this patient who is not actively bleeding. (C) This previously bleeding ulcer is now covered by an adherent clot. (D) This flat, pigmented spot identifies the site of a nonbleeding peptic ulcer. Image courtesy of Professor Enders KW Ng and Dr RS Tang.

controlled trials showed a reduction in high-risk stigmas of bleeding and need for endoscopic therapy in patients receiving intravenous PPI before endoscopy.[26] Randomized controlled trials and recent meta-analysis have shown a reduction in rebleeding, need for operation, transfusion requirement, and duration of hospital stay in patients receiving high-dose intravenous PPI bolus, followed by intravenous PPI infusion for 72 hours after successful endoscopic treatment of bleeding ulcers and high-risk stigmas of recent hemorrhage (e.g. nonbleeding visible vessel and adherent clot).[27-29]

Besides acid suppression, the use of antifibrinolytic agents has been suggested to enhance clot function. Tranexamic acid has been evaluated in multiple trials and two meta-analyses. Although one meta-analysis showed a reduction in mortality and need for operation with tranexamic acid, there is still insufficient evidence to support routine use of antifibrinolytic agents in patients with acute upper GI bleeding.[30]

When the acute bleeding episode subsides, patients should be tested for *H. pylori* infection. An ulcer associated with *H. pylori* should be treated with a course of combination antibiotic therapy. Successful eradication of *H. pylori* significantly reduces the occurrence of recurrent ulceration and bleeding and obviates the need for maintenance of acid suppression therapy.[31,32]

Endoscopic Hemostasis

Various endoscopic hemostasis modalities have been used in the treatment of ulcer bleeding. In the last two decades, injection therapy, cautery devices, and mechanical therapies have become widely accepted as the firstline

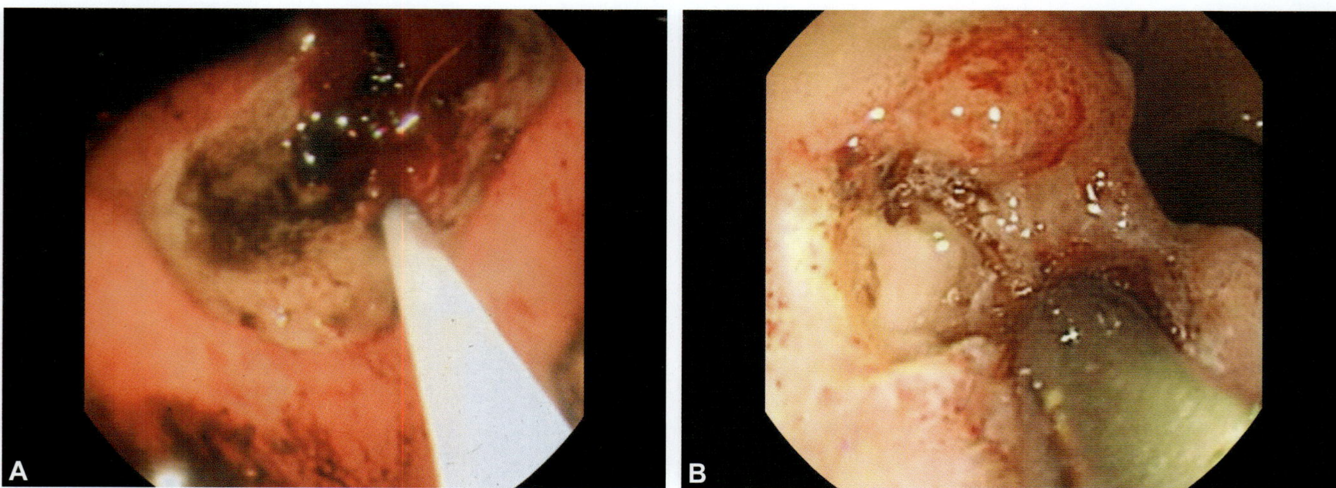

Figs. 73.4A and B: Endoscopic hemostasis. (A) Epinephrine injection into and around the site of bleeding. (B) Heat probe coagulation is applied by pressing on the vessel before activating coagulation. Image courtesy of Professor Enders K W Ng.

treatment for bleeding ulcers.[25,33] Combination therapy (injection therapy + cautery device or mechanical therapy) is the preferred approach to endoscopic hemostasis. A pooled analysis of 16 randomized controlled trials showed that combination therapy reduces rebleeding, need for operation, and mortality rate in patients with bleeding peptic ulcer.[34]

Injection Therapy: This method is illustrated in Figure 73.4A. Endoscopic injection of epinephrine (adrenaline) (1:10,000 dilution) is performed in 0.5–1.0 mL aliquots (up to 10–15 mL) into and around the ulcer bleeding point. Debate exists as to whether the hemostatic effect is a result of local tamponade produced by the volume injected or of vasoconstriction and platelet aggregation caused by epinephrine. Absorption of epinephrine into the systemic circulation has been documented, but without any important effect on the hemodynamic status of the patients.[35]

Epinephrine injection is an effective, cheap, easy-to-learn method of hemostasis and has acquired worldwide popularity. Other sclerosants such as polidocanol, alcohol, and sodium tetradecyl sulfate have been used but cause more tissue necrosis and local complications when large volumes are used.

Cautery Devices: Cautery devices include heater probes, bipolar probes, argon plasma coagulation, and neodymium: yttrium-aluminum-garnet (Nd:YAG) lasers. Heater probes and bipolar probes achieve hemostasis by coaptive coagulation (Fig. 73.4B). This method uses direct pressure and heat energy (heater probe) or electrocoagulation (bipolar probe) to weld the walls of the artery together.[33] Occasionally, it is not possible to obtain a direct frontal view of the bleeding ulcer, particularly if it is on the lesser curve or the posterior wall of the duodenal bulb. In this situation, direct pressure cannot be applied and the failure rate of coaptive coagulation is higher.

Argon plasma coagulation represents a noncontact cautery device for superficial tissue. Nd:YAG laser is another noncontact thermal method for ulcer hemostasis. The interaction between laser energy and tissue generates heat, but its use has declined in recent years because of the lack of a tamponade effect and the prohibitive cost of the machine.[25]

Mechanical Therapies: These are devices that cause physical tamponade of a bleeding site and include endoclips, endoloops, and rubber band ligation. The most widely used mechanical therapy for bleeding ulcer is an endoclip (Fig. 73.5). Endoclips are designed to grasp the submucosa, to seal bleeding vessels, or to approximate the sides of lesions, and typically slough off within days to weeks after placement.[33] The efficacy of endoclips in achieving hemostasis is comparable to that of thermocoagulation.[36]

New Modalities: Recently several newer modalities such as nanopowder hemostatic agent (Hemospray), over-the-scope-clip, and endoscopic suturing devices have become available. A pilot study of 20 patients showed that Hemospray was safe and effective in achieving acute hemostasis in active ulcer bleeding (Forrest Ia and Ib).[37] At this point, much of the experience in use of these modalities originates from selected expert centers. More data would be needed before these newer modalities become established therapy for treatment of ulcer bleeding.

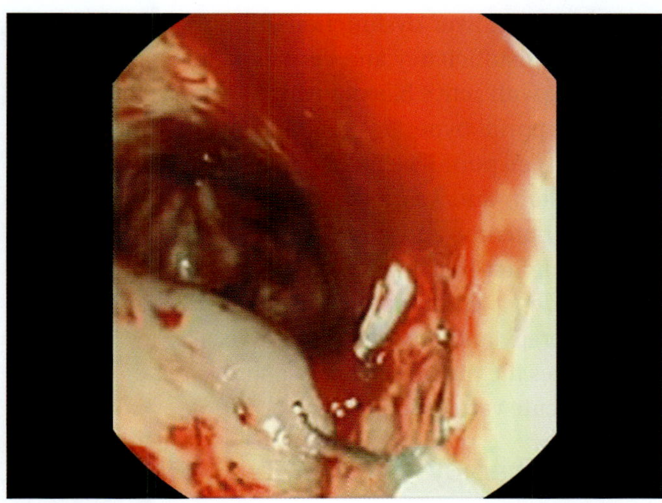

Fig. 73.5: Endoclip use in the treatment of bleeding gastric ulcer.

Angiographic Embolization

In patients with massive GI bleeding in whom primary endoscopic hemostasis fails or in those with recurrent bleeding after initial endoscopic hemostasis, angiographic embolization may be an alternative to surgery if local expertise is available. Data from retrospective studies comparing angiographic embolization to operation in patients who did not respond to endoscopic hemostasis have shown a higher rate of recurrent bleeding, but a lower rate of treatment-related complications in the angiographic embolization group. There is no difference in mortality rate between the two groups.[4,38]

Flowchart 73.1: Combined approach to the management of acute ulcer bleeding.

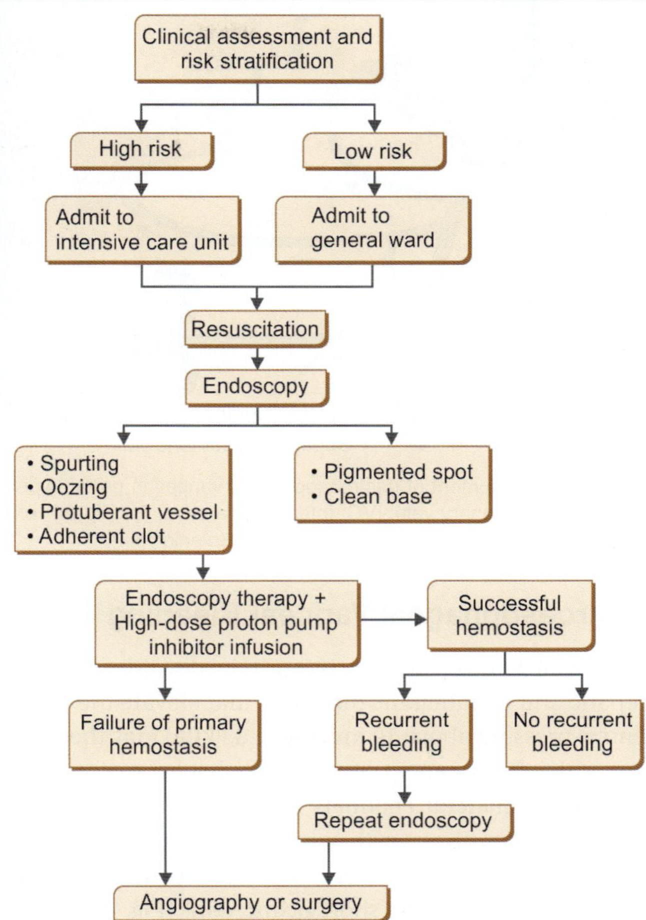

Operative Treatment

Operative treatment remains the most definitive method of treatment for ulcer bleeding. However, there is little agreement on the exact indications and best timing for surgical intervention. Surgical operation is generally performed if endoscopy fails to control bleeding or an ulcer rebleeds after endoscopic hemostasis (Flowchart 73.1). The overall mortality rate of emergency surgery for GI bleeding ranges from 10% to 20%. This is partly due to delayed surgical intervention after repeated failure of endoscopic hemostasis. The results of operation are better if it is carried out early, especially for those over 60 years of age.[39] Early operation should also be considered for patients who are bleeding from the gastroduodenal artery or a large gastric ulcer.

The surgical management depends upon the location of the bleeding ulcer. Oversewing the ulcer bed in the duodenum through a pylorotomy and ligation of the gastroduodenal artery may be necessary to control the bleeding. In the past, a definitive operation such as vagotomy with pyloroplasty or Billroth II gastrectomy was often performed to prevent ulcer recurrence, but this is probably unnecessary in the modern age of effective antiulcer drugs. With a major bleed from the gastroduodenal artery, a good case can be made for formal ligation of the vessel close to its origin from the hepatic artery rather than relying solely on under-running the vessel in the ulcer base.

Bleeding from a gastric ulcer often required excision of the ulcer with a definitive procedure (i.e. either partial gastrectomy or vagotomy and drainage). Now that the link between *H. pylori* infection and peptic ulceration has been recognized, the need for acid-reducing procedures must be re-evaluated. The approach of simple oversewing of the bleeding point and subsequent treatment of *H. pylori* infection may be adequate in selected patients.

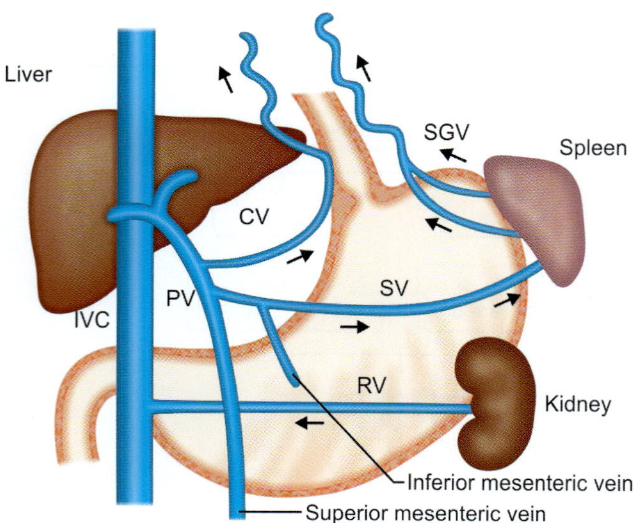

Fig. 73.6: Development of gastroesophageal varices in portal hypertension. (CV: Coronary vein; IVC: Inferior vena cava; PV: Portal vein; RV: Renal vein; SGV: Short gastric vein; SV: Splenic vein).

Gastroesophageal Variceal Bleeding

The portal venous system is entirely devoid of valves. Hepatic and extrahepatic disorders that elevate the portal venous pressure above 10 mm Hg (1.33 kPa) may therefore lead to the development of gastroesophageal varices. Portosystemic collateral channels connecting the cardioesophageal venous plexus with splenic or hepatic veins dilate. The most important of these channels are the coronary (left gastric vein) and the short gastric veins (Fig. 73.6).[40]

Gastroesophageal varices can be found in approximately 50% of patients with cirrhosis. The presence of varices correlates with the severity of the liver disease, ranging from 40% in Child's class A cirrhosis to 85% in Child's class C cirrhosis.[41] Variceal bleeding occurs at a yearly rate of 5–15%.[42] Fifty percent of patients with cirrhosis develop variceal bleeding during their lifetime. Large varix size, presence of red wale signs on endoscopy, and decompensated cirrhosis are predictors of variceal hemorrhage.[43] About 40% of patients stop bleeding spontaneously at the time of presentation, but 30–60% of patients rebleed during hospitalization.[44-46] The 1-year rate of recurrent variceal bleeding is approximately 60%.[41] Recurrent bleeding often occurs during the first 5–14 days after the initial episode of bleeding, resulting in high morbidity and mortality rates.[45,46] Therefore, prevention of early rebleeding is mandatory to improve patient survival.

The 6-week mortality is 15–20% per episode of variceal bleeding.[44,45] This figure is higher than that of other causes of upper GI bleeding, and it is highest for patients who have advanced liver dysfunction and other organ failure (e.g. renal insufficiency and cardiac failure) and patients presenting with active bleeding during endoscopy. Patients who have portal hypertension, but relatively normal liver function (i.e. portal vein thrombosis, idiopathic portal hypertension, and schistosomiasis), have a much more favorable outcome and survival.

Current first-line management of acute variceal bleeding includes a combination of vasoactive drugs, endoscopic therapy and antibiotic prophylaxis.[41] Flowchart 73.2 summarizes the multidisciplinary approach to the management of acute variceal bleeding.

Medical Therapy

Resuscitation with blood and fluid replacement should be implemented promptly, with the goals of maintaining hemodynamic stability and a hemoglobin level around 8 g/dL.[41] Caution should be taken not to over-transfuse or over-volume expand as variceal rebleeding may be precipitated.

Vasoactive drugs such as somatostatin and its analogs (octreotide, vapreotide), or terlipressin (a synthetic analog of vasopressin with a longer biological activity and fewer side effects) are most commonly used.[41] Octreotide is thought to act through its inhibitory effect on vasodilator hormones and direct splanchnic vasocontriction. Terlipressin exerts its effect by causing nonspecific arteriolar vasoconstriction. The vasoactive drugs are usually infused for 2–5 days. In a recent meta-analysis of 15 trials comparing vasoactive drugs and emergency endoscopic sclerotherapy, similar efficacy with fewer side effects was found in the vasoactive drugs group.[47] Thus, octreotide or terlipressin should be initiated early in the management when variceal bleeding is suspected.

The incidence of bacterial infections in patients with cirrhosis and acute upper GI bleeding is high. The use of prophylactic antibiotics for 5–7 days in this setting has been shown to reduce the rate of bacterial infections (including spontaneous bacterial peritonitis), the risk of variceal rebleeding, and mortality.[48] The antibiotic of choice is a third-generation cephalosporin, or a fluoroquinolone if the patient is allergic to cephalosporin or penicillin.

Endoscopic Therapy

Timely endoscopy (within 12 hours of presentation) should be performed in patients with suspected variceal bleeding.[41] Options for endoscopic therapies include endoscopic variceal band ligation (EVL), sclerotherapy,

Flowchart 73.2: Combined approach to the management of acute variceal bleeding. (EVL: Endoscopic variceal ligation; TIPSS: Transjugular intrahepatic portosystemic shunt).

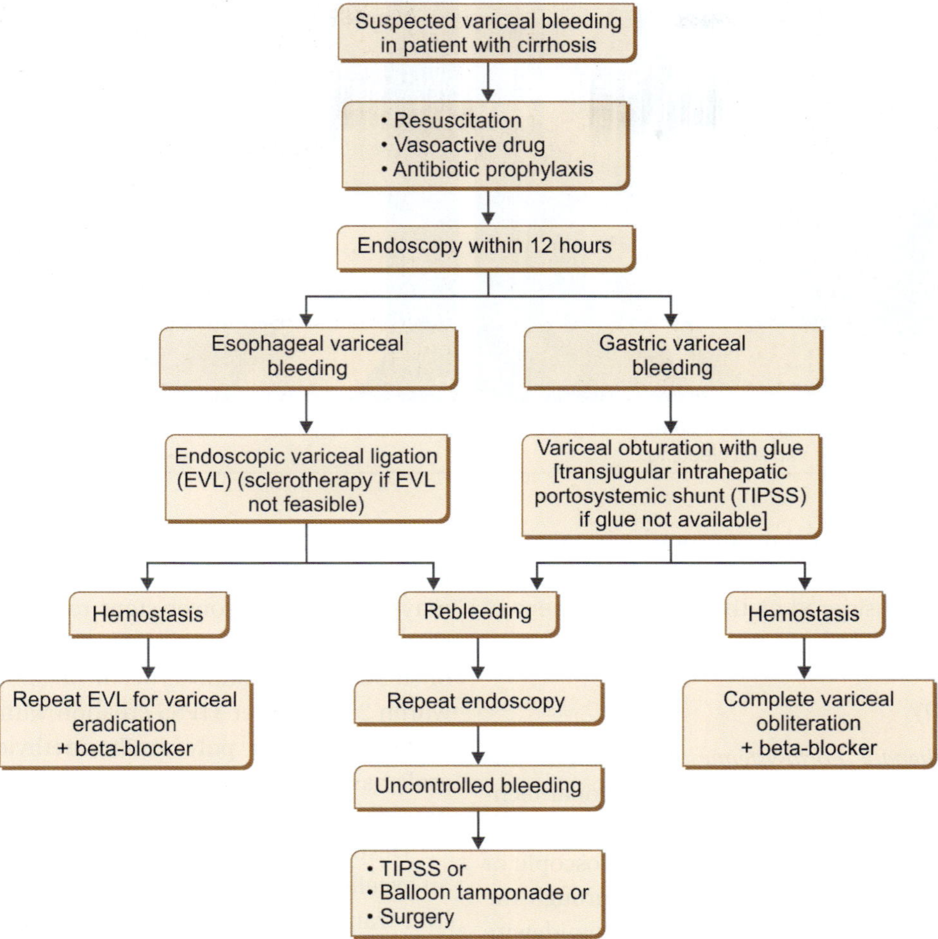

and endoscopic variceal obturation with a tissue adhesive (glue) (Figs. 73.7A and B). Choice of therapy depends on the location of varices and the availability of local expertise. The availability of a multiband variceal ligation device has greatly facilitated the management of variceal bleeding. The multiband ligation device is fitted at the tip of a gastroscope. The varix is then suctioned into the plastic hood of the device, followed by deployment of elastic bands. Sclerotherapy refers to injection of sclerosants (e.g. ethanolamine, sodium tetradecyl sulfate, sodium morrhuate, and polidocanol) into the variceal lumen (intravariceal) or adjacent esophageal mucosa (paravariceal). Hemostasis is achieved by sealing of bleeding points due to the local pressure effects of the sclerosants and thrombosis of the varices secondary to inflammation. Variceal obturation refers to injection of a tissue adhesive (e.g. *N*-Butyl-2-cyanoacrylate) directly into the variceal lumen (intravariceal) causing obliteration of varix.

For bleeding esophageal varices, EVL is the endoscopic treatment of choice, with a success rate of 70–90%.[41] Data from randomized trials and meta-analysis showed that EVL is more effective than sclerotherapy in initial control of bleeding and is associated with fewer side effects.[49,50] However, sclerotherapy is an alternative for patients in whom EVL is not feasible (e.g. those with extensive scarring from prior EVL).

Gastric varices are present in 20% of patients with cirrhosis. Bleeding from gastric varices is usually more severe and with a higher mortality when compared to esophageal variceal bleeding.[41] If expertise is available, variceal obturation with tissue adhesive (e.g. N-Butyl-2-cyanoacrylate or 2-octyl cyanoacrylate) is the recommended treatment.[41] In a randomized trial comparing variceal obturation with N-Butyl-2-cyanoacrylate and EVL, the initial success in bleeding control was similar in both groups, while there was less rebleeding in the group treated with variceal

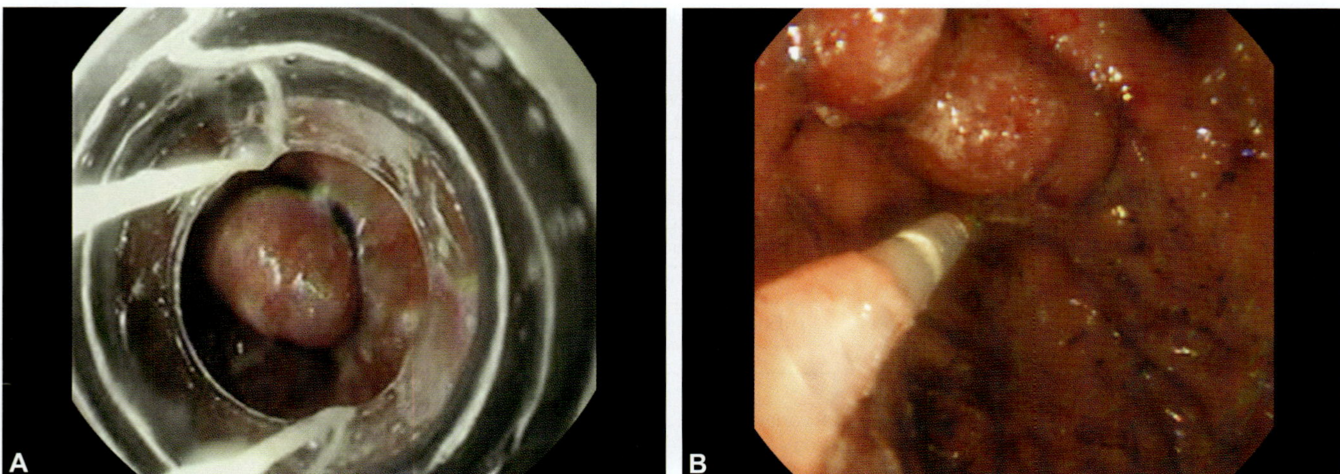

Figs. 73.7A and B: Endoscopic therapy for variceal bleeding. (A) Endoscopic variceal ligation of esophageal varices. (B) Variceal obturation with N-butyl-2-cyanoacrylate for gastric variceal bleeding.

obturation with glue.[50] When glue or expertise is not available, then transjugular intrahepatic portosystemic shunt (TIPSS) should be considered as the initial treatment of bleeding gastric varices.[41]

Rescue Therapy

Transjugular Intrahepatic Portosystemic Shunt: A TIPSS is a portacaval shunt performed using interventional techniques. The hepatic vein is first cannulated by a transjugular approach. A needle is advanced under fluoroscopic or sonographic guidance from the hepatic vein through the liver parenchyma to a branch of the portal vein. A guidewire is next advanced into the superior mesenteric vein. An angioplasty balloon is passed over the guidewire to expand the liver parenchyma. Finally, a self-expanding metal stent is placed to connect the hepatic vein to the portal vein. Successful shunting is confirmed by lowering of portal pressure and flow of radiologic contrast from the portal vein through the shunt into the systemic circulation.

Transjugular intrahepatic portosystemic shunt is widely accepted as one of the salvage therapies for unsuccessful endoscopic control of variceal bleeding. In patients with bleeding gastric varices, TIPSS should be the first-line therapy for bleeding gastric varices when endoscopic variceal obturation with glue is not available.[41] The bleeding control rate is more than 90% in uncontrolled bleeding from gastric varices.[41] A prospective study reported equal efficacy of emergency TIPSS placement for both gastric variceal bleeding and esophageal variceal bleeding.[51]

Hepatic encephalopathy and TIPSS stenosis over time have been two major concerns after treatment. Hepatic encephalopathy occurs in 25–35% of patients after TIPSS placement.[52] Patients who develop severe encephalopathy may require a narrower stent to reduce the size of the shunt or total occlusion of the first stent. Stent occlusion or stenosis by thrombosis occurs in about half the patients within 2 years after TIPSS creation with bare metal stent-grafts.[53] A newer polytetrafluoroethylene-covered stent graft has been reported to increase TIPSS patency, with patency rates greater than 70% in 2 years.[54,55]

Despite the two aforementioned concerns, TIPSS offers an excellent temporary treatment for potential orthotopic liver transplant recipients as it does not interfere with the extrahepatic anatomy and the portal system.[56]

Balloon Tamponade: Balloon tamponade is considered a temporary bridge to more definitive therapy for control of variceal bleeding when primary endoscopic hemostasis fails or expertise for emergency TIPSS placement is not available.[41] Several designs of equipment are available: Sengstaken–Blakemore tube, Minnesota tube, and Linton–Nachlas tube. The patient should be admitted to the intensive care unit with intubation for airway protection before insertion of the balloon tamponade system. The inflation of the balloon generally should not exceed 24 hours. The rebleeding rate is high after balloon deflation. Complications of balloon tamponade include aspiration pneumonia, esophageal perforation, tissue necrosis, and acute laryngeal obstruction.

Surgical Treatment

Operative treatment may be necessary if rebleeding occurs soon after nonoperative treatment. The mortality

Table 73.2 Surgical procedures for the treatment of variceal hemorrhage.

Procedure	Advantages	Disadvantages
Nonshunt procedures		
Esophageal transection	Controls active bleeding	High rebleeding rate
Sugiura procedure	No encephalopathy; preserve hepatic perfusion	Inconsistent results
Nonselective shunts		
End-to-side portacaval shunt	Low rebleeding rate	Encephalopathy
Side-to-side portacaval shunt	Low rebleeding rate	Liver hypoperfusion
Mesocaval shunt (H-graft)	Low rebleeding rate	Shunt thrombosis
Proximal splenorenal shunt plus splenectomy	Low rebleeding rate	Infection
Selective shunt		
Distal splenorenal shunt	Few develop encephalopathy	Technically more difficult
Liver transplantation	Best outcome	Immunosuppression

and morbidity rates of operation in patients with acute variceal hemorrhage is high because most of them are high-risk surgical candidates who have advanced and complicated liver disease. Surgical therapies for variceal bleeding can be classified into four groups (Table 73.2): esophageal transection, nonselective shunting, selective shunting, and orthotopic liver transplantation.

Esophageal Transection: Transection of the esophagus is an effective method for controlling active variceal bleeding. The procedure is performed via a left subcostal approach. The left hemiliver is retracted and the esophagus is mobilized. A staple gun is passed into the distal esophagus through a gastrostomy. The esophagus is transected. A complete ring of about 1 cm is removed, and the two ends are reanastomosed by the stapler. Care should be taken to avoid injuring the vagus nerves. The success rate is comparable to that of sclerotherapy.[57] However, rebleeding eventually occurs in 50% of patients after simple esophageal transection without devascularization.

The Sugiura operation incorporates esophageal transection with devascularization procedures: division of the coronary vein, splenectomy, pyloroplasty, and devascularization of the distal 8–10 cm of esophagus plus the greater and lesser curve of the stomach. This procedure has produced excellent results in Japan, but these have been difficult to reproduce in other countries.[58]

Nonselective Shunting: Most surgeons do not use shunt surgery as treatment for acute variceal hemorrhage.[59] However, shunting is the best way to prevent rebleeding. The most effective shunt for portal decompression is an end-to-side portacaval shunt. This is also the easiest shunt to perform technically. A side-to-side portacaval shunt requires mobilization of the portal vein and, sometimes, interposition of a vascular prosthesis (H-graft).

Both types of portacaval shunt produce total diversion of hepatopedal portal venous blood to the inferior vena cava and decompression of the splanchnic circulation. A side-to-side portacaval shunt may also steal blood retrogradely from the hepatic artery, causing further deprivation of hepatic perfusion. A small side-to-side portacaval H-graft (8-mm diameter) may provide a controlled decompression of the portal circulation, reducing the risk of hepatic encephalopathy.

A mesocaval shunt is performed by transposing a vascular prosthesis between the superior mesenteric vein and the inferior vena cava. It functions much like a side-to-side portacaval shunt. Its use is usually limited to patients who have a thrombosed portal vein in whom the superior mesenteric vein remains patent. It may also be helpful in patients in whom the approach to the porta hepatis may be too bloody and hazardous due to previous cholecystectomy or gastrectomy. A mesocaval shunt may be complicated by problems with graft kinking, occlusion of the superior mesenteric vein, clotting and infection of the prosthesis.

A proximal splenorenal shunt involves anastomosis of the proximal splenic vein to the left renal vein together with splenectomy. The risk of shunt thrombosis is high because the proximal splenic vein is usually of small caliber. Splenectomy also increases the risk of overwhelming infection in children.

Selective Shunting: The distal splenorenal shunt aims to selectively decompress the variceal channels while maintaining the high pressure and hepatopedal blood flow in the rest of the portal system. It involves anastomosis of the distal end (splenic end) of the divided splenic vein to the left renal vein and ligation of all collateral pathways between the gastrosplenic circulation and the mesenteric system. However, the shunt will eventually be functionally converted into a side-to-side portacaval shunt as collateral veins develop around the pancreas draining into the distal splenic vein.

Prospective randomized studies have demonstrated that shunting procedures are more effective than endoscopic therapy but do not improve survival.[60,61] Hepatic encephalopathy is more common after all types of shunting procedures but seems to be less of a problem with distal splenorenal shunts.[62]

Orthotopic Liver Transplantation: Liver transplantation is the only treatment that changes the natural history of portal hypertension and prolongs patient survival.[63] Liver transplantation cannot be carried out if there is acute variceal bleeding, but it is the best treatment to prevent rebleeding from varices. Potential candidates for liver transplantation should not be given portacaval shunts as they jeopardize the chance of successful transplantation.

LOWER GASTROINTESTINAL BLEEDING

Diagnosis and Management

Lower GI bleeding arises from a source distal to the ligament of Treitz. It accounts for 10–20% of acute GI bleeding. Common causes include diverticular hemorrhage, angiodysplasia, colonic polyps and carcinoma, Meckel's diverticulum, and inflammatory bowel disease.

Patients who have lower GI bleeding often present with hematochezia. However, bleeding from the proximal colon may also present with melena or a combination of melena and hematochezia. Lower GI bleeding often stops spontaneously. About 10% of patients have more severe bleeding that results in hemodynamic instability and requires urgent treatment.

A detailed history is helpful in diagnosing the cause of GI bleeding. Patients with a chronic history of recurrent bleeding episodes may have angiodysplasia, diverticular bleeding, or inflammatory bowel disease. Abdominal pain is common for patients who have ischemic colitis and Crohn's disease. The presence of a prosthetic aortic graft suggests a possible aortoenteric fistula, and a history of radiotherapy in the pelvic organs suggests radiation colitis/proctitis.

Anoscopy

Patients with hematochezia should be examined by anoscopy (proctoscopy). The finding of an obvious bleeding lesion in the rectum (e.g. hemorrhoid, rectal ulcer, fissure, or tumor) may obviate the need for further investigation.

Colonoscopy

Colonoscopy allows direct examination of the mucosa of the colon and terminal ileum if blood can be evacuated from the bowel. An accurate diagnosis of angiodysplasia, diverticular bleeding, and postpolypectomy bleeding is possible if bleeding continues; however, brisk bleeding may obscure the colonoscopic view. The risk of perforation during urgent colonoscopy is increased if the visibility of the colonic lumen is poor due to torrential bleeding and poor bowel preparation.

Urgent colonoscopy provides potential therapeutic intervention for actively bleeding lesions. If urgent colonoscopy is considered, an oral bowel purge with polyethylene glycol is recommended.[64,65] The diagnostic yield of colonoscopy in severe hematochezia ranges from 48% to 90%.[65] If a bleeding site is identified but hemostasis cannot be achieved endoscopically, localization of the bleeding site by placement of endoclips or injection of tattoo during colonoscopy may aid subsequent management of bleeding by angiographic embolization or operation.

Selective Visceral Angiography

Selective visceral angiography is most often used for patients who have a brisk GI hemorrhage when endoscopy fails to identify the precise location of the bleeding. Angiographic diagnosis of acute GI bleeding is based upon direct visualization of contrast extravasation into the intestinal lumen (Figs. 73.8A and B). The small bowel and colon receive their blood supply from branches of the superior and inferior mesenteric arteries. The rectum and anus receive their blood supply from the superior hemorrhoidal branches of the inferior mesenteric, the middle hemorrhoidal branches of the internal iliac, and the inferior hemorrhoidal branches of the internal pudendal arteries. These are the vessels that need careful examination in angiography.

The most common causes of lower GI bleeding diagnosed by angiography are diverticular bleeding and angiodysplasia.[66] As GI bleeding is often intermittent, the timing of angiography is important. Patients must be bleeding actively as the contrast injection is given, and the rate of bleeding has to be at least 0.5 mL/min for successful location of the source of bleeding.[67] Patients who have slower bleeding are more likely to have a positive result with scintigraphy.

Angiography may reveal abnormal vasculature even if extravasation of contrast is not seen. As the feeding vessels to the bleeding lesion can go into spasm at the time

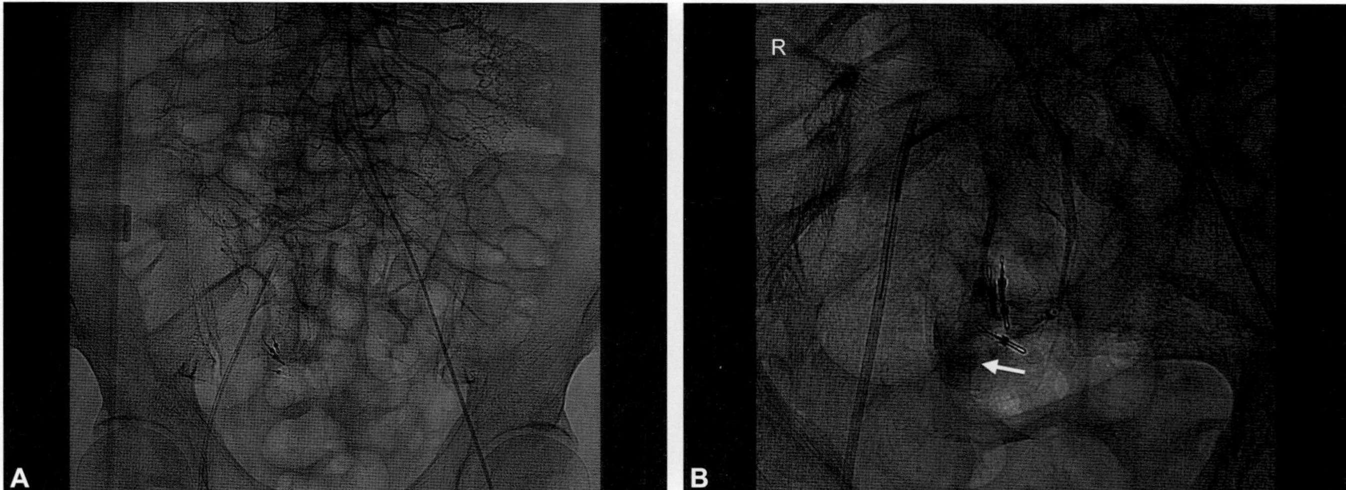

Figs. 73.8A and B: Selective visceral angiography. (A) Arteriogram of superior mesenteric artery initially did not show obvious contrast extravasation in a patient with GI bleeding from the distal ileum found on retrograde push enteroscopy. (B) Superselective catheterization of the small branches of the ileocolic artery (guided by location of hemoclips placed during retrograde push enteroscopy) showed contrast extravasation in distal ileum (arrow).

of bleeding, making the abnormal vasculature invisible on angiography, repeating the procedure with recurrent episodes of GI bleeding may increase the diagnostic yield of this investigation.[68]

Arterial embolization of the bleeding vessel can also be used to control GI bleeding and is useful for life-threatening lower GI bleeding in patients with comorbidities that are considered to contraindicate operation. Bowel ischemia is the most serious potential complication after mesenteric embolization, but superselective cannulation of the bleeding vessel can minimize this complication. A recent long-term outcome study reported that if extravasation of contrast into the gut lumen was identified, angiographic embolization was often effective with a relatively low rate of ischemic complication (10%).[69] However, not all urgent angiographic examinations are diagnostic. Another recent study reported that only 47% of patients with lower GI bleeding had angiography showing a source of bleeding.[70]

Scintigraphy

Nuclear scintigraphy is a sensitive noninvasive study for detecting active GI bleeding. Two techniques are available: technetium-99m sulfur colloid scan and technetium-99m-labeled red cell scan.[71]

A technetium-99m sulfur colloid scan is highly sensitive and detects bleeding as slow as 0.1 mL/min. The test is specific in diagnosing GI bleeding. If the test is positive, there is an excellent chance that the bleeding site can be localized by angiography.[72] However, the patient must be actively bleeding at the time of study as technetium-99m sulfur colloid is rapidly cleared from the bloodstream. A bleeding site near the liver and spleen may be obscured by the overlying activity of these organs.

As red blood cells are not readily cleared from the circulation, a technetium-99m-labeled red cell scan allows imaging for an extended period (Figs. 73.9A to C). This technique may reveal intermittent bleeding, but at the cost of reduced sensitivity. Furthermore, when extravasation is noted only on delayed images, it is difficult to determine the origin of the bleeding because blood moves in both an antegrade and retrograde direction in the gut. Vascular organs such as liver, spleen, and kidney may also interfere with the study.

A technetium-99m pertechnetate scan, also called Meckel's scan, is a useful tool in the investigation of lower GI bleeding in those <30 years of age. An intravenous administration of technetium-99m pertechnetate is concentrated and then excreted by mucus-producing cells of the gastric mucosa. Meckel's diverticulum, which is usually found in the distal ileum, is revealed as an area of increased uptake of technetium-99m in the right lower quadrant of the abdomen. The specificity of this scan can be improved by pentagastrin stimulation.[73]

Computed Tomography and Barium Studies

Modern multidetector CT may be helpful for the diagnosis of an aortoenteric fistula in selected patients with severe

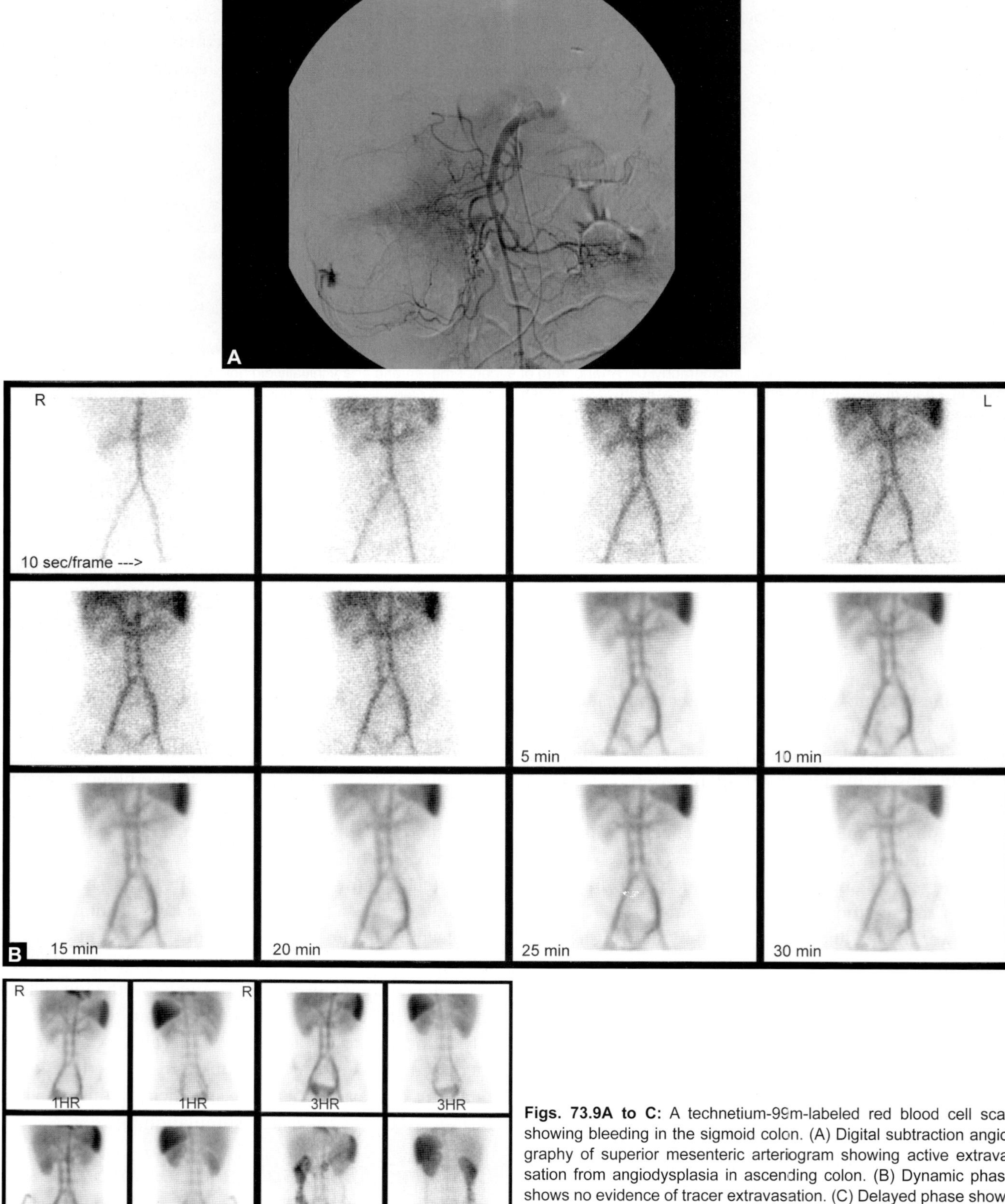

Figs. 73.9A to C: A technetium-99m-labeled red blood cell scan showing bleeding in the sigmoid colon. (A) Digital subtraction angiography of superior mesenteric arteriogram showing active extravasation from angiodysplasia in ascending colon. (B) Dynamic phase shows no evidence of tracer extravasation. (C) Delayed phase shows tracer extravasation that outlines the caecum and ascending colon. Image courtesy of Professor S Yu.

vascular disease (e.g. known abdominal aortic aneurysm) and persistent severe hematochezia, if colonoscopy and push enteroscopy do not identify a bleeding site.

Barium studies of the colon have little to offer in the diagnosis of acute lower GI bleeding. Diagnoses such as diverticular bleeding and angiodysplasia are often missed by barium enema. Radiologic changes of ischemic colitis, ulcerative colitis, and irradiation colitis are difficult to distinguish from each other without histologic proof. Barium left in the colon precludes the use of angiography.

Emergency Surgery

Surgical intervention should be considered if patients have persistent shock despite resuscitation, a large transfusion requirement, severe active bleeding with no diagnosis on endoscopy, or bleeding that cannot be controlled by endoscopy or angiography.[65]

Diverticular Hemorrhage

Diverticulosis is common in elderly people. Colonic diverticula are false or pseudodiverticula consisting of mucosa and serosa with no intervening muscular coat. They are acquired with advancing age and are most commonly found in the sigmoid and descending colon. In Asia, however, right-sided diverticula are more common.[74] At least 80% of individuals with diverticulosis never present with symptoms. Diverticular bleeding presents as a painless rectal bleed, which can be massive and lead to hypovolemic shock. Spontaneous cessation of bleeding occurs in 80% of patients. Urgent colonoscopy after rapid bowel purge should be attempted first, if possible, since stigmas of recent hemorrhage on a diverticulum may sometimes be identified and treated endoscopically with clipping or cautery. Radionuclide scan and angiography may locate the site of bleeding, for which selective embolization may be performed. If the bleeding fails to stop, surgical resection of the bleeding bowel loop is necessary. It should be performed only after the site of bleeding has been identified. Diverticular bleeding can arise from the right or left colon; therefore, a "blind" hemicolectomy should be avoided.

Angiodysplasia

Angiodysplasia is a vascular lesion of the digestive tract that accounts for about 6% of cases of lower GI bleeding.[75] In most cases, it is detected in the cecum and ascending colon, but in about 30% of cases the lesions are found in the small intestine. Macroscopically, they appear as a cluster of cherry spots or fern-like vascular lesions.

Histologically, angiodysplasia consists of dilated thin-walled vascular channels in the mucosa or submucosa of the intestinal wall. The cause is unknown, but most cases are probably acquired as a result of degenerative processes of aging. It has been claimed that angiodysplasia occurs more frequently in patients with renal failure, von Willebrand's disease, pulmonary disease, and aortic stenosis, but these associations are mostly unsubstantiated.

The natural history of angiodysplasia is incompletely understood. Most patients present with recurrent, but often mild, bleeding, which usually stops by the time the patients arrive in hospital.[76] In those few patients who have brisk bleeding, angiography may demonstrate extravasation of contrast.

Symptomatic angiodysplasia is often treated by endoscopic methods such as argon plasma coagulation, heater probe, and bipolar cautery, with satisfactory results and low complication rates.[65,76] If symptomatic angiodysplasia is refractory to endoscopic therapy, surgical resection of the involved bowel segment can be considered.

Meckel's Diverticulum

Meckel's diverticulum is the most common congenital anomaly of the GI tract, occurring in 1–3% of the population; it is caused by failure of the vitelline (omphalomesenteric) duct to obliterate completely. Meckel's diverticulum is a blind-ended segment of intestine usually found at the antimesenteric border of the ileum within 100 cm of the ileocecal valve. It derives its blood supply from the superior mesenteric artery. About half of all cases contain ectopic gastric epithelium.

Most Meckel's diverticula remain asymptomatic. Bleeding is the most common complication as a result of peptic ulceration adjacent to the ectopic gastric mucosa. The most common presentation is painless dark-red colored (redcurrant jelly) stool in patients <30 years of age. The diagnosis is best confirmed by Meckel's scan, or angiography if actively bleeding. Surgical resection is the treatment of choice.

GASTROINTESTINAL BLEEDING OF OBSCURE ORIGIN

Obscure GI bleeding refers to bleeding of unknown origin that persists or recurs after initial negative upper endoscopy and colonoscopy.[77] Because upper endoscopy and colonoscopy usually provide a detailed examination of the esophagus, stomach, duodenum, and colon, bleeding that

Flowchart 73.3: Suggested algorithm for overt obscure gastrointestinal bleeding.

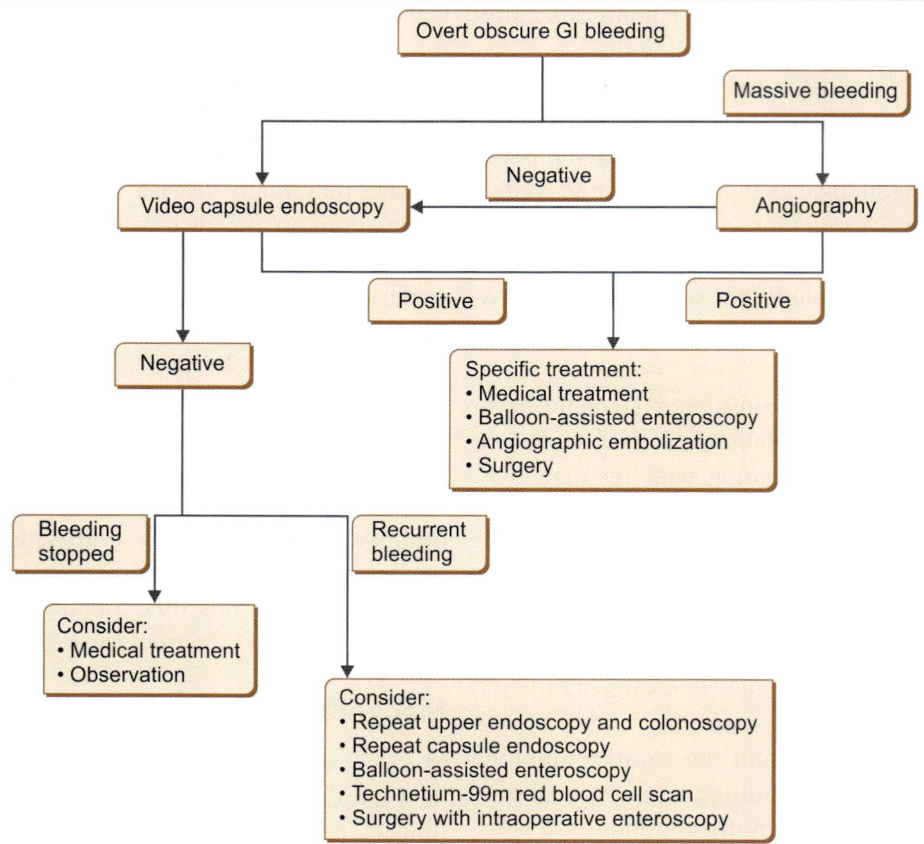

is unidentified after these procedures is likely to originate from the small intestine. The presentation of obscure GI bleeding may be overt or occult. The discussion below will focus on management of overt obscure GI bleeding.

In patients with obscure GI bleeding, missed lesions in the upper GI tract or colon during prior endoscopies are possible. Repeat upper endoscopy and/or colonoscopy should be considered in the initial evaluation if clinical presentation suggests. Push enteroscopy with passage of a pediatric colonoscope into the jejunum could be helpful if lesion in the proximal 60-80 cm of the jejunum is suspected. The diagnostic yield for push enteroscopy ranges from 24–56%.[77,78]

Small bowel video capsule endoscopy (VCE) allows visualization of the entire small bowel and may guide subsequent management decision (e.g. the route of balloon-assisted enteroscopy). A meta-analysis of 14 prospective studies comparing VCE and push enteroscopy or small bowel follow-through showed a significantly higher diagnostic yield for VCE (56% in VCE vs. 26% in push enteroscopy and 6% in small bowel follow-through).[79] In a study comparing VCE with CT angiography and standard angiography, VCE was reported to detect more sources of bleeding than the other two modalities.[80] Rebleeding rate in patients with a negative VCE was reported to be low.[81]

Deep enteroscopy can be achieved by balloon-assisted enteroscopy (the double balloon or single balloon systems), or enteroscopy with a spiral overtube.[77] When balloon-assisted enteroscopy system is used, total enteroscopy is possible by combining the antegrade and retrograde approaches. When compared to VCE, deep enteroscopy has the benefit of therapeutic and tissue sampling potential. Findings on VCE can be used to guide the initial route of deep enteroscopy.

If the bleeding rate is more than 0.5 mL/min, then selective visceral angiography may be helpful, with the potential for embolization of the bleeding vessel. Computed tomographic angiography is an alternative, but it lacks the therapeutic potential. Scintigraphy can be considered if the bleeding rate is at least 0.1 mL/min. Although sensitive, scintigraphy may only be able to provide a general location of the possible bleeding point.

If the source of bleeding is still unclear in patients with massive overt obscure GI bleeding despite evaluation by the aforementioned modalities, then intraoperative enteroscopy during laparotomy should be performed. At laparotomy, gross examination by inspection, palpation, and transillumination of the intestine against strong light will often help to identify the site of bleeding. Intraoperative enteroscopy is very useful for locating the source of bleeding before resection.[82,83] The endoscope can be passed through the anus or the mouth. The tip of the endoscope is guided up from the colon or down from the duodenum into the small intestine by the surgeon, who telescopes the bowel onto the endoscope. The bowel should be manipulated gently by the surgeon to avoid mucosal trauma. The endoscopist should try to keep the bowel lumen in the center of the endoscopic view. After the endoscope has been fully inserted, the room light is switched off. The lumen of the intestine is examined by the endoscopist, while the external surface of the transilluminated bowel is inspected simultaneously by the surgeon. A proposed algorithm for investigating overt obscure GI bleeding is given in Flowchart 73.3.

REFERENCES

1. Silverstein FE, Gilbert DA, Tedesco FJ, et al. The National ASGE survey on upper gastrointestinal bleeding I. Study design and baseline data. Gastrointest Endosc. 1981;27:73-9.
2. Silverstein FE, Gilbert DA, Tedesco FJ, et al. The National ASGE survey on upper gastrointestinal bleeding II. Clinical prognostic factors. Gastrointest Endosc. 1981;27:80-93.
3. Rockall T, Logan R, Devlin H, et al. Incidence and mortality from acute upper gastrointestinal haemorrhage in the United Kingdom. BMJ. 1995;311:222-6.
4. Lau JY, Barkun A, Fan DM, et al. Challenges in the management of acute peptic ulcer bleeding. Lancet. 2013;381(9882):2033-43.
5. Marshall BJ, Warren JR. Unidentified curved bacilli in the stomach of patients with gastritis and peptic ulceration. Lancet. 1984;323:1311-15.
6. Malfertheiner P, Megraud F, O'Morain CA, et al. Management of Helicobacter pylori infection: the Maastricht IV/ Florence Consensus Report. Gut. 2012;61(5): 646-64.
7. Gabriel SE, Jaakkimainen L, Bombardier C. Risk for serious gastrointestinal complications related to use of nonsteroidal anti-inflammatory drugs. A meta-analysis. Ann Intern Med. 1991;115:787-96.
8. Garcia Rodriguez LA, Barreales TL. Risk of upper gastrointestinal complications among users of traditional NSAIDs and COXIBs in the general population. Gastroenterology. 2007;132:498-506.
9. Wang YR, Richter JE, Dempsey DT. Trends and outcomes of hospitalization for peptic ulcer disease in the United States, 1993–2006. Ann Surg. 2010;251:251-8.
10. Hearnshaw SA, Logan RFA, Palmer KR, et al. Outcomes following early red blood transfusion in acute upper gastrointestinal hemorrhage. Aliment Pharmacol Ther. 2010;32:215-24.
11. Villanueva C, Colomo A, Bosch A, et al. Transfusion strategies for acute upper gastrointestinal bleeding. N Engl J Med. 2013;368:11-21.
12. Sung JJ, Lau JY, Ching JY, et al. Continuation of low-dose aspirin therapy in peptic ulcer bleeding: a randomized trial. Ann Intern Med. 2010;152:1-9.
13. Rockall TA, Logan RF, Devlin HB, et al. Risk assessment after acute upper gastrointestinal hemorrhage. Gut. 1996;38:316-21.
14. Blatchford O, Murray WR, Blatchford M. A risk score to predict need for treatment for upper gastrointestinal hemorrhage. Lancet. 2000;356:1318-21.
15. Cook DJ, Guyatt GH, Salena BJ, et al. Endoscopic therapy for acute non-variceal upper gastrointestinal hemorrhage: a meta-analysis. Gastroenterology. 1992;102:139-48.
16. Lin HJ, Wang K, Perng CL, et al. Early or delayed endoscopy for patients with peptic ulcer bleeding: a prospective randomized study. J Clin Gastroenterol. 1996;22:267-71.
17. Spiegel BMR, Vakil NB, Ofman JJ. Endoscopy for acute nonvariceal upper gastrointestinal tract hemorrhage: is sooner better? A systematic review. Arch Intern Med. 2001;161:1393-404.
18. Bjorkman DJ, Zaman A, Fennerty MB, et al. Urgent vs. elective endoscopy for acute non-variceal upper-GI bleeding: an effectiveness study. Gastrointest Endosc. 2004;60:1-8.
19. Swain CP, Storey DW, Bown SG, et al. Nature of the bleeding vessel in recurrently bleeding gastric ulcers. Gastroenterology. 1986;90:595-608.
20. Swain CP, Lai KC, Kalabakas A, et al. A comparison of size and pathology of vessel and ulcer in patients dying from bleeding gastric and duodenal ulcers [Abstract]. Gastroenterology. 1993;104:A202.
21. National Institutes of Health Consensus Conference. Therapeutic endoscopy and bleeding ulcers. JAMA. 1989;262:1369-72.
22. Fleischer D. Etiology and prevalence of severe persistent upper gastrointestinal bleeding. Gastroenterology. 1983;84:538-43.
23. Forrest JAH, Finlayson NDC, Shearman DJC. Endoscopy of upper gastrointestinal bleeding. Lancet. 1974;ii:394-7.
24. Laine L, Peterson WL. Bleeding peptic ulcer. N Engl J Med. 1994;331:717-27.
25. Kovacs TO, Jensen DM. Complications of peptic ulcer disease. In: Dimarino AJ, Jr, Benjamin SB (Eds). Gastrointestinal Disease: An Endoscopic Approach. Thorofare, NJ: Slack; 2002. pp. 411-38.
26. Sreedharan A, Martin J, Leontiadis GI, et al. Proton pump inhibitor treatment initiated prior to endoscopic diagnosis in upper gastrointestinal bleeding. Cochrane Database Syst Rev. 2010;7:CD005415.
27. Lau JY, Sung JJ, Lee KK, et al. Effects of intravenous omeprazole on recurrent bleeding after endoscopic treatment of bleeding peptic ulcers. N Engl J Med. 2000;343:310-6.
28. Leontiadis GI, McIntyre L, Sharma VK, et al. Proton pump inhibitor treatment for acute peptic ulcer bleeding. Cochrane Database Syst Rev. 2006;1:CD002094.

29. Sung JJ, Barkun A, Kuipers EJ, et al. Intravenous esomeprazole for prevention of recurrent peptic ulcer bleeding: a randomized trial. Ann Intern Med. 2009;150(7):455-64.
30. Jensen DM, Kovacs TO, Jutabha R, et al. Randomized trial of medical or endoscopic therapy to prevent recurrent ulcer hemorrhage in patients with adherent clots. Gastroenterology. 2002;123:407-13.
31. Santander C, Gravalos RG, Cedenilla AG, et al. Maintenance treatment versus Helicobacter pylori eradication therapy in preventing rebleeding of the peptic ulcer disease. A clinical trial and follow-up for 2 years. Am J Gastroenterol. 1996;91:1549-52.
32. Sung JJY, SCS Chung, Leung VKS, et al. H. pylori eradication or maintenance H2-blockade in preventing recurrent ulcer bleeding [Abstract]. Gastrointest Endosc. 1996;43:A273.
33. Hwang JH, Fisher DA, Ben-Menachem, et al. ASGE guideline: the role of endoscopy in the management of acute non-variceal upper GI bleeding. Gastrointest Endosc. 2012;75(6):1132-8.
34. Calvet X, Vergara M, Brullet E, et al. Addition of a second endoscopic treatment following epinephrine injection improves outcome in high risk bleeding ulcers. Gastroenterology. 2004;126:441-50.
35. Sung JJ, Chung SC, Low J, et al. Systemic absorption of epinephrine after submucosal injection in patients with bleeding peptic ulcers. Gastrointest Endosc. 1993;39:20-2.
36. Kovacs TO, Jensen DM. Endoscopic treatment of ulcer bleeding. Curr Treat Options Gastroenterol. 2007;10:143-8.
37. Sung JJ, Luo D, Wu JC, et al. Early clinical experience of the safety and effectiveness of Hemospray in achieving hemostasis in patients with acute peptic ulcer bleeding. Endoscopy. 2011;43(4):291-5.
38. Wong TC, Wong KT, Chiu PW, et al. A comparison of angiographic embolization with surgery after failed endoscopic hemostasis to bleeding peptic ulcers. Gastrointest Endosc. 2011;73:900-8.
39. Morris DL, Hawker PC, Brearley S, et al. Optimal timing of operation for bleeding peptic ulcer: prospective randomized trial. Br Med J. 1984;288:1277-80.
40. Lebrec D, De Fleury P, Rueff B, et al. Portal hypertension, size of esophageal varices, and risk of gastrointestinal bleeding in alcoholic cirrhosis. Gastroenterology. 1980;79:1139-44.
41. Garcia-Tsao G, Sanyal AJ, Grace ND, et al. Prevention and management of gastroesophageal varices and variceal hemorrhage in cirrhosis. Hepatology. 2007;46(3):922-8.
42. D'Amico G, Pagliaro L, Bosch J. Pharmacological treatment of portal hypertension: an evidence-based approach. Semin Liver Dis. 1999;19:475-505.
43. The North Italian Endoscopic Club for the Study and Treatment of Esophageal Varices. Prediction of the first variceal hemorrhage in patients with cirrhosis of the liver and esophageal varices. A prospective multicenter study. N Engl J Med. 1988;319:983-9.
44. D'Amico G, de Franchis R. Upper digestive bleeding in cirrhosis. Posttherapeutic outcome and prognostic indicators. Hepatology. 2003;38:599-612.
45. Carbonell N, Pauwels A, Serfaty L, et al. Improved survival after variceal bleeding in patients with cirrhosis over the past two decades. Hepatology. 2004;40:652-9.
46. Graham DY, Smith J. The course of patients after variceal hemorrhage. Gastroenterology. 1981;80:800-9.
47. D'Amico G, Pietrosi G, Tarantino I, et al. Emergency sclerotherapy versus vasoactive drugs for variceal bleeding in cirrhosis: a Cochrane meta-analysis. Gastroenterology. 2003; 124:1277-91.
48. Bernard B, Grange JD, Khac EN, et al. Antibiotic prophylaxis for the prevention of bacterial infections in cirrhotic patients with gastrointestinal bleeding: a meta-analysis. Hepatology. 1999;29:1655-61.
49. Villanueva C, Piqueras M, Aracil C, et al. A randomized controlled trial comparing ligation and sclerotherapy as emergency endoscopic treatment added to somatostatin in acute variceal bleeding. J Hepatol. 2006;45:560-7.
50. Tan PC, Hou MC, Lin HC, et al. A randomized trial of endoscopic treatment of acute gastric variceal hemorrhage: N-butyl-2-cyanoacrylate injection versus band ligation. Hepatology. 2006;43:690-7.

Additional references appear in the online version of this book.

74

Acute Abdomen and Peritonitis

Sarah Goodbrand, Chris Deans

Key Points

- Evaluation of the acute abdomen is challenging and should involve experienced clinicians throughout the process.
- Reorganization of emergency surgical services, which includes the creation of a dedicated surgical "emergency team," establishment of a surgical admission unit and timely access to investigations and operating theatres, is associated with improved patient outcomes.
- A standardized approach to the acute abdomen should be followed routinely to identify unwell patients who require urgent resuscitation, operation, and/or critical care input.
- Thorough clinical assessment by means of a detailed history and examination will provide the likely diagnosis in many situations. Appropriate investigations can then be performed to confirm the diagnosis.
- Repeated clinical assessment, keeping an open mind and taking advice from colleagues when necessary, are the hallmarks of a good clinician in the difficult emergency setting.

INTRODUCTION

The "acute abdomen" is a clinical condition characterized by new-onset abdominal pain (and often other abdominal symptoms) that usually arises as a consequence of intra-abdominal pathology, such as infection, perforation, or infarction. The acute abdomen is a common presentation in emergency general surgery and frequently provides diagnostic and management challenges for the clinician. Evaluation of the acute abdomen is often difficult and requires careful initial and repeated clinical assessment, which should be complemented with blood tests and radiological investigations (and other investigations) where necessary.

The decision-making process relating to the acute abdomen may be challenging, especially when deciding whether or not the patient requires emergency operation. The emergency laparotomy network in the United Kingdom has demonstrated that the 30-day mortality rate from emergency surgery is in the region of 15% for all patient groups[1]; therefore, the decision to operate must be certain to be of clear benefit. For the emergency surgeon, these problems are likely to increase as numbers of acute hospital admissions continue to rise and patient expectations increase.[2] In addition, there are challenges of an increasing aging patient population: many patients now present with increasing complexity related to coexisting medical conditions that have to be managed during the acute episode. Retrospective studies have shown that older patients are twice as likely to undergo surgical intervention following emergency admission, with associated higher morbidity and mortality rates, especially in the over-80 age group.[3-5] The mortality rate for emergency surgery in older patients is 24%, with the precipitant likely to be coexisting disease.[1] Other groups that require special consideration are the immunocompromised patient (either as a consequence of disease or medical therapy) and the pregnant patient. In each case, the physiological response and disease presentation may be atypical, and this should be borne in mind during the assessment.

There is little doubt that the challenges of modern emergency surgery are best managed by experienced clinicians who ideally would be working as part of a dedicated "emergency team." There is clear evidence that such teams staffed by senior clinicians who are free from elective duties and other responsibilities provide a safer and higher standard of patient care in the emergency setting, together with improved outcomes.[6]

Reorganization of other hospital departments is also required to maximize the effectiveness of the emergency surgical team. A dedicated surgical admissions area is required to allow rapid assessment of acute admissions and enable repeated clinical assessment of patients by the on-call team. In this way, changes in the clinical status of the patients can be readily detected and promptly managed. Ready access to an appropriately staffed emergency theatre with 24-hour availability is essential to avoid unnecessary delays in accessing, theatre, and it reduces the need for out-of-hours operating.[7] Such theatres should be fully staffed with senior anesthetic colleagues. There must be timely access to radiological investigations, such as ultrasound and computed tomography (CT), along with availability of interventional radiological procedures if required. Critical care support and availability is vital for optimal management of the unwell patient. Finally, appropriate liaison with other colleagues, departments, and subspecialties may be necessary in complex situations.

This chapter describes (1) the general principles surrounding the approach to the "acute abdomen", including the initial assessment of patients and the early management of some of the common causes of the acute abdomen (many of these conditions will be covered in more detail elsewhere in this book); (2) the importance of regular clinical review of patients by the same surgical team; and (3) the pathophysiology underlying the acute abdomen and peritonitis. Understanding these processes enables the clinician to appreciate the clinical relevance of the symptoms and signs displayed by the patient presenting with an acute abdomen.

CAUSES OF ACUTE ABDOMINAL PAIN

Many conditions can present with an acute abdomen. Some of the most common causes (Table 74.1) emerge from an audit of almost 1,200 patients presenting as a general surgery emergency with acute abdominal pain to a UK hospital, and the findings are likely to be representative of other centers in Europe and North America.[8] Acute appendicitis and intestinal obstruction are the most commonly identified conditions, with most other conditions responsible individually for 5% or less. Since urological, gynecological, and vascular causes constitute almost 10% of the causes in total, these conditions should be borne in mind when assessing patients with an acute abdomen. In addition, the patient may have an underlying medical diagnosis, such as a pneumonia or diabetic crisis, which may have been incorrectly interpreted as a surgical abdomen. Advice from other specialists should be sought if these conditions are regarded as the likely diagnosis. What is also evident from these data is that some conditions are more likely in different age groups. As is also shown in Table 74.1, acute appendicitis, abdominal trauma, urological and gynecological causes are commoner in the younger patient (<60 years). Conversely, intestinal obstruction, gallstone-related conditions (including pancreatitis), peptic ulcer disease, diverticular disease, and abdominal malignancy are more likely in the older population (>60 years). The data presented in this chapter exclude children, and the pattern of disease in this age group differs from that of an adult population (*see* Chapter 125, "Gastrointestinal Surgery in Children").

Geographical location is also an important determinant of the likely cause of acute abdominal pain. Certain disease processes are commoner in certain parts of the world and reflect racial and cultural differences in epidemiology of disease. In addition, some conditions may be endemic in certain locations. Table 74.2 lists the causes of acute abdominal pain in patients presenting as an emergency to an African hospital (in Ghana) over a 7-year period.[9] There are some similarities when compared with a UK population. Acute appendicitis and intestinal obstruction are among the commonest causes of acute abdominal pain. In contrast to the UK data, abdominal trauma and perforated peptic ulcer disease are more prevalent, whereas nonspecific abdominal pain (NSAP) and gallstone

Table 74.1 Causes of acute abdominal pain presenting as emergency surgical admissions in the UK.

Diagnosis	*Prevalence (%)*	*Age (years)*
Nonspecific abdominal pain	35	<60
Acute appendicitis	17	<60
Intestinal obstruction	15	>60
Urological	6	<60
Cholelithiasis	5	>60
Diverticular disease	4	>60
Abdominal trauma	3	<60
Abdominal malignancy	3	>60
Peptic ulcer disease	4	>60
Acute pancreatitis	2	>60
Vascular (ruptured aortic aneurysm, mesenteric vascular occlusion)	2	>60
Medical (gastroenteritis, pneumonia, myocardial infarction, etc.)	2	ns
Gynecological	1	<60
Inflammatory bowel disease	1	ns
Miscellaneous	1	ns

Source: Irvin T. Abdominal pain: a surgical audit of 1190 emergency admissions. Br J Surg. 1989;76:1121-5.

Table 74.2 Causes of acute abdominal pain presenting as emergency admissions in Africa [*n* = 3114].

Diagnosis	*Prevalence (%)*
Acute appendicitis	22
Typhoid ileal perforation	16
Intestinal obstruction	13
Perforated peptic ulcer	11
Nonspecific abdominal pain	10
Abdominal trauma	8
Acute cholecystitis	3
Miscellaneous	17

Source: Ohene-Yeboah M. Acute surgical admissions for abdominal pain in adults in Kumasi, Ghana. ANZ J Surg. 2006;76(10):898-903.

disease are less prevalent. Typhoid disease resulting in ileal perforation is endemic to the region and constitutes a common cause of acute abdominal emergencies in this region. Table 74.3 presents the causes of acute abdominal in over 500 patients presenting to a regional hospital in Pakistan.[10] It is important to appreciate that these data exclude abdominal trauma and urological and gynecological emergencies. Although intestinal obstruction is common as in the United Kingdom, tuberculous strictures are responsible for many of these cases as opposed to strangulated hernia and adhesions. Hepatic abscesses are another important cause of acute abdominal pain in Africa, often with an amebic etiology.[11]

Clinicians will become familiar with diseases that are more prevalent within their locale.

Nonspecific Abdominal Pain

Nonspecific abdominal pain is responsible for approximately one third of the causes of acute abdominal pain in Europe and North America and to a lesser extent in other countries (Tables 74.1 to 74.3). The label of NSAP is applied when no diagnosis for the acute abdominal pain has been established. The proportion of patients with this condition will, therefore, be dependent upon the extent of investigation undertaken to establish a diagnosis, given that symptoms will often settle before further investigations are undertaken and a diagnosis has been achieved. In some instances, NSAP is functional; some studies have shown an association with other functional conditions such as irritable bowel syndrome.[12] Another study identified gluten sensitivity in 10% of patients labeled with NSAP.[13] A subsequent gluten exclusion diet was associated with resolution of symptoms. The authors propose that all patients with a diagnosis of NSAP should undergo celiac

Table 74.3 Causes of acute abdominal pain presenting as emergency admissions in Pakistan (excluding abdominal trauma) [*n* = 586].

Diagnosis	*Prevalence (%)*
Acute appendicitis	35
Intestinal obstruction (including TB strictures)	28
GI tract perforation (peptic ulcer, typhoid, etc.)	23
Acute cholecystitis	7
Hepatic abscess	5

Source: Memon A, Bhutto A, Shaikh G, et al. Spectrum of diseases in patients with nontraumatic acute abdomen. J Liaquat Univ Med Health Sci. 2008;180-83.

Box 74.1 Possible causes of nonspecific abdominal pain.

- Gluten enteropathy/food intolerance
- Functional bowel disorders (e.g., irritable bowel syndrome)
- Viral infections
- Abdominal wall pain (e.g., peripheral neuralgia and costochondritis)
- Psychosomatic pain

serology testing. Other conditions implicated as possible causes of NSAP are listed in Box 74.1 and include viral infections, abdominal wall pain, and psychosomatic conditions.[14]

The principal concern with the term NSAP is missing underlying serious pathology. Several studies have investigated longer-term outcomes of patients with an original diagnosis of NSAP. Jess and colleagues followed 230 patients for 5 years and found that 77% of patients were healthy and symptom free,[15] while the others had further admissions with abdominal complaints and 1% of patients (4% of patients over 50 years of age) were subsequently diagnosed with a malignant condition. Another group similarly followed 104 patients for 5 years following a diagnosis of NSAP and found that 28% of patients had recurring abdominal pain 5 years after the initial presentation.[16] No patients were diagnosed with a malignancy during the study period but the patient population was young, with a median age of 29 years. The use of diagnostic laparoscopy in the investigation of NSAP has been shown to increase the rates of establishing a definitive diagnosis.[17] A recent Cochrane review examined the role of laparoscopy in the management of acute lower abdominal pain in women of reproductive age. The authors concluded that when compared with observation alone, laparoscopy was associated with more diagnoses being made, reduced hospital stay, and earlier return to work.[18] There were no increased adverse events associated with laparoscopy.

It is the authors' view that every reasonable effort should be undertaken to establish a definitive diagnosis for acute abdominal pain in all patients. This is particularly important for those patients with persistent or recurrent symptoms and especially among older patients who are more at risk of serious underlying pathology.

GENERAL APPROACH TO THE ACUTE ABDOMEN

It is crucial to recognize the acutely unwell patient. The clinician has to be able to identify which patients are unwell and would benefit from urgent resuscitation and emergency operation, which patients require urgent resuscitation and critical care, and which only require repeated assessment and delayed investigation. One of the key decisions to be made is whether or not the patient requires an operation.

The initial assessment of an emergency surgical patient should follow the "ABC" principles. By following this, standardized approach of unwell patients may be readily identified and appropriately managed. For those patients who do not require urgent resuscitation, a thorough history and examination should be undertaken. Box 74.2 outlines the primary goals of this stepwise approach to the acute abdomen.

Clinical Assessment

History

A systematic history is the most important tool during the evaluation of the acute abdomen. A carefully taken history improves diagnostic accuracy and reduces the utilization of useless or harmful investigations. The history can be augmented by computer- or algorithm-aided decision making, which has been shown to have a positive impact on reducing hospital admissions, length of hospital stay and perhaps most importantly, unnecessary laparotomies, which can be associated with appreciable morbidity and mortality rates.[19] The introduction of standardized history data collection forms has also been shown to improve diagnostic accuracy by 20% over history taking alone.[20] Some clinical features are highly suggestive of certain conditions and should therefore be sought.

Box 74.2	Primary goals of a stepwise approach to the acute abdomen.
Resuscitate the patient in accordance with "ABC" principles	
Establish a differential diagnosis	
Instigate an appropriate management plan to confirm or refute the above differential diagnosis	
Identify high-risk patient groups	
Ascertain if the patient requires surgery and the timing of such.	
Differentiating those patients who require active observation	
Minimize morbidity and mortality	

Abdominal Pain

Abdominal pain is often the predominant symptom of the acute abdomen. Understanding the physiology underlying the generation of pain is important to appreciate the clinical relevance of the patient's symptoms and signs. Abdominal pain is nociceptive and can be derived in one of three ways:

1. *Somatic*: The parietal peritoneum (which includes the interior surface of the diaphragm) derives sensory fibers from somatic nerves T6 to L1. They are the same nerves that supply the overlying skin and muscle. The central part of the diaphragm is innervated by the phrenic nerve, the peripheral part by the lower six thoracic nerves. Most of the pelvic parietal peritoneum is innervated by the obturator nerve. Unilateral myelinated afferent pain fibers transmit the painful stimulus to specific dorsal root ganglia on the same side and dermatome level as the origin of the pain. The parietal peritoneum is sensitive to pain, temperature, touch, and pressure. Inflammation and ischemia are normally associated with pain arising from the parietal peritoneum, and this is the type of pain associated with peritonitis. Pain from the parietal peritoneum can be localized to the region of the painful stimulus. It is typically sharp, asymmetrical, constant, and aggravated by movement.
2. *Visceral*: The abdominal viscera and its associated peritoneum receive sensory fibers from the T5 to L3 sympathetic chain. Visceral pain fibers are bilateral, unmyelinated, and enter the spinal cord at multiple levels. The sensory fibers are sparse, and thus the cause of visceral pain is secondary to stretching of the muscle fibers or capsule of the organ. Visceral pain is usually vague, diffuse, and can be localized to the epigastrium, mid, or lower abdomen (foregut, midgut, and hindgut distribution).
3. *Referred pain*: This results from the convergence of visceral neurons from different locations entering the spinal cord at the same level as the somatic structures experiencing the pain. Three nerves are of particular

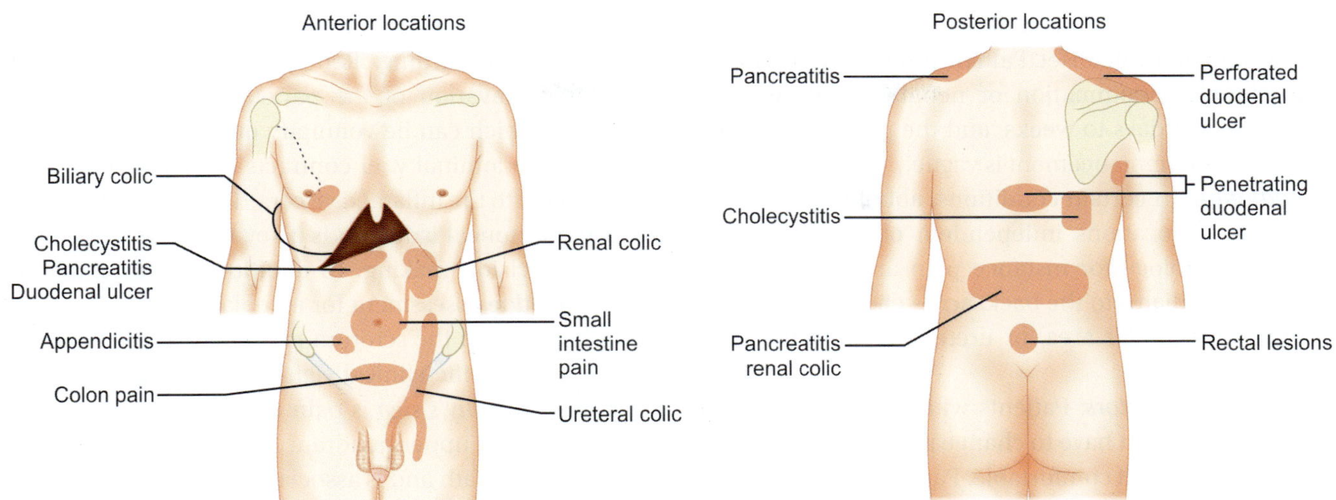

Fig. 74.1: Locations for pain related to conditions causing an acute abdomen. Biliary colic may radiate to the back or shoulder (dotted line).

clinical significance in the assessment of the acute abdomen. Irritation of the diaphragm results in activation of the phrenic nerve and pain is referred to the shoulder (C3–C5). Retroperitoneal pathology such as retrocecal appendicitis or retroperitoneal perforation of the duodenum can result in pain in the labia or testis secondary to irritation of the genitofemoral nerve (L1–L2). An obturator hernia irritates the obturator nerve to produce pain in the medial aspect of the upper thigh (L2–L4).

A number of key questions relating to the features of abdominal pain will help guide the initial appraisal and allow the clinician to formulate a preliminary differential diagnosis.

- *Character*: Many terms can be used to describe abdominal pain. It may be intermittent, constant, dull, cramping, or sharp. Intermittent pain is usually associated with colic, for instance in intestinal obstruction when the bowel contracts vigorously against the obstruction, or in renal colic when the ureter contracts against a stone. It is a misnomer that the pain related to gallstones is colicky, because there is actually no regular peristalsis in the gallbladder, which lacks a strong muscular coat. It is actually perceived as a constant dull pain that can crescendo if an obstructed gallbladder contracts against a large stone impacted in Hartmann's pouch or against a stone within the cystic duct. Constant pain can be correlated with conditions causing ischemia or inflammation of the peritoneum. For instance, the pain from intestinal obstruction will change from intermittent to continuous when ischemia ensues. Dull or aching abdominal pain is associated with distension or edema of the wall of a hollow viscus. Pain from the liver or splenic capsule stretching can also be comprehended in this way.
- *Location*: The localization of pain to certain regions of the abdomen can indicate the potential organs involved (Fig. 74.1). Epigastric pain is associated with structures innervated by T6–T8, including the stomach, duodenum, pancreas, liver, and biliary tree along with the associated parietal peritoneum (foregut). Periumbilical pain can arise from small intestine, appendix, and upper ureters that are innervated from T9 to T10 (midgut). Lower abdominal pain originates from structures innervated by T11 and T12 including the colon, lower ureters, bladder, and uterus (hindgut). Although this general distribution holds true, pain can shift during the patient's presentation as is well exemplified in acute appendicitis. It is, therefore, imperative to ascertain the location of the pain at onset and not just at presentation. The location of pain can also be atypical because of the underlying neuronal and pathological mechanisms, so that the clinician should only use it as an approximate guide to diagnosis.
- *Onset*: Abdominal pain may be of sudden, rapid, or gradual onset. Sudden pain is normally associated with an organ rupturing or giving way, such as a ruptured ovarian cyst, ruptured abdominal aortic aneurysm (AAA), or perforated viscus. The patient can normally recall the exact time and mode of onset. Pain of rapid onset is typically associated with conditions that are not only secondary to inflammation such as appendicitis, diverticulitis, and pancreatitis but also intestinal obstruction. The onset of pain is over seconds to hours.

The patient often finds it difficult to recall the precise time and mode of onset. Pain of gradual onset is linked to chronic inflammation or neoplasms; it generally occurs over days to weeks, and the patient's recollection of its commencement is vague.

- *Radiation*: In certain conditions, abdominal pain will radiate to locations independent of the site of primary pathology for instance pain arising from pancreatitis radiates to the back, acute cholecystitis to the right subscapular area, or ureteric colic to the groin (Fig. 74.1).
- *Aggravating factors*: Patients with colic are unable to lie still and often have to change position frequently in an attempt to get comfortable. Patients with peritonitis will prefer to lie still. Eating may precipitate an episode of biliary colic.

In addition to pain, there may be a number of associated symptoms that should be elicited as part of the history process, for example, constipation and abdominal distension secondary to large bowel obstruction or hematuria secondary to a renal tract calculus. This process should involve not only a detailed assessment of the gastrointestinal system but also a detailed history of the urological and gynecological systems. It is also essential to determine any relevant comorbidities, establish a drug history, and perform a functional assessment by determining performance status in patients who may be of borderline fitness for surgical intervention.

Examination

Following a detailed systematic history, a thorough examination should be undertaken. Steps should initially be taken early to ensure that are no signs of physiological compromise and that the patient is comfortable. There is good evidence to support the early administration of opiate analgesia and to show that it has no impact on further clinical assessment.[21] It is, therefore, no longer acceptable to withhold analgesia from any patient for the purposes of clinical assessment. Initially, the general appearance and the observations should be noted, although the measurement of temperature is relatively nondiscriminatory in the early assessment of the acute abdomen.[22] A full general examination should then be performed, including the cardiovascular, respiratory, and neurological systems in addition to the gastrointestinal and genitourinary systems. The general principles of examination should be followed, namely inspection, palpation, percussion, and auscultation. An exhaustive inspection and palpation of the abdomen is then performed to elicit any signs of rebound tenderness or guarding. Rebound tenderness occurs if there is aggravation of the parietal peritoneum, while guarding (which can be voluntary or involuntary) occurs when the abdominal wall contracts in response to pressure applied to the inflamed viscera. The presence of these signs of peritoneal irritation is a key factor in influencing surgical decision making. In addition, the examination should include assessment for an enlarged bladder, AAA, groin hernia, and the scrotum to exclude a testicular torsion. Some specific clinical signs suggest the underlying diagnosis. *Murphy's sign* is pain that is elicited on palpation in the right upper quadrant (RUQ) when the patient takes a deep breath and is associated with acute cholecystitis. *Rovsing's sign* may be present in acute appendicitis when palpation in the left iliac fossa produces pain in the right iliac fossa. In severe acute pancreatitis, bruising and skin discoloration in the flanks (Grey Turner's sign) or around the umbilicus (Cullen's sign) reflect retroperitoneal hemorrhage.

It is the authors' opinion that a routine rectal examination in all patients with an acute abdomen adds little to the clinical assessment unless there is a specific indication, such as evaluating rectal bleeding or palpating for a pelvic collection.[23]

Investigations

Timely investigations are arranged to aid the diagnostic process and confirm or refute the differentials. Appropriate access to the necessary tests is essential and likewise senior interpretation of scans and other results where applicable. It is important that surgical treatment is not delayed at the expense of performing needless or even potentially harmless investigations.

Blood Tests

Although individual blood tests have a limited influence on decision making in the acute abdomen, individual results are helpful as baseline references and trends over time may be monitored as the clinical condition changes.[24] A full blood count will show a low hemoglobin that requires correction prior to surgical intervention. Leukocytosis (raised white cell count) supports the presence of infection or inflammation. Serum urea and electrolytes are essential in patients who may be hypovolemic and require fluid and electrolyte replacement. Liver function tests (LFTs) are often useful in the decision making of acute hepatobiliary disease and may suggest either obstructive or

Table 74.4 Conditions that may be associated with elevated serum amylase concentration.

Pancreatic disease	Acute pancreatitis Pancreatic trauma Pancreatic cancer
Intra-abdominal pathology	Bowel obstruction Peptic ulcer disease Acute cholecystitis Appendicitis Mesenteric ischemia
Medical conditions	Pneumonia Myocardial infarction Renal failure Diabetic crisis
Malignancy	Lung Ovary Breast
Head injury	
Drugs	Ciprofloxacin, aspirin, codeine
Macroamylasemia	

hepatocellular etiology. Serum amylase is probably the one blood investigation with true diagnostic value. Elevated serum amylase concentrations may be diagnostic of acute pancreatitis, but lesser values may be nonspecific and may be elevated due to other conditions that are listed in Table 74.4. It is also possible that serum amylase concentration may have returned to within the normal range after 48 hours of onset of acute pancreatitis and the diagnostic "peak" will be missed. In these circumstances, urinary amylase or lipase may be diagnostic or cross-sectional imaging may be of value.

Inflammatory markers, such as C-reactive protein (CRP), suggest infection or inflammations and have some value in monitoring response to treatment and disease progression. There is evidence that monitoring trends in serum CRP concentrations improves prognostication in patients with acute pancreatitis and helps predict complications.[25] Serum calcium measurement is also useful in the prognostication of patients with acute pancreatitis; hypercalcemia may be associated with abdominal pain, renal tract calculi, and paraneoplastic syndromes. Coagulation tests are not routinely required unless there is suspicion of a coagulopathy or another clinical indication, such as measurement of International Normalized Ratio (INR) in patients receiving warfarin therapy. Other blood tests may be necessary in certain situations; for example, serum troponin should be measured if there is suspected myocardial ischemia and blood glucose measurement is required in all diabetic patients and in those with pancreatitis or suspected new diabetes. A sample of blood should be sent for cross-match or "group and save" if there is a suspicion of bleeding or there is a likelihood that operation will be required.

Blood cultures should be collected in patients with fever or suspected sepsis, ideally prior to commencement of antimicrobial treatment. Arterial blood gas analysis provides useful information on levels of oxygenation and acid-base status in acutely unwell patients. Lactate concentrations in particular can be useful in assessing the severity of sepsis, diagnosing mesenteric ischemia and also as a guide to aid fluid resuscitation.

Urinalysis

Routine dipstick urinalysis should be performed on all patients with acute abdominal pain. Detection of nitrites, leucocytes, protein, or blood may suggest a urinary tract infection, and a formal urine specimen should then be obtained for culture. In instances where there is suspected urinary sepsis, an urgent microscopy and Gram stain is indicated. This may be of particular relevance in pregnant patients. Hematuria supports a diagnosis of renal tract calculi or malignancy. Glycosuria and the presence of ketones may confirm a case of diabetic ketoacidosis, which can mimic an acute surgical abdomen. In addition, a pregnancy test should be performed in all women of reproductive age as a matter of routine. It should be remembered that in the initial stages of pregnancy the urinary pregnancy test may still be negative, so if an ectopic pregnancy is considered a formal serum pregnancy test should be requested.

Radiological Investigations

Radiological investigations have an increasingly central role in the management of patients with an acute abdomen. There are extensive data to show that radiological investigations such as plain X-rays, ultrasound, and CT scan help in the decision-making process as well as reduce unnecessary operations and surgical admissions.[26]

Plain X-rays

An erect chest X-ray should be performed in all cases of suspected luminal perforation.[27] Approximately 50% of patients with a perforated peptic ulcer will have a pneumoperitoneum visible on an erect chest X-ray (Figs. 74.2A and B).[28] Chest X-ray is also indicated where there is suspicion of lung pathology, such as a pneumonia or pleural effusion, conditions that can present with upper abdominal

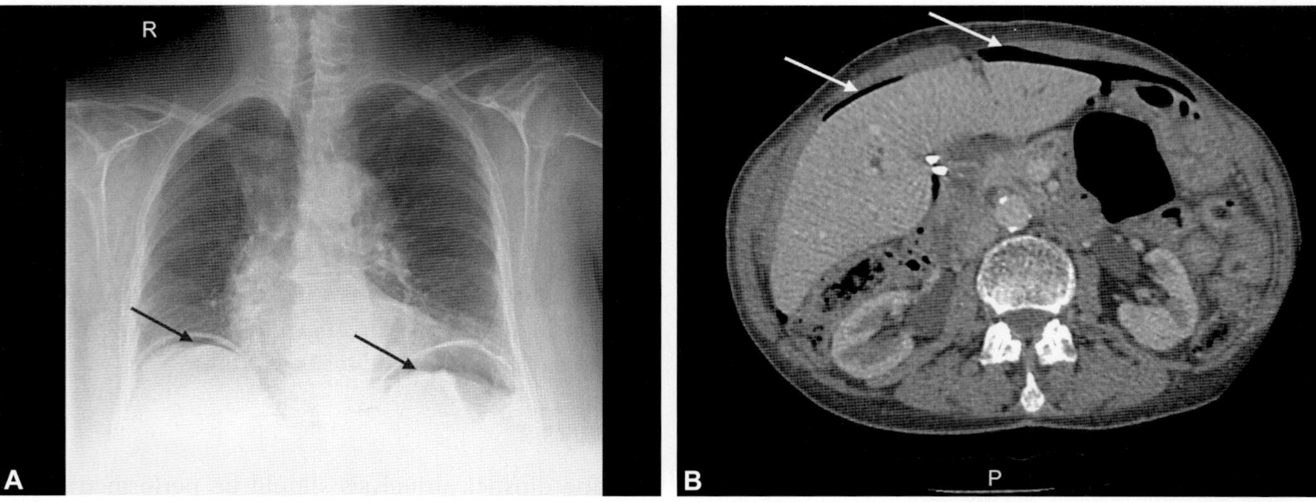

Figs. 74.2A and B: (A) Erect chest X-ray (CXR) demonstrating free subdiaphragmatic gas due to a perforated duodenal ulcer (arrow). (B) An abdominal CT scan showing free gas also in a patient with a perforated duodenal ulcer (arrow), but this patient had no gas visible on the erect CXR.

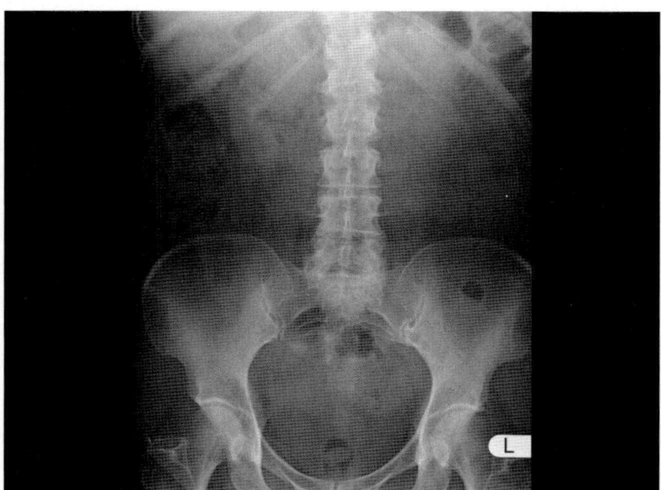

Fig. 74.3: A supine abdominal X-ray (AXR) showing dilated loops of central small bowel suggesting small bowel obstruction.

pain or may arise as a consequence of intra-abdominal pathology, for example, pleural effusion in acute pancreatitis or aspiration pneumonia in intestinal obstruction. The indications for an abdominal X-ray are suspected perforation, acute colitis/toxic megacolon and intestinal obstruction.[27] A supine film is usually sufficient to reveal dilated bowel loops associated with bowel obstruction (*see* below), but an erect film may be required to demonstrate the air-fluid levels within the bowel more clearly (Fig. 74.3). A KUB (plain X-ray of kidney-ureter-bladder) should be requested when a ureteric calculus is suspected, although this test has largely been replaced by low-dose CT-KUB.

Contrast Radiology

Contrast may be administered into the gastrointestinal tract to provide further information regarding the structure and function of the bowel. In the acute setting, water-soluble contrast, such as Gastromiro or Gastrografin, is preferred to barium, which is an irritant to the peritoneal cavity and lungs, if there is a risk of aspiration. Contrast may be given orally, via a nasogastric tube or rectally depending upon the clinical situation. The main role of contrast investigations is in adhesive small bowel obstruction, large bowel obstruction, and perforated peptic ulcer, although in many circumstances contrast radiology has largely been superseded by CT scan.

In adhesive small bowel obstruction, a water-soluble contrast follow-through has been shown to help identify which patients may settle without the need for surgical intervention. Failure of the contrast to reach the colon within 24 hours is predictive for the need of operation in 96% of patients (Figs. 74.4A and B).[29] The use of water-soluble contrast in this clinical setting also promotes faster resolution of symptoms, with a lesser requirement for surgical intervention and reduced length of hospital stay.[30] A water-soluble contrast enema is useful in differentiating mechanical obstruction from pseudo-obstruction in patients with large bowel obstruction, although a CT scan with rectal contrast is now often the preferred investigation.

Since not all perforated peptic ulcers will display a pneumoperitoneum on an erect CXR, if there is a high clinical suspicion then a water-soluble contrast meal and follow-through will help to confirm or refute this diagnosis

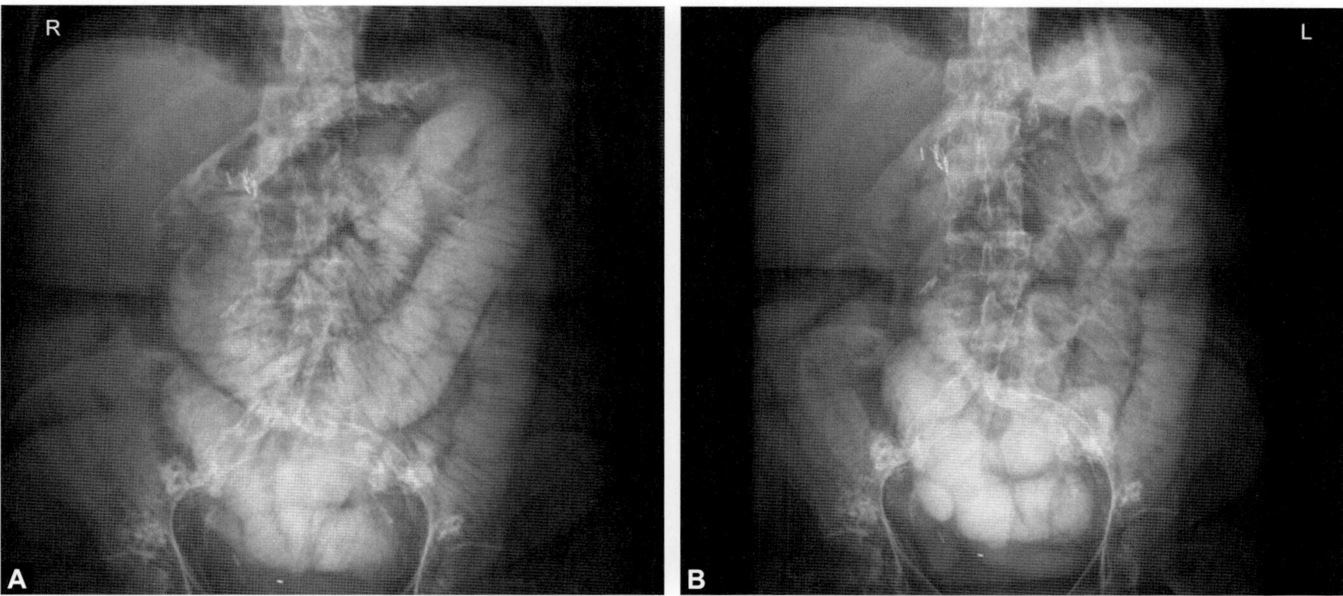

Figs. 74.4A and B: Abdominal X-ray taken (A) 90 minutes and (B) 4 hours after oral administration of water soluble contrast. The contrast demonstrates the dilated small bowel loops. After 4 hours the contrast has failed to reach the cecum suggesting complete obstruction. This patient required a laparotomy where small bowel obstruction secondary to adhesions was confirmed.

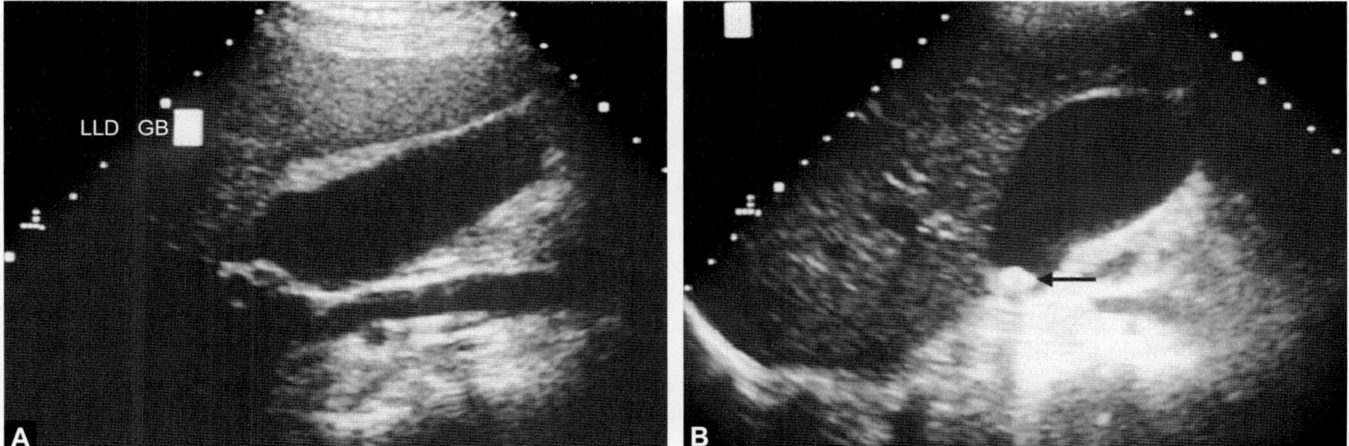

Figs. 74.5A and B: Normal and stone-containing gallbladders. Ultrasounds of the right upper quadrant. (A) Normal gallbladder without stones. (B) Gallbladder containing stones (arrow), as demonstrated by sonographic echogenicity, the thickened gallbladder wall and pericholecystic fluid.

as well as showing if the perforation has sealed. It is now well recognized that some patients who present with a perforated peptic ulcer may be managed conservatively.[31]

Ultrasound Scan

Ultrasonography (USS) is one of the mainstays for investigating the acute abdomen. Some of the benefits are that it is noninvasive, relatively cheap and does not involve a radiation dose. However, USS is highly operator-dependent, meaningful results reflecting the experience of the radiologist performing the test.

Ultrasonography is the first line of investigation for acute biliary disease, with sensitivity > 95% for acute cholecystitis (Figs. 74.5A and B).[32] Ultrasound scan has also been shown to detect an acutely inflamed but nonperforated appendix, with a sensitivity of 81% and specificity of 100% in some studies (Fig. 74.6).[33] For perforated appendicitis, this diagnostic accuracy falls to 29%.[34] Ultrasound is particularly useful for the detection of free intra-abdominal fluid which may be associated with perforated viscera, appendicitis, ruptured ovarian cysts, or trauma. Ultrasound also has a role in assessing the pelvis in females to examine

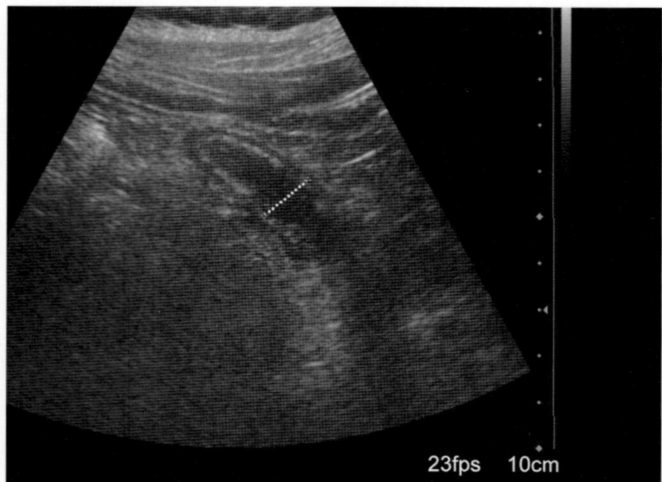

Fig. 74.6: Abdominal ultrasound scan demonstrating a thick-walled, distended tubular structure lying within the right iliac fossa. Acute appendicitis was confirmed at laparoscopy.

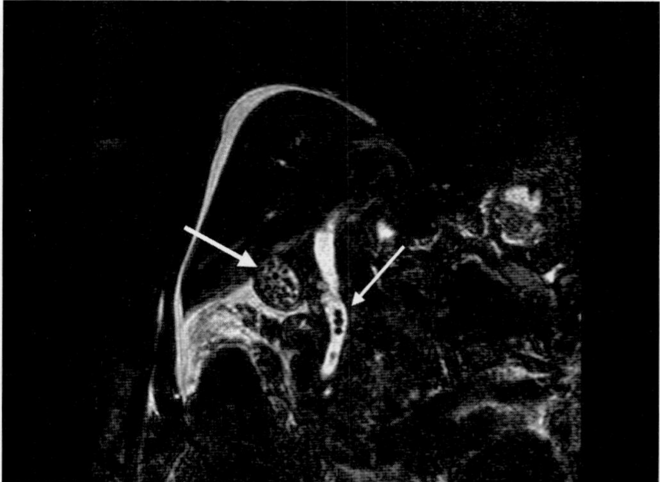

Fig. 74.7: Magnetic resonance cholangiopancreatography (MRCP) is the investigation of choice for imaging the biliary tree. This image demonstrates gallstones within a thick-walled gallbladder (thick arrow) and stones lying within the common bile duct (thin arrow).

the gynecological organs, the abdominal wall for hernias, and in the assessment of aortic and iliac aneurysms.

Computed Tomography

With the development of multislice scanners that produce high-quality images, CT scan is used increasingly in the investigation of acute abdominal pain. It is, however, costly and exposes the patient to an appreciable dose of radiation. Computed tomography can accurately identify free intraperitoneal gas, acute appendicitis, bowel ischemia, and diverticulitis (Fig. 74.2B). It is useful in the diagnosis of large and small bowel obstruction, when enteric or rectal contrast will often identify the underlying cause. Computed tomography is used to confirm acute pancreatitis when there is diagnostic uncertainty, and it also enables detection of associated pancreatic complications such as necrosis or pseudocyst formation. Computed tomography is valuable in the diagnosis of ruptured AAAs and ureteric calculi. The rapid processing of multiple high-quality images obtained with modern scanners has made CT a vital investigation for trauma patients. In fact, CT is now regarded as the standard for victims of trauma who do not require immediate surgical intervention.[35]

The routine use of early abdominal CT scanning in patients presenting with acute abdominal pain has been investigated. Early CT scanning (within 24 hours of admission) resulted in superior diagnostic certainty when compared with standard practice, but this did not translate into reduced length of hospital stay or improved clinical outcomes.[36] These findings, together with the concerns regarding radiation exposure, support the continued selective use of CT scan in the investigation of acute abdominal pain.

Magnetic Resonance Imaging

Magnetic resonance imaging (MRI) has the advantage over CT scan in that there is no radiation exposure. However, there are certain contraindications to scanning, such as possession of a pacemaker and a proportion of patients are unable to tolerate the scanning process due to claustrophobia. However, MRI does have a role in the investigation of the acute abdomen. Magnetic resonance cholangiopancreatography (MRCP) is the investigation of choice for imaging the biliary tree (Fig. 74.7). MRI has a role in the diagnosis of small bowel abnormalities, such as Crohn's disease. Due to absence of radiation exposure, MRI may also be useful in the investigation of pregnant patients where there is diagnostic doubt.[37]

Peritoneal Aspiration

Sampling of peritoneal fluid by paracentesis is indicated in cases of suspected spontaneous bacterial peritonitis or in peritoneal dialysis patients where there is concern that the dialysis fluid is infected. Samples should be sent for urgent gram stain and culture.

Endoscopy

Gastroscopy is indicated in patients with upper abdominal pain in whom peptic ulcer disease is suspected or in upper gastrointestinal bleeding. Endoscopic examination of the lower gastrointestinal tract by flexible sigmoidoscopy or colonoscopy is required for sigmoid volvulus; it allows decompression of the bowel under vision and inspection of the condition of the underlying mucosa. Sigmoidoscopy is also mandatory for examination of the anorectal region in cases of large bowel obstruction. Gentle colonoscopy may be necessary in patients with colitis to visualize the extent of disease involvement and to obtain biopsies for diagnostic purposes.

Laparoscopy

Laparoscopy has the advantage of combining a diagnostic role with the potential for therapeutic intervention. However, it requires the patient to undergo general anesthesia. Many studies have shown that diagnostic laparoscopy improves surgical decision making, especially when it is unclear if an operation is required or not, and when clinical assessment and noninvasive methods have failed to delineate pathology.[38] Two studies have shown that using laparoscopy as a diagnostic tool reduces length of hospital stay and increases levels of patient satisfaction.[39,40] Laparoscopy is particularly useful in the evaluation of lower abdominal pain in women in whom there is often diagnostic difficulty in distinguishing gynecological pathology from acute appendicitis.[41] The value of diagnostic laparoscopy in patients with NSAP has been described previously in this chapter.

DIAGNOSIS AND MANAGEMENT OF SPECIFIC CONDITIONS

This chapter so far has outlined the general approach to the assessment and investigation of the acute abdomen. The remainder of this chapter focuses on some of the more common conditions associated with acute abdominal pain. For a more detailed description the reader is directed to the relevant chapters elsewhere in this book.

Acute Appendicitis

Acute appendicitis is the commonest cause of acute abdominal pain in Europe, North America, Africa, and Pakistan (Tables 74.1 to 74.3).

Clinical Features

Typically vague periumbilical pain migrates to the right lower quadrant several hours after the onset associated with nausea, vomiting, and anorexia. As the inflammation progresses, pain and tenderness intensify at McBurney's point, one third of the way from the anterior superior iliac spine to the umbilicus, although the position of the appendix is variable. Since appendicitis tends to be progressive over 24–36 hours, a different diagnosis should be considered for patients who have had a waxing and waning course over for >36–48 hours.

There can be additional signs: Rovsing's sign is referred pain in the right iliac fossa when the left lower quadrant is palpated. The psoas sign is tested by asking the patient to raise his or her leg against the pressure of the examiner's hand placed on the anterior tibial surface; pain suggests an inflammatory process near the psoas muscle, such as retrocecal appendicitis. The obturator sign is tested by passively internally rotating the hip with both the hip and knee flexed to 90°; pain is elicited if there is inflammation near the obturator internus muscle. Rectal examination may reveal right-sided tenderness with pelvic appendicitis.

Rebound tenderness and guarding signify inflammation of the parietal peritoneum. An inflamed appendix lying deep in the pelvis or retrocecally may produce few anterior abdominal signs.

Differential Diagnoses

Acute appendicitis often does not present in a classical fashion. There are many mimicking conditions, several of which do not require surgical intervention including gastroenteritis, mesenteric lymphadenitis, Meckel's diverticulitis, right-sided diverticulitis coli, terminal ileitis, and ureteral calculi. In males, an "acceptable" rate for finding a normal appendix operation is 10–15%.[42] In females, additional possibilities include acute salpingitis, ectopic pregnancy, endometriosis, mittelschmerz, and complications of an ovarian cyst.

Investigation

Laboratory tests are of limited value in the diagnosis. White blood cell count and inflammatory markers may be normal at first. Urinalysis is essential to exclude urinary tract infection. In a woman of reproductive age, a pregnancy test is mandatory to exclude an ectopic pregnancy.

Imaging studies are occasionally helpful. A fecalith is visible in the right lower quadrant on plain AXR in 7% of patients with acute appendicitis. Ultrasonography can detect an acutely inflamed but nonperforated appendix with a sensitivity of 81% and specificity of 100% in some studies (Fig. 74.6),[33] although the true accuracy will depend upon the radiologist performing the scan. Ultrasound scan is especially useful if the diagnosis is unclear and to assess the female pelvis. Computed tomography can also be helpful in difficult cases; the diagnostic accuracy is 98%.[43]

Management

Patients presenting with the classic symptoms and signs of appendicitis should be taken to the operating room for emergency appendicectomy after adequate hydration and antibiotic administration (*see* Chapter 68, "Appendix"). Diagnostic laparoscopy should be considered if there is clinical concern but a remaining degree of diagnostic uncertainty. If acute appendicitis is confirmed, the appendix may be removed laparoscopically. Delay in diagnosis may result in perforation, which occurs in about 20% of patients who have appendicitis and 40–75% of patients over 60 years of age.[44] The mortality rate of appendicectomy for nonperforated appendicitis is $<0.2\%$, but this increases 10-fold following perforation. Perforation tends to occur more frequently at the extremes of age and is associated with mortality rates of 1% for patients under 50 years of age, 4.5% for those aged 50–70 years, and 16.2% for those who are 70–90 years of age. Untreated, perforation leads to peritonitis and abscess formation.

In patients with an appendix mass conservative treatment with a course of antibiotics is appropriate, although imaging should be undertaken to exclude an abscess that may be suitable for percutaneous drainage. Appendicectomy on these patients is unnecessary and associated with increased complication rates.[45] An interval colonoscopy should be arranged to exclude an underlying cecal malignancy in older patients.

The diagnosis of acute appendicitis in pregnant patients is particularly challenging, particularly after the first trimester, because anorexia, nausea, vomiting, and diffuse abdominal pains frequently accompany pregnancy. In addition, physical examination of the abdomen of a pregnant female is often compromised by the enlarging uterus and the laxity of the abdominal wall. As the uterus enlarges, the cecum and appendix move from the right lower quadrant to the RUQ. The appendix is also displaced from contact with the anterior abdominal wall, reducing the likelihood of being able to demonstrate parietal peritoneal inflammation. The omentum is less likely to migrate toward the inflamed appendix to seal a perforation, resulting in a higher incidence of diffuse peritonitis than in nonpregnant females or males. Pursuing the diagnosis in pregnant females should be as aggressive as in the nonpregnant population because delay in the diagnosis resulting in the development of peritonitis carries a substantial risk of premature labor. An abdominal MRI may be useful in cases of diagnostic uncertainty, especially in the earlier stages of pregnancy.[37] Appendicitis is considered in greater detail in Chapter 68, "Appendix".

Small Bowel Obstruction

Mechanical small bowel obstruction is most commonly due to adhesions (which may or may not have arisen from previous surgery) or herniae. In the older patient a cecal neoplasm should be considered. Other causes include inflammatory strictures, such as Crohn's disease, and in endemic regions, complete small bowel obstruction requires urgent surgical intervention to minimize the requirement for bowel resection and to prevent complications, especially in the context of strangulation (*see* Chapter 61, "Inflammatory Colorectal Conditions"). Small bowel obstruction secondary to an incarcerated hernia always requires surgical intervention.

Clinical Features

The transition from intermittent pain to continuous pain, as well as localized abdominal tenderness on examination, is ominous sign of bowel ischemia and imminent bowel perforation. The abdomen should be carefully inspected for scars and there should be a thorough examination for incisional, umbilical, and groin hernias. Bowel sounds on auscultation are hyperactive early in small bowel obstruction and may be described as "tinkling" or "high pitched." Later, as the bowel fills with fluid, the bowel sounds may be absent.

Differential Diagnoses

Mechanical small bowel obstruction should be distinguished from large bowel obstruction and from functional small bowel obstruction (paralytic ileus). Abdominal distension and constipation are earlier features of large bowel obstruction but vomiting rather later; investigation helps to differentiate between the two. In functional small bowel obstruction, colicky pain and bowel sounds are usually absent.

Investigation

Routine blood tests are necessary to identify electrolyte disturbances from vomiting and fluid loss. Radiologic examinations are of key importance. A supine abdominal X-ray demonstrates distended loops of small bowel and air-fluid levels appearing as a "stepladder" plus a paucity of colonic gas (Fig. 74.3); an erect film is sometimes helpful. The absence of distended bowel loops does not rule out bowel obstruction because in individuals who have a closed loop obstruction the obstructed loop is filled with fluid, which will not be visible. Contrast radiology may help differentiate between complete and incomplete small bowel obstruction (Fig. 74.4). Failure of enteric contrast to reach the colon within 24 hours indicates that surgical intervention will likely be required.[46] Computed tomography is often the investigation of choice in small bowel obstruction, where not only will the diagnosis be confirmed, but also the likely underlying pathology (Fig. 74.8).

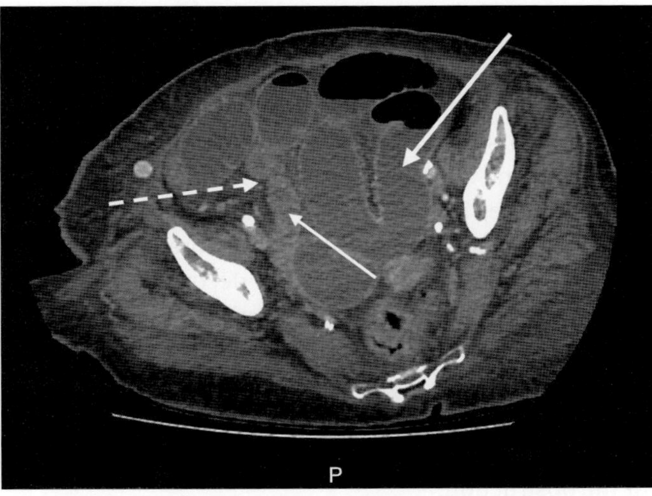

Fig. 74.8: An abdominal CT scan showing small bowel obstruction. Dilated small bowel loops can be seen (thick arrow) with adjacent collapsed small bowel (thin arrow). The adhesive band that was responsible can also be appreciated (interrupted arrow).

Management

Initial management should involve resuscitation with fluid and electrolyte replacement and accurate fluid balance. A nasogastric tube helps decompress the bowel and reduce the risk of aspiration. Adhesive obstruction that fails to settle with conservative strategies or where there is concern about bowel ischemia (strangulation) demands operation. Bowel obstruction secondary to hernia incarceration should always undergo surgical intervention. Laparoscopy may be used successfully in the management of adhesive small bowel obstruction.[47]

Large Bowel Obstruction

The primary causes of colonic obstruction are carcinoma, diverticular stricture of the sigmoid colon, and sigmoid or cecal volvulus.

Clinical Features

Colonic obstruction usually presents with a history of several days to weeks of increasing abdominal distension, colicky abdominal pain, and constipation. Pain is a less frequent presenting symptom of colonic obstruction than of small bowel obstruction. Vomiting is usually lates.

Carcinoma of the colon is typically associated with a change in bowel habit and evidence of blood in the stool before the acute onset of the abdominal pain and distension. Volvulus of the sigmoid colon or cecum is potentially life-threatening, as there is a high risk of colonic ischemia and perforation, which occur more rapidly than with an obstructing carcinoma. Absolute constipation is the rule because each type of volvulus causes complete luminal obstruction. Sigmoid volvulus is much more frequent than cecal volvulus, and it leads to gross abdominal distension. It generally affects in patients over 65 years of age, especially those who reside in long-term care facilities or who are bedridden. Abdominal tenderness is a grave sign suggesting underlying bowel ischemia or perforation. Bowel signs may be high pitched. The rectum is empty and devoid of feces.

Differential Diagnoses

Small bowel obstruction and functional large bowel obstruction (pseudo-obstruction) are the likely alternative diagnoses. Investigations are also directed to identify the underlying cause of colonic obstruction.

Investigation

Colonic dilatation may be seen on plain abdominal X-ray. A distinct cutoff may be visible, with absence of colonic gas distally. When the diameter of the cecum approaches 12 cm, there is a major risk of perforation. Patients with an incompetent ileocecal valve may small bowel dilatation on X-ray. The classic radiologic finding on abdominal radiography in either sigmoid or cecal volvulus is a large air-filled loop of bowel taking up the entire abdomen. It appears as a "bent inner tube," with the "beak" in the left lower quadrant in the sigmoid volvulus and in the right lower quadrant in cecal volvulus (Fig. 74.9).

A water-soluble contrast enema or, increasingly CT scan with rectal contrast, should confirm the diagnosis of mechanical large bowel obstruction and will often identify the underlying cause.

Management

As with small bowel obstruction, correction of fluid and electrolyte disturbances and nasogastric intubation are useful initial steps. Flexible sigmoidoscopy can be both diagnostic and therapeutic in sigmoid volvulus. During the procedure, it is important to assess the viability of the bowel at the site of obstruction before advancing the scope to allow the closed loop to decompress. Patients with malignant large bowel obstruction require a colonic resection. There is good evidence that patient outcomes are better if the procedure is performed by a colorectal specialist.[48] In some situations, a colonic stent may be used either as a bridge to surgery or as definitive treatment for the obstruction.[49]

Acute Gallstone Disease

Acute calculous cholecystitis occurs when a gallstone obstructs the cystic duct resulting in congestion, gallbladder wall edema, and secondary bacterial infection. This condition may progress to empyema and gangrene (*see* Chapter 55, "Gallbladder and Biliary Tree") (Figs. 74.10A and B).

Clinical Features

The typical symptom of cholelithiasis is biliary colic: postprandial pain in the RUQ that often radiates to the right shoulder or interscapular area of the back. Although described as "colic," the pain is typically constant in nature lasting 30–120 minutes and associated with nausea and vomiting. Between episodes of biliary colic, most patients are completely symptom free. In acute cholecystitis, there are features of inflammation and infection. There is tenderness in the RUQ and the patient may display Murphy's sign. There may be tachycardia, fever, and leukocytosis.

Acute acalculous cholecystitis is rare, accounting for only 3% of the conditions for which biliary tract operations are completed. Affected patients are particularly likely to have comorbid conditions such as a recent operation on a different organ system, cardiac surgery requiring cardiopulmonary bypass, thermal burns, or major trauma. The cause of the condition is multifactorial, including bile stasis because of prolonged periods of fasting, sphincter of Oddi contraction by narcotic analgesics and cystic duct obstruction due to edema.

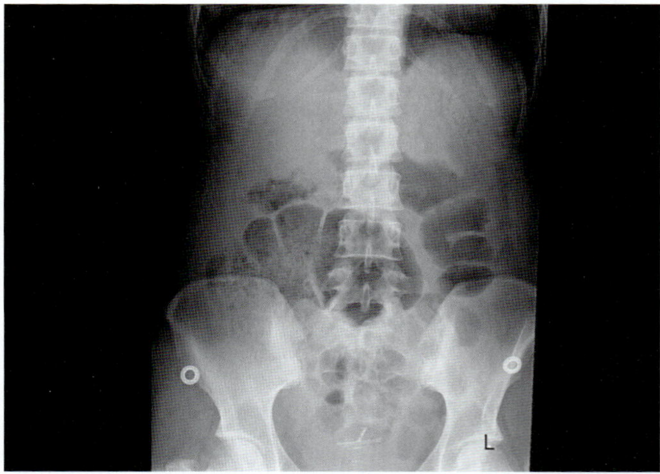

Fig. 74.9: A supine abdominal X-ray showing a cecal volvulus. A large gas-filled sigmoid is visible emerging from the pelvis.

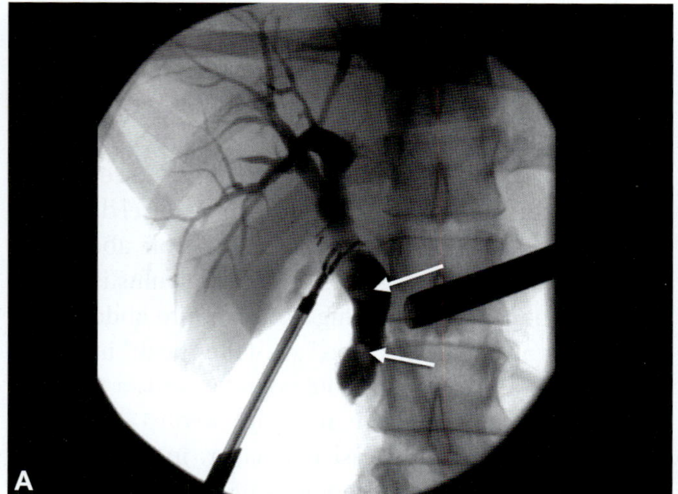

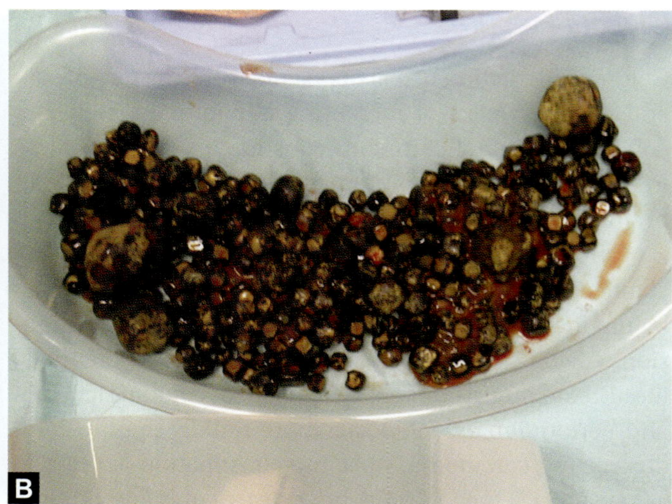

Figs. 74.10A and B: (A) An intraoperative cholangiogram demonstrating stones within the common bile duct (arrows). These were removed following a choledochotomy and bile duct clearance. (B) Multiple stones were removed from the bile duct and gallbladder from this patient.

Differential Diagnoses

Other conditions that need to be considered are peptic ulcer disease (including acute perforation), acute hepatitis, acute pancreatitis, and acute pyelonephritis.

Investigation

An ultrasound of the abdomen should be the first diagnostic study (Fig. 74.5). Gallstones are revealed with 95% accuracy. The study may also demonstrate a dilated common bile duct, a thickened gallbladder wall, fluid around the gallbladder (pericholecystic fluid), and sonolucency of the abdominal wall. Pain elicited over the gallbladder during ultrasound examination, referred to as the ultrasonic Murphy's sign, is a feature in 90% of patients with acute cholecystitis.[50] In patients with an equivocal USS result or residual diagnostic uncertainty, CT scan may confirm the diagnosis by demonstration of pericholecystic fluid, air in the gallbladder wall (in emphysematous cholecystitis) perforation of the gallbladder, or abscess formation. However, CT scan is not a good modality for demonstrating gallstones with certainty.

Derangement of LFTs raises the possibility of stones within the common bile duct. g-Glutamyl transferase (GGT) has the highest accuracy for predicting choledocholithiasis.[51] Magnetic resonance cholangiopancreatography is the investigation of choice for imaging the biliary tree and has replaced endoscopic retrograde cholangiopancreatography (ERCP) as an investigative tool in this situation (Fig. 74.7).

Management

Fit patients should be offered a cholecystectomy for symptomatic gallstone disease (biliary colic or acute cholecystitis). Management of suspected bile duct stones will vary according to the preference and capabilities of the surgeon. Some surgeons will undertake an intraoperative cholangiogram at the time of cholecystectomy and proceed to bile duct exploration if required. Others will prefer to ensure that the bile duct is clear by ERCP prior to cholecystectomy. Unfit patients should be treated with systemic antibiotics with or without percutaneous drainage (cholecystostomy).

Acute Pancreatitis

Clinical Features

The clinical presentation reflects the severity of acute pancreatitis and ranges from mild self-limiting pain with hyperamylasemia to fulminant life-threatening hemorrhagic pancreatic necrosis (*see* Chapter 56, "Pancreas"). As the pancreas is retroperitoneal and overlies the celiac plexus, pain can radiate from the epigastrium to the back; the patient often prefers to sit forward to try and alleviate the pain. Anorexia and nausea are common. In the fulminant form of acute pancreatitis, there may be evidence of cardiovascular instability, respiratory difficulty, and renal failure.

On examination, the patient may exhibit signs of cardiorespiratory compromise. Palpation and percussion reveal abdominal tenderness either in the epigastrium or throughout the abdomen. Grey Turner's sign and Cullen's sign may be visible (*see* above).

Differential Diagnoses

The main diagnoses to consider are (perforated) peptic ulcer disease, cholecystitis, and a ruptured AAA.

Investigation

An elevated serum amylase concentration is diagnostic of acute pancreatitis. However, the half-life of amylase is just over 2 hours, so the serum concentration may have returned to normal should the patient present late. Also, conditions other than acute pancreatitis may be associated with a modest elevation in serum amylase concentration (*see* Table 74.4). In case of diagnostic uncertainty, serum lipase levels may be helpful because concentrations remain elevated for longer than serum amylase; alternatively, CT scan will show pancreatic edema and adjacent fat stranding in-keeping with acute inflammation. Later in the disease process CT scan may identify complications such as pancreatic necrosis and pseudocyst formation. An abdominal ultrasound can detect the gallstones that are so often the etiological cause as well as a dilated bile duct.

The magnitude of elevation of serum amylase does not correlate with the severity or the outcome for patients who have pancreatitis. Several "scoring systems" that have been developed as an attempt to identify patients at increased risk of complications and poor outcome (*see* Chapter 56, "Pancreas"); the latest Atlanta classification has recently been revised.[52]

Management

Resuscitation is the initial priority. Aggressive fluid resuscitation and organ support are necessary in a severe attack. Liaison with critical care teams at an early stage is vital to maximize the chances of a favorable outcome. The management of acute pancreatitis is mainly supportive. However, there is evidence that an early ERCP may improve outcome in patients with acute severe pancreatitis secondary to choledocholithiasis, particularly if associated with cholangitis.[53]

Peptic Ulcer Disease

If untreated, at least 10% of gastric or duodenal ulcers perforate. An anterior perforation of the stomach or duodenum produces acute peritonitis. A posterior perforation of the duodenum may result in pancreatitis or a hepatic abscess, whereas a posterior perforation of the stomach is likely to result in a lesser sac abscess.

Clinical Features

Acute perforation results in severe abdominal pain of sudden onset. The patient can usually time the exact minute of onset. There may or may not be a preceding history of ulcer-like symptoms, such as epigastric pain before or after a meal or pain awakening the patient at night.

Patients with an acute perforation usually look unwell, lie still on the bed and are reluctant to move, with tachycardia and fever. The abdominal examination classically reveals "board-like" rigidity. The abdominal musculature moves little with respiration, and breathing is often shallow. Bowel sounds may be diminished. Free air in the peritoneal cavity may be evident by loss of liver dullness on abdominal percussion. Early diagnosis is important because survival is affected by any delay in diagnosis, particularly if longer than 24 hours.

Differential Diagnoses

Other diagnoses to consider are acute pancreatitis, mesenteric ischemia, and acute gallstone disease.

Investigation

Approximately 50% of patients with a perforated peptic ulcer have a pneumoperitoneum visible on erect chest X-ray (Fig. 74.2A).[13] Computed tomography can confirm free gas in many of the rest, but it is poor at distinguishing colonic perforation from peptic ulcer perforation (Fig. 74.2B). A water-soluble meal and follow-through may be of use in patients where it is suspected that the perforation has sealed and operation might be avoidable.[54]

Management

Early fluid resuscitation and adequate analgesia are essential. A nasogastric tube should be passed, and broad-spectrum antibiotics should be administered in addition to an intravenous proton pump inhibitor. Most patients with an acute perforation will require laparotomy and repair of the perforation. A simple omental patch repair is generally all that is required. All gastric ulcers should be biopsied at the time of surgery to exclude an underlying malignancy. Thorough peritoneal lavage is of paramount importance to reduce the chance of postoperative abscess formation. If the duodenum is particularly scarred or friable or there is a large defect, it may not be possible to simply patch the perforation but rather to perform a partial gastrectomy. Closure of the diseased duodenal stump may be challenging and require drainage over a Foley catheter or T-tube (*see* Chapter 48, "Peptic Ulcer Disease"). In a subset of patients, the perforation may seal spontaneously. It is acceptable to manage these patients nonoperatively providing the patient remains well and without evidence of peritonitis.[31]

Acute Diverticulitis

Acute diverticulitis is commoner in older patient groups from Western societies and usually affects the sigmoid colon. The right colon is more commonly affected in Asian populations. Simple acute diverticulitis may be complicated by perforation, bleeding, or abscess formation.

Clinical Features

Most patients complain of pain in the lower abdomen either in the midline or in the left (or right) iliac fossa. There may be associated constipation, although mucus or pus may sometimes be passed per rectum. There may be systemic upset with fevers and chills. On examination, the abdomen tends to be mildly distended, with tenderness will be localized in the lower quadrants. There may be peritoneal signs, particularly if there is an extraluminal fluid collection with peritoneal inflammation.

Differential Diagnoses

Alternative diagnoses include colitis in general, pyelonephritis, and acute appendicitis (for right-sided diverticulitis).

Investigation

White cell count is usually elevated. Ultrasound scan may demonstrate colonic wall thickening or an associated abscess. Computed tomography is the best investigation: the diagnosis is confirmed by the appearance of diverticula, thickening of the bowel wall and fat stranding in the mesocolon. Computed tomography will also identify associated complications, such as abscess formation or perforation.

Management

Unwell patients require resuscitation. Broad-spectrum antibiotics with activity against gram-negative organisms and anaerobes are given intravenously. Radiologically directed percutaneous drainage should be performed for discrete abscesses. Patients with a colonic perforation will require a laparotomy and colonic resection, with or without a primary anastomosis. The decision to perform a primary anastomosis will depend on the condition of the bowel, the condition of the patient, and surgeon experience. If in doubt, the safer option is always to perform a Hartmann's resection. There is some evidence that laparoscopic washout and drainage may provide an alternative to laparotomy and acute resection for some patients.[55]

Small Bowel Conditions

Meckel's Diverticulitis

Meckel's diverticulum (persistent vitellointestinal duct) is the commonest congenital anomaly of the small bowel. It occurs in 2% of the population, it is found 2 ft (60 cm) from the ileocecal valve on the antimesenteric wall of the terminal ileum, and is about 2 in. (5 cm) long. It may contain ectopic pancreatic tissue or gastric mucosa that secretes acid to cause ulceration within the diverticulum with resultant bleeding and pain (*see* Chapter 61, "Inflammatory Colorectal Conditions").

The signs and symptoms produced by Meckel's diverticulitis can mimic those of appendicitis. The diagnosis is suggested by symptoms of partial small bowel obstruction and tenderness that is relatively poorly localized, more medial and higher than McBurney's point. The condition may be difficult to distinguish from acute appendicitis or Crohn's disease.

Although CT scan can be suggestive, acute Meckel's diverticulitis is generally diagnosed at the time of operation for suspected acute appendicitis.

Crohn's Disease

When localized to the terminal ileum, Crohn's disease is referred to as terminal ileitis. It too can present with signs and symptoms similar to those of appendicitis. Clues for distinguishing it from appendicitis involve knowledge that the patient has pre-existing Crohn's disease, partial small bowel obstruction, or a history of weight loss or diarrhea. Computed tomography should show ileal thickening. A small bowel MRI has largely superseded contrast radiology and can indicate the extent of disease. Colonoscopy with intubation of the terminal ileum allows biopsies to be taken for histological confirmation of the diagnosis.

If the diagnosis of Crohn's disease is suspected for the first time at operation, whether laparoscopic or open, visualization of the terminal ileum allows the surgeon to diagnose of "terminal ileitis" if the appendix is normal and the terminal ileum is thickened with "creeping mesenteric fat." Appendicectomy should be carried out unless the cecal wall is so inflamed that the stump closure would be precarious. Further details on Crohn's disease are given in Chapter 61, "Inflammatory Colorectal Conditions".

Gynecological Conditions Associated with Acute Abdominal Pain

Acute inflammatory or ischemic changes in the female pelvic organs often produce signs and symptoms that mimic those of acute appendicitis. A thorough menstrual and sexual history must be obtained to maximize diagnostic accuracy. A pregnancy test is mandatory for any female of childbearing age who complains of acute abdominal pain. Diagnostic laparoscopy is often helpful in assessing this group of patients.

Mittelschmerz

Mittelschmerz refers to pelvic pain caused by bleeding from a ruptured ovarian follicle at the time of ovulation. Patients describe a sudden onset of lower abdominal or pelvic pain in the middle of their menstrual cycle. If the pain is localized to the right side of the abdomen, the findings can mimic those of acute appendicitis. Pain may also be referred to the shoulder (Kehr's sign). The patient may have a mild fever and leukocytosis, but does not appear to be ill. Pain and tenderness are mild. Similar pain may be experienced with a ruptured corpus luteum cyst occurring near the onset of menstruation.

Pelvic Inflammatory Disease

This term refers to acute salpingitis, tubo-ovarian abscess, or hydrosalpinx. Perhaps more than any other condition, these conditions pose the greatest dilemma to the surgeon or gynecologist evaluating a woman with acute abdominal pain. Each condition can present with right-sided abdominal or pelvic pain accompanied by nausea, vomiting, anorexia, fever, and tachycardia. In contrast to acute appendicitis, the pain may be bilateral and evolves over several days.

On bimanual examination, the cervix may be inflamed and a vaginal discharge may be noted. Vaginal swabs should be collected for culture and sensitivity. Common pathogens include streptococcus, gonococcus, and chlamydia. Treatment consists of antibiotics.

Ruptured Ectopic Pregnancy

Implantation of the fertilized ovum outside the uterine cavity occurs in approximately 1 in 200 pregnancies. The commonest site for ectopic implantation is the fallopian tube. The developing trophoblast invades the tubal wall, which eventually ruptures, typically at about 6 weeks of gestation.

Pelvic pain is the commonest presentation and may be associated with abnormal uterine bleeding in 50–80%. Rupture produces sudden pain and may be associated with hemodynamic shock secondary to hemorrhage. Ectopic pregnancy should be considered in women with a previous history of ectopic pregnancy, pelvic inflammatory disease, use of an intrauterine device, or endometriosis. It should be noted whether the patient missed her previous menstrual period. It may be necessary to perform a serum pregnancy test (human chorionic gonadotropin) in the early stages of pregnancy to confirm the diagnosis.

Adnexal Torsion

Torsion can complicate a benign ovarian cyst, a dermoid cyst, or the fallopian tube itself. The onset of the pain is sudden, nearly always associated with vomiting and tends to be worse than in appendicitis.

Adnexal tenderness on bimanual pelvic examination is usually greater than in appendicitis, and a mass may be palpable. Localized peritonitis is usually present because torsion interrupts the blood supply to the ovary, leading to infarction irritation of the overlying parietal peritoneum. Laparoscopy helps to distinguish adnexal torsion from appendicitis.

Vascular Emergencies Associated with the Acute Abdomen

Acute mesenteric arterial or venous occlusion, nonocclusive mesenteric ischemia, and either an expanding or leaking AAA should be considered in the differential diagnosis of the patient who presents with acute abdominal pain (*see* Chapter 96, "Surgical Emergencies Resulting from Aortic Aneurysms or Dissections").

Mesenteric Ischemia

Acute arterial occlusion may result from embolization of clot, most frequently from a cardiac source, or from rupture of an atheromatous plaque. The physician should have a high index of suspicion for this condition in patients with atrial fibrillation or those recovering from myocardial infarction or with known anatomic cardiac defects. The site of embolization tends to be distal to the origin of the superior mesenteric artery, where either the pancreaticoduodenal or middle colic artery originate. Venous occlusion results in vascular congestion of the bowel as a consequence of outflow obstruction due to venous thrombosis. Nonocclusive mesenteric ischemia may be secondary to low cardiac output, hypovolemia, dehydration or the use of pharmacologic agents known to have vasoconstrictor effects, including digoxin and diuretics. This condition usually affects the "watershed" areas of the bowel, such as the distal transverse colon.

Patients develop acute severe epigastric or central abdominal pain, vomiting and diarrhea and are usually able to pinpoint the exact time of the onset of the pain. The abdomen may be mildly distended and diffusely tender. Bowel sounds may be hypoactive. Abdominal signs are often minimal in comparison to the degree of pain. Peritoneal signs and bloody diarrhea usually herald bowel infarction.

The diagnosis is usually confirmed by CT scan, which demonstrates thickening of the bowel wall, bowel dilatation and lack of bowel enhancement; in more advanced cases there may be evidence of gas within the bowel wall (pneumatosis intestinalis) or gas within the portal venous system. The site of vascular occlusion (arterial or venous) may also be identified on contrast-enhanced CT scan (Fig. 74.11). Laparotomy and resection of the diseased bowel is required, and it may be necessary to delay attempts at anastomosis until a further re-look laparotomy confirms bowel viability. Some cases may be suitable for embolectomy or revascularization and expertise should be sought from vascular specialists.

Abdominal Aortic Aneurysm

Acute onset of severe back, flank or abdominal pain is characteristic of a leaking, rupturing or acutely expanding AAA (*see* Chapter 96, "Surgical Emergencies Resulting from Aortic Aneurysms or Dissections"). In fact, this condition should be considered in all elderly (male) patients who present with back, loin, or groin pain. Pain on palpation

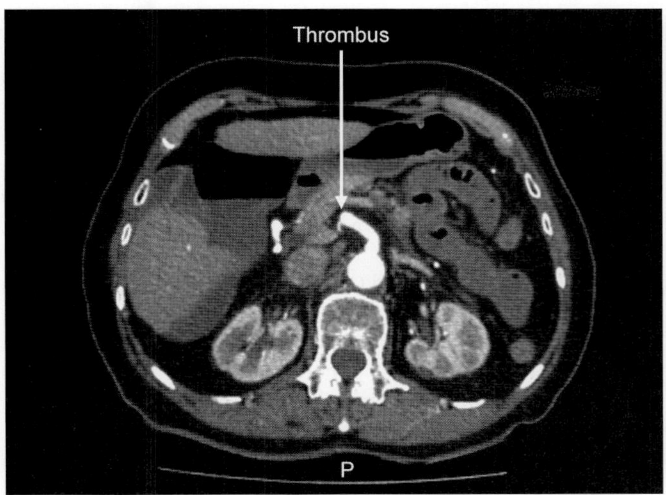

Fig. 74.11: Abdominal CT angiogram demonstrating complete occlusion near the origin of the superior mesenteric artery secondary to an acute thrombus (arrow). There is also free fluid present around the liver. This patient underwent a successful embolectomy and did not require bowel resection.

Fig. 74.12: A noncontrast CT-KUB showing a ureteric calculus impacted at the left vesicoureteric junction (arrow). The stone eventually passed with relief of symptoms.

of an epigastric or left flank expansive mass suggests an AAA that is threatening rupture. The pain of a leaking or rupturing aneurysm may be pulsatile initially and present for hours to days before rupture; it is usually not associated with nausea or vomiting. Patients with whom clinical findings plus evidence of hemodynamic shock should be considered to have a ruptured AAA and should be taken directly to the operating room. A portable ultrasound may be undertaken provided that it does not delayed operation.

For those patients who are not in shock, an abdominal CT scan is the study of choice, as it provides an accurate size and location of the aneurysm and demonstrates evidence of rupture.

Urological Conditions Associated with Acute Abdominal Pain

Calculous disease of the urinary tract may cause pain that is indistinguishable from other causes of an acute abdomen (*see* Chapter 138, "Case Study: Mohs Resection—How Can I Close this Defect?"). Pyelonephritis or acute hydronephrosis are associated with flank pain and exquisite loin angle tenderness. The pain of renal colic is severe, originating in the flank with radiation through the lateral abdomen and into the scrotum or labia; there may be hyperesthesia of the abdominal wall, and nausea and vomiting are common. As the smooth muscle of the ureter is contracting against an obstruction, the pain is a true colic. The patient can be writhing with pain and unable to find a comfortable position by contrast with peritonitis, in which the patient remains quiet and avoids movement. Dysuria, urgency, and frequency of micturition are common features of urinary tract infection.

Urinalysis demonstrates microscopic hematuria, proteinuria, or pyuria. A KUB radiograph allows visualization of a kidney stone in 80% of cases. A noncontrast CT-KUB has replaced intravenous pyelography as the diagnostic modality of choice to demonstrate kidney stones and confirm ureteral dilation or hydronephrosis (Fig. 74.12).

Testicular Torsion

Torsion of the testis generally affects teenagers. There may be a preceding history of minor trauma or episodes of minor testicular pain related to partial torsion. There is sudden-onset scrotal pain associated with vomiting and scrotal swelling and making it difficult to walk. Pain may also be referred to the loin or lower abdomen and conversely, any young male presenting with acute abdominal pain should undergo a testicular examination routinely to exclude testicular torsion. On examination, the testicle is tender and described as "high lying" due to its elevated position within the scrotum. Examination of the untwisted testis may demonstrate a horizontal lie because of the bilateral nature of the predisposing anatomical anomaly ("bell-clapper" testis). Scrotal erythema implies incipient or actual infarction of the testis. The diagnosis is made on clinical ground with or without ultrasound scan; urgent scrotal exploration should not be delayed pending investigation (*See* Chapter 142, "Testis and Scrotum").

Other Causes of an Acute Abdomen

Primary Peritonitis

Primary peritonitis is an uncommon condition characterized by spontaneous bacterial peritonitis secondary to either gut translocation of organisms or blood-borne spread. It is mostly found in patients with ascites (e.g., those with chronic liver disease or nephrotic syndrome) and patients with chronic renal failure undergoing peritoneal dialysis. A sample of peritoneal fluid should be sent for gram stain and culture and sensitivity, and the patient should be started on appropriate antibiotics. In some cases, laparoscopy or a laparotomy is required to exclude an underlying intra-abdominal source of the infection.

Sickle Cell Anemia

A sickle cell crisis may be brought on by a variety of factors including hypoxia and infections, whether bacterial or viral. Abdominal pain is associated with fever, chills, and backache. The pathogenesis of the crisis involves multiple intravascular thrombi resulting in small infarcts in the spleen and other intra-abdominal organs. The abdominal pain is usually sudden in onset and diffuse, and it may be associated with nausea and vomiting. Physical examination is often unremarkable, although the sclerae may be icteric due to increased hemolysis.

Laboratory data reveal anemia, reticulocytosis, and elevations in lactate dehydrogenase and bilirubin. Most patients have experienced a previous crisis. It is essential to determine whether the clinical situation is mimicking the "normal crisis" or whether there are aspects of the presentation, signs, and symptoms that suggest another diagnosis. Treatment involves adequate analgesia, hydration, and blood transfusion where necessary.

Acute Porphyria

This rare condition may be characterized by episodes of diffuse abdominal pain and urinary symptoms. The pain tends to move from one location in the abdomen to another, without localization. Occasionally, the abdominal examination may reveal rigidity and rebound tenderness making it indistinguishable from overt peritonitis. It is not uncommon to find that these patients have had previous abdominal surgery for similar symptoms, but that no organic cause was found.

REFERENCES

1. Saunders DI, Murray D, Pichel AC, et al.; UK Emergency Laparotomy Network. Variations in mortality after emergency laparotomy: the first report of the UK Emergency Laparotomy Network. Br J Anaesth. 2012;109(3):368-75.
2. Campbell WB, Lee EJK, Van de Sijpe K, et al. A 25-year study of emergency surgical admissions. Ann R Coll Surg Engl. 2002;84(4):273-7.
3. Marco CA, Schoenfeld CN, Keyl PM, et al. Abdominal pain in geriatric emergency patients: variables associated with adverse outcomes. Acad Emerg Med. 1998;5:1163-8.
4. Kizer KW, Vassar MJ. Emergency department diagnosis of abdominal disorders in the elderly. Am J Emerg Med. 1998;16:357-62.
5. Brewer BJ, Golden GT, Hitch DC, et al. Abdominal pain. An analysis of 1,000 consecutive cases in a University Hospital emergency room. Am J Surg. 1976;131:219-23.
6. Campling EA, Devlin HB, Hoile RW, et al. Report of the National Confidential Enquiry into Perioperative Deaths 1990. London: HMSO; 1992.
7. Calder FR, Jadhav V, Hale JE. The effect of a dedicated emergency theatre facility on emergency operating patterns. J R Coll Surg Edinb. 1998;43:17-9.
8. Irvin T. Abdominal pain: a surgical audit of 1190 emergency admissions. Br J Surg. 1989;76:1121-5.
9. Ohene-Yeboah M. Acute surgical admissions for abdominal pain in adults in Kumasi, Ghana. ANZ J Surg. 2006;76(10):898-903.
10. Memon A, Bhutto A, Shaikh G, et al. Spectrum of diseases in patients with nontraumatic acute abdomen. J Liaquat Univ Med Health Sci. 2008;180-83.
11. Qazi AR, Hussain NaqviI SQ, et al. Liver abscess: diagnosis and treatment. Pak J Surg. 2008:24(3):203-7.
12. Doshi K, Heaton W. Irritable bowel syndrome in patients discharged from surgical wards with non-specific abdominal pain. Br J Surg. 1994:81;1216-8.
13. Sanders D, Azmy IAF, Hurlstone DO. A new insight into non-specific abdominal pain. Ann RCS Eng. 2006;88(2):92-4.
14. Gray DWR, Collin J. Non-specific abdominal pain as a cause of acute admission to hospital. Br J Surg. 1987;74:239-42.
15. Jess P, Bjerregaard B, Brynitz S, et al. Prognosis of acute nonspecific abdominal pain: a prospective study. Am J Surg. 1982;144(3):338-40.
16. Banz VM, Sperisen O, de Moya M, et al. A 5-year follow-up of patients discharged with non-specific abdominal pain: out of sight, out of mind? Int Med J. 2012;42(4):395-401.
17. Paterson-Brown S. The acute abdomen: the role of laparoscopy. In: Williamson RCN, Thompson JN (EDs). Baillière's clinical gastroenterology: gastrointestinal emergencies, Part 1. London: Baillière Tindall; 1991. pp. 691-703.
18. Gaitan HG, Reveiz L, Farquhar C. Laparoscopy for the management of acute abdominal pain in women of childbearing age (Review). Cochrane Collaboration. 2011;Issue 1.
19. Adams ID, Chan M, Clifford PC, et al. Computer aided diagnosis of acute abdominal pain: a multi-centre study. Br Med J. 1986;293:800-4.

20. Paterson-Brown S, Vipond MN, Simms K, et al. Clinical decision-making and laparoscopy versus computer prediction in the management of the acute abdomen. Br J Surg. 1989;76:10113.
21. Attard AR, Corlett MJ, Kidner NJ, et al. Safety of early pain relief for acute abdominal pain. Br Med J. 1992;305:554-6.
22. Howie CR, Gunn AA. Temperature: a poor diagnostic indicator in abdominal pain. J R Coll Surg. 2000;87:49-52.
23. Dixon JM, Elton RA, Rainey JB, et al. Rectal examination in patients with pain in the right lower quadrant of the abdomen. Br Med J. 1991;302:386-8.
24. Andersson REB. Meta-analysis of the clinical and laboratory diagnosis of appendicitis. Br J Surg. 2004;91:28-37.
25. UK Working Party on Acute Pancreatitis. UK guidelines for the management of acute pancreatitis. Gut. 2005;54:1-9.
26. Cochrane RA, Edwards AT, Crosby DL, et al. Senior surgeons and radiologists should assess emergency patients on presentation: a prospective randomised controlled trial. J R Coll Surg Edinb. 1998;43:324-7.
27. Royal College of Radiologists working party. Making the Best Use of a Department of Clinical Radiology: Guidelines for Doctors, 5th edition. London: Royal College of Radiologists; 2003.
28. Wellwood JM, Wilson AN, Hopkinson BR. Gastrograffin as an aid to the diagnosis of perforated paptic ulcer. Br J Surg. 1971;58:245-9.
29. Chen SC, Lin FY, Lee PH, et al. Water-soluble contrast study predicts the need for early surgery in adhesive small bowel obstruction. Br J Surg. 1998;85:1692-4.
30. Lee JF-Y, Meng WC-S, Leung K-L, et al. Water soluble contrast follow through in the management of adhesive small bowel obstruction: a prospective randomized trial. Ann Coll Surg HK. 2004;8:120-6.
31. Crofts TJ, Park KGM, Steele RJC, et al. A randomized trial of non-operative treatment for perforated peptic ulcer. N Engl J Med. 1989;320:970-3.
32. Samuels BL, Freitas JE, Bree RL, et al. A comparison of radionuclide hepatobiliary imaging and real time ultrasound for the detection of acute cholecystitis. Radiology. 1983;47:207-10.
33. Puylaert IBCM, Rutgers PF, Lalisang RI, et al. A prospective study of ultrasonography in the diagnosis of appendicitis. N Engl J Med. 1987;317:666-9.
34. Gallego MG, Fadrique B, Nieto MA, et al. Evaluation of ultrasonography and clinical diagnostic scoring in suspected appendicitis. Br J Surg. 1998;85:37-40.
35. Huber-Wagner S, Lefering R, Qvick LM, et al. Effect of whole-body CT during trauma resuscitation on survival: a retrospective, multicentre study. Lancet. 2009;373:1455-61.
36. Sala E, Watson CJ, Beadsmoore C, et al. A randomized, controlled trial of routine early abdominal computed tomography in patients presenting with non-specific acute abdominal pain. Clin Radiol. 2007;62(10):961-9.
37. Birchard KR, Brown MA, Hyslop WB, et al. MRI of acute abdominal and pelvic pain in pregnant patients. AJR Am J Roentgenol. 2005;184(2):452-8.
38. Paterson-Brown S. Emergency laparoscopic surgery. Br J Surg. 1993;80:279-83.
39. Decadt B, Sussman L, Lewis MPN, et al. Randomised clinical trial of early laparoscopy in the management of acute non-specific abdominal pain. Br J Surg. 1999;86:1383-6.
40. Morino M, Pellegrino L, Castagna E, et al. Acute non-specific abdominal pain: a randomized controlled trial comparing early laparoscopy versus clinical observation. Ann Surg. 2006;244:881-8.
41. Paterson-Brown S, Thompson JN, Eckersley JRT, et al. Which patient with suspected appendicitis should undergo laparoscopy? Br Med J. 1988;296:1363-4.
42. Wen SW, Naylor CD. Diagnostic accuracy and short-term surgical outcomes in cases of suspected appendicitis. Can Med Assoc J. 1995;152:1617-26.
43. Rao PM, Rhea JT, Novelline RA, et al. Effect of computed tomography of the appendix on treatment of patients and use of hospital resources. N Engl J Med. 1998;338:141-6.
44. Temple CL, Huchcroft SA, Temple WJ. The natural history of appendicitis in adults: a prospective study. Ann Surg. 1995;221:278-81.
45. De U, Ghosh S. Acute appendicectomy for appendicular mass: a study of 87 patients. Ceylon Med J. 2002:47; 117-8.
46. Assalia A, Schein M, Kopelman D, et al. Therapeutic effect of oral Gastrografin on adhesive, partial small bowel obstruction: a prospective randomized trial. Surgery. 1994;115: 433-7.
47. Zerey M, Sechrist CW, Kercher KW, et al. The laparoscopic management of small-bowel obstruction. Am J Surg. 2007;194(6):882-7.
48. Zorcolo L, Covotta L, Carlomagno N, et al. Safety of primary anastomosis in emergency colorectal surgery. Colorectal Disease. 2003;262-9.
49. Sebastian S, Johnston S, Geoaghegan T, et al. Pooled analysis of the efficacy and safety of self-expanding metal stenting in malignant colorectal obstruction. Am J Gastroenterology. 2004;9:2051-7.
50. Ralls PW, Colletti PM, Lapin SA, et al. Real-time sonography in suspected acute cholecystitis: prospective evaluation of primary and secondary signs. Radiology. 1985;155:767-71.

Additional references appear in the online version of this book.

75

Intestinal Obstruction

Abeezar I Sarela

Key Points

- Think of intestinal obstruction according to whether or not there has been a previous abdominal operation.
- In early postoperative "ileus", peritonitis due to a "missed" enterotomy or another source of enteric leakage should always be considered.
- In a previously operated abdomen, adhesions are the commonest cause of mechanical obstruction, but alternative diagnoses should always be considered.
- Non-operative treatment should be limited to adhesional obstruction and non-mechanical (paralytic) obstruction.
- Consider the use of laparoscopy when an operation is required.
- Consider self-expanding metallic stents for left-sided colonic obstruction.

INTRODUCTION

Intestinal obstruction has been recognized and described since classical times. The late 19th and early 20th centuries saw major advances in the understanding and clinical management of bowel obstruction. Treves's seminal publication in 1884[1] dealt with the pathological basis, diagnosis, and management of the condition. Along with the evolution in the management of intestinal obstruction, the relative frequencies of various causes of obstruction have also changed. Large series from the late 19th and early 20th centuries showed incarcerated hernias to be responsible for intestinal obstruction in up to 50% of cases.[2,3] In contrast, case-series during the past 40 years report that postoperative adhesions are now the most common cause of obstruction.

Obstruction of the intestine may be broadly categorized as (1) mechanical, i.e., caused by a structural blockage to the lumen of the bowel or (2) nonmechanical, often referred to as paralytic or adynamic ileus, which implies failure of the propulsive activity of the bowel. Mechanical obstruction will be considered separately for the small intestine and the large intestine, because of important differences in etiology, clinical features, and management options. Ileus is dealt with in the separate section on early postoperative intestinal obstruction; in this situation it is particularly necessary to distinguish between mechanical and nonmechanical causes. However, ileus can also occur in situations unrelated to recent operation, such as electrolyte disturbances associated with a systemic medical disorder, trauma with retroperitoneal bleeding, or acute pancreatitis; in such situations, the primary management is that of the underlying disorder.

ETIOLOGY

Mechanical obstruction may be classified as partial or complete, depending upon whether or not the obstructing lesion permits the passage of some intestinal content. (Table 75.1) Open-loop obstruction—obstruction at only

Table 75.1 Classification of mechanical intestinal obstruction.

Classification	*Division*
Etiology	Intraluminal Intramural Extrinsic
Location within the gastrointestinal tract	Small bowel (proximal or distal) Large bowel
Speed of onset	Acute Subacute Chronic
Degree	Partial or complete
Progression	Open versus closed loop Simple versus strangulated

Table 75.2 Causes of small bowel obstruction.

Site of obstruction	*Cause*
Luminal	Intussusception Meconium Polypoid tumor Gallstone Bezoar (trichobezoar, phytobezoar) Parasites Feces
Mural	Stricture (e.g., caused by inflammatory bowel disease, radiation) Small bowel tumor (benign, malignant) Congenital (atresia, stenosis, duplication)
Extrinsic	Adhesion Hernia (external, internal) Volvulus Malignant or inflammatory mass

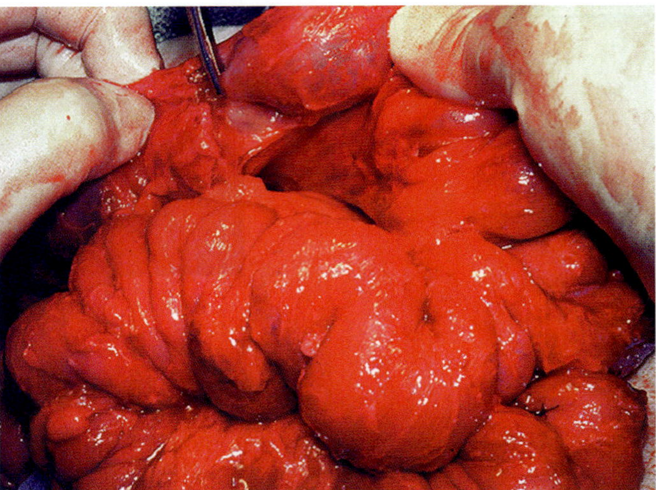

Fig. 75.1: Grade 4 fibrous adhesions between loops of small bowel. Typical appearance at operation.

one level in the intestine—allows some decompression by progressive distention of proximal bowel and vomiting. In contrast, with closed-loop obstruction, there is obstruction at two levels, e.g., volvulus of the colon or colonic obstruction with a competent ileocecal valve. Herein, there is no decompression of the obstructed bowel, which may result in rapid distention and high luminal pressure leading to ischemia and perforation of the bowel wall. Strangulation occurs if the blood supply to the obstructed bowel is compromised. The blood supply may be impaired by external compression of the bowel wall, as in incarcerated hernias; compression or twisting of the mesentery, as in a volvulus or intussusception; and high pressure within the obstructed bowel, as in a closed-loop obstruction.

The etiology of mechanical obstruction may be conceptually divided into factors that occur in the lumen of the intestine (intraluminal), in the wall of the intestine (intramural), or extrinsic (extramural) (Table 75.2). In practice, the etiology of obstruction is best considered in terms of frequency of incidence and separately for the small intestine versus the colon. Intestinal obstruction in the early period after an abdominal operation is dealt with as a third, separate entity.

Small Intestine

In dealing with mechanical obstruction of the small intestine, it is useful to categorize patients in two separate groups: those who have had previous abdominal surgery and those with an unoperated or "virgin" abdomen.

Previous Abdominal Surgery

In case of small intestinal obstruction in patients who have previously undergone an abdominal operation, the most frequent cause is peritoneal adhesions (Fig. 75.1). Adhesions form because of fibrin deposition at the site of peritoneal injury—a part of the normal healing mechanism. Insufficient fibrinolysis during the early postoperative period (48 hours) leads to infiltration of the fibrin deposits with cells, which comprise a variable population of smooth muscle, nerve, and endothelium, and the entire assembly, is covered with a mesothelial lining (Flowchart 75.1). Formation of adhesions is promoted by repeated operations, intra-abdominal infection, blood, debris, and technical trauma.[4]

There are sparse data on the frequency with which adhesions occur after abdominal surgery, but available evidence suggests that at least some adhesions form in up to 100% of cases. The relevant issue is the proportion of patients who suffer adverse consequences from adhesions: either direct consequences (intestinal obstruction, chronic abdominal pain, or female infertility) or indirect consequences (difficulty during subsequent unrelated operations). Some insightful information on the consequences of adhesions comes from a Scottish population-based study of about 30,000 patients, with 10 years of follow-up.[5] Following abdominal or pelvic surgery, one in three patients was readmitted to hospital at least twice during the subsequent 10 years for a problem that was directly or possibly caused by adhesions or for an unrelated operation that was complicated by the presence of

Flowchart 75.1: Pathophysiology of postoperative adhesions.

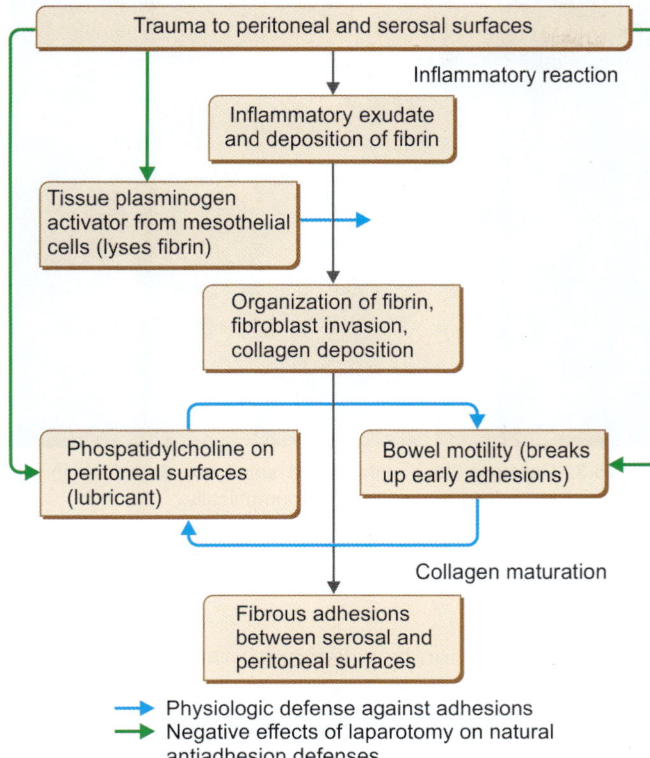

adhesions: about 55% of these patients had 1 readmission, 40% had 2–5 readmissions, and 5% had 6 or more readmissions, resulting in an overall incidence of 70 readmissions for every 100 laparotomies. Patients are most likely to be readmitted in the first year after operation (20% of all readmissions), but the incidence of readmission does continue steadily thereafter. About 12% of patients with abdominal surgery had reoperation for reasons directly or possibly related to adhesions, and about 25% of patients had nonoperative management of problems directly or possibly related to adhesions.[5] The frequency of readmission and number of admissions are higher with midgut or hindgut operations as compared with foregut or gynecological operations. It appears logical to assume that laparoscopy is associated with fewer and less problematic adhesions than conventional, open operation. However, long-term follow-up of patients in a clinical trial of laparoscopic versus open colorectal resection indicates a similar incidence of intestinal obstruction with either approach.[6]

Whilst adhesions are the commonest cause of obstruction in the previously operated abdomen, it is important to remember other conditions:

- Abdominal wall hernia (at the site of a laparotomy incision or laparoscopy port-site). It can be particularly difficult in obese patients to detect such hernias by clinical examination.
- Internal hernia of the intestine through an iatrogenically-created defect or space in the mesentery or mesocolon.
- Stenosis of an intestinal anastomosis.
- Recurrence of recrudescence of disease for which laparotomy had been performed, e.g. cancer or Crohn's disease.
- Any one of the causes of obstruction discussed in the section below on a "virgin" abdomen can occur also in the previously operated abdomen.

The index of suspicion and diagnosis of a causative factor, other than adhesions, will depend on the constellation of history, symptoms, physical signs, and radiological findings. The distinction is important because (as discussed subsequently) a trial of nonoperative treatment is usually only applicable to patients with adhesive obstruction.

"Virgin" Abdomen

In case of small intestinal obstruction in the absence of previous abdominal surgery, an abdominal wall hernia is the most likely cause. Of all cases of hernia-related obstruction, about 50% result from inguinal hernias, 25% from femoral hernias, and 25% from ventral hernias. Compared with adhesive obstruction, hernia obstruction is more likely to be complete, less likely to resolve nonoperatively (unless the hernia can be reduced), and more likely to strangulate. Femoral hernias are especially prone to obstruction and strangulation; 50% of all strangulated groin hernias are femoral.[7,8]

If there is no hernia on clinical examination, the differential diagnosis should consider the following causes:

Congenital

Adhesions, malrotation of the intestine, or internal hernias of the intestine through a naturally occurring defect in the mesentery, mesocolon, or omentum.

Cancer

Primary cancers of the small intestine—adenocarcinoma, gastrointestinal stromal tumor, lymphoma, and neuroendocrine carcinoma—are all uncommon but may present with features of obstruction. Adenocarcinoma of caecum, presenting with features of small intestinal obstruction, is probably more common than primary small bowel cancer. Peritoneal metastasis from a nonintestinal cancer, e.g., stomach or pancreas, also may present with small intestinal obstruction.

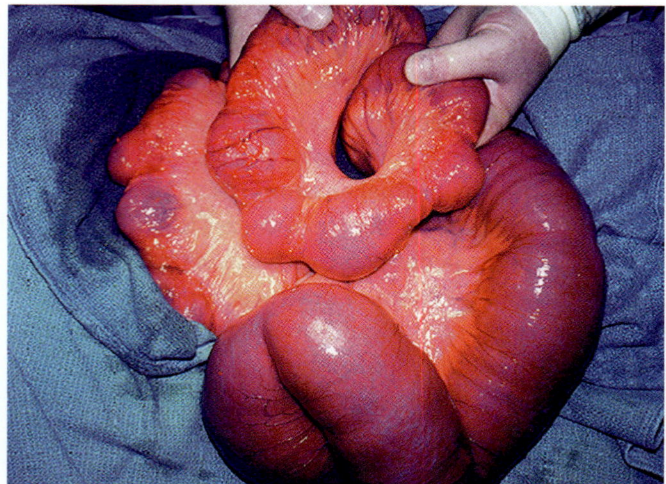

Fig. 75.2: Multiple small bowel strictures in Crohn's disease. These are causing marked distention of the proximal bowel.

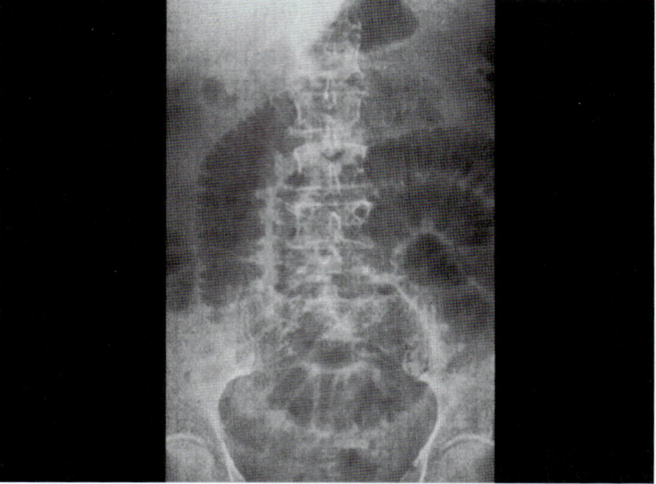

Fig. 75.3: Gallstone ileus with dilated small bowel and air in the biliary tree. No gallstone was seen radiographically.
Source: Courtesy of David Einstein.

Crohn's Disease

The small bowel is the most common site of obstruction caused by Crohn's disease: the terminal ileum and ileocecal regions are especially affected (Fig. 75.2). The obstruction may result from either the acute inflammatory process or the fibrosis and scarring of the bowel wall that occurs with persistence or healing of the acute process. Obstruction associated with the acute phase of the disease usually responds to nonoperative therapy with bowel rest, corticosteroids, and 5-aminosalicylate compounds; urgent operation is rarely required. Failure to respond to an appropriate trial of anti-inflammatory medication and inability to withdraw high levels of corticosteroids without recurrence of symptoms are indications for surgical intervention. Small bowel strictures are usually suspected on clinical grounds and are best confirmed by small bowel contrast studies such as an enteroclysis or small bowel series.

Radiation Enteritis

Radiation injury to the bowel produces a characteristic pattern of damage. There is an acute phase of injury, in which the rapidly dividing mucosal cells are damaged, and a later phase, characterized by obliteration of the small end arterioles. This endarteritis obliterans produces an ischemia-like injury with fibrosis and stricture, and these features are pronounced in the small intestine. Injury is especially common after irradiation for uterine or cervical cancer. The commonly injured sites are the ileum, rectosigmoid, and rectum.

Gallstone Ileus

Intestinal obstruction by gallstones is rare, being responsible for about 1% of all cases of small bowel obstruction and occurring in only a very small proportion of the patients who have cholelithiasis. Large gallstones can erode from the gallbladder or bile duct into the duodenum. Patients are often not known to have gallstones. Symptoms are dependent upon the site of impaction of the gallstone: most commonly, the terminal ileum, followed by the second portion of the duodenum, and the sigmoid colon. Abdominal plain radiographs may show features of intestinal obstruction, air in the biliary tree (Fig. 75.3), and a gallstone within the intestine (all three signs constitute Rigler's triad, which is present in $<10\%$ of cases); computed tomography CT scan can demonstrate similar features.

Intussusception

Intussusception is the invagination of a more proximal segment of bowel (intussusceptum) into a more distal segment of bowel (intussuscipiens). It is a rare cause of bowel obstruction in adults, unlike in children, who comprise the vast majority of patients with intussusception. In most adult cases, an intraluminal lesion forms the leading edge of the intussusceptum, which by peristalsis is invaginated into the distal bowel lumen (Fig. 75.4). As the intussusceptum passes progressively further distally, its mesentery enters the intussuscipiens and may be compressed, which compromises the vascular supply and leads to edema, ischemia, and ultimately gangrene. Small bowel intussusception is approximately twice as common as large bowel intussusception. The stool of a patient with intussuception has been described to have a "red currant jelly" appearance because of the presence of blood and mucosal slough. Diagnosis may be confirmed with either small bowel series, a barium enema, or a CT scan, but it is often made at operation or at colonoscopy (Figs. 75.5A to C).

Large Intestine

In case of colonic obstruction, the commonest cause is carcinoma, followed by benign strictures (diverticular or ischemia) and volvulus of the sigmoid colon.

Early Postoperative Obstruction

An operation on the abdomen may result in temporary cessation or paralysis of the propulsive activity of the gastrointestinal tract; this condition often is referred to as "ileus." The term ileus is derived from a Greek word that means "to roll." The commonest cause of an ileus is a laparotomy, following which there is a predictable decrease in intestinal motility. The response is not uniform throughout the intestinal tract: the small bowel migrating motor complexes usually return first, with activity seen as early as 6 hours after laparotomy; gastric tone takes up to 1 day to return, and colonic motility may take 2–3 days.

The etiology of postoperative ileus is multifactorial: surgical stress, secretion of inflammatory mediators and endogenous opioids in the gastrointestinal tract, changes in hormone levels, and electrolyte and fluid imbalance. The frequency and severity of ileus can differ enormously, according to the nature of the procedure and clinical management of the perioperative pathway.[9] One of the major benefits of recently popularized enhanced recovery pathways is to speed intestinal recovery.[10] "Bowel rest" is no longer considered to be an essential part of the postoperative period, and early introduction of oral intake, in fact, is advantageous.

There is a typical duration of ileus following different procedures: for example, following an uneventful laparoscopic cholecystectomy, immediate resumption of intake

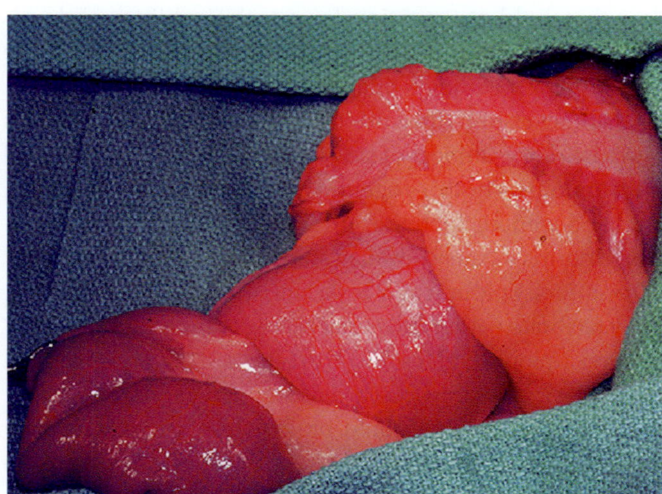

Fig. 75.4: Adult ileocecal intussusception secondary to a terminal ileal polyp. Terminal ileum (left) intussuscepting into cecum (right), intraoperative appearance.

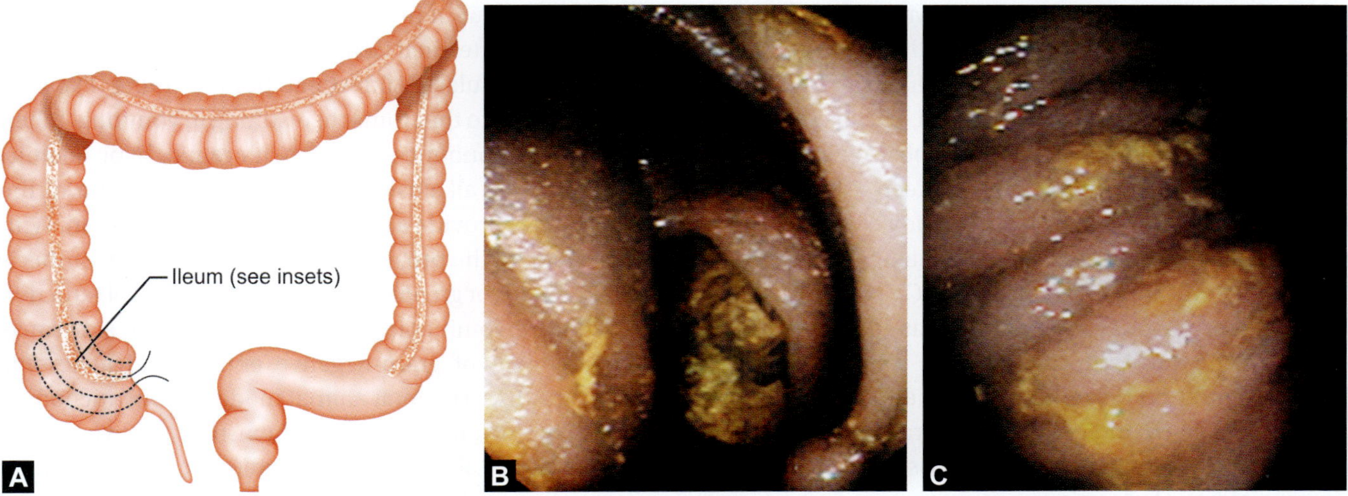

Figs. 75.5A to C: Colonoscopic appearance of ileocecal intussusception shown in Figure 75.4. Ileum (intussusceptum) has intussuscepted into the cecum (intussuscipiens).

of solid food is expected, whereas full recovery of bowel function (i.e., toleration of solid food and passage of flatus and stool) takes an average of 5 days after colonic resection.[11] Prolonged postoperative ileus—failure of recovery of intestinal function in the usual time-frame—is an issue of concern. There are no threshold intervals for intestinal recovery, which will vary by nature of the procedure and individual surgical practice. For example, in colonic resections, prolonged ileus—defined as need for insertion of a nasogastric tube during the postoperative period or a complication related to bowel dysfunction—occurs in about 15% of patients.[11]

In the case of prolonged ileus, it is critical to keep a low threshold of suspicion for a technical intra-abdominal catastrophe—such as iatrogenic perforation of the intestine or bleeding—that may be the cause of ileus.

Strategies to reduce the duration of postoperative ileus have been the subject of much effort. It is well recognized that opioids—both exogenously administered analgesia and endogenous secretions in response to the stress of surgical trauma—cause bowel dysfunction by action on enteric μ receptors. Epidural analgesia with a local anesthetic agent may facilitate earlier intestinal recovery than that with parenteral opioid analgesia.[12] Also, there is now substantial evidence that alvimopan, a synthetic μ receptor antagonist that does not cross the blood-brain barrier, can significantly enhance bowel recovery.[13] The recommended dose is one 12 mg capsule just before operation and another 12 mg dose twice daily for up to 7 days, but not exceeding 15 doses. Gum chewing[14] and coffee consumption[15] also have been reported to reduce the duration of postoperative ileus.

The possibility of mechanical obstruction must be considered in the postoperative patient with delayed recovery of bowel function. It is difficult to distinguish clinically between mechanical and nonmechanical obstruction, during the early postoperative period, because the typical symptoms and signs of mechanical obstruction are often absent. It is, therefore, prudent to keep a high index of suspicion for mechanical obstruction (and for intra-abdominal catastrophes, such as bleeding or peritonitis) and a low threshold for requesting a CT scan of the abdomen. Adhesions may cause problems in the early postoperative period. With laparoscopic surgery, a port-site hernia should be borne in mind. If an anastomosis has been constructed, then early postoperative stenosis due to a technical error or excessive fibrosis is another possibility. In case of bowel resection or anastomosis, an early postoperative internal hernia through a defect in the mesentery may cause obstruction.

PATHOPHYSIOLOGY AND CLINICAL FEATURES

The classic presenting symptoms of intestinal obstruction are abdominal distension, vomiting, constipation or obstipation (failure to pass flatus or stool), and colic-like abdominal pain. The prominence of any symptom is likely to vary according to the site and degree of the obstruction.

Accumulation of fluid and air leads to progressive dilation of the intestine proximal to the site of obstruction, with consequent distension of the abdomen. There may be little or no distension of the abdomen in case of obstruction in the proximal jejunum. The gas that accumulates proximal to an obstructed segment of bowel is largely from swallowed air, reflected in its high nitrogen content (70–80%); the contribution of bacterial gas is small. The increased luminal pressure decreases absorption and increases secretion of water and electrolytes by the bowel wall. Sequestration of fluid within the bowel is particularly important in case of a distal site of obstruction; conversely, with proximal obstruction, loss of fluid by vomiting may be greater. In each case, substantial amounts of fluid are lost from the extracellular space. A mild acidosis is often observed, as a result of the systemic hypovolemia.

The proximal intestine initially attempts forceful, spasmodic contractions in order to overcome the obstruction, resulting in episodes of colic that correspond to the contractions, with intermittent pain relief during muscular relaxation. If the obstruction is not relieved, there is progressive failure of smooth muscular activity; the colic-like pain resolves and may be replaced with a constant dull ache. It is important to remember that constant pain that is severe and out of proportion to physical signs is highly suggestive of intestinal ischemia.

The accumulated intestinal fluid is quite likely to decompress into the stomach, resulting in vomiting. When vomiting is pronounced, a hypochloremic, hypokalemic, and metabolic alkalosis may develop. The nature of the vomitus may provide a clue to the site of obstruction. With obstruction of the proximal small intestine, the vomitus is usually bilious or greenish in color. As the site of obstruction moves distal, vomitus acquires a feculent character because of overgrowth of gram-negative enteric and anaerobic organisms. Experimental animal models of obstruction, in the absence of bacteria, fail to demonstrate the hypersecretion and reduce absorption of fluid and electrolytes. Further, obstruction predisposes to intravascular translocation of bacteria and endotoxins, which may be responsible for some of the systemic septic consequences of bowel obstruction.

Box 75.1	The four cardinal features of strangulation
1. Persistence of pain after nasogastric decompression.	
2. Local abdominal tenderness.	
3. Tachycardia.	
4. Leukocytosis.	

Note: Not all of these features are present in every case, and the surgeon should have a low threshold for urgent operation if there is any suspicion of strangulation. One seldom regrets this course and sometimes small bowel infarction is present despite very little clinical evidence.

Obstipation is most likely with distal colonic obstruction. When the site of obstruction is more proximal, passage of small volumes of fecal matter or gas (from the distal segment of the intestine) may continue for some days despite complete obstruction of the lumen. Similarly, if there is only partial obstruction of the lumen of the intestine, passage of flatus and stools may continue and all symptoms may be attenuated.

CLINICAL EVALUATION AND INVESTIGATIONS

Clinical evaluation of a patient with obstruction should aim to answer the following questions:

- Are the symptoms and signs consistent with bowel obstruction?
- Is the obstruction partial or complete?
- Is there obstruction of the small or large intestine?
- Is there evidence of strangulation or perforation (*see* Box 75.1)?
- What is the likely etiology of the obstruction?
- How severe is the fluid deficit and electrolyte imbalance?

Examination

Inspection of the abdomen should make note of operation scars, all hernial orifices and the presence or absence of distension. Palpation aims to reveal signs of localized or generalized peritonitis (involuntary guarding, rebound, and tenderness), abdominal masses, and tender hernial masses. Auscultation may reveal classic high-pitched "tinkling" bowel sounds, which often accompany the colicky pain, but bowel sounds may be entirely absent—a "silent" abdomen—at a late stage. Gentle percussion can be used to detect tenderness, suggestive of localized or generalized peritonitis. Rectal examination is an essential part of the clinical examination to diagnose an obstructing rectal lesion, usually a carcinoma.

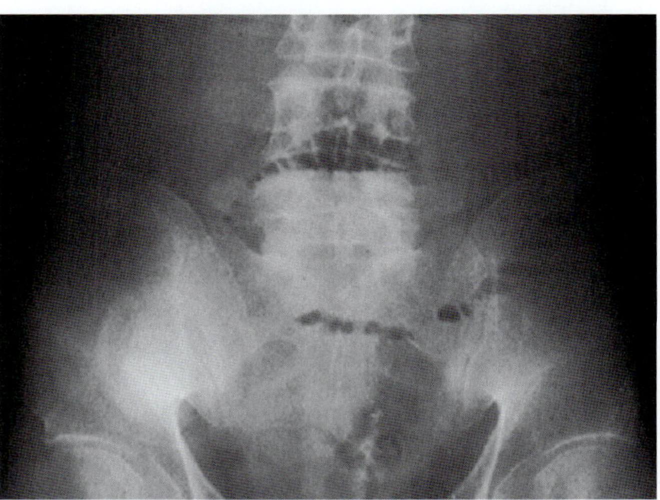

Fig. 75.6: String of pearls or string of beads sign. This is a classic upright plain radiograph seen in small bowel obstruction.
Source: Courtesy of David Einstein.

Investigations

Laboratory Investigations

Laboratory investigations aim to assess the degree of dehydration and electrolyte imbalance. Laboratory evidence of bowel ischemia also may be present, but no single test is specific or sensitive enough to be of consistent value. Leukocytosis, metabolic acidosis, and increased serum lactate levels are indicators of bowel ischemia and may be used to help with decision-making.

Radiology

Plain X-rays: Radiological evaluation traditionally starts with three plain X-rays films: erect chest view and erect as well as supine abdomen views. The upper limit of normal small bowel caliber on a plain radiograph is 3 cm. In the upright or decubitus radiograph, the interface between gas and fluid in the bowel forms a straight, horizontal margin, or an "air-fluid level"; more than two air-fluid levels are considered to be abnormal. Distinction of the small bowel from the large bowel can be difficult: small bowel has a central location within the abdomen and circumferential, fine valvulae conniventes, in contrast to the more peripheral colon with its thicker and incomplete haustral markings. Sometimes, the bowel contains mostly fluid with little air, especially if the patient has a nasogastric tube. On an upright radiograph, such fluid-filled bowel may produce a "string of beads" appearance, with small gas bubbles in an oblique line (Fig. 75.6); however, if there is no gas, the fluid-filled loops may be difficult to appreciate.

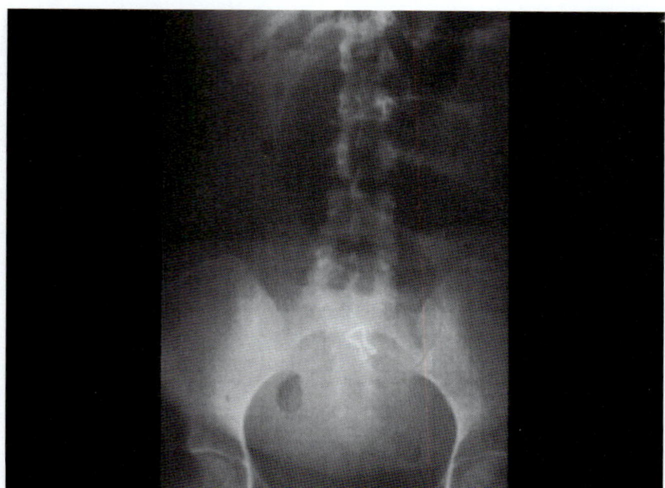

Fig. 75.7: Dilated loops of small bowel. Typical appearance of small bowel obstruction on supine film with dilated loops in the left upper quadrant (incidental overlying metallic object in pelvis).
Source: Courtesy of David Einstein.

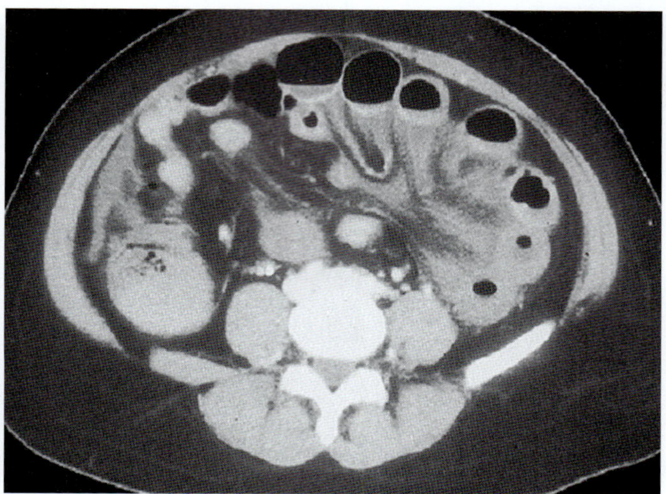

Fig. 75.8: Closed-loop obstruction. This CT scan shows thickening of the small bowel wall (most pronounced in the left gutter) with edema or hemorrhage into the mesentery.
Source: Courtesy of David Einstein.

The number and position of dilated small bowel loops can give some information about the level of obstruction. Jejunal obstruction may produce only a few dilated loops of small bowel, high in the central or upper left quadrants of the abdomen. As additional loops are affected, these tend to be placed one below the other, progressing from the left upper to the right lower quadrants, as dictated by the attachment of the base of the mesentery, giving a "step-ladder" pattern. The presence of gas in the colon in the setting of a small bowel obstruction may suggest that the obstruction is partial, although after the onset of complete small bowel obstruction it may take 1–2 days for air to clear from the colon (Fig. 75.7). A gas-filled, closed-loop obstruction, assuming the shape of a coffee bean, may be apparent on a plain radiograph. However, a closed loop is usually filled with fluid only and this may be difficult to see unless outlined by other gas-distended loops of bowel. This "pseudotumor" sign suggests a closed loop, especially if it remains in the same position with different projections. The complications of strangulation are occasionally noted on a plain radiograph: free fluid may separate adjacent loops of bowel; mural necrosis may produce gas within the bowel wall or in the portal venous system; and perforation can lead to the presence of free air within the abdomen.

It is radiologically difficult to distinguish between adynamic ileus and mechanical small bowel obstruction. With ileus, gas is expected to be present in both the small and large intestine but, as mentioned above, in complete small bowel obstruction gas may take up to 48 hours to clear from the colon; hence, clinical correlation and repeat radiographs are important.

Single contrast enema studies: If obstruction of the left colon is suspected by plain X-rays, a water-soluble contrast enema study may be used to distinguish between pseudo-obstruction and mechanical obstruction. Contrast studies confirm a plain x-ray diagnosis of mechanical obstruction in only about 2 out of 3 patients.[16] CT scan can confirm a diagnosis of obstruction or pseudo-obstruction in over 90% of cases and will avoid the need for a contrast enema.

Computed tomography scan: There are several limitations and fallacies in plain radiology evaluation, and CT scan should be the primary imaging modality for decision-making. CT scan with intravenous contrast can diagnose bowel ischemia plus the site and cause of obstruction with fairly high accuracy. CT scan findings of obstruction are distended bowel, with a transition area to collapsed bowel, and failure of oral contrast to progress beyond the transition zone (Fig. 75.8). Localization of the site of obstruction by CT scanning is particularly valuable if the intent is to perform laparoscopic surgery.[17] CT scan is also useful to diagnose metastatic disease in cases of large bowel cancer; such staging can result in important changes in the management plan.

CONSERVATIVE OR OPERATIVE MANAGEMENT?

A critical decision is whether an operation should be performed immediately or whether the patient should

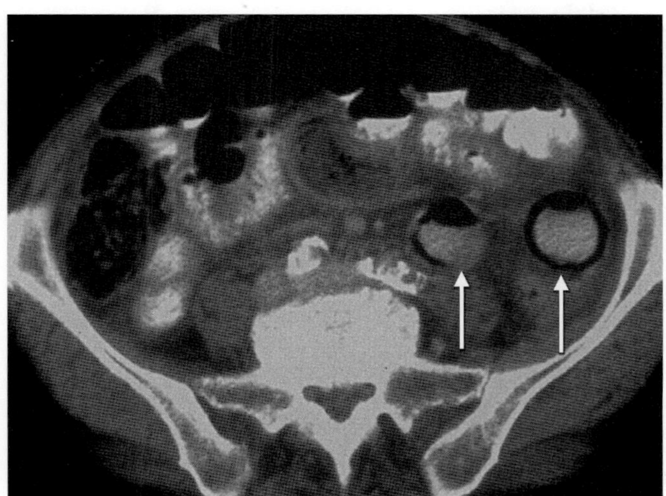

Fig. 75.9: Obstructed loop of small bowel in the left lower quadrant with strangulation causing pronounced pneumatosis in both limbs of this loop (arrows).
Source: Courtesy of David Einstein.

have an initial trial of nonoperative treatment. A trial of nonoperative management is mainly relevant for patients in whom the suspected etiology is adhesions. Patients with clinical features of peritonitis or ischemia, such as constant pain, tachycardia, leukocytosis, guarding, metabolic acidosis, or CT features of bowel ischemia (Fig. 75.9), should undergo an urgent operation. It is salutary to remember that clinical and radiological diagnoses of ischemia are subject to various inaccuracies. There have been attempts to devise composite models to predict the risk of strangulation, but none is able to replace clinical wisdom. In view of the disastrous and potentially lethal consequences of strangulation, it is sensible to maintain a low threshold for early operation. CT evidence of a disease, e.g., a tumor, that will inevitably require an operation for relief of obstruction, also should prompt early operation.

The incidence of successful nonoperative management is higher in cases of partial or low-grade obstruction of the lumen of the intestine (as judged by CT scan) as opposed to complete or high-grade obstruction. The initial management of patients with complete small bowel obstruction remains controversial, but nonoperative care is not absolutely contraindicated. Standard nonoperative management comprises decompression of the upper gastrointestinal tract by a nasogastric tube and administration of appropriate fluid and electrolytes ("suck and drip").

If intestinal obstruction does not resolve by the end of a 48-hour period of nonoperative management, it is recommended that the patient should undergo a water soluble contrast study.[18] In a meta-analysis of 14 prospectively conducted studies, appearance of contrast in the colon within 4–24 hours predicted resolution of obstruction without an operation in 99% of patients. On the other hand, if contrast does not reach the colon within the specified time period, then about 90% of patients are likely to need an operation. The pooled sensitivity and specificity approached 100%, indicating that water-soluble contrast is a very accurate indicator. In addition, water-soluble contrast may have a therapeutic role, possibly by reducing bowel wall edema through osmotic drawing of intramural fluid into the lumen; it significantly reduces the need for operation (20% in patients who had contrast versus 29% without contrast) and shortens hospital stay. Irrespective of a contrast study, failure to resolve by 5 days indicates the need for operation.[19] Apart from a contrast study, various predictive models[20] and single-agent markers[21] have been proposed to estimate the success of nonoperative treatment and the optimum threshold for operation.

Decision-making about operative versus continued nonoperative management can be particularly difficult in terminally ill patients and in those with incurable, often recurrent, intra-abdominal malignancy of gastrointestinal or gynecological origin. Operations for acute bowel obstruction in the face of such advanced intra-abdominal cancer are associated with very high morbidity and mortality rates and a median postoperative survival of no more than 6 months. Further, relief of symptoms by operation can vary greatly between 40% and 80%, and there is high risk of reobstruction (10–50%).[22] Careful staging of the cancer and consideration of the natural history of disease is necessary for thoughtful decision-making; discussion with the oncologist in charge of the case is usually very helpful. Conversely, adhesions may be the causative factor in patients who have had previous abdominal surgery for cancer, so cancer recurrence should not automatically be assumed to be the cause of obstruction in such patients.

Serious consideration should be given to a nonoperative approach, such as endoscopic percutaneous gastrostomy for decompression plus pharmacologic treatment of symptoms. Symptoms of obstruction may be greatly relieved by opioids, phenothiazine antiemetics, anticholinergics (to reduce colic) and somatostatin analogs (to reduce intestinal secretions), corticosteroids,[23] and dietary manipulation (low residue). Consultation with a palliative care team is valuable in these circumstances. If an operation is undertaken, the least extensive procedure should be undertaken, e.g., bypass of an obstructed area in preference to resection.

TREATMENT OF INTESTINAL OBSTRUCTION

Surgical management of obstructing lesions in the small intestine and right side of the colon are considered together because emergency resection and reconstruction of the right colon appears to have risks that are similar to those of elective operation. In contrast, it has been historically perceived that operating on an obstructing left-sided colonic lesion is associated with much higher risks than those of an elective operation; hence, surgical management of left-sided colonic obstruction, which is most often due to malignancy, is considered separately. Irrespective of the site of obstruction, adequate resuscitation and replenishment of fluid and electrolyte deficiencies is vital before any operation.

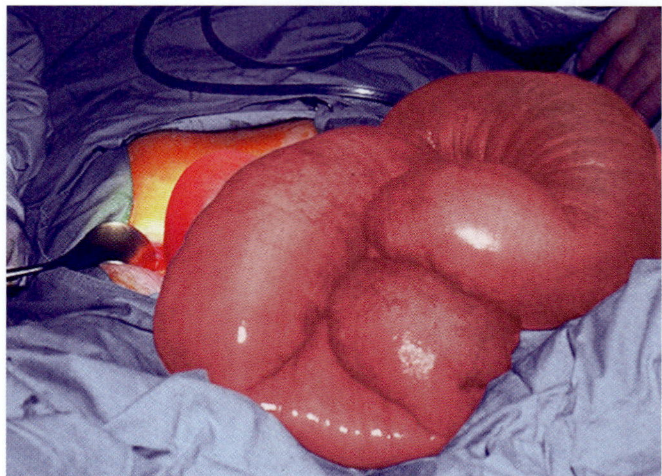

Fig. 75.10: Massive small bowel distention. This was secondary to adhesive obstruction, and the loops required decompression before adhesiolysis could be safely carried out.

Obstruction of Small Bowel and Right Colon

Several special situations and areas of debate are considered separately.

Approach: Laparoscopic versus Open?

Laparoscopic surgery has been considered particularly for adhesions, but the general considerations may be extrapolated to other causes of obstruction. Laparoscopic adhesiolysis has substantial potential benefit[24] and should be undertaken according to the expertise and experience of the operator. There are no absolute contraindications to laparoscopy, although it is useful to bear in mind the greater technical difficulty in case of substantially distended bowel because of limited intra-abdominal space and risk of iatrogenic perforation during manipulation (Fig. 75.10). If laparoscopic expertise is available, it is sensible to attempt laparoscopy liberally, provided that there is not excessive concern for safe access, and then make a decision, according to the laparoscopic findings, about continuing with laparoscopic dissection or converting to laparotomy.[25,26] For example, dense or diffuse adhesions are likely to be associated with high incidence of iatrogenic perforation, in which case it would be prudent to convert early to laparotomy.[27] In general, it is sensible to opt for early conversion to open operation in case of difficulty or failure to progress rather than be compelled to convert in order to deal with an iatrogenic injury.

Limited versus Complete Dissection of Small Intestine

An occasional intraoperative dilemma in case of adhesional obstruction is whether to limit adhesiolysis to the site of the likely obstruction or to dissect the entire small intestine. A single-band adhesion that demarcates distended from collapsed bowel provides a discrete target and an easy decision; the effectiveness of adhesiolysis may be confirmed by visual decompression of the distended proximal bowel and entry of the fluid into the collapsed segment. If an obvious cause of obstruction is not apparent, then a useful technique is to identify collapsed ileum close to the ileocecal valve and follow the collapsed intestine to identify the site of obstruction. Such a strategy minimizes the handling of dilated bowel, with the associated risk of perforation. The surgeon's confidence in effective relief of obstruction may be less if there are complex or matted adhesions, and some studies have reported a high incidence of reoperations because of misrecognition at the initial operation. However, on balance, it appears prudent to "do less rather than more" and limit adhesiolysis to the area of obstruction rather than undertake complete adhesiolysis of the entire length of the small intestine.[17] Ultimately, however, clinical discretion must be applied on a case-by-case basis.

Routine Manual Decompression

Conventional teaching is to decompress the distended small intestine into either the stomach or the colon or via an enterotomy. However, there is some evidence that "milking" of the small intestine does not appear to confer benefit.[28] Whilst decompression may not necessarily benefit physiological recovery of the intestine, it can be of considerable technical help in facilitating closure of the abdomen after a laparotomy.

Determination of Intestinal Viability

Determination of viability of bowel that appears to have impaired blood supply—variously described as dusky, mottled, or bluish-back—can be exceedingly difficult. The initial approach is to wrap the bowel in warm, moist pads for about 15 minutes and then reexamine the bowel. If doubt persists, the use of intravenous fluorescein with an ultraviolet light source or a Doppler probe to check for arterial pulsation in the bowel wall may help. Short segments of questionable bowel should be excised, but if removal of all doubtful bowel would leave insufficient intestine for effective enteral nutrition, then only clearly dead bowel should be removed and a second-look laparotomy should be performed within 12–24 hours. Early postoperative institution of parenteral feeding may prevent nutritional depletion in such patients.

Anti-adhesion Measures

Several adhesion-prevention barrier agents have been tried, but none can be definitively recommended at present. Hyaluronic acid-carboxymethyl cellulose membrane (Seprafilm™) appears to reduce the severity of adhesions but not the incidence of intestinal obstruction, and it may increase the incidence of anastomotic leakage and intra-abdominal abscesses.[29] Meticulous dissection with minimal trauma is a fundamental strategy to minimize adhesions; no single technique—scissors, scalpel, ultrasonic dissection, etc.—has an overriding advantage.

Hernia

Patients who present with obstruction and an incarcerated hernia must be carefully examined; the findings of redness, marked tenderness, and irreducibility strongly suggest strangulation. In such a case, immediate operation is indicated. In the absence of findings suggestive of strangulation, reduction of the hernia may be attempted. If reduction of the hernia relieves pain and obstructive symptoms, then early elective repair should be performed. Failure to achieve reduction requires prompt surgical intervention. In the case of inguinal hernias, a standard inguinal incision is made and the bowel within the hernia sac is assessed. If following the release of the constriction (usually at the neck of the hernia sac) the bowel appears viable, it may be reduced and a standard hernia repair is performed. Nonviable bowel should be excised, and this can sometimes easily be achieved through the groin incision. However, if there is any difficulty or concern about reduced loops of bowel, it is safer to perform a laparotomy (or laparoscopy). Incarcerated femoral hernias may be approached low in the groin, as for an elective repair, but if resection of bowel is required a formal laparotomy is needed. Alternatively, the Lotheissen approach through the posterior wall of the inguinal canal or the McEvedy preperitoneal approach allows hernia repair and access to the peritoneal cavity through a single incision. Immediate closure of the hernia-defect with a mesh is advisable, provided that there is no peritonitis. In case of infection, a simple suture repair is recommended, with acceptance of a high risk of recurrence.

Intussusception

Hydrostatic or air enema reduction in children may be sufficient; only a small proportion of intussusceptions recur or fail to reduce. In adults, there is usually a pathological lead point of the intussusception, which predisposes to recurrence and may be malignant, and operation is indicated. At operation it is usually not advisable to reduce the intussusception because of the possibility of a perforated malignant lead point. Resection is the procedure of choice, with either anastomosis or diversion as appropriate for the site and severity of the obstruction.

Gallstone Ileus

Operative removal of the stone is usually required, at which time the rest of the intestine should be carefully palpated for further stones. The calculus should be gently milked back for a few centimeters to allow enterotomy through healthy small bowel. Removal of an impacted duodenal stone may necessitate cholecystectomy to allow mobilization of the duodenum, as may bleeding from the biliary-enteric fistula, but in other cases cholecystectomy is usually deferred. If the gallbladder is left in place, there is a small incidence of recurrence of gallstone obstruction;[30] hence, interval cholecystectomy is performed for most patients.

Crohn's Disease

There may be multiple strictures, and management has evolved from liberal resection to bypass of diseased segments to limited resection and strictureplasty. Strictureplasty may be of the Heineke-Mikulicz or Finney variety, depending upon the length of the stricture. Strictureplasty is safe, durable, and need extend only beyond macroscopic disease.[31] Indeed, stricureplasty is now described in segments of active disease, and depending on the experience of the surgeon, quite long strictures over 20 cm and longer can be dealt with safely, especially when there is a need to preserve intestinal length. Resections are reserved for segments with multiple strictures, ileocecal disease, severely malnourished patients, and segments of bowel involved with an abscess.

Colonic Crohn's strictures are less common than small bowel strictures and require resection when there is a tight stenosis that causes symptoms. It is also essential to exclude malignancy in those strictures that do not warrant resection (6–7% of all strictures);[32] colonoscopic biopsy is the procedure of choice. Ileocolic and ileorectal anastomoses are also prone to restricturing: up to two thirds of cases become symptomatic after long-term follow-up.[33] Not only may an anastomosis be affected, but it is also common for the preanastomotic or prestomal intestine to develop recurrent strictures. This process may require further operation or endoscopic balloon dilatation for selected short strictures.

Radiation Enteritis

Treatment of radiation enteritis can be very difficult as the irradiation can induce dense adhesions and the affected bowel is scarred and liable to heal poorly if injured or anastomosed (Fig. 75.11). Resection of affected bowel up to the junction with normal bowel is the treatment of choice; an alternative is to perform a short-segment bypass.

Left-Sided Large Bowel Obstruction

The underlying causes of large bowel obstruction differ from those of small bowel obstruction in that adhesions and hernias are very unusual. Malignancy, volvulus, and diverticular stricture account for approximately 90% of cases of mechanical obstruction of the colon. Over 50% of colonic obstructions and most rectal obstructions are malignant in nature, with primary colorectal cancer as the predominant cause. Less common causes of large bowel obstruction include inflammatory bowel disease, radiation stricture, fecal impaction, intussusception, and ischemic stricture.

The common presenting complaints are pain and distension. Distension may be gross, and it affects the flanks rather than the central abdomen as in small bowel obstruction. Vomiting is less common because of the distal nature of the obstruction. Pain is not usually of a colicky nature, as seen with small bowel obstruction. Diarrhea is not uncommon with an incomplete obstruction.

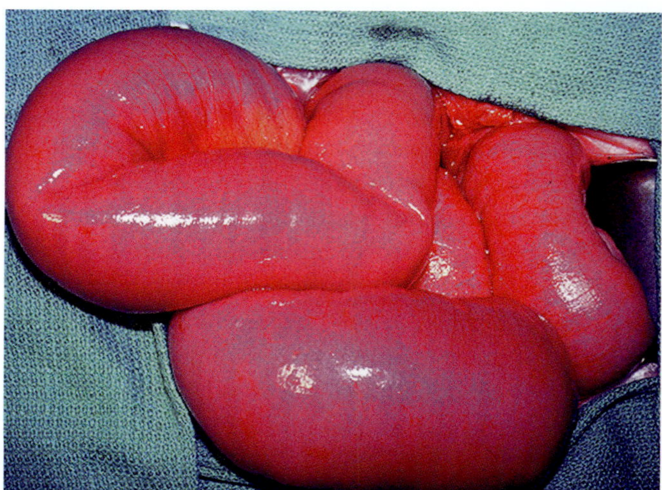

Fig. 75.11: Distended small bowel proximal to a loop of small bowel that shows scarring and narrowing caused by previous irradiation for a gynecologic malignancy.

Rectal examination and rigid proctoscopy should be carried out in all instances, although colonoscopy with insufflation of air may exacerbate symptoms. Plain radiographs may suggest the level of the obstruction, and water-soluble contrast enemas may be useful to localize accurately the site and completeness of obstruction; however, CT scanning is the radiological test of choice to determine the cause of obstruction and to detect metastasis.

Since the consistency of the stool changes from liquid in the cecum to progressively more solid in the left colon and rectum, it is not surprising that about three quarters of obstructing colon cancers are distal to the splenic flexure. Complete colonic obstruction with a competent ileocecal valve requires urgent decompression as this is a closed-loop obstruction that can result in massive dilatation and perforation, especially of the cecum.

Colonic Stents

Self-expanding metallic stents (SEMS) came into use for relief of obstruction, as a palliative measure, in patients with large bowel obstruction from cancer and distant metastasis that rendered the disease incurable. Self-expanding metallic stents provide an attractive option in such patients because of the avoidance of a potentially high-risk operation, creation of a permanent stoma, and improved quality of life.[34,35] Clearly, SEMS will not be suitable for patients with associated complications, such as perforation or suspicion of colonic ischemia.

Self-expanding metallic stents can be used also in order to avoid emergency surgery and serve as a "bridge" to an elective operation after thorough staging and evaluation.

If facilities are available, SEMS should be considered for all patients who present with acute left-sided (distal to the splenic flexure) colonic obstruction and do not have features of perforation. There is limited experience with SEMS for obstructing tumors in the right or transverse colon. In a recent meta-analysis, the technical and clinical success of stenting, as a bridge to operation, was about 70%.[36] The incidence of clinically evident perforation was 7% and that of silent perforation was 14%. The group with SEMS had a higher proportion of successful primary anastomosis and a lower overall stoma rate, with no difference in mortality.[36]

Resection

Operative treatment is necessary for colonic obstruction if stenting is unavailable, technically unfeasible, or if there is a perforation. Right-sided (proximal to the splenic flexure) malignant colonic obstruction may be generally treated by resection with primary anastomosis because the technical safety of this procedure appears similar in the emergency and elective situations. However, the operative treatment of malignant left-sided large bowel obstruction remains controversial.[37] Conventionally, two- or three-stage procedures have been recommended, in preference to a single-stage resection and anastomosis, because of a perception of increased safety. A two-stage operation (often referred to as a Hartman's procedure) entails resection of the tumor, creation of an end stoma of the proximal colon and closure of the rectal stump; on a subsequent occasion, usually after several months, the stoma may be excised and the proximal colon is anastomosed to the rectum. In a three-stage procedure, the emergency operation is limited to the creation of a loop stoma of the transverse colon, in order to relieve the obstruction. The second stage involves resection of the tumor, whilst retaining the stoma, and at the third and final stage, the stoma is excised and proximal colon is anastomosed to distal colon or rectum.

There is now robust evidence that single-stage resection and anastomosis for malignant left-sided large bowel obstruction is associated with low morbidity and mortality rates similar to those for two- or three-stage procedures.[38] Staged procedures carry the risk of morbidity and mortality during the subsequent operation and entail a substantially longer overall stay in hospital. Moreover, a substantially higher proportion of patients with staged operations will remain with a permanent stoma. Thus, primary resection and anastomosis is the preferred modern surgical treatment for left-sided obstruction; however, staged operations should not be considered obsolete and may be used judiciously, particularly in complicated situations, e.g., peritonitis, ischemia, or excessively high perioperative risk, including the use of a covering loop ileostomy. However, the latter is not an easy maneuver in the obese patient.

Segmental colonic resection and subtotal colectomy are equally safe options.[16] Generally, subtotal colectomy is preferred if there is cecal ischemia or perforation, more than one (synchronous) tumor or the need to perform anastomosis to the rectum. Segmental colectomy may be undertaken according to the surgeon's preference when there is a realistic choice of procedures. If segmental resection is undertaken, performance of on-table colonic lavage does not confer significant benefit in terms of reduced morbidity or mortality but does add to the operating time. On-table lavage and manual decompression appear to be equally effective. One important reason for avoiding primary anastomosis in the emergency situation was that preoperative bowel preparation was believed to be critical for anastomotic integrity. With current evidence that bowel preparation can, in fact, be harmful and should be avoided for elective operations, similar considerations may be extended to the emergency situation.

Volvulus

Volvulus is a less common cause of colonic obstruction than cancer, being responsible for about 10–15% of all cases. Almost two-thirds of cases involve the sigmoid colon and about one-third the cecum; a few cases involve the transverse colon or the flexures. Patients are usually elderly, and features common to all types of colonic volvulus are excessive mobility or redundancy of the affected segment of the colon. Diagnosis may be suspected on clinical grounds, and the plain radiographs are often characteristic (Fig. 75.12). Contrast studies show a characteristic cut-off at the point of twist of the bowel.

Endoscopic decompression is usually successful with sigmoid volvulus (Fig. 75.13). Failure of decompression, recurrence, or suspected gangrene or perforation requires operation. At operation, nonviable colon should be resected with or without primary anastomosis. Viable colon may be fixed along the inner aspect of the abdominal wall, or its mesenteric attachment may be broadened by mesosigmoid plasty to prevent recurrence. However, colpopexy and mesosigmoid plasty, although less extensive procedures, are associated with an appreciable incidence of recurrence, and in all but the most frail of patients a resection should be performed.

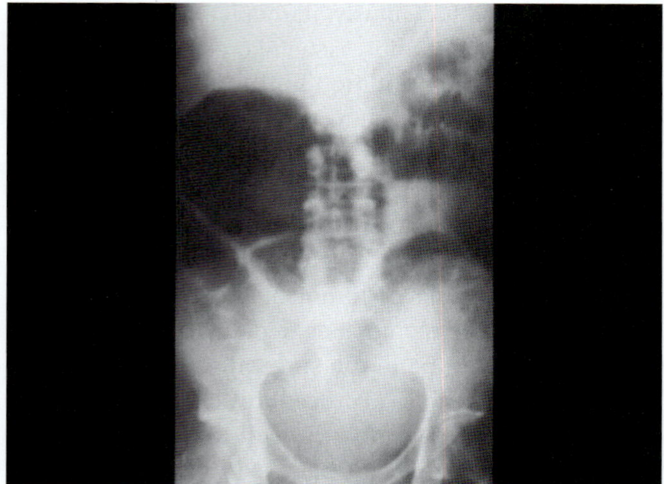

Fig. 75.12: Cecal volvulus appears as a large gas-filled structure in the right upper quadrant (often may appear in the left upper quadrant also).

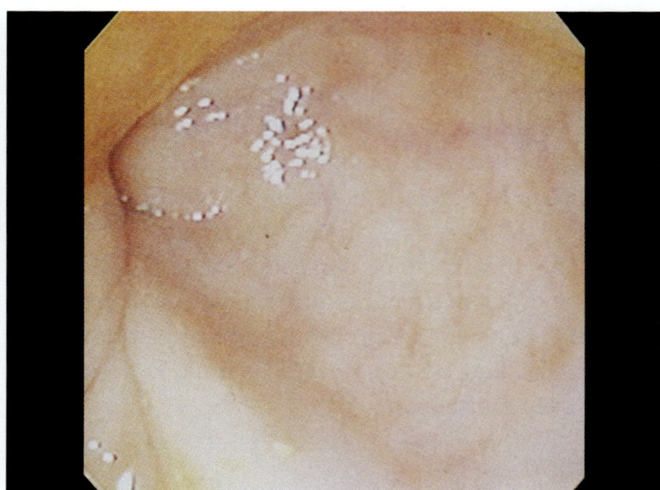

Fig. 75.13: Endoscopic view of site of obstruction in sigmoid volvulus.

Diverticular Strictures

Repeated attacks of diverticulitis may lead to obstruction from scarring and fibrosis. Clinically, it can be very difficult to distinguish this latter obstruction from malignant obstruction, but previous attacks of documented diverticulitis may help. Contrast enemas show an area of stricture, which is usually longer than the relatively short malignant stricture, and there may be preservation of a normal mucosal pattern. However, on occasion diverticular strictures mimic cancer and the distinction can be made only by colonoscopy or, if this is not possible because the stricture is too tight, at operation. Even if a malignancy can be excluded, fibrotic diverticular strictures usually require an elective resection because they do not respond to nonoperative measures. In addition, adherence of a loop of small bowel to a "diverticuloma" can cause obstruction at this level.

Colonic Pseudo-obstruction

In 1948, Sir Heneage Ogilvie described two cases of colonic obstruction without an obvious underlying mechanical cause on barium enema. Acute colonic pseudo-obstruction or Ogilvie's syndrome, as this condition has also come to be known, has been recognized with increasing frequency in recent years. Many conditions are associated with acute colonic pseudo-obstruction (Table 75.3).The common pathway whereby this diverse group of conditions leads to decreased colonic motility is still not well defined. A neurologic basis is an attractive theory, since control of colonic motility is mainly dependent upon the intrinsic neural plexus and a tonic supply by the parasympathetic nerves. Current evidence, in particular the effectiveness of neostigmine (an anticholinesterase that potentiates cholinergic parasympathetic effects), suggests that suppression of the tonic parasympathetic supply may be the most important cause.

Table 75.3 Causes of acute colonic pseudo-obstruction.

Etiology	*Examples*
Metabolic	Diabetes mellitus, hypothyroidism, renal failure, electrolyte imbalance
Pharmacologic	Opiates, tricylics, anticholinergics, phenothiazines, ganglion blockers
Systemic illness	Amyloid, congestive cardiac failure, hypoxia
Surgical	Abdominal surgery, nonabdominal surgery (especially orthopedic, cardiac, and neurosurgery)
Neurologic	Multiple sclerosis, myotonic dystrophy, Chagas' disease
Autoimmune	Lupus, scleroderma, dermatomyositis
Infective	Systemic sepsis
Miscellaneous	Nonabdominal trauma, especially head and spinal injuries

Clinical Features

Abdominal distention, noncolicky abdominal pain and failure to pass flatus or stool in conjunction with one of the known predisposing factors are the classic features of Ogilvie's syndrome. Examination usually reveals a markedly distended quiet abdomen, which is tympanic to percussion. Localized tenderness, guarding, or rebound and tenderness are absent, unless perforation is present or imminent, and must be carefully excluded on repeated physical examinations. Rectal examination is usually normal.

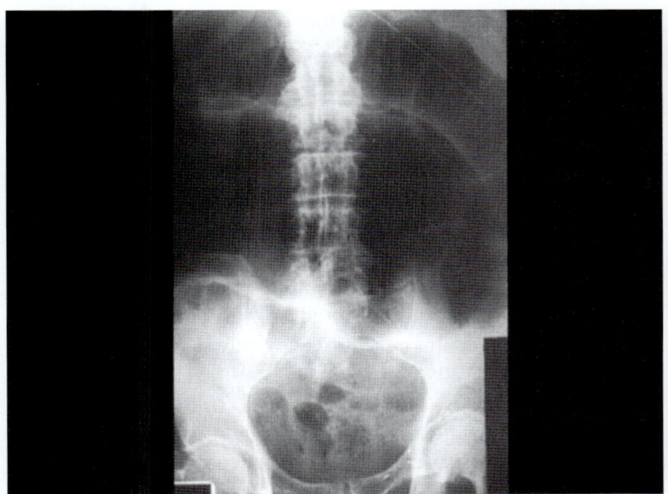

Fig. 75.14: Plain radiograph showing Ogilvie's syndrome following a knee replacement.

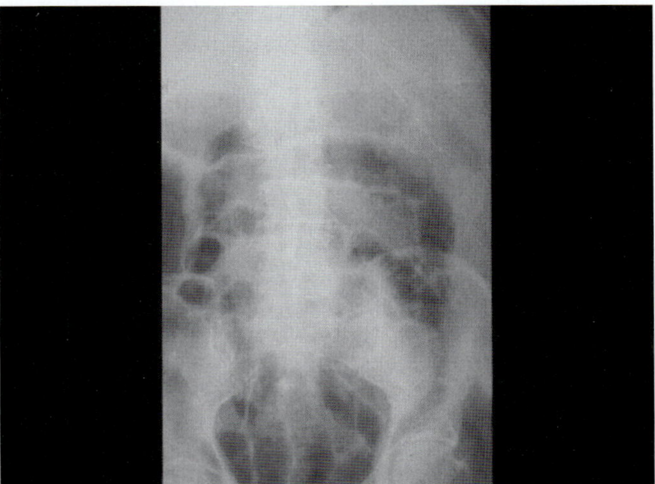

Fig. 75.15: Postcolonoscopic appearance of the patient shown in Figure 75.14.

Pseudo-obstruction must be distinguished from true mechanical obstruction, and this is often possible on clinical grounds. The typical abdominal radiographs of pseudo-obstruction show dilatation of part of or the entire colon, usually with a normal small bowel pattern (Fig. 75.14). If only part of the colon is dilated, an abrupt cut-off may be seen; this most commonly occurs at the splenic flexure but sometimes at the hepatic flexure or rectosigmoid. The colon may become massively dilated and usually the cecum shows the greatest enlargement. A water-soluble contrast enema excludes mechanical obstruction in cases where there is doubt; at times it may be therapeutic.

Management

Initial management involves the removal, where possible, of instigating or potentiating factors, such as opiates or tricyclic drugs. Metabolic or endocrine abnormalities, such as hypokalemia, uremia, or hypothyroidism, should be corrected. Gentle stimulation with suppositories or enemas may be helpful.

Colonoscopy is indicated if conservative management fails and there is either no resolution or worsening of colonic dilatation. Success depends upon expertise in colonoscopy with minimal insufflation of air, and rates of decompression of 70–90% can be expected (Fig. 75.15). The recurrence rate after colonoscopy is 10–20%, although this can often be treated successfully by repeat colonoscopy. Pharmacologic treatment with neostigmine (an anticholinesterase), in patients who fail to respond to conservative management, can rapidly decompress the colon.[39] Neostigmine may be administered in a dose of 2 mg intravenously over 3 minutes. Patients are monitored with electrocardiography, and bradycardia may require treatment with atropine. It is vital to have excluded mechanical distal obstruction, either by colonoscopy or contrast enema, before using this approach.[40] Operative management may be required if there is failure to respond to medical or endoscopic therapy or in case of development of signs of perforation. A colostomy or resection with proximal ileostomy and mucous fistula may be performed.

REFERENCES

1. Treves F. Intestinal obstruction: its varieties WTP, diagnosis and treatment. Philadelphia: HC Lea's Son; 1884.
2. Gibson CL. II. A study of one thousand operations for acute intestinal obstruction and gangrenous hernia. Ann Surg. 1900;32(4):486-514.
3. Vick RM. Statistics of acute intestinal obstruction. Br Med J.(Clin Res Ed) 1932;2(3741):546-8.
4. Ouaissi M, Gaujoux S, Veyrie N, et al. Post-operative adhesions after digestive surgery: their incidence and prevention: review of the literature. J Visc Surg. 2012;149(2): e104-14.
5. Ellis H, Moran BJ, Thompson JN, et al. Adhesion-related hospital readmissions after abdominal and pelvic surgery: a retrospective cohort study. Lancet. 1999;353(9163): 1476-80.
6. Taylor GW, Jayne DG, Brown SR, et al. Adhesions and incisional hernias following laparoscopic versus open surgery for colorectal cancer in the CLASICC trial. Br J Surg. 2010;97(1):70-8.
7. Gallegos NC, Dawson J, Jarvis M, et al. Risk of strangulation in groin hernias. Br J Surg. 1991;78(10):1171-3.

8. Stewardson RH, Bombeck CT, Nyhus LM. Critical operative management of small bowel obstruction. Ann Surg. 1978; 187(2):189-93.
9. Mattei P, Rombeau JL. Review of the pathophysiology and management of postoperative ileus. World J Surg. 2006;30(8): 1382-91.
10. Chestovich PJ, Lin AY, Yoo J. Fast-track pathways in colorectal surgery. Surg Clin North Am. 2013;93(1):21-32.
11. Wolff BG, Viscusi ER, Delaney CP, et al. Patterns of gastrointestinal recovery after bowel resection and total abdominal hysterectomy: pooled results from the placebo arms of alvimopan phase III North American clinical trials. J Am Coll Surg. 2007;205(1):43-51.
12. Marret E, Remy C, Bonnet F. Meta-analysis of epidural analgesia versus parenteral opioid analgesia after colorectal surgery. Br J Surg. 2007;94(6):665-73.
13. Delaney CP, Wolff BG, Viscusi ER, et al. Alvimopan, for postoperative ileus following bowel resection: a pooled analysis of phase III studies. Ann Surg. 2007;245(3):355-63.
14. Noble EJ, Harris R, Hosie KB, et al. Gum chewing reduces postoperative ileus? A systematic review and meta-analysis. Int J Surg. 2009;7(2):100-5.
15. Muller SA, Rahbari NN, Schneider F, et al. Randomized clinical trial on the effect of coffee on postoperative ileus following elective colectomy. Br J Surg. 2012;99(11):1530-8.
16. Finan PJ, Campbell S, Verma R, et al. The management of malignant large bowel obstruction: ACPGBI position statement. Colorectal Dis. 2007;9(Suppl 4):1-17.
17. Vettoretto N, Carrara A, Corradi A, et al. Laparoscopic adhesiolysis: consensus conference guidelines. Colorectal Dis. 2012;14(5):e208-15.
18. Maung AA, Johnson DC, Piper GL, et al. Evaluation and management of small-bowel obstruction: an eastern association for the surgery of trauma practice management guideline. J Trauma Acute Care Surg. 2012;73(5 Suppl 4):S362-9.
19. Schraufnagel D, Rajaee S, Millham FH. How many sunsets? Timing of surgery in adhesive small bowel obstruction: a study of the nationwide inpatient sample. J Trauma Acute Care Surg. 2013;74(1):181-7; discussion 187-9.
20. Zielinski MD, Eiken PW, Heller SF, et al. Prospective, observational validation of a multivariate small-bowel obstruction model to predict the need for operative intervention. J Am Coll Surg. 2011;212(6):1068-76.
21. Cosse C, Regimbeau JM, Fuks D, et al. Serum procalcitonin for predicting the failure of conservative management and the need for bowel resection in patients with small bowel obstruction. J Am Coll Surg.2013;216(5):997-1004.
22. Feuer DJ, Broadley KE, Shepherd JH, et al. Systematic review of surgery in malignant bowel obstruction in advanced gynecological and gastrointestinal cancer. The systematic review steering committee. Gynecol Oncol. 1999;75(3):313-22.
23. Feuer DJ, Broadley KE. Systematic review and meta-analysis of corticosteroids for the resolution of malignant bowel obstruction in advanced gynaecological and gastrointestinal cancers. Systematic review steering committee. Ann Oncol. 1999;10(9):1035-41.
24. Mancini GJ, Petroski GF, Lin WC, et al. Nationwide impact of laparoscopic lysis of adhesions in the management of intestinal obstruction in the US. J Am Coll Surg. 2008; 207(4):520-6.
25. O'Connor DB, Winter DC. The role of laparoscopy in the management of acute small-bowel obstruction: a review of over 2,000 cases. Surg Endosc. 2012;26(1):12-7.
26. Li MZ, Lian L, Xiao LB, et al. Laparoscopic versus open adhesiolysis in patients with adhesive small bowel obstruction: a systematic review and meta-analysis. Am J Surg. 2012; 204(5):779-86.
27. Johnson KN, Chapital AB, Harold KL, et al. Laparoscopic management of acute small bowel obstruction: evaluating the need for resection. J Trauma Acute Care Surg. 2012;72(1):25-30; discussion 30-1; quiz 317.
28. Ezer A, Torer N, Colakoglu T, et al. Clinical outcomes of manual bowel decompression (milking) in the mechanical small bowel obstruction: a prospective randomized clinical trial. Am J Surg. 2012;203(1):95-100.
29. Zeng Q, Yu Z, You J, et al. Efficacy and safety of seprafilm for preventing postoperative abdominal adhesion: systematic review and meta-analysis. World J Surg. 2007;31(11):2125-31; discussion 2132.
30. Reisner RM, Cohen JR. Gallstone ileus: a review of 1001 reported cases. Am Surg. 1994;60(6):441-6.
31. Dehn TC, Kettlewell MG, Mortensen NJ, et al. Ten-year experience of strictureplasty for obstructive Crohn's disease. Br J Surg. 1989;76(4):339-41.
32. Yamazaki Y, Ribeiro MB, Sachar DB, et al. Malignant colorectal strictures in Crohn's disease. Am J Gastroenterol. 1991;86(7):882-5.
33. Trnka YM, Glotzer DJ, Kasdon EJ, et al. The long-term outcome of restorative operation in Crohn's disease: influence of location, prognostic factors and surgical guidelines. Ann Surg. 1982;196(3):345-55.
34. Nagula S, Ishill N, Nash C, et al. Quality of life and symptom control after stent placement or surgical palliation of malignant colorectal obstruction. J Am Coll Surg. 2010;210(1):45-53.
35. Watt AM, Faragher IG, Griffin TT, et al. Self-expanding metallic stents for relieving malignant colorectal obstruction: a systematic review. Ann Surg. 2007;246(1):24-30.
36. Tan CJ, Dasari BVM, Gardiner K. Systematic review and meta-analysis of randomized clinical trials of self-expanding metallic stents as a bridge to surgery versus emergency surgery for malignant left-sided large bowel obstruction. Br J Surg. 2012;99(4):469-76.
37. De Salvo GL, Gava C, Pucciarelli S, et al. Curative surgery for obstruction from primary left colorectal carcinoma: primary or staged resection? Cochrane Database Syst Rev. 2002;(1):CD002101.
38. Breitenstein S, Rickenbacher A, Berdajs D, et al. Systematic evaluation of surgical strategies for acute malignant left-sided colonic obstruction. Br J Surg. 2007;94(12):1451-60.
39. Ponec RJ, Saunders MD, Kimmey MB. Neostigmine for the treatment of acute colonic pseudo-obstruction. N Engl J Med. 1999;341(3):137-41.
40. St John PH, Radcliffe AG. Contraindication for the use of neostigmine in colonic pseudo-obstruction. Br J Surg. 1997; 84(10):1481-2.

Case Study: 76

Use of Synthetic Mesh such as Polypropylene in Hernia Repair in the Presence of Contamination

Andrew de Beaux

THE PROBLEM

It is not unusual with hernia repair, especially incisional hernia repair, for there to be a degree of contamination during the operation. This problem may relate to ulcerated skin, the presence of a stoma, inadvertent enterotomy if dense adhesions are encountered, or indeed the need to resect bowel if the primary indication for operation is a strangulated hernia or the hernia is present but unrelated to the acute abdomen. The use of mesh is considered to give a more durable repair of the hernia, but there are concerns about leaving a permanent foreign body in the presence of intraoperative contamination, whether the procedure be clean-contaminated, contaminated, or dirty.

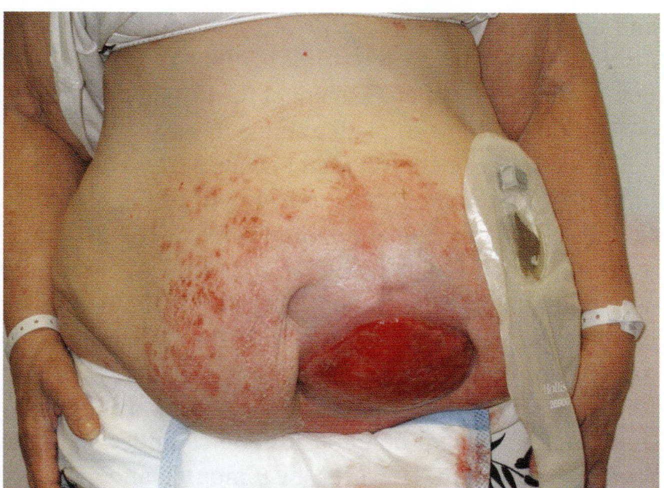

Fig. 76.1: Preoperative photograph.

THE TYPICAL CASE

A 70-year-old woman had undergone an emergency Hartmann's resection for perforated diverticular disease 7 months ago. She had made a good recovery in terms of only a short time in the high dependency unit, as her sepsis-related organ dysfunction had been mild and short lived. She did develop a major wound infection, which resulted in a partial superficial and deep wound dehiscence requiring a vacuum-assisted closure type dressing for several months. Figure 76.1 shows her current state, with an area of granulation tissue overlying an incisional hernia, a colostomy with an associated parastomal hernia, and erythematous patches consistent with her known psoriasis. Understandably, she wished to have re-epithelialization of her anterior abdominal wall, with reversal of her stoma as well as repair of the abdominal wall.

DIAGNOSTIC DILEMMAS

The patient's wishes as noted above really identify the three goals of the operation(s) on this abdomen. (1) There is a need for skin closure, which could be achieved by secondary intention with long-term nursing care alone—probably over many more months—or the option of skin grafting. The downside of waiting until secondary closure is the ongoing need for daily dressing, which greatly limits this lady's independence. The downside of grafting is the comorbidity of the donor site along with the risk of failure of the skin graft. (2) Reversal of the stoma is possible as a first option, but primary closure of the abdomen afterward is unlikely to be easy. An alternative would be excision of the area of granulation tissue and attempting primary abdominal wall closure leaving the stoma as it is, but this is not an easy option either. (3) The third surgical option is to undertake all three goals at one operation. Finally, avoiding any operation at all could be another potential course.

MANAGEMENT OPTIONS

There are benefits, risks, and alternatives to most surgical strategies. Clearly this type of operation is quality of life surgery, so dialogue with the patient and family is important. In general, the longer the better in terms of the time interval between the original and subsequent operation, to allow the resolution of inflammatory/vascular adhesions. Most surgeons would want to wait at least 4 months, if not 6 months or more from the time of the Hartmann's procedure.

The patient needs to be in as good shape as possible for the operation, so attention should focus on controlling any comorbidity, optimizing nutrition if there are oral intake issues, minimizing infective complications such as methicillin-resistant *Staphylococcus aureus,* screening and decolonization as far as possible, encouraging weight loss (as this reduces the risk of loss of domain issues), cessation of smoking, and assessment of the distal bowel length and condition if contemplating stoma reversal.

The surgical operation then becomes freestyle (*secundum artem*), adapting the surgical plan to the operative findings. Access to the abdominal cavity is the first challenge. In general, one should start as far away from the contamination as reasonably possible, without making the incision too long. This maneuver should allow access to the abdominal cavity away from major adhesions, and further opening of the abdominal wall will permit assessment of the bowel or omental adherence underneath the area of granulation. However, by 9 months and certainly by 1 year, it is remarkable how easily such adhesions can be taken down with a combination of blunt and sharp dissection. At this stage, try *not* to excise any of the abdominal wall or the hernial sac—you might need it later!

Reversal of a stoma or otherwise will be based on the patient's condition once the abdomen has been opened, the length of the bowel available and how easily it can be mobilized to provide a well-vascularized tension-free anastomosis. There may be a degree of compromise between how well the bowel can be mobilized versus tension, as dividing mesentery to gain length to the bowel may reduce the blood supply to the mobilized bowel end.

Abdominal wall reconstruction is the final big decision. Again, how well is the patient so far, how much contamination has occurred, and what is the quality of the abdominal wall? Very rarely, if the operation has been difficult and prolonged, leaving the abdomen open with some sort of vacuum-assisted dressing, along the principles of damage-limitation surgery, is appropriate. Rarely, it is sensible to suture close the abdominal wall, with or without skin closure, and repair the likely subsequent incisional hernia another day. However, if the operation is going as planned, consideration of mesh repair is likely. The questions are what type of mesh, and in what position? The three main mesh positions are onlay, sublay, or intraperitoneal (please refer to Chapter 70, "Abdominal Wall Hernia," for a detailed explanation of mesh position). In a situation like this, raising skin flaps and performing a colonic mobilization and anastomosis make the degree of contamination highest for the onlay and intraperitoneal spaces. Thus, making use of the retromuscular or sublay space is attractive. This technique places mesh into a space that was not contaminated at the beginning or during the operation, and is relatively well vascularized as the mesh will sit very close to the bellies of the rectus muscles.

In this case, stoma reversal, sublay polypropylene mesh reinforcement of both the incisional and parastomal hernias, and the primary skin closure were all achieved at a single operation (Fig. 76.2). The patient subsequently underwent an abdominoplasty (Fig. 76.3).

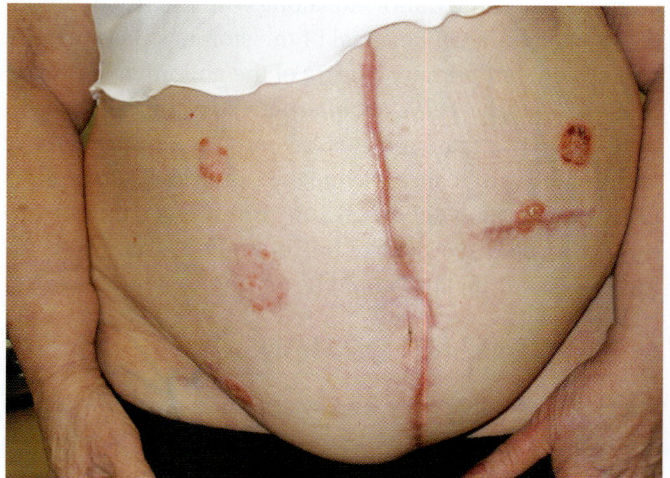

Fig. 76.2: Post repair.

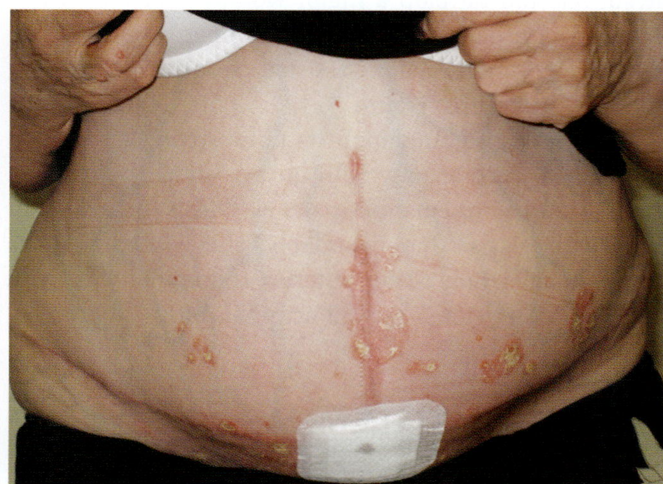

Fig. 76.3: Post abdominoplasty.

Why not use a biological mesh in this context? Biological meshes have been strongly promoted as the current answer to the small but real problems associated with synthetic meshes in the contaminated situation. Although such mesh material is very expensive, many surgeons have jumped on this bandwagon. However, the risk of mesh infection requiring re-exploration appears to have been overstated with more modern, large-pore synthetic meshes. Moreover, biological meshes do not seem to reduce surgical site infections, and the short-term recurrence rate of the hernia appears to be higher than with synthetic meshes. In addition, the 5-year outcomes in terms of hernia recurrence or major bulging (pseudo recurrence) appear to be unacceptably high when compared to synthetic meshes.

FURTHER READING

1. Abdelfatah MM, Rostambeigi N, Podgaetz E, et al. Long-term outcomes (>5-year follow-up) with porcine acellular dermal matrix (PermacolTM) in incisional hernias at risk of infection. Hernia. 2015;19:135-40..
2. Carbonell AM, Criss CN, Cobb WS, et al. Outcomes of synthetic mesh in contaminated ventral hernia repairs. J Am Coll Surg. 2013;217:991-8.
3. Cole WC, Balent EM, Masella PC, et al. An experimental comparison of the effects of bacterial colonization on biologic and synthetic meshes. Hernia. 2015;19:197-205.
4. Deerenberg EB, Mulder IM, Grotenhuis N, et al. Experimental study on synthetic and biological mesh implantation in a contaminated environment. Br J Surg. 2012;99:1734-41.
5. Primus FE, Harris HW. A critical review of biologic mesh use in ventral hernia repairs under contaminated conditions. Hernia. 2013;17:21-30.

77

Case Study: Small Bowel Obstruction in the "Virgin" Abdomen

Andrew de Beaux

THE PROBLEM

Small bowel obstruction in the "virgin" abdomen, that is, an abdomen with no previous operations, is relatively unusual. In the elderly, especially in the presence of anemia, malignancy is likely. But in the young, malignancy is less likely. Nevertheless, because of a perceived high incidence of underlying malignant lesions in such patients, the old surgical idiom was that the sun should not set on small bowel obstruction in a virgin abdomen.

THE TYPICAL CASE

A 28-year-old man self-presented to the accident and emergency department with 3 days of severe colicky abdominal pain and bilious vomiting. Six weeks earlier, while playing soccer, he had received an inadvertent blow from an opponent's knee into his abdomen. Shortly afterward, he developed episodes of abdominal pain that came and went, associated with the occasional episode of vomiting. His weight had been stable. There was minimal systemic upset, and he felt well between his bouts of abdominal pain until 3 days before admission.

Clinical examination revealed a mildly tender, mildly distended abdomen with quiet bowel sounds. His inflammatory markers revealed a white cell count just above the upper limit of normal with a normal C-reactive protein, and the other blood tests were normal.

A computed tomography (CT) scan showed small bowel obstruction to the level of the distal jejunum, where there was an identifiable transition point. The bowel wall was markedly thickened in this region in association with multiple enlarged mesenteric nodes (Fig. 77.1). There was no free fluid of note.

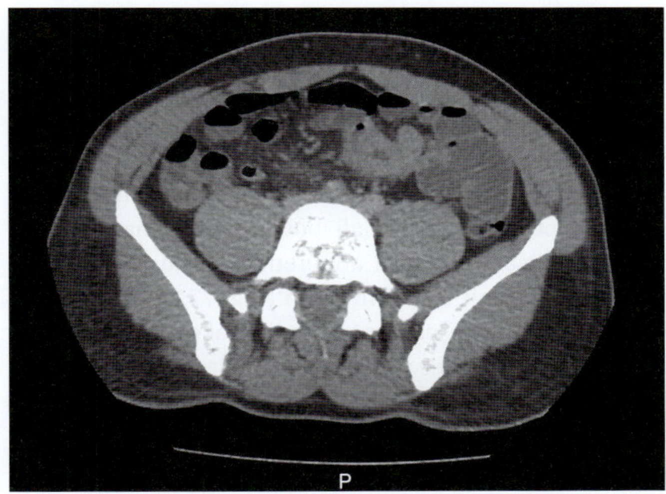

Fig. 77.1: CT slice of thickened bowel with a very small lumen in the middle of the abdominal cavity with dilated fluid-filled small bowel to the left of the abdominal cavity.

DIAGNOSTIC DILEMMAS

Thickened bowel with lymphadenopathy would raise concerns about the presence of malignant pathology. However, the lack of a discrete mass lesion would also raise the possibility of inflammatory bowel disease such as Crohn's disease. While there was no evidence of sepsis, and the inflammatory markers were normal, an "inflammatory process" was still considered possible.

MANAGEMENT OPTIONS

Three questions arose: (1) Would the obstruction settle with supportive measures only? (2) Would any drug therapy be required? and/or (3) Would operation be necessary and, if so, whether on an emergency or elective basis?

A period of nasogastric suction, intravenous hydration, and bowel rest was an option. The downside of such management is that the diagnosis remains unclear and the concern of malignancy remains, while spontaneous resolution of the bowel obstruction is unlikely.

Although the patient appeared reasonably well nourished on admission, it was likely that without relief of obstruction oral nutrition would soon become a concern.

Parenteral nutrition combined with systemic steroid therapy for suspected inflammatory bowel disease seemed another reasonable management option, but again it would not address the concern about malignancy or indeed any other mechanical cause of obstruction.

Since the patient's clinical condition did not merit emergency surgery on day of admission, he underwent laparoscopy on the following day. It was not possible to identify the cause of the obstruction at laparoscopy, although it was evident that there was a clear-cut problem at the site of the bowel obstruction: collapsed distal bowel and distended proximal bowel could be traced to this region. The operation was thus converted to an open procedure, although the incision was only 10 cm long as the laparoscopy had identified the correct location for the incision. Mid small bowel obstruction was evident, with a short segment of thickened small bowel double-backed and matted to itself and with adherent omentum. This area was delivered out of the incision (Fig. 77.2), and a limited small bowel resection was undertaken with primary anastomosis. Recovery was uneventful.

The pathology report of the resected specimen noted marked mucosal ulceration with a fibroinflammatory process in the mesentery, but no evidence of malignancy, and the resection ends were normal. The working diagnosis was unclear, but in view of the recent history of abdominal trauma, the most likely explanation of the pathological findings was thought to be a localized small bowel perforation into the mesentery, with a resultant inflammatory reaction leading to progressive distortion and narrowing of the bowel lumen.

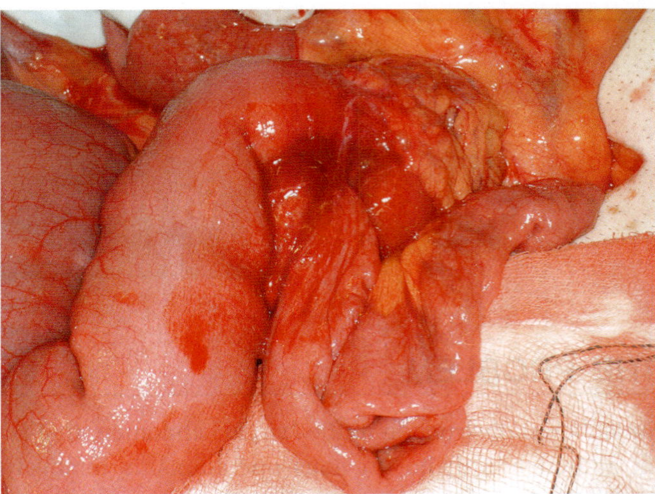

Fig. 77.2: Intraoperative photograph of dilated and collapsed small bowel with region of obstructing pathology delivered though a small laparotomy wound.

FURTHER READING

1. Beardsley C, Furtado R, Mosse C, et al. Small bowel obstruction in the virgin abdomen: the need for a mandatory laparotomy explored. Am J Surg. 2014;208:243-8.
2. Davies SW, Gillen JR, Guidry CA, et al. A comparative analysis between laparoscopic and open adhesiolysis at a tertiary care center. Am Surg. 2014;80:261-9.
3. Felder S, Margel D, Murrell Z, et al. Usefulness of bowel sound auscultation: a prospective evaluation. J Surg Educ. 2014;71:768-73.
4. O'Leary EA, Desale SY, Yi WS, et al. Letting the sun set on small bowel obstruction: can a simple risk score tell us when nonoperative care is inappropriate. Am Surg. 2014;80:572-9.

Index

Page numbers followed by *f* refer to figures; those followed by *t* refer to tables.

A

B

C

D

E

F

G

H

I

J

K

L

M

N

O

P

Q

R

S

T

U

V

W

X

Y

Z